MEDICINE
MCQs for Medical Professionals

Celebrating 50 Years
Passion, Quality and Innovation in Healthcare Publishing

MEDICINE
MCQs for Medical Professionals

Based on 20th Edition of Harrison's Principles of Internal Medicine

Fifth Edition

Ajay Mathur
Senior Professor of Medicine
SMS Medical College and Hospital
Jaipur, Rajasthan, India

JAYPEE

JAYPEE BROTHERS MEDICAL PUBLISHERS
The Health Sciences Publisher
New Delhi | London

Jaypee Brothers Medical Publishers (P) Ltd

Headquarters
Jaypee Brothers Medical Publishers (P) Ltd
4838/24, Ansari Road, Daryaganj
New Delhi 110 002, India
Phone: +91-11-43574357
Fax: +91-11-43574314
Email: jaypee@jaypeebrothers.com

Overseas Office
J.P. Medical Ltd
83 Victoria Street, London
SW1H 0HW (UK)
Phone: +44 20 3170 8910
Fax: +44 (0)20 3008 6180
Email: info@jpmedpub.com

Website: www.jaypeebrothers.com
Website: www.jaypeedigital.com

Medicine MCQs for Medical Professionals

First Edition: 2007

Second Edition: 2010

Third Edition: 2013

Reprint: 2014

Fourth Edition: *2017*

Fifth Edition 2020

ISBN 978-93-89776-98-0

Printed at Sanat Printers

FOREWORD

As a professional, who has been practicing medicine for over four decades now, I appreciate the value this book brings to the table in times like today. As we move from a largely descriptive era to the bullet-point generation, this academic initiative appears even more relevant than its first three earlier editions.

Many refinements have been made in this book bearing in mind the reception it has received in the last few years. The book has been a reference point for many medical entrance examinations and has left an impact on medical professionals who look for high quality of academic material.

Harrison's Principles of Internal Medicine, published by The McGraw-Hill Companies, Inc. is an epic in the world of medical science. This book serves as a faithful companion to the epic by assisting the readers draw most out of it in the service of mankind.

Knowledge is a more processed form of information. Prof. Ajay Mathur stays true to his pledge by presenting well-digested bytes of knowledge across different fields of medicine. He relies on good old word-of-mouth to make this book a success rather than blitzkrieg marketing. I recommend that you make this a must-have without an iota of doubt.

Prof. Ramesh Roop Rai
Senior Professor & Head, Gastroenterology (Retd.)
SMS Medical College and Hospital, Jaipur, Rajasthan, India
Past President, Indian Society of Gastroenterology (2008)

PREFACE

Medicine, in all its vastness, needs to be understood in a way that makes most sense to how it is applied today. Memorizing each word is elusive and therefore, testing knowledge of a discipline remains an evergreen challenge.

It is a widely accepted fact that taking a quiz soon after studying helps one retain information and knowledge better. The brain works in mysterious ways but a sure way of holding onto what the mind has already digested is to put lessons to test. Multiple Choice Questions are a quick and effective way of remembering the gist of the matter. This is precisely the reason why most examinations today follow this format. This book is committed to hone your skills for retaining knowledge; it is only axiomatic that excellence will follow when you acquire knowledge properly.

In its fifth edition, this book incorporates the recent advances in medicine as well as my personal insights on how to learn better. Based on earlier and the 20th edition of Harrison's Principles of Internal Medicine, published by The McGraw-Hill Companies, Inc., this book also comprises relevant studies from the leading medical journals from the world over.

This book caters to medical professionals at all levels. Not only can this be used by aspiring doctors to prepare for medical entrance examinations but by seasoned medical professionals to update knowledge long after it has been acquired. The book is sign-posted with resources and references should the reader require elaboration on any given topic.

Over 15,000 questions and still counting; I take it upon myself to continually refine the content of the book and chronicle the advances of medical science.

The chapters and page numbers mentioned is the same as in 20th edition of Harrison's Principles of Internal Medicine.

Prof. Ajay Mathur
Senior Professor of Medicine
SMS Medical College and Hospital
Jaipur, Rajasthan, India

CONTENTS

Hematology 1

Anemia and Polycythemia

1. According to WHO, anemia is defined as a hemoglobin level of?
Harrison's 20th Ed. Chapter 59 Page 386

A. < 14 g/dL in men & <13 g/dL in women
B. < 13 g/dL in men & <12 g/dL in women
C. < 12 g/dL in men & <11 g/dL in women
D. < 11 g/dL in men & <10 g/dL in women

The World Health Organization (WHO) defines anemia as a hemoglobin level <13 g/dL in men and < 12 g/dL in women.

2. Hematopoietic stem cell produce which of the following?
Harrison's 20th Ed. Chapter 59 Page 385

A. Red cells
B. All classes of granulocytes
C. Cells of the immune system
D. All of the above

Stem cells are capable of producing red cells, all classes of granulocytes, monocytes, platelets, and the cells of the immune system.

3. Erythroid cells develop with the expression of?
Harrison's 20th Ed. Chapter 59 Page 385

A. GATA -1
B. BATA -1
C. TATA -1
D. SATA -1

Erythroid cells come from a common erythroid/megakaryocyte progenitor that does not develop in the absence of expression of the GATA - 1 and FOG- 1 (friend of GATA- 1) transcription factors.

4. In the absence of erythropoietin (EPO), committed erythroid progenitor cells undergo?
Harrison's 20th Ed. Chapter 59 Page 385

A. Stunted growth
B. Halting of growth
C. Programmed cell death (apoptosis)
D. Change to other series of hematopoietic cell

For RBC production, EPO is the regulatory hormone. It is required for maintenance of committed erythroid progenitor cells which undergoes programmed cell death (apoptosis) if EPO is absent.

5. How many mature red cells are produced from a pronormoblast?
Harrison's 20th Ed. Chapter 59 Page 385

A. 1 to 16
B. 16 to 32
C. 32 to 48
D. 48 to 64

Pronormoblast is the first morphologically recognizable erythroid precursor In bone marrow. Pronormoblast undergoes 4–5 cell divisions resulting in the production of 16–32 mature RBC's.

6. Regulation of EPO production is linked to?
Harrison's 20th Ed. Chapter 59 Page 385

A. O_2
B. CO_2
C. Red cell mass
D. Hemoglobin concentration

The regulation of EPO production is linked to O_2 availability and tissue oxygenation.

7. Which of the following about mature red cell is false?
Harrison's 20th Ed. Chapter 59 Page 385

A. Diameter is 8 μm
B. Anucleate
C. Discoid in shape
D. None of the above

Mature RBC is 8 μ in diameter, anucleate, discoid in shape, and extremely pliable for it to negotiate microcirculation successfully.

8. What percentage of all circulating RBC's is replaced daily?
Harrison's 20th Ed. Chapter 59 Page 385

A. 0.2 to 0.4%
B. 0.4 to 0.6%
C. 0.6 to 0.8%
D. 0.8 to 1%

Since the average red cell lives for 100–120 days, normal red cell production results in the daily replacement of 0.8–1% of all circulating red cells in the body,

9. Term "erythron" best relates to?
Harrison's 20th Ed. Chapter 59 Page 385

A. Erythroid/megakaryocyte progenitor
B. Red cell destruction
C. Organ responsible for red cell production
D. Red blood cell mass

The organ responsible for red cell production is called "erythron" which consists of a rapidly proliferating pool of marrow erythroid precursor cells & the mass of mature circulating RBCs.

10. Erythropoietin is a?
Harrison's 20th Ed. Chapter 59 Page 386

A. Peptide hormone
B. Glycoprotein hormone
C. Steroid hormone
D. None of the above

EPO is a glycoprotein hormone that acts by binding to specific receptors on surface of marrow erythroid precursors, inducing them to proliferate & mature when iron is adequately available.

11. Erythropoietin is produced and released by?
Harrison's 20th Ed. Chapter 59 Page 386

A. Glomerular capillaries
B. Proximal tubular cells
C. Peritubular capillary lining cells of kidney
D. All of the above

Physiologic regulator of RBC production, glycoprotein hormone EPO, is produced & released by highly specialized epithelial-like peritubular capillary lining cells within kidney.

12. Erythropoietin is also produced by?
Harrison's 20th Ed. Chapter 59 Page 386

A. Pancreas
B. Spleen
C. Hepatocytes
D. Al of the above

A small amount of EPO is produced by hepatocytes.

13. Key to EPO gene regulation is?
Harrison's 20th Ed. Chapter 59 Page 386

A. (HIF)-1α
B. (EIF)-1α
C. (RIF)-1α
D. (GIF)-1α

Key to EPO gene regulation is hypoxia-inducible factor (HIF)-1α In the presence of oxygen, HIF-1α is hydroxylated at a key proline allowing HIF-1α to be ubiquitinated and degraded via the proteasome pathway.

14. EPO production is increased in?
Harrison's 20th Ed. Chapter 59 Page 386

A. Anemia
B. Hypoxemia
C. Renal artery stenosis
D. All of the above

The fundamental stimulus for EPO production is the availability of O_2 for tissue metabolic needs. Anemia, hypoxemia, or renal artery stenosis can raise EPO production.

15. Normal level of Plasma EPO is?
Harrison's 20th Ed. Chapter 59 Page 386

A. 10 to 25 U/L
B. 25 to 50 U/L
C. 50 to 75 U/L
D. 75 to 100 U/L

Normal EPO level in plasma is 10–25 U/L.

16. Plasma EPO levels increase when hemoglobin falls below?
Harrison's 20th Ed. Chapter 59 Page 386 Figure 59-2

A. 10 to 12 g/dL
B. 8 to 10 g/dL
C. 6 to 8 g/dL
D. 4 to 6 g/dL

When the hemoglobin level falls to 12 g/dL, plasma EPO levels increase logarithmically. When hemoglobin concentration falls below 10–12 g/dL, plasma EPO levels increase in proportion to the severity of anemia.

17. In circulation, EPO has a half-clearance time of?
Harrison's 20th Ed. Chapter 59 Page 386

A. 1 to 3 hours
B. 3 to 6 hours
C. 6 to 9 hours
D. 9 to 12 hours

In circulation, EPO has a half-clearance time of 6 - 9 hours.

18. The mean hematocrit value for adult males is?
Harrison's 20th Ed. Chapter 59 Page 386

A. 42%
B. 45%
C. 47%
D. 49%

Mean hematocrit value for adult males is 47% (± SD 7) and for adult females is 42% (± 5).

19. Anemia is most often recognized by?
Harrison's 20th Ed. Chapter 59 Page 386

A. Attendant symptoms
B. Attendant signs
C. Abnormal screening laboratory tests
D. All of the above

Anemia is most often recognized by (incidental) abnormal screening laboratory tests.

20. O_2–hemoglobin dissociation curve relates to which of the following?
Harrison's 20th Ed. Chapter 59 Page 386

A. Claude effect
B. Bohr effect
C. Charles effect
D. Bennett effect

Bohr effect refers to enhanced O_2 delivery through changes in O_2–hemoglobin dissociation curve mediated by a decreased pH or increased CO_2.

21. Signs of vascular instability appear with acute blood loss of?
Harrison's 20th Ed. Chapter 59 Page 386

A. 5 to 10% of total blood volume
B. 10 to 15% of total blood volume
C. 15 to 20% of total blood volume
D. 20 to 25% of total blood volume

Signs of vascular instability appear with acute losses of 10 - 15% of the total blood volume.

22. Hypovolemic shock results if volume of blood lost is?
Harrison's 20th Ed. Chapter 59 Page 386

A. > 25%
B. > 30%
C. > 35%
D. > 40%

If the volume of blood lost is >40% (>2 L in average-sized adult), signs of hypovolemic shock including confusion, dyspnea, diaphoresis, hypotension and tachycardia appear.

23. Intravascular hemolysis with release of free hemoglobin may be associated with?
Harrison's 20th Ed. Chapter 59 Page 386

A. Acute back pain
B. Acute pain in lower limbs
C. Acute pain in upper limbs
D. Acute headache

Intravascular hemolysis with release of free hemoglobin may be associated with acute back pain, free hemoglobin in the plasma and urine, and renal failure.

24. Organs that are relatively rich in blood supply include?

Harrison's 20th Ed. Chapter 59 Page 386

A. Kidney
B. Gut
C. Skin
D. All of the above

Organs that are relatively rich in blood supply are kidney, gut and skin. In anemia, protection of O_2 delivery to vital organs is achieved by the shunting of blood away from these organs.

25. Which of the following may be associated with autoimmune hemolysis?

Harrison's 20th Ed. Chapter 59 Page 386

A. Chronic lymphocytic leukemia
B. Infection
C. Rheumatoid arthritis
D. All of the above

Chronic inflammatory states (infection, rheumatoid arthritis, cancer) are associated with mild to moderate anemia, whereas lymphoproliferative disorders (chronic lymphocytic leukemia and certain other B cell neoplasms) may be associated with autoimmune hemolysis.

26. If palmar creases are lighter in color than surrounding skin, hemoglobin level is usually?

Harrison's 20th Ed. Chapter 59 Page 387

A. < 10 g/dL
B. < 8 g/dL
C. < 6 g/dL
D. < 4 g/dL

If the palmar creases are lighter in color than the surrounding skin with hyperextended hand, the hemoglobin level is usually <8 g/dL.

27. Femtoliters is the unit of expression of which of the following?

Harrison's 20th Ed. Chapter 59 Page 387 Table 59-2

A. Mean cell volume (MCV)
B. Mean cell hemoglobin (MCH)
C. Mean concentration of Hb per volume of RBCs (MCHC)
D. None of the above

Mean cell volume (MCV)-femtoliters, mean cell hemoglobin (MCH)-picograms per cell, and mean concentration of hemoglobin per volume of red cells (MCHC)-grams per liter.

28. Which of the following reflects iron supply?

Harrison's 20th Ed. Chapter 59 Page 387

A. Serum iron
B. Total iron-binding capacity (TIBC)
C. Serum ferritin
D. All of the above

Serum iron, total iron-binding capacity (TIBC), and serum ferritin are measurements of iron supply.

29. Which of the following is not included in the red blood cell count?

Harrison's 20th Ed. Chapter 59 Page 387 Table 59–1

A. Hemoglobin
B. Hematocrit
C. Reticulocyte count
D. Red cell distribution width (RDW)

30. Red blood cell indices includes all except?

Harrison's 20th Ed. Chapter 59 Page 387 Table 59–1

A. Mean cell volume (MCV)
B. Mean cell hemoglobin (MCH)
C. Mean cell hemoglobin concentration (MCHC)
D. Hematocrit

31. Which of the following formula estimates MCV?

Harrison's 20th Ed. Chapter 59 Page 387 Table 59–2

A. (Hematocrit × 10)/(red cell count × 106)
B. (Hemoglobin × 10)/(red cell count × 106)
C. (Hemoglobin × 10)/hematocrit
D. (Hematocrit × 10)/hemoglobin

Microcytosis is reflected by a lower than normal MCV (<80), whereas high values (>100) reflect macrocytosis. Mean cell hemoglobin (MCH) is derived from the formula (hemoglobin × 10)/(red cell count × 106). Mean cell hemoglobin concentration (MCHC) is derived from the formula (hemoglobin × 10)/hematocrit or MCH/MCV.

32. Anisocytosis is related to which feature of RBC?

Harrison's 20th Ed. Chapter 59 Page 387

A. Size
B. Shape
C. Number
D. Colour

Variations in red cell size is called anisocytosis.

33. Poikilocytosis is related to which feature of RBC?

Harrison's 20th Ed. Chapter 59 Page 387

A. Size
B. Shape
C. Number
D. Colour

Variations in red cell shape is called poikilocytosis. Poikilocytosis suggests a defect in the maturation of red cell precursors in bone marrow or fragmentation of circulating red cells.

34. RDW correlates with?

Harrison's 20th Ed. Chapter 59 Page 387

A. Anisocytosis
B. Poikilocytosis
C. Polychromasia
D. All of the above

Degree of anisocytosis correlates with increases in RDW or the range of cell sizes.

35. Upon staining with supravital dye, reticulocytes are identified by what colour of punctate spots?

Harrison's 20th Ed. Chapter 59 Page 387

A. Red
B. Blue
C. Green
D. Yellow

Reticulocytes are larger red cells, grayish blue in color on Wright-Giemsa stain, that are recently released from bone marrow & their color represents residual amounts of ribosomal RNA.

36. Reliable estimate of red cell production is provided by?
Harrison's 20th Ed. Chapter 59 Page 387

A. EPO levels
B. Reticulocyte count
C. RDW
D. Polychromasia

Reticulocyte count provides a reliable measure of red cell production.

37. "Shift" cells refer to?
Harrison's 20th Ed. Chapter 59 Page 389

A. Older RBC's
B. Prematurely released reticulocytes
C. Normoblasts
D. Any of the above

In anemia, polychromatophilic macrocytes in PBF represent prematurely released reticulocytes referred to as "shift" cells.

38. Erythroid cells take about how many days to mature?
Harrison's 20th Ed. Chapter 59 Page 390 Figure 59-13

A. 2.5
B. 3.5
C. 4.5
D. 5.5

Erythroid cells take ~4.5 days to mature. At normal hematocrit levels, they are released to the circulation with ~1 day left as reticulocytes.

39. Absolute reticulocyte count is calculated by?
Harrison's 20th Ed. Chapter 59 Page 389 Table 59-4

A. Reticulocyte count × (Hemoglobin ÷ expected hemoglobin)
B. Reticulocyte count × (Hemoglobin + Hematocrit)
C. Reticulocyte count × (Hemoglobin × Hematocrit)
D. Reticulocyte count/(Hemoglobin + Hematocrit)

40. Which of the following about macrocytes is false?
Harrison's 20th Ed. Chapter 59 Page 388 Figure 59-5

A. Red cells are larger than a small lymphocyte
B. Well hemoglobinized red cells
C. Often oval shaped
D. None of the above

Macrocytes are red blood cells that are larger than a small lymphocyte and are well hemoglobinized. Often macrocytes are oval shaped (macro-ovalocytes).

41. Howell-Jolly bodies best relate to which of the following?
Harrison's 20th Ed. Chapter 59 Page 388 Figure 59-6

A. Uremia
B. Nuclear remnants
C. Foreign bodies in the circulation
D. All of the above

Howell-Jolly bodies refer to tiny nuclear remnants that are not removed from red cells due to absence of a functional spleen (splenectomy) and with maturation/dysplastic disorders (excess production). They remain as small homogeneously staining blue inclusions on Wright stain.

42. Teardrop-shaped red cells best relates to?
Harrison's 20th Ed. Chapter 59 Page 388 Figure 59-7

A. Uremia
B. Myelofibrosis
C. Thalassemia
D. Liver disease

Teardrop-shaped red cells are seen in myelofibrosis and extramedullary hematopoiesis.

43. Target red cells best relates to?
Harrison's 20th Ed. Chapter 59 Page 389 Figure 59-8

A. Uremia
B. Myelofibrosis
C. Thalassemia
D. Acute hemolysis

Target red cells have a bull's-eye appearance & are seen in thalassemia and liver disease.

44. Target cells are seen in?
Harrison's 20th Ed. Chapter 59 Page 389 Figure 59-8

A. Liver disease
B. Thalassemia
C. Hemoglobin C disease
D. All of the above

Target cells are recognized by the bull's-eye appearance of the red cell. Small numbers of target cells are seen with liver disease & thalassemia. Larger numbers are typical of hemoglobin C disease.

45. Thermal injury may produce which of the following?
Harrison's 20th Ed. Chapter 59 Page 389 Figure 59-9

A. Target cells
B. Burr cells
C. Howell-Jolly bodies
D. Red cell fragmentation

Presence of foreign bodies in the circulation (mechanical heart valves), or thermal injury may cause red cell fragmentation.

46. Burr cells are also called?
Harrison's 20th Ed. Chapter 59 Page 389 Figure 59-10

A. Echinocytes
B. Acanthocytes
C. Elliptocytes
D. Spherocytes

Burr cells are also called echinocytes. Echinocytes have small, uniform, and evenly spaced membrane projections.

47. Echinocytes are found in patients with?
Harrison's 20th Ed. Chapter 59 Page 389 Figure 59-10

A. Severe uremia
B. Glycolytic red cell enzyme defects
C. Microangiopathic hemolytic anemia
D. All of the above

Echinocytes are found in patients with severe uremia, in glycolytic red cell enzyme defects, and in microangiopathic hemolytic anemia.

48. Acanthocytes are present in which of the following conditions?
Harrison's 20th Ed. Chapter 59 Page 389 Figure 59-11

A. Severe liver disease
B. Abetalipoproteinemia
C. Patients with McLeod blood group
D. All of the above

Acanthocytes are contracted dense cells with irregular membrane projections that vary in length and width. Acanthocytes are present in severe liver disease, in patients with abetalipoproteinemia, and in rare patients with McLeod blood group.

49. Dacrocytes are seen in?
Harrison's 20th Ed. Chapter 58 Page 379

A. Hemolytic anemias
B. Severe iron deficiency
C. Myelodysplastic syndromes
D. All of the above

Dacrocytes are teardrop-shaped cells that can be seen in hemolytic anemias, severe iron deficiency, thalassemias, myelofibrosis and myelodysplastic syndromes.

50. Helmet-shaped red blood cells are called?
Harrison's 20th Ed. Chapter 58 Page 379

A. Echinocytes
B. Acanthocytes
C. Schistocytes
D. Stomatocytes

Schistocytes are helmet-shaped cells that reflect microangiopathic hemolytic anemia or fragmentation on an artificial heart valve.

51. The best place to examine blood cell morphology is?
Harrison's 20th Ed. Chapter 58 Page 379

A. Thick, blunt initial edge of blood smear
B. Middle uniform layer of blood smear
C. Feathered edge of the blood smear
D. Any of the above

The best place to examine blood cell morphology is the feathered edge of the blood smear where red cells lie in a single layer, side by side and not overlapping.

52. While examining the peripheral blood smear, which of the following should be looked at first?
Harrison's 20th Ed. Chapter 58 Page 379

A. Platelets
B. Red blood cells
C. White blood cells
D. Reticulocytes

While looking at PBF, correct approach is to look at the smallest cellular elements, platelets first and then work up in size to red cells and then white cells.

53. Red cell distribution width (RDW) is calculated from?
Harrison's 20th Ed. Chapter 58 Page 379

A. MCV
B. MCH
C. MCHC
D. Reticulocyte index

Red cell distribution width (RDW) is calculated from the MCV. It is derived from the curve displaying the frequency of cells at each volume also called the distribution. The width of red cell volume distribution curve is what determines the RDW.

54. The RDW is calculated as?
Harrison's 20th Ed. Chapter 58 Page 379

A. (Standard deviation of MCV/mean MCV) × 100
B. (Mean MCV/standard deviation of MCV) × 100
C. (Standard error of MCV/mean MCV) × 100
D. (Mean MCV/standard error of MCV) × 100

The RDW is calculated as (standard deviation of MCV/mean MCV) x 100.

55. The normal serum iron range is?
Harrison's 20th Ed. Chapter 59 Page 390

A. 10 to 50 μg/dL
B. 50 to 150 μg/ dL
C. 150 to 250 μg/dL
D. 250 to 450 μg/dL

Normal serum iron ranges from 50–150 μg/dL

56. The normal serum TIBC range is?
Harrison's 20th Ed. Chapter 59 Page 390

A. 100 to 150 μg/dL
B. 150 to 300 μg/dL
C. 300 to 360 μg/dL
D. 350 to 450 μg/dL

Normal TIBC is 300–360 μg/dL.

57. Percent transferrin saturation is calculated by?
Harrison's 20th Ed. Chapter 59 Page 390

A. (TIBC × 100) ÷ Serum iron
B. (Serum iron + TIBC) ÷ 100
C. (Serum iron × 100) ÷ TIBC
D. (Serum iron ÷ TIBC) x 100

Percent transferrin saturation is derived by dividing serum iron level (x 100) by TIBC. Normal transferrin saturation ranges from 25 - 50%.

58. Adult males have average serum ferritin levels of about?
Harrison's 20th Ed. Chapter 59 Page 390

A. 10 μg/L
B. 50 μg/L
C. 100 μg/L
D. 200 μg/L

Serum ferritin is used to evaluate total-body iron stores. Adult males have serum ferritin levels that average ~100 μg/L, corresponding to iron stores of ~1 gram. Serum ferritin level of 10 - 15 μg/L represents depletion of body iron stores.

59. Adult females have average serum ferritin levels of about?
Harrison's 20th Ed. Chapter 59 Page 390

A. 10 μg/L
B. 30 μg/L
C. 60 μg/L
D. 90 μg/L

Adult females have serum ferritin levels averaging 30 μg/L, reflecting lower iron stores (300 mg).

60. Ferritin is also an?

Harrison's 20th Ed. Chapter 59 Page 390

A. Enzyme
B. Cytokine
C. Chemokine
D. Acute-phase reactant

Ferritin is also an acute-phase reactant.

61. Erythroblasts containing what are called sideroblasts?

Harrison's 20th Ed. Chapter 59 Page 391

A. Hemosiderin
B. Ferritin
C. Residual RNA
D. All of the above

In bone marrow smears, developing erythroblasts with small ferritin granules are sideroblasts.

62. Hemolysis is most likely cause if reticulocyte production index is more than?

Harrison's 20th Ed. Chapter 59 Page 391

A. 2.5
B. 3.5
C. 4.5
D. 5.5

Reticulocyte production index of >2.5 indicates that hemolysis is most likely.

63. Which of the following anemias is most frequent?

Harrison's 20th Ed. Chapter 59 Page 391

A. Hypoproliferative
B. Maturation Disorders
C. Hemoglobinopathies
D. Hemolytic

At least 75% of all cases of anemia are hypoproliferative in nature. Hemolytic disease is among the least common forms of anemia.

64. A hypoproliferative anemia can result from?

Harrison's 20th Ed. Chapter 59 Page 391

A. Marrow damage
B. Iron deficiency
C. Inadequate EPO stimulation
D. All of the above

Majority of hypoproliferative anemias are due to mild to moderate iron deficiency or inflammation. They result from marrow damage, iron deficiency or inadequate EPO stimulation.

65. Which of the following is the iron regulatory hormone?

Harrison's 20th Ed. Chapter 59 Page 392

A. Erythropoietin
B. Transferrin
C. Hepcidin
D. All of the above

Hepcidin is the iron regulatory hormone that is increased in inflammation.

66. Nuclear maturation defects of RBC's result from all except?

Harrison's 20th Ed. Chapter 59 Page 392

A. Vitamin B_{12} deficiency
B. Folic acid deficiency
C. Iron deficiency
D. Methotrexate therapy

Nuclear maturation defects result from vitamin B_{12} or folic acid deficiency, drug damage (methotrexate or alkylating agents), myelodysplasia and alcohol.

67. Cytoplasmic maturation defects of RBC's result from?

Harrison's 20th Ed. Chapter 59 Page 392

A. Severe iron deficiency
B. Abnormalities in heme synthesis
C. Abnormalities in globin synthesis
D. Any of the above

Cytoplasmic maturation defects result from 'severe' iron deficiency or abnormalities in globin or heme synthesis.

68. Increased red cell mass is present when hematocrit in men is?

Harrison's 20th Ed. Chapter 59 Page 393

A. > 45%
B. > 50%
C. > 55%
D. > 60%

PCV >60% in men & >55% in women are invariably associated with an increased red cell mass.

69. Gaisbock's syndrome relates to?

Harrison's 20th Ed. Chapter 59 Page 393

A. Spurious polycythemia
B. High altitude polycythemia
C. Ectopic EPO production
D. Familial polycythemia

Gaisbock's syndrome refers to spurious polycythemia due to a decrease in plasma volume.

70. Tests that support the diagnosis of polycythemia vera include?

Harrison's 20th Ed. Chapter 59 Page 393

A. Elevated white blood cell count
B. Increased absolute basophil count
C. Thrombocytosis
D. All of the above

Tests that support the diagnosis of polycythemia vera include elevated white blood cell count, increased absolute basophil count and thrombocytosis.

71. EPO-producing neoplasms include?

Harrison's 20th Ed. Chapter 59 Page 394

A. Hepatoma
B. Uterine leiomyoma
C. Cerebellar hemangiomas
D. All of the above

EPO-producing neoplasms include hepatoma, uterine leiomyoma, renal cancer or cysts and cerebellar hemangiomas.

Disorders of Granulocytes and Monocytes

72. Which of the following is a leukocyte?
Harrison's 20th Ed. Chapter 60 Page 394

A. Natural killer (NK) cell
B. B lymphocyte
C. Monocyte
D. All of the above

Leukocytes include neutrophils, T and B lymphocytes, natural killer (NK) cells, monocytes, eosinophils, and basophils.

73. Which of the following statements about leukocytes is false?
Harrison's 20th Ed. Chapter 60 Page 394

A. Derived from common stem cell in bone marrow
B. Three-fourths of nucleated cells of bone marrow are committed to leukocyte production
C. Their maturation in marrow is regulated by colony-stimulating factors & interleukins
D. None of the above

Leukocytes are derived from a common stem cell in bone marrow. Three-fourths of nucleated cells of bone marrow are committed to production of leukocytes. Leukocyte maturation in the marrow is under the regulatory control of colony-stimulating factors (CSFs) & interleukins (ILs).

74. Minimum number of stem cells necessary to support hematopoiesis is?
Harrison's 20th Ed. Chapter 60 Page 394

A. 100 to 200
B. 200 to 300
C. 300 to 400
D. 400 to 500

Minimum number of stem cells necessary to support hematopoiesis is 400 - 500 at any one time.

75. Colony-stimulating factors are produced by?
Harrison's 20th Ed. Chapter 60 Page 394

A. Monocytes
B. Tissue macrophages
C. Stromal cells
D. All of the above

Human blood monocytes, tissue macrophages & stromal cells produce CSFs, hormones required for growth of monocytes & neutrophils in bone marrow.

76. In a 80 kg person, how many neutrophils are produced by hematopoietic system per day?
Harrison's 20th Ed. Chapter 60 Page 394

A. $\sim 0.3 \times 10^{11}$
B. $\sim 1.3 \times 10^{11}$
C. $\sim 2.3 \times 10^{11}$
D. $\sim 3.3 \times 10^{11}$

In a 80 kg person, $\sim 1.3 \times 10^{11}$ neutrophils are produced by hematopoietic system per day.

77. Maturation from metamyelocyte to neutrophil takes how many days?
Harrison's 20th Ed. Chapter 60 Page 394

A. 2 days
B. 5 days
C. 7 days
D. 10 days

Proliferation phase through the metamyelocyte takes ~1 week, while maturation phase from metamyelocyte to mature neutrophil takes ~1 week.

78. Which of the following is the largest cell in size?
Harrison's 20th Ed. Chapter 60 Page 395 Figure 60-2

A. Myeloblast
B. Promyelocyte
C. Myelocyte
D. Metamyelocyte

79. Primary or azurophil granules are present in?
Harrison's 20th Ed. Chapter 60 Page 395

A. Myeloblast
B. Promyelocyte
C. Myelocyte
D. All of the above

Classic lysosomal granules called the primary or azurophil granules are found in promyelocyte.

80. Primary or azurophil granules contain?
Harrison's 20th Ed. Chapter 60 Page 395

A. Hydrolases
B. Cathepsin G
C. Myeloperoxidase
D. All of the above

Primary granules contain hydrolases, elastase, myeloperoxidase, cathepsin G, cationic proteins, bactericidal/permeability-increasing protein & defensins.

81. Which of the following azurophil granules has broad antimicrobial activity against bacteria, fungi & certain enveloped viruses?
Harrison's 20th Ed. Chapter 60 Page 395

A. Hydrolases
B. Cathepsin G
C. Myeloperoxidase
D. Defensins

Defensins in azurophil granules have a broad antimicrobial activity against bacteria, fungi, and certain enveloped viruses.

82. Specific or secondary granules are present in?
Harrison's 20th Ed. Chapter 60 Page 395

A. Myeloblast
B. Promyelocyte
C. Myelocyte
D. All of the above

83. Secondary granules contain all except?

Harrison's 20th Ed. Chapter 60 Page 395

A. Acid hydrolases
B. Lactoferrin
C. Vitamin B_{12} binding protein
D. Histaminase

Myelocyte synthesises specific or secondary granules which contains lactoferrin, vitamin B_{12} binding protein, membrane components of reduced nicotinamide-adenine dinucleotide phosphate (NADPH) oxidase, histaminase, and laminin. Secondary granules do not contain acid hydrolases.

84. Packaging of secondary granule contents during myelopoiesis is controlled by?

Harrison's 20th Ed. Chapter 60 Page 395

A. CCAAT/enhancer binding protein-α
B. CCAAT/enhancer binding protein-β
C. CCAAT/enhancer binding protein-γ
D. CCAAT/enhancer binding protein-ε

Packaging of secondary granule contents during myelopoiesis is controlled by CCAAT/enhancer binding protein-ε.

85. Excessive segmentation of nucleus of neutrophils is a manifestation of?

Harrison's 20th Ed. Chapter 60 Page 395

A. Folate or vitamin B_{12} deficiency
B. Iron deficiency
C. Thalassemia
D. Repeated blood transfusion

Nucleus of neutrophils normally contains up to four segments. Excessive segmentation (>5 nuclear lobes) is seen in folate or vitamin B_{12} deficiency & congenital neutropenia syndrome of warts, hypogammaglobulinemia, infections & myelokathexis (WHIM).

86. Which of the following is false about 'Pelger-Huet anomaly'?

Harrison's 20th Ed. Chapter 60 Page 395 Figure 60-5

A. Benign disorder
B. Majority of granulocytes are bilobed
C. Nucleus has spectacle-like configuration
D. None of the above

Pelger-Hüet anomaly is a benign inherited disorder. Majority of granulocytes are bilobed (hyposegmented neutrophils). Nucleus has a spectacle-like, or "pince-nez" configuration. Acquired bilobed nuclei, pseudo Pelger-Huet anomaly, can occur with acute infections or in myelodysplastic syndromes.

87. In neutrophils, which of the following is seen in severe acute bacterial infections?

Harrison's 20th Ed. Chapter 60 Page 395

A. Toxic granulations
B. Dohle bodies
C. Large neutrophil vacuoles
D. All of the above

In severe acute bacterial infection toxic granulations (immature or abnormally staining azurophil granules), Döhle bodies (cytoplasmic inclusions which are fragments of ribosome-rich endoplasmic reticulum) & large neutrophil vacuoles (pinocytosed or internalized membrane) are seen.

88. Which of the following is false about 'Dohle body'?

Harrison's 20th Ed. Chapter 60 Page 395 Figure 60-3

A. Discrete, blue-staining nongranular areas found in periphery of cytoplasm of neutrophils
B. Found in infections and other toxic states
C. Aggregates of rough endoplasmic reticulum
D. None of the above

Döhle bodies are discrete, blue-staining nongranular areas found in periphery of cytoplasm of neutrophil in infections & toxic states. They are aggregates of rough endoplasmic reticulum.

89. Under normal conditions, what proportion of neutrophil pool is in the bone marrow?

Harrison's 20th Ed. Chapter 60 Page 395

A. ~ 20%
B. ~ 50%
C. ~ 70%
D. ~ 90%

90. Under normal conditions, what proportion of neutrophil pool is in the circulation?

Harrison's 20th Ed. Chapter 60 Page 395

A. ~ 2%
B. ~ 20%
C. ~ 50%
D. ~ 90%

Normally, ~90% of the neutrophil pool is in bone marrow, 2 - 3% in circulation (freely flowing & marginated), & remainder in tissues.

91. Marginated leukocytes are maximum in?

Harrison's 20th Ed. Chapter 60 Page 395

A. Lungs
B. Spleen
C. Liver
D. Kidneys

Circulating pool of neutrophils exists in two dynamic compartments: one freely flowing and one marginated. Freely flowing pool is ~half the neutrophils in basal state and is composed of those cells that are in the blood and not in contact with endothelium. Marginated leukocytes are those that are in close physical contact with endothelium. Due to extensive capillary bed (~1000 capillaries per alveolus) in pulmonary circulation, margination occurs because the capillaries are about the same size as a mature neutrophil.

92. "Rolling" of the neutrophil along the endothelial surface is a function of?

Harrison's 20th Ed. Chapter 60 Page 396

A. Selectins
B. Integrins
C. Intercellular adhesion molecules
D. Opsonins

Selectins are glycoproteins expressed on neutrophils & endothelial cells and cause a low-affinity interaction resulting in "rolling" of neutrophil along the endothelial surface.

93. Neutrophils "stick" to the endothelium through?

Harrison's 20th Ed. Chapter 60 Page 396

A. Selectins
B. Integrins
C. Intercellular adhesion molecules
D. Opsonins

In response to chemotactic stimuli from injured tissues or bacterial products, neutrophil adhesiveness increases and they "stick" to the endothelium through integrins. Integrins are leukocyte glycoproteins that bind to specific endothelial receptors [intercellular adhesion molecules (ICAM) 1 & 2].

94. Diapedesis involves which of the following?

Harrison's 20th Ed. Chapter 60 Page 396

A. PECAM 1
B. Anaphylatoxins
C. Vascular endothelial growth factor (VEGF)
D. Prostaglandins E & I

Process of migration into tissues is called diapedesis and involves crawling of neutrophils between postcapillary endothelial cells that open junctions between adjacent cells to permit leukocyte passage. Diapedesis involves platelet/endothelial cell adhesion molecule (PECAM) 1 (CD31) expressed on emigrating leukocyte & endothelial cells.

95. In the healthy adult, most neutrophils leave the body by?

Harrison's 20th Ed. Chapter 60 Page 397

A. Migration through mucous membrane of GI tract
B. Apoptosis
C. Phagocytosis
D. All of the above

In the healthy adult, most neutrophils leave the body by migration through the mucous membrane of the gastrointestinal tract.

96. Normally, neutrophils spend how much time in circulation?

Harrison's 20th Ed. Chapter 60 Page 397

A. 2 to 3 hours
B. 6 to 7 hours
C. 12 to 24 hours
D. 24 to 36 hours

Normally, neutrophils spend a short time in circulation (half-life, 6 - 7 hours).

97. Senescent neutrophils are cleared from the circulation by macrophages in?

Harrison's 20th Ed. Chapter 60 Page 397

A. Kidneys
B. Lung
C. GI tract
D. Thymus

Senescent neutrophils are cleared from the circulation by macrophages in the lung and spleen.

98. Characteristic green color to pus is due to?

Harrison's 20th Ed. Chapter 60 Page 397

A. Collagenase
B. Elastase
C. Myeloperoxidase
D. All of the above

Myeloperoxidase confers the characteristic green color to pus and may participate in turning off the inflammatory process by inactivating chemoattractants and immobilizing phagocytic cells.

99. Which of the following is not a group of chemokines?

Harrison's 20th Ed. Chapter 60 Page 397

A. C
B. CC
C. CCC
D. CXC

Four major groups of chemokines are recognized based on cysteine structure near N terminus: C, CC, CXC, and CXXXC. C chemokine (lymphotactin) is T cell tropic. CC chemokines (MIP-1) attract lymphocytes, monocytes, eosinophils, & basophils. CXC cytokines (IL-8) attract neutrophils. CXXXC chemokine (fractalkine) attracts neutrophils, monocytes, & T cells.

100. Which of the following infection is rare in patients with congenital phagocyte defects?

Harrison's 20th Ed. Chapter 60 Page 397

A. Skin infection
B. Upper and lower respiratory tract infection
C. Osteomyelitis
D. Meningitis

Patients with congenital phagocyte cell defects can have infections within the first few days of life. Skin, ear, upper and lower respiratory tract and bone infections are common. Sepsis and meningitis are rare.

101. Susceptibility to infectious diseases increases sharply when neutrophil counts fall below?

Harrison's 20th Ed. Chapter 60 Page 397

A. 1000 cells/μL
B. 2000 cells/μL
C. 3000 cells/μL
D. 4000 cells/μL

Susceptibility to infectious diseases increases sharply when neutrophil counts fall <1000 cells/μL.

102. Inflammatory process is absent, when absolute neutrophil count (ANC) falls below?

Harrison's 20th Ed. Chapter 60 Page 397

A. < 100 cells/μL
B. < 200 cells/μL
C. < 500 cells/μL
D. < 1000 cells/μL

When absolute neutrophil count (band forms & mature neutrophils combined) is <200/μL, the inflammatory process is absent.

103. Neutropenia can be due to?

Harrison's 20th Ed. Chapter 60 Page 397

A. Depressed production
B. Increased peripheral destruction
C. Excessive peripheral pooling
D. All of the above

Neutropenia can be due to depressed production, increased peripheral destruction, or excessive peripheral pooling.

104. Which of the following drugs cause neutropenia due to decreased production?

Harrison's 20th Ed. Chapter 60 Page 398 Page Table 60–1

A. Carbamazepine
B. Clozapine
C. Antithyroid drugs
D. All of the above

Drugs cause neutropenia due to decreased production include alkylating agents (nitrogen mustard, busulfan, chlorambucil, cyclophosphamide), antimetabolites (methotrexate, 6-mercaptopurine, 5-flucytosine), antibiotics (chloramphenicol, penicillins, sulfonamides), phenothiazines, tranquilizers (meprobamate), anticonvulsants (carbamazepine), antipsychotics (clozapine), certain diuretics, anti-inflammatory agents, antithyroid drugs.

105. Which of the following drugs act as haptens to cause neutropenia due to peripheral destruction?
Harrison's 20th Ed. Chapter 60 Page 398 Table 60–1

A. Alpha methyldopa
B. Phenylbutazone
C. Mercurial diuretics
D. All of the above

Drugs that act as haptens to cause neutropenia due to peripheral destruction include aminopyrine, alpha methyldopa, phenylbutazone, mercurial diuretics, some phenothiazines.

106. Which of the following is a cause of neutropenia due to peripheral pooling (Transient neutropenia)?
Harrison's 20th Ed. Chapter 60 Page 398 Table 60–1

A. Overwhelming bacterial infection (acute endotoxemia)
B. Hemodialysis
C. Cardiopulmonary bypass
D. All of the above

107. Congenital forms of neutropenia include?
Harrison's 20th Ed. Chapter 60 Page 398

A. Kostmann's syndrome
B. Shwachman-Diamond syndrome
C. WHIM syndrome
D. All of the above

Congenital forms of neutropenia include Kostmann's syndrome, cartilage-hair hypoplasia syndrome, Shwachman-Diamond syndrome, WHIM syndrome and hereditary cyclic neutropenia.

108. Kostmann's syndrome is due to mutations in?
Harrison's 20th Ed. Chapter 60 Page 398

A. Potassium voltage-gated channel gene KCNA1
B. PKD-1 gene
C. Anti-apoptosis gene HAX-1
D. GJB2 gene

Kostmann's syndrome is due to mutations in anti-apoptosis gene HAX-1.

109. Which of the following is associated with pancreatic insufficiency?
Harrison's 20th Ed. Chapter 60 Page 398

A. Kostmann's syndrome
B. Shwachman-Diamond syndrome
C. WHIM syndrome
D. All of the above

Shwachman-Diamond syndrome is associated with pancreatic insufficiency and is due to mutations in the Shwachman-Bodian-Diamond syndrome gene SBDS.

110. Felty's syndrome include all except?
Harrison's 20th Ed. Chapter 60 Page 398

A. Rheumatoid arthritis
B. Hepatomegaly
C. Splenomegaly
D. Neutropenia

Rheumatoid arthritis, splenomegaly & neutropenia form the triad of Felty's syndrome. Neutropenia is due to antibodies produced by spleen that shorten neutrophil life span, while large granular lymphocytes (LGL) can attack marrow neutrophil precursors.

111. Neutrophilia results from?
Harrison's 20th Ed. Chapter 60 Page 398

A. Increased neutrophil production
B. Increased marrow release
C. Defective margination
D. All of the above

Neutrophilia is due to increased neutrophil production & marrow release or defective margination.

112. Persistent neutrophilia with what level of raised cell counts is called leukemoid reaction?
Harrison's 20th Ed. Chapter 60 Page 398

A. > 10000 to 30000/μL
B. > 30000 to 50000/μL
C. > 50000 to 75000/μL
D. > 75000 to 100000/μL

113. Which of the following is false about leukemoid reaction?
Harrison's 20th Ed. Chapter 60 Page 398

A. Neutrophil cell count > 30000 to 50000/μL
B. Circulating neutrophils are mature
C. Circulating neutrophils are clonally derived
D. None of the above

Persistent neutrophilia with cell counts of 30,000 - 50,000/μL is called a leukemoid reaction. In leukemoid reaction, circulating neutrophils are usually mature & not clonally derived.

114. Which of the following drugs can cause neutrophilia?
Harrison's 20th Ed. Chapter 60 Page 399 Table 60–2

A. Meprobamate
B. Lithium
C. Phenothiazines
D. Phenylbutazone

Epinephrine, glucocorticoids, nonsteroidal anti-inflammatory agents, lithium, , granulocyte colony-stimulating factor (G-CSF) can cause neutrophilia.

115. Which of the following about leukocyte adhesion deficiency (LAD) 1 & 2 is false?
Harrison's 20th Ed. Chapter 60 Page 399

A. Autosomal dominant traits
B. Inability of neutrophils to exit circulation
C. Leukocytosis
D. Increased susceptibility to infection

LAD 1 & 2 are autosomal recessive traits leading to inability of neutrophils to exit circulation to sites of infection, leukocytosis & increased susceptibility to infection.

116. Patients with leukocyte adhesion deficiency 1 (LAD 1) have mutations in?
Harrison's 20th Ed. Chapter 60 Page 399

A. CD18
B. CD31
C. CD34
D. CD62

Patients with LAD1 have mutations in CD18. CD18 gene is located on distal chromosome 21q.

117. Which of the following is called "Congenital disorder of glycosylation IIc (CDGIIc)"?

Harrison's 20th Ed. Chapter 60 Page 399

A. Leukocyte adhesion deficiency 1 (LAD 1)
B. Leukocyte adhesion deficiency 2 (LAD 2)
C. Leukocyte adhesion deficiency 3 (LAD 3)
D. None of the above

LAD 2 is also known as congenital disorder of glycosylation IIc (CDGIIc) due to mutation in a GDP-fucose transporter (SLC35C1).

118. Which of the following is caused by mutations in the gene FERMT3?

Harrison's 20th Ed. Chapter 60 Page 399

A. Leukocyte adhesion deficiency 1 (LAD 1)
B. Leukocyte adhesion deficiency 2 (LAD 2)
C. Leukocyte adhesion deficiency 3 (LAD 3)
D. None of the above

LAD 3 is caused by mutations in the gene FERMT3.

119. For lymphocytes, "CD" stands for?

Harrison's 20th Ed. Chapter 60 Page 397 Table 60–8

A. Clonal determinant
B. Cluster determinant
C. Capsule determinant
D. Cell determinant

CD = Cluster determinant.

120. The most common neutrophil defect is?

Harrison's 20th Ed. Chapter 60 Page 399

A. Myeloperoxidase deficiency
B. Chediak-Higashi syndrome (CHS)
C. Leukocyte adhesion deficiency 1 (LAD 1)
D. Leukocyte adhesion deficiency 2 (LAD 2)

The most common neutrophil defect is myeloperoxidase deficiency. It is an autosomal recessive primary granule defect (incidence is ~1 in 2000). Isolated myeloperoxidase deficiency is not associated with clinically compromised defenses, because other defense systems.

121. Patients with myeloperoxidase deficiency are more susceptible to?

Harrison's 20th Ed. Chapter 60 Page 399

A. Malaria
B. Subacute bacterial endocarditis
C. Candida infections
D. Enteric fever

Patients with myeloperoxidase deficiency and diabetes are more susceptible to Candida infections.

122. Acquired form of myeloperoxidase deficiency occurs in?

Harrison's 20th Ed. Chapter 60 Page 399

A. Acute myeloid leukemia
B. Chronic myeloid leukemia
C. Polycythemia vera
D. Sarcoidosis

An acquired form of myeloperoxidase deficiency occurs in myelomonocytic leukemia and acute myeloid leukemia.

123. Which of the following is false about Chédiak-Higashi syndrome (CHS)?

Harrison's 20th Ed. Chapter 60 Page 399

A. Autosomal recessive inheritance
B. Defects in lysosomal transport protein LYST
C. Abnormal packaging & disbursement of granules
D. None of the above

CHS is a systemic disease with autosomal recessive inheritance due to defects in the lysosomal transport protein LYST required for normal packaging and disbursement of granules, encoded by the gene CHS1 at 1q42. Characterized by the presence of giant lysosomes within leukocytes.

124. Patients with Chédiak-Higashi syndrome (CHS) may have which of the following?

Harrison's 20th Ed. Chapter 60 Page 399

A. Seizure
B. Blindness
C. Nystagmus
D. Tremors

Patients with CHS have nystagmus, partial oculocutaneous albinism, and an increased frequency of infections. Patients may develop a severe disabling peripheral neuropathy in adulthood. Vitamin C supplementation is useful in Chédiak-Higashi syndrome. Hematopoietic cell transplantation can cure patients of CHS.

125. Leukocytes from patients with chronic granulomatous disease (CGD) have severely diminished production of?

Harrison's 20th Ed. Chapter 60 Page 401

A. Hydrogen peroxide
B. Nitric oxide
C. IL-1
D. TNF-alpha

Leukocytes from patients with CGD have severely diminished hydrogen peroxide production.

126. Frequency of which of the following is increased in CGD?

Harrison's 20th Ed. Chapter 60 Page 401

A. Immune thrombocytopenic purpura (ITP)
B. Juvenile rheumatoid arthritis
C. Discoid lupus
D. All of the above

127. Mononuclear phagocyte system is composed of?

Harrison's 20th Ed. Chapter 60 Page 401

A. Monoblasts
B. Promonocytes
C. Monocytes
D. All of the above

Mononuclear phagocyte system is composed of monoblasts, promonocytes, monocytes and tissue macrophages.

128. Monocytes have a half-life in the blood of?

Harrison's 20th Ed. Chapter 60 Page 401

A. 1 to 3 hours
B. 6 to 7 hours
C. 12 to 24 hours
D. 24 to 36 hours

Monocytes have a half-life in blood of 12–24 hours.

129. "Big eaters" is the term used for?
Harrison's 20th Ed. Chapter 60 Page 401

A. Neutrophils
B. Monocytes
C. Macrophages
D. None of the above

Macrophages are called "big eaters". They differentiate from blood monocytes that arrive in tissues.

130. Function of macrophage secreted product - IL-1 is?
Harrison's 20th Ed. Chapter 60 Page 401

A. Initiating fever in hypothalamus
B. Mobilizing leukocytes from bone marrow
C. Activating lymphocytes & neutrophils
D. All of the above

Functions of IL-1 include initiating fever in hypothalamus, mobilizing leukocytes from bone marrow and activating lymphocytes & neutrophils.

131. TNF-α duplicates the function of which of the following?
Harrison's 20th Ed. Chapter 60 Page 401

A. IL-1
B. IL-8
C. IL-12
D. IL-18

TNF-α is a pyrogen that duplicates many actions of IL-1. It plays significant role in the pathogenesis of gram-negative shock.

132. Monocytosis is associated with?
Harrison's 20th Ed. Chapter 60 Page 402

A. Tuberculosis
B. Brucellosis
C. Subacute bacterial endocarditis
D. All of the above

133. Monocytosis is associated with?
Harrison's 20th Ed. Chapter 60 Page 402

A. Malaria
B. Visceral leishmaniasis (kala azar)
C. Hemolytic anemias
D. All of the above

Monocytosis is associated with TB, brucellosis, SABE, Rocky Mountain spotted fever, malaria, visceral leishmaniasis (kala azar), leukemias, myeloproliferative syndromes, hemolytic anemias, chronic idiopathic neutropenias & granulomatous diseases like sarcoidosis & regional enteritis.

134. Monocytopenia occurs with?
Harrison's 20th Ed. Chapter 60 Page 402

A. Acute infections
B. Glucocorticoid therapy
C. Aplastic anemia
D. All of the above

135. Monocytopenia occurs with?
Harrison's 20th Ed. Chapter 60 Page 402

A. Hairy cell leukemia
B. Acute myeloid leukemia
C. Stress
D. All of the above

Monocytopenia occurs with acute infections, stress, glucocorticoid use, aplastic anemia, hairy cell leukemia, acute myeloid leukemia & use of myelotoxic drugs.

136. "TRAPS" stands for?
Harrison's 20th Ed. Chapter 60 Page 402

A. Tumour associated periodic syndromes
B. TNF-α receptor associated periodic syndromes
C. Thyroid associated periodic syndromes
D. T receptor associated periodic syndromes

Gain-of-function mutations in TNF-α receptor cause TNF-a receptor-associated periodic syndrome (TRAPS) characterized by recurrent fever without infection (persistent stimulation of TNF-a receptor).

137. Familial Mediterranean fever due to mutations in PYRIN is due to abnormal regulation of?
Harrison's 20th Ed. Chapter 60 Page 402

A. IL-1
B. IL-8
C. IL-12
D. IL-18

Diseases with abnormal IL-1 regulation leading to fever include familial Mediterranean fever due to mutations in PYRIN.

138. Mutations in cold-induced autoinflammatory syndrome 1 (CIAS1) lead to?
Harrison's 20th Ed. Chapter 60 Page 402

A. Neonatal-onset multisystem autoinflammatory disease
B. Familial cold urticaria
C. Muckle-Wells syndrome
D. All of the above

Mutations in cold-induced autoinflammatory syndrome 1 (CIAS1) lead to neonatal-onset multisystem autoinflammatory disease, familial cold urticaria, and Muckle-Wells syndrome.

139. Mutations in CD2BP1 cause which of the following?
Harrison's 20th Ed. Chapter 60 Page 402

A. PAPA syndrome
B. Muckle-Wells syndrome
C. Familial cold urticaria
D. Familial Mediterranean fever

The syndrome of pyoderma gangrenosum, acne, and sterile pyogenic arthritis (PAPA syndrome) is caused by mutations in CD2BP1.

140. Which of the following is a TNF-α antagonist?
Harrison's 20th Ed. Chapter 60 Page 402

A. Infliximab
B. Adalimumab
C. Etanercept
D. All of the above

TNF-α antagonists are infliximab, adalimumab, certolizumab, golimumab and etanercept.

141. Specific chemokine expressed by eosinophils is?

Harrison's 20th Ed. Chapter 60 Page 402

A. Eotaxin
B. Eosinotaxin
C. Eosinophilotaxin
D. All of the above

Eosinophils express a specific chemokine EOTAXIN.

142. Which of the following is false about eosinophils?

Harrison's 20th Ed. Chapter 60 Page 402

A. Shorter half life than neutrophils
B. Eosinophils can recirculate
C. During most infections, eosinophils are not important
D. Central role in defense against invasive helminthic infections

Eosinophils have a longer half life than neutrophils. Unlike neutrophils, tissue eosinophils can recirculate. During most infections, eosinophils are not important but plays a central role in host defense in invasive helminthic infections (hookworm, schistosomiasis, strongyloidiasis, toxocariasis, trichinosis, filariasis, echinococcosis and cysticercosis).

143. Which of the following is false about eosinophil granule?

Harrison's 20th Ed. Chapter 60 Page 402

A. Arginine-rich protein content
B. Histaminase activity
C. Contain eosinophil peroxidase
D. None of the above

Eosinophil granule contains arginine-rich protein in its crystalline core which has histaminase activity, eosinophil peroxidase that catalyzes oxidation by hydrogen peroxide.

144. Charcot-Leyden crystal protein in eosinophil cytoplasm is?

Harrison's 20th Ed. Chapter 60 Page 402

A. Hyaluronidase
B. Phospholipase
C. Lysophospholipase
D. Immunoglobulin E

Eosinophil cytoplasm contains Charcot-Leyden crystal protein which is a lysophospholipase.

145. Eosinophilia refers to how many eosinophils per microliter of blood?

Harrison's 20th Ed. Chapter 60 Page 402

A. > 200
B. > 300
C. > 400
D. > 500

Eosinophilia is the presence of >500 eosinophils per μL of blood.

146. Eosinophilia is due to allergic reaction which of the following drugs?

Harrison's 20th Ed. Chapter 60 Page 402

A. Iodides
B. Aspirin
C. Nitrofurantoin
D. All of the above

147. Eosinophilia is associated with which of the following diseases?

Harrison's 20th Ed. Chapter 60 Page 402

A. Serum sickness
B. Eczema
C. Pemphigus
D. All of the above

148. Eosinophilia is associated with which of the following malignancies?

Harrison's 20th Ed. Chapter 60 Page 403

A. Cancer pancreas
B. Cancer ovary
C. Cancer uterus
D. All of the above

Eosinophilia occurs in allergic reaction to drugs (iodides, aspirin, sulfonamides, nitrofurantoin, penicillins & cephalosporins), allergies (hay fever, asthma, eczema, serum sickness, allergic vasculitis, & pemphigus), collagen vascular diseases (RA, eosinophilic fasciitis, allergic angiitis & PAN), malignancies (Hodgkin's disease; mycosis fungoides; CML, Ca. lung, stomach, pancreas, ovary, uterus), Job's syndrome & CGD, and helminthic infections.

149. Which of the following is the dominant eosinophil growth factor?

Harrison's 20th Ed. Chapter 60 Page 403

A. IL-1
B. IL-3
C. IL-5
D. All of the above

IL-5 is the dominant eosinophil growth factor.

150. Which of the following is false about eosinophilia-myalgia syndrome?

Harrison's 20th Ed. Chapter 60 Page 403

A. Eosinophil count > 1000/μL
B. Caused by ingesting contaminants in L-tryptophan containing products
C. Responds to glucocorticoids
D. None of the above

151. Which of the following is an adverse effect of eosinopenia?

Harrison's 20th Ed. Chapter 60 Page 403

A. Cardiac arrhythmias
B. Myopathy
C. Pulmonary fibrosis
D. None of the above

There is no known adverse effect of eosinopenia.

152. Which of the following is false about hyperimmunoglobulin E–recurrent infection (HIE) syndrome?

Harrison's 20th Ed. Chapter 60 Page 403

A. Also called Job's syndrome
B. 'Cold' skin abscesses
C. Kyphoscoliosis
D. Obstructive lung disease

Hyperimmunoglobulin E - recurrent infection syndrome is also called Job's syndrome, characte-rized by typical facies with broad nose, kyphoscoliosis, osteoporosis & eczema. Primary teeth erupt normally but do not deciduate requiring extraction. Patients develop recurrent sinopulmonary & cutaneous infections much less inflamed than expected ("cold abscesses").

153. Which of the following is performed to assess bone marrow reserves?

Harrison's 20th Ed. Chapter 60 Page 403

A. Steroid challenge test

B. Epinephrine challenge test

C. Endotoxin challenge test

D. All of the above

Assessment of bone marrow reserves of WBC's is done by steroid challenge test. Epinephrine challenge test is for marginated circulating pool of cells & endotoxin challenge test is for their marginating ability.

154. In vivo assessment of inflammation is done by?

Harrison's 20th Ed. Chapter 60 Page 403

A. Rebuck skin window test

B. Nitroblue tetrazolium (NBT) dye test

C. Dihydrorhodamine (DHR) oxidation test

D. All of the above

In vivo assessment of inflammation is done by Rebuck skin window test or skin blister assay, which measures the ability of leukocytes & inflammatory mediators to accumulate locally in skin. NBT & DHR tests are for detecting deficiencies of oxidative metabolism.

155. Which of the following drugs is useful to restore myelopoiesis in neutropenia due to impaired production?

Harrison's 20th Ed. Chapter 60 Page 403

A. Androgens

B. Glucocorticoids

C. Lithium

D. All of the above

Apart from recombinant G-CSF, androgens, glucocorticoids, lithium & immunosuppressive therapy are used to restore myelopoiesis in patients with neutropenia due to impaired production.

Bleeding and Thrombosis

156. In the human hemostatic system, procoagulant forces include?
Harrison's 20th Ed. Chapter 61 Page 404

A. Platelet adhesion
B. Platelet aggregation
C. Fibrin clot formation
D. All of the above

In the human hemostatic system, procoagulant forces include platelet adhesion and aggregation and fibrin clot formation.

157. The major components of the hemostatic system are?
Harrison's 20th Ed. Chapter 61 Page 404

A. Platelets, monocytes and red cells
B. Plasma proteins
C. Vessel wall
D. All of the above

Major components of the hemostatic system platelets & other formed elements of blood (monocytes & RBCs), plasma proteins (coagulation & fibrinolytic factors & inhibitors) and vessel wall.

158. Formed element of blood that is not a component of the hemostatic system is?
Harrison's 20th Ed. Chapter 61 Page 404

A. Neutrophil
B. Monocyte
C. Red cell
D. Platelet

Major components of hemostatic system are platelets, monocytes & red cells, plasma proteins (coagulation & fibrinolytic factors & inhibitors) and vessel wall itself.

159. Platelet adhesion is mediated primarily by?
Harrison's 20th Ed. Chapter 61 Page 404

A. von Willebrand factor (vWF)
B. Gp IIb/IIIa
C. Gp Ia/IIa
D. Fibronectin

Platelet adhesion is mediated primarily by von Willebrand factor (vWF). Platelet adhesion is also facilitated by direct binding to subendothelial collagen through specific platelet membrane collagen receptors.

160. Which of the following is termed as "molecular glue"?
Harrison's 20th Ed. Chapter 61 Page 404

A. von Willebrand factor (vWF)
B. Gp IIb/IIIa
C. Gp Ia/IIa
D. Fibronectin

161. Which of the following is false about von Willebrand factor (vWF)?
Harrison's 20th Ed. Chapter 61 Page 404

A. Large multimeric protein
B. Present in plasma
C. Present in extracellular matrix of subendothelial vessel wall
D. None of the above

von Willebrand factor (VWF) is a large multimeric protein present in both plasma & extracellular matrix of subendothelial vessel wall. It serves as the primary "molecular glue" to withstand high levels of shear stress that would detach platelets due to flow of blood.

162. Which of the following is first to happen?
Harrison's 20th Ed. Chapter 61 Page 404

A. Platelet activation
B. Platelet adhesion
C. Platelet aggregation
D. Platelet accumulation

Platelet adhesion results in subsequent platelet activation and aggregation.

163. Which of the following is released from activated platelets?
Harrison's 20th Ed. Chapter 61 Page 404

A. Epinephrine
B. Thrombin
C. Adenosine diphosphate
D. All of the above

Platelet adhesion is followed by platelet activation and aggregation which is enhanced & amplified by humoral mediators in plasma (epinephrine, thrombin), mediators released from activated platelets (adenosine diphosphate, serotonin) & vessel wall extracellular matrix constituents that come in contact with adherent platelets (collagen, VWF).

164. Most abundant receptor on the platelet surface is?
Harrison's 20th Ed. Chapter 61 Page 404

A. Gp Ia/IIa
B. Gp Ib/IX
C. Gp IIb/IIIa
D. Gp VI

Platelet glycoprotein (Gp) IIb/IIIa (aIIbb3) complex is the most abundant receptor on platelet surface.

165. Platelet surface receptor GpIIB/IIIa binds to?
Harrison's 20th Ed. Chapter 61 Page 404

A. Thrombospondin
B. Fibrinogen
C. Collagen
D. All of the above

Platelet activation converts the normally inactive GpIIb/IIIa receptor into an active receptor enabling its binding to fibrinogen and vWF.

166. Surface of each platelet has how many GpIIb/IIIa binding sites?
Harrison's 20th Ed. Chapter 61 Page 404

A. ~ 10,000
B. ~ 25,000
C. ~ 50,000
D. ~ 100,000

Surface of each platelet has ~50,000 GpIIb/IIIa binding sites.

167. Which of the following is the key mediator of platelet aggregation?

Harrison's 20th Ed. Chapter 61 Page 404

A. Gp Ia/IIa
B. Gp Ib/IX
C. GpIIb/IIIa
D. Gp VI

Platelet glycoprotein GpIIb/IIIa receptor is the key mediator of platelet aggregation and is therefore the key target for antiplatelet therapy.

168. Structure of Fibrinogen is?

Harrison's 20th Ed. Chapter 61 Page 405 Figure 61-2

A. Uninodular
B. Binodular
C. Trinodular
D. Quadrinodular

Fibrinogen is a trinodular.

169. Which of the following about Fibrinogen is correct?

Harrison's 20th Ed. Chapter 61 Page 405 Figure 61-2

A. Binodular structure with two D domains & one E domain
B. Binodular structure with one D domain & two E domains
C. Trinodular structure with one D domain & two E domains
D. Trinodular structure with two D domains & one E domain

Fibrinogen is a trinodular structure consisting of two D domains and one E domain.

170. Cross-linking of the D domains on adjacent fibrinogen molecules is done by?

Harrison's 20th Ed. Chapter 61 Page 405 Figure 61-2

A. FX
B. FXI
C. FXII
D. FXIIIa

Cross-linking of D domains on adjacent fibrinogen molecules is done by FXIIIa.

171. Which of the following about D-Dimers is false?

Harrison's 20th Ed. Chapter 61 Page 405 Figure 61-2

A. Product of complete lysis of fibrin
B. Released when plasmin acts on fibrin
C. Relatively specific test of fibrin degradation
D. Relatively specific test of fibrinogen degradation

D-Dimers are the product of complete lysis of fibrin, maintaining the cross-linked D domains. When plasmin acts on covalently cross-linked fibrin, D-dimers are released. D-dimers in plasma are as a relatively specific test of fibrin rather than fibrinogen degradation. D-Dimer assays are a sensitive marker of blood clot formation and coagulation activation.

172. Normal level of D-Dimer in blood is?

Arch Intern Med. 1999;159:1569-1572

A. < 500 pg/mL
B. < 500 ng/mL
C. < 500 μg/mL
D. < 500 mg/mL

Normal level of D-Dimer in blood is < 500 ng/mL.

173. Plasma level of D-Dimer is?

Arch Intern Med. 1999;159:1569-1572

A. 0.22–0.74 mg/mL
B. 0.22–0.74 μg/mL
C. 0.22–0.74 ng/mL
D. 0.22–0.74 pg/mL

Plasma level of D-Dimer is 0.22–0.74 μg/mL or 220–740 ng/mL FEU.

174. D-dimer levels increase in patients with?

Arch Intern Med. 1999;159:1569-1572

A. Myocardial infarction
B. Pneumonia
C. II or III trimester of pregnancy
D. All of the above

D-dimer levels increase in myocardial infarction, pneumonia, intestinal ischemia, sepsis, cancer, postoperative state, initial infusion of human or humanized antibodies (rituximab, gemtuzumab, trastuzumab), and second or third trimester of pregnancy. D-dimer elevation is not as predictive of DVT in cancer patients as it is in patients without cancer.

175. Coagulation initiation and activation take place on?

Harrison's 20th Ed. Chapter 61 Page 404

A. Endothelial cell
B. Smooth muscle cells
C. Activated platelet surface
D. Fibroblasts

Coagulation initiation and activation reactions take place on phospholipid surfaces, usually the activated platelet surface.

176. Tissue factor (TF) is present on?

Harrison's 20th Ed. Chapter 61 Page 404

A. Subendothelial cellular components of vessel wall
B. Circulating microparticles from monocytes
C. Circulating microparticles from platelets
D. All of the above

TF is expressed on surfaces of subendothelial cellular components of vessel wall (smooth-muscle cells & fibroblasts). TF is present in circulating microparticles shed from monocytes & platelets.

177. Which of the following is a serine protease factor?

Harrison's 20th Ed. Chapter 61 Page 404

A. III
B. VIIa
C. IX
D. X

TF binds serine protease factor VIIa and their complex (TF+VIIa) activates factor X to factor Xa. Factor IXa also activates factor X to factor Xa.

178. Thrombin activates which of the following factor by positive feedback?

Harrison's 20th Ed. Chapter 61 Page 404

A. Factor V
B. Factor VII
C. Factor X
D. Factor XI

Factor XI is activated by positive feedback activation by thrombin. Factor XIa then activates Factor IX to IXa. Factor XIa functions in the "propagation and amplification", rather than in the initiation, of the coagulation cascade.

179. Thrombin activates which of the following?
Harrison's 20th Ed. Chapter 61 Page 404

A. Factor XI
B. Factor VIII
C. Factor V
D. All of the above

Thrombin activates Factor XI, Factor VIII and Factor V. Thrombin also activates factor XIII (fibrin-stabilizing factor) to factor XIIIa, which covalently cross-links & stabilizes the fibrin clot. Thrombin also activates Protein C which then becomes an anticoagulant by cleaving and inactivating activated factors V and VIII.

180. Factor Xa is formed through the action of?
Harrison's 20th Ed. Chapter 61 Page 404

A. TF/Factor VIIa complex
B. Factor IXa
C. Factor VIIIa
D. All of the above

Factor Xa is formed through the actions of either TF/factor VIIa complex or factor IXa (with factor VIIIa as a cofactor) and converts prothrombin to thrombin.

181. Essential cofactor for conversion of prothrombin to thrombin is?
Harrison's 20th Ed. Chapter 61 Page 404

A. Va
B. VIIa
C. IX
D. X

Factor Xa converts prothrombin to thrombin, the pivotal protease of the coagulation system. The essential cofactor for this reaction is factor Va. Factor Va is produced by thrombin-induced limited proteolysis of factor V.

182. Which of the following in endothelial cells has antithrombotic effect?
Harrison's 20th Ed. Chapter 61 Page 405

A. Prostacyclin
B. Nitric oxide
C. EctoADPase/CD39
D. All of the above

Prostacyclin, nitric oxide & ectoADPase/CD39 produced from endothelial cells act to inhibit platelet binding, secretion and aggregation.

183. Anticoagulant factor produced by endothelial cells is?
Harrison's 20th Ed. Chapter 61 Page 405

A. Heparan proteoglycans
B. Antithrombin
C. Thrombomodulin
D. All of the above

Endothelial cells produce anticoagulant factors like heparan proteoglycans, antithrombin, TF pathway inhibitor and thrombomodulin.

184. Which of the following produced by endothelial cells acts as an anticoagulant?
Harrison's 20th Ed. Chapter 61 Page 405

A. Plasminogen activator inhibitor
B. Thrombomodulin
C. Prostacyclin
D. Nitric oxide

185. Endothelial cells activate fibrinolytic mechanisms through the production of?
Harrison's 20th Ed. Chapter 61 Page 405

A. Tissue plasminogen activator 1
B. Urokinase
C. Plasminogen activator inhibitor
D. All of the above

Endothelial cells activate fibrinolytic mechanisms through the production of tissue plasminogen activator 1, urokinase, plasminogen activator inhibitor & annexin-2.

186. Which of the following best relates to heparin?
Harrison's 20th Ed. Chapter 61 Page 405

A. Antithrombin III
B. Protein C
C. Protein S
D. All of the above

Antithrombin III inhibits thrombin by forming inactivating complexes that increase several folds in the presence of heparin.

187. Which of the following becomes an anticoagulant when it is activated by thrombin?
Harrison's 20th Ed. Chapter 61 Page 405

A. Antithrombin III
B. Protein C
C. Protein S
D. Tissue factor pathway inhibitor (TFPI)

Protein C is a plasma glycoprotein that becomes an anticoagulant when activated by thrombin.

188. Which of the following about thrombomodulin is false?
Harrison's 20th Ed. Chapter 61 Page 405

A. Transmembrane proteoglycan binding site for thrombin on endothelial cell surface
B. Thrombin-induced activation of protein C occurs physiologically on thrombomodulin
C. Anticoagulant factor from endothelial cell
D. None of the above

Thrombomodulin expressed on the surface of endothelial cells binds thrombin at low concentrations and inhibits coagulation through activation of the protein C pathway, leading to enhanced catabolism of clotting factors Va and VIIIa, thereby combating thrombus formation.

189. Activated protein C acts as an anticoagulant by cleaving and inactivating which of the following activated factor?
Harrison's 20th Ed. Chapter 61 Page 405

A. II
B. V
C. VI
D. X

Activated protein C acts as an anticoagulant by cleaving & inactivating activated factors V & VIII.

190. Which of the following relates to protein S?
Harrison's 20th Ed. Chapter 61 Page 405

A. Cofactor
B. Glycoprotein
C. Vitamin K dependent posttranslational modification
D. All of the above

Glycoprotein Protein S is a cofactor that undergoes vitamin K dependent posttranslational modification. It accelerates the reaction of activated protein C with factors V and VIII.

191. Which of the following inhibits TF/FVIIa/FXa complex?
Harrison's 20th Ed. Chapter 61 Page 405

A. Activated protein C
B. Protein S
C. Tissue factor pathway inhibitor (TFPI)
D. All of the above

Tissue factor pathway inhibitor (TFPI) is a plasma protease inhibitor that regulates the TF–induced extrinsic pathway of coagulation. TFPI inhibits the TF/FVIIa/FXa complex.

192. Tissue factor pathway inhibitor (TFPI) be released by?
Harrison's 20th Ed. Chapter 61 Page 405

A. Heparin
B. Streptokinase
C. Urokinase
D. All of the above

TFPI is bound to lipoprotein and can also be released by heparin from endothelial cells, where it is bound to glycosoaminoglycans, and from platelets.

193. Plasminogen activators (tPA & uPA) cleave which bond of plasminogen to generate the active enzyme plasmin?
Harrison's 20th Ed. Chapter 61 Page 406

A. Arg460 – Val461
B. Arg560 – Val561
C. Arg660 – Val661
D. Arg760 – Val761

Plasminogen activators (tissue type plasminogen activator & urokinase type plasminogen activator cleave Arg560-Val561 bond of plasminogen to generate the active enzyme plasmin which is the major protease enzyme of the fibrinolytic system, acting to digest fibrin to fibrin degradation products.

194. "Fibrin specific" activity of plasmin is due to its?
Harrison's 20th Ed. Chapter 61 Page 406

A. Arginine-binding sites
B. Lysine-binding sites
C. Valine-binding sites
D. Leucine-binding sites

The lysine-binding sites of plasmin (and plasminogen) permit it to bind specifically to fibrin and therefore physiologic fibrinolysis is "fibrin specific".

195. Which of the following antiplasmin inhibits plasmin?
Harrison's 20th Ed. Chapter 61 Page 406 Figure 61-4

A. α1 antiplasmin
B. α2 antiplasmin
C. α3 antiplasmin
D. α4 antiplasmin

PAI1 is the primary inhibitor of tPA & uPA and α2 antiplasmin is the main inhibitor of plasmin in human plasma, inactivating any nonfibrin clot associated plasmin.

196. Physiologic regulation of fibrinolysis is done by?
Harrison's 20th Ed. Chapter 61 Page 406

A. Plasminogen activator inhibitors (PAI-1 & PAI-2)
B. Thrombin-activatable fibrinolysis inhibitor (TAFI)
C. α2-antiplasmin
D. All of the above

Physiologic regulation of fibrinolysis occurs primarily at three levels - plasminogen activator inhibitors (PAI-1 & PAI-2) which inhibit physiologic plasminogen activators, thrombin-activatable fibrinolysis inhibitor (TAFI) that limits fibrinolysis and alpha-2 antiplasmin which inactivates any nonfibrin clot-associated plasmin.

197. Which of the following is due to defect of platelet adhesion?
Harrison's 20th Ed. Chapter 61 Page 407 Table 61-1

A. Glanzmann's thrombasthenia
B. Bernard-Soulier syndrome
C. Scott's syndrome
D. All of the above

198. Which of the following is due to defect of platelet aggregation?
Harrison's 20th Ed. Chapter 61 Page 407 Table 61-1

A. Glanzmann's thrombasthenia
B. Bernard-Soulier syndrome
C. Scott's syndrome
D. All of the above

199. Epistaxis is the most common symptom in?
Harrison's 20th Ed. Chapter 61 Page 407

A. Hemophilia A
B. Ehlers-Danlos syndrome
C. Hereditary hemorrhagic telangiectasia
D. Cushing's syndrome

Epistaxis is the most common symptom in hereditary hemorrhagic telangiectasia & in boys with VWD.

200. How much blood per cycle is lost in menorrhagia?
Harrison's 20th Ed. Chapter 61 Page 407

A. > 50 mL
B. > 60 mL
C. > 70 mL
D. > 80 mL

Menorrhagia is defined quantitatively as a loss of >80 mL of blood per cycle.

201. Menorrhagia is a common symptom in women with?
Harrison's 20th Ed. Chapter 61 Page 407

A. VWD
B. Factor XI deficiency
C. Symptomatic carriers of hemophilia
D. All of the above

Menorrhagia is a common symptom in women with underlying bleeding disorders. It is seen in majority of women with VWD & factor XI deficiency & in symptomatic carriers of hemophilia.

202. Which of the following is called a "life-threatening site of bleeding"?

Harrison's 20th Ed. Chapter 61 Page 407

A. Bleeding into oropharynx
B. Bleeding into central nervous system
C. Bleeding into retroperitoneum
D. All of the above

Life-threatening sites of bleeding include bleeding into oropharynx, into central nervous system, and into retroperitoneum.

203. Which of the following about clopidogrel is false?

Harrison's 20th Ed. Chapter 61 Page 407

A. Thienopyridine
B. Inhibits ADP-mediated platelet aggregation
C. Can precipitate or exacerbate bleeding symptoms
D. None of the above

Thienopyridines (clopidogrel and prasugrel) inhibit ADP-mediated platelet aggregation and like NSAIDs can precipitate or exacerbate bleeding symptoms.

204. Herb with potential anti-platelet activity is?

Harrison's 20th Ed. Chapter 61 Page 408 Page Table 61–2

A. Ginger
B. Turmeric
C. Garlic
D. All of the above

Herbs with potential anti-platelet activity include Ginkgo, Garlic, Bilberry, Ginger, Dong quai, Feverfew, Asian, Siberian & American ginseng, Turmeric, Meadowsweet and Willow.

205. Which of the following is a coumarin containing herb?

Harrison's 20th Ed. Chapter 61 Page 408 Table 61–2

A. Motherwort
B. Chamomile
C. Horse chestnut
D. All of the above

Coumarin containing herbs include Motherwort (Leonurus cardiaca), Chamomile (Matricaria recutita, Chamaemelum mobile), Horse chestnut (Aesculus hippocastanum) Red clover (Trifolium pratense) Fenugreek (Trigonella foenum-graecum).

206. Bruising or mucosal bleeding may be the presenting complaint in?

Harrison's 20th Ed. Chapter 61 Page 407

A. Liver disease
B. Severe renal impairment
C. Hypothyroidism
D. All of the above

Bruising or mucosal bleeding may be the presenting complaint in liver disease, severe renal impairment, hypothyroidism, paraproteinemias or amyloidosis & bone marrow failure.

207. All coagulation factors are synthesized in?

Harrison's 20th Ed. Chapter 61 Page 407

A. Liver
B. Kidney
C. Lungs
D. None of the above

All coagulation factors are synthesized in liver & hepatic failure results in combined factor deficiencies.

208. Which of the following coagulation factors is dependent on vitamin K for posttranslational modification?

Harrison's 20th Ed. Chapter 61 Page 408

A. Factor II
B. Factor VII
C. Factor IX
D. All of the above

209. Which of the following proteins is dependent on vitamin K for posttranslational modification?

Harrison's 20th Ed. Chapter 61 Page 408

A. Protein C
B. Protein S
C. Protein Z
D. All of the above

Coagulation factors II, VII, IX, X and proteins C, S, and Z are dependent on vitamin K for posttranslational modification.

210. Normal blood platelet count is?

Harrison's 20th Ed. Chapter 61 Page 408

A. 50,000 to 100,000/μL
B. 100,000 to 250,000/μL
C. 150,000 to 450,000/μL
D. 250,000 to 550,000/μL

Normal blood platelet count is 150,000 to 450,000/μL.

211. Thrombocytopenia results from?

Harrison's 20th Ed. Chapter 61 Page 408

A. Decreased production of platelets
B. Increased destruction of platelets
C. Sequestration of platelets
D. Any of the above

Thrombocytopenia results from decreased production, increased destruction, &/or sequestration.

212. Bleeding rarely occurs in isolated thrombocytopenia at counts?

Harrison's 20th Ed. Chapter 61 Page 408

A. > 50000/μL
B. > 80000/μL
C. > 100000/μL
D. > 150000/μL

Bleeding rarely occurs in isolated thrombocytopenia at counts > 50000/μL.

213. Most procedures can be performed in patients with a platelet count of?

Harrison's 20th Ed. Chapter 61 Page 408

A. 50000/μL
B. 80000/μL
C. 100000/μL
D. 150000/μL

Most procedures can be performed in patients with a platelet count of 50,000/μL. For major surgery, a count of about 80,000/μL is likely to be sufficient.

214. The major risk factor for arterial thrombosis is?

Harrison's 20th Ed. Chapter 61 Page 408

A. Atherosclerosis
B. Hyperhomocysteinemia
C. Dysfibrinogenemia
D. Hormonal therapy

The major risk factor for arterial thrombosis is atherosclerosis. Risk factors for venous thrombosis are immobility, surgery, underlying medical conditions, malignancy, hormonal therapy, obesity, and genetic predispositions.

215. Most coagulation assays are performed in plasma anticoagulated with?

Harrison's 20th Ed. Chapter 61 Page 409

A. Ethylenediamine tetraacetic acid (EDTA)
B. Sodium citrate
C. Heparin
D. Any of the above

Most coagulation assays are performed in sodium citrate anticoagulated plasma that is recalcified for the assay.

216. PT assesses the factors except?

Harrison's 20th Ed. Chapter 61 Page 409

A. Factor I
B. Factor II
C. Factor V
D. Factor VIII

PT assesses factors I (fibrinogen), II (prothrombin), V, VII, and X. PT only measures one aspect of hemostasis affected by liver dysfunction.

217. International normalized ratio (INR) is calculated by?

Harrison's 20th Ed. Chapter 61 Page 409

A. PT ratio × International Sensitivity Index (ISI)
B. PT ratio ÷ International Sensitivity Index (ISI)
C. PT ratio + International Sensitivity Index (ISI)
D. (PT ratio)International Sensitivity Index (ISI)

International normalized ratio (INR) is calculated by the formula: INR = (PTpatient/PTnormal mean)ISI.

218. Activated partial thromboplastin time (aPTT) assesses which of the following factors?

Harrison's 20th Ed. Chapter 61 Page 409

A. Factor VIII
B. Factor IX
C. Factor X
D. All of the above

aPTT assesses the intrinsic & common coagulation pathways, factors XI, IX, VIII, X, V, II, fibrinogen, and also prekallikrein, high-molecular-weight kininogen & factor XII.

219. Platelet interaction with vascular collagen is stabilized by?

Harrison's 20th Ed. Chapter 61 Page 409

A. Gp Ia/IIa
B. Gp VI
C. von Willebrand factor (vWF)
D. FcRg

von Willebrand factor (vWF) is an adhesive glycoprotein that allows platelets to remain attached to the vessel wall despite the high shear forces generated within the vascular lumen by stabilizing interaction between platelets with collagen.

220. Platelet surface receptor GpIb/IX binds to?

Harrison's 20th Ed. Chapter 61 Page 410

A. vWF
B. Fibrinogen
C. Collagen
D. All of the above

221. vWF forms a link between collagen fibrils & which of the following platelet receptor?

Harrison's 20th Ed. Chapter 61 Page 405 Figure 61-2

A. Gp Ia/IIa
B. Gp Ib/IX
C. Gp VI
D. All of the above

GpIb/IX complex binds vWF. Adhesion of platelets with vessel wall is stabilized by von Willebrand factor, which forms a bridge between collagen fibrils in the vessel wall & receptors on platelet glycoprotein Ib/IX. Similarly, platelet aggregation is mediated by fibrinogen, which links adjacent platelets via receptors on the platelet glycoprotein IIb/IIIa complex.

222. Formation of thromboxane A2 (TXA2) from arachidonic acid is mediated by enzyme?

Harrison's 20th Ed. Chapter 61 Page 410

A. Phospholipase C
B. Phospholipase A2
C. Cyclooxygenase
D. All of the above

Formation of TXA2 from arachidonic acid is mediated by the enzyme cyclooxygenase.

223. Platelet surface receptor GpIa/IIa binds to?

Harrison's 20th Ed. Chapter 61 Page 410

A. vWF
B. Fibrinogen
C. Collagen
D. All of the above

GpIa/IIa binds collagen.

224. Platelet surface receptor GpVI/FcγRIIa binds to?

Harrison's 20th Ed. Chapter 61 Page 410

A. vWF
B. Fibrinogen
C. Collagen
D. All of the above

GpVI/FcγRIIa binds collagen.

225. After leaving bone marrow, what proportion of platelets are sequestered in spleen?

Harrison's 20th Ed. Chapter 61 Page 410

A. One-third
B. One-half
C. Two-thirds
D. Three-fourths

226. The life span of platelets in circulation is about?
Harrison's 20th Ed. Chapter 61 Page 410

A. 1 to 3 days
B. 3 to 5 days
C. 5 to 7 days
D. 7 to 10 days

After leaving bone marrow, ~one-third of platelets are sequestered in spleen, while the other two-thirds circulate for 7 to 10 days.

227. During menstrual cycle, platelet count rise at what time?
Harrison's 20th Ed. Chapter 61 Page 410

A. Following ovulation
B. At the onset of menses
C. After completion of menstrual flow
D. Before ovulation

228. During menstrual cycle, platelet count fall at what time?
Harrison's 20th Ed. Chapter 61 Page 410

A. Following ovulation
B. At the onset of menses
C. After completion of menstrual flow
D. Before ovulation

Platelet count varies in menstrual cycle, rising following ovulation & falling at onset of menses.

229. Platelet counts are decreased in which of the following deficiencies?
Harrison's 20th Ed. Chapter 61 Page 410

A. Severe Iron deficiency
B. Folic acid deficiency
C. Vitamin B12 deficiency
D. All of the above

Platelet count are decreased in severe iron, folic acid or vitamin B12 deficiency.

230. Secondary or reactive thrombocytosis is due to which property of platelets?
Harrison's 20th Ed. Chapter 61 Page 410

A. Hormonal
B. Acute-phase reactant
C. Enzymatic
D. All of the above

Platelets are acute-phase reactants. Secondary or reactive thrombocytosis refers to an increase in platelet counts in patients with systemic inflammation, tumors, bleeding & mild iron deficiency.

231. Which of the following cytokines interleukins stimulate platelet production in acute inflammation?
Harrison's 20th Ed. Chapter 61 Page 410

A. IL-3
B. IL-6
C. IL-11
D. All of the above

Cytokines interleukin IL-3, IL-6 & IL-11 stimulate platelet production in acute inflammation.

232. Mechanism of thrombocytopenia include?
Harrison's 20th Ed. Chapter 61 Page 410

A. Decreased bone marrow production
B. Increased splenic sequestration
C. Accelerated destruction
D. All of the above

Thrombocytopenia is caused by decreased bone marrow production or increased splenic sequestration or accelerated destruction of platelets.

233. TAR syndrome means?
Harrison's 20th Ed. Chapter 61 Page 410

A. Thrombocytopenia with absent reticulocytes
B. Thrombocytopenia with absent renin
C. Thrombocytopenia with absent radii
D. Thrombocytopenia with abnormal vessels

Congenital amegakaryocytic hypoplasia & thrombocytopenia with absent radii (TAR syndrome) produce a selective decrease in megakaryocyte production.

234. Acute ITP is common in?
Harrison's 20th Ed. Chapter 61 Page 410

A. Children
B. Adults
C. Elderly
D. All of the above

Acute ITP is a severe thrombocytopenia following recovery from a viral exanthem or upper respiratory illness. It is common in children & is responsible 90% of pediatric cases of immunologic thrombocytopenia. >90% cases recover within 3 to 6 months.

235. Which of the following appear in the red cells of asplenic individuals?
Harrison's 20th Ed. Chapter 61 Page 410

A. Macroovalocytes
B. Basophilic stippling
C. Howell-Jolly bodies
D. Target cells

Howell-Jolly bodies are tiny nuclear remnants that are normally removed by spleen. They appear in blood after splenectomy & with maturation/dysplastic disorders.

236. Rituximab is what type of a monoclonal antibody?
Harrison's 20th Ed. Chapter 61 Page 410

A. Anti-CD19
B. Anti-CD20
C. Anti-CD21
D. Anti-CD22

Rituximab is an anti-CD20 monoclonal antibody. Efficacy is established in ITP. It eliminates normal B cells that produce antiplatelet antibody.

Enlargement of Lymph Nodes and Spleen

237. Which of the following palpable lymph nodes are considered normal in adults?

Harrison's 20th Ed. Chapter 62 Page 411

A. Palpable upper cervical nodes of up to 2 cm
B. Palpable lower cervical nodes of up to 2 cm
C. Palpable inguinal nodes of up to 2 cm
D. Palpable axillary nodes of up to 2 cm

Soft, flat submandibular nodes (< 1 cm) are often palpable in healthy children and young adults. Healthy adults may have palpable inguinal nodes of up to 2 cm, which are considered normal.

238. Generalized adenopathy means involvement of how many noncontiguous lymph node areas?

Harrison's 20th Ed. Chapter 62 Page 412

A. One or more
B. Two or more
C. Three or more
D. Four or more

Generalized adenopathy is defined as involvement of three or more noncontiguous lymph node areas. Localized or regional adenopathy implies involvement of a single anatomic area.

239. Which of the following is a cause of generalized lymphadenopathy?

Harrison's 20th Ed. Chapter 62 Page 412

A. AIDS
B. Systemic lupus erythematosus (SLE)
C. Mixed connective tissue disease
D. All of the above

Generalized lymphadenopathy is frequently associated with infectious mononucleosis (EBV) or cytomegalovirus (CMV), toxoplasmosis, AIDS, systemic lupus erythematosus (SLE), and mixed connective tissue disease. Acute and chronic lymphocytic leukemias and malignant lymphomas also produce generalized adenopathy in adults.

240. Occipital lymphadenopathy accompanies which of the following?

Harrison's 20th Ed. Chapter 62 Page 412

A. Scalp infection
B. Ear infection
C. Conjunctival infections
D. Tooth infection

Occipital adenopathy often reflects infection of the scalp.

241. Preauricular lymphadenopathy accompanies which of the following?

Harrison's 20th Ed. Chapter 62 Page 412

A. Scalp infection
B. Ear infection
C. Conjunctival infections
D. Tooth infection

Preauricular adenopathy accompanies conjunctival infections and cat-scratch disease.

242. Most frequent site of regional lymphadenopathy is?

Harrison's 20th Ed. Chapter 62 Page 412

A. Axilla
B. Neck
C. Groin
D. Abdominal

Most frequent site of regional lymphadenopathy is neck.

243. Which of the following about lymphadenopathy is false?

Harrison's 20th Ed. Chapter 62 Page 412

A. Most frequent site of regional lymphadenopathy is neck
B. Enlargement of supraclavicular and scalene nodes is always abnormal
C. Virchow's node is enlarged right supraclavicular node
D. Sarcoidosis can cause supraclavicular adenopathy

Virchow's node is an enlarged left supraclavicular node infiltrated with metastatic cancer from a gastrointestinal primary.

244. Metastases to supraclavicular nodes occur from?

Harrison's 20th Ed. Chapter 62 Page 412

A. Lung
B. Breast
C. Testis
D. Any of the above

Metastases to supraclavicular nodes occur from lung, breast, testis or ovarian cancers.

245. Which of the following is a cause of supraclavicular adenopathy?

Harrison's 20th Ed. Chapter 62 Page 412

A. Tuberculosis
B. Sarcoidosis
C. Toxoplasmosis
D. All of the above

TB, sarcoidosis & toxoplasmosis are causes of supraclavicular adenopathy.

246. Benign lymphadenopathy is assumed when lymph node area is?

Harrison's 20th Ed. Chapter 62 Page 412

A. < 0.25 cm^2
B. < 0.50 cm^2
C. < 0.75 cm^2
D. < 1.00 cm^2

Lymph nodes <1.0 cm^2 in area (1 × 1 cm or less) are almost always secondary to benign, nonspecific reactive causes. Lymph node size of 2.25 cm^2 (1.5 × 1.5 cm) is the best size limit to differentiate malignant or granulomatous from other causes of lymphadenopathy.

247. Tenderness of lymph node is due to?
Harrison's 20th Ed. Chapter 62 Page 412

A. Inflammation of capsule
B. Rupture of capsule
C. Stretching of capsule
D. All of the above

Lymph node tenderness occurs when the capsule is stretched during its rapid enlargement, usually secondary to an inflammatory process.

248. Which of the following is not a characteristic of enlarged lymph nodes in lymphoma?
Harrison's 20th Ed. Chapter 62 Page 412

A. Discrete
B. Asymmetric
C. Rubbery
D. Nontender

Lymph nodes involved by lymphoma tend to be large, discrete, symmetric, rubbery, firm, mobile, and nontender.

249. Which of the following is characteristic of enlarged lymph nodes in metastatic cancer?
Harrison's 20th Ed. Chapter 62 Page 412

A. Hard
B. Nonmovable
C. Nontender
D. All of the above

Lymph nodes containing metastatic cancer are hard, nontender & nonmovable.

250. Which of the following can cause unilateral paratracheal lymph node involvement?
Harrison's 20th Ed. Chapter 62 Page 412

A. Histoplasmosis
B. Infectious mononucleosis
C. Sarcoidosis
D. All of the above

Histoplasmosis can cause unilateral paratracheal lymph node involvement.

251. Which parameter is used in ultrasonography of cervical nodes for distinguishing benign from malignant nodes?
Harrison's 20th Ed. Chapter 62 Page 412

A. Area
B. Volume
C. Ratio of long to short axis (L/S ratio)
D. Sonodensity

On Ultrasonography of cervical nodes, a ratio of long to short axis of <2.0 is useful in distinguishing benign & malignant nodes in patients with head & neck cancer.

252. Winterbottom's sign is a classic finding of?
Harrison's 20th Ed. Chapter 16 Page 108 Table 16-1

A. Giardiasis
B. Toxoplasmosis
C. Human African Trypanosomiasis
D. Balantidiasis

253. In Winterbottom's sign, location of lymph node enlargement is?
Harrison's 20th Ed. Chapter 16 Page 108 Table 16-1

A. Axilla
B. Posterior cervical triangle
C. Submental
D. Inguinal

Lymphadenopathy of the posterior cervical triangle, or Winterbottom's sign, is a classic finding in T. b. gambiense trypanosomiasis.

254. Romaña's sign is a feature of?
Harrison's 20th Ed. Chapter 222 Page 1603 Table 222-1

A. Acute Chagas' disease
B. Cutaneous leishmaniasis
C. Visceral leishmaniasis
D. Babesiosis

Romaña's sign is a classic finding in acute Chagas' disease, and consists of unilateral painless edema of palpebrae & periocular tissues when conjunctiva is the portal of entry. Generalized lymphadenopathy & hepatosplenomegaly may develop.

255. Enlarged, grayish yellow or orange tonsils are pathognomonic of?
Harrison's 20th Ed. Chapter 400 Page 2899

A. Waldenström's macroglobulinemia
B. Polycythemia vera
C. Wolman disease
D. Tangier disease

Tangier disease is associated with cholesterol accumulation in reticuloendothelial system with hepatosplenomegaly & enlarged, grayish yellow or orange tonsils.

256. Accessory spleens are seen in what percentage of persons?
Harrison's 20th Ed. Chapter 62 Page 413

A. 5%
B. 10%
C. 15%
D. 20%

Embryologic origin of spleen is in dorsal mesogastrium at about 5 weeks' gestation as a series of hillocks that migrates to left upper quadrant. When these hillocks fail to unify into a single tissue mass, accessory spleens may develop in ~20% of persons.

257. Which of the following about structure of spleen is false?
Harrison's 20th Ed. Chapter 62 Page 413 Figure 62-1

A. White pulp is lymphoid in nature
B. To return to circulation, RBCs traverse sinusoidal pores
C. Pulp cords are dead ends
D. None of the above

Spleen comprises many units of red and white pulp centered around small branches of splenic artery, called central arteries. White pulp is lymphoid in nature & contains B cell follicles, a marginal zone around the follicles, and T cell rich areas sheathing arterioles. Red pulp areas include pulp sinuses & pulp cords. Cords are dead ends. In order to regain access to the circulation, red blood cells must traverse tiny openings in the sinusoidal lining. Stiff, damaged, or old red cells cannot enter the sinuses.

258. Weight of a normal spleen is?
Harrison's 20th Ed. Chapter 62 Page 414

A. < 150 grams
B. < 250 grams
C. < 350 grams
D. < 450 grams

Normal spleen weighs <250 grams.

259. Which of the following is false about spleen?
Harrison's 20th Ed. Chapter 62 Page 414

A. Decreases in size with age
B. Lies entirely within rib cage
C. Maximum cephalocaudad diameter is 13 cm by USG
D. Maximum width of 14 cm by radionuclide scan

Spleen decreases in size with age, lies entirely within rib cage, has a maximum cephalocaudad diameter of 13 cm by USG or maximum length of 12 cm and/or width of 7 cm by radionuclide scan, and is normally not palpable.

260. Middleton maneuver is used for splenic?
Harrison's 20th Ed. Chapter 62 Page 414

A. Inspection
B. Palpation
C. Percussion
D. Auscultation

Palpation of spleen can be done by bimanual palpation, ballotment, and palpation from above (Middleton maneuver). Bimanual palpation in the right lateral decubitus position adds nothing to the supine examination.

261. Which of the following is false in spleen examination?
Harrison's 20th Ed. Chapter 62 Page 414

A. Auscultation may reveal venous hum or friction rub
B. Bimanual palpation in right lateral decubitus position adds nothing to supine examination
C. Reproducibility among examiners is better for palpation than percussion
D. None of the above

262. Nixon, Castell, or Barkun methods are used for splenic?
Harrison's 20th Ed. Chapter 62 Page 414

A. Inspection
B. Palpation
C. Percussion
D. Auscultation

Percussion for splenic dullness is accomplished with either Nixon, Castell, or Barkun technique.

263. In Nixon's method, splenic enlargement is indicated when upper border of dullness above costal margin is?
Harrison's 20th Ed. Chapter 62 Page 414

A. > 4 cm
B. > 8 cm
C. > 12 cm
D. > 16 cm

In Nixon's method, patient is in right decubitus. Percussion begins at lower level of pulmonary resonance in posterior axillary line & proceeds toward lower midanterior costal margin. Upper border of dullness is normally 6-8 cm above costal margin. Dullness >8 cm in adult indicates splenic enlargement.

264. In Castell's method, percussion in the lowest intercostal space is done in?
Harrison's 20th Ed. Chapter 62 Page 414

A. Midclavicular line
B. Anterior axillary line
C. Midaxillary line
D. Posterior axillary line

In Castell's method, patient is supine, percussion is done in lowest intercostal space in anterior axillary line. A dull percussion note on full inspiration suggests splenomegaly.

265. Which of the following is a 'Red cell inclusion body'?
Harrison's 20th Ed. Chapter 62 Page 414

A. RBC parasites
B. Howell-Jolly bodies
C. Heinz bodies
D. All of the above

Red cell inclusion bodies like parasites, nuclear residua (Howell-Jolly bodies, or denatured hemoglobin - Heinz bodies) are pinched off while passing through slits, a process called pitting.

266. Which of the following is false about spleen?
Harrison's 20th Ed. Chapter 62 Page 414

A. Normal spleen contains ~one-third of total body platelets
B. Normal spleen contains significant no. of marginated neutrophils
C. Spleen is in the portal circulation
D. None of the above

267. Katayama fever is characterized by all except?
Harrison's 20th Ed. Chapter 229 Page 1638

A. Fever
B. Generalized lymphadenopathy
C. Lymphocytosis
D. Hepatosplenomegaly

Symptomatic acute schistosomiasis is called Katayama fever. It is a serum sickness like syndrome with fever, generalized lymphadenopathy, hepatosplenomegaly & high peripheral blood eosinophilia.

268. Massive splenomegaly is defined as spleen extending?
Harrison's 20th Ed. Chapter 62 Page 415

A. > 2 cm below left costal margin
B. > 4 cm below left costal margin
C. > 6 cm below left costal margin
D. > 8 cm below left costal margin

269. Massive splenomegaly is defined as spleen that weighs?
Harrison's 20th Ed. Chapter 62 Page 415

A. > 250 gram
B. > 500 gram
C. > 750 gram
D. > 1000 gram

Massive splenomegaly refers to spleen that extends >8 cm below left costal margin and/or weighs (drained) more than 1000 grams.

270. Causes of massive splenomegaly include?
Harrison's 20th Ed. Chapter 62 Page 416 Table 62-3

A. Chronic myelogenous leukemia
B. Lymphomas
C. Hairy cell leukemia
D. All of the above

271. Causes of massive splenomegaly include?
Harrison's 20th Ed. Chapter 62 Page 416 Table 62-3

A. Myelofibrosis with myeloid metaplasia
B. Polycythemia vera
C. Gaucher's disease
D. All of the above

272. Causes of Massive splenomegaly include?
Harrison's 20th Ed. Chapter 62 Page 416 Table 62-3

A. Chronic lymphocytic leukemia
B. Sarcoidosis
C. Autoimmune hemolytic anemia
D. All of the above

Causes of massive splenomegaly fall into four main categories: infectious diseases such as chronic malaria, kala-azar, and leishmaniasis; infiltrative diseases such as Gaucher's disease and Niemann-Pick disease; portal hypertension; and hematologic diseases, including myeloproliferative and lymphoproliferative disorders (N Engl J Med. 2001:345, 682).

273. 'Abscopal effect' refers to?
Harrison's 20th Ed. Chapter 62 Page 416

A. Ultrafiltration of abnormal RBCs
B. Regression of systemic disease after splenectomy
C. Increased tendency of enlarged splenic rupture
D. Peritoneal seeding of splenic fragments

274. Term "splenosis" best relates to?
Harrison's 20th Ed. Chapter 62 Page 416

A. Regression of systemic disease after splenectomy
B. Ultrafiltration of abnormal RBCs
C. Iatrogenic splenic rupture
D. Ectopic spleen tissue

At times in patients with splenic rupture, peritoneal seeding of splenic fragments can lead to splenosis i.e. presence of multiple collections of spleen tissue not connected to portal circulation. This ectopic spleen tissue may cause pain or gastrointestinal obstruction, as in endometriosis.

275. Which out of the following is a contraindication for splenectomy?
Harrison's 20th Ed. Chapter 62 Page 416

A. Iatrogenic splenic rupture
B. Thrombocytopenia
C. Presence of bone marrow failure
D. Hairy cell leukemia

The only contraindication to splenectomy is the presence of marrow failure, in which the enlarged spleen is the only source of hematopoietic tissue.

276. Chronic manifestations of splenectomy include?
Harrison's 20th Ed. Chapter 62 Page 416

A. Howell-Jolly bodies
B. Heinz bodies
C. Basophilic stippling
D. All of the above

Chronic manifestations of splenectomy include anisocytosis, poikilocytosis, presence of Howell-Jolly bodies (nuclear remnants), Heinz bodies (denatured hemoglobin), basophilic stippling.

277. Frequency of a serious infection following splenectomy is highest within?
Harrison's 20th Ed. Chapter 62 Page 416

A. First 6 months
B. First 1 year
C. First 3 years
D. First 5 years

Frequency of a serious infection following splenectomy is highest within first 3 years.

278. Which of the following is false in postsplenectomy period?
Harrison's 20th Ed. Chapter 62 Page 416

A. Increased susceptibility to capsulated bacterial infections
B. No increased risk of viral infection
C. Increased susceptibility to babesiosis
D. None of the above

279. In elective splenectomy, pneumococcal vaccine should be administered how many weeks before surgery?
Harrison's 20th Ed. Chapter 62 Page 416

A. 1 week
B. 2 weeks
C. 3 weeks
D. 4 weeks

Pneumococcal vaccine (23-valent polysaccharide vaccine) should be administered to all patients 2 weeks before elective splenectomy.

280. Splenectomized patients are more susceptible to which of the following?
Harrison's 20th Ed. Chapter 62 Page 417

A. Leishmaniasis
B. Babesiosis
C. Trypanosomiasis
D. Ehrlichiosis

Splenectomized patients are more susceptible to the parasitic disease babesiosis.

Iron Deficiency and Other Hypoproliferative Anemias

281. Which of the following is false about hypoproliferative anemias?

Harrison's 20th Ed. Chapter 93 Page 683

A. Normocytic RBC's
B. Normochromic RBC's
C. Reticulocyte index < 2.0–2.5
D. None of the above

Anemias associated with normocytic and normochromic red cells and an inappropriately low reticulocyte response (reticulocyte index <2.0–2.5) are hypoproliferative anemias.

282. Which of the following is a hypoproliferative anemia?

Harrison's 20th Ed. Chapter 93 Page 683

A. Anemia of acute and chronic inflammation
B. Anemia of hypometabolic states
C. Anemias from marrow damage
D. All of the above

Hypoproliferative anemias include early iron deficiency, acute and chronic inflammation, renal disease, hypometabolic states (protein malnutrition & endocrine deficiencies), and anemias from marrow damage.

283. Most common anemia among hypoproliferative anemias is?

Harrison's 20th Ed. Chapter 93 Page 683

A. Anemias associated with renal disease
B. Anemias associated with inflammation
C. Anemias associated with cancer
D. Anemias associated with hypometabolic states

Anemia associated with inflammation is the most common of the above mentioned hypoproliferative anemias. All these are characterized by an abnormal erythropoietin response to the anemia.

284. Which of the following is called iron transport protein?

Harrison's 20th Ed. Chapter 93 Page 683

A. Ferritin
B. Transferrin
C. Divalent metal transporter 1 (DMT1)
D. All of the above

Iron absorbed from the diet or released from stores circulates in the plasma bound to transferrin, the iron transport protein.

285. Turnover or half-clearance time of transferrin-bound iron is?

Harrison's 20th Ed. Chapter 93 Page 683

A. 5 – 10 minutes
B. 10 – 30 minutes
C. 30 – 60 minutes
D. 60 – 90 minutes

Turnover or half-clearance time of transferrin-bound iron is 60 - 90 minutes.

286. Which of the following has the highest affinity for transferrin receptors?

Harrison's 20th Ed. Chapter 93 Page 683

A. Monoferric transferrin
B. Diferric transferrin
C. Apotransferrin
D. All of the above

Iron-transferrin complex in plasma interacts with specific transferrin receptors on marrow erythroid cell surface. Diferric transferrin has the highest affinity for transferrin receptors. Apotransferrin does not carry iron and has very little affinity for transferrin receptors.

287. Iron is crucial to which of the following biologic functions?

N Engl J Med 2015;372:1832-43

A. Energy production
B. DNA synthesis
C. Cell proliferation
D. All of the above

Iron is crucial to biologic functions, including respiration, energy production, DNA synthesis, and cell proliferation.

288. Daily requirement of dietary iron in adult man is?

Harrison's 20th Ed. Chapter 93 Page 683 Figure 93-1

A. 1 mg
B. 2 mg
C. 3 mg
D. 4 mg

Normally, an adult male needs ~1 mg of elemental iron daily, while females in childbearing years need 1.4 mg/day.

289. Transferrin-receptor complex is internalized via?

Harrison's 20th Ed. Chapter 93 Page 683

A. Etharin-coated pits
B. Megalin-coated pits
C. Clathrin-coated pits
D. Azalin-coated pits

Transferrin-receptor complex is internalized via clathrin-coated pits and transported to an acidic endosome, where iron is released at a low pH.

290. In erythroid cell, excess iron binds to which of the following to form ferritin?

Harrison's 20th Ed. Chapter 93 Page 684

A. Apoferritin
B. Transferritin
C. Coferritin
D. Endoferritin

In erythroid cell, excess iron binds to Apoferritin to form ferritin.

291. What proportion of red cells turn over each day?

Harrison's 20th Ed. Chapter 93 Page 684

A. 0.2 to 0.4%
B. 0.4 to 0.6%
C. 0.6 to 0.8%
D. 0.8 to 1.0%

Normally, average RBC life span is 120 days. Thus, 0.8 –1.0% of red cells turn over each day.

292. Each milliliter of red cells contain how much elemental iron?
Harrison's 20th Ed. Chapter 93 Page 684

A. 1 mg
B. 2 mg
C. 3 mg
D. 4 mg

Each milliliter of red cells contains 1 mg of elemental iron.

293. An adult has a red cell mass of?
Harrison's 20th Ed. Chapter 93 Page 684

A. 2 Liters
B. 3 Liters
C. 4 Liters
D. 5 Liters

An adult has a red cell mass of 2 Liters.

294. 1000 calories of diet contains how much elemental iron?
Harrison's 20th Ed. Chapter 93 Page 684

A. ~ 6 mg
B. ~ 9 mg
C. ~ 12 mg
D. ~ 15 mg

Dietary iron content is closely related to total caloric intake. 1000 calories of diet contains ~6 mg of elemental iron.

295. What percentage of iron intake is absorbed in an average male?
Harrison's 20th Ed. Chapter 93 Page 684

A. ~ 1%
B. ~ 3%
C. ~ 6%
D. ~ 9%

296. What percentage of iron intake is absorbed in an average female?
Harrison's 20th Ed. Chapter 93 Page 684

A. ~ 8%
B. ~ 10%
C. ~ 12%
D. ~ 15%

In United States, average iron intake in an adult male is 15 mg/day with 6% absorption. In an average female, daily intake is 11 mg/day with 12% absorption. Those with iron deficiency can increase iron absorption to ~20% of iron present in a meat containing diet but only 5 - 10% of iron in a vegetarian diet.

297. Phytates and phosphates in food reduce iron absorption by?
Harrison's 20th Ed. Chapter 93 Page 684

A. ~ 25%
B. ~ 50%
C. ~ 75%
D. ~ 90%

Phytates and phosphates in food stuff reduce iron absorption by ~ 50%.

298. During the last two trimesters of pregnancy, daily iron requirements increase to?
Harrison's 20th Ed. Chapter 93 Page 684

A. 2 to 3 mg
B. 3 to 4 mg
C. 4 to 5 mg
D. 5 to 6 mg

During the last two trimesters of pregnancy, daily iron requirements increase to 5 - 6 mg/day.

299. Iron absorption takes place largely in?
Harrison's 20th Ed. Chapter 93 Page 684

A. Stomach
B. Proximal small intestine
C. Distal small intestine
D. Large intestine

Iron absorption takes place largely in proximal small intestine through a carefully regulated process.

300. Reduction of ferric (Fe^{+++}) to ferrous (Fe^{++}) iron at brush border membrane of duodenal enterocytes is done by?
Harrison's 20th Ed. Chapter 93 Page 684

A. Duodenal hepcidin
B. Duodenal ferroportin
C. Duodenal hephaestin
D. Duodenal cytochrome B (Dcytb)

Dietary inorganic iron traverses brush border membrane of duodenal enterocytes via DMT1 after reduction of ferric (Fe^{3+}) to ferrous (Fe^{2+}) iron by duodenal cytochrome B (Dcytb) - a ferrireductase.

301. Iron transport across the enteric absorptive cell membrane is accomplished by?
Harrison's 20th Ed. Chapter 93 Page 684

A. Duodenal cytochrome B (Dcytb)
B. Hephaestin
C. Ferroportin
D. Divalent metal transporter type 1 (DMT-1)

Iron transport across enteric absorptive cell membrane is achieved by divalent metal transporter type 1 (DMT-1). DMT-1 is a general cation transporter and is also known as natural resistance macrophage-associated protein type 2 (Nramp 2) or DCT-1.

302. Iron in gut cell is transported through its basolateral surface to plasma transferrin through?
Harrison's 20th Ed. Chapter 93 Page 684

A. Duodenal cytochrome B (Dcytb)
B. Hephaestin
C. Ferroportin (FPN)
D. Divalent metal transporter 1 (DMT-1)

In gut cell, iron may be stored as ferritin or released at basolateral surface to plasma transferrin through membrane - embedded iron exporter, ferroportin (FPN).

303. Which of the following is called "iron regulatory hormone"?
Harrison's 20th Ed. Chapter 93 Page 684

A. Ferritin
B. Transferrin
C. Erythropoietin
D. Hepcidin

304. Hepcidin principally acts on which of the following?
Harrison's 20th Ed. Chapter 93 Page 684

A. Duodenal cytochrome B (Dcytb)
B. Hephaestin
C. Ferroportin
D. Divalent metal transporter 1 (DMT-1)

Hepcidin (principal iron regulatory hormone) is involved in regulation of iron uptake by enterocytes & iron release by RE cells. Hepcidin represses ferroportin at basolateral surface as well as iron release from macrophages & serves as a central regulator of body iron traffic. It is a crucial molecule in iron metabolism, linking body stores with intestinal iron absorption. Thus, the function of ferroportin is negatively regulated by hepcidin. In iron deficiency, hepcidin levels are low and iron is much more efficiently absorbed, contrary is true in states of secondary iron overload.

305. Which of the following about Hepcidin is false?
N Engl J Med 2015;372:1832-43

A. Hepcidin is a peptide hormone
B. Synthesized primarily in the liver
C. Functions as an acute-phase reactant
D. None of the above

306. Which of the following oxidizes iron to ferric form for transferrin binding at the basolateral surface of gut cell?
Harrison's 20th Ed. Chapter 93 Page 684

A. Duodenal cytochrome B (Dcytb)
B. Hephaestin
C. Ferroportin
D. Divalent metal transporter 1 (DMT-1)

Iron moves from enterocyte into circulation via a process requiring basolateral iron exporter ferroportin (FPN) & iron oxidase hephaestin (Heph) - which oxidizes iron to ferric form for transferrin binding.

307. Hephaestin is similar to which of the following?
Harrison's 20th Ed. Chapter 93 Page 684

A. Ferritin
B. Erythropoietin
C. C-reactive protein
D. Ceruloplasmin

Hephaestin is similar to ceruloplasmin, the copper-carrying protein.

308. Hepcidin is derived from?
Harrison's 20th Ed. Chapter 93 Page 684

A. Bone marrow
B. Liver
C. Duodenum
D. Spleen

Hepcidin is a 25-amino-acid peptide made by the liver.

309. Hepcidin responds to signals mediated by?
Harrison's 20th Ed. Chapter 93 Page 684

A. HFE
B. TfR2 (transferrin receptor 2)
C. Hemojuvelin (HJV)
D. All of the above

Hepcidin responds to changes in body iron requirements by signals mediated by HFE, TfR2 & hemojuvelin (HJV). Mutations in the genes encoding HFE, TfR2, hemojuvelin, and hepcidin lead to decreased hepcidin release and increased iron absorption, resulting in hemochromatosis.

310. Globally, iron deficiency accounts for what percentage of anemia?
Harrison's 20th Ed. Chapter 93 Page 684

A. 25%
B. 50%
C. 75%
D. 90%

Globally, 50% of anemia is attributable to iron deficiency.

311. Bone marrow iron stores are absent when serum ferritin level is?
Harrison's 20th Ed. Chapter 93 Page 685

A. < 15 µg/L
B. < 25 µg/L
C. < 35 µg/L
D. < 45 µg/L

Bone marrow iron stores are absent when the serum ferritin level is <15 µg/L.

312. Hemoglobin synthesis is impaired when transferrin saturation falls to?
Harrison's 20th Ed. Chapter 93 Page 685

A. 10 to 15%
B. 15 to 20%
C. 20 to 25%
D. 25 to 30%

Once the transferrin saturation falls to 15 - 20%, hemoglobin synthesis becomes impaired. This is a period of iron-deficient erythropoiesis. When transferrin saturation is 10 - 15%, hemoglobin & hematocrit begin to fall, reflecting iron-deficiency anemia.

313. Which of the following about iron-deficient erythropoiesis is false?
Harrison's 20th Ed. Chapter 93 Page 685

A. Impaired hemoglobin synthesis
B. Microcytic RBCs first appear in PBF
C. Hyperchromic reticulocytes in circulation
D. Transferrin saturation between 15 to 20%

When transferrin saturation is between 15 to 20%, hemoglobin synthesis is impaired. This is a period of iron-deficient erythropoiesis. Peripheral blood smear reveals the first appearance of microcytic cells and hypochromic reticulocytes in circulation.

314. Microcytic RBC's & hypochromic reticulocytes first appear in circulation in which of the following stages?
Harrison's 20th Ed. Chapter 93 Page 685

A. Negative iron balance
B. Iron-deficient erythropoiesis
C. Iron-deficiency anemia
D. All of the above

Hb synthesis is impaired in iron-deficient erythropoiesis and PBF shows microcytic RBCs and hypochromic reticulocytes.

315. Iron-deficient erythropoiesis is recognized by?
Harrison's 20th Ed. Chapter 93 Page 685 Figure 93-2

A. Percent transferrin saturation
B. Pattern of marrow sideroblasts
C. RBC protoporphyrin level
D. All of the above

Iron-deficient erythropoiesis is recognized from additional abnormalities in the serum iron (SI), percent transferrin saturation, the pattern of marrow sideroblasts and the red blood cell (RBC) protoporphyrin level. Patients with iron-deficiency demonstrate all the same abnormalities plus hypochromic microcytic anemia.

316. Appearance of iron deficiency in an adult male means?
Harrison's 20th Ed. Chapter 93 Page 685

A. Acute inflammation
B. Chronic inflammation
C. Gastrointestinal blood loss
D. Blood malignancy

317. Iron deficiency in adult male usually means?
Harrison's 20th Ed. Chapter 93 Page 685

A. Inadequate iron in diet
B. Inadequate iron absorption
C. Gastrointestinal blood loss
D. All of the above

As a rule, iron deficiency in adult male means gastrointestinal blood loss until proved otherwise.

318. Which of the following is a sign of advanced tissue iron deficiency?
Harrison's 20th Ed. Chapter 93 Page 685

A. Fatigue
B. Pallor
C. Reduced exercise capacity
D. Cheilosis

Usual signs of iron deficiency anemia are fatigue, pallor & reduced exercise capacity. Cheilosis (fissures at corners of mouth) & koilonychia are signs of advanced tissue iron deficiency.

319. Which of the following is an indirect measure of circulating transferrin?
Harrison's 20th Ed. Chapter 93 Page 685

A. Serum Iron
B. Total Iron-Binding Capacity (TIBC)
C. Transferrin saturation
D. Serum Ferritin

TIBC is an indirect measure of circulating transferrin.

320. Normal range for serum iron is?
Harrison's 20th Ed. Chapter 93 Page 685

A. 10 to 40 μg/dL
B. 20 to 80 μg/dL
C. 30 to 100 μg/dL
D. 50 to 150 μg/dL

321. Normal range for TIBC is?
Harrison's 20th Ed. Chapter 93 Page 685

A. 180 to 250 μg/dL
B. 300 to 360 μg/dL
C. 450 to 700 μg/dL
D. 750 to 1050 μg/dL

322. Normal Transferrin saturation is?
Harrison's 20th Ed. Chapter 93 Page 685

A. 12 to 18%
B. 15 to 28%
C. 25 to 50%
D. 45 to 70%

Normal range for serum iron is 50–150 μg/dL. Normal range for TIBC is 300–360 μg/dL. Transferrin saturation is normally 25–50%.

323. Which of the following is the formula for calculating transferrin saturation?
Harrison's 20th Ed. Chapter 93 Page 685

A. (Serum iron × 100) ÷ TIBC
B. (TIBC × 100) ÷ Serum iron
C. (Serum iron ÷ 100) × TIBC
D. (TIBC ÷ 100) × Serum iron

Transferrin saturation is calculated by as serum iron × 100 ÷ TIBC.

324. Iron deficiency state is present when transferrin saturation is below?
Harrison's 20th Ed. Chapter 93 Page 685

A. 6%
B. 10%
C. 14%
D. 20%

Iron-deficiency is associated with transferrin saturation levels < 20%.

325. Serum iron level represents the amount of?
Harrison's 20th Ed. Chapter 93 Page 685

A. Circulating free iron
B. Circulating iron bound to transferrin
C. Circulating free iron + iron bound to transferrin
D. Any of the above

Serum iron level represents amount of circulating iron bound to transferrin.

326. Within cells, iron is stored complexed to protein as?
Harrison's 20th Ed. Chapter 93 Page 685

A. Apoferritin
B. Protoporphyrin
C. Hemosiderin
D. Any of the above

Within cells, iron is stored complexed to protein as ferritin or hemosiderin. Apoferritin binds to free ferrous iron and stores it in the ferric state. As ferritin accumulates within cells of the RE system, protein aggregates are formed as hemosiderin. Iron in ferritin or hemosiderin can be extracted for release by the RE cells.

327. Adult males have serum ferritin values averaging about?
Harrison's 20th Ed. Chapter 93 Page 685

A. 100 μg/L
B. 200 μg/L
C. 300 μg/L
D. 400 μg/L

328. Adult females have serum ferritin values averaging about?
Harrison's 20th Ed. Chapter 93 Page 685

A. 10 μg/L
B. 20 μg/L
C. 30 μg/L
D. 40 μg/L

Serum ferritin level correlates with total body iron stores. Normal value for adult males & females average ~100 and 30 μg/L respectively.

329. Sideroblasts have granules consisting of?

Harrison's 20th Ed. Chapter 93 Page 685

A. Ferritin

B. Transferrin

C. Glycogen

D. All of the above

330. Sideroblasts are?

Harrison's 20th Ed. Chapter 93 Page 685

A. Developing erythroblasts

B. Developing myeloblasts

C. Defective erythroblasts

D. Defective myeloblasts

331. Normal percentage of sideroblasts in bone marrow is?

Harrison's 20th Ed. Chapter 93 Page 685

A. 5%

B. 10%

C. 40%

D. 75%

When the marrow smear is stained for iron, 20 - 40% of developing erythroblasts will have visible ferritin granules in their cytoplasm. These are called sideroblasts. This represents iron in excess of that needed for hemoglobin synthesis.

332. In 'ringed sideroblasts', the accumulation of iron is around?

Harrison's 20th Ed. Chapter 93 Page 686

A. Cell membrane

B. Nucleus

C. Mitochondria

D. Endoplasmic reticulum

333. Sideroblastic anemia usually points to the diagnosis of?

Harrison's 20th Ed. Chapter 93 Page 686

A. Aplastic anemia

B. Myelodysplasia

C. Pernicious anemia

D. All of the above

Ringed sideroblasts are seen in myelodysplastic syndromes due to mitochondrial dysfunction. Iron accumulates in mitochondria in a necklace fashion around the nucleus of erythroblast.

334. Normal value of red cell protoporphyrin is?

Harrison's 20th Ed. Chapter 93 Page 686

A. < 30 μg/dL

B. < 60 μg/dL

C. < 90 μg/dL

D. < 120 μg/dL

Normal value of red cell protoporphyrin is < 30 μg/dL. Most common causes of increased red cell protoporphyrin levels are absolute or relative iron deficiency and lead poisoning. In iron deficiency, values in excess of 100 μg/dL are seen.

335. Which of the following is false about transferrin receptor protein (TRP)?

Harrison's 20th Ed. Chapter 93 Page 686

A. Serum levels of TRP reflect total erythroid marrow mass

B. TRP is released by erythroid cells into circulation

C. TRP levels are elevated in absolute iron deficiency

D. None of the above

Serum levels of transferrin receptor protein (TRP) is 4–9 μg/L. It along with serum ferritin, distinguishes between iron deficiency & anemia of inflammation.

336. Which of the following is a cause of hypochromic microcytic anemia?

Harrison's 20th Ed. Chapter 93 Page 686

A. Iron deficiency

B. Thalassemia

C. Sideroblastic anemia

D. All of the above

337. Which of the following is false about thalassemias?

Harrison's 20th Ed. Chapter 93 Page 686

A. Hypochromic microcytic anemia

B. Normal or increased serum iron levels

C. Normal or increased serum transferrin saturation

D. Elevated red blood cell distribution width (RDW) index

Characteristics of thalassemia include hypochromic microcytic anemia, normal or increased serum iron levels & transferrin saturation with small RDW index which is elevated in iron deficiency.

338. Which of the following is false about anemia of chronic inflammation?

Harrison's 20th Ed. Chapter 93 Page 686

A. Normocytic and normochromic anemia

B. Normal or increased serum ferritin levels

C. Below normal serum transferrin saturation

D. Normal TIBC

Anemia of chronic inflammation with inadequate iron supply is normocytic and normochromic. Ferritin level is normal or increased and percent transferrin saturation & TIBC are typically below normal.

339. Elemental iron per day for iron replacement therapy is?

Harrison's 20th Ed. Chapter 93 Page 686

A. ~ 30 mg

B. ~ 100 mg

C. ~ 200 mg

D. ~ 300 mg

For iron replacement therapy, ~200 mg of elemental iron is given per day.

340. Ideally, oral iron preparations should be taken?

Harrison's 20th Ed. Chapter 93 Page 686

A. Empty stomach

B. Just before a meal

C. Along with meals

D. Following meals

Since foods may inhibit oral iron absorption, iron preparations should be taken on empty stomach.

341. How many days after initiation of oral iron therapy, reticulocyte count begin to increase?
Harrison's 20th Ed. Chapter 93 Page 687

A. 4 – 7 days
B. 7 – 14 days
C. 14 – 21 days
D. 21 – 28 days

Typically, reticulocyte count begin to increase within 4 - 7 days after initiation of oral iron therapy and peak at 1½ weeks.

342. In normal iron tolerance test, 2 hours after 2 iron tablets, serum iron increases by?
Harrison's 20th Ed. Chapter 93 Page 687

A. 10 μg/dL
B. 500 μg/dL
C. 75 μg/dL
D. 100 μg/dL

In normal iron tolerance test, 2 hours after 2 iron tablets on an empty stomach, serum iron increases by at least 100 μg/dL indicating patient's ability to absorb iron adequately.

343. Amount of parenteral iron needed is calculated by?
Harrison's 20th Ed. Chapter 93 Page 687

A. Weight (kg) × 0.3 × (15 - patients Hb) + 500 or 1000 mg
B. Weight (kg) × 1.3 × (15 - patients Hb) + 500 or 1000 mg
C. Weight (kg) × 2.3 × (15 - patients Hb) + 500 or 1000 mg
D. Weight (kg) × 3.3 × (15 - patients Hb) + 500 or 1000 mg

Amount of parenteral iron needed is calculated by weight (kg) × 2.3 × (15-patients Hb in grams/dL) + 500 or 1000 mg (for stores).

344. Which of the following intravenous iron preparations has most chances of anaphylaxis?
Harrison's 20th Ed. Chapter 93 Page 687

A. Iron dextran
B. Ferric carboxymaltose
C. Sodium ferric gluconate
D. Iron sucrose

345. Infusion of iron must be stopped immediately if which of the following develops?
Harrison's 20th Ed. Chapter 93 Page 687

A. Chest pain
B. Wheezing
C. Fall in blood pressure
D. Any of the above

Early in the infusion of iron, if chest pain, wheezing, a fall in blood pressure, or other systemic symptoms occur, the infusion of iron should be stopped immediately.

346. Endogenous erythropoietin production is inadequate for the degree of anemia in?
Harrison's 20th Ed. Chapter 93 Page 687

A. Chronic inflammation
B. Renal disease
C. Hypometabolism
D. All of the above

With chronic inflammation, renal disease, or hypometabolism, endogenous EPO production is inadequate for the degree of anemia observed.

347. Appropriate elevations in endogenous EPO levels are typically found in which of the following hypoproliferative anemias?
Harrison's 20th Ed. Chapter 93 Page 687

A. Chronic inflammation
B. Renal disease
C. Hypometabolism
D. Marrow damage

348. Which of the following is a feature of anemia of chronic disease?
Harrison's 20th Ed. Chapter 93 Page 687

A. Increased red cell protoporphyrin
B. Hypoproliferative marrow
C. Normal or increased serum ferritin
D. All of the above

Features of anemia of chronic disease are a low serum iron, increased red cell protoporphyrin, hypoproliferative marrow, transferrin saturation of 15 - 20%, & normal or increased serum ferritin.

349. Which of the following is the most distinguishing feature between true iron-deficiency anemia & iron-deficient erythropoiesis associated with inflammation?
Harrison's 20th Ed. Chapter 93 Page 688

A. Low serum iron
B. Increased red cell protoporphyrin
C. Normal or increased serum ferritin
D. Hypoproliferative marrow

Serum ferritin level is the most distinguishing feature between true iron-deficiency anemia & iron-deficient erythropoiesis associated with inflammation which increase threefold over basal levels in inflammation due to effects of inflammatory cytokines & hepcidin.

350. Which of the following is true in anemia of chronic inflammation?
Harrison's 20th Ed. Chapter 93 Page 688

A. Increased Interleukin 1 (IL - 1)
B. Increased tumor necrosis factor (TNF)
C. Increased Hepcidin
D. All of the above

Anemia of chronic disorders or anemia of inflammation is a multifactorial anemia associated with increased cytokine production, up-regulation of hepcidin, and abnormal iron homeostasis.

351. Which of the following gene is related to Iron-refractory iron-deficiency anemia (IRIDA)?
N Engl J Med 2015;372:1832-43

A. GATA- 1
B. TCNL
C. MTHFR
D. TMPRSS6

352. Which of the following about Iron-refractory iron-deficiency anemia (IRIDA) is false?

N Engl J Med 2015;372:1832-43

A. Autosomal recessive disorder

B. Caused by a mutation in TMPRSS6

C. High production of hepcidin

D. None of the above

Iron-refractory iron-deficiency anemia (IRIDA) is a rare autosomal recessive disorder. Iron-deficiency anemia is defined as "refractory" when there is an absence of hematologic response (an increase of <1 g of hemoglobin) after 4 to 6 weeks of treatment with oral iron. IRIDA is caused by a loss-of-function mutation in TMPRSS6, the gene encoding transmembrane protease, serine 6, also known as matriptase-2, which inhibits the signaling pathway that activates hepcidin. High production of hepcidin blocks the intestinal absorption of iron thus unresponsive to treatment with oral iron. Typical findings include a striking microcytosis and extremely low transferrin saturation in the presence of normal or borderline-low ferritin levels and high hepcidin levels. The diagnosis ultimately requires sequencing of TMPRSS6.

353. A typical unit of packed RBC increases hemoglobin by?

Harrison's 20th Ed. Chapter 93 Page 689

A. 0.5 g/dL

B. 0.75 g/dL

C. 1 g/dL

D. 1.25 g/dL

A typical unit of packed red cells increases the hemoglobin level by 1 g/dL.

354. A unit of packed RBCs contains how much iron?

Harrison's 20th Ed. Chapter 93 Page 689

A. 25 to 30 mg

B. 100 to 150 mg

C. 150 to 250 mg

D. 250 to 300 mg

355. Inadequate erythropoietin response is due to?

Harrison's 20th Ed. Chapter 93 Page 689

A. Iron depletion

B. Aluminum toxicity

C. Hyperparathyroidism

D. All of the above

A fall in Hb during EPO therapy signifies infection or iron depletion. Aluminum toxicity and hyperparathyroidism can also compromise EPO response.

356. Normal blood level of erythropoietin is?

N Engl J Med 2006;354:2034-45

A. 10 mU per milliliter

B. 20 mU per milliliter

C. 30 mU per milliliter

D. 40 mU per milliliter

Normal blood level of erythropoietin is 20 mU per milliliter.

357. Which of the following is the longer-acting preparation of erythropoietin?

Harrison's 20th Ed. Chapter 93 Page 689

A. Rubropoetin alpha

B. Telepoetin alpha

C. Darbepoetin alpha

D. All of the above

Darbepoetin alpha is a molecularly modified longer-acting preparations of EPO.

Disorders of Hemoglobin

358. Hemoglobinopathies are disorders that affect which of the following parameters of hemoglobin?
Harrison's 20th Ed. Chapter 94 Page 690

A. Structure
B. Function
C. Production
D. All of the above

Hemoglobinopathies are disorders affecting the structure, function, or production of hemoglobin.

359. The major adult hemoglobin, HbA, has the structure?
Harrison's 20th Ed. Chapter 94 Page 690

A. $\alpha 2\beta 2$
B. $\alpha 2\gamma 2$
C. $\alpha 2\delta 2$
D. None of the above

360. Structure of HbF is?
Harrison's 20th Ed. Chapter 94 Page 690

A. $\alpha 2\beta 2$
B. $\alpha 2\gamma 2$
C. $\alpha 2\delta 2$
D. None of the above

361. Structure of HbA2 is?
Harrison's 20th Ed. Chapter 94 Page 690

A. $\alpha 2\beta 2$
B. $\alpha 2\gamma 2$
C. $\alpha 2\delta 2$
D. None of the above

362. Which of the following about human hemoglobins is false?
Harrison's 20th Ed. Chapter 94 Page 690 Figure 94-1

A. α-like globin genes are on chromosome 16
B. β-like globin genes on chromosome 11
C. LCR controlling α globin gene is modulated by ATRX
D. None of the above

Gene clusters encoding human hemoglobins are alpha-like globin genes (on chromosome 16), and beta-like genes (on chromosome 11). Locus control region (LCR) LCR controlling the alpha-globin gene cluster is modulated by ATRX.

363. Which of the following is false?
Harrison's 20th Ed. Chapter 94 Page 690

A. Normal individual has four α globin genes
B. Normal individual has two β globin genes
C. γ and δ are β-like genes
D. None of the above

A normal individual has 4 α globin genes on short arm of chromosome 16 (two genes per chromosome -αα/αα) & two β globin genes on short arm of chromosome 11 (one per chromosome, or β/β). The β-like genes (α & δ) are nearby on chromosome 11.

364. Heme consists of which of the following protoporphyrin ring?
Harrison's 20th Ed. Chapter 94 Page 690

A. IX
B. X
C. XI
D. XII

Each globin chain has a single heme moiety, consisting of a protoporphyrin IX ring complexed with a single iron atom in ferrous state (Fe^{2+}).

365. Every molecule of hemoglobin can transport how many oxygen molecules?
Harrison's 20th Ed. Chapter 94 Page 690

A. 1
B. 2
C. 3
D. 4

Each heme moiety can bind a single oxygen molecule. One molecule of hemoglobin can transport up to four oxygen molecules.

366. Severe fetal hydrops is related to which of the following?
Cleveland clinic J of Med 2015;82(3):156

A. Ballantyne syndrome
B. Mirror syndrome
C. Triple oedema syndrome
D. All of the above

Ballantyne syndrome is also known as mirror syndrome and Triple oedema syndrome.

367. Oxygen equilibrium curve is shaped like?
Harrison's 20th Ed. Chapter 94 Page 690

A. V
B. S
C. Z
D. W

Sigmoid, cooperative oxygen binding curve of Hb only observed in the presence of 2,3-BPG.

368. Hemoglobin-oxygen dissociation curve is between which of the two parameters?
Harrison's 20th Ed. Chapter 94 Page 691 Figure 94-2

A. Tissue PO_2 and% saturation of Hb
B. Alveolar PO_2 and% saturation of Hb
C. Tissue PCO_2 and% saturation of Hb
D. Alveolar PCO_2 and% saturation of Hb

369. Hemoglobin-oxygen dissociation curve is between percent saturation of Hb and?
Harrison's 20th Ed. Chapter 94 Page 691 Figure 94-2

A. pH
B. Tissue PO_2
C. Alveolar PO_2
D. Tissue PCO_2

Hemoglobin-oxygen dissociation curve is between percent saturation of Hb and tissue PO_2.

370. Modulator of O_2 affinity of heme molecules is?
Harrison's 20th Ed. Chapter 94 Page 691 Figure 94-2

A. 2,3-bisphosphoglycerate (2,3-BPG)
B. pH
C. Temperature
D. CO_2

Blood pH is the most important modulator of O_2 affinity (Bohr effect after Christian Bohr, father of Neil Bohr, the atomic physicist).

371. As oxygen is bound to the hemoglobin tetramer, which of the following is expelled?
Harrison's 20th Ed. Chapter 94 Page 691 Figure 94-2

A. 2,3-bisphosphoglycerate (2,3-BPG)
B. H+
C. HCO_3
D. All of the above

As oxygen is bound to the hemoglobin tetramer, 2,3-bisphosphoglycerate (2,3-BPG) and carbon dioxide (CO_2) are expelled. 2,3-BPG binds at a site distant from the Fe where oxygen binds, it is called an allosteric effector.

372. Bohr effect is the ability of hemoglobin to deliver more oxygen to tissues at?
Harrison's 20th Ed. Chapter 94 Page 690

A. Low pH
B. Neutral pH
C. High pH
D. Any of the above

The Bohr effect is the ability of hemoglobin to deliver more oxygen to tissues at low pH. $HbO_2 + H^+ = H.Hb + O_2$

373. Which of the following about 2,3-BPG is false?
Harrison's 20th Ed. Chapter 94 Page 690

A. Intermediate compound in glycolytic pathway
B. Formed in human erythrocytes from 1,3-BPG
C. Is a negative allosteric effector of oxygen binding to Hb
D. None of the above

2,3-BPG is an intermediate compound in glycolytic pathway. It is formed in human erythrocytes from 1,3-BPG. Like oxygen and carbon dioxide, 2,3-BPG is a negative allosteric effector of oxygen binding to hemoglobin. In hypoxic states, production of 2,3-BPG is increased which enhances release of oxygen from oxyhemoglobin. In its absence, oxygen will not be released from oxyhemoglobin and oxygen dissociation curve will shift to the left.

374. Which of the following favours delivery of more O_2?
Harrison's 20th Ed. Chapter 94 Page 691 Figure 94-2

A. Decrease in pH
B. Increase in 2,3-BPG
C. Increase in temperature
D. All of the above

375. In which week of gestation red cells first appear in foetus?
Harrison's 20th Ed. Chapter 94 Page 690

A. About 2 weeks
B. About 4 weeks
C. About 6 weeks
D. About 8 weeks

Red cells first appear at about 6 weeks after conception.

376. Which of the following is an embryonic hemoglobin?
Harrison's 20th Ed. Chapter 94 Page 690

A. Hb Portland
B. Hb Gower I
C. Hb Gower II
D. All of the above

Embryonic hemoglobins are Hb Portland, Hb Gower I and Hb Gower II.

377. In which week of gestation does fetal hemoglobin become predominant?
Harrison's 20th Ed. Chapter 94 Page 690

A. About 6 weeks
B. About 10 weeks
C. About 18 weeks
D. About 24 weeks

At 10–11 weeks, fetal hemoglobin (HbF) becomes predominant.

378. Almost exclusive synthesis of adult hemoglobin (HbA) in foetus occurs at about?
Harrison's 20th Ed. Chapter 94 Page 690

A. 28 weeks
B. 30 weeks
C. 34 weeks
D. 38 weeks

Nearly exclusive synthesis of adult hemoglobin (HbA) occurs at ~38 weeks.

379. When mutations alter the amino acid sequence of a globin chain, which of the following hemoglobinopathies occur?
Harrison's 20th Ed. Chapter 94 Page 691

A. Structural hemoglobinopathies
B. Thalassemia syndromes
C. Hereditary persistence of fetal hemoglobin (HPFH)
D. Acquired hemoglobinopathies

Structural hemoglobinopathies occur when mutations alter the amino acid sequence of a globin chain therby altering physiologic properties of the variant hemoglobins (sickle cell anemia - the most common structural hemoglobinopathy).

380. Which of the following transcription factors play a pivotal role in transition from HbF to HbA?
Harrison's 20th Ed. Chapter 94 Page 690

A. RUNX1
B. PHF6
C. Bcl11a
D. WTI

Transcription factor Bcl11a plays a pivotal role in transition of HbF to HbA. Small amounts of HbF are produced during postnatal life.

381. HbF levels tend to rise in which of the following conditions?
Harrison's 20th Ed. Chapter 94 Page 690

A. Bone marrow transplantation
B. Sickle cell anemia
C. Thalassemia
D. All of the above

Profound erythroid stresses as in severe hemolytic anemias, bone marrow transplantation or cancer chemotherapy cause more of the F-potent BFU-e to be recruited. HbF levels thus tend to rise in some patients with sickle cell anemia or thalassemia.

382. When mutations impair production or translation of globin mRNA, which of the following hemoglobinopathies occur?
Harrison's 20th Ed. Chapter 94 Page 690

A. Structural hemoglobinopathies
B. Thalassemia syndromes
C. Hereditary persistence of fetal hemoglobin (HPFH)
D. Acquired hemoglobinopathies

Thalassemia syndromes arise from mutations that impair production or translation of globin mRNA, leading to deficient globin chain biosynthesis.

383. Which of the following statements about hemoglobinopathies is false?
Harrison's 20th Ed. Chapter 94 Page 690

A. Common in malaria endemic areas
B. Thalassemia children more susceptible to infection with nonlethal Plasmodium vivax
C. Thalassemia naturally protects against infection with Plasmodium falciparum
D. None of the above

384. In sickle cell syndrome, HbS is best illustrated as?
Harrison's 20th Ed. Chapter 94 Page 692

A. $\alpha 2\beta 2^{3\ Glu \rightarrow Va1}$
B. $\alpha 2\beta 2^{4\ Glu \rightarrow Va1}$
C. $\alpha 2\beta 2^{5\ Glu \rightarrow Va1}$
D. $\alpha 2\beta 2^{6\ Glu \rightarrow Va1}$

The sickle cell syndromes are caused by a mutation in the beta-globin gene that changes the sixth amino acid from glutamic acid to valine. Whereas thalassemias are caused by gene mutations resulting in decreased production of alpha or beta globin chains, the sickle cell disorders are hemoglobinopathies caused by mutations in the beta globin gene resulting in the production of a structurally abnormal beta globin chain.

385. Which of the following is not a characteristic of Sickle Cell Syndromes?
Harrison's 20th Ed. Chapter 94 Page 692

A. Microvascular vasoocclusion
B. Premature RBC destruction
C. Stiff RBC membrane
D. None of the above

386. HbC is best illustrated as?
Harrison's 20th Ed. Chapter 94 Page 692

A. $\alpha 2\beta 2^{3\ Glu \rightarrow Lys}$
B. $\alpha 2\beta 2^{4\ Glu \rightarrow Lys}$
C. $\alpha 2\beta 2^{5\ Glu \rightarrow Lys}$
D. $\alpha 2\beta 2^{6\ Glu \rightarrow Lys}$

387. Provocative factors of painful crises in sickle cell syndromes include?
Harrison's 20th Ed. Chapter 94 Page 692

A. Infection
B. Abrupt changes in temperature
C. Hypoxia
D. All of the above

Provocative factors include infection, fever, excessive exercise, anxiety, abrupt changes in temperature, hypoxia or hypertonic dyes.

388. Which of the following occurs in sickle cell syndromes?
Harrison's 20th Ed. Chapter 94 Page 693

A. Renal papillary necrosis
B. Retinal hemorrhage
C. Aseptic necrosis of bone
D. All of the above

389. Which of the following occurs in sickle cell syndromes?
Harrison's 20th Ed. Chapter 94 Page 693

A. Stroke in children
B. Priapism
C. Chronic lower leg ulcers
D. All of the above

390. Renal papillary necrosis produces which of the following?
Harrison's 20th Ed. Chapter 94 Page 693

A. Isosthenuria
B. Painless hematuria
C. Urethral obstruction
D. All of the above

Renal papillary necrosis invariably produces isosthenuria (nonconcentrated urine, isosmotic with plasma). Painless hematuria is due to papillary necrosis. Sloughing of papillae with urethral obstruction may occur.

391. Hand-foot syndrome is related to which of the following?
Harrison's 20th Ed. Chapter 94 Page 693

A. Tietze Syndrome
B. Hypertrophic Osteoarthropathy
C. Sickle cell disease
D. Syringomyelia

Sickle cell dactylitis or hand-foot syndrome caused by painful infarcts of digits & dactylitis is seen in sickle cell disease & sickle cell thalassemia below the age 4 or 5 years & not in adults.

392. Bone pain in sickle cell crisis is due to?
Harrison's 20th Ed. Chapter 94 Page 693

A. Fracture
B. Bone & bone marrow infarction
C. Hyperuricemia
D. Osteoporosis

The bone pain in sickle cell crisis is due to bone and bone marrow infarction.

393. Acute chest syndrome is due to which of the following?
Harrison's 20th Ed. Chapter 94 Page 693

A. Transient coronary spasm
B. Transient intercostal muscle spasm
C. Sickling within the lung
D. Pulmonary embolic shower

Acute chest syndrome is a medical emergency and is due to in-situ sickling within the lung, producing pain and temporary pulmonary dysfunction. It manifests by chest pain, tachypnea, fever, cough and arterial oxygen desaturation. Repeated episodes of acute chest pain correlate with reduced survival.

394. On Hemoglobin Electrophoresis, HbS : A ratio is 40 : 60 in which of the following?
Harrison's 20th Ed. Chapter 94 Page 693 Table 94-2

A. Sickle cell trait
B. Sickle cell anemia
C. S/β+ thalassemia
D. Hemoglobin SC

395. On Hemoglobin Electrophoresis, HbS : A ratio is 100 : 0 in which of the following?
Harrison's 20th Ed. Chapter 94 Page 693 Table 94-2

A. Sickle cell trait
B. Sickle cell anemia
C. S/β+ thalassemia
D. Hemoglobin SC

396. On Hemoglobin Electrophoresis, HbS : A ratio is 100 : 0 in which of the following?
Harrison's 20th Ed. Chapter 94 Page 693 Table 94-2

A. Sickle cell trait
B. S/β0 thalassemia
C. S/β+ thalassemia
D. Hemoglobin SC

397. Which of the following is true for Hemoglobin SC disease?
Harrison's 20th Ed. Chapter 94 Page 693

A. Lesser degree of hemolytic anemia
B. Greater propensity for retinopathy
C. Greater propensity for aseptic necrosis of bones
D. None of the above

Hemoglobin SC disease is a common variant of sickle cell anemia and is frequently marked by lesser degrees of hemolytic anemia, a greater propensity for development of retinopathy and aseptic necrosis of bones.

398. In Sickle cell syndromes, factors associated with increased morbidity & reduced survival include ?
Harrison's 20th Ed. Chapter 94 Page 694

A. More than three crises requiring hospitalization per year
B. Chronic neutrophilia
C. Second episodes of acute chest syndrome
D. All of the above

Factors associated with increased morbidity and reduced survival include >three crises requiring hospitalization per year, chronic neutrophilia, history of splenic sequestration or hand-foot syndrome and second episodes of acute chest syndrome.

399. Which of the following is useful in the treatment of sickle cell disease?
Harrison's 20th Ed. Chapter 94 Page 694

A. Anagrelide
B. Danazol
C. IFN-alpha
D. Hydroxyurea

Hydroxyurea (10 - 30 mg/kg per day) increases fetal hemoglobin within a few months, has favourable effects on RBC hydration, vascular wall adherence, and suppresses granulocyte & reticulocyte counts.

400. Which of the following drugs may elevate HbF?
Harrison's 20th Ed. Chapter 94 Page 694

A. Hydroxyurea
B. 5-azacytidine
C. Decitabine
D. All of the above

Antitumor drug 5-azacytidine was the first agent found to elevate HbF. Its widespread use has been prevented because of concerns about acute toxicity & carcinogenesis. Low doses of 5-deoxyazacytidine (decitabine) can elevate HbF with more acceptable toxicity.

401. Which of the following is best related to unstable hemoglobins?
Harrison's 20th Ed. Chapter 94 Page 695

A. Thalassemia
B. Methemoglobinemia
C. Heinz bodies
D. Pseudoanemia

Amino acid substitutions result in unstable hemoglobins that precipitate forming inclusion bodies injurious to the RBC membrane. Inclusion Heinz bodies are clinically detectable by staining with supravital dyes such as crystal violet.

402. Which of the following is a high-affinity hemoglobin?
Harrison's 20th Ed. Chapter 94 Page 695 Table 94-3

A. Hb Yakima
B. Hb Kansas
C. Hb Koln
D. Hb M Iwata

403. Pseudoanemia relates best with?
Harrison's 20th Ed. Chapter 94 Page 695 Table 94-3

A. Hb Yakima
B. Hb Kansas
C. Hb Koln
D. Hb M Iwata

404. Polycythemia is the main clinical manifestation of?
Harrison's 20th Ed. Chapter 94 Page 695 Table 94-3

A. Hb Yakima
B. Hb Kansas
C. Hb Koln
D. Hb M Iwata

High-affinity hemoglobin Hb Yakima binds oxygen more readily but deliver less to tissues at normal capillary PO_2 levels. Mild tissue hypoxia ensues that stimulates RBC production and erythrocytosis.

405. Southeast Asian poplulation is affected with which of the following abnormal hemoglobins?

Harrison's 20th Ed. Chapter 94 Page 695 Table 94-3

A. S
B. C
C. E
D. All of the above

406. Muddy appearance of freshly drawn blood is characteristic of which of the following?

Harrison's 20th Ed. Chapter 94 Page 695 Table 94-3

A. Sickle cell anemia
B. Methemoglobinemia
C. Thalassemia
D. All of the above

Muddy appearance of freshly drawn blood is characteristic of Methemoglobinemia. Methemoglobin is generated by oxidation of the heme iron moieties to the ferric state, causing a characteristic bluish-brown muddy color resembling cyanosis. Methemoglobin has such high oxygen affinity that virtually no oxygen is delivered.

407. Which of the following abnormal hemoglobins is related to congenital methemoglobinemia?

Harrison's 20th Ed. Chapter 94 Page 695 Table 94-3

A. Hb Yakima
B. Hb Kansas
C. Hb Koln
D. Hb M Iwata

408. Which of the following is a test for diagnosing unstable hemoglobins?

Harrison's 20th Ed. Chapter 94 Page 695

A. Acid glycerol lysis test
B. Isopropanol or heat stability test
C. Competitive-binding luminescence assay (CBLA)
D. Osmotic fragility

Many unstable Hb variants are electrophoretically silent. A normal electrophoresis does not rule out the diagnosis. The two best tests for diagnosing unstable hemoglobins are the Heinz body preparation and the isopropanol or heat stability test. Mass spectroscopy or direct gene analysis will provide a definitive diagnosis.

409. Which of the following is a cause of "saturation gap"?

Cleveland clinic J of Med 2015;82(3):156

A. Methemoglobinemia
B. Cyanide poisoning
C. Carbon monoxide poisoning
D. All of the above

Saturation gap refers to the discrepancy between oxyhemoglobin levels and oxygen saturation by pulse oximetry. Causes of "saturation gap" are Methemoglobinemia, cyanide poisoning and carbon monoxide poisoning. Saturation gap of >5% between the oxygen saturation by pulse oximetry and blood gas analysis is abnormal.

410. What is the normal level of methemoglobin in the blood?

Cleveland clinic J of Med 2015;82(3):156, Harrison's 20th Ed. Chapter 94 Page 695

A. < 1% of the total hemoglobin
B. < 2% of the total hemoglobin
C. < 3% of the total hemoglobin
D. < 4% of the total hemoglobin

Methemoglobin is normally present in the blood (< 1% of the total hemoglobin). Methemoglobinemia often causes symptoms of cerebral ischemia at levels >15%, while levels >60% are usually lethal.

411. Which of the following is important for binding of oxygen to iron in hemoglobin?

Cleveland clinic J of Med 2015;82(3):156

A. NADH-cytochrome b5 reductase
B. NADH dehydrogenase 2
C. NADH oxidase
D. Phosphofructokinase

Methemoglobinemia is rarely caused by a congenital deficiency of NADH-cytochrome b5 reductase.

412. Which of the following drugs can cause methemoglobinemia?

Cleveland clinic J of Med 2015;82(3):156

A. Acetaminophen
B. Primaquine
C. Nitroglycerin
D. All of the above

Common agents that can cause acquired methemoglobinemia include Antibiotics (Dapsone, trimethoprim-sulfamethoxazole, sulfonamide), Anesthetics (Benzocaine, lidocaine, procaine, prilocaine), Analgesics (Acetaminophen), Antimalarials (Primaquine, chloroquine), Anticancer agents (Cyclophosphamide, flutamide), Nitroglycerin, sodium nitroprusside, mesalamine and rasburicase. Acetaminophen, Dapsone, Benzocaine, Primaquine, chloroquine, nitroglycerin, and sulfonamides are common culprits for causing acquired methemoglobinemia. Potentially fatal methemoglobinemia has been reported in patients with a deficiency of G-6-phosphate dehydrogenase (G6PD) who received rasburicase, a recombinant version of urate oxidase enzyme used to prevent and treat tumor lysis syndrome. Methemoglobinemia has been reported in patients with inflammatory bowel disease treated with mesalamine.

413. Regular pulse oximetry measures light absorbance at?

Cleveland clinic J of Med 2015;82(3):156

A. 360 and 640 nm
B. 460 and 740 nm
C. 560 and 840 nm
D. 660 and 940 nm

Regular pulse oximetry works by measuring light absorbance at two distinct wavelengths i.e. 660 and 940 nm, to calculate the ratio of oxyhemoglobin to deoxyhemoglobin. Methemoglobin absorbs light at both these wavelengths, thus lowering the pulse oximetry values. In contrast, oxygen saturation of arterial blood gas (oxyhemoglobin) is calculated indirectly from the concentration of dissolved oxygen in the blood and does not include oxygen bound to hemoglobin. Therefore, the measured arterial oxygen saturation is often normal in patients with methemoglobinemia since it relies only on inspired oxygen content and is independent of the methemoglobin concentration.

414. Which of the following is related to the action of methylene blue?

Cleveland clinic J of Med 2015;82(3):156

A. Unimethylene blue
B. Amylomethylene blue
C. Leukomethylene blue
D. Tryptomethylene blue

Methylene blue is converted to its reduced form, leukomethylene blue, by NADPH-methemoglobin reductase. As it is oxidized, leukomethylene blue reduces methemoglobin to hemoglobin.

415. What is the initial intravenous dose of methylene blue?

Cleveland clinic J of Med 2015;82(3):156

A. 1 mg/kg
B. 2 mg/kg
C. 3 mg/kg
D. 4 mg/kg

Methylene blue is given in a dose of 1 mg/kg intravenously initially. Improvement in symptoms occurs within 30 to 60 minutes. If MethHb levels remain high, the dose can be repeated 1 hour later. Methylene blue therapy should be avoided in patients with complete G6PD deficiency. Methylene blue works through the enzyme NADPH-methemoglobin reductase, and since patients with G6PD deficiency lack this enzyme, methylene blue is ineffective. Milder cases and follow-up of severe cases can be treated orally with methylene blue (60 mg three to four times each day) or ascorbic acid (300-600 mg/day).

Thalassemia Syndromes

416. Which of the following about Thalassemias is false?
N Engl J Med 2014;371:1908-16

A. Inherited disorders of hemoglobin synthesis
B. Reduced production of globin chains of hemoglobin
C. Monogenic diseases
D. None of the above

Thalassemias are the most common human monogenic diseases. These inherited disorders of hemoglobin synthesis are characterized by a reduced production of globin chains of hemoglobin.

417. What percentage of the population worldwide carry an alpha-thalassemia variant?
N Engl J Med 2014;371:1908-16

A. 1%
B. 5%
C. 10%
D. 15%

It has been estimated that about 5% of the population worldwide carry an a-thalassemia variant.

418. Which of the following represents fetal hemoglobin?
N Engl J Med 2014;371:1908-16

A. $\alpha 2\beta 2$
B. $\alpha 2\delta 2$
C. $\alpha 2\gamma 2$
D. $\alpha 2\varepsilon 2$

Normal adult hemoglobin consists of pairs of alpha and beta chains ($\alpha 2\beta 2$), and fetal hemoglobin has two alpha chains and two gamma chains ($\alpha 2\gamma 2$).

419. Which of the following is false?
N Engl J Med 2014;371:1908-16

A. $\alpha\alpha/\alpha\alpha$
B. $\beta\beta/\beta\beta$
C. $\gamma\gamma/\gamma\gamma$
D. β/β

The genes for the alpha chains and gamma chains are duplicated (αα/αα, γγ/γγ), whereas the β chains are encoded by a single gene locus (β/β).

420. In fetus, defective production of a chains is reflected by the presence of excess?
N Engl J Med 2014;371:1908-16

A. α chains
B. β chains
C. γ chains
D. δ chains

421. In adults, defective production of a chains is reflected by the presence of excess?
N Engl J Med 2014;371:1908-16

A. α chains
B. β chains
C. γ chains
D. δ chains

In the fetus, defective production of alpha chains is reflected by the presence of excess gamma chains, which form gamma4 tetramers, called hemoglobin Bart's. In adults, excess beta chains form beta4 tetramers, called hemoglobin H (HbH). These two tetramers have very high oxygen affinity and consequently cannot transport oxygen. Instability of HbH leads to production of inclusion bodies in red cells and a variable degree of hemolytic anemia.

422. α-thalassemia 1 is now called?
N Engl J Med 2014;371:1908-16

A. α0 thalassemia
B. α1 thalassemia
C. α+ thalassemia
D. α- thalassemia

423. α-thalassemia 2 is now called?
N Engl J Med 2014;371:1908-16

A. α0 thalassemia
B. α1 thalassemia
C. α+ thalassemia
D. α- thalassemia

On the basis of the numbers of α-globin genes lost by deletion or totally or partially inactivated by point mutations, α-thalassemias are classified into two main subgroups: α+-thalassemia (formerly called α-thalassemia 2) and α0-thalassemia (formerly called α-thalassemia 1). In α+-thalassemia, one pair of genes is deleted or inactivated by a point mutation (-α/αα or ααND/αα, with ND denoting nondeletion). In α0-thalassemia, both pairs of α-globin genes on the same chromosome are deleted (--/αα).

424. Which of the following is not associated with hemoglobin Bart's hydrops fetalis syndrome?
N Engl J Med 2014;371:1908-16

A. Severe anemia of pregnancy
B. Preeclampsia
C. Polyhydramnios
D. Small placenta

Congenital malformations and maternal complications that accompany hemoglobin Bart's hydrops fetalis syndrome include severe anemia of pregnancy, preeclampsia, polyhydramnios, & extreme difficulty in delivery of both fetus and hugely enlarged placenta.

425. α-thalassemia is associated with which of the following syndromes?
Harrison's 20th Ed. Chapter 94 Page 696, Cold Spring Harb Perspect Med 2012;2:a011759

A. ATR-X syndrome
B. ATR-16 syndrome
C. ATMDS
D. All of the above

There are two syndromes in which α-thalassemia is associated with mental retardation (ATR syndromes). ATR-16 and ATR-X, are characterized by α-thalassemia in association with multiple developmental abnormalities including mental retardation. ATMDS (Alpha thalassemia myelodysplasia syndrome), is an acquired disorder in which α-thalassemia arises in the context of myelodysplasia.

426. α-thalassemia is highly protective against which of the following?

N Engl J Med 2014;371:1908-16

A. Dengue
B. Scrub typhus
C. Severe malaria
D. All of the above

a-thalassemia is highly protective against severe malaria.

427. DALY stands for?

N Engl J Med 2014;371:1908-16

A. Disease-adjusted life-years
B. Disability-adjusted life-years
C. Drug-adjusted life-years
D. Diagnosis-adjusted life-years

DALY stands for Disability-adjusted life-years.

428. Which of the following facies is typical of thalassemia?

Harrison's 20th Ed. Chapter 94 Page 696

A. Plethoric moon facies
B. Leonine facies
C. Chipmunk facies
D. Elfin facies

In thalassemic children, characteristic "chipmunk" facies occurs due to maxillary marrow hyperplasia & frontal bossing.

429. In α-thalassemia-2 trait, how many of the four α-globin loci are deleted?

Harrison's 20th Ed. Chapter 94 Page 696

A. 1
B. 2
C. 3
D. 4

430. In α-thalassemia-1 trait, how many of the four α-globin loci are deleted?

Harrison's 20th Ed. Chapter 94 Page 696

A. 1
B. 2
C. 3
D. 4

431. In hydrops fetalis with Hb Bart's, how many of the four α-globin loci are deleted?

Harrison's 20th Ed. Chapter 94 Page 696

A. 1
B. 2
C. 3
D. 4

432. In HbH disease, how many of the four α-globin loci are deleted?

Harrison's 20th Ed. Chapter 94 Page 696

A. 1
B. 2
C. 3
D. 4

The four classic alpha thalassemias are alpha-thalassemia-2 trait (one of the four α-globin loci is deleted), alpha-thalassemia-1 trait (with two deleted loci), HbH disease (with three loci deleted) and hydrops fetalis with Hb Bart's (all four loci deleted).

433. Which of the following α-thalassemia resembles β-thalassemia minor?

Harrison's 20th Ed. Chapter 94 Page 696

A. α-thalassemia-1 trait
B. α-thalassemia-2 trait
C. HbH disease
D. Hydrops fetalis with Hb Bart's

α-thalassemia-1 trait resembles β-thalassemia minor. α-thalassemia-2 trait is an asymptomatic, silent carrier state.

434. Hb Barts is designated as?

Harrison's 20th Ed. Chapter 94 Page 696

A. $\alpha 4$
B. $\beta 4$
C. $\gamma 4$
D. $\delta 4$

Hb Barts is designated as $\gamma 4$

435. Which of the following is not a feature of thalassemia?

Harrison's 20th Ed. Chapter 94 Page 696

A. Avascular necrosis
B. Osteomalacia
C. Osteopenia
D. Microfractures

Avascular necrosis is not a feature of thalassemia because there is no sickling of red cells leading to thrombosis and infarction.

436. Which of the following joints is most frequently involved in beta thalassemia?

Harrison's 20th Ed. Chapter 367 Page 2641

A. Ankles
B. Knees
C. Hips
D. Shoulders

In patients with beta thalassemia, symmetric ankle arthropathy occurs frequently, characterized by a dull aching pain aggravated by weight bearing. Onset is in the second or third decade of life.

437. Which of the following has been reported in thalassemia?

Harrison's 20th Ed. Chapter 410 Page 3003

A. Orotic Aciduria
B. Myoadenylate Deaminase Deficiency
C. Adenylosuccinate Lyase Deficiency
D. Acquired pyrimidine 5'-nucleotidase deficiency

Acquired pyrimidine 5'-nucleotidase deficiency has been reported in lead poisoning and in thalassemia.

438. In sickle cell disease, presence of palpable spleen after what age suggests a coexisting thalassemia?

Harrison's 20th Ed. Chapter 62 Page 417

A. 5 years
B. 10 years
C. 15 years
D. 20 years

Presence of a palpable spleen in sickle cell disease after age 5 years suggests a coexisting hemoglobinopathy like thalassemia.

439. Which of the following is a cause of microcytic erythrocytosis?

Harrison's 20th Ed. Chapter 99 Page 734

A. β-Thalassemia trait
B. Hypoxic erythrocytosis
C. Polycythemia vera (PV)
D. All of the above

Only 3 conditions cause microcytic erythrocytosis – β-thalassemia trait, hypoxic erythrocytosis & PV. RDW is normal in beta-thalassemia, while it is elevated in hypoxic erythrocytosis & PV.

440. Target cells in PBF can be seen in which of the following conditions?

Harrison's 20th Ed. Chapter 94 Page Figure 94-13

A. Thalassemia
B. Iron deficiency
C. Cholestatic liver disease
D. All of the above

Target cells (area of central pallor with dense center or bull's eye) is typical of thalassemia, but can be seen in iron deficiency, cholestatic liver disease or as an artifact. Larger numbers are typical of hemoglobin C disease.

441. Geographic distributions of which of the following closely resemble that of falciparum malaria?

Harrison's 20th Ed. Chapter 219 Page 1577

A. Sickle cell disease
B. Thalassemia
C. Glucose-6-phosphate dehydrogenase (G6PD) deficiency
D. All of the above

Geographic distributions of sickle cell disease, hemoglobins C and E, hereditary ovalocytosis, thalassemia, and glucose-6-phosphate dehydrogenase (G6PD) deficiency closely resemble that of falciparum malaria

442. Which of the following is normal or increased in thalassemia?

Harrison's 20th Ed. Chapter 94 Page 696

A. Serum iron level
B. Transferrin saturation
C. Serum ferritin level
D. All of the above

Normal or increased serum iron & ferritin levels and transferrin saturation are characteristic of the thalassemias. Red blood cell distribution width (RDW) index is generally normal in thalassemia.

443. Cooley's anemia refers to?

Harrison's 20th Ed. Chapter 94 Page 696

A. Beta thalassemia minor
B. Beta thalassemia intermedia
C. Beta thalassemia major
D. Any of the above

In β-thalassemia, the β globin chains are structurally normal but quantitatively reduced.

444. Variant hemoglobins that may be co-inherited with β-thalassemia are?

Harrison's 20th Ed. Chapter 94 Page 697

A. Hemoglobin S
B. Hemoglobin E
C. Hemoglobin C
D. All of the above

Variant hemoglobins that may be co-inherited with β-thalassemia are Hemoglobin S, Hemoglobin E and Hemoglobin C.

445. Which of the following is referred to as a "thalassemic hemoglobinopathy"?

Am J Pathol. 1983;113(3):396-409

A. Hemoglobin S
B. Hemoglobin E
C. Hemoglobin C
D. All of the above

Hemoglobin E is referred to as a "thalassemic hemoglobinopathy" because in addition to being structurally abnormal it is produced in reduced quantities. Patient who inherits a HbE mutation from one parent and a β-thalassemia mutation from another (HbE/β-thalassemia) will clinically be similar to a patient with β-thalassemia intermedia or major.

446. Features of thalassemia include all except?

N Engl J Med 2005;353:1135-46

A. Hypopituitarism
B. Hypogonadism
C. Hypoparathyroidism
D. Diabetes insipidus

447. Features of thalassemia include all except?

N Engl J Med 2005;353:1135-46

A. Cardiomyopathy
B. Excessive melanin skin pigmentation
C. Pulmonary fibrosis
D. Diabetes mellitus

448. Which of the following about Hepcidin is false?

N Engl J Med 2005;353:1135-46

A. Inhibits iron absorption in small bowel
B. Levels increase when iron stores are elevated
C. Levels are high in patients with thalassemia major
D. Also called "Storage iron regulator"

Hepcidin is a small peptide that inhibits iron absorption in small bowel. Hepcidin levels normally increase when iron stores are elevated. Hepcidin levels are inappropriately low in thalassemia intermedia & thalassemia major.

449. Which of the following findings rules out thalassemia and no additional thalassemia testing is required?

Harrison's 20th Ed. Chapter 94 Page 697

A. MCV > 80 fL, MCH > 27 pg, normal Hb electrophoresis
B. MCV > 90 fL, MCH > 27 pg, normal Hb electrophoresis
C. MCV > 100 fL, MCH > 27 pg, normal Hb electrophoresis
D. MCV > 110 fL, MCH > 27 pg, normal Hb electrophoresis

The finding of a normal MCV (>= 80 fL) with normal MCH (>= 27 pg) and normal Hb electrophoresis or HPLC rules out most cases of thalassemia and requires no additional thalassemia testing.

450. Patients with β-thalassemia trait have an elevated HbA2 of?
Harrison's 20th Ed. Chapter 94 Page 697

A. > 0.5%
B. > 1.5%
C. > 2.5%
D. > 3.5%

Patients with β-thalassemia trait have an elevated HbA2 of > 3.5%.

451. Which of the following is not applicable for estimating iron overload in thalassemia patients? *N Engl J Med 2005;353:1135-46*

A. Serum ferritin
B. Magnetic susceptometry (SQUID)
C. Labile plasma iron estimation
D. CT of liver

452. A unit (250–300 mL) of packed RBCs contains how much iron?
Harrison's 20th Ed. Chapter 94 Page 697

A. 50 – 100 mg
B. 100 – 150 mg
C. 150 – 250 mg
D. 250 – 300 mg

A unit (250–300 mL) of packed RBCs contains 250–300 mg of iron (1 mg/mL).

453. Patients develop hemosiderosis after how many units of packed RBCs? *Harrison's 20th Ed. Chapter 94 Page 698*

A. > 50 units
B. > 100 units
C. > 200 units
D. > 500 units

Patients who receive >100 units of packed RBCs usually develop hemosiderosis.

454. Which of the following is an not an oral iron-chelating agent?
N Engl J Med 2005;353:1135-46

A. Deferoxamine
B. Deferiprone
C. Deferasirox
D. None of the above

Deferoxamine is iron-chelating agent & requires parenteral administration.

455. Which of the following promotes high levels of HbF synthesis?
Harrison's 20th Ed. Chapter 94 Page 698

A. Hydroxyurea
B. Butyrates
C. Cytarabine
D. All of the above

Reestablishing high levels of HbF synthesis can ameliorate symptoms of thalassemia. Hydroxyurea & cytarabine promote high levels of HbF synthesis by stimulating proliferation of F cell progenitors. Butyrates also stimulate HbF production.

456. Lucarelli classification is used to classify?
N Engl J Med 2005;353:1135-46

A. Porphyria
B. Hemolytic anemia
C. Thalassemia
D. Anemia

Lucarelli classification assess risk factors that predict outcome & prognosis in thalassemia.

457. Which of the following should be avoided in an iron excess state? *Harrison's 20th Ed. Chapter 94 Page 698*

A. Vitamin C
B. Vitamin E
C. Folic acid
D. Plant flavonoids

Vitamin C should not be supplemented in iron excess states because it generates free radicals.

458. Heinz bodies is best related to?
N Engl J Med 2005;353:1135-46

A. Precipitates of unpaired β globin chains
B. Precipitates of unpaired α globin chains
C. Precipitates of unpaired α & β globin chains
D. Any of the above

Precipitates of unpaired β chains form single large inclusions known as Heinz bodies.

459. Which parameter in fetal ultrasound is used to assess risk of hemoglobin Bart's hydrops fetalis?
N Engl J Med 2005;353:1135-46

A. Abdominal circumference
B. Nuchal translucency
C. Cardiothoracic ratio
D. Ventricular system of fetal brain

Cardiothoracic ratio in fetal ultrasound is used to assess risk of hemoglobin Bart's hydrops fetalis (normal < 0.53).

460. Estimated 5-year survival rate following allogeneic bone marrow transplantation is?
Harrison's 20th Ed. Chapter 110 Page 821

A. 30%
B. 50%
C. 70%
D. 90%

Estimated 5-year survival rate following allogeneic bone marrow transplantation is 90% if done before they develop hepatomegaly or portal fibrosis and if given adequate iron chelation therapy.

461. Best outcomes of marrow transplantation in patients with thalassemia major is expected before they develop?
Harrison's 20th Ed. Chapter 110 Page 821

A. Skeletal deformities
B. Cardiomegaly
C. Portal fibrosis
D. Splenomegaly

Although prolonged survival can be achieved with aggressive chelation therapy, transplantation is the only curative treatment for thalassemia. Marrow transplantation from an HLA-identical sibling with preparative busulfan & cyclophosphamide can cure 80-90% of patients with thalassemia major. Best outcomes are expected before patients develop hepatomegaly or portal fibrosis.

462. Aplastic crises in patients with hemoglobinopathies is caused by infection with?
Harrison's 20th Ed. Chapter 94 Page 698

A. Parvovirus B I9A
B. Epstein-Barr virus
C. Human herpes virus 6
D. All of the above

Aplastic crises in hemolytic anemias and some PRCAs is caused by infection with parvovirus - B I9A.

Megaloblastic Anemias

463. Element found at the center of corrin ring in cobalamin is?
Harrison's 20th Ed. Chapter 95 Page 699

A. Copper
B. Cadmium
C. Cobalt
D. Calcium

All forms of Cobalamin (vit. B12) have a cobalt atom at the center of corrin ring.

464. Which of the following form of cobalamin is located in mitochondria?
Harrison's 20th Ed. Chapter 95 Page 699

A. Methylcobalamin
B. 2-deoxyadenosyl (ado)
C. Hydroxocobalamin
D. All of the above

In nature, cobalamin is mainly in 2-deoxyadenosyl (ado) form which is located in mitochondria.

465. 2-deoxyadenosyl (ado) form of cobalamin is a cofactor for which enzyme?
Harrison's 20th Ed. Chapter 95 Page 699

A. Methionine synthase
B. Methylmalonyl coenzyme A (CoA) mutase
C. Cystathionine synthase
D. Serine - glycine hydroxymethylase

2-deoxyadenosyl (ado) form is the cofactor for enzyme methylmalonyl coenzyme A (CoA) mutase.

466. Which form of cobalamin is present in human plasma & in cell cytoplasm?
Harrison's 20th Ed. Chapter 95 Page 699

A. Cobalamin
B. Methylcobalamin
C. Hydroxocobalamin
D. Adocobalamin

Cobalamin (vitamin B12) exists in a number of different chemical forms. Methylcobalamin is the form of cobalamin in human plasma & in cell cytoplasm.

467. Methylcobalamin is the cofactor for?
Harrison's 20th Ed. Chapter 95 Page 699

A. Cystathionine synthase
B. Methionine synthase
C. Serine - glycine hydroxymethylase
D. All of the above

Methylcobalamin is the cofactor for methionine synthase. Vitamin B12 is a cofactor for only two enzymes: methionine synthase and L-methylmalonyl–coenzyme A mutase.

468. Which of the following about cobalamin is false?
Harrison's 20th Ed. Chapter 95 Page 699

A. Copper atom is situated within a corrin ring
B. Cannot be synthesized in human body
C. Only dietary source is animal products
D. Daily requirement is ~ 1 - 3 μg

Cobalamin is a complex organometallic compound in which a "cobalt" atom is situated within a corrin ring. It cannot be synthesized in human body & must be supplied in diet of animal products (meat, fish, and dairy products). Daily requirement for cobalamin is ~ 1 - 3 μg.

469. Body stores of cobalamin can suffice for how many years after supplies are completely cut off?
Harrison's 20th Ed. Chapter 95 Page 699

A. 1 to 2 years
B. 2 to 3 years
C. 3 to 4 years
D. 5 to 7 years

Body stores of 2 - 3 mg are sufficient for 3 - 4 years if supplies are completely cut off essentially due to enterohepatic cycle & size of liver stores. There is a permanent liver reserve of 1 mg.

470. Normal active physiologic mechanism of cobalamin absorption occurs in?
Harrison's 20th Ed. Chapter 95 Page 699

A. Buccal mucosa
B. Duodenal mucosa
C. Ileal mucosa
D. All of the above

Cobalamin absorption can be passive through buccal, duodenal & ileal mucosa. More efficient normal physiologic active mechanism is through ileum mediated by gastric intrinsic factor (IF).

471. Which of the following is a family of cobalamin-binding proteins?
Harrison's 20th Ed. Chapter 95 Page 699

A. Glucocorrins
B. Enterocorrins
C. Haptocorrins
D. All of the above

Dietary cobalamin combines rapidly with a salivary glycoprotein that belongs to the family of cobalamin-binding proteins known as haptocorrins (HCs).

472. In intestine, haptocorrin is digested by which of the following enzyme?
Harrison's 20th Ed. Chapter 95 Page 699

A. Pancreatic trypsin
B. Pancreatic amylase
C. Pancreatic lipase
D. Pancreatic colipase

In intestine, haptocorrin is digested by pancreatic trypsin to release cobalamin which is transferred to IF.

473. Intrinsic factor (IF) is produced in?
Harrison's 20th Ed. Chapter 95 Page 699

A. Gastric parietal cells
B. Gastric chief cells
C. Gastric endocrine cells
D. Gastric enterochromaffin cells

IF is produced in the acid-secreting gastric parietal cells located in oxyntic gland of fundus & body of stomach.

474. Gene for IF is on which chromosome?

Harrison's 20th Ed. Chapter 95 Page 699

A. 6
B. 8
C. 9
D. 11

Gene for IF is on chromosome II q13.

475. Secretion of gastric intrinsic factor (IF) parallels that of?

Harrison's 20th Ed. Chapter 95 Page 699

A. Gastrin
B. Potassium
C. Hydrochloric acid
D. Bicarbonate

Secretion of gastric intrinsic factor (IF) parallels that of hydrochloric acid.

476. Name of the receptor that mediates intestinal absorption of cobalamin-IF complex is?

Harrison's 20th Ed. Chapter 95 Page 699

A. Spirulin
B. Humulin
C. Cubulin
D. Cobalin

Cubilin is a specific receptor on microvillus membrane of enterocytes. IF-cobalamin attaches to it and enters the ileal cell, where IF is destroyed..

477. Endocytic receptor protein related to cubulin is?

Harrison's 20th Ed. Chapter 95 Page 699

A. Amnionless (AMN)
B. Leptin receptor
C. Asialo-GM1
D. Glycophorin A

Cubulin acts through amnionless (AMN), an endocytic receptor protein that directs sublocalization and endocytosis of cubulin with its ligand IF-cobalamin complex.

478. Cubilin also is present in?

Harrison's 20th Ed. Chapter 95 Page 699

A. Cardiomyocyte
B. Renal proximal tubular epithelium
C. Islet of Langerhans
D. All of the above

Cubilin also is present in yolk sac and renal proximal tubular epithelium.

479. Gastric R binder is found in which of the following secretions?

Am J Gastroenterol. 1985;80(11):841-52

A. Saliva
B. Gastric juice
C. Bile
D. All of the above

Cobalamin in food is released and forms a stable complex with gastric R binder that is found in secretions like saliva, milk, gastric juice and bile.

480. Intrinsic factor (IF) catalyzes the conversion?

Am J Gastroenterol. 1985;80(11):841-52

A. Methionine to homocysteine
B. Homocysteine to methionine
C. Serine to glycine
D. Glycine to serine

On entering the duodenum, the cobalamin-R binder complex is digested, releasing the cobalamin, which then binds to intrinsic factor (IF), a 50-kDa glycoprotein which catalyzes the conversion of homocysteine to methionine.

481. Most circulating cobalamin is bound to?

Harrison's 20th Ed. Chapter 95 Page 699

A. Gastric R binder
B. Transcobalamin (TC) I
C. Transcobalamin (TC) II
D. Intrinsic factor (IF)

TC I is derived from specific granules in neutrophils. Normally, it is ~ two-thirds saturated with cobalamin, which it binds tightly. TC I does not enhance cobalamin entry into tissues.

482. Which of the following is not related to "absorption" of cobalamin in humans?

Harrison's 20th Ed. Chapter 95 Page 699

A. Gastric R binder
B. Intrinsic factor (IF)
C. Transcobalamin (TC) I
D. Transcobalamin (TC) II

Two main cobalamin transport proteins in human plasma are TC I & TC II. TC II carries cobalamin in plasma & gives up cobalamin to marrow, placenta, and other tissues.

483. Cobalamin-binding haptocorrin - TC I is derived primarily from?

Harrison's 20th Ed. Chapter 95 Page 699

A. Saliva
B. Reticuloendothelial cells
C. Liver
D. Neutrophils

Cobalamin-binding haptocorrin - TC I is derived primarily from the specific granules in neutrophils.

484. The gene for cobalamin-binding haptocorrin - TC I is?

Harrison's 20th Ed. Chapter 95 Page 699

A. TSC2
B. TCNL
C. PTCH-1
D. MGMT

The gene for cobalamin-binding haptocorrin - TC I is TCNL at chromosome 11q11-q12.3.

485. TC II is synthesized by?

Harrison's 20th Ed. Chapter 95 Page 699

A. Saliva
B. Reticuloendothelial cells
C. Liver
D. Neutrophils

TC II is synthesized by liver, macrophages, ileum and vascular endothelium.

486. The common name for pteroylmonoglutamic acid is?
Harrison's 20th Ed. Chapter 95 Page 699

A. Folic acid
B. Vitamin B12
C. Ascorbic acid
D. Pyridoxine

Folic acid is the common name for pteroylmonoglutamic acid.

487. Which of the following is primary dietary source of folic acid?
Harrison's 20th Ed. Chapter 95 Page 699

A. Fruits and vegetables
B. Eggs
C. Milk
D. Meat

Fruits and vegetables are the primary dietary source of folic acid. Folate concentrations is highest in liver, yeast, spinach, other greens, and nuts.

488. Which of the following is the major body store of folic acid?
Harrison's 20th Ed. Chapter 95 Page 699

A. Liver
B. Bone marrow
C. Spleen
D. Kidney

Total-body folate in the adult is ~10 mg, liver containing the largest store.

489. Normally, minimum daily requirement of folic acid is about?
Harrison's 20th Ed. Chapter 95 Page 699

A. 100 μg
B. 200 μg
C. 300 μg
D. 400 μg

Daily requirement is normally about 100 μg, but this may be increased several fold during periods of enhanced metabolic demand such as pregnancy, infancy, malignancy, increased hematopoiesis (chronic hemolytic anemias), chronic exfoliative skin disorders, hemodialysis.

490. Body stores of folate can suffice for how many months after supplies are completely cut off?
Harrison's 20th Ed. Chapter 95 Page 699

A. 1 to 2 months
B. 2 to 3 months
C. 3 to 4 months
D. 5 to 7 months

Total-body folate in adult is ~10 mg. Daily adult requirement is ~100 μg, so stores are sufficient for 3 - 4 months, if severe folate deficiency develops rapidly.

491. Site of absorption of Folic acid is?
Harrison's 20th Ed. Chapter 95 Page 699

A. Stomach
B. Proximal jejunum
C. Terminal Ileum
D. Colon

Folates in food are largely conjugated to a chain of glutamic acid residues which impair its intestinal absorption. Conjugases (g-glutamyl carboxypeptidases) in gut lumen convert polyglutamates to mono- & diglutamates, which are readily absorbed in proximal jejunum.

492. All dietary folates are converted to which of the following before entering portal plasma?
Harrison's 20th Ed. Chapter 95 Page 699

A. N5-methyltetrahydrofolate
B. N10-methyltetrahydrofolate
C. N15-methyltetrahydrofolate
D. N20-methyltetrahydrofolate

Plasma folate is primarily in the form of N5-methyltetrahydrofolate. All dietary folates are converted to 5-methyl THF (5-MTHF) within small-intestinal mucosa before entering portal plasma.

493. N5-methyltetrahydrofolate is a type of?
Harrison's 20th Ed. Chapter 95 Page 699

A. Monoglutamate
B. Diglutamate
C. Triglutamate
D. Polyglutamate

N5-methyltetrahydrofolate is a monoglutamate.

494. Monoglutamates are actively transported across the enterocyte by?
Harrison's 20th Ed. Chapter 95 Page 699

A. SCFT
B. PCFT
C. CCFT
D. TCFT

Monoglutamates are actively transported across enterocyte by a proton-coupled folate transporter (PCFT, SCL46A1) situated at the apical brush border. Genetic mutations of this protein underlie hereditary malabsorption of folate.

495. Which of the following is related to transportation of folate?
Harrison's 20th Ed. Chapter 95 Page 700

A. RFC
B. FR2
C. FR3
D. All of the above

Folate is transported in plasma - ~one-third loosely bound to albumin and two-thirds unbound as 5-MTHF in monoglutamate form. Three types of folate-binding protein are involved. RFC & SLC19A1 deliver plasma folate (5-MTHF) to cells. Two folate receptors, FR2 & FR3 embedded in cell membrane by a glycosyl phosphatidylinositol anchor, transport folate into the cell via receptor mediated endocytosis. The third protein, PCFT transports folate at low pH from the vesicle to the cell cytoplasm.

496. The prime function of folate compounds is?
Harrison's 20th Ed. Chapter 95 Page 700

A. To transfer single-carbon moieties to organic compounds
B. Factor for methionine synthase & methylmalonyl coenzyme A (CoA) synthase
C. Conversion of methylmalonyl CoA to succinyl CoA
D. Conversion of succinyl CoA to methylmalonyl CoA

Primary function of folate compounds is to transfer single carbon moieties such as methyl and formyl groups to various organic compounds. The sources of these 1-carbon moieties is usually serine which reacts with tetrahydrofolate to produce glycine and N5,10 methylenetetrahydrofolate.

497. Which of the following drugs inhibit DHF reductase?
Harrison's 20th Ed. Chapter 95 Page 700

A. Methotrexate
B. Pyrimethamine
C. Trimethoprim
D. All of the above

5,10-methylene-THF is oxidized to DHF (dihydrofolate). Enzyme DHF reductase converts DHF to THF. Methotrexate, pyrimethamine, and trimethoprim inhibit DHF reductase that prevents formation of active THF coenzymes from DHF.

498. Gamma-glutamyl carboxypeptidases in gut lumen convert?
Harrison's 20th Ed. Chapter 95 Page 700

A. Polyglutamates to mono & diglutamates
B. Diglutamates to monoglutamates
C. Polysaccharides to mono and disaccharides
D. Disaccharides to monosaccharides

Conjugases (g-glutamyl carboxypeptidases) in the gut lumen convert polyglutamates to mono- and diglutamates, which are readily absorbed in the proximal jejunum.

499. Folate is essential for the de-novo synthesis of?
Harrison's 20th Ed. Chapter 95 Page 700

A. Purines
B. Deoxythymidylate monophosphate (dTMP)
C. Methionine
D. All of the above

Folate is essential for the de novo synthesis of purines, deoxythymidylate monophosphate (dTMP), and methionine, serving as an intermediate carrier of 1-carbon fragments used in the biosynthesis of these compounds.

500. Which of the following is universal methyl donor?
Harrison's 20th Ed. Chapter 95 Page 700

A. 5-Methyl tetrahydrofolate
B. 5,10-Methylene tetrahydrofolate
C. S-Adenosylhomocysteine (SAH)
D. S-adenosylmethionine (SAM)

Methionine, a product of methionine synthase reaction, is the precursor for S-adenosylmethionine (SAM), the universal methyl donor involved in > 100 methyltransferase reactions.

501. In deficiencies of either folate or cobalamin, there is failure to convert?
Harrison's 20th Ed. Chapter 95 Page 700

A. dUMP to dTMP
B. dTMP to dUMP
C. dUMP to dUTP
D. dUTP to dUMP

The common feature of all megaloblastic anemias is a defect in DNA synthesis that affects rapidly dividing cells in the bone marrow. In deficiencies of either folate or cobalamin, there is failure to convert deoxyuridine monophosphate (dUMP) to deoxythymidine monophosphate (dTMP), the precursor of dTTP because folate is needed as the coenzyme 5,10-methylene - THF polyglutamate for conversion of dUMP to dTMP.

502. Active form of folic acid is?
Harrison's 20th Ed. Chapter 95 Page 700

A. Dihydrofolate
B. Trihydrofolate
C. Tetrahydrofolate
D. Pentahydrofolate

Active form of folate is tetrahydrofolate (THF).

503. Folate coenzymes are essential in which of the following biochemical reactions?
Harrison's 20th Ed. Chapter 95 Page 700 Table 95–2

A. Purine synthesis
B. Pyrimidine synthesis
C. Serine - glycine interconversion
D. All of the above

Folate coenzymes are essential in formate activation, Purine synthesis (formation of glycinamide ribonucleotide and formylation of aminoimidazole carboxamide ribonucleotide (AICAR), Pyrimidine synthesis (Methylation of deoxyuridine monophosphate (dUMP) to thymidine monophosphate (dTMP), Amino acid interconversion (serine - glycine interconversion, homocysteine to methionine and forminoglutamic acid to glutamic acid in histidine catabolism).

504. Which of the following about megaloblastic anemias is false?
Harrison's 20th Ed. Chapter 95 Page 700

A. Caused by impaired DNA synthesis
B. Hematopoietic precursors & GI epithelial cells affected
C. Megaloblastic cells have increased DNA to RNA ratio
D. Ineffective erythropoiesis

Megaloblastic anemias are caused by impaired DNA synthesis in cells with rapid turnover like hematopoietic precursors & gastrointestinal epithelial cells. Cell division becomes sluggish but cytoplasmic development progresses normally, so megaloblastic cells tend to be large, with an increased ratio of RNA to DNA. Megaloblastic erythroid progenitors are destroyed in marrow whose cellularity is increased but production of RBC is decreased (ineffective erythropoiesis).

505. Which of the following is a cobalamin-requiring reaction?
Harrison's 20th Ed. Chapter 95 Page 700

A. Purines synthesis
B. Deoxythymidylate monophosphate (dTMP) synthesis
C. Methionine synthesis
D. All of the above

THF acquires 1-carbon fragment from serine which is converted to glycine. For purine synthesis, the 1-carbon fragment is first oxidized to the level of formic acid, then transferred to substrate. For methionine synthesis, a cobalamin-requiring reaction, the 1-carbon fragment is first reduced to the level of a methyl group, then transferred to homocysteine. In these reactions the cofactor is released as THF, which can immediately participate in another 1-carbon transfer cycle. During the production of dTMP from dUMP, the 1-carbon fragment is reduced from formaldehyde to a methyl group during transfer reaction. Hydrogen atoms used for this reduction come from the cofactor, which is released, not as THF, but as dihydrofolate (DHF). To participate further in the 1-carbon transfer cycle, DHF has to be re-reduced to THF, a reaction catalyzed by dihydrofolate reductase.

506. Methylmalonyl CoA isomerization requires which of the following?
Harrison's 20th Ed. Chapter 95 Page 700

A. Adocobalamin
B. Methylcobalamin
C. 5-MTHF
D. All of the above

Methylmalonyl CoA isomerization requires adocobalamin, and the methylation of homocysteine to methionine requires both methylcobalamin and 5-MTHF. An elevated level of methylmalonic acid is reasonably specific for vitamin B12 deficiency, and the level always decreases with vitamin B12 therapy.

507. Which of the following abnormalities of folate metabolism occur in cobalamin deficiency?

Harrison's 20th Ed. Chapter 95 Page 700

A. High serum folate
B. Low cell folate
C. Positive purine precursor aminoimidazole carboxamide ribonucleotide (AICAR) excretion
D. All of the above

Abnormalities of folate metabolism that occur in cobalamin deficiency include high serum folate, low cell folate and positive purine precursor aminoimidazole carboxamide ribonucleotide (AICAR) excretion.

508. Which of the following symptoms is marked in megaloblastic anemias?

Harrison's 20th Ed. Chapter 95 Page 700

A. Anorexia
B. Weight loss
C. Constipation
D. Diarrhea

Main clinical features of severe cases of megaloblastic anemias are those of anemia. Anorexia is usually marked. There may be weight loss, diarrhea or constipation, glossitis, angular cheilosis, a mild fever, unconjugated jaundice and reversible melanin skin hyperpigmentation.

509. In megaloblastic anemias, thrombocytopenia leading to bruising may be aggravated by?

Harrison's 20th Ed. Chapter 95 Page 700

A. Vitamin A deficiency
B. Vitamin C deficiency
C. Vitamin D deficiency
D. Vitamin K deficiency

Thrombocytopenia sometimes leads to bruising and this may be aggravated by vitamin C deficiency or alcohol in malnourished patients.

510. In megaloblastic anemias, anemia and low leukocyte count may predispose to?

Harrison's 20th Ed. Chapter 95 Page 700

A. Skin infection
B. Gastrointestinal tract infection
C. Urinary tract infection
D. All of the above

The anemia and low leukocyte count may predispose to infections particularly of the respiratory and urinary tracts. Cobalamin deficiency may impair bactericidal function of phagocytes.

511. Which of the following statements about megaloblastic anemia due to folate deficiency is true?

Harrison's 20th Ed. Chapter 95 Page 700

A. Raised serum methylmalonic acid, elevated homocysteine
B. Reduced serum methylmalonic acid, reduced homocysteine
C. Normal serum methylmalonic acid, reduced homocysteine
D. Normal serum methylmalonic acid, elevated homocysteine

512. Which of the following statements about megaloblastic anemia due to cobalamin deficiency is true?

Harrison's 20th Ed. Chapter 95 Page 700

A. Raised serum methylmalonic acid, elevated homocysteine
B. Reduced serum methylmalonic acid, reduced homocysteine
C. Raised serum methylmalonic acid, reduced homocysteine
D. Reduced serum methylmalonic acid, elevated homocysteine

513. Most frequently affected tissue in cobalamin and folate deficiencies is?

Harrison's 20th Ed. Chapter 95 Page 702

A. Epithelial cell surfaces of the mouth
B. Bone marrow
C. Peripheral nerves
D. Epithelial cell surfaces of the small intestine

Most frequently affected tissue in cobalamin and folate deficiencies is the bone marrow followed by the epithelial cell surfaces of the mouth, stomach, and small intestine and the respiratory, urinary, and female genital tracts.

514. Folate deficiency & cobalamin deficiency have been implicated in?

Harrison's 20th Ed. Chapter 95 Page 702

A. Infertility
B. Recurrent fetal loss
C. Neural tube defects
D. All of the above

Infertility is common in both men & women with folate deficiency & cobalamin deficiency. Maternal folate deficiency has been implicated as a cause of prematurity and both folate deficiency & cobalamin deficiency have been implicated in recurrent fetal loss & neural tube defects.

515. To prevent neural tube defects, folic acid supplements must be started at?

Harrison's 20th Ed. Chapter 95 Page 702

A. Conception
B. First 4 weeks of pregnancy
C. First 8 weeks of pregnancy
D. First 12 weeks of pregnancy

To prevent neural tube defects, folic acid supplements must be started at the time of conception and in the first 12 weeks of pregnancy. It reduces the incidence of neural tube defects (NTDs) (anencephaly, meningomyelocele, encephalocele, and spina bifida) in the fetus by 70%.

516. What dose of folic acid provides protective effect against Neural Tube Defects (NTDs) at conception?

Harrison's 20th Ed. Chapter 95 Page 702

A. 0.1 mg daily
B. 0.2 mg daily
C. 0.3 mg daily
D. 0.4 mg daily

0.4 mg daily of folic acid provides protective effect against NTDs at conception. Folic acid (400 μg daily, should be given as a supplement before and throughout pregnancy. In women who have had a previous fetus with a neural tube defect, 5 mg daily is recommended when pregnancy is contemplated and throughout the subsequent pregnancy.

517. In NTD fetuses, which of the following maternal folate metabolic abnormality has been identified?

Harrison's 20th Ed. Chapter 95 Page 702

A. Mutations in methionine synthase
B. Mutations in serine - glycine hydroxymethylase
C. Autoantibodies to folate receptors
D. Reduced activity of 5,10-methylene-THF reductase (MTHFR)

In NTD fetuses, reduced activity of the enzyme 5,10-methylene-THF reductase (MTHFR) caused by a common C677T polymorphism in the MTHFR gene has been identified as the maternal folate metabolic abnormality. Maternal TC II receptor polymorphisms are associated with increased risk of NTD births.

518. Incidence of which of the following can be reduced by prophylactic folic acid?

Harrison's 20th Ed. Chapter 95 Page 702

A. Cleft palate
B. Colour blindness
C. Pes cavus
D. Omphalocoele

The incidence of cleft palate and harelip also can be reduced by prophylactic folic acid.

519. Deficiency of which of the following enzymes can cause homocystinuria?

Harrison's 20th Ed. Chapter 95 Page 702

A. Methionine synthase
B. MTHFR
C. Cystathionine synthase
D. All of the above

Severe homocystinuria (≥100 μmol/L) may be due to deficiency of methionine synthase, MTHFR, or cystathionine synthase. Homocystinuria is a rare metabolic defect in the conversion of homocysteine to cystathionine. Folate deficiency is due to excessive utilization because of compensatory increased conversion of homocysteine to methionine.

520. Individuals with which of the following enzyme deficiency have an increased risk of vascular disease?

Harrison's 20th Ed. Chapter 95 Page 702

A. Methionine synthase
B. MHTFR
C. Cystathionine synthase
D. All of the above

Children with deficiency of enzyme methionine synthase, MHTFR or cystathionine synthase have an increased risk of vascular disease, ischemic heart disease, cerebrovascular disease or pulmonary embolus.

521. Meta-analysis has suggested that folic acid supplementation reduces the risk of stroke by?

Harrison's 20th Ed. Chapter 95 Page 702

A. 4%
B. 8%
C. 18%
D. 25%

Meta-analysis has suggested that folic acid supplementation reduces the risk of stroke by 18%.

522. Prophylactic folic acid in pregnancy reduces subsequent incidence of which of the following?

Harrison's 20th Ed. Chapter 95 Page 702

A. Acute lymphoblastic leukemia (ALL)
B. Hodgkin's lymphoma
C. Astrocytoma
D. Hemangioma

Prophylactic folic acid in pregnancy reduces the subsequent incidence of acute lymphoblastic leukemia (ALL) in childhood.

523. Clinical features of cobalamin deficiency involve which of the following?

Harrison's 20th Ed. Chapter 95 Page 702

A. Blood
B. Gastrointestinal tract
C. Nervous system
D. All of the above

The clinical features of cobalamin deficiency involve the blood, the gastrointestinal tract, and the nervous system.

524. Hematologic manifestations of cobalamin deficiency are due to?

Harrison's 20th Ed. Chapter 95 Page 700

A. Anemia
B. Leucopenia
C. Thrombocytopenia
D. All of the above

The hematologic manifestations are almost entirely the result of anemia, although very rarely purpura may appear, due to thrombocytopenia.

525. Which of the following pathological situations can be seen in cobalamin deficiency?

Harrison's 20th Ed. Chapter 95 Page 700

A. Demyelination
B. Axonal degeneration
C. Neuronal death
D. All of the above

Initial pathology is demyelination, followed by axonal degeneration & eventual neuronal death.

526. Involvement of which of the following structures is uncommon in cobalamin deficiency?

Harrison's 20th Ed. Chapter 95 Page 701

A. Peripheral nerves
B. Spinal cord
C. Cerebellum
D. Cerebrum

Cobalamin deficiency may cause a bilateral peripheral neuropathy or degeneration (demyelination) of posterior & pyramidal tracts of spinal cord & less frequently optic atrophy or cerebral symptoms.

527. Earliest neurologic manifestation of cobalamin deficiency is?

Harrison's 20th Ed. Chapter 95 Page 701

A. Numbness and paresthesia in extremities
B. Motor weakness
C. Ataxia
D. Sphincter disturbances

Signs and symptoms of cobalamin deficiency include numbness and paresthesia in the extremities (the earliest neurologic manifestations), weakness, and ataxia. There may be sphincter disturbances.

528. Cobalamin deficiency is diagnosed by?

Harrison's 20th Ed. Chapter 95 Page 706

A. Serum gastrin level
B. Tests for antibodies to IF or parietal cells
C. Serum methylmalonic acid (MMA) measurement
D. All of the above

529. What value of MCV is diagnostic of megaloblastic anemia?
Harrison's 20th Ed. Chapter 95 Page 702

A. > 70 fL
B. > 80 fL
C. > 90 fL
D. > 100 fL

Many symptomless patients are detected through the finding of a raised mean corpuscular volume (MCV) on a routine blood count. Significant & marked macrocytosis (MCV > 100 fL) suggests presence of a megaloblastic anemia. PBF shows marked anisocytosis & poikilocytosis, with oval macrocytes, which are large, oval, fully hemoglobinized erythrocytes typical of megaloblastic anemias. Macrocytosis is less marked with concurrent iron deficiency or thalassemia. Reticulocyte index is low, & leukocyte and platelet count may also be decreased, particularly in severely anemic patients.

530. Neutrophils with > 5 nuclear lobes is suggestive of?
Harrison's 20th Ed. Chapter 95 Page 702

A. Megaloblastic anemia
B. CML
C. AML
D. Multiple myeloma

Hypersegmented nuclei of neutrophils is a characteristic finding of megaloblastic anemia. A single cell with a nucleus of six lobes or more raises suspicion of a megaloblastic anemia.

531. Causes of macrocytosis include all except?
Harrison's 20th Ed. Chapter 95 Page 702

A. Hemolysis
B. Aplastic anemia
C. Liver disease
D. Hyperthyroidism

Macrocytosis occurs in hemolysis, liver disease, alcoholism, hypothyroidism & aplastic anemia.

532. Megaloblastoid morphologic picture of RBC series is seen in?
Harrison's 20th Ed. Chapter 95 Page 702

A. Hemolysis
B. Pernicious anemia
C. Myelodysplasia
D. All of the above

Myelodysplasia produces a distinct morphologic picture most apparent in orthochromatic normoblasts in which a megaloblastic nucleus is associated with severely hypochromic cytoplasm. This variant is called "megaloblastoid" meaning presence of both nuclear & cytoplasmic maturation defects. "Megaloblastoid" does not mean "mildly megaloblastic."

533. Megaloblastic anemia is seen in all except?
Harrison's 20th Ed. Chapter 95 Page 708

A. Hereditary TC I deficiency
B. TC II deficiency
C. Orotic aciduria
D. Imerslund-Gräsbeck disease

534. Which of the following is not a finding in bone marrow examination in folate or B12 deficiency megaloblastic anemia?
Harrison's 20th Ed. Chapter 95 Page 702

A. Hypercellularity
B. Increased myeloid/erythroid ratio
C. Nuclear-cytoplasmic asynchrony in RBC precursors
D. Fenestrated nuclear chromatin in RBC precursors

In B12 deficiency megaloblastic anemia, bone marrow is hypercellular with decreased myeloid/erythroid ratio & abundant stainable iron. RBC precursors are abnormally large & have nuclei that appear much less mature than would be expected from the development of cytoplasm (nuclear-cytoplasmic asynchrony). Nuclear chromatin is more dispersed & it condenses in a peculiar fenestrated pattern that is very characteristic of megaloblastic erythropoiesis. Abnormal mitoses may be seen. Granulocyte precursors are also affected appearing as giant bands and metamyelocytes. Megakaryocytes are decreased & show abnormal morphology.

535. Which of the following is a bone marrow examination finding in folate or B12 deficiency megaloblastic anemia?
Harrison's 20th Ed. Chapter 95 Page 702

A. Hypercellular marrow
B. Giant & abnormally shaped metamyelocytes
C. Enlarged hyperpolyploid megakaryocytes
D. All of the above

In megaloblastic anemia, the bone marrow is hypercellular with accumulation of primitive cells due to selective death by apoptosis of more mature forms (may mimic acute myeloid leukemia). Erythroblast nucleus maintains a primitive appearance despite maturation and hemoglobinization of cytoplasm. Cells are larger than normoblasts and an increased number of cells with eccentric lobulated nuclei or nuclear fragments may be present. Giant & abnormally shaped metamyelocytes and enlarged hyperpolyploid megakaryocytes are characteristic. In severe cases.

536. Which of the following provides evidence of ineffective erythropoiesis?
Harrison's 20th Ed. Chapter 95 Page 703

A. Reduced haptoglobins
B. Positive urine hemosiderin
C. Raised serum lactate dehydrogenase
D. All of the above

Raised urine urobilinogen, reduced haptoglobins and positive urine hemosiderin, and a raised serum lactate dehydrogenase provides evidence of ineffective erythropoiesis.

537. Deficiency of cobalamin is almost always due to?
Harrison's 20th Ed. Chapter 95 Page 703

A. Dietary deficiency
B. Malabsorption
C. Alcohol abuse
D. Specific congenital enzyme deficiencies

Dietary intake of cobalamin is more than adequate for body's requirements, except in complete vegetarians & their breast-fed infants. Deficiency of cobalamin is almost always due to malabsorption.

538. Incidence of pernicious anemia is increased in?
Harrison's 20th Ed. Chapter 95 Page 703

A. Graves' disease
B. Myxedema
C. Thyroiditis
D. All of the above

539. Incidence of pernicious anemia is increased in?
Harrison's 20th Ed. Chapter 95 Page 703

A. Addison's disease
B. Vitiligo
C. Hypoparathyroidism
D. All of the above

Incidence of pernicious anemia is increased in patients with other diseases of immunologic origin like Graves' disease, myxedema, thyroiditis, Addison's disease, vitiligo & hypoparathyroidism.

540. Which of the following about IF immunoglobulin G antibody is false?
Harrison's 20th Ed. Chapter 95 Page 704

A. Type I antibody prevents combination of IF & cobalamin
B. Type II antibody prevents attachment of IF to ileal mucosa
C. IF antibodies do not cross the placenta
D. Type I antibody occurs in sera of ~55% patients

Two types of IF immunoglobulin G antibody may be found in the sera of patients with PA. Type I or "blocking" antibody prevents combination of IF and cobalamin. Type II or the "binding" antibody prevents attachment of IF to ileal mucosa. Type I occurs in sera of ~55% of patients, and type II in 35%. IF antibodies cross the placenta and may cause temporary IF deficiency in a newborn infant. Patients with PA also show cell-mediated immunity to IF.

541. Which of the following about pernicious anemia is false?
Harrison's 20th Ed. Chapter 95 Page 704

A. Gastric atrophy does not affect antrum of stomach
B. 90% of patients have antiparietal cell antibody
C. ~80% of patients have anti-IF antibody in gastric juice
D. None of the above

~90% patients with PA have antiparietal cell antibody directed against gastric proton pump H+,K+-ATPase, while IF antibodies are detected in gastric juice in ~80%. In patients with gastric atrophy without pernicious anemia, parietal cell antibody is found in 50%, but anti-IF antibody is usually absent. Antiparietal cell antibody is found in 10 - 15% of random patient population.

542. Which of the following about pernicious anemia is false?
Harrison's 20th Ed. Chapter 95 Page 704

A. Hypergastrinemia
B. Pentagastrin-fast achlorhydria
C. Relatives have increased incidence of disease
D. It is uncommon in patients with agammaglobulinemia

PA is associated with hypogammaglobulinemia, with premature graying or blue eyes, and in persons of blood group A. Gastric output of hydrochloric acid, pepsin, and IF is severely reduced. Serum gastrin level is raised, and serum pepsinogen I levels are low.

543. Which of the following is false about pernicious anemia?
Harrison's 20th Ed. Chapter 95 Page 704

A. Rare under the age of 30 years
B. Average age of presentation is 60 years
C. Men more affected than women
D. Caused by the absence of IF

Pernicious anemia is the most common cause of cobalamin deficiency. It is caused by absence of IF, due to atrophy of gastric mucosa or autoimmune destruction of parietal cells. Ratio of incidence of PA in men and women among whites is 1:1.6. Average age of presentation is 60 (disease of elderly) & is rare < 30 years of age.

544. Which of the following about pernicious anemia is false?
Harrison's 20th Ed. Chapter 95 Page 704

A. Unusually common in agammaglobulinemia
B. Helicobacter pylori infection is infrequent
C. Gastric atrophy spares the antrum
D. None of the above

Pernicious anemia is unusually common in patients with agammaglobulinemia. Helicobacter pylori does not cause parietal cell destruction in pernicious anemia. Most characteristic finding in pernicious anemia is gastric atrophy affecting the acid- and pepsin-secreting portion of the stomach while sparing the antrum.

545. Which of the following about pernicious anemia is false?
Harrison's 20th Ed. Chapter 95 Page 704

A. Gastric epithelium atypia common
B. Hypergastrinemia common
C. Gastric polyps common
D. None of the above

Abnormalities in gastric epithelium appear as cellular atypia that must be distinguished from cytologic abnormalities of gastric malignancy. Hypergastrinemia & pentagastrin-fast achlorhydria occur secondary to gastric atrophy. Incidence of gastric polyps & stomach cancer is increased.

546. Which of the following about juvenile pernicious anemia is false?
Harrison's 20th Ed. Chapter 95 Page 704

A. Gastric atrophy
B. Achlorhydria
C. Serum IF antibodies present
D. Parietal cell antibodies present

In Juvenile PA, gastric atrophy, achlorhydria and serum IF antibodies are present, but parietal cell antibodies are usually absent.

547. Which of the following is not a feature of congenital IF deficiency?
Harrison's 20th Ed. Chapter 95 Page 704

A. Autosomal dominant inheritance
B. Normal gastric mucosa
C. Normal gastric secretion of acid
D. Parietal cell & IF antibodies are absent

The inheritance is autosomal recessive in congenital IF deficiency.

548. Removal of what length of terminal ileum causes malabsorption of cobalamin?
Harrison's 20th Ed. Chapter 95 Page 704

A. 0.2 meter
B. 0.5 meter
C. 0.8 meter
D. 1.2 meter

Removal of 1.2 meters of terminal ileum causes malabsorption of cobalamin.

549. Disease due to mutation in cubulin receptor leading to selective defect in cobalamin absorption is?
Harrison's 20th Ed. Chapter 95 Page 704

A. Stickler syndrome
B. Imerslund-Gräsbeck syndrome
C. Cogan's syndrome
D. Menkes' syndrome

Imerslund-Gräsbeck syndrome is a congenital disorder (autosomal recessive) of selective defect in cobalamin absorption accompanied by nonspecific proteinuria but renal functions are normal. Mutation occurs in cubulin receptor that mediates intestinal absorption of cobalamin-IF complex. Patients have normal amounts of IF & gastric acid as are other tests of intestinal absorption.

550. Combined deficiencies of cobalamin and folic acid is seen in which of the following conditions?
Harrison's 20th Ed. Chapter 95 Page 704

A. Gastric achlorhydria
B. Tropical sprue
C. Regional enteritis
D. Pregnancy

Combined deficiencies of cobalamin & folic acid is seen in tropical sprue. Gastric achlorhydria produces cobalamin deficiency by malabsorption due to defective release of cobalamin from food. Regional enteritis produces cobalamin deficiency by malabsorption due to terminal ileum malfunctioning. Pregnancy produces folate deficiency due to increased requirements.

551. Fish tapeworm - D. latum causes megaloblastic anemia due to?
Harrison's 20th Ed. Chapter 95 Page 705

A. Defective release of cobalamin from food
B. Inadequate production of intrinsic factor (IF)
C. Competition for cobalamin
D. Intestinal stasis

Megaloblastic anemia or cobalamin neuropathy is seen in persons heavily infested by fish tapeworm, Diphyllobothrium latum, due to competition by the worm for cobalamin. Individuals acquire the worm by eating raw or partly cooked fish. Destruction of the worm eliminates the problem.

552. Infestations by fish tapeworm "Diphyllobothrium latum" is common in which of the following countries?
Harrison's 20th Ed. Chapter 95 Page 705

A. South East Asia
B. Scandinavia
C. South Africa
D. South America

Individuals acquire fish tapeworm, Diphyllobothrium latum by eating raw or partly cooked fish. Infestation is common around the lakes of Scandinavia, Germany, Japan, North America & Russia.

553. In severe chronic pancreatitis, concentration of which of the following in ileum falls below the level needed to maintain normal cobalamin absorption?
Harrison's 20th Ed. Chapter 95 Page 705

A. Iron
B. Magnesium
C. Calcium
D. Zinc

In severe chronic pancreatitis and in Zollinger-Ellison syndrome, lack of trypsin causes dietary cobalamin attached to gastric non-IF (R) binder to be unavailable for absorption. Also, in pancreatitis, concentration of calcium ions in the ileum falls below the level needed to maintain normal cobalamin absorption.

554. Acute megaloblastic anemia can be seen after?
Harrison's 20th Ed. Chapter 95 Page 705

A. Nitrous oxide anesthesia
B. Halothane anesthesia
C. Chloroform anesthesia
D. Ether anesthesia

Nitrous oxide irreversibly oxidizes methylcobalamin to an inactive precursor which inactivates methionine synthase.

555. Malabsorption of folate is seen with which of the following drugs?
Harrison's 20th Ed. Chapter 95 Page 706

A. Salazopyrine
B. Cholestyramine
C. Triamterene
D. All of the above

Malabsorption of folate occurs in patients receiving salazopyrine, cholestyramine & triamterene. Antifolate drugs include anticonvulsant drugs (phenytoin, primidone, barbiturates), sulphasalazine, Nitrofurantoin, and tetracycline.

556. Neonatal folate level falls rapidly to the lowest values at?
Harrison's 20th Ed. Chapter 95 Page 706

A. 6 weeks of age
B. 12 weeks of age
C. 24 weeks of age
D. 32 weeks of age

Neonatal folate level falls rapidly to the lowest values at about 6 weeks of age.

557. Folic acid deficiency is due to?
Harrison's 20th Ed. Chapter 95 Page 706

A. Inadequate intake
B. Increased demand
C. Malabsorption
D. All of the above

558. Conditions that increase demand of folic acid are all except?
Harrison's 20th Ed. Chapter 95 Page 706

A. Chronic hemolytic anemias
B. Pregnancy
C. Hemodialysis
D. Tropical sprue

The mechanism of folic acid deficiency in tropical sprue is malabsorption. Rest of the above conditions lead to increased folic acid requirements and cause megaloblastic anemia.

559. Folate deficiency frequently occurs in which of the following?
Harrison's 20th Ed. Chapter 95 Page 706

A. Sickle cell disease
B. Autoimmune hemolytic anemia
C. Congenital spherocytosis
D. All of the above

Folate deficiency frequently occurs in chronic hemolytic anemia, particularly in sickle cell disease, autoimmune hemolytic anemia, and congenital spherocytosis.

560. Alcohol causes folic acid deficiency by which of the following mechnism?
Harrison's 20th Ed. Chapter 95 Page 706

A. Inadequate intake
B. Increased requirements
C. Malabsorption
D. Impaired metabolism

Alcohol interferes with folate metabolism. Distilled spirits are devoid of folic acid, while beer and wine do not contain enough of vitamin for daily requirement.

561. Which of the following drugs is an inhibitor of dihydrofolate reductase?

Harrison's 20th Ed. Chapter 95 Page 706

A. Zidovudine
B. Methotrexate
C. Azathioprine
D. All of the above

562. Which of the following drugs is an inhibitor of dihydrofolate reductase?

Harrison's 20th Ed. Chapter 95 Page 706

A. Methotrexate
B. Trimethoprim
C. Pyrimethamine
D. All of the above

Drugs that inhibit DHF reductase include methotrexate, pyrimethamine & trimethoprim. Methotrexate has the most powerful action against the human enzyme, whereas trimethoprim is most active against the bacterial enzyme and is only likely to cause megaloblastic anemia when used in conjunction with sulphamethoxazole in patients with preexisting folate or cobalamin deficiency. The activity of pyrimethamine is intermediate.

563. In megaloblastic anemia due to folate antagonists, which of the following is given?

Harrison's 20th Ed. Chapter 95 Page 706

A. Folic acid
B. Folinic acid
C. Pyridoxine
D. All of the above

Megaloblastic anemia due to folate antagonists that inhibit dihydrofolate reductase can be counteracted by folinic acid [5-formyl tetrahydrofolate (THF)] in a dose of 100 to 200 mg/day, which circumvents the block in folate metabolism by providing a form of folate that can be converted to 5,10-methylene THF. For the megaloblastic forms of sideroblastic anemia, pyridoxine in pharmacologic doses (~300 mg/day) can be tried. Folinic Acid (5-Formyl-THF) is a stable form of fully reduced folate. It is given orally or parenterally to overcome the toxic effects of methotrexate or other DHF reductase inhibitors.

564. The normal range of cobalamin in serum is?

Harrison's 20th Ed. Chapter 95 Page 706

A. 5 to 50 ng/L
B. 60 to 100 ng/L
C. 160 to 1000 ng/L
D. 1200 to 1400 ng/L

The normal range of serum cobalamin in serum is 160–200 ng/L. Values between 100 & 200 ng/L are regarded as borderline.

565. Levels of which of the following is raised in patients with cobalamin deficiency?

Harrison's 20th Ed. Chapter 95 Page 706

A. Calcium
B. Iron
C. Serum methylmalonate (MMA)
D. Glycine

In patients with cobalamin deficiency sufficient to cause anemia or neuropathy, serum methylmalonate (MMA) level is raised.

566. Serum homocysteine is raised in all except?

Harrison's 20th Ed. Chapter 95 Page 706

A. Chronic renal disease
B. Hyperthyroidism
C. Alcoholism
D. Pyridoxine deficiency

Serum homocysteine is raised in early cobalamin & folate deficiency, CKD, alcoholism, smoking, pyridoxine deficiency, hypothyroidism, steroid & cyclosporine therapy. Levels are higher in serum than in plasma, in men than in premenopausal women, in women taking HRT or oral contraceptives. Homocysteine levels are not used for diagnosis of cobalamin or folate deficiency.

567. Normal serum folic acid levels are?

Harrison's 20th Ed. Chapter 95 Page 706

A. 6 to 20 ng/mL
B. 30 to 40 ng/mL
C. 60 to 80 ng/mL
D. 80 to 100 ng/mL

568. Normal range of serum folate is?

Harrison's 20th Ed. Chapter 95 Page 706

A. 2 to 15 μg/L
B. 12 to 25 μg/L
C. 25 to 45 μg/L
D. 42 to 75 μg/L

Normal range of serum folate is 2 to 15 μg/L.

569. Serum folate rises in?

Harrison's 20th Ed. Chapter 95 Page 707

A. Severe cobalamin deficiency
B. Intestinal stagnant loop syndrome
C. In newborn infant
D. All of the above

Serum folate rises in severe cobalamin deficiency because of the block in conversion of MTHF to THF inside cells. Raised levels are also seen in intestinal stagnant loop syndrome due to absorption of bacterially synthesized folate. A newborn infant, whether full term or premature, has higher serum and red cell folate concentrations than does an adult.

570. Serum folate level is affected by?

Harrison's 20th Ed. Chapter 95 Page 707

A. Sleep
B. Exercise
C. Recent diet
D. All of the above

Serum folate level reflects recent diet. Red cell folate assay is less affected than the serum assay by recent diet and traces of hemolysis.

571. In normal adults, red cell folate levels are?

Harrison's 20th Ed. Chapter 95 Page 707

A. 160 – 640 μg/L
B. 600 – 940 μg/L
C. 1080 – 1640 μg/L
D. 1650 – 2640 μg/L

In normal adults, red cell folate concentrations range from 160 - 640 μg/L of packed red cells.

572. In folate deficiency due to drugs inhibiting dihydrofolate reductase, tissue folate concentrations are?

Harrison's 20th Ed. Chapter 95 Page 707

A. Normal
B. Elevated
C. Reduced
D. Any of the above

Various drugs can inhibit dihydrofolate reductase thereby producing folate deficiency. However, tissue folate concentrations remain normal.

573. What value of folic acid is diagnostic of folate deficiency?

Harrison's 20th Ed. Chapter 95 Page 707

A. ≤ 1 ng/mL
B. ≤ 2 ng/mL
C. ≤ 3 ng/mL
D. ≤ 4 ng/mL

574. Which is a better index of folate stores?

Harrison's 20th Ed. Chapter 95 Page 707

A. Serum folate level
B. RBC folate level
C. WBC folate level
D. Platelet folate level

Normal serum folic acid ranges from 6 to 20 ng/mL. Values ≤4 ng/mL are considered diagnostic of folate deficiency. Measurement of RBC folate level is not subject to short-term fluctuations in folate intake & is better than serum folate as an index of folate stores.

575. For cobalamin maintenance therapy, 1000 µg of hydroxocobalamin IM is given?

Harrison's 20th Ed. Chapter 95 Page 707

A. Once a month
B. Once every 2 months
C. Once every 3 months
D. Once every 6 months

576. For cobalamin maintenance therapy, 1000 µg of cyanocobalamin IM is given?

Harrison's 20th Ed. Chapter 95 Page 707

A. Once a month
B. Once every 2 months
C. Once every 3 months
D. Once every 6 months

Replenishment of body stores of cobalamin is complete with six 1000-µg IM injections of hydroxocobalamin given at 3- to 7-day intervals. For maintenance therapy, 1000 µg hydroxocobalamin IM once every 3 months is satisfactory. Because of the poorer retention, cyanocobalamin is given 1000 µg IM, monthly.

577. Vitamin B12 injections are used in?

Harrison's 20th Ed. Chapter 95 Page 707

A. Multiple sclerosis
B. Chronic fatigue syndrome
C. Myalgic encephalomyelitis (ME)
D. All of the above

578. Oral dose of folic acid in folate deficiency is?

Harrison's 20th Ed. Chapter 95 Page 707

A. 5 – 15 mg for ~ 1 month
B. 5 – 15 mg for ~ 4 months
C. 5 – 15 mg for ~ 8 months
D. 5 – 15 mg for ~ 12 months

Oral dose of folic acid in folate deficiency is 5 - 15 mg daily for ~4 months because all folate-deficient RBC's will be eliminated in this time.

579. Long-term folic acid therapy is required in which of the following?

Harrison's 20th Ed. Chapter 95 Page 708

A. Chronic dialysis
B. Hemolytic anemias
C. Gluten-induced enteropathy
D. All of the above

Long-term folic acid therapy is required in chronic dialysis, hemolytic anemias and gluten-induced enteropathy that does not respond to gluten-free diet.

580. Which of the following is false about folic acid therapy?

Harrison's 20th Ed. Chapter 95 Page 708

A. Exclude cobalamin deficiency
B. Measure serum cobalamin levels regularly
C. Encourage improvement in diet
D. None of the above

581. Adenosylcobalamin is required for the conversion of?

Harrison's 20th Ed. Chapter 95 Page 700

A. Methylmalonyl CoA to succinyl CoA
B. Succinyl CoA to Methylmalonyl CoA
C. Propionyl CoA to Methylmalonyl CoA
D. Methylmalonyl CoA to Propionyl CoA

Adenosylcobalamin is required for the conversion of methylmalonyl CoA to succinyl CoA. Lack of this cofactor leads to large increases in the tissue levels of methylmalonyl CoA and its precursor, propionyl CoA. As a consequence, nonphysiologic fatty acids containing an odd number of carbon atoms are synthesized and incorporated into neuronal lipids. This biochemical abnormality may also contribute to the neurologic complications of cobalamin deficiency.

582. Pathway deranged in cobalamin deficiency is?

Harrison's 20th Ed. Chapter 95 Page 700

A. Methyltetrahydrofolate to tetrahydrofolate
B. N5-methenyltetrahydrofolate to N5-methylenetetrahydrofolate
C. N5-methylenetetrahydrofolate to Dihydrofolate
D. Dihydrofolate to tetrahydrofolate

Due to IF deficiency, cobalamine is deficient thereby impairing conversion of homocysteine to methionine. Cobalamin is essential for the conversion of methyltetrahydrofolate to tetrahydrofolate. Its absence deranges folate metabolism. Defect in DNA synthesis and megaloblastic maturation pattern in patients who are deficient in cobalamin is due to this mechanism (Folate trap hypothesis).

583. Which of the following about cobalamin is false?

Harrison's 20th Ed. Chapter 95 Page 700

A. Cobalamin is an essential cofactor for methionine synthase & methylmalonyl-CoA synthase
B. Methylcobalamin and adenosylcobalamin are metabolically active forms
C. Therapeutically available as cyanocobalamin
D. Cyanocobalamin is biologically active

584. Cobalamin deficiency without anemia is common in?
Harrison's 20th Ed. Chapter 95 Page 707

A. Infants
B. Adolescents
C. Adults
D. Elderly

585. Which isoenzyme of plasma lactic acid dehydrogenase is increased in enhanced intramedullary destruction of erythroblasts?
Harrison's 20th Ed. Chapter 95 Page 707

A. Isoenzyme 1
B. Isoenzyme 2
C. Isoenzyme 3
D. Isoenzyme 4

Enhanced intramedullary destruction of erythroblasts results in an increase in unconjugated bilirubin and lactic acid dehydrogenase (isoenzyme 1) in plasma.

586. Which of the following manifestations occur with cobalamin deficiency but not with folic acid deficiency?
Nutrients. 2013;5(11):4521–4539

A. Gastrointestinal
B. Neurologic
C. Hematologic
D. All of the above

Patients with folic acid deficiency are more malnourished than those with cobalamin deficiency. Gastrointestinal, hematologic manifestations are similar. Neurologic abnormalities do not occur with folic acid deficiency.

587. Folic acid supplementation is required in patients on chronic hemodialysis because?
Nutrients. 2013;5(11):4521–4539

A. Folate is lost in dialysate
B. Heparin reduces folate levels in blood
C. Protamine reduces folate levels in blood
D. All of the above

Patients on chronic hemodialysis require folate supplementation to replace that lost in dialysate.

588. Normally, what percentage of RBC precursors are destroyed in bone marrow?
Nutrients. 2013;5(11):4521–4539

A. 10 – 15%
B. 25 – 30%
C. 50 – 60%
D. 75 – 80%

Megaloblastic anemias are characterized by ineffective erythropoiesis. In a severely megaloblastic patient, as many as 90% of RBC precursors may be destroyed before they are released into the bloodstream, compared with 10 to 15% in normal individuals.

589. Clinically significant deficiency of cobalamin is present when its levels are?
Nutrients. 2013;5(11):4521–4539

A. < 100 pg/mL
B. < 200 pg/mL
C. < 300 pg/mL
D. < 400 pg/mL

Values <200 pg/mL indicate clinically significant cobalamin deficiency.

590. Reticulocytosis after intramuscular cyanocobalamin therapy for megaloblastic anemia due to cobalamin deficiency peaks at about?
Nutrients. 2013;5(11):4521–4539

A. Day 3
B. Day 5
C. Day 7
D. Day 10

Reticulocytosis begins 4 to 5 days after intramuscular cyanocobalamin therapy is started & peaks at ~ day 7. If reticulocytosis does not occur, or if it is less brisk than expected from the level of hematocrit, other factors contributing to anemia (infection, coexisting iron and/or folate deficiency, or hypothyroidism) need to be looked.

Hemolytic Anemias

591. The triad for the diagnosis of hemolytic anemia includes all except?

Harrison's 20th Ed. Chapter 96 Page 714

A. Normomacrocytic anemia
B. Splenomegaly
C. Reticulocytosis
D. Hyperbilirubinemia

For the diagnosis of hemolytic anemia, the triad of normomacrocytic anemia, reticulocytosis, and hyperbilirubinemia is useful.

592. Which of the following is called Biermer's anemia?

Journal of Medical Case Reports, 2017; 11(1): 250

A. Hereditary spherocytosis
B. Hereditary elliptocytosis
C. Pernicious anemia
D. Acute posthemorrhagic anemia (APHA)

Biermer, in 1872, coined the term pernicious anemia for a fatal condition previously described by Addison. Biermer's anemia refers to a gastropathy resulting from a defective IF secretion and not as a vague synonym for vitamin B12 deficiency or for megaloblastic anemia.

593. The most abundant red cell membrane proteins is?

Harrison's 20th Ed. Chapter 96 Page 710

A. Band 1
B. Band 2
C. Band 3
D. Band 4

594. The main cytoskeletal protein is?

Harrison's 20th Ed. Chapter 96 Page 711

A. Band 3
B. Band 4.1
C. Glycophorin
D. Spectrin

RBC cell membrane (7 nm thick) is a lipid bilayer. Most abundant of the membrane proteins are glycophorins & band 3 (anion transporter). Main cytoskeletal protein is spectrin, the basic unit of which is a dimer of a-spectrin and β-spectrin. Membrane is physically linked to cytoskeleton by proteins (ankyrin, band 4.1 & band 4.2). Spectrin, actin with bands 4.1 & 4.2 together form a fibrillar, weblike network on inner surface of RBC membrane.

595. Which is the largest component of RBC cell membrane?

Sci Rep. 2017; 7: 39661

A. Protein
B. Lipid
C. Carbohydrate
D. Others

RBC cell membrane contain ~52% protein, 40% lipid & 8% carbohydrate by weight.

596. Enzyme required for the production & utilization of ATP in RBC cell membrane is?

Sci Rep. 2017; 7: 39661

A. Aldolase
B. Glyceraldehyde-3 phosphate dehydrogenase (G-3PD)
C. Phosphoglycerate kinase
D. All of the above

A three-enzyme sequence concerned with ATP production is membrane bound - aldolase, glyceraldehyde-3 phosphate dehydrogenase (G-3PD) & phosphoglycerate kinase. Together, they convert fructose diphosphate to 3-phosphoglycerate with production of ATP.

597. Phospholipid of RBC membrane is?

Sci Rep. 2017; 7: 39661

A. Phosphatidylcholine (lecithin)
B. Phosphatidylethanolamine
C. Sphingomyelin
D. All of the above

Most of phospholipid of RBC membrane is phosphatidylcholine (lecithin), phosphatidylethanol-amine, sphingomyelin & phosphatidylserine. Lecithin & sphingomyelin can substitute each other.

598. What is the estimated frequency of hereditary spherocytosis (HS)?

Harrison's 20th Ed. Chapter 96 Page 711

A. 1 in 1000
B. 1 in 5000
C. 1 in 10,000
D. 1 in 100,000

Estimated frequency of hereditary spherocytosis (HS) is 1 in 5000.

599. Main clinical finding of hereditary spherocytosis is?

Harrison's 20th Ed. Chapter 96 Page 711

A. Jaundice
B. Splenomegaly
C. Gallstones
D. All of the above

The main clinical findings of hereditary spherocytosis are jaundice, enlarged spleen and often gallstones.

600. In hemolysis, level of unconjugated bilirubin never exceeds?

Harrison's 20th Ed. Chapter 96 Page 711

A. 1 to 2 mg/dL
B. 2 to 3 mg/dL
C. 3 to 4 mg/dL
D. 4 to 5 mg/dL

In patients with hemolysis, the level of unconjugated bilirubin never exceeds 4 to 5 mg/dL unless liver function is impaired.

601. Condition in which mean corpuscular hemoglobin concentration (MCHC) is increased is?

Harrison's 20th Ed. Chapter 96 Page 712

A. Polycythemia vera
B. Acute myeloid leukemia
C. Hereditary spherocytosis
D. Thalassemia

An increased mean corpuscular hemoglobin concentration (MCHC) on an ordinary blood count report should raise the suspicion of HS, because HS is almost the only condition in which this abnormality occurs.

602. Gene responsible for production of Band 3 is?

Harrison's 20th Ed. Chapter 96 Page 711 Table 96-3

A. ANK1
B. SLC4A1
C. SPTA1
D. EPB41

SLC4A1 is located on 17q21 and produces protein Band 3 which is also known as as AE (anion exchanger) or AE1.

603. Which of the following gene mutation accounts for majority of autosomal dominant hereditary spherocytosis (HS)?

Harrison's 20th Ed. Chapter 96 Page 711 Table 96-3

A. ANK1
B. SPTA1
C. SLC4A1
D. EPB41

Mutations in ANK1 gene on chromosome 8p11.2 producing ankyrin protein accounts for majority of autosomal dominant hereditary spherocytosis (HS).

604. Which of the following gene mutation accounts for majority of autosomal dominant hereditary elliptocytosis (HE)?

Harrison's 20th Ed. Chapter 96 Page 711 Table 96-3

A. SPTA 1
B. SPTB
C. EPB41
D. All of the above

Mutations of SPTA1 gene account for ~65% of hereditary elliptocytosis (HE). Mutations of SPTB gene account for ~30% of HE. Mutations of EPB41 account for ~5% of HE.

605. Which of the following is false about hereditary spherocytosis?

Harrison's 20th Ed. Chapter 96 Page 712

A. Increased ratio of RBC surface area to volume
B. Splenomegaly is very common
C. Mean corpuscular volume usually normal
D. Mean corpuscular hemoglobin concentration increased

Anemia in HS is normocytic. Increase in MCHC is a characteristic feature. HS is the only condition in which high MCHC is seen.

606. Which of the following is false about hereditary spherocytosis?

Harrison's 20th Ed. Chapter 96 Page 712

A. Due to defect in ankyrin/protein 3/spectrin/palladin
B. Pigmented gallstones are common
C. RBC survival after splenectomy is normal
D. None of the above

Main clinical findings of HS are jaundice, an enlarged spleen, and gallstones. Splenectomy is regarded as an obligatory therapeutic measure in HS.

607. Spherocytes are seen in?

Harrison's 20th Ed. Chapter 96 Page 712

A. Cirrhosis liver
B. Clostridial infections
C. Snake envenomations
D. All of the above

608. Which of the following laboratory investigations is helpful in diagnosis of hereditary spherocytosis (HS)?

Harrison's 20th Ed. Chapter 96 Page 712

A. Acid glycerol lysis test
B. Eosin-5'-maleimide (EMA)-binding test
C. SDS-gel electrophoresis of membrane proteins
D. All of the above

Laboratory investigations hereditary spherocytosis (HS) are osmotic fragility, acid glycerol lysis test, eosin-5'-maleimide (EMA)-binding test, SDS-gel electrophoresis of membrane proteins and molecular studies demonstrating a mutation in one of the genes underlying HS.

609. Pink test is a modified version of which of the following?

Eur J Haematol. 1989;42(2):217

A. RBC absolute values
B. Red cell survival study
C. Osmotic fragility test
D. Schilling test

A modified version of osmotic fragility test is called the "pink test".

610. Splenectomy is strongly contraindicated in which of the following conditions?

Harrison's 20th Ed. Chapter 96 Page 713

A. Xerocytosis
B. Stomatocytosis
C. Cryohydrocytosis
D. All of the above

In stomatocytosis, splenectomy is strongly contraindicated because it has been followed by severe thromboembolic complications.

611. Which of the following is false about pyruvate kinase deficiency?

Harrison's 20th Ed. Chapter 96 Page 714

A. High reticulocytosis
B. Oxygen delivery to tissues is increased
C. Oral folic acid should be given constantly
D. None of the above

Metabolic block at the last step in glycolysis increase bisphosphoglycerate (or DPG), a major effector of hemoglobin-oxygen dissociation curve. Thus, oxygen delivery to tissues is increased.

612. Which of the following protects RBC's against oxidant stress?

Harrison's 20th Ed. Chapter 96 Page 714

A. Glutathione
B. Glucose-6-phosphate dehydrogenase (G6PD)
C. Pyruvate
D. Erythropoietin (EPO)

G6PD protects RBC's proteins from oxidative damage by generating NADPH, which maintains high levels of reduced glutathione. Glutathione protects RBC's against oxidant stress.

613. Glucose-6-phosphate dehydrogenase (G6PD) is related to which of the following pathways?

Harrison's 20th Ed. Chapter 96 Page 709 Figure 96-1

A. Embden-Meyerhof pathway
B. Hexose monophosphate shunt
C. Purine salvage pathway
D. All of the above

G6PD is a HMP shunt enzyme. The hexose monophosphate shunt generates NADPH that is used to reduce glutathione, which protects the red cell against oxidant stress.

614. Which of the following reactions is related to G6PD?
Harrison's 20th Ed. Chapter 96 Page 715

A. ATP to ADP
B. ADP to ATP
C. NADP to NADPH
D. NADPH to NADP

G6PD reduces NADP to NADPH while oxidizing glucose-6-phosphate (G6P) to 6-phosphogluconate (6PG). NADPH then provides the reducing power that converts oxidized glutathione (GSSG) to reduced glutathione (GSH). Reduced glutathione protects against oxidant injury by catalyzing breakdown of oxidant compounds like H_2O_2.

615. Which of the following protects the patient from malaria?
Harrison's 20th Ed. Chapter 96 Page 714

A. G6PD deficiency
B. Hemoglobin S
C. Hereditary ovalocytosis
D. All of the above

616. The G6PD gene is located on?
Harrison's 20th Ed. Chapter 96 Page 714

A. X chromosome
B. Y chromosome
C. Autosome
D. Any of the above

Gene for G6PD is located on X chromosome (Xq28). Mode of transmission of G6PD deficiency is X-linked recessive. It is the most common enzymatic disorder of RBC's in humans. Defect is expressed in all erythrocytes of the affected male. In heterozygous female, two populations of red cells, some deficient, others normal, are present owing to random inactivation of the X chromosomes. It follows that males are more vulnerable to oxidant injury than females are.

617. Which of the following is the most prevalent of the enzyme deficiency states?
Harrison's 20th Ed. Chapter 96 Page 709 Figure 96-1

A. Glucose 6- phosphate dehydrogenase (G6PD)
B. Pyruvate kinase
C. Glucose-6-phosphate isomerase
D. Cytochrome b5 reductase

Enzyme deficiency states in order of prevalence are glucose 6- phosphate dehydrogenase (G6PD) > pyruvate kinase > glucose-6-phosphate isomerase.

618. The enzymatically active form of G6PD is a?
Harrison's 20th Ed. Chapter 96 Page 714

A. Monomer
B. Dimer
C. Trimer
D. All of the above

Enzymatically active form of G6PD is either a dimer or a tetramer of a single protein subunit of 514 amino acids.

619. The normal G6PD is designated as?
Harrison's 20th Ed. Chapter 96 Page 714

A. Type A (+)
B. Type A (–)
C. Type B
D. Any of the above

Most common normal "wild type" G6PD enzyme is designated as G6PD-B. Two variants, designated G6PD A- ((10 - 60% of activity) and G6PD Mediterranean (<10% of normal activity), lead to clinically significant hemolysis. A- type is present in ~10% of American blacks, G6PD Mediterranean is found in Middle East, G6PD Vianchan & G6PD Mahidol in Southeast Asia, G6PD Canton in China, and G6PD Union worldwide.

620. Which of the following 'vitamins' can cause hemolysis in G6PD deficient subjects?
Harrison's 20th Ed. Chapter 96 Page 716 Table 96-5

A. Vitamin A
B. Vitamin D
C. Vitamin E
D. Vitamin K

Vitamins that G6PD deficient persons should avoid include vitamin C & K. Vitamin E is protective.

621. Which of the following 'antimalarials' can cause hemolysis in G6PD deficient subjects?
Harrison's 20th Ed. Chapter 96 Page 716 Table 96-5

A. Chloroquine
B. Quinine
C. Primaquine
D. Mefloquine

Deficiency of G6PD protects against malaria due to Plasmodium falciparum. It was primaquine (PQ) that led to the discovery of G6PD deficiency.

622. Which of the following can precipitate an episode of hemolysis in G6PD deficient subjects?
Harrison's 20th Ed. Chapter 96 Page 716 Table 96-5

A. Viral & bacterial infections
B. Naphthalene
C. Metabolic acidosis
D. All of the above

623. Which of the following is a peripheral blood finding of hemolysis in G6PD deficiency?
Harrison's 20th Ed. Chapter 96 Page 717

A. Heinz bodies
B. Bite cells or blister cells
C. Spherocytes
D. All of the above

Hemolysis in G6PD deficiency is both intravascular & extravascular. Exposure to oxidants causes oxidation of sulfhydryl groups of globin chains leading to denaturation of hemoglobin & formation of precipitates (Heinz bodies) which damage RBC membrane to cause intravascular hemolysis. Heinz bodies decrease RBC deformability, macrophages pluck out or bite Heinz bodies, giving rise to "bite cells". Membrane damage induces formation of spherocytes. Bizarre poikilocytes with RBC's having unevenly distributed hemoglobin are called hemighosts.

624. Which of the following is false about acute hemolytic anemia due to G6PD deficiency?
Harrison's 20th Ed. Chapter 96 Page 717

A. Hemoglobinemia
B. Hemoglobinuria
C. Raised plasma haptoglobin
D. Raised LDH

Acute hemolytic anemia due to G6PD deficiency leads to anisocytosis, poikilocytosis, polychromasia, spherocytes, reticulocytosis, unconjugated hyperbilirubinemia, hemoglobinemia, hemoglobinuria, low or absent plasma haptoglobin, raised LDH, gallstones, splenomegaly.

625. Which of the following is false about CNSHA?
Harrison's 20th Ed. Chapter 96 Page 716

A. Patient is always a male
B. History of neonatal jaundice (NNJ)
C. Chronic hemolysis
D. None of the above

Chronic nonspherocytic hemolytic anemia (CNSHA) is a severe clinical phenotype of G6PD deficiency, always in a male, with history of NNJ.

626. Which population of RBC is rapidly destroyed during hemolysis in G6PD deficient subjects?
Harrison's 20th Ed. Chapter 96 Page 718 Table 96-6

A. Immature
B. Mature
C. Older
D. All of the above

G6PD enzyme activity is normal in reticulocytes, but older RBC's are markedly deficient. Exposure to oxidants induces hemolysis of older red cells but not of younger ones.

627. Which of the following element is essential for the activity of glutathione peroxidase (GSHPx)?
Harrison's 20th Ed. Chapter 96 Page 717

A. Cobalt
B. Zinc
C. Mercury
D. Selenium

Infantile poikilocytosis is due to deficiency of glutathione peroxidase (GSHPx) due to nutritional deficiency of selenium which is an essential element for the activity of GSHPx.

628. Basophilic stippling is a highly distinctive feature of?
Harrison's 20th Ed. Chapter 96 Page 717

A. Autoimmune Hemolytic Anemia (AIHA)
B. Familial Hemolytic Uremic Syndrome (HUS)
C. Pyrimidine 5'-Nucleotidase (P5N) Deficiency
D. All of the above

P5N is a key enzyme in catabolism of nucleotides arising from degradation of nucleic acids that takes place in final stages of RBC maturation. Basophilic stippling is highly distinctive feature of P5N deficiency. HA caused by lead poisoning is also characterized by basophilic stippling.

629. Drug that can cause hemolysis by depletion of ATP is?
Antiviral Res. 2017;146:153-160

A. Dapsone
B. Ribavirin
C. Cisplatin
D. Methyldopa

Ribavirin causes hemolysis by depletion of ATP. Hyperbaric oxygen, nitrates, chlorates, methylene blue, dapsone, cisplatin cause hemolysis by their oxidative potential. Penicillin acts as a hapten & induces antibody production leading to hemolysis. Methyldopa, through mimicry, produces of an antibody (Rhesus antibody anti-e) against RBC antigen causing hemolysis.

630. Which of the following about HUS due to Shiga toxin producing Escherichia coli O157:H7 is false?
Harrison's 20th Ed. Chapter 96 Page 717

A. Nonimmune [Coombs test (–)] hemolytic anemia
B. Microangiopathic hemolytic anemia
C. Thrombocytopenia
D. Leucopenia

Shiga toxin producing Escherichia coli O157:H7 is an etiologic agent of HUS, more common in children, developing several days after diarrhea. HUS is a nonimmune [Coombs test (–)] hemolytic anemia with classical triad - microangiopathic hemolytic anemia, thrombocytopenia & acute renal failure due to thrombosis of glomerular capillaries. Leucocytosis occurs in HUS.

631. In which of the following, hemolysis results from an inherited defect external to red cells?
Harrison's 20th Ed. Chapter 96 Page 717

A. Hemoglobinopathies
B. Paroxysmal nocturnal hemoglobinuria (PNH)
C. Familial (atypical) hemolytic uremic syndrome
D. Hereditary spherocytosis (HS)

All other inherited HAs are due to intrinsic red cell abnormalities, atypical HUS (aHUS) is unique in that hemolysis results from an inherited defect external to red cells.

632. Which of the following is not a feature of familial (atypical) hemolytic-uremic syndrome?
Harrison's 20th Ed. Chapter 96 Page 717

A. Microangiopathic HA
B. Fragmented RBCs in PBF
C. Thrombocytosis
D. Acute renal failure

Familial (atypical) hemolytic-uremic syndrome mostly affects children and is characterized by microangiopathic HA with presence of fragmented RBCs in peripheral blood smear, thrombocytopenia (usually mild) and acute renal failure. It is due to mutations in genes encoding complement regulatory proteins like complement factor H (CFH), CD46 or membrane cofactor protein (MCP), complement factor 1 (CFI), complement component C3, complement factor B (CFB) and thrombomodulin.

633. Direct Coombs test is also called?
Harrison's 20th Ed. Chapter 96 Page 718

A. Direct antiglobulin test
B. Direct agglutination test
C. Direct antigen test
D. Direct antibody test

Direct Coombs test is also called Direct antiglobulin test (DAT). The antiglobulin test was first described by Coombs in 1945. It is performed to detect either erythrocyte directed IgG in plasma or IgG or complement coating on surface of circulating erythrocytes. Neither of these molecules can cause direct agglutination of erythrocytes, so, to detect their presence, monoclonal antihuman globulin (AHG) with specificity for IgG or various complement proteins is added to a suspension of erythrocytes. The AHG reagent is sufficiently large to cause agglutination of erythrocytes that are coated with IgG or complement.

634. A positive direct antiglobulin test (DAT) indicates the presence of which of the following bound to the red cell membrane?
British Journal of Haematology, 2017, 176, 395–411

A. IgG
B. IgM
C. IgA
D. Any of the above

A positive direct antiglobulin test (DAT) indicates the presence of immunoglobulin (Ig)G, IgM, IgA or complement (usually C3d) bound to the red cell membrane.

635. Which of the following is false about direct antiglobulin test (DAT)?

British Journal of Haematology, 2017, 176, 395–411

A. Reflects in-vivo antibody sensitization of RBCs
B. Reflects in-vitro antibody sensitization of RBCs
C. Erythrocytes are washed before the test
D. Anti-IgG antihuman globulin (AHG) reagent is used

DAT reflects in-vivo antibody sensitization of RBCs. RBCs are washed to remove unbound Ab's & anti-IgG AHG reagent is then added. IgG antibodies cannot cause direct RBC agglutination, but if RBC's are coated with IgG antibodies, AHG reagent will cause them to agglutinate.

636. Which of the following is false about indirect antiglobulin test (IAT)?

British Journal of Haematology, 2017, 176, 395–411

A. Used to detect IgG antibodies in serum
B. Reflects in-vitro antibody sensitization of RBC's
C. Reagent RBC's are incubated in with serum
D. Anti-IgG antihuman globulin reagent is not used

Indirect antiglobulin test (IAT) is used to detect the presence of IgG antibodies in serum (in-vitro sensitization). Reagent RBC's are incubated with serum that potentially contains antibodies. If Ab's are present, they bind to their target antigens on reagent RBC's. After an incubation period, RBC's are washed to remove unbound antibodies. Anti-IgG AHG reagent is then added and will cause IgG-coated RBC's to agglutinate.

637. Cold Autoimmune Hemolytic Anemia (AIHA) is caused by?

Harrison's 20th Ed. Chapter 96 Page 719 Table 96-7

A. IgA antibody
B. IgG antibody
C. IgM antibody
D. ANy of the above

AIHA is usually classified on the basis of thermal amplitude of the autoantibody. Warm AIHA is caused by IgG antibody, whereas cold AIHA is caused by an IgM antibody that fixes complement to the surface of the RBC.

638. Conditions associated with hemolysis and a negative DAT result include all except?

Harrison's 20th Ed. Chapter 96 Page 719 Table 96-7

A. Hemoglobinopathies
B. Systemic lupus erythematosus (SLE)
C. Thrombotic thrombocytopenic purpura (TTP)
D. Disseminated intravascular coagulation (DIC)

Antierythrocyte membrane autoantibodies in SLE have positive direct Coombs' test (60% prevalence). Some may develop overt hemolysis. Conditions associated with hemolysis and a negative DAT result are Microangiopathic hemolytic anemias (TTP, DIC), Hypersplenism, Liver disease, Hemoglobinopathies (sickle cell disease, thalassemia), Erythrocyte membranopathies (spherocytosis), Erythrocyte enzymopathies (G-6-PD deficiency, pyruvate kinase deficiency), Infectious diseases (Clostridium difficile infection), Erythrocyte trauma (mechanical heart valves).

639. Which of the following is a cause of positive DAT?

British Journal of Haematology, 2017, 176, 395–411

A. Intravenous immunoglobulin (IVIg)
B. Antithymocyte globulin
C. Systemic lupus erythematosus (SLE)
D. All of the above

A positive DAT is not specific and is also associated with a wide range of non-haemolytic disease states, possibly through passive deposition of immunoglobulins or immune complexes; examples include liver disease, chronic infection, malignancy, systemic lupus erythematosus (SLE), renal disorders and drugs such as intravenous immunoglobulin (IVIg) or antithymocyte globulin.

640. Which of the following should be considered in differential diagnosis of chronic Coombs-negative HA?

Harrison's 20th Ed. Chapter 96 Page 714

A. Drug-induced hemolytic anemias
B. Enzymopathies
C. Paroxysmal Cold Hemoglobinuria (PCH)
D. Acute hemolytic transfusion reaction

Enzymopathies (G-6-PD deficiency, pyruvate kinase deficiency) should be considered in the differential diagnosis of any chronic Coombs-negative HA.

641. Most common form of acquired hemolytic anemia in areas where malaria is not endemic is?

British Journal of Haematology, 2017, 176, 395–411

A. Paroxysmal Nocturnal Hemoglobinuria (PNH)
B. Paroxysmal Cold Hemoglobinuria (PCH)
C. Autoimmune Hemolytic Anemia (AIHA)
D. Hemolytic Uremic Syndrome (HUS)

Autoimmune Hemolytic Anemia (AIHA) is the most common form of acquired hemolytic anemia in areas where malaria is not endemic.

642. Which of the following is true for Autoimmune Hemolytic Anemia (AIHA)?

British Journal of Haematology, 2017, 176, 395–411

A. Compensated acquired haemolysis
B. Decompensated acquired haemolysis
C. Compensated hereditary haemolysis
D. Decompensated hereditary haemolysis

AIHA is a decompensated acquired haemolysis caused by the host's immune system acting against its own red cell antigens. The incidence is ~1 per 100,000/year. It can occur at any age but incidence rises with increasing age.

643. Which of the following is the most common form of Autoimmune Hemolytic Anemia (AIHA)?

British Journal of Haematology, 2017, 176, 395–411

A. Warm type
B. Cold type
C. Mixed AIHA
D. None of the above

Serologically, AIHA cases are divided into warm type (65%), cold type (29% cold haemagglutinin disease [CHAD], 1% paroxysmal cold haemoglobinuria) or mixed AIHA (5%). Approximately half are primary (idiopathic) AIHA and half are secondary to associated disorders.

644. Which of the following is the most common presenting feature of AIHA?

British Journal of Haematology, 2017, 176, 395–411

A. Dizziness
B. Dyspnoea
C. Jaundice
D. Dark urine

Patients with AIHA may present with symptoms of anaemia (weakness 88%, dizziness 50%, dyspnoea 9%), haemolysis (jaundice 21%, dark urine 3%) or symptoms of an underlying disorder.

645. Blood film in patients with autoimmune haemolytic anaemia shows which of the following?

British Journal of Haematology, 2017, 176, 395–411

A. Spherocytes
B. Agglutination
C. Polychromasia
D. All of the above

646. Paroxysmal cold hemoglobinuria (PCH) was more frequent when which of the following disease was prevalent?

Harrison's 20th Ed. Chapter 96 Page 719

A. Tuberculosis
B. Tertiary syphilis
C. Gonorrhoea
D. Protein calorie malnutrition

647. Antibody in Paroxysmal cold hemoglobinuria (PCH) is?

Harrison's 20th Ed. Chapter 96 Page 719

A. Anti-Jo-1 antibody
B. Anti-Smith antibody
C. Ki-67 monoclonal antibody
D. Donath-Landsteiner antibody

Antibody in PCH is Donath-Landsteiner antibody which has anti-P specificity and binds to RBC's only at a low temperature (~4°C), and in the presence of complement when temperature becomes 37°C, lysis of RBC's, intravascular hemolysis & hemoglobinuria occurs.

648. Cold Agglutinin Disease (CAD) is related to which of the following?

Harrison's 20th Ed. Chapter 96 Page 719

A. Familial cold autoinflammatory syndrome (FCAS)
B. Cold urticaria
C. Waldenström macroglobulinemia (WM)
D. Systemic mastocytosis

CAD is a form of chronic AIHA & affects elderly. Autoantibody (IgM with anti-I specificity) reacts with RBC's strongly at lower temperatures (cold exposure), not at all at 37°C. Antibody is produced by expanded clone of B lymphocytes and may show as a spike in plasma protein electrophoresis resembling monoclonal gammopathy and may be related to Waldenström macroglobulinemia (WM).

649. Which of the following is a feature of Paroxysmal Nocturnal Hemoglobinuria (PNH)?

Harrison's 20th Ed. Chapter 96 Page 719

A. Hemolysis
B. Pancytopenia
C. Tendency to venous thrombosis
D. All of the above

PNH is an acquired chronic HA characterized by persistent intravascular hemolysis subject to recurrent exacerbations. The triad of PNH is hemolysis, pancytopenia and tendency to venous thrombosis.

650. Which of the following is false about Paroxysmal Nocturnal Hemoglobinuria (PNH)?

Harrison's 20th Ed. Chapter 96 Page 719

A. Intracorpuscular defect acquired at stem cell level
B. Hemolytic anemia
C. Arterial thrombosis
D. Bone marrow failure

PNH has three attributes—complement-dependent acquired chronic intravascular hemolytic anemia, venous thrombosis & bone marrow failure which preceds overt PNH. Hemolysis often occurs during sleep, when decline in blood pH triggers activation of complement components. Urine is black when patient awakens. Hemoglobin-drenched renal tubules lock iron of Hb into hemosiderin and continuous sloughing of these cells into urine culminates in iron deficiency.

651. Which of the following is false about Paroxysmal Nocturnal Hemoglobinuria (PNH)?

Harrison's 20th Ed. Chapter 96 Page 719

A. Hemolysis due to activation of complement
B. Hemosiderinuria is usually absent
C. Granulocytopenia & thrombocytopenia
D. May present as Budd-Chiari syndrome

In PNH, RBC's have an increased susceptibility to complement (C) due to the deficiency on their surface of CD59 & CD55 proteins that normally protect RBC's from activated C. When thrombosis affects hepatic veins, Budd-Chiari syndrome occurs. The hemoglobin-drenched renal tubules lock iron of hemoglobin into hemosiderin, and the continuous sloughing of these cells into the urine culminates in iron deficiency.

652. Which of the following is the most important protective RBC membrane protein?

Harrison's 20th Ed. Chapter 96 Page 721

A. CD29
B. CD39
C. CD49
D. CD59

CD59 (membrane inhibitor of reactive lysis) is a protective RBC membrane protein.

653. Which of the following is diagnostic of PNH?

Harrison's 20th Ed. Chapter 96 Page 721

A. CD59–, CD55–
B. CD59+, CD55–
C. CD59–, CD55+
D. CD59+, CD55+

Discrete population of cells that is CD59–, CD55– is diagnostic of PNH.

654. Which of the following is the action of CD59?

Harrison's 20th Ed. Chapter 96 Page 721

A. Inhibits insertion of C9 into cell membrane
B. Binds C3b
C. Inhibiting C3 convertase
D. All of the above

Erythrocytes defend themselves from membrane attack complexes with two membrane-bound proteins, CD55 (decay-accelerating factor), which binds C3b, and CD59, which inhibits the insertion of C9 polymers into the membrane.

655. In paroxysmal nocturnal hemoglobinuria, name of the defective gene is?

Harrison's 20th Ed. Chapter 96 Page 721

A. HNF4a
B. PIG-A
C. BRCA1
D. CFTR

PNH results from clonal expansion of hematopoietic stem cells that have somatic mutations in the X-linked gene called PIG-A (phosphatidylinositol glycan class A). PIG-A mutations cause an early block in the synthesis of glycosylphosphatidyl-inositol (GPI) anchors, which tether many proteins to the cell surface. Consequently, the blood cells in PNH have a partial deficiency (type II) or a complete deficiency (type III) of GPI-linked proteins. Intravascular hemolysis is the consequence of absence of GPI-linked complement regulatory protein CD59. CD59 blocks the formation of terminal complement complex (membrane-attack complex) on the cell surface, thereby preventing erythrocyte lysis and in vitro platelet activation.

656. Which of the following tests is useful in diagnosing Paroxysmal Nocturnal Hemoglobinuria?

Harrison's 20th Ed. Chapter 96 Page 721

A. Acidified serum lysis test (Ham's test)
B. Sucrose lysis test
C. Flow cytometry
D. All of the above

Thomas Hale Ham (1938) developed Ham's test at Thorndike Laboratory of Boston City Hospital and reported that RBC's in PNH are highly susceptible to lysis in an acidic environment. CD55 is called decay-accelerating factor (DAF).

657. Pathway of activation of the complement system is called?

N Engl J Med 2001;344:1058

A. Classical pathway
B. Mannose-binding lectin pathway
C. Alternative pathway
D. All of the above

There are three pathways of activation of the complement system - the classical, mannose-binding lectin and alternative pathways. Terminal pathway is common to these three pathways leads to membrane attack complex that lyses cells.

658. Pathways of activation of the complement system converge at the point of cleavage of?

N Engl J Med 2001;344:1058

A. C3
B. C4
C. C5
D. C6

3 activation pathways of complement converge to generate C3 convertase that cleaves C3.

659. Eculizumab binds specifically to?

N Engl J Med 2004;350:553

A. C1
B. C3
C. C4
D. C5

Eculizumab is a recombinant humanized monoclonal antibody that binds specifically to terminal complement protein C5, inhibiting its cleavage into C5a and C5b, thereby preventing release of inflammatory mediator C5a & formation of the cytolytic pore C5b–C9. Blockade of complement cascade at C5 preserves early components of complement that are essential for opsonization of microorganisms & clearance of immune complexes.

660. Which of the following is false about 'Haptoglobin'?

Harrison's 20th Ed. Chapter 96 Page 720

A. α globulin
B. Binds to heme in hemoglobin
C. Decreased in hepatocellular disease
D. Increased in inflammatory states

Haptoglobin binds specifically to the globin in hemoglobin.

661. Which of the following is false about 'Haptoglobin'?

Harrison's 20th Ed. Chapter 96 Page 720

A. Serum concentration is ~1.0 g/L
B. Low or absent is significant hemolysis
C. Hemoglobin-haptoglobin complex is cleared rapidly by mononuclear phagocyte system
D. None of the above

662. Prussian blue is useful in the treatment of which of the following internal contaminations?

Harrison's 20th Ed. Chapter 449 Page 3300

A. Strontium
B. Molybdenum
C. Thallium
D. Radium

Prussian blue prevents absorption of Thallium and is given orally at 250 mg/kg in divided doses.

663. Drug that cause immunohemolytic anemia is?

Harrison's 20th Ed. Chapter 96 Page 719 Table 96-7

A. α-methyldopa
B. Penicillin
C. Ceftriaxone
D. All of the above

Drugs causing warm antibody immunohemolytic anemia are α-methyldopa, penicillin & ceftriaxone.

664. Which of the following can directly parasitize RBC's & cause severe hemolysis?

Am Fam Physician. 2004;69(11):2599-2607

A. Bartonellosis
B. Malaria
C. Babesiosis
D. All of the above

Bartonellosis, malaria & babesiosis directly parasitize RBC & cause severe hemolysis.

665. Spur cell anemia is due to?

Harrison's 20th Ed. Chapter 59 Page 389

A. Clostridium welchii infection
B. HELLP syndrome
C. Severe hepatocellular disease
D. Hemolytic-uremic syndrome

Spur cells are irregularly spiculated acanthocytes. Spur cell anemia is a hemolytic anemia with bizarre-shaped RBC occurring in severe hepatocellular disease (Laennec's cirrhosis). Hemolytic anemia with spur cells and acanthocytes called Zieve's syndrome can occur in patients with severe alcoholic hepatitis.

666. Surface membrane of a spur cell (acanthocytes) contain excess of?

Harrison's 20th Ed. Chapter 59 Page 389

A. Phospholipid
B. Cholesterol
C. Triglyceride
D. Glycoprotein

Surface membrane of a spur cell contains 50 to 70% excess cholesterol, but its total phospholipid content is normal. This decreases membrane fluidity & cell deformability forbiding their passage through filtering system of spleen.

667. 'Burr cells' are found in?

Harrison's 20th Ed. Chapter 59 Page 389

A. Severe hepatocellular disease
B. Uremia
C. DIC
D. HELLP syndrome

Burr cells or echinocytes are seen in uremia. In such RBC's numerous, regularly spaced, small spiny projections are seen. Echinocytes are a frequent artifact in PBF. Echinocytes are found in patients with severe uremia, glycolytic red cell enzyme defects and microangiopathic hemolytic anemia.

Bone Marrow Failure Syndromes Including Aplastic Anemia and Myelodysplasia

668. Which of the following is not a hypoproliferative anemia?

Harrison's 20th Ed. Chapter 98 Page 723

A. Aplastic anemia
B. Myelodysplasia (MDS)
C. Pure red cell aplasia (PRCA)
D. Congenital dyserythropoietic anemia

Hypoproliferative anemia is a prominent feature of bone marrow failure states like aplastic anemia, myelodysplasia (MDS), pure red cell aplasia (PRCA) and myelophthisis.

669. First case description of aplastic anemia was published by?

N Engl J Med 2018;379:1643-56

A. Paul Ehrlich
B. Louis Henri Vaquez
C. Richard C. Cabot
D. None of the above

The first case description of aplastic anemia was published by Paul Ehrlich in 1888. Term "anemia aplastique" originated with Louis Henri Vaquez in 1904, and clinical features were described by Richard C. Cabot.

670. In aplastic anemia, age mostly affected is?

Harrison's 20th Ed. Chapter 98 Page 724

A. Children
B. Teens
C. Young adults
D. Teens & twenties and older adults

In aplastic anemia, men & women are affected equally. The age distribution is biphasic, with the major peak in the teens and twenties and a second rise in older adults.

671. Most cases of aplastic anemia are?

Harrison's 20th Ed. Chapter 98 Page 724

A. Idiopathic
B. Due to drug exposure
C. Due to immune diseases
D. Due to inherited disorders

Most cases of aplastic anemia are idiopathic.

672. Which of the following is not a late effect of irradiation?

Harrison's 20th Ed. Chapter 98 Page 725

A. Aplastic anemia
B. MDS
C. Leukemia
D. All of the above

MDS & leukemia, but probably not aplastic anemia, are late effects of radiation.

673. Which of the following has consistent association with aplastic anemia?

Harrison's 20th Ed. Chapter 98 Page 725 Table 98-3

A. Benzene
B. Chloramphenicol
C. Carbamazapine
D. All of the above

674. Which of the following has consistent association with aplastic anemia?

Harrison's 20th Ed. Chapter 98 Page 725 Table 98-3

A. Gold
B. Phenylbutazone
C. Cimetidine
D. All of the above

Benzene, hydantoins, carbamazapine, quinacrine, gold, cimetidine, chloramphenicol, phenylbutazone show most consistent association with AA.

675. Which of the following hepatitis virus infections most often precede posthepatitis marrow failure?

Harrison's 20th Ed. Chapter 98 Page 725

A. A
B. B
C. C
D. None of the above

Posthepatitis aplastic anemia is typically seronegative (non-A, non-B, non-C, non-G) & probably due to as yet undiscovered infectious agent.

676. Cause of transient aplastic crisis in hemolytic anemias is?

Harrison's 20th Ed. Chapter 98 Page 725

A. Hepatitis
B. Infectious mononucleosis
C. Parvovirus B19
D. All of the above

Parvovirus B19 is the cause of transient aplastic crisis in hemolytic anemias.

677. Aplastic anemia is strongly associated with which of the following collagen vascular syndrome?

Harrison's 20th Ed. Chapter 98 Page 725

A. Polyarteritis nodosa
B. Schnitzler's syndrome
C. Wegener's granulomatosis
D. Eosinophilic fasciitis

Aplastic anemia is strongly associated with eosinophilic fasciitis which is characterized by painful induration of subcutaneous tissues.

678. Aplastic anemia is strongly associated with which of the following?

Harrison's 20th Ed. Chapter 98 Page 725

A. Transfusion-associated graft-versus-host disease (GVHD)
B. Eosinophilic fasciitis
C. Systemic lupus erythematosus (SLE)
D. All of the above

679. Aplastic anemia is related to?
Harrison's 20th Ed. Chapter 98 Page 725

A. Fanconi's anemia
B. Paroxysmal nocturnal hemoglobinuria
C. Dyskeratosis congenita
D. All of the above

Fanconi's anemia presents as progressive pancytopenia. Bone marrow from PNH patients show evidence of defective hematopoiesis and may later develop frank marrow aplasia & pancytopenia. In Dyskeratosis congenita, aplastic anemia develops during childhood.

680. Which of the following about Fanconi's anemia is false?
Harrison's 20th Ed. Chapter 98 Page 725

A. Autosomal dominant disorder
B. Short stature, café au lait spots
C. Type A is due to mutation in FANCA
D. Increased risk of malignancy

Fanconi's anemia is an autosomal recessive disorder.

681. Dyskeratosis congenita is characterized by all except?
Harrison's 20th Ed. Chapter 98 Page 725

A. Abnormal skin pigmentation
B. Pancreatic insufficiency
C. Nail dystrophy
D. Mucosal leucoplakia

Dyskeratosis congenita is an inherited bone-marrow-failure syndrome in childhood & presents with the triad of reticular hyperpigmentation, nail dystrophy and mucous membrane leukoplasia.

682. Dyskeratosis is due to mutations in which of the following genes?
Harrison's 20th Ed. Chapter 98 Page 726

A. DKC1
B. TERC
C. TERT
D. Any of the above

Dyskeratosis congenita is due to mutations in genes of the telomere repair complex that maintain telomere length in replicating cells: The X-linked variety is due to mutations in DKC1 (dyskerin) gene. the autosomal dominant type is due to mutation in TERC, which encodes an RNA template, and TERT, which encodes the catalytic reverse transcriptase, telomerase. Mutations in TNF2, a component of the shelterin, proteins that bind the telomere DNA, also occur in dyskeratosis.

683. Shwachman-Diamond syndrome features include all except?
Harrison's 20th Ed. Chapter 98 Page 726

A. Pancreatic insufficiency
B. Malabsorption
C. Eosinophilia
D. Risk of aplastic anemia

Schwachman-Diamond syndrome is an autosomal recessive disorder characterised by pancreatic exocrine dysfunction, malabsorption, metaphyseal dysostosis, and bone marrow failure due to compound heterozygous mutations in SBDS.

684. Which cell in the bone marrow is helpful in differentiating aplastic anaemia from hypoplastic myelodysplastic syndromes?
Harrison's 20th Ed. Chapter 98 Page 726, Lancet 2005;365:1647–56

A. CD34 positive stem cells
B. CD38 positive stem cells
C. CD42 positive stem cells
D. CD46 positive stem cells

Bone marrow failure results from severe damage to hematopoietic cell compartment. In AA, cells bearing CD34 antigen, a marker of early hematopoietic cells, are greatly diminished, committed & primitive progenitor cells are virtually absent.

685. Which of the following is the most common early symptom in aplastic anemia?
Harrison's 20th Ed. Chapter 98 Page 726

A. Bleeding
B. Infection
C. Weight loss
D. Jaundice

Aplastic anemia can have abrupt or insidious onset. Most common early symptom is bleeding. Systemic complaints and weight loss should point to other etiologies of pancytopenia.

686. Which of the following is unusual in aplastic anemia?
Harrison's 20th Ed. Chapter 98 Page 727

A. Infection on presentation
B. Lymphadenopathy
C. Splenomegaly
D. All of the above

Infection on presentation, lymphadenopathy & splenomegaly are atypical of aplastic anemia.

687. Which of the following is not a feature of blood smear in aplastic anemia?
Harrison's 20th Ed. Chapter 98 Page 727

A. Decreased mean corpuscular volume (MCV)
B. Few or absent reticulocytes
C. Normal lymphocyte number
D. Reduced platelets and granulocytes

In AA, PBF shows large erythrocytes & reduced platelets & granulocytes. MCV is commonly increased. Reticulocytes are absent or few & lymphocyte numbers may be normal or reduced. No immature myeloid forms and abnormal platelets.

688. Which of the following is not a feature of bone marrow cytology in aplastic anemia?
Harrison's 20th Ed. Chapter 98 Page 727

A. Dilute aspirate
B. Hematopoietic cells occupying < 50% of marrow
C. Megakaryocytes greatly reduced/absent
D. Mild megaloblastic erythropoiesis

In AA, bone marrow is readily aspirated but dilute on smear. BM biopsy shows mainly fat under the microscope, with hematopoietic cells occupying <25% of marrow space.

689. Which of the following is false?
Harrison's 20th Ed. Chapter 98 Page 727

A. Aplastic anemia is a disease of the young
B. Agranulocytosis is more frequent in elderly & women
C. In single lineage failure syndromes, progression to pancytopenia or leukemia is unusual
D. None of the above

Aplastic anemia is a disease of young. In all the single lineage failure syndromes, progression to pancytopenia or leukemia is unusual.

690. Severe aplastic anemia is defined by?
Harrison's 20th Ed. Chapter 98 Page 727

A. Absolute neutrophil count < 500/μL
B. Platelet count < 20,000/μL
C. Absolute reticulocyte count < 60,000/μL
D. All of the above

Severe AA is defined by the presence of two of three parameters : absolute neutrophil count <500/μL, platelet count <20,000/μL & corrected reticulocyte count <1% (or absolute reticulocyte count <60,000/μL). Very severe disease is defined as absolute neutrophil count <200/μL.

691. Which of the following about aplastic anemia is false?
Lancet 2005;365:1647–56

A. CD34+ cells greatly reduced
B. Immunological deficiencies are common
C. Normal lymphocyte count
D. Complete recovery can occur with effective immunosuppressive therapy

692. Which of the following have no value in treating severe acquired aplastic anemia?
Harrison's 20th Ed. Chapter 98 Page 727

A. Hematopoietic growth factors (HGFs)
B. Glucocorticoids
C. Antithymocyte globulin (ATG)
D. Bone Marrow Transplantation

Treatment options in severe acquired aplastic anemia are replacement of the absent hematopoietic cells by stem cell transplant, or suppression of immune system. Hematopoietic growth factors (HGFs) are not recommended as initial therapy for severe aplastic anemia, and even their roles as adjuncts to immunosuppression are not clear. Glucocorticoids are of no value.

693. Which of the following is used along with ALG or ATG to increase response rates in aplastic anemia?
Harrison's 20th Ed. Chapter 98 Page 728

A. Azithromycin
B. Zinc
C. Cyclosporine
D. Vitamin E

Addition of cyclosporine to ALG (antilymphocyte globulin) or ATG (antithymocyte globulin) increases response rates in AA.

694. With standard regimen of ATG + cyclosporine for AA, improvement in granulocyte number is generally apparent within?
Harrison's 20th Ed. Chapter 98 Page 728

A. 1 month of treatment
B. 2 months of treatment
C. 3 months of treatment
D. 4 months of treatment

With standard regimen of ATG + cyclosporine for AA, improvement in granulocyte number is generally apparent within 2 months of treatment.

695. In aplastic anemia treatment responders, MDS develops in what percentage of patients?
Harrison's 20th Ed. Chapter 98 Page 728

A. 10%
B. 15%
C. 20%
D. 25%

In aplastic anemia treatment responders, MDS develops in 15% of patients.

696. In adults, initial oral dose of cyclosporine in treatment of aplastic anemia is?
Blood. 2012;120(6):1185–1196

A. 2 mg/kg per day
B. 8 mg/kg per day
C. 12 mg/kg per day
D. 20 mg/kg per day

Cyclosporine is administered orally at an initial dose of 12 mg/kg per day in adults

697. Trough blood levels of cyclosporine in treatment of aplastic anemia should be between?
Blood. 2012;120(6):1185–1196

A. 150 and 200 ng/mL
B. 250 and 400 ng/mL
C. 450 and 600 ng/mL
D. 650 and 800 ng/mL

Trough cyclosporine blood levels in treatment of AA should be between 150 - 200 ng/mL.

698. Most important side effects of chronic cyclosporine treatment include all except?
Harrison's 20th Ed. Chapter 98 Page 728

A. Nephrotoxicity
B. Hepatotoxicity
C. Hypertension
D. Seizures

Most important side effects of chronic cyclosporine treatment are nephrotoxicity, hypertension, seizures & opportunistic infections especially Pneumocystis jiroveci..

699. Dose of Horse ATG in treatment of aplastic anemia is?
Harrison's 20th Ed. Chapter 98 Page 728

A. 40 mg/kg per day for 1 day
B. 40 mg/kg per day for 2 days
C. 40 mg/kg per day for 3 days
D. 40 mg/kg per day for 4 days

Horse ATG is given at 40 mg/kg per day for 4 days.

700. The single best method of preventing the spread of infection while treating patients of aplastic anemia is?
Harrison's 20th Ed. Chapter 98 Page 728

A. Prompt institution of parenteral, broad-spectrum antibiotics
B. Handwashing
C. Nonabsorbed antibiotics for gut decontamination
D. Total reverse isolation

Handwashing, the single best method of preventing the spread of infection, but remains a neglected practice.

701. In chronic anemia, iron chelators are given after how many blood transfusions?

Harrison's 20th Ed. Chapter 98 Page 728

A. 10
B. 20
C. 40
D. 50

In chronic anemia, iron chelators (deferoxamine & deferasirox) are given at around the fiftieth transfusion to avoid secondary hemochromatosis.

702. PRCA is characterized by?

Harrison's 20th Ed. Chapter 98 Page 728

A. Anemia
B. Reticulocytopenia
C. Absent or rare erythroid precursor cells in bone marrow
D. All of the above

PRCA is characterized by anemia, reticulocytopenia & absent or rare erythroid precursor cells in bone marrow.

703. Congenital pure red cell aplasia is known as?

Harrison's 20th Ed. Chapter 98 Page 729

A. Fanconi's anemia
B. Shwachman-Diamond syndrome
C. Kostmann's Syndrome
D. Diamond-Blackfan anemia

Diamond-Blackfan anemia or congenital PRCA is diagnosed at birth or in early childhood & often responds to glucocorticoid treatment. A minority of patients have etiologic mutations in a ribosomal RNA processing gene called RPS19.

704. Congenital pure red cell aplasia (Diamond-Blackfan syndrome) is which variety of PRCA?

Harrison's 20th Ed. Chapter 98 Page 729 Table 98–4

A. Fetal red blood cell aplasia
B. Hereditary pure red cell aplasia
C. Acquired pure red cell aplasia
D. Idiopathic

705. Drug that may cause PRCA is?

Harrison's 20th Ed. Chapter 98 Page 729 Table 98–4

A. Phenytoin
B. Chloramphenicol
C. Isoniazid
D. All of the above

Drug that may cause PRCA include phenytoin, azathioprine, chloramphenicol, procainamide, isoniazid and erythropoietin.

706. PRCA may be associated with which of the following?

Harrison's 20th Ed. Chapter 98 Page 729

A. Thymoma
B. Chronic lymphocytic leukemia
C. Subcutaneous administration of erythropoietin
D. All of the above

PRCA may be associated with thymoma, large granular lymphocytosis, chronic lymphocytic leukemia, hypogammaglobulinemic and subcutaneous administration of erythropoietin.

707. Pathognomonic cell in bone marrow of PRCA patients with B19 parvovirus infection is?

Harrison's 20th Ed. Chapter 98 Page 729

A. Uninuclear megakaryocyte
B. Giant megakayroblast
C. Giant pronormoblast
D. Ringed sideroblast

Bone marrow in PRCA due to chronic parvovirus infection shows red cell aplasia & giant pronormoblasts, which is the cytopathic sign of B19 parvovirus infection.

708. B19 parvovirus tropism for human erythroid progenitor cells is due to its use of which erythrocyte antigen?

Harrison's 20th Ed. Chapter 98 Page 730

A. L
B. M
C. P
D. S

B19 parvo viral tropism for human erythroid progenitor cells is due to its use of erythrocyte P antigen as a cellular receptor for entry.

709. PRCA patients with persistent B19 parvovirus infection respond best to?

Harrison's 20th Ed. Chapter 98 Page 730

A. Glucocorticoids
B. Intravenous immunoglobulin therapy
C. Cyclosporine
D. Daclizumab

Almost all patients with PRCA due to persistent B19 parvovirus infection respond to IV Ig therapy (0.4 gram/kg daily for 5 days). Majority of patients with idiopathic PRCA respond favorably to immunosuppression with glucocorticoids, cyclosporine, ATG, azathioprine, cyclophosphamide, and daclizumab (antibody to IL-2 receptor).

Transfusion Biology and Therapy

710. Production of antibodies directed against blood group antigens of another individual are called?
Harrison's 20th Ed. Chapter 109 Page 809

A. Alloantibodies
B. Heteroantibodies
C. Autoantibodies
D. Oligoantibodies

RBC's and other cellular blood elements & plasma proteins are antigenic and can result in alloimmunization i.e. production of antibodies directed against blood group antigens of another individual. These antibodies are called alloantibodies.

711. Antibodies resulting from "natural" exposure are?
Harrison's 20th Ed. Chapter 109 Page 809

A. IgG
B. IgM
C. IgA
D. IgE

Antibodies directed against RBC antigens resulting from "natural" exposure are of IgM isotype.

712. Antibodies that result from allogeneic exposure like transfusion or pregnancy are usually?
Harrison's 20th Ed. Chapter 109 Page 809

A. IgG
B. IgM
C. IgA
D. IgE

Blood transfusion or pregnancy (allogeneic exposure) result in IgG antibody formation. IgG antibodies can cross placenta resulting in hemolytic disease of the newborn, or hydrops fetalis.

713. A and B antigens are?
Harrison's 20th Ed. Chapter 109 Page 809

A. Carbohydrates
B. Proteins
C. Lipids
D. None of the above

A or B antigens are carbohydrates attached to a precursor backbone. They are found on cellular membrane either as glycosphingolipids or glycoproteins, and are secreted into plasma and body fluids as glycoproteins.

714. Immediate precursor upon which A & B antigen are added is?
Harrison's 20th Ed. Chapter 109 Page 809

A. H substance
B. P substance
C. Z substance
D. K substance

H substance is the immediate precursor on which the A and B antigens are added.

715. In the formation of H substance, the essential substance is?
Harrison's 20th Ed. Chapter 109 Page 809

A. Fucose
B. Galactose
C. Fructose
D. Mannose

H substance is formed by the addition of fucose to the glycolipid or glycoprotein backbone.

716. Addition of N-acetylgalactosamine to H substance creates?
Harrison's 20th Ed. Chapter 109 Page 809

A. A antigen
B. B antigen
C. Rh antigen
D. None of the above

717. Addition of galactose to H substance creates?
Harrison's 20th Ed. Chapter 109 Page 809

A. A antigen
B. B antigen
C. Rh antigen
D. None of the above

Addition of N-acetylgalactosamine creates A antigen, while addition of galactose produces B antigen.

718. Genes that determine A & B phenotypes are found on chromosome?
Harrison's 20th Ed. Chapter 109 Page 809

A. 6 p
B. 7 p
C. 8 p
D. 9 p

719. Genes that determine the A and B phenotypes are expressed in?
Harrison's 20th Ed. Chapter 109 Page 809

A. Mendelian dominant manner
B. Mendelian recessive manner
C. Mendelian codominant manner
D. None of the above

The genes that determine the A and B phenotypes are found on chromosome 9p and are expressed in a Mendelian codominant manner.

720. Which of the following "transferases" contributes to the formation of A or B blood groups?
Harrison's 20th Ed. Chapter 109 Page 809

A. N-acetyl transferase (NAT)
B. Glutathione-S-transferase
C. Histone acetyl transferase (HAT)
D. Glycosyl transferases

Glycosyl transferases are gene products which confer enzymatic capability of attaching specific antigenic carbohydrate. Individuals who lack "A" and "B" transferases are phenotypically type "O" while those who inherit both transferases are type "AB".

721. Naturally occurring anti-A and anti-B antibodies are termed?
Harrison's 20th Ed. Chapter 109 Page 810

A. Isoagglutinins
B. Homoagglutinins
C. Naturoagglutinins
D. AB agglutinins

Naturally occurring anti-A & anti-B antibodies are termed isoagglutinins.

722. Isoagglutinin found in type AB individuals is?
Harrison's 20th Ed. Chapter 109 Page 810

A. Anti-A
B. Anti-B
C. Anti-A + Anti-B
D. None of the above

723. Isoagglutinin found in type O individuals is?
Harrison's 20th Ed. Chapter 109 Page 810

A. Anti-A
B. Anti-B
C. Anti-A + Anti-B
D. None of the above

Type A individuals produce anti-B, while type B individuals make anti-A isoagglutinins. Neither isoagglutinin is found in type AB individuals. Type O individuals produce both anti-A & anti-B.

724. Individuals with Bombay phenotype produce antibodies to?
Harrison's 20th Ed. Chapter 109 Page 810

A. H substance
B. A antigens
C. B antigens
D. All of the above

Individuals with Bombay phenotype produce antibodies to H substance as well as to both A & B antigens and are therefore compatible only with other hh donors.

725. Nonsecretors of A & B antigens by cells in the circulation are susceptible to?
Harrison's 20th Ed. Chapter 109 Page 810

A. Hemolysis
B. Malignancy
C. Infections
D. All of the above

A & B antigens are secreted by cells in the circulation. Nonsecretors are susceptible to infections (C. albicans, N. meningitidis, S. pneumoniae, H. influenzae) as they may bind to polysaccharides on cells. Soluble blood group antigens block this binding.

726. Gene determining Rh phenotypes is found on chromosome?
Harrison's 20th Ed. Chapter 109 Page 810

A. 1
B. 2
C. 3
D. 4

727. Which of the following is Rh antigen?
Harrison's 20th Ed. Chapter 109 Page 810

A. C
B. D
C. E
D. All of the above

The three Rh genes, E/e, D, and C/c, are arranged in tandem on chromosome 1 and inherited as a haplotype, i.e., cDE or Cde.

728. What percentage of of people lack the D antigen?
Harrison's 20th Ed. Chapter 109 Page 810

A. About 15%
B. About 20%
C. About 25%
D. About 30%

~15% of individuals lack D alloantigen.

729. Which of the following is not a RBC blood group system?
Harrison's 20th Ed. Chapter 109 Page 810 Table 109–1

A. Lewis
B. Smith
C. Kell
D. Duffy

RBC blood group systems are Rh (D, C/c, E/e), Lewis (Lea, Leb), Kell (K/k), Duffy (Fya/Fyb), Kidd (Jka/Jkb), I/i and MNSsU.

730. The Lewis gene is located on?
Harrison's 20th Ed. Chapter 109 Page 810

A. Chromosome 10
B. Chromosome 12
C. Chromosome 15
D. Chromosome 19

Lewis gene product is a fucosyl transferase and maps to chromosome 19.

731. Which of the following statements about antibodies to Lewis antigens is false?
Harrison's 20th Ed. Chapter 109 Page 810

A. Usually IgM type
B. Can cross placenta
C. Cause incompatibility during pretransfusion screening
D. None of the above

Lewis antigens cannot cross placenta.

732. Paroxysmal Cold Hemoglobinuria (PCH) is related to?
Harrison's 20th Ed. Chapter 109 Page 810

A. Lewis system
B. P system
C. MNSsU system
D. I system

In PCH, autoantibody with biphasic properties (Donath-Landsteiner antibodies) to P is produced that binds to RBCs in cold & fixes complement upon warming.

733. Which of the following antigen is the cellular receptor for Plasmodium vivax?
Harrison's 20th Ed. Chapter 109 Page 810

A. Lewis antigen
B. Kidd antigen
C. P antigen
D. Duffy antigen

Duffy antigens serve as receptors for Plasmodium vivax. >70% of persons in malaria-endemic areas lack these antigens.

734. In Plasmodium falciparum infection, which of the following microbial ligand interacts with host receptor Glycophorin A?
Harrison's 20th Ed. Chapter 109 Page 867 Table 116–1

A. Erythrocyte-binding protein 165 (EBA-165)
B. Erythrocyte-binding protein 175 (EBA-175)
C. Erythrocyte-binding protein 185 (EBA-185)
D. Erythrocyte-binding protein 195 (EBA-195)

735. Which of the following antigen is the cellular receptor of parvovirus B19?
Harrison's 20th Ed. Chapter 109 Page 810

A. Lewis antigen
B. Kidd antigen
C. P antigen
D. Duffy antigen

The P antigen is the cellular receptor of parvovirus B19.

736. Which of the following gene is present on the X chromosome?
Harrison's 20th Ed. Chapter 109 Page 810

A. AB
B. Rh
C. Kell
D. Lewis

Kell precursor protein is controlled by a gene on X.

737. Virtually every donor is incompatible because nearly all persons express?
Harrison's 20th Ed. Chapter 109 Page 810

A. M
B. N
C. S
D. U

Anti-U antibodies are rare but problematic. Virtually every donor is incompatible because nearly all persons express U.

738. After ABO and Rh systems, which of the following RBC blood group system is most immunogenic?
Harrison's 20th Ed. Chapter 109 Page 810

A. Lewis
B. MNSsU
C. Kell
D. Duffy

The immunogenicity of Kell is third behind the ABO and Rh systems.

739. McLeod syndrome is related to which of the following blood group antigens?
Harrison's 20th Ed. Chapter 109 Page 810

A. Lewis
B. Kidd
C. Kell
D. Duffy

McLeod syndrome is due to absence of Kell precursor protein that leads to acanthocytosis, shortened RBC survival & progressive form of muscular dystrophy that includes cardiac defects.

740. Collection of multiple units of platelets from a single donor is called?
Harrison's 20th Ed. Chapter 109 Page 811

A. Thrombopheresis technology
B. Hyperpheresis technology
C. Neopheresis technology
D. Apheresis technology

Collection of multiple units of platelets from a single donor is done by Apheresis technology.

741. Which of the following is not a processed component of whole blood?
Harrison's 20th Ed. Chapter 109 Page 811

A. Packed RBC (PRBC)
B. Platelets
C. Heat precipitate
D. Cryoprecipitate

Blood products intended for transfusion are routinely collected as whole blood (450 mL) in various anticoagulants. Most donated blood is processed into following components - PRBCs, platelets, and fresh-frozen plasma (FFP) or cryoprecipitate. By slow centrifugation, whole blood is first separated into PRBCs & platelet-rich plasma (PRP). Platelet-rich plasma is then centrifuged at high speed to yield one unit of random donor (RD) platelets & one unit of FFP. Cryoprecipitate is produced by thawing FFP to precipitate the plasma proteins, then separated by centrifugation.

742. Single-donor apheresis platelets (SDAP) is equivalent to how many units of random donor (RD) platelets?
Harrison's 20th Ed. Chapter 109 Page 811

A. 2
B. 4
C. 5
D. 8

Single-donor apheresis platelets (SDAP) contain platelets equivalent to ~5 units of random donor (RD) platelets.

743. Threshold for prophylactic platelet transfusion in patients without fever or infections is?
Harrison's 20th Ed. Chapter 109 Page 812

A. 5,000/μL
B. 10,000/μL
C. 25,000/μL
D. 50,000/μL

Threshold for prophylactic platelet transfusion in patients without fever or infections is 5,000/μL. 50000/μL for those undergoing invasive procedures.

744. Refractoriness to rise in post-transfusion platelet counts is investigated by?

Harrison's 20th Ed. Chapter 109 Page 812

A. Anti-HLA antibodies in recipient's serum
B. Anti-Jk antibodies in recipient's serum
C. Anti-U antibodies in recipient's serum
D. Anti-I autoantibodies in recipient's serum

Refractoriness to rise in post transfusion platelet counts is investigated by detecting anti-HLA antibodies in the recipient's serum.

745. Fresh-Frozen Plasma (FFP) contains all except?

Harrison's 20th Ed. Chapter 109 Page 812

A. Fibrinogen
B. Prothrombin
C. Antithrombin
D. Proteins C and S

FFP contains stable coagulation factors and plasma proteins like fibrinogen, antithrombin, albumin, and proteins C and S.

746. Cryoprecipitate is a source of?

Harrison's 20th Ed. Chapter 109 Page 812

A. Fibrinogen
B. Factor VIII
C. von Willebrand factor (vWF)
D. All of the above

Cryoprecipitate is a source of fibrinogen, factor VIII & von Willebrand factor (vWF).

747. Each unit of cryoprecipitate contains how much of factor VIII?

Harrison's 20th Ed. Chapter 109 Page 812

A. ~ 20 units
B. ~ 80 units
C. ~ 200 units
D. ~ 800 units

Each unit of cryoprecipitate contains ~80 units of factor VIII.

748. Infectious agents rarely associated with transfusion include?

Harrison's 20th Ed. Chapter 109 Page 813 Table 109–3

A. West Nile virus
B. Hepatitis A virus
C. Treponema pallidum
D. All of the above

Infectious agents rarely associated with transfusion include West Nile virus, hepatitis A virus, parvovirus B-19, Babesia microti (babesiosis), Borrelia burgdorferi (Lyme disease), Anaplasma phagocytophilum (human granulocytic ehrlichiosis), Trypanosoma cruzi (Chagas disease), Treponema pallidum, and human herpesvirus-8.

749. Laboratory evaluation for post-transfusion hemolysis includes?

Harrison's 20th Ed. Chapter 109 Page 812

A. Haptoglobin
B. Lactate dehydrogenase (LDH)
C. Indirect bilirubin
D. All of the above

Laboratory evaluation for posttransfusion hemolysis includes the measurement of serum haptoglobin, lactate dehydrogenase (LDH), and indirect bilirubin levels.

750. Most frequent reaction associated with transfusion of cellular blood components is?

Harrison's 20th Ed. Chapter 109 Page 813

A. Febrile Nonhemolytic Transfusion Reaction (FNHTR)
B. Allergic Reactions
C. Anaphylactic Reaction
D. Graft-versus-host disease (GVHD)

Most frequent reaction associated with transfusion of cellular blood components is a febrile nonhemolytic transfusion reaction (FNHTR). Antibodies directed against donor leukocyte & HLA antigens & cytokines released from cells within stored blood components mediate these reactions.

751. Risk of TRALI after blood transfusion is?

Harrison's 20th Ed. Chapter 109 Page 813 Table 109-3

A. 1 : 1000
B. 1 : 5000
C. 1 : 10000
D. 1 : 50000

TRALI refers to transfusion-related acute lung injury. Its risk is 1 : 5000.

752. Which of the following infection is most frequent with blood transfusion?

Harrison's 20th Ed. Chapter 109 Page 813 Table 109-3

A. HIV-1, -2
B. Hepatitis B
C. Hepatitis C
D. Malaria

753. Urticarial reactions are related to which of the following components of transfused blood?

Harrison's 20th Ed. Chapter 109 Page 813

A. RBC
B. Platelets
C. Plasma proteins
D. Leucocytes

Urticarial reactions are related to plasma proteins found in transfused components.

754. Patients with which of the following are at risk for anaphylactic reactions associated with plasma transfusion?

Harrison's 20th Ed. Chapter 109 Page 813

A. IgA deficiency
B. IgG deficiency
C. IgE deficiency
D. IgM deficiency

Patients who are IgA-deficient are at risk for anaphylactic reactions associated with plasma transfusion and should therefore receive only IgA-deficient plasma and washed cellular blood components.

755. Alloantibodies directed against which of the following RBC antigens does not result in hemolysis?

Harrison's 20th Ed. Chapter 109 Page 813 Page Table 109-1

A. Rh
B. Kell
C. I
D. Duffy

I and i are not allelic pairs but are carbohydrate antigens. Alloantibodies directed against other RBC antigens like Rh, Kell, and Duffy may result in hemolysis.

756. Which of the following can occur after blood/blood product transfusion?

Harrison's 20th Ed. Chapter 109 Page 813

A. Graft-versus-host disease (GVHD)
B. Hypothermia
C. Thrombocytopenia
D. All of the above

No transfusion is a zero-risk event. Predominantly in women, thrombocytopenia may occur 7 - 10 days after platelet transfusion. Platelet-specific antibodies are found in recipient's serum, and most frequently recognized antigen is HPA-1a found on the platelet glycoprotein IIIa receptor. Antibodies react to both donor & recipient platelets, hence the delay. Treatment with IVIg neutralizes the effector antibodies. Plasmapheresis can be used to remove the antibodies.

757. Transfusion-associated GVHD (TA-GVHD) is characterized by?

Harrison's 20th Ed. Chapter 109 Page 813

A. Marrow aplasia & pancytopenia
B. Resistance to immunosuppressive therapies
C. Clinical manifestations appear at 8 - 10 days
D. All of the above

TA-GVHD is characterized by marrow aplasia & pancytopenia. It is highly resistant to treatment with immunosuppressive therapies like glucocorticoids, cyclosporine, antithymocyte globulin & ablative therapy followed by allogeneic bone marrow transplantation. Clinical manifestations appear at 8 - 10 days and death occurs at 3 - 4 weeks posttransfusion.

758. Transfusion-related acute lung injury (TRALI) occurs within how many hours after blood transfusion?

Harrison's 20th Ed. Chapter 109 Page 813

A. 6 hours
B. 12 hours
C. 24 hours
D. 48 hours

TRALI, an acute respiratory distress syndrome, occurs within 6 hours after blood transfusion & is characterized by dyspnea & hypoxia due to noncardiogenic pulmonary edema.

759. Cause of TRALI usually is?

Harrison's 20th Ed. Chapter 109 Page 814

A. High-titer anti-HLA antibodies in recepient plasma
B. Low-titer anti-HLA antibodies in donor plasma
C. High-titer anti-HLA antibodies in donor plasma
D. HPA-1a on the platelet glycoprotein IIIa receptor

TRALI usually results from the transfusion of donor plasma that contains high-titer anti-HLA class II antibodies that bind recipient leukocytes which aggregate in pulmonary vasculature & release mediators that increase capillary permeability.

760. Iron content in each unit of RBCs transfusion is?

Harrison's 20th Ed. Chapter 109 Page 815

A. 100 to 125 mg of iron
B. 125 to 150 mg of iron
C. 150 to 200 mg of iron
D. 200 to 250 mg of iron

Each unit of RBCs contains 200 - 250 mg of iron.

761. Symptoms and signs of iron overload are common after how many units of RBCs transfusion?

Harrison's 20th Ed. Chapter 109 Page 815

A. 10
B. 20
C. 50
D. 100

Symptoms and signs of iron overload (endocrine, hepatic, cardiac) are common after 100 units of RBC transfusion (total-body iron load of 20 grams).

762. Transient hypotension during blood transfusion is more common in those taking?

Harrison's 20th Ed. Chapter 109 Page 815

A. Angiotensin-converting enzyme (ACE) inhibitors
B. Beta blockers
C. Calcium channel blockers
D. All of the above

Transient hypotension is noted in transfused patients taking ACE inhibitors due to increased bradykinin levels. Blood products contain bradykinin that is normally degraded by ACE.

763. Nucleic acid amplification testing (NAT) is used to prevent which of the following complications of transfusion?

Harrison's 20th Ed. Chapter 109 Page 815

A. Transfusion-associated GVHD
B. Infectious complications
C. Transfusion-related acute lung injury (TRALI)
D. All of the above

764. Which of the following carries the least risk of transmission through blood transfusion?

Harrison's 20th Ed. Chapter 109 Page 813 Table 109-3

A. Hepatitis B
B. Hepatitis C
C. HIV-1
D. Malaria

No cases of HIV-2 infection have been reported in the United States since 1992. Other infectious agents rarely associated with transfusion include - Hepatitis A virus, parvovirus B-19, Babesia microti (babesiosis), Borrelia burgdorferi (Lyme disease), Trypanosoma cruzi (Chagas disease), and Treponema pallidum , human herpesvirus-8 and hepatitis G virus.

765. To detect HIV-1 infection, donor blood is tested for?

Harrison's 20th Ed. Chapter 109 Page 815

A. p24 antigen
B. Glycoprotein 120
C. Glycoprotein 41
D. All of the above

Donated blood is tested for antibodies to HIV-1, HIV-1 p24 antigen, and HIV RNA using Nucleic acid amplification testing (NAT). Risk of HIV-1 infection per transfusion episode is 1 in 2 million.

766. Bacteria most commonly implicated in contamination of red cells during blood transfusion is?

Harrison's 20th Ed. Chapter 109 Page 815

A. Staphylococcus aureus
B. Klebsiella pneumoniae
C. Yersinia enterocolitica
D. Staphylococcus epidermidis

Organism most commonly causing bacterial contamination of RBCs is Yersinia enterocolitica. Yersinia, Pseudomonas, Serratia, Acinetobacter, and Escherichia species have all been implicated in infections related to PRBC transfusion.

767. Parasitic diseases that can be transmitted by blood transfusion include?

Harrison's 20th Ed. Chapter 109 Page 815

A. Malaria
B. Babesiosis
C. Chagas' disease
D. All of the above

Parasitic diseases that can be transmitted by blood transfusion include malaria, babesiosis, Chagas disease. Dengue, chikungunya virus, variant Creutzfeldt-Jakob disease, Anaplasma phagocytophilum, and yellow fever vaccine virus can also be transmitted by blood transfusion.

768. Perfluorocarbons are best known as?

N Engl J Med 2005;353:2042-55

A. Oxygen-carrying blood substitutes
B. Protein substitutes
C. Fat substitutes
D. Iron chelators

Oxygen-carrying blood substitutes, such as perfluorocarbons and aggregated hemoglobin solution, are presently in various stages of clinical trials.

769. Specialized tissues that sense local oxygen tension include?

N Engl J Med 2005;353:2042-55

A. Glomus cells of the carotid body
B. Neuroepithelial bodies in the lungs
C. Chromaffin cells of the fetal adrenal medulla
D. All of the above

770. Specialized tissues that sense local oxygen tension include?

N Engl J Med 2005;353:2042-55

A. Smooth-muscle cells of the resistance pulmonary arteries
B. Fetoplacental arteries
C. Ductus arteriosus
D. All of the above

771. What are Howell–Jolly bodies?

N Engl J Med 2005;353:498-507

A. Nuclear fragments
B. Hemosiderin-containing granules
C. Altered ribosomes
D. All of the above

772. What are Pappenheimer bodies?

N Engl J Med 2005;353:498-507

A. Nuclear fragments
B. Hemosiderin-containing granules
C. Altered ribosomes
D. All of the above

773. What is basophilic stippling or punctate basophilia?

N Engl J Med 2005;353:498-507

A. Nuclear fragments
B. Hemosiderin-containing granules
C. Altered ribosomes
D. All of the above

774. Microspherocytes can be found in?

N Engl J Med 2005;353:498-507

A. Spherocytic hemolytic anemia
B. Microangiopathic hemolytic anemia
C. Burns
D. All of the above

Disorders of Platelets and Vessel Wall

775. Major regulator of platelet production - thrombopoietin (TPO) is synthesized in?
Harrison's 20th Ed. Chapter 111 Page 823

A. Kidney
B. Liver
C. Muscle
D. Adipose tissue

Thrombopoietin (TPO) is a hormone synthesized in liver that regulates platelet production.

776. Synthesis of thrombopoietin is increased specifically by?
Harrison's 20th Ed. Chapter 111 Page 823

A. Interleukin 6
B. Prostaglandin D2
C. TNF alpha
D. Interferon beta

Synthesis is increased with inflammation and specifically by interleukin 6.

777. Average life span of platelets in circulation is?
Harrison's 20th Ed. Chapter 111 Page 823

A. 1 – 3 days
B. 3 – 7 days
C. 7 – 10 days
D. 11 – 18 days

Average life span of platelets in circulation is 7-10 days. Platelets were identified in 1865 and their function was elucidated by Giulio Bizzozero in 1882.

778. What proportion of platelets reside in the spleen?
Harrison's 20th Ed. Chapter 111 Page 823

A. One-third
B. Half
C. Two-third
D. Three-fourth

Approximately one-third of the platelets reside in the spleen

779. Which of the following statements is false?
Harrison's 20th Ed. Chapter 111 Page 823

A. TPO binds to its receptor on platelets
B. TPO binds to its receptor on megakaryocytes
C. Platelets are anucleate
D. None of the above

TPO binds to its receptor on platelets and megakaryocytes and is thus removed from the circulation. Therefore, a reduction in platelet and megakaryocyte mass increases the level of TPO, which then stimulates platelet production.

780. Which of the following statements is false?
Harrison's 20th Ed. Chapter 111 Page 823

A. Nitric oxide is a platelet inhibitor
B. Endothelin is a platelet activator
C. Platelets adhere to exposed intimal surface through VWF
D. None of the above

Endothelium-derived vasodilator nitric oxide is a platelet inhibitor. Endothelium-derived vasoconstrictor endothelin is a platelet activator.

781. Pseudothrombocytopenia is due to?
Harrison's 20th Ed. Chapter 111 Page 823

A. Exercise
B. Laboratory artifact
C. Cold weather
D. Fasting

Pseudothrombocytopenia is an in vitro artifact resulting by blood collection.

782. Pseudothrombocytopenia is most likely when blood is collected with which of the following anticoagulants?
Harrison's 20th Ed. Chapter 111 Page 823

A. EDTA
B. Sodium citrate
C. Heparin
D. All of the above

Pseudothrombocytopenia is an in vitro artifact resulting from platelet agglutination via antibodies when the calcium content is decreased by blood collection in ethylenediamine tetraacetic (EDTA) anticoagulated blood tubes.

783. Which of the following is the most common cause of thrombocytopenia?
Harrison's 20th Ed. Chapter 111 Page 823

A. Inherited disorders
B. Myelodysplasia
C. Drugs
D. Pseudothrombocytopenia

Drugs are the most common cause of thrombocytopenia.

784. What is the platelet count required to maintain vascular integrity in the microcirculation?
Harrison's 20th Ed. Chapter 111 Page 823

A. 5000 – 10,000/μL
B. 15000 – 20,000/μL
C. 25000 – 40,000/μL
D. 50000 – 100,000/μL

A platelet count of ~5000 - 10,000 is required to maintain vascular integrity in microcirculation.

785. Which of the following statements about petechiae is false?
Harrison's 20th Ed. Chapter 111 Page 823

A. Nonblanching hemorrhages
B. First appear in areas of increased venous pressure
C. Pinpoint
D. Sign of a platelet dysfunction

Petechiae first appear in areas of increased venous pressure and are pinpoint, nonblanching hemorrhages and are usually a sign of a decreased platelet number and not platelet dysfunction. Excessive bruising is seen in disorders of both platelet number and function.

786. In wet purpura, blood blisters form on?
Harrison's 20th Ed. Chapter 111 Page 823

A. Sole
B. Palm
C. Oral mucosa
D. Scalp

Wet purpura, blood blisters that form on the oral mucosa denote an increased risk of life-threatening hemorrhage in the thrombocytopenic patient.

787. Immune-mediated thrombocytopenia (ITP2) in children usually follows which of the following?
Harrison's 20th Ed. Chapter 111 Page 823

A. Bacterial infection
B. Viral infection
C. Drug ingestion
D. Any of the above

Immune-mediated thrombocytopenia (ITP2) in children usually follows a viral infection and almost always resolves spontaneously.

788. Which out of the following drugs is most capable of inducing drug-dependent antibodies?
Harrison's 20th Ed. Chapter 111 Page 825

A. Amiadarone
B. Cephalosporin
C. Digoxin
D. Quinine

Classic drug-dependent antibodies are antibodies that react with specific platelet surface antigens and result in thrombocytopenia only when the drug is present. They are more common with quinine, quinidine, rifampicin, and trimethoprim-sulphamethoxazole.

789. Drug induced thrombocytopenia usually resolves how many days after drug withdrawal?
Harrison's 20th Ed. Chapter 111 Page 825

A. 1 – 3 days
B. 3 – 7 days
C. 7 – 10 days
D. 14 - 21 days

Drug induced thrombocytopenia typically occurs after a period of initial exposure (median length 21 days), or upon reexposure, and usually resolves in 7-10 days after drug withdrawal.

790. Which of the following is false about Heparin-Induced Thrombocytopenia (HIT)?
Harrison's 20th Ed. Chapter 111 Page 825

A. HIT is not usually severe
B. HIT is not associated with bleeding
C. HIT markedly increases risk of thrombosis
D. None of the above

791. In Heparin-Induced Thrombocytopenia (HIT), antibody formation is against which of the following?
Harrison's 20th Ed. Chapter 111 Page 825

A. Platelet factor 4 (PF4)
B. Heparin
C. Platelet factor 4 (PF4) and heparin complex
D. Endothelial cells

HIT results from antibody formation to a complex of platelet-specific protein platelet factor 4 (PF4) and heparin. Anti-heparin/PF4 antibody can activate platelets through FcgRIIa receptor and also activate monocytes and endothelial cells.

792. As compared to LMWH, HIT is how many times more common with the use of UFH?
Harrison's 20th Ed. Chapter 111 Page 825

A. Twice
B. Thrice
C. 5 times
D. 10 times

HIT is about 10 times more common with the use of unfractionated heparin (UFH) than after exposure to low-molecular-weight heparin (LMWH).

793. Most patients develop HIT after exposure to heparin for how many days?
Harrison's 20th Ed. Chapter 111 Page 825

A. 1 – 3 days
B. 3 – 5 days
C. 5 –14 days
D. 14 – 21 days

Most patients develop HIT after exposure to heparin for 5 – 14 days.

794. Which of the following statements about HIT is false?
Harrison's 20th Ed. Chapter 111 Page 825

A. Occurs earlier if heparin given within past 3 months
B. More common in medical than in surgical patients
C. HIT is more frequent in females than in males
D. Platelet count rarely fall to <20000/μL

HIT is more common in surgical patients than in medical patients

795. Which of the following about HIT is false?
Harrison's 20th Ed. Chapter 111 Page 825

A. Most specific diagnostic test is serotonin release assay
B. Venous thrombosis more common than arterial thrombosis
C. Platelet transfusions are not advised
D. None of the above

796. Which of the following drugs is effective in the treatment of Heparin induced thrombocytopenia and thrombosis (HITT)?
Harrison's 20th Ed. Chapter 111 Page 825

A. Argatroban
B. Lepirudin
C. Danaparoid
D. All of the above

Early recognition, prompt discontinuation of heparin and use of alternative anticoagulants is key in treatment of HIT. Argatroban, Lepirudin, Danaparoid, Bivalirudin & Fondaparinux are effective in HITT.

797. Secondary immune thrombocytopenic purpura is associated with which of the following diseases?

Harrison's 20th Ed. Chapter 111 Page 825

A. Systemic lupus erythematosis (SLE)

B. HIV

C. Hepatitis C

D. All of the above

Immune/idiopathic thrombocytopenic purpura ITP is termed secondary if it is associated with an underlying disorder like systemic lupus erythematosis (SLE), HIV and hepatitis C

798. Evans's syndrome refers to?

Harrison's 20th Ed. Chapter 111 Page 826

A. Autoimmune hemolytic anemia with ITP

B. SLE with ITP

C. HIV with ITP

D. Hepatitis C with ITP

Autoimmune hemolytic anemia with ITP is termed as Evans's syndrome.

799. Which of the following is not consistent with the diagnosis of hemolytic anemia?

N Engl J Med 2013;369:2032-43

A. Raised lactate dehydrogenase

B. Raised indirect bilirubin

C. Raised haptoglobin

D. Dark urine

Raised levels of lactate dehydrogenase & indirect bilirubin and low haptoglobin levels favour diagnosis of hemolytic anemia.

800. Secondary causes of Evans Syndrome is?

N Engl J Med 2013;369:2032-43

A. Systemic lupus erythematosus

B. Antiphospholipid antibody syndrome

C. Sjogren's syndrome

D. All of the above

Evans syndrome is characterized by thrombocytopenia and auto-immune haemolytic anaemia (AIHA). Autoimmune diseases that can secondarily cause Evans Syndrome include Systemic lupus erythematosus, Antiphospholipid antibody syndrome and Sjogren's syndrome.

801. Thrombocytopenia related mortality increases with platelet counts less than?

Harrison's 20th Ed. Chapter 111 Page 826

A. 30,000/μL

B. 50,000/μL

C. 75,000/μL

D. 100,000/μL

Patients with platelet counts >30,000/μL appear not to have increased mortality related to the thrombocytopenia.

802. All IVIgG immunoglobulin preparations are derived from?

Harrison's 20th Ed. Chapter 111 Page 826

A. Human plasma

B. Horse plasma

C. Bovine plasma

D. Pig plasma

All IVIgG immunoglobulin preparations are derived from human plasma.

803. In ITP, total dose of IVIgG is?

Harrison's 20th Ed. Chapter 111 Page 826

A. 1 gram/kg

B. 2 gram/kg

C. 3 gram/kg

D. 4 gram/kg

In ITP, total dose of IVIgG is 2 gram/kg.

804. Which of the following drugs is useful in refractory ITP?

Harrison's 20th Ed. Chapter 111 Page 826

A. Rituximab

B. Romiplostim

C. Eltrombopag

D. All of the above

Rituximab, an anti-CD20 (B cell) antibody, has shown efficacy in the treatment of refractory ITP. Two thrombopoietin receptor agonists - one administered subcutaneously (romiplostim) and another orally (eltrombopag), have shown response in many patients with refractory ITP.

805. Large platelets is a feature of which of the following?

Harrison's 20th Ed. Chapter 111 Page 826

A. May-Hegglin anomaly

B. Sebastian syndrome

C. Epstein's syndrome

D. All of the above

May-Hegglin anomaly, and Sebastian, Epstein's, and Fechtner syndromes have thrombocytopenia with large platelets & are inherited as autosomal dominant & are associated with mutations in nonmuscle myosin heavy chain MYH9 gene.

806. Autosomal recessive inherited thrombocytopenic disorders include?

Harrison's 20th Ed. Chapter 111 Page 826

A. Congenital amegakaryocytic thrombocytopenia

B. Thrombocytopenia with absent radii

C. Bernard Soulier syndrome

D. All of the above

Autosomal recessive inherited thrombocytopenic disorders include congenital amegakaryocytic thrombocytopenia, thrombocytopenia with absent radii and Bernard Soulier syndrome.

807. Which of the following is inherited as X-linked pattern in inherited thrombocytopenia?

Harrison's 20th Ed. Chapter 111 Page 826

A. May-Hegglin anomaly

B. Wiskott-Aldrich syndrome

C. Fechtner syndrome

D. Bernard-Soulier syndrome

X-linked inherited thrombocytopenic disorders include Wiskott-Aldrich syndrome.

808. Which of the following is false regarding thrombotic thrombocytopenic microangiopathies?

Harrison's 20th Ed. Chapter 111 Page 826

A. Thrombocytopenia
B. Laboratory evidence of hemolysis
C. Abnormal PT and aPTT
D. Microvascular thrombosis

Thrombotic thrombocytopenic microangiopathies are characterized by thrombocytopenia, microangiopathic hemolytic anemia, laboratory evidence of hemolysis & microvascular thrombosis. It includes thrombotic thrombocytopenic purpura (TTP) & hemolytic uremic syndrome (HUS). PT & aPTT are characteristically normal in TTP or HUS and is used to differentiate TTP from DIC. Despite thrombocytopenia, severe bleeds are uncommon. Neurologic changes are common in TTP, renal failure in HUS & neurologic or renal changes are absent in HELLP.

809. Thrombotic thrombocytopenic purpura (TTP) was first described by?

Harrison's 20th Ed. Chapter 111 Page 826

A. Balint
B. Eli Moschcowitz
C. Verner-Morrison
D. Wiskott-Aldrich

TTP was initially described by Dr Eli Moschcowitz at the Mount Sinai Hospital in New York City in 1924. Thrombotic thrombocytopenic purpura (TTP) is also called Moschcowitz disease.

810. Which of the following is not a feature of TTP?

Harrison's 20th Ed. Chapter 111 Page 826

A. Microangiopathic hemolytic anemia
B. Renal failure
C. Hepatic failure
D. Neurologic dysfunction

TTP is characterized by a pentad of findings that include microangiopathic hemolytic anemia, thrombocytopenia, renal failure, neurologic findings, and fever. Schistocytes are typically seen in PBF.

811. Upshaw-Schulman syndrome is related to?

Harrison's 20th Ed. Chapter 111 Page 826

A. Multiple transfusions
B. Thrombotic thrombocytopenic purpura
C. Uremia
D. CHF

Upshaw Schulman syndrome is due to a hereditary deficiency of a metalloprotease that cleaves vWF which is normally secreted as ultra-large multimers. It is cleaved by ADAMTS13. Persistence of ultra-large vWF molecules produces pathogenic platelet adhesion & aggregation.

812. Upshaw-Schulman syndrome is best related to?

Harrison's 20th Ed. Chapter 111 Page 826

A. Idiopathic TTP
B. Inherited TTP
C. Medication-related TTP
D. TTP in pregnant women

Hereditary form of TTP is called Upshaw-Schulman syndrome. It is due to inherited deficiency of or antibodies to the plasma metalloprotease ADAMTS13. 5-10% of all TTP cases are due to Upshaw-Schulman syndrome.

813. TTP is due to deficiency in the activity of?

Harrison's 20th Ed. Chapter 111 Page 826

A. ADAMTS 11
B. ADAMTS 12
C. ADAMTS 13
D. ADAMTS 14

ADAMTS 13 is a member of ADAMTS (a disintegrin with thrombospondin type 1 motifs) zinc metalloproteinase family that cleaves vWF complexes & prevents vWF-platelet interaction. Severe deficiency of ADAMTS causes TTP.

814. Which of the following is related to TTP?

Harrison's 20th Ed. Chapter 111 Page 826

A. ADAMTS-10
B. ADAMTS-11
C. ADAMTS-12
D. ADAMTS-13

Plasma metalloprotease ADAMTS-13 (vWF-cleaving protease) is responsible for proteolytic cleavage of large hemostatically hyperactive vWf multimers that are synthesized and secreted by endothelial cells in plasma into smaller less adhesive multimers. ADAMTS-13 prevents inappropriate microvascular platelet aggregation. Deficiency of ADAMTS-13 results in TTP. The relationship of reduced ADAMTS13 to the pathogenesis of TTP is known as the Furlan-Tsai hypothesis.

815. Which of the following is false about ADAMTS-13?

Harrison's 20th Ed. Chapter 111 Page 826

A. ADAMTS-13 prevents inappropriate microvascular platelet aggregation
B. Deficiency of ADAMTS-13 is a finding for TTP
C. vWf multimers is the physiologic substrate for ADAMTS-13
D. None of the above

Various studies support the clinical diagnosis of TTP when ADAMTS-13, the vWf-cleaving protease, activity is less than 5% of the activity in normal human plasma.

816. Which of the following is false about ADAMTS-13?

Harrison's 20th Ed. Chapter 111 Page 826

A. ADAMTS refers to "A Disintegrin-like And Metalloprotease with ThromboSpondin type 1 motif"
B. Human ADAMTS-13 gene is on chromosome 9q34
C. ADAMTS-13 molecule depends upon zinc and calcium ions for activity
D. None of the above

817. Idiopathic TTP is more common in?

Harrison's 20th Ed. Chapter 111 Page 826

A. Women
B. HIV infection
C. Pregnant women
D. All of the above

Idiopathic TTP is more common in women, HIV infection & in pregnant women.

818. Which of the following antiplatelet agent has been implicated in the causation of TTP?

Harrison's 20th Ed. Chapter 111 Page 826

A. Aspirin
B. Ticlopidine
C. Carvadilol
D. All of the above

Medication-related TTP may be secondary to antibody formation (ticlopidine and possibly c1opidogrel) or direct endothelial toxicity (cyclosporine, mitomycin C, tacrolimus, quinine).

819. In TTP, hyaline thrombi without inflammatory changes in vessel wall may be found in?

Harrison's 20th Ed. Chapter 111 Page 826

A. Arterioles
B. Capillaries
C. Venules
D. All of the above

Presence of hyaline thrombi in arterioles, capillaries & venules without any inflammatory changes in the vessel wall is diagnostic of TTP.

820. Severity of TTP is estimated by the degree of?

Harrison's 20th Ed. Chapter 111 Page 826

A. Anemia
B. Thrombocytopenia
C. Serum LDH level
D. All of the above

Findings to support the TTP diagnosis include an increased lactate dehydrogenase and indirect bilirubin, decreased haptoglobin and increased reticulocyte count with a negative direct antiglobulin test. The peripheral smear shows schistocytes, polychromasia.

821. Which of the following is not a feature of TTP?

Harrison's 20th Ed. Chapter 111 Page 826

A. Severe Coombs-positive hemolytic anemia
B. Near normal prothrombin time
C. Near normal fibrinogen level
D. Near normal FDP level

Presence of severe Coombs-negative hemolytic anemia with schistocytes or fragmented RBC's in PBF, with thrombocytopenia & minimal activation of coagulation system confirm diagnosis of TTP.

822. Which of the following supports the diagnosis of TTP?

Harrison's 20th Ed. Chapter 111 Page 827

A. Increased lactate dehydrogenase
B. Increased indirect bilirubin
C. Decreased haptoglobin
D. All of the above

Findings that support the diagnosis of TTP include increased LDH, increased indirect bilirubin, decreased haptoglobin, increased reticulocyte count, negative direct antiglobulin test, schistocytes in PBF and polychromasia.

823. Which of the following laboratory finding does not support diagnosis of TTP?

Harrison's 20th Ed. Chapter 111 Page 827

A. Increased lactate dehydrogenase
B. Increased direct bilirubin
C. Decreased haptoglobin
D. Increased reticulocyte count

Laboratory finding that support diagnosis of TTP include increased LDH, increased "indirect bilirubin", decreased haptoglobin, increased reticulocyte count with negative direct antiglobulin test. PBF shows schistocytes and polychromasia.

824. Mainstay of treatment of idiopathic TTP is?

Harrison's 20th Ed. Chapter 111 Page 827

A. Rituximab
B. IV Ig
C. Plasma exchange
D. Splenectomy

Plasma exchange remains the mainstay of treatment of ITP idiopathic TTP.

825. Which of the following is false about TTP?

Harrison's 20th Ed. Chapter 111 Page 827

A. TTP is more common in HIV patients and pregnant women
B. Coagulation studies are essentially normal in TTP
C. Severe bleeds are usually absent
D. None of the above

826. Which of the following is false about Weibel-Palade bodies?

Blood. 2011;117(19):5033–5043

A. Are organelles in the vascular endothelium
B. Major constituents of Weibel-Palade bodies are von Willebrand factor (vWF) and P-selectin
C. George Emil Palade won the Nobel Prize in Physiology or Medicine in 1974
D. None of the above

827. Which of the following is false about Weibel-Palade bodies (WPBs)?

Blood. 2011;117(19):5033–5043

A. Weibel-Palade bodies play a dual role in blood coagulation hemostasis and inflammation
B. Weibel-Palade bodies are the main source of vWF
C. Weibel-Palade bodies are secretory organelles used for post-synthesis storage in endothelial cells.
D. None of the above

828. Findings in TTP include?

N Engl J Med 2006;354:1927-35

A. Abdominal pain, nausea, vomiting and weakness
B. Seizures and fluctuating focal deficits
C. Thrombocytopenia without leukopenia
D. All of the above

829. Which of the following is not used in the treatment of TTP?

Harrison's 20th Ed. Chapter 111 Page 827

A. Platelet concentrates
B. Plasma exchange
C. Fresh-frozen plasma (FFP)
D. Solvent/detergent-treated plasma (SD-FFP)

Plasma exchange remains the mainstay of treatment of TTP. Use of platelet concentrates and Desmopressin, or DDAVP in the treatment of TTP is contraindicated as it leads to extensive platelet aggregation in the CNS.

830. Immunomodulatory therapies reported to be successful in refractory or relapsing TTP include?

Harrison's 20th Ed. Chapter 111 Page 827

A. Rituximab
B. Vincristine
C. Cyclophosphamide
D. All of the above

Immunomodulatory therapies reported to be successful in refractory or relapsing TTP include rituximab, vincristine, cyclophosphamide, and splenectomy.

831. Hemolytic Uremic Syndrome is a disease of?
Harrison's 20th Ed. Chapter 111 Page 827

A. Infancy and early childhood
B. Adolescence
C. Adults
D. Elderly

HUS is seen predominantly in children.

832. Features of Hemolytic Uremic Syndrome include all except?
Harrison's 20th Ed. Chapter 111 Page 827

A. Chronic renal failure
B. Microangiopathic hemolytic anemia (MAHA)
C. Thrombocytopenia
D. Frequently preceded by an episode of diarrhea

HUS is a syndrome characterized by acute renal failure, microangiopathic hemolytic anemia (MAHA), and thrombocytopenia. In most cases is preceded by an episode of (hemorrhagic) diarrhea. Plasma exchange treatment is not appropriate for hemolytic-uremic syndrome.

833. In the United States and Europe, the most common STEC strain is?
Harrison's 20th Ed. Chapter 111 Page 827

A. OH147:H7
B. OH157:H7
C. OH167:H7
D. OH177:H7

In the United States and Europe, the most common Shiga toxin-producing Escherichia coli (STEC) strain is O157:H7. After entry into the circulation, Shiga toxin binds to the glycolipid surface receptor globotriaosylceramide (Gb3) which is richly expressed on cells of the renal microvasculature. Upon binding the toxin enters the cells, inducing inflammatory cytokines (interleukin 8, monocyte chemotactic protein 1, and stromal cell-derived factor 1 and chemokine receptors CXCR4 and CXCR7. This action results in platelet aggregation and microangiopathic provess.

834. STEC HUS is caused by the Shiga toxins (Stx1 and Stx2) which are called?
Harrison's 20th Ed. Chapter 111 Page 827

A. Verotoxins
B. Merotoxins
C. Xerotoxins
D. Shigatoxins

Shiga toxin-producing Escherichia coli (STEC) HUS is caused by the Shiga toxins (Stx1 and Stx2) which are also referred to as verotoxins. STEC) HUS is also known as D+HUS or enterohemorrhagic E. coli (EHEC) HUS.

835. In HUS, which of the following is not present?
Harrison's 20th Ed. Chapter 111 Page 827

A. Abdominal pain
B. Cramping
C. Vomiting
D. Fever

Abdominal pain, cramping and vomiting are frequent whereas fever is typically absent.

836. Thrombocytosis is due to deficiency of?
Harrison's 20th Ed. Chapter 111 Page 827

A. Vitamin B12
B. Folic acid
C. Iron
D. Calcium

Thrombocytosis is almost always due to iron deficiency, reactive thrombocytosis (inflammation, cancer, infection) or underlying myeloproliferative process (essential thrombocythemia or PV) and rarely in the 5q- myelodysplastic process.

837. In which of the following disorders, there is absence of the platelet GpIIb/IIIa receptor?
Harrison's 20th Ed. Chapter 111 Page 827

A. Glanzmann's thrombasthenia
B. Bernard-Soulier syndrome
C. Hermansky-Pudlak syndrome
D. Heyde's syndrome

Autosomal recessive inherited qualitative disorders of platelet function include Glanzmann's thrombasthenia (absence of the platelet GpIIb/IIIa receptor) and Bernard Soulier syndrome (absence of the platelet GpIb-IX-V receptor). Edward Glanzmann - Swiss physician (1918)

838. Bleeding symptoms or prevention of bleeding in patients in inherited disorders of platelet dysfunction include?
Harrison's 20th Ed. Chapter 111 Page 827

A. Prestorage leukodepleted platelets transfusion
B. Desmopressin (DDAVP)
C. EACA or tranexamic acid
D. All of the above

In platelet transfusion, risk of alloimmunization can be limited by using prestorage leukodepleted platelets. Desmopressin (DDAVP) increases plasma vWF & FVIII levels. Antifibrinolytic therapy (EACA or tranexamic acid) is used alone or in conjunction with DDAVP or platelet therapy.

839. Acquired platelet dysfunction can occur in?
Harrison's 20th Ed. Chapter 111 Page 827

A. Uremia
B. High dose penicillins
C. With cardiopulmonary bypass
D. All of the above

840. Acquired platelet dysfunction due to uremia, respond to?
Harrison's 20th Ed. Chapter 111 Page 828

A. Dialysis
B. DDAVP
C. Conjugated estrogens
D. All of the above

841. Most common inherited bleeding disorder is?
Harrison's 20th Ed. Chapter 111 Page 828

A. Glanzmann's thrombasthenia
B. Bernard-Soulier syndrome
C. von Willebrand Disease
D. Hemophilia

von Willebrand Disease (vWD) is the most common inherited bleeding disorder with prevalence of ~1%. vWD affects both males & females, while hemophilia mainly affects males.

842. Nationality of Dr. Erik von Willebrand was?
N Engl J Med 2004;351:683-94

A. French
B. Finnish
C. Spanish
D. Danish

In 1925, Dr. Erik von Willebrand of Finland observed a disorder that was due to a disturbed function of thrombocytes and a general lesion of capillary walls and called it "pseudohemophilia".

843. von Willebrand factor gene is located on which chromosome?
N Engl J Med 2004;351:683-94

A. 10
B. 11
C. 12
D. 13

von Willebrand factor is a large multimeric glycoprotein that is encoded by a gene spanning 178 kb of genomic DNA on chromosome 12.

844. Most common type of vWD is?
Harrison's 20th Ed. Chapter 111 Page 828

A. Type 1
B. Type 2A
C. Type 2B
D. Type 3

vWD is classified into three major types 1, 2 and 3. Type 2 has four subtypes (A,B,M,N). Most common type of VWD is type 1 disease, with a parallel decrease in VWF protein, VWF function and FVIII levels accounting for at least 80% of cases.

845. Which of the following vWD is not inherited as autosomal dominant trait?
Harrison's 20th Ed. Chapter 111 Page 828

A. Type I
B. Type IIA
C. Type IIB
D. Type III

Except type III vWF disease, all forms are inherited as autosomal dominant traits.

846. vWF precursor subunit is synthesized in?
Harrison's 20th Ed. Chapter 111 Page 828

A. Endothelial cells
B. Platelets
C. Vascular subendothelium
D. All of the above

A single large vWF precursor subunit is synthesized in endothelial cells & megakaryocytes, where it is cleaved & assembled into disulfide-linked multimers in plasma, platelets, & subendothelium.

847. vWF protein levels are lowest in which of the following blood groups?
Harrison's 20th Ed. Chapter 111 Page 828

A. A
B. B
C. AB
D. O

Patients with "O" blood group have vWF protein levels about one-half those of patients with AB blood type.

848. Platelet count are modestly reduced in which of the following types of vWD?
Harrison's 20th Ed. Chapter 111 Page 829

A. Type 1
B. Type 2N
C. Type 2B
D. Type 3

Platelet counts are within the normal range in vWD except in type 2B vWD where mild thrombocytopenia may be seen and may be misdiagnosed as autoimmune thrombocytopenia. RIPA (Ristocetin induced platelet aggregation) shows a low to absent response in all vWD types except type 2B vWD where a brisk platelet aggregation is seen even at low concentrations.

849. Which type of vWD reflects mutations in vWF that affect binding of FVIII?
Harrison's 20th Ed. Chapter 111 Page 829

A. Type 2A
B. Type 2B
C. Type 2M
D. Type 2N

Type 2N vWD reflects mutations in vWF that preclude binding of FVIII.

850. Which type of vWD is termed "autosomal hemophilia"?
Harrison's 20th Ed. Chapter 111 Page 829

A. Type 2A
B. Type 2B
C. Type 2M
D. Type 2N

In type 2N vWD, FVIII has a very short half-life and level is markedly decreased. This is termed autosomal hemophilia. Type 2N vWD is due to abnormal FVIII binding sites. It is distinguished from haemophilia A by the finding of normal vWF:Ag levels and limitation of the disorder to males in inherited haemophilia A.

851. What is the nature of "Ristocetin"?
N Engl J Med 2004;351:683-94

A. Analgesic
B. Antibiotic
C. Uterine relaxant
D. Digestive enzyme

852. Which of the following vWD type is most severe?
Harrison's 20th Ed. Chapter 111 Page 829

A. Type 1
B. Type 2A
C. Type 2B
D. Type 3

Type III vWF disease is a very severe form of vWD with no detectable vWF antigen or activity and and FVIII levels < 10%. Patients are usually the offspring of two parents (usually asymptomatic) with mild type I disease.

853. Which of the following vWD is due to a defect in factor VIII binding site of vWF?
Harrison's 20th Ed. Chapter 111 Page 828 Table 111-2

A. Type 1
B. Type 2A
C. Type 2N
D. Type 3

Type 2N vWD is due to a defect in factor VIII binding site of vWF.

854. In which of the following vWD, vWF: Ag is normal?

Harrison's 20th Ed. Chapter 111 Page 828 Figure 111-5

A. Type 1
B. Type 2A
C. Type 2B
D. Type 3

855. In which of the following vWD, vWF: Ag is normal?

Harrison's 20th Ed. Chapter 111 Page 828 Figure 111-5

A. Type 2M
B. Type 2N
C. Type 2B
D. Type 3

Normal vWF:Ag levels does not exclude vWD. vWF levels are just below normal in type 1, normal in type 2A and 2M, usually decreased in 2B and 2N and nearly to completely absent in type 3 vWD.

856. vWD may be acquired in which of the following situations?

Harrison's 20th Ed. Chapter 111 Page 829

A. Monoclonal gammopathies of undetermined significance
B. Waldenström's macroglobulinemia
C. Multiple myeloma
D. All of the above

Acquired vWD is mostly seen in patients with underlying lymphoproliferative disorders like MGUS, multiple myeloma & Waldenstrom's macroglobulinemia. Also seen in patients with aortic valvular disease.

857. Acquired vWD is seen most commonly in?

Harrison's 20th Ed. Chapter 111 Page 829

A. Monoclonal gammopathies of undetermined significance
B. Multiple myeloma
C. Waldenström's macroglobulinemia
D. None of the above

Acquired vWD is seen most commonly in MGUS.

858. Which of the following best relates to Heyde's syndrome?

Harrison's 20th Ed. Chapter 111 Page 829

A. Cirrhosis of liver
B. Angiodysplasia of gastrointestinal tract
C. Pancreatic neoplasis
D. Ectopic spleen

Heyde's syndrome refers to aortic stenosis with gastrointestinal bleeding due to presence of angiodysplasia of gastrointestinal tract in patients with aortic stenosis. Shear stress on blood passing through stenotic aortic valve produces change in vWF, making it susceptible to serum proteases with loss of large multimer forms, leading to acquired type 2 vWD.

859. In Heyde's syndrome, which of the following is a feature apart from aortic stenosis?

Harrison's 20th Ed. Chapter 111 Page 829

A. Raynaud's phenomenon
B. Gastrointestinal bleeding
C. Clubbing
D. Pes cavus

Heyde's syndrome refers to aortic stenosis with GI bleeding due to angiodysplasia of GI tract.

860. Which of the following is false in von Willebrand Disease?

Harrison's 20th Ed. Chapter 111 Page 829

A. Prolonged BT
B. Normal platelet count
C. Decreased plasma vWF concentration
D. None of the above

Laboratory findings in vWD are variable. Most common diagnostic pattern is prolonged BT, normal platelet count, CT, PT, increased APTT, decreased plasma vWF concentration, reduction in its vWF biologic activity (ristocetin cofactor assay) and reduced FVIII activity. Bleeding time is normal in hemophilia A.

861. Which of the following is false in diagnostic pattern of vWD?

Harrison's 20th Ed. Chapter 111 Page 828 Table 111-2

A. Prolonged clotting time
B. Reduced vWF concentration
C. Reduced vWF biologic activity
D. Reduced factor VIII activity

Lab. diagnostic findings in vWD are prolonged BT, reduction in plasma vWF level, a parallel reduction in vWF biologic activity by ristocetin cofactor assay and reduced factor VIII activity.

862. Patients of which type of vWD are the best candidates for desmopressin therapy?

Harrison's 20th Ed. Chapter 111 Page 829

A. Type I
B. Type IIA
C. Type IIB
D. Type III

Patients with type I vWD are the best candidates for desmopressin therapy which results in release of vWF and FVIII from endothelial stores.

863. Desmopressin acts through which of the following vasopressin receptors?

N Engl J Med 2004;351:683-94

A. Type 1
B. Type 2
C. Type 3
D. Type 4

Desmopressin is a synthetic derivative of antidiuretic hormone that acts through type 2 vasopressin receptors. It has no activity on type 1 receptors.

864. Dose of Desmopressin is?

N Engl J Med 2004;351:683-94

A. 0.3 μg/kg body weight IV infusion
B. 3.0 μg/kg body weight IV infusion
C. 30 μg/kg body weight IV infusion
D. 300 μg/kg body weight IV infusion

Desmopressin is given in a dose of 0.3 μg/kg body weight IV infusion. Peak activity occurs ~30 minutes after intravenous infusion. DDAVP is a synthetic hormone and can be given by high-concentration intranasal spray (1.5 mg/mL) that peaks in activity after two hours. Repeated dosing of DDAVP results in tachyphylaxis. More than three consecutive doses become ineffective and if further therapy is indicated, FVIII replacement is required to achieve hemostasis.

865. Major side effect of DDAVP is?
Harrison's 20th Ed. Chapter 111 Page 829

A. Peptic ulcer
B. Seizure
C. Hyperkalemia
D. Hyponatremia

Major side effect of DDAVP is hyponatremia due to decreased free water clearance. This occurs most commonly in the very young and the very old, but fluid restriction should be advised for all patients for the 24 hours following each dose.

866. DDAVP, or desmopressin is not indicated in which type of von Willebrand disease?
Harrison's 20th Ed. Chapter 111 Page 829

A. Type 1
B. Type 2A
C. Type 2B
D. Type 2M

Desmopressin or DDAVPis not recommended in type 2B where it is known to aggravate thrombocytopenia. Types 2A and 2M vWD respond to DDAVP.

867. Antifibrinolytic amino acids like Aminocaproic acid or tranexamic acid used in treatment of vWD can cause which of the following complications?
Harrison's 20th Ed. Chapter 111 Page 829

A. Cholelithiasis
B. Ureteral obstruction
C. Glaucoma
D. Alopecia

Antifibrinolytic amino acids are contraindicated in patients with upper UTI or gross hematuria because clots that do not lyse may cause ureteral obstruction.

868. In type 3 vWD, which of the following is the treatment of first choice in patients with alloantibodies?
N Engl J Med 2004;351:683-94

A. Desmopressin
B. Factor VIII–von Willebrand factor concentrates
C. Recombinant factor VIII
D. Platelet concentrates

869. Cryoprecipitate is a source of which of the following?
Harrison's 20th Ed. Chapter 111 Page 829

A. Fibrinogen
B. Factor VIII
C. von Willebrand factor (VWF)
D. All of the above

Cryoprecipitate is a source of fibrinogen, factor VIII, von Willebrand factor (VWF) & Cold-insoluble plasma proteins. Virally inactivated vWF-containing factor concentrates are safer than cryoprecipitate as the replacement product.

870. In which of the following diseases, platelets are deficient or defective in Gp IIb/IIIa complex?
Harrison's 20th Ed. Chapter 111 Page 829

A. Bernard-Soulier syndrome
B. Glanzmann's thrombasthenia
C. Hermansky-Pudlak syndrome
D. Chediak-Higashi syndrome

871. In which of the following diseases, platelets have deficiency or dysfunction of the Gp Ib-IX-V complex?
Harrison's 20th Ed. Chapter 111 Page 829

A. Bernard-Soulier syndrome
B. Glanzmann's thrombasthenia
C. Hermansky-Pudlak syndrome
D. Chediak-Higashi syndrome

Inherited platelet function qualitative disorders include autosomal recessive disorders like Glanzmann's thrombasthenia (absence of platelet GpIIbIIIa receptor) & Bernard Soulier syndrome (absence of platelet GpIb-IX-V receptor). Both present with bleeding symptoms in childhood.

872. Which of the following is not an autosomal recessive trait?
Harrison's 20th Ed. Chapter 111 Page 829

A. Bernard-Soulier syndrome
B. Glanzmann's thrombasthenia
C. von Willebrand's disease Type II
D. Congenital amegakaryocytic thrombocytopenia

873. Which of the following is a platelet aggregation agonist?
Harrison's 20th Ed. Chapter 61 Page 404

A. ADP
B. Thrombin
C. Epinephrine
D. All of the above

Platelet activation & then aggregation occurs after platelet adhesion. This process is promoted by humoral mediators (epinephrine, thrombin), mediators from activated platelets (ADP, serotonin) & vessel wall extracellular matrix constituents in contact with adherent platelets (collagen, vWF).

874. In platelet granules, which of the following is "adhesive glycoprotein"?
Harrison's 20th Ed. Chapter 113 Page 839

A. Thrombospondin
B. Fibronectin
C. vWF
D. All of the above

Formation of a thrombus is initiated by adherence of platelets to damaged vessel wall. Damage exposes subendothelial components responsible for triggering platelet reactivity, including collagen, vWF, fibronectin and other adhesive proteins like vitronectin & thrombospondin.

875. Which of the following vWD is inherited as autosomal recessive trait?
N Engl J Med 2004;351:683-94

A. Type 1
B. Type 2A
C. Type 2B
D. Type 3

Type 3 vWD, which accounts for 1–5% percent of cases, is transmitted as an autosomal recessive trait in homozygous or compound heterozygous persons.

876. Which of the following is a Primary Vasculitis Syndrome?
Harrison's 20th Ed. Chapter 111 Page 829

A. Wegener's granulomatosis
B. Churg-Strauss syndrome
C. Henoch-Schönlein purpura
D. All of the above

Primary vasculitis syndromes include Wegener's granulomatosis, Churg-Strauss syndrome, Henoch-Schönlein purpura, Polyarteritis nodosa, Microscopic polyangiitis, Giant cell arteritis, Takayasu's arteritis, Idiopathic cutaneous vasculitis, Essential mixed cryoglobulinemia, Behçet's syndrome, Isolated vasculitis of CNS, Cogan's syndrome & Kawasaki disease.

877. Henoch-Schönlein purpura is also referred to as?
Harrison's 20th Ed. Chapter 111 Page 829

A. Anaphylactoid purpura
B. Purple purpura
C. Emergent purpura
D. Sympathetic purpura

Henoch-Schönlein purpura is also referred to as anaphylactoid purpura.

878. Henoch-Schönlein purpura is best related to?
Harrison's 20th Ed. Chapter 111 Page 829

A. Leukocytoclastic vasculitis (LCV)
B. Livedoid vasculitis
C. Necrotizing vasculitis
D. Systemic vasculitis

Henoch-Schönlein purpura (HSP) is a subtype of acute leukocytoclastic vasculitis (LCV).

879. Henoch-Schönlein purpura lesions are most commonly distributed over?
Harrison's 20th Ed. Chapter 356 Page 2586

A. Buttocks and lower extremities
B. Neck and upper limbs
C. Chest and abdomen
D. Face

In Henoch-Schönlein purpura, palpable purpura lesions are most commonly distributed over buttocks and lower extremities.

880. Henoch-Schönlein purpura is often preceded by?
Harrison's 20th Ed. Chapter 111 Page 829

A. Trauma
B. Conjunctivitis
C. Upper respiratory infection
D. Exercise

Henoch-Schönlein purpura is often preceded by an upper respiratory infection (streptococcal pharyngitis) or is triggered by drug or food allergies.

881. Henoch-Schönlein purpura is a?
Harrison's 20th Ed. Chapter 111 Page 829

A. Small vessel vasculitis
B. Medium vessel vasculitis
C. Large vessel vasculitis
D. All of the above

Henoch-Schönlein purpura is a small-vessel vasculitis. Patients have an acute inflammatory reaction with IgA and complement components in capillaries, mesangial tissues and small arterioles leading to increased vascular permeability and localized hemorrhage.

882. Which of the following is false about Henoch-Schönlein purpura?
Harrison's 20th Ed. Chapter 111 Page 829

A. Mostly in age between 4–7 years
B. Male-to-female ratio is 1.5:1
C. Peak incidence in spring
D. None of the above

Most patients of HSP are between 4 - 7 years of age. Male-to-female ratio is 1.5:1. Peak incidence in spring has been noted. All coagulation tests are normal, but renal impairment may occur.

883. In Henoch-Schönlein purpura, the antibody class most often seen in the immune complexes is?
Harrison's 20th Ed. Chapter 111 Page 829

A. IgA
B. IgG
C. IgM
D. IgE

IgA is the antibody class most often seen in immune complexes and demonstrated in renal biopsies of HSP patients. IgA levels are elevated in ~half of patients.

884. In pediatric patients, which of the following is the most common presentation in HSP?
Harrison's 20th Ed. Chapter 111 Page 829

A. Palpable purpura
B. Gastrointestinal involvement
C. Glomerulonephritis
D. Arthritis

In pediatric HSP, palpable purpura is seen in virtually all patients. HSP is a subtype of acute LCV. Livedoid vasculitis represents a combination of a vasculopathy plus intravascular thrombosis.

885. Which of the following statements about renal involvement in Henoch-Schönlein purpura is false?
Harrison's 20th Ed. Chapter 111 Page 829

A. Proteinuria
B. Microscopic hematuria
C. Red blood cell casts
D. Progressive glomerulonephritis frequent

886. Which of the following statements about renal involvement in Henoch-Schönlein purpura is false?
Harrison's 20th Ed. Chapter 111 Page 829

A. Usually resolves spontaneously without therapy
B. Progressive glomerulonephritis rare
C. Renal failure is the most common cause of death
D. None of the above

Renal involvement occurs in 10 –50% of HSP patients. Mild glomerulonephritis, proteinuria, microscopic hematuria, with RBC casts occurs in the majority. it resolves spontaneously without therapy. Rarely, a progressive glomerulonephritis will develop.

887. Which of the following statements about gastrointestinal involvement in Henoch-Schönlein purpura is false?

Harrison's 20th Ed. Chapter 111 Page 829

A. Colicky abdominal pain

B. Blood and mucus per rectum

C. Bowel intussusception

D. None of the above

888. In Henoch-Schönlein purpura, mesangial immune deposits consists of?

Harrison's 20th Ed. Chapter 111 Page 829

A. IgA

B. IgG

C. C3

D. All of the above

889. In Henoch-Schönlein purpura, immune deposits may be found in?

Harrison's 20th Ed. Chapter 111 Page 829

A. Mesangial and paramesangial areas

B. Peripheral glomerular capillary wall

C. Small arterioles

D. All of the above

HSP patients have an acute inflammatory reaction with IgA and complement components in capillaries, mesangial tissues, and small arterioles, leading to increased vascular permeability and localized hemorrhage.

Coagulation Disorders

890. Factor X or Stuart-Prower factor is named after?
Med J Armed Forces India. 2015;71(Suppl 1):S184–S186

A. Patients– Ms. Audrey Prower & Mr. Rufus Stuart
B. Doctors– Ms. Audrey Prower & Mr. Rufus Stuart
C. Scientists– Ms. Audrey Prower & Mr. Rufus Stuart
D. Politicians– Ms. Audrey Prower & Mr. Rufus Stuart

Factor X, or Stuart-Prower factor was identified in Ms. Audrey Prower of London, who had life-long bleeding tendency. An American group identified the same factor in Mr. Rufus Stuart (1957).

891. Coagulation-related protein prekallikrein is also called?
Ann Clin Lab Sci. 1985;15(4):279-85

A. Fletcher Factor
B. Fitzgerald Factor
C. MacFarlane Factor
D. Furie Factor

Fletcher Factor and Fitzgerald Factor are coagulation-related proteins prekallikrein and high-molecular-weight kininogen respectively.

892. Factor IX or Christmas Factor is named after?
Ann Clin Lab Sci. 1985;15(4):279-85

A. Patient - Stephen Christmas
B. Doctor - Stephen Christmas
C. Scientist - Stephen Christmas
D. Politician - Stephen Christmas

Stephen Christmas (1947-1993) of Canada sufferd from hemophilia B. He died due to transfusion-related AIDS. Christmas factor (factor IX) was the first coagulation protein to be named after a patient.

893. An isolated abnormal prothrombin time (PT) suggests deficiency of?
Harrison's 20th Ed. Chapter 112 Page 830

A. FV
B. FVI
C. FVII
D. FVIII

894. Prolonged activated partial thromboplastin time indicates?
Harrison's 20th Ed. Chapter 112 Page 830

A. FII deficiency
B. FV deficiency
C. FVIII deficiency
D. FX deficiency

895. Prolongation of both PT & aPTT suggests deficiency of?
Harrison's 20th Ed. Chapter 112 Page 830

A. FV
B. FX
C. FII
D. All of the above

An isolated abnormal prothrombin time (PT) suggests FVII deficiency. A prolonged activated partial thromboplastin time (aPTT) indicates most commonly hemophilia or FXI deficiency. The prolongation of both PT & aPTT suggests deficiency of FV, FX, FII or fibrinogen abnormalities. Patients with hemophilia have normal bleeding times & platelet counts.

896. Which of the following is a test for blood coagulation?
Harrison's 20th Ed. Chapter 112 Page 830

A. PT
B. aPTT
C. Thrombin time (TT)
D. All of the above

897. Which of the following is an example of acquired deficiencies of plasma coagulation?
Harrison's 20th Ed. Chapter 112 Page 830

A. Hemorrhagic diathesis of liver disease
B. Disseminated intravascular coagulation (DIC)
C. Vitamin K deficiency
D. All of the above

Acquired deficiencies of plasma coagulation factors are more frequent than congenital disorders. Most common disorders include hemorrhagic diathesis of liver disease, disseminated intravascular coagulation (DIC), and vitamin K deficiency. Blood coagulation is hampered by the deficiency of more than one clotting factor.

898. Which of the following could lead to a prolonged aPTT and normal PT?
N Engl J Med 2009;361:1887-94

A. Deficiency of factor VIII, IX, or XI
B. von Willebrand's disease
C. Unfractionated heparin
D. All of the above

Deficiency of factor VIII, IX, or XI, Inhibitor of factor VIII, IX, or XI, Von Willebrand's disease, Unfractionated heparin and Direct thrombin inhibitors cause a prolonged aPTT and normal PT.

899. Which of the following could lead to a prolonged PT and normal aPTT?
N Engl J Med 2009;361:1887-94

A. Deficiency of factor VII
B. Vitamin K deficiency
C. Warfarin therapy
D. All of the above

Deficiency of factor VII, Inhibitor of factor VII, Vitamin K deficiency, Liver disease and Warfarin therapy could lead to a prolonged PT and normal aPTT.

900. Which of the following could lead to a prolonged aPTT and prolonged PT?
N Engl J Med 2009;361:1887-94

A. Deficiency of prothrombin, fibrinogen, factor V or X
B. Supratherapeutic doses of heparin or warfarin
C. Disseminated intravascular coagulation
D. All of the above

Deficiency of prothrombin, fibrinogen, factor V, or factor X, Inhibitor of prothrombin, fibrinogen, factor V, or factor X, Supratherapeutic doses of heparin or warfarin, Liver disease, Disseminated intravascular coagulation and Argatroban could lead to a prolonged aPTT and prolonged PT

901. Which of the following is a disorder of primary hemostasis?
N Engl J Med 2009;361:1887-94

A. Thrombocytopenia
B. Qualitative platelet disorders
C. von Willebrand's disease
D. All of the above

902. Which of the following royal persons was a clinically normal carrier of hemophilia?
N Engl J Med 2001;344:1773

A. Queen Marie
B. Queen Elizabeth I
C. Queen Victoria
D. Queen Harper

Queen Victoria, a clinically normal carrier of hemophilia, had one son, Leopold, who had hemophilia and two daughters, Alice and Beatrice, who were carriers and who, in turn, transmitted the disease to the Russian, Prussian, and Spanish royal families.

903. World Hemophilia Day is observed on?

A. April 17
B. May 17
C. June 17
D. July 17

904. What is the prevalence of hemophilia?
Harrison's 20th Ed. Chapter 112 Page 830

A. 1 in 10,000 males worldwide
B. 1 in 100.000 males worldwide
C. 1 in 10,00000 males worldwide
D. 1 in 10,000000 males worldwide

Hemophilia is an X-linked recessive hemorrhagic disease due to mutations in the F8 gene (hemophilia A or classic hemophilia) or F9 gene (hemophilia B). The disease affects 1 in 10,000 males worldwide, in all ethnic groups.

905. Most common hemophilia A F8 mutations results from?
Harrison's 20th Ed. Chapter 112 Page 831

A. Inversion of intron 22 DNA sequence
B. Inversion of intron 23 DNA sequence
C. Inversion of intron 24 DNA sequence
D. Inversion of intron 25 DNA sequence

40 to 50 percent of the mutations causing severe hemophilia A are due to an inversion of DNA sequences in intron 22 that disrupts factor VIII gene.

906. Family history of hemophilia is absent in what percentage of cases of hemophilia?
Harrison's 20th Ed. Chapter 112 Page 830

A. ~10%
B. ~20%
C. ~30%
D. ~40%

Hemophilia affects males, women, who carry a single mutated gene, are generally asymptomatic. Family history of the disease is absent in ~30% of cases and arise from a spontaneous mutation..

907. The minimal level of most clotting factors needed for adequate hemostasis is?
Harrison's 20th Ed. Chapter 112 Page 831

A. 5%
B. 10%
C. 15%
D. 25%

Those with residual FVIII or FIX activity >25% of normal, hemophilia is discovered only by bleeding after major trauma or during presurgery laboratory tests.

908. Clinically, hemophilia is classified as severe when residual activity of FVIII is?
Harrison's 20th Ed. Chapter 112 Page 831

A. < 1%
B. < 2%
C. < 3%
D. < 4%

When residual activity of FVIII or FIX is < 1%, hemophilia is classified as severe. Between 1 - 5%, it is moderate. Between 6–30%, it is mild.

909. Which of the following is a laboratory finding in hemophilia?
Harrison's 20th Ed. Chapter 112 Page 831

A. Prolonged aPTT
B. Normal bleeding time
C. Normal platelet count
D. All of the above

Patients with hemophilia have prolongation of aPTT, normal bleeding time and normal platelet count. Diagnosis is made by specific determination of FVIII or FIX clotting activity.

910. Which of the following is related to hemophilia?
Harrison's 20th Ed. Chapter 112 Page 831

A. Target joint
B. Compartment syndrome
C. Pseudotumor syndrome
D. All of the above

Recurrent bleeding episodes in a joint results in clinically recognized "target joint" with a vicious cycle of bleeding, resulting in progressive joint deformity. Hematomas into muscle of distal parts of the limbs may lead to external compression of arteries, veins or nerves that can evolve to a compartment syndrome. Retroperitoneal hemorrhages can accumulate large quantities of blood with formation of masses with calcification & inflammatory tissue reaction (pseudotumor syndrome) and also result in damage to the femoral nerve. Pseudotumors can also form in bones, especially long bones of the lower limbs.

911. One unit of factor VIII is defined as the amount of factor VIII present in?
Harrison's 20th Ed. Chapter 112 Page 832

A. 1 mL normal plasma
B. 10 mL normal plasma
C. 100 mL normal plasma
D. 1000 mL normal plasma

One unit is by definition the amount of FVIII (100 ng/mL) or FIX (5 µg/mL) in 1 mL of normal plasma. One unit of FVIII per kilogram of body weight increases the plasma FVIII level by 2%.

912. To increase FVIII levels to 100% in a 70-kg severe hemophilia patient (<1%), how many units of FVIII will be required?

Harrison's 20th Ed. Chapter 112 Page 832

A. 2500
B. 3500
C. 4500
D. 5500

To increase FVIII levels to 100% in a 70-kg severe hemophilia patient (< 1%), 3500 units of FVIII will be required. The formula is FVIII dose (IU) = (Target FVIII levels - FVIII baseline levels) x body weight (kg) × 0.5 unit/kg.

913. Factor VIII has a half-life of?

Harrison's 20th Ed. Chapter 112 Page 832

A. 1 to 4 hours
B. 4 to 8 hours
C. 8 to 12 hours
D. 12 to 16 hours

FVIII half-life of 8 to 12 hours, therefore requires twice a day administration to maintain therapeutic levels. Half-life of FIX is about 24 hours.

914. Oral antifibrinolytic drug is coupled with Factor VIII replacement in which of the following?

Harrison's 20th Ed. Chapter 112 Page 832

A. Hemarthroses
B. Bleeds into deep muscles
C. Prophylactic replacement
D. Oral surgery

Oral surgery is associated with extensive tissue damage that usually requires factor replacement for 1 -3 days coupled with oral antifibrinolytic drugs.

915. Which of the following is false about antihemophilic factor (AHF)?

Harrison's 20th Ed. Chapter 112 Page 832

A. Multiple-chain protein
B. Synthesized in liver
C. Circulates complexed to vWF protein
D. None of the above

916. Which of the following is false about antihemophilic factor (AHF)?

Harrison's 20th Ed. Chapter 112 Page 832

A. Regulates activation of factor X
B. Gene for factor VIII is on the X chromosome
C. Symptomatic patients have factor VIII levels of < 5%
D. None of the above

917. Which of the following is false about hemophilia A?

Harrison's 20th Ed. Chapter 112 Page 832

A. Severe iron-deficiency anemia is uncommon
B. Patients with type I inhibitor should not receive factor VIII
C. Prenatal diagnosis from chorionic villus biopsy or amniocentesis possible
D. None of the above

918. Which of the following medicines is useful in managing bleeding in hemophilia patients?

Harrison's 20th Ed. Chapter 112 Page 832

A. Desmopressin (DDAVP)
B. ε-aminocaproic acid (EACA)
C. Tranexamic acid
D. All of the above

DDAVP is a synthetic vasopressin analogue that causes a transient rise in FVIII and vWF, but not FIX, in patients with mild to moderate hemophilia A but not in severe hemophilia A as there are no stores to release. Repeated dosing of DDAVP results in tachyphylaxis. Oral antifibrinolytic drugs such as ε-aminocaproic acid (EACA) or tranexamic acid enhance local hemostasis.

919. Laboratory test required to confirm presence of an inhibitor alloantibodies to FVIII is?

Harrison's 20th Ed. Chapter 112 Page 832

A. PT mixed with normal plasma
B. PT mixed with patients plasma
C. aPTT mixed with normal plasma
D. aPTT mixed with patients plasma

Laboratory test for confirming presence of an inhibitor is aPTT mixed with normal plasma. In hemophilia, a 1:1 mix with normal plasma corrects aPTT. In inhibitor patients, aPTT on a 1:1 mix is abnormally prolonged, as inhibitor neutralizes FVIII clotting activity of normal plasma.

920. Alloantibody inhibitor formation to FVIII occurs after how many cumulative days of exposure?

Harrison's 20th Ed. Chapter 112 Page 832

A. 10
B. 20
C. 30
D. 40

Formation of alloantibodies to FVIII or FIX is a major complication of hemophilia treatment with a prevalence of 5-10%. Inhibitors appear early in life & after 10 cumulative days of exposure.

921. Which of the following assay is used to define the specificity of the inhibitor and its titer?

Harrison's 20th Ed. Chapter 112 Page 832

A. Minnesota assay
B. Bethesda assay
C. Glasgow assay
D. Athens assay

Bethesda assay defines the specificity of the inhibitor and its titer. One Bethesda unit (BU) is the amount of antibody that neutralizes 50% of FVIII or FIX present in normal plasma after 2 hours of incubation at 37°C.

922. Control of bleeding episodes in high-responder inhibitor patients can be achieved by?

Harrison's 20th Ed. Chapter 112 Page 833

A. Prothrombin complex concentrates (PCCs)
B. Activated prothrombin complex concentrates (aPCCs)
C. Recombinant activated Factor VII (FVIIa)
D. All of the above

High-responder inhibitor patients are those with initial inhibitor titer of >10 BU & do not respond to FVIII or FIX concentrates. Control of bleeding is achieved by using concentrates enriched for prothrombin, FVII, FIX, FX (prothrombin complex concentrates), recombinant activated Factor VII (Bypass agents).

923. Which of the following is not effective for eradication of the inhibitory antibody in hemophiliacs?
Harrison's 20th Ed. Chapter 112 Page 833

A. Immunosuppression
B. Immune tolerance induction (ITI)
C. Anti-CD20 monoclonal antibody (rituximab)
D. None of the above

For eradication of the inhibitory antibody, immunosuppression is not effective. Most effective strategy is immune tolerance induction (ITI). Addition of anti-CD20 monoclonal antibody (rituximab) as a coadjuvant to ITI is beneficial.

924. Which of the following is the major cause of morbidity and second leading cause of death in hemophilia patients exposed to older clotting factor concentrates?
Harrison's 20th Ed. Chapter 112 Page 833

A. Hepatitis A virus
B. Hepatitis B virus
C. Hepatitis C virus
D. Hepatitis E virus

Hepatitis C virus (HCV) infection is the major cause of morbidity and the second leading cause of death in hemophilia patients exposed to older clotting factor concentrates.

925. Factor IX is activated to IXa by?
Harrison's 20th Ed. Chapter 112 Page 833

A. Factor IIa
B. Factor Va
C. Factor XIa
D. Factor Xa

Factor XI is a zymogen of an active serine protease (FXIa) in the intrinsic pathway of blood coagulation that activates FIX to FIXa.

926. Which of the following is false about Factor IX?
Harrison's 20th Ed. Chapter 112 Page 833

A. Synthesized in liver
B. Requires vitamin K for biologic activity
C. Factor IX gene is on X chromosome
D. None of the above

927. In liver, Vitamin K is converted into its active form called?
Harrison's 20th Ed. Chapter 112 Page 834

A. Hydroxide
B. Sulphide
C. Butyrate
D. Epoxide

Following absorption, vitamin K is converted to an active epoxide in liver microsomes & serves as a cofactor in enzymatic carboxylation of glutamic acid residues on prothrombin complex proteins.

928. Vitamin K deficiency is due to?
Harrison's 20th Ed. Chapter 112 Page 834

A. Inadequate dietary intake
B. Intestinal malabsorption
C. Loss of storage in liver
D. All of the above

Three major causes of vitamin K deficiency are inadequate dietary intake, intestinal malabsorption, and loss of storage sites due to hepatocellular disease.

929. Which of the following clotting factors has the shortest half-life?
Harrison's 20th Ed. Chapter 112 Page 834

A. Factor II
B. Factor VII
C. Factor IX
D. Factor X

930. Purpura fulminans is related best to?
Harrison's 20th Ed. Chapter 112 Page 834

A. Hemophilia
B. Christmas disease
C. Disseminated intravascular coagulation (DIC)
D. Vitamin K deficiency

Purpura fulminans is a severe form of DIC resulting from thrombosis of extensive areas of skin following viral or bacterial infection, more in children. It is more common in those with inherited or acquired hypercoagulability due to deficiencies of components of protein C pathway.

931. Which of the following is the mechanism of DIC?
Harrison's 20th Ed. Chapter 112 Page 834

A. Uncontrolled generation of thrombin
B. Suppression of physiologic anticoagulant mechanisms
C. Abnormal fibrinolysis
D. All of the above

DIC is the result of uncontrolled generation of thrombin by exposure of blood to pathologic levels of tissue factor. Simultaneous suppression of physiologic anticoagulant mechanisms and abnormal fibrinolysis further accelerate the process. Together these abnormalities contribute to systemic fibrin deposition in small and mid-sized vessels.

932. Which of the following is the first phase in DIC?
Harrison's 20th Ed. Chapter 112 Page 835

A. Thrombotic phase
B. Procoagulant consumption phase
C. Secondary fibrinolysis phase
D. None of the above

The early thrombotic phase of DIC is followed by a phase of procoagulant consumption and secondary fibrinolysis.

933. The most sensitive test for DIC is?
Harrison's 20th Ed. Chapter 112 Page 835

A. Prolongation of PT and/or aPTT
B. Platelet counts <100,000/mm^3
C. Elevated levels of FDP
D. Presence of schistocytes (fragmented red cells) in PBF

Findings in DIC include the prolongation of PT and/or aPTT, platelet counts <100,000/mm^3, presence of schistocytes (fragmented RBCs) in PBF, and elevated levels of fibrin degradation products (FDPs). The most sensitive test for DIC is the FDP level. D-dimer test is more specific for detection of fibrin, but not fibrinogen degradation products.

934. Chronic DIC can occur in?
Harrison's 20th Ed. Chapter 112 Page 836

A. Giant hemangioma
B. Metastatic carcinoma
C. Dead fetus syndrome
D. All of the above

Low-grade, compensated DIC can occur in giant hemangioma, metastatic carcinoma, or the dead fetus syndrome.

935. Findings evident in chronic DIC are all except?
Harrison's 20th Ed. Chapter 112 Page 836

A. Normal platelet count
B. Normal aPTT
C. Normal levels of plasma FDP or D-dimers
D. Normal fibrinogen

In chronic compensated DIC, plasma levels of FDP or D-dimers are elevated. aPTT, PT, and fibrinogen values are within normal range or high. Normal platelet counts is a common finding.

936. Laboratory findings in DIC include?
Harrison's 20th Ed. Chapter 112 Page 835

A. Thrombocytopenia
B. Schistocytes
C. Prolonged thrombin time
D. All of the above

937. Laboratory findings in DIC include?
Harrison's 20th Ed. Chapter 112 Page 835

A. Reduced fibrinogen level
B. Elevated fibrin degradation products (FDP)
C. Positive D dimer immunoassay
D. All of the above

Laboratory features of DIC include thrombocytopenia, schistocytes or fragmented RBC's, prolonged PT, PTT & thrombin time, reduced fibrinogen level, elevated fibrin degradation products (FDP) and positive D dimer immunoassay.

938. Which of the following predict more bleeding in DIC?
Harrison's 20th Ed. Chapter 112 Page 835

A. Thrombocytopenia
B. Schistocytes
C. Prolonged thrombin time
D. Reduced fibrinogen level

Low fibrinogen levels in DIC predict more bleeding. Because fibrinogen has a prolonged half life, plasma levels diminish acutely only in severe cases of DIC.

939. Inhibitor of coagulation is?
Harrison's 20th Ed. Chapter 112 Page 836

A. Antithrombin III
B. Protein C
C. Protein S
D. All of the above

Coagulation inhibitors include protein C, protein S and antithrombin III.

940. Which of the following has no role in the management of hemorrhagic symptoms of DIC?
Harrison's 20th Ed. Chapter 112 Page 836

A. FFP
B. Cryoprecipitate
C. Clotting factor concentrates
D. Platelet concentrates

Clotting factor concentrates are not recommended for control of bleeding in DIC because of the limited efficacy afforded by replacement of single factors and high risk of products containing traces of activated blood proteases (aPCCs), which further aggravates the disease.

941. Low doses of continuous heparin infusion may be effective in patients with low-grade DIC due to?
Harrison's 20th Ed. Chapter 112 Page 836

A. Purpura fulminans
B. During removal of a dead fetus
C. During surgical resection of giant hemangiomas
D. All of the above

Heparin is indicated for the treatment of purpura fulminans, during the surgical resection of giant hemangiomas, and during removal of a dead fetus.

942. Vitamin K-dependent proteins include which of the following?
Harrison's 20th Ed. Chapter 112 Page 836

A. Proteins found in bone, lung and kidney
B. Proteins found in placenta
C. Clotting factor proteins
D. All of the above

Vitamin K-dependent proteins are a heterogenous group, including clotting factor proteins and also proteins found in bone, lung, kidney and placenta.

943. Which of the following is the enzyme involved in vitamin K metabolism?
Harrison's 20th Ed. Chapter 112 Page 836

A. VKORC1
B. VKORC2
C. VKORC3
D. VKORC4

Vitamin K mediates posttranslational modification of glutamate residues to g-carboxylglutamatefor vitamin K-dependent proteins calcium binding & proper assembly to phospholipid membranes. GGCX or VKORC1 are enzymes involved in vitamin K metabolism.

944. Which of the following is the earliest finding in vitamin K-deficient patients?
Harrison's 20th Ed. Chapter 112 Page 836

A. Prolongation of aPTT
B. Prolongation of PT
C. Prolongation of bleeding time
D. Prolongation of clotting time

Prolongation of PT values is the most common & earliest finding in vitamin K-deficient patients due to reduction in prothrombin, FVII, FIX and FX levels.

945. Parenteral administration of what total dose of vitamin K is sufficient to restore normal levels of clotting factors?
Harrison's 20th Ed. Chapter 112 Page 836

A. 1 mg
B. 5 mg
C. 10 mg
D. 20 mg

Parenteral administration of vitamin K at a total dose of 10 mg is sufficient to restore normal levels of clotting factor within 8–10 hours.

946. Parenteral administration of what total dose of vitamin K is sufficient for reversal of excessive anticoagulant therapy with warfarin?

Harrison's 20th Ed. Chapter 112 Page 837

A. 1 mg
B. 5 mg
C. 10 mg
D. 20 mg

Reversal of excessive anticoagulant therapy with warfarin or warfarin like drugs can be achieved by minimal doses of vitamin K (1 mg orally or by intravenous injection) for asymptomatic patients.

947. Laboratory findings in patients with liver disease include?

Harrison's 20th Ed. Chapter 112 Page 837

A. Prolonged PT
B. Prolonged PTT
C. Thrombocytopenia
D. All of the above

948. Which of the following is the site of clearance of most procoagulant & natural anticoagulant proteins?

Harrison's 20th Ed. Chapter 112 Page 837

A. Kidney
B. Liver
C. Spleen
D. Bone marrow

Liver is the site of synthesis & clearance of most procoagulant and natural anticoagulant proteins and of essential components of the fibrinolytic system.

949. Liver failure is associated with a high risk of bleeding due to?

Harrison's 20th Ed. Chapter 112 Page 837

A. Deficient synthesis of procoagulant factors
B. Enhanced fibrinolysis
C. Thrombocytopenia
D. All of the above

High risk of bleeding in liver failure is due to deficient synthesis of procoagulant factors, enhanced fibrinolysis & thrombocytopenia. Dysfibrinogenemia is also common due to impaired fibrin polymerization as in DIC concomitant to chronic liver disease.

950. Patients with liver disease have which of the following?

Harrison's 20th Ed. Chapter 112 Page 837

A. Prolonged PT
B. Prolonged aPTT
C. Prolonged TT
D. All of the above

Typically, patients with liver disease have prolonged PT, aPTT and TT. Presence of prolonged TT and normal fibrinogen and FDP levels suggest dysfibrinogenemia.

951. Fibrinogen levels are diminished in which of the following?

Harrison's 20th Ed. Chapter 112 Page 837

A. Fulminant hepatitis
B. Decompensated cirrhosis or advanced liver disease
C. Presence of DIC
D. All of the above

Fibrinogen levels are diminished only in fulminant hepatitis, decompensated cirrhosis or advanced liver disease or in the presence of DIC.

952. A decreased level of factor VIII in patients with liver failure suggests which of the following?

Harrison's 20th Ed. Chapter 112 Page 837

A. Hepatocellular carcinoma
B. Ascending cholangitis
C. Superimposing DIC
D. Any of the above

FVIII levels are often normal or elevated in patients with liver failure and decreased levels suggest superimposing DIC.

953. Which of the following is not a vitamin K -dependent protein?

Harrison's 20th Ed. Chapter 112 Page 837

A. FV
B. FVII
C. FIX
D. FX

Because FV is only synthesized in hepatocyte & is not a vitamin K-dependent protein, reduced levels of FV indicates hepatocyte failure. Normal levels of FV & decreased levels of FVII suggest vitamin K deficiency.

954. Vitamin K levels are reduced in patients with liver failure due to?

Harrison's 20th Ed. Chapter 112 Page 837

A. Compromised storage in hepatocellular disease
B. Changes in bile acids
C. Cholestasis which diminishes absorption of vitamin K
D. All of the above

Vitamin K levels may be reduced in patients with liver failure due to compromised storage in hepatocellular disease, changes in bile acids or cholestasis that can diminish absorption of vitamin K.

955. Which of the following is the most common & earliest finding in vitamin K-deficient patients?

Harrison's 20th Ed. Chapter 112 Page 837

A. Prolongation of PT
B. Prolongation of aPTT
C. Prolongation of TT
D. All of the above

Prolongation of PT values is the most common and earliest finding in vitamin K-deficient patients due to reduction in prothrombin, FVII, FIX and FX levels.

956. Bleeding in liver disease is best managed with?

Harrison's 20th Ed. Chapter 112 Page 837

A. Fresh-frozen plasma
B. Prothrombin complex concentrates
C. Fibrinogen concentrates
D. Anticoagulation with heparin

FFP is the most effective way to correct hemostasis in patients with liver failure. FFP infusion (5-10 mL/kg) is sufficient. FFP, even high doses, does not correct PT or aPTT.

957. Which of the following is not advocated in management of patients of liver failure?

Harrison's 20th Ed. Chapter 112 Page 837

A. Platelet concentrates
B. Vitamin K infusion
C. Cryoprecipitate
D. Prothrombin complex concentrate infusion

Platelet concentrates for thrombocytopenia & cryoprecipitate for decreased fibrinogen levels are indicated in patients with liver failure. Prothrombin complex concentrate infusion should be avoided due to the high risk of thrombotic complications.

958. Patients with liver disease develop which of the following?

Harrison's 20th Ed. Chapter 112 Page 837

A. Portal vein thrombosis
B. Mesenteric vein thrombosis
C. Deep vein thrombosis
D. All of the above

A big mistake will be to exclude thrombosis in patients with advanced liver disease even in the presence of prolongation of routine clotting times. Caution should be exercised on overcorrection of these laboratory abnormalities.

959. Which of the following is not a part of Virchow's triad?

Harrison's 20th Ed. Chapter 112 Page 837

A. Inflammation
B. Thrombosis
C. Hypercoagulability
D. Endothelial injury

Virchow's triad consists of inflammation, hypercoagulability and endothelial injury.

960. Acquired inhibitor is most common against which of the following clotting factors?

Harrison's 20th Ed. Chapter 112 Page 837

A. FV
B. FVIII
C. FIX
D. FX

An acquired inhibitor is an immune-mediated disease characterized by presence of an autoantibody against a specific clotting factor. FVIII is the most common target of antibody formation (acquired hemophilia A), but inhibitors to prothrombin, FV, FIX, FX and FXI are also known.

961. Acquired inhibitor to FVIII occurs in?

Harrison's 20th Ed. Chapter 112 Page 837

A. Older adults
B. Pregnant women
C. Postpartum women
D. All of the above

Acquired inhibitor to FVIII occurs predominantly in older adults, in pregnant or postpartum women.

962. Which of the following time is prolonged in patients with acquired inhibitor to FVIII?

Harrison's 20th Ed. Chapter 112 Page 838

A. PT
B. aPTT
C. TT
D. All of the above

The diagnosis is based on the prolonged aPTT with normal PT and TT.

963. Which of the following treatment is advised in patients with acquired inhibitor to FVIII?

Harrison's 20th Ed. Chapter 112 Page 838

A. Cyclophosphamide
B. Intravenous gammaglobulin
C. Anti-CD20 monoclonal antibody
D. All of the above

964. Lupus anticoagulant interferes with the clotting activity of?

Harrison's 20th Ed. Chapter 112 Page 838

A. FVIII
B. FIX
C. FXII
D. All of the above

Lupus anticoagulant interferes with the clotting activity of many factors (FVIII, FIX, FXII, FXI), whereas acquired inhibitors are specific to a single factor.

Arterial and Venous Thrombosis

965. Which of the following is not a key factor in hemostasis & thrombosis?

Harrison's 20th Ed. Chapter 113 Page 839

A. Red blood corpuscles
B. Platelets
C. Vessel wall
D. Coagulation proteins

Hemostasis and thrombosis primarily involve the interplay among three factors : vessel wall, coagulation proteins and platelets.

966. Which of the following has lesser role in venous thrombosis?

Harrison's 20th Ed. Chapter 113 Page 839

A. Defects in coagulation and/or fibrinolysis proteins
B. Platelets
C. Abnormalities of blood vessels
D. Abnormalities of blood flow

In venous thrombosis, primary hypercoagulable states reflecting defects in coagulation and/or fibrinolysis proteins, or secondary hypercoagulable states involving abnormalities of blood vessels and blood flow or stasis lead to thrombosis. Arterial thrombosis is highly dependent on state of vessel wall, platelet and factors related to blood flow.

967. Which of the following about platelets is false?

Harrison's 20th Ed. Chapter 113 Page 839

A. Disc-shaped
B. Lack nucleus
C. Average lifespan of 7 to 10 days
D. None of the above

968. Which of the following is present in platelet dense-granules?

Harrison's 20th Ed. Chapter 113 Page 840

A. Adenosine diphosphate (ADP)
B. Soluble coagulation proteins
C. Growth factors
D. Integrins

The two types of platelet granules are alpha and dense. Alpha-granules contain soluble coagulation proteins, adhesion molecules, growth factors, integrins, cytokines & inflammatory modulators. Platelet dense-granules contain high concentrations of adenosine diphosphate (ADP) and serotonin, that influence platelet aggregation.

969. Which of the following subendothelial components trigger platelet reactivity?

Harrison's 20th Ed. Chapter 113 Page 840

A. Vitronectin
B. Fibronectin
C. Thrombospondin
D. All of the above

Exposed subendothelial components that trigger platelet reactivity favouring adhesion include collagen, von Willebrand factor, fibronectin, vitronectin and thrombospondin.

970. Which of the following expressed on platelet surface regulate collagen-induced platelet adhesion?

Harrison's 20th Ed. Chapter 113 Page 840

A. GP IV
B. GP VI
C. Integrin α2β1
D. All of the above

Certain proteins are expressed on the platelet surface that regulate collagen-induced platelet adhesion. These include glycoprotein (GP) IV, GPVI, and integrin α2β1.

971. Which of these is central to platelet adhesion and to the initiation of platelet activation?

Harrison's 20th Ed. Chapter 113 Page 840

A. GPIIb-IX-VII
B. GPIb-IX-VII
C. GPIb-IX-V
D. GPIIb-IX-V

The platelet GPIb-IX-V complex adhesive receptor is central both to platelet adhesion and to the initiation of platelet activation. GPIb-IX-V complex binds to the exposed von Willebrand factor, causing platelets to adhere. vWF–bound GPIb-IX-V transforms the GPIIb/IIIa receptor from an inactive low-affinity state to an active high-affinity receptor for fibrinogen.

972. On activation, platelets release which of the following?

Harrison's 20th Ed. Chapter 113 Page 839 Figure 113-1

A. Thromboxane A2
B. Serotonin (5-HT)
C. Adenosine diphosphate (ADP)
D. All of the above

Adhesion leads to activation of platelet and synthesis & release of thromboxane A2, serotonin (5-HT) and adenosine diphosphate (ADP).

973. Which of the following seven transmembrane receptors is found on platelets?

Harrison's 20th Ed. Chapter 113 Page 840

A. Prostaglandin receptors
B. Lipid receptors
C. Chemokine receptors
D. All of the above

Seven transmembrane receptors are found on platelets include ADP receptors, prostaglandin receptors, lipid receptors and chemokine receptors.

974. Which of the following receptors is present on platelets?

Harrison's 20th Ed. Chapter 113 Page 840

A. PAR1
B. PAR2
C. PAR4
D. All of the above

On platelets, seven transmembrane receptors for thrombin comprise the protease activation receptor 1 (PAR1) which involves specific cleavage of N-terminus of thrombin which in turn acts as a ligand for the receptor. Other PAR receptors present on platelets include PAR2 (not activated by thrombin) and PAR4.

975. Which of the following signal transduction events occur on activation of platelets?

Harrison's 20th Ed. Chapter 113 Page 840

A. Tyrosine kinase
B. Serine/threonine kinase
C. Lipid kinase
D. All of the above

Activation of platelets results in a rapid series of signal transduction events, including tyrosine kinase, serine/threonine kinase and lipid kinase activation.

976. Which of the following integrins is expressed on platelets?

Harrison's 20th Ed. Chapter 113 Page 840

A. α4β7
B. α6β4
C. GPIIb/IIIa
D. All of the above

Integrins are cell-surface adhesion molecules that affect attachment between ce11s and the extracellular matrix and mediate signal transduction that reflects the chemical composition of the cell environment. Integrin α4β7 is an accessory receptor for HIV and plays an important role in the transmission of HIV at mucosal surfaces such as the genital tract and gut. integrin GPIIb/IIIa is only expressed on platelets.

977. ADP binds to which of the following receptors on the platelet surface?

Harrison's 20th Ed. Chapter 113 Page 840

A. Purinergic receptors
B. Muscarinic receptors
C. Peptidergic receptors
D. All of the above

Adenosine receptors are responsible for transduction of ADP-induced signaling events, which are initiated by the binding of ADP to purinergic receptors on the platelet surface.

978. P2X1, P2Y1, and P2Y12 are which variety of receptors?

Harrison's 20th Ed. Chapter 113 Page 840

A. ADP receptors
B. Prostaglandin receptors
C. Lipid receptors
D. Chemokine receptors

Receptors found on platelets regulate their functions. They include the ADP receptors, prostaglandin receptors, lipid receptors, and chemokine receptors. ADP receptors are classified as P2X1, P2Y1, and P2Y12. Activation of both P2Y12 & P2Y1 receptors is essential for ADP-induced platelet aggregation. Thienopyridine derivatives, clopidogrel & prasugrel, are clinically utilized inhibitors of ADP-induced platelet aggregation.

979. Under which of the following conditions, people are at higher risk of myocardial infarction & thrombotic stroke?

Harrison's 20th Ed. Chapter 113 Page 840

A. Acute upper respiratory infections
B. Cholelithiasis
C. Fracture neck of femur
D. Conjunctivitis

In the setting of acute upper respiratory infections, people are at higher risk of myocardial infarction and thrombotic stroke.

980. P-selectin glycoprotein ligand 1 (PSGL-1) best relates with?

Harrison's 20th Ed. Chapter 113 Page 840

A. Platelet surface receptor
B. Leukocyte receptor
C. Endothelial receptor
D. All of the above

Activated platelets adhere to circulating leukocytes. Platelets bind via P-selectin (CD62P) expressed on the surface of activated platelets to the leukocyte receptor, P-selectin glycoprotein ligand 1 (PSGL-1). This association leads to increased expression of CD11b/CD18 (Mac-1) on leukocytes.

981. Risk of developing a venous thromboembolic event doubles after air travel lasting how many hours?

Harrison's 20th Ed. Chapter 113 Page 842

A. 4 hours
B. 6 hours
C. 8 hours
D. 10 hours

The risk of developing a venous thromboembolic event doubles after air travel lasting 4 hours, although the absolute risk remains low (1 in 6000).

982. Homozygous protein C or protein S deficiencies may lead to?

Harrison's 20th Ed. Chapter 113 Page 842

A. Thrombotic thrombocytopenic purpura
B. Leukocytoclastic vasculitis
C. Purpura fulminans
D. All of the above

Homozygous protein C or protein S deficiencies may lead to fatal purpura fulminans.

983. Activated protein C impairs coagulation by proteolytic degradation of?

Harrison's 20th Ed. Chapter 113 Page 843

A. FVa
B. FXa
C. FXIa
D. FXIIIa

Activated protein C impairs coagulation by proteolytic degradation of FVa. Patients resistant to the activity of activated protein C may have a point mutation in the FV gene located on chromosome 1, a mutant denoted as factor V Leiden.

984. Which of the following is not a component of Virchow's triad?

BMJ 2014;349:g4387

A. Thrombophilia
B. Ischemia
C. Stasis
D. Abnormalities of the vessel wall

Thrombophilia refers to an abnormality of blood coagulation that increases the risk of thrombosis. They may be heritable or acquired.

985. Which of the following is a naturally occurring anticoagulant?

BMJ 2014;349:g4387

A. Antithrombin
B. Protein C
C. Protein S
D. All of the above

986. Which of the following is an acquired thrombophilic disorder?
BMJ 2014;349:g4387

A. Antiphospholipid syndrome
B. Non-O blood group
C. Sickle cell disorder
D. All of the above

Genetic deficiencies of the naturally occurring anticoagulants like antithrombin, protein C & protein S, "gain of function" genetic polymorphisms like factor V Leiden and prothrombin gene mutation, non-O blood group and sickle cell disorders lead to heritable thrombophilia. Most heritable thrombophilias are heterozygous defects. Antiphospholipid syndrome is an acquired thrombophilic disorder.

987. Factor V Leiden is essentially not found in?
BMJ 2014;349:g4387

A. South East Asia
B. Japan
C. Sub-Saharan Africa
D. All of the above

Factor V Leiden is essentially not found in South East Asia, Japan, and sub-Saharan Africa, or in indigenous Australian populations.

988. Leiden University is situated in?
BMJ 2014;349:g4387

A. Sweden
B. Netherlands
C. Denmark
D. Greece

Leiden University is situated in the Netherlands.

989. Which of the following is a vitamin K dependent glycoprotein?
BMJ 2014;349:g4387

A. Protein C
B. Protein S
C. Antithrombin
D. All of the above

Protein C and protein S are vitamin K dependent glycoproteins.

Antiplatelet, Anticoagulant, and Fibrinolytic Drugs

990. Which of the following class of drugs come under the category of antithrombotic drugs?
Harrison's 20th Ed. Chapter 114 Page 844

A. Antiplatelet drugs
B. Anticoagulants
C. Fibrinolytic agents
D. All of the above

Antithrombotic drugs target the components of thrombi and include antiplatelet drugs, anticoagulants and fibrinolytic agents.

991. Circulating platelets are maintained in an inactive state by?
Harrison's 20th Ed. Chapter 114 Page 844

A. Nitric oxide (NO)
B. Prostacyclin
C. CD39
D. All of the above

Circulating platelets are maintained in an inactive state by nitric oxide (NO) and prostacyclin released by endothelial cells lining the blood vessels. Endothelial cells also express CD39 on their surface, a membrane-associated ecto-adenosine diphosphatase (ADPase) that degrades ADP released from activated platelets.

992. Thromboxane A2 (TxA2) plays a role in?
Thrombosis Research 2007;120: 337–346

A. Activating platelets
B. Constricting blood vessels
C. Promoting atherogenesis by inducing proliferation of vascular smooth muscle cells
D. All of the above

993. Which of the following statements is false?
Lancet 2006; 367: 606–17

A. NSAIDs (ibuprofen/diclofenac) are reversible inhibitors of COX
B. In mature human platelets, COX-2 are absent
C. Thromboxane A2 can be produced in monocytes and macrophages
D. None of the above

994. Which of the following drugs is used in arterial disease management?
Harrison's 20th Ed. Chapter 114 Page 844

A. That inhibit platelet activation & aggregation
B. That inhibit thrombin generation
C. That inhibit fibrin generation
D. All of the above

Drugs that inhibit platelet activation & aggregation play a primary role in arterial disease manage-ment while drugs that inhibit thrombin & fibrin generation play a primary role in venous disease.

995. At what dose, aspirin also inhibits COX-2?
Harrison's 20th Ed. Chapter 114 Page 844

A. ~ 325 mg/day
B. ~ 500 mg/day
C. ~ 750 mg/day
D. ~ 1000 mg/day

Aspirin produces its antithrombotic effect by irreversibly acetylating and inhibiting platelet cyclooxygenase COX-1. At high doses (~1000 mg/day), aspirin also inhibits COX-2.

996. Aspirin can produce antithrombotic effect at a dose of?
Harrison's 20th Ed. Chapter 114 Page 844

A. 20 mg/day
B. 30 mg/day
C. 40 mg/day
D. 50 mg/day

997. The major thrombin receptor on human platelets is?
Harrison's 20th Ed. Chapter 114 Page 845 Figure 114-3

A. Glycoprotein (GP) IIb/IIIa
B. Integrin α2β1
C. Protease-activated receptor-1 (PAR-1)
D. GPIb-IX-V

Protease-activated receptor-1 (PAR-1) is the major thrombin receptor on human platelets.

998. Compared with placebo, aspirin produces a reduction in the risk of cardiovascular death, MI, or stroke by?
Harrison's 20th Ed. Chapter 114 Page 844

A. 5%
B. 15%
C. 25%
D. 35%

Compared with placebo, aspirin led to a 25% reduction in risk of CV death, MI, or stroke.

999. For most indications, recommended daily dose of aspirin is?
Harrison's 20th Ed. Chapter 114 Page 845

A. 40 – 75 mg
B. 75 – 100 mg
C. 100 – 150 mg
D. 150 – 300 mg

Daily aspirin doses of 75–100 mg are recommended for most indications.

1000. Ticlopidine, clopidogrel, and prasugrel irreversibly block which of the following?
Harrison's 20th Ed. Chapter 114 Page 845

A. P2X 12
B. P2Y12
C. P2X 21
D. P2Y21

Thienopyridines (Ticlopidine, clopidogrel, and prasugrel) irreversibly block P2Y12, a key ADP receptor on the platelet surface. Cangrelor and ticagrelor are reversible inhibitors of P2Y12.

1001. Which of the following is a prodrug?
Harrison's 20th Ed. Chapter 114 Page 845

A. Ticlopidine
B. Clopidogrel
C. Prasugrel
D. All of the above

1002. Compared with aspirin, clopidogrel produces a reduction in the risk of cardiovascular death, MI, or stroke by?
Harrison's 20th Ed. Chapter 114 Page 845

A. 2.5%
B. 8.7%
C. 13.5%
D. 18.2%

When compared with aspirin in patients with recent ischemic stroke, MI, or peripheral arterial disease, clopidogrel reduced the risk of cardiovascular death, MI, and stroke by 8.7%.

1003. Which of the following drugs is known to produce thrombotic thrombocytopenic purpura (TTP)?
Harrison's 20th Ed. Chapter 114 Page 845

A. Ticlopidine
B. Clopidogrel
C. Quinine
D. All of the above

Ticlopidine produces TTP by inducing an autoantibody to ADAMTS13. Side effects of ticlopidine are gastrointestinal and hematologic. Neutropenia, thrombocytopenia, and thrombotic thrombocytopenic purpura usually occur within the first few months of starting treatment. Clopidogrel rarely precipitates TTP.

1004. Which of the following drugs can produce TTP?
Harrison's 20th Ed. Chapter 114 Page 845

A. Ticlopidine
B. Dipyridamole
C. Tirofiban
D. Aspirin

1005. Which of the following represents the final common pathway of platelet activation?
Harrison's 20th Ed. Chapter 114 Page 845 Figure 114-3

A. Cyclooxygenase (COX)
B. Adenosine diphosphate (ADP) receptors
C. Gp Ib
D. Gp IIb/IIIa

Expression of functionally active GpIIb/IIIa on platelet surfaces is the final common pathway of platelet activation regardless of initial stimulus.

1006. Which drug was studied in the 'CAPRIE trial'?
Harrison's 20th Ed. Chapter 114 Page 846

A. Aspirin
B. Ticlopidine and clopidogrel
C. Clopidogrel
D. All of the above

Clopidogrel was compared to aspirin in CAPRIE (Clopidogrel versus Aspirin in Patients at Risk of Ischemic Events) trial for effect on ischemic events in patients with recent stroke or MI and in those with symptomatic peripheral arterial disease.

1007. Subjects with which of the following allele exhibit decreased responsiveness to clopidogrel?
Harrison's 20th Ed. Chapter 114 Page 846

A. CYP2C17*2
B. CYP2C18*2
C. CYP2C19*2
D. CYP2C20*2

*Subjects with loss-of-function CYP2C19*2 allele exhibit decreased responsiveness to clopidogrel.*

1008. Which of the following about ticagrelor is false?
Harrison's 20th Ed. Chapter 114 Page 846

A. Not a prodrug
B. Produces reversible inhibition of ADP receptor
C. Inhibits P2Y12
D. None of the above

Ticagrelor is an orally active inhibitor of P2Y12. It does not require metabolic activation and produces reversible inhibition of ADP receptor. Ticagrelor inhibits P2Y12.

1009. Which of the following is a common side effect of ticagrelor?
Harrison's 20th Ed. Chapter 114 Page 846

A. Pruritis
B. Dysgeusia
C. Dyspnea
D. Diarrhoea

Besides bleeding, the most common side effects of ticagrelor are dyspnea, which can occur in up to 15% of patients and asymptomatic ventricular pauses.

1010. Which of the following is a platelet membrane glycoprotein receptor?
The Lancet 2000;355:1531

A. Glycoprotein Ia-IIa
B. Glycoprotein Ib-V-IX
C. Glycoprotein IIb-IIIa
D. All of the above

On platelets, Glycoprotein Ia-IIa is an active receptor for collagen, Glycoprotein Ib-V-IX is an active receptor for insoluble von Willebrand factor while the most abundant surface protein Glycoprotein IIb-IIIa requires conformational change during platelet activation to express receptor function, mainly for fibrinogen.

1011. Which of the following is a GPIIb/IIIA receptor antagonist?
Harrison's 20th Ed. Chapter 114 Page 847

A. Abciximab
B. Eptifibatide
C. Tirofiban
D. All of the above

Parenteral GPIIb/IIIa receptor antagonists are abciximab, eptifibatide, and tirofiban.

1012. Which of the following is false about GPIIb/IIIa adhesion receptors?
Harrison's 20th Ed. Chapter 114 Page 847, The Lancet 2000;355:1531

A. Found on surface of platelets & megakaryocytes
B. About 80,000 per platelet
C. GPIIb/IIIa is inactive on resting platelets
D. None of the above

Per platelet, the number of GP Ia-IIa receptors is 900–2300 molecules, GP Ib-V-IX receptors is 25000 molecules, GP IIb-IIIa receptors is 80000 molecules.

1013. Once activated, GPIIb/IIIa binds which of the following?
Harrison's 20th Ed. Chapter 114 Page 847

A. Thrombin
B. RBC
C. Fibrinogen
D. WBC

Once activated, GPIIb/IIIa binds fibrinogen. Also, it binds to von Willebrand factor, fibronectin, vitronectin and and thrombospondin.

1014. Deficiency of which of the following results in Glanzmann's thrombasthenia?
The Lancet 2000;355:1533

A. Glycoprotein IIb-IIIa
B. Glycoprotein Ia-IIa
C. Glycoprotein Ib-V-IX
D. All of the above

Patients with Glanzmann's thrombasthenia have undetectable platelet glycoprotein IIb-IIIa.

1015. Which of the following target the GPIIb/IIIa receptor?
Harrison's 20th Ed. Chapter 114 Page 847

A. Abciximab
B. Eptifibatide
C. Tirofiban
D. All of the above

Abciximab, eptifibatide and tirofiban—all target the GPIIb/IIIa receptor.

1016. Which of the following is a Fab fragment of a humanized murine monoclonal antibody?
Harrison's 20th Ed. Chapter 114 Page 847

A. Abciximab
B. Eptifibatide
C. Tirofiban
D. All of the above

Abciximab is a Fab fragment of a humanized murine monoclonal antibody that binds to the activated GPIIb/IIIa receptor with high affinity and blocks the binding of adhesive molecules like fibrinogen.

1017. Abciximab inhibits which of the following?
Harrison's 20th Ed. Chapter 114 Page 847

A. Gp IIb/IIIa
B. αvβ3 receptor
C. αMβ2 receptor
D. All of the above

Eptifibatide & tirofiban are specific for Gp IIb/IIIa. Abciximab also inhibits αvβ3 receptor, which binds vitronectin and αMβ2 receptor, a leukocyte integrin. Inhibition of αvβ3 and αMβ2 may endow abciximab with anti-inflammatory and/or antiproliferative properties besides platelet inhibition.

1018. Which of the following GPIIb/IIIa antagonists are given as an IV bolus followed by an infusion?
Harrison's 20th Ed. Chapter 114 Page 847

A. Abciximab
B. Eptifibatide
C. Tirofiban
D. All of the above

All of the GPIIb/IIIa antagonists are given as an IV bolus followed by an infusion.

1019. Most serious complication of GPIIb/IIIa antagonist therapy is?
Harrison's 20th Ed. Chapter 114 Page 847

A. Anemia
B. Leucopenia
C. Thrombocytopenia
D. All of the above

Immune-mediated thrombocytopenia is the most serious complication of GPIIb/IIIa therapy.

1020. Which of the following is an inhibitor of protease-activated receptor 1 (PAR-1)?
Harrison's 20th Ed. Chapter 114 Page 847

A. Cangrelor
B. Rivaroxaban
C. Apixaban
D. Vorapaxar

1021. Which of the following can be administered orally?
Harrison's 20th Ed. Chapter 114 Page 854

A. Cangrelor
B. Lepirudin
C. Dabigatran etexilate
D. Fondaparinux

Parenteral anticoagulants include heparin, low-molecular-weight heparin (LMWH), fondaparinux, lepirudin, desirudin, bivalirudin and argatroban. Only available oral anticoagulant is warfarin. Dabigatran etexilate is an oral thrombin inhibitor, and rivaroxaban, apixaban and edoxaban are oral Factor Xa inhibitors.

1022. Commercial unfractionated heparin (UFH) is obtained from which of the following sources?
Harrison's 20th Ed. Chapter 114 Page 848

A. Porcine lung
B. Porcine intestinal mucosa
C. Porcine liver
D. Porcine bone marrow

Commercial UFH is obtained from porcine intestinal mucosa. Heparin is a sulfated polysaccharide and is isolated from mammalian tissues rich in mast cells. Most commercial heparin is a polymer of alternating D-glucuronic acid and N-acetyl-d-glucosamine residues.

1023. Antithrombin is a member of?
Harrison's 20th Ed. Chapter 114 Page 848

A. Ornithine protease inhibitor
B. Cystine protease inhibitor
C. Glycine protease inhibitor
D. Serine protease inhibitor

Antithrombin is a plasma cofactor for heparin. It is a member of serine protease inhibitor (serpin) superfamily.

1024. Which unique sequence of UFH molecule binds to antithrombin?
Harrison's 20th Ed. Chapter 114 Page 848

A. Pentasaccharide
B. Hexasaccharide
C. Heptasaccharide
D. Decasaccharide

Heparin acts as an anticoagulant exclusively by activating antithrombin III. Presence of antithrombin III is mandatory for its action. Heparin binds to antithrombin III via a unique pentasaccharide sequence that is found on one-third of the chains of commercial heparin.

1025. Antithrombin is synthesized in?
Harrison's 20th Ed. Chapter 114 Page 848

A. Kidney
B. Liver
C. Intestinal mucosa
D. Lung

Antithrombin is synthesized in liver and acts as a suicide substrate for its target enzymes.

1026. UFH-antithrombin complex inactivates which of the following?
Harrison's 20th Ed. Chapter 114 Page 848

A. Factor IX
B. Factor X
C. Factor Xa
D. Factor II

Once bound to antithrombin III, heparin induces a conformational change in reactive center loop of antithrombin that makes it readily accessible to its target proteases. This conformational change enhances the rate at which antithrombin inhibits factor Xa by at least two orders of magnitude but has little effect on the rate of thrombin inhibition by antithrombin. To catalyze thrombin inhibition, heparin serves as a template that binds antithrombin & thrombin simultaneously. Formation of this ternary complex brings the enzyme in close apposition to the inhibitor, thereby promoting the formation of a stable covalent thrombin-antithrombin complex.

1027. For thrombin inhibition, heparin of what nature simultaneously binds to antithrombin and thrombin?
Harrison's 20th Ed. Chapter 114 Page 848

A. At least 16 saccharide units, molecular weight 5400
B. At least 17 saccharide units, molecular weight 5400
C. At least 18 saccharide units, molecular weight 5400
D. At least 19 saccharide units, molecular weight 5400

For thrombin inhibition, heparin chain of at least 18 saccharide units (molecular weight 5400) simultaneously binds to antithrombin and thrombin.

1028. What is the mean molecular weight of heparin?
Harrison's 20th Ed. Chapter 114 Page 848

A. 15,000
B. 20,000
C. 25,000
D. 30,000

Heparin has a mean molecular weight of 15,000.

1029. Which of the following statements about tissue factor pathway inhibitor (TFPI) is false?
Harrison's 20th Ed. Chapter 114 Page 848

A. Derived from endothelium
B. Factor Xa–dependent
C. Contribute to antithrombotic activity of heparin
D. None of the above

Heparin causes the release of tissue factor pathway inhibitor (TFPI) from the endothelium contributing to the antithrombotic activity of heparin.

1030. In the circulation, heparin binds to?
Harrison's 20th Ed. Chapter 114 Page 848

A. Endothelium
B. Macrophages
C. Platelet factor 4 (PF4)
D. All of the above

In the circulation, heparin binds to the endothelium, antithrombin, macrophages, acute-phase reactants, platelet factor 4 (PF4).

1031. Plasma half-life of heparin given as IV bolus (100 U/kg) is?
Harrison's 20th Ed. Chapter 114 Page 848

A. 60 minutes
B. 120 minutes
C. 180 minutes
D. 240 minutes

Plasma half-life of heparin ranges from 30 - 60 minutes with bolus IV doses of 25 and 100 U/kg, respectively.

1032. Which of the following internalize & depolymerize long heparin chains & secrete shorter chains back into the circulation?
Harrison's 20th Ed. Chapter 114 Page 848

A. Endothelium
B. Macrophages
C. Platelets
D. RBCs

Heparin binds to macrophages, which internalize and depolymerize the long heparin chains and secrete shorter chains back into the circulation.

1033. Which of the following statements about heparin is false?
Harrison's 20th Ed. Chapter 114 Page 848

A. Heparin must be given parenterally
B. Clearance is mainly renal
C. Platelet factor 4 can neutralize anticoagulant activity of heparin
D. Anti-factor Xa levels is used to monitor heparin therapy

Clearance of heparin is mainly extrarenal.

1034. For therapeutic anticoagulation, after IV bolus of 70 units/kg, heparin is infused at rate of?
Harrison's 20th Ed. Chapter 114 Page 849

A. 12 – 15 units/kg per hour
B. 25 – 30 units/kg per hour
C. 30 – 50 units/kg per hour
D. 50 – 65 units/kg per hour

For therapeutic anticoagulation, after IV bolus of 70 units/kg, heparin is infused at rate of 12–15 units/kg per hour.

1035. One USP unit of heparin is defined as the concentration of heparin that prevents 1 mL of citrated sheep plasma from clotting for 1 hour after addition of?
Harrison's 20th Ed. Chapter 114 Page 849

A. Calcium
B. Sodium
C. Potassium
D. Citrate

One USP unit of heparin is defined as the concentration of heparin that prevents 1 mL of citrated sheep plasma from clotting for 1 hour after addition of calcium.

1036. Which of the following is not a side effect of heparin?
Harrison's 20th Ed. Chapter 114 Page 849

A. Thrombocytopenia
B. Osteoporosis
C. Elevated levels of transaminases
D. Leucopenia

The most common side effect of heparin is bleeding. Other complications include thrombocytopenia, osteoporosis, and elevated levels of transaminases.

1037. Protamine sulfate is isolated from?
Harrison's 20th Ed. Chapter 114 Page 849

A. Horse urine
B. Horse serum
C. Salmon sperm
D. Bovine urine

Protamine sulfate, a mixture of basic polypeptides isolated from salmon sperm. Protamine binds heparin with high affinity, and the resultant protamine-heparin complexes are then cleared.

1038. 1 mg of protamine sulfate neutralizes how many units of heparin?
Harrison's 20th Ed. Chapter 114 Page 849

A. 100
B. 200
C. 300
D. 400

1 mg of protamine sulfate neutralizes 100 units of heparin.

1039. Mode of administration of protamine sulfate is?
Harrison's 20th Ed. Chapter 114 Page 849

A. Subcutaneous
B. Intramuscular
C. Intravenous
D. Any of the above

Protamine sulfate is given as a slow IV infusion. Anaphylactoid reactions can occur.

1040. Which of the following best relates to Heparin-induced thrombocytopenia (HIT)?
Harrison's 20th Ed. Chapter 114 Page 849

A. Antibodies of the IgM isotype
B. Antibodies against neoantigens on PF4
C. More common in medical than surgical patients
D. More frequent in males than in females

HIT is an antibody-mediated process triggered by antibodies directed against neoantigens on PF4 that are exposed when heparin binds to this protein. These antibodies are of the IgG isotype and bind simultaneously to heparin-PF4 complex and to platelet Fc receptors which activates platelets & generates platelet microparticles. Circulating microparticles are prothorombotic because they express anionic phospholipids on their surface and can bind clotting factors and promote thrombin generation. HIT is more common in surgical patients than in medical patients and, like many autoimmune disorders, occurs more frequently in females than in males.

1041. HIT occurs how many days after initiation of heparin therapy?
Harrison's 20th Ed. Chapter 114 Page 849

A. 1 to 3 days
B. 2 to 5 days
C. 5 to 14 days
D. 12 to 25 days

HIT occurs 5 to 14 days after initiation of heparin therapy.

1042. Which of the following about Heparin-induced thrombocytopenia (HIT) is false?
Harrison's 20th Ed. Chapter 114 Page 849

A. Thrombocytopenia is not severe
B. Not associated with bleeding
C. Increased risk of thrombosis
D. None of the above

1043. Anti-heparin/PF4 antibody can activate platelets through which of the following?
Harrison's 20th Ed. Chapter 111 Page 825

A. FcαRIIa
B. FcβRIIa
C. FcγRIIa
D. FcδRIIa

HIT results from antibody formation to a complex of the platelet-specific protein platelet factor 4 (PF4) and heparin. The anti-heparin/PF4 antibody can activate platelets through the FcγRIIa receptor and also activate monocytes and endothelial cells.

1044. Which of the following is not part of the 4T's used in diagnosis of HIT?
Harrison's 20th Ed. Chapter 111 Page 825

A. Thrombocytopenia
B. Timing of platelet count drop
C. Thrombosis and other sequelae
D. Other evident causes of thrombocytopenia

The "4T's" is recommended to be used in a diagnostic algorithm for HIT. They are thrombocytopenia, timing of platelet count drop, thrombosis and other sequelae such as localized skin reactions and other causes of thrombocytopenia not evident.

1045. The most specific diagnostic test for diagnosis of HIT is?
Harrison's 20th Ed. Chapter 111 Page 825

A. ELISA for antibodies against heparin-PF4 complexes
B. Platelet activation assays
C. Serotonin release assay
D. None of the above

The diagnosis of HIT is established using enzyme-linked assays to detect antibodies against heparin-PF4 complexes or with platelet activation assays. But, the most specific diagnostic test is the serotonin release assay. This test is performed by quantifying serotonin release when washed platelets loaded with labeled serotonin are exposed to patient serum in the absence or presence of varying concentrations of heparin. If the patient serum contains the HIT antibody, heparin addition induces platelet activation and serotonin release

1046. Which of the following drugs is useful in HIT?
Harrison's 20th Ed. Chapter 111 Page 825

A. Lepirudin
B. Bivalirudin
C. Fondaparinux
D. All of the above

Heparin must be stopped in suspected or documented HIT. Alternative anticoagulant to prevent or treat thrombosis is started like parenteral direct thrombin inhibitors (lepirudin, argatroban, or bivalirudin), or factor Xa inhibitors (fondaparinux). Danaparoid, a mixture of glycosaminoglycans with anti-Xa activity, is used for the treatment of HITT. LMWH should not be used to treat HIT patients because most HIT antibodies exhibit cross-reactivity with LMWH.

1047. In HIT, warfarin therapy should be overlapped with?
Harrison's 20th Ed. Chapter 111 Page 825

A. Argatroban
B. Bivalirudin
C. Fondaparinux
D. Any of the above

Introduction of warfarin alone in the setting of H IT or HITT may precipitate thrombosis, particularly venous gangrene, presumably due to clotting activation and severely reduced levels of proteins C and S. Warfarin therapy should be overlapped with a DTI (Lepirudin, argatroban or bivalirudin) or factor Xa inhibitor fondaparinux and started after resolution of the thrombocytopenia and lessening of the prothrombotic state.

1048. "White clot syndrome" is also called?
Eur J Vasc Endovasc Surg 2018;55:404

A. Heparin-induced thrombosis
B. Warfarin-induced thrombosis
C. Phenytoin-induced thrombosis
D. Thiazide-induced thrombosis

Heparin-induced thrombosis is also called "white clot syndrome".

1049. Which of the following drugs does not cause thrombocytopenia?
Harrison's 20th Ed. Chapter 114 Page 849

A. Unfractionated Heparin
B. Sulfonamides
C. Danazol
D. Thiazide diuretics

1050. What is the mean molecular weight of LMWH?
Harrison's 20th Ed. Chapter 114 Page 850

A. 4000
B. 5000
C. 6000
D. 7500

LMWH have a mean molecular weight of 5000.

1051. LMWH have a mean molecular mass of?
Harrison's 20th Ed. Chapter 114 Page 850

A. ~5 saccharide units
B. ~17 saccharide units
C. ~30 saccharide units
D. ~45 saccharide units

LMWH have a mean molecular weight of 5000 (~ 17 saccharide units)

1052. LMWHs have an anti-factor Xa:antithrombin activity ratio of?
Harrison's 20th Ed. Chapter 114 Page 850

A. 0.2 : 1
B. 0.5 : 1
C. 1:1
D. 2:1

LMWH accelerates factor Xa inhibition by antithrombin. It has little effect on thrombin inhibition. LMWH have anti-factor Xa to anti-factor IIa ratios ranging from 2:1 - 4:1.

1053. Plasma half-life of LMWH is?
Harrison's 20th Ed. Chapter 114 Page 850

A. 4 hour
B. 6 hour
C. 8 hour
D. 12 hour

LMWH has a plasma half-life of ~4 hours and is cleared almost exclusively by kidneys.

1054. Which of the following statements about LMWH is false?
Harrison's 20th Ed. Chapter 114 Page 850

A. LMWH cannot be administered IV
B. LMWH is prepared from unfractionated heparin
C. LMWH is cleared by kidneys
D. Resistance to LMWH is rare

Usually given SC, LMWH can be administered IV if a rapid anticoagulant response is needed.

1055. Coagulation monitoring with LMWH is done by?
Harrison's 20th Ed. Chapter 114 Page 851

A. PT
B. aPTT
C. Anti-factor Xa levels
D. Any of the above

If required, LMWH coagulation monitoring is done by anti-factor Xa levels because most LMWH preparations have little effect on aPTT.

1056. Range of therapeutic anti-factor Xa levels with LMWH is?
Harrison's 20th Ed. Chapter 114 Page 851

A. 0.5 –1.2 units/mL
B. 1.5 – 2.2 units/mL
C. 2.5 – 3.2 units/mL
D. 3.5 – 4.2 units/mL

Therapeutic anti-factor Xa levels with LMWH range from 0.5 - 1.2 units/mL, 3-4 hours later.

1057. Peak anti-factor Xa levels required when LMWH is given in prophylactic doses is?
Harrison's 20th Ed. Chapter 114 Page 851

A. 0.1 – 0.3 units/mL
B. 0.2 – 0.5 units/mL
C. 0.5 – 0.8 units/mL
D. 0.8 – 1.0 units/mL

When LMWH is given in prophylaxis, peak anti-factor Xa levels of 0.2 - 0.5 units/mL are desirable.

1058. Indications for LMWH monitoring include?
Harrison's 20th Ed. Chapter 114 Page 851

A. Renal insufficiency
B. Obesity
C. Pregnancy
D. All of the above

Indications for LMWH monitoring include renal insufficiency, obesity, pregnancy (III trimester), mechanical heart valves, infants or children.

1059. In unstable angina, dose of LMWH is?

Harrison's 20th Ed. Chapter 114 Page 851

A. 30 – 50 units/kg
B. 50 – 80 units/kg
C. 80 – 100 units/kg
D. 100 – 120 units/kg

In unstable angina, LMWH is given SC, twice-daily, at a dose of 100 - 120 units/kg.

1060. Which of the following statements about LMWH is false?

Harrison's 20th Ed. Chapter 114 Page 851

A. Major complication of LMWH is bleeding
B. Protamine sulfate completely reverses anti-factor IIa activity of LMWH
C. Patients at high risk for bleeding are more safely treated with continuous IV UFH than with SC LMWH
D. None of the above

1061. Fondaparinux has a molecular weight of?

Harrison's 20th Ed. Chapter 114 Page 851

A. 1728
B. 2728
C. 3728
D. 4728

Fondaparinux has a molecular weight of 1728. Fondaparinux binds only to antithrombin and is too short to bridge thrombin to antithrombin. Consequently, fondaparinux catalyzes factor Xa inhibition by antithrombin and does not enhance the rate of thrombin inhibition.

1062. Which of the following about Fondaparinux is false?

Harrison's 20th Ed. Chapter 114 Page 851

A. Bioavailability of SC Fondaparinux is 100%
B. Plasma half-life of Fondaparinux is 17 hours
C. Fondaparinux does not cause HIT
D. None of the above

Fondaparinux does not cause HIT because it does not bind to PF4. Also, there is no cross-reactivity of fondaparinux with HIT antibodies, hence can be used for the treatment of HIT. There is no antidote for fondaparinux.

1063. Which of the following drugs used for thromboprophylaxis has longest duration of action?

N Engl J Med 2005;353:1028-40

A. Fondaparinux
B. Idraparinux
C. Ximelagatran
D. Argatroban

Idraparinux is a long-acting pentasaccharide with a half-life of 130 hours. This facilitates once-weekly dosing for primary and/or secondary prevention of thromboembolic events.

1064. Which of the following is a natural anticoagulant?

N Engl J Med 2005;353:1028-40

A. Tissue factor pathway inhibitor
B. Protein C and S
C. Antithrombin
D. All of the above

Coagulation cascade is regulated by natural anticoagulants like tissue factor pathway inhibitor, protein C & protein S & antithrombin. They restrict formation of hemostatic plug to the site of injury.

1065. Which of the following is related to the action of direct thrombin inhibitors?

N Engl J Med 2005;353:1028-40, Harrison's 19th Ed. 753

A. Thrombocite
B. Platesite
C. Exosite
D. Natusite

Recombinant forms of hirudin, lepirudin and desirudin are bivalent direct thrombin inhibitors that interact with the active site and exosite 1, the substrate-binding site on thrombin.

1066. Which of the following "Direct Thrombin Inhibitors" is cleared by liver?

Harrison's 20th Ed. Chapter 114 Page 852, N Engl J Med 2005;353:1028-40

A. Melagatran
B. Argatroban
C. Ximelagatran
D. Recombinant Hirudins

Argatroban is predominantly cleared by hepatic metabolism and requires dose adjustments in patients with hepatic dysfunction. Rest of the above DTI's are cleared by kidney.

1067. Which of the following statements about Direct Thrombin Inhibitors is false?

N Engl J Med 2005;353:1028-40

A. Activity of DTIs is independent of antithrombin
B. DTIs can bind to and inhibit the activity of soluble thrombin and also thrombin bound to fibrin
C. DTIs also have an antiplatelet effect
D. None of the above

1068. aPTT is used to monitor the anticoagulant effect of all except?

Harrison's 20th Ed. Chapter 114 Page 852

A. Heparin
B. Lepirudin
C. Low-molecular-weight heparin
D. Argatroban

If monitoring is necessary in patients receiving LMWH, anti-factor Xa levels must be measured because most LMWH preparations have little effect on the aPTT.

1069. Which of the following target factor Xa for the anticoagulant activity?

Harrison's 20th Ed. Chapter 114 Page 852

A. Rivaroxaban
B. Apixaban
C. Edoxaban
D. All of the above

New oral anticoagulants include dabigatran, which targets thrombin and rivaroxaban, apixaban and edoxaban, which target factor Xa.

1070. Which of the following is an oral anticoagulant?
Harrison's 20th Ed. Chapter 114 Page 852

A. Dabigatran etexilate
B. Rivaroxaban
C. Apixaban
D. All of the above

Dabigatran etexilate is an oral thrombin inhibitor. Rivaroxaban and apixaban are oral factor Xa inhibitors.

1071. Warfarin was initially developed as a?
Harrison's 20th Ed. Chapter 114 Page 852

A. Diuretic
B. Antibiotic
C. Sedative
D. Rodenticide

Warfarin was initially developed as a rodenticide.

1072. Which of the following is a vitamin K - dependent coagulation protein?
Harrison's 20th Ed. Chapter 114 Page 852

A. Factor VII
B. Factor X
C. Prothrombin
D. All of the above

Warfarin interferes with the synthesis of the vitamin K–dependent clotting proteins like prothrombin (factor II) and factors VII, IX, and X. Synthesis of the vitamin K–dependent anticoagulant proteins, proteins C and S, is also reduced by vitamin K antagonists.

1073. Warfarin acts by inhibiting which of the following?
Harrison's 20th Ed. Chapter 114 Page 852

A. Vitamin K epoxide reductase (VKOR)
B. Vitamin K reductase
C. Vitamin K carboxylase
D. Vitamin K hydrolase

Warfarin is a water-soluble vitamin K antagonist. It inhibits vitamin K epoxide reductase (VKOR) thereby interfering with the synthesis of the vitamin K dependent clotting proteins (factor II, VII, IX, and X). Synthesis of vitamin K dependent anticoagulant proteins (proteins C & S) is also reduced by vitamin K antagonists..

1074. All of the vitamin K dependent clotting factors possess which amino acid residues at their N termini?
Harrison's 20th Ed. Chapter 114 Page 852

A. Leucine
B. Isoleucine
C. Glutamic acid
D. Tryptophan

All of the vitamin K–dependent clotting factors possess glutamic acid residues at their N termini.

1075. Warfarin is a racemic mixture of which of the following isomers?
Harrison's 20th Ed. Chapter 114 Page 853

A. C and D
B. M and N
C. R and S
D. X and Y

Warfarin is a racemic mixture of R and S isomers, more active being the S isomer. In liver, CYP2C9 mediates oxidative metabolism of S isomer.

1076. Antithrombotic effect of warfarin depends on reduction in the functional level of?
Harrison's 20th Ed. Chapter 114 Page 853

A. Factor VIII
B. Factor IX
C. Factor X
D. Factor XI

Antithrombotic effect of warfarin depends on reduction in functional levels of factor X & prothrombin.

1077. The half-life of warfarin in plasma is?
Harrison's 20th Ed. Chapter 114 Page 853

A. ~ 12 hours
B. ~ 24 hours
C. ~ 36 hours
D. ~ 60 hours

Racemic warfarin has a plasma half-life of 36 - 42 hours. >97% of circulating warfarin is bound to albumin so only a small fraction of unbound warfarin is biologically active.

1078. INR in patients with prosthetic mechanical heart valves should be?
Harrison's 20th Ed. Chapter 114 Page 853

A. 1.5 to 2.0
B. 2.0 to 3.0
C. 2.5 to 3.5
D. 3.5 to 4.0

For most indications, warfarin is administered in doses that produce a target INR of 2.0 - 3.0. For patients with mechanical heart valves, a target INR of 2.5 - 3.5 is recommended.

1079. In atrial fibrillation, the risk of cardioembolic stroke increases at what level of INR?
Harrison's 20th Ed. Chapter 114 Page 853

A. < 1.7
B. < 1.9
C. < 2.1
D. < 2.3

1080. In atrial fibrillation, the risk of bleeding increases at what level of INR?
Harrison's 20th Ed. Chapter 114 Page 853

A. > 3.0
B. > 3.5
C. > 4.0
D. > 4.5

In atrial fibrillation, there occurs an increased risk of cardioembolic stroke when the INR falls to <1.7 and an increase in bleeding with INR values >4.5.

1081. Initial treatment with warfarin is supported by concomitant administration of which of the following?
Harrison's 20th Ed. Chapter 114 Page 853

A. Heparin
B. LMWH
C. Fondaparinux
D. Any of the above

Initial treatment with warfarin is supported by concomitant administration of either heparin, LMWH or fondaparinux. A minimum 5 day course of parenteral anticoagulation is recommended.

1082. Which of the following statements about warfarin is false?
Harrison's 20th Ed. Chapter 114 Page 853

A. Warfarin is usually started at a dose of 5-10 mg.
B. Warfarin crosses the placenta
C. Warfarin does not pass into the breast milk
D. None of the above

1083. Patients on warfarin with serious bleeding are treated with?
Harrison's 20th Ed. Chapter 114 Page 854

A. IV Vitamin K infusion
B. Fresh-frozen plasma
C. Prothrombin complex concentrates
D. Any of the above

Patients on warfarin with serious bleeding should be given 10 mg of vitamin K by slow IV infusion till INR is in normal range. Treatment with vitamin K should be supplemented with fresh-frozen plasma (FFP) as a source of the vitamin K dependent clotting proteins. For life-threatening bleeds, prothrombin complex concentrates can be used.

1084. Warfarin-induced skin necrosis occurs in which week of therapy?
Harrison's 20th Ed. Chapter 114 Page 854

A. First week
B. Second week
C. Third week
D. Fourth week

Skin necrosis due to warfarin therapy is seen 2 - 5 days after initiation of therapy.

1085. Warfarin-induced skin necrosis is seen in patients with congenital or acquired deficiencies of?
Harrison's 20th Ed. Chapter 114 Page 854

A. Tissue factor pathway inhibitor
B. Protein C or S
C. Antithrombin
D. All of the above

Warfarin-induced skin necrosis is seen in patients with congenital or acquired deficiencies of protein C or protein S.

1086. In pregnant women, risk of warfarin embryopathy is greatest in which trimester of pregnancy?
Harrison's 20th Ed. Chapter 114 Page 854

A. First
B. Second
C. Third
D. Any of the above

Warfarin embryopathy consists of nasal hypoplasia and stippled epiphyses. Risk of embryopathy is highest if warfarin is given in the first trimester of pregnancy.

1087. CNS abnormalities can occur with exposure to coumarins during which trimester of pregnancy?
Harrison's 20th Ed. Chapter 114 Page 854

A. First
B. Second
C. Third
D. Any of the above

CNS abnormalities can occur with exposure to coumarins at any time during pregnancy.

1088. For prevention or treatment of thrombosis, which of the following can be given during pregnancy?
Harrison's 20th Ed. Chapter 114 Page 854

A. Heparin
B. LMWH
C. Fondaparinux
D. Any of the above

1089. "Purple-toe syndrome" is seen in patients receiving warfarin with?
BMJ Case Rep. 2014; 2014: bcr2014205320

A. Atherosclerotic vascular disease
B. Hypertension
C. Diabetes mellitus
D. Porphyria

"Purple-toe syndrome" presents with atheroembolic symptoms like ischemic (purple) toes, livedo reticularis, gangrene, abdominal pain, or symptoms of renal infarction. Skin biopsy reveals cholesterol emboli in the purple-toe syndrome.

1090. Warfarin embryopathy is due to effect of warfarin on which bone matrix protein?
Harrison's 20th Ed. Chapter 114 Page 854

A. Osteocalcin
B. Osteotensin
C. Osteophysin
D. Osteogenin

Osteocalcin is a vitamin K–dependent bone matrix protein.

1091. Recombinant derivative of recombinant tissue-type plasminogen activator (rt-PA) is?
Harrison's 20th Ed. Chapter 114 Page 857

A. Anistreplase
B. Alteplase
C. Tenecteplase
D. Activase

Approved fibrinolytic agents are streptokinase, acylated plasminogen streptokinase activator complex (anistreplase), urokinase, recombinant tissue-type plasminogen activator (rt-PA), also known as alteplase or activase & two recombinant derivatives of rt-PA, tenecteplase & reteplase.

1092. Which of the following is a fibrin-specific plasminogen activator?
Harrison's 20th Ed. Chapter 114 Page 857

A. Streptokinase
B. Alteplase
C. Anistreplase
D. Urokinase

Alteplase, tenecteplase and reteplase are fibrin-specific plasminogen activators while streptokinase, anistreplase and urokinase are nonspecific plasminogen activators.

1093. Which of the following is false about 'Streptokinase'?
Harrison's 20th Ed. Chapter 114 Page 856

A. Obtained from cultures of β-hemolytic streptococci
B. By itself, it has no plasminogen activator (PA) activity
C. Not fibrin-selective
D. None of the above

1094. Streptokinase binds to which of the following?
Harrison's 20th Ed. Chapter 114 Page 856

A. Plasmin
B. Plasminogen
C. Fibrin
D. All of the above

Streptokinase is not an enzyme and does not directly convert plasminogen to plasmin. Instead, streptokinase forms a 1:1 stoichiometric complex with plasminogen. This complex induces a conformational change in plasminogen that exposes its active site which then converts additional plasminogen molecules to plasmin to induce a systemic lytic state.

1095. Which of the following is false about 'Streptokinase'?
Harrison's 20th Ed. Chapter 114 Page 856

A. Acts only when complexed with plasminogen
B. Streptokinase has no affinity for fibrin
C. Antigenic and anaphylactogenic
D. None of the above

1096. Urokinase is derived from?
Harrison's 20th Ed. Chapter 114 Page 857

A. Cultured fetal kidney cells
B. Horse's urine
C. Cow's urine
D. All of the above

Urokinase is a two-chain serine protease derived from cultured fetal kidney cells with a molecular weight of 34,000. Urokinase converts plasminogen to plasmin directly by cleaving the Arg560-Val561 bond.

1097. The half-life of Urokinase is?
Harrison's 20th Ed. Chapter 114 Page 857

A. ~ 5 minutes
B. ~ 10 minutes
C. ~ 15 minutes
D. ~ 20 minutes

Half-life of Urokinase is ~20 minutes.

1098. Half-life of tissue-type plasminogen activator (t-PA) is?
Harrison's 20th Ed. Chapter 114 Page 857

A. ~ 5 minutes
B. ~ 10 minutes
C. ~ 15 minutes
D. ~ 20 minutes

The half-life of t-PA is ~5 minutes.

1099. Which of the following is a direct fibrinolytic agent?
Drugs R D. 2008;9(3):185-90

A. Alfimeprase
B. Staphylokinase
C. TNK-rt-PA
D. Streptokinase

Alfimeprase is a metalloproteinase enzyme (isolated from venom of southern copperhead snake) that degrades fibrin & fibrinogen in a plasmin-independent fashion. In circulation, alfimeprase is inhibited by a2-macroglobulin. Alfimeprase must be delivered via a catheter directly into the thrombus.

1100. Risk of intracranial hemorrhage with use of thrombolytic agents is increased in all except?
Harrison's 20th Ed. Chapter 114 Page 857

A. Older age
B. Female sex
C. Higher body weight
D. Hypertension

1101. Which of the following is a "bolus fibrinolytic" agent?
Harrison's 20th Ed. Chapter 114 Page 857

A. Tenecteplase (TNK)
B. Streptokinase
C. Urokinase
D. Tissue plasminogen activator

TNK and rPA are referred to as bolus fibrinolytics.

1102. Paget-Schroetter syndrome relates to?
Lancet 2005; 365: 1163–74

A. Acute deep vein thrombosis in cancer patients
B. Deep vein thrombosis of arms
C. Deep vein thrombosis in pregnant women
D. Recurrent ipsilateral deep vein

ANSWERS

1. B	43. C	85. A	127. D	169. D	211. D
2. D	44. D	86. D	128. C	170. D	212. A
3. A	45. D	87. D	129. C	171. D	213. A
4. C	46. A	88. D	130. D	172. B	214. A
5. B	47. D	89. D	131. A	173. B	215. B
6. A	48. D	90. A	132. D	174. D	216. D
7. D	49. D	91. A	133. D	175. C	217. D
8. D	50. C	92. A	134. D	176. D	218. D
9. C	51. C	93. B	135. D	177. B	219. C
10. B	52. A	94. A	136. B	178. D	220. A
11. C	53. A	95. A	137. A	179. D	221. B
12. C	54. A	96. B	138. D	180. D	222. C
13. A	55. B	97. B	139. A	181. A	223. C
14. D	56. C	98. C	140. D	182. D	224. C
15. A	57. C	99. C	141. A	183. D	225. A
16. A	58. C	100. D	142. A	184. B	226. D
17. C	59. B	101. A	143. D	185. D	227. A
18. C	60. D	102. B	144. C	186. A	228. B
19. C	61. B	103. D	145. D	187. B	229. D
20. B	62. A	104. D	146. D	188. D	230. B
21. B	63. A	105. D	147. D	189. B	231. D
22. D	64. D	106. D	148. D	190. D	232. D
23. A	65. C	107. D	149. C	191. C	233. C
24. D	66. C	108. C	150. D	192. A	234. A
25. A	67. D	109. B	151. D	193. B	235. C
26. B	68. D	110. B	152. D	194. B	236. B
27. A	69. A	111. D	153. A	195. B	237. C
28. D	70. D	112. B	154. A	196. D	238. C
29. D	71. D	113. C	155. D	197. B	239. D
30. D	72. D	114. B	156. D	198. A	240. A
31. A	73. D	115. A	157. D	199. C	241. C
32. A	74. D	116. A	158. A	200. D	242. B
33. B	75. D	117. B	159. A	201. D	243. C
34. A	76. B	118. C	160. A	202. D	244. D
35. B	77. C	119. B	161. D	203. D	245. D
36. B	78. B	120. A	162. B	204. D	246. D
37. B	79. B	121. C	163. C	205. D	247. C
38. C	80. D	122. A	164. C	206. D	248. B
39. A	81. D	123. D	165. B	207. A	249. D
40. D	82. C	124. C	166. C	208. D	250. A
41. B	83. A	125. A	167. C	209. D	251. C
42. B	84. D	126. D	168. C	210. C	252. C

ANSWERS

253. B
254. A
255. D
256. D
257. D
258. B
259. D
260. B
261. D
262. C
263. B
264. B
265. D
266. D
267. C
268. D
269. D
270. D
271. D
272. D
273. B
274. D
275. C
276. D
277. C
278. D
279. B
280. B
281. D
282. D
283. B
284. B
285. D
286. B
287. D
288. A
289. C
290. A
291. D
292. A
293. A
294. A
295. C
296. C
297. B
298. D
299. B
300. D
301. D
302. C
303. D
304. C
305. D
306. B
307. D
308. B
309. D
310. B
311. A
312. B
313. C
314. B
315. D
316. C
317. C
318. D
319. B
320. D
321. B
322. C
323. A
324. D
325. B
326. C
327. A
328. C
329. A
330. A
331. C
332. B
333. B
334. A
335. D
336. D
337. D
338. D
339. C
340. A
341. A
342. D
343. C
344. A
345. D
346. D
347. D
348. D
349. C
350. D
351. D
352. D
353. C
354. D
355. D
356. B
357. C
358. D
359. A
360. B
361. C
362. D
363. D
364. A
365. D
366. D
367. B
368. A
369. B
370. B
371. A
372. A
373. D
374. D
375. C
376. D
377. B
378. D
379. A
380. C
381. D
382. B
383. D
384. D
385. D
386. D
387. D
388. D
389. D
390. D
391. C
392. B
393. C
394. A
395. B
396. B
397. D
398. D
399. D
400. D
401. C
402. A
403. B
404. A
405. C
406. B
407. D
408. B
409. D
410. A
411. A
412. D
413. D
414. C
415. A
416. D
417. B
418. C
419. B
420. C
421. B
422. A
423. C
424. D
425. D
426. C
427. B
428. C
429. A
430. B
431. D
432. C
433. A
434. C
435. A
436. A
437. D
438. A
439. D
440. D
441. D
442. D
443. C
444. D
445. B
446. D
447. C
448. C
449. A
450. D
451. D
452. D
453. B
454. A
455. D
456. C
457. A
458. A
459. C
460. D
461. C
462. A
463. C
464. B
465. B
466. B
467. B
468. A
469. C
470. C
471. C
472. A
473. A
474. D
475. C
476. C
477. A
478. B
479. D
480. B
481. B
482. C
483. D
484. B
485. C
486. A
487. A
488. A
489. A
490. C
491. B
492. A
493. A
494. B
495. D
496. A
497. D
498. A
499. D
500. D
501. A
502. C
503. D
504. C

ANSWERS

505. C	547. A	589. B	631. C	673. D	715. A
506. A	548. D	590. C	632. C	674. D	716. A
507. D	549. B	591. B	633. A	675. D	717. B
508. A	550. B	592. C	634. D	676. C	718. D
509. B	551. C	593. C	635. B	677. D	719. C
510. C	552. B	594. D	636. D	678. D	720. D
511. D	553. C	595. A	637. C	679. D	721. A
512. A	554. A	596. D	638. B	680. A	722. D
513. B	555. D	597. D	639. D	681. B	723. C
514. D	556. A	598. B	640. B	682. D	724. D
515. A	557. D	599. D	641. C	683. C	725. C
516. D	558. D	600. D	642. B	684. A	726. A
517. D	559. D	601. C	643. A	685. A	727. D
518. A	560. D	602. B	644. A	686. D	728. A
519. D	561. B	603. A	645. D	687. A	729. B
520. D	562. D	604. A	646. D	688. B	730. D
521. C	563. B	605. A	647. D	689. D	731. B
522. A	564. C	606. D	648. C	690. D	732. B
523. D	565. C	607. D	649. D	691. B	733. D
524. A	566. B	608. D	650. C	692. B	734. B
525. D	567. A	609. C	651. B	693. C	735. C
526. C	568. A	610. B	652. D	694. B	736. C
527. A	569. D	611. D	653. A	695. B	737. D
528. D	570. C	612. A	654. A	696. C	738. C
529. D	571. A	613. B	655. B	697. A	739. C
530. A	572. A	614. C	656. D	698. B	740. D
531. D	573. D	615. D	657. D	699. D	741. C
532. C	574. B	616. A	658. A	700. B	742. C
533. A	575. C	617. A	659. D	701. D	743. A
534. B	576. A	618. B	660. B	702. D	744. A
535. D	577. D	619. C	661. D	703. D	745. B
536. D	578. B	620. D	662. C	704. B	746. D
537. B	579. D	621. C	663. D	705. D	747. B
538. D	580. D	622. D	664. D	706. D	748. D
539. D	581. A	623. D	665. C	707. C	749. D
540. C	582. A	624. C	666. B	708. C	750. A
541. D	583. D	625. D	667. B	709. B	751. B
542. D	584. D	626. C	668. D	710. A	752. B
543. C	585. A	627. D	669. A	711. B	753. C
544. D	586. B	628. C	670. D	712. A	754. A
545. D	587. A	629. B	671. A	713. A	755. C
546. D	588. A	630. D	672. A	714. A	756. D

ANSWERS

757. D	799. C	841. C	883. A	925. C	967. D
758. A	800. D	842. B	884. A	926. D	968. A
759. C	801. A	843. C	885. D	927. D	969. D
760. D	802. A	844. A	886. D	928. D	970. D
761. D	803. B	845. D	887. D	929. B	971. C
762. A	804. D	846. A	888. D	930. C	972. D
763. B	805. D	847. D	889. D	931. D	973. D
764. D	806. D	848. C	890. A	932. A	974. D
765. A	807. B	849. D	891. A	933. C	975. D
766. C	808. C	850. D	892. A	934. D	976. C
767. D	809. B	851. B	893. C	935. C	977. A
768. A	810. C	852. D	894. C	936. D	978. A
769. D	811. B	853. C	895. D	937. D	979. A
770. D	812. B	854. B	896. D	938. D	980. B
771. A	813. C	855. A	897. D	939. D	981. A
772. B	814. D	856. D	898. D	940. C	982. C
773. C	815. D	857. A	899. D	941. D	983. A
774. D	816. D	858. B	900. D	942. D	984. B
775. B	817. D	859. B	901. D	943. A	985. D
776. A	818. B	860. D	902. C	944. B	986. A
777. C	819. D	861. A	903. A	945. C	987. D
778. A	820. D	862. A	904. A	946. A	988. B
779. D	821. A	863. B	905. A	947. D	989. C
780. D	822. D	864. A	906. C	948. B	990. D
781. B	823. B	865. D	907. D	949. D	991. D
782. A	824. C	866. C	908. A	950. D	992. D
783. C	825. D	867. B	909. D	951. D	993. D
784. A	826. D	868. C	910. D	952. C	994. A
785. D	827. D	869. D	911. A	953. A	995. D
786. C	828. D	870. B	912. B	954. D	996. B
787. B	829. A	871. A	913. C	955. A	997. C
788. D	830. D	872. C	914. D	956. A	998. C
789. C	831. A	873. D	915. A	957. D	999. B
790. D	832. A	874. D	916. D	958. D	1000. B
791. C	833. B	875. D	917. D	959. B	1001. D
792. D	834. A	876. D	918. D	960. B	1002. B
793. C	835. D	877. A	919. C	961. D	1003. D
794. B	836. C	878. A	920. A	962. B	1004. A
795. D	837. A	879. A	921. B	963. D	1005. D
796. D	838. D	880. C	922. D	964. D	1006. C
797. D	839. D	881. A	923. A	965. A	1007. C
798. A	840. D	882. D	924. C	966. B	1008. D

ANSWERS

1009. C	1025. B	1041. C	1057. B	1073. C	1089. A
1010. D	1026. C	1042. D	1058. D	1074. C	1090. A
1011. D	1027. C	1043. C	1059. D	1075. C	1091. C
1012. D	1028. A	1044. D	1060. D	1076. C	1092. C
1013. C	1029. D	1045. C	1061. A	1077. C	1093. D
1014. A	1030. D	1046. D	1062. D	1078. C	1094. B
1015. D	1031. A	1047. D	1063. B	1079. A	1095. D
1016. A	1032. B	1048. A	1064. D	1080. D	1096. A
1017. B	1033. B	1049. C	1065. C	1081. D	1097. D
1018. D	1034. A	1050. B	1066. B	1082. D	1098. A
1019. C	1035. A	1051. B	1067. D	1083. D	1099. A
1020. D	1036. D	1052. D	1068. C	1084. A	1100. C
1021. C	1037. C	1053. A	1069. D	1085. B	1101. A
1022. B	1038. A	1054. A	1070. D	1086. A	1102. B
1023. D	1039. C	1055. C	1071. D	1087. D	
1024. A	1040. B	1056. A	1072. A	1088. D	

Cardiology 2

Dyspnea

1. Which of the following about dyspnea is false?

Harrison's 20th Ed. Chapter 33 Page 226

A. Self-reported
B. Subjective experience of breathing discomfort
C. Qualitatively distinct sensations that vary in intensity
D. None of the above

Dyspnea is a symptom. American Thoracic Society (ATS) defines dyspnea as a "subjective experience of breathing discomfort that consists of qualitatively distinct sensations that vary in intensity. Dyspnea can be perceived only by the person experiencing it and, therefore, must be self-reported.

2. Which of the following features of breathing define dyspnea?

S Afr Med J. 2016;106(1):32-36

A. Abnormal
B. Uncomfortable
C. Awareness
D. All of the above

Normally, at rest, one is unaware of the act of breathing. With exercise, though aware of breathing, discomfort is expected to be transient. Dyspnea is defined with prefixes before awareness of breathing i.e. abnormally uncomfortable.

3. Which of the following is a sign of increased work of breathing?

Harrison's 20th Ed. Chapter 33 Page 226

A. Tachypnea
B. Use of accessory muscles of respiration
C. Intercostal retraction
D. All of the above

4. Which of the following can cause dyspnea?

Harrison's 20th Ed. Chapter 33 Page 226

A. Pulmonary diseases
B. Cardiac diseases
C. Neurologic diseases
D. All of the above

Dyspnea, like hunger or thirst, is a "synthetic sensation" as it often arises from multiple sources of information rather than from stimulation of a single neural receptor.

5. Which of the following best relates to dyspnea?

Harrison's 20th Ed. Chapter 33 Page 226

A. Efferent - afferent mismatch
B. Efferent - reafferent mismatch
C. Afferent - reefferent mismatch
D. All of the above

Three main components contribute to dyspnea - afferent signals, efferent signals and central information processing. Dyspnea arises when there is a mismatch in integrative signaling between afferent signals from the respiratory system and efferent signals from the CNS. This is termed as "neuro-mechanical" or "efferent-reafferent mismatch".

6. Neural signal termed "corollary discharge" is sent to?

Harrison's 20th Ed. Chapter 33 Page 226

A. Sensory cortex
B. Motor cortex
C. Ventilatory muscles
D. All of the above

The sensory cortex is simultaneously activated when motor signals are sent to the chest wall, resulting in the conscious sensation of muscular effort and breathlessness. When there is increased work of breathing, increased neural output from the motor cortex is sensed via a neural signal, termed corollary discharge, is sent to the sensory cortex at the same time that motor output is directed to the ventilatory muscles. Corollary discharges are important in shaping the sense of respiratory effort.

7. Chemoreceptors in the carotid bodies and medulla are activated by?

Harrison's 20th Ed. Chapter 33 Page 226

A. Hypoxemia
B. Acute hypercapnia
C. Acidemia
D. All of the above

Chemoreceptors in the carotid bodies and medulla are activated by hypoxemia, acute hypercapnia, and acidemia.

8. The sense of air hunger arises from?

Harrison's 20th Ed. Chapter 33 Page 226

A. Stimulation of chemoreceptors
B. J-receptors
C. Pulmonary vascular receptors
D. All of the above

Sensation of air hunger arises from a combination of stimuli that increase drive to breathe such as hypoxemia or hypercapnia (mediated by signals from chemoreceptors in the carotid body and aortic arch), acute hypercapnia or acidemia (mediated by signals from peripheral & central chemoreceptors), airway & interstitial inflammation (mediated by pulmonary afferents), and pulmonary vascular receptors.

9. J (juxtacapillary) receptors are found in?

N Engl J Med. 2008;358:1054-9

A. Bronchi
B. Terminal brochiole
C. Alveolar interstitial space
D. All of the above

Pulmonary "J Receptors" are sensory cells located within alveolar septa and are "juxtaposed" to the pulmonary capillaries. These cells are activated by physical engorgement of the pulmonary capillaries (left heart dysfunction) or increased pulmonary interstitial volume (pulmonary edema). Dyspnea results from transudation of pulmonary fluid & stretching of pulmonary interstitial juxtacapillary receptors due to combination of increased pulmonary arterial blood flow in concert with elevated pulmonary venous pressures.

10. Irritant receptors around the epithelial cells of bronchial walls are activated by?

Am J Respir Crit Care Med. 1999;159:321-340

A. Tactile stimulation in the bronchial mucosa
B. High rates of air flow
C. Increases in bronchial smooth muscle tone
D. All of the above

Pulmonary irritant receptors are sensors present within the respiratory epithelium which can sense and respond to a variety of chemical irritants.

11. J-receptors are sensitive to?

Harrison's 19th Ed. 47e-1

A. Changes in pulmonary artery pressure
B. Acidemia
C. Interstitial edema
D. Hypercapnia

J-receptors or pulmonary C-fiber receptors are sensitive to interstitial edema.

12. The sensation of chest tightness results from?
Harrison's 20th Ed. Chapter 33 Page 226

A. Chemoreceptors in medulla
B. Mechanoreceptors in lungs
C. Chemoreceptors in aortic and carotid bodies
D. Afferent fibers in the phrenic nerves

Mechanoreceptors in the lungs, when stimulated by bronchospasm, lead to a sensation of chest tightness.

13. Metaboreceptors are located in?
Harrison's 20th Ed. Chapter 33 Page 226, J Physiol. 2007;585(Pt 1):165-174

A. Medulla
B. Carotid bodies
C. Skeletal muscle
D. All of the above

Metaboreceptors are located in skeletal muscle. During exercise, accumulation of metabolites within the active skeletal muscle, stimulates group III & IV afferent neurons which evoke a reflex increase in muscle sympathetic nerve activity (MSNA), known as the muscle metaboreflex.

14. Which of the following is an ischemic metabolite?
J Physiol. 2007;585(Pt 1):165-174

A. Lactic acid
B. Adenosine
C. Bradykinin
D. All of the above

Muscle metaboreceptors regulate sympathetic activation during exercise. This reflex is activated by lactic acid, phosphate, K+, H+, adenosine, prostaglandins, and bradykinin released from exercising skeletal muscle. These ischemic metabolites stimulate groups III and IV chemosensitive afferents.

15. Which of the following is used to measure dyspnea?
Am J Respir Crit Care Med. 1999;159:321-340

A. Medical Research Council (MRC) Scale
B. Baseline dyspnea index
C. Oxygen Cost Diagram (OCD) scale
D. All of the above

16. Modified Medical Research Council Dyspnea Scale classifies dyspnea into how many grades?
Harrison's 20th Ed. Chapter 33 Page 228 Table 33-1

A. 3
B. 4
C. 5
D. 6

Modified Medical Research Council Dyspnea Scale classifies dyspnea into 5 grades i.e. 0 to 4. This scale has been incorporated into GOLD 2017 guidelines as a tool for rating dyspnea in COPD.

17. What is the grade of dyspnea if one has to stop to rest after walking 100 meters on level ground?
Harrison's 20th Ed. Chapter 33 Page 228 Table 33-1

A. 1
B. 2
C. 3
D. 4

18. Chronic dyspnea is defined as symptoms lasting longer than?
Harrison's 20th Ed. Chapter 33 Page 226

A. 1 month
B. 3 months
C. 6 months
D. 12 months

Chronic dyspnea is defined as symptoms lasting longer than 1 month.

19. What proportion of patients have multifactorial reasons underlying dyspnea?
Harrison's 20th Ed. Chapter 33 Page 226

A. 10%
B. 25%
C. 33%
D. 50%

As many as one-third of patients may have multifactorial reasons underlying dyspnea.

20. Breathing discomfort during exercise in anemia is due to stimulation of?
Harrison's 20th Ed. Chapter 33 Page 228 Table 33-2

A. Chemoreceptors
B. Mechanoreceptors
C. Metaboreceptors
D. All of the above

21. Increased work of breathing (WOB) is the possible mechanism underlying dyspnea in?
Harrison's 20th Ed. Chapter 33 Page 228 Table 33-2

A. COPD
B. Interstitial lung disease
C. Kyphoscoliosis
D. All of the above

22. Orthopnea is seen in?
Harrison's 20th Ed. Chapter 33 Page 227

A. Congestive heart failure
B. Asthma triggered by esophageal reflux
C. Mechanical impairment of diaphragm in obesity
D. All of the above

23. "Nocturnal dyspnea" is a feature of which of the following?
Harrison's 20th Ed. Chapter 33 Page 227

A. Chronic heart failure
B. Myocardial ischemia
C. Interstitial lung disease
D. COPD

CHF or asthma cause nocturnal dyspnea. Circadian variations increase bronchial sensitivity between 2 AM & 4 AM in asthma patients leading to episodes of nocturnal dyspnea.

24. Which of the following is most characteristic feature of severe paroxysmal dyspnea of left ventricular failure?
N Engl J Med. 2010; 363:1464-1469

A. Nocturnal episodes
B. Sudden and unexpected
C. Orthopnea
D. All of the above

Nocturnal episodes of dyspnea are a typical feature of left ventricular failure. Sudden & unexpected dyspneic episodes at rest is more typical of pulmonary embolization, spontaneous pneumothorax, anxiety. Orthopnea is characteristic of congestive heart failure. The differential diagnosis of orthopnea and paroxysmal nocturnal dyspnea includes ischemic heart disease, nonischemic cardiomyopathies, valvular heart disease, constrictive pericarditis, and infiltrative cardiomyopathies.

25. Acute intermittent episodes of dyspnea are due to?
Harrison's 20th Ed. Chapter 33 Page 227

A. Myocardial ischemia
B. Bronchospasm
C. Pulmonary embolism
D. All of the above

Acute intermittent episodes of dyspnea are more likely to reflect episodes of myocardial ischemia, bronchospasm or pulmonary embolism.

26. Chronic persistent dyspnea is typical of?
Harrison's 20th Ed. Chapter 33 Page 227

A. COPD
B. Interstitial lung disease
C. Chronic thromboembolic disease
D. All of the above

Chronic persistent dyspnea is typical of COPD, interstitial lung disease and chronic thromboembolic disease.

27. Platypnea is dyspnea that occurs in which position?
Harrison's 20th Ed. Chapter 33 Page 228

A. Upright
B. Sitting
C. Supine
D. Lateral

Platypnea is dyspnea that occurs only in upright position with relief in supine position.

28. Platypnea is a feature of?
Harrison's 20th Ed. Chapter 33 Page 227

A. Hepatopulmonary syndrome
B. Emphysema
C. Ankylosing spondylitis
D. Psychogenic

29. Platypnea is a feature of?
Harrison's 20th Ed. Chapter 33 Page 227

A. Obesity
B. Left atrial myxoma
C. Interstitial lung disease
D. Chronic thromboembolic disease

Left atrial myxoma and hepatopulmonary syndrome are the causes of platypnea.

30. Trepopnea most often occurs in patients with?
N Engl J Med. 1970; 283:266

A. Asthma
B. COPD
C. Heart disease
D. Pleural effusion

Trepopnea is dyspnea that occurs only in a lateral decubitus position, most often in patients with heart disease due to positional alterations in ventilation-perfusion relationships. Most cardiac patients seem to prefer sleeping on the right side. The reasons given for this preference include "awareness of the heart" and dyspnea. The feature common to most patients seems to be cardiomegaly, and the mechanism of the dyspnea is thought to be positional compression of pulmonary veins. Perhaps trepopnea explains why unilateral pulmonary edema and unilateral pleural effusions, when they occur in these patients, are almost always just on the right.

31. Which of the following is called "cardiac asthma"?
Harrison's 20th Ed. Chapter 252 Page 1766

A. Paroxysmal nocturnal dyspnea (PND)
B. Orthopnea
C. Platypnea
D. Trepopnea

PND is also called cardiac asthma. During night, with recumbency, total blood volume is increased due to fluid mobilization from edematous areas leading to pulmonary congestion.

32. Presence of resting hypoxemia suggests?
Harrison's 20th Ed. Chapter 33 Page 228

A. Ventilation-perfusion mismatch
B. Shunt
C. Impairment in diffusion capacity
D. All of the above

33. Which of the following indicate increased work of breathing?
Harrison's 20th Ed. Chapter 33 Page 228

A. Supraclavicular retractions
B. Use of accessory muscles of ventilation
C. Tripod position
D. All of the above

Increased work of breathing is evidenced by supraclavicular retractions, use of accessory muscles of ventilation and tripod position (sitting with hands braced on knees). It is indicative of increased airway resistance or stiffness of the lungs & chest wall.

34. Paradoxical movement of the abdomen during breathing is suggestive of?
Harrison's 20th Ed. Chapter 33 Page 229

A. Abdominal hernia
B. Diaphragmatic weakness
C. Pulmonary edema
D. Acute asthma

35. Rounding of the abdomen during exhalation is suggestive of?
Harrison's 20th Ed. Chapter 33 Page 229

A. Abdominal hernia
B. Diaphragmatic weakness
C. Pulmonary edema
D. Acute asthma

Rounding of the abdomen during exhalation is suggestive of pulmonary edema.

36. Low lung volumes on a chest radiograph suggests?
Harrison's 20th Ed. Chapter 33 Page 229

A. Interstitial edema or fibrosis
B. Diaphragmatic dysfunction
C. Impaired chest wall motion
D. All of the above

37. On a chest radiograph, prominent pulmonary vasculature in the upper lung zones indicates?
Harrison's 20th Ed. Chapter 33 Page 229

A. Pulmonary arterial hypertension
B. Pulmonary venous hypertension
C. Pulmonary embolism
D. Any of the above

38. On a chest radiograph, enlarged central pulmonary arteries indicates?

Harrison's 20th Ed. Chapter 33 Page 229

A. Pulmonary arterial hypertension
B. Pulmonary venous hypertension
C. Pulmonary embolism
D. Any of the above

39. In cardiopulmonary exercise test (CPET), which of the following suggests respiratory system as the cause of dyspnea?

Harrison's 20th Ed. Chapter 33 Page 229

A. Patient achieves predicted maximal ventilation
B. Demonstrates an increase in dead space or hypoxemia
C. Develops bronchospasm
D. All of the above

40. In cardiopulmonary exercise test (CPET), which of the following suggests cardiovascular system as the cause of dyspnea?

Harrison's 20th Ed. Chapter 33 Page 229

A. If the heart rate is >85% of the predicted maximum
B. If the anaerobic threshold occurs early
C. If the BP is excessively high or decreases during exercise
D. All of the above

At peak exercise in CPET, if heart rate is >85% of the predicted maximum, if anaerobic threshold occurs early, if BP becomes excessively high or decreases during exercise, if O_2 pulse falls, or if there are ischemic changes on ECG, an abnormality of cardiovascular system is likely cause of dyspnea.

41. Cardiopulmonary exercise testing (CPET) provides assessment of the integrative exercise responses involving?

Postgrad Med J. 2007;83(985):675-682

A. Pulmonary
B. Cardiovascular
C. Skeletal muscle systems
D. All of the above

Cardiopulmonary exercise testing (CPET) provides assessment of the integrative exercise responses involving the pulmonary, cardiovascular, hematopoietic, neuropsychological, and skeletal muscle systems, which are not adequately reflected through the measurement of individual organ system function.

42. Exercise tolerance is determined by?

Postgrad Med J. 2007;83(985):675-682

A. Pulmonary gas exchange
B. Cardiovascular performance
C. Skeletal muscle metabolism
D. All of the above

Peak exercise capacity is defined as "the maximum ability of the cardiovascular system to deliver oxygen to exercising skeletal muscle and of the exercising muscle to extract oxygen from the blood".

43. Oxygen uptake (VO_2) is calculated by?

Postgrad Med J. 2007;83(985):675-682

A. Bernoulli equation
B. Fick equation
C. Friedewald equation
D. Henderson-Hasselbalch equation

44. One metabolic equivalent (MET) is the resting oxygen uptake in a sitting position and equals?

Postgrad Med J. 2007;83(985):675-682

A. 1.5 mL/kg/minute
B. 2.5 mL/kg/minute
C. 3.5 mL/kg/minute
D. 4.5 mL/kg/minute

Oxygen uptake (VO_2) equals cardiac output times the arterial minus mixed venous oxygen content or $VO_2 = (SV \times HR) \times (CaO_2 - CvO_2)$, where SV is the stroke volume, HR is the heart rate, CaO_2 is the arterial oxygen content, and CvO_2 is the mixed venous oxygen content.

45. In dyspnea, supplemental O_2 should be administered if?

Harrison's 20th Ed. Chapter 33 Page 230

A. Resting O_2 saturation is ≤ 88%
B. If patient's saturation drops to ≤ 88% with activity
C. If patient's saturation drops to ≤ 88% with sleep
D. All of the above

46. Which of the following may have a role in managing dyspnea?

Harrison's 20th Ed. Chapter 33 Page 230

A. Opioids
B. Anxiolytics
C. Inhaled furosemide
D. All of the above

Hypoxia and Cyanosis

47. Pasteur's effect relates to?

Harrison's 20th Ed. Chapter 36 Page 234

A. Switch from aerobic to anaerobic metabolism
B. Abnormal hemoglobin derivative
C. Pulmonary arteriovenous fistulae
D. Flow rate in vessels

Pasteur's effect refers to switch from aerobic to anaerobic metabolism.

48. Severe hypoxia with inadequate production of ATP leads to?

Harrison's 20th Ed. Chapter 36 Page 234

A. Uncontrolled Ca++ influx in cells
B. Activation of Ca++ dependent phospholipases
C. Activation of Ca++ dependent proteases
D. All of the above

49. Which of the following gene is upregulated in adaptation to hypoxia?

Harrison's 20th Ed. Chapter 36 Page 234

A. Phosphoglycerate kinase
B. Phosphofructokinase
C. Glucose transporters Glut-1 and Glut-2
D. All of the above

Adaptations to hypoxia are mediated by upregulation of genes encoding glycolytic enzymes like phosphoglycerate kinase & phosphofructokinase & glucose transporters Glut-1 & Glut-2, and by growth factors like vascular endothelial growth factor (VEGF) & erythropoietin (EPO).

50. During hypoxia systemic arterioles dilate by opening of?

Harrison's 20th Ed. Chapter 36 Page 234

A. NaATP channels in vascular smooth-muscle cells
B. KATP channels in vascular smooth-muscle cells
C. ClATP channels in vascular smooth-muscle cells
D. All of the above

In hypoxia systemic arterioles dilate by opening of KATP channels in vascular smooth-muscle cells.

51. During hypoxia, pulmonary vascular smooth-muscle cells contract due to inhibition of?

Harrison's 20th Ed. Chapter 36 Page 234

A. Na^+ channels
B. K^+ channels
C. Cl^- channels
D. All of the above

In pulmonary vascular smooth-muscle cells, inhibition of K^+ channels causing contraction.

52. Acute hypoxia causes a clinical picture resembling?

Harrison's 20th Ed. Chapter 36 Page 235

A. Partial seizure
B. Peripheral neuropathy
C. Acute alcoholism
D. Migraine

Clinically, acute hypoxia resembles acute alcoholism (impaired judgment, motor incoordination).

53. Headache in high-altitude illness is caused by?

Harrison's 20th Ed. Chapter 36 Page 235

A. Cerebral vasodilation
B. Pulmonary arterial constriction
C. Pulmonary venous constriction
D. All of the above

High-altitude illness is characterized by headache secondary to cerebral vasodilation, gastrointestinal symptoms, dizziness, insomnia, fatigue or somnolence. High-altitude cerebral edema (HACE) is manifest by severe headache and papilledema and can cause coma.

54. In severe hypoxia, death usually results from?

Harrison's 20th Ed. Chapter 36 Page 235

A. Respiratory failure
B. Cardiac arrhythmia
C. Seizure
D. Autonomic failure

In severe hypoxia, centers of brainstem are affected & death results from respiratory failure.

55. When hypoxia occurs consequent to respiratory failure, hemoglobin-oxygen dissociation curve is displaced to?

Harrison's 20th Ed. Chapter 36 Page 235

A. Right
B. Left
C. Center
D. Any of the above

When hypoxia occurs due to respiratory failure, PaO_2 declines, $PaCO_2$ rises & Hb-O_2 dissociation curve is displaced to right, with greater quantities of O_2 released at any level of tissue PO_2.

56. Most common cause of respiratory hypoxia is?

Harrison's 20th Ed. Chapter 36 Page 235

A. Hypoventilation
B. Ventilation-perfusion mismatch
C. Intrapulmonary right-to-left shunting
D. None of the above

Most common cause of respiratory hypoxia is ventilation-perfusion mismatch.

57. High-altitude illness develops when a person ascends rapidly to a height of?

Harrison's 20th Ed. Chapter 36 Page 235

A. 1000 meters
B. 2000 meters
C. 3000 meters
D. 4000 meters

High-altitude illness develops when a person ascends rapidly to a height of 3000 meters or ~10,000 feet. At this altitude, the reduction of O_2 content of inspired air (FIO_2) leads to a decrease in alveolar PO_2 to ~60 mm Hg.

58. In which of the following conditions, PaO_2 cannot be restored to normal with inspiration of 100% O_2?

Harrison's 20th Ed. Chapter 36 Page 235

A. Tetralogy of Fallot (TOF)
B. Transposition of great arteries (TGA)
C. Eisenmenger's syndrome
D. All of the above

Hypoxia due to congenital cardiac malformations (TOF, TGA & Eisenmenger's syndrome) resembles intrapulmonary right-to-left shunting & PaO_2 cannot be restored to normal with 100% O_2.

59. In anemic hypoxia, the PaO_2 is?

Harrison's 20th Ed. Chapter 36 Page 235

A. Normal
B. Decreased
C. Increased
D. Any of the above

In anemic hypoxia, PaO_2 is normal but due to reduction of Hb concentration, absolute quantity of O_2 transported per unit volume of blood is diminished.

60. Which of the following is false about in anemic hypoxia?

Harrison's 20th Ed. Chapter 36 Page 235

A. Absolute quantity of O_2 transported per unit volume of blood is diminished
B. Usual quantity of O_2 is removed from blood in capillaries
C. PO_2 & saturation in venous blood decline to a greater extent
D. None of the above

61. In which of the following hypoxia's, venous blood tends to have a high O_2?

Harrison's 20th Ed. Chapter 36 Page 235

A. Excercise induced
B. Circulatory hypoxia
C. Cyanide poisoning
D. Carbon monoxide intoxication

62. Example of "Histotoxic hypoxia" is?

Harrison's 20th Ed. Chapter 36 Page 235

A. Severe exercise
B. Cyanide poisoning
C. Raynaud's phenomenon
D. High altitude hypoxia

Cyanide causes cellular hypoxia because tissues are unable to utilize O_2. As a result, venous blood tends to have a high O_2 tension. This condition is called histotoxic hypoxia.

63. Special chemosensitive cells that determine respiratory response to hypoxia are located in?

Harrison's 20th Ed. Chapter 36 Page 235

A. Carotid bodies
B. Aortic bodies
C. Respiratory center in the brainstem
D. All of the above

64. Which of the following is a feature of chronic mountain sickness?

Harrison's 20th Ed. Chapter 36 Page 236

A. Reduced ventilation
B. Cyanosis
C. Right ventricular enlargement
D. All of the above

In persons with chronic hypoxemia secondary to prolonged residence at a high altitude (>13000 feet or 4200 meters), chronic mountain sickness develops. This is characterized by a blunted respiratory drive, reduced ventilation, erythrocytosis, cyanosis, weakness, right ventricular enlargement secondary to pulmonary hypertension and even stupor.

65. Cyanosis is usually most marked in?

Harrison's 20th Ed. Chapter 36 Page 236

A. Nail beds
B. Ears
C. Malar eminences
D. All of the above

Cyanosis is usually most marked in the lips, nail beds, ears, and malar eminences.

66. The degree of cyanosis is modified by?

Harrison's 20th Ed. Chapter 36 Page 236

A. Color of the cutaneous pigment
B. Thickness of the skin
C. State of the cutaneous capillaries
D. All of the above

67. Cyanosis is apparent when the mean capillary concentration of reduced hemoglobin exceeds?

Harrison's 20th Ed. Chapter 36 Page 236

A. 2 gram / dL
B. 3 gram / dL
C. 4 gram / dL
D. 5 gram / dL

It is the absolute rather than relative quantity of reduced Hb that produces cyanosis. As concentration of total Hb is markedly reduced in severe anemia, absolute quantity of reduced Hb is still small and patients may not become cyanotic even with marked arterial desaturation.

68. Central and peripheral cyanosis may be present in?

Harrison's 20th Ed. Chapter 36 Page 236

A. Shock
B. Congestive failure
C. Peripheral vascular disease
D. Cardiogenic shock with pulmonary edema

69. Cyanosis occurs upon ascent to an altitude of?

Harrison's 20th Ed. Chapter 36 Page 236

A. 2000 meters
B. 3000 meters
C. 4000 meters
D. 5000 meters

Cyanosis is manifest in an ascent to 4000 m (13,000 ft). At this height, FIO_2 & alveolar PO_2 are about 85 & 50 mm Hg, respectively & SaO_2 is ~75% leaving more reduced Hb in arterial blood.

70. Cyanosis can be observed in all except?

Harrison's 20th Ed. Chapter 36 Page 237

A. Marked polycythemia
B. Carboxyhemoglobin (COHb)
C. Methemoglobin
D. Sulfhemoglobin

Patients with marked polycythemia become cyanotic at higher levels of SaO_2 than patients with normal hematocrit values. Cyanosis is also observed when nonfunctional hemoglobin (methemoglobin or sulfhemoglobin) is present in blood.

71. Most common congenital cardiac lesion associated with cyanosis in adult is?

Harrison's 20th Ed. Chapter 234 Page 1667

A. Tetralogy of Fallot
B. Patent ductus arteriosus
C. Ventricular septal defect
D. Atrial septal defect

Most common congenital cardiac lesion with cyanosis in the adult is tetralogy of Fallot.

72. Differential cyanosis is a feature of?

Harrison's 20th Ed. Chapter 234 Page 1667

A. Tetralogy of Fallot
B. Patent ductus arteriosus
C. Ventricular septal defect
D. Atrial septal defect

In patent ductus arteriosus, pulmonary hypertension and right-to-left shunt, differential cyanosis results, that is, cyanosis occurs in the lower but not in the upper extremities.

73. Which of the following is suspected when blood remains brown after mixing in test tube & exposed to air?

Harrison's 20th Ed. Chapter 94 Page 695

A. Marked polycythemia
B. Carboxyhemoglobin (COHb)
C. Methemoglobin
D. Sulfhemoglobin

Diagnosis of methemoglobinemia is suspected if blood remains brown after mixing in a test tube & exposure to air. Spectroscopy confirms the diagnosis.

74. Acquired methemoglobinemia may occur on exposure to?

N Engl J Med. 2000;343:337

A. Dapsone
B. Nitrates
C. Sulfonamides
D. All of the above

Acquired methemoglobinemia is a rare consequence of the exposure of normal red cells to oxidizing drugs such as benzocaine, dapsone, nitrates, primaquine and sulfonamides.

75. Symptomatic methemoglobinemia should be treated with?

N Engl J Med. 1992;327:1461

A. Methylcobalamin
B. Hexamethylene diisocyanate
C. Methylene blue
D. Toluene diisocyanate

Symptomatic methemoglobinemia should be treated with intravenous injection of methylene blue (1 to 2 mg per kilogram) or oral methylene blue (60 mg three to four times each day) or ascorbic acid (300 - 600 mg/day).

76. Which of the following is false in Eisenmenger syndrome?

Harrison's 20th Ed. Chapter 264 Page 1838

A. Cyanosis
B. Elevated pulmonary vascular resistance
C. Intracardiac communication
D. Pulmonic stenosis

Elevated pulmonary vascular resistance that produces cyanosis in the presence of intra- & extracardiac communications without pulmonic stenosis is termed Eisenmenger syndrome.

77. In peripheral cyanosis of extremities, the arterial blood is?

Harrison's 20th Ed. Chapter 36 Page 237

A. Normally saturated with oxygen
B. Over saturated with oxygen
C. Under saturated with oxygen
D. Any of the above

78. Clubbing without cyanosis is frequent in?

Harrison's 20th Ed. Chapter 36 Page 237

A. Infective endocarditis
B. Inflammatory bowel disease
C. Jackhammer operators
D. All of the above

Clubbing without cyanosis is frequent in infective endocarditis, inflammatory bowel disease & in Jackhammer operators.

Edema

79. Edema is defined as a clinically apparent increase in?
Harrison's 20th Ed. Chapter 37 Page 237

A. Intracellular fluid volume
B. Plasma volume
C. Interstitial fluid volume
D. All of the above

Edema is defined as a clinically apparent increase in interstitial fluid volume.

80. Which of the following statements is false?
Harrison's 20th Ed. Chapter 37 Page 237

A. ~ Two-thirds of total body water is intracellular
B. ~ One-third of total body water is extracellular
C. ~ One-fourth of extracellular water is in the plasma and the remainder comprises the interstitial fluid
D. None of the above

81. Which of the following about movement of water & diffusible solutes from plasma to interstitium is false?
Harrison's 20th Ed. Chapter 37 Page 237

A. Promoted by hydrostatic pressure within the capillaries
B. Promoted by colloid oncotic pressure in the interstitial fluid
C. Most prominent at the arterial origin of the capillary
D. None of the above

82. Fluid is returned from the interstitial space into the vascular system largely through?
Harrison's 20th Ed. Chapter 37 Page 237

A. Arterial system
B. Venous system
C. Lymphatic system
D. All of the above

Fluid is returned from the interstitial space into the vascular system largely through the lymphatic system.

83. Development of edema occurs due to?
Harrison's 20th Ed. Chapter 37 Page 237

A. Inadequate lymphatic drainage
B. Damage to capillary endothelial barrier
C. Increase in the oncotic pressure in interstitial space
D. All of the above

Development of edema occurs due to an increase in intracapillary hydrostatic pressure, inadequate lymphatic drainage, reductions in oncotic pressure in plasma, damage to capillary endothelial barrier and increases in the oncotic pressure in interstitial space.

84. Which of the following is referred to as "tissue tension"?
Harrison's 19th Ed. 250

A. Hydrostatic pressure within the vascular system
B. Colloid oncotic pressure within the vascular system
C. Hydrostatic pressure within the interstitial fluid
D. All of the above

Plasma & interstitial fluid are two components of extracellular fluid regulate by Starling forces. Hydrostatic pressure within interstitial fluid is referred to as the tissue tension which promotes the movement of fluid into the vascular compartment.

85. Movement of water & diffusible solutes from vascular space into the interstitial space occurs at?
Harrison's 20th Ed. Chapter 37 Page 237

A. Arteriolar end of capillaries
B. Venous end of capillaries
C. Lymphatics
D. All of the above

Movement of water & diffusible solutes from vascular space into interstitial space occurs at the arteriolar end of capillaries. Fluid is returned from interstitial space into vascular system at the venous end of capillary & by way of lymphatics.

86. Which of the following about renal juxtaglomerular cells is false?
Harrison's 20th Ed. Chapter 37 Page 237

A. Secrete renin
B. Specialized myoepithelial cells
C. Surround the afferent renal arteriole
D. None of the above

87. Which of the following best define renin?
Harrison's 20th Ed. Chapter 37 Page 237

A. Enzyme
B. Pro-hormone
C. Hormone
D. Cofactor

Renin is an enzyme with a molecular weight of ~40,000 secreted by juxtaglomerular cells.

88. Conditions that reduce effective arterial blood volume cause constriction of which of the following?
Harrison's 20th Ed. Chapter 37 Page 237

A. Renal afferent arteriolar constriction
B. Renal efferent arteriolar constriction
C. Renal glomerular capillary constriction
D. All of the above

Heart failure, nephrotic syndrome & cirrhosis reduce effective arterial blood volume and cause renal efferent arteriolar constriction.

89. Which of the following stimulates renin release?
Harrison's 20th Ed. Chapter 37 Page 237

A. Diminished stretch of the juxtaglomerular cells
B. Low sodium chloride load in distal renal tubules
C. Circulating catecholamines
D. All of the above

Diminished renal blood flow resulting in diminished stretch of juxtaglomerular cells lowers sodium chloride load reaching distal renal tubules signals juxtaglomerular cells to secrete renin. Activation of β-adrenergic receptors in juxtaglomerular cells by sympathetic nervous system & circulating catecholamines stimulates renin release.

90. Angiotensinogen is synthesized by?
Harrison's 20th Ed. Chapter 37 Page 237

A. Kidney
B. Liver
C. Pancreas
D. Lung

Angiotensinogen, an α2 globulin, is synthesized by liver. Renin converts angiotensinogen to a decapeptide angiotensin I, which is broken down to an octapeptide angiotensin II.

91. Renal effects of Angiotensin II are mediated by activation of which type of Angiotensin II receptors?
Harrison's 20th Ed. Chapter 37 Page 238

A. Type 1
B. Type 2
C. Type 3
D. Type 4

Angiotensin II produces renal vasoconstriction & salt and water retention. These renal effects are mediated by activation of Angiotensin II type 1 receptors.

92. Which of the following stimulates the production of aldosterone?
Harrison's 20th Ed. Chapter 37 Page 238

A. Angiotensinogen
B. Angiotensin I
C. Angiotensin II
D. All of the above

93. Aldosterone is produced by?
Harrison's 20th Ed. Chapter 37 Page 238

A. Juxtaglomerular cells of kidney
B. Macula densa cells of kidney
C. Zona glomerulosa of adrenal cortex
D. Zona reticularis of adrenal cortex

Aldosterone is produced by zona glomerulosa of adrenal cortex & its release is stimulated by Angiotensin II. It is metabolized by liver.

94. Site of action of aldosterone is?
Harrison's 20th Ed. Chapter 37 Page 238

A. Proximal convoluted tubule
B. Loop of Henle
C. Distal convoluted tubule
D. Collecting tubule

95. Blockade of the action of aldosterone can be done by?
Harrison's 20th Ed. Chapter 37 Page 238

A. Spironolactone
B. Eplerenone
C. Amiloride
D. All of the above

96. In heart failure, aldosterone secretion is elevated due to?
Harrison's 20th Ed. Chapter 37 Page 238

A. Prolongation of biologic half-life
B. Increased secretion
C. Reduced hepatic catabolism
D. All of the above

In heart failure, levels of aldosterone are raised due to increased secretion, prolonged biologic half-life & reduced hepatic catabolism due to reduced hepatic blood flow, secondary to reduction in cardiac output.

97. Activation of Renin-Angiotensin-Aldosterone (RAA) system is most striking in which of the following?
Harrison's 20th Ed. Chapter 37 Page 238

A. Acute, severe heart failure
B. Chronic heart failure
C. Stable heart failure
D. Compensated heart failure

Activation of RAA system is seen conspicuously in early phase of acute, severe heart failure & is less intense in patients with chronic, stable, compensated heart failure.

98. Mineralocorticoid escape phenomenon is best explained by?
Harrison's 20th Ed. Chapter 37 Page 238

A. Deficit in effective arterial blood volume
B. Aldosterone antagonism
C. Pressure natriuresis
D. Blocking of epithelial sodium channels

Administration of potent mineralocorticoids (deoxycorticosterone acetate or fludrocortisone) leads to salt & water retention. This accumulation is self-limiting, despite continued exposure to steroid, a phenomenon known as mineralocorticoid escape wherein edema does not develop. It is due to an increase in GFR (pressure natriuresis).

99. Arginine vasopressin (AVP) is best related to?
Harrison's 20th Ed. Chapter 37 Page 238

A. V1 receptors
B. V2 receptors
C. V3 receptors
D. V4 receptors

Secretion of arginine vasopressin (AVP) occurs in response to increased intracellular osmolar concentration. By stimulating V2 receptors, AVP increases the reabsorption of free water in the distal tubules and collecting ducts of the kidneys, thereby increasing total-body water.

100. Which of the following is an effect of Endothelin-1?
Harrison's 20th Ed. Chapter 37 Page 238

A. Renal vasoconstriction
B. Sodium retention
C. Edema
D. All of the above

Endothelin-1 is a potent peptide vasoconstrictor released by endothelial cells. Its concentration in the plasma is elevated in patients with severe heart failure and contributes to renal vasoconstriction, sodium retention and edema.

101. Atrial natriuretic peptide (ANP) is stored in secretory granules within?
Harrison's 20th Ed. Chapter 37 Page 238

A. Sinoatrial node
B. Atrial myocytes
C. Pulmonary veins
D. All of the above

Polypeptide ANP is secreted by atrial myocytes secondary to atrial distention and/or sodium load. Its actions are excretion of sodium & water by increasing GFR, inhibiting sodium reabsorption in PCT & inhibiting release of renin & aldosterone. It also antagonizes vasoconstrictor actions of Angiotensin II, AVP & sympathetic stimulation causing arteriolar & venous dilatation.

102. Brain natriuretic peptide (BNP) is present in?
Harrison's 20th Ed. Chapter 37 Page 238

A. Cardiac ventricular myocardium
B. Cerebral cortex
C. Cerebellum
D. All of the above

BNP is stored in cardiac ventricular myocardium & is released when ventricular diastolic pressure rises. Its actions are similar to ANP. Circulating levels of ANP & BNP are elevated in CHF.

103. Released ANP & BNP bind to?
Harrison's 20th Ed. Chapter 37 Page 238

A. Natriuretic receptor-A
B. Natriuretic receptor-B
C. Natriuretic receptor-C
D. Natriuretic receptor-D

Released ANP & BNP bind to the natriuretic receptor-A.

104. Which of the following is an action of ANP and BNP?
Harrison's 20th Ed. Chapter 37 Page 238

A. Excretion of sodium & water
B. Inhibiting sodium reabsorption
C. Inhibiting release of renin & aldosterone
D. All of the above

Released ANP and BNP lead to excretion of sodium & water by augmenting glomerular filtration rate, inhibiting sodium reabsorption in proximal tubule and inhibiting release of renin & aldosterone.

105. ANP and BNP antagonize the vasoconstrictor actions of?
Harrison's 20th Ed. Chapter 37 Page 238

A. Angiotensin II
B. Arginine vasopressin
C. Sympathetic stimulation
D. All of the above

Released ANP and BNP also cause dilation of arterioles & venules by antagonizing the vasoconstrictor actions of AII, AVP and sympathetic stimulation. Thus, elevated levels of natriuretic peptides have the capacity to oppose sodium retention in hypervolemic and edematous states.

106. Which of the following is a form of edema?
Harrison's 20th Ed. Chapter 37 Page 238

A. Anasarca
B. Ascites
C. Hydrothorax
D. All of the above

Anasarca refers to gross, generalized edema. Ascites and hydrothorax refer to accumulation of excess fluid in the peritoneal and pleural cavities, respectively and are considered special forms of edema.

107. Which of the following about edema of renal disease is false?
Harrison's 20th Ed. Chapter 37 Page 239

A. Hypertension
B. Without considerable cardiac enlargement
C. Develop orthopnea
D. Normal cardiac output

108. NSAIDs and cyclosporine cause edema due to?
Harrison's 20th Ed. Chapter 37 Page 239

A. Renal vasoconstriction
B. Arteriolar dilation
C. Augmented renal sodium reabsorption
D. Capillary damage

109. Refeeding edema best relates to?
Harrison's 20th Ed. Chapter 37 Page 239

A. Calcium
B. Insulin
C. Paratharmone
D. Oxytocin

Refeeding edema may be linked to increased release of insulin which directly increases tubular sodium reabsorption.

110. Which of the following is involved in the edema of starvation?
Harrison's 20th Ed. Chapter 37 Page 239

A. Hyponatremia
B. Hypokalemia
C. Hypocalcemia
D. Hypomagnesemia

In addition to hypoalbuminemia, hypokalemia and caloric deficits may be involved in the edema of starvation.

111. Edema of hypothyroidism best relates to?
Harrison's 20th Ed. Chapter 37 Page 240

A. Glutamic acid
B. Aggrecan
C. Hyaluronic acid
D. Lubricin

Nonpitting edema of hypothyroidism (myxedema) due to deposition of hyaluronic acid.

112. Causes of facial edema include?
Harrison's 20th Ed. Chapter 37 Page 240

A. Trichinosis
B. Hypoproteinemia
C. Myxedema
D. All of the above

Apart from hypoproteinemia, causes of facial edema include trichinosis (Trichinella spiralis), allergic reactions & myxedema. Trichinosis can also lead to membranous glomerulopathy, proliferative glomerulonephritis & acute pericarditis. Trichinosis is a cause of FUO.

113. Antihypertensive agents associated with edema formation include all except?
Harrison's 20th Ed. Chapter 37 Page 240 Table 37-2

A. Minoxidil
B. Hydralazine
C. Clonidine
D. Atenolol

114. Antihypertensive agents associated with edema formation include all except?
Harrison's 20th Ed. Chapter 37 Page 240 Table 37-2

A. Methyldopa
B. Calcium channel antagonists
C. ACE Inhibitors
D. Alpha adrenergic antagonists

115. Steroid hormones associated with edema formation include all except?

Harrison's 20th Ed. Chapter 37 Page 240 Table 37-2

A. Glucocorticoids
B. Mineralocorticoids
C. Anabolic steroids
D. Estrogens / Progestins

116. Which of the following is associated with edema formation?

Harrison's 20th Ed. Chapter 37 Page 240 Table 37-2

A. Cyclosporine
B. Growth hormone
C. Interleukin 2
D. All of the above

117. Which of the following is false about idiopathic edema?

N Engl J Med. 1960; 263:1342-1345

A. Occurs in women
B. Edema unrelated to menstrual cycle
C. Occurs after upright posture
D. None of the above

Idiopathic cyclic edema occurs almost exclusively in women, is characterized by periodic episodes of edema (unrelated to menstrual cycle), frequently accompanied by abdominal distention orthostatic retention of sodium & water after upright posture.

118. Venous pressure in upper extremities is elevated in all except?

Harrison's 20th Ed. Chapter 37 Page 240

A. Advanced heart failure
B. Constrictive pericarditis
C. Tricuspid stenosis
D. Cirrhosis liver

Venous pressure in upper extremities is elevated in advanced heart failure, constrictive pericarditis or tricuspid stenosis but is normal in cirrhosis. In hepatic cirrhosis, JVP is normal.

Palpitations

119. Palpitations are often noted when the patient is?
Harrison's 20th Ed. Chapter 39 Page 249

A. Exercising
B. Quietly resting
C. Sleeping
D. Post prandial

Palpitations are often noted when the patient is quietly resting, when other stimuli are minimal.

120. Positional palpitations can be due to?
Harrison's 20th Ed. Chapter 39 Page 249

A. Atrial myxoma
B. HOCM
C. Supravalvular aortic stenosis
D. All of the above

Positional palpitations are generally due to a structural process within (atrial myxoma) or adjacent to (mediastinal mass, diaphragmatic hernia, gastric volvulus) the heart.

121. Psychiatric illnesses contribute to what proportion of cases of palpitations?
Harrison's 20th Ed. Chapter 39 Page 249

A. ~ 10%
B. ~ 20%
C. ~ 30%
D. ~ 40%

Palpitations are caused by cardiac (43%), psychiatric (31%), miscellaneous (10%), and unknown (16%) causes.

122. Which of the following is a cause of palpitation?
Harrison's 20th Ed. Chapter 39 Page 249

A. Mitral valve prolapse
B. Aortic insufficiency
C. Pulmonary embolism
D. All of the above

Cardiovascular causes of palpitation include premature atrial and ventricular contractions, supraventricular and ventricular arrhythmias, mitral valve prolapse (with or without associated arrhythmias), aortic insufficiency, atrial myxoma, myocarditis, and pulmonary embolism.

123. Irregular, sustained palpitations can be caused by?
Harrison's 20th Ed. Chapter 39 Page 249

A. Atrial fibrillation
B. Premature atrial contractions
C. Premature ventricular contractions
D. Supraventricular tachycardias

Irregular, sustained palpitations can be caused by atrial fibrillation.

124. Palpitation with rapid and irregular rhythm suggest?
N Engl J Med. 1998;338(19):1369

A. Atrial fibrillation
B. Atrial flutter
C. Tachycardia with variable block
D. Any of the above

125. Which of the following statements about palpitations is false?
Harrison's 20th Ed. Chapter 39 Page 249

A. Most arrhythmias are not associated with palpitations
B. Palpitations are common among athletes
C. Palpitations due to psychiatric causes have a longer duration of the sensation (>15 minutes)
D. None of the above

126. Which of the following enhances the strength of myocardial contraction and cause palpitations?
Harrison's 20th Ed. Chapter 39 Page 249

A. Tobacco
B. Cocaine
C. Amphetamines
D. All of the above

Tobacco, caffeine, aminophylline, atropine, thyroxine, cocaine, and amphetamines enhance the strength of myocardial contraction and can cause palpitations.

127. Which of the following conditions frequently lead to the sensation of palpitations? *Harrison's 20th Ed. Chapter 39 Page 249*

A. Aortic stenosis
B. Aortic regurgitation
C. HOCM
D. All of the above

Hyperdynamic cardiovascular states caused by catecholaminergic stimulation as in exercise, stress, or pheochromocytoma can lead to palpitations. Enlarged ventricle of aortic regurgitation & accompanying hyperdynamic precordium frequently lead to the sensation of palpitations.

128. Which of the following is the most common structural heart disease leading to palpitations? *Am Fam Physician. 2011;84(1):63-69*

A. Mitral stenosis
B. Mitral regurgitation
C. Mitral valve prolapse
D. Atrial septal defect

Mitral valve prolapse is the most common structural heart disease leading to palpitations and is likely caused by papillary muscle fibrosis.

129. Which of the following arrhythmia has been described with mitral-valve prolapse? *N Engl J Med. 1998;338(19):1369*

A. Supraventricular arrhythmia
B. Ventricular premature depolarizations
C. Nonsustained ventricular tachycardia
D. All of the above

Virtually every type of supraventricular arrhythmia, as well as ventricular premature depolarizations and nonsustained ventricular tachycardia, has been described with mitral-valve prolapse, and palpitations are nearly ubiquitous in mitral-valve prolapse.

130. Which of the following is a cause of palpitations?
Harrison's 20th Ed. Chapter 39 Page 249

A. Ethanol
B. Pheochromocytoma
C. Systemic mastocytosis
D. All of the above

Thyrotoxicosis, drugs (aminophylline, atropine, thyroxine, cocaine, amphetamines), ethanol, spontaneous skeletal muscle contractions of chest wall, pheochromocytoma & systemic mastocytosis cause palpitations.

Basic Biology of the Cardiovascular System

131. Cardiac embryogenesis best relates to?
Harrison's 20th Ed. Chapter 232 Page 1651

A. Anterior splanchnic mesoderm
B. Posterior splanchnic mesoderm
C. Medial splanchnic mesoderm
D. Lateral splanchnic mesoderm

Early cardiac progenitors arise within crescent-shaped fields of lateral splanchnic mesoderm and migrate to midline to form the linear heart tube which is a single layer of endocardium and a single layer of cardiomyocyte precursors.

132. "Cardiac jelly" which accumulates within the endocardial cushions best relates to?
Harrison's 20th Ed. Chapter 232 Page 1651

A. Folic acid
B. Hyaluronic acid
C. Citric acid
D. Lactic acid

Early in development, the single layer of myocardial cells secretes an extracellular matrix rich in hyaluronic acid or "cardiac jelly" which is the precursor of the cardiac valves.

133. Proepicardial organ is a derivative of?
Harrison's 20th Ed. Chapter 232 Page 1651

A. Septum transversum
B. Anterior conal septum
C. Septum pellucidum
D. All of the above

Epicardial cells arise in the transient embryonic structure called proepicardial organ which is a derivative of septum transversum. Septum transversum separates the embryo's thorax from its abdomen, and to the diaphragm and liver. Proepicardial cells contribute smooth-muscle to coronary arteries and are required for proper coronary patterning.

134. Neural crest cells are sensitive to which of the following vitamins?
Harrison's 20th Ed. Chapter 232 Page 1652

A. A
B. C
C. D
D. E

Neural crest cells are sensitive to both vitamin A and folic acid, and congenital heart disease involving abnormal remodeling of aortic arch arteries associates with their maternal deficiencies.

135. Neural crest cells form components of?
N Engl J Med. 2010;363:1638-47

A. Peripheral nervous system
B. Craniofacial regions
C. Cardiac outflow tract
D. All of the above

136. Which of the following cells contribute to cardiac morphogenesis?
N Engl J Med. 2010;363:1638-47

A. Neural-crest cells
B. Cells arising from the second heart field
C. Epicardial progenitors
D. All of the above

137. Which of the following is a second-heart–field cardiac defect?
N Engl J Med. 2010;363:1638-47

A. Pulmonic stenosis
B. Tetralogy of Fallot
C. Ebstein's anomaly
D. All of the above

138. Second-heart–field progenitors that express which of the following?
N Engl J Med. 2010;363:1638-47

A. Islet 1
B. Islet 2
C. Islet 3
D. Islet 4

Second-heart–field progenitors that express islet 1 are multipotent cells that can give rise to smooth-muscle cells at the base of aorta and pulmonary arteries, to endothelial cells, or to myocardium. Cells in second heart field migrate first to pharyngeal regions and express specific marker genes, including the transcription factor islet 1.

139. Which of the following statements is false?
N Engl J Med. 2010;363:1638-47

A. Cells that give rise to sinus node express fetal TBX18 gene
B. Cells that give rise to atrioventricular node & Purkinje system express NKX2-5 transcription factor
C. Development of pulmonary-vein myocardium requires PITX2 transcription factor
D. None of the above

140. Cells from which of the following help in repair of damaged or aging arteries?
Harrison's 20th Ed. Chapter 232 Page 1652

A. Neural crest
B. Mesodermal structures
C. Bone marrow derived endothelial progenitors
D. All of the above

Bone marrow derived endothelial progenitors may aid repair of damaged or aging arteries.

141. Adventitia of arteries consists of?
Harrison's 20th Ed. Chapter 232 Page 1652

A. Fibroblasts
B. Mast cells
C. Nerve terminals
D. All of the above

142. Pericytes best relate to?
Harrison's 20th Ed. Chapter 232 Page 1652

A. Endothelial cells
B. Smooth-muscle-like cells
C. Fibroblasts
D. All of the above

The smallest blood vessels i.e. capillaries consist of a monolayer of endothelial cells on a basement membrane, adjacent to a discontinuous layer of smooth-muscle-like cells known as pericytes.

143. Vasa vasorum nourishes which of the following?
Harrison's 20th Ed. Chapter 232 Page 1652

A. Tunica intima
B. Tunica media
C. Tunica adventitia
D. All of the above

Larger arteries the vasa vasorum which nourishes the tunica media.

144. Which of the following about blood vessels is false?
Harrison's 20th Ed. Chapter 232 Page 1653 Figure 232-2

A. Veins have thin medias and thicker adventitias
B. Small muscular artery has a prominent tunica media
C. Larger elastic arteries have cylindrical layers of elastic tissue alternating with concentric rings of smooth muscle cells
D. None of the above

145. "Capillary leak" occurs in?
Harrison's 20th Ed. Chapter 232 Page 1653

A. Hypertension
B. Renal disease
C. Sepsis
D. All of the above

"Capillary leak" occur in atherosclerosis, hypertension, renal disease, pulmonary edema & sepsis.

146. Endogenous substance produced by endothelial cells is?
Harrison's 20th Ed. Chapter 231 Page 1653

A. Prostacyclin
B. Nitric oxide (NO)
C. Hydrogen peroxide (H_2O_2)
D. All of the above

Endogenous substances produced by endothelial cells are prostacyclin, endothelium-derived hyperpolarizing factor, nitric oxide (NO), and hydrogen peroxide (H_2O_2). These provide tonic vasodilatory stimuli under physiologic conditions in vivo.

147. Potent vasoconstrictor substance produced by endothelial cells is?
Harrison's 20th Ed. Chapter 232 Page 1653

A. Cathelin
B. Endoglin
C. Endothelin
D. All of the above

Potent vasoconstrictor substance produced by endothelial cells is endothelin.

148. Which of the following, elaborated by endothelial cells, can inhibit smooth-muscle proliferation?
Harrison's 20th Ed. Chapter 232 Page 1653

A. Heparan sulfate proteoglycan
B. Heparan sulfate glycosaminoglycan
C. Dermatan sulfate proteoglycan
D. Dermatan sulfate glycosaminoglycan

Heparan sulfate glycosaminoglycans elaborated by endothelial cells inhibits smooth-muscle proliferation.

149. Endothelial cells can produce which of the following?
Harrison's 20th Ed. Chapter 232 Page 1653

A. Plasminogen activator inhibitor 1 (PAI-1)
B. Platelet-derived growth factor
C. Heparan sulfate glycosaminoglycan
D. All of the above

150. Which of the following is a neurotransmitter of peptidergic neuronal class?
Harrison's 20th Ed. Chapter 232 Page 1654

A. Substance P
B. Vasoactive intestinal peptide
C. Calcitonin gene-related peptide
D. All of the above

151. Which of the following about cardiomyocyte is false?
Harrison's 20th Ed. Chapter 232 Page 1655

A. Normally, 60–140 μm in length & 17–25 μm in diameter
B. Each cardiomyocyte contains multiple myofibrils
C. Myofibrils are composed of repeating sarcomeres
D. None of the above

152. The structural & functional unit of contraction is?
Harrison's 20th Ed. Chapter 232 Page 1655

A. Cardiomyocyte
B. Myofibril
C. Sarcomere
D. All of the above

Sarcomere is the structural & functional unit of contraction. It lies between adjacent Z lines. The distance between Z lines ranges between 1.6 and 2.2 μm.

153. What is the length of the dark A band?
Harrison's 20th Ed. Chapter 232 Page 1655

A. 0.5 μm
B. 1.0 μm
C. 1.5 μm
D. 2.0 μm

154. With muscle contraction, which of the following occurs?
Harrison's 20th Ed. Chapter 232 Page 1655

A. A band remains constant in length
B. I band shortens
C. Z lines move toward one another
D. All of the above

155. Double helix of two chains of actin molecules are wound on?
Harrison's 20th Ed. Chapter 232 Page 1655

A. Tropomyosin
B. Titin
C. Actin
D. Dystrophin

156. Which of the following connects myosin to the Z line?
Harrison's 20th Ed. Chapter 232 Page 1655

A. Tropomyosin
B. Titin
C. Actin
D. Dystrophin

Flexible myofibrillar protein, Titin connects myosin to the Z line.

157. During activation of the cardiac myocyte, Ca++ binds to which of the following?
Harrison's 20th Ed. Chapter 232 Page 1655

A. Troponin C
B. Troponin I
C. Troponin T
D. All of the above

During activation of the cardiac myocyte, Ca^{++} binds troponin C, resulting in conformational changes in the regulatory protein tropomyosin and exposing actin cross-bridge interaction sites.

158. The extracellular concentration of calcium is how many times more than the intracellular concentration?
N Engl J Med. 2006;355:608

A. 2000 times
B. 5000 times
C. 10000 times
D. 20000 times

159. Stretching capability of which myofibrillar protein contributes to the elasticity of heart?
Harrison's 20th Ed. Chapter 232 Page 1655

A. Titin
B. Myosin
C. Actin
D. All of the above

160. During activation of the myocyte, Ca^{2+} becomes attached to?
Harrison's 20th Ed. Chapter 232 Page 1655

A. Troponin C
B. Troponin I
C. Troponin T
D. All of the above

161. Acceleration of cardiac relaxation occurs by phosphorylation by cyclic AMP of which protein?
Harrison's 20th Ed. Chapter 232 Page 1655

A. Troponin C
B. Troponin I
C. Troponin T
D. All of the above

162. Which of the following gene encods titin?
N Engl J Med. 2012; 366:619-628

A. TIN
B. TTN
C. TNN
D. TTT

TTN gene encodes the sarcomere protein titin.

163. Which of the following is the largest human protein?
N Engl J Med. 2012; 366:619-628

A. Dystrophin
B. Titin
C. Myosin
D. Actin

Titin is the largest human protein, composed of ~33,000 amino acids. It is the third most abundant striated-muscle protein. Titin molecules are anchored at the Z-line and M-line. TTN truncating mutations are the most common known genetic cause of dilated cardiomyopathy.

164. Drugs that enhance relaxation of myocardium are called?
Harrison's 20th Ed. Chapter 232 Page 1658

A. Dromotropic
B. Ionotropic
C. Lusitropic
D. Cathotropic

165. Which of the following is termed as the "disease of the sarcomere"?
N Engl J Med. 2011;364:1643-1656

A. Dilated cardiomyopathy
B. Hypertrophic cardiomyopathy
C. Arrhythmogenic Right Ventricular Cardiomyopathy (ARVC)
D. All of the above

166. Which of the following enzyme is responsible for maintaining correct calcium homeostasis in cardiomyocyte?
N Engl J Med. 2011; 364:1643-1656

A. Diacylglycerol (DAG)
B. Phosphatidylinositol 4,5-bisphosphate
C. Sarcoplasmic reticulum Ca^{++}ATPase (SERCA)
D. Inositol 1,4,5-trisphosphate (IP3)

167. SERCA is regulated by?
N Engl J Med. 2011; 364:1643-1656

A. Calsequestrin
B. Phospholamban
C. Calstabin 2
D. All of the above

In cardiac muscle, SERCA (sarco(endo)plasmic reticulum Ca^{++}-ATPase) is regulated by phospholamban (PLB), a small inhibitory phosphoprotein that decreases the Ca^{++} affinity of SERCA and attenuates contractile strength. cAMP-dependent phosphorylation of PLB reverses Ca^{++}-ATPase inhibition.

168. Which of the following about protein phospholamban is false?
Harrison's 20th Ed. Chapter 232 Page 1657

A. Situated on the membrane of sarcoplasmic reticulum
B. Activated by cAMP
C. Controls rate of uptake of calcium into sarcoplasmic reticulum
D. None of the above

Activated by cAMP, protein phospholamban, situated on membrane of sarcoplasmic reticulum (SR), controls the rate of uptake of calcium into SR. The latter effect explains enhanced relaxation (lusitropic effect).

169. Cyclic adenosine monophosphate (cAMP) acts via?
Harrison's 20th Ed. Chapter 232 Page 1657

A. Nuclear factor-κB
B. Protein kinase A
C. Calcium-dependent calcineurin
D. Phospholipase C

Cyclic adenosine monophosphate (cAMP) or the second messenger acts via protein kinase A to stimulate metabolism and phosphorylate the Ca^{++} channel protein.

170. Ca^{++} is stored in the sarcoplasmic reticulum by forming a complex with?

Harrison's 20th Ed. Chapter 232 Page 1657

A. Calsequestrin
B. Phospholamban
C. Calstabin 2
D. All of the above

171. Inactive cardiac cell has a transmembrane potential of?

Harrison's 20th Ed. Chapter 232 Page 1657

A. –40 to –60 mV
B. –60 to –80 mV
C. –80 to –100 mV
D. –100 to –120 mV

Inactive cardiac cell has a transmembrane potential (Vm) of –80 to –100 mV. The interior being negatively charged relative to outside of cell.

172. Plateau phase of action potential corresponds to?

Harrison's 20th Ed. Chapter 232 Page 1657

A. Phase 1
B. Phase 2
C. Phase 3
D. Phase 4

173. Ca^{++}-induced Ca^{++} release occurs in?

Harrison's 20th Ed. Chapter 232 Page 1657

A. Sarcolemma
B. Sarcoplasmic reticulum
C. Nuclear membrane
D. All of the above

Absolute quantity of Ca^{++} entering sarcolemma & T tubules is modest and insufficient to activate contraction fully. However, this Ca^{++} current, through Ca^{++}-induced Ca^{++} release, triggers substantial Ca^{++} release from the sarcoplasmic reticulum, inducing contraction.

174. Ryanodine receptor (RyR2) best relate to?

Harrison's 20th Ed. Chapter 232 Page 1657

A. Sarcolemma
B. Sarcoplasmic reticulum
C. Nuclear membrane
D. All of the above

Ca^{++} is released from sarcoplasmic reticulum through a Ca^{++} release channel, a cardiac isoform of ryanodine receptor (RyR2).

175. Which of the following inhibits ryanodine receptor (RyR2)?

Harrison's 20th Ed. Chapter 232 Page 1657

A. Calsequestrin
B. Phospholamban
C. Calstabin 2
D. All of the above

Calstabin 2 inhibits RyR2 and thus Ca^{++} release from sarcoplasmic reticulum.

176. Ca^{++} released from sarcoplasmic reticulum interacts with?

Harrison's 20th Ed. Chapter 232 Page 1657

A. Troponin C
B. Troponin I
C. Troponin T
D. All of the above

177. Myocardial contractile force is optimal at a sarcomere length of?

Harrison's 20th Ed. Chapter 232 Page 1657

A. ~ 1.8 µm
B. ~ 2.0 µm
C. ~ 2.2 µm
D. ~ 2.4 µm

Preload determines sarcomere length at the onset of contraction. Myocardial contractile force is optimal at a sarcomere length of ~2.2 µm where myofilament Ca^{++} sensitivity is maximal. Starling's law of the heart states that within limits, the ventricular contraction force depends on end-diastolic length of cardiac muscle which relates closely to the ventricular end-diastolic volume.

178. In Starling's law of heart, the force of ventricular contraction is a function of?

Harrison's 20th Ed. Chapter 232 Page 1658

A. End-diastolic length of cardiac muscle
B. End-systolic length of cardiac muscle
C. Mid-diastolic length of cardiac muscle
D. Mid-systolic length of cardiac muscle

179. Afterload is determined by?

Harrison's 20th Ed. Chapter 232 Page 1658

A. Aortic pressure
B. LV volume
C. Thickness of LV wall
D. All of the above

180. Which of the following parameter is included in Laplace's law?

Harrison's 20th Ed. Chapter 232 Page 1658

A. Intracavitary ventricular pressure
B. Ventricular radius
C. Wall thickness
D. All of the above

181. Laplace's law indicates?

Harrison's 20th Ed. Chapter 232 Page 1658

A. Length of myocardial fiber
B. Tension of myocardial fiber
C. Diameter of myocardial fiber
D. All of the above

182. Aortic pressure depends on?

Harrison's 20th Ed. Chapter 232 Page 1658

A. Peripheral vascular resistance
B. Biomechanics of the arterial tree
C. Volume of blood at the onset of ejection
D. All of the above

183. During exercise, which of the following parameters show relatively little change?

Harrison's 20th Ed. Chapter 232 Page 1659

A. LV end-diastolic pressure
B. Cardiac output
C. Aortic flow velocity
D. Rate of ventricular pressure development

184. Ejection fraction is the?
Harrison's 20th Ed. Chapter 232 Page 1659

A. Ratio of stroke volume to end-systolic volume
B. Ratio of stroke volume to end-diastolic volume
C. Ratio of end-systolic volume to stroke volume
D. Ratio of end-diastolic volume to stroke volume

185. Normal value of ejection fraction is?
Harrison's 20th Ed. Chapter 232 Page 1659

A. 47 ± 8%
B. 57 ± 8%
C. 67 ± 8%
D. 77 ± 8%

186. Normal value of ventricular end-diastolic volume is?
Harrison's 20th Ed. Chapter 232 Page 1659

A. 55 ± 20 mL/m^2
B. 65 ± 20 mL/m^2
C. 75 ± 20 mL/m^2
D. 85 ± 20 mL/m^2

187. Normal value of ventricular end-systolic volume is?
Harrison's 20th Ed. Chapter 232 Page 1659

A. 15 ± 7 mL/m^2
B. 25 ± 7 mL/m^2
C. 35 ± 7 mL/m^2
D. 45 ± 7 mL/m^2

188. Which of the following is of value in the clinical assessment of myocardial function?
Harrison's 20th Ed. Chapter 232 Page 1659

A. Echocardiography
B. Radionuclide scintigraphy
C. Cardiac magnetic resonance imaging (MRI)
D. All of the above

189. Which of the following strongly influence the measurements of CO, EF and ventricular volumes?
Harrison's 20th Ed. Chapter 232 Page 1659

A. Heart rate
B. Ventricular loading
C. Arterial oxygen saturation
D. All of the above

190. Cardiac function variable that is influenced by ventricular loading conditions is?
Harrison's 20th Ed. Chapter 232 Page 1659

A. Cardiac output
B. Ejection fraction
C. Ventricular volumes
D. All of the above

191. Which of the following does not depend on preload and afterload?
Harrison's 20th Ed. Chapter 232 Page 1659

A. End-systolic left ventricular pressure-volume relationship
B. End-diastolic left ventricular pressure-volume relationship
C. Cardiac output
D. Ejection fraction

192. Which of the following best relates to myocardial relaxation?
Harrison's 20th Ed. Chapter 232 Page 1660

A. Rate of uptake of Na^+ by the SR
B. Rate of uptake of K^+ by the SR
C. Rate of uptake of Ca^{++} by the SR
D. All of the above

193. The heart requires a continuous supply of energy (ATP) for?
Harrison's 20th Ed. Chapter 232 Page 1660

A. Mechanical contraction
B. Maintaining ionic homeostasis
C. Maintaining biochemical homeostasis
D. All of the above

194. Which of the following is a determinant of the heart's energy needs?
Harrison's 20th Ed. Chapter 232 Page 1660

A. Ventricular wall tension
B. Frequency of contraction
C. Myocardial contractility
D. All of the above

195. Which of the following statements is false?
Harrison's 20th Ed. Chapter 232 Page 1661

A. Energy substrates of heart are glucose & free fatty acids
B. Oxidation of glucose & FFA produce acetyl coenzyme A in cytoplasm
C. In fasted, resting state, FFA furnish ~70% of heart's acetyl-CoA
D. In the fed state, glucose furnish heart's acetyl-CoA

These two principal sources of acetyl coenzyme A in cardiac muscle i.e. glucose & FFA, vary reciprocally. Glucose is broken down in cytoplasm into pyruvate, which passes into mitochondria, where it is metabolized to acetyl-CoA, and undergoes oxidation. FFAs are converted to acyl-CoA in cytoplasm and acetyl-CoA in mitochondria. Acetyl-CoA enters the citric acid (Krebs) cycle to produce ATP. ATP enters cytoplasm from mitochondrial compartment.

196. Myocardial energy is stored as?
Harrison's 20th Ed. Chapter 232 Page 1661

A. Calsequestrin
B. Creatine phosphate
C. Phospholamban
D. All of the above

Myocardial energy is stored as creatine phosphate (CP) or phosphocreatine, which is in equilibrium with ATP, the immediate energy source.

Electrocardiography

197. ECG leads displays?
Harrison's 20th Ed. Chapter 235 Page 1675

A. Instantaneous differences in electrical potential between electrodes
B. Differences in electrical potential between electrode and neutral
C. Differences in electrical potential between electrode & maximum positive charge
D. Differences in electrical potential between electrode & maximum negative charge

ECG leads display instantaneous differences in potential between electrodes.

198. Electric currents that spread through the heart can be produced by?
Harrison's 20th Ed. Chapter 235 Page 1675

A. Cardiac pacemaker cells
B. Specialized conduction tissue
C. Heart muscle
D. All of the above

Depolarization of the heart is the initiating event for cardiac contraction. The electric currents that spread through the heart are produced by cardiac pacemaker cells, specialized conduction tissue, and heart muscle. The ECG records only the depolarization (stimulation) and repolarization (recovery) potentials generated by the atrial and ventricular myocardium.

199. AV junction is constituted by?
Harrison's 20th Ed. Chapter 235 Page 1675

A. Atrioventricular (AV) node
B. AV node and His-bundle
C. AV node, His-bundle and fascicles
D. AV node, His-bundle, fascicles & Purkinje fibres

AV nodal region & His-bundle area together constitute AV junction.

200. Ventricular repolarization is represented by?
Harrison's 20th Ed. Chapter 235 Page 1675

A. ST segment
B. T wave
C. U wave
D. ST-T-U complex

QRS complex represents ventricular depolarization & ST-T-U complex (ST segment, T wave & U wave) represents ventricular repolarization.

201. J point is the junction between?
Harrison's 20th Ed. Chapter 235 Page 1675

A. End of P wave & beginning of QRS complex
B. End of QRS complex & beginning of ST segment
C. End of ST segment & beginning of T wave
D. End of T wave & beginning of U wave

J point is the junction between the end of QRS complex and the beginning of ST segment.

202. Atrial repolarization wave may become apparent in?
Harrison's 20th Ed. Chapter 235 Page 1675

A. Acute pericarditis
B. Cardiomyopathy
C. PSVT
D. Wandering pacemaker

203. Atrial repolarization wave may become apparent in?
Harrison's 20th Ed. Chapter 235 Page 1675

A. Acute rheumatic fever
B. Cardiomyopathy
C. PSVT
D. Atrial infarction

204. Atrial repolarization wave may become apparent in?
Harrison's 20th Ed. Chapter 235 Page 1675

A. Acute pericarditis
B. Atrial infarction
C. AV heart block
D. All of the above

Atrial repolarization is usually too low in amplitude to be detected, but it may become apparent in acute pericarditis, atrial infarction and AV heart block.

205. Rapid upstroke of the action potential that corresponds to the onset of QRS is called?
Harrison's 20th Ed. Chapter 235 Page 1675

A. Phase 0
B. Phase 1
C. Phase 2
D. Phase 3

206. Plateau of the action potential that corresponds to isoelectric ST segment is called?
Harrison's 20th Ed. Chapter 235 Page 1675

A. Phase 0
B. Phase 1
C. Phase 2
D. Phase 3

The QRS-T waveforms of the surface ECG correspond with the different phases of simultaneously obtained ventricular action potentials. Rapid upstroke (phase 0) of the action potential corresponds to the onset of QRS. Plateau (phase 2) corresponds to the isoelectric ST segment, and active repolarization (phase 3) corresponds to the inscription of the T wave.

207. Which of the following prolong phase 2 of the cardiac muscle action potential and increase the QT interval?
Harrison's 20th Ed. Chapter 235 Page 1675

A. Hyperkalemia
B. Amiodarone
C. Digitalis
D. Hypercalcemia

Factors that decrease slope of phase 0 by impairing influx of Na^+ (hyperkalemia & flecainide) tend to increase QRS duration. Conditions that prolong phase 2 (amiodarone, hypocalcemia) increase QT interval. Shortening of ventricular repolarization (phase 2) by digitalis administration or hypercalcemia, abbreviates ST segment.

208. The action potential of the His-Purkinje system and ventricular myocardium has?
Harrison's 20th Ed. Chapter 235 Page 1675

A. Two phases
B. Three phases
C. Four phases
D. Five phases

Action potential of the His-Purkinje system has five phases.

209. Resting membrane potential in ventricular myocardium is?
Harrison's 20th Ed. Chapter 235 Page 1675

A. Phase 1
B. Phase 2
C. Phase 3
D. Phase 4

Rapid depolarizing current (phase 0) is due to influx of Na+ into myocardial cells followed by influx of Ca^{++}. Repolarization phases of action potential (phases 1 to 3) are due to outward flux of K^{+}. Resting membrane potential is phase 4.

210. Which of the following intervals is used to calculate heart rate?
Harrison's 20th Ed. Chapter 235 Page 1676

A. RR
B. PR
C. QRS
D. QT

Heart rate can be computed from the interbeat (RR) interval by dividing number of large (0.20 second) time units between consecutive R waves into 300 or the number of small (0.04 second) units into 1500.

211. Which of the following statements is false?
Harrison's 20th Ed. Chapter 235 Page 1676

A. Normal PR interval is 120 – 200 ms
B. Normal QRS interval is <100 – 110 ms
C. Normal QT interval is ≤ 0.44 s
D. None of the above

212. Which of the following statements is false?
Harrison's 20th Ed. Chapter 235 Page 1676

A. QT interval varies inversely with the heart rate
B. Rate-related ("corrected") QT interval is calculated as QT/√RR
C. Upper normal limits of QTc is 0.45 s in men & 0.46 s in women
D. None of the above

213. Rate-related ("corrected") QT interval (QTc) is calculated by?
N Engl J Med. 1993; 328:287

A. Alwyn's formula
B. Bazett's formula
C. Frank's formula
D. Donald's formula

Original formula for QTc was published in 1920 by Bazett based on the study of 39 patients.

214. Rate-related ("corrected") QT interval (QTc) is calculated by?
Circ J. 2010;74(8):1663-9

A. Fridericia's formula
B. Holter's formula
C. Grobbee's formula
D. Wilde's formula

Fridericia's is a cube-root formula while Bazett's is a square-root formula.

215. Which of the following is the more appropriate measure of ventricular cell repolarization?
N Engl J Med. 1993; 328:287

A. RT interval
B. JT interval
C. RU interval
D. JU interval

JT interval, the more appropriate measure of ventricular cell repolarization, which is the point of attack for most influences altering QT intervals.

216. Automaticity is characteristic of?
Harrison's 20th Ed. Chapter 238 Page 1717

A. Sinoatrial (SA)
B. Coronary sinus
C. Pulmonary veins
D. All of the above

Automaticity is characteristic of pacemaking cells in the sinoatrial (SA) and atrioventricular (AV) nodes, His-Purkinje system, coronary sinus and pulmonary veins. It is the property of a cardiac cell that causes it to depolarize spontaneously during phase 4 of the action potential leading to the generation of an impulse.

217. PR interval is related to?
Harrison's 20th Ed. Chapter 235 Page 1676

A. Atrial musculature conduction
B. AV node
C. AV junction area
D. All of the above

PR interval measures the time (normally 120 - 200 ms) between atrial & ventricular depolarization, which includes the physiologic delay imposed by stimulation of cells in the AV junction area.

218. Extremity ECG leads record potentials transmitted onto?
Harrison's 20th Ed. Chapter 235 Page 1676

A. Frontal plane
B. Vertical plane
C. Horizontal plane
D. Diagonal plane

219. ECG chest leads record potentials transmitted onto?
Harrison's 20th Ed. Chapter 235 Page 1676

A. Frontal plane
B. Vertical plane
C. Horizontal plane
D. Diagonal plane

Six extremity leads record potentials transmitted onto the frontal plane & the six chest leads record potentials transmitted onto the horizontal plane.

220. Which of the following statements about each ECG lead is false?

Harrison's 20th Ed. Chapter 235 Page 1676 Figure 235-4

A. Each ECG lead has a specific spatial orientation
B. Each ECG lead has a specific polarity
C. Positive pole of lead I is labeled as 0°
D. None of the above

The positive pole of each lead axis and the negative pole are designated by their angular position relative to the positive pole of lead I (0°) in increments of 30°.

221. In the hexaxial diagram representing frontal plane (limb or extremity) leads, 0° corresponds to which lead?

Harrison's 20th Ed. Chapter 235 Page 1676 Figure 235-4

A. Lead I
B. Lead II
C. Lead III
D. Any of the above

Each lead axis is designated by their angular position relative to the positive pole of lead I (0°).

222. Additional posterior leads are placed on the same horizontal plane as?

Harrison's 20th Ed. Chapter 235 Page 1676 Figure 235-5

A. V3
B. V4
C. V5
D. V6

Additional posterior leads are sometimes placed on the same horizontal plane as V4.

223. Which chest lead is placed in posterior axillary line?

Harrison's 20th Ed. Chapter 235 Page 1676 Figure 235-5

A. V6
B. V7
C. V8
D. V9

224. Number of intercostal spaces used for placing unipolar chest leads in ECG are?

Harrison's 20th Ed. Chapter 235 Page 1676

A. 1
B. 2
C. 3
D. 4

IV and V intercostal spaces.

225. In ECG, if the mean orientation of the depolarization vector is at right angles to a given lead axis, which of the following will happen?

Harrison's 20th Ed. Chapter 235 Page 1676

A. Positive wave will be recorded
B. Negative wave will be recorded
C. Biphasic wave will be recorded
D. Flat wave will be recorded

ECG leads are configured so that a positive (upright) deflection is recorded in a lead if a wave of depolarization spreads toward the positive pole of that lead, and a negative deflection if the wave spreads toward the negative pole. If the mean orientation of depolarization vector is at right angles to a given lead axis, a biphasic (equally positive & negative) deflection is recorded.

226. ECG leads I, II, and III are called?

Harrison's 20th Ed. Chapter 235 Page 1676

A. Unipolar leads
B. Bipolar leads
C. Tripolar leads
D. Multipolar leads

227. ECG leads aVR, aVL, and aVF are called?

Harrison's 20th Ed. Chapter 235 Page 1676

A. Unipolar leads
B. Bipolar leads
C. Tripolar leads
D. Multipolar leads

Six extremity leads are 3 bipolar leads (I, II & III) and 3 unipolar leads (aVR, aVL & aVF) leads. Each bipolar lead measures the difference in potential between electrodes at two extremities.

228. Bipolar lead I measures the difference in potential between?

Harrison's 20th Ed. Chapter 235 Page 1676

A. Left arm-right arm voltages
B. Left leg-right arm voltages
C. Left leg-left arm voltages
D. Left leg-right leg voltages

229. Bipolar lead II measures the difference in potential between?

Harrison's 20th Ed. Chapter 235 Page 1676

A. Left arm-right arm voltages
B. Left leg-right arm voltages
C. Left leg-left arm voltages
D. Left leg-right leg voltages

230. Bipolar lead III measures the difference in potential between?

Harrison's 20th Ed. Chapter 235 Page 1676

A. Left arm-right arm voltages
B. Left leg-right arm voltages
C. Left leg-left arm voltages
D. Left leg-right leg voltages

Each bipolar lead measures the difference in potential between electrodes at two extremities: lead I = left arm–right arm voltages, lead II = left leg–right arm, and lead III = left leg–left arm.

231. In unipolar leads, the lowercase "a" stands for?

Harrison's 20th Ed. Chapter 235 Page 1676

A. Added
B. Augmented
C. Arithmatic
D. Apparent

232. Electrical augmentation of unipolar potentials in unipolar leads is by?

Harrison's 20th Ed. Chapter 235 Page 1676

A. 25%
B. 50%
C. 75%
D. 100%

The lowercase "a" indicates that these unipolar potentials are electrically augmented by 50%. The right leg electrode functions as a ground. Unipolar leads measure the voltage at one locus relative to an electrode (called central terminal or indifferent electrode) that has approximately zero potential. Thus, aVR = right arm, aVL = left arm, and aVF = left leg.

233. The normal atrial depolarization vector is oriented?
Harrison's 20th Ed. Chapter 235 Page 1676

A. Downward and toward left
B. Upward and toward left
C. Downward and toward right
D. Upward and toward right

Normal atrial depolarization vector (P wave) is oriented downward & toward left, indicating spread of depolarization from sinus node to right & then left atrial myocardium. Since this vector points toward the negative pole of lead aVR, normal P wave will be negative in aVR. Opposite will occur if an ectopic pacemaker is in the lower part of either atrium or in the AV junction region.

234. QRS vector 1 points towards?
Harrison's 20th Ed. Chapter 235 Page 1677 Figure 235-6

A. Leftward and posteriorly
B. Leftward and anteriorly
C. Rightward and posteriorly
D. Rightward and anteriorly

235. QRS vector 2 points towards?
Harrison's 20th Ed. Chapter 235 Page 1677 Figure 235-6

A. Leftward and posteriorly
B. Leftward and anteriorly
C. Rightward and posteriorly
D. Rightward and anteriorly

QRS complex represents depolarization of ventricles. Its first phase (vector 1) is depolarization of interventricular septum from left to right & anteriorly. Second phase (vector 2) results from the simultaneous depolarization of right & left ventricles that points leftward & posteriorly due to the more massive left ventricle.

236. Above what degree of QRS axis is left axis deviation defined?
Harrison's 20th Ed. Chapter 235 Page 1676

A. – 10º
B. – 20º
C. – 30º
D. – 40º

237. Above what degree of QRS axis is called right axis deviation?
Harrison's 20th Ed. Chapter 235 Page 1676

A. + 80º
B. + 90º
C. + 100º
D. + 110º

Normally, the QRS axis ranges from –30º to +100º. QRS axis more negative than – 30º is referred to as left axis deviation, while an axis more positive than + 100º is referred to as right axis deviation.

238. Left axis deviation occurs in?
Harrison's 20th Ed. Chapter 235 Page 1676

A. As a normal variant
B. Left ventricular hypertrophy
C. Inferior myocardial infarction
D. All of the above

Left axis deviation may occur as a normal variant but is more commonly associated with left ventricular hypertrophy, left anterior fascicular hemiblock, or inferior myocardial infarction.

239. Right axis deviation occurs in?
Harrison's 20th Ed. Chapter 235 Page 1676

A. Due to reversal of left and right arm electrodes
B. Right ventricular overload
C. Infarction of lateral wall of left ventricle
D. All of the above

240. Right axis deviation (RAD) occurs in?
Harrison's 20th Ed. Chapter 235 Page 1676

A. Dextrocardia
B. Left pneumothorax
C. Left posterior hemiblock
D. All of the above

RAD may occur as a normal variant (in children & young adults), as a spurious finding due to reversal of left & right arm electrodes, or in right ventricular overload (acute or chronic), infarction of lateral wall of left ventricle, dextrocardia, left pneumothorax or left posterior fascicular block.

241. An abnormal increase in U-wave amplitude is due to which of the following drugs?
Harrison's 20th Ed. Chapter 235 Page 1677

A. Quinidine
B. Dofetilide
C. Amiodarone
D. All of the above

242. An abnormal increase in U-wave amplitude is due which of the following electrolyte disturbance?
Harrison's 20th Ed. Chapter 235 Page 1677

A. Hyponatremia
B. Hyperkalemia
C. Hypokalemia
D. All of the above

Abnormal increase in U-wave amplitude is mostly due to hypokalemia or drugs like dofetilide, amiodarone, sotalol, quinidine.

243. Very prominent U waves are a marker of increased susceptibility to which of the following?
Harrison's 20th Ed. Chapter 235 Page 1677

A. Torsades de pointes (TDP)
B. AIVR
C. Ventricular flutter
D. Any of the above

Very prominent U waves are a marker of increased susceptibility to TDP type of ventricular tachycardia. Inversion of U wave in precordial leads is abnormal & may be a subtle sign of ischemia.

244. P wave amplitude of how many millimeter suggests right atrial overload?
Harrison's 20th Ed. Chapter 235 Page 1677

A. ≥ 1.0 mm
B. ≥ 1.5 mm
C. ≥ 2.0 mm
D. ≥ 2.5 mm

Right atrial overload (acute or chronic) may lead to an increase in P wave amplitude (≥ 2.5 mm).

245. Ventricular "strain" pattern is due to which abnormality in hypertrophied muscle?
Harrison's 20th Ed. Chapter 235 Page 1677

A. Depolarization
B. Repolarization
C. Repolarization & depolarization
D. None of the above

Ventricular "strain" pattern is due to repolarization abnormalities in hypertrophied muscle.

246. Which of the following is not a common feature in right ventricular hypertrophy due to pressure load?
Harrison's 20th Ed. Chapter 235 Page 1677

A. R ≥ S wave in lead V1
B. Right axis deviation
C. Incomplete or complete right bundle branch block pattern
D. ST depression, T-wave inversion in (R) to midprecordial leads

RVH due to a pressure load (PS, PHT) is characterized by tall R wave in lead V1 (R > S wave), with right axis deviation. ST depression and T-wave inversion in right to midprecordial leads are also often present (ventricular strain pattern). Right ventricular hypertrophy with right ventricular volume overload (ostium secundum ASD) is commonly associated with incomplete or complete right bundle branch block pattern with a rightward QRS axis.

247. In acute cor pulmonale due to pulmonary embolism, which of the following is the most common arrhythmia?
Harrison's 20th Ed. Chapter 235 Page 1677

A. Sinus tachycardia
B. Atrial fibrillation
C. Atrial flutter
D. PSVT

Acute cor pulmonale due to pulmonary embolism may be associated with a normal ECG. Sinus tachycardia is the most common arrhythmia. Atrial fibrillation or flutter may occur.

248. S1Q3T3 pattern is seen in?
Harrison's 20th Ed. Chapter 235 Page 1677

A. Acute cor pulmonale due to pulmonary embolism
B. Right bundle branch block
C. Severe mitral stenosis
D. Acute dissection of aorta

S1Q3T3 pattern i.e. prominence of S wave in lead I, Q wave in lead III, T-wave inversion in lead III, is seen in acute cor pulmonale due to pulmonary embolism.

249. Poor R-wave progression seen in chronic cor pulmonale due to obstructive lung disease is due to?
Harrison's 20th Ed. Chapter 235 Page 1677

A. Hyperaeration of lungs
B. Downward displacement of diaphragm and heart
C. Myocardial ischemia
D. All of the above

Poor R-wave progression is noted in chronic cor pulmonale due to obstructive lung disease despite right ventricular hypertrophy. This is due to downward displacement of diaphragm and heart. Low-voltage complexes are commonly present, owing to hyperaeration of the lungs.

250. In ECG, SV1 + (RV5 or RV6) ≥ 35 mm indicates?
Harrison's 20th Ed. Chapter 235 Page 1677

A. Right ventricular hypertrophy
B. Left ventricular hypertrophy
C. Biventricular hypertrophy
D. None of the above

SV1 + (RV5 or RV6) ≥ 35 mm indicate LVH by voltage criteria.

251. In ECG, RaVL ≥ 11 to 13 mm, RaVF ≥ 20 mm or R1 + SIII ≥ 25 mm indicates?
Harrison's 20th Ed. Chapter 235 Page 1677

A. Right ventricular hypertrophy
B. Left ventricular hypertrophy
C. Biventricular hypertrophy
D. None of the above

RaVL ≥ 11 to 13 mm, RaVF ≥ 20 mm, R1+SIII ≥ 25 mm, with or without increased precordial voltage, indicates left ventricular hypertrophy.

252. Which of the following statements about left ventricular hypertrophy (LVH) is false?
Harrison's 20th Ed. Chapter 235 Page 1677

A. Left atrial abnormality increases likelihood of underlying LVH
B. LVH often progresses to incomplete or complete LBBB
C. Sensitivity of conventional voltage criteria for LVH is decreased in thin persons
D. ECG evidence of LVH is a marker of sudden cardiac death

Presence of left atrial abnormality increases the likelihood of underlying LVH. LVH often progresses to incomplete or complete LBBB. Sensitivity of conventional voltage criteria for LVH is decreased in obese persons & in smokers. ECG evidence for LVH is a major noninvasive marker of increased risk of cardiovascular morbidity & mortality, including sudden cardiac death.

253. Which of the following about bundle branches is true?
J Interv Card Electrophysiol. 2014;39(1):45-56

A. Left is narrow & cable-like, right is a broad sheet of fibers
B. Left is a broad sheet of fibers & right is narrow & cable-like
C. Left & right bundle branches are broad sheets of fibers
D. Left & right bundle branches are narrow & cable-like

Bundle of His gives rise to a broad sheet of fibers that course over the left side of interventricular septum to form left bundle branch & a narrow cable-like structure on the right side that forms the right bundle branch.

254. The infrahisian conduction system is insulated by?
J Interv Card Electrophysiol. 2014;39(1):45-56

A. Mucopolysaccharide
B. Elastin
C. Collagen
D. All of the above

The infrahisian conduction system originates at bundle of His and ends at individual Purkinje cell–ventricular myocyte junctions. It is insulated by collagen, which is thick & fibrous in proximal portions, and gradually diminishes such that a delicate insulating layer is seen to surround individual Purkinje fibers.

255. The conduction velocity in His-Purkinje system is?
J Interv Card Electrophysiol. 2014;39(1):45-56

A. 1.3 m/s
B. 2.3 m/s
C. 3.3 m/s
D. 4.3 m/s

The His-Purkinje system is specialized for rapid conduction, with conduction velocities of 2.3 m/s as compared to 0.75 m/s in ventricular muscle.

256. Muscle of Lancisi best relates to?
J Interv Card Electrophysiol. 2014;39(1):45-56

A. Septal papillary muscle of the mitral valve
B. Septal papillary muscle of the tricuspid valve
C. Septal papillary muscle of the pulmonary valve
D. Septal papillary muscle of the aortic valve

Lancisi's muscle is the main muscle of medial papillary complex, tension apparatus supporting the antero-septal commissure of the tricuspid valve.

257. With complete bundle branch blocks the QRS interval is?
Harrison's 20th Ed. Chapter 235 Page 1678

A. ≥ 90 ms in duration
B. ≥ 100 ms in duration
C. ≥ 110 ms in duration
D. ≥ 120 ms in duration

With complete bundle branch blocks the QRS interval is ≥ =120 ms in duration. With incomplete blocks, the QRS interval is between 100 and 120 ms.

258. In RBBB, the terminal QRS vector is oriented?
Harrison's 20th Ed. Chapter 235 Page 1678

A. Anteriorly and to right
B. Anteriorly and to left
C. Posteriorly and to right
D. Posteriorly and to left

In bundle branch blocks, QRS vector is oriented in the direction of myocardial region where depolarization is delayed. In RBBB, the terminal QRS vector is oriented anteriorly and to the right (rSR′ in V1 & qRS in V6).

259. In LBBB, the major QRS vector is oriented?
Harrison's 20th Ed. Chapter 235 Page 1678

A. Anteriorly and to right
B. Anteriorly and to left
C. Posteriorly and to right
D. Posteriorly and to left

LBBB alters both early & later phases of ventricular depolarization. Major QRS vector is directed to left & posteriorly. Normal early left to right pattern of septal activation is disrupted so septal depolarization proceeds from right to left. LBBB has wide, predominantly negative (QS) complexes in lead V1 & entirely positive (R) complexes in lead V6. A pattern identical to that of LBBB, preceded by a sharp spike, is seen in cases of electronic right ventricular pacing because of the relative delay in left ventricular activation.

260. Which of the following about bundle branch blocks is false?
Harrison's 20th Ed. Chapter 235 Page 1678

A. Without structural heart disease, LBBB is more common than RBBB
B. Bundle branch blocks may be chronic or intermittent
C. Bundle branch block may be rate-related
D. LBBB pattern is seen in electronic right ventricular pacing

In subjects without structural heart disease, RBBB is seen more commonly than LBBB.

261. Left bundle branch block is often a marker of?
Harrison's 20th Ed. Chapter 235 Page 1679

A. Coronary heart disease
B. Severe aortic valve disease
C. Cardiomyopathy
D. All of the above

LBBB is a marker of increased risk of cardiovascular morbidity & mortality (coronary heart disease, hypertensive heart disease, aortic valve disease, and cardiomyopathy).

262. Examples of bifascicular block include?
Harrison's 20th Ed. Chapter 235 Page 1679

A. RBBB and LPHB
B. RBBB with LAHB
C. Complete LBBB
D. All of the above

263. Alternation of right & left bundle branch block is a sign of?
Harrison's 20th Ed. Chapter 235 Page 1679

A. Bifascicular disease
B. Trifascicular disease
C. Complete heart block
D. AV Dissociation

Alternation of RBBB & LBBB is a sign of trifascicular disease.

264. Trifascicular block is the combination of?
Harrison's 20th Ed. Chapter 235 Page 1679

A. Right bundle branch block
B. Left anterior or posterior fascicular block
C. First-degree AV block
D. All of the above

265. Which of the following statements is false?
Harrison's 20th Ed. Chapter 235 Page 1679

A. Discordance of QRS–T-wave vectors seen in BBB
B. Primary repolarization abnormalities are independent of QRS changes
C. Primary and secondary T-wave changes may coexist
D. None of the above

266. Intraventricular conduction delays can be caused by?
Harrison's 20th Ed. Chapter 235 Page 1679

A. Hyperkalemia
B. Tricyclic antidepressants
C. Phenothiazines
D. All of the above

Intraventricular conduction delays can be caused by toxic factors that slow ventricular conduction (hyperkalemia, class 1 antiarrhythmic agents, tricyclic antidepressants, phenothiazines).

267. Which of the following is diagnostic of Wolff-Parkinson-White syndrome?
Harrison's 20th Ed. Chapter 235 Page 1679

A. Wide QRS complex
B. Relatively short PR interval
C. Slurring of initial part of QRS (delta wave)
D. All of the above

Prolongation of QRS duration does not necessarily indicate a conduction delay but may be due to A form of ventricular preexcitation via a bypass tract, Wolff-Parkinson-White (WPW) syndrome is diagnosed by a triad consisting of a wide QRS complex associated with a relatively short PR interval and slurring of the initial part of the QRS (delta wave), with the latter effect being due to aberrant activation of ventricular myocardium.

268. Which of the following about myocardial ischemia is false?
Harrison's 20th Ed. Chapter 235 Page 1679

A. Complex time-dependent effects on electrical properties of myocardial cells
B. Severe, acute ischemia lengthens duration of action potential
C. Cause a voltage gradient between normal & ischemic zones
D. Leads to flow of currents of injury

Severe, acute ischemia lowers the resting membrane potential & shortens duration of action potential.

269. Wellens T waves are usually associated with?
Harrison's 20th Ed. Chapter 235 Page 1680 Figure 235-12, N Engl J Med. 2015; 372:66

A. Stenosis of left anterior descending coronary artery
B. Stenosis of posterior descending coronary artery
C. Stenosis of left circumflex coronary artery
D. Stenosis of right coronary artery

Severe anterior wall ischemia (with or without infarction) may cause prominent T-wave inversions in the precordial leads. This pattern referred to as Wellens T waves is usually associated with a high-grade stenosis of the left anterior descending coronary artery.

270. Wellen's syndrome criteria consists of?
J Emerg Trauma Shock. 2009;2(3):206-208

A. Normal ECG or mild ST ↑ or ↓ during chest pain
B. Deeply inverted or biphasic T-waves in V2 & V3 when pain free
C. Cardiac enzymes are normal or mildly elevated
D. All of the above

Wellen's syndrome criteria consists of prior history of chest pain, EKG is normal or with mild ST elevation or depression during chest pain, or with terminal negative deflection of the T wave in V1 and V2, cardiac enzymes are normal or mildly elevated, no pathologic precordial Q-waves, no loss of precordial R-waves, deeply inverted or biphasic T-waves in V2 and V3, possibly V1, V4, V5 and/or V6 when pain free.

271. Deep T-wave inversions are seen in which of the following ECG leads in severe obstruction in left anterior descending coronary artery?
Harrison's 20th Ed. Chapter 235 Page 1679

A. I
B. aVL
C. V1 - V4
D. All of the above

272. ST elevation in lead aVR is seen in?
Harrison's 20th Ed. Chapter 235 Page 1679

A. Ischemia of subendocardium
B. Transmural ischemia
C. Wellen's syndrome
D. Takostubo syndrome

273. Which of the following may exactly simulate the patterns of STEMI or non-STEMI?
Harrison's 20th Ed. Chapter 235 Page 1679

A. Wellen's syndrome
B. Takostubo syndrome
C. Brugada angina
D. Gorlin's syndrome

Takostubo syndrome may exactly simulate the patterns of STEMI or non-STEMI.

274. Which of the following is false about Prinzmetal's angina?
Harrison's 20th Ed. Chapter 235 Page 1680

A. Reversible transmural ischemia
B. Coronary vasospasm
C. Transient ST-segment ↑ without development of Q waves
D. None of the above

275. Which of the following statements is false?
Harrison's 20th Ed. Chapter 235 Page 1680

A. Transmural infarcts may occur without Q waves
B. Subendocardial infarcts may be associated with Q waves
C. Complete normalization of ECG after Q-wave infarction may occur in smaller infarcts
D. None of the above

276. Atrial infarction may be associated with?
Harrison's 20th Ed. Chapter 235 Page 1680

A. PR-segment deviations
B. Changes in P-wave morphology
C. Atrial arrhythmias
D. All of the above

Atrial infarction may be associated with PR-segment deviations due to an atrial current of injury, changes in P-wave morphology, or atrial arrhythmias.

277. Diagnostic changes of acute or evolving ischemia are masked by?
Harrison's 20th Ed. Chapter 235 Page 1680

A. Left bundle branch block
B. Electronic ventricular pacemaker patterns
C. Wolff-Parkinson-White preexcitation
D. All of the above

Diagnostic changes of acute or evolving ischemia can be masked by presence of LBBB, electronic ventricular pacemaker patterns & WPW preexcitation.

278. Osborn wave in ECG is found in?
Harrison's 20th Ed. Chapter 235 Page 1681 Table 235-1

A. Heat stroke
B. Hypothermia
C. Cerebrovascular accident
D. Pneumothorax

Systemic hypothermia also prolongs repolarization, usually with a distinctive convex elevation or "hump" at the J point referred to as Osborn wave. It is due to altered ventricular action potential characteristics.

279. ST-segment elevations simulating ischemia may occur with?
Harrison's 20th Ed. Chapter 235 Page 1681 Table 235-1

A. Hypercalcemia
B. Hyperkalemia
C. Hypothermia
D. All of the above

280. ST-segment elevations simulating ischemia may occur with?
Harrison's 20th Ed. Chapter 235 Page 1681 Table 235-1

A. Acute pericarditis
B. Myocarditis
C. Brugada syndrome
D. All of the above

281. Tall, positive T waves are seen in?
Harrison's 20th Ed. Chapter 235 Page 1681

A. Hyperkalemia
B. Cerebrovascular injury
C. Left ventricular volume overload (MR or AR)
D. All of the above

Tall, positive T waves may be seen in hyperacute ischemic changes, normal variants, hyperkalemia, cerebrovascular injury & left ventricular volume overload due to mitral or aortic regurgitation.

282. The first ECG change in hyperkalemia is?
Harrison's 20th Ed. Chapter 235 Page 1681

A. Diminution in P-wave amplitude
B. Narrowing & peaking (tenting) of T waves
C. Widening of QRS interval
D. AV conduction disturbances

ECG changes in hyperkalemia usually begin with narrowing and peaking (tenting) of the T waves. Further elevation of extracellular K^+ leads to AV conduction disturbances, diminution in P-wave amplitude, and widening of the QRS interval. Severe hyperkalemia causes a slow sinusoidal type of mechanism ("sine-wave" pattern) followed by asystole.

283. ECG changes in hypertrophic cardiomyopathy may simulate?
Harrison's 20th Ed. Chapter 235 Page 1681

A. Anterior MI
B. Lateral MI
C. Inferior MI
D. All of the above

284. QRS & QT prolongation along with sinus tachycardia can be seen in?
Harrison's 20th Ed. Chapter 235 Page 1682 Figure 235-15

A. Tricyclic antidepressant overdose
B. Quinidine excess
C. Subarachnoid hemorrhage
D. Hyperkalemia

Drugs that prolong QT are quinidine, disopyramide, procainamide, tricyclic antidepressants, phenothiazines, amiodarone, sotalol, ibutilide. QRS & QT prolongation along with sinus tachycardia occur in tricyclic antidepressant overdose.

285. "CVA T-wave" pattern consists of all except?
Harrison's 20th Ed. Chapter 235 Page 1681

A. Marked QT prolongation
B. Marked PR prolongation
C. Deep T-wave inversions
D. Wide T-wave inversions

Marked QT prolongation, with deep & wide T-wave inversions occur with intracranial bleeds, particularly subarachnoid hemorrhage and are called as "CVA T-wave" pattern.

286. Systemic hypothermia prolongs?
Harrison's 20th Ed. Chapter 235 Page 1681

A. Depolarization
B. Repolarization
C. Depolarization + repolarization
D. None of the above

Systemic hypothermia also prolongs repolarization with a distinctive convex elevation of the J point called Osborn wave.

287. Which of the following prolongs the QT interval?
Harrison's 20th Ed. Chapter 235 Page 1681

A. Hypothermia
B. Hypokalemia
C. Hypocalcemia
D. All of the above

288. Abbreviation of ST segment and shortening of QT interval is found in?
Harrison's 20th Ed. Chapter 235 Page 1681

A. Hypocalcemia
B. Hypercalcemia
C. Hyponatremia
D. Hyperkalemia

Hypocalcemia typically prolongs the QT interval (ST portion), while hypercalcemia shortens it.

289. Which of the following shortens the QT interval?
Harrison's 20th Ed. Chapter 235 Page 1681

A. Digitalis
B. Disopyramide
C. Ibutilide
D. Procainamide

Digitalis glycosides also shorten the QT interval, often with a characteristic "scooping" of the ST–T-wave complex (digitalis effect).

290. Low QRS voltage is defined as peak-to-trough QRS amplitudes of?
Harrison's 20th Ed. Chapter 235 Page 1681

A. ≤ 5 mm in 3 limb leads
B. ≤ 5 mm in 4 limb leads
C. ≤ 5 mm in 5 limb leads
D. ≤ 5 mm in 6 limb leads

Low QRS voltage is arbitrarily defined as peak-to-trough QRS amplitudes of ≤5 mm in the six limb leads and/or ≤10 mm in the chest leads.

291. Q waves in ECG can be seen in all of the following except?
Harrison's 20th Ed. Chapter 235 Page 1681

A. Sarcoidosis
B. Scleroderma
C. SLE
D. Chagas' disease

292. Q waves in ECG can be seen in all of the following except?
Harrison's 20th Ed. Chapter 235 Page 1681

A. Left pneumothorax
B. Dextrocardia
C. Long QT syndrome
D. Wolff-Parkinson-White syndrome

293. In ECG, transient nonspecific repolarization changes occur following all except?
Harrison's 20th Ed. Chapter 235 Page 1681

A. Meals
B. Postural (orthostatic) change
C. Hyperventilation
D. Sleep

Transient nonspecific ST–T-wave repolarization changes may occur following a meal or with postural (orthostatic) change, hyperventilation, or exercise in healthy individuals.

294. In ECG, total electrical alternans (P-QRS-T) with sinus tachycardia is a relatively specific sign of?

Harrison's 20th Ed. Chapter 235 Page 1683

A. Myocardial ischemia

B. Myocarditis

C. Pericardial effusion

D. Pneumothorax

Total electrical alternans (P-QRS-T) with sinus tachycardia (beat-to-beat alternation in one or more components of ECG) is a relatively specific sign of pericardial effusion with cardiac tamponade due to periodic swinging motion of heart in effusion at a frequency exactly half of heart rate.

295. Repolarization (ST-T or U wave) alternans is a sign of?

Harrison's 20th Ed. Chapter 235 Page 1683

A. Mechanical instability of heart

B. Electrical instability of heart

C. Serious pulmonary disease

D. Serious hepatic disease

Repolarization (ST-T or U wave) alternans is a sign of electrical instability & may precede ventricular tachyarrhythmias.

296. Chronic renal failure (CRF) is suspected if ECG shows?

Acta Cardiol Sin. 2015;31(1):83-86

A. Peaked T waves

B. Long QT

C. Left ventricular hypertrophy (LVH)

D. All of the above

CRF can have the following ECG features as a triad - peaked T waves (hyperkalemia), long QT due to ST segment lengthening (hypocalcemia) & LVH (systemic hypertension).

297. "Persistent juvenile T-wave pattern" consists of?

Heart. 2018;104:A63

A. T-wave inversions in leads V_1 - V_3

B. T-wave inversions in leads V_1 - V_4

C. T-wave inversions in leads V_1 - V_5

D. T-wave inversions in leads V_1 - V_6

The juvenile ECG pattern is defined as T wave inversion in 2 contiguous anterior leads (V1 to V3) in individuals <16 years of age. This is due to electrical predominance of right ventricle in infancy which gradually resolves with normalisation of T waves post-puberty. Anterior TWI is also the hallmark of arrhythmogenic cardiomyopathy.

298. Yamaguchi's syndrome best relates to?

Acta Cardiol Sin. 2015;31(1):83-86

A. Scleroderma

B. Long QT syndrome

C. Apical HCM

D. Dextrocardia

LVH with deep T-wave inversions in limb leads, striking T-wave inversions in precordial leads suggest apical HCM (Yamaguchi's syndrome).

Principles of Electrophysiology

299. Electrocardiogram (ECG) was developed by?
Harrison's 20th Ed. Chapter 238 Page 1716

A. Hewlet
B. Judkin
C. Einthoven
D. White

ECG was developed by Einthoven at the turn of the twentieth century.

300. Body surface ECG is the timed sum of the cellular action potentials in the?
Harrison's 20th Ed. Chapter 238 Page 1716

A. Atria
B. Ventricles
C. Atria and ventricles
D. None of the above

Body surface ECG is the timed sum of the cellular action potentials in the atria & ventricles.

301. Sinoatrial (SA) node is located at the junction of?
Harrison's 20th Ed. Chapter 238 Page 1716

A. Right atrium and superior vena cava
B. Right atrium and inferior vena cava
C. Right atrium and left atrium
D. Right atrium and coronary sinus

SA node is composed of a cluster of small fusiform cells located in sulcus terminalis on epicardial surface of heart at right atrial - superior vena caval junction where they envelop SA nodal artery.

302. PR interval of ECG represents time needed for activation of?
Harrison's 20th Ed. Chapter 238 Page 1716

A. Both atria
B. Atrioventricular node (AVN)
C. Both atria + Atrioventricular node (AVN)
D. Both atria + AVN + His Purkinje system

Electrical impulse from SA node is transmitted slowly through nodal tissue to atria, and rapidly on to atrioventricular node (AVN), resulting in the P wave of the ECG.

303. Which of the following statements is false?
Harrison's 20th Ed. Chapter 238 Page 1716

A. Body surface ECG is the timed sum of cellular action potentials in atria & ventricles
B. Repolarization occurs first on endocardium then proceeds to epicardium
C. Activation of atria & AV node is PR interval
D. QT interval is duration of activation & recovery of ventricles

Repolarization occurs first on the epicardial surface, then proceeds to the endocardium.

304. Electrophysiologically, there are how many phases of action potential in cardiac myocyte?
Circ Arrhythmia Electrophysiol. 2009;2:185-194

A. 3
B. 4
C. 5
D. 6

305. Which of the following phase represents resting potential?
Circ Arrhythmia Electrophysiol. 2009;2:185-194

A. 0
B. 2
C. 3
D. 4

Phase 4, or the resting potential, is stable at (-)90 mV in normal working myocardial cells.

306. Which of the following phase represents plateau phase?
Circ Arrhythmia Electrophysiol. 2009;2:185-194

A. 0
B. 2
C. 3
D. 4

Phase 2, a plateau phase, is the longest phase. It is unique among excitable cells and marks the phase of calcium entry into the cell.

307. Which of the following is a category of cardiac K^+ channel?
Circ Arrhythmia Electrophysiol. 2009;2:185-194

A. Voltage gated
B. Inward rectifier channels
C. Background K+ currents
D. All of the above

Cardiac K^+ channels fall into 3 broad categories: Voltage gated (Ito, IKur, IKr, and IKs), inward rectifier channels (IK1, IKAch, and IKATP), and the background K^+ currents (TASK-1, TWIK-1/2).

308. Duration of action potential in cardiac myocytes is?
Harrison's 20th Ed. Chapter 238 Page 1716

A. 20 – 40 ms
B. 80 – 1600 ms
C. 200 – 400 ms
D. 500 – 800 ms

Cardiac myocytes have a characteristically long action potential (200–400 ms) compared to neurons or skeletal muscle cells (1–5 ms).

309. Which of the following participate in the cardiac myocyte action potential?
Harrison's 20th Ed. Chapter 238 Page 1716

A. Ion channels
B. Pumps, transporters
C. Exchangers
D. All of the above

The action potential of cardiac myocyte results from the activity of multiple distinctive time- and voltage-dependent ionic currents. The currents in turn are carried by transmembrane proteins that passively conduct ions down their electrochemical gradients through selective pores (ion channels), actively transport ions against their electrochemical gradient (pumps, transporters), or electrogenically exchange ionic species (exchangers).

310. Diastole corresponds to which phase of action potentials?
Harrison's 20th Ed. Chapter 238 Page 1717 Figure 238-1

A. Phase 1
B. Phase 2
C. Phase 3
D. Phase 4

Phase 0 is rapid upstroke, phase 1 is early repolarization, phase 2 is plateau, phase 3 is late repolarization, and phase 4 is diastole.

311. Which of the following gene is responsible for ventricular repolarization?
Harrison's 20th Ed. Chapter 238 Page 1717 Figure 238-1

A. KCNJ2
B. SCN5A
C. CACNA1C
D. SLC8A1

312. Which of the following is principal current during phase 4?
Harrison's 20th Ed. Chapter 238 Page 1717 Figure 238-1

A. I_{K1}
B. I_{to}
C. I_{Kr}
D. I_{Ks}

313. Which of the following determines the resting membrane potential of the myocyte?
Harrison's 20th Ed. Chapter 238 Page 1717 Figure 238-1

A. I_{K1}
B. I_{to}
C. I_{Kr}
D. I_{Ks}

Potassium current (IK1) is the principal current during phase 4 and determines the resting membrane potential of the myocyte.

314. Which of the following causes phase 3 repolarization?
Harrison's 20th Ed. Chapter 238 Page 1717 Figure 238-1

A. Inactivation of the calcium current
B. Persistent activation of I_{Kr}
C. Persistent activation of I_{Ks}
D. All of the above

Inactivation of the calcium current with persistent activation of potassium currents (predominantly IKr and IKs) causes phase 3 repolarization.

315. Sodium-calcium exchanger transports how many Na^+ for one Ca^{2+}?
Harrison's 20th Ed. Chapter 238 Page 1716

A. 1
B. 2
C. 3
D. 4

Electrogenic sodium-calcium exchanger transports three Na^+ for one Ca^{2+}.

316. Reestablishing of the negative resting membrane potential of the heart cells is done by?
Harrison's 20th Ed. Chapter 238 Page 1716

A. Inactivation of Na channel
B. Inactivation of Ca channel
C. Activation of K channel
D. All of the above

317. Automaticity is a property of?
Harrison's 20th Ed. Chapter 238 Page 1717

A. Sinoatrial (SA) node
B. His-Purkinje system
C. Coronary sinus
D. All of the above

Property of automaticity (pacemaking i.e. spontaneous diastolic depolarization) is characteristic of sinoatrial (SA) & atrioventricular (AV) nodes, His-Purkinje system, coronary sinus & pulmonary veins.

318. Abnormal automaticity may produce which of the following?
Harrison's 20th Ed. Chapter 238 Page 1717

A. Atrial tachycardia
B. Accelerated idioventricular rhythms
C. Ventricular tachycardia
D. All of the above

Abnormal automaticity may produce atrial tachycardia, accelerated idioventricular rhythms, and ventricular tachycardia, particularly associated with ischemia and reperfusion.

319. Triggered automaticity refers to impulse initiation that is dependent on?
Harrison's 20th Ed. Chapter 238 Page 1718

A. Entrance block
B. Overdrive suppression
C. Afterdepolarizations
D. All of the above

Triggered automaticity or activity refers to impulse initiation that is dependent on afterdepolarizations which are membrane voltage oscillations that occur during (early afterdepolarizations, EADs) or after (delayed afterdepolarizations, DADs) an action potential.

320. Early afterdepolarizations occur during?
Harrison's 20th Ed. Chapter 238 Page 1718

A. Phases 0 and 1 of the action potential
B. Phases 1 and 2 of the action potential
C. Phases 2 and 3 of the action potential
D. Phases 3 and 4 of the action potential

321. Delayed afterdepolarizations occur after completion of?
Harrison's 20th Ed. Chapter 238 Page 1718

A. Phase 1 of action potential
B. Phase 2 of action potential
C. Phase 3 of action potential
D. Phase 4 of action potential

Afterdepolarizations are spontaneous depolarizations due to membrane voltage oscillations in cardiac myocytes. Early afterdepolarizations (EAD) occur before the end of the action potential (phases 2 and 3), interrupting repolarization. Delayed afterdepolarizations (DAD) occur during phase 4 of the action potential after completion of repolarization.

322. Cellular feature common to induction of DADs is the presence of?
Harrison's 20th Ed. Chapter 238 Page 1718

A. Increased Ca^{2+} load in the cytosol
B. Increased Na^{+} load in the cytosol
C. Increased K^{+} load in the cytosol
D. Increased Mg^{2+} load in the cytosol

The cellular feature common to induction of DADs is the presence of an increased Ca^{2+} load in the cytosol and sarcoplasmic reticulum.

323. Which of the following enhance Ca^{2+} loading sufficiently to produce DADs?
Harrison's 20th Ed. Chapter 238 Page 1718

A. Digitalis glycoside toxicity
B. Catecholamines
C. Myocardial ischemia
D. All of the above

Digitalis glycoside toxicity, catecholamines, and ischemia all can enhance Ca^{2+} loading sufficiently to produce DADs.

324. Which of the following about connexins is false?
Harrison's 20th Ed. Chapter 30, 438, 238 Page 1718

A. Gap junction membrane-spanning protein
B. CMT1X is caused by mutations in connexin 32 gene
C. Mutations in connexin 26 causes progressive hearing loss
D. None of the above

Connexins are gap junction membrane-spanning structural proteins that are important in cell-to-cell communication. They pair across adjacent cells.

325. Which of the following is the principal connexin expressed in the heart?
Circ Arrhythmia Electrophysiol. 2009;2:185-194

A. Connexin 40
B. Connexin 43
C. Connexin 45
D. All of the above

Three types of connexins are expressed in heart and are defined on the basis of their molecular weight: connexin 40, connexin 43, and connexin 45. Connexin 43 is the principal connexin expressed in the heart.

326. Chronically ischemic myocardium exhibits a downregulation of?
Harrison's 20th Ed. Chapter 238 Page 1719

A. Connexin 26
B. Connexin 31
C. Connexin 32
D. Connexin 43

Chronically ischemic myocardium exhibits a downregulation of the gap junction channel protein (connexin 43) that carries intercellular ionic current.

327. Epsilon waves in ECG are a feature of?
Harrison's 20th Ed. Chapter 238 Page 1720

A. Wolff-Parkinson-White (WPW) syndrome
B. Long QT syndrome
C. Arrhythmogenic right ventricular dysplasia
D. Brugada syndrome

328. Right precordial ST-segment abnormalities in ECG are a feature of?
Harrison's 20th Ed. Chapter 238 Page 1720

A. Wolff-Parkinson-White (WPW) syndrome
B. Long QT syndrome
C. Arrhythmogenic right ventricular dysplasia
D. Brugada syndrome

329. Delta waves in ECG are a feature of?
Harrison's 20th Ed. Chapter 238 Page 1720

A. Wolff-Parkinson-White (WPW) syndrome
B. Long QT syndrome
C. Arrhythmogenic right ventricular dysplasia
D. Brugada syndrome

330. Ventricular tachyarrhythmias occur more frequently in patients with?
Harrison's 20th Ed. Chapter 238 Page 1720

A. Ventricular systolic dysfunction
B. Hypertrophic cardiomyopathy
C. Sarcoidosis
D. All of the above

Ventricular tachyarrhythmias occur more frequently in patients with ventricular systolic dysfunction and chamber dilation, in hypertrophic cardiomyopathy, and in infiltrative diseases like sarcoidosis.

331. Supraventricular arrhythmias may be associated with?
Harrison's 20th Ed. Chapter 238 Page 1720

A. Transposition of the great arteries
B. Ebstein's anomaly
C. Ostium primum atrial septal defect (ASD)
D. Ventricular septal defects (VSD)

Supraventricular arrhythmias may be associated with Ebstein's anomaly.

332. Which of the following is a response to Head-up tilt (HUT)?
Harrison's 20th Ed. Chapter 238 Page 1720

A. Initial increase in heart rate
B. Drop in blood pressure
C. Late reduction in heart rate
D. All of the above

Exaggerated activation of a central reflex in response to Head-up tilt (HUT) testing produces a stereotypic response of an initial increase in heart rate, then a drop in blood pressure followed by a reduction in heart rate characteristic of neurally mediated hypotension.

333. Head-up tilt (HUT) is a useful tool in the diagnosis of and therapy for?
Harrison's 20th Ed. Chapter 238 Page 1720

A. Recurrent idiopathic vertigo
B. Chronic fatigue syndrome
C. Recurrent transient ischemic attacks
D. All of the above

HUT is used most often in patients with recurrent syncope. HUT is also a useful tool in the diagnosis of and therapy for recurrent idiopathic vertigo, chronic fatigue syndrome, recurrent transient ischemic attacks, and repeated falls of unknown etiology in the elderly.

334. Head-up tilt (HUT) testing is relatively contraindicated in?

Harrison's 20th Ed. Chapter 238 Page 1720

A. Aortic stenosis
B. Severe mitral stenosis
C. Severe cerebrovascular disease
D. All of the above

HUT is relatively contraindicated in the presence of severe CAD with proximal coronary stenoses, severe cerebrovascular disease, severe mitral stenosis, and obstruction to left ventricular outflow (aortic stenosis).

335. Nationality of Miles Vaughan Williams was?

Circulation. 2018;138:1879-1896

A. American
B. British
C. Canadian
D. Swedish

Miles Vaughan Williams (1918–2016) was a British cardiac pharmacologist and worked at Hertford College, University of Oxford. Miles was born in Bangalore, India.

336. Which of the following best relates to classification of antiarrhythmic drug therapy?

European Heart Journal 1991;12(10):1112-1131

A. Queen's Gambit
B. Sicilian Gambit
C. Roman Gambit
D. Danish Gambit

Sicilian Gambit is a new approach to classify antiarrhythmic drugs. It correlated information on molecular targets, cellular mechanisms, functional targets & clinical arrhythmias for individual drugs with similarities and differences in their effects, accommodating their multiple actions.

337. Which of the following relates best with Vaughan-Williams class I class of antiarrhythmic drugs?

Harrison's 20th Ed. Chapter 238 Page 1721

A. Local anesthetic effect due to blockade of Na^+ current
B. Interference of catecholamine action at β-adrenergic receptor
C. Delayed repolarization by K^+ current inhibition or activation of depolarizing current
D. Interference with calcium conductance

338. Which of the following relates best with Vaughan-Williams class II class of antiarrhythmic drugs?

Harrison's 20th Ed. Chapter 238 Page 1721

A. Local anesthetic effect due to blockade of Na^+ current
B. Interference of catecholamine action at β-adrenergic receptor
C. Delayed repolarization by K^+ current inhibition or activation of depolarizing current
D. Interference with calcium conductance

339. Which of the following relates best with Vaughan-Williams class III class of antiarrhythmic drugs?

Harrison's 20th Ed. Chapter 238 Page 1721

A. Local anesthetic effect due to blockade of Na^+ current
B. Interference of catecholamine action at β-adrenergic receptor
C. Delayed repolarization by K^+ current inhibition or activation of depolarizing current
D. Interference with calcium conductance

340. Which of the following relates best with Vaughan-Williams class IV class of antiarrhythmic drugs?

Harrison's 20th Ed. Chapter 238 Page 1721

A. Local anesthetic effect due to blockade of Na^+ current
B. Interference of catecholamine action at β-adrenergic receptor
C. Delayed repolarization by K^+ current inhibition or activation of depolarizing current
D. Interference with calcium conductance

Class I exert their antiarrhythmic action by local anesthetic effect by blockade of Na+ current, class II interfere with the action of catecholamines at β-adrenergic receptor, class III cause delay of repolarization due to inhibition of K^+ current or activation of depolarizing current and class IV interfere with calcium conductance.

341. Which of the following is a class Ia antiarrhythmic agent?

Harrison's 20th Ed. Chapter 238 Page 1721

A. Lidocaine
B. Mexiletine
C. Procainamide
D. Propafenone

Class I antiarrhythmics have been further subdivided based on the kinetics and potency of Na+ channel binding. Class Ia agents (quinidine, procainamide) have moderate potency & intermediate kinetics. Class Ib agents (lidocaine, mexiletine) have low potency and rapid kinetics while class Ic drugs (flecainide, propafenone) have high potency and the slowest kinetics. Class I drugs produce moderate (Ia), weak (Ib), or marked (Ic) Na+ channel block and reduce AP phase 0 slope & overshoot while increasing, reducing, or conserving AP duration (APD) and effective refractory period (ERP), respectively.

342. Which of the following is a Class 0 antiarrhythmic agent?

Circulation. 2018;138:1879-1896

A. Ajmaline
B. Ivabradine
C. Dronedarone
D. Dofetilide

343. Which of the following about Ivabradine is false?

Circulation. 2018;138:1879-1896

A. Inhibits I_f current
B. Acts through hyperpolarization activated cyclic nucleotide-gated channel (HCN)
C. Reduces sinus node automaticity
D. None of the above

344. Which of the following is a Class 1a antiarrhythmic agent?

Circulation. 2018;138:1879-1896

A. Quinidine
B. Ajmaline
C. Disopyramide
D. All of the above

345. Which of the following is a nonselective K^+ channel blocker?

Circulation. 2018;138:1879-1896

A. Ambasilide
B. Amiodarone
C. Dronedarone
D. All of the above

346. Which of the following is a Kv11.1 (HERG) channel–mediated rapid K^+ current (IKr) blocker?

Circulation. 2018;138:1879-1896

A. Dofetilide
B. Ibutilide
C. Sotalol
D. All of the above

347. Which of the following is a Kv1.5 channel–mediated, ultrarapid K^+ current (IKur) blocker?

Circulation. 2018;138:1879-1896

A. Bepridil
B. Nicorandil
C. Vernakalant
D. All of the above

348. Which of the following is an intracellular Ca^{++} channel blocker?

Circulation. 2018;138:1879-1896

A. Flecainide
B. Diltiazem
C. Verapamil
D. Bepridil

349. First catheter ablation using a DC energy source was performed in the early 1980s by?

Harrison's 20th Ed. Chapter 238 Page 1721

A. Scheinman
B. Hille
C. Josephson
D. Zipes

First catheter ablation using a DC energy source was performed in the early 1980s by Scheinman and colleagues.

350. Which of the following produces a reversible local conduction block in catheter-based ablation in the heart?

Harrison's 20th Ed. Chapter 238 Page 1721

A. Lasers
B. Ultrasound
C. Cryoablation
D. Radio frequency

351. Which of the following increases mortality rates in patients after myocardial infarction?

Can J Cardiol. 2010;26(6):303-312

A. Late potentials
B. T wave alternans (TWA) at low heart rates
C. Decrease in heart rate variability (HRV)
D. All of the above

352. Which of the following methods is related to autonomic nervous system influence on the heart?

Europace. 2016;18(6):925-944

A. Late potentials
B. T wave alternans (TWA) at low heart rates
C. QT interval variability (QTV)
D. All of the above

Heart rate variability (HRV) & QT interval variability (QTV) provide noninvasive methods to assess autonomic nervous system influence on heart. A decrease in HRV is associated with increased sympathetic nervous system tone and increased mortality rates in patients after myocardial infarction.

353. 1 metabolic equivalent (MET) is?

BMJ. 2002;324(7345):1084-1087

A. 1.5 mL oxygen / kg per minute
B. 2.5 mL oxygen / kg per minute
C. 3.5 mL oxygen / kg per minute
D. 4.5 mL oxygen / kg per minute

1 MET is 3.5 mL oxygen/kg per minute, which is the oxygen consumption of an average individual at rest.

354. To carry out the activities of daily living an exercise intensity of at least how many METs is required?

BMJ. 2002;324(7345):1084-1087

A. 2 METs
B. 3 METs
C. 4 METs
D. 5 METs

To carry out the activities of daily living an exercise intensity of at least 5 METs is required.

355. In stage 1 of Bruce protocol, energy expenditure is estimated to be?

BMJ. 2002;324(7345):1084-1087

A. 2.8 METs
B. 3.8 METs
C. 4.8 METs
D. 5.8 METs

In stage 1 of Bruce protocol, the patient walks at 1.7 mph (2.7 km) up a 10% incline. Energy expenditure is estimated to be 4.8 METs (metabolic equivalents) during this stage.

356. For men, the maximum predicted heart rate in exercise stress testing is calculated as?

BMJ. 2002;324(7345):1084-1087

A. 200 minus the patient's age
B. 210 minus the patient's age
C. 220 minus the patient's age
D. 230 minus the patient's age

By convention, the maximum predicted heart rate in exercise stress testing is calculated as 220 (210 for women) minus the patient's age.

357. Which of the following is a normal electrocardiographic change during exercise?

BMJ. 2002;324(7345):1084-1087

A. P wave increases in height
B. R wave decreases in height
C. T wave decreases in height
D. All of the above

358. Which of the following is a normal electrocardiographic change during exercise?

BMJ. 2002;324(7345):1084-1087

A. J point becomes depressed
B. ST segment becomes sharply upsloping
C. Q-T interval shortens
D. All of the above

Normal electrocardiographic changes during exercise include P wave increases in height, R wave decreases in height, J point becomes depressed, ST segment becomes sharply upsloping, Q-T interval shortens and T wave decreases in height.

359. Which of the following is an abnormal electrocardiographic change during exercise?

BMJ. 2002;324(7345):1084-1087

A. ST segment depression of >1 mm (horizontal or downsloping)
B. ST elevation of >1 mm
C. Inversion of the U wave
D. All of the above

360. In exercise stress testing, findings suggesting high probability of coronary artery disease include?

BMJ. 2002;324(7345):1084-1087

A. Early positive response within six minutes
B. Persistence of ST depression for > 6 minutes into recovery
C. ST segment depression in five or more leads
D. All of the above

Findings suggesting high probability of coronary artery disease include horizontal ST segment depression of < 2 mm, downsloping ST segment depression, early positive response within six minutes, persistence of ST depression for > 6 minutes into recovery, ST segment depression in ≥5 leads and exertional hypotension.

361. Contraindications to exercise stress testing include?

BMJ. 2002;324(7345):1084-1087

A. Severe aortic stenosis
B. Rest angina within 48 hours
C. Active infective endocarditis
D. All of the above

362. Contraindications to exercise stress testing include?

BMJ. 2002;324(7345):1084-1087

A. Acute myocardial infarction (within 4–6 days)
B. Deep vein thrombosis
C. Systolic BP > 220 mm Hg/diastolic BP >120 mm Hg
D. All of the above

The Bradyarrhythmias: Disorders of the Sinoatrial Node

363. Electrical activation of the heart can originate in?
Harrison's 20th Ed. Chapter 239 Page 1722

A. Atrioventricular (AV) node
B. Specialized conducting system
C. Muscle
D. All of the above

Electrical activation of the heart normally originates in sinoatrial (SA) node, the predominant pacemaker. Other subsidiary pacemakers in atrioventricular (AV) node, specialized conducting system and muscle may initiate electrical activation if SA node is dysfunctional or suppressed.

364. Which of the following is false about nodal cells?
Harrison's 20th Ed. Chapter 239 Page 1722

A. Less negative resting membrane potential
B. Most rapid phase 4 depolarization
C. Slow action potential upstrokes (phase 0)
D. Action potential mediated by Na^+ rather than Ca^{++}

In nodal cells, action potential mediated by Ca^{++} rather than Na^+ current.

365. Nodal cell action potentials exhibit which of the following?
Harrison's 20th Ed. Chapter 239 Page 1723 Figure 239-1

A. More depolarized resting membrane potentials
B. Slower phase 0 upstrokes
C. Slower phase 4 diastolic depolarization
D. All of the above

Nodal cell action potentials exhibit more depolarized resting membrane potentials, slower phase 0 upstrokes, and phase 4 diastolic depolarization.

366. Which of the following is not a depolarizing current?
Harrison's 20th Ed. Chapter 239 Page 1723 Figure 239-2

A. $I_{Ca\text{-}L}$
B. $I_{Ca\text{-}T}$
C. I_f
D. I_{KACh}

367. Which of the following is a repolarizing current?
Harrison's 20th Ed. Chapter 239 Page 1723 Figure 239-2

A. I_K
B. I_{K1}
C. I_{KACh}
D. All of the above

368. Which of the following is the location of SA node?
Harrison's 20th Ed. Chapter 239 Page 1723

A. Coronal sulcus
B. Superior sulcus
C. Sulcus terminalis
D. Sulcus fusiform

SA node is composed of a cluster of small fusiform cells in sulcus terminalis on the epicardial surface of heart at the right atrial - superior vena caval junction, where they envelop the SA nodal artery.

369. Which of the following is not a feature of SA nodal cells?
Harrison's 20th Ed. Chapter 239 Page 1723

A. Fewer myofibrils
B. No intercalated disks
C. Well developed sarcoplasmic reticulum
D. No T-tubules

SA nodal cells have fewer distinct myofibrils than surrounding atrial myocardium, no intercalated disks, poorly developed sarcoplasmic reticulum, and no T-tubules. There is a relative absence of inward rectifier potassium current (I_{K1}) and absence of available fast sodium current (I_{Na}).

370. Intrinsic discharge rate is highest of which of the following potential cardiac pacemakers?
Harrison's 20th Ed. Chapter 239 Page 1723

A. Sinus node
B. Specialized fibers of His-Purkinje system
C. Some specialized atrial fibers
D. None of the above

SA node is normally the dominant cardiac pacemaker because its intrinsic discharge rate is the highest of all potential cardiac pacemakers.

371. In majority, SA nodal artery arises from?
Harrison's 20th Ed. Chapter 239 Page 1723

A. Right coronary artery
B. Left anterior descending artery
C. Left circumflex artery
D. Posterior descending artery

SA nodal artery arises from RCA in 55 - 60% and left circumflex artery in 40 - 45% of persons.

372. Membrane potential of SA nodal cells is?
Harrison's 20th Ed. Chapter 239 Page 1723

A. –20 to –40 mV
B. –40 to –60 mV
C. –60 to –80 mV
D. –80 to –100 mV

The action potentials of SA nodal cells are characterized by a relatively depolarized membrane potential of –40 to –60 mV, slow phase 0 upstroke, and relatively rapid phase 4 diastolic depolarization compared to the action potentials recorded in cardiac muscle cells.

373. In SA node, which of the following is modulated by β-adrenergic stimulation?
Harrison's 20th Ed. Chapter 239 Page 1723

A. $I_{Ca\text{-}L}$
B. $I_{Ca\text{-}T}$
C. I_f
D. All of the above

374. In SA node, which of the following is modulated by vagal stimulation?
Harrison's 20th Ed. Chapter 239 Page 1723

A. $I_{Ca\text{-}L}$
B. I_{Na}
C. I_{K1}
D. I_{KAch}

$I_{Ca\text{-}L}$, $I_{Ca\text{-}T}$, and If are modulated by β-adrenergic stimulation and I_{KACh} by vagal stimulation.

375. Cushing's response is best related to?
Harrison's 20th Ed. Chapter 239 Page 1724

A. Visual blurring
B. Accelerated hypertension
C. Increased intracranial pressure
D. Dermopathy

Increased intracranial pressure producing SA nodal dysfunction is called Cushing's response.

376. Which of the following is a cause of extrinsic SA node dysfunction?
Harrison's 20th Ed. Chapter 239 Page 1724

A. Sleep apnea
B. Increased intracranial pressure
C. Hypothyroidism
D. All of the above

Most common causes of extrinsic SA node dysfunction are drugs & autonomic nervous system influences.

377. Which of the following is associated with SA nodal disease?
Harrison's 20th Ed. Chapter 239 Page 1724

A. Pericarditis
B. Myocarditis
C. Rheumatic heart disease
D. All of the above

378. Which of the following is associated with SA nodal disease?
Harrison's 20th Ed. Chapter 239 Page 1724

A. Systemic lupus erythematosus (SLE)
B. Rheumatoid arthritis (RA)
C. Mixed connective tissue disorders (MCTDs)
D. All of the above

379. Acute myocardial infarction in which location is associated with transient SA nodal dysfunction?
Harrison's 20th Ed. Chapter 239 Page 1724-5

A. Anterior
B. Inferior
C. Lateral
D. All of the above

Sinus bradycardia is common in patients with acute inferior or posterior MI and can be exacerbated by vagal activation induced by pain or the use of morphine. Ischemia of the SA nodal artery occurs in acute coronary syndromes due to involvement with right coronary artery, and even with infarction, the effect on SA node function is transient.

380. Senile amyloidosis causing intrinsic sinus node dysfunction typically presents in which decade of life?
Harrison's 20th Ed. Chapter 239 Page 1724

A. 6th
B. 7th
C. 8th
D. 9th

Senile amyloidosis is an infiltrative disorder and causes Intrinsic sinus node dysfunction in patients typically in the ninth decade of life.

381. Tachycardia-bradycardia variant of sick-sinus syndrome is referred to as?
Harrison's 20th Ed. Chapter 239 Page 1724

A. SSS1
B. SSS2
C. SSS3
D. SSS4

Autosomal dominant sinus node dysfunction in conjunction with supraventricular tachycardia - tachycardia-bradycardia variant of sick-sinus syndrome is referred to as SSS2.

382. Tachycardia-bradycardia variant of sick-sinus syndrome is related to which of the following gene?
Harrison's 20th Ed. Chapter 239 Page 1724

A. SCN5A
B. HCN4
C. MYH6
D. APC

Tachycardia-bradycardia variant of sick-sinus syndrome has been linked to mutations in the pacemaker current (I_f) subunit gene HCN4 on chromosome 15.

383. Autosomal recessive form of SSS1 is related to which of the following gene?
Harrison's 20th Ed. Chapter 239 Page 1724

A. SCN5A
B. HCN4
C. MYH6
D. APC

An autosomal recessive form of SSS1 with prominent feature of atrial inexcitability and absence of P waves on the electrocardiogram (ECG) is caused by mutations in the cardiac sodium channel gene, SCN5A, on chromosome 3.

384. Which of the following neuromuscular disease produce SA node disease?
Harrison's 20th Ed. Chapter 239 Page 1724

A. Myasthenia gravis
B. Botulism
C. Lambert-Eaton syndrome
D. Kearns-Sayre syndrome

Neuromuscular diseases like Kearns-Sayre syndrome (ophthalmoplegia, pigmentary degeneration of retina & cardiomyopathy) & myotonic dystrophy produce conducting system & SA node disease.

385. Patients with the tachycardia-bradycardia variant of SSS are at risk for?
Harrison's 20th Ed. Chapter 239 Page 1724

A. Ventricular fibrillation
B. Thromboembolism
C. Myocardial infarction
D. All of the above

Patients with tachycardia-bradycardia variant of SSS, similar to patients with atrial fibrillation, are at risk for thromboembolism. In such patients, overall longevity is not compromised in absence of other significant comorbid conditions.

386. Sinus rate of how much in awake state & in absence of physical conditioning generally is considered abnormal?

Harrison's 20th Ed. Chapter 239 Page 1724

A. < 40 beats / minute
B. < 50 beats / minute
C. < 60 beats / minute
D. < 70 beats / minute

A sinus rate of <40 beats/minute in awake state in the absence of physical conditioning generally is considered abnormal.

387. Which of the following statements is false?

Harrison's 20th Ed. Chapter 239 Page 1724

A. Sinus pause result from failure of SA node to discharge
B. Sinus arrest result from failure of SA node to discharge
C. Sinus pauses of up to 3 seconds are common in awake athletes
D. None of the above

388. Sinus bradycardia is associated with all except?

Harrison's 20th Ed. Chapter 239 Page 1724

A. Hypothyroidism
B. Advanced liver disease
C. Trypnosomiasis
D. Brucellosis

389. Sinus bradycardia is associated with all except?

Harrison's 20th Ed. Chapter 239 Page 1724

A. Typhoid fever
B. Acute hypertension
C. Hypercapnia
D. Alkalosis

390. Sinus arrest means?

Harrison's 20th Ed. Chapter 239 Page 1724

A. Failure of sinus impulse formation
B. Block of conduction of sinus impulses to atrial tissue
C. Block of conduction of sinus impulses at AV node
D. Block of conduction of sinus impulses beyond AV node

391. Sinus exit block means?

Harrison's 20th Ed. Chapter 239 Page 1724

A. Failure of sinus impulse formation
B. Failure of conduction of sinus impulses to surrounding atrial tissue
C. Failure of conduction of sinus impulses at AV node
D. Failure of conduction of sinus impulses beyond AV node

Sinus pauses & sinus arrest result from failure of SA node to discharge, causing a pause without P waves visible on ECG. Intermittent failure of conduction from SA node produces sinus exit block.

392. Electrocardiographic manifestations of SA node dysfunction include?

Harrison's 20th Ed. Chapter 239 Page 1724

A. Sinus pauses
B. Sinus exit block
C. Alternating supraventricular tachycardia & bradycardia
D. All of the above

Electrocardiographic manifestations of SA node dysfunction include sinus bradycardia, sinus pauses, sinus arrest, sinus exit block, tachycardia (in SSS), and chronotropic incompetence.

393. Which of the following is false about tachycardia-bradycardia variant of SSS?

Harrison's 20th Ed. Chapter 239 Page 1724

A. Are at risk for thromboembolism
B. May have concurrent AV conduction disease
C. Symptoms may be related to slow & fast heart rates
D. SA node dysfunction is associated with increased mortality

SA node dysfunction is not associated with increased mortality rates.

394. Intermittent absence of P waves on ECG is due to?

Harrison's 20th Ed. Chapter 239 Page 1724

A. Second-degree SA block
B. Sinus exit block
C. Sinus arrest
D. Sick sinus syndrome

395. A prolongation of conduction time from SA node to surrounding atrial tissue is called?

Harrison's 20th Ed. Chapter 239 Page 1724

A. First-degree sinoatrial exit block
B. Second-degree sinoatrial exit block
C. Third-degree sinoatrial exit block
D. None of the above

396. The intermittent failure of conduction of sinus impulses to the surrounding atrial tissue is called?

Harrison's 20th Ed. Chapter 239 Page 1724

A. First-degree sinoatrial exit block
B. Second-degree sinoatrial exit block
C. Third-degree sinoatrial exit block
D. None of the above

397. Lack of atrial activity or the presence of an ectopic subsidiary atrial pacemaker is called?

Harrison's 20th Ed. Chapter 239 Page 1724

A. First-degree sinoatrial exit block
B. Second-degree sinoatrial exit block
C. Third-degree sinoatrial exit block
D. None of the above

Type I second-degree SA block results from progressive prolongation of SA node conduction with intermittent failure of the impulses originating in the sinus node to conduct to the surrounding atrial tissue. Second-degree SA block appears on the ECG as an intermittent absence of P waves. In type II second-degree SA block, there is no change in SA node conduction before the pause. Complete or third-degree SA block results in no P waves on the ECG.

398. Sick sinus syndrome refers to a combination of all except?

Harrison's 20th Ed. Chapter 239 Page 1724

A. Sinus bradycardia
B. Sinoatrial block
C. Sinus arrest
D. Sinus arrhythmia

ECG manifestations of SA node dysfunction include sinus bradycardia, sinus pauses, sinus arrest, sinus exit block, tachycardia (in SSS), and chronotropic incompetence (inability to increase heart rate in response to exercise or other stress appropriately).

399. In sinus arrest and in sinus exit block, atrial asystole is of what duration?

Harrison's 20th Ed. Chapter 239 Page 1724

A. > 1 seconds
B. > 1.5 seconds
C. > 2.5 seconds
D. > 3 seconds

Sinus pauses of up to 3 seconds are common in the awake athlete, & pauses of this duration or longer may be observed in asymptomatic elderly subjects.

400. In Tachycardia-bradycardia syndrome, which of the following is the most common tachycardia?

Harrison's 20th Ed. Chapter 239 Page 1724

A. Atrial tachycardia
B. Atrial flutter
C. Atrial fibrillation
D. Any of the above

Tachycardia-bradycardia syndrome manifests as alternating sinus bradycardia & atrial tachyarrhythmias. Although atrial tachycardia, atrial flutter, and atrial fibrillation may be observed, the latter is the most common tachycardia.

401. Which of the following is false about Mobitz type I SA nodal exit block?

Harrison's 20th Ed. Chapter 239 Page 1725 Figure 239-4

A. Regularly irregular heart rhythm
B. Decreasing P-P intervals before the pause
C. Pause less than twice the cycle length of last sinus interval
D. None of the above

In Mobitz type I SA nodal exit block, there is grouped beating producing a regularly irregular heart rhythm. SA node rate is constant with progressive delay in exit from the node and activation of atria. This produces subtly decreasing P-P intervals before the pause, and the pause is less than twice the cycle length of the last sinus interval.

402. Chronotropic incompetence is failure to reach what percentage of predicted maximal heart rate at peak exercise?

Harrison's 20th Ed. Chapter 239 Page 1725

A. 55%
B. 65%
C. 75%
D. 85%

Exercise testing is useful in discriminating chronotropic incompetence from resting bradycardia. Failure to increase the heart rate with exercise is called chronotropic incompetence. Alternatively defined as a failure to reach 85% of predicted maximal heart rate at peak exercise or failure to achieve a heart rate >100 beats/minute with exercise or a maximal heart rate with exercise less than two standard deviations below that of an age-matched control population.

403. Normal values of intrinsic heart rate are calculated by the formula?

Harrison's 20th Ed. Chapter 239 Page 1725

A. 116.2 – (0.53 × age) beats per minute
B. 117.2 – (0.53 × age) beats per minute
C. 118.2 – (0.53 × age) beats per minute
D. 119.2 – (0.53 × age) beats per minute

Determining the intrinsic heart rate (IHR) may distinguish SA node dysfunction from slow heart rates resulting from high vagal tone. Normal IHR after administration of 0.2 mg/kg propranolol & 0.04 mg/kg atropine is 117.2 – (0.53 x age) in beats/minute. Low IHR is indicative of SA disease.

404. Which of the following conditions do not require electrophysiologic tests for diagnosis in 'symptomatic' patients with ECG documentation of?

Harrison's 20th Ed. Chapter 239 Page 1725

A. Asystole
B. Sinoatrial block or arrest
C. Bradycardia-tachycardia syndrome
D. All of the above

Symptomatic patients with ECG documentation of asystole, sinoatrial block or arrest, or the bradycardia-tachycardia syndrome do not require electrophysiologic tests for diagnosis.

405. Which of the following is a sensitive and specific indicator of intrinsic SA node disease?

Harrison's 20th Ed. Chapter 239 Page 1725

A. Sinus node recovery time (SNRT)
B. Sinoatrial conduction time (SACT)
C. Intrinsic heart rate (IHR)
D. All of the above

Sinus node recovery time (SNRT) is defined as the longest pause after cessation of overdrive pacing of right atrium near SA node (normal <1500 msec. or, corrected for sinus cycle length, <550 msec.). Sinoatrial conduction time (SACT) is defined as one-half the difference between intrinsic sinus cycle length and a noncompensatory pause after a premature atrial stimulus (normal <125 msec.). Combination of an abnormal SNRT, an abnormal SACT, and a low IHR is a sensitive and specific indicator of intrinsic SA node disease.

406. In susceptible individual, SA node dysfunction may become manifest in the presence of which of the following?

Harrison's 20th Ed. Chapter 239 Page 1725

A. Cardiac glycosides
B. Amiodarone
C. Calcium channel blockers
D. All of the above

Cardiac glycosides, beta-blockers, calcium channel blockers, amiodarone may unmask evidence of sinus node dysfunction in susceptible individuals.

407. Which of the following pharmacologic agents may improve SA node function?

Harrison's 20th Ed. Chapter 239 Page 1725

A. Class I Antiarrhythmics
B. Class III Antiarrhythmics
C. Calcium channel blockers
D. Digitalis

Beta blockers and calcium channel blockers increase SNRT in patients with SA node dysfunction, and antiarrhythmic drugs with class I and III action may promote SA node exit block. Digitalis shortens SNRT in SA node dysfunction. Isoproterenol or atropine administered IV may increase sinus rate acutely. Theophylline increases heart rate.

408. How many letter codes are used for describing pacemaker modes & function?

Harrison's 20th Ed. Chapter 239 Page 1725

A. 3
B. 4
C. 5
D. 6

Pacemaker modes & function are named using a five-letter code.

409. The first letter in the pacing code indicates?

Harrison's 20th Ed. Chapter 239 Page 1725

A. Chamber(s) paced
B. Chamber in which electrical activity is sensed
C. The response to a sensed electric signal
D. Programmability and rate modulation

410. The second letter in the pacing code indicates?

Harrison's 20th Ed. Chapter 239 Page 1725

A. Chamber(s) paced
B. Chamber in which electrical activity is sensed
C. The response to a sensed electric signal
D. Programmability and rate modulation

411. The third letter in the pacing code indicates?

Harrison's 20th Ed. Chapter 239 Page 1725

A. Chamber(s) paced
B. Chamber in which electrical activity is sensed
C. The response to a sensed electric signal
D. Programmability and rate modulation

412. The fourth letter in the pacing code indicates?

Harrison's 20th Ed. Chapter 239 Page 1725

A. Chamber(s) paced
B. Chamber in which electrical activity is sensed
C. The response to a sensed electric signal
D. Programmability and rate modulation

In pacing code, the first letter indicates the chamber(s) that is paced (O, none; A, atrium; V, ventricle; D, dual; S, single), the second letter indicates the chamber(s) in which sensing occurs (O, none; A, atrium; V, ventricle; D, dual; S, single), the third letter indicates the response to a sensed event (O, none; I, inhibition; T, triggered; D, inhibition + triggered), the fourth letter refers to the programmability or rate response (R, rate responsive), and the fifth refers to the existence of antitachycardia functions if present (O, none; P, antitachycardia pacing; S, shock; D, pace + shock).

413. Twiddler's syndrome best relates to?

Harrison's 20th Ed. Chapter 239 Page 1726

A. Failing battery of pacemaker
B. Interference by external stimuli on pacemaker
C. Rotation of pacemaker pulse generator in its pocket
D. All of the above

Rotation of the pacemaker pulse generator in its subcutaneous pocket, either intentionally or inadvertently, often referred to as "twiddler's syndrome" producing dislodgment with failure to sense or pace the heart.

414. Pacemaker syndrome is associated in those?

Harrison's 20th Ed. Chapter 239 Page 1726

A. Who do not maintain AV synchrony
B. Who do not have adequate cardiac output
C. Who have chronic illnesses (HTN, DM)
D. All of the above

Pacemaker syndrome is a constellation of signs and symptoms associated with any mode of pacing that does not maintain or restore AV synchrony.

415. Pacemaker syndrome includes which of the following?

Harrison's 20th Ed. Chapter 239 Page 1726

A. Cough
B. Confusion
C. Third heart sound
D. All of the above

Pacemaker syndrome includes neck pulsation, fatigue, palpitations, cough, confusion, exertional dyspnea, dizziness, syncope, elevation in jugular venous pressure, canon A waves, and stigmata of congestive heart failure, including edema, rales, and a third heart sound.

416. Class I indication for pacing in SA node dysfunction include all except?

Harrison's 20th Ed. Chapter 239 Page 1726

A. Documented symptomatic bradycardia
B. Syncope of unexplained origin with major abnormalities of SA node dysfunction
C. Sinus node dysfunction associated long-term drug therapy for which there is no alternative
D. Symptomatic chronotropic incompetence

Class I indications for pacing in SA node dysfunction include documented symptomatic bradycardia, sinus node dysfunction associated long-term drug therapy for which there is no alternative, or symptomatic chronotropic incompetence.

The Bradyarrhythmias : Disorders of the Atrioventricular Node

417. Phase 0 depolarization in cells in AV node is mediated by?
Harrison's 20th Ed. Chapter 240 Page 1727

A. Sodium
B. Potassium
C. Calcium
D. All of the above

Cells in AV node have slower phase 0 depolarization, mediated by calcium influx in nodal tissue rather than mediated by sodium influx as seen in ventricular tissue.

418. Transient AV conduction block is common in?
Harrison's 20th Ed. Chapter 240 Page 1727

A. Infants
B. Young
C. Middle age
D. Elderly

Transient AV conduction block is common in the young and is most likely the result of high vagal tone found in ~10% of young adults.

419. AV conduction axis consists of?
Harrison's 20th Ed. Chapter 240 Page 1727

A. Atria
B. Ventricles
C. AV node
D. All of the above

AV conduction axis involves the atria and ventricles as well as the AV node.

420. Which of the following about AV node is false?
Harrison's 20th Ed. Chapter 240 Page 1727

A. Subendocardial structure
B. Located in the posterior-inferior right atrium
C. Measure ~1 × 3 × 5 mm
D. None of the above

421. The AV node lies at the?
Harrison's 20th Ed. Chapter 240 Page 1727

A. Base of interatrial septum just above tricuspid annulus and anterior to coronary sinus
B. Base of interatrial septum just below tricuspid annulus and anterior to coronary sinus
C. Base of interatrial septum just above tricuspid annulus and posterior to coronary sinus
D. Base of the interventricular septum just above tricuspid annulus and anterior to coronary sinus

422. Which of the following statements is false?
Harrison's 20th Ed. Chapter 240 Page 1727

A. Compact AV node continues as the penetrating AV bundle
B. Superior, medial, & posterior transitional atrionodal bundles converge on the compact AV node
C. Located at the apex of triangle of Koch
D. None of the above

423. Intra-atrial conduction system of the heart consists of?
Cardiology Journal 2011;18 (3):337

A. Anterior interatrial band or Bachmann's bundle
B. Middle internodal tract or Wenckebach's bundle
C. Posterior internodal tract of Thorel
D. All of the above

424. Boundaries of triangle of Koch include all except?
Harrison's 20th Ed. Chapter 240 Page 1727

A. Coronary sinus ostium
B. Septal tricuspid valve annulus
C. Septal mitral valve annulus
D. Tendon of Todaro

Triangle of Koch is bordered by coronary sinus ostium posteriorly, septal tricuspid valve annulus anteriorly & tendon of Todaro superiorly.

425. The penetrating AV bundle is in close proximity to?
Harrison's 20th Ed. Chapter 240 Page 1727

A. Aortic valve annuli
B. Mitral valve annuli
C. Tricuspid valve annuli
D. All of the above

426. First septal perforator of left anterior descending coronary artery supplies?
Harrison's 20th Ed. Chapter 240 Page 1727

A. Penetrating AV bundle
B. Left bundle branch
C. Right bundle branch
D. All of the above

Bundle branches also have a dual blood supply from the septal perforators of left anterior descending coronary artery & branches of posterior descending coronary artery.

427. In decremental conduction, with increasingly rapid rates of stimulation, the conduction?
Harrison's 20th Ed. Chapter 240 Page 1727

A. Slows
B. Becomes faster
C. No change
D. Any of the above

Atrionodal transitional connections exhibit decremental conduction, defined as slowing of conduction with increasingly rapid rates of stimulation.

428. Myocytes that constitute the compact node have a resting membrane potential of about?
Harrison's 20th Ed. Chapter 240 Page 1727

A. - 50 mV
B. - 60 mV
C. - 70 mV
D. - 80 mV

Myocytes that constitute the compact node are depolarized with a resting membrane potential of about –60 mV. Action potentials have low amplitudes, slow upstrokes of phase 0 (<10 V/s), and phase 4 diastolic depolarization, high-input resistance and relative insensitivity to external [K⁺].

429. AV nodal cells lack which of the following?
Harrison's 20th Ed. Chapter 240 Page 1727

A. I_{Na}
B. $I_{Ca\text{-}L}$
C. $I_{Ca\text{-}T}$
D. I_f

AV nodal cells lack I_{K1} and INa. $I_{Ca\text{-}L}$ is responsible for phase 0. Phase 4 depolarization reflects the composite activity of the depolarizing currents If, $I_{Ca\text{-}L}$, $I_{Ca\text{-}T}$, and INCX and the repolarizing currents IKr and IKAch.

430. Which of the following connexin is present in gap junction channels between cells in the AV node?
Harrison's 20th Ed. Chapter 240 Page 1727

A. Connexin-23
B. Connexin-32
C. Connexin-40
D. Connexin-43

431. Which of the following about His bundle & bundle branches is false?
Harrison's 20th Ed. Chapter 240 Page 1727

A. Minimally influenced by autonomic tone
B. Have most rapid conduction in heart
C. Insulated from ventricular myocardium
D. None of the above

432. Which of the following about His bundle & bundle branches is false?
Harrison's 20th Ed. Chapter 240 Page 1727

A. Very rapid upstrokes (phase 0)
B. Prolonged plateaus (phase 2)
C. Modest automaticity (phase 4 depolarization)
D. None of the above

433. Normal AV node in vivo possesses?
Harrison's 19th Ed. 1470

A. Automaticity always
B. Automaticity sometimes
C. No automaticity
D. None of the above

434. Which of the following is associated with SA node slowing and AV conduction block?
Harrison's 20th Ed. Chapter 240 Page 1728

A. Carotid sinus hypersensitivity
B. Cough
C. Micturition syncope
D. All of the above

Heightened vagal tone during sleep or in well-conditioned individuals can lead to all grades of AV block. Carotid sinus hypersensitivity, vasovagal syncope, and cough and micturition syncope may be associated with SA node slowing and AV conduction block.

435. Conditions that can produce AV conduction block include?
Harrison's 20th Ed. Chapter 240 Page 1728 Table 240-1

A. Hypothyroidism
B. Hypermagnesemia
C. Adrenal insufficiency
D. All of the above

436. Drugs that can produce atrioventricular block include?
Harrison's 20th Ed. Chapter 240 Page 1728 Table 240-1

A. Lithium
B. Adenosine
C. Antiarrhythmics (class I and III)
D. All of the above

437. Conditions that can produce AV conduction block include?
Harrison's 20th Ed. Chapter 240 Page 1728 Table 240-1

A. Tuberculosis
B. Lyme disease
C. Diphtheria
D. All of the above

438. Conditions that can produce AV conduction block include?
Harrison's 20th Ed. Chapter 240 Page 1728 Table 240-1

A. Chagas disease
B. Toxoplasmosis
C. Syphilis
D. All of the above

439. Conditions that can produce AV conduction block include?
Harrison's 20th Ed. Chapter 240 Page 1728 Table 240-1

A. Sarcoidosis
B. Systemic lupus erythematosus
C. Rheumatoid arthritis
D. All of the above

Infectious diseases that lead to conducting system disturbances include Lyme disease, Chagas' disease, and syphilis. Autoimmune and infiltrative diseases like SLE, RA, MCTD, scleroderma, amyloidosis (primary & secondary), sarcoidosis, and hemochromatosis may produce AV conduction block

440. AV conduction block has been associated with which of the following?
Harrison's 20th Ed. Chapter 240 Page 1728 Table 240-1

A. Kearns-Sayre syndrome
B. Myotonic dystrophy
C. Facioscapulohumeral muscular dystrophy
D. All of the above

441. Mutation in which of the following gene causes accelerated forms of progressive familial heart block?
Harrison's 20th Ed. Chapter 240 Page 1728

A. KCNQ1
B. KCNH2 (HERG)
C. SCN5A
D. ANK2

Accelerated forms of progressive familial heart block have been identified in families with mutations in cardiac sodium channel gene (SCN5A).

442. Congenital AV block may be seen in which of the following?

Harrison's 20th Ed. Chapter 240 Page 1728

A. Transposition of the great arteries
B. Ostium primum atrial septal defect
C. Ventricular septal defect
D. All of the above

Congenital AV block may be observed in complex congenital cardiac anomalies such as transposition of the great arteries, ostium primum atrial septal defects (ASDs), ventricular septal defects (VSDs), endocardial cushion defects and some single-ventricle defects.

443. Congenital AV block in a structurally normal heart is seen in children born to mothers with?

Harrison's 20th Ed. Chapter 240 Page 1728

A. SLE
B. Sarcoidosis
C. Rheumatoid arthritis
D. Hemochromatosis

Congenital AV block in a structurally normal heart is seen in children born to mothers with SLE.

444. In acute MI, AV block transiently develops in what percentage of patients?

Harrison's 20th Ed. Chapter 240 Page 1728

A. 5 - 10%
B. 10 - 25%
C. 20 - 35%
D. 30 - 45%

In acute MI, AV block transiently develops in 10 - 25% of patients.

445. Level of AV block in inferior MI tends to be in?

Harrison's 20th Ed. Chapter 240 Page 1728

A. AV node
B. Distal AV nodal complex
C. His bundle
D. Bundle branches

Level of AV block in inferior MI tends to be in AV node with more stable, narrow escape rhythms. Acute anterior MI is associated with block in distal AV nodal complex, His bundle or bundle branches & results in wide complex, unstable escape rhythms & a worse prognosis with high mortality rates.

446. First-degree AV block is determined by?

Harrison's 20th Ed. Chapter 240 Page 1728

A. Atrial activation
B. AV nodal activation
C. His-Purkinje activation
D. All of the above

I° AV block (PR interval > 200 ms) is a slowing of conduction through AV "junction". The site of delay is typically in AV node but may be in atria, AV node bundle of His, or His-Purkinje system.

447. I° AV block with wide QRS suggests delay in?

Harrison's 20th Ed. Chapter 240 Page 1728

A. Proximal AV node
B. Mid AV node
C. Distal AV node
D. Distal conduction system

I° AV block with wide QRS is suggestive of delay in the distal conduction system, whereas a narrow QRS suggests delay in the AV node proper or, less commonly, in the bundle of His.

448. Nationality of Woldemar Mobitz was?

Circulation. 2004;110:1162-1167

A. Russian German
B. British American
C. Spanish
D. Anglo Indian

Woldemar Mobitz (1889-1951) was a Russian-German physician.

449. Mobitz Type I is also named after?

Circulation. 2004;110:1162-1167

A. Karel Frederik Wenckebach
B. John Hay
C. Robert Silverman
D. Jack Upshaw

450. Mobitz Type II is also named after?

Circulation. 2004;110:1162-1167

A. Karel Frederik Wenckebach
B. John Hay
C. Robert Silverman
D. Jack Upshaw

451. In presence of a normal duration QRS complex, delay within AV node is the cause of prolonged PR interval if it is?

Harrison's 20th Ed. Chapter 240 Page 1728

A. > 0.21 second
B. > 0.22 second
C. > 0.23 second
D. > 0.24 second

452. When some atrial impulses fail to conduct to ventricles, the type of AV block is?

Harrison's 20th Ed. Chapter 240 Page 1728

A. First-degree heart block
B. Second-degree heart block
C. Third-degree heart block
D. Sick sinus syndrome

In II° AV block there is an intermittent failure of electrical impulse conduction from atrium to ventricle.

453. Which of the following statements about Mobitz type I, second degree AV block is false?

Harrison's 20th Ed. Chapter 240 Page 1728

A. Also called AV Wenckebach block
B. Progressive PR prolongation prior to block of an atrial impulse
C. Pause that follows is fully compensatory
D. PR interval of first conducted impulse is shorter than last conducted atrial impulse prior to blocked P wave

In Mobitz type 1 II° AV block, periodic failure of conduction occurs characterized by a progressively lengthening PR interval, shortening of RR interval, & a pause that is < 2 times the immediately preceding RR interval. ECG complex after the pause exhibits a shorter PR interval that immediately preceding the pause.

454. Which of the following statements about Mobitz type I second degree AV block is false?
Harrison's 20th Ed. Chapter 240 Page 1728

A. Usually the difference between the longest & shortest PR intervals exceeds 100 mseconds
B. Block is almost always localized to AV node
C. Usually associated with a normal QRS duration
D. Amiodarone therapy is a frequent cause

455. Which of the following statements about Mobitz type I second degree AV block is false?
Harrison's 20th Ed. Chapter 240 Page 1728

A. Most often occurs transiently with inferior MI
B. Due to digitalis, β-blockers, and Ca^{++} channel blockers
C. Seen in normal individuals with heightened vagal tone
D. Leads to complete heart block

In Mobitz type 1 II° AV block, difference between the longest & shortest PR intervals exceeds 100 mseconds. It is almost always localized to AV node & associated with a normal QRS duration. It is seen most often as a transient abnormality with inferior wall infarction or with drug intoxication (digitalis, beta and calcium channel blockers) or in normal individuals with heightened vagal tone. Progression to complete heart block is uncommon, except in acute inferior wall myocardial infarction. Even when it does, this heart block is well tolerated because the escape pacemaker usually arises in the proximal His bundle & provides a stable rhythm & rarely requiring aggressive therapy.

456. Which of the following statements about Mobitz type II second degree AV block is false?
Harrison's 20th Ed. Chapter 240 Page 1728

A. Conduction fails suddenly and unexpectedly without a preceding change in PR intervals
B. Due to disease of His-Purkinje system and associated with prolonged QRS duration
C. When Mobitz type II block occurs with a normal QRS duration, an intra-AV node block should be expected
D. High incidence of progression to complete heart block with an unstable, slow, lower escape pacemaker

457. Which of the following statements about Mobitz type II second degree AV block is false?
Harrison's 20th Ed. Chapter 240 Page 1728

A. Occur in anteroseptal myocardial infarction
B. Occur in primary or secondary sclerodegenerative or calcific disorders of fibrous skeleton of heart
C. Block is usually in AV node
D. Block is usually in His-Purkinje system

458. Which of the following statements about Mobitz type II second degree AV block is false?
Harrison's 20th Ed. Chapter 240 Page 1728

A. Intermittent failure of conduction of the P wave without changes in the preceding PR intervals
B. Intermittent failure of conduction of the P wave without changes in the preceding RR intervals
C. Typically occurs in distal or infra-His conduction system
D. None of the above

Type 2 II° AV block is characterized by intermittent failure of conduction of the P wave without changes in the preceding PR or RR intervals. It typically occurs in distal or infra-His conduction system, is often associated with intraventricular conduction delays (bundle branch block), and is more likely to proceed to higher grades of AV block.

459. It may be difficult to distinguish between type I from type II block when AV block is?
Harrison's 20th Ed. Chapter 240 Page 1728

A. 2 : 1
B. 3 : 1
C. 4 : 1
D. 5 : 1

When AV block is 2:1, it may be difficult to distinguish type I from type II block. The finding of a His bundle electrogram after every atrial electrogram indicates that block is occurring in the distal conduction system. Must obtain a long rhythm strip or use atropine to induce 3:2 block.

460. Which of the following about Type II second-degree AV block is false?
Harrison's 20th Ed. Chapter 240 Page 1728

A. Occurs in distal or infra-His conduction system
B. Associated with intraventricular conduction delays
C. May proceed to higher grades of AV block
D. None of the above

Type II second-degree AV block typically occurs in distal or infra-His conduction system and is often associated with intraventricular conduction delays (bundle branch block). It is more likely to proceed to higher grades of AV block than is type I second-degree AV block.

461. "Paroxysmal AV block" best relates to?
Harrison's 20th Ed. Chapter 240 Page 1729

A. Self correcting AV block
B. Series of nonconducted P waves
C. P waves buried in QRS complex
D. P waves following QRS complex

Second-degree AV block (particularly type II) may be associated with a series of nonconducted P waves, referred to as paroxysmal AV block. It implies significant conduction system disease and is an indication for permanent pacing.

462. AV block that is intermediate between second degree & third degree is referred to as?
Harrison's 20th Ed. Chapter 240 Page 1729

A. High-grade AV block
B. Pre third degree AV block
C. Post second degree AV block
D. Paroxysmal AV block

AV block that is intermediate between second degree & third degree is referred to as high-grade AV block and like CHB implies advanced AV conduction system disease.

463. Which of the following about Third-degree AV block is false?
Harrison's 20th Ed. Chapter 240 Page 1729

A. No atrial impulse propagates to ventricles
B. Congenital complete AV block is localized to AV node
C. In AV nodal block, QRS duration is prolonged
D. In His bundle block, QRS duration is prolonged

Complete failure of conduction from atrium to ventricle is called complete or third-degree AV block. It is most often distal to the AV node. A wide QRS escape rhythm implies block in the distal His or bundle branches, while a narrow QRS rhythm implies block in the AV node or proximal His and an escape rhythm originating in the AV junction.

464. Which of the following argue that the site of block is in the AV node?
Harrison's 20th Ed. Chapter 240 Page 1729

A. Mobitz I
B. Junctional escape (narrow QRS), faster rate
C. HR responds to atropine/exercise, vagal
D. All of the above

AH becomes progressively long if blockage is in the AV node.

465. Which of the following argue that the site of block is in the bundle branch / fascicle?

Harrison's 20th Ed. Chapter 240 Page 1729

A. Concomitant BBB
B. Slower escape rhythm with wide QRS
C. No response to Atropine
D. All of the above

466. Which of the following about Lev's disease is false?

Ann Intern Med. 1983;98(3):414

A. Calcification & sclerosis of fibrous cardiac skeleton
B. Frequently involves pulmonary & tricuspid valves
C. Involves central fibrous body & summit of ventricular septum
D. Produces AV block

Lev's disease occurs in older people with progressive fibrosis of the left side of cardiac skeleton. It also involves the mitral and aortic rings.

467. Which of the following about Lenegre's disease is false?

Ann Intern Med. 1983;98(3):414

A. Primary sclerodegenerative disease in conducting system
B. No involvement of myocardium
C. Involves fibrous skeleton of heart
D. Cause of isolated chronic heart block in adults

Lenegre's disease, caused by SCN5A gene mutation, is a progressive sclerosis of the cardiac conduction system in young patients.

468. Which of the following improve conduction through AV node & impair infranodal conduction?

Harrison's 20th Ed. Chapter 240 Page 1729

A. Atropine
B. Isoproterenol
C. Exercise
D. All of the above

Atropine, isoproterenol & exercise improve conduction through AV node & impair infranodal conduction.

469. Which of the following is false?

Harrison's 20th Ed. Chapter 240 Page 1729

A. First-degree AV block is intranodal
B. Mobitz type 1 second-degree AV block is intranodal
C. Mobitz type 2 second-degree block is infranodal
D. None of the above

470. To obtain a recording from the bundle of His, the electrode catheter is positioned?

Harrison's 20th Ed. Chapter 240 Page 1729

A. Across the pulmonary valve
B. Superior margin of the tricuspid valve
C. In coronary sinus
D. In superior vena cava

Recording of His bundle electrogram by a catheter positioned at superior margin of tricuspid valve annulus provides information about conduction at all levels of AV conduction axis.

471. Normal AH interval in the His bundle recording is?

Harrison's 20th Ed. Chapter 240 Page 1729

A. 10 to 50 ms
B. 60 to 130 ms
C. 130 to 180 ms
D. 180 to 250 ms

472. AH interval in the His bundle recording represents an indirect method of assessing?

Harrison's 20th Ed. Chapter 240 Page 1729

A. AV nodal conduction time
B. Atrial conduction time
C. Sinus node activation time
D. None of the above

Time from the most rapid deflection of the atrial electrogram in the His bundle recording to the His electrogram (AH interval) represents conduction through the AV node and is normally <130 ms.

473. HV interval in the His bundle recording represents conduction time through?

Harrison's 20th Ed. Chapter 240 Page 1729

A. AV node
B. His bundle
C. His-Purkinje system
D. Endocardium to epicardium

474. Normal HV interval in the His bundle recording is?

Harrison's 20th Ed. Chapter 240 Page 1730

A. 10 to 20 ms
B. 15 to 35 ms
C. 35 to 55 ms
D. 60 to 75 ms

The time from the His electrogram to the earliest onset of the QRS on the surface ECG (HV interval) represents the conduction time through the His-Purkinje system and is normally ≤55 ms.

475. Normal PA interval in the His bundle recording is?

Harrison's 19th Ed. 1474

A. 30 ms
B. 40 ms
C. 50 ms
D. 60 ms

PA interval is the time from the earliest onset of P wave on surface ECG to onset of atrial deflection on His bundle catheter. It is an index of intra-atrial conduction time & should be 50 ms.

476. Pacemaker implantation should be performed in any patient with?

Harrison's 20th Ed. Chapter 240 Page 1731

A. Symptomatic bradycardia
B. Irreversible second degree AV block
C. Irreversible third degree AV block
D. All of the above

Pacemaker implantation should be performed in any patient with symptomatic bradycardia and irreversible second- or third-degree AV block, regardless of the cause or level of block in the conducting system.

477. Anisotropic conduction means impulse propagation is more rapid?

Harrison's 19th Ed. 1474

A. Parallel to fiber orientation than transverse to it
B. Transverse to fiber orientation than parallel to it
C. In a particular fiber type
D. In a particular fiber length

Impulse propagation is more rapid parallel to fiber orientation than transverse to it. This property is termed anisotropic conduction.

478. "Effective" refractory period is defined as that portion of action potential during which?

Harrison's 19th Ed. 1474

A. No stimulus can evoke another response
B. Stimulus can evoke a local, nonpropagated response
C. Stronger stimulus is required to evoke a response
D. Weaker stimulus can evoke a response

Effective refractory period is that part of the action potential during which a stimulus can evoke only a local, nonpropagated response.

479. To obtain a recording of left atrial activity, the electrode catheter is positioned?

Harrison's 19th Ed. 1474

A. Across the pulmonary valve
B. Across the tricuspid valve
C. In the coronary sinus
D. In the superior vena cava

Left atrial activity is recorded directly via a catheter placed across a patent foramen ovale or indirectly using a catheter inserted into the coronary sinus.

480. Escape pacemaker following AV nodal block is usually in?

A. His bundle
B. Bundle branches
C. Purkinje fibres
D. Ventricular myocardium

Escape pacemaker following AV nodal block is usually in the His bundle.

481. Which of the following statements about escape pacemaker in His bundle is false?

A. Has a rate of 40 to 60 beats per minute
B. Is associated with a QRS complex of normal duration
C. Is the escape pacemaker following AV nodal block
D. Is unstable

Escape pacemaker in His bundle is stable with discharge rate of 40 to 60 beats/minute, associated with a QRS complex of normal duration.

482. Which of the following statements about escape pacemaker in distal His-Purkinje system is false?

A. Has a rate of 25 to 45 beats per minute
B. Wide QRS complex of prolonged duration
C. Is the escape pacemaker following AV nodal block
D. Is unstable

Escape rhythms arising in the distal His-Purkinje system have lower intrinsic rates (25 to 45 beats/minute), manifest wide QRS complexes with prolonged duration and are unstable.

Approach to Supraventricular Tachyarrhythmias

483. Which of the following produces a wide QRS complex during supraventricular tachycardia?
Harrison's 20th Ed. Chapter 241 Page 1733

A. Conduction block in the left bundle branch
B. Conduction block in the right bundle branch
C. Activation of ventricles from an accessory pathway
D. All of the above

484. Which of the following is a pathologic supraventricular tachycardia?
Harrison's 20th Ed. Chapter 241 Page 1733

A. Reentrant arrhythmias dependent on AV nodal conduction
B. Large reentry circuits within atrial tissue alone
C. Focal atrial tachycardias due to automaticity or reentry circuits
D. All of the above

Mechanisms of pathologic supraventricular tachycardia can be reentrant arrhythmias dependent on AV nodal conduction (AV reentry), large reentry circuits within atrial tissue alone (atrial flutter) or focal atrial tachycardias due to automaticity or small reentry circuits.

485. Paroxysmal supraventricular tachycardia (PSVT) refers to?
Harrison's 20th Ed. Chapter 241 Page 1733

A. AV node reentry
B. AV reentry using an accessory pathway
C. Atrial tachycardia
D. All of the above

Paroxysmal supraventricular tachycardia (PSVT) refers to a family of tachycardias including AV node reentry, AV reentry using an accessory pathway and atrial tachycardia.

486. The most common supraventricular tachycardia is?
Harrison's 20th Ed. Chapter 241 Page 1733

A. Physiologic sinus tachycardia
B. Inappropriate sinus tachycardia
C. Focal atrial tachycardia (AT)
D. Atrial fibrillation

The most common supraventricular tachycardia is sinus tachycardia in response to physiologic stress, such as exercise, but it can also be a manifestation acute illness.

487. Which of the following is a tachycardia not originating from the atrium?
Harrison's 20th Ed. Chapter 241 Page 1733 Table 241-1

A. Atrial flutter
B. Atrial fibrillation
C. Preexcited tachycardia
D. Multifocal atrial tachycardia

488. Which of the following is the most common sustained cardiac arrhythmia in older adults?
Harrison's 20th Ed. Chapter 241 Page 1733 Table 241-1

A. Atrial flutter
B. Atrial fibrillation
C. Preexcited tachycardia
D. Multifocal atrial tachycardia

489. Which of the following is the mostly seen in patients with pulmonary disease?
Harrison's 20th Ed. Chapter 241 Page 1733 Table 241-1

A. Atrial flutter
B. Atrial fibrillation
C. Preexcited tachycardia
D. Multifocal atrial tachycardia

490. Which of the following is the most common paroxysmal sustained tachycardia in healthy young adults?
Harrison's 20th Ed. Chapter 241 Page 1733 Table 241-1

A. AV nodal reentry tachycardia (AVNRT)
B. Atrial fibrillation
C. Preexcited tachycardia
D. Multifocal atrial tachycardia

491. Which of the following is a wide QRS tachycardia with QRS morphology similar to VT?
Harrison's 20th Ed. Chapter 241 Page 1733 Table 241-1

A. AV nodal reentry tachycardia (AVNRT)
B. Atrial fibrillation
C. Preexcited tachycardia
D. Multifocal atrial tachycardia

492. Which of the following is a preexcited tachycardia?
Harrison's 20th Ed. Chapter 241 Page 1733 Table 241-1

A. AV nodal reentry tachycardia (AVNRT)
B. Orthodromic AV reentry tachycardia
C. Antidromic AV reentry tachycardia
D. All of the above

493. Multiple discrete P waves are seen in which of the following?
Harrison's 20th Ed. Chapter 241 Page 1733 Table 241-1

A. Atrial flutter
B. Orthodromic AV reentry tachycardia
C. Antidromic AV reentry tachycardia
D. Multifocal atrial tachycardia

494. Sawtooth waves are seen in which of the following?
Harrison's 20th Ed. Chapter 241 Page 1733 Table 241-1

A. Atrial flutter
B. Orthodromic AV reentry tachycardia
C. Antidromic AV reentry tachycardia
D. Multifocal atrial tachycardia

495. Supraventricular arrhythmia may precipitate cardiac arrest in?
Harrison's 20th Ed. Chapter 241 Page 1733

A. Wolff-Parkinson-White syndrome
B. Eisenmenger's syndrome
C. Marfan's syndrome
D. Osler Weber-Rendu syndrome

Rarely, supraventricular arrhythmia may precipitate cardiac arrest in patients with Wolff-Parkinson-White syndrome or hypertrophic cardiomyopathy.

496. In narrow complex tachycardia, regular atrial rate is seen in all except?

Harrison's 20th Ed. Chapter 241 Page 1734 Figure 241-1

A. AV nodal reentry tachycardia (AVNRT)
B. Junctional tachycardia
C. Multifocal atrial tachycardia
D. Atrial flutter

497. AV node blockade with vagal maneuvers, adenosine, verapamil or beta blockers may terminate tachycardia in?

Harrison's 20th Ed. Chapter 241 Page 1734 Figure 241-2

A. AV nodal reentry tachycardia (AVNRT)
B. Orthodromic AV reentry tachycardia (ORT)
C. Focal atrial tachycardia (AT)
D. All of the above

498. Short R-P tachycardia best relates to?

Harrison's 20th Ed. Chapter 241 Page 1735 Table 241-2

A. AV nodal reentry tachycardia (AVNRT)
B. Orthodromic AV reentry tachycardia (ORT)
C. Focal atrial tachycardia (AT)
D. All of the above

Physiologic and Nonphysiologic Sinus Tachycardia

499. Crista terminalis is located in?

Harrison's 20th Ed. Chapter 242 Page 1735

A. Right atrium
B. Left atrium
C. Right ventricle
D. Left ventricle

Crista terminalis is a thick ridge of muscle and is a natural anatomic barrier of conduction. It is the vertical crest on interior wall of right atrium that separates nontrabeculated posterior right atrium from rest of the trabeculated right atrium.

500. Which of the following is an anatomic ridge in heart?

Harrison's 18th Ed. 1887

A. Crista terminalis
B. Valve annuli
C. Limbus of fossa ovalis
D. All of the above

Anatomic ridges of heart are crista terminalis, valve annuli or limbus of the fossa ovalis.

501. Tachyarrhythmias typically refer to?

Harrison's 19th Ed. 1476

A. Isolated premature complexes (depolarizations)
B. Nonsustained forms of tachycardia originating from myocardial foci or reentrant circuits
C. Sustained forms of tachycardia originating from myocardial foci or reentrant circuits
D. All of the above

502. Sinus P waves are characterized by all except?

Harrison's 20th Ed. Chapter 242 Page 1735

A. Frontal plane axis directed inferiorly & rightward
B. Positive in leads II, III & aVF
C. Negative in aVR
D. Initially positive biphasic P wave in V1

Sinus P waves are characterized by a frontal plane axis directed inferiorly & leftward, with positive P waves in leads II, III & aVF, a negative P wave in aVR and an initially positive biphasic P wave in V1.

503. In sinus tachycardia, the ventricular rate should be?

Harrison's 20th Ed. Chapter 242 Page 1735

A. > 90 beats/minute
B. > 100 beats/minute
C. > 110 beats/minute
D. > 120 beats/minute

Normal sinus rhythm has a rate of 60-100 beats/minute. Definition of tachycardia is rhythm that produces a ventricular rate >100 beats/minute.

504. In sinus bradycardia, the ventricular rate should be?

Harrison's 20th Ed. Chapter 242 Page 1735

A. < 70 beats/minute
B. < 60 beats/minute
C. < 50 beats/minute
D. < 40 beats/minute

Sinus bradycardia is defined as rates less than 60 beats/minute. Bradycadia can be normal during sleep and in fit individuals.

505. In sinus tachycardia, P waves become taller in which of the following ECG leads?

Harrison's 20th Ed. Chapter 242 Page 1735

A. aVR
B. II, III, aVF
C. V_1 - V_3
D. V_4 - V_6

In sinus tachycardia, the rate of spontaneous depolarization of sinus node increases & focus of earliest activation within the node shifts more leftward & closer to superior septal aspect of crista terminalis, producing taller P waves in the inferior limb leads when compared to normal sinus rhythm.

506. Which of the following is false for physiologic sinus tachycardia?

Harrison's 20th Ed. Chapter 242 Page 1735

A. Present when heart rate exceeds 100 beats/min
B. Heart rate rarely exceeds 200 beats/min
C. Has a gradual onset and offset
D. Carotid sinus pressure produces slowing with sudden return to previous rate upon cessation

Sinus tachycardia, carotid sinus pressure produces modest & transient slowing but no abrupt termination.

507. Which of the following conditions can cause physiologic sinus tachycardia?

Harrison's 20th Ed. Chapter 242 Page 1735 Table 242-1

A. Pulmonary insufficiency
B. Hyperthyroidism
C. Pheochromocytoma
D. All of the above

508. Which of the following drugs can cause physiologic sinus tachycardia?

Harrison's 20th Ed. Chapter 242 Page 1735 Table 242-1

A. Tricyclic antidepressants
B. Theophylline
C. Nifedipine
D. All of the above

509. Which of the following about inappropriate sinus tachycardia is false?

Harrison's 20th Ed. Chapter 242 Page 1735

A. Heart rate increases spontaneously
B. Heart rate increases out of proportion to stress/exercise
C. Therapy is ineffective or poorly tolerated
D. Anxiolytics are the treatment of choice

In inappropriate sinus tachycardia, heart rate increases either spontaneously or out of proportion to the degree of physiologic stress/exercise. It must be distinguished from appropriate sinus tachycardia and from focal atrial tachycardia.

510. Which of the following about inappropriate sinus tachycardia is false?

Harrison's 20th Ed. Chapter 242 Page 1735

A. Sinus rate increases spontaneously at rest
B. Sinus rate out of proportion to physiologic stress or exertion
C. Affects women in third or fourth decade of life
D. None of the above

In "inappropriate sinus tachycardia" the sinus rate increases spontaneously at rest or out of proportion to physiologic stress or exertion. Affected individuals are often women in third or fourth decade of life. It must be distinguished from appropriate sinus tachycardia and from focal atrial tachycardia. Therapy is often ineffective or poorly tolerated with beta blockers and/or calcium channel blockers, clonidine, serotonin reuptake inhibitors and Ivabradine.

511. Which of the following drugs block the current that causes sinus node depolarization?

Harrison's 20th Ed. Chapter 242 Page 1736

A. Digoxin
B. Mexiletine
C. Ivabradine
D. Midodrine

Ivabradine blocks the I_f current that causes sinus node depolarization.

512. Postural orthostatic tachycardia syndrome (POTS) is diagnosed when on standing heart rate increases by?

Harrison's 20th Ed. Chapter 242 Page 1736

A. 10 beats / minute
B. 20 beats / minute
C. 30 beats / minute
D. 40 beats / minute

513. Postural orthostatic tachycardia syndrome (POTS) is diagnosed when on standing heart rate increases to?

Harrison's 20th Ed. Chapter 242 Page 1736

A. > 100 beats / minute
B. > 110 beats / minute
C. > 120 beats / minute
D. > 130 beats / minute

Postural orthostatic tachycardia syndrome (POTS) is characterized by symptomatic orthostatic intolerance without OH, accompanied by either an increase in heart rate to > 120 beats/minute or an increase of 30 beats/minute within 10 minutes of standing. It may occur after a viral illness and resolve spontaneously over 3 - 12 months (postviral dysautonomia).

514. Which of the following drugs is of use in postural orthostatic tachycardia syndrome (POTS)?

Harrison's 20th Ed. Chapter 242 Page 1736

A. Fludrocortisone
B. Midodrine
C. Volume expansion with salt supplementation
D. All of the above

Volume expansion with salt supplementation, oral fludrocortisone, compression stockings, alpha-agonist midodrine, can be helpful in POTS. Reconditioning and exercise training also improves symptoms.

Focal Atrial Tachycardia

515. Focal Atrial Tachycardia can be due to?
Harrison's 20th Ed. Chapter 243 Page 1736

A. Abnormal automaticity
B. Triggered automaticity
C. Small reentry circuit
D. All of the above

516. Atrial tissue may extend into?
Harrison's 20th Ed. Chapter 243 Page 1736

A. Pulmonary vein
B. Coronary sinus
C. Vena cava
D. All of the above

Focal atrial tachycardia (AT) can be due to abnormal automaticity, triggered automaticity or a small reentry circuit confined to atrium or atrial tissue extending into a pulmonary vein, the coronary sinus or vena cava.

517. Focal Atrial Tachycardia can be?
Harrison's 20th Ed. Chapter 243 Page 1736

A. Sustained
B. Nonsustained
C. Paroxysmal or incessant
D. Any of the above

518. Which of the following is false about focal AT?
Harrison's 20th Ed. Chapter 243 Page 1736

A. May lead to atrial fibrillation and flutter
B. Due to atrial fibrosis
C. Sympathetic stimulation is a promoting factor
D. None of the above

519. Incessant AT can cause?
Harrison's 20th Ed. Chapter 243 Page 1736

A. Complete heart block
B. CHF
C. Tachycardia-induced cardiomyopathy
D. All of the above

Incessant AT can cause tachycardia-induced cardiomyopathy.

520. Which of the following is false about focal AT?
Harrison's 20th Ed. Chapter 243 Page 1736

A. AT will not terminate with AV block
B. Accelerated warm-up or cool-down phase
C. P waves are often discrete
D. R-P interval shorter than the P-R interval

In focal AT, P-R interval is shorter than the R-P interval. P-wave morphology differs depending on the location of the focus.

521. Focal AT tends to originate in?
Harrison's 20th Ed. Chapter 243 Page 1736

A. Crista terminalis
B. Valve annuli
C. Atrial septum
D. Any of the above

Focal AT tends to originate in areas of complex atrial anatomy like crista terminalis, valve annuli, atrial septum and atrial muscle extending along cardiac thoracic veins (superior vena cava, coronary sinus and pulmonary veins). The location can be estimated by P-wave morphology.

522. In focal AT, P wave will resemble that of sinus tachycardia when the focus originates in?
Harrison's 20th Ed. Chapter 243 Page 1736

A. Superior aspect of crista terminalis
B. Superior pulmonary veins
C. Left atrium
D. Ostium of the coronary sinus

AT from the right atrium has a positive P-wave morphology in lead 1 and biphasic P-wave morphology in lead V1. AT from the atrial septum will frequently have a narrower P-wave duration than sinus rhythm. AT from the left atrium will usually have a monophasic, positive P wave in lead V1. AT that originates from superior atrial locations, such as the superior vena cava or superior pulmonary veins, will be positive in the inferior limb leads II, III and aVF, whereas AT from a more inferior location, such as the ostium of the coronary sinus, will inscribe negative P waves in these same leads. When the focus is in the superior aspect of the crista terminalis, close to the sinus node, however, the P wave will resemble that of sinus tachycardia.

523. Focal ATs can be distinguished by?
Harrison's 20th Ed. Chapter 243 Page 1736

A. Response to adenosine
B. Response to amiodarone
C. Response to verapamil
D. All of the above

Focal ATs can be distinguished by observations made at AT initiation & in response to adenosine.

524. Which of the following drugs is used to terminate reentrant SVT involving AV node?
Harrison's 20th Ed. Chapter 243 Page 1738 Table 243-1

A. Amiodarone
B. Adenosine
C. Digoxin
D. All of the above

525. Which of the following drugs is indicated in Long QT syndrome?
Harrison's 20th Ed. Chapter 243 Page 1738 Table 243-1

A. Amiodarone
B. Verapamil
C. Digoxin
D. Metoprolol

526. Which of the following drugs is indicated in Long QT syndrome?

Harrison's 20th Ed. Chapter 243 Page 1738 Table 243-2

A. Atenolol
B. Acebutolol
C. Metoprolol
D. All of the above

527. Which of the following drugs is indicated in exercise induced VT?

Harrison's 20th Ed. Chapter 243 Page 1738 Table 243-1

A. Amiodarone
B. Verapamil
C. Digoxin
D. Metoprolol

528. Which of the following drugs is indicated for prevention of atrial fibrillation?

Harrison's 20th Ed. Chapter 243 Page 1738 Table 243-2

A. Dofetilide
B. Dronedarone
C. Disopyramide
D. All of the above

529. Long QT and Torsades des pointes is the proarrhythmic toxicity of which of the following antiarrhythmic agent?

Harrison's 20th Ed. Chapter 243 Page 1738 Table 243-3

A. Ibutilide
B. Amiodarone
C. Procainamide
D. All of the above

530. Ataxia, tremor, gait disturbances is the toxicity of which of the following antiarrhythmic agent?

Harrison's 20th Ed. Chapter 243 Page 1738 Table 243-3

A. Mexiletine
B. Propafenone
C. Procainamide
D. Disopyramide

531. Acute urinary retention is the toxicity of which of the following antiarrhythmic agent?

Harrison's 20th Ed. Chapter 243 Page 1738 Table 243-3

A. Mexiletine
B. Propafenone
C. Procainamide
D. Disopyramide

532. Taste disturbance is the toxicity of which of the following antiarrhythmic agent?

Harrison's 20th Ed. Chapter 243 Page 1738 Table 243-3

A. Mexiletine
B. Propafenone
C. Procainamide
D. Disopyramide

533. Lupus erythematosus–like syndrome is the toxicity of which of the following antiarrhythmic agent?

Harrison's 20th Ed. Chapter 243 Page 1738 Table 243-3

A. Mexiletine
B. Propafenone
C. Procainamide
D. Disopyramide

Paroxysmal Supraventricular Tachycardias

534. Supraventricular tachycardia (SVT) refers?

Am Fam Physician. 2015;92(9):793-800

A. Atrioventricular nodal reentrant tachycardia (AVNRT)
B. Atrioventricular reciprocating tachycardia (AVRT)
C. Atrial tachycardia
D. All of the above

Supraventricular tachycardia (SVT) refers to rapid rhythms that originate and are sustained in atrial or atrioventricular nodal tissue, and then transmit through bundle of His and cause rapid ventricular response. Although atrial flutter, atrial fibrillation, and multifocal atrial tachycardia also arise from this area, in practice, SVT refers to atrioventricular nodal reentrant tachycardia (AVNRT), atrioventricular reciprocating tachycardia (AVRT), and atrial tachycardia.

535. Which of the following about AV nodal reentry tachycardia (AVNRT) is false?

Harrison's 20th Ed. Chapter 244 Page 1739

A. Most common paroxysmal regular SVT
B. More common in men than in women
C. Typically manifests in II to IV decades of life
D. Occur in the absence of structural heart disease

AV nodal reentrant tachycardia is the most common paroxysmal regular SVT. It is more common in women than in men (>2:1). Typically manifests in second to fourth decades of life and tends to occur in the absence of structural heart disease, it is usually well tolerated.

536. AVNRT is more common during?

Am Fam Physician. 2015;92(9):793-800

A. Follicular phase of the menstrual cycle
B. Luteal phase of the menstrual cycle
C. Pregnancy
D. All of the above

AVNRT incidence in women is twice that in men. It is correlated with lower estrogen levels & higher progesterone levels, and is therefore more common during luteal phase of the menstrual cycle and less common during pregnancy.

537. Most forms of AVNRT utilize which of the following AV nodal pathway?

Harrison's 20th Ed. Chapter 244 Page 1739

A. Right inferior extension
B. Left inferior extension
C. Right superior extension
D. Left superior extension

Most forms of AVNRT utilize a slowly conducting (α) AV nodal pathway (right inferior extension) that extends from the compact AV node near His bundle, inferiorly along the tricuspid valve annulus to floor of coronary sinus. The reentry wavefront propagates up this slowly conducting pathway to the compact AV node and then exits from the fast pathway at the top of the AV node. The path back to the slow pathway probably involves the left atrial septum which has connections to the coronary sinus musculature.

538. Which of the following is false about atrioventricular nodal reentrant tachycardia?

N Engl J Med. 2016; 374:e17

A. Regular tachycardia
B. Narrow QRS complex
C. Narrow P waves deforming the terminal QRS complex
D. None of the above

539. Which of the following is false about atrioventricular nodal reentrant tachycardia (AVNRT)?

Am Fam Physician. 2015;92(9):793-800

A. Antegrade conduction down in slow AV nodal pathway
B. Retrograde conduction up in the fast AV nodal pathway
C. Pseudo–R wave in lead V1 is the P wave
D. None of the above

540. Which of the following is false about atrioventricular nodal reentrant tachycardia (AVNRT)?

N Engl J Med. 2016; 374:e17

A. Re-entrant rhythm confined to the AV node
B. Fast (β) pathway has fast conduction & long refractory period
C. Slow (α) pathway has slow conduction & short refractory period
D. None of the above

The fast and slow fibres form the circuit for AVNRT. Each revolution of the circuit generates an impulse that exits the AV node via the His bundle to activate the ventricles. Because atria and ventricles are activated simultaneously the P wave is either buried within the QRS complex or inscribed just after it. The P wave is narrower than in sinus rhythm because left and right atria are activated simultaneously not sequentially.

541. Which of the following relate to atrioventricular nodal reentrant tachycardia?

Harrison's 20th Ed. Chapter 244 Page 1739

A. Pseudo-S wave
B. Pseudo-r' wave
C. Canon A waves
D. All of the above

In typical forms, the conduction time from the compact AV node region to atrium is similar to that from compact node to His bundle and ventricles. Therefore, atrial activation occurs at about the same time as ventricular activation. P wave is seen at the end of the QRS complex as a pseudo-r' (r' prime) in lead V1 (an appearance similar to incomplete RBBB) and pseudo-S waves in leads II, III, and aVF, typical of slow-fast AVNRT.

542. "Frog sign" is best related to?

N Engl J Med. 2016; 374:e17

A. Arterial pulse
B. Jugular veins
C. Abdominal pulsations
D. Nail beds

543. "Frog sign" is best related to?

N Engl J Med. 2016; 374:e17

A. Atrial fibrillation
B. Atrioventricular nodal reentrant tachycardia
C. Ventricular tachycardia
D. All of the above

In atrioventricular nodal reentrant tachycardia, the characteristic flapping or bulging appearance of the neck vein pulsations are felt due to simultaneous atrial & ventricular contraction, and a "frog sign" is identified on physical examination during arrhythmia.

544. Which of the following is a symptom of AVNRT?
Harrison's 20th Ed. Chapter 244 Page 1739

A. Polydipsia
B. Polyuria
C. Anorexia
D. Polyphagia

Elevated venous pressures in AVNRT may lead to release of natriuretic peptides that cause post-tachycardia diuresis.

545. Which of the following is a type of AVNRT?
https://www.ncbi.nlm.nih.gov/books/NBK499936

A. Slow-Fast AVNRT
B. Fast-Slow AVNRT
C. Slow-Slow AVNRT
D. All of the above

A Slow-Fast AVNRT accounts for 90% of AVNRTs with anterograde conduction by the slow AV nodal pathway and retrograde conduction by the fast AV nodal pathway.

546. Pseudo-S wave in II, III, AVF and Pseudo-R' in V1 are a feature of?
https://www.ncbi.nlm.nih.gov/books/NBK499936

A. Slow-Fast AVNRT
B. Fast-Slow AVNRT
C. Slow-Slow AVNRT
D. All of the above

547. P waves between QRS and T waves (QRS-P-T complexes) is a feature of?
https://www.ncbi.nlm.nih.gov/books/NBK499936

A. Slow-Fast AVNRT
B. Fast-Slow AVNRT
C. Slow-Slow AVNRT
D. All of the above

548. Late P waves after a QRS, appearing as atrial tachycardia is a feature of?
https://www.ncbi.nlm.nih.gov/books/NBK499936

A. Slow-Fast AVNRT
B. Fast-Slow AVNRT
C. Slow-Slow AVNRT
D. All of the above

The anatomy of re-entrant circuit defines the type of AVNRT. A Slow-Fast AVNRT accounts for 90% of AVNRTs with anterograde conduction by slow AV nodal pathway & retrograde conduction by fast AV nodal pathway. Fast-slow AVNRT represents ~5 - 10% of AVNRTs with anterograde conduction by fast AV nodal pathway and retrograde conduction by slow AV nodal pathway. Slow-slow AVNRTs account 1 - 5% of AVNRTs with anterograde conduction by slow AV nodal pathways and retrograde conduction by slow atrial fibers.

549. Which of the following can cause a regular, narrow QRS complex tachycardia?
https://www.ncbi.nlm.nih.gov/books/NBK499936

A. Intra-atrial reentrant tachycardia
B. Sinoatrial nodal reentrant tachycardia
C. Junctional ectopic tachycardia
D. All of the above

A regular, narrow QRS complex tachycardia can be caused by Atrioventricular nodal reentrant tachycardia, Atrioventricular reentrant tachycardia, Intraatrial reentrant tachycardia, Sinoatrial nodal reentrant tachycardia, Junctional ectopic tachycardia, Atrial tachycardia, Atrial flutter, Sinus tachycardia and Inappropriate sinus tachycardia

550. Atrial-His / His-atrial ratio (AH/HA) in typical (slow-fast) AVNRT is?
Circulation. 2016;134:1655-1663

A. > 0.25
B. > 0.50
C. > 0.75
D. > 1.00

551. HA interval in typical (slow-fast) AVNRT is?
Circulation. 2016;134:1655-1663

A. ≤ 70 ms
B. ≤ 90 ms
C. ≤ 110 ms
D. ≤ 130 ms

Typical (slow-fast) AVNRT was defined by an atrial-His/His-atrial ratio (AH/HA) >1, and HA interval ≤70 ms. Atypical AVNRT was defined by delayed retrograde atrial activation with HA>70 ms. If the AH was <200 ms and the AH<HA, the atypical form was characterized as fast-slow. If AH >200 ms and AH>HA, the atypical form is considered slow-slow. Tachycardias with a prolonged AH interval >200 ms but AH<HA, or with AH<200 ms and AH>HA, or with variable intervals during the same or different episodes, are classified as indeterminate.

552. Which of the following about AVNRT is false?
Harrison's 20th Ed. Chapter 244 Page 1739

A. Fast pathway has a longer refractory period
B. Slow pathway lower in the AV node region
C. During sinus rhythm, conduction is through both pathways
D. None of the above

Fast pathway is in superior part of AV node and has a longer refractory period, whereas pathway lower in AV node region conducts more slowly and has a shorter refractory period. During sinus rhythm, conduction is through both pathways.

553. Which of the following occurs in a typical AV nodal reentrant tachycardia?
Harrison's 20th Ed. Chapter 244 Page 1739

A. Repetitive activation up slow and down fast pathway
B. Repetitive activation down slow and up fast pathway
C. Repetitive activation down slow pathway
D. Repetitive activation down fast pathway

Repetitive activation down the slow and up the fast pathway results in typical AV nodal reentrant tachycardia.

554. Atrioventricular nodal reentrant tachycardia is caused by a reentrant loop that involves atrioventricular node and?
N Engl J Med. 2012;367:1438-48

A. Atrial tissue
B. Ventricular tissue
C. Bundle of His
D. Fascicles

Atrioventricular nodal reentrant tachycardia is caused by a reentrant loop that involves the atrioventricular node and the atrial tissue.

555. P waves immediately precede the QRS complex in all except?
N Engl J Med. 2012;367:1438-48

A. Atrial tachycardia
B. Multifocal atrial tachycardia
C. Atrioventricular nodal reentrant tachycardia
D. Multiple atrial premature contractions

P waves immediately precede the QRS complex in sinus tachycardia, atrial tachycardia, multifocal atrial tachycardia, and multiple atrial premature contractions. P waves follow the QRS complex in atrioventricular nodal reentrant tachycardia and atrioventricular reciprocating tachycardia.

556. Junctional ectopic tachycardia (JET) is due to automaticity within the?
Harrison's 20th Ed. Chapter 244 Page 1739

A. AV node
B. Bundle of His
C. Bundle branch
D. Purkinje fibers

Junctional ectopic tachycardia (JET) is due to automaticity within the AV node.

557. Which of the following about junctional ectopic tachycardia (JET) is false?
Harrison's 20th Ed. Chapter 244 Page 1739

A. Narrow QRS tachycardia
B. Often with ventriculoatrial (VA) block
C. May be seen after administration of isoproterenol
D. None of the above

558. What is the heart rate in accelerated junctional rhythm?
Harrison's 20th Ed. Chapter 244 Page 1739

A. 40 to 60 beats / minute
B. 50 to 100 beats / minute
C. 100 to 120 beats / minute
D. 120 to 160 beats / minute

Accelerated junctional rhythm is a junctional automatic rhythm between 50 and 100 beats/minute.

559. Which of the followig resembles AVNRT at a slow rate?
Harrison's 20th Ed. Chapter 244 Page 1739

A. First degree heart block
B. Torsade de pointes
C. Multifocal atrial tachycardia
D. Accelerated junctional rhythm

560. Which of the following is false about automatic atrial tachycardias?
Harrison's 19th Ed. 1479

A. Respond to adenosine
B. Provoked by isoproterenol infusion
C. First P wave of AT has same morphology as remaining waves
D. None of the above

Automatic ATs start with a "warm-up" period over the first 3 - 10 complexes and slow in rate before termination. They may respond to adenosine. Initiation of automatic ATs frequently can be provoked by isoproterenol infusion. First P wave of tachycardia has same morphology as remaining waves.

561. Which of the following is false about focal reentrant atrial tachycardias?
Harrison's 19th Ed. 1479

A. Initiate with spontaneous premature beats
B. P wave initiating tachycardia has different morphology than P wave during sustained AT
C. Do not slow and/or terminate with adenosine
D. None of the above

Focal reentrant AT initiate with programmed atrial stimulation or spontaneous premature beats. P wave initiating tachycardia has a different morphology than P wave during sustained AT. P wave in AT is characteristically distinct from the sinus P-wave morphology. With adenosine, reentrant ATs will produce AV block but typically do not slow and/or terminate.

562. Which of the following arrhythmia may be a manifestation of digoxin toxicity?
Harrison's 18th Ed. 1888

A. Multifocal atrial tachycardia
B. Focal atrial tachycardias
C. AV junctional tachycardias
D. AV nodal reentrant tachycardia

563. Junctional tachycardia due to abnormal automaticity can be treated pharmacologically with?
Harrison's 18th Ed. 1888

A. Digitalis
B. Beta blockers
C. Calcium channel blockers
D. All of the above

Junctional tachycardia due to abnormal automaticity can be treated with beta blockers.

564. AV bypass tracts are associated with which of the following?
Harrison's 20th Ed. Chapter 244 Page 1739

A. Narrow-complex PSVT
B. Wide-complex tachycardias
C. Sudden death
D. All of the above

565. Accessory pathways (APs) are associated with which of the following?
Harrison's 20th Ed. Chapter 244 Page 1739

A. Ebstein's anomaly of the tricuspid valve
B. Forms of HCM including PRKAG2 mutations
C. Danon's disease
D. All of the above

566. AV bypass tracts are associated with which of the following congenital abnormalities?
Harrison's 20th Ed. Chapter 244 Page 1739

A. ASD
B. VSD
C. TOF
D. Ebstein's anomaly

Accessory pathways (APs) are associated with Ebstein's anomaly of the tricuspid valve and forms of hypertrophic cardiomyopathy including PRKA G2 mutations, Danon's disease and Fabry's disease.

567. Which of the following statements about accessory pathways (APs) is false?
Harrison's 20th Ed. Chapter 244 Page 1739

A. Abnormal connections
B. Allow conduction between atrium & ventricles across AV ring
C. Present from birth
D. None of the above

568. The most common accessory pathway (AP) connects which of the following?
Harrison's 20th Ed. Chapter 244 Page 1740

A. Left atrium to left ventricle
B. Right atrium to right ventricle
C. Left atrium to right ventricle
D. Right atrium to left ventricle

The most common AP connects the left atrium to the left ventricle, followed by posterior septal, right free wall, and anterior septal APs.

569. Accessory pathways (APs) occur most frequently between?
Harrison's 20th Ed. Chapter 244 Page 1740

A. Left atrium and free wall of left ventricle
B. Left atrium and posteroseptal
C. Left atrium and anteroseptal
D. Left atrium and right free wall

APs are abnormal connections that allow conduction between the atrium and ventricles across the AV ring. They are present from birth and are due to failure of complete partitioning of atrium and ventricle by the fibrous AV rings. APs occur across either an AV valve annulus or septum, most frequently between the left atrium and free wall of left ventricle, followed by posteroseptal, right free wall and anteroseptal locations.

570. Which of the following occurs when ventricles are "preexcited" during sinus rhythm?
Harrison's 20th Ed. Chapter 244 Page 1740

A. Short P-R interval (<0.12 second)
B. Slurred initial portion of the QRS (delta wave)
C. Prolonged QRS duration
D. All of the above

If the impulse from sinus node conducts through AP to ventricle (antegrade) before the impulse conducts through AV node & His bundle, the ventricles are "preexcited" during sinus rhythm, and ECG shows a short P-R interval (<0.12 second), slurred initial portion of QRS (delta wave), and prolonged QRS duration produced by slow conduction through direct activation of ventricular myocardium over the AP.

571. The morphology of the QRS and delta wave is determined by?
Harrison's 20th Ed. Chapter 244 Page 1740

A. Thickness of accessory pathway
B. Length of accessory pathway
C. Location of accessory pathway
D. All of the above

The morphology of the QRS and delta wave is determined by the AP location and the degree of fusion between the excitation wave fronts from conduction over the AV node and conduction over the AP.

572. Which of the following is false about right-sided accessory pathways?
Harrison's 20th Ed. Chapter 244 Page 1740

A. Create marked preexcitation
B. Preexcite the right ventricle
C. Produce an LBBB like configuration in lead V1
D. None of the above

Right-sided pathways preexcite right ventricle, produce a left bundle branch block–like configuration in lead V1, and often create marked preexcitation because of relatively close proximity of the AP to sinus node.

573. Which of the following is false about left-sided accessory pathways?
Harrison's 20th Ed. Chapter 244 Page 1740

A. Produce a right bundle branch like configuration in lead V_1
B. Produce a negative delta wave in aVL
C. Preexcitation may be minimal or absent
D. None of the above

Left-sided pathways preexcite left ventricle & produce a right bundle branch–like configuration in lead V1 and a negative delta wave in aVL, due to initial depolarization of lateral portion of left ventricle. Due to a relatively large distance between sinus node & left free wall APs, preexcitation may be minimal or absent on 12-lead ECG.

574. Delta waves may be negative in leads III and aVF when preexcitation due to an AP is at?
Harrison's 20th Ed. Chapter 244 Page 1740

A. Left lateral wall
B. Right lateral wall
C. Diaphragmatic surface
D. All of the above

Preexcitation due to an AP at the diaphragmatic surface of heart produces delta waves that are negative in leads III & aVF, mimicking q waves of inferior wall infarction.

575. Preexcitation can be intermittent and disappear during?
Harrison's 20th Ed. Chapter 244 Page 1740

A. Sleep
B. Hyperventilation
C. Exercise
D. All of the above

Preexcitation can be intermittent & disappear during exercise as conduction over AV node accelerates and may take over ventricular activation completely.

576. Which of the following rhythms is associated with WPW syndrome?
Harrison's 20th Ed. Chapter 244 Page 1741 Figure 244-3

A. Sinus rhythm - antegrade AP conduction
B. Orthodromic AV reentry - retrograde AP conduction
C. Antidromic AV reentry - antegrade AP conduction
D. All of the above

Most common rhythms associated with WPW syndrome are sinus rhythm with antegrade conduction over AP & AV node, orthodromic AVRT using retrograde conduction over AP and antegrade conduction over AV node and antidromic AVRT using retrograde conduction over AV node and antegrade conduction over AP.

577. Which of the following about concealed accessory pathways is false?
Harrison's 20th Ed. Chapter 244 Page 1740

A. Allow only retrograde conduction, from ventricle to atrium
B. No preexcitation is present during sinus rhythm
C. SVT can occur
D. None of the above

578. Which of the following statements about accessory pathways (APs) is correct?
Harrison's 20th Ed. Chapter 244 Page 1740

A. APs connect the atria with the ventricles
B. There may be no delta wave in the ECG of concealed APs
C. More than 50% of APs are located at the left free wall
D. All of the above

579. Pseudopreexcitation syndrome is related to which of the following?
Cleveland Clinic J of Medicine 2018;85(7):508

A. Hypoplastic left heart syndrome
B. Atrioventricular canal defect
C. Ebstein anomaly
D. All of the above

A short PR interval with or without delta waves can also be seen in the absence of an accessory pathway, e.g. in hypoplastic left heart syndrome, atrioventricular canal defect, and Ebstein anomaly. These conditions are termed pseudopreexcitation syndrome.

580. Wolff-Parkinson-White (WPW) syndrome is defined as?
Harrison's 20th Ed. Chapter 244 Page 1740

A. A preexcited QRS
B. During sinus rhythm
C. Episodes of PSVT
D. All of the above

581. WPW pattern is defined by preexcitation findings on ECG without?

Cleveland Clinic J of Medicine. 2018;85(7):508

A. Family history
B. Genetic predisposition
C. Symptomatic arrhythmias
D. All of the above

WPW pattern is defined only by preexcitation findings on ECG without symptomatic arrhythmias. Patients with WPW syndrome can present with palpitation, dizziness, and syncope resulting from underlying arrhythmia. This is not seen in patients with WPW pattern.

582. WPW pattern can be unmasked by?

Cleveland Clinic J of Medicine. 2018;85(7):508

A. Anesthesia
B. Sympathomimetic drugs
C. Postoperatively
D. All of the above

WPW pattern can be unmasked by anesthesia, sympathomimetic drugs, and postoperatively.

583. Which of the following about atriofascicular accessory pathways is false?

Harrison's 20th Ed. Chapter 244 Page 1740

A. Originate from the right atrium
B. Conduct more slowly
C. Has decremental antegrade conduction
D. None of the above

584. Which of the following is an accessory pathway?

Circulation. 2016;133(14):e506-74

A. Nodo-fascicular
B. Nodo-ventricular
C. Fasciculoventricular
D. All of the above

Accessory pathways include atriofascicular, nodo-fascic ular, nodo-ventricular, and fasciculoventricular pathways.

585. Which of the following accessory pathway do not cause arrhythmia?

Harrison's 20th Ed. Chapter 244 Page 1740

A. Atriofascicular
B. Fasciculoventricular
C. Atrioventricular
D. None of the above

Fasciculoventricular connections between the His bundle and ventricular septum produce preexcitation but do not cause arrhythmia, probably because the circuit is too short to promote reentry.

586. Which of the following best relates to connection between right atrium to fascicles of the right bundle branch?

Harrison's 20th Ed. Chapter 244 Page 1740

A. James fibers
B. Bundle of Kent
C. Mahaim fibers
D. Brechenmacher fibers

There are several types of accessory pathways. The classic accessory pathway is the AV bypass tract or bundle of Kent in WPW that directly connects atrial and ventricular myocardium, bypassing the AV node/His-Purkinje system. James fibers or atrionodal tracts, connect atrium to distal or compact AV node. Brechenmacher fibers (atrio-Hisian tracts) connect the atrium to His bundle. Atriofascicular pathways, also known as Mahaim fibers, probably represent a duplicate AV node and His-Purkinje system that connect the right atrium to fascicles of the right bundle branch and conduct slowly only in the anterograde direction.

587. Wolff-Parkinson-White syndrome is best related to?

N Engl J Med. 1987; 317:109-111

A. James fibers
B. Bundle of Kent
C. Mahaim fibers
D. Brechenmacher fibers

Preexcitation through an AV bypass tract, the bundle of Kent, produces the ECG pattern described by Wolff, Parkinson, and White in 1930. Bundle of Kent in WPW directly connects atrial & ventricular myocardium, bypassing the AV node/His-Purkinje system. AV conduction is nondecremental and more rapid through the accessory pathway than through the AV node, a difference that is increased at fast heart rates. Decremental conduction means increase in conduction time of the impulse propagating through the AV node as the cycle length shortens (heart rate increased).

588. Classic electrocardiographic triad in WPW syndrome includes all except?

N Engl J Med. 2003;349:1787

A. Short PR interval
B. Slurred QRS upstroke (delta wave)
C. Prolonged QRS complex
D. Prolonged QT interval

In WPW syndrome, classic electrocardiographic triad is a short PR interval, a slurred QRS upstroke (delta wave), and a prolonged QRS complex.

589. Most common arrhythmia associated with WPW syndrome is?

N Engl J Med. 2003;349:1787

A. Atrioventricular reciprocating tachycardia
B. Atrioventricular nodal reentrant tachycardia
C. Atrial tachycardia
D. Multifocal atrial tachycardia

Most common arrhythmia associated with WPW syndrome is atrioventricular reciprocating tachycardia.

590. The following are ECG features of WPW syndrome except?

Harrison's 20th Ed. Chapter 244 Page 1740

A. Presence of delta wave
B. Shortened PR interval of < 0.12 seconds
C. PR depression
D. Prolonged QRS interval of > 0.12 seconds

591. Which of the following are known conditions associated with WPW syndrome?

Harrison's 20th Ed. Chapter 244 Page 1740

A. ST elevation myocardial infarction
B. Ebstein anomaly
C. Acute pericarditis
D. Marfan's syndrome

592. The WPW ECG may mimic the following?

Harrison's 20th Ed. Chapter 244 Page 1740

A. Left ventricular hypertrophy
B. Right ventricular hypertrophy
C. Bundle branch block
D. All of the above

593. AV bypass tract in ventricular preexcitation are composed of?
Harrison's 20th Ed. Chapter 244 Page 1740

A. Atrial-like muscle
B. Ventricular-like muscle
C. Specialized conduction tissue
D. All of the above

594. Which of the following is not a feature of Wolff-Parkinson-White (WPW) syndrome?
Harrison's 20th Ed. Chapter 244 Page 1740

A. Short PR interval (< 0.12 sec.)
B. Slurred upstroke of QRS complex (delta wave)
C. Wide QRS complex
D. Prolonged QT interval

595. Which of the following is not true regarding Wolff-Parkinson-White syndrome?
Harrison's 20th Ed. Chapter 244 Page 1740

A. During PSVT in WPW, impulse is conducted antegradely over normal AV system and retrogradely through bypass tract
B. Atrial flutter and AF are common
C. Ventricular responses during atrial flutter or fibrillation is unusually rapid and may cause VF
D. Quinidine or flecainide slow conduction and increase refractoriness primarily of the AV node

596. In AV reentry tachycardia, relation between P wave and QRS complex is?
Harrison's 20th Ed. Chapter 244 Page 1740

A. P waves are simultaneous with a narrow QRS complex
B. P waves always precede the QRS
C. P waves always follow the QRS
D. Any of the above

Unlike typical AVNRT, in AVRT, P waves always follow QRS & are never simultaneous with QRS complex because ventricles must be activated before reentry wavefront reaches AP and conducts back to atrium.

597. Most common tachycardia caused by an accessory pathway is?
Harrison's 20th Ed. Chapter 244 Page 1740

A. Macroreentrant atrial tachycardia
B. Antidromic AV reentry
C. Orthodromic AV reentry
D. Permanent junctional reciprocating tachycardia (PJRT)

The most common tachycardia caused by an AP is the PSVT designated orthodromic AV reentry. The circulating reentry wavefront propagates from the atrium anterogradely over the AV node and His-Purkinje system to the ventricles and then reenters the atria via retrograde conduction over the AP.

598. Which of the following about permanent junctional reciprocating tachycardia (PJRT) is false?
Harrison's 20th Ed. Chapter 244 Page 1741

A. Slow AP conduction
B. Incessant tachycardia
C. Tachycardia-induced cardiomyopathy
D. None of the above

599. Which of the following about permanent junctional reciprocating tachycardia (PJRT) is false?
Circulation. 2016;134:1655-1663

A. Incessant orthodromic AVRT
B. Involves a slowly conducting, concealed, usually posteroseptal accessory pathway
C. Produces delayed atrial activation & a long RP interval
D. None of the above

600. Which of the following is the most common mechanism in preexcited tachycardia? *Harrison's 20th Ed. Chapter 244 Page 1741*

A. Macrorerentrant atrial tachycardia
B. Antidromic AV reentry
C. Orthodromic AV reentry
D. Paroxysmal junctional reciprocating tachycardia (PJRT)

601. Which of the following tachycardia is indistinguishable from monomorphic ventricular tachycardia?
Harrison's 20th Ed. Chapter 244 Page 1741

A. Macrorerentrant atrial tachycardia
B. Antidromic AV reentry
C. Orthodromic AV reentry
D. Paroxysmal junctional reciprocating tachycardia (PJRT)

Preexcitated tachycardia occurs when the ventricles are activated by antegrade conduction over the AP. The most common is antidromic AV reentry in which activation propagates from atrium to ventricle via the AP and then conducts retrogradely to the atria via the His-Purkinje system and the AV node.

602. Which of the following is false about preexcited tachycardia?
Harrison's 20th Ed. Chapter 244 Page 1741

A. Presence of preexcitation in sinus rhythm
B. Atrium to ventricle activation via the AP
C. Ventricle to atrium activation via the AV node
D. None of the above

603. Preexcited tachycardia occurs if an AP allows antegrade conduction to ventricles during?
Harrison's 20th Ed. Chapter 244 Page 1741

A. AT
B. Atrial flutter
C. Atrial fibrillation
D. All of the above

604. Which of the following is contraindicated during preexcited AF?
Harrison's 20th Ed. Chapter 244 Page 1741

A. Diltiazem
B. Intravenous adenosine
C. Intravenous amiodarone
D. All of the above

Administration of AV nodal blocking agents like oral or intravenous verapamil, diltiazem, beta blockers, intravenous adenosine, and intravenous amiodarone are contraindicated during preexcited AF.

605. Rapid preexcited tachycardia should be treated with?
Harrison's 20th Ed. Chapter 244 Page 1741

A. Electrical cardioversion
B. Intravenous procainamide
C. Intravenous ibutilide
D. Any of the above

Rapid preexcited tachycardia should be treated with electrical cardioversion or intravenous procainamide or ibutilide, which may terminate the arrhythmia or slow the ventricular rate.

606. In preexcited atrial fibrillation, what duration of shortest R-R interval indicate a risk of sudden death?

Harrison's 20th Ed. Chapter 244 Page 1741

A. < 250 ms
B. < 300 ms
C. < 350 ms
D. < 400 ms

In preexcited atrial fibrillation, shortest R-R intervals between preexcited QRS complexes of <250 ms indicate a risk of sudden death.

607. Patients with WPW syndrome may have wide-complex tachycardia due to?

Harrison's 20th Ed. Chapter 244 Page 1741

A. Antidromic AV reentry
B. Orthodromic AV with bundle branch block
C. Preexcited tachycardia
D. Any of the above

Patients with WPW syndrome may have wide-complex tachycardia due to antidromic AV reentry, orthodromic AV with bundle branch block, or a preexcited tachycardia, and treatment depends on the underlying rhythm.

608. Which of the following is a complication of catheter ablation?

Harrison's 20th Ed. Chapter 244 Page 1742

A. AV block
B. Cardiac tamponade
C. Thromboemboli
D. All of the above

Serious complications of catheter ablation occur in <3% of patients and include AV block, cardiac tamponade, thromboemboli, coronary artery injury, and vascular access complications. Procedure mortality is <1 in 1000 patients.

609. Which of the following rhythms is associated with WPW syndrome?

Harrison's 20th Ed. Chapter 244 Page 1741 Figure 244-3

A. Sinus rhythm demonstrating antegrade conduction over the AP and AV node
B. Orthodromic AVRT using retrograde conduction over the AP and antegrade conduction over the AV node
C. Antidromic AVRT using retrograde conduction over the AV node and antegrade conduction over the AP
D. All of the above

Three most common rhythms associated with WPW syndrome: sinus rhythm demonstrating antegrade conduction over the AP and AV node; orthodromic AVRT using retrograde conduction over the AP and antegrade conduction over the AV node; and antidromic AVRT using retrograde conduction over the AV node and antegrade conduction over the AP.

610. Which of the following can cause Wide–QRS Complex Tachycardia?

Circulation. 2016;134:1655-1663

A. SVT with aberrant conduction
B. SVT with pre-existing bundle-branch block
C. Paced rhythm
D. All of the above

Causes of Wide–QRS Complex Tachycardia are Ventricular tachycardia, SVT with pre-existing bundle-branch block or intraventricular conduction defect, SVT with aberrant conduction due to tachycardia (normal QRS when in sinus rhythm), SVT with wide QRS related to electrolyte or metabolic disorder, SVT with conduction over an accessory pathway (pre-excitation), Paced rhythm, Artifact.

611. Wide-complex tachycardia includes which of the following?

Harrison's 20th Ed. Chapter 244 Page 1742

A. Ventricular tachycardia
B. PSVT with bundle branch block aberrancy
C. Preexcited tachycardia
D. All of the above

Wide-complex tachycardia includes ventricular tachycardia, PSVT with bundle branch block aberrancy and preexcited tachycardia.

612. Very irregular wide-complex tachycardia should be managed with?

Harrison's 20th Ed. Chapter 244 Page 1742

A. Cardioversion
B. Intravenous procainamide
C. Intravenous ibutilide
D. Any of the above

Very irregular wide-complex tachycardia should be managed with cardioversion, intravenous procainamide or ibutilide, which presumes preexcited atrial fibrillation or flutter.

613. Intravenous adenosine terminates PSVT episodes by transiently blocking conduction in?

Harrison's 20th Ed. Chapter 244 Page 1742

A. AV node
B. Accessory pathway
C. AV node + accessory pathway
D. None of the above

Intravenous adenosine terminates PSVT episodes by transiently blocking conduction in the AV node.

Common Atrial Flutter, Macroreentrant, and Multifocal Atrial Tachycardias

614. Which of the following statements is false about macroreentrant arrhythmias?
Harrison's 20th Ed. Chapter 245 Page 1743

A. Macroreentrant arrhythmias involving atrial myocardium are called AFL
B. Nonfocal source of an atrial arrhythmia
C. AFL is poorly tolerated than AF
D. None of the above

Macroreentrant nonfocal arrhythmias involving the atrial myocardium are referred to collectively as AFL.

615. Cavotricuspid isthmus-dependent atrial flutter is known as?
Harrison's 20th Ed. Chapter 245 Page 1743

A. Common right atrial flutter
B. Left atrial flutter
C. Perimitral left atrial tlutter
D. None of the above

Common right atrial flutter is also known as sub-Eustachian or cavotricuspid isthmus flutter. Macroreentrant atrial tachycardia is due to a large reentry circuit, often associated with areas of scar in the atria. Common or typical right atrial futter is due to a circuit that revolves around the tricuspid valve annulus, bounded anteriorly by the annulus and posteriorly by functional conduction block in the crista terminalis. The wavefront passes through an isthmus between the inferior vena cava and the tricuspid valve annulus, known as the sub-Eustachian or cavotricuspid isthmus.

616. Atrial flutter is a form of atrial reentry localized to the?
Harrison's 20th Ed. Chapter 245 Page 1743

A. Right atrium
B. Left atrium
C. Both atria
D. Both atria and AV node

617. Typical AFL circuit rotates around?
Harrison's 20th Ed. Chapter 245 Page 1743

A. Mitral valve annulus
B. Tricuspid valve annulus
C. Aortic valve annulus
D. Pulmonary valve annulus

618. In ECG, flutter waves of atrial flutter are most prominent in?
Harrison's 20th Ed. Chapter 245 Page 1743

A. Inferior leads
B. Anterior leads
C. Posterior leads
D. Lateral leads

Typical AFL circuit rotates in right atrium around tricuspid valve annulus. Counterclockwise right AFL with superiorly directed activation of interatrial septum produces saw-toothed appearance of P waves in ECG leads II, III and aVF. Clockwise rotation of right atrial circuit produces predominantly positive P waves in leads II, III, and aVF.

619. In atrial flutter, the atrial rate is?
Harrison's 20th Ed. Chapter 245 Page 1743

A. 150 and 240 bpm
B. 240 and 300 bpm
C. 300 and 400 bpm
D. 400 and 550 bpm

Classic or typical right AFL has an atrial rate of 240 - 300 beats/minute with a ventricular response at 2:1 or 120 - 150 beats/minute.

620. Which of the following is not an ECG feature of common right atrial flutter?
Harrison's 20th Ed. Chapter 245 Page 1744 Figure 245-1

A. Atrial rate 240–300 beats/minute
B. Positive P waves in lead V_1
C. Negative "sawtooth" pattern in lead II
D. QRS duration > 0.12 seconds

Common right atrial flutter or cavotricuspid isthmus flutter, shows on ECG positive P waves in lead V1 & negative "sawtooth" pattern in lead II, typical of counterclockwise rotation relative to the tricuspid valve annulus.

621. Which of the following is false about atypical atrial flutter?
Harrison's 20th Ed. Chapter 245 Page 1743

A. Not dependent on conduction through cavotricuspid isthmus
B. Can occur in either atrium
C. Almost always associated with areas of atrial scar
D. None of the above

622. Atypical atrial flutter can be difficult to distinguish from?
Harrison's 20th Ed. Chapter 245 Page 1743

A. Atrial fibrillation
B. Focal AT
C. Paroxysmal supraventricular tachycardia
D. AV Nodal reentrant tachycardia

623. Which of the following drugs is particularly effective for conversion of atrial flutter to sinus rhythm?
Harrison's 20th Ed. Chapter 245 Page 1743

A. Ibutilide
B. Beta blocker
C. Calcium antagonist
D. Digitalis

In AFL, rate control with calcium antagonists (diltiazem, verapamil), beta blockers, and/or digoxin is difficult. In patients with high anesthetic risk, pharmacologic cardioversion with procainamide, amiodarone or ibultilide is appropriate. Antiarrhythmic drug therapy may enhance efficacy of direct current cardioversion & maintenance of sinus rhythm after cardioversion.

624. Which of the following drugs is useful in preventing recurrences of atrial flutter?
Harrison's 20th Ed. Chapter 245 Page 1743

A. Dofetilide
B. Sotalol
C. Amiodarone
D. All of the above

For recurrent episodes, antiarrhythmic drug therapy with sotalol, dofetilide, disopyramide and amiodarone is effective.

625. Which of the following statements about multifocal atrial tachycardia (MAT) is false?

Harrison's 20th Ed. Chapter 245 Page 1745

A. Defined as ≥ 3 consecutive P waves of different morphologies at rates >100 beats/minute
B. Common following theophylline administration
C. Irregular ventricular rate
D. High incidence of VF

There is a high incidence of AF in patients with MAT.

626. Which of the following is the signature tachycardia of significant pulmonary disease?

Harrison's 20th Ed. Chapter 245 Page 1745

A. Atrial flutter
B. Atrial fibrillation
C. Multifocal atrial tachycardia
D. AV Nodal reentrant tachycardia

Multifocal AT (MAT) is the signature tachycardia of patients with significant pulmonary disease.

627. Which of the following about multifocal atrial tachycardia is false?

Harrison's 20th Ed. Chapter 245 Page 1745

A. Signature tachycardia of significant pulmonary disease
B. Clear isoelectric intervals between P waves on ECG
C. Absence of any intervening sinus rhythm
D. None of the above

Macroreentrant ATs represent continuous atrial activation and isoelectric baseline between P waves is frequently absent.

628. Electrical cardioversion has no effect in which of the following?

Harrison's 20th Ed. Chapter 245 Page 1745

A. Atrial flutter
B. Atrial fibrillation
C. Multifocal atrial tachycardia
D. Paroxysmal supraventricular tachycardia

Atrial Fibrillation

629. Which of the following is characteristic of Atrial fibrillation?
Harrison's 20th Ed. Chapter 246 Page 1746

A. Disorganized, rapid, and irregular atrial activation
B. Loss of atrial contraction
C. Irregular ventricular rate determined by AV nodal conduction
D. All of the above

Atrial fibrillation (AF) is characterized by disorganized, rapid, and irregular atrial activation with loss of atrial contraction and an irregular ventricular rate that is determined by AV nodal conduction. Patients with high vagal tone or AV nodal conduction disease have slow ventricular rates.

630. Which of the following is characteristic of Atrial fibrillation?
Harrison's 20th Ed. Chapter 246 Page 1746 Figure 246-1

A. Paroxysmal AF is initiated by premature beats
B. Persistent AF is associated with atrial structural and electrophysiologic remodeling
C. Triggering foci are an important cause of AF
D. All of the above

631. In atrial fibrillation, the ventricular rate is usually?
Harrison's 20th Ed. Chapter 246 Page 1746

A. 120 and 160 bpm
B. 150 and 180 bpm
C. 200 and 260 bpm
D. 250 and 280 bpm

AF produces disorganized, rapid & irregular atrial activation with irregular ventricular response. Depending on conduction properties of AV junction, rate varies between 120 & 160 beats/minute.

632. Which of the following is the most common sustained arrhythmia?
Harrison's 20th Ed. Chapter 246 Page 1746

A. Atrial flutter
B. Atrial fibrillation
C. AV nodal reentrant tachycardia (AVNRT)
D. None of the above

AF is the most common sustained arrhythmia.

633. Which of the following about AF is false?
Harrison's 20th Ed. Chapter 246 Page 1746

A. ~95% of AF patients are older than 60 years
B. Prevalence by age 80 years is ~10%
C. Lifetime risk of developing AF over 40 years is ~25%
D. None of the above

634. Risk factor for developing AF is?
Harrison's 20th Ed. Chapter 246 Page 1746

A. Hypertension
B. Diabetes mellitus
C. Sleep apnea
D. All of the above

AF is a marker for heart disease. Risk factors for developing AF are age, hypertension, diabetes mellitus, cardiac disease, obesity and sleep apnea.

635. AF is associated with increased risk of?
Harrison's 20th Ed. Chapter 246 Page 1746

A. Heart failure
B. Stroke
C. Dementia
D. All of the above

AF is associated with increased risk of mortality, heart failure, stroke and dementia.

636. AF is associated with?
Harrison's 20th Ed. Chapter 246 Page 1746

A. Hyperthyroidism
B. Acute alcohol intoxication
C. Pulmonary embolism
D. All of the above

AF is associated with an acute precipitating factor such as hyperthyroidism, acute alcohol intoxication or an acute illness including myocardial infarction or pulmonary embolism.

637. Paroxysmal AF is defined by episodes that start spontaneously & stop within?
Harrison's 20th Ed. Chapter 246 Page 1746

A. 24 hours of onset
B. 3 days of onset
C. 7 days of onset
D. 14 days of onset

Paroxysmal AF is defined by episodes that start spontaneously and stop within 7 days of onset.

638. Long-standing persistent AF is defined as?
Harrison's 20th Ed. Chapter 246 Page 1746

A. AF > 7 days
B. AF > 1 month
C. AF > 3 months
D. AF > 1 year

Long-standing persistent AF (>1 year), significant fibrosis is usually present and it is difficult to restore and maintain sinus rhythm.

639. Paroxysmal AF is triggered by automatic foci located in?
Harrison's 20th Ed. Chapter 246 Page 1746

A. Left atrium
B. Right atrium
C. Pulmonary veins
D. Left atrial appendage

640. Which of the following relates best to AF initiation & maintenance?
Harrison's 20th Ed. Chapter 246 Page 1746

A. Atrial scarring
B. Atrialized musculature that enters pulmonary veins
C. Accessory atrio-ventricular tracts
D. All of the above

Drivers responsible for initiation and maintenance of AF originate from atrialized musculature that enters the pulmonary veins.

641. AF, episodes are often initiated by rapidly firing foci within?
Harrison's 20th Ed. Chapter 246 Page 1746

A. Pulmonary veins
B. Myocardial sleeves around superior vena cava (SVC)
C. Myocardial sleeves around coronary sinus
D. All of the above

642. Persistent AF is associated with?
Harrison's 20th Ed. Chapter 246 Page 1746

A. Atrial structural remodeling
B. Atrial electrophysiologic remodeling
C. Triggering foci in many patients
D. All of the above

Persistent AF is associated with atrial structural, electrophysiologic remodeling and triggering foci in many patients.

643. It is difficult to convert AF to sinus rhythm and/or maintain it, despite therapy, when the left atrial diameter exceeds?
Harrison's 19th Ed. 1487

A. 2.5 cm
B. 3.5 cm
C. 4.5 cm
D. 5.5 cm

644. Clinical consequences of AF are related to?
Harrison's 20th Ed. Chapter 246 Page 1746

A. Rapid ventricular rates
B. Loss of atrial contribution to ventricular filling
C. Predisposition to thrombus formation in left atrial appendage
D. All of the above

Clinical consequences of AF are related to rapid ventricular rates, loss of atrial contribution to ventricular filling, and predisposition to thrombus formation in the left atrial appendage with potential embolization.

645. Treatment for AF is primarily guided by?
Harrison's 20th Ed. Chapter 246 Page 1746

A. Patients' symptoms
B. Hemodynamic effect of AF
C. Duration of AF
D. All of the above

Treatment for AF is primarily guided by patients' symptoms, the hemodynamic effect of AF, the duration of AF, the risk of stroke and the underlying heart disease.

646. Electric cardioversion is done in patients of new-onset AF who have?
Harrison's 20th Ed. Chapter 246 Page 1746

A. Severe hypotension
B. Pulmonary edema
C. Angina
D. All of the above

647. In AF, if a patient's clinical status is severely compromised, which of the following is the treatment of choice?
Harrison's 20th Ed. Chapter 246 Page 1746

A. β adrenergic blocker
B. Calcium channel antagonist
C. Digitalis
D. Electrical cardioversion

648. Electrical cardioversion for new-onset AF is accomplished through delivery of?
Harrison's 20th Ed. Chapter 246 Page 1746

A. 40 J
B. 100 J
C. 200 J
D. 400 J

New-onset AF that produces severe hypotension, pulmonary edema, or angina should be electrically cardioverted starting with a QRS synchronous shock of 200 J, ideally after sedation or anesthesia. Anticoagulation strategies for new-onset AF are debated.

649. In AF, pretreatment with which of the following drugs facilitates cardioversion?
Harrison's 20th Ed. Chapter 246 Page 1746

A. Ibutilide
B. Beta blocker
C. Calcium antagonist
D. Digitalis

IV ibutilide may be used in selected patients to facilitate termination with direct current (DC) cardioversion. It should not be used in patients with prolonged QT interval or severe LV dysfunction because of a significant risk of torsades de Pointes.

650. Anticoagulation must be commenced before cardioversion, if the duration of AF is?
Harrison's 20th Ed. Chapter 246 Page 1747

A. > 3 hours
B. > 6 hours
C. > 12 hours
D. > 48 hours

If the duration of AF is unclear or is known to be >48 hours, anticoagulation must be commenced before cardioversion.

651. The major source of thromboembolism & stroke in AF is formation of thrombus in?
Harrison's 20th Ed. Chapter 246 Page 1747

A. Left atrial appendage
B. Left atrium
C. Left ventricle
D. All of the above

The major source of thromboembolism & stroke in AF is formation of thrombus in the left atrial appendage where flow is relatively stagnant.

652. Which of the following patients undergoing cardioversion to restore sinus rhythm are at high risk for stroke?
Harrison's 20th Ed. Chapter 246 Page 1747

A. Rheumatic mitral stenosis
B. Hypertrophic cardiomyopathy
C. Marked left atrial enlargement
D. All of the above

Patients with a prior history of embolic events, rheumatic mitral stenosis, or hypertrophic cardiomyopathy with marked left atrial enlargement are at high risk for stroke when undergoing cardioversion to restore sinus rhythm.

653. In AF, conversion to sinus rhythm by cardioversion should be done after proper anticoagulation for?
Harrison's 20th Ed. Chapter 246 Page 1747

A. 1 week
B. 2 weeks
C. 3 weeks
D. 4 weeks

654. In AF, following cardioversion, anticoagulation must be maintained for? *Harrison's 20th Ed. Chapter 246 Page 1747*

A. 1 week
B. 2 weeks
C. 3 weeks
D. 4 weeks

For patients who do not warrant early cardioversion of AF, anticoagulation should be maintained for at least 3 weeks with the INR confirmed to be >1.8 on at least two separate occasions prior to attempts at cardioversion and maintained for a minimum of 4 weeks after cardioversion.

655. Ventricular rate control for acute AF is best established with?
Harrison's 20th Ed. Chapter 246 Page 1747

A. Adenosine
B. Beta blockers
C. Amiodarone
D. All of the above

Ventricular rate control for acute AF is best established with beta blockers and/or calcium channel blocking agents, verapamil or diltiazem. Digoxin may add to the rate-controlling benefit of other agents but is uncommonly used as a stand-alone agent, especially in acute AF.

656. Goal of acute rate control in AF is to reduce ventricular rate to?
Harrison's 20th Ed. Chapter 246 Page 1747

A. < 70 / minute
B. < 80 / minute
C. < 90 / minute
D. < 100 / minute

The goal of acute rate control in AF is to reduce the ventricular rate to <100/minute.

657. 'Tachycardia-induced cardiomyopathy' is caused by?
Harrison's 20th Ed. Chapter 246 Page 1747

A. Digitalis
B. Atrial Fibrillation
C. Thyrotoxicosis
D. Acute alcoholic intoxication

658. In CHA_2DS_2-VASc Score, 2 refers to?
Harrison's 20th Ed. Chapter 246 Page 1748 Table 246-1

A. Age and angina
B. Stroke and sex
C. Two points for age and stroke
D. Half points for age and stroke

659. In AF, anticoagulation is recommended for a CHA_2DS_2-VASc score of?
Harrison's 20th Ed. Chapter 246 Page 1748

A. ≥ 1
B. ≥ 2
C. ≥ 3
D. ≥ 4

Anticoagulation is recommended for a CHA_2DS_2-VASc score of ≥2.

660. In high-risk patients with AF, which of the following is not advised?
Harrison's 20th Ed. Chapter 246 Page 1748

A. Dabigatran
B. Aspirin and clopidogrel
C. Rivaroxaban
D. Apixaban

Antiplatelet agents (aspirin and clopidogrel) are not given in high-risk patients with AF because they have substantially less effect. Major options for anticoagulation are antithrombin inhibitor dabigitran, factor Xa inhibitors rivaroxaban, apixaban, and edoxaban, vitamin K antagonist warfarin.

661. Which of the following anticoagulant is preferred for patients with rheumatic mitral stenosis or mechanical heart valves?
Harrison's 20th Ed. Chapter 246 Page 1748

A. Dabigatran
B. Warfarin
C. Rivaroxaban
D. Apixaban

Warfarin is the agent required for patients with rheumatic mitral stenosis or mechanical heart valves.

662. Which of the following newer oral anticoagulants have renal excretion?
Harrison's 20th Ed. Chapter 246 Page 1748

A. Dabigatran
B. Rivaroxaban
C. Apixaban
D. All of the above

Dabigatran, rivaroxaban and apixaban have renal excretion and cannot be used with severe renal insufficiency.

663. Which of the following is a thrombin inhibitor?
Harrison's 20th Ed. Chapter 246 Page 1749

A. Warfarin
B. Dabigatran
C. Rivaroxaban
D. Apixaban

664. Which of the following oral anticoagulants has no reversal agent for bleeding?
Harrison's 20th Ed. Chapter 246 Page 1749

A. Dabigatran
B. Rivaroxaban
C. Apixaban
D. All of the above

665. Which of the following is a reversal agent of anticoagulants?
Harrison's 20th Ed. Chapter 246 Page 1749

A. Idarucizumab
B. Andexanet alfa
C. Ciraparantag
D. All of the above

A reversal agent, idarucizumab, is available for dabigatran and reversal agents for the Xa inhibitors like andexanet alfa and ciraparantag are being evaluated.

666. Risk factors for bleeding in patients on chronic anticoagulation include?

Harrison's 20th Ed. Chapter 246 Page 1749

A. Heart failure
B. Renal insufficiency
C. Excessive alcohol consumption
D. All of the above

Risk factors for bleeding in patients on chronic anticoagulation include age >65-75 years, heart failure, renal insufficiency, excessive alcohol or nonsteroidal anti-inflammatory, aspirin and a thienopyridine drug use.

667. AF is associated with?

Harrison's 20th Ed. Chapter 246 Page 1749

A. Obesity
B. Hypertension
C. Sleep apnea
D. All of the above

AF is associated with obesity, hypertension, excessive alcohol use and sleep apnea.

668. Which of the following is false about rhythm control strategy with antiarrhythmic medications?

Harrison's 20th Ed. Chapter 246 Page 1749

A. Did not improve survival or symptoms
B. Drug therapy group had more hospitalizations
C. More likely to be beneficial in younger patients
D. None of the above

669. A rhythm control strategy is usually selected for patients with?

Harrison's 20th Ed. Chapter 246 Page 1749

A. Symptomatic paroxysmal AF
B. Recurrent episodes of symptomatic persistent AF
C. AF with difficult rate control
D. All of the above

A rhythm control strategy is usually selected for patients with symptomatic paroxysmal AF, recurrent episodes of symptomatic persistent AF, AF with difficult rate control, and AF that has resulted in depressed ventricular function or that aggravates heart failure.

670. Which drug is preferred in AF to maintain sinus rhythm in patients without evidence of structural heart disease?

Harrison's 20th Ed. Chapter 246 Page 1749

A. Sotalol
B. Flecainide
C. Amiodarone
D. Dofetilide

In AF patients without evidence of structural heart disease, use of flecainide, disopyramide or propafenone (class I sodium channel-blocking agents) is well tolerated and does not have significant proarrhythmia risk.

671. Which drug is preferred in AF to maintain sinus rhythm in patients with evidence of structural heart disease?

Harrison's 20th Ed. Chapter 246 Page 1749

A. Disopyramide
B. Flecainide
C. Propafenone
D. Dofetilide

Class III agents sotalol and dofetilide can be given to patients with coronary artery disease or structural heart disease but have a ~3% risk of inducing excessive QT prolongation and torsades des pointes.

672. The Cox-MAZE procedure is a surgical approach to cure?

Harrison's 20th Ed. Chapter 246 Page 1749

A. AF
B. VT
C. PSVT
D. All of the above

Most ablation strategies isolate atrial muscle sleeves entering the pulmonary veins which are a source of triggers responsible for initiation of AF. Risks include pulmonary vein stenosis, atrioesophageal fistula, systemic embolic events & perforation/tamponade. The Cox-Maze procedure is designed to interrupt all macroreentrant circuits that might potentially develop in the atria, thereby precluding the ability of the atria to fibrillate.

673. Exogenous digoxin-like immunoreactive substances include?

N Engl J Med. 2018;378:1931-8

A. Spironolactone
B. Canrenone
C. Chinese herbal medications
D. All of the above

Exogenous digoxin-like immunoreactive substances include spironolactone, canrenone and Chinese herbal medications.

674. Which of the following is related to digoxin toxicity?

N Engl J Med. 2018;378:1931-8

A. Chloropsia
B. Erythropsia
C. Cyanopsia
D. Xanthopsia

Xanthopsia refers to yellow vision.

675. Adverse events associated with use of digoxin immune Fab include?

N Engl J Med. 2018;378:1931-8

A. Heart failure
B. Hypokalemia
C. Hypersensitivity to ovine Fab epitopes
D. All of the above

Adverse events associated with the use of digoxin immune Fab include heart failure, hypokalemia, and hypersensitivity to ovine Fab epitopes.

676. Vortex keratopathy is an ocular side effect of which of the following?

S Afr Fam Pract. 2014;56(1):8-14

A. Amiodarone
B. Corticosteroids
C. Chloroquine
D. Acetazolamide

Vortex keratopathy refers to innocuous corneal deposits.

677. Toxic optic neuropathy, with loss of central and colour vision is an ocular side effect of?

S Afr Fam Pract. 2014;56(1):8-14

A. Streptomycin
B. Ethambutol
C. Isoniazid
D. All of the above

678. Which of the following is not an ocular finding in Marfan's syndrome?

S Afr Fam Pract. 2014;56(1):8-14

A. Myopia
B. Retinal haemorrhage
C. Dislocated lens
D. Retinal detachment

679. Which of the following is an ocular manifestation of ankylosing spondylitis?

S Afr Fam Pract. 2014;56(1):8-14

A. Uveitis
B. Scleritis, episcleritis
C. Keratitis
D. All of the above

680. Electrical cardioversion for atrial flutter is accomplished through delivery of?

Harrison's 19th Ed. 1487

A. 20 – 40 J
B. 50 – 100 J
C. 100 – 150 J
D. 150 – 300 J

Organized atrial flutter activity can frequently be terminated with low-energy external cardioversion of 50 - 100 J.

681. Electrical cardioversion for atrioventricular nodal reentrant tachycardia (AVNRT) is accomplished through delivery of?

Harrison's 19th Ed. 1487

A. 20 – 40 J
B. 50 – 100 J
C. 100 – 200 J
D. 200 – 300 J

R wave synchronous DC cardioversion using 100 - 200 J can terminate atrioventricular nodal reentrant tachycardia (AVNRT).

682. Which of the following statements is false?

Harrison's 19th Ed. 1486

A. Pacing does not provoke automatic rhythms
B. Pacing provoke tachycardias due to triggered activity
C. Abnormal automaticity is responsible for APCs & VPCs
D. None of the above

683. Abnormal impulse formation due to triggered activity is related to?

Harrison's 18th Ed. 1879

A. Reentry
B. Extra pathways
C. Myocardial ion channel abnormalities
D. Cellular afterdepolarizations

Abnormal impulse formation is due to the development of triggered activity. Triggered activity is related to cellular afterdepolarizations that occur at the end of the action potential, during phase 3 (early afterdepolarizations), or after the action potential, during phase 4 (late afterdepolarizations).

684. Afterdepolarizations are due to an increase in?

Harrison's 18th Ed. 1879

A. Intracellular calcium accumulation
B. Altered sodium transport
C. Altered potassium transport
D. Intracellular potassium deficiency

Afterdepolarizations are attributable to an increase in intracellular calcium accumulation.

685. Early afterdepolarizations are responsible for?

Harrison's 18th Ed. 1879

A. Catecholamine-sensitive VT
B. Atrial tachyarrhythmias caused by digoxin toxicity
C. Torsades des pointes
D. All of the above

Early afterdepolarizations may be responsible for VPCs that trigger torsades des pointes (TDP). Late afterdepolarizations are responsible for atrial, junctional & fascicular tachyarrhythmias caused by digoxin toxicity and for catecholamine-sensitive VT originating in the outflow tract.

686. Late afterdepolarizations in digoxin toxicity may lead to?

Harrison's 18th Ed. 1879

A. Atrial tachyarrhythmias
B. Junctional tachyarrhythmias
C. Fascicular tachyarrhythmias
D. All of the above

Late afterdepolarizations caused by digoxin toxicity may lead to atrial, junctional, and fascicular tachyarrhythmias.

687. Inhomogeneities in myocardial conduction and/or recovery leading to reentry is exaggerated by?

Harrison's 18th Ed. 1879

A. Presence of extra pathways
B. Myocardial ion channel abnormalities
C. Myocardial fibrosis
D. All of the above

Reentry is due to inhomogeneities in myocardial conduction and/or recovery properties. Inhomogeneities can be exaggerated by the presence of extra pathways (WPW syndrome), generalized genetically determined myocardial ion channel abnormalities (long QT syndrome) or by the interruption of normal myocardial patterns of activation due to the development of fibrosis.

688. Which of the following is a genetically determined ion channel abnormality?

Harrison's 18th Ed. 1879

A. Brugada syndrome
B. LQTS
C. Catecholaminergic polymorphic VT
D. All of the above

689. Which of the following statements about mechanism of sustained paroxysmal tachyarrhythmia is false?

Harrison's 19th Ed. 1486

A. Electrophysiologic inhomogeneity
B. Unidirectional block in one pathway
C. Fast conduction over an alternative pathway
D. Reexcitation of the initially blocked pathway

690. Which of the following statements about mechanism of tachyarrhythmia is false?
Harrison's 19th Ed. 1486

A. Reentrant arrhythmias can be reproducibly initiated and terminated by premature complexes and rapid stimulation
B. Myocardial cells do not possess pacemaker activity
C. Tachycardia caused by automaticity cannot be started or stopped by pacing
D. Triggered activity is caused by early afterdepolarizations only

691. Which of the following statements about atrial premature complexes (APCs) is false?
Harrison's 16th Ed. 1342

A. Can be found in over 90% of normal adults
B. May originate from any location in either atrium
C. P wave of APC differs from sinus P wave morphology
D. Conduct to ventricles when they occur late in cardiac cycle

692. Which of the following statements about atrial premature complexes (APCs) is false?
Harrison's 16th Ed. 1342

A. Sum of pre and postextrasystolic PP intervals is less than the sum of two sinus PP intervals
B. QRS complex following most APCs is normal
C. Alcohol, tobacco or adrenergic stimulants precipitate APCs
D. None of the above

693. Which of the following about APCs is false?
Harrison's 18th Ed. 1880

A. Most common arrhythmia
B. Frequently increases with age & structural heart disease
C. Asymptomatic
D. None of the above

694. APCs from which of the following may mimic the sinus P wave morphology?
Harrison's 18th Ed. 1880

A. Right atrial appendage
B. Superior vena cava (SVC)
C. Superior aspect of crista terminalis
D. All of the above

P wave contour differs from that seen during sinus rhythm. APCs from right atrial appendage, superior vena cava (SVC) and superior aspect of the crista terminalis in the region of sinus node may mimic sinus P wave morphology.

695. Which of the following about APCs is false?
Harrison's 18th Ed. 1880

A. APCs characteristically reset the sinus node
B. Sum of pre- & post-APC RR is < 2 sinus PP intervals
C. Class IC antiarrhythmic agents may eliminate APCs
D. None of the above

APCs characteristically reset the sinus node. The resulting sum of the pre- and post-APC RR interval is less than two sinus PP intervals. Class IC antiarrhythmic agents may eliminate the APCs but should be avoided if structural heart disease is present.

696. Which of the following about junctional premature complexes is false?
Harrison's 18th Ed. 1880

A. Extremely uncommon
B. Originate from AV node & His bundle region
C. Produce retrograde atrial activation
D. None of the above

JPCs are extremely uncommon. Complexes originate from AV node & His bundle region & may produce retrograde atrial activation with P wave distorting the initial or terminal portions of QRS complex producing pseudo Q or S waves in leads II, III, and aVF.

697. Incidence of supraventricular tachycardia (SVT) is about?
N Engl J Med. 2006;354:1039-51

A. 35 cases per 100,000 persons per year
B. 70 cases per 100,000 persons per year
C. 100 cases per 100,000 persons per year
D. 150 cases per 100,000 persons per year

698. Prevalence of supraventricular tachycardia is about?
N Engl J Med. 2006;354:1039-51

A. 2.25 per 1000
B. 5 per 1000
C. 10 per 1000
D. 20 per 1000

699. Which of the following symptoms is uncommon in supraventricular tachycardia?
N Engl J Med. 2006;354:1039-51

A. Palpitations
B. Dyspnea
C. Light-headedness
D. Syncope

700. Which of the following statements about SVT is false?
N Engl J Med. 2006;354:1039-51

A. Most have a reentry mechanism
B. Classified according to location of reentry circuit
C. ~ 60% are due to AV nodal reentry circuit
D. SVT is usually associated with structural heart disease

701. In SVT, adenosine is contraindicated in patients with?
N Engl J Med. 2006;354:1039-51

A. In heart-transplant recipients
B. In patients with severe obstructive lung disease
C. In patients with tachycardia with a wide QRS complex
D. All of the above

702. Which of the following drugs are used in treatment of SVT?
N Engl J Med. 2006;354:1039-51

A. Adenosine
B. Intravenous verapamil
C. Intravenous beta-blocker
D. All of the above

703. Which of the following drugs are used in treatment of SVT?
N Engl J Med. 2006;354:1039-51

A. Intravenous Procainamide
B. Intravenous Ibutilide
C. Intravenous Propafenone
D. All of the above

704. Danger of radiofrequency catheter ablation of accessory pathway in SVT is?
N Engl J Med. 2006;354:1039-51

A. Atrioventricular block that requires pacemaker therapy
B. Damage to an artery, bleeding, arteriovenous fistula
C. Coronary venous thrombosis
D. All of the above

705. Danger of radiofrequency catheter ablation of accessory pathway in SVT is?
N Engl J Med. 2006;354:1039-51

A. Pulmonary embolism
B. Myocardial perforation
C. Valvular damage
D. All of the above

706. Characteristic of radiofrequency current used for catheter ablation of accessory pathways in SVT is?
N Engl J Med. 2006;354:1039-51

A. Low-voltage, high-frequency form of electrical energy
B. High-voltage, low-frequency form of electrical energy
C. High-voltage, high-frequency form of electrical energy
D. Low-voltage, low-frequency form of electrical energy

Catheter ablation, directed at elimination or modification of slow pathway conduction, is very effective in permanently eliminating AVNRT.

707. Which of the following statements about SVT is false?
Harrison's 19th Ed. 1486

A. Most common cause is AV nodal reentrant tachycardia
B. More commonly observed in women
C. Presents as regular narrow QRS complex tachycardia @ 120 to 250 bpm
D. APCs that initiate the SVT has a normal PR interval

APC initiating AVNRT is characteristically followed by a long PR interval consistent with conduction via the slow pathway.

708. Which of the following about sinus tachycardia is false?
N Engl J Med. 2012;367:1438-48

A. Sudden in onset and recession
B. Regular
C. Rate < 220 bpm minus the patient's age
D. P waves precede the QRS complex

Sinus tachycardia is gradual in onset and recession. The heart rate is regular and classically does not exceed 220 beats per minute minus the patient's age. In sinus tachycardia, P waves precede the QRS complex.

709. Atrial flutter results from a reentrant circuit around?
N Engl J Med. 2012;367:1438-48

A. Mitral valve
B. Tricuspid valve
C. Aortic valve
D. Pulmonary valve

Atrial flutter, the second most common pathologic supraventricular tachycardia, results from a reentrant circuit around the tricuspid valve in the right atrium.

710. Which of the following parameter helps distinguish atrial flutter from other supraventricular tachycardias?
N Engl J Med. 2012;367:1438-48

A. Regularity
B. Rate
C. Blood pressure
D. Jugular venous pulsations

Atrial flutter is an organized regular rhythm that is characterized by an atrial rate of 280 to 300 beats per minute and with 2:1 conduction in AV node results in a ventricular rate of 140 to 150 beats per minute. Flutter waves are usually obscured by T waves, making the surface ECG tracing for this tachycardia difficult to distinguish from that of other supraventricular tachycardias. However, a heart rate of 150 beats per minute is highly suggestive of this tachyarrhythmia.

711. Which of the following occurs more frequently in the pediatric population?
N Engl J Med. 2012;367:1438-48

A. Atrioventricular nodal reentrant tachycardia
B. Atrioventricular reciprocating tachycardia
C. Atrial tachycardia
D. Atrial flutter

Atrioventricular nodal reentrant tachycardia is most common in persons >20 years of age, whereas atrioventricular reciprocating tachycardia occurs more frequently in pediatric population.

712. Regular supraventricular tachycardias include all except?
N Engl J Med. 2012;367:1438-48

A. Atrial tachycardia (AT)
B. Atrioventricular nodal reentrant tachycardia (AVNRT)
C. Atrioventricular reciprocating tachycardia (AVRT)
D. Multifocal atrial tachycardia (MAT)

Regular supraventricular tachycardias include sinus tachycardia, atrial flutter (AFL), atrioventricular nodal reentrant tachycardia (AVNRT), atrioventricular reciprocating tachycardia (AVRT), and atrial tachycardia (AT). Orthodromic AVRT is more common than antidromic AVRT. Irregular supraventricular tachycardias include atrial fibrillation (AF), AFL when it occurs in a patient with variable AV block, multifocal atrial tachycardia (MAT) & sinus rhythm with multiple atrial premature beats.

713. Which of the following arrhythmias are seen with bypass tracts?
N Engl J Med. 2012;367:1438-48

A. Orthodromic AV reentry
B. Antidromic AV reentry
C. Wide irregular QRS complex (atrial fibrillation)
D. All of the above

Three arrhythmias are seen with bypass tracts: a narrow regular QRS complex (orthodromic; conduction down the atrioventricular node and retrograde conduction through the bypass tract), a wide regular QRS complex (antidromic; conduction down the bypass tract and retrograde conduction through the atrioventricular node), and a wide irregular QRS complex (atrial fibrillation).

714. Heart rate regularity is defined as beat-to-beat timing variation of less than?

N Engl J Med. 2012;367:1438-48

A. 5%
B. 10%
C. 15%
D. 20%

Regularity is defined as variation of less than 10% in beat-to-beat timing, but most regular tachycardias actually vary by less than 5%.

715. Which of the following is a wide-complex tachycardia?

N Engl J Med. 2012;367:1438-48

A. Ventricular tachycardia
B. Ventricular fibrillation
C. Torsades de pointes
D. All of the above

Wide-complex tachycardias are caused by ventricular arrhythmia (ventricular tachycardia, ventricular fibrillation, and torsades de pointes or polymorphic ventricular tachycardia) or supraventricular tachycardias with aberrant conduction resulting from disease in His–Purkinje system (left or right bundle-branch block), a bypass tract (Wolff–Parkinson–White syndrome), with depolarization of ventricle from bypass tract; and a ventricular paced rhythm from a pacemaker.

716. Vagomimetic maneuvers include?

N Engl J Med. 2012;367:1438-48

A. Carotid sinus massage
B. Valsalva maneuver
C. Immersion of face in cold water (dive response)
D. All of the above

Vagal maneuvers include Valsalva maneuver, carotid sinus massage, bearing down, and immersion of the face in ice water They increase vagal tone and block the atrioventricular node.

717. Adenosine terminates which of the following?

N Engl J Med. 2012;367:1438-48

A. Atrioventricular nodal reentrant tachycardias
B. Atrioventricular reciprocating tachycardias
C. Atrial tachycardias
D. All of the above

Adenosine, a very short-acting endogenous nucleotide that blocks atrioventricular nodal conduction, terminates nearly all atrioventricular nodal reentrant tachycardias and atrioventricular reciprocating tachycardias as well as up to 80% of atrial tachycardias.

718. Adenosine should not be given in?

N Engl J Med. 2012;367:1438-48

A. Regular wide-complex tachycardias
B. Irregular wide-complex tachycardias
C. Atrioventricular nodal reentrant tachycardias
D. Atrioventricular reciprocating tachycardias

Adenosine is also useful in the differential diagnosis and treatment of wide-complex tachycardias, but it should be given only when these tachycardias are regular, since irregular wide-complex tachycardias may be rendered unstable after the administration of adenosine.

719. Arrhythmias that cause which of the following require urgent electrical cardioversion?

N Engl J Med. 2012;367:1438-48

A. Hypotension
B. Heart failure
C. Coronary ischemia
D. All of the above

Arrhythmias causing hemodynamic instability (hypotension, heart failure, or coronary ischemia) require urgent electrical cardioversion.

720. If hemodynamic compromise is present, which of the following is preferred to terminate atrioventricular nodal reentrant tachycardia?

Harrison's 19th Ed. 1486

A. Intravenous adenosine
B. Intravenous beta blockade
C. Intravenous calcium channel therapy
D. R-wave synchronous DC cardioversion (100 - 200 J)

If hemodynamic compromise is present, R-wave synchronous DC cardioversion using 100–200 J can terminate atrioventricular nodal reentrant tachycardia.

721. Which of the following drugs slow conduction in the antegrade slow pathway in atrioventricular nodal reentrant tachycardia?

Harrison's 19th Ed. 1486

A. Digitalis
B. Beta blockers
C. Calcium channel blockers
D. All of the above

AVNRT prevention may be achieved with drugs that slow conduction in the antegrade slow pathway, such as digitalis, beta blockers, and calcium channel blockers.

722. Which of the following drugs is useful in preventing exercise-precipitated atrioventricular nodal reentrant tachycardia?

Harrison's 19th Ed. 1486

A. Digitalis
B. Beta blockers
C. Calcium channel blockers
D. All of the above

In patients who have a history of exercise-precipitated AVNRT, use of beta blockers frequently eliminates symptoms.

723. Which of the following drugs slow conduction in the antegrade slow pathway in atrioventricular nodal reentrant tachycardia?

Harrison's 19th Ed. 1486

A. Digitalis
B. Beta blockers
C. Calcium channel blockers
D. Flecainide

In patients who do not respond to drug therapy directed at antegrade slow pathway, treatment with class IA or IC agents directed at altering conduction of the fast pathway may be considered.

724. Which of the following is false for carotid sinus massage?

Harrison's 19th Ed. 1486

A. Not performed in patients with carotid arterial bruits
B. Massage one carotid bulb at a time
C. Performed by applying firm pressure just underneath the angle of jaw for up to 10 seconds
D. Patient should be supine with neck extended

Approach to Ventricular Arrhythmias

725. Ventricular arrhythmias originate from?
Harrison's 20th Ed. Chapter 247 Page 1750

A. A focus of myocardial cells
B. A focus of Purkinje cells
C. Reentry through areas of scar
D. All of the above

Ventricular arrhythmias originate from a focus of myocardial or Purkinje cells capable of automaticity, or triggered automaticity, or from reentry through areas of scar or a diseased Purkinje system.

726. Which of the following statements is false?
Harrison's 20th Ed. Chapter 247 Page 1750

A. QRS complex during ventricular arrhythmias is wide (>0.12 s)
B. Two consecutive ventricular beats are ventricular couplets
C. Arterial pressure following premature beats is attenuated
D. None of the above

727. VT is defined as ≥3 consecutive ventricular beats @?
Harrison's 20th Ed. Chapter 247 Page 1750

A. ≥ 90 beats/minute
B. ≥ 100 beats/minute
C. ≥ 120 beats/minute
D. ≥ 150 beats/minute

728. Which of the following statements is false?
Harrison's 20th Ed. Chapter 247 Page 1750

A. Idioventricular rhythm is ≥3 consecutive ventricular beats @ <100 beats/minute
B. Non-sustained VT terminates spontaneously within 30 sec.
C. Sustained VT persists >30 sec. or is terminated by an active intervention
D. None of the above

729. Which of the following is false about ventricular tachycardia (VT) of right ventricular outflow tract origin?
Harrison's 20th Ed. Chapter 247 Page 1751 Figure 247-2

A. Has a left bundle branch block pattern
B. Inferior axis
C. Tall QRS complexes in inferior leads
D. None of the above

730. Which of the following about monomorphic VT is false?
Harrison's 20th Ed. Chapter 247 Page 1750

A. VT that originate from right ventricle produce LBBB like configuration
B. VT that originate from septum produce LBBB like configuration
C. VT that originate from free wall of left ventricle produce RBBB like configuration
D. None of the above

731. Very rapid monomorphic VT is also called?
Harrison's 20th Ed. Chapter 247 Page 1750

A. Ventricular flutter
B. Ventricular fibrillation
C. Idioventricular rhythm
D. Torsade de Pointes

Very rapid monomorphic VT has a sinusoidal appearance and is also called ventricular flutter, because it is not possible to distinguish the QRS complex from the T wave.

732. Relatively slow sinusoidal VTs with wide QRS can be caused by?
Harrison's 20th Ed. Chapter 247 Page 1750

A. Hyperkalemia
B. Toxicity from sodium channel blockers
C. Severe global myocardial ischemia
D. All of the above

Relatively slow sinusoidal VTs with wide QRS indicate slowed ventricular conduction. It can be caused by hyperkalemia, toxicity from sodium channel blockers (flecainide, propafenone, or tricyclic antidepressants) and severe global myocardial ischemia.

733. Polymorphic VT is also called?
Harrison's 20th Ed. Chapter 247 Page 1750

A. Ventricular flutter
B. Ventricular fibrillation
C. Idioventricular rhythm
D. Torsade de Pointes

734. Which of the following about ventricular fibrillation is false?
Harrison's 20th Ed. Chapter 247 Page 1750

A. Continuous irregular activation
B. No discrete QRS complexes
C. Monomorphic or polymorphic VT may transition to VF
D. None of the above

735. Which of the following about idiopathic ventricular arrhythmias is false?
Harrison's 20th Ed. Chapter 247 Page 1750

A. PVCs / VT that occurs without structural heart disease
B. Not associated with a genetic syndrome
C. Not associated with a risk of sudden death
D. None of the above

736. Which of the following can cause syncope?
Harrison's 20th Ed. Chapter 247 Page 1750

A. An episode of VT
B. Neuro-cardiogenic (vasovagal) reflex
C. Orthostatic hypotension
D. All of the above

737. Medications that prolong the QT interval predispose to?
Harrison's 20th Ed. Chapter 247 Page 1752

A. Monomorphic VT
B. Polymorphic VT
C. Idioventricular rhythm
D. All of the above

Medications that prolong the QT interval predispose to polymorphic VT.

738. Which of the following suggests a genetic arrhythmia syndrome?
Harrison's 20th Ed. Chapter 247 Page 1752

A. Dysbiotic features
B. Biochemical features
C. Dysmorphic features
D. Systemic features

Stigmata of neuromuscular disease or dysmorphic features may suggest a genetic arrhythmia syndrome.

739. Which of the following is a genetic arrhythmia syndrome?
Harrison's 20th Ed. Chapter 247 Page 1752

A. Long QT syndrome
B. Brugada syndrome
C. Short QT syndrome
D. All of the above

740. Which of the following is the first choice of therapy for most ventricular arrhythmias?
Harrison's 20th Ed. Chapter 247 Page 1753

A. Beta-adrenergic Blockers
B. Calcium Channel Blockers
C. Sodium Channel Blocking Agents
D. Potassium Channel Blocking Agents

741. Which of the following is a sodium channel blocker?
Harrison's 20th Ed. Chapter 247 Page 1753

A. Quinidine
B. Disopyramide
C. Propafenone
D. All of the above

742. Which of the following is a sodium channel blocker?
Harrison's 20th Ed. Chapter 247 Page 1753

A. Mexiletine
B. Flecainide
C. Propafenone
D. All of the above

743. Which of the following sodium channel blocking agents has a potassium channel blocking effect?
Harrison's 20th Ed. Chapter 247 Page 1753

A. Quinidine
B. Disopyramide
C. Procainamide
D. All of the above

744. Which of the following is false about Dronedarone?
Harrison's 20th Ed. Chapter 247 Page 1754

A. No iodine moiety
B. Efficacy for ventricular arrhythmias is poor
C. Increases mortality in patients with heart failure
D. None of the above

745. Which of the following is a toxicity of amiodarone?
Harrison's 20th Ed. Chapter 247 Page 1754

A. Hyper or hypothyroidism
B. Pneumonitis or pulmonary fibrosis
C. Neuropathy and ocular toxicity
D. All of the above

Premature Ventricular Beats, Non-sustained Ventricular Tachycardia, and Idioventricular Rhythm

746. Which of the following statements about premature ventricular contractions (PVCs) is false?

Harrison's 20th Ed. Chapter 248 Page 1755

A. Can be due to automaticity or reentry
B. Can be a sign of increased sympathetic tone
C. Can be a harbinger of sustained VT or VF
D. None of the above

747. Which of the following statements about PVCs is false?

Harrison's 20th Ed. Chapter 248 Page 1755

A. Smooth uninterrupted contours & sharp QRS deflections suggest an ectopic focus in relatively normal myocardium
B. Broad notching & slurred QRS deflections suggest a diseased myocardial substrate
C. Those with RBBB configuration are more likely to be associated with structural heart disease
D. None of the above

748. Most ventricular arrhythmias that are not associated with structural heart disease have?

Harrison's 20th Ed. Chapter 248 Page 1756

A. Left bundle branch block like configuration
B. Right bundle branch block like configuration
C. Left anterior hemiblock like configuration
D. Left posterior hemiblock like configuration

Most ventricular arrhythmias that are not associated with structural heart disease have a left bundle branch block like configuration.

749. Which of the following about nonsustained VT is false?

Harrison's 20th Ed. Chapter 248 Page 1756

A. Usually monomorphic
B. Rate < 200 beats / minute
C. Lasts less than 8 beats
D. None of the above

Nonsustained VT is usually monomorphic with rates < 200 beats/minute and typically lasts < 8 beats.

750. Which of the following features of nonsustained VT has ominous prognosis?

Harrison's 20th Ed. Chapter 248 Page 1756

A. Very rapid
B. Polymorphic
C. First beat that occurs prior to peak of T-wave ("short-coupled")
D. All of the above

Nonsustained VT that is very rapid, polymorphic, or with a first beat that occurs prior to the peak of the T-wave ("short-coupled") should prompt careful evaluation for underlying disease or genetic syndromes associated with sudden death.

751. Genetic syndromes associated with sudden death include?

Harrison's 20th Ed. Chapter 248 Page 1756

A. Cardiomyopathy
B. Long QT syndrome
C. Arrhythmogenic right ventricular cardiomyopathy
D. All of the above

Genetic syndromes associated with sudden death include cardiomyopathy, long QT syndrome, and arrhythmogenic right ventricular cardiomyopathy.

752. Which of the following is included in 'Genetically determined arrhythmia syndrome'?

Harrison's 20th Ed. Chapter 248 Page 1756

A. Long QT syndrome
B. Brugada syndrome
C. Hypertrophic cardiomyopathy
D. All of the above

753. Which of the following 'Genetically determined arrhythmia syndromes' have autosomal dominant inheritance?

Harrison's 20th Ed. Chapter 248 Page 1756

A. Long QT syndrome
B. Brugada syndrome
C. Hypertrophic cardiomyopathy
D. All of the above

754. Repolarization abnormalities are seen in which of the following genetically determined syndromes ?

Harrison's 20th Ed. Chapter 248 Page 1756

A. Long QT syndrome
B. Brugada syndrome
C. Arrhythmogenic right ventricular cardiomyopathy (ARVC)
D. All of the above

Repolarization abnormalities are seen in genetically determined syndromes associated with sudden death. These include long QT syndrome, Brugada syndrome, arrhythmogenic right ventricular cardiomyopathy (ARVC) and hypertrophic cardiomyopathy.

755. Following recovery from acute MI, which of the following is a marker for depressed ventricular function and increased mortality?

Harrison's 20th Ed. Chapter 248 Page 1756

A. > 10 PVCs per hour
B. Repetitive PVCs with couplets
C. Nonsustained VT
D. All of the above

Following recovery from acute MI, frequent PVCs (> 10 PVCs per hour), repetitive PVCs with couplets and nonsustained VT are markers for depressed ventricular function and increased mortality, but routine antiarrhythmic drug therapy to suppress these arrhythmias is not warranted.

756. Which of the following is a potassium channel blocker?

Harrison's 20th Ed. Chapter 248 Page 1757

A. Mexiletine
B. Quinidine
C. Disopyramide
D. Dofetilide

Antiarrhythmic drugs that block cardiac sodium channel are flecainide, propafenone, mexiletine, quinidine and disopyramide. Antiarrhythmic drug that block cardiac potassium channel blocker is dofetilide.

757. Depression of ventricular function occurs when PVCs account for?

Harrison's 20th Ed. Chapter 248 Page 1757

A. > 1– 2% of total beats over a 24-hour period
B. > 2 – 5% of total beats over a 24-hour period
C. > 5 – 10% of total beats over a 24-hour period
D. > 15 – 20% of total beats over a 24-hour period

Depression of ventricular function rarely occurs unless PVCs account for more than 15–20% of total beats over a 24-hour period.

758. Idioventricular rhythms are commonly associated with?

Harrison's 20th Ed. Chapter 248 Page 1757

A. Acute MI
B. Cardiomyopathies
C. Sleep apnea
D. All of the above

Sustained Ventricular Tachycardia

759. Which of the following is a feature of sustained monomorphic ventricular tachycardia (VT)?
Harrison's 20th Ed. Chapter 249 Page 1757

A. Wide QRS tachycardia
B. Same QRS configuration from beat to beat
C. Originates from a stable focus or reentry circuit
D. All of the above

760. Clinical presentation of sustained ventricular tachycardia depends on?
Harrison's 20th Ed. Chapter 249 Page 1757

A. Rate of arrhythmia
B. Underlying cardiac function
C. Autonomic adaptation in response to arrhythmia
D. All of the above

761. Sustained monomorphic VT can mimic which of the following?
Harrison's 20th Ed. Chapter 249 Page 1757

A. SVT with left / right bundle branch block aberrant conduction
B. SVT conducted to ventricles over an accessory pathway
C. Rapid cardiac pacing in patient with ICD
D. All of the above

Sustained monomorphic VT has to be distinguished from other causes of uniform wide QRS tachycardia. These include supraventricular tachycardia with left or right bundle branch block aberrant conduction, supraventricular tachycardias conducted to ventricles over an accessory pathway and rapid cardiac pacing in a patient with a pacemaker or defibrillator.

762. Which of the following favor the diagnosis of sustained monomorphic VT?
Harrison's 20th Ed. Chapter 249 Page 1757

A. Presence of AV dissociation
B. Monophasic R wave or Rs complex in AVR
C. Concordance from V1 to V6 of monophasic R or S waves
D. All of the above

763. Which of the following is rarely a cause of sustained monomorphic VT?
Harrison's 20th Ed. Chapter 249 Page 1758

A. Nonischemic cardiomyopathy
B. Acute MI
C. Arrhythmogenic right ventricular cardiomyopathy
D. Long QT syndrome

Acute MI is rarely a cause of sustained monomorphic VT.

764. Scars in myocardium is suggested by?
Harrison's 20th Ed. Chapter 249 Page 1758

A. Pathologic Q-waves on ECG
B. Segmental LV or RV wall motion abnormalities on 2D echo
C. Areas of delayed gadolinium enhancement in MR imaging
D. All of the above

765. Scars that cause VT are often located adjacent to?
Harrison's 20th Ed. Chapter 249 Page 1758

A. Apex
B. Papillary muscle
C. Valve annulus
D. Interventricular septum

Scars that cause VT are often located adjacent to a valve annulus and can occur in either ventricle.

766. Which of the following is associated with monomorphic VT?
Harrison's 20th Ed. Chapter 249 Page 1758

A. Chagas' disease
B. Leishmaniasis
C. Babesiosis
D. All of the above

Cardiac sarcoidosis, Chagas' disease and cardiomyopathy due to Lamin A/C genetic cardiomyopathy are particularly associated with monomorphic VT due to intramural or sub-epicardial scars.

767. VT in the absence of structural heart disease is called?
Harrison's 20th Ed. Chapter 249 Page 1758 Table 249-1

A. Functional VT
B. Idiopathic VT
C. Casual VT
D. Benign VT

VT in the absence of structural heart disease is called idiopathic VT.

768. Long QT syndrome is complicated by?
Harrison's 20th Ed. Chapter 249 Page 1758 Table 249-1

A. Torsade de Pointes VT
B. Polymorphic VT or bidirectional VT
C. Ventricular fibrillation
D. All of the above

769. Brugada syndrome is complicated by?
Harrison's 20th Ed. Chapter 249 Page 1758 Table 249-1

A. Torsade de Pointes VT
B. Polymorphic VT or bidirectional VT
C. Ventricular fibrillation
D. All of the above

770. Which of the following is due to mutation in genes encoding for cardiac desmosomal proteins?
Harrison's 20th Ed. Chapter 249 Page 1758

A. Arrhythmogenic right ventricular cardiomyopathy (ARVC)
B. Naxos disease
C. Carvajal syndrome
D. All of the above

771. Epsilon wave is an ECG feature of?
Harrison's 20th Ed. Chapter 249 Page 1758

A. Arrhythmogenic right ventricular cardiomyopathy (ARVC)
B. Naxos disease
C. Carvajal syndrome
D. All of the above

772. Location of epsilon wave in ECG is?
Harrison's 20th Ed. Chapter 249 Page 1758

A. Deflection at the beginning of QRS
B. Deflection at the end of QRS
C. Deflection at the beginning of T
D. Deflection at the end of T

773. Which of the following is related to arrhythmogenic RV cardiomyopathy (ARVC)?
Harrison's 20th Ed. Chapter 249 Page 1758

A. Genetically determined
B. After viral myocarditis
C. Sporadic
D. Any of the above

ARVCM/D due to a genetically determined dysplastic process or after a suspected viral myocarditis is also associated with VT/VF. Sporadic nonfamilial/nondysplastic form of RV cardiomyopathy is also seen.

774. Epsilon wave is characteristic ECG finding of?
Harrison's 20th Ed. Chapter 249 Page 1758

A. Arrhythmogenic RV cardiomyopathy
B. Brugada syndrome
C. Long QT syndrome (LQTS)
D. Digoxin toxicity

Epsilon wave is the terminal notching of QRS complex & is separated from the QRS complex. It is seen in ARVCM/D. Epsilon waves are due to marked delay in ventricular activation in RV free wall near the base of tricuspid & pulmonic valves which undergo extensive fibrosis.

775. In arrhythmogenic RV cardiomyopathy (ARVC), ventricles have an excess of?
Harrison's 20th Ed. Chapter 249 Page 1758

A. Fat
B. Glycogen
C. Mucopolysaccharide
D. All of the above

MRI in arrhythmogenic RV cardiomyopathy/dysplasia (ARVCM/D) shows fibrosis and fibro-fatty replacement of the ventricle, thinning of the RV free wall with increased fibrosis, and associated wall motion abnormalities.

776. Echocardiographic finding in arrhythmogenic RV cardiomyopathy (ARVC) is?
Harrison's 20th Ed. Chapter 249 Page 1758

A. RV enlargement
B. RV wall motion abnormalities
C. RV apical aneurysm formation
D. All of the above

In patients with ARVCM/D, echocardiography shows RV enlargement with RV wall motion abnormalities and RV apical aneurysm formation.

777. Which of the following about Naxos disease is false?
Harrison's 20th Ed. Chapter 254 Page 1781 Table 254-3

A. Arrhythmogenic RV dysplasia
B. Palmar-plantar keratosis
C. Autosomal dominant inheritance
D. Woolly hair

Naxos disease, an autosomal recessive cardio-cutaneous syndrome, consists of arrhythmogenic RV dysplasia with palmar-plantar keratosis & woolly hair with a high risk of SCD in adolescents & young adults.

778. Which of the following is false about bundle branch reentry VT?
Harrison's 20th Ed. Chapter 249 Page 1759

A. Reentry circuit revolves retrograde via left bundle
B. Reentry circuit revolves anterograde via right bundle
C. Usually associated with severe underlying heart disease
D. None of the above

Reentry through the Purkinje system occurs in ~5% of patients with monomorphic VT in the presence of structural heart disease. Catheter ablation of the right bundle branch abolishes this VT.

779. In ECG, bundle branch reentrant VT presents as?
Harrison's 20th Ed. Chapter 249 Page 1759

A. Right bundle block
B. Left bundle block
C. Complete heart block
D. Any of the above

In sinus rhythm, bundle branch reentrant VT presents as left bundle block.

780. Sudden death due to VT is rare in which of the following conditions?
Harrison's 20th Ed. Chapter 249 Page 1759

A. Premature ventricular beats and nonsustained VT
B. Idiopathic VT
C. Genetically determined syndromes
D. Depressed ventricular function

781. Which of the following about idiopathic outflow tract VTs is false?
Harrison's 20th Ed. Chapter 249 Page 1759

A. Produces monophasic R waves in leads II, III & aVF
B. Occur as repeated bursts of nonsustained bursts of VT
C. Provoked by exercise or emotional upset
D. Most originate in the left ventricular outflow tract

Acute medical therapy for idiopathic outflow tract VT is rarely required because the VT is hemodynamically tolerated and is typically nonsustained. Most originate in the right ventricular outflow tract.

782. Which of the following can be induced by exercise?
Harrison's 20th Ed. Chapter 249 Page 1759

A. Anaphylaxis
B. Asthma
C. Arrhythmia
D. All of the above

783. Which of the following can terminate the idiopathic outflow tract ventricular tachycardia?
Harrison's 20th Ed. Chapter 249 Page 1759

A. IV lidocaine
B. IV procainamide
C. IV amiodarone
D. IV beta blockers

Intravenous beta blockers frequently terminate idiopathic outflow tract ventricular tachycardia.

784. Which of the following VT can be terminated by intravenous verapamil?

Harrison's 20th Ed. Chapter 249 Page 1759

A. Idiopathic VT
B. Bundle branch reentry VT
C. LV intrafascicular VT
D. All of the above

785. Which of the following about LV intrafascicular VT is false?

Harrison's 20th Ed. Chapter 249 Page 1759

A. Right bundle branch block-like configuration
B. Exercise-induced
C. Reentry in or near septal ramifications of LV Purkinje system
D. None of the above

LV intrafascicular VT presents with sustained VT that has a right bundle branch block-like configuration. It is often exercise-induced and occurs more often in men than women. The mechanism is reentry in or near the septal ramifications of the LV Purkinje system. This VT can be terminated by intravenous administration of verapamil.

Polymorphic Ventricular Tachycardia and Ventricular Fibrillation

786. Which of the following is a potential mechanism for polymorphic ventricular tachycardia?

Harrison's 20th Ed. Chapter 250 Page 1759

A. Reentry with continually changing reentrant paths
B. Spiral wave reentry
C. Multiple automatic foci
D. All of the above

Sustained polymorphic VT is seen with any form of structural heart disease, but does not always indicate a structural abnormality or focus of automaticity. Potential mechanisms include reentry with continually changing reentrant paths, spiral wave reentry and multiple automatic foci.

787. Polymorphic VT is typically seen in association with?

Harrison's 20th Ed. Chapter 250 Page 1759

A. Acute myocardial infarction or ischemia
B. Ventricular hypertrophy
C. Genetic mutations that affect cardiac ion channels
D. All of the above

788. What percentage of patients with acute MI develop VT that degenerates to VF?

Harrison's 20th Ed. Chapter 250 Page 1759

A. 1%
B. 3%
C. 5%
D. 10%

Approximately 10% of patients with acute MI develop VT that degenerates to VF, related to reentry through the infarct border zone. The risk is greatest in the first hour of acute MI.

789. Patients who survive primary VF within first 48 hours of onset of acute infarction have?

Harrison's 20th Ed. Chapter 250 Page 1759

A. Good short-term prognosis
B. Good long-term prognosis
C. Poor long-term prognosis
D. None of the above

Polymorphic VT & VF that occur within the first 48 h of acute MI are associated with greater in-hospital mortality but those who survive past hospital discharge are not at increased risk for arrhythmic sudden death.

790. "Pause-dependent" phrase best relates to?

Harrison's 20th Ed. Chapter 250 Page 1760

A. Short QT syndrome
B. Brugada syndrome
C. Torsade de pointes
D. Early repolarization syndrome

Polymorphic VT Torsade de pointes has a characteristic initiation sequence of a premature ventricular beat that induces a pause, followed by a sinus beat that has a longer QT interval and interruption of the T wave by the PVC that is the first beat of the polymorphic VT. This characteristic initiation is termed "pause-dependent".

791. Bazett's formula for the calculation of QTc is?

N Engl J Med. 1993;328:287

A. QT / Square root of PR
B. QT / Square root of RR
C. QT x Square root of PR
D. QT x Square root of RR

QT interval is from the onset of QRS complex to the end of the T wave. Bazett's formula (QT interval is adjusted for heart rate) for the calculation of QTc is QT interval (in seconds) divided by the square root of the RR interval (in seconds). Bazett's formula, however, overcorrects QT interval at fast heart rates & undercorrects it at low heart rates. Fridericia, Hodges or Framingham formula can be used instead.

792. Which of the following about congenital long QT syndromes is false?

Harrison's 20th Ed. Chapter 250 Page 1760

A. Type 1 has reduced repolarizing current I_{Ks}
B. Type 2 has reduced repolarizing current I_{Kr}
C. Type 3 has delayed inactivation of the I_{Na}
D. None of the above

793. Which of the following do not cause QT prolongation?

Harrison's 20th Ed. Chapter 250 Page 1761 Table 250-3

A. Ibutilide
B. Sotalol
C. Lidocaine
D. Disopyramide

Class IB antiarrhythmic agents (lidocaine) do not cause QT prolongation. Class IA (Quinidine, Disopyramide and Procainamide) and Class III antiarrhythmic agents (Sotalol, Dofetilide, Ibutilide and almokalant) prolong QT interval and may precipitate torsades de pointes.

794. Which of the following prolong QT interval?

Harrison's 20th Ed. Chapter 250 Page 1761 Table 250-3

A. Hypocalcemia
B. Hypomagnesemia
C. Hypokalemia
D. All of the above

795. Which of the following prolong QT interval?

Harrison's 20th Ed. Chapter 250 Page 1761 Table 250-3

A. Hyperparathyroidism
B. Pheochromocytoma
C. Hyperaldosteronism
D. All of the above

796. Which of the following intracranial disorders prolong QT interval?

Harrison's 20th Ed. Chapter 250 Page 1761 Table 250-3

A. Subarachnoid hemorrhage
B. Thalamic hematoma
C. Encephalitis
D. All of the above

797. Long QT syndrome (LQTS) was first described by?
Circulation. 2006;113:783-790

A. Romano and Ward
B. Levine and Woodworth
C. Jervell and Lange-Nielsen
D. Moss and Schwartz

In 1957, Anton Jervell and Fred Lange-Nielsen first described a family with long QT syndrome (LQTS). The family consisted of unrelated parents and their six children, four of whom were deaf with frequent fainting attacks precipitated by acute emotional arousal and exercise. Three of the four deaf children died suddenly while playing at the ages of 4, 5, and 9 years. In 1963 and 1964, Romano and Ward respectively, reported separate families with QT prolongation in one parent and several children, all of whom possessed normal hearing but experienced recurrent syncope and sudden death (autosomal dominant mode of inheritance). In 1979 Moss and Schwartz established the prospective International LQTS Registry for enrollment and follow-up of proband-identified LQTS families.

798. Syncope in long-QT syndrome is attributed to?
N Engl J Med. 2008;358:169-76

A. Emotional or physical stress
B. Electrolyte disturbances
C. Torsades de pointes
D. Lack of sleep

Syncope in patients with the long-QT syndrome is generally attributed to the form of polymorphic ventricular tachycardia called torsades de pointes. Death is usually due to ventricular fibrillation.

799. LQT1-specific trigger is?
N Engl J Med. 2008;358:169-76

A. Emotional stress
B. Physical stress
C. Diving and swimming
D. All of the above

800. Schwartz scoring system for diagnosis of LQTS includes all except?
N Engl J Med. 2008;358:169-76

A. Genetic information
B. ECG features
C. Personal history
D. Family history

Schwartz scoring system for LQTS includes ECG features, personal & family history, but does not take into account genetic information.

801. Which of the following is not useful in diagnosis of LQTS?
N Engl J Med. 2008;358:169-76

A. Echocardiography
B. Holter monitoring
C. Electrophysiological testing
D. All of the above

Physical examination, echocardiography, MRI, Holter monitoring and electrophysiological testing show no abnormalities in LQTS.

802. Most powerful predictor of risk in LQTS is?
N Engl J Med. 2008;358:169-76, Harrison's 17th Ed. 1441

A. QTc duration
B. Family history
C. History of syncope
D. Gender

The most powerful predictor of risk is the QTc duration. Marked lengthening of the QT interval to > 500 ms is clearly associated with a greater arrhythmia risk in patients with the LQTS. In LQT2, females fared worse than their males, while opposite was true in LQT3, and no sex bias occurs in LQT1. Syncope and sudden death are most frequent in childhood and adolescence. The risk of cardiac events is higher in males before puberty and higher in females during adulthood.

803. Which of the following is false about LQT1?
Harrison's 20th Ed. Chapter 250 Page 1760

A. Most common genotypic abnormality in LQTS
B. QT interval fails to shorten with exercise
C. T wave is broad
D. None of the above

804. Which of the following is false about LQT1?
Harrison's 20th Ed. Chapter 250 Page 1760

A. Exercise is the most common trigger for arrhythmias
B. Respond to beta blocker therapy
C. Due to mutation in potassium-channel gene (KCNQ1) on chromosome 11
D. None of the above

805. Which of the following is false about LQT2?
Harrison's 20th Ed. Chapter 250 Page 1760

A. T wave is low amplitude, notched and bifid
B. Emotional stress /startle triggers arrhythmias
C. Sleep or auditory stimulation triggers arrhythmias
D. None of the above

806. Which of the following is false about LQT2?
Harrison's 20th Ed. Chapter 250 Page 1760

A. Risk of syncope & sudden death increased in postpartum period
B. Respond to beta blocker therapy
C. Due to a mutation in a potassium-channel gene on chromosome 7 (KCNH2 or HERG)
D. None of the above

807. Which of the following is false about LQT3?
Harrison's 20th Ed. Chapter 250 Page 1760

A. Due to a mutation in cardiac sodium channel gene on chromosome 3
B. Late-onset peaked biphasic/asymmetric T waves
C. Prognosis for LQT3 is the poorest of all LQTs
D. None of the above

808. Which of the following is false about LQT3?
Harrison's 20th Ed. Chapter 250 Page 1760

A. Beta blockers are not recommended
B. Exercise is not restricted in LQT3
C. QT shortening occurs with mexiletine
D. None of the above

809. Which of the following is false about LQT3?
Harrison's 20th Ed. Chapter 250 Page 1760

A. Most events in LQT3 patients occur during sleep
B. LQT3 is caused by a mutation in sodium channel gene on chromosome 3 (SCN5A)
C. Male patients have worst prognosis in LQT3
D. None of the above

810. In short QT syndrome, QT interval is?
Harrison's 20th Ed. Chapter 250 Page 1760

A. < 300 ms
B. < 340 ms
C. < 360 ms
D. < 380 ms

Usually, a QT interval < 300 ms is required to establish the diagnosis of Short QT syndrome.

811. Mutations in which of the following gene is the cause of short QT syndrome?
Harrison's 20th Ed. Chapter 250 Page 1760

A. HERG
B. KvLQT1
C. KCNJ2
D. Any of the above

Mutations in the HERG, KvLQT1 & KCNJ2 genes cause of Short QT syndrome due to a gain of function of the potassium channel (IK) or reduced inward depolarizing currents.

812. Which of the following is a feature of short QT syndrome?
Harrison's 20th Ed. Chapter 250 Page 1760

A. Short PR interval
B. Flat P waves
C. Tall and peaked T waves
D. Prominent U waves

In Short QT syndrome, T waves tends to be tall and peaked especially in leads V2 to V4 and may be interpreted as R waves by an implantable cardioverter-defibrillator. Patients with the syndrome are predisposed to both AF and VF.

813. Which of the following can shorten QT interval?

A. Hypercalcemia
B. Hyperkalemia
C. Acidosis
D. All of the above

Conditions that can shorten QT interval include hypercalcemia (with an accompanying prolonged PR interval and a wide QRS complex), hyperkalemia, acidosis, increased vagal tone, after ventricular fibrillation (due to increased intracellular calcium), digitalis use, androgen use. Interestingly, a shorter-than-expected QT interval was noted in patients with chronic fatigue syndrome. Quinidine is helpful.

814. Which of the following is a repolarization abnormality?

A. Brugada syndrome
B. Arrhythmogenic right ventricular cardiomyopathy
C. Short QT syndrome
D. All of the above

Besides LQTS, other repolarization abnormalities are Brugada syndrome (opposite of LQT3), arrhythmogenic right ventricular cardiomyopathy, & short QT syndrome.

815. In Brugada syndrome, ST segment elevation in V1 - V3 may be?
Harrison's 19th Ed. 1497

A. Manifest
B. Transient
C. Concealed
D. Any of the above

816. ECG manifestations of Brugada syndrome are provoked with?
Harrison's 19th Ed. 1497

A. Ajmaline
B. Flecainide
C. Procainamide
D. All of the above

The major clinical features of autosomal dominant Brugada syndrome include manifest, transient, or concealed ST segment elevation in V1 to V3 that can typically be provoked with sodium channel-blocking drugs ajmaline, flecainide & procainamide & a risk of polymorphic ventricular arrhythmias.

817. Which of the following is false about Brugada syndrome?
Harrison's 19th Ed. 1497

A. Left bundle branch block pattern
B. ST elevation leads $V_1 - V_3$
C. Terminal T-wave inversion in leads $V_1 - V_3$
D. Due to mutation in cardiac sodium channel SCN5A

In ECG, right bundle-branch block (rSR') and downsloping ST-segment elevation in lead V1 is typical of Brugada syndrome. It is syndrome of RBBB & nonischemic ST-segment elevations.

818. Which of the following is false about Brugada syndrome?
Harrison's 19th Ed. 1497

A. Most common in young Asian male
B. Affected region is RV outflow tract epicardium
C. Patients do not benefit from beta blocker therapy
D. Procainamide & flecainide are beneficial

Procainamide & flecainide exacerbate Brugada syndrome. Quinidine is successful in suppressing frequent episodes of VT.

819. Which of the following statements about PVCs is false?
Harrison's 20th Ed. Chapter 248 Page 1755

A. May occur in up to 80% of patients with previous MI
B. On ECG show wide (usually > 0.12 s), bizarre QRS complexes not preceded by P waves
C. When they arise in specialized conduction system (fascicles), they may be < 0.12 s in duration
D. They result in a fully compensatory pause

PVCs are associated with a "fully compensatory pause" i.e. duration between last QRS before PVC and next QRS complex is equal to twice the sinus rate. PVC produces slow ventricular activation and a wide QRS complex that is typically >140 ms in duration.

820. Which of the following statements about PVCs is false?
Harrison's 19th Ed. 1490

A. When fixed coupling is not present and interval between PVCs has a common denominator, ventricular parasystole is said to be present
B. Trigeminy means two sinus beats followed by a PVC
C. Two successive PVCs are termed pairs or couplets
D. ≥3 consecutive PVCs are termed ventricular tachycardia when the rate exceeds 160 beats/minute

PVCs may occur in patterns of bigeminy, in which every sinus beat is followed by a PVC, or trigeminy, in which two sinus beats are followed by a PVC. PVCs may have different morphologies and are thus referred to as multiformed. Two successive PVCs are termed pairs or couplets. Three or more consecutive PVCs are termed VT when the rate is >100 beats/minute.

821. Which of the following statements about PVCs is false?
Harrison's 19th Ed. 1490

A. Ventricular impulses are never conducted retrogradely to atrium
B. PVC that does not produce retrograde concealed conduction and fails to influence oncoming sinus impulse is termed interpolated PVC
C. Antiarrhythmic agents can produce lethal arrhythmias
D. Prophylactic antiarrhythmic therapy is recommended only for young patients with complicated MI

PVC typically does not conduct to the atrium. Occasionally PVC can occur early enough & conduct retrograde to atrium to reset the sinus node. Pause that results will be less than compensatory. PVCs that fail to influence the oncoming sinus impulse are termed interpolated PVCs.

822. QRS duration of a premature ventricular complex (PVC) is?
Harrison's 19th Ed. 1490

A. > 110 ms
B. > 120 ms
C. > 130 ms
D. > 140 ms

A PVC has a wide QRS complex that is typically >140 ms in duration.

823. Sustained ventricular tachycardia is defined as VT that persists for?
Harrison's 19th Ed. 1490

A. > 10 seconds
B. > 15 seconds
C. > 20 seconds
D. > 30 seconds

A time duration of 30 seconds is frequently used to distinguish sustained from nonsustained VT. Hemodynamically unstable VT that requires termination before 30 seconds or VT that is terminated by therapy from an implantable defibrillator is also typically classified as sustained.

824. Which of the following is not true for sustained VT?
Harrison's 19th Ed. 1490

A. Almost always symptomatic
B. Mostly associated with marked hemodynamic compromise
C. Almost always leads to development of myocardial ischemia
D. Acute ischemia is responsible for most recurrent episodes of sustained uniform VT

825. The heart rate in ventricular flutter usually is?
Harrison's 19th Ed. 1490

A. 100 to 150 beats/minute
B. 150 to 300 beats/minute
C. 300 to 450 beats/minute
D. 450 to 600 beats/minute

Ventricular flutter appears as a sine wave on the ECG and has a rate of >250 beats/minute.

826. It is not possible to assign a specific morphology to which of the following arrhythmia?
Harrison's 19th Ed. 1490

A. Atrial flutter
B. Ventricular flutter
C. Torsades de pointes
D. WPW syndrome with AF

A rapid rate with sine wave oscillations of ventricular flutter make it impossible to assign it a specific morphology and in some cases to distinguish it from rapid VT.

827. VT that shows an alternation in QRS axis is called?
Harrison's 19th Ed. 1491

A. Monomorphic VT
B. Polymorphic VT
C. Bidirectional tachycardia
D. Torsades de pointes

828. Torsades de pointes occurs most often in the setting of?
Harrison's 19th Ed. 1491

A. Slow heart rate
B. QT prolongation
C. Hypokalemia
D. All of the above

TDP occurs most often with slow heart rates, QT prolongation & hypokalemia or hypomagnesemia and at the time of conversion from atrial fibrillation to sinus rhythm.

829. Characteristics ECG findings that suggest VT are all except?
Harrison's 19th Ed. 1491, Figure 233-10, Table 233–6

A. QRS complex > 0.20 seconds
B. AV dissociation
C. Inferior QRS frontal plane axis
D. Concordance of QRS pattern in all precordial leads

Ventricular tachycardia on ECG shows AV dissociation, wide QRS >200 ms, superior frontal plane axis, slurring of initial portion of QRS, and large S wave in V6.

830. Which of the following always produce hemodynamic collapse if allowed to continue?
Harrison's 19th Ed. 1491

A. Polymorphic ventricular arrhythmias
B. Ventricular flutter
C. Ventricular fibrillation
D. All of the above

Polymorphic ventricular arrhythmias, ventricular flutter, and VF always produce hemodynamic collapse if allowed to continue.

831. Characteristics ECG findings that suggest VT are all except?
Harrison's 19th Ed. 1491

A. Superior and rightward QRS frontal plane axis
B. Bizarre QRS complex mimiking LBBB or RBBB
C. Slurring of the initial portion of QRS
D. AV dissociation

VT on ECG is suggested by presence of QRS duration >140 ms in the absence of drug therapy, superior & rightward QRS frontal plane axis, bizarre QRS complex that does not mimic the characteristic QRS pattern associated with LBBB or RBBB, and slurring of initial portion of QRS.

832. Which of the following about idiopathic ventricular arrhythmias is false?
Harrison's 20th Ed. Chapter 248 Page 1756

A. ~80% of outflow tract VTs originate in LV
B. Not associated with SCD
C. Vagal maneuvers terminate them
D. Adenosine & beta blockers terminate them

~80% of outflow tract VTs originate in RV & ~20% in LV outflow tract regions.

833. Idioventricular rhythm is defined as?

Harrison's 20th Ed. Chapter 248 Page 1757

A. 2 or more ventricular beats at a rate <100 beats/minute
B. 3 or more ventricular beats at a rate <100 beats/minute
C. 4 or more ventricular beats at a rate <100 beats/minute
D. 5 or more ventricular beats at a rate <100 beats/minute

Three or more ventricular beats at a rate slower than 100 beats/minute are termed idioventricular rhythm. Automaticity is the likely mechanism.

834. Accelerated idioventricular rhythm (AIVR) has overlap features with?

Harrison's 19th Ed. 1490

A. Monomorphic VT
B. Polymorphic VT
C. Slow VT
D. None of the above

By definition there is an overlap between AIVR and "slow" VT.

835. Which of the following about AIVR is false?

Harrison's 19th Ed. 1490

A. Heart rate ranges from 60 to 120 beats/min
B. Occurs in acute MI
C. Usually transient
D. Treatment consists of b blockers

AIVR refers to a ventricular rhythm that is characterized by three or more complexes at a rate >40 and <120 beats/minute due to abnormal automaticity. Transient AIVR is frequently seen in acute myocardial infarction, cocaine intoxication, acute myocarditis, digoxin intoxication & postoperative cardiac surgery. Sustained AIVR is seen in acute MI & postoperatively. Treatment consists of atropine and atrial pacing.

836. Which of the following is the cause of ST-segment elevation?

N Engl J Med. 2003;349:2128-35

A. Acute pericarditis
B. Hyperkalemia
C. Pulmonary embolism
D. All of the above

837. ST-segment elevation in normal healthy young men (male pattern) is seen in?

N Engl J Med. 2003;349:2128-35

A. V1
B. V2
C. V3
D. V4

Concave ST-segment elevation of 1–3 mm seen in ~90% of healthy young men (male pattern) is most marked in V2.

838. ST-segment elevation in early repolarization is seen in?

N Engl J Med. 2003;349:2128-35

A. V1
B. V2
C. V3
D. V4

ST-segment elevation due to early repolarization is most marked in V4, with notching at J point, tall, upright T waves, reciprocal ST depression in aVR, not in aVL, when limb leads are involved.

839. Which of the following is an ECG marker of abnormality in repolarization?

N Engl J Med. 2001;345:1476

A. PR-interval dispersion
B. QT-interval dispersion
C. J-point dispersion
D. All of the above

Two ECG markers of abnormalities in repolarization are QT-interval dispersion & T-wave alternans. They identify patients who are at risk for sudden death from arrhythmia. QT-interval dispersion refers to difference between maximal & minimal QT intervals from various leads on standard ECG. T-wave alternans is defined as alternating T-wave amplitude from beat to beat on special ECG recording techniques.

840. Catecholaminergic polymorphic VT is best related to?

Harrison's 19th Ed. 1498

A. Ang II type I receptor
B. B2-Bradykinin receptor
C. Ryanodine receptor
D. All of the above

In catecholaminergic polymorphic VT there occurs a mutation of myocardial ryanodine release channel, which creates a "leak" in calcium from sarcoplasmic reticulum (SR). Accumulation of intracellular calcium potentiates delayed afterdepolarizations and triggered activity. Ca^{2+} is released from SR through a Ca^{2+} release channel-ryanodine receptor (RyR2), which controls intracytoplasmic $[Ca^{2+}]$ and leads to local changes in intracellular $[Ca^{2+}]$ called calcium sparks. Regulatory protein, calsequestin 2 inhibit RyR2 and thereby release of Ca^{2+} from SR. PKA dissociates calstabin from RyR2, enhancing Ca^{2+} release and thereby myocardial contractility. Excessive plasma catecholamine levels and cardiac sympathetic neuronal release of norepinephrine cause hyperphosphorylation of PKA, leading to calstabin 2–depleted RyR2. The latter depletes SR Ca^{2+} stores and thereby impairs cardiac contraction, leading to heart failure, and also triggers ventricular arrhythmias.

841. Patients of catecholaminergic polymorphic VT may present with?

Harrison's 19th Ed. 1498

A. Bidirectional VT
B. Precipitated by exercise & emotional stress
C. Polymorphic VT resembles that seen with digitalis toxicity
D. Any of the above

Patients of catecholaminergic polymorphic VT can manifest bidirectional VT, nonsustained polymorphic VT, or recurrent VF resembling that seen with digitalis toxicity. The arrhythmias are precipitated by exercise & emotional stress. Treatment with beta blockers & ICD implantation is recommended.

Electrical Storm and Incessant Ventricular Tachycardia (VT)

842. Electrical storm refers to the occurrence of ≥3 episodes of VT or ventricular fibrillation (VF) within?

Harrison's 20th Ed. Chapter 251 Page 1762

A. 1 hour
B. 3 hours
C. 12 hours
D. 24 hours

Electrical storm or ventricular tachycardia (VT) storm refers to the occurrence of three or more episodes of VT or ventricular fibrillation (VF) within 24 hours.

843. Repeated VT episodes requiring defibrillation is called?

Harrison's 20th Ed. Chapter 251 Page 1762

A. VT storm
B. VT paroxysm
C. VT battle
D. VT flow

844. "VT storm" or "electrical storm" is most commonly encountered in patients with?

Harrison's 20th Ed. Chapter 251 Page 1762

A. ICDs
B. Myocardial infarction
C. Cardiomyopathy
D. Cardiac surgery

Repeated VT episodes requiring external cardioversion/defibrillation or repeated appropriate ICD shock therapy are referred to as VT storm. "VT storm" or "electrical storm" refers to three or more separate episodes of VT within 24 hours most commonly encountered in patients with ICDs.

845. If QT prolongation causes torsades de pointes, which of the following is useful?

Harrison's 20th Ed. Chapter 251 Page 1762

A. Intravenous magnesium
B. Intravenous beta blocker
C. Intravenous amiodarone
D. Intravenous quinidine

If QT prolongation causing torsades de pointes is possible intravenous magnesium should be administered and bradycardia treated.

846. In Brugada syndrome, polymorphic VT/VF episode is managed with?

Harrison's 20th Ed. Chapter 251 Page 1762

A. Intravenous lidocaine
B. Intravenous beta blocker
C. Intravenous amiodarone
D. Intravenous quinidine

If QT interval is not prolonged & Brugada syndrome is possible, administration of quinidine and/or isoproterenol may abolish recurrent polymorphic VT/VF episodes.

847. VT is designated incessant when VT continues to recur shortly after?

Harrison's 20th Ed. Chapter 251 Page 1762

A. Electrical conversion to sinus rhythm
B. Pharmacologic conversion to sinus rhythm
C. Spontaneous conversion to sinus rhythm
D. Any of the above

VT is designated incessant when VT continues to recur shortly after electrical, pharmacologic, or spontaneous conversion to sinus rhythm.

848. Which of the following about sotalol is false?

Harrison's 20th Ed. Chapter 251 Page 1762

A. Class III antiarrhythmic drug, non-selective β-blocker
B. Blocks repolarizing potassium currents, prolongs QT
C. Excreted via the kidneys
D. None of the above

849. Which of the following should be considered for polymorphic VT storm?

Harrison's 19th Ed. 1498

A. Intravenous beta blocker
B. Intravenous calcium channel blocker
C. Intravenous nitroglycerine
D. Intravenous digoxin

Intravenous beta blockade therapy should be considered for polymorphic VT storm.

850. Which of the following is available as intravenous formulation?

Harrison's 19th Ed. 1498

A. Lidocaine
B. Quinidine
C. Procainamide
D. All of the above

Lidocaine, quinidine and procainamide are available as intravenous formulations.

851. Which of the following can prevent recurrences in patients with recurrent monomorphic VT?

Harrison's 19th Ed. 1491

A. IV lidocaine
B. IV procainamide
C. IV amiodarone
D. Any of the above

In patients with recurrent monomorphic VT, acute IV administration of lidocaine, procainamide, or amiodarone can prevent recurrences.

852. Verapamil is least effective / contraindicated in which of the following?

Harrison's 19th Ed. 1498

A. Idiopathic LV septal VT
B. Ventricular tachycardia
C. Accessory pathway mediated tachycardias
D. Atrial fibrillation

Most VTs do not respond to carotid sinus massage, Valsalva maneuver or adenosine administration. IV administration of verapamil and/or adenosine is not recommended as a diagnostic test. Verapamil is associated with hemodynamic collapse when administered to patients with structural heart disease and VT.

853. Which of the following is unique in its suppression with verapamil?
Harrison's 19th Ed. 1498

A. Idiopathic LV septal VT
B. VT associated with LV dilated cardiomyopathy
C. Bundle branch reentrant VT
D. All of the above

Idiopathic LV septal VT responds uniquely to IV verapamil.

854. Which of the following drug exhibits properties consistent with multiple classes in Vaughan-Williams classification?
Harrison's 19th Ed. 1498

A. Quinidine
B. Amiodarone
C. Mexiletine
D. Propafenone

Amiodarone is consistent with multiple classes.

855. Which of the following antiarrhythmic drugs is used to treat painful sensory neuropathy?
Harrison's 19th Ed. 2682

A. Mexiletine
B. Flecainide
C. Propafenone
D. Amiodarone

856. Which of the following antiarrhythmic drugs is used to treat myotonia?
Harrison's 19th Ed. 462e-18

A. Mexiletine
B. Flecainide
C. Propafenone
D. Amiodarone

Mexiletine is helpful in patients with significant myotonia in paramyotonia congenita (PC).

857. Which of the following antiarrhythmic drugs is least likely to produce bradycardia?
Harrison's 19th Ed. 1498

A. Mexiletine
B. Flecainide
C. Propafenone
D. Amiodarone

858. Which of the following is not an adverse effect of amiodarone?
Harrison's 19th Ed. 1498

A. Pulmonary infiltrates
B. Hepatitis
C. Photosensitivity
D. Bronchospasm

859. Which of the following is an adverse effect of amiodarone?
Harrison's 19th Ed. 1498

A. Photosensitivity
B. Neuropathy
C. Ocular toxicity
D. All of the above

860. Vaughan-Williams classification is used to classify?
Harrison's 19th Ed. 273e-5

A. Cardiotonic drugs
B. Antiarrhythmic drugs
C. Vasodilator drugs
D. Vasopressor drugs

Antiarrhythmic agents classification scheme was proposed in 1970 by Vaughan-Williams and later modified by Singh and Harrison. The classes of antiarrhythmic action are class I - local anesthetic effect due to blockade of Na+ current; class II - interference with the action of catecholamines at the β-adrenergic receptor; class III - delay of repolarization due to inhibition of K+ current or activation of depolarizing current; and class IV - interference with calcium conductance. Class I antiarrhythmics have been further subdivided based on the kinetics and potency of Na+ channel binding. Class Ia agents (quinidine, procainamide) have moderate potency and intermediate kinetics; class Ib agents (lidocaine, mexiletine) have low potency and rapid kinetics; and class Ic drugs (flecainide, propafenone) have high potency and the slowest kinetics.

861. Which of the following drug does not fit in Vaughan-Williams classification of antiarrhythmic drugs?
Harrison's 19th Ed. 1480, Table 276-3

A. Ibutilide
B. Adenosine
C. Bretylium
D. Propafenone

Adenosine does not fit into VW classification.

862. Class III antiarrhythmics exert their action through?
Harrison's 19th Ed. 1480, Table 276-4

A. Cardiac cellular excitatory current
B. Action potential duration
C. Automaticity
D. All of the above

863. Class I and IV antiarrhythmics exert their action through?
Harrison's 19th Ed. 1480, Table 276-4

A. Cardiac cellular excitatory current
B. Action potential duration
C. Automaticity
D. All of the above

864. Which of the following antiarrhythmic drugs can cause 'Lupus erythematosus like syndrome'?
Harrison's 19th Ed. 1480 Table 276-5

A. Procainamide
B. Bretylium
C. Lidocaine
D. Mexiletine

865. Which of the following antiarrhythmic drugs can cause 'Lupus erythematosus like syndrome'?
Harrison's 19th Ed. 2134

A. Procainamide
B. Disopyramide
C. Propafenone
D. All of the above

866. Which of the following antiarrhythmic drugs can cause true myositis?

Harrison's 19th Ed. 2199

A. Procainamide
B. Ibutilide
C. Propafenone
D. Bretylium

D-Penicillamine, procainamide and statins may produce a true myositis resembling PM or necrotizing myositis.

867. Which of the following antiarrhythmic drugs can cause seizures?

Harrison's 19th Ed. 1480 Table 276-5

A. Procainamide
B. Disopyramide
C. Lidocaine
D. Mexiletine

868. Which of the following antiarrhythmic drugs can cause congestive heart failure?

Harrison's 19th Ed. 1480 Table 276-5

A. Procainamide
B. Disopyramide
C. Lidocaine
D. Mexiletine

869. Which of the following antiarrhythmic drugs can cause taste disturbance?

Harrison's 19th Ed. 1480 Table 276-5

A. Procainamide
B. Disopyramide
C. Propafenone
D. Sotalol

870. Which of the following antiarrhythmic drugs can cause bronchospasm?

Harrison's 19th Ed. 1480 Table 276-5

A. Procainamide
B. Disopyramide
C. Propafenone
D. Sotalol

871. Most uniform sustained VT associated with LV dilated cardiomyopathy can be mapped to?

Harrison's 18th Ed. 1895

A. Mitral valvular region
B. Tricuspid valvular region
C. Pulmonary valvular region
D. All of the above

VT associated with LV dilated cardiomyopathy may be mono- or polymorphic. Myopathic process has a predilection for fibrosis around mitral & aortic valvular regions. Most uniform sustained VT are mapped to these regions.

872. WPW syndrome is observed in patients with hypertrophic cardiomyopathy associated with which mutation?

Harrison's 19th Ed. 433e-2, Table 433e-1

A. ACTN2
B. S135L mutation
C. PRKAG2 mutation
D. CRYAB

WPW syndrome is seen in patients with hypertrophic cardiomyopathy associated with PRKAG2 mutations.

873. Infiltrative / Inflammatory & neuromuscular disorders associated with increased ventricular arrhythmia risk include?

Harrison's 18th Ed. 1896, Table 233-7

A. Sarcoidosis
B. Myotonic muscular dystrophy
C. Kearn-Sayre syndrome
D. All of the above

874. Infiltrative / Inflammatory & disorders associated with increased ventricular arrhythmia risk include?

Harrison's 18th Ed. 1896, Table 233-7

A. Chagas disease
B. Fabry disease
C. Amyloidosis
D. All of the above

875. Infiltrative / Inflammatory & neuromuscular disorders associated with increased ventricular arrhythmia risk include?

Harrison's 18th Ed. 1896, Table 233-7

A. Becker's muscular dystrophy
B. Hemochromatosis
C. Friedreich's ataxia
D. All of the above

876. Neuromuscular disorders associated with increased ventricular arrhythmia risk include all except?

Harrison's 18th Ed. 1896, Table 233-7

A. Facioscapulohumeral muscular dystrophy
B. Emery-Dreyfuss muscular dystrophy
C. Limb-girdle muscular dystrophy
D. Duchenne's muscular dystrophy

Characteristically, FSH muscular dystrophy does not involve other organ systems. Labile hypertension & nerve deafness is common. Coats' disease (telangiectasia, exudation & retinal detachment) also occurs.

877. Ventricular fibrillation can occur due to?

N Engl J Med. 2003;349:2128-35

A. Antiarrhythmic drugs
B. Torsades de pointes
C. WPW syndrome with AF
D. All of the above

IHD is mostly responsible for VF which also occur with antiarrhythmic drugs, TDP and WPW syndrome who develop AF with an extremely rapid ventricular response.

878. Which of the following about digoxin toxicity is false?
N Engl J Med. 2003;349:2128-35

A. Myocardial cell calcium overload
B. Bidirectional VT from left anterior & posterior fascicles
C. Narrow QRS right bundle branch configuration
D. None of the above

The signature VT associated with digoxin toxicity is bidirectional VT due to triggered activity associated with calcium overload resulting from inhibition of Na^+/K^+ ATPase by digoxin. Bidirectional VT originates from left anterior & posterior fascicles creating a relatively narrow QRS right bundle branch configuration with beat-to-beat alternating right & left frontal plane QRS axis.

879. Which of the following is an ECG feature of acute pericarditis?
N Engl J Med. 2003;349:2128-35

A. Diffuse ST-segment elevation
B. Reciprocal ST-segment depression in aVR, not in aVL
C. PR-segment depression
D. All of the above

In acute pericarditis, ECG shows diffuse ST-segment elevation (seldom >5 mm), reciprocal ST-segment depression in aVR, not in aVL and PR-segment depression.

880. Which of the following is not an ECG feature of hyperkalemia?
N Engl J Med. 2003;349:2128-35

A. Widened QRS
B. Tall, peaked, tented T waves
C. Low-amplitude or absent P waves
D. ST segment usually upsloping

In Hyperkalemia, ECG shows widened QRS, tall, peaked, tented T waves, low-amplitude or absent P waves, with ST segment usually downsloping.

881. Which of the following "Channelopathies" can cause Ventricular Fibrillation–Induced Cardiac Arrest?
N Engl J Med. 2005;353:2492-501

A. Long-QT syndrome
B. Short-QT syndrome
C. Brugada syndrome
D. All of the above

882. Noncardiac causes of Ventricular Fibrillation Induced Cardiac Arrest include?
N Engl J Med. 2005;353:2492-501

A. Bronchospasm
B. Sleep apnea
C. Seizure
D. All of the above

Noncardiac causes of Ventricular Fibrillation Induced Cardiac Arrest are Respiratory (Bronchospasm, Aspiration, Sleep apnea, Primary pulmonary hypertension, Pulmonary embolism), Metabolic or toxic (Electrolyte disturbances, Medications or drug ingestion, Environmental poisoning, Sepsis) and Neurologic (Seizure, Cerebrovascular accident: intracranial hemorrhage, or ischemic stroke).

883. Who, from the following, was one of the inventors of cardiac defibrillator?
N Engl J Med. 2001;344:1311

A. Mickey Isenberg
B. Bardy GH
C. Claude Beck
D. Terry Mengert

Claude Beck is one of the inventors of cardiac defibrillation.

884. The first intervention in the "chain of survival" is?
N Engl J Med. 2001;344:1311

A. Rapid access
B. Rapid cardiopulmonary resuscitation
C. Rapid defibrillation
D. Rapid advanced care

The sequence of rapid access, rapid cardiopulmonary resuscitation, rapid defibrillation, and rapid advanced care is termed the chain of survival.

885. In cardiopulmonary resuscitation, chest compression should be administered in the center of the chest on the?
N Engl J Med. 2001;344:1311

A. Upper half of the sternum
B. Middle of the sternum
C. Lower half of the sternum
D. Any of the above

In cardiopulmonary resuscitation, chest compression should be administered in the center of the chest on the lower half of the sternum.

886. In cardiopulmonary resuscitation in adults, the depth of chest compression should be?
N Engl J Med. 2001;344:1311

A. 2 to 3 cm
B. 3 to 4 cm
C. 4 to 5 cm
D. 5 to 6 cm

In CPR in adults, the depth of chest compression should be 4 to 5 cm in adults.

887. In cardiopulmonary resuscitation in adults, the rate of chest compression should be approximately?
N Engl J Med. 2001;344:1311

A. 30 per minute
B. 50 per minute
C. 75 per minute
D. 100 per minute

888. In cardiopulmonary resuscitation performed by two persons, the ratio of compressions to breaths is?
N Engl J Med. 2001;344:1311

A. 10 : 1
B. 10 : 2
C. 15 : 1
D. 15 : 2

When cardiopulmonary resuscitation is performed by two persons, the ratio of chest compressions to breaths remains 15:2 with pause during ventilations. After endotracheal intubation, the ratio should be five compressions to one ventilation, and there should be no pause in chest compressions for the ventilatory breath.

889. In ventricular fibrillation, initial shock with a monophasic wave-form defibrillator should be?
N Engl J Med. 2001;344:1311

A. 100 J
B. 200 J
C. 300 J
D. 360 J

When a monophasic wave-form defibrillator is used for ventricular fibrillation, the initial shock should be 200 J. If the arrhythmia persists, a second shock of 200 to 300 J should be given, followed by a third shock of 360 J if still necessary. All three shocks should be given in quick succession.

890. What energy should be used for initial attempts at terminating VF?

N Engl J Med. 2001;344:1311

A. At least 100 W
B. At least 200 W
C. At least 300 W
D. At least 400 W

891. Paddle diameter for external cardioversion is?

N Engl J Med. 2001;344:1311

A. 10 cm
B. 12 cm
C. 18 cm
D. 24 cm

892. One paddle during external cardioversion is placed at?

N Engl J Med. 2001;344:1311

A. Fourth ICS, midclavicular line
B. Fifth ICS, midclavicular line
C. Fourth ICS, left anterior axillary line
D. Fifth ICS, left anterior axillary line

893. One paddle during external cardioversion is placed at?

N Engl J Med. 2001;344:1311

A. Right parasternally at the level of first rib
B. Right parasternally at the level of second rib
C. Right parasternally at the level of third rib
D. Right parasternally at the level of fourth rib

Heart Failure: Pathophysiology and Diagnosis

894. Which of the following is false about heart failure (HF)?
Harrison's 20th Ed. Chapter 252 Page 1763

A. Cardinal clinical symptoms are dyspnea & fatigue
B. Cardinal clinical signs are edema and rales
C. Term "congestive heart failure" is preferred over HF
D. None of the above

Because many patients present without signs or symptoms of volume overload, term "heart failure" is preferred over the older term "congestive heart failure".

895. Which of the following is false about heart failure (HF)?
Harrison's 20th Ed. Chapter 252 Page 1763

A. Complex clinical syndrome
B. Due to structural or functional impairment of ventricular filling
C. Due to structural or functional impairment of ejection of blood
D. None of the above

896. Overall prevalence of HF in adult population in developed countries is?
Harrison's 20th Ed. Chapter 252 Page 1763

A. 0.3%
B. 0.5%
C. 1%
D. 2%

Overall prevalence of HF in the adult population in developed countries is 2%.

897. Prevalence of HF in people aged > 65 years is?
Harrison's 20th Ed. Chapter 252 Page 1763

A. 2 - 4%
B. 4 - 6%
C. 6 - 10%
D. 10 - 13%

Prevalence of HF in people aged > 65 years is 6 - 10%.

898. What percentage of patients who develop Heart failure (HF) have normal or preserved EF?
Harrison's 20th Ed. Chapter 252 Page 1763

A. ≥ 10%
B. ≥ 20%
C. ≥ 35%
D. ≥ 50%

Epidemiologic studies show that approximately one-half of patients who develop HF have a normal or preserved EF (EF ≥ 50%) i.e. diastolic failure.

899. Which of the following is a category of HF?
Harrison's 20th Ed. Chapter 252 Page 1763

A. HF with a reduced EF (HFrEF)
B. HF with a preserved EF (HRpEF)
C. Borderline or mid-range EF
D. All of the above

900. LV ejection fraction is considered depressed if it is?
Harrison's 20th Ed. Chapter 252 Page 1763 Table 252-1

A. < 60%
B. < 50%
C. < 40%
D. < 30%

901. Which of the following is a cadiac cytoskeletal protein?
Harrison's 20th Ed. Chapter 252 Page 1763

A. Desmin
B. Myosin
C. Vinculin
D. All of the above

902. Which of the following is not a cadiac cytoskeletal protein?
Harrison's 20th Ed. Chapter 252 Page 1763

A. Desmin
B. Myosin
C. Vinculin
D. Laminin

Cytoskeletal proteins include desmin, cardiac myosin & vinculin. Laminin is a nuclear membrane protein.

903. Which of the following condition does not lead to HF in a normal heart?
Harrison's 20th Ed. Chapter 252 Page 1763

A. Hypertension
B. Infiltrative disorders
C. Chagas' disease
D. Arteriovenous fistula

Conditions that lead to a high cardiac output like arteriovenous fistula and anemia seldom lead to HF in a normal heart.

904. Dilated cardiomyopathy is associated with which of the following muscular dystrophies?
Harrison's 20th Ed. Chapter 252 Page 1764

A. Duchenne's
B. Becker's
C. Limb-girdle
D. All of the above

Dilated cardiomyopathy is associated with Duchenne's, Becker's and limb-girdle muscular dystrophies.

905. Chagas' disease is a major cause of HF in?
Harrison's 20th Ed. Chapter 252 Page 1764

A. Africa
B. South America
C. Western Europe
D. South east Asia

906. Which of the following is the single most common cause of HF?
Harrison's 20th Ed. Chapter 252 Page 1764

A. Hypertension
B. Diabetes mellitus
C. CAD
D. Anemia

CAD is the single most common cause of HF.

907. New York Heart Association (NYHA) classification was introduced in which year?
Harrison's 20th Ed. Chapter 252 Page 1764 Table 252-2

A. 1960
B. 1964
C. 1968
D. 1972

New York Heart Association Inc., Diseases of the Heart and Blood Vessels: Nomenclature and Criteria for Diagnosis, 6th ed. Boston, Little Brown, 1964, p. 114.

908. In heart failure, which of the following compensatory mechanisms is activated after an index event?
Harrison's 20th Ed. Chapter 252 Page 1764 Figure 252-1

A. Adrenergic nervous system
B. Renin-angiotensin-aldosterone system
C. Cytokine system
D. All of the above

Heart failure begins after an index event produces an initial decline in the heart's pumping capacity. After this initial decline in pumping capacity, a compensatory mechanisms are activated that includes adrenergic nervous system, renin-angiotensin-aldosterone system and cytokine system.

909. Which of the following is a vasodilatory molecule?
Harrison's 20th Ed. Chapter 252 Page 1764

A. Atrial and brain natriuretic peptides (ANP & BNP)
B. Prostaglandins (PGE_2 & PGI_2)
C. Nitric oxide (NO)
D. All of the above

In HF, there is activation of a family of compensatory vasodilatory molecules like atrial & brain natriuretic peptides (ANP & BNP), prostaglandins (PGE_2 & PGI_2) and nitric oxide (NO), that oppose excessive peripheral vascular vasoconstriction.

910. Which of the following is false about neprilysin?
Harrison's 20th Ed. Chapter 252 Page 1764

A. Membrane-bound peptidase
B. Degrades natriuretic peptides
C. Degrades bradykinin
D. None of the above

911. Which of the following clinical trials studied neprilysin inhibition in HF?
Heart 2016;102:1342-1347

A. Consensus
B. Titration
C. Paradigm-HF
D. Overture

912. Neprilysin is found in high concentrations in?
Heart 2016;102:1342-1347

A. Kidney
B. Lungs
C. Heart
D. Liver

Neprilysin is found in a number of tissues but in especially high concentrations in the kidney.

913. Which of the following are cleaved & inactivated by neprilysin?
Heart 2016;102:1342-1347

A. ANP
B. BNP
C. CNP
D. All of the above

ANP, BNP, CNP and urodilatin are cleaved & inactivated by a membrane bound endopeptidase, neprilysin. Natriuretic peptides are also cleared via the natriuretic peptide clearance receptor (NPRC & NPRC3).

914. Neprilysin breaks down which of the following?
Heart 2016;102:1342-1347

A. Angiotensin II
B. Vasopressin
C. Bradykinin
D. All of the above

915. Carperitide is related to which of the following?
Heart 2016;102:1342-1347

A. ANP
B. BNP
C. CNP
D. All of the above

Carperitide is a recombinant ANP.

916. Nesiritide is related to which of the following?
Heart 2016;102:1342-1347

A. ANP
B. BNP
C. CNP
D. All of the above

Nesiritide is a recombinant human BNP.

917. Urodilatin is related to which of the following?
Heart 2016;102:1342-1347

A. ANP
B. BNP
C. CNP
D. All of the above

Urodilatin is structurally related to ANP, and is derived from kidneys.

918. Which of the following is a combined ACE and neprilysin inhibitor?
Heart 2016;102:1342-1347

A. Racecodotril
B. Omapatrilat
C. Candoxatrilat
D. Ecadotril

The combined ACE and neprilysin inhibitor omapatrilat was studied in the Omapatrilat Versus Enalapril Randomized Trial of Utility in Reducing Events (OVERTURE) trial. Both ACE & neprilysin break down bradykinin and omapatrilat also inhibits aminopeptidase P which also catabolises bradykinin resulting in high rates of serious angio-oedema.

919. Adaptive changes in the myocardium or LV remodeling is due to increasing activation of?
Harrison's 20th Ed. Chapter 252 Page 1764

A. Neurohormonal system
B. Adrenergic system
C. Cytokine system
D. All of the above

920. Baroreceptors are located in which of the following locations?
Harrison's 20th Ed. Chapter 252 Page 1765 Figure 252-2

A. Left ventricle
B. Carotid sinus
C. Aortic arch
D. All of the above

High-pressure baroreceptors are located in left ventricle, carotid sinus and aortic arch.

921. Which of the following mechanism may be responsible in the development of HF with preserved EF (HRpEF)?
Harrison's 20th Ed. Chapter 252 Page 1764

A. Diastolic dysfunction
B. Increased vascular stiffness
C. Impaired renal function
D. All of the above

922. Which of the following contribute to LV remodeling?
Harrison's 20th Ed. Chapter 252 Page 1765

A. Myocyte hypertrophy
B. Altered contractile properties of myocyte
C. Progressive loss of myocytes
D. All of the above

Adaptive changes within the myocardium is collectively referred to as LV remodeling. LV remodeling is a result of myocyte hypertrophy, altered contractile properties of myocyte, progressive loss of myocytes through necrosis, apoptosis, and autophagic cell death, beta-adrenergic desensitization, abnormal myocardial energetics and metabolism and reorganization of extracellular matrix (organized structural collagen around myocytes being replaced by interstitial collagen matrix that is unable to provide structural support to myocytes).

923. Activation of renin-angiotensin-aldosterone system causes?
Harrison's 20th Ed. Chapter 252 Page 1765 Figure 252-2

A. Cardiomyocyte hypertrophy
B. Cardiomyocyte cell death
C. Myocardial fibrosis
D. All of the above

Activation of the renin-angiotensin-aldosterone system promotes salt and water retention and leads to vasoconstriction of the peripheral vasculature, myocyte hypertrophy, myocyte cell death and myocardial fibrosis.

924. Which of the following act as a biologic stimuli in LV remodeling?
Harrison's 20th Ed. Chapter 252 Page 1765

A. Mechanical stretch of myocyte
B. Circulating neurohormones
C. Circulating inflammatory cytokines
D. All of the above

Biologic stimuli leading to LV remodeling include mechanical stretch of myocyte, circulating neurohormones (norepinephrine, angiotensin II), inflammatory cytokines (tumor necrosis factor), peptides and growth factors (endothelin) and reactive oxygen species (superoxide).

925. Which of the following is best related to a failing cardiac myocyte?
Harrison's 20th Ed. Chapter 252 Page 1765

A. NCK-adaptor protein
B. SERCA2A
C. CD2-associated protein (CD2AP)
D. Giant cell line-derived neutrophilic factor (GDNF)

Changes that regulate excitation-contraction include decreased function of sarcoplasmic reticulum Ca^{2+} adenosine triphosphatase (SERCA2A), resulting in decreased calcium uptake into SR, and hyperphosphorylation of ryanodine receptor, leading to calcium leakage from SR.

926. In HF, which of the following changes occur in cross-bridges?
Harrison's 20th Ed. Chapter 252 Page 1765

A. Decreased expression of α-myosin heavy chain
B. Increased expression of β-myosin heavy chain
C. Myocytolysis
D. All of the above

927. Which of the following is false about myocardial relaxation?
Harrison's 20th Ed. Chapter 252 Page 1765

A. Adenosine triphosphate (ATP)-dependent process
B. Regulated by uptake of cytoplasmic calcium into the SR by SERCA2A
C. Regulated by extrusion of calcium by sarcolemmal pumps
D. None of the above

928. Left ventricular remodeling refers to changes in which of the following?
Harrison's 20th Ed. Chapter 252 Page 1766

A. LV mass
B. LV volume
C. LV shape
D. All of the above

Left ventricular remodeling refers to changes in LV mass, volume, and shape and the composition of heart that occur after cardiac injury and/or abnormal hemodynamic loading conditions. LV remodeling can be reversed following medical and device therapy.

929. In HF, which of the following changes occur in heart?
Harrison's 20th Ed. Chapter 252 Page 1766

A. Increase in LV end-diastolic volume
B. LV wall thinning
C. Functional afterload mismatch
D. All of the above

930. High end-diastolic wall stress leads to?
Harrison's 20th Ed. Chapter 252 Page 1766

A. Hypoperfusion of the subendocardium
B. Increased oxidative stress
C. Sustained expression of hypertrophic signaling pathways
D. All of the above

931. Dyspnea in HF is best related to?
Harrison's 20th Ed. Chapter 252 Page 1766

A. Juxtacapillary J receptors
B. Juxtacapillary K receptors
C. Juxtacapillary L receptors
D. Juxtacapillary M receptors

Most important mechanism of dyspnea in HF is pulmonary congestion with accumulation of interstitial or intra-alveolar fluid, which activates juxtacapillary J receptors, which in turn stimulate the rapid, shallow breathing characteristic of cardiac dyspnea.

932. Which of the following factors contribute to dyspnea on exertion in HF?
Harrison's 20th Ed. Chapter 252 Page 1766

A. Reductions in pulmonary compliance
B. Increased airway resistance
C. Respiratory muscle &/or diaphragm fatigue
D. All of the above

933. Dyspnea in HF may become less frequent with the onset of?
Harrison's 20th Ed. Chapter 252 Page 1766

A. Mitral regurgitation
B. Tricuspid regurgitation
C. Aortic regurgitation
D. Pulmonary regurgitation

Dyspnea in HF may become less frequent with the onset of right ventricular (RV) failure and tricuspid regurgitation.

934. Which of the following is a symptom of HF?
Harrison's 20th Ed. Chapter 252 Page 1766

A. Nocturia
B. Nocturnal cough
C. Early satiety
D. All of the above

935. Orthopnea is caused due to redistribution of fluid from?
Harrison's 20th Ed. Chapter 252 Page 1766

A. Coronary circulation
B. Pulmonary circulation
C. Splanchnic circulation
D. Cerebral circulation

Orthopnea (dyspnea occurring in recumbent position), results from redistribution of fluid from splanchnic circulation and lower extremities into central circulation during recumbency, with a resultant increase in pulmonary capillary pressure.

936. Orthopnea may occur in patients with?
Harrison's 20th Ed. Chapter 252 Page 1766

A. Heart failure
B. Abdominal obesity or ascites
C. Pulmonary disease
D. All of the above

937. Which of the following about orthopnea in HF is false?
Harrison's 20th Ed. Chapter 252 Page 1766

A. Later manifestation of HF
B. Relatively specific symptom of HF
C. Due to increase in pulmonary capillary pressure
D. None of the above

938. In HF, paroxysmal nocturnal dyspnea (PND) occurs how many hours after the patient retires?
Harrison's 20th Ed. Chapter 252 Page 1766

A. 15 - 30 minutes
B. 1 - 3 hours
C. 3 - 4 hours
D. 5 - 6 hours

PND refers to acute episodes of severe shortness of breath and coughing that awaken the patient from sleep, usually 1 - 3 hours after the patient retires.

939. Paroxysmal nocturnal dyspnea (PND) may manifest as?
Harrison's 20th Ed. Chapter 252 Page 1766

A. Severe shortness of breath
B. Persistent coughing even after assuming upright position
C. Persistent wheezing even after assuming upright position
D. All of the above

940. Paroxysmal nocturnal dyspnea (PND) is caused by?
Harrison's 20th Ed. Chapter 252 Page 1766

A. Increased pressure in bronchial arteries causing airway compression
B. Interstitial pulmonary edema
C. Increased airway resistance
D. All of the above

941. Which of the following is false for cardiac asthma?
Harrison's 20th Ed. Chapter 252 Page 1766

A. Closely related to PND
B. Wheezing
C. Bronchospasm
D. None of the above

Cardiac asthma is closely related to PND & is characterized by wheezing secondary to bronchospasm.

942. Cheyne-Stokes respiration is due to increased sensitivity of respiratory center to?
Harrison's 20th Ed. Chapter 252 Page 1766

A. Arterial PCO_2
B. Venous PCO_2
C. Arterial PO_2
D. Venous PCO_2

943. Cheyne-Stokes respiration is associated with?
Harrison's 20th Ed. Chapter 252 Page 1766

A. Increased intravascular volume
B. Low cardiac output
C. Cerebral vasoconstriction
D. All of the above

In early 19th century, John Cheyne & William Stokes described cyclical episodes of apnea & hyperventilation. Cheyne-Stokes respiration (periodic respiration or cyclic respiration) is present in 40% of patients with advanced HF and usually is associated with low cardiac output. Cheyne-Stokes respiration is caused by an increased sensitivity of the respiratory center to arterial $PC0_2$. There is an apneic phase, during which arterial PO_2 falls and arterial $PC0_2$ rises. These changes in the arterial blood gas content stimulate the respiratory center, resulting in hyperventilation and hypocapnia, followed by recurrence of apnea. Ventilation length in Cheyne-Stokes respiration is >40 seconds compared to <40 seconds in central sleep apnea. Also, relative duration of hyperventilation is more than apnea duration.

944. In HF, which of the following is caused by excessive adrenergic activity?
Harrison's 20th Ed. Chapter 252 Page 1766

A. Sinus tachycardia
B. Cool peripheral extremities
C. Cyanosis of lips and nail beds
D. All of the above

945. Jugular venous pressure is quantified in which of the following units?

Harrison's 20th Ed. Chapter 252 Page 1766

A. Centimeters of water
B. Centimeters of blood
C. Centimeters of mercury
D. Any of the above

Jugular venous pressure is quantified in centimeters of water (normal ≤8 cm) by estimating height of venous column of blood above the sternal angle in centimeters and then adding 5 cm.

946. Which of the following is false about pleural effusions in HF?

Harrison's 20th Ed. Chapter 252 Page 1766

A. Due to elevation of pleural capillary pressure
B. Due to transudation of fluid into the pleural cavities
C. Pleural veins drain into the systemic & pulmonary veins
D. None of the above

947. Which of the following is false about pleural effusions in HF?

Harrison's 20th Ed. Chapter 252 Page 1766

A. Occur most commonly with biventricular failure
B. Often bilateral in HF
C. If unilateral, more frequently in the right pleural space
D. None of the above

948. Protodiastolic gallop best relates to?

Harrison's 20th Ed. Chapter 252 Page 1767

A. S1
B. S2
C. S3
D. S4

S3 or protodiastolic gallop is mostly present in HF patients with volume overload who have tachycardia & tachypnea. It signifies severe hemodynamic compromise.

949. In bedridden HF patients, edema may be found in?

Harrison's 20th Ed. Chapter 252 Page 1767

A. Interscapular region
B. Scrotum
C. Nape of the neck
D. All of the above

In bedridden HF patients, edema may be found in sacral area (presacral edema) and scrotum.

950. Which of the following is a late manifestation of HF?

Harrison's 20th Ed. Chapter 252 Page 1767

A. Orthopnea
B. Ascites
C. Jaundice
D. All of the above

951. Which of the following statements is false?

Harrison's 20th Ed. Chapter 252 Page 1767

A. A normal ECG excludes LV systolic dysfunction
B. Majority of patients with chronic HF do not have evidence of pulmonary HT, interstitial edema, and/or pulmonary edema
C. Magnetic resonance imaging (MRI) is the gold standard for assessing LV mass & volumes
D. None of the above

Majority of patients with chronic HF do not have evidence of pulmonary hypertension, interstitial edema, and/or pulmonary edema due to increased capacity of the lymphatics to remove interstitial and/or pulmonary fluid.

952. Which of the following denotes ejection fraction?

Harrison's 20th Ed. Chapter 252 Page 1767

A. End-diastolic volume - End-systolic volume
B. End-diastolic volume / End-systolic volume
C. Stroke volume / End-diastolic volume
D. Stroke volume / End-systolic volume

953. Which of the following is superior to EF as a measure of LV function?

Eur Heart J. 2016;37(15):1196-1207

A. Global circumferential strain by speckle-tracking echocardiography
B. Global longitudinal strain by speckle-tracking echocardiography
C. Global diagonal strain by speckle-tracking echocardiography
D. All of the above

In echocardiography, the term 'strain' is used to describe local shortening, thickening & lengthening of the myocardium as a measure of regional LV function. Strain in myocardium can be measured by tissue Doppler imaging (TDI) or by speckle-tracking echocardiography (STE). Most laboratories record LV strain in long axis & use global longitudinal strain (GLS) calculated as average from all segments, as a measure of global LV function.

954. Which of the following is useful in HF patients with a preserved EF?

Harrison's 20th Ed. Chapter 252 Page 1767

A. B-type natriuretic peptide (BNP)
B. N-terminal pro-BNP
C. Left atrial dilation by 2D Echo
D. All of the above

By 2-D echocardiogram/Doppler, presence of left atrial dilation and LV hypertrophy, together with abnormalities of LV diastolic filling is useful for the assessment of HF with a preserved EF. B-type natriuretic peptide (BNP) and N-terminal pro-BNP are elevated in HF patients with a preserved EF, although to a lesser degree.

955. Natriuretic peptide levels are more in?

Harrison's 20th Ed. Chapter 252 Page 1767

A. Aged
B. Renal impairment
C. Women
D. All of the above

Natriuretic peptide levels increase with age & renal impairment, are more elevated in women, and can be elevated in right HF from any cause.

956. Natriuretic peptide levels can be falsely low in?

Harrison's 20th Ed. Chapter 252 Page 1767

A. Lean individuals
B. Obese individuals
C. Post meal
D. Fasting

Natriuretic peptide levels can be falsely low in obese patients.

957. Which of the following is a biomarker used for determining the prognosis of HF patients?

Harrison's 20th Ed. Chapter 252 Page 1767

A. Galectin-1
B. Galectin-2
C. Galectin-3
D. Galectin-4

Newer biomarkers that can be used for determining the prognosis of HF patients are soluble ST-2 and galectin-3. Galectin-3 as a biomarker of fibrosis and inflammation has been implicated in the development and progression of HF, and may predict increased morbidity and mortality. Galectin-3 is a strong independent predictor of mortality in patients with chronic heart failure.

958. What level of peak oxygen uptake (VO_2) is associated with a relatively poor prognosis in HF?

Harrison's 20th Ed. Chapter 252 Page 1767

A. <3 mL/kg per minute
B. <7 mL/kg per minute
C. <14 mL/kg per minute
D. <21 mL/kg per minute

A peak oxygen consumption (vo2) <14 mL/kg per minute is associated with a relatively poor prognosis in HF. They have better survival when transplanted than when treated medically.

959. Which of the following is known as pulmonary heart disease?

Harrison's 20th Ed. Chapter 252 Page 1767

A. Asthma
B. Pulmonary hypertension
C. Cor pulmonale
D. Pulmonary thromboembolism

960. Cor pulmonale is triggered by?

Harrison's 20th Ed. Chapter 252 Page 1768

A. Hypoxia
B. Hypercarbia
C. Pulmonary hypertension
D. All of the above

Cor pulmonale or pulmonary heart disease is defined as altered RV structure and/or function in the context of chronic lung disease and is triggered by the onset of pulmonary hypertension. Although RV dysfunction is also an important sequela of HFpEF and HFrEF, this is not considered as cor pulmonale.

961. Normally, mean pulmonary artery pressure is?

Harrison's 20th Ed. Chapter 252 Page 1768

A. ~ 5 mm Hg
B. ~ 10 mm Hg
C. ~ 15 mm Hg
D. ~ 20 mm Hg

Normally, mean pulmonary artery pressure is ~ 15 mm Hg.

962. Trigger for acute decompensation of previously compensated chronic cor pulmonale is?

Harrison's 20th Ed. Chapter 252 Page 1768

A. Acidemia
B. Acute pulmonary embolus
C. Atrial tachyarrhythmia
D. All of the above

Triggers for acute decompensation of previously compensated chronic cor pulmonale are worsening hypoxia (pneumonia), acidemia (exacerbation of COPD), acute pulmonary embolus, atrial tachyarrhythmia, hypervolemia and mechanical ventilation that leads to compressive forces on alveolar blood vessels.

963. Decompensation of chronic cor pulmonale is aggravated by?

Harrison's 20th Ed. Chapter 252 Page 1768

A. Obesity hypoventilation syndrome (OHS)
B. Acute pulmonary emboli
C. Positive-pressure (mechanical) ventilation
D. All of the above

Decompensation of chronic cor pulmonale can be aggravated by events that induce pulmonary vasoconstriction and RV afterload.

964. Which of the following is the most common symptom of chronic cor pulmonale?

Harrison's 20th Ed. Chapter 252 Page 1768

A. Dyspnea
B. Orthopnea
C. PND
D. All of the above

Orthopnea and PND are rarely symptoms of isolated right HF and usually point toward concurrent left heart dysfunction.

965. Which of the following about Tei index is false?

Harrison's 20th Ed. Chapter 252 Page 1769, J Cardiol. 1995; 26: 357-366

A. Ratio of time intervals
B. Independent of ventricular geometry
C. Independent of blood pressure, heart rate and age
D. None of the above

966. Formula for Tei index is?

J Cardiol. 1995; 26: 357-366

A. (IVCT + IVRT) / ET
B. (IVCT + IVRT) x ET
C. ET / (IVCT + IVRT)
D. ET / (IVCT x IVRT)

Isovolumic contraction time (IVCT, Isovolumic relaxation time (IVRT), Ejection time (ET).

Heart Failure: Management

967. Which of the following is a syndrome of heart failure?
Harrison's 20th Ed. Chapter 253 Page 1769

A. Heart failure with reduced ejection fraction (HFrEF)
B. Heart failure with preserved ejection fraction (HFpEF)
C. Acute decompensated heart failure (ADHF)
D. All of the above

Syndromes of heart failure include heart failure with reduced ejection fraction (HFrEF), heart failure with preserved ejection fraction (HFpEF), acute decompensated heart failure (ADHF) and advanced heart failure.

968. Lusitropic effect best relates to?
Harrison's 20th Ed. Chapter 232 Page 1658 Figure 232-7

A. Enhanced velocity
B. Enhanced rate
C. Enhanced relaxation
D. Enhanced contraction

969. Which of the following trials were done on HFpEF patients?
Harrison's 20th Ed. Chapter 253 Page 1769

A. Charm
B. Seniors
C. I-Preserve
D. All of the above

Candesartan in Heart Failure-Assessment of Mortality and Morbidity (CHARM) Preserved study, Irbesartan in Heart Failure with Preserved Systolic Function (I-PRESERVE) trial, Digitalis Investigation Group (DIG) trial, Study of the Effects of Nebivolol Intervention on Outcomes and Rehospitalization in Seniors with Heart Failure (SENIORS) trial, Phosphodiesterase-5 Inhibition to Improve Clinical Status and Exercise Capacity in Diastolic Heart Failure (RELAX), Aldosterone Antagonist Therapy in Adults with Preserved Ejection Fraction Congestive Heart Failure (TOPCAT) trial and Aldosterone Receptor Blockade in Diastolic Heart Failure (ALDO-DHF) study were done on HFpEF patients.

970. Which of the following is an endopeptidase inhibitor?
Harrison's 20th Ed. Chapter 253 Page 1769

A. LCZ596
B. LCZ696
C. LCZ796
D. LCZ896

A unique molecule that hybridizes an ARB with an endopeptidase inhibitor, LCZ696, increases the generation of myocardial cyclic guanosine 3'5'-monophosphate, enhances myocardial relaxation, and reduces ventricular hypertrophy. This dual blocker has been shown to reduce circulating natriuretic peptides and reduce left atrial size to a significantly greater extent than valsartan alone in patients with HFpEF.

971. Which of the following is a precipitating cause of acute decompensated HF (ADHF)?
Harrison's 20th Ed. Chapter 253 Page 1770

A. Infection
B. Pulmonary embolism
C. Occult myocardial ischemia
D. All of the above

Precipitating causes of acute decompensated HF (ADHF) include infection, arrhythmias, dietary indiscretion, pulmonary embolism, infective endocarditis, occult myocardial ischemia/infarction, and environmental and/or emotional stress.

972. Which of the following is a component of heterogeneous clinical syndrome ADHF?
Harrison's 20th Ed. Chapter 253 Page 1770

A. Decreased cardiac performance
B. Renal dysfunction
C. Alterations in vascular compliance
D. All of the above

ADHF is a heterogeneous clinical syndrome that increases need for hospitalization due to confluence of interrelated abnormalities of decreased cardiac performance, renal dysfunction, & alterations in vascular compliance.

973. Which of the following is associated with worse outcomes in ADHF?
Harrison's 20th Ed. Chapter 253 Page 1770

A. BUN level >43 mg/dL
B. Systolic blood pressure <115 mm Hg
C. Serum creatinine level >2.75 mg/dL
D. All of the above

974. Which of the following provides a synergistic effect in patients receiving long-term therapy with loop diuretic agents?
Harrison's 20th Ed. Chapter 253 Page 1771

A. Spironolactone
B. Eplerenone
C. Triamterene
D. Metolazone

Addition of a thiazide diuretic agent such as metolazone in combination provides a synergistic effect in patients receiving long-term therapy with loop diuretic agents.

975. Which of the following is false about cardiorenal syndrome?
Harrison's 20th Ed. Chapter 253 Page 1771

A. Complication of ADHF
B. Most patients have a preserved cardiac output
C. Due to complex interplay of neurohormonal factors
D. None of the above

976. Which of the following trials pertain to cardiorenal syndrome?
Harrison's 20th Ed. Chapter 253 Page 1771

A. Carress-HF trial
B. Relax-AHF trial
C. Revive II trial
D. Survive trial

977. Which of the following is false about Ultrafiltration (UF)?
Harrison's 20th Ed. Chapter 253 Page 1771

A. Controlled rates of fluid removal
B. Neutral effects on serum electrolytes
C. Decreased neurohormonal activity
D. None of the above

Ultrafiltration (UF) or aquapheresis is an invasive fluid removal technique.

978. Which of the following drugs exerts dilating effect on arterial resistance and venous capacitance vessels?
Harrison's 20th Ed. Chapter 253 Page 1772

A. Nitroglycerin
B. Nitroprusside
C. Nesiritide
D. All of the above

By stimulating guanylyl cyclase within smooth-muscle cells, nitroglycerin, nitroprusside, and nesiritide exert dilating effects on arterial resistance and venous capacitance vessels.

979. Recombinant human relaxin-2 or serelaxin is upregulated in?
Harrison's 20th Ed. Chapter 253 Page 1772

A. High altitude
B. Atheletes
C. Pregnancy
D. All of the above

Recombinant human relaxin-2 or serelaxin is a peptide upregulated in pregnancy and examined in ADHF patients with a normal or elevated blood pressure.

980. Nesiritide is best related to?
Harrison's 20th Ed. Chapter 253 Page 1772

A. Atrial-type natriuretic peptide
B. Brain-type natriuretic peptide
C. Phosphodiesterase III inhibitor
D. Endogenous catecholamine

Nesiritide is a recombinant form of brain-type natriuretic peptide, which is an endogenous peptide secreted primarily from LV in response to an increase in wall stress.

981. Which of the following is an inotropic agent?
Harrison's 20th Ed. Chapter 253 Page 1772

A. Dopamine
B. Dobutamine
C. Tolvaptan
D. All of the above

Dobutamine is an inotropic agent for the treatment of acute HF. It exerts its effects by stimulating β_1 and β_2 receptors, with little effect on α_1 receptors.

982. Which of the following is a phosphodiesterase III inhibitor?
Harrison's 20th Ed. Chapter 253 Page 1772

A. Dopamine
B. Dobutamine
C. Tolvaptan
D. Milrinone

Milrinone is a phosphodiesterase III inhibitor that leads to increased cyclic AMP by inhibiting its breakdown.

983. Dopamine stimulates which of the following?
Harrison's 20th Ed. Chapter 253 Page 1772

A. α_1 receptors
B. β_1 receptors
C. Dopaminergic receptors
D. All of the above

Dopamine is an endogenous catecholamine that stimulates α_1 and β_1 receptors and dopaminergic receptors (DA_1 and DA_2) in the heart and circulation.

984. Which of the following is administered orally?
Harrison's 20th Ed. Chapter 253 Page 1772

A. Nesiritide
B. Nitroprusside
C. Tolvaptan
D. Milrinone

985. TRUE-AHF trial evaluated which of the following in ADHF?
Harrison's 20th Ed. Chapter 253 Page 1772

A. Nesiritide
B. Urodilatin
C. Serelaxin
D. Milrinone

986. Which of the following is a calcium sensitizer that provides inotropic activity?
Harrison's 20th Ed. Chapter 253 Page 1772

A. Serelaxin
B. Milrinone
C. Levosimendan
D. Nesiritide

Levosimendan is a calcium sensitizer that provides inotropic activity and also possesses phosphodiesterase-3 inhibition properties that are vasodilators in action.

987. Which of the following is a selective myosin activator?
Harrison's 20th Ed. Chapter 253 Page 1772

A. Serelaxin
B. Omecamtiv mecarbil
C. Tolvaptan
D. Rolofylline

Omecamtiv mecarbil functions as a selective myosin activator. It prolongs ejection period and increases fractional shortening. Distinctively, the force of contraction is not increased and it does not increase myocardial oxygen demand.

988. Which of the following beta blockers is proven to improve survival in HFrEF clinical trials?
Harrison's 20th Ed. Chapter 253 Page 1773

A. Carvedilol
B. Bisoprolol
C. Metoprolol succinate
D. All of the above

989. Aldosterone antagonism reduces mortality in which symptomatic NYHA class of HFrEF?
Harrison's 20th Ed. Chapter 253 Page 1773

A. Class II
B. Class III
C. Class IV
D. All of the above

Aldosterone antagonism is associated with a reduction in mortality in all stages of symptomatic NYHA class II to IV HFrEF.

990. ASTRONAUT trial tested which of the following drug?
Harrison's 20th Ed. Chapter 253 Page 1773

A. Aliskiren
B. Eplerenone
C. Spironolactone
D. Ivabradine

Aliskiren Trial on Acute Heart Failure Outcomes (ASTRONAUT) tested the direct renin inhibitor, aliskiren, in addition to other heart failure medications, within a week after hospital discharge for decompensated HFrEF. No significant difference in cardiovascular death or hospitalization at 6 or 12 months was noted.

991. Bosentan is best related to?
Harrison's 20th Ed. Chapter 253 Page 1773

A. Centrally acting sympatholytic agent
B. Endothelin antagonist
C. Endopeptidase inhibitor
D. Anticytokine agent

992. Moxonidine is best related to?
Harrison's 20th Ed. Chapter 253 Page 1774

A. Centrally acting sympatholytic agent
B. Endothelin antagonist
C. Endopeptidase inhibitor
D. Anticytokine agent

993. Omapatrilat is best related to?
Harrison's 20th Ed. Chapter 253 Page 1774

A. Centrally acting sympatholytic agent
B. Endothelin antagonist
C. Endopeptidase inhibitor
D. Anticytokine agent

Omapatrilat hybridizes an ACEI with a neutral endopeptidase inhibitor.

994. Sacubitril-valsartan is best related to?
Harrison's 20th Ed. Chapter 253 Page 1774

A. Centrally acting sympatholytic agent
B. Endothelin antagonist
C. Endopeptidase inhibitor
D. Angiotensin Receptor Neprilysin Inhibitor

995. Which of the following is false about Ivabradine?
Harrison's 20th Ed. Chapter 253 Page 1774

A. Inhibitor of the I_f current in sinoatrial node
B. Slows heart rate
C, No negative inotropic effect
D. None of the above

Ivabradine is an inhibitor of the I_f current in the sinoatrial node. It slows the heart rate without a negative inotropic effect.

996. Which of the following is false about digitalis glycosides?
Harrison's 20th Ed. Chapter 253 Page 1775

A. Inotropic
B. Attenuate carotid sinus baroreceptor activity
C. Sympatho-inhibitory
D. None of the above

Digitalis glycosides exert a mild inotropic effect, attenuate carotid sinus baroreceptor activity and are sympathoinhibitory.

997. Digitalis glycosides decrease which of the following?
Harrison's 20th Ed. Chapter 253 Page 1775

A. Serum norepinephrine levels
B. Plasma renin levels
C. Plasma aldosterone levels
D. All of the above

Digitalis glycosides decrease serum norepinephrine levels, plasma renin levels and aldosterone levels.

998. Levels of which of the following may be elevated in HF?
Harrison's 20th Ed. Chapter 253 Page 1775

A. C-reactive protein
B. TNF receptors
C. Uric acid
D. All of the above

Levels of troponin T and I, C-reactive protein, TNF receptors, and uric acid, may be elevated in HF and provide important prognostic information.

999. Loop diuretics increase fractional excretion of sodium by?
J Clin Diagn Res. 2015;9(4):OC01-OC3

A. 5 - 10%
B. 10 - 20%
C. 20 - 25%
D. 25 - 50%

FENa, an indicator of diuretic resistance, is the fraction of the filtered sodium load that is reabsorbed by the tubules. FENa depends on sodium intake, effective intravascular volume, GFR, and intact tubular reabsorptive mechanisms. Loop diuretics increase the fractional excretion of sodium by 20 - 25%. Thiazide diuretics increase it by 5 - 10%.

1000. Which of the following diuretics lead to hyperkalemia?
Harrison's 20th Ed. Chapter 253 Page 1775

A. Spironolactone
B. Eplerenone
C. Triamterene
D. All of the above

1001. Which of the following can attenuate the effects of ACE inhibitors?
Harrison's 20th Ed. Chapter 253 Page 1775

A. Anxiety
B. Physical exercise
C. Fluid retention
D. All of the above

Fluid retention can attenuate the effects of ACE inhibitors. It is preferable to optimize the dose of diuretic before starting the ACE inhibitor.

1002. Nonproductive cough as a side effect of ACE inhibitors is related to?
Harrison's 20th Ed. Chapter 253 Page 1775

A. Stimulating guanylyl cyclase
B. Interference with adrenergic nervous system
C. Kinin potentiation
D. All of the above

The side effects of ACE inhibitors related to kinin potentiation include a nonproductive cough (10 - 15%) and angioedema (1%).

1003. Which of the following statements about beta blockers in HF is false?

Harrison's 20th Ed. Chapter 253 Page 1775

A. Should be initiated in low doses
B. Upward titration at 2-week intervals
C. Maximum dose as reported effective in clinical trials
D. None of the above

1004. Aldosterone antagonists are not recommended when?

Harrison's 20th Ed. Chapter 253 Page 1773

A. Serum creatinine is > 2.5 mg/dL
B. Creatinine clearance is < 30 mL/minute
C. Serum potassium is > 5 mmol/L
D. Any of the above

1005. Amiodarone increases the level of which of the following?

Harrison's 20th Ed. Chapter 63 Page 425

A. Quinidine
B. Digoxin
C. Warfarin
D. All of the above

1006. Most patients with acute pulmonary edema belong to which of the following profiles?

Int J Crit Care Emerg Med. 2017;3:023

A. Profile A
B. Profile B
C. Profile C
D. Profile L

Patients with acute HF present with one of four basic hemodynamic profiles. Profile A - normal LV filling pressure with normal perfusion, Profile B - elevated LV filling pressure with normal perfusion, Profile C - elevated LV filling pressures with decreased perfusion and Profile L - normal or low LV filling pressure with decreased tissue perfusion. Profile B includes most patients with acute pulmonary edema.

1007. Cyanide toxicity in nitroprusside therapy occurs at doses?

Ann Thorac Surg. 2015;99:1432-4

A. > 150 µg / minute for over 24 hours
B. > 150 µg / minute for over 48 hours
C. > 250 µg / minute for over 24 hours
D. > 250 µg / minute for over 48 hours

Cyanide toxicity (gastrointestinal & central nervous system) in nitroprusside therapy occurs at doses > 250 µg / minute for over 48 hours.

1008. Most common cause of right-heart failure is?

European Society of Cardiology. 2016;14(32)

A. Pulmonary parenchymal disease
B. Pulmonary vascular disease
C. Left heart failure
D. Any of the above

Most common cause of right-heart failure is not pulmonary parenchymal or vascular disease but left heart failure.

Cardiomyopathy and Myocarditis

1009. Cardiomyopathy is disease of?
Harrison's 20th Ed. Chapter 254 Page 1779

A. Cardiac muscle
B. Cardiac microvasculature
C. Cardiac interstitium
D. All of the above

Cardiomyopathy is disease of the heart muscle. As of 2006, cardiomyopathies are defined as "a heterogeneous group of diseases of the myocardium associated with mechanical and/or electrical dysfunction that usually (but not invariably) exhibit inappropriate ventricular hypertrophy or dilatation and are due to a variety of causes that frequently are genetic".

1010. Cardiomyopathy can be a result of which of the following?
Harrison's 20th Ed. Chapter 254 Page 1779

A. Hypertension
B. Congenital or acquired valvular abnormality
C. Pericardial abnormalities
D. None of the above

Cardiomyopathies are a group of diseases that affect heart muscle itself & are not the result of hypertension or congenital or acquired valvular, coronary or pericardial abnormalities.

1011. In the diagnosis of restrictive cardiomyopathy, which of the following has most relevance?
Harrison's 20th Ed. Chapter 254 Page 1779

A. Atrial size
B. Left ventricular diastolic dimension
C. Left ventricular wall thickness
D. Arrhythmia

Prominent atrial enlargement is a distinguishing feature of restrictive cardiomyopathy.

1012. Which of the following is a cause of primary cardiomyopathy?
Harrison's 20th Ed. Chapter 254 Page 1779

A. Genetic
B. Mixed genetic and acquired
C. Acquired
D. All of the above

The primary cardiomyopathy causes are divided into genetic, mixed genetic and acquired, and acquired.

1013. All three types of cardiomyopathy can be associated with?
Harrison's 20th Ed. Chapter 254 Page 1779

A. Atrioventricular valve regurgitation
B. Typical and atypical chest pain
C. Atrial and ventricular tachyarrhythmias
D. All of the above

All three types of cardiomyopathy (dilated, restrictive and hypertrophic) can be associated with atrioventricular valve regurgitation, typical and atypical chest pain, atrial and ventricular tachyarrhythmias, and embolic events.

1014. Which of the following is the "right-sided symptom" in heart failure?
Harrison's 20th Ed. Chapter 254 Page 1780, Table 254-1

A. Dyspnea on exertion
B. Discomfort on bending
C. Orthopnea
D. Paroxysmal nocturnal dyspnea

Left-sided symptoms of pulmoary congestlon are dyspnea on exertion, orthopnea, paroxysmal nocturnal dyspnea. Right-sided symptoms of systemic venous congestion are hepatic and abdominal distention, discomfort on bending and peripheral edema.

1015. What proportion of dilated cardiomyopathy are familial?
Harrison's 20th Ed. Chapter 254 Page 1779

A. 10%
B. 20%
C. 30%
D. 40%

Up to one-third of cases of dilated cardiomyopathy may be familial.

1016. Most familial cardiomyopathies are inherited in which of the following pattern?
Harrison's 20th Ed. Chapter 254 Page 1779

A. Autosomal dominant
B. Autosomal recessive
C. X-linked inheritance
D. Any of the above

Most familial cardiomyopathies are inherited in an autosomal dominant pattern, with occasional autosomal recessive and X-linked inheritance.

1017. Which of the following is most common in cardiomyopathy?
Harrison's 20th Ed. Chapter 254 Page 1779

A. Deletions of an entire exon or gene
B. Duplications of an entire exon or gene
C. Missense mutations with amino acid substitutions
D. All of the above

Missense mutations with amino acid substitutions are the most common in cardiomyopathy.

1018. Which of the following is false about cardiomyopathy?
Harrison's 20th Ed. Chapter 254 Page 1779

A. Defining phenotype of CMP is rarely present at birth
B. Genetic CMP is characterized by age dependence
C. Genetic CMP is characterized by incomplete penetrance
D. None of the above

1019. Most commonly recognized genetic causes of dilated cardiomyopathy are structural mutations of?
Harrison's 20th Ed. Chapter 254 Page 1780

A. Dystrophin
B. Desmin
C. Titin
D. All of the above

The most commonly recognized genetic causes of dilated cardiomyopathy are structural mutations of the giant protein titin, encoded TTN, which maintains sarcomere structure and acts as a key signaling molecule.

1020. Defects in sarcomeric proteins are mostly associated with?
Harrison's 20th Ed. Chapter 254 Page 1779

A. Dilated cardiomyopathy
B. Restrictive cardiomyopathy
C. Hypertrophic cardiomyopathy
D. All of the above

Defects in sarcomeric proteins of myosin, actin, and troponin are mostly associated with hypertrophic cardiomyopathy.

1021. The most commonly recognized genetic causes of DCM are truncating mutations of?
Harrison's 20th Ed. Chapter 254 Page 1780

A. Actin
B. Myosin
C. Tropomyosin
D. Titin

The most commonly recognized genetic causes of DCM are truncating mutations of titin, encoded by TTN, which maintains sarcomere structure and acts as a key signaling molecule.

1022. Most of the identified genetic defects in the Z-disk and cytoskeleton are associated with?
Harrison's 20th Ed. Chapter 254 Page 1780

A. Dilated cardiomyopathy
B. Restrictive cardiomyopathy
C. Hypertrophic cardiomyopathy
D. All of the above

Desmin forms intermediate filaments that connect the nuclear and plasma membranes, Z-lines, and the intercalated disks between muscle cells. Desmin mutations impair the transmission of force and signaling for both cardiac & skeletal muscle leading to a peripheral myopathy and a dilated cardiomyopathy. Most of the identified genetic defects in the Z-disk and cytoskeleton are associated with dilated cardiomyopathy.

1023. Which of the following is a sarcomeric protein?
Harrison's 20th Ed. Chapter 254 Page 1782 Figure 254-1

A. Actin
B. Myosin
C. Tropomyosin
D. All of the above

1024. Which of the following is related to "myocyte stabilizing and connecting the cell membrane to intracellular structures"?
Harrison's 20th Ed. Chapter 254 Page 1782 Figure 254-1

A. Sarcomeric proteins
B. Dystrophin complex
C. Desmosome complex
D. All of the above

1025. Which of the following is related to "cell-cell connections and myocyte stability"?
Harrison's 20th Ed. Chapter 254 Page 1782 Figure 254-1

A. Sarcomeric proteins
B. Dystrophin complex
C. Desmosome complex
D. All of the above

Sarcomeric proteins include actin, myosin, tropomyosin, and the associated regulatory proteins. Dystrophin complex stabilizes and connects the cell membrane to intracellular structures. Desmosome complexes are associated with cell-cell connections and stability.

1026. Abnormal dystrophin can be acquired during infection by?
Harrison's 20th Ed. Chapter 254 Page 1780

A. Coxsackie virus
B. Varicella-zoster virus
C. Herpes simplex virus (HSV) type 1
D. Epstein-Barr virus

Abnormal dystrophin can be acquired when Coxsackie virus cleaves dystrophin in viral myocarditis.

1027. Mutations in which of the following genes is associated with Brugada syndrome?
Harrison's 20th Ed. Chapter 254 Page 1780

A. SCN5A
B. ACTN2
C. DES
D. TTN

Mutations in SCN5A, distinct from those that cause the Brugada or long-QT syndromes, have been implicated in dilated cardiomyopathy with conduction disease.

1028. Which of the following about nuclear membrane protein defects in cardiac muscle is false?
Harrison's 20th Ed. Chapter 254 Page 1780

A. Occurs in autosomal (lamin A/C) pattern
B. Occurs in X-linked (emerin) pattern
C. High prevalence of atrial arrhythmias & conduction system disease
D. None of the above

1029. "Arrhythmogenic cardiomyopathy" is best related to?
Harrison's 20th Ed. Chapter 254 Page 1780

A. Cellular metabolism
B. Nuclear membrane
C. Mitochondria
D. Desmosome

1030. Which of the following diseases can affect heart without mutation of genes expressed in heart?
Harrison's 20th Ed. Chapter 254 Page 1780

A. Fabry's disease
B. Familial amyloidosis
C. Becker's muscle dystrophy
D. Long QT syndrome

Familial amyloidosis and hemochromatosis can affect heart without mutation of genes expressed in heart.

1031. Mostly, familial forms of DCM are due to mutations in?
Harrison's 20th Ed. Chapter 254 Page 1780

A. Genes encoding nuclear envelope protein lamin A/C
B. Genes encoding sarcomeric proteins
C. Mitochondrial genes
D. None of the above

Most commonly, familial forms of DCM are due to mutations in genes encoding sarcomeric proteins like alpha-cardiac actin, beta- & alpha-myosin, heavy chain alpha-tropomyosin & troponins T, I, and C. Mutations in gene encoding nuclear envelope protein lamin A/C are responsible for DCM associated with atrioventricular (AV) conduction disorder that may cause sudden cardiac death (SCD). Mutations in mitochondrial genes have also been reported in DCM.

1032. Upper limit of normal of the weight of human heart is?
Harrison's 20th Ed. Chapter 254 Page 1783 Figure 254-2

A. 320 grams
B. 340 grams
C. 360 grams
D. 380 grams

Upper limit of normal of the weight of human heart is 360 grams.

1033. Histopathological feature of a dilated cardiomyopathy specimen is?
Harrison's 20th Ed. Chapter 254 Page 1783 Figure 254-4

A. Interstitial fibrosis
B. Increased myocyte size
C. Enlarged, irregular nuclei
D. All of the above

Microscopically, a dilated cardiomyopathy specimen would show nonspecific changes of interstitial fibrosis and myocyte hypertrophy characterized by increased myocyte size and enlarged, irregular nuclei.

1034. What proportion of patients with new-onset cardiomyopathy have substantial spontaneous recovery?
Harrison's 20th Ed. Chapter 254 Page 1782

A. 20%
B. 30%
C. 40%
D. 50%

Almost half of all patients with new-onset cardiomyopathy have substantial spontaneous recovery.

1035. Which of the following is a feature of cardiac remodeling?
Circulation. 2000;102:Iv-14–Iv-23

A. Impaired ventricular systolic pump function
B. Cardiac enlargement
C. Cardiac hypertrophy
D. All of the above

Left and/or right ventricular systolic pump function is impaired, leading to progressive cardiac enlargement and hypertrophy, a process called remodeling.

1036. Myocardial damage leading to dilated cardiomyopathy can be produced by which of the following?
Circulation. 2000;102:Iv-14–Iv-23

A. Toxic agents
B. Metabolic factors
C. Infectious agents
D. All of the above

DCM is either familial or the end result of myocardial damage produced by known or unknown infectious, metabolic, or toxic agents.

1037. In which of the following conditions, dilated cardiomyopathy is reversible?
Circulation. 2000;102:Iv-14–Iv-23

A. Alcohol abuse
B. Pregnancy
C. Thyroid disease
D. All of the above

Reversible form of dilated cardiomyopathy may be found with alcohol abuse, pregnancy, thyroid disease, cocaine use, and chronic uncontrolled tachycardia. Obesity & sleep apnea increases the risk of developing heart failure.

1038. ECG of a DCM patient may show all of the following except?
Circulation. 2000;102:Iv-14–Iv-23

A. Atrial fibrillation
B. Ventricular arrhythmias
C. High voltage
D. Intraventricular conduction defects

ECG in a case of DCM shows sinus tachycardia or atrial fibrillation, ventricular arrhythmias, left atrial abnormality, diffuse nonspecific ST-T-wave abnormalities & sometimes intraventricular conduction defects and low voltage.

1039. Which of the following should be avoided in dilated cardiomyopathy?
Circulation. 2000;102:Iv-14–Iv-23

A. Alcohol
B. Calcium channel blockers
C. Nonsteroidal anti-inflammatory drugs
D. All of the above

Alcohol, calcium channel blockers & NSAIDs should be avoided in DCM.

1040. Which of the following drugs should be avoided in a patient of dilated cardiomyopathy?
Circulation. 2000;102:Iv-14–Iv-23

A. Digitalis
B. Beta adrenergic blocker
C. Calcium channel blocker
D. Spironolactone

Standard therapy of heart failure with salt restriction, ACE inhibitors or angiotensin II receptor blocker, diuretics, and digitalis produces symptomatic improvement. Most patients should be treated with a beta adrenergic blocker. Spironolactone should be added for most patients with recent or current advanced heart failure.

1041. Cardiac involvement is common in which of the following conditions?
Harrison's 20th Ed. Chapter 254 Page 1784

A. Duchenne's progressive muscular dystrophy
B. Myotonic dystrophy
C. Friedreich's ataxia
D. All of the above

Cardiac involvement is common in Duchenne's progressive muscular dystrophy, Myotonic dystrophy and Friedreich's ataxia.

1042. Cardiomyopathy-neutropenia syndrome is also called?
Am J Med Genet Part C Semin Med Genet 163C:198–205

A. Pompe disease
B. Barth syndrome
C. Holt-Oram syndrome
D. Fraser syndrome

Barth syndrome (BTHS) is named after Dr. Peter Barth (Netherlands). It is found exclusively in males. It is also known as 3-Methylglutaconic aciduria type II and Cardiomyopathy-neutropenia syndrome. It is due to mutations in BTHS gene, tafazzin (TAZ) located at Xq28, the long arm of X chromosome and is associated with cardiolipin molecules in the electron transport chain & mitochondrial membrane structure. Syndrome consists of metabolism distortion, delayed motor skills, stamina deficiency, hypotonia, chronic fatigue, delayed growth, cardiomyopathy, and compromised immune system.

Myocarditis

1043. Infective agents injure myocardium through?
Harrison's 20th Ed. Chapter 254 Page 1783

A. Direct invasion
B. Production of cardiotoxic substances
C. Chronic inflammation with or without persistent infection
D. All of the above

Myocarditis is commonly attributed to infective agents that injure myocardium through direct invasion, production of cardiotoxic substances or chronic inflammation with or without persistent infection.

1044. Infectious myocarditis is most commonly associated with?
Harrison's 20th Ed. Chapter 254 Page 1783

A. Borrelia burgdorferi
B. HIV
C. Trypanosoma cruzi
D. Diphtheria

Infectious myocarditis is reported with almost all types of infective agents but is most commonly associated with viruses and the protozoan Trypanosoma cruzi.

1045. Which of the following receptor on heart cells has enhanced expression in viral-induced myocarditis?
Harrison's 20th Ed. Chapter 254 Page 1783

A. Epidermal growth receptor 2
B. β-adrenergic receptor
C. Coxsackie-adenovirus receptor
D. All of the above

Viral-induced myocarditis is due to abnormalities in cell surface receptors, such as coxsackie-adenovirus receptor, that bind viral proteins. Human coxsackievirus and adenovirus receptor (CAR) is a common receptor for two of the most common viral causes of myocarditis (coxsackieviruses B3 and B4, and adenoviruses 2 and 5). Increased expression of CAR has been reported in patients with DCM and myocarditis.

1046. Ventricular tachyarrhythmias may be a feature of?
Harrison's 20th Ed. Chapter 254 Page 1784

A. Viral myocarditis
B. Sarcoidosis
C. Giant cell myocarditis
D. All of the above

Ventricular tachyarrhythmias dominate the presentation in viral myocarditis, sarcoidosis and giant cell myocarditis.

1047. On auscultation in a case of myocarditis, which of the following murmur is frequently heard?
Harrison's 20th Ed. Chapter 254 Page 1784

A. Mitral stenosis
B. Mitral regurgitation
C. Aortic stenosis
D. Aortic regurgitation

Auscultatory findings in a case of myocarditis include muffled S1 with S3 & a murmur of mitral regurgitation. Pericardial rub may be heard in patients with associated pericarditis.

1048. Criteria used for myocarditis on endomyocardial biopsy is?
Harrison's 20th Ed. Chapter 254 Page 1784

A. American
B. Boston
C. Chicago
D. Dallas

Dallas Criteria for myocarditis on endomyocardial biopsy include lymphocytic infiltrate with evidence of myocyte necrosis.

1049. Which of the following viruses most often produces clinically significant acute myocarditis?
Harrison's 20th Ed. Chapter 254 Page 1785

A. Influenza
B. Toxoplasma gondii
C. Coxsackievirus
D. HIV

While almost every infectious agent is capable of producing myocarditis, clinically significant acute myocarditis in USA is caused by viruses, especially coxsackievirus B.

1050. Myocarditis can result from?
Harrison's 20th Ed. Chapter 254 Page 1785

A. Infectious process
B. Hypersensitivity to drugs
C. Radiation
D. All of the above

Myocarditis results from infections, drug hypersensitivity, radiation, chemicals or physical agents.

1051. In HIV myocarditis, the most common finding is?
Harrison's 20th Ed. Chapter 254 Page 1785

A. Pericarditis
B. Left ventricular dysfunction
C. Right ventricular dysfunction
D. Conduction abnormalities

In HIV patients, the most common finding is left ventricular dysfunction that in some cases appears to be due to infiltration of myocardium by virus.

1052. Chagas disease is caused by?
Harrison's 20th Ed. Chapter 254 Page 1786

A. Toxoplasma gondii
B. Trypanosoma cruzi
C. Schistosoma haematobium
D. Dermatobia hominis

Chagas disease caused by protozoan Trypanosoma cruzi is transmitted by the bite of insect vector reduvid bug.

1053. Protozoan Trypanosoma cruzi can be transmitted by?
Harrison's 20th Ed. Chapter 254 Page 1786

A. Blood transfusion
B. Organ donation
C. Mother to fetus
D. All of the above

Transmission of protozoan T. cruzi can also occur through blood transfusion, organ donation, from mother to fetus, and occasionally orally.

1054. Which of the following is a typical feature of Chagas' disease in ECG?
Harrison's 20th Ed. Chapter 254 Page 1786

A. Atrial fibrillation
B. Ventricular tachyarrhythmias
C. Conduction system abnormalities
D. Nonspecific ST-T abnormalities

Features typical of Chagas' disease are conduction system abnormalities, particularly sinus node and atrioventricular (AV) node dysfunction and right bundle branch block. Atrial fibrillation and ventricular tachyarrhythmias also occur.

1055. Multiple left ventricular aneurysm formation is a feature of which of the following?
Harrison's 20th Ed. Chapter 254 Page 1786

A. Diphtheritic myocarditis
B. Myocarditis in patients with HIV
C. Chagas disease
D. Lyme carditis

Cardiac involvement in Chagas heart disease is characterized by dilatation of cardiac chambers, fibrosis & thinning of ventricular wall, aneurysm formation in left ventricular apex and mural thrombi that may embolize to pulmonary and systemic circulations.

1056. Which of the following drug is used in the treatment of Chagas' disease?
Harrison's 20th Ed. Chapter 254 Page 1786

A. Pentamidine
B. Benznidazole
C. Suramin
D. Melarsoprol

Antiparasitic therapy for Chagas' disease include benznidazole and nifurtimox.

1057. West African trypanosomiasis is caused by?
Harrison's 20th Ed. Chapter 254 Page 1786

A. Trypanosoma brucei gambiense
B. Trypanosoma brucei rhodesiense
C. Trypanosoma cruzi
D. All of the above

African trypanosomiasis infection results from the tsetse fly bite. The West African form is caused by Trypanosoma brucei gambiense while the East African form is caused by Trypanosoma brucei rhodesiense.

1058. Toxoplasmosis can cause which of the following?
Harrison's 20th Ed. Chapter 254 Page 1786

A. Myocarditis
B. Pericardial effusion
C. Constrictive pericarditis
D. All of the above

Toxoplasmosis may present with encephalitis or chorioretinitis and, in the heart, can cause myocarditis, pericardial effusion, constrictive pericarditis and heart failure.

1059. Multidrug antituberculous regimens are effective in the treatment of?
Harrison's 20th Ed. Chapter 254 Page 1787

A. Brucellosis
B. Whipple's disease
C. Clostridial infections
D. Psittacosis

Multidrug antituberculous regimens are effective in the treatment of Whipple's disease caused by Tropheryma whipplei.

1060. Most common cardiac abnormality in Lyme disease is?
Harrison's 20th Ed. Chapter 254 Page 1787

A. Myopericarditis
B. Left ventricular dysfunction
C. Right ventricular dysfunction
D. Conduction abnormalities

In Lyme disease, conduction abnormalities are the most common manifestations of cardiac involvement.

1061. Giant cell myocarditis may occur in association with?
Harrison's 20th Ed. Chapter 254 Page 1787

A. Thymoma
B. Thyroiditis
C. Pernicious anemia
D. All of the above

Associated conditions of giant cell myocarditis are thymomas, thyroiditis, pernicious anemia, other autoimmune diseases.

1062. Myocarditis may result from hypersensitivity to which of the following drugs?
Harrison's 20th Ed. Chapter 254 Page 1788

A. Thiazides
B. Antibiotics
C. Methyldopa
D. All of the above

Myocarditis may result from hypersensitivity to antibiotics, thiazides, anticonvulsants, indomethacin, and methyldopa.

1063. Peripartum cardiomyopathy (PPCM) usually develops in which trimester of pregnancy?
Harrison's 20th Ed. Chapter 254 Page 1788

A. First
B. Second
C. Third
D. All of the above

Cardiac dilatation & CHF of unexplained cause may develop during last trimester of pregnancy or within 6 months after delivery.

1064. Likelihood of peripartum cardiomyopathy (PPCM) is more in?
Harrison's 20th Ed. Chapter 254 Page 1788

A. Malnutrition
B. Increased maternal age & parity
C. Use of tocolytic therapy for premature labor
D. All of the above

1065. Risk factor for peripartum cardiomyopathy (PPCM) is?
Harrison's 20th Ed. Chapter 254 Page 1788

A. Blood group AB
B. Recurrent UTI
C. Preeclampsia or toxemia of pregnancy
D. All of the above

Risk factors are increased maternal age, increased parity, twin pregnancy, malnutrition, use of tocolytic therapy for premature labor and preeclampsia or toxemia of pregnancy.

1066. Pregnancy-associated cardiomyopathy (PACM) refers to?
Harrison's 20th Ed. Chapter 254 Page 1788

A. Heart failure occuring in successive pregnancies
B. Heart failure presenting earlier in pregnancy
C. Heart failure occuring after miscarriage
D. Any of the above

Heart failure presenting earlier in pregnancy has been termed pregnancy-associated cardiomyopathy (PACM).

1067. Which of the following statements is false?
Harrison's 20th Ed. Chapter 254 Page 1788

A. Chagas' disease is the most common infective cause of cardiomyopathy
B. Granulomatous myocarditis is the most common cause of noninfective inflammation
C. Alcohol is the most common toxin implicated in chronic DCM
D. None of the above

1068. Polymorphisms of which of the following genes increases the likelihood of alcoholic cardiomyopathy?
Harrison's 20th Ed. Chapter 254 Page 1788

A. Angiotensin-converting enzyme
B. β_1 - adrenergic receptor
C. β_2 - adrenergic receptor
D. All of the above

Polymorphisms of the genes encoding alcohol dehydrogenase and the angiotensin-converting enzyme increase the likelihood of alcoholic cardiomyopathy.

1069. Alcohol consumption necessary to produce cardiomyopathy is?
Harrison's 20th Ed. Chapter 254 Page 1788

A. 1 ounce of pure ethanol daily for 5 - 10 years
B. 2 ounces of pure ethanol daily for 5 - 10 years
C. 3 ounces of pure ethanol daily for 5 - 10 years
D. 4 ounces of pure ethanol daily for 5 - 10 years

Alcohol consumption necessary to produce cardiomyopathy in an otherwise normal heart is about 4 ounces of pure ethanol (five to six drinks) daily for 5 - 10 years.

1070. "Holiday heart syndrome" is the term used for cardiotoxicity produced by?
Harrison's 20th Ed. Chapter 254 Page 1788

A. Alcohol
B. Tobacco
C. Cocaine
D. Amphetamine

Holiday heart syndrome is a state of alcoholic cardiotoxicity presenting as recurrent supraventricular or ventricular tachyarrhythmias without overt heart failure due to alcoholic binge drinking.

1071. Which of the following arrhythmias is most frequent in "Holiday heart syndrome"?
Harrison's 20th Ed. Chapter 254 Page 1788

A. Atrial flutter
B. Atrial fibrillation
C. Ventricular premature depolarizations
D. Ventricular tachycardia

In holiday heart syndrome, atrial fibrillation is the most common arrhythmia, followed by atrial flutter and ventricular premature depolarizations.

1072. What quantity of alcohol consumption has been shown to be cardio-protective?
Genes Nutr. 2010;5:111-120

A. 10 - 20 grams / day
B. 20 - 30 grams / day
C. 30 - 40 grams / day
D. 40 - 50 grams / day

Alcohol consumption in moderate quantity (20 - 30 grams/day) appears to be cardio-protective.

1073. Pathologic findings in CMP due to cocaine resemble those of?
Harrison's 20th Ed. Chapter 254 Page 1788

A. Beri-beri heart disease
B. Diabetes
C. Pheochromocytoma
D. Hyperthyroidism

Cocaine & amphetamine related cardiomyopathy reveals microinfarcts due to small vessel ischemia, similar to those seen with pheochromocytoma.

1074. Which of the following about cocaine is false?
Harrison's 20th Ed. Chapter 447 Page 3287

A. Vasospastic
B. Enhances sympathetic activity
C. Psychostimulant
D. None of the above

1075. Which of the following can lead to adrenergic crisis due to catecholamine excess?
Harrison's 20th Ed. Chapter 271 Page 1906

A. Amphetamine overdose
B. Clonidine withdrawal
C. Interaction of tyramine-containing food with MAO inhibitors
D. All of the above

Adrenergic crisis due to catecholamine excess may be related to pheochromocytoma, cocaine or amphetamine overdose, clonidine withdrawal, acute spinal cord injuries, and an interaction of tyramine-containing compounds with monoamine oxidase inhibitors.

1076. Which of the following drugs should be avoided while treating cocaine-induced cardiotoxicity?
Harrison's 20th Ed. Chapter 447 Page 3287

A. Nitrates
B. Calcium channel blockers
C. Beta-adrenergic blockers
D. Benzodiazepines

Nitrates, calcium channel blockers (to reduce coronary spasm) & benzodiazepines are used to treat cocaine-induced cardiotoxicities. Beta-adrenergic blockers should be avoided.

1077. Which of the following is the explanation for myocyte injury & fibrosis with use of doxorubicin?
Harrison's 20th Ed. Chapter 254 Page 1788

A. Generation of ROS involving 5-lipoxygenase
B. Generation of ROS involving heme compounds
C. Generation of ROS involving vascular endothelial growth factor
D. Generation of ROS involving matrix metalloproteinase

Generation of reactive oxygen species (ROS) involving heme compounds is currently the favored explanation for myocyte injury and fibrosis with the use of anthracyclines like doxorubicin. Antineoplastic activity of anthracyclines is almost exclusively due to the ability to bind to DNA and act as a poison to topoisomerase II by inducing lethal double-strand DNA breaks.

1078. Which of the following is a cardioprotective agent when doxorubicin (Adriamycin) is given to a patient?

Cancer Management and Research 2014:6 357–363

A. Erythropoietin
B. Dexrazoxone
C. Amiodarone
D. Cyclophosphamide

Iron chelator dexrazoxone is cardioprotective and reduces risk of doxorubicin (Adriamycin) cardiotoxicity. Recovery of cardiac function occurs with aggressive use of ACE inhibitors.

1079. Dexrazoxane best relates to which of the following?

Cancer Management and Research 2014:6 357–363

A. British anti-Lewisite (BAL)
B. Ethylene diamine tetraacetic acid (EDTA)
C. Dimercaptosuccinic acid (DMSA)
D. Penicillamine

Dexrazoxane is a water-soluble ring-closed analog of iron chelator ethylenediaminetetraacetic acid (EDTA). Unlike EDTA, dexrazoxane easily passes into cells. Upon hydrolysis, dexrazoxane opens into its EDTA-like form, ADR-925, which is a strong iron chelator that has the ability to displace iron from the anthracycline.

1080. Which of the following drug is an anthracycline?

Cancer Management and Research 2014:6 357–363

A. Doxorubicin
B. Epirubicin
C. Daunorubicin
D. All of the above

1081. Which of the following drug is an anthracenedione?

Cancer Management and Research 2014:6 357–363

A. Etoposide
B. Teniposide
C. Mitoxantrone
D. All of the above

Etoposide and teniposide are podophyllotoxins.

1082. Dexrazoxane is a catalytic inhibitor of?

Cancer Management and Research 2014:6 357–363

A. DNA Topoisomerase I
B. DNA topoisomerase II
C. DNA topoisomerase IV
D. All of the above

Dexrazoxane is a catalytic inhibitor of DNA topoisomerase II that is the same target as the DNA topoisomerase II poisonous anticancer agents like anthracyclines, anthracenediones and podophyllotoxins. Dexrazoxane does not induce lethal DNA double-strand breaks as do the topoisomerase poisons.

1083. Trastuzumab interferes with?

Harrison's 20th Ed. Chapter 254 Page 1788

A. Human epidermal growth receptor 2
B. Vascular endothelial growth receptor
C. Peptide receptor radionuclides
D. All of the above

Trastuzumab (Herceptin) is a monoclonal antibody that interferes with human epidermal growth receptor 2 (HER2) crucial for some tumor growth and for cardiac adaptation.

1084. Which of the following drug causes dilated cardiomyopathy?

Harrison's 20th Ed. Chapter 254 Page 1789

A. Trastuzumab
B. Ifosfamide
C. Cyclophosphamide
D. All of the above

1085. Which of the following chemotherapeutic agents can cause recurrent coronary spasm?

Harrison's 20th Ed. Chapter 254 Page 1789

A. Cyclophosphamide
B. Ifosfamide
C. Cisplatin
D. All of the above

5-Fluorouracil, cisplatin, and some other alkylating agents can cause recurrent coronary spasm.

1086. Which of the following drugs can cause cardiotoxicity with chronic use?

Harrison's 20th Ed. Chapter 254 Page 1789

A. Hydroxychloroquine
B. Chloroquine
C. Emetine
D. All of the above

1087. Which of the following about a patient of pheochromocytoma is false?

Harrison's 20th Ed. Chapter 254 Page 1789

A. Very labile blood pressure & heart rate
B. Episodic palpitations
C. Postural hypotension
D. None of the above

1088. Heart failure with "preserved" ejection fraction best applies to?

Harrison's 20th Ed. Chapter 254 Page 1789

A. Hyperthyroidism
B. Hypothyroidism
C. Obesity
D. Diabetes

Diabetes is a typical factor, along with hypertension, advanced age, and female gender, in heart failure with "preserved" ejection fraction.

1089. Which of the following conditions is associated with a high risk of death in patients with viral myocarditis?

Harrison's 20th Ed. Chapter 254 Page 1789

A. Pulmonary hypertension
B. Pericarditis
C. Arrhythmias
D. Heart failure

Patients with viral myocarditis & pulmonary hypertension are at a particularly high risk of death.

1090. Deficiency of which of the following plays a pathogenetic role in peripartum cardiomyopathy?

Harrison's 20th Ed. Chapter 254 Page 1789

A. Gold
B. Zinc
C. Copper
D. Selenium

Pathogenetic factors in peripartum cardiomyopathy include low socioeconomic status, high parity, prolonged lactation, excessive dietary salt intake & selenium deficiency.

1091. "Wet beri-beri heart disease" is characterized by all except?
Harrison's 20th Ed. Chapter 254 Page 1789

A. Third heart sound
B. Cold extremities
C. Reduced ECG voltage
D. Prolongation of QT interval

"Wet beri-beri heart disease" is characterized by high cardiac output failure state & is associated with tachycardia, wide pulse pressure, S3, & warm extremities. ECG shows reduced voltage, diffuse T-wave abnormalities & prolongation of QT interval.

1092. While treating "wet beri-beri heart disease" with thiamine, which of the following drugs should be given?
Harrison's 20th Ed. Chapter 254 Page 1789

A. Digoxin
B. Theophylline
C. Quinidine
D. Diuretics

Response to thiamine in "wet beri-beri heart disease" is dramatic & must be accompanied by diuretics.

1093. Which of the following diseases is associated with selenium deficiency?
Harrison's 20th Ed. Chapter 254 Page 1789

A. Keshan Disease
B. Kallmann syndrome
C. Liddle's syndrome
D. Tay–Sachs disease

Specific diseases associated with selenium deficiency are Keshan Disease, Kashin-Beck Disease (Big Bone disease) and Myxedematous Endemic Cretinism. Keshan disease is an endemic cardiomyopathy found in children and young women residing in regions of China where dietary intake of selenium is low.

1094. Which of the following is best absorbed & utilized form of selenium?
J Am College of Nutr. 2001;20:1-4

A. Selenothiamine
B. Selenoarginine
C. Selenoleucine
D. Selenomethionine

Selenomethionine is considered to be the best absorbed and utilized form of selenium.

1095. Recommended Dietary Allowances (RDA) for selenium for adults is?
J Am College of Nutr. 2001;20:1-4

A. 50 μg/day
B. 500 μg/day
C. 5000 μg/day
D. 50000 μg/day

Recommended Dietary Allowances (RDA) for selenium for adults is 50-200 μg/day.

1096. Clinical syndrome of Hemochromatosis includes?
Harrison's 20th Ed. Chapter 254 Page 1789

A. Cirrhosis
B. Diabetes
C. Hypogonadism
D. All of the above

The clinical syndrome of Hemochromatosis includes cirrhosis, diabetes & hypogonadism.

1097. Which of the following is false about Hemochromatosis?
Harrison's 20th Ed. Chapter 254 Page 1789

A. May be due to iron overload as in hemolytic anemia
B. Iron deposited in perinuclear area of cardiomyocytes
C. Transferrin saturation > 60% for men
D. None of the above

1098. In right ventricular dysplasia, there is progressive replacement of right ventricular wall with?
Harrison's 20th Ed. Chapter 254 Page 1790

A. Elastic tissue
B. Collagen tissue
C. Adipose tissue
D. Mucopolysaccharides

RV dysplasia is a familial cardiomyopathy marked by progressive replacement of right ventricular wall with adipose tissue. Ventricular arrhythmias are common & sudden death is a constant threat.

1099. Which of the following is false about arrhythmogenic ventricular dysplasia?
Harrison's 20th Ed. Chapter 254 Page 1790

A. Can affect right ventricle
B. Can affect left ventricle
C. Can affect both ventricles
D. None of the above

Arrhythmogenic ventricular dysplasia can affect either or both ventricles.

1100. Which of the following is mostly affected in Arrhythmogenic Right Ventricular Dysplasia (ARVD)
Harrison's 20th Ed. Chapter 254 Page 1790

A. Nuclear membrane
B. Endoplasmic reticulum
C. Mitochondria
D. Desmosomes

ARVC/D is an autosomal dominant disorder caused by multiple mutations of several genes encoding proteins that constitute desmosomes, structures that maintain normal contacts between cells leading to detachment of myocytes with consequent myocyte apoptosis and fibrofatty replacement.

1101. Which of the following best relates to genetic defect in the desmosomal protein?
Harrison's 20th Ed. Chapter 254 Page 1790

A. Strabismus
B. Gait disturbance
C. Woolly hair
D. Cyanosis

Genetic defects in proteins of the desmosomal complex disrupt myocyte junctions & adhesions, leading to replacement of myocardium by deposits of fat. This same protein also affects hair & skin, leading to a distinct syndrome of "woolly hair" and thickened palms and soles.

1102. Drooping eyelids is a feature of?
Neurol Genet 2018;4:e230, Harrison's 19th Ed. 207

A. Hemochromatosis
B. Duchenne's and Becker's dystrophy
C. Mitochondrial myopathies
D. Hypothyroidism

Mitochondrial myopathies show the characteristic "ragged red fiber" appearance. Some patients with mitochondrial myopathy have characteristic drooping eyelids.

1103. Cardinal clinical feature of left ventricular noncompaction is?
Harrison's 20th Ed. Chapter 254 Page 1790

A. Ventricular arrhythmias
B. Embolic events
C. Heart failure
D. All of the above

The three cardinal clinical features of left ventricular noncompaction are ventricular arrhythmias, embolic events, and heart failure.

1104. Which of the following is false about Left Ventricular Noncompaction (LVNC)?
Harrison's 20th Ed. Chapter 254 Page 1790

A. Congenital cardiomyopathy
B. Abnormal embryogenesis
C. Multiple deep trabeculations into myocardium
D. None of the above

Left ventricular noncompaction (LVNC) is a congenital cardiomyopathy that may present at any age with symptoms of CHF, thromboembolism or ventricular arrhythmias due to arrest of normal embryogenesis, with persistence of multiple deep trabeculations into myocardium communicating with ventricular cavity, 2 layered structure of endomyocardium leading to LV contractile dysfunction. It is diagnosed echocardiographically.

1105. Left ventricular noncompaction is best related to?
Harrison's 20th Ed. Chapter 254 Page 1790

A. Restanin
B. Tafazzin
C. Gibazin
D. Frufin

Diagnostic criteria of left ventricular noncompaction includes presence of multiple trabeculations in left ventricle distal to papillary muscles, creating a "spongy" appearance of apex. It is associated with multiple genetic variants in sarcomeric and other proteins such as tafazzin.

1106. What does "tako tsubo" in Japanese language mean?
Harrison's 20th Ed. Chapter 254 Page 1790, Q J Med 2003; 96:563–573

A. Japanese baloon
B. Japanese parachute
C. Japanese pot for fishing octopus
D. Japanese fishing net

"Tako-tsubo" in Japanese language refers to a Japanese pot for fishing for octopus.

1107. Which of the following is false about Tako-Tsubo cardiomyopathy?
Harrison's 20th Ed. Chapter 254 Page 1790

A. Also known as apical ballooning syndrome
B. Severe chest discomfort preceded by stressful emotional or physical event
C. Occurs mostly in women >50 years
D. None of the above

Also known as apical ballooning syndrome, Tako-Tsubo (stress) cardiomyopathy is characterized by abrupt & severe chest discomfort preceded by a stressful emotional or physical event. It occurs mostly in women >50 years.

1108. Which of the following is false about Tako-Tsubo cardiomyopathy?
Harrison's 20th Ed. Chapter 254 Page 1790

A. ST elevations &/or T-wave inversions in chest leads
B. Normal coronary angiography
C. ECG & Echo CG changes revert in 3-7 days
D. None of the above

ECG in Tako-Tsubo (stress) cardiomyopathy shows ST-segment elevations and/or deep T-wave inversions in chest leads. Coronary angiography shows no obstruction in epicardial arteries. Severe akinesia of distal portion of left ventricle with EF reduction occurs. Troponins are mildly elevated. Changes are reversible in 3 - 7 days without consequences.

1109. Which of the following can present as dilated or restrictive disease?
Harrison's 20th Ed. Chapter 254 Page 1791

A. Sarcoidosis
B. Fabry's disease
C. Carcinoid syndrome
D. Amyloidosis

Sarcoidosis and hemochromatosis can present as dilated or restrictive disease.

1110. Overlapping types of cardiomyopathy are more common with?
Harrison's 20th Ed. Chapter 254 Page 1791

A. Inflammatory myocarditis
B. Toxic myocarditis
C. Nutritional deficiencies
D. Inherited metabolic disorders

Overlaps are particularly common with the inherited metabolic disorders, which can present as any of the three major phenotypes.

1111. Fabry's disease results from a deficiency of?
Harrison's 20th Ed. Chapter 254 Page 1791

A. Alpha-galactosidase A
B. Beta-galactosidase
C. Sphingomyelinase
D. Neuraminidase

Fabry's disease results from a deficiency of the lysosomal enzyme alpha-galactosidase A.

1112. Which of the following about Fabry's disease is false?
Harrison's 20th Ed. Chapter 254 Page 1791

A. Autosomal dominant disorder
B. Disorder of glycosphingolipid metabolism
C. Leg lymphedema without hypoproteinemia
D. Enzyme therapy useful

Fabry's disease is an X-linked recessive disorder that may also cause clinical disease in female carriers. Clinically, it manifests with angiokeratomas (telangiectatic skin lesions), hypohidrosis, corneal & lenticular opacities, acroparesthesia; & small-vessel disease of kidney, heart & brain.

1113. Which of the following about angiokeratomas in Fabry's disease is false?
Harrison's 20th Ed. Chapter 411 Page 3007

A. Do not blanch with pressure
B. Mostly between umbilicus & knees "bathing suit area"
C. Punctate, dark red to blue-black
D. Asymmetric

Angiokeratomas are punctate, dark red to blue-black, flat or slightly raised, and usually symmetric; they do not blanch with pressure. They range from barely visible to several millimeters in diameter and have a tendency to increase in size and number with age. They are most dense between umbilicus & knees - the "bathing suit area". Angiokeratomas also occur in Fordyce scrotal angiokeratoma and several other very rare lysosomal storage diseases.

1114. Cardiac Danon's Disease is due to mutations in?
Harrison's 20th Ed. Chapter 254 Page 1791

A. LAMP1
B. LAMP2
C. LAMP3
D. LAMP4

Cardiac Danon Disease is caused by mutations in an X-linked lysosome-associated membrane protein (LAMP2).

1115. Extreme left ventricular hypertrophy is seen in?
Harrison's 20th Ed. Chapter 254 Page 1791

A. Fabry's disease
B. Gaucher's disease
C. Glycogen storage disease type III
D. Danon's disease

Danon's disease consists of skeletal myopathy, mental retardation and hepatic dysfunction. Extreme left ventricular hypertrophy appears early, often in childhood, and can progress rapidly to end-stage heart failure with low ejection fraction.

1116. ECG of which of the following inherited metabolic cardiomyopathies with LVH shows ventricular preexcitation?
Harrison's 20th Ed. Chapter 254 Page 1791

A. Fabry Disease
B. Friedreich's Ataxia
C. Cardiac Danon Disease
D. Glycogen Storage Cardiomyopathy

ECG in Cardiac Danon Disease shows severe LV hypertrophy & ventricular preexcitation. Deficiencies of LAMP2 and protein kinase, adenosine monophosphate (AMP)-activated gamma 2 noncatalytic subunit (PRKAG2) result in the accumulation of glycogen in heart and skeletal muscle. Their electrophysiologic abnormalities, particularly ventricular preexcitation and conduction defects distinguish them from patients with hypertrophic cardiomyopathy resulting from defects in sarcomere-protein genes.

Restrictive Cardiomyopathy

1117. The hallmark of the late secondary restrictive cardiomyopathies is an abnormal?
Harrison's 20th Ed. Chapter 254 Page 1791

A. Systolic dysfunction
B. Diastolic dysfunction
C. Systolic + diastolic dysfunction
D. Any of the above

Hallmark of restrictive cardiomyopathies is abnormal diastolic function. Ventricular walls are excessively rigid & impede ventricular filling due to myocardial fibrosis, hypertrophy or infiltration. Infiltrative diseases leading to secondary RCM may show impairment of systolic function.

1118. Which of the following is a feature of restrictive cardiomyopathy?
Harrison's 20th Ed. Chapter 254 Page 1791

A. Both atria are enlarged
B. End-diastolic pressures are elevated in both ventricles
C. Preserved cardiac output
D. All of the above

1119. Restrictive cardiomyopathy more commonly presents with clinical features related to?
Harrison's 20th Ed. Chapter 254 Page 1791

A. Right heart
B. Left heart
C. Both ventricles
D. Any of the above

Restrictive cardiomyopathy presents with relatively more right-sided symptoms, such as edema, abdominal discomfort, and ascites, although filling pressures are elevated in both ventricles.

1120. Which of the following is a clinical feature of restrictive cardiomyopathy?
Harrison's 20th Ed. Chapter 254 Page 1791

A. S4 more common than S3
B. Rapid Y descent in jugular venous examination
C. Positive Kussmaul's sign
D. All of the above

1121. Restrictive cardiomyopathies are due to?
Harrison's 20th Ed. Chapter 254 Page 1792

A. Infiltration of abnormal substances between myocytes
B. Storage of abnormal metabolic products within myocytes
C. Fibrotic endomyocardial injury
D. Any of the above

Most restrictive cardiomyopathies are due to infiltration of abnormal substances between myocytes, storage of abnormal metabolic products within myocytes, or fibrotic injury.

1122. Which of the following is the more common cause of secondary restrictive cardiomyopathy?
Harrison's 20th Ed. Chapter 254 Page 1792

A. Amyloidosis
B. Sarcoidosis
C. Scleroderma
D. Hemochromatosis

Myocardial involvement with amyloid is a common cause of secondary RCM, although restriction is also seen in the transplanted heart, in hemochromatosis, glycogen deposition, endomyocardial fibrosis, sarcoidosis, hypereosinophilic disease, and scleroderma, following mediastinal irradiation, and in neoplastic infiltration.

1123. Familial amyloidosis results from an autosomal dominant mutation in?
Harrison's 20th Ed. Chapter 254 Page 1792

A. Calcitonin
B. Gelsolin
C. Transthyretin
D. Amyloid β protein

Familial amyloidosis results from an autosomal dominant mutation in transthyretin, a carrier protein for thyroxine and retinol.

1124. Amyloidosis is best related to which of the following?
Harrison's 20th Ed. Chapter 254 Page 1793 Figure 254-14

A. Glycosphingolipid
B. Congo red stain
C. Mucopolysaccharidoses
D. Hypereosinophilic syndrome

Congo red stain can be used to highlight amyloid.

1125. Amyloid fibrils infiltrate the myocardium, especially around?
Harrison's 20th Ed. Chapter 254 Page 1793

A. Cardiomyocyte
B. Coronary vessels
C. Lymphatics
D. Entry of SVC, IVC

Amyloid fibrils infiltrate myocardium, especially around conduction system & coronary vessels.

1126. Typical feature of amyloidosis is?
Harrison's 20th Ed. Chapter 254 Page 1793

A. Conduction block
B. Autonomic neuropathy
C. Renal involvement
D. All of the above

Typical clinical features are conduction block, autonomic neuropathy, renal involvement, and occasionally thickened skin lesions.

1127. 2D echocardiogram that shows refractile brightness in the septum is suggestive of?
Harrison's 20th Ed. Chapter 254 Page 1793

A. Endomyocardial fibrosis
B. Eosinophilic endomyocardial disease
C. Primary cardiac amyloidosis
D. All of the above

2D echocardiogram that shows a characteristic refractile brightness in the septum suggestive of cardiac amyloidosis.

1128. Which of the following go in favour of amyloidosis?
Harrison's 20th Ed. Chapter 254 Page 1792

A. Low voltage ECG
B. Hyperrefractile "glittering" of myocardium on 2D Echo
C. Both atria are dilated
D. All of the above

1129. Best overall prognosis is in which of the following?
Harrison's 20th Ed. Chapter 254 Page 1793

A. Primary amyloid
B. Immunoglobulin-associated amyloid
C. Abnormal transthyretin-associated cardiac amyloid
D. Senile cardiac amyloid

The prognosis is worst for primary amyloid with a median survival of 6-12 months after symptoms of heart failure. Senile cardiac amyloid has the slowest progression and best overall prognosis.

1130. Which of the following is beneficial in the treatment of AL amyloidosis?
Blood 2011 118:827-828

A. Rituximab
B. Bortezomib
C. Etoposide
D. Dasatinib

Bortezomib has the highest activity that has ever been recorded for a single agent in AL amyloidosis.

1131. Differentiation of constrictive pericarditis from restrictive cardiomyopathies is done by which of the following?
N Engl J Med. 1997;336:273

A. Apex impulse
B. Mitral regurgitation
C. Pericardial calcification
D. All of the above

Apex impulse is easily palpable & mitral regurgitation is more common in RCM. Pericardial calcification on Chest X-ray/CT/MRI occurs commonly in constrictive pericarditis.

1132. Löffler's endocarditis best relates to?
Harrison's 20th Ed. Chapter 254 Page 1793

A. Postcardiac injury syndrome
B. Hypoplastic left heart syndrome
C. Hypereosinophilic syndrome
D. Straight back syndrome

Löffler's endocarditis is associated with a history of chronic hypereosinophilic syndrome, which is more common in men than women. Pericardial effusions are not common. Eosinophilic myocarditis or Löffler's endocarditis can lead to endomyocardial fibrosis.

1133. In chronic hypereosinophilic syndrome, there is persistent hypereosinophilia of >1500 eos/μL for at least?
Harrison's 20th Ed. Chapter 254 Page 1793

A. 3 months
B. 6 months
C. 9 months
D. 12 months

In chronic hypereosinophilic syndrome, there is persistent hypereosinophilia of >1500 eos/μL for at least 6 months.

1134. Endomyocardial fibrosis most commonly affects which of the following age groups?
Harrison's 20th Ed. Chapter 254 Page 1793

A. Children and young adults
B. Middle aged
C. Elderly
D. Any of the above

Endomyocardial fibrosis is a progressive disease of unknown cause that occurs mostly in children & young adults residing in tropical & subtropical Africa, particularly Uganda & Nigeria.

1135. Fibrous endocardial lesions in endomyocardial fibrosis involve which of the following areas of heart?
Harrison's 20th Ed. Chapter 254 Page 1793

A. Inflow portion of right or left atria (or both)
B. Outflow portion of right or left atria (or both)
C. Inflow portion of right or left ventricle (or both)
D. Outflow portion of right or left ventricle (or both)

Endomyocardial fibrosis is characterized by fibrous endocardial lesions of inflow portion of right or left ventricle (or both) & often involves atrioventricular valves, producing valvular regurgitation.

1136. Endocardial fibrosis results from which of the following?
Harrison's 20th Ed. Chapter 254 Page 1793

A. Carcinoid syndrome
B. Fenfluramine
C. Phentermine
D. All of the above

Carcinoid syndrome, use of anorexic agents like fenfluramine & phentermine result in endocardial fibrosis & stenosis and/or regurgitation of the tricuspid and/or pulmonary valve.

Hypertrophic Cardiomyopathy (HCM)

1137. Hypertrophic cardiomyopathy is associated with?
Harrison's 20th Ed. Chapter 254 Page 1793

A. Hypertension
B. Aortic valve disease
C. Systemic infiltrative or storage diseases
D. None of the above

Hypertrophic cardiomyopathy is defined as left ventricular hypertrophy that develops in absence of causative hemodynamic factors like hypertension, aortic valve disease, or systemic infiltrative or storage diseases.

1138. Hypertrophic cardiomyopathy (HCM) is also called?
Harrison's 20th Ed. Chapter 254 Page 1793

A. Hypertrophic obstructive cardiomyopathy (HOCM)
B. Asymmetric septal hypertrophy (ASH)
C. Idiopathic hypertrophic subaortic stenosis (IHSS)
D. All of the above

The accepted terminology presently is hypertrophic cardiomyopathy with or without obstruction.

1139. Which of the following about HCM is false?
Harrison's 20th Ed. Chapter 254 Page 1794

A. Autosomal dominant pattern of inheritance
B. Mutation in either MYH7 or MYBPC3
C. Age-dependent and incomplete penetrance
D. None of the above

HCM is caused by mutations in β myosin heavy chain (MYH7) or myosin-binding protein C gene (MYBPC3).

1140. The defining phenotype of HCM is?
Harrison's 20th Ed. Chapter 254 Page 1794

A. Asymmetric septal hypertrophy
B. Left ventricular outflow tract obstruction
C. Left ventricular hypertrophy
D. Endocardial fibrosis

Defining phenotype of left ventricular hypertrophy is rarely present at birth & usually develops later in life.

1141. In MYBPC3 mutation carriers, the average age of HCM development is?
Harrison's 20th Ed. Chapter 254 Page 1794

A. 20 years
B. 30 years
C. 40 years
D. 50 years

In MYBPC3 mutation carriers, the average age of HCM disease development is 40 years.

1142. Hypertrophic cardiomyopathy mutations lead to?
Harrison's 20th Ed. Chapter 254 Page 1794

A. Enhanced calcium sensitivity
B. Maximal force generation
C. ATPase activity
D. All of the above

At the level of sarcomere, HCM mutations lead to enhanced calcium sensitivity, maximal force generation, and ATPase activity. All of these lead to abnormal energetics & impaired relaxation.

1143. Hypertrophic cardiomyopathy is characterized by?
Harrison's 20th Ed. Chapter 254 Page 1794

A. Misaligned, disarrayed enlarged myofibrils & myocytes
B. Interstitial fibrosis
C. Microinfarction of hypertrophied myocardium
D. All of the above

Hypertrophic cardiomyopathy is characterized by misalignment and disarray of the enlarged myofibrils and myocytes.

1144. Hypertrophic cardiomyopathy is characterized by?
Harrison's 20th Ed. Chapter 254 Page 1794

A. Hypertrophy
B. Interstitial fibrosis
C. Microvascular disease
D. All of the above

Interstitial fibrosis is detectable before overt hypertrophy develops in HCM.

1145. In HCM, maximal hypertrophy is seen in?
Harrison's 20th Ed. Chapter 254 Page 1795

A. Interventricular septum
B. Midventricle
C. Ventricular apex
D. All of the above

The interventricular septum is the typical location of maximal hypertrophy in HCM.

1146. Apical HCM (ApHCM) is also referred as?
Acta Cardiol Sin 2015;31:8386, Harrison's 19th Ed. 269e-10

A. Ishimura syndrome
B. Yamaguchi's syndrome
C. Nishiyama syndrome
D. Takatsu syndrome

Yamaguchi's syndrome is also called "Japanese heart disease".

1147. Which of the following is false about Yamaguchi's syndrome?
Acta Cardiol Sin. 2015;31:8386.

A. Apical nonobstructive type of HCM
B. Giant T wave negativity in left precordial leads in ECG
C. "Ace of Spade" like configuration of LV cavity at end-diastole on left ventriculography
D. None of the above

Typical features of apical nonobstructive type of HCM (Yamaguchi's syndrome, relatively common in Japan) include an audible fourth heart sound, giant T wave negativity in left precordial leads in ECG, a "Ace of spade" like configuration of left ventricular cavity at end-diastole on left ventriculography.

1148. Which of the following accompanies obstructive HCM?
Harrison's 20th Ed. Chapter 254 Page 1795

A. AS
B. AR
C. MS
D. MR

In HCM, mitral leaflet coaptation may lead to posteriorly directed mitral regurgitation.

1149. Which of the following is the most common monogenic cardiovascular disorder?
N Engl J Med. 2018;379:655-68

A. Hypertrophic Cardiomyopathy
B. Marfan's syndrome
C. Sudden death associated with a prolonged QT syndrome
D. Monogenic hypertension

About 65% of human monogenic disorders are autosomal dominant, 25% are autosomal recessive and 5% are X-linked. HCM is the most common monogenic cardiovascular disorder. Each child of a parent with HCM has a 50% chance of inheriting the condition. Spontaneous (de novo) mutations probably accounts for this disease burden. Sporadic (nonfamilial) HCM (i.e., sarcomere mutations in a patient without a family history of HCM) may be more common than currently thought. Genetic testing is the only reliable way to identify unaffected family members who may need to be screened for sudden death risk factors.

1150. Which of the following is false about HCM?
Cleveland Clinic J of Medicine 2018;85(5):399

A. Dynamic obstruction of LV outflow tract is a key pathophysiologic mechanism
B. Transthoracic echocardiography is the first-line imaging test
C. β-blockers are the 1st line drugs for treating symptoms of HCM
D. None of the above

1151. Which of the following diseases can mimic HCM?
N Engl J Med. 2018;379:655-68

A. Lysosome-associated membrane protein 2 cardiomyopathy
B. Fabry's disease
C. Amyloidosis
D. All of the above

Genetic testing can identify metabolic & storage phenocopies like lysosome-associated membrane protein 2 (LAMP2) cardiomyopathy, Fabry's disease, Pompe disease, PRKAG2, Danon disease and amyloidosis, that mimic HCM.

1152. Which of the following laboratory test will help differentiate HCM from Fabry disease?
Cleveland Clinic J of Medicine 2018;85(5):399

A. Liver function tests
B. Renal function tests
C. Creatine kinase
D. Blood glucose levels

Derangements in liver function & glucose levels will be evident in patients with glycogen storage disorders (Pompe disease). Renal dysfunction (serum creatinine) will be seen in patients with Fabry disease or amyloidosis. Creatine kinase may be elevated in patients with Danon disease.

1153. Which of the following is related to cellular metabolism?
Harrison's 20th Ed. Chapter 254 Page 1781 Table 254-3

A. PRKAG2
B. MYH7
C. MYBPC3
D. All of the above

1154. Gene defect in which of the following can cause HCM?
Harrison's 20th Ed. Chapter 254 Page 1781 Table 254-3

A. Sarcomere
B. Z-disk and Cytoskeleton
C. Cellular Metabolism
D. All of the above

1155. HCM⁺ refers to?
Harrison's 20th Ed. Chapter 254 Page 1781 Table 254-3

A. HCM with preexcitation
B. HCM with dilated cardiomyopathy
C. HCM with restrictive cardiomyopathy
D. Any of the above

HCM+ refers to HCM with preexcitation.

1156. Which of the following gene products is related to HCM⁺?
Harrison's 20th Ed. Chapter 254 Page 1781 Table 254-3

A. PRKAG2 (γ-subunit of AMP kinase)
B. LAMP2 (lysosomal associated X-linked membrane protein)
C. GLA (α-galactosidase-A)
D. All of the above

1157. HCMc refers to?
Harrison's 20th Ed. Chapter 254 Page 1781 Table 254-3

A. HCM with cardiomyopathy
B. Congenital HCM
C. HCM with coronary artery disease
D. HCM with conduction disease

HCMc refers to HCM with conduction disease.

1158. Clinical diagnosis of HCM is based on which of the following?
N Engl J Med. 2018;379:655-68

A. Hypertrophied, nondilated left ventricle
B. Identified by echocardiography or MRI
C. Absence of another cardiac, systemic, metabolic, or syndromic disease
D. All of the above

Clinical diagnosis of HCM is based on a hypertrophied, nondilated left ventricle, identified by means of echocardiography or magnetic resonance imaging (MRI) in the absence of another cardiac, systemic, metabolic, or syndromic disease. HCM is not characteristically a progressive disorder. Two or more major (but treatable) complications develop in only 10% of affected patients during their lifetime.

1159. Which of the following is false about HCM?
Harrison's 20th Ed. Chapter 254 Page 1794

A. Found in ~1 in 500 of general population
B. Systolic anterior motion of mitral valve is characteristic
C. Myocardial perfusion defects on thallium 201 radionuclide scintigraphy frequent
D. None of the above

HCM is found in ~1 in 500 of the general population. Dynamic LV subaortic outflow tract pressure gradient due to midsystolic proximity of anterior mitral valve leaflet against hypertrophied septum is typical of obstructive HCM. Radionuclide scintigraphy with thallium 201 frequently shows myocardial perfusion defects even in asymptomatic patients.

1160. Which of the following is the most common cause of sudden death among young athletes?
Harrison's 20th Ed. Chapter 254 Page 1794, N Engl J Med. 2003;349:1064-75.

A. Mitral valve prolapse syndrome
B. Hypertrophic cardiomyopathy
C. Thyrotoxicosis
D. Anxiety

Hypertrophic cardiomyopathy is the most common cause of sudden death among young athletes.

1161. Which of the following is the most common cause of SCD in young competitive athletes?

Harrison's 20th Ed. Chapter 254 Page 1794

A. MVP
B. Long QT syndrome
C. HCM
D. Tetralogy of Fallot

HCM is the most common cause of SCD in young competitive athletes.

1162. Established risk marker for sudden death in cases of HCM is?

N Engl J Med. 2018;379:655-68

A. Unexplained syncope
B. Extreme left ventricular wall thickness
C. HCM-related sudden death in a first-degree relative
D. All of the above

Established risk markers for sudden death in cases of HCM are unexplained syncope, extreme left ventricular wall thickness, HCM-related sudden death in a first-degree relative, and multiple or prolonged episodes of nonsustained ventricular tachycardia.

1163. Differential diagnosis of large negative T-waves in ECG include?

The American Journal of Medicine 2014;127(1):31

A. Acute coronary syndrome
B. Cocaine toxicity
C. Subarachnoid hemorrhage
D. All of the above

Differential diagnosis of large negative T-waves in ECG include acute coronary syndrome, cocaine toxicity, neurological disorders (subarachnoid hemorrhage), and electrolyte abnormalities.

1164. In ECG, causes of giant T-wave inversion include?

Cleveland Clinic J of Medicine 2013;80(3):139

A. Elevated intracranial pressure
B. Acute pancreatitis
C. Wolff-Parkinson-White syndrome
D. All of the above

In ECG, causes of giant T-wave inversion include Apical hypertrophic obstructive cardiomyopathy, Subarachnoid hemorrhage, Cocaine abuse, Non-Q-wave myocardial infarction, Acute abdomen (acute pancreatitis), Complete heart block, Severe right ventricular hypertrophy, Elevated intracranial pressure, Post-pacemaker syndrome, Wolff-Parkinson-White syndrome.

1165. Systolic murmur in obstructive HCM is best heard at?

Cleveland Clinic J of Medicine 2018;85(5):399

A. A_1 area
B. A_2 area
C. Pulmonary area
D. Lower left sternal border

Hallmark of obstructive HCM is a systolic murmur which is typically harsh, diamond-shaped & begins after S1, since ejection is unimpeded early in systole. Murmur is best heard at lower left sternal border as well as at apex, where it is often more holosystolic & blowing in quality due to mitral regurgitation that usually accompanies obstructive HCM.

1166. In HCM, physical findings include?

Cleveland Clinic J of Medicine 2018;85(5):399

A. Fourth heart sound
B. Systolic murmurs
C. Bifid carotid pulse
D. All of the above

In HCM, physical findings are nonspecific and include systolic murmurs, bifid carotid pulse, a fourth heart sound, and a hyperdynamic precordium. Valsalva maneuver helps distinguish the murmur of left ventricular outflow tract obstruction in HCM from a murmur related to aortic stenosis by auscultation.

1167. Which of the following is the preferred method to provoke left ventricular outflow gradients?

N Engl J Med. 2018;379:655-68

A. Amyl nitrite inhalation
B. Valsalva maneuver
C. Isoproterenol infusion
D. Exercise (stress) echocardiography

1168. Maneuvers that increase the murmur of obstructive HCM include all except?

Harrison's 20th Ed. Chapter 254 Page 1795

A. Valsalva maneuver
B. Tachycardia
C. Sudden standing
D. Passive leg raising

1169. Maneuvers that decrease the murmur of obstructive HCM include all except?

Harrison's 20th Ed. Chapter 254 Page 1795

A. Squatting
B. Sustained handgrip
C. Nitroglycerin
D. Passive leg raising

Interventions that increase myocardial contractility like exercise, sympathomimetic amines & digitalis glycosides, and those that reduce ventricular volume like Valsalva maneuver, sudden standing, nitroglycerin, amyl nitrite or tachycardia, may all cause an increase in the gradient & the murmur. Conversely, elevation of arterial pressure by phenylephrine, squatting, sustained handgrip, augmentation of venous return by passive leg raising & expansion of the blood volume all increase ventricular volume & ameliorate the gradient & murmur.

1170. Left ventricular outflow tract obstruction is defined as a resting peak gradient of?

Cleveland Clinic J of Medicine 2018;85(5):399

A. 10 mm Hg
B. 20 mm Hg
C. 30 mm Hg
D. 40 mm Hg

Left ventricular outflow tract obstruction is defined as a resting peak gradient of 30 mm Hg or higher.

1171. In HCM, ubiquitous pathophysiologic abnormality is?

Harrison's 20th Ed. Chapter 254 Page 1795

A. Systolic dysfunction
B. Diastolic dysfunction
C. Systolic + diastolic dysfunction
D. None of the above

Ubiquitous pathophysiologic abnormality in HCM is diastolic dysfunction, characterized by increased stiffness of hypertrophied muscle. This results in elevated diastolic filling pressures & is present despite of a hyperdynamic left ventricle.

1172. In HCM, most common mutations occur in which of the following genes?
The American Journal of Medicine 2016;129:148-152

A. Cardiac alpha-myosin heavy chain gene
B. Cardiac beta-myosin heavy chain gene
C. Cardiac myosin light chain gene
D. Cardiac troponins C, I, and T gene

In HCM, most common are mutations of the cardiac beta-myosin heavy chain gene and cardiac myosin-binding protein C gene. Others involve alpha-myosin heavy chains, cardiac troponins C, I, and T, actin, myosin light chains & titin.

1173. In HCM, most common mutations of cardiac beta-myosin heavy chain gene is on?
The American Journal of Medicine 2016;129:148-152

A. Chromosome 10
B. Chromosome 12
C. Chromosome 14
D. Chromosome 16

In HCM, most common mutations of cardiac beta-myosin heavy chain gene is on chromosome 14.

1174. At what age, full genetic expression occurs in first-degree relatives of patients with familial HCM?
The American Journal of Medicine 2016;129:148-152

A. 5 years
B. 10 years
C. 20 years
D. 30 years

Echocardiographic studies have confirmed that by age 20 years, full genetic expression occurs in about half of the first-degree relatives of patients with familial HCM.

1175. What proportion of first-degree relatives of patients with familial HCM have evidence of the disease?
The American Journal of Medicine 2016;129:148-152

A. One-fourth
B. One-third
C. One-half
D. Three-fourth

Echocardiographic studies have confirmed that about one-third of the first-degree relatives of patients with familial HCM have evidence of disease.

1176. Hypertrophic cardiomyopathy commonly "masquerades" as?
The American Journal of Medicine 2016;129:148-152

A. Asthma
B. Mitral prolapse
C. Coronary artery disease
D. All of the above

Hypertrophic cardiomyopathy is cardiology's "great masquerader."

1177. In symptomatic HCM, the most common complaint is?
The American Journal of Medicine 2016;129:148-152

A. Dyspnea
B. Palpitation
C. Angina pectoris
D. Syncope

In symptomatic HCM patients, most common complaint is dyspnea, due to diastolic ventricular dysfunction which impairs ventricular filling & leads to elevated LV diastolic, left atrial & pulmonary capillary pressures. Other symptoms include syncope, angina pectoris & fatigue. Symptoms are not closely related to the presence or severity of an outflow pressure gradient.

1178. Mendelian transmission of single-gene defects may occur in?
Harrison's 20th Ed. Chapter 231 Page 1650

A. Hypertrophic cardiomyopathy
B. Marfan syndrome
C. Long QT syndrome
D. All of the above

Familial clustering due to Mendelian transmission of single-gene defects may occur in hypertrophic cardiomyopathy, Marfan syndrome & sudden death associated with a prolonged QT syndrome. Essential hypertension or coronary atherosclerosis are often polygenic disorders.

1179. Risk of sudden death in HCM correlates with all except?
Harrison's 20th Ed. Chapter 254 Page 1794

A. Ventricular tachycardia on ambulatory monitoring
B. Marked ventricular septal hypertrophy (>30 mm)
C. Abnormal blood pressure response to exercise
D. Severity of symptoms

HCM patients at higher risk of sudden death are those with a history of resuscitation from sudden cardiac death, ventricular tachycardia on ambulatory monitoring or at electrophysiologic testing, marked ventricular hypertrophy (ventricular septal thickness >30 mm), syncope (in children), genetic mutations associated with an increased risk, abnormal blood pressure response to exercise & a family history of sudden death. There is no correlation between the risk of sudden death and the severity of symptoms, but there is an increased risk of death in patients with outflow gradients.

1180. Left ventricular cavity in HCM is typically?
Harrison's 20th Ed. Chapter 254 Page 1794

A. Small
B. Normal
C. Large
D. Any of the above

Left ventricular cavity typically is small in HCM, with vigorous posterior wall motion but reduced septal excursion.

1181. In a hypertrophic cardiomyopathy phenotype, which of the following pathologic feature is possible?
The American Journal of Medicine 2016;129:148-152

A. Abnormal anterior papillary muscle position in LV cavity
B. Mitral valve leaflets elongated and redundant
C. Narrowing of intramural small coronary arteries
D. All of the above

Systolic anterior motion (SAM) of the mitral valve results not from a Venturi effect, as previously believed, but rather from an early systolic flow interaction with the abnormally elongated anterior mitral valve leaflet pushing it into the left ventricular outflow tract.

1182. Differential diagnosis of hypertrophic cardiomyopathy include?
Cleveland Clinic J of Medicine 2018;85(5):399

A. Noncompaction cardiomyopathy
B. Hemochromatosis
C. 'Athlete's heart'
D. All of the above

Differential diagnosis of hypertrophic cardiomyopathy include hypertensive cardiomyopathy, Aortic valvulopathy (Aortic stenosis, Supra-aortic or subaortic membranes), Infiltrative cardiomyopathy like Amyloidosis, Fabry disease, Lysosomal diseases (Danon disease), Glycogen storage disorders (Pompe disease), Hemochromatosis, 'Athlete's heart' and Noncompaction cardiomyopathy.

1183. In echocardiography of HCM, interventricular septum is how many times thicker than high posterior left ventricular free wall?

Cleveland Clinic J of Medicine 2018;85(5):399

A. 0.5 times
B. 0.8 times
C. 1.1 times
D. 1.3 times

HCM echocardiogram, demonstrates LVH, with septum 1.3 or more times the thickness of high posterior left ventricular free wall.

1184. Which of the following investigation is best for accurate measurements of regional hypertrophy and in identifying sites of regional fibrosis?

Harrison's 20th Ed. Chapter 254 Page 1794

A. ECG
B. Echocardiography
C. CMRI
D. LV Angiography

Cardiac MRI is superior to echocardiography in providing accurate measurements of regional hypertrophy and in identifying sites of regional fibrosis.

1185. Which of the following electrocardiographic findings can be seen in patients of HCM?

Cleveland Clinic J of Medicine 2018;85(5):399

A. Left ventricular hypertrophy
B. Pseudoinfarct pattern with Q waves in anterolateral leads
C. Repolarization abnormalities
D. All of the above

More than 90% of HCM patients have ECG abnormalities. Common findings include Left ventricular hypertrophy, pseudoinfarct pattern with Q waves in anterolateral leads, repolarization changes like T-wave inversions & horizontal or down-sloping ST segments. Apical HCM presents with giant T-wave inversion (> 10 mm) in anterolateral leads, most prominent in V4, V5, and V6.

1186. In HCM patients with circulatory shock requiring vasopressor support, which of the following should be used?

Cleveland Clinic J of Medicine 2018;85(5):399

A. Digoxin
B. Phenylephrine
C. Norepinephrine
D. Dobutamine and Dopamine

Positive inotropic effect of vasopressors increases contractility & increases left ventricular outflow tract gradient. Therefore, Digoxin, Norepinephrine, dobutamine and dopamine should be avoided. In patients with circulatory shock requiring vasopressor support, pure alpha-agonists like phenylephrine is preferred, as they increase peripheral resistance without an inotropic effect.

1187. Complications of HCM include?

N Engl M Med. 2004;350:1320-7

A. Atrial fibrillation
B. Infective endocarditis
C. Sudden death
D. All of the above

Propensity for sudden death in HCM is genetic. Other complications include atrial fibrillation, infective endocarditis & end-stage heart failure.

1188. Which of the following calcium channel blockers should be avoided in cases of obstructive HCM?

Harrison's 20th Ed. Chapter 254 Page 1796

A. Verapamil
B. Diltiazem
C. Nifedipine
D. All of the above

Verapamil & diltiazem reduces stiffness of ventricle, reduces elevated diastolic pressures, increase exercise tolerance & reduces severity of outflow tract pressure gradients. Nifedipine should be avoided. Dihydropyridine calcium channel blockers should be avoided altogether, as they produce even more peripheral vasodilation and afterload reduction than nondihydropyridine calcium channel blockers.

1189. Which of the following drugs should be avoided in cases of obstructive HCM?

Harrison's 20th Ed. Chapter 254 Page 1796

A. Digitalis
B. Diuretics
C. Nitrates
D. All of the above

Digitalis, diuretics, nitrates, vasodilators are best avoided, particularly in patients with known left ventricular outflow tract pressure gradients. Any medication that causes afterload reduction, peripheral vasodilation, intravascular volume depletion, or positive inotropy can worsen the dynamic left ventricular outflow tract obstruction in a patient with HCM and should be avoided.

1190. Which out of the following drugs should not be used in a case of obstrutive HCM?

Harrison's 20th Ed. Chapter 254 Page 1796

A. Beta-blockers
B. Digitalis
C. Nondihydropyridine calcium blockers
D. Disopyramide

Beta blockers block the effects of catecholamines that exacerbate outflow tract obstruction & to slow the heart rate so that diastolic filling is enhanced. Disopyramide exerts negative inotropic effects that decreases the outflow gradient and thereby improve symptoms. Digitalis increases left ventricular outflow tract pressure gradients by increasing myocardial contractility.

1191. Which of the following drug is protective against SCD in HCM?

N Engl J Med. 2018;379:655-68

A. Amiodarone
B. Beta-adrenergic blockers
C. Disopyramide
D. Diltiazem

Amiodarone is effective in reducing the frequency of supraventricular as well as life-threatening ventricular arrhythmias and anecdotal data suggest that it may reduce the risk of SCD.

1192. Which of the following is the treatment for nonobstructive HCM with heart failure?

N Engl J Med. 2018;379:655-68

A. Heart transplantation
B. Implantable cardioverter – defibrillator (ICD) placement
C. Surgical septal myectomy
D. Alcohol septal ablation

1193. Which of the following surgery can be considered for obstructive HCM?

Cleveland Clinic J of Medicine 2018;85(5):399

A. Ventricular septal myectomy
B. Alcohol septal ablation
C. Papillary muscle reorientation surgery
D. All of the above

1194. What is meant by "burned out HCM"?

Harrison's 20th Ed. Chapter 254 Page 1796

A. HCM not manifesting in offsprings
B. HCM disappearing with advancing age
C. HCM progressing to DCM with disappearance of preexisting outflow pressure gradient
D. HCM with AR

Progression of HCM to left ventricular dilatation & dysfunction (DCM) with wall thinning & disappearance of a preexisting outflow pressure gradient is called burned out HCM. It occurs in 5 - 10% of patients & may be associated with nonresponsive CHF requiring cardiac transplantation.

Aortic Valve Disease

1195. The accelerated natural history of rheumatic valvular disease in Indian subcontinent is due to?

Harrison's 20th Ed. Chapter 256 Page 1802

A. Genetic predisposition
B. Nutritional deficiencies
C. Repeated infections with rheumatogenic streptococci
D. All of the above

Repeated infections with more virulent strains of rheumatogenic streptococci is perhaps the cause of accelerated natural history of rheumatic valvular disease in Indian subcontinent and in Southeast Asia.

1196. Severe aortic stenosis (AS) affects what percentage of the population above 75 years of age?

Harrison's 20th Ed. Chapter 256 Page 1802

A. 1.5%
B. 2.5%
C. 3.5%
D. 4.5%

Severe aortic stenosis (AS) is estimated to affect 3.5% of the population aged >75 years.

1197. Which of the following studies estimated the prevalence of moderate or severe mitral & aortic valve disease in US?

Harrison's 20th Ed. Chapter 256 Page 1802 Figure 256-2

A. Coronary Artery Risk Development in Young Adults (CARDIA)
B. The Atherosclerosis Risk in Communities (ARIC)
C. The Cardiovascular Health Study (CHS)
D. All of the above

1198. Aortic stenosis (AS) occurs in what percentage of all patients with chronic valvular heart disease?

Harrison's 20th Ed. Chapter 256 Page 1803

A. 10%
B. 15%
C. 25%
D. 33%

Aortic stenosis (AS) occurs in ~ one-fourth of all patients with chronic valvular heart disease.

1199. What percentage of adult patients with symptomatic valvular AS are male?

Harrison's 20th Ed. Chapter 256 Page 1803

A. 30%
B. 50%
C. 60%
D. 80%

80% of adult patients with symptomatic valvular AS are male.

1200. Degenerative calcification in AS occurs most commonly over and above which of the following?

Harrison's 20th Ed. Chapter 256 Page 1803

A. Bicuspid aortic valve (BAV)
B. Chronic trileaflet aortic valve deterioration
C. Previous rheumatic inflammation of aortic valve
D. All of the above

AS in adults is due to degenerative calcification of the aortic cusps and occurs most commonly on an existing disease like bicuspid aortic valve, chronic trileaflet deterioration, or previous rheumatic inflammation. Out of these, most cases have bicuspid aortic valve (BAV) disease.

1201. Process of aortic valve deterioration and calcification shares many features with?

Harrison's 20th Ed. Chapter 256 Page 1803

A. Atherosclerosis
B. Apoptosis
C. Mitochondrial diseases
D. Neoplasia

The process of aortic valve deterioration & calcification shares many features with vascular atherosclerosis, including endothelial dysfunction, lipid accumulation, inflammatory cell activation, cytokine release, and upregulation of several signaling pathways.

1202. Which of the following is central in the pathogenesis of aortic valve deterioration & calcification?

Harrison's 20th Ed. Chapter 256 Page 1803

A. Foam cell
B. Myofibroblast
C. Endothelial cell
D. Macrophage

In aortic valve deterioration & calcification, valvular myofibroblasts differentiate phenotypically into osteoblasts and actively produce bone matrix proteins that allow for the deposition of calcium hydroxyapatite crystals.

1203. Genetic polymorphisms involving which of the following is linked to the development of calcific AS?

Harrison's 20th Ed. Chapter 256 Page 1803

A. Vitamin D receptor
B. Estrogen receptor
C. Apolipoprotein E4
D. All of the above

Genetic polymorphisms involving the vitamin D receptor, the estrogen receptor in postmenopausal women, interleukin 10 and apolipoprotein E4 have been linked to the development of calcific AS and a strong familial clustering of cases.

1204. Polymorphism & elevated levels of which of the following is associated with aortic-valve calcification and incident aortic stenosis?

N Engl J Med. 2014;371:744-56

A. HDLc
B. Triglycerides
C. Lipoprotein(a)
D. All of the above

In a genome wide linkage meta-analysis of three large population-based studies, a specific lipoprotein(a) polymorphism was shown to be associated with elevated serum levels of lipoprotein(a), aortic-valve calcification, and incident aortic stenosis.

1205. Population-based studies have shown associations between calcific valve disease and?

N Engl J Med. 2014;371:744-56

A. Male sex
B. Elevated levels of serum low-density lipoprotein cholesterol
C. Elevated levels of serum lipoprotein(a)
D. All of the above

Population-based studies have shown associations between calcific valve disease and older age, male sex, elevated serum levels of low-density lipoprotein (LDL) cholesterol & lipoprotein(a), hypertension, smoking, diabetes, and metabolic syndrome.

1206. Specific populations at increased risk for aortic stenosis include?

N Engl J Med. 2014;371:744-56

A. Mediastinal irradiation
B. Renal failure
C. Disorders of calcium metabolism
D. All of the above

Specific populations at increased risk for aortic stenosis include patients with a history of mediastinal irradiation, renal failure, familial hypercholesterolemia, or disorders of calcium & phosphate metabolism.

1207. Which of the following is false about aortic valve sclerosis?

Harrison's 20th Ed. Chapter 256 Page 1803

A. Focal thickening of the leaflets
B. Focal calcification of the leaflets
C. No obstruction
D. None of the above

Aortic valve sclerosis means focal thickening and calcification of the leaflets not severe enough to cause obstruction.

1208. What percentage of persons over 65 years exhibit aortic valve sclerosis?

Harrison's 20th Ed. Chapter 256 Page 1803

A. 30%
B. 50%
C. 60%
D. 80%

1209. What percentage of persons over 65 years exhibit frank aortic stenosis?

Harrison's 20th Ed. Chapter 256 Page 1803

A. 2%
B. 4%
C. 8%
D. 10%

About 30% of persons older than 65 years exhibit aortic valve sclerosis, whereas 2% exhibit frank stenosis.

1210. Among persons older than age 65, presence of aortic valve sclerosis is associated with an excess risk of?

Harrison's 20th Ed. Chapter 256 Page 1803

A. Hypertension
B. Myocardial infarction
C. Left ventricular hypertrophy
D. Cardiomyopathy

Presence of aortic valve sclerosis is associated with an excess risk of cardiovascular death and myocardial infarction (MI) among persons older than age 65.

1211. What is the prevalence of aortic stenosis among adults between the ages of 50 and 59 years?

N Engl J Med. 2014;371:744-56

A. About 0.1%
B. About 0.2%
C. About 0.3%
D. About 0.4%

The prevalence of aortic stenosis is only about 0.2% among adults between the ages of 50 and 59 years.

1212. What is the prevalence of AS among octogenarians?

N Engl J Med. 2014;371:744-56

A. About 10%
B. About 20%
C. About 30%
D. About 40%

The prevalence of aortic stenosis is about 9.8% in octogenarians. Overall prevalence is 2.8% in adults older than 75 years of age.

1213. What is the rate of death at 2 years in patients with symptomatic aortic-valve disease?

N Engl J Med. 2014;371:744-56

A. Over 30%
B. Over 40%
C. Over 50%
D. Over 60%

Although mortality is not increased when aortic stenosis is asymptomatic, the rate of death is >50% at 2 years in patients with symptomatic aortic-valve disease unless aortic-valve replacement is performed promptly.

1214. A rheumatic etiology of aortic stenosis is favored by?

Harrison's 20th Ed. Chapter 256 Page 1803

A. History of rheumatic fever
B. Rheumatic involvement of mitral valve
C. Associated AR
D. All of the above

Rheumatic AS is almost always associated with involvement of the mitral valve and with AR.

1215. Autotaxin is involved in which of the following in the pathogenesis of calcific aortic stenosis?

Harrison's 20th Ed. Chapter 256 Page 1804 Figure 256-3

A. Lipid infiltration
B. Inflammation
C. Fibro-calcific response
D. All of the above

Valvular interstitial cells (VIC) are critical participants in the formation of disorganized collagen (fibrosis) and calcium hydroxyapatite (bone) deposition in the pathogenesis of calcific aortic stenosis.

1216. Which of the following is the most common congenital heart valve defect?

Harrison's 20th Ed. Chapter 256 Page 1803

A. Congenital pulmonic stenosis
B. Bicuspid aortic valve (BAV)
C. Congenital mitral stenosis
D. Congenital tricuspid stenosis

A bicuspid aortic valve (BAV) is the most common congenital heart valve defect and occurs in 0.5–1.4% of the population with a 2—4:1 male to female predominance.

1217. Inheritance pattern of bicuspid aortic valve disease is?
Harrison's 20th Ed. Chapter 256 Page 1803

A. Autosomal recessive with incomplete penetrance
B. Autosomal recessive with complete penetrance
C. Autosomal dominant with incomplete penetrance
D. Autosomal dominant with complete penetrance

Inheritance pattern of bicuspid aortic valve disease is autosomal dominant with incomplete penetrance.

1218. Bicuspid aortic valve disease may be associated with?
Harrison's 20th Ed. Chapter 256 Page 1803

A. Ellis-van Creveld syndrome
B. Noonan syndrome
C. Holt-Oram syndrome
D. Turner's syndrome

X-linked inheritance is suggested by prevalence of BAV disease in patients with Turner's syndrome.

1219. Prevalence of BAV disease among first-degree relatives of an affected individual is?
Harrison's 20th Ed. Chapter 256 Page 1803

A. ~ 5%
B. ~ 10%
C. ~ 15%
D. ~ 20%

Prevalence of BAV disease among 1° relatives of an affected individual is ~10%.

1220. Mutation in which of the following gene may be associated with BAV disease?
Harrison's 20th Ed. Chapter 256 Page 1803

A. NOTCH1
B. NOTCH2
C. NOTCH3
D. NOTCH4

Mutation in NOTCH1 gene on chromosome 9q34-35 has been described in some families suffering from BAV disease. Abnormalities in endothelial nitric oxide synthase and NKX2.5 have been implicated as well.

1221. Which of the following occur commonly among patients with BAV disease?
Harrison's 20th Ed. Chapter 256 Page 1803

A. Aortic coarctation
B. Ascending aortic aneurysm
C. Aortic dissection
D. All of the above

1222. In BAV disease, which of the following is the most common bicuspid variant?
Harrison's 20th Ed. Chapter 256 Page 1803

A. Left-right cusp fusion
B. Right-left cusp fusion
C. Lateral-medial cusp fusion
D. Medial-lateral cusp fusion

Right-left cusp fusion is the most common bicuspid variant.

1223. Shone's complex consists of all except?
Harrison's 20th Ed. Chapter 256 Page 1803

A. Parachute like mitral valve
B. Supravalvular mitral ring
C. Asymmetric septal hypertrophy
D. Coarctation of aorta

Shone's complex is a rare congenital heart disease (Shone, 1963) typically consisting of four obstructive left heart lesions namely parachute like mitral valve, supravalvular mitral ring, subaortic stenosis, and coarctation of aorta. BAV can be a component of Shone's complex. The severity of mitral obstruction is the most significant indicator of survival and long-term prognosis.

1224. Shone's complex or Shone's anomaly is found in what percentage of all congenital heart diseases?
Heart Views. 2016;17(1):23-26

A. 0.1%
B. 0.3%
C. 0.6%
D. 0.9%

Shone's complex or Shone's anomaly is 0.6% of all congenital heart diseases.

1225. Heyde's syndrome best relates to?
N Engl J Med. 2014;371:744-56

A. Thromboxane A2
B. Prostacyclin I2
C. von Willebrand factor
D. Angiotensin II

In some patients with aortic stenosis, angiodysplastic gastrointestinal bleeding is seen in association with an acquired deficiency of von Willebrand factor multimers, a condition known as Heyde's syndrome. Unfolding of the von Willebrand multimers owing to abnormal shear stress as blood passes through the narrow valve results in cleavage by a specific plasma metalloproteinase. Low levels of von Willebrand factor also affect platelet function and may confer a predisposition to angiogenesis. These abnormalities typically normalize after valve replacement.

1226. Lp(a) is best related to?
Harrison's 20th Ed. Chapter 400 Page 2890 Table 400-1

A. ApoB-48
B. ApoC- III
C. ApoB-100
D. ApoE

Lp(a) is a cholesterol-rich particle lipoprotein similar to LDL consisting of a covalently linked molecule of apolipoprotein B100 with a molecule of apolipoprotein(a). Apo(a) is synthesized in the liver and attached to apoB- 100 by a disulfide linkage. The major site of clearance of Lp(a) is liver.

1227. Which of the following produce obstruction to LV outflow?
Harrison's 20th Ed. Chapter 256 Page 1803

A. Hypertrophic obstructive cardiomyopathy
B. Fibromuscular / membranous subaortic stenosis
C. Supravalvular aortic stenosis
D. All of the above

Hypertrophic obstructive cardiomyopathy, discrete fibromuscular / membranous subaortic stenosis and supravalvular AS produce obstruction to LV outflow.

1228. Laplace relation is?
Harrison's 20th Ed. Chapter 256 Page 1803

A. Systolic wall stress = (Pressure x Radius) / Wall thickness
B. Systolic wall stress = (Pressure x Wall thickness) / Radius
C. Systolic wall stress = (Wall thickness x Radius) / Pressure
D. Systolic wall stress = (Pressure + Radius) / Wall thickness

Systolic stress developed by myocardium is predicted by Laplace relation ($S = Pr/h$, where S = systolic wall stress, P = pressure, r = radius, and h = wall thickness).

1229. In normal sized adults, severe obstruction to LV outflow is considered when effective aortic orifice area is?

Harrison's 20th Ed. Chapter 256 Page 1803

A. 0.6 cm^2/m^2 body surface area
B. 0.8 cm^2/m^2 body surface area
C. 1.0 cm^2/m^2 body surface area
D. 1.2 cm^2/m^2 body surface area

A mean systolic pressure gradient >40 mm Hg with a normal CO or an effective aortic orifice area < ~1.0 cm^2 (or ~<0.6 cm^2/m^2 body surface area in a normal-sized adult) i.e., < ~ one-third of the normal orifice is considered to represent severe obstruction to LV outflow.

1230. In AS, hypertrophied LV compresses coronary arteries causing ischemia of?

Harrison's 20th Ed. Chapter 256 Page 1804

A. Subendocardium
B. Myocardium
C. Epicardium
D. All of the above

Hypertrophied LV in AS causes an increase in myocardial oxygen requirements. Capillary density is reduced relative to wall thickness, compressive forces are increased, and the elevated LV end-diastolic pressure reduces the coronary driving pressure. Subendocardium is especially vulnerable to ischemia by this mechanism.

1231. Which of the following is not a cardinal symptom of aortic stenosis?

Harrison's 20th Ed. Chapter 256 Page 1804

A. Exertional dyspnea
B. Angina pectoris
C. Syncope
D. Palpitation

Exertional dyspnea, angina pectoris and syncope are the three cardinal symptoms in patients with pure or predominant AS.

1232. Which of the following excludes the possibility of pure or predominant severe aortic stenosis?

Harrison's 20th Ed. Chapter 256 Page 1804

A. Atrial fibrilation
B. Absence of systolic thrill
C. Bisferiens pulse
D. All of the above

AF in AS suggests the possibility of associated mitral valve disease.

1233. In aortic stenosis, systolic thrill is generally present at?

Harrison's 20th Ed. Chapter 256 Page 1805

A. Base of heart
B. In suprasternal notch
C. Along carotid arteries
D. All of the above

Systolic thrill is present at the base of heart, in suprasternal notch & along carotid arteries (commonly left).

1234. Which of the following is false about aortic stenosis murmur?

Harrison's 20th Ed. Chapter 256 Page 1805

A. High pitched
B. Rough & rasping in character
C. Ejection systolic
D. Loudest in second right intercostal space

Murmur of AS is ejection (mid) systolic murmur commencing shortly after S1, increasing in intensity to reach a peak toward middle of ejection & ending just before aortic valve closure. It is characteristically low-pitched, rough & rasping in character & loudest at the base of heart in 2nd right intercostal space. It is transmitted along carotid arteries.

1235. In Gallavardin effect, murmur of AS radiates to which of the following?

Harrison's 20th Ed. Chapter 256 Page 1805

A. Apex
B. Carotids
C. Back
D. None of the above

Occasionally, murmur of AS may be transmitted downward to the apex, where it is loudest with musical quality (Gallavardin effect) and may be confused with systolic murmur of MR. In almost all patients with severe obstruction & preserved CO, the murmur of AS is at least grade III/VI.

1236. Intensity of a cardiac murmur is graded (1-6) according to?

Am J Cardiol. 2008;102(8):1107-10

A. Morrison scale
B. Mogagni scale
C. Levine scale
D. Osler scale

Murmurs were described first by Laennec in 1819. The intensity of a cardiac murmur is graded according to the Levine scale of 1 to 6 grades of intensity.

1237. Echocardiographically, which of the following is characteristic of congenitally bicuspid valves?

Harrison's 20th Ed. Chapter 256 Page 1805

A. Leaflet calcification and restriction
B. Eccentric closure of the aortic valve cusps
C. Distortion of the subvalvular apparatus
D. All of the above

The key findings on TTE in AS are thickening, calcification, and reduced systolic opening of the valve leaflets and LV hypertrophy. Eccentric closure of the aortic valve cusps is characteristic of congenitally bicuspid valves.

1238. Aortic stenosis is called "mild", when the aortic valve area is?

Harrison's 20th Ed. Chapter 256 Page 1805

A. 1.0–1.5 cm^2
B. 1.5–2.0 cm^2
C. 2.0–2.5 cm^2
D. 2.5–3.0 cm^2

1239. Aortic stenosis is called "moderate", when the aortic valve area is?

Harrison's 20th Ed. Chapter 256 Page 1805

A. 1.0 – 1.5 cm^2
B. 1.5 – 2.0 cm^2
C. 2.0 – 2.5 cm^2
D. 2.5 – 3.0 cm^2

Mitral stenosis is called "moderate", when the mitral valve orifice is 1.0 cm^2–1.5 cm^2.

1240. Aortic stenosis is called "severe", when aortic valve area is?

Harrison's 20th Ed. Chapter 256 Page 1805

A. < 1.5 cm^2
B. < 1.0 cm^2
C. < 0.5 cm^2
D. < 0.2 cm^2

1241. Aortic sclerosis is defined echocardiographically as focal thickening or calcification of valve cusps with a peak Doppler transaortic velocity of?
Harrison's 20th Ed. Chapter 256 Page 1805

A. ≤ 2.5 meters/second
B. ≤ 3.5 meters/second
C. ≤ 4.5 meters/second
D. ≤ 5.5 meters/second

Aortic sclerosis is defined echocardiographically as focal thickening or calcification of the valve cusps with a peak Doppler transaortic velocity of ≤2.5 meters/second at a peak gradient <25 mm Hg.

1242. Which of the following chest X-ray findings indicate that valvular AS is not severe?
Harrison's 20th Ed. Chapter 256 Page 1805

A. Little overall cardiac enlargement
B. Proximal ascending aorta not dilated
C. Absence of valvular calcification
D. Absence of pulmonary congestion

In chest X-ray, absence of valvular calcification in adults suggests that severe valvular AS is not present.

1243. Following onset of symptoms in AS, which of the following leads to early death?
Harrison's 20th Ed. Chapter 256 Page 1806

A. Angina pectoris
B. Syncope
C. Congestive heart failure
D. None of the above

After onset of symptoms in AS, life expectancy in angina pectoris & syncope is 3 years, dyspnea - 2 years and congestive heart failure - 1.5 to 2 years.

1244. Endocarditis prophylaxis is advised to AS patients with?
Harrison's 20th Ed. Chapter 256 Page 1807

A. Significant LV hypertrophy
B. Associated aortic regurgitation
C. Prior history of endocarditis
D. All of the above

The need for endocarditis prophylaxis is restricted to AS patients with a prior history of endocarditis.

1245. Operation is indicated in patients with severe AS who are?
Harrison's 20th Ed. Chapter 256 Page 1807

A. Symptomatic severe AS
B. LV systolic dysfunction (EF <50%)
C. BAV disease
D. All of the above

1246. Very severe AS is defined by?
Harrison's 20th Ed. Chapter 256 Page 1807

A. Mean gradient > 30 mm Hg
B. Mean gradient > 40 mm Hg
C. Mean gradient > 50 mm Hg
D. Mean gradient > 60 mm Hg

Very severe AS is defined by an aortic valve jet velocity >5 m/s or mean gradient >60 mm Hg.

1247. Long-term postoperative survival correlates with?
Harrison's 20th Ed. Chapter 256 Page 1807

A. Aortic valve area
B. Duration of symptoms
C. Preoperative LV function
D. All of the above

Long-term postoperative survival correlates with preoperative LV function.

1248. Dobutamine stress echocardiography is considered positive if after dobutamine challenge, there is?
Harrison's 20th Ed. Chapter 256 Page 1807

A. ≥ 5% increase in stroke volume
B. ≥ 10% increase in stroke volume
C. ≥ 20% increase in stroke volume
D. ≥ 30% increase in stroke volume

Dobutamine stress echocardiography is considered positive by an ≥20% increase in stroke volume after dobutamine challenge.

1249. Homograft AVR is usually reserved for patients with?
Harrison's 20th Ed. Chapter 256 Page 1807

A. Rheumatic valvulitis
B. Aortic valve endocarditis
C. Traumatic aortic valve
D. All of the above

Homograft AVR is usually reserved for patients with aortic valve endocarditis.

1250. Transcatheter aortic valve replacement (TAVR) is associated with postprocedural?
Harrison's 20th Ed. Chapter 256 Page 1807

A. Stroke
B. Paravalvular AR
C. Heart block
D. All of the above

1251. Paradoxical, low-flow, low-gradient severe aortic stenosis is staged as?
Harrison's 20th Ed. Chapter 256 Page 1806 Figure 256-4

A. D1
B. D2
C. D3
D. D4

With aortic stenosis, stage D1 refers to symptomatic patients with severe AS and a high valve gradient (>40 mm Hg mean gradient). Stage D2 refers to patients with symptomatic, severe, low flow, low-gradient aortic stenosis and low LVEF. Stage D3 characterizes patients with symptomatic, severe, low-flow, low gradient AS and preserved LVEF (paradoxical, low-flow, low-gradient severe aortic stenosis).

1252. Which of the following trials relate to aortic valve replacement?
Harrison's 20th Ed. Chapter 256 Page 1808 Figure 256-6

A. CORP-2 trial
B. PARTNER I trial
C. SYNTAX trial
D. FREEDOM trial

Aortic Regurgitation

1253. Severe LV hypertrophy is present when a wall thickness is?
Harrison's 19th Ed. 1532

A. > 5 mm
B. > 10 mm
C. > 15 mm
D. > 20 mm

Severe LV hypertrophy is present when a wall thickness is > 15 mm.

1254. Aortic regurgitation can occur due to?
Harrison's 20th Ed. Chapter 257 Page 1809

A. Membranous subaortic stenosis
B. Ventricular septal defect
C. Myxomatous degeneration
D. All of the above

1255. Which of the following is the cause of aortic regurgitation due to primary valve disease?
Harrison's 20th Ed. Chapter 257 Page 1809, Table 257-1

A. Aortic dissection
B. Hypertension
C. Ankylosing spondylitis
D. Marfan's syndrome

1256. Which of the following is the cause of aortic regurgitation due to both primary valve disease & primary aortic root disease?
Harrison's 20th Ed. Chapter 257 Page 1809, Table 257-1

A. Aortitis
B. Bicuspid aortic valve
C. Marfan's syndrome
D. Rheumatic fever

Causes of AR due to primary valve disease include congenital (bicuspid), endocarditis, rheumatic fever, myxomatous (prolapse), traumatic, syphilis and ankylosing spondylitis. Causes of AR due to primary aortic root disease include aortic dissection, cystic medial degeneration (Marfan's syndrome, bicuspid aortic valve, nonsyndromic familial aneurysm), aortitis and hypertension.

1257. Coexistence of hemodynamically significant AS with AR occurs in which of the following?
Harrison's 20th Ed. Chapter 257 Page 1810

A. Congenital AR
B. Syphilis
C. Marfan's syndrome
D. All of the above

Coexistence of hemodynamically significant AS with AR occurs almost exclusively in patients with rheumatic or congenital AR.

1258. Which of the following is the cause of aortic regurgitation due to both primary valve disease & primary aortic root disease?
Harrison's 20th Ed. Chapter 257 Page 1810

A. Syphilis
B. Bicuspid aortic valve
C. Ankylosing spondylitis
D. All of the above

Both syphilis & ankylosing spondylitis affect aortic valves. They may also be associated with cellular infiltration & scarring of media of thoracic aorta, leading to aortic dilation, aneurysm formation, & severe aortic regurgitation.

1259. Which of the following condition predisposes to AR?
Harrison's 20th Ed. Chapter 257 Page 1810

A. Marfan syndrome
B. Ankylosing spondylitis
C. Bicuspid aortic valve
D. All of the above

Conditions that predispose to AR are bicuspid aortic valve, IE, Marfan syndrome, or ankylosing spondylitis.

1260. At autopsy, heart of which of the following lesions is heaviest?
Harrison's 20th Ed. Chapter 257 Page 1810

A. Chronic AS
B. Chronic AR
C. HOCM
D. Dilated cardiomyopathy

At autopsy, hearts of patients with chronic AR may be among the largest encountered sometimes weighing >1000 grams.

1261. Early sign of LV dysfunction in chronic AR is?
Harrison's 20th Ed. Chapter 257 Page 1810

A. Elevation of LA pressure
B. Reduction in LVEF
C. Elevation of PA wedge pressure
D. Elevation of LV end-diastolic pressure

In chronic AR, both LV preload & afterload increase. When adaptive measures fail, LV function deteriorates, end-diastolic volume rises further and the forward stroke volume and EF decline. An early sign of LV dysfunction is a reduction in the EF. Deterioration of LV function often precedes the development of symptoms.

1262. A large fraction of coronary blood flow occurs during?
Harrison's 20th Ed. Chapter 257 Page 1810

A. Systole
B. Diastole
C. Systole + diastole
D. Any of the above

A large fraction of coronary blood flow occurs during diastole.

1263. Myocardial ischemia occurs in AR because of?
Harrison's 20th Ed. Chapter 257 Page 1810

A. LV dilation
B. Elevated LV systolic tension
C. Low arterial pressure
D. All of the above

Myocardial ischemia, particularly of the subendocardium, occurs in AR because of myocardial oxygen requirements are elevated by LV dilation, hypertrophy, and elevated LV systolic tension, and coronary blood flow may be compromised due to low arterial pressure.

1264. Which of the following is a cause of acute severe AR?
Harrison's 20th Ed. Chapter 257 Page 1810

A. Infective endocarditis
B. Aortic dissection
C. Nonpenetrating cardiac injury
D. All of the above

Acute severe AR results from infective endocarditis, aortic dissection, or trauma (Nonpenetrating cardiac injury leading to rupture or avulsion of the aortic valve).

1265. Which of the following about AR is false?
Harrison's 20th Ed. Chapter 257 Page 1810

A. 3/4th of patients with predominant valvular AR are men
B. Primary valvular AR with rheumatic mitral valve disease more common in women
C. Exertional dyspnea is the first symptom of diminished cardiac reserve
D. None of the above

1266. Which of the following is a symptom of chronic severe AR?
Harrison's 20th Ed. Chapter 257 Page 1810

A. Vomiting
B. Gait disturbance
C. Vertigo
D. Diaphoresis

Exertional dyspnea is followed by orthopnea, paroxysmal nocturnal dyspnea, and excessive diaphoresis. Nocturnal angina that does not respond satisfactorily to sublingual nitroglycerin may be accompanied by marked diaphoresis.

1267. Diaphoresis is a predominant symptom of which of the following valvular heart disease?
Harrison's 20th Ed. Chapter 257 Page 1810

A. AS
B. AR
C. MS
D. MR

1268. In free AR, booming "pistol-shot" sound heard over femoral arteries is called?
Harrison's 20th Ed. Chapter 257 Page 1810

A. Corrigan's pulse
B. Quincke's pulse
C. Traube's sign
D. Duroziez's sign

In free AR, booming "pistol-shot" sound heard over femoral arteries is termed as Traube's sign.

1269. Large-volume 'collapsing' water hammer peripheral pulse seen in AR is named after?
J Postgrad Med. 2008;54:163-5

A. Corrigan
B. Watson
C. de Musset
D. Duroziez

Large-volume 'collapsing' water hammer peripheral pulse seen in AR is named after Watson. Other peripheral signs of AR include Corrigan's pulse (rapid upstroke & collapse of carotid artery pulse), de Musset's sign (head nodding in time with heart beat), Quincke's sign (pulsation of capillary bed in nails), Traube's sign (systolic & diastolic murmurs described as 'pistol shots' heard over femoral artery when it is gradually compressed), Duroziez's sign (a double sound heard over femoral artery when it is compressed distally), Lighthouse sign (blanching & flushing of forehead), Landolfi's sign (alternating constriction & dilatation of pupil), Becker's sign (pulsations of retinal vessels), Müller's sign (pulsations of uvula), Mayen's sign (diastolic drop of BP >15 mm Hg with arm raised), Rosenbach's sign (pulsatile liver), Gerhardt's sign (enlarged spleen), Hill's sign - a >20 mm Hg difference in popliteal & brachial systolic cuff pressures in chronic severe AR, Lincoln sign (pulsatile popliteal artery), Sherman sign (dorsalis pedis pulse is quickly located & unexpectedly prominent in age >75 years).

1270. Which of the following is a feature of murmur of chronic AR?
Harrison's 20th Ed. Chapter 257 Page 1811

A. High-pitched, blowing
B. Decrescendo diastolic murmur
C. Heard best in III intercostal space along left sternal border
D. All of the above

As the severity of AR increases, decrescendo brief diastolic murmur becomes louder and longer and becomes holodiastolic.

1271. Decrescendo diastolic murmur of AR is best heard with?
Harrison's 20th Ed. Chapter 257 Page 1811

A. Patient sitting up
B. Patient leaning forward
C. Breath held in forced expiration
D. All of the above

When the murmur of AR is soft, it can be heard best with the diaphragm of the stethoscope and with the patient sitting up, leaning forward, and with the breath held in forced expiration.

1272. The murmur of AR is typically heard best in?
Harrison's 20th Ed. Chapter 257 Page 1811

A. II left ICS parasternally
B. III left ICS parasternally
C. IV left ICS parasternally
D. V left ICS parasternally

Murmur of chronic AR is typically high-pitched, blowing, decrescendo diastolic murmur, heard best in 3rd intercostal space along left sternal border. It seldom causes thrill.

1273. When murmur of AR is heard best along right sternal border, it suggests that AR is?
Harrison's 20th Ed. Chapter 257 Page 1811

A. Accompanied by significant MS
B. Accompanied by Infective endocarditis
C. Due to aneurysmal dilatation of aortic root
D. Due to severe hypertension

When murmur of AR is heard best along right sternal border, it suggests that AR is caused by aneurysmal dilatation of aortic root.

1274. "Cooing" or musical diastolic murmurs of AR suggests?
Harrison's 20th Ed. Chapter 257 Page 1811

A. Vegetations of the aortic leaflet
B. Fenestrations in the aortic leaflet
C. Eversion of an aortic cusp
D. Any of the above

"Cooing" or musical diastolic murmur of AR suggest eversion of aortic cusp vibrating in regurgitant stream.

1275. Austin Flint (1812-86) was a physician of which country?
N Engl J Med. 2010;363:2164

A. American
B. United Kingdom
C. Australia
D. Canada

Austin Flint, an American physician (1812-1886) was a pioneer in the use of the stethoscope. His "A Treatise on the Principles and Practice of Medicine" (1866) was a leading textbook of medicine.

1276. Which of the following murmur is heard in chronic AR?
Harrison's 20th Ed. Chapter 257 Page 1811

A. Decrescendo diastolic murmur
B. Mid-systolic ejection murmur
C. Mid-to-late diastolic murmur
D. All of the above

1277. The auscultatory features of AR are intensified by?
Harrison's 20th Ed. Chapter 257 Page 1811

A. Inhalation of amyl nitrite
B. Strenuous and sustained handgrip
C. Valsalva maneuver
D. All of the above

The auscultatory features of AR are intensified by strenuous and sustained handgrip, which augments systemic vascular resistance.

1278. Which of the following is a hemodynamic effect of amly nitrite?
N Engl J Med. 1966;275:1007

A. Decrease in systemic arterial pressure
B. Decrease in duration of contraction of left ventricle
C. Increase in heart rate
D. All of the above

Major hemodynamic effects of amly nitrite include a decrease in systemic arterial pressure, vascular resistance, stroke work, circulation time and duration of contraction of the left ventricle, ejection and diastolic filling period; an increase in heart rate, cardiac index and ejection velocity; and no change in stroke volume or minute work.

1279. Which of the following is a feature of acute severe AR?
Harrison's 20th Ed. Chapter 257 Page 1811

A. Soft S_1
B. Pulse pressure not wide
C. Soft, short, early diastolic murmur of AR
D. All of the above

1280. Most common pathologic condition associated with aortic aneurysm is?
N Engl J Med. 2004;351:1539-46

A. Syphilis
B. Atherosclerosis
C. Tuberculosis
D. Marfan's syndrome

1281. In ECG of patient with AR, which of the following findings usually signify a poor prognosis?
Harrison's 20th Ed. Chapter 257 Page 1811

A. No electrocardiographic abnormalities
B. ST depression & T-wave inversion in I, aVL
C. ST depression & T-wave inversion in V_5 & V_6
D. QRS prolongation

Left axis deviation and/or QRS prolongation denote diffuse myocardial disease and signify a poor prognosis.

1282. On echocardiogram, which of the following can be found in a patient of AR?
Harrison's 20th Ed. Chapter 257 Page 1811

A. Increased systolic excursion of posterior LV wall
B. High-frequency diastolic fluttering of anterior mitral leaflet
C. Dilatation of aortic annulus
D. All of the above

A rapid, high-frequency fluttering of the anterior mitral leaflet produced by the impact of the regurgitant jet is a characteristic finding in 2D echocardiogram of AR patient.

1283. Which of the following findings in color flow Doppler imaging suggest severe AR?
Harrison's 20th Ed. Chapter 257 Page 1811

A. Central jet width > 65% of left ventricular outflow tract
B. Regurgitant volume > 60 mL/beat
C. Regurgitant fraction > 50%
D. All of the above

With severe AR, central jet width assessed by color flow Doppler imaging exceeds 65% of left ventricular outflow tract, regurgitant volume is ≥60 mL/beat, regurgitant fraction is >=50%, and diastolic flow reversal in the proximal descending thoracic aorta is seen.

1284. In chronic severe AR, the apex is displaced?
Harrison's 20th Ed. Chapter 257 Page 1811

A. Downward
B. Leftward
C. Posteriorly
D. All of the above

1285. Which of the following is contraindicated in the treatment of acute aortic regurgitation?
Harrison's 20th Ed. Chapter 257 Page 1811

A. Intravenous diuretics
B. Vasodilators (sodium nitroprusside)
C. Intra-aortic balloon counterpulsation
D. Surgery

Patients with acute severe AR may respond to IV diuretics and vasodilators like sodium nitroprusside. Surgery is the treatment of choice and is usually necessary within 24 hours of diagnosis. Intraaortic balloon counterpulsation is contraindicated. Beta blockers are also best avoided as they may reduce CO further.

1286. In AR, which of the following drugs can delay the need for surgery?
Harrison's 20th Ed. Chapter 257 Page 1811

A. Digitalis glycosides
B. Diuretics
C. Nondihydropyridine calcium channel blockers
D. Long-acting nifedipine

1287. In AR, operation should be carried out in?
Harrison's 20th Ed. Chapter 257 Page 1811

A. LVEF < 50%
B. LV end-systolic dimension > 50 mm
C. Acute, severe AR
D. All of the above

Surgery should be carried out in asymptomatic patients with severe AR and progressive LV dysfunction defined by an LVEF <50%, an LV end-systolic dimension >50 mm or end-systolic volume >55 mL/m², or an LV diastolic dimension >65 mm.

1288. In "55 rule" for gauging the timing of surgery for AR, 55 refers to?
N Engl J Med. 1997;337:37

A. Ejection fraction
B. Shortening fraction
C. Mean pressure gradient
D. Maximum velocity

"55 rule" has been useful in gauging the timing of surgery for AR. Aortic-valve surgery should be performed before the ejection fraction falls below 55 percent or the endsystolic dimension exceeds 55 mm.

Mitral Stenosis

1289. Which of the following condition affects the mitral valve?
Circulation. 2004;109:e38-e41

A. Obstruction
B. Leakage
C. Bulging backward during valve closure
D. All of the above

There are 3 main conditions that affect the valve: Obstruction (stenosis), leakage (regurgitation), and bulging backward during valve closure (prolapse). Prolapse is the most common, occurring in up to 5% of the population, whereas stenosis is the least common, accounting for <1% of cardiac diagnoses in the US, although it is more frequently seen in developing nations.

1290. Which of the following is not a cause of obstruction to left atrial outflow?
Harrison's 20th Ed. Chapter 258 Page 1813

A. Systemic lupus erythematosus
B. Rheumatoid arthritis
C. Wegener's granulomatosis
D. Cor triatriatum

Rheumatic fever is the leading cause of mitral stenosis (MS). Other less common etiologies of obstruction to left atrial outflow include congenital mitral valve stenosis, cor triatriatum, mitral annular calcification with extension onto the leaflets, systemic lupus erythematosus, rheumatoid arthritis, left atrial myxoma, and infective endocarditis with large vegetations.

1291. What proportion of all patients with rheumatic heart disease & a history of rheumatic fever have pure or predominant MS?
Harrison's 20th Ed. Chapter 258 Page 1814

A. 10%
B. 20%
C. 30%
D. 40%

Pure or predominant MS occurs in ~40% of all patients with rheumatic heart disease and a history of rheumatic fever.

1292. Which of the following is a component of Shone's Syndrome?
Am J Cardiol. 1963; 11:714–25

A. Parachute mitral valve
B. Subaortic stenosis
C. Coarctation of aorta
D. All of the above

Shone syndrome is a collection of eight left-sided obstructive heart lesions. These affect blood flow to and from the left ventricle. The lesions are Cor Triatriatum, Supramitral Ring, Parachute mitral valve, Subaortic stenosis, Bicuspid Aortic Valve, Coarctation of the Aorta, Hypoplastic (stiff) left ventricle and Small Aortic Arch.

1293. What proportion of all patients with mitral stenosis are female?
Circulation. 2004;109:e38-e41

A. One-fourth
B. One-third
C. Two-third
D. Three-fourth

1294. The mitral valve (MV) apparatus comprises of?
Arch Cardiovasc Dis. 2013;106:111-5

A. Mitral valve annulus
B. Anterior and posterior MV leaflets
C. Chordae, and anteromedial & posterolateral papillary muscles
D. All of the above

The mitral valve (MV) apparatus is comprised of the mitral valve annulus, anterior and posterior MV leaflets, chordae, and anteromedial and posterolateral papillary muscles.

1295. Which of the following statements is false?
Arch Cardiovasc Dis. 2013;106:111-5

A. Anterior & posterior leaflets have roughly the same area
B. Annulus is a saddle-shaped structure
C. Posterior leaflet occupies two thirds of the annulus
D. None of the above

1296. Which of the following statements about MS is false?
Arch Cardiovasc Dis. 2013;106:111-5

A. Congenital MS is a disease of newborn and infancy
B. Rheumatic MS typically presents in III & IV decades of life
C. Degenerative MS presents in the VII & VIII decades of life
D. None of the above

1297. Which of the following statements about MS is false?
Arch Cardiovasc Dis. 2013;106:111-5

A. Degenerative MS has more annular & basal leaflet calcification
B. Calcification in rheumatic MS primarily affects leaflet tips
C. Calcification in congenital MS is minimal or absent
D. None of the above

The hallmark of degenerative MS is mitral annular calcification (MAC).

1298. Which of the following statements about MS is false?
Arch Cardiovasc Dis. 2013;106:111-5

A. In rheumatic MS, commissural fusion is the norm
B. In degenerative MS, the commissures are open
C. In congenital MS, commissures are absent
D. None of the above

1299. In rheumatic MS, chronic inflammation leads to?
Harrison's 20th Ed. Chapter 258 Page 1814

A. Fusion of mitral commissures
B. Fusion & shortening of chordae tendineae
C. Rigidity of valvular cusps
D. All of the above

1300. Which of the following term define the appearance of valve orifice in MS?

Harrison's 20th Ed. Chapter 258 Page 1814

A. Pigeon chest
B. Parrot peek
C. Camel back
D. Fish-mouth

In rheumatic MS, chronic inflammation leads to diffuse thickening of valve leaflets with fibrosis often with calcific deposits. Mitral commissures fuse, chordae tendineae fuse and shorten, valvular cusps become rigid, and the pathologic process eventually leads to narrowing at apex of the funnel-shaped ("fish-mouth") valve.

1301. In patients of MS without atrial fibrillation (AF), thrombi arise more frequently from?

Harrison's 20th Ed. Chapter 258 Page 1814

A. Mitral valve leaflets
B. Chordae tendineae
C. Left atrial appendage
D. Mitral commissures

1302. In patients of MS with atrial fibrillation (AF), thrombi arise more frequently from?

Harrison's 20th Ed. Chapter 258 Page 1814

A. Mitral valve leaflets
B. Chordae tendineae
C. Left atrial appendage
D. Mitral commissures

Thrombus formation & arterial embolization may arise from calcific valve itself, but in patients with atrial fibrillation (AF), thrombi arise more frequently from the dilated left atrium (LA), particularly from within the left atrial appendage.

1303. The mitral valve's annulus is shaped more like a?

BJA Education. 2017; 17(1):1-9

A. M
B. D
C. O
D. Any of the above

The mitral valve's annulus is a saddle-shaped structure which is shaped more like a 'D' than an 'O'.

1304. Which of the following coronary artery is closest to the annulus of the mitral valve?

BJA Education. 2017;17(1):1-9

A. Right coronary artery
B. Left circumflex artery
C. Left anterior descending artery
D. Posterior descending artery

The left circumflex artery follows the line of annulus as it passes anteriorly around base of the heart, a position that places it at risk during any mitral valve surgery.

1305. Which of the following regarding papillary muscles and chorda tendinae is false?

BJA Education. 2017;17(1):1-9

A. Anterolateral muscle receives a dual blood supply from left anterior descending and circumflex artery
B. Posteromedial muscle is supplied by right coronary artery
C. Primary chordae are attached to free edge of valve leaflet, and secondary chordae are attached to ventricular surface of leaflet
D. None of the above

1306. Number of discrete segments or scallops on posterior mitral leaflet is?

BJA Education. 2017;17(1):1-9

A. 1
B. 2
C. 3
D. 4

There are three discrete segments or scallops on anterior leaflet (A1, A2, and A3) and posterior leaflet (P1, P2, and P3).

1307. In normal adults, which of the following parameter of the mitral valve orifice is 4-6 cm^2?

Harrison's 20th Ed. Chapter 258 Page 1814

A. Diameter
B. Circumference
C. Area
D. Radius

In normal adults, the area of the mitral valve orifice is 4-6 cm^2.

1308. Significant obstruction of mitral valve orifice is considered when the orifice is less than approximately?

Harrison's 20th Ed. Chapter 258 Page 1814

A. 1 cm^2
B. 2 cm^2
C. 3 cm^2
D. 4 cm^2

Mitral valve orifice area of < ~2 cm^2 is considered "significant obstruction" because blood can flow from LA to LV only if propelled by an abnormally elevated left atrioventricular pressure gradient.

1309. Mitral stenosis is called "severe", when the mitral valve opening is reduced to?

Harrison's 20th Ed. Chapter 258 Page 1814

A. < 1.5 cm^2
B. < 1 cm^2
C. < 0.5 cm^2
D. < 0.2 cm^2

When the mitral valve opening is reduced to < 1.5 cm^2 it is referred to as "severe" MS. When the mitral valve opening is reduced to < 1 cm^2 it is referred to as "very severe" MS.

1310. In severe MS, LA pressure required to maintain a normal cardiac output is?

Harrison's 20th Ed. Chapter 258 Page 1814

A. ~ 10 mm Hg
B. ~ 15 mm Hg
C. ~ 20 mm Hg
D. ~ 25 mm Hg

In severe MS, LA pressure of ~25 mm Hg is required to maintain a normal cardiac output.

1311. Hemodynamic variable of importance in mitral stenosis is?
Harrison's 20th Ed. Chapter 258 Page 1814

A. Transvalvular pressure gradient
B. Cardiac output
C. Heart rate
D. All of the above

Hemodynamic severity of MS depends on transvalvular pressure gradient and the flow rate which depends on the cardiac output and heart rate.

1312. Clinical and hemodynamic features of MS are influenced importantly by?
Harrison's 20th Ed. Chapter 258 Page 1814

A. Cardiac output
B. Heart rate
C. Transvalvular pressure gradient
D. Pulmonary arterial pressure (PAP)

The clinical and hemodynamic features of MS are influenced importantly by the level of the PAP.

1313. "Second stenosis" refers to which of the following?
Harrison's 20th Ed. Chapter 258 Page 1814

A. Passive backward transmission of elevated LA pressure
B. Pulmonary arteriolar constriction
C. Interstitial edema in walls of small pulmonary vessels
D. Organic obliterative changes in pulmonary vascular bed

Pulmonary hypertension results from passive backward transmission of elevated LA pressure; pulmonary arteriolar constriction ("second stenosis"), interstitial edema in walls of small pulmonary vessels and organic obliterative changes in pulmonary vascular bed.

1314. Severe pulmonary hypertension results in?
Harrison's 20th Ed. Chapter 258 Page 1814

A. RV enlargement
B. Secondary tricuspid regurgitation (TR)
C. Pulmonic regurgitation (PR)
D. All of the above

Severe pulmonary hypertension results in RV enlargement, secondary tricuspid regurgitation (TR) and pulmonic regurgitation (PR), as well as right-sided heart failure.

1315. Which of the following about mitral stenosis is false?
Harrison's 20th Ed. Chapter 258 Page 1814

A. Latent period between initial attack of rheumatic carditis & development of symptoms due to MS is ~ 2 decades
B. Infective endocarditis is rare in isolated MS
C. Hemoptysis is rarely fatal
D. None of the above

1316. Most patients of MS begin to experience disability in?
Harrison's 20th Ed. Chapter 258 Page 1814

A. II decade of life
B. III decade of life
C. IV decade of life
D. V decade of life

1317. Once MS patient becomes seriously symptomatic, MS progresses inexorably to death within?
Harrison's 20th Ed. Chapter 258 Page 1814

A. 6 months to 1 year
B. 1– 2 years
C. 2–5 years
D. 5–7 years

Once MS patient becomes seriously symptomatic, MS progresses inexorably to death within 2–5 years.

1318. LA pressure gets markedly elevated by sudden changes in?
Harrison's 20th Ed. Chapter 258 Page 1814

A. Heart rate
B. Volume status
C. Cardiac output
D. All of the above

1319. Which of the following marks a turning point in the disease course of MS?
Harrison's 20th Ed. Chapter 258 Page 1814

A. Development of orthopnea
B. Development of paroxysmal nocturnal dyspnea
C. Development of paroxysmal AF
D. Development of persistent AF

Development of persistent AF marks a turning point in the course of an MS patient. It is associated with acceleration of the rate at which symptoms progress.

1320. In MS, hemoptysis results from rupture of?
Harrison's 20th Ed. Chapter 258 Page 1814

A. Alveolar capillaries
B. Pulmonary arterioles
C. Bronchial arterioles
D. Pulmonary-bronchial venous connections

Hemoptysis results from rupture of pulmonary-bronchial venous connections secondary to pulmonary venous hypertension in patients who have elevated LA pressures without markedly elevated pulmonary vascular resistances and is rarely fatal.

1321. In MS, hemoptysis results from?
Harrison's 20th Ed. Chapter 258 Page 1814

A. Pulmonary-bronchial venous connections
B. Recurrent pulmonary emboli
C. Pulmonary infections
D. All of the above

1322. Which of the following occurs in the pulmonary vascular bed MS?
Harrison's 20th Ed. Chapter 258 Page 1814

A. Fibrous thickening of the walls of alveoli
B. Fibrous thickening of the walls of pulmonary capillaries
C. Interstitial edema in walls of small pulmonary vessels
D. All of the above

1323. Which of the following PFT variable is reduced in MS?
Harrison's 20th Ed. Chapter 258 Page 1814

A. Vital capacity
B. Total lung capacity
C. Maximal breathing capacity
D. All of the above

In addition to interstitial edema in walls of small pulmonary vessels and organic obliterative changes in pulmonary vascular bed, fibrous thickening of walls of alveoli & pulmonary capillaries occurs commonly in MS. Vital capacity, total lung capacity, maximal breathing capacity, and oxygen uptake per unit of ventilation are reduced.

1324. The incidence of systemic embolization in MS is?

Harrison's 20th Ed. Chapter 258 Page 1814

A. 1–2%
B. 2–5%
C. 5–10%
D. 10–20%

The incidence of systemic embolization is 10–20% in MS.

1325. In MS, systemic embolization occurs more frequently in?

Harrison's 20th Ed. Chapter 258 Page 1814

A. Patients with AF
B. In older patients
C. In those with a reduced cardiac output
D. All of the above

Thrombi form in left atria, particularly in enlarged atrial appendages of patients with MS. Systemic embolization, incidence of which is 10–20%, occurs more frequently in patients with AF, in older patients (>65 years), and in those with a reduced CO.

1326. Which of the following may rarely be present in MS?

Harrison's 20th Ed. Chapter 258 Page 1815

A. Malar flush with pinched and blue facies
B. Prominent a waves in jugular venous pulse
C. Diastolic thrill at cardiac apex
D. Parasternal heave

1327. Which of the following is false about auscultation in MS?

Harrison's 20th Ed. Chapter 258 Page 1815

A. S_1 is accentuated and delayed
B. OS follows A_2 by 0.05–0.12 seconds
C. A_2 - OS interval varies directly with severity of MS
D. None of the above

A2 - OS time interval varies inversely with the severity of the MS.

1328. Which of the following correlates with the severity of mitral stenosis?

Harrison's 20th Ed. Chapter 258 Page 1815

A. Loudness of opening snap
B. Duration of mid-diastolic murmur
C. Duration of presystolic accentuation
D. All of the above

Duration of low-pitched, rumbling, diastolic murmur correlates with the severity of the stenosis in patients with preserved CO. The A2 - OS time interval varies inversely with the severity of MS.

1329. In patients with MS with RV failure, pleural effusion is on which side?

Harrison's 20th Ed. Chapter 258 Page 1815

A. Right
B. Left
C. Bilateral
D. Any of the above

Pleural effusion, particularly in right pleural cavity, may occur in patients with MS and RV failure.

1330. In MS, which of the following findings can be found along left sternal border?

Harrison's 20th Ed. Chapter 258 Page 1815

A. Pansystolic murmur
B. High-pitched, diastolic, decrescendo blowing murmur
C. Soft, grade I or II/VI systolic murmurs
D. All of the above

With severe pulmonary hypertension, a pansystolic murmur, louder during inspiration, produced by functional TR may be audible along the left sternal border. Graham Steell murmur of PR, a high-pitched, diastolic, decrescendo blowing murmur along the left sternal border, results from dilation of pulmonary valve ring due to severe pulmonary hypertension. Soft, grade I or II/VI systolic murmurs are commonly heard at the apex or along the left sternal border in patients with pure MS and do not necessarily signify the presence of MR.

1331. Carvallo's sign best relates to?

Harrison's 20th Ed. Chapter 258 Page 1815

A. Right heart murmur
B. Phases of breathing
C. Elicited along the left sternal border
D. All of the above

1332. Which of the following is found in the ECG of a patient of MS?

Harrison's 20th Ed. Chapter 258 Page 1815

A. Tall and peaked P wave in lead II
B. Upright P wave in lead V1
C. Normal QRS complex
D. All of the above

1333. Which of the following echocardiographic technique is most useful in evaluating a patient of MS?

Harrison's 20th Ed. Chapter 258 Page 1815

A. M-mode Echocardiography
B. 2D Echocardiography with Color Doppler studies
C. Transthoracic echocardiography (TTE) with color flow and spectral Doppler imaging
D. All of the above

Transthoracic echocardiography (TTE) with color flow and spectral Doppler imaging provides critical information in evaluation of a patient of MS.

1334. Transesophageal echocardiography (TEE) in MS is especially indicated to exclude?

Harrison's 20th Ed. Chapter 258 Page 1815

A. Left atrial myxoma
B. Presence of LA thrombus
C. Presence of LV thrombus
D. All of the above

TEE is especially indicated to exclude the presence of LA thrombus prior to percutaneous mitral balloon valvotomy (PMBV). TEE is utilised to perform precise 3D reconstruction of the MV and its apparatus. Cardiac computed tomography (CCT) has also emerged as a valuable tool for studying cardiac calcifications including calcific valvular lesions.

1335. Which of the following is a chest X-ray sign of pulmonary venous hypertension in MS?

A. Stag's antler sign
B. Hands-up sign
C. Inverted moustache sign
D. All of the above

On CxR, in pulmonary venous hypertension, prominence of upper lobe pulmonary veins is seen and is called Stag's antler sign. It is the earliest sign of pulmonary venous hypertension. This sign is also known as hands-up sign or inverted moustache sign.

1336. In MS, Kerley B lines on X-ray chest are apparent when the resting mean LA pressure exceeds approximately?
Harrison's 20th Ed. Chapter 258 Page 1815

A. 10 mm Hg
B. 15 mm Hg
C. 20 mm Hg
D. 25 mm Hg

Kerley B lines are fine, dense, opaque, horizontal lines most prominent in the lower and mid-lung fields resulting from distention of interlobular septae and lymphatics with edema when resting mean LA pressure > ~20 mm Hg.

1337. Which of the following about Kerley's A lines is false?
Circulation. 1972;XLV:1323

A. Linear opacities on CxR chest
B. Extend from periphery to hila
C. Caused by distention of anastomotic channels between peripheral & central lymphatics
D. None of the above

Kerley's A lines are linear opacities extending from periphery to hila caused by distention of anastomotic channels between peripheral & central lymphatics. They do not bifurcate and they do not follow the normal branching pattern of bronchi and vessels. These lines are most commonly seen in the upper lobes, are slightly curved rather than straight.

1338. Which of the following about Kerley's B lines is false?
Circulation. 1972;XLV:1323

A. Short horizontal lines on CxR chest
B. Situated perpendicularly to pleural surface at lung base
C. Represent edema of interlobular septa
D. None of the above

Kerley's B lines are short horizontal lines situated perpendicularly to pleural surface at lung base. They represent edema of the interlobular septa. B lines are "short, sharp lines seen only at the bases, usually less than an inch long and running transversely outward to touch the pleural margin. These are the most commonly recognized of the Kerley lines.

1339. Which of the following about Kerley's C lines is false?
Circulation. 1972;XLV:1323

A. Reticular opacities at lung base
B. Represent Kerley's B lines en face
C. Suggest cardiogenic pulmonary edema
D. None of the above

Kerley's C lines are reticular opacities at the lung base, representing Kerley's B lines en face suggesting cardiogenic pulmonary edema. C lines are "fine interlacing lines givinlg a network appearance.

1340. Which of the following is false about Austin Flint murmur?
Harrison's 20th Ed. Chapter 258 Page 1815

A. Apical
B. Mid-diastolic
C. Not intensified in presystole
D. None of the above

Apical mid-diastolic murmur associated with severe AR (Austin Flint murmur) is differentiated from MS because it is not intensified in presystole & becomes softer with administration of amyl nitrite.

1341. Which of the following features differentiates atrial septal defect from MS?
Harrison's 20th Ed. Chapter 258 Page 1815

A. Absence of LA enlargement
B. Absence of Kerley B lines
C. Fixed splitting of S_2
D. All of the above

Atrial septal defect may be mistaken for MS as in both conditions there is clinical, ECG, and chest X-ray evidence of RV enlargement and accentuation of pulmonary vascularity. Absence of LA enlargement and of Kerley B lines and the demonstration of fixed splitting of S2 with a grade 2 or 3 mid-systolic murmur at the mid to upper left sternal border all favor atrial septal defect over MS.

1342. Auscultatory findings change markedly with body position in which of the following?
Harrison's 20th Ed. Chapter 258 Page 1815

A. Mitral stenosis
B. Tricuspid stenosis
C. Left atrial myxoma
D. Atrial septal defect

The auscultatory findings in left atrial myxoma change markedly with body position.

1343. Levels of which of the following is elevated in left atrial myxoma?
Harrison's 20th Ed. Chapter 258 Page 1815

A. Interleukin 2 (IL-2)
B. Interleukin 4 (IL-4)
C. Interleukin 6 (IL-6)
D. Interleukin 8 (IL-8)

In LA myxoma, elevated levels of serum IgG and interleukin 6 (IL-6) are found.

1344. Which of the following is a feature of left atrial myxoma?
Harrison's 20th Ed. Chapter 258 Page 1815

A. Systemic manifestations
B. Elevated serum IgG
C. Echo-producing mass in the LA with TTE
D. All of the above

1345. Anticoagulants are administered for how long to MS patients who have suffered systemic and/or pulmonary embolization?
Harrison's 20th Ed. Chapter 258 Page 1816

A. At least 3 months
B. At least 6 months
C. At least 1 year
D. Life long

1346. Anticoagulants should be administered for how long to patients with MS who have atrial fibrillation?
Harrison's 20th Ed. Chapter 258 Page 1816

A. At least 3 months
B. At least 6 months
C. At least 1 year
D. Life long

1347. In MS with AF of relatively recent origin, cardioversion is undertaken after patient has had anticoagulant treatment for?
Harrison's 20th Ed. Chapter 258 Page 1816

A. 1 week
B. 2 weeks
C. 3 weeks
D. 4 weeks

Cardioversion should be undertaken after the patient has had at least 3 consecutive weeks of anticoagulant treatment to a therapeutic INR.

1348. In patients with MS and AF, conversion to sinus rhythm is rarely sustained when?

Harrison's 20th Ed. Chapter 258 Page 1816

A. LA is enlarged
B. AF has been present for more than 1 year
C. Severe MS
D. All of the above

Conversion to sinus rhythm is rarely successful or sustained in patients with severe MS, particularly those in whom the LA is especially enlarged or in whom AF has been present for more than 1 year.

1349. Mitral valvotomy is indicated in the symptomatic patient with isolated MS whose effective orifice is less than?

Harrison's 20th Ed. Chapter 258 Page 1816

A. 1.0 cm^2/m^2 body surface area
B. 1.5 cm^2/m^2 body surface area
C. 2.0 cm^2/m^2 body surface area
D. 2.5 cm^2/m^2 body surface area

Mitral valvotomy is indicated in symptomatic patients with isolated MS whose effective orifice is < ~1.0 cm^2/m^2 body surface area or <1.5 cm^2 in normal-sized adults.

1350. In pregnant patient with MS, percutaneous mitral balloon valvuloplasty (PMBV) is performed with?

Harrison's 20th Ed. Chapter 258 Page 1816

A. CT
B. MRI
C. TEE
D. Any of the above

In the pregnant patient with MS not responding to intensive medical treatment, PMBV is the preferred strategy and is performed with TEE and no or minimal X-ray exposure.

1351. Successful mitral valvotomy is defined as a reduction in the mean mitral valve gradient by?

Harrison's 20th Ed. Chapter 258 Page 1817

A. 10%
B. 20%
C. 30%
D. 50%

Successful mitral valvotomy is defined by a 50% reduction in the mean mitral valve gradient and a doubling of the mitral valve area.

1352. Operative mortality is maximum in which of the following?

Harrison's 20th Ed. Chapter 258 Page 1817 Table 258-2

A. Aortic valve replacement with coronary artery bypass
B. Mitral valve replacement with coronary artery bypass
C. Mitral valve replacement
D. Aortic valve replacement

1353. Operative mortality is maximum in which of the following?

Harrison's 20th Ed. Chapter 258 Page 1817 Table 258-2

A. Aortic valve repair
B. Mitral valve repair
C. Tricuspid valve surgery
D. Pulmonic valve replacement

Mitral Regurgitation

1354. Which of the following is a component of mitral valve apparatus?
Harrison's 20th Ed. Chapter 259 Page 1818

A. Chordae tendineae
B. Papillary muscles
C. Subjacent myocardium
D. All of the above

Five functional components of the mitral valve apparatus are leaflets, annulus, chordae tendineae, papillary muscles, and subjacent myocardium. Dysfunction in any of these may cause MR.

1355. Which of the following is used to classify Mitral Regurgitation?
J Thorac Cardiovasc Surg. 1980;79:338-48

A. Gorman
B. Miller
C. Carpentier
D. Lamas

1356. Modified Carpentier classification of mitral regurgitation is based on?
J Thorac Cardiovasc Surg. 1980;79:338-48

A. Regurgitant volume
B. Regurgitant fraction
C. Leaflet motion
D. All of the above

Carpentier et al. introduced a pathophysiologic classification of MR. The basis of this classification is mitral leaflet motion. MR with normal motion is type I, with increased motion is type II and with restricted motion is type III.

1357. Acute MR can occur in which of the following?
Harrison's 20th Ed. Chapter 259 Page 1818

A. Infective endocarditis
B. Acute myocardial infarction with papillary muscle rupture
C. Blunt chest wall trauma
D. All of the above

Acute MR can occur in infective endocarditis, papillary muscle rupture (post Acute MI), following blunt chest wall trauma, and rupture of chordae tendineae in MVP & IE.

1358. Which of the following statements is false?
Harrison's 20th Ed. Chapter 259 Page 1818

A. Posteromedial papillary muscle has singular blood supply
B. Transient, acute MR can occur during angina pectoris
C. In acute MI, anterolateral papillary muscle is involved much more frequently
D. None of the above

With acute MI, posteromedial papillary muscle is involved much more frequently than anterolateral papillary muscle because of its singular blood supply.

1359. Which of the following is a cause of chronic primary MR?
Harrison's 20th Ed. Chapter 259 Page 1818 Table 259-1

A. Ischemic cardiomyopathy
B. Dilated cardiomyopathy
C. Radiation
D. HOCM (with SAM)

Causes of chronic primary MR i.e. those (affecting leaflets & chordae) include myxomatous, rheumatic fever, IE (healed), congenital and radiation. Causes of chronic secondary MR include ischemic cardiomyopathy, dilated cardiomyopathy, HOCM (with SAM) and chronic AF with LA enlargement and annular dilatation.

1360. In secondary (functional) MR, regurgitation is caused by?
Harrison's 20th Ed. Chapter 259 Page 1818

A. Left ventricular remodeling with annular enlargement
B. Papillary muscle displacement
C. Leaflet tethering
D. All of the above

In secondary (functional) MR, leaflets & chordae tendineae are usually normal but regurgitation is caused by LV remodeling with annular enlargement, papillary muscle displacement, leaflet tethering, or their combination.

1361. Chronic MR can result from all except?
Harrison's 20th Ed. Chapter 259 Page 1818

A. Ankylosing spondylitis
B. Hypertrophic obstructive cardiomyopathy (HOCM)
C. Mitral valve prolapse (MVP)
D. Dilated cardiomyopathy

Chronic MR can result from rheumatic disease, mitral valve prolapse (MVP), extensive mitral annular calcification, congenital valve defects, hypertrophic obstructive cardiomyopathy (HOCM), and dilated cardiomyopathy.

1362. Which of the following about functional (secondary) MR is false?
Harrison's 20th Ed. Chapter 259 Page 1818

A. Leaflets are structurally normal
B. Chordae tendineae are structurally normal
C. Annular enlargement
D. None of the above

1363. MR associated with which of the following is dynamic in nature?
Harrison's 20th Ed. Chapter 259 Page 1818

A. HOCM
B. Acute myocardial infarction
C. Dilated cardiomyopathy
D. All of the above

The MR associated with both MVP and HOCM is usually dynamic in nature.

1364. Chronic MR is frequently secondary to?
Harrison's 20th Ed. Chapter 259 Page 1818

A. Ventricular remodeling
B. Leaflet tethering
C. Fibrosis of a papillary muscle
D. All of the above

Chronic MR is frequently secondary to ischemia and may occur as a consequence of ventricular remodeling, papillary muscle displacement, and leaflet tethering or with fibrosis of a papillary muscle in patients with healed MI and ischemic cardiomyopathy.

1365. MR occurs universally in patients with nonischemic forms of dilated cardiomyopathy when left ventricular end-diastolic dimension is?

Harrison's 20th Ed. Chapter 259 Page 1818

A. 3.0 cm
B. 4.0 cm
C. 5.0 cm
D. 6.0 cm

Annular dilatation and ventricular remodeling contribute to MR that occurs universally among patients with nonischemic forms of dilated cardiomyopathy once the left ventricular end-diastolic dimension reaches 6.0 cm.

1366. In severe chronic MR, enlargement of LA places tension on?

Harrison's 20th Ed. Chapter 259 Page 1818

A. Anterior mitral leaflet
B. Posterior mitral leaflet
C. Chordae tendineae
D. All of the above

Chronic severe MR is progressive since enlargement of LA places tension on posterior mitral leaflet, pulling it away from the mitral orifice & thereby aggravating valvular dysfunction.

1367. Significant pulmonary hypertension at rest is defined as?

J Am Heart Assoc. 2014;3:e000748

A. Pulmonary artery systolic pressure [PASP] >20 mm Hg
B. Pulmonary artery systolic pressure [PASP] >30 mm Hg
C. Pulmonary artery systolic pressure [PASP] >40 mm Hg
D. Pulmonary artery systolic pressure [PASP] >50 mm Hg

Significant pulmonary hypertension is defined as pulmonary artery systolic pressure (PASP) >50 mm Hg at rest or >60 mm Hg with exercise.

1368. Which of the following defines severe MR?

Harrison's 20th Ed. Chapter 259 Page 1818

A. Regurgitant volume ≥ 60 mL/beat
B. Regurgitant fraction (RF) ≥ 50%
C. Effective regurgitant orifice area ≥ 0.40 cm^2
D. All of the above

Severe nonischemic MR is defined by a regurgitant volume ≥60 mL/beat, regurgitant fraction (RF) ≥50%, and effective regurgitant orifice area ≥0.40 cm^2. Severe ischemic MR is usually associated with an effective regurgitant orifice area of >0.3 cm^2.

1369. Acute severe MR & chronic severe MR are differentiated by?

Harrison's 20th Ed. Chapter 259 Page 1819

A. V wave in the LA pressure pulse
B. Frequency of acute pulmonary edema
C. Decrescendo configuration of systolic murmur
D. All of the above

In acute severe MR, v wave in LA pressure pulse is prominent. Acute pulmonary edema is common. Murmur is early in timing and decrescendo in configuration. In chronic severe MR, LA v wave is relatively less prominent. Murmur is classically holosystolic in timing and plateau in configuration.

1370. In mitral regurgitation due to papillary muscle dysfunction, the systolic murmur commences in?

Harrison's 20th Ed. Chapter 259 Page 1819

A. Early systole
B. Midsystole
C. Late systole
D. All of the above

1371. Which of the following is not ordinarily heard with isolated MR?

Harrison's 20th Ed. Chapter 259 Page 1819

A. Holosystolic murmur
B. S_3
C. S_4
D. Presystolic murmur

In chronic MR, S1 is generally absent, soft, or buried in the holosystolic murmur. In severe MR, aortic valve may close prematurely, resulting in wide but physiologic splitting of S2. Low-pitched S3 occurring 0.12–0.17 seconds after A2 is caused by sudden tensing of papillary muscles, chordae tendineae and valve leaflets. Short, rumbling, mid-diastolic murmur, even in the absence of structural MS may follow. S4 is heard in acute severe MR in sinus rhythm. A presystolic murmur is not ordinarily heard with isolated MR.

1372. Systolic murmur of MR, transmitted to base of heart indicates primary involvement of?

Harrison's 20th Ed. Chapter 259 Page 1819

A. Anterior mitral leaflet
B. Posterior mitral leaflet
C. Both mitral leaflets
D. Mitral valve annulus

In patients with ruptured chordae tendineae or primary involvement of the posterior mitral leaflet with prolapse or flail, regurgitant jet is eccentric, directed anteriorly, & strikes LA wall adjacent to aortic root. In this situation, systolic murmur is transmitted to base of heart.

1373. In patients with which of the following, systolic murmur may have a cooing or "seagull" quality?

Harrison's 20th Ed. Chapter 259 Page 1819

A. Mitral valve prolapse (MVP)
B. Ruptured chordae tendineae
C. Acute rheumatic fever
D. HOCM

In patients with ruptured chordae tendineae, systolic murmur of MR may have a cooing or "sea gull" quality.

1374. In patients with which of the following, systolic murmur may have a musical quality?

Harrison's 20th Ed. Chapter 259 Page 1819

A. Mitral valve prolapse (MVP)
B. Ruptured chordae tendineae
C. Acute rheumatic fever
D. HOCM

In patients with a flail leaflet, murmur of MR may have a musical quality. Systolic murmur of chronic MR not due to MVP is intensified by isometric exercise (handgrip) but is reduced during the strain phase of the Valsalva maneuver.

1375. Rheumatic heart disease is the cause of chronic MR in what percentage of cases?

Harrison's 17th Ed. 1469

A. 25%
B. 33%
C. 50%
D. 66%

Rheumatic heart disease is the cause of chronic MR in only about one-third of cases and occurs more frequently in males.

1376. Which of the following best relates to Cabot - Locke murmur?

N Engl J Med. 2010;363:22

A. Hyperthyroidism
B. Anemia
C. Pericarditis
D. Endocarditis

Cabot - Locke murmur is a diastolic murmur heard best at the left sternal border. It sounds similar to aortic insufficiency but does not have a decrescendo. Murmur resolves with treatment of anemia. Richard Cabot was an American physician and Frank Locke was his colleague.

Mitral Valve Prolapse

1377. Barlow's syndrome refers to?
Harrison's 20th Ed. Chapter 260 Page 1821

A. Bicuspid aortic stenosis
B. Atrial myxoma
C. Mitral valve prolapse
D. HOCM

MVP is also termed systolic click-murmur syndrome, Barlow's syndrome, floppy-valve syndrome, and billowing mitral leaflet syndrome.

1378. John Barlow belonged to which country?
N Engl J Med. 2010;363:22

A. South Africa
B. United Kingdom
C. Australia
D. Canada

South African physician John Barlow first submitted his work on mitral-valve prolapse to the journal Circulation, but the manuscript was refused for its "overstated conclusion." After considerable abbreviation of the paper, it was finally accepted & published in 1968 by British Heart Journal.

1379. Which of the following statements about MVP is false?
Harrison's 20th Ed. Chapter 260 Page 1822

A. Reduced production of type III collagen
B. Increased concentrations of acid mucopolysaccharide
C. Posterior leaflet is more affected than anterior
D. None of the above

1380. Mitral valve prolapse has association with heritable disorder like?
Harrison's 20th Ed. Chapter 260 Page 1822

A. Down syndrome
B. Osteogenesis imperfecta
C. Turner syndrome
D. Hemophilia

MVP is a frequent finding in patients with heritable disorders of connective tissue, including Marfan syndrome, osteogenesis imperfecta & Ehler-Danlos syndrome.

1381. Mitral valve prolapse (MVP) may occur as a sequel to?
Harrison's 20th Ed. Chapter 260 Page 1822

A. Acute rheumatic fever
B. Ischemic heart disease
C. Various cardiomyopathies
D. All of the above

MVP may occur as a sequel to acute rheumatic fever, in ischemic heart disease, and in various cardiomyopathies.

1382. Mitral valve prolapse (MVP) is associated with which of the following?
Harrison's 20th Ed. Chapter 260 Page 1822

A. Ostium primum atrial septal defect
B. Ostium secundum atrial septal defect
C. Ventricular septal defect
D. Patent ductus arteriosus

Mitral valve prolapse (MVP) is associated with 20% of patients with ostium secundum ASD.

1383. Which of the following may be an associated feature of MVP?
Harrison's 20th Ed. Chapter 260 Page 1822

A. Inguinal hernias
B. Joint dislocations
C. Meniscal tears
D. All of the above

1384. Which of the following valve may be affected in MVP?
Harrison's 20th Ed. Chapter 260 Page 1822

A. Mitral valve
B. Tricuspid valve
C. Aortic valve
D. All of the above

1385. Ventricular arrhythmias in MVP result from stress placed on?
Harrison's 20th Ed. Chapter 260 Page 1822

A. Mitral annulus
B. Posterior mitral leaflet
C. Chordae tendineae
D. Papillary muscles

MVP causes ventricular arrhythmias due to excessive stress on papillary muscles which lead to dysfunction & ischemia of papillary muscles and subjacent ventricular myocardium.

1386. Which of the following valvular heart disease is more common in male?
Harrison's 20th Ed. Chapter 260 Page 1822

A. Rheumatic MR
B. Mitral stenosis (MS)
C. MVP
D. AR with associated mitral valve disease

1387. Which of the following valvular heart disease is more common in female?
Harrison's 20th Ed. Chapter 260 Page 1822

A. Rheumatic MR
B. MVP
C. Adult patients with symptomatic valvular AS
D. Patients with pure or predominant valvular AR

1388. Which of the following valvular heart disease is more common in female?
Harrison's 20th Ed. Chapter 260 Page 1822

A. Rheumatic MR
B. Tricuspid Stenosis
C. Adult patients with symptomatic valvular AS
D. Patients with pure or predominant valvular AR

1389. Sudden death occurs most often in MVP patients with?
Harrison's 20th Ed. Chapter 260 Page 1822

A. Severe MR
B. Depressed left ventricle (LV) systolic function
C. Flail leaflet
D. All of the above

Sudden death is a very rare complication of MVP and occurs most often in patients with severe MR & depressed left ventricle systolic function or among patients with a flail leaflet.

1390. In MVP, nonejection systolic click occurs how many seconds after S1?

Harrison's 20th Ed. Chapter 260 Page 1822

A. 0.11 seconds
B. 0.12 seconds
C. 0.13 seconds
D. 0.14 seconds

In MVP, the mid- or late (nonejection) systolic click occurs 0.14 seconds or more after S1 and is due to sudden tensing of slack, elongated chordae tendineae or due to prolapsing mitral leaflet when it reaches its maximum excursion.

1391. Which of the following about MVP is false?

Harrison's 20th Ed. Chapter 260 Page 1822

A. Systolic clicks may be multiple
B. High-pitched, late systolic crescendo-decrescendo murmur
C. Late systolic murmur heard best at apex
D. None of the above

In MVP, the late systolic murmur is high-pitched, crescendo-decrescendo configuration ("whooping" or "honking") and is heard best at the apex.

1392. Systolic click & murmur of MVP occur earlier in all of the following except?

Harrison's 20th Ed. Chapter 260 Page 1822

A. Standing
B. Squatting
C. During the strain phase of Valsalva maneuver
D. All of the above

In MVP, systolic click & murmur occur earlier with standing, during strain phase of Valsalva maneuver, and with any intervention that decreases LV volume. Conversely, squatting & isometric exercises, which increase LV volume, diminish click-murmur complex of MVP thus moving it away from S1.

1393. Most frequent serious sequelae of mitral valve prolapse is?

Harrison's 20th Ed. Chapter 260 Page 1822

A. Infective endocarditis
B. Sudden cardiac death
C. Severe mitral regurgitation
D. None of the above

Sudden death is a rare complication & occurs in patients with severe MR & depressed LV systolic function. MVP is the commonest cause of isolated severe MR requiring surgical treatment.

1394. Which view in echocardiography is best to diagnose mitral valve prolapse?

Harrison's 20th Ed. Chapter 260 Page 1822

A. Parasternal long-axis view
B. Parasternal short-axis view
C. Four-chamber view
D. All of the above

1395. "Classic" mitral valve prolapse is defined as?

Harrison's 20th Ed. Chapter 260 Page 1823

A. Prolapse of mitral valve
B. Prolapse > 2 mm beyond long-axis annular plane
C. Thickening of the valve leaflets
D. All of the above

Echocardiographic definition of MVP is systolic displacement (in the parasternal long axis view) of mitral valve leaflets by at least 2 mm into LA superior to the plane of the mitral annulus.

1396. Which of the following is true in mitral valve prolapse syndrome?

Lancet. 2005;365:507

A. Expansion of spongiosa layer by proteoglycans
B. Structural alterations of collagen in all components of leaflet
C. Structurally abnormal chordae tendinae
D. All of the above

1397. Non-prolapse related systolic clicks are documented in?

Lancet. 2005;365:507

A. Bicuspid aortic stenosis
B. Atrial myxoma
C. Pericarditis
D. All of the above

1398. Which of the following echocardiographic parameters is useful to risk stratify patients with mitral valve prolapse?

Lancet. 2005;365:507

A. Leaflet thickness
B. Redundancy
C. Increased left-ventricular diameter
D. All of the above

1399. Transthoracic echocardiography (TTE) does not exclude?

Lancet. 2005;365:507

A. Medial scallop prolapse
B. Middle scallop prolapse
C. Lateral scallop prolapse
D. None of the above

1400. Patients with mitral valve prolapse at increased risk of complications are?

Lancet. 2005;365:507

A. Depressed left ventricular systolic function
B. Moderate-severe mitral regurgitation
C. Mitral leaflet thickness greater than 5 mm
D. All of the above

1401. In MVP, which of the following echocardiographic finding predicts a greater risk of severe MR?

Lancet. 2005;365:507

A. Presence of thickened leaflets
B. Posterior leaflet prolapse
C. Increased left ventricular dimensions
D. All of the above

Tricuspid Valve Disease

1402. Which of the following about tricuspid stenosis is false?
Harrison's 20th Ed. Chapter 261 Page 1823

A. Generally congenital in origin
B. More common in women than men
C. Does not occur as an isolated lesion
D. Rheumatic TS commonly associated with TR

Tricuspid stenosis (TS) is generally rheumatic in origin and more common in women than men. It does not occur as an isolated lesion and is usually associated with MS. Rheumatic TS is commonly associated with some degree of TR. Nonrheumatic causes of TS are rare.

1403. Systemic venous congestion sets in when mean RA - RV diastolic pressure gradient is?
Harrison's 20th Ed. Chapter 261 Page 1823

A. 1 mm Hg
B. 2 mm Hg
C. 3 mm Hg
D. 4 mm Hg

A diastolic pressure gradient between the RA and RV defines TS. A mean diastolic pressure gradient of 4 mm Hg is usually sufficient to elevate the mean RA pressure to levels that result in systemic venous congestion (hepatomegaly, ascites, edema).

1404. In Tricuspid stenosis (TS), jugular veins may show?
Harrison's 20th Ed. Chapter 261 Page 1824

A. Giant 'a' wave
B. Less conspicuous 'v' wave
C. Slow 'y' descent
D. All of the above

In TS with sinus rhythm, jugular veins are distended with giant "a" waves. "v" waves are less conspicuous with a slow "y" descent.

1405. Which of the following statements is false?
Harrison's 20th Ed. Chapter 261 Page 1824

A. Development of MS precedes that of TS
B. Presence of TS can mask clinical features of MS
C. TS is almost always accompanied by significant TR
D. None of the above

Presence of TS can mask hemodynamic & clinical features of MS. Development of MS generally precedes that of TS. TS is almost always accompanied by significant TR.

1406. Murmur of which of the following valvular heart disease is heard best over the xiphoid process?
Harrison's 20th Ed. Chapter 261 Page 1824

A. TS
B. TR
C. VSD
D. All of the above

Murmur of TS is best heard along left lower sternal margin and over xiphoid process.

1407. In sinus rhythm, murmur of TS is most prominent during?
Harrison's 20th Ed. Chapter 261 Page 1824

A. Early diastole
B. Mid systole
C. Presystole
D. All of the above

Murmur of TS is most prominent during presystole in patients with sinus rhythm. It is augmented during inspiration, reduced during expiration and during the strain phase of Valsalva maneuver.

1408. Which of the following is false about combined MS & TS?
Harrison's 20th Ed. Chapter 261 Page 1824

A. Absence of ECG evidence of RVH
B. Prominence of RA & SVC without enlarged PA on CxR
C. Less evidence of pulmonary vascular congestion
D. None of the above

In combined MS & TS there is absence of ECG evidence of right ventricular hypertrophy (RVH) in a patient with right-sided heart failure. Chest X-ray shows prominence of RA & superior vena cava without much enlargement of PA with less evidence of pulmonary vascular congestion.

1409. Severe TS is characterized by a valve area of?
Harrison's 20th Ed. Chapter 261 Page 1824

A. $\leq 2\ cm^2$
B. $\leq 1.5\ cm^2$
C. $\leq 1\ cm^2$
D. $\leq 0.5\ cm^2$

Severe TS is characterized by a valve area $\leq 1\ cm^2$ or pressure half-time of ≥ 190 ms.

1410. Thromboembolic complications are most when mechanical valves are used for which valve replacement?
Harrison's 20th Ed. Chapter 261 Page 1824

A. Mitral
B. Tricuspid
C. Aortic
D. Pulmonary

Mechanical valves in the tricuspid position are more prone to thromboembolic complications than in other positions.

1411. Functional tricuspid regurgitation (TR) may be observed in?
Harrison's 20th Ed. Chapter 261 Page 1824

A. Inferior MI
B. Ischemic cardiomyopathy
C. Idiopathic dilated cardiomyopathy
D. All of the above

1412. Severe pulmonary artery hypertension is defined when pulmonary artery systolic pressure is?
Harrison's 20th Ed. Chapter 261 Page 1824

A. > 25 mm Hg
B. > 35 mm Hg
C. > 45 mm Hg
D. > 55 mm Hg

Severe pulmonary artery hypertension is defined when pulmonary artery systolic pressure is > 55 mm Hg.

1413. Carcinoid heart disease predominantly affects which of the following heart valves?

Harrison's 20th Ed. Chapter 261 Page 1824

A. Mitral
B. Tricuspid
C. Aortic
D. Pulmonary

Infarction of RV papillary muscles, tricuspid valve prolapse, carcinoid heart disease, endomyocardial fibrosis, radiation, infective endocarditis, and trauma may produce TR.

1414. Carcinoid syndrome may cause?

Harrison's 20th Ed. Chapter 261 Page 1824

A. Tricuspid regurgitation
B. Pulmonic stenosis
C. Pulmonic regurgitation
D. All of the above

Carcinoid syndrome may cause TR, pulmonic stenosis and/or regurgitation.

1415. Which of the following is seen in jugular venous pulsations in tricuspid regurgitation?

Harrison's 20th Ed. Chapter 261 Page 1824

A. No x descent
B. Prominent c-v wave
C. Rapid y descent
D. All of the above

In severe TR, RA pressure pulse shows no x descent during early systole but a prominent c-v wave with a rapid y descent.

1416. In RA pressure pulse, prominent c-v wave with rapid y descent is typical of?

Harrison's 20th Ed. Chapter 261 Page 1824

A. Ebstein's anomaly
B. Tricuspid regurgitation
C. Constrictive pericarditis
D. All of the above

In severe TR, RA pressure pulse may exhibit no x descent during early systole but a prominent c-v wave with a rapid y descent.

1417. Carvallo's sign is related to which of the following?

Harrison's 20th Ed. Chapter 261 Page 1825

A. Aortic regurgitation
B. Mitral regurgitation
C. Tricuspid regurgitation
D. Pericarditis

A prominent RV pulsation along the left parasternal region and a blowing holosystolic murmur along the lower left sternal margin, which may be intensified during inspiration & reduced during expiration or the strain of the Valsalva maneuver (Carvallo's sign), are characteristic findings of TR.

1418. A positive hepatojugular reflex is seen in?

Harrison's 20th Ed. Chapter 261 Page 1825

A. TS
B. TR
C. PS
D. All of the above

In TR, systemic venous congestion causes right-sided heart failure manifesting as marked hepatomegaly, ascites, pleural effusions, edema, systolic pulsations of liver, and a positive hepatojugular reflex.

1419. Hepatic vein systolic flow reversal on Doppler echocardiography is a feature of?

Harrison's 20th Ed. Chapter 261 Page 1825

A. TS
B. TR
C. PS
D. All of the above

1420. On Doppler examination, "hepatic vein systolic flow reversal" is a feature of?

Harrison's 20th Ed. Chapter 261 Page 1825

A. Constrictive pericarditis
B. Tricuspid regurgitation
C. SVC obstruction
D. All of the above

On Doppler examination, severe TR is accompanied by hepatic vein systolic flow reversal.

Pulmonic Valve Disease

1421. Which of the following about pulmonic valve stenosis (PS) is false?

Harrison's 20th Ed. Chapter 262 Page 1826

A. Essentially a congenital disorder
B. Pulmonic valve is typically domed
C. Very rarely affected by the rheumatic process
D. None of the above

1422. Dysplastic pulmonic valves are seen as part of which of the following syndrome?

Harrison's 20th Ed. Chapter 262 Page 1826

A. Down syndrome
B. Parkes-Weber syndrome
C. Noonan syndrome
D. Williams syndrome

Dysplastic pulmonic valves are seen as part of the Noonan syndrome.

1423. Severe PS is defined by a peak systolic gradient across the pulmonic valve of?

Harrison's 20th Ed. Chapter 262 Page 1826

A. > 30 mm Hg
B. > 40 mm Hg
C. > 50 mm Hg
D. > 60 mm Hg

1424. PS rarely progresses in patients with peak gradients of?

Harrison's 20th Ed. Chapter 262 Page 1826

A. < 30 mm Hg
B. < 40 mm Hg
C. < 50 mm Hg
D. < 60 mm Hg

Severe PS is defined by a peak systolic gradient across the pulmonic valve of > 50 mm Hg. PS rarely progresses in patients with peak gradients <30 mm Hg.

1425. Which of the following is a right-sided acoustic event that decreases in intensity with inspiration?

Harrison's 20th Ed. Chapter 262 Page 1826

A. Third heart sound
B. Fourth heart sound
C. Systolic murmur
D. Ejection sound (click)

The ejection sound is the only right-sided acoustic event that decreases in intensity with inspiration.

1426. Which of the following heart valves is least affected by infective endocarditis?

Harrison's 20th Ed. Chapter 262 Page 1826

A. Mitral
B. Tricuspid
C. Aortic
D. Pulmonary

Pulmonic valve is affected by rheumatic fever far less frequently than the other valves, and it is uncommonly a nidus for infective endocarditis.

1427. Which of the following is false about 'Graham Steell murmur'?

Harrison's 20th Ed. Chapter 262 Page 1827

A. High-pitched
B. Decrescendo, diastolic
C. Along left sternal border
D. None of the above

Graham Steell murmur due to severe pulmonary hypertension is a high-pitched, decrescendo, diastolic blowing murmur along the left sternal border.

1428. Pulmonic regurgitation occurs universally among patients who have undergone which of the following?

Harrison's 20th Ed. Chapter 262 Page 1827

A. Mustard operation
B. Repair of tetralogy of Fallot
C. Senning operation
D. Ross procedure

Pulmonic regurgitation occurs universally among patients who have undergone childhood repair of tetralogy of Fallot with reconstruction of the RV outflow tract.

Multiple and Mixed Valvular Heart Disease

1429. Which of the following drug can cause aortic insufficiency?
Harrison's 20th Ed. Chapter 262 Page 1827

A. Methysergide
B. Fenfluramine
C. Penicillin
D. Cisplatin

Aortic insufficiency can be caused by serotonin reuptake inhibitors, specifically medications containing fenfluramine or dexfenfluramine isotopes, and dopamine agonists.

1430. Which of the following can produce mixed valve lesions?
Harrison's 20th Ed. Chapter 262 Page 1827

A. Mediastinal radiation
B. Carcinoid heart disease
C. Marfan's syndrome
D. All of the above

1431. An enlarged azygos vein in the frontal projection indicates?
Harrison's 20th Ed. Chapter 262 Page 1829

A. RA hypertension
B. LA hypertension
C. Increased pulmonary vascular resistance (PVR)
D. All of the above

An enlarged azygos vein in the frontal projection indicates RA hypertension.

1432. Bioprosthetic valves are indicated in?
Harrison's 20th Ed. Chapter 262 Page 1829

A. Elderly (> 65 years)
B. Women who expect to become pregnant
C. In whom anticoagulation is contraindicated
D. All of the above

Bioprostheses are preferred for patients >65 years, for women who expect to become pregnant & for those who refuse to take anticoagulation or for whom anticoagulation is contraindicated.

Congenital Heart Disease in the Adult

1433. Pregnant women with certain CHD, may not tolerate?
Harrison's 20th Ed. Chapter 264 Page 1831

A. Elevated pulmonary artery (PA) pressures
B. Decreased ventricular function
C. Symptomatic left-sided obstructive lesions
D. All of the above

1434. Which of the following agents are teratogenic and contraindicated during pregnancy?
Harrison's 20th Ed. Chapter 264 Page 1831

A. Angiotensin converting enzyme (ACE) inhibitors
B. Angiotensin receptor blockers
C. Endothelin-receptor blockers
D. All of the above

1435. Which of the following occurs in pregnancy?
British Medical Bulletin. 2008;85:151-180

A. 50% expansion in blood volume & cardiac output
B. Increase in heart rate from 6th week, peaking at III trimester
C. Decrease in systemic vascular resistance (SVR)
D. All of the above

1436. Which of the following can occur during pregnancy in woman with CHD?
British Medical Bulletin. 2008;85:151-180

A. Endocarditis
B. Arrhythmias
C. Aortic dissection
D. All of the above

1437. Which of the following condition can lead to aortic dissection during pregnancy in woman with CHD?
British Medical Bulletin. 2008;85:151-180

A. Coarctation of aorta
B. Bicuspid aortic valve
C. Marfan syndrome
D. All of the above

Potential risk of adverse cardiovascular events during pregnancy in woman with CHD include arrhythmias, thromboembolic events, heart failure or pulmonary oedema, aortic dissection (for patients with coarctation of aorta, bicuspid aortic valve and Marfan syndrome), endocarditis and even death.

1438. A fetal echocardiogram is advised for parents with CHD between?
Harrison's 20th Ed. Chapter 264 Page 1831, British Medical Bulletin. 2008;85:151-180

A. 12 and 14 weeks of gestation
B. 14 and 18 weeks of gestation
C. 18 and 22 weeks of gestation
D. 22 and 25 weeks of gestation

A fetal echocardiogram between 18 and 22 weeks of gestation is advised for parents with CHD.

1439. The heart starts to form in which week of gestation?
Harrison's 20th Ed. Chapter 264 Page 1831

A. II
B. III
C. IV
D. V

1440. The heart is nearly fully formed by which week of gestation?
Harrison's 20th Ed. Chapter 264 Page 1831

A. VII
B. VIII
C. IX
D. X

The heart starts to form in the third week of gestation, and is nearly fully formed by 8 weeks' gestation.

1441. Cells of the second heart field contribute to the formation of?
Harrison's 20th Ed. Chapter 264 Page 1831

A. Atria
B. RV
C. Outflow tract
D. All of the above

1442. Which of the following is essential for septation of the outflow tracts and formation of the semilunar valves?
Harrison's 20th Ed. Chapter 264 Page 1831

A. Mesodermal precardiac cells
B. Cells of the second heart field
C. Cardiac neural crest cells
D. All of the above

1443. The most common birth defects have origin in?
Harrison's 20th Ed. Chapter 264 Page 1831

A. Cardiovascular system
B. Central nervous system
C. Gastrointestinal system
D. Urogenital system

The most common birth defects are cardiovascular in origin.

1444. Which of the following is the most commonly occurring birth defect?
Harrison's 20th Ed. Chapter 264 Page 1831

A. Cleft palate
B. Flat foot
C. Congenital heart disease
D. Strabismus

CHD is the most commonly occurring birth defect.

1445. What percentage of children born with Trisomy 21 have a CHD?
Harrison's 20th Ed. Chapter 264 Page 1832

A. 10%
B. 25%
C. 50%
D. 75%

Children born with Trisomy 21 have a 50% chance of having CHD, most commonly defects in the atrioventricular canal.

1446. DiGeorge syndrome is characterized by?
Harrison's 20th Ed. Chapter 264 Page 1832

A. Conotruncal defects
B. Psychiatric disorders
C. Disabilities in cognitive function
D. All of the above

1447. Noonan syndrome is characterized by?
Harrison's 20th Ed. Chapter 264 Page 1832

A. Dysplastic pulmonary valve
B. Facial abnormalities
C. Lymphatic abnormalities
D. All of the above

1448. Hypercalcemia is a feature of?
Harrison's 20th Ed. Chapter 264 Page 1832

A. Down syndrome
B. DiGeorge syndrome
C. Noonan syndrome
D. Williams syndrome

1449. Mutation in PTPN11 gene causes which of the following?
Harrison's 20th Ed. Chapter 264 Page 1832

A. Williams syndrome
B. Down syndrome
C. Noonan syndrome
D. DiGeorge/velocardiofacial syndrome

1450. Which of the following is a congenital etiology for right heart dilation?
Harrison's 20th Ed. Chapter 264 Page 1832 Table 264-3

A. Ebstein anomaly
B. Arrhythmogenic RV cardiomyopathy
C. Uhl's anomaly
D. All of the above

1451. Which of the following is a feature of Uhl's anomaly?
Ann Pediatr Card. 2015;8:71-3

A. Absence of myocardium in parietal wall of right ventricle
B. Apposition of endocardium & epicardium, no adipose tissue
C. Papillary muscles of tricuspid valve are normally musculerized
D. All of the above

Uhl's Anomaly is a rare cardiac condition in which there is total absence of right ventricular myocardium resulting in apposition of the endocardium and epicardium. The septal wall, septomarginal trabeculation and the papillary muscles of the tricuspid valve are normally muscularized.

1452. Which of the following shunt lesions cause right heart dilation?
Harrison's 20th Ed. Chapter 264 Page 1832 Table 264-3

A. Gerbode defect
B. Coronary sinus septal defect
C. Partial anomalous pulmonary venous return
D. All of the above

1453. In Gerbode defect, abnormal shunting occurs between?
Harrison's 20th Ed. Chapter 264 Page 1832 Table 264-3

A. RV - LA
B. LV - RA
C. LV - RV
D. LA - RA

Gerbode defect is defined as abnormal shunting between the left ventricle and right atrium resulting from either a congenital defect or prior cardiac insults. Surgeon Frank Gerbode at Stanford University described it as "the lesion consists of a high ventricular septal defect associated with a defect of the septal leaflet of the tricuspid valve which allows left ventricular blood to enter the right atrium".

1454. In Gerbode defect, physical examination finding include?
J Clin Diagn Res. 2015;9(9):OD06–OD08

A. Pansystolic murmur similar to that of a VSD
B. Unvarying with respiration
C. Thrill along the left sternal border
D. All of the above

1455. Congenital heart disease complicates what percentage of all live births?
British Medical Bulletin. 2008;85:151-180

A. ~ 1%
B. ~ 2%
C. ~ 3%
D. ~ 4%

CHD complicates ~1% of all live births in general population, but occurs in 4% of offspring of women with CHD.

1456. Which of the following arches develop as the internal carotid arteries?
Circulation. 2006;114:1873-1882

A. 1
B. 2
C. 3
D. 4

Truncus arteriosus & aortic sac initially develop six paired symmetric arches. Development of arch 3 results in internal carotid arteries, left arch 4 as the aortic arch and right subclavian artery, and part of arch 6 as the patent ductus arteriosus.

1457. Sinus venosus receives which of the following veins?
Circulation. 2006;114:1873-1882

A. Umbilical vein
B. Vitelline vein
C. Common cardinal vein
D. All of the above

Sinus venosus receives the umbilical, vitelline, and common cardinal veins.

1458. Which of the following congenital heart disease is more common in females?

N Engl J Med. 2000;342:256-263

A. ASD
B. Congenital valvular AS
C. Coarctation of aorta
D. Complete transposition of great vessels

ASD occurs more frequently in females. Congenital valvular AS, Coarctation of aorta and Complete transposition of great vessels is more frequent in males.

1459. Which of the following ASD type is false?

N Engl J Med. 2000;342:256-263

A. Ostium secundum is in the region of the fossa ovalis
B. Ostium primum is in the lower part of the atrial septum
C. Sinus venosus is in the upper atrial septum
D. None of the above

Ostium secundum defects make up 75 percent of all atrial septal defects, ostium primum defects make up 15 percent, and sinus venosus defects make up 10 percent.

1460. Which of the following ASD type is associated with anomalous pulmonary venous connection?

N Engl J Med. 2000;342:256-263

A. Sinus venosus ASD
B. Ostium primum ASD
C. Ostium secundum ASD
D. Patent foramen ovale

ASD in sinus venosus type is high up in the atrial septum near the entry of superior vena cava into right atrium. It is associated frequently with anomalous pulmonary venous connection from the right lung to the superior vena cava or right atrium.

1461. ASD occurs in the basal portion of the interventricular septum in which of the following?

N Engl J Med. 2000;342:256-263

A. Sinus venosus ASD
B. Ostium primum ASD
C. Ostium secundum ASD
D. Patent foramen ovale

1462. Mitral-valve prolapse occurs with?

N Engl J Med. 2000;342:256-263

A. Sinus venosus ASD
B. Ostium primum ASD
C. Ostium secundum ASD
D. Patent foramen ovale

Additional cardiac abnormalities may occur with each type of defect; these include mitral-valve prolapse (with ostium secundum defects), mitral regurgitation (due to a cleft in the anterior mitral-valve leaflet, which occurs with ostium primum defects), and partial anomalous drainage of the pulmonary veins into the right atrium or venae cavae (with sinus venosus defects).

1463. Which of the following ASD is more common in Down syndrome?

Harrison's 19th Ed. 1520

A. Sinus venosus ASD
B. Ostium primum ASD
C. Ostium secundum ASD
D. Patent foramen ovale

1464. Which out of the following ASD is most common ?

Harrison's 20th Ed. Chapter 264 Page 1832

A. Sinus venosus ASD
B. Ostium primum ASD
C. Ostium secundum ASD
D. Patent foramen ovale

1465. Which out of the following ASD is in the region of fossa ovalis?

Harrison's 20th Ed. Chapter 264 Page 1832

A. Sinus venosus ASD
B. Ostium primum ASD
C. Ostium secundum ASD
D. Patent foramen ovale

1466. Patent foramen ovale (PFO) persists in what proportion of adults?

Harrison's 20th Ed. Chapter 264 Page 1832

A. 5%
B. 15%
C. 25%
D. 35%

Patent foramen ovale (PFO) is the persistence of patency of the flap valve of fossa ovalis. It is not associated with right-sided cardiac dilation. PFO persists in ~25% of adults.

1467. ASD is considered a large shunt, with substantial hemodynamic consequences, when its diameter is more than?

N Engl J Med. 2000;342:256-263

A. 0.5 cm
B. 1.0 cm
C. 1.5 cm
D. 2.0 cm

A small ASD (<0.5 cm in diameter) is associated with a small shunt and no hemodynamic sequelae. A sizable defect (>2 cm in diameter) may be associated with a large shunt, with substantial hemodynamic consequences.

1468. A small ASD is characterized by a ratio of pulmonary to systemic flow of less than?

N Engl J Med. 2000;342:256-263

A. 0.5
B. 1.0
C. 1.5
D. 2.0

A small defect with minimal left-to-right shunting (characterized by a ratio of pulmonary to systemic flow of <1.5) usually causes no symptoms or hemodynamic abnormalities and therefore does not require closure.

1469. Flow across the atrial septal defect itself produces which of the following murmur?

N Engl J Med. 2000;342:256-263

A. Systolic
B. Diastolic
C. Continuous
D. No murmur

Flow across the atrial septal defect itself does not produce a murmur.

1470. Mid-diastolic rumbling murmur in ASD is loudest at?
N Engl J Med. 2000;342:256-263

A. 3rd intercostal space, along left sternal border
B. 3rd intercostal space, along right sternal border
C. 4th intercostal space, along left sternal border
D. 4th intercostal space, along right sternal border

1471. Which of the following cardiac murmurs can be heard in various types of compensated ASD?
N Engl J Med. 2000;342:256-263

A. Midsystolic pulmonary outflow murmur
B. Mid-diastolic left parasternal murmur
C. Apical holosystolic murmur
D. All of the above

Increased flow across the pulmonic valve is responsible for a midsystolic pulmonary outflow murmur. Mid-diastolic murmur at fourth intercostal space and along left sternal border indicates increased flow across tricuspid valve. In ostium primum ASD, apical holosystolic murmur indicates associated mitral or tricuspid regurgitation or a ventricular septal defect (VSD).

1472. In ASD, second heart sound is widely split and is relatively fixed in relation to?
Harrison's 20th Ed. Chapter 264 Page 1832

A. Respiration
B. Posture
C. Heart rate
D. All of the above

In ASD, second heart sound is widely split and is relatively fixed in relation to respiration.

1473. Which of the following is key to wide and fixed splitting of the second heart sound in ASD?
N Engl J Med. 2000;342:256-263

A. No respiratory changes in right & left atrial stroke volumes
B. No respiratory changes in right & left ventricular stroke volumes
C. No respiratory changes in pulmonary artery
D. No respiratory changes in pulmonary vasculature

Wide & fixed splitting of S2 in ASD is due to prolonged RV ejection and increased PA capacitance which delays pulmonary valve closure. Splitting of S2 is fixed because phasic changes in systemic venous return to right atrium during respiration are accompanied by reciprocal changes in volume of shunted blood from left atrium to the right atrium, thereby minimizing the respiratory changes in right & left ventricular stroke volumes that are normally responsible for physiologic splitting.

1474. In adults with an ASD and atrial fibrillation, the physical findings may be confused with? *Harrison's 19th Ed. 1521*

A. Mitral stenosis
B. Tricuspid stenosis
C. Pulmonary stenosis
D. Mitral regurgitation

In adults with an ASD and atrial fibrillation, physical findings may be confused with mitral stenosis with pulmonary hypertension because the tricuspid diastolic flow murmur and widely split second heart sound may be mistakenly thought to represent the diastolic murmur of mitral stenosis and the mitral "opening snap," respectively.

1475. Which of the following statements about ostium secundum type of ASD is false?
Harrison's 20th Ed. Chapter 264 Page 1832

A. ECG shows left axis deviation
B. S_2 widely split and relatively fixed
C. Middiastolic rumbling murmur
D. Midsystolic pulmonary ejection murmur

In ostium secundum ASD, ECG shows right-axis deviation and an rSr' pattern in right precordial leads representing enlargement of the RV outflow tract.

1476. In ECG of cases of ostium primum ASD, which of the following is true?
N Engl J Med. 2000;342:256-263

A. Right-axis deviation
B. Left superior axis deviation
C. Left inferior axis deviation
D. Left-axis deviation

1477. In ECG of cases of ostium primum ASD, which of the following is true?
N Engl J Med. 2000;342:256-263

A. Clockwise rotation of frontal plane QRS loop
B. Counterclockwise rotation of frontal plane QRS loop
C. Clockwise rotation of sagittal plane QRS loop
D. Counterclockwise rotation of sagittal plane QRS loop

In ostium primum ASD, the RV conduction defect is accompanied by left superior axis deviation and counterclockwise rotation of the frontal plane QRS loop.

1478. Which of them is a finding in echocardiogram of a patient of ASD?
N Engl J Med. 2000;342:256-263

A. Pulmonary arterial dilatation
B. RV and RA dilatation
C. Abnormal (paradoxical) ventricular septal motion
D. All of the above

In ASD, echocardiography reveals pulmonary arterial and RV and RA dilatation with abnormal (paradoxical) ventricular septal motion in the presence of a significant right heart volume overload. ASD may be visualized directly by two-dimensional imaging, color-flow imaging, or echocontrast.

1479. Which of the following about atrial septal defect is false?
N Engl J Med. 2000;342:256-263

A. Sinus venosus ASD cases rarely die before 5th decade
B. Ostium secundum ASD cases rarely die before 5th decade
C. Risk of infective endocarditis in ASD is low
D. None of the above

Closure by an appropriate method should be advised in uncomplicated secundum ASD with significant left-to-right shunting, i.e., pulmonary-to-systemic flow ratios 2:1. Patients with sinus venosus or ostium secundum ASDs rarely die before the fifth decade. Risk of infective endocarditis is quite low unless ASD is complicated by valvular regurgitation or has recently been repaired with a patch or device.

1480. Ebstein's anomaly is a disease of?
Harrison's 20th Ed. Chapter 264 Page 1832

A. Right atrium
B. Right ventricle
C. Right ventricular outflow tract
D. All of the above

Ebstein's anomaly is a disease of the entire right ventricle.

1481. Ebstein anomaly is the result of?
Harrison's 20th Ed. Chapter 264 Page 1832

A. Failure of delamination of TV leaflets from ventricular myocardium
B. Failure of delamination of TV leaflets from atrial myocardium
C. Failure of septation of ventricular myocardium
D. Failure of septation of atrial myocardium

Ebstein anomaly is due to embryologic failure of delamination or "peeling away" of tricuspid valve leaflets from the ventricular myocardium, resulting in adherence of the valve leaflets to the underlying myocardium.

1482. Which of the following about Ebstein anomaly is false?
Harrison's 20th Ed. Chapter 264 Page 1832

A. Apical & posterior displacement of dilated TV annulus
B. Dilation of the "atrialized" portion of the RV
C. Fenestrations, redundancy & tethering of anterior leaflet of TV
D. None of the above

Ebstein anomaly consists of apical & posterior displacement of dilated tricuspid valve annulus, dilation of "atrialized" portion of RV, and fenestrations, redundancy & tethering of anterior leaflet of tricuspid valve.

1483. Most common finding in Ebstein's anomaly is?
Harrison's 20th Ed. Chapter 264 Page 1832

A. MS
B. MR
C. TS
D. TR

Ebstein's Anomaly is characterized by a downward displacement of tricuspid valve into right ventricle, due to anomalous attachment of dysplastic tricuspid leaflets. This results in tricuspid regurgitation.

1484. Which of the following signs is related to Ebstein anomaly?
Harrison's 20th Ed. Chapter 264 Page 1832

A. McConnell's sign
B. Broadbent's sign
C. Sail sign
D. Ewart's sign

In Ebstein anomaly, there are few hemodynamic correlates for the observed auscultatory events. Multiple components of the first sound and "ejection" sounds are frequently described. 'Sail sound' in patients with Ebstein's anomaly is not simply a closing sound of tricuspid valve, but a complex closing sound which includes a sudden stopping sound after the redundant anterior and/or other tricuspid leaflets balloon out at systole.

1485. An interatrial communication is present in what percentage of patients with Ebstein's anomaly?
Circulation. 2007;115:277-285

A. 50% – 60%
B. 60% – 70%
C. 70% – 80%
D. 80% – 90%

An interatrial communication is present in 80% to 94% of patients with Ebstein's anomaly.

1486. Which of the following is false about Ebstein anomaly?
Circulation. 2007;115:277-285

A. Jugular venous pulse rarely shows a large V wave
B. Widely split S2 and several added sounds
C. Marked enlargement of the right atrium
D. None of the above

On examination, the jugular venous pulse rarely shows a large V wave despite severe regurgitation of the tricuspid valve because the large right atrium engulfs the increased volume. S1 & S2 heart sounds are widely split, and a S3 or S4 heart sound is often present, resulting in a "triple" or "quadruple" rhythm.

1487. Patients with Ebstein's anomaly and an interatrial communication are at risk for?
N Engl J Med. 2000;342(5):334-342

A. Paradoxical embolization
B. Brain abscess
C. Sudden death
D. All of the above

1488. Which of the following is false about ECG in Ebstein anomaly?
Circulation. 2007;115:277-285

A. Tall and broad P waves
B. Complete or incomplete right bundle-branch block
C. Complete heart block is rare
D. None of the above

1489. On CxR, cardiac silhouette of typical Ebstein's anomaly is similar to that of?
Circulation. 2007;115:277-285

A. Mitral stenosis
B. Pericardial effusion
C. Partially anomalous pulmonary venous drainage
D. Tetralogy of Fallot

The cardiac silhouette may vary from almost normal to the typical Ebstein's anomaly configuration consisting of a globe-shaped heart (due to right atrial enlargement) with a narrow waist similar to that seen with pericardial effusion. Vascularity of pulmonary fields is either normal or decreased. Cardiothoracic ratio 0.65 carries a poor prognosis.

1490. Wolff–Parkinson–White syndrome occurs frequently in which of the following CHD?
Harrison's 20th Ed. Chapter 264 Page 1832, British Medical Bulletin. 2008;85:151-180

A. Tetralogy of Fallot
B. Ebstein's anomaly
C. ASD
D. All of the above

Wolff–Parkinson–White syndrome occurs in ~20% of patients with Ebstein's anomaly.

1491. Most common congenital cardiac anomaly recognized at birth is?
Harrison's 20th Ed. Chapter 264 Page 1833

A. ASD
B. VSD
C. PDA
D. Coarctation of the Aorta

VSD are the most common congenital anomaly recognized at birth. However, they account for only ~10% of CHD in the adult, due to the high rate of spontaneous closure of small VSDs during the early years of life.

1492. Which of the following about ventricular septal defect is false?
N Engl J Med. 2000;342:256-263

A. Occur with similar frequency in boys and girls
B. 25%–40% close spontaneously by the age of 2 years
C. 90% close by the age of 10 years
D. None of the above

1493. Which of the following about ventricular septal defect is false?
N Engl J Med. 2000;342:256-263

A. 70% are located in membranous portion of IVS
B. 20% are located in muscular portion of IVS
C. 5% are located just below the aortic valve
D. None of the above

VSD located just below the aortic valve undermine the valve annulus and cause aortic regurgitation. 5% of VSD are located near the junction of mitral & tricuspid valves (atrioventricular canal defects).

1494. The risk associated with surgery for VSD is prohibitive once the ratio of pulmonary to systemic vascular resistance exceeds?
N Engl J Med. 2000;342:256-263

A. 0.6
B. 0.7
C. 0.8
D. 0.9

Once the ratio of pulmonary to systemic vascular resistance exceeds 0.7, the risk associated with surgery is prohibitive.

1495. Which of the following gene can cause septal defects?
Circulation. 2006;114:2190-2197

A. TBX5
B. GATA4
C. NKX2.5
D. All of the above

1496. Which of the following is false about VSD?
Circulation. 2006;114:2190-2197

A. Smaller defects are loudest and may have a thrill
B. Murmurs are typically holosystolic or pansystolic
C. Large defects with no shunt do not have a VSD murmur
D. None of the above

1497. Which of the following is false about VSD?
Circulation. 2006;114:2190-2197

A. Endocarditis is a lifelong risk in unoperated patients
B. Chamber enlargement is a measure of the degree of shunting
C. Small VSD have no apparent ECG & radiographic abnormality
D. None of the above

1498. Which of the following about ductus arteriosus is false?
Harrison's 20th Ed. Chapter 264 Page 1834

A. Originates from bifurcation of pulmonary artery
B. Ends at aorta just distal to left subclavian artery
C. Continuous murmur best heard at upper left sternal edge
D. None of the above

Patent ductus arteriosus (PDA) is a vascular structure that connects the proximal descending aorta to the roof of the main pulmonary artery near the origin of the left branch pulmonary artery.

1499. Incidence of PDA is higher than average in?
N Engl J Med. 2000;342:256-263

A. Pregnancies complicated by persistent perinatal hypoxemia
B. Maternal rubella infection
C. Infants born at high altitude or prematurely
D. All of the above

Rubella infection during the first trimester of pregnancy, particularly in the first 4 weeks, is associated with a high incidence of PDA. It has been reported to be associated with fetal valproate syndrome.

1500. PDA occurs with increased frequency in which of the following genetic syndromes?
Circulation. 2006;114:1873-1882

A. Trisomy 21
B. Carpenter's syndrome
C. Holt-Oram syndrome
D. All of the above

PDA occurs with increased frequency in trisomy 21, 4p- syndrome, Carpenter's syndrome, Holt-Oram syndrome, and incontinentia pigmenti.

1501. Which of the following about moderate or large patent ductus arteriosus is false?
N Engl J Med. 2000;342:256-263

A. Bounding peripheral arterial pulses
B. Widened pulse pressure
C. Hyperdynamic left ventricular impulse
D. None of the above

1502. Which of the following about continuous "machinery" or Gibson's murmur of PDA is false?
N Engl J Med. 2000;342:256-263

A. Heard in second left anterior intercostal space
B. Begins shortly after S1
C. Peaks in intensity at or immediately after S2
D. None of the above

In PDA, S1 heart sound is normal. A continuous "machinery" murmur, audible in II left anterior intercostal space, begins shortly after S1, peaks in intensity at or immediately after S2 (thereby obscuring it), and declines in intensity during diastole. As pulmonary vascular obstruction and hypertension develop, the continuous murmur decreases in duration and intensity and eventually disappears and a pulmonary ejection click and a diastolic decrescendo murmur of pulmonary regurgitation may appear.

1503. Differential cyanosis is best related to?
Harrison's 20th Ed. Chapter 234 Page 1667

A. ASD
B. VSD
C. Patent ductus arteriosus
D. Tetralogy of Fallot

In PDA, severe pulmonary vascular disease results in reversal of flow through ductus therby unoxygenated blood is shunted to descending aorta leading to cyanosis and clubbing of the toes, but not fingers because the right-to-left ductal shunting is distal to the subclavian arteries. This is called differential cyanosis.

1504. Which of the following about patent ductus arteriosus is false?
N Engl J Med. 2000;342:256-263

A. Rarely closes spontaneously after infancy
B. Elevated risk of infective endocarditis
C. May become aneurysmal & calcified leading to rupture
D. None of the above

1505. Infective endocarditis involves which of the following in a case of PDA?
N Engl J Med. 2000;342:256-263

A. Aortic side of ductus arteriosus
B. Pulmonary side of ductus arteriosus
C. Mid portion of ductus arteriosus
D. Any of the above

Infective endocarditis involves the pulmonary side of the ductus arteriosus or the pulmonary artery opposite the duct orifice, from which septic pulmonary emboli may arise.

1506. Leading cause of death in adults with PDA is?
N Engl J Med. 2000;342:256-263

A. Infective endarteritis
B. Cardiac arrhythmia
C. Brain abscess
D. Restrictive lung disease

Leading causes of death in adults with patent ductus are cardiac failure & infective endarteritis.

1507. Which of the following is the most common form of cyanotic CHD after infancy?
Harrison's 20th Ed. Chapter 264 Page 1834

A. Tetralogy of Fallot (TOF)
B. Ebstein's Anomaly
C. Transposition of the Great Arteries
D. Eisenmenger's syndrome

1508. Which of the following about Tetralogy of Fallot is false?
Cleveland Clinic J of Medicine. 2010;77(11):822-828

A. Occurs in ~1 in 3,600 live births
B. Occurs in 3.5% of infants born with congenital heart disease
C. Accounts for 10% of all cases
D. None of the above

Tetralogy of Fallot occurs in approximately 1 in 3,600 live births or 3.5% of infants born with congenital heart disease. It is the most common type of cyanotic congenital heart disease, accounting for 10% of all cases.

1509. Which of the following is a component of Tetralogy of Fallot?
Harrison's 20th Ed. Chapter 264 Page 1835

A. Right ventricular hypertrophy
B. Overriding aorta
C. Membranous ventricular septal defect
D. All of the above

The four components of Tetralogy of Fallot are right ventricular hypertrophy, overriding aorta, membranous ventricular septal defect, and right ventricular outflow tract obstruction.

1510. In Tetralogy of Fallot, severity of which of the following determines the clinical presentation?
Harrison's 20th Ed. Chapter 264 Page 1835

A. Size of VSD
B. Aortic override of the VSD
C. RV outflow obstruction
D. RV hypertrophy

The four components of the tetralogy of Fallot are malaligned VSD, obstruction to RV outflow, aortic override of the VSD, and RV hypertrophy due to the RV's response to aortic pressure via the large VSD. The severity of RV outflow obstruction determines the clinical presentation.

1511. "Pink tetralogy of Fallot" refers to?
J Cardiovasc Comput Tomogr. 2010;4(1):58-61

A. Noncyanotic TOF
B. Pulmonary stenosis is mild
C. Ventricular septal defect is in balance
D. All of the above

"Pink tetralogy of Fallot" refers to the the noncyanotic patient in whom pulmonary stenosis is mild and ventricular septal defect is in balance.

1512. Tetrology of Fallot may be seen in?
International Journal of Current Advanced Research. 2018;07(5):12979-12981

A. CATCH 22
B. DiGeorge syndrome
C. Shprintzen syndrome
D. All of the above

1513. Which of the following abnormalities may occur in association with tetralogy of Fallot?
N Engl J Med. 2000;342(5):334-342

A. Right aortic arch
B. Atrial septal defect
C. Coronary arterial anomalies
D. All of the above

Abnormalities that may occur in association with tetralogy of Fallot include right aortic arch (25%), atrial septal defect (10%) -so called pentalogy of Fallot, and coronary arterial anomalies (10%).

1514. Which of the following is not a part of Trilogy of Fallot?
J Pract Cardiovasc Sci. 2016;2:114-9

A. Atrial septal defect
B. Valvular pulmonary stenosis
C. Infundibular pulmonary stenosis
D. Right ventricular hypertrophy

1515. Which of the following coronary artery is anomalous in TOF?
Harrison's 20th Ed. Chapter 264 Page 1835

A. Right coronary artery
B. Left anterior descending coronary artery
C. Left circumflex coronary artery
D. Posterior descending coronary artery

~7% of patients with TOF have an anomalous coronary artery, most commonly, anomalous left anterior descending coronary artery from the right coronary cusp.

1516. Which of the following affect the magnitude of right-to-left shunting in TOF?
N Engl J Med. 2000;342(5):334-342

A. Changes in pulmonary vascular resistance
B. Changes in systemic vascular resistance
C. Size of VSD
D. All of the above

Since the resistance to flow across right ventricular outflow tract is relatively fixed, changes in systemic vascular resistance affect the magnitude of right-to-left shunting. A decrease in systemic vascular resistance increases right-to-left shunting, whereas an increase in systemic resistance decreases right-to-left shunting.

1517. Which of the following about TOF is false?
N Engl J Med. 2000;342(5):334-342

A. Most patients have cyanosis from birth or beginning in first year
B. Hypoxic "spells" do not occur in adolescents or adults
C. Without surgical intervention, most patients die in childhood
D. None of the above

1518. In TOF, hypoxic "spells" are characterized by?

N Engl J Med. 2000;342(5):334-342

A. Tachypnea
B. Hyperpnea
C. Worsening cyanosis
D. All of the above

1519. Which of the following about TOF is false?

J Pract Cardiovasc Sci. 2016;2:114-9

A. Normal JVP
B. Aortic ejection sound
C. Congestive heart failure rare
D. None of the above

1520. Which of the following is a complication of chronic cyanosis?

N Engl J Med. 2000;342(5):334-342

A. Abnormalities of hemostasis
B. Cerebral abscesses or stroke
C. Endocarditis
D. All of the above

Complications of chronic cyanosis include erythrocytosis, hyperviscosity, abnormalities of hemostasis, cerebral abscesses or stroke, and endocarditis.

1521. Which of the following may also be present in TOF?

N Engl J Med. 2000;342(5):334-342

A. Pulmonary valve stenosis
B. Unilateral absence of a pulmonary artery
C. Right-sided aortic arch & descending thoracic aorta
D. All of the above

In tetralogy of Fallot, severity of hypoplasia of the RV outflow tract varies from mild to complete (pulmonary atresia). Pulmonary valve stenosis and supravalvular and peripheral pulmonary arterial obstruction may coexist. Rarely, there is unilateral absence of a pulmonary artery (usually left). A right-sided aortic arch and descending thoracic aorta occur in 25%.

1522. Which of the following is a clinical finding in TOF?

N Engl J Med. 2000;342(5):334-342

A. Normal S1
B. Single S2
C. Systolic ejection murmur along the left sternal border
D. All of the above

In TOF, second heart sound is single, since its pulmonary component is inaudible.

1523. Which of the following about ECG findings in Tetralogy of Fallot is false?

N Engl J Med. 2000;342(5):334-342

A. Right-axis deviation
B. Right ventricular hypertrophy
C. T wave inversion very rare
D. None of the above

1524. Which of the following about chest X-ray findings in Triology of Fallot is false?

J Pract Cardiovasc Sci. 2016;2:114-9

A. Cardiomegaly
B. Dilated PA
C. Normal shape of the heart
D. None of the above

1525. Which of the following about chest X-ray findings in Tetralogy of Fallot is false?

N Engl J Med. 2000;342(5):334-342

A. Enlarged heart
B. Boot-shaped heart (coeur en sabot)
C. Oligemic lung fields
D. Concavity in the region of pulmonary conus

In Tetralogy of Fallot, chest X-ray shows a normal-sized or small heart, boot-shaped (coeur en sabot) with a prominent right ventricle and a concavity in the region of pulmonary conus. Pulmonary vascular markings are typically diminished, and the aortic arch and knob may be on the right side.

1526. Which of the following is an operative procedure for Tetralogy of Fallot?

N Engl J Med. 2000;342(5):334-342

A. Waterston operation
B. Potts operation
C. Blalock–Taussig operation
D. All of the above

Procedures for correction of TOF involve anastomosis of a systemic artery to a pulmonary artery. Waterston operation (a side-to-side anastomosis of ascending aorta and right pulmonary artery), Potts operation (a side-to-side anastomosis of the descending aorta to the left pulmonary artery), and Blalock–Taussig operation (end-to-side anastomosis of the subclavian artery to the pulmonary artery).

1527. Which of the following about treatment in TOF is false?

Harrison's 20th Ed. Chapter 264 Page 1835

A. Reoperation in adults is mostly for severe PR
B. Ventricular and atrial arrhythmias common
C. Aortic regurgitation common
D. Endocarditis risk eliminated after surgical repair

Most adults with tetralogy of Fallot have had some form of previous surgical intervention. Reoperation in adults is most commonly for severe pulmonary regurgitation. Ventricular & atrial arrhythmias require treatment. Aortic root has a medial tissue defect & it is commonly enlarged & associated with aortic regurgitation. Endocarditis remains a risk despite surgical repair.

1528. On a resting ECG, QRS duration of what duration is associated with ↑ risk of VT & sudden death in patients with repaired TOF?

Harrison's 20th Ed. Chapter 264 Page 1835

A. ≥ 100 ms
B. ≥ 120 ms
C. ≥ 160 ms
D. ≥ 180 ms

On a resting ECG, QRS duration of ≥ 180 ms is associated with ↑ risk of VT & sudden death in patients with repaired TOF.

1529. On a resting ECG, what rate of change in QRS duration is associated with ↑ risk of VT & sudden death in patients with TOF?

Cleveland Clinic J of Medicine. 2010;77(11):822-828

A. > 1.5 ms/year
B. > 2.5 ms/year
C. > 3.5 ms/year
D. > 4.5 ms/year

In TOF, a relatively rapid increase (> 3.5 ms/year) in QRS duration is strongly associated with ventricular arrhythmias & sudden death, even if the QRS duration is not markedly prolonged. Reduced heart rate variability also is a marker of risk of sudden cardiac death in TOF.

1530. The most common re-intervention in a repaired TOF patient is?
Harrison's 20th Ed. Chapter 264 Page 1835

A. Closure of residual VSDs
B. Dilation and/or stenting of the RVOT
C. Pulmonary valve replacement (PVR)
D. Catheter ablation for arrhythmias

The most common re-intervention in a repaired TOF patient is pulmonary valve replacement (PVR).

1531. Which of the following is false about Transposition of the great arteries (TGA)?
Harrison's 20th Ed. Chapter 264 Page 1835

A. Aorta arises from the RV and the PA arises from the LV
B. D-loop TGA is the more common form of TGA
C. VSD is the most common additional congenital defect in TGA
D. None of the above

1532. Which communication in TGA provides compatibility with life?
Harrison's 20th Ed. Chapter 264 Page 1835

A. Atrial septal defect (ASD)
B. Ventricular septal defect (VSD)
C. Patent ductus arteriosus (PDA)
D. All of the above

Without interchamber or intravascular communications, this circulation is incompatible with life. Presence of ASD, VSD or PDA, allow for some interchamber or intravascular mixing, and provide partial relief of cyanosis and sustenance of life, at the expense of increased pulmonary blood flow.

1533. Which is the most common communication in complete transposition of the great arteries?
Harrison's 20th Ed. Chapter 264 Page 1835

A. ASD
B. VSD
C. PDA
D. All of the above

Most patients of complete transposition of the great arteries have an interatrial communication, two-thirds have a patent ductus arteriosus, and about one-third have an associated VSD.

1534. Which of the following procedure is used for correction of TGA?
Harrison's 20th Ed. Chapter 264 Page 1835

A. Mustard procedure
B. Senning procedure
C. Rastelli procedure
D. All of the above

1535. Which of the following about L-loop TGA is false?
Harrison's 20th Ed. Chapter 264 Page 1836

A. Also called congenitally corrected TGA
B. Atrioventricular discordance
C. Ventriculoarterial discordance
D. None of the above

1536. Associated congenital anomaly with L-loop TGA is?
Harrison's 20th Ed. Chapter 264 Page 1836

A. Dextrocardia
B. ASDs
C. Pulmonary stenosis
D. All of the above

Patients with L-loop TGA commonly have associated congenital anomalies, including dextrocardia, ASDs, a dysplastic tricuspid valve and pulmonary stenosis.

1537. Transposition of great arteries is associated with which of the following genetic syndromes?
Front Pediatr. 2013;1:11

A. Turner
B. Noonan
C. Williams
D. None of the above

Transposition of great arteries is very rarely associated with the most frequent genetic syndromes, such as Turner, Noonan, Williams or Marfan syndromes, and in Down syndrome, it is virtually absent.

1538. The only genetic syndrome with a strong relation with TGA is?
Front Pediatr. 2013;1:11

A. Kartagener syndrome
B. Heterotaxy syndrome
C. Patau syndrome
D. Edward syndrome

The only genetic syndrome with a strong relation with TGA is the Heterotaxy. Heterotaxy is defined as an abnormality where the internal thoraco-abdominal organs demonstrate abnormal arrangement across the left-right axis of the body.

1539. Which of the following is a form of trisomy?
Front Pediatr. 2013;1:11

A. Down syndrome
B. Edward syndrome
C. Patau syndrome
D. All of the above

Trisomy 21 (Down syndrome), Trisomy 18 (Edward syndrome) and Trisomy 13 (Patau syndrome).

1540. The incidence of Coarctation of the aorta is?
Harrison's 20th Ed. Chapter 271 Page 1899

A. 0.1–4 per 1000 live births
B. 0.8–4 per 1000 live births
C. 1–8 per 1000 live births
D. 5–18 per 1000 live births

Coarctation of the aorta was first described by Morgagni in 1760.

1541. Coarctation of the aorta occurs in what percentage of patients with congenital heart disease?
World J Cardiol. 2015;7(11):765-775

A. 1%
B. 3%
C. 7%
D. 9%

Narrowing or constriction of the lumen of the aorta may occur anywhere along its length but is most common distal to the origin of the left subclavian artery near the insertion of the ligamentum arteriosum. Coarctation of the aorta occurs in 7% of patients with congenital heart disease and is more common in males than females.

1542. Coarctation less commonly involves which of the following?
Harrison's 20th Ed. Chapter 264 Page 1837

A. Ascending aortic arch
B. Transverse aortic arch
C. Abdominal aorta
D. None of the above

Coarctation less commonly involves the transverse aortic arch.

1543. Which of the following is most common concomitant lesion with coarctation of the aorta?
Harrison's 20th Ed. Chapter 264 Page 1839 Figure 264-10

A. Aortic regurgitation
B. Bicuspid aortic valve
C. ASD
D. VSD

Bicuspid aortic valve is most common concomitant lesion with coarctation of the aorta.

1544. Which of the following is commonly associated with coarctation of the aorta?
Harrison's 20th Ed. Chapter 264 Page 1837, 1899

A. Turner syndrome
B. Bicuspid aortic valve
C. Circle of Willis aneurysms
D. All of the above

Coarctation of the aorta is frequent in patients with gonadal dysgenesis (Turner syndrome) and is associated with bicuspid aortic valve (75%) and Circle of Willis aneurysms. Coarctation of the aorta is usually sporadic but occurs in 35% of children with Turner's syndrome.

1545. Blood pressure difference in both arms is > 10 mm Hg in?
Harrison's 20th Ed. Chapter 234 Page 1669

A. Supravalvular aortic stenosis
B. Aortic coarctation
C. Aortic dissection
D. All of the above

Blood pressure difference in both arms should be <10 mm Hg. A blood pressure differential that exceeds this threshold may be associated with atherosclerotic or inflammatory subclavian artery disease, supravalvular aortic stenosis, aortic coarctation, or aortic dissection.

1546. In aortic coarctation, a blowing systolic murmur may be heard in?
Harrison's 20th Ed. Chapter 271 Page 1899

A. Posterior right interscapular area
B. Posterior left interscapular area
C. Left axilla
D. Left occiput

In aortic coarctation, a blowing systolic murmur may be heard in the posterior left interscapular areas or along the course of one or more ribs.

1547. In coarctation of the aorta, enlarged and pulsatile collateral vessels may be palpated in?
World J Cardiol. 2015;7(11):765-775

A. Intercostal spaces
B. Axillae
C. Interscapular area
D. All of the above

In coarctation of the aorta, enlarged and pulsatile collateral vessels may be palpated in the intercostal spaces anteriorly, in the axillae, or posteriorly in the interscapular area.

1548. In Chest X-ray, "3" sign relates to which of the following?
World J Cardiol. 2015;7(11):765-775

A. Patent ductus arteriosus
B. Supravalvular Aortic Stenosis
C. Coarctation of the aorta
D. Tetralogy of Fallot

Chest X-ray in coarctation of the aorta shows a dilated left subclavian artery high on the left mediastinal border and a dilated ascending aorta. Indentation of the aorta at the site of coarctation with pre- and poststenotic dilatation ("3" sign) along left paramediastinal shadow are pathognomonic.

1549. In coarctation of the aorta, radiographic notching of which of the following ribs is seen?
World J Cardiol. 2015;7(11):765-775

A. 3rd to 5th ribs
B. 3rd to 7th ribs
C. 3rd to 9th ribs
D. 3rd to 12th ribs

In coarctation of the aorta, notching of the third to ninth ribs is an important radiographic sign. This is due to inferior rib erosion by dilated collateral vessels.

1550. Which of the following is the hazard of coarctation of aorta?
Harrison's 20th Ed. Chapter 264 Page 1839 Figure 264-10

A. Cerebral aneurysms and hemorrhage
B. Aortic dissection and rupture
C. Premature coronary arteriosclerosis
D. All of the above

In coarctation of the aorta, the chief hazards of proximal aortic severe hypertension include cerebral aneurysms and hemorrhage, aortic dissection and rupture, premature coronary arteriosclerosis, and LV failure.

1551. Which of the following best relates to Fontan circulation?
Harrison's 20th Ed. Chapter 264 Page 1837

A. Surgical removal of RV outflow tract obstruction
B. Surgical removal of the atrial septum
C. Absence of a pumping chamber to pulmonary artery
D. Physiologically corrected transposition of the great arteries

1552. Which of the following relates to single ventricle heart disease?
Harrison's 20th Ed. Chapter 264 Page 1837

A. Tricuspid atresia
B. Double inlet LV
C. Hypoplastic left heart syndrome
D. All of the above

1553. In Eisenmenger's syndrome, a large communication between systemic and pulmonary circulation exists at?
Harrison's 20th Ed. Chapter 264 Page 1838

A. Aortopulmonary level
B. Ventricular level
C. Atrial level
D. Any of the above

Eisenmenger's syndrome refers to a large communication between systemic and pulmonary circulations at the aortopulmonary, ventricular, or atrial levels. Flow is bidirectional or predominantly right-to-left because of high resistance and obstructive pulmonary hypertension.

1554. In Eisenmenger syndrome, symptoms in adult life consist of?
N Engl J Med. 2000;342(5):334-342

A. Chest pain
B. Syncope
C. Hemoptysis
D. All of the above

In patients with Eisenmenger syndrome, symptoms in adult life consist of exertional dyspnea, chest pain, syncope, and hemoptysis. Hemoptysis occurs as a result of pulmonary infarction or rupture of dilated pulmonary arteries, arterioles, or aorticopulmonary collateral vessels.

1555. In patients with Eisenmenger syndrome, right-to-left shunt leads to?
N Engl J Med. 2000;342(5):334-342

A. Cyanosis
B. Clubbing
C. Erythrocytosis
D. All of the above

In patients with Eisenmenger syndrome, right-to-left shunt leads to cyanosis, clubbing, and erythrocytosis.

1556. The murmur of which of the following disappears when Eisenmenger's syndrome develops?
N Engl J Med. 2000;342(5):334-342

A. Ventricular septal defect
B. Patent ductus arteriosus
C. Atrial septal defect
D. All of the above

The murmur caused by a ventricular septal defect, patent ductus arteriosus, or atrial septal defect disappears when Eisenmenger's syndrome develops.

1557. Which of the following can occur in Eisenmenger's syndrome?
N Engl J Med. 2000;342(5):334-342

A. Decrescendo diastolic murmur of pulmonary regurgitation
B. Holosystolic murmur of tricuspid regurgitation
C. Right-sided fourth heart sound
D. None of the above

Many patients of Eisenmenger's syndrome have a decrescendo diastolic murmur of pulmonary regurgitation or a holosystolic murmur of tricuspid regurgitation. A right-sided S4 is usually present. The lungs are clear.

1558. Pulmonary vascular disease does not progress after operative correction of shunt, if pulmonary vascular resistance is less than systemic vascular resistance by?
N Engl J Med. 2000;342(5):334-342

A. One-third
B. One-half
C. Two-third
D. Three-fourth

The degree to which pulmonary vascular resistance is elevated before operation is a critical factor determining prognosis. If the pulmonary vascular resistance is one-third or less of the systemic value, progression of pulmonary vascular disease after operation is unusual.

1559. Which of the following pulmonary vascular morphologic changes is irreversible in Eisenmenger's syndrome?
N Engl J Med. 2000;342(5):334-342

A. Plexiform lesions
B. Medial hypertrophy of pulmonary arterioles
C. Intimal proliferation and fibrosis
D. Occlusion of capillaries & small arterioles

1560. Which of the following is a pulmonary vasodilator?
N Engl J Med. 2000;342(5):334-342

A. Oxygen
B. Intravenous adenosine
C. Intravenous epoprostenol
D. All of the above

Pulmonary vasodilators such as oxygen, inhaled nitrous oxide, or intravenous adenosine or epoprostenol are administered to assess the reversibility of pulmonary hypertension.

1561. Eisenmenger's syndrome, which of the following portend a poor outcome?
N Engl J Med. 2000;342(5):334-342

A. A history of syncope
B. Clinically evident right ventricular systolic dysfunction
C. Severe hypoxemia
D. All of the above

A history of syncope, clinically evident right ventricular systolic dysfunction, low cardiac output, and severe hypoxemia portend a poor outcome in Eisenmenger's syndrome.

1562. Which of the following should be avoided in Eisenmenger syndrome?
N Engl J Med. 2000;342(5):334-342

A. Anticoagulants
B. Antiplatelet agents
C. Vasodilators
D. All of the above

Anticoagulants and antiplatelet agents should be avoided in Eisenmenger syndrome, since they exacerbate the hemorrhagic diathesis.

1563. Which of the following is a consequence of chronic hypoxemia in cyanotic CHD?
N Engl J Med. 2000;342(5):334-342

A. Secondary erythrocytosis
B. Abnormal hemostasis
C. Hyperviscosity
D. All of the above

1564. Which of the following is a symptom of hyperviscosity?
N Engl J Med. 2000;342(5):334-342

A. Visual disturbances
B. Fatigue, headache, dizziness
C. Paresthesias
D. All of the above

1565. Cerebrovascular accidents in Eisenmenger syndrome may occur as a result of?
N Engl J Med. 2000;342(5):334-342

A. Paradoxical embolization
B. Venous thrombosis of cerebral vessels
C. Intracranial hemorrhage
D. All of the above

1566. Which of the following is aortic root - to - right-heart shunt?
Harrison's 19th Ed. 1523

A. Congenital aneurysm of aortic sinus of Valsalva with fistula
B. Coronary arteriovenous fistula
C. Anomalous origin of LCA from pulmonary trunk
D. All of the above

The three most common causes of aortic root–to-right-heart shunts are congenital aneurysm of an aortic sinus of Valsalva with fistula, coronary arteriovenous fistula, and anomalous origin of the left coronary artery (LCA) from the pulmonary trunk.

1567. Which of the following is not a feature of Williams-Beuren syndrome?
N Engl J Med. 2010;362:239-52

A. "Elfin" facies
B. Mental retardation with retained language skills
C. Supravalvular aortic stenosis
D. Transient hyperkalemia

Supravalvular aortic stenosis is associated cardiac defect in Williams-Beuren syndrome, typically comprising of "elfin" facies, low nasal bridge, cheerful demeanor, mental retardation with retained language skills and love of music, and transient hypercalcemia.

1568. Genetic defect for Williams-Beuren syndrome is located on which chromosome?
N Engl J Med. 2010;362:239-52

A. 5
B. 6
C. 7
D. 8

In most patients, a genetic defect for Williams-Beuren syndrome is located in the same chromosomal region as elastin on chromosome 7. Williams syndrome is associated with interstitial deletions of the long arm of chromosome 7 (7ql 1 .23).

1569. Which of the following is a microdeletion disorder?
N Engl J Med. 2010;362:239-52

A. DiGeorge syndrome
B. Williams-Beuren syndrome
C. Pseudohypoparathyroidism IB (PHP-IB)
D. All of the above

PHP-Ib is caused by microdeletions within or upstream of the GNAS locus located on chromosome 20q 13.3. Men with oligospermia/azoospermia frequently have microdeletions on the long arm of the Y chromosome that involve one more of the azoospermla factor (AZF) genes. DiGeorge/velocardiofacial syndromes is associated with interstitial deletions of the long arm of chromosome 22 (22q 1 1 .2). Genetic mutations involving microdeletions at the elastin locus gene on chromosome 7 may play a role in the pathogenesis of Williams-Beuren syndrome.

1570. Which of the following is a facial feature of Williams–Beuren syndrome children?
N Engl J Med. 2010;362:239-52

A. Flat nasal bridge, short upturned nose
B. Periorbital puffiness & full cheeks
C. Long philtrum and delicate chin
D. All of the above

Facial feature of Williams–Beuren syndrome children include a flat nasal bridge, short upturned nose, periorbital puffiness, long philtrum, and delicate chin. Older patients have slightly coarse features, with full lips, a wide smile, and a full nasal tip.

1571. Which of the following is a finding in Williams–Beuren syndrome?
N Engl J Med. 2010;362:239-52

A. Hypercalcemia
B. Supravalvular aortic stenosis
C. Premature graying of the hair
D. All of the above

1572. Which of the following is a finding in Williams–Beuren syndrome?
N Engl J Med. 2010;362:239-52

A. Diverticulosis
B. Diabetes mellitus
C. Sensorineural hearing loss
D. All of the above

1573. Which of the following gene is implicated in Williams–Beuren syndrome?
N Engl J Med. 2010;362:239-52

A. SH
B. ELN
C. STAT1
D. HRP2

1574. No endocarditis prophylaxis is required in which of the following CHD?
British Medical Bulletin. 2008;85:151-180, N Engl J Med. 2000;342:256-263

A. Mitral valve prolapse without regurgitation
B. Pulmonary stenosis
C. Isolated secundum atrial septal defect
D. All of the above

Prophylaxis against infective endocarditis is not recommended for patients with atrial septal defects (repaired or unrepaired) unless a concomitant valvular abnormality is present.

1575. Endocarditis prophylaxis indicated in which of the following CHD?
British Medical Bulletin. 2008;85:151-180

A. Tetralogy of Fallot
B. Transposition of the great arteries (TGA)
C. Prosthetic heart valves
D. All of the above

1576. Heritable syndromes with associated ASD include?
Circ Res. 2013;112:707-720

A. Patau
B. Holt-Oram
C. Ellis-van Creveld
D. All of the above

1577. Heritable syndromes with associated VSD include?
Circ Res. 2013;112:707-720

A. Cri-Du-Chat
B. Okihiro syndrome
C. Kabuki syndrome
D. All of the above

1578. Heritable syndromes with associated PDA include?
Circ Res. 2013;112:707-720

A. Char
B. 1p36 Deletion
C. Cri-Du-Chat
D. All of the above

1579. Heritable syndromes that are associated with Tetralogy of Fallot include?
Circ Res. 2013;112:707-720

A. 22q11 Deletion
B. Cat Eye
C. CHARGE
D. All of the above

1580. Heritable syndrome with associated supravalvular aortic stenosis is?
Circ Res. 2013;112:707-720

A. Kartagener
B. Laurence-Moon-Biedl-Bardet
C. Williams
D. Crouzon

1581. Chromosomal abnormalities with associated VSD include?
Circ Res. 2013;112:707-720

A. Cri du chat
B. Holt-Oram
C. Okihiro syndrome
D. All of the above

1582. Which of the following heritable syndromes is associated with ASD?
Circ Res. 2013;112:707-720

A. Ellis-van Creveld syndrome
B. Patau
C. Holt-Oram syndrome
D. All of the above

1583. Which of the following heritable syndromes is associated with PDA?
Circ Res. 2013;112:707-720

A. Char
B. 1p36 Deletion
C. Cri-Du-Chat
D. All of the above

1584. Which of the following connective tissue disorders is associated with supravalvular aortic stenosis?
Harrison's 20th Ed. Chapter 406 Page 2976

A. Marfan's
B. Osteogenesis imperfecta
C. Pseudoxanthoma elasticum
D. Cutis laxa

1585. Which of the following chromosomal disorders is associated with Tetralogy of Fallot?
Circ Res. 2013;112:707-720

A. 22q11 Deletion
B. CHARGE
C. Okihiro syndrome
D. All of the above

1586. Which of the following chromosomal disorders is associated with coarctation of aorta?
Circ Res. 2013;112:707-720

A. Turner syndrome
B. Down syndrome
C. Trisomy 18
D. Cri du chat syndrome

1587. Which of the following heritable syndromes is associated with supravalvular aortic stenosis?
Circ Res. 2013;112:707-720

A. Turner syndrome
B. Catch-22 syndrome
C. Shprintzen syndrome
D. Williams syndrome

1588. Which genetic condition has clinical features overlapping those of Noonan syndrome?
Circ Res. 2013;112:707-720

A. Turner syndrome
B. LEOPARD syndrome
C. Ellis-van Creveld syndrome
D. Holt-Oram syndrome

Pericardial Disease

1589. Cardiac tamponade occurs when fluid in pericardial space reaches a pressure exceeding?
Cleveland Clinic Journal of Medicine. 2013;80(2):109

A. Lymphatic pressure
B. Intrapleural pressure
C. Central venous pressure
D. Pulmonary artery wedge pressure

Cardiac tamponade occurs when fluid in pericardial space reaches a pressure that exceeds central venous pressure (CVP).

1590. Pericardial cavity normally contains how much fluid?
Harrison's 20th Ed. Chapter 265 Page 1841

A. 5 to 10 mL of fluid
B. 10 to 20 mL of fluid
C. 15 to 50 mL of fluid
D. 50 to 100 mL of fluid

Normal pericardium is a double-layered sac. Visceral pericardium is a serous membrane that is separated by a small quantity (15 to 50 mL) of fluid, an ultrafiltrate of plasma, from the fibrous parietal pericardium.

1591. Which of the following is a function of normal pericardium?
Harrison's 20th Ed. Chapter 265 Page 1841

A. Prevents sudden dilation of the cardiac chambers
B. Restricts anatomic position of the heart
C. Retards spread of infections from lungs & pleural cavities
D. All of the above

1592. In partial left pericardial defects, which of the following may bulge through the defect?
Harrison's 20th Ed. Chapter 265 Page 1841

A. Aorta
B. Left atrium
C. Left ventricle
D. Pulmonary vein

In partial left pericardial defects, main pulmonary artery & left atrium may bulge through the defect.

1593. Effusive-constrictive pericarditis is a type of?
Harrison's 20th Ed. Chapter 265 Page 1841 Table 265-1

A. Acute pericarditis
B. Subacute pericarditis
C. Chronic pericarditis
D. All of the above

1594. Which of the following is a type of chronic pericarditis?
Harrison's 20th Ed. Chapter 265 Page 1841 Table 265-1

A. Constrictive pericarditis
B. Effusive pericarditis
C. Adhesive (nonconstrictive) pericarditis
D. All of the above

1595. Which of the following is a type of familial pericarditis?
Harrison's 20th Ed. Chapter 265 Page 1841 Table 265-1

A. Wolman disease
B. Vici syndrome
C. Mulibrey nanism
D. Stauffer's syndrome

Mulibrey nanism is an autosomal recessive syndrome characterized by growth failure, muscle hypotonia, hepatomegaly, ocular changes, enlarged cerebral ventricles, mental retardation, ventricular hypertrophy and chronic constrictive pericarditis.

1596. Dressler's syndrome best relates to?
Harrison's 20th Ed. Chapter 265 Page 1841 Table 265-1

A. Post-myocardial infarction
B. Post-pericardiotomy
C. Post-traumatic
D. All of the above

1597. Most common cause of acute pericarditis is?
N Engl J Med. 2004;351:2195-202

A. Viral or unknown (idiopathic)
B. Trauma to the chest
C. Neoplastic invasion of the pericardium
D. Tuberculosis

1598. Pain of pleural pericarditis is referred to the shoulder and neck is related to?
Harrison's 20th Ed. Chapter 265 Page 1841

A. Sensory fibers originating in the first cervical segment
B. Sensory fibers originating in the second cervical segment
C. Sensory fibers originating in the third cervical segment
D. Sensory fibers originating in the fourth cervical segment

Owing to the overlapping sensory supply of the central diaphragm via the phrenic nerve with somatic sensory fibers originating in the third to fifth cervical segments, the pain of pleural pericarditis is often referred to the shoulder and neck. Involvement of the pleural surface of the lateral diaphragm can lead to pain in the upper abdomen. Radiation to the trapezius ridge is characteristic of pericardial pain and does not usually occur with angina.

1599. Which of the following mainly influences the clinical presentation of cardiac tamponade?
Cleveland Clinic Journal of Medicine. 2013;80(2):109

A. Quantity of pericardial fluid
B. Rate at which pericardial fluid accumulates
C. Left ventricular ejection fraction
D. All of the above

1600. Rapid accumulation of pericardial fluid is characterized more by?
Cleveland Clinic Journal of Medicine. 2013;80(2):109

A. Edema
B. Hypotension
C. Dyspnea
D. All of the above

Rate at which pericardial fluid accumulates influences the clinical presentation of cardiac tamponade, particularly edema. Thus, edema & dyspnea are more prominent clinical presentations of cardiac tamponade, when there is a slow accumulation and hence slow rise in pericardial pressure. Rapid accumulation is characterized more by hypotension than by edema.

1601. Which of the following favors the diagnosis of cardiac tamponade?
Cleveland Clinic Journal of Medicine. 2013;80(2):109

A. Hypotension
B. Tachycardia
C. Jugular venous distention
D. All of the above

1602. Chest pain is often absent in which of the following?
Harrison's 20th Ed. Chapter 265 Page 1841

A. Postirradiation pericarditis
B. Neoplastic pericarditis
C. Uremic pericarditis
D. All of the above

Chest pain is absent in slowly developing TB, postirradiation, neoplastic & uremic pericarditis.

1603. Which of the following statements about chest pain of acute pericarditis is false?
Harrison's 20th Ed. Chapter 265 Page 1841

A. Retrosternal and left precordial
B. Exacerbated by inspiration
C. Worse when the patient sits upright and leans forward and improves in supine position
D. Pain may radiate to one or both trapezius muscle ridges

Pain of acute pericarditis is often severe, retrosternal & left precordial, referred to neck, arms, or left shoulder. Often pain is pleuritic, aggravated by inspiration, coughing & changes in body position. Pericardial pain is relieved by sitting up & leaning forward & is intensified by lying supine.

1604. Pericardial friction rub is best heard at?
Harrison's 20th Ed. Chapter 265 Page 1841

A. Apex
B. Left lower sternal border
C. Right sternal border
D. All of the above

Pericardial friction rub is high-pitched, elicited sometimes only at the left lower sternal border at end-expiration with the patient upright & leaning forward throughout the respiratory cycle.

1605. "Triphasic" pericardial friction rub is heard in about?
N Engl J Med. 2004;351:2195-202

A. 100% of patients
B. 75% of patients
C. 50% of patients
D. 25% of patients

1606. Which of the following is a component of "triphasic" pericardial friction rub?
N Engl J Med. 2004;351:2195-202

A. Ventricular systole
B. Rapid early diastolic filling
C. Late presystolic filling after atrial contraction
D. All of the above

The three components of "Triphasic" pericardial friction rub are ventricular systole, rapid early diastolic filling and late presystolic filling after atrial contraction in patients in sinus rhythm.

1607. Atrial repolarization (STa and Ta) may become apparent in?
N Engl J Med. 2004;351:2195-202

A. Atrial infarction
B. Pre-excitation syndrome
C. Constrictive pericarditis
D. STEMI

Atrial repolarization (STa and Ta) is usually too low in amplitude to be detected, but it may become apparent in conditions such as acute pericarditis and atrial infarction.

1608. PR-segment depression is seen in which stage of acute pericarditis?
Harrison's 20th Ed. Chapter 265 Page 1841

A. Stage I
B. Stage II
C. Stage III
D. Stage IV

PR-segment deviation (opposite in polarity to the ST segment) due to a concomitant atrial injury current.

1609. Widespread T-wave inversions are found in which stage of acute pericarditis?
Harrison's 20th Ed. Chapter 265 Page 1842

A. Stage I
B. Stage II
C. Stage III
D. Stage IV

ECG in acute pericarditis evolves through 4 stages. In stage 1, there is widespread elevation of ST segments with upward concavity, involving two or three standard limb leads and V2 to V6, as well as PR-segment depression with no significant changes in QRS. In stage 2, ST segments return to normal and then T waves become inverted (stage 3). Weeks or months later, ECG returns to normal in stage 4.

1610. In acute pericarditis, reciprocal depression is seen in?
Harrison's 20th Ed. Chapter 265 Page 1842

A. aVR
B. aVL
C. aVF
D. All of the above

ECG in stage 1 of acute pericarditis shows widespread elevation of ST segments, with upward concavity, involving two or three standard limb leads and V2 to V6, with reciprocal depressions only in aVR and sometimes V1, as well as depression of the PR segment below the TP segment reflecting atrial involvement without significant changes in QRS complexes.

1611. The most reliable ECG distinguishing feature between acute pericarditis and acute myocardial infarction is?
N Engl J Med. 2004;351:2195-202

A. Ratio of ST segment elevation to T-wave height in V_6 of > 0.16
B. Ratio of ST segment elevation to T-wave height in V_6 of > 0.20
C. Ratio of ST segment elevation to T-wave height in V_6 of > 0.24
D. Ratio of ST segment elevation to T-wave height in V_6 of > 0.28

In early repolarization, T waves are usually tall and the ST/T ratio is <0.25, this ratio is higher in acute pericarditis.

1612. Which of the following about ECG changes in pericarditis is false?
Harrison's 20th Ed. Chapter 265 Page 1842

A. ST-segment elevation
B. Diffuse lead involvement not corresponding to a specific coronary anatomic distribution
C. PR-segment depression
D. None of the above

In patients with ST-segment elevation, the presence of diffuse lead involvement not corresponding to a specific coronary anatomic distribution and PR-segment depression can aid in distinguishing pericarditis from acute MI.

1613. Auenbrugger's sign in cases of pericardial effusion best relates to?
American Review of Respiratory Disease. 1961;84(3):458

A. Retraction of thoracic wall, synchronous with cardiac systole
B. Epigastric prominence
C. Percussion dullness in fifth right intercostal space
D. Dullness on auscultation beneath angle of left scapula

Named after Joseph Leopold Auenbrugger, Auenbrugger's sign is a bulging of epigastrium noticed cases of severe pericardial effusion. Compression of this bulge may cause hemodynamic compromise & cardiac tamponade.

1614. Patch of dullness on auscultation beneath angle of left scapula in pericardial effusion is called?
Harrison's 20th Ed. Chapter 265 Page 1842

A. Auenbrugger's sign
B. Ewart's Sign
C. Broadbent's sign
D. Ebstein's sign

Patch of dullness on auscultation with egophony and bronchial breathing beneath angle of left scapula due to compressive atelectasis of left lung base by pericardial fluid is called Ewart's Sign (William Ewart, UK). Also known as Bamberger-Pins-Ewart Sign or Pins' Syndrome. Ewart's second sign - A large pericardial effusion makes the first rib more prominent along sternal border. Conner's sign - Dullness at the right lower lung field. Bamberger's sign - Disappearance of Ewart's or Conner's signs when patient sits up & leans forward. Dressler's sign - dullness to percussion of lower one half of sternum. Sansom's sign - Percussible dullness in left third intercostal space. Greene's sign - Lateral displacement of percussed cardiac border with expiration. Auenbrugger's sign - epigastric prominence seen in marked pericardial effusion. Broadbent's sign - retraction of thoracic wall, synchronous with cardiac systole, visible in left posterior axillary line is a sign of adherent pericardium. Ebstein's sign - obtuseness of the cardio-hepatic angle on percussion. Friedreich's sign - sudden collapse of previously distended veins of neck at each diastole. Rotch's sign - percussion dullness in fifth intercostal space on the right. Heim-Kreysig sign - in drawing of the intercostal spaces, synchronous with cardiac systole.

1615. Which of the following is not a part of Moschcowitz triad?
JAMA. 1933;100(21):1663-1664

A. Widening of the area of cardiac flatness
B. Abrupt transition from pulmonary resonance to cardiac flatness
C. Widening of cardiac dulness in second intercostal space
D. Percussion dullness in fifth right intercostal space

1616. Which of the following is the name given to the configuration of the cardiac silhouette in pericardial effusion?
Harrison's 20th Ed. Chapter 265 Page 1842

A. Hour glass
B. Water bottle
C. Dust bin
D. Tear drop

Chest roentgenogram in pericardial effusion may show a "water bottle" configuration of the cardiac silhouette but may be normal.

1617. Which of the following is concentrated in and interferes with the migration of neutrophils?
Harrison's 20th Ed. Chapter 265 Page 1843

A. Aspirin
B. Indomethacin
C. Colchicine
D. Glucocorticoids

Colchicine is concentrated in and interferes with the migration of neutrophils. In acute idiopathic pericarditis, colchicine should be administered for 3 months.

1618. In acute idiopathic pericarditis, full-dose corticosteroids should be given for what length of time?
Harrison's 20th Ed. Chapter 265 Page 1843

A. 2–4 days
B. 2 weeks
C. 1 month
D. 3 months

In acute idiopathic pericarditis, if the patient does not respond to or cannot tolerate NSAIDs and colchicine, glucocorticoids are indicated. However, since they increase the risk of subsequent recurrence, full-dose corticosteroids should be given for only 2–4 days and then tapered.

1619. Which of the following is an IL-1β receptor antagonist?
Harrison's 20th Ed. Chapter 265 Page 1843

A. Anakinra
B. Azathioprine
C. Colchicine
D. None of the above

1620. Which of the following drugs is not indicated in treatment of idiopathic acute pericarditis?
Harrison's 20th Ed. Chapter 265 Page 1843

A. Phenylbutazone
B. Colchicine
C. Prednisone
D. Ibuprofen

If treatment with aspirin is ineffective, colchicine is used. Colchicine may prevent recurrences.

1621. Azathioprine or anakinra is used in acute idiopathic pericarditis when?
Harrison's 20th Ed. Chapter 265 Page 1843

A. Multiple, frequent, disabling recurrences for > 2 years
B. No response with continuing NSAIDs & colchicine
C. No response with glucocorticoids
D. All of the above

1622. Which out of the following is the less common cause of cardiac tamponade?
Harrison's 20th Ed. Chapter 265 Page 1843

A. Neoplastic disease
B. Tuberculosis
C. Idiopathic pericarditis
D. Renal failure

3 commonest causes of tamponade are neoplastic disease, idiopathic pericarditis & renal failure.

1623. In cardiac tamponade, Beck's triad consists of all except?
Harrison's 20th Ed. Chapter 265 Page 1843

A. Hypotension
B. Soft or absent heart sounds
C. Pulsus paradoxus
D. Jugular venous distention with a prominent "x" descent but an absent "y" descent

Three main features of acute cardiac tamponade (Beck's triad) are hypotension, soft, muffled or absent heart sounds, and jugular venous distention (JVD) with a prominent "x" descent but an absent "y" descent. Beck triad for chronic tamponade consists of increased CVP (JVD), ascites, and a small quiet heart (muffled heart sounds).

1624. Presence of which of the following should raise suspicion of cardiac tamponade?
Harrison's 20th Ed. Chapter 265 Page 1843

A. Reduction in amplitude of QRS complexes
B. Electrical alternans of P wave
C. Electrical alternans of QRS or T waves
D. All of the above

1625. In ECG, electrical alternans may be present in?
Harrison's 20th Ed. Chapter 265 Page 1844 Table 265-2

A. Cardiac tamponade
B. Constrictive pericarditis
C. Restrictive cardiomyopathy
D. Right ventricular myocardial infarction (RVMI)

1626. Kussmaul's sign is absent in which of the following?
Harrison's 20th Ed. Chapter 265 Page 1844 Table 265-2

A. Cardiac tamponade
B. Constrictive pericarditis
C. Restrictive cardiomyopathy
D. Right ventricular myocardial infarction (RVMI)

When jugular veins are distended and venous pressure fails to decline during inspiration is called Kussmaul's sign. It is absent in cardiac tamponade and is seen in chronic pericarditis, tricuspid stenosis, right ventricular infarction, and restrictive cardiomyopathy.

1627. Right ventricular size is small in which of the following?
Harrison's 20th Ed. Chapter 265 Page 1844 Table 265-2

A. Cardiac tamponade
B. Constrictive pericarditis
C. Restrictive cardiomyopathy
D. Right ventricular myocardial infarction (RVMI)

1628. On echocardiography, right atrial collapse and right ventricular diastolic collapse (RVDC) is present in which of the following?
Harrison's 20th Ed. Chapter 265 Page 1844 Table 265-2

A. Cardiac tamponade
B. Constrictive pericarditis
C. Restrictive cardiomyopathy
D. Right ventricular myocardial infarction (RVMI)

1629. Prominent "y" descent is usually present in which of the following condition?
Harrison's 20th Ed. Chapter 265 Page 1844 Table 265-2

A. Cardiac tamponade
B. Constrictive pericarditis
C. Restrictive cardiomyopathy
D. Right ventricular myocardial infarction (RVMI)

1630. Prominent "x" descent is rare in?
Harrison's 20th Ed. Chapter 265 Page 1844 Table 265-2

A. Cardiac tamponade
B. Constrictive pericarditis
C. Restrictive cardiomyopathy
D. Right ventricular myocardial infarction (RVMI)

In constrictive pericarditis, right & left atrial pressure pulses display an M-shaped contour, with prominent x and y descents. y descent, which is absent or diminished in cardiac tamponade, is the most prominent deflection in constrictive pericarditis. It reflects rapid early filling of the ventricles. y descent is interrupted by a rapid rise in atrial pressure during early diastole, when ventricular filling is impeded by constricting pericardium. In constrictive pericarditis, ventricular pressure pulses in both ventricles exhibit characteristic "square root" signs during diastole.

1631. Pericardial knock is often present in?
Harrison's 20th Ed. Chapter 265 Page 1844 Table 265-2

A. Cardiac tamponade
B. Constrictive pericarditis
C. Restrictive cardiomyopathy
D. RVMI

An early third heart sound i.e., a pericardial knock, occurring at the cardiac apex 0.09–0.12 s after aortic valve closure, is often conspicuous in constrictive pericarditis. It is due to an abrupt cessation of ventricular filling.

1632. Pulsus paradoxus is defined as a decrease in systolic arterial pressure of?
Harrison's 20th Ed. Chapter 265 Page 1843

A. > 10 mm Hg with inspiration
B. > 20 mm Hg with inspiration
C. > 30 mm Hg with inspiration
D. > 40 mm Hg with inspiration

The presence of cardiac tamponade consists of a greater than normal (10 mm Hg) inspiratory decline in systolic arterial pressure.

1633. Pulsus paradoxus is most common in?
Harrison's 20th Ed. Chapter 265 Page 1843

A. Cardiac tamponade
B. Constrictive pericarditis
C. Restrictive cardiomyopathy
D. All of the above

Paradoxical pulse occurs not only in cardiac tamponade but also in approximately one-third of patients with constrictive pericarditis.

1634. Pulsus paradoxus is observed in which of the following condition?
Harrison's 20th Ed. Chapter 265 Page 1843

A. Hypovolemic shock
B. Acute and chronic obstructive airways disease
C. Pulmonary embolus
D. All of the above

Pulsus paradoxus is not pathognomonic of pericardial disease as it may be observed in some cases of hypovolemic shock, acute & chronic obstructive airways disease & pulmonary embolus.

1635. The term pulsus paradoxus was coined by?
Cleveland Clinic Journal of Medicine. 2013;80(2):109

A. Korotkoff
B. Bainbridge
C. Kussmaul
D. Meyers

In 1873, term pulsus paradoxus was coined by Adolph Kussmaul. This was the time when physicians could even measure blood pressure.

1636. Factors that can oppose pulsus paradoxus include?
Cleveland Clinic Journal of Medicine. 2013;80(2):109

A. Positive pressure ventilation
B. Severe aortic regurgitation
C. Atrial septal defect
D. All of the above

1637. Factors that can oppose pulsus paradoxus include?
Cleveland Clinic Journal of Medicine. 2013;80(2):109

A. Severe left ventricular hypertrophy
B. Severe left ventricular dysfunction
C. Intravascular volume depletion
D. All of the above

1638. Doppler ultrasound in cardiac tamponade shows marked increase in flow velocities during inspiration across?
Harrison's 20th Ed. Chapter 265 Page 1843

A. Pulmonic valve
B. Pulmonic vein
C. Mitral valve
D. Aortic valve

In cardiac tamponade, Doppler ultrasound shows that tricuspid & pulmonic valve flow velocities increase markedly during inspiration, whereas pulmonic vein, mitral & aortic flow velocities diminish.

1639. Pericardiocentesis is done by which of the following approaches?
Harrison's 20th Ed. Chapter 265 Page 1844

A. Apical
B. Parasternal
C. Subxiphoid
D. Any of the above

1640. Which of the following about pericardiocentesis in cardiac tamponade is false?
Harrison's 20th Ed. Chapter 265 Page 1844

A. Pericardiocentesis must not be delayed
B. Pericardial fluid should be drained as completely as possible
C. Small, multiholed catheter may be left in place
D. None of the above

1641. Viral or idiopathic acute pericarditis occurs most commonly in?
Harrison's 20th Ed. Chapter 265 Page 1845

A. Infants
B. Young adult males
C. Menopausal females
D. Elderly males

Viral or idiopathic acute pericarditis occurs at all ages but is most common in young adult males.

1642. In viral or idiopathic acute pericarditis, fever & precordial pain develop how many days after a presumed viral illness?
Harrison's 20th Ed. Chapter 265 Page 1845

A. 3–5 days
B. 10–12 days
C. 14–21 days
D. 21–30 days

In viral or idiopathic acute pericarditis, almost simultaneous development of fever & precordial pain occurs 10 - 12 days after a presumed viral illness.

1643. Recurrent pericarditis after acute idiopathic pericarditis occurs in what percentage of patients?
Harrison's 20th Ed. Chapter 265 Page 1845

A. 5%
B. 10%
C. 25%
D. 50%

The most frequent complication of acute idiopathic pericarditis is recurrent (relapsing) pericarditis, which occurs in about one-fourth of patients.

1644. Abnormal T waves may persist for what length of time after acute idiopathic pericarditis?
Harrison's 20th Ed. Chapter 265 Page 1845

A. 3 months
B. 1 year
C. 3 years
D. Several years

1645. Which of the following is false about postcardiac injury syndrome?
Harrison's 20th Ed. Chapter 265 Page 1845

A. Clinical picture mimics acute viral or idiopathic pericarditis
B. Usually develops 1–4 weeks after the cardiac injury
C. Cardiac tamponade is rare
D. None of the above

Postcardiac injury syndrome results from a hypersensitivity reaction to antigens originating from injured myocardial tissue and/or pericardium.

1646. Which out of the following collagen vascular diseases is commonly complicated by pericarditis?
Harrison's 20th Ed. Chapter 265 Page 1845

A. Systemic lupus erythematosus (SLE)
B. Rheumatoid arthritis
C. Scleroderma
D. Polyarteritis nodosa

1647. In which of the following conditions, pericarditis may be of the fibrinous variety?
Harrison's 20th Ed. Chapter 265 Page 1845

A. Postcardiac injury syndrome
B. Uremic pericarditis
C. Dialysis-associated pericarditis
D. All of the above

1648. In rheumatoid arthritis, pericardial fluid has which of the following features?
Harrison's 20th Ed. Chapter 265 Page 1845

A. Exudate
B. Decreased concentrations of complement and glucose
C. Elevated cholesterol
D. All of the above

1649. In constrictive pericarditis, right & left atrial pressure pulses display a contour of the shape of?
Harrison's 20th Ed. Chapter 265 Page 1846

A. A - shape
B. M - shape
C. V - shape
D. W - shape

In constrictive pericarditis, right & left atrial pressure pulses show M-shaped contour, with prominent x and y descents. The y descent, reflects rapid early filling of ventricles (absent or diminished in cardiac tamponade) is the most prominent deflection in constrictive pericarditis. The y descent is interrupted by a rapid rise in atrial pressure during early diastole, when ventricular filling is impeded by the constricting pericardium.

1650. Kussmaul's sign is not seen in?
Harrison's 20th Ed. Chapter 265 Page 1846

A. Tricuspid stenosis
B. Right ventricular infarction
C. Restrictive cardiomyopathy
D. Cor pulmonale

Kussmaul's sign refers to failure of venous pressure to decline during inspiration. It is common in chronic pericarditis but may occur in tricuspid stenosis, right ventricular infarction & restrictive cardiomyopathy. In cor pulmonale, Kussmaul's sign is negative.

1651. Broadbent's sign is a feature of?
Harrison's 20th Ed. Chapter 265 Page 1846

A. Cardiac tamponade
B. Constrictive pericarditis
C. Restrictive cardiomyopathy
D. Right ventricular myocardial infarction (RVMI)

In chronic constrictive pericarditis, apical pulse is reduced & may retract in systole - Broadbent's sign.

1652. Pericardial calcification is most common in?
Harrison's 20th Ed. Chapter 265 Page 1846

A. Dialysis-associated pericarditis
B. Tuberculous pericarditis
C. Pericarditis due to systemic lupus erythematosus
D. Scleroderma

Pericardial calcification is most common in tuberculous pericarditis.

1653. Which of the following is a feature of chronic constrictive pericarditis?
Harrison's 20th Ed. Chapter 265 Page 1846

A. Jaundice
B. Intractable ascites
C. Splenomegaly
D. All of the above

1654. Which of the following is less accurate to definitively establish or exclude the diagnosis of constrictive pericarditis?
Harrison's 20th Ed. Chapter 265 Page 1846

A. Doppler echocardiography
B. CT
C. MRI
D. All of the above

1655. Which of the following may simulate chronic constrictive pericarditis?
Harrison's 20th Ed. Chapter 265 Page 1846

A. Cor pulmonale
B. Tricuspid stenosis
C. Restrictive cardiomyopathy
D. All of the above

1656. Which of the following can cause subacute effusive-constrictive pericarditis?
Harrison's 20th Ed. Chapter 265 Page 1846

A. Tuberculosis
B. Multiple attacks of acute idiopathic pericarditis
C. Renal failure
D. All of the above

1657. Tuberculous pericarditis may present as?
Harrison's 20th Ed. Chapter 265 Page 1846

A. Pericardial effusion
B. Chronic constrictive pericarditis
C. Subacute effusive constrictive pericarditis
D. Any of the above

1658. The possible sequelae of pericarditis include?
N Engl J Med. 2004;351:2195-202

A. Cardiac tamponade
B. Recurrent pericarditis
C. Pericardial constriction
D. All of the above

1659. The presence of which of the following is most sensitive indicator of cardiac tamponade?
N Engl J Med. 2004;351:2195-202

A. Systemic arterial hypotension
B. Tachycardia
C. Elevated jugular venous pressure
D. Pulsus paradoxus

1660. The appearance of cardiomegaly on chest radiography indicates a pericardial effusion of?
N Engl J Med. 2004;351:2195-202

A. > 150 mL
B. > 250 mL
C. > 350 mL
D. > 450 mL

1661. Drugs implicated in the causation of pericarditis include?
N Engl J Med. 2004;351:2195-202

A. Dantrolene
B. Doxorubicin
C. Hydralazine
D. All of the above

1662. Drugs implicated in the causation of pericarditis include?
N Engl J Med. 2004;351:2195-202

A. Isoniazid
B. Methysergide
C. Pergolide
D. All of the above

1663. Drugs implicated in the causation of pericarditis include?
N Engl J Med. 2004;351:2195-202

A. Phenylbutazone
B. Phenytoin
C. Procainamide
D. All of the above

Procainamide, hydralazine, phenytoin, isoniazid, minoxidil, anticoagulants, methysergide can cause pericarditis.

1664. Plasma troponin concentrations are elevated in what percent of patients with pericarditis?
N Engl J Med. 2004;351:2195-202

A. 10 to 15 percent
B. 20 to 25 percent
C. 35 to 50 percent
D. 50 to 60 percent

1665. Which of the following is a complication of rapid pericardiocentesis?
Cleveland Clinic Journal of Medicine. 2013;80(2):109

A. Hypotension
B. Pulmonary embolism
C. Pulmonary edema
D. All of the above

The mechanism of pulmonary edema occuring after rapid pericardiocentesis is a sudden increase in right ventricular stroke volume and resultant left ventricular filling after excess pericardial fluid is removed, before systemic arteries, which constrict to keep the systemic blood pressure up during cardiac tamponade, have had time to relax.

1666. A large pericardial effusion is diagnosed if the echo-free space on 2D echocardiography is?
N Engl J Med. 2004;351:2195-202

A. > 10 mm
B. > 20 mm
C. > 30 mm
D. > 40 mm

1667. Which of the following endocrine diseases can cause cardiac tamponade?
Cleveland Clinic Journal of Medicine. 2013;80(2):109

A. Hyperthyroidism
B. Hypothyroidism
C. Conn's syndrome
D. Addison's syndrome

1668. Pericardial fluid is turbid, like gold paint in which of the following conditions?
Cleveland Clinic Journal of Medicine. 2013;80(2):109

A. Mycobacterial infection
B. Rheumatoid arthritis
C. Myxedema
D. All of the above

1669. Interferon alpha is reported to be beneficial in pericarditis caused by?
Cleveland Clinic Journal of Medicine. 2013;80(2):109

A. Cytomegalovirus
B. Coxsackie B
C. Adenovirus
D. Parvovirus

1670. Hyperimmune globulin is reported to be beneficial in pericarditis caused by?
Cleveland Clinic Journal of Medicine. 2013;80(2):109

A. Cytomegalovirus
B. Adenovirus
C. Parvovirus
D. All of the above

Hyperimmune globulin is beneficial in cytomegalovirus, adenovirus & parvovirus pericarditis, while interferon alpha has been reported to be so in coxsackie B pericarditis.

1671. Cardiac manifestation of systemic lupus erythematosus is?
Harrison's 20th Ed. Chapter 349 Page 2520

A. Pericarditis
B. Libman-Sacks endocarditis
C. Myocarditis
D. All of the above

Pericarditis, Libman-Sacks endocarditis, myocarditis, arterial and venous thrombosis are the cadriac manifestation of systemic lupus erythematosus.

Atrial Myxoma and Other Cardiac Tumors

1672. Cardiac masses include which of the following?
Harrison's 20th Ed. Chapter 266 Page 1847

A. Vegetation
B. Thrombus
C. Myocardial hypertrophy
D. All of the above

1673. Which of the following imaging modality may differentiate tumor from thrombus?
Harrison's 20th Ed. Chapter 266 Page 1847 Table 266-1

A. Transesophageal echocardiography (TEE)
B. Cardiac MRI with gadolinium contrast
C. Gated cardiac CT
D. FDG-PET

1674. Which of the following imaging modality allows better assessment of cardiac calcified lesions?
Harrison's 20th Ed. Chapter 266 Page 1847 Table 266-1

A. Transesophageal echocardiography (TEE)
B. Cardiac MRI with gadolinium contrast
C. Gated cardiac CT
D. FDG-PET

1675. Which of the following imaging modality allows better assessment of cardiac neuroendocrine tumors?
Harrison's 20th Ed. Chapter 266 Page 1847 Table 266-1

A. Transesophageal echocardiography (TEE)
B. Cardiac MRI with gadolinium contrast
C. Gated cardiac CT
D. FDG-PET

1676. Which of the following is the most common primary tumor of heart in adults?
Harrison's 20th Ed. Chapter 266 Page 1847

A. Myxoma
B. Rhabdomyoma
C. Fibroma
D. Hemangioma

Myxomas are the most common type of primary cardiac tumor in all age groups, most commonly in third to sixth decade, with a female predilection.

1677. Which of the following is the most common primary tumor of heart in adults?
Harrison's 20th Ed. Chapter 266 Page 1847

A. Lipoma
B. Myocytic hamartoma
C. Myxoma
D. Inflammatory psuedotumor

1678. Which of the following statements is false?
Harrison's 20th Ed. Chapter 266 Page 1847

A. 75% of primary tumors of heart are benign
B. Almost all primary cardiac malignant tumors are sarcomas
C. All cardiac tumors have life-threatening complications
D. None of the above

1679. Which of the following statements about cardiac myxoma is false?
Harrison's 20th Ed. Chapter 266 Page 1847, J Thorac Dis 2014;6(S1):S32-S38

A. Most common in third and sixth decades of life
B. Female predilection
C. Myxomas can originate from any of the heart chambers
D. Most myxomas are familial

Myxomas represent the most common primary cardiac tumors. They can appear in almost all age groups but most commonly between III & VI decades of life with a female predilection. Myxomas can originate from any of the heart chambers, most commonly from left atrium. Right atrial myxomas and heart valve myxomas are rare. Most myxomas are single and sporadic although familiar cases are also well known.

1680. Which of the following statements about familial cardiac myxoma is false?
Harrison's 20th Ed. Chapter 266 Page 1847, J Thorac Dis 2014;6(S1):S32-S38

A. Tend to occur in elderly individuals
B. Often multiple
C. May be ventricular in location
D. More likely to recur after initial resection

Familial myxomas tend to occur in younger individuals, are often multiple, may be ventricular in location, and are more likely to recur after initial resection. Myxomas recur in 12–22% of familial cases but in only 1–2% of sporadic cases.

1681. Cardiac myxoma in the left atrium originate from?
Harrison's 20th Ed. Chapter 266 Page 1847, J Thorac Dis 2014;6(S1):S32-S38

A. Left atrial appendage
B. Mitral valve annulus
C. Interatrial septum near or on the fossa ovalis
D. Any of the above

Cardiac myxoma most commonly occurs in the left atrium, originating from the interatrial septum near or on the fossa ovalis.

1682. Which of the following statements about sporadic cardiac myxoma is false?
Harrison's 20th Ed. Chapter 266 Page 1847, J Thorac Dis 2014;6(S1):S32-S38

A. Solitary
B. Often pedunculated on a fibrovascular stalk
C. Arise from interatrial septum in the vicinity of fossa ovalis
D. None of the above

Most sporadic tumors are solitary, arise from the interatrial septum in the vicinity of the fossa ovalis (particularly in the left atrium), and are often pedunculated on a fibrovascular stalk.

1683. Carney syndrome is characterized by all except?
Harrison's 20th Ed. Chapter 266 Page 1847

A. Spotty skin pigmentation
B. Myxomas
C. Cataract
D. Pituitary adenomas

Carney complex comprises of myxomas (cardiac, skin, and/or breast), lentigines and/or pigmented nevi and endocrine overactivity (primary nodular adrenal cortical disease with or without Cushing's syndrome, testicular tumors, and/or pituitary adenomas with gigantism or acromegaly).

1684. NAME syndrome includes all except?
Harrison's 20th Ed. Chapter 266 Page 1847

A. Nevi
B. Atrial myxoma
C. Myxoedema
D. Ephelides

NAME syndrome consists of nevi, atrial myxoma, myxoid neurofibroma and ephelides.

1685. LAMB syndrome includes all except?
Harrison's 20th Ed. Chapter 266 Page 1847

A. Lentigines
B. Atrial myxoma
C. Melanoma
D. Blue nevi

LAMB syndrome consists of lentigines, atrial myxoma and blue nevi.

1686. Myxoma can occur in?
Harrison's 20th Ed. Chapter 266 Page 1847

A. Left atrium
B. Left ventricle
C. Right ventricle
D. All of the above

Myxomas most commonly arise from left atrium, usually from a stalk attached to the atrial septum, 75% in the left atrium, up to 20% in the right atrium, and around 8% in the ventricles.

1687. Which of the following gene best relates to Carney complex?
Harrison's 20th Ed. Chapter 266 Page 1847

A. MEN1
B. NF1
C. PRKAR1A
D. VHL

The genetic basis of Carney complex is inactivating mutations in the tumor-suppressor gene PRKAR1A, which encodes protein kinase A type I-α regulatory subunit.

1688. Which of the following statements about "tumor plop" is false?
Harrison's 20th Ed. Chapter 266 Page 1848, N Engl J Med. 2018; 379:e26

A. Low-pitched sound on cardiac auscultation
B. Early or mid-diastole
C. Due to impact of tumor against mitral valve or ventricular wall
D. None of the above

1689. Mechanism of symptoms of cardiac tumors is?
J Thorac Dis 2014;6(S1):S32-S38

A. Intracardiac obstruction
B. Systematic embolization of tumor fragments
C. Constitutional symptoms
D. All of the above

1690. The most common presenting symptom of myxoma is?
J Thorac Dis 2014;6(S1):S32-S38

A. Dyspnoea
B. Chest pain
C. Pain and paraesthesia of the limbs
D. Weight loss

The most common presenting symptom of myxoma is dyspnoea.

1691. Differential diagnosis of myxoma include?
Harrison's 20th Ed. Chapter 266 Page 1848

A. Endocarditis
B. Collagen vascular disease
C. Paraneoplastic syndrome
D. All of the above

Constitutional signs and symptoms in myxoma include fever, weight loss, cachexia, malaise, arthralgias, rash, clubbing and Raynaud's phenomenon.

1692. Most common tumor of the cardiac valves is?
Harrison's 20th Ed. Chapter 266 Page 1848

A. Lipoma
B. Papillary fibroelastoma
C. Sarcoma
D. Cardiac metastases

Papillary fibroelastomas are the most common tumors of the cardiac valves.

1693. Which of the following best relates to papillary fibroelastoma?
Harrison's 20th Ed. Chapter 266 Page 1848

A. Cardiac trauma
B. Irradiation
C. Cytomegalovirus
D. Folic acid deficiency

Remnants of cytomegalovirus have been recovered from papillary fibroelastoma, raising the possibility that they arise as a result of chronic viral endocarditis.

1694. Which of the following is the most common primary tumor of heart in infants and children?
Harrison's 20th Ed. Chapter 266 Page 1848

A. Myxoma
B. Rhabdomyoma
C. Lipoma
D. Hemangioma

Rhabdomyomas and fibromas are the most common cardiac tumors in infants and children and usually occur in ventricles. Rhabdomyomas are strongly associated with tuberous sclerosis.

1695. Which of the following about cardiac rhabdomyoma is false?
Harrison's 20th Ed. Chapter 266 Page 1848

A. Multiple in 90% of cases
B. Strongly associated with tuberous sclerosis
C. Have a tendency to regress completely or partially
D. None of the above

1696. Which of the following cardiac tumors are universally ventricular in location?
Harrison's 20th Ed. Chapter 266 Page 1849

A. Fibroma
B. Rhabdomyoma
C. Lipoma
D. Hemangioma

Fibromas are usually single, universally ventricular in location, often calcified, tend to grow and cause arrhythmias and obstructive symptoms, and should be completely resected when possible.

1697. Which of the following heart tumor is located in the roof of the left atrium?
Harrison's 20th Ed. Chapter 266 Page 1849

A. Chemodectoma
B. Neurilemoma
C. Granular cell myoblastoma
D. Paraganglioma

Paragangliomas represent extra-adrenal pheochromocytomas. Most are located in roof of left atrium. They are highly vascular and may be hormonally active, resulting in uncontrolled hypertension.

1698. Which of the following heart tumour is intramyocardial in location?
Harrison's 20th Ed. Chapter 266 Page 1849

A. Myxoma
B. Rhabdomyoma
C. Lipoma
D. Hemangioma

Hemangiomas and mesotheliomas most often are intramyocardial in location, and may cause atrioventricular (AV) conduction disturbances.

1699. Which of the following about cardiac sarcoma is false?
Harrison's 20th Ed. Chapter 266 Page 1849

A. Almost all malignant primary cardiac tumors are sarcomas
B. Angiosarcomas are the most common type in adults
C. Rhabdomyosarcomas are the most common type in children
D. None of the above

1700. Which of the following cardiac sarcoma may respond to a combination of chemo- and radiotherapy?
Harrison's 20th Ed. Chapter 266 Page 1849

A. Angiosarcoma
B. Lymphosarcoma
C. Rhabdomyosarcoma
D. None of the above

1701. Relative incidence of cardiac metastases is highest in which of the following malignancies?
Harrison's 20th Ed. Chapter 266 Page 1849

A. Leukemia
B. Lymphoma
C. Malignant melanoma
D. None of the above

Relative incidence of cardiac metastases is high in malignant melanoma.

1702. Most common primary originating site of cardiac metastases is?
Harrison's 20th Ed. Chapter 266 Page 1849

A. Carcinoma breast
B. Carcinoma thyroid
C. Carcinoma pancreas
D. Carcinoma testes

Most common primary originating sites of cardiac metastases are carcinoma of breast & lung.

1703. In cardiac metastases, which of the following is least involved?
Harrison's 20th Ed. Chapter 266 Page 1849

A. Pericardium
B. Myocardium
C. Endocardium
D. Any of the above

Cardiac metastases occur via hematogenous or lymphangitic spread or by direct tumor invasion. Pericardium is most often involved, followed by myocardial and rarely by involvement of endocardium or cardiac valves.

1704. Which of the following investigation is most useful in diagnostic evaluation of cardiac metastases & cardiac tumors?
Harrison's 20th Ed. Chapter 266 Page 1849

A. Echocardiography
B. CT
C. Cardiac MRI
D. Angiography

Cardiac MRI plays a central role in diagnostic evaluation of cardiac metastases & cardiac tumors.

1705. Characteristic endocardial lesions of SLE (Libman & Sacks) are most often located at?
Harrison's 16th Ed. 1424

A. Atria
B. Ventricular surface of mitral valve
C. Left ventricular outflow tract
D. Right ventricular outflow tract

1706. What is meant by "commotio cordis"?
N Engl J Med. 2010;362:917-27

A. Impact to chest wall overlying heart
B. Torsion injury of heart
C. Kinking of coronary artery
D. Aneurysmal rupture of coronary artery

Blunt, nonpenetrating injuries to chest that trigger ventricular fibrillation is referred to as commotio cordis (Latin: agitation of the heart). Impact to chest wall overlying heart during the susceptible phase of repolarization just prior to peak of T wave is the cause. Prompt defibrillation saves life.

1707. In Commotio Cordis, which of the following is injured?
N Engl J Med. 2010;362:917-27

A. Ribs
B. Sternum
C. Heart
D. None of the above

In Commotio Cordis, there is no damage to the ribs, sternum, or heart. Also, there is no underlying cardiovascular disease in the patient. In cardiac contusion, high-impact blows result in traumatic damage to myocardial tissue and the overlying thorax.

1708. Which of the following is the most frequent cardiovascular cause of sudden death in young athletes?
N Engl J Med. 2010;362:917-27

A. Hypertrophic cardiomyopathy
B. Congenital coronary-artery anomalies

C. Commotio Cordis
D. Cardiac contusion

Commotio Cordis is among the most frequent cardiovascular causes of sudden death in young athletes, after hypertrophic cardiomyopathy and congenital coronary-artery anomalies.

1709. Which of the following about Commotio cordis is false?

N Engl J Med. 2010;362:917-27

A. Predilection for children and adolescents
B. Rarely been reported in blacks or in girls or women
C. Most victims are white
D. None of the above

1710. Broken-Heart Syndrome refers to?

Tex Heart Inst J. 2007;34(1):76-79

A. Commotio cordis
B. Takotsubo syndrome
C. Cardiac contusion
D. Any of the above

Takotsubo cardiomyopathy mimics acute coronary syndrome and is accompanied by reversible left ventricular apical ballooning in the absence of angiographically significant coronary artery stenosis. In Japanese, "Takotsubo" means "fishing pot for trapping octopus," and the left ventricle of a patient diagnosed with this condition resembles that shape. Takotsubo cardiomyopathy, which is transient and typically precipitated by acute emotional stress, is also known as "stress cardiomyopathy" or "broken-heart syndrome" or Gebrochenes-Herz syndrome.

1711. Which of the following is false about Takotsubo syndrome?

Tex Heart Inst J. 2007;34(1):76-79

A. Sudden emotional trauma
B. Hyperdynamic function at ventricular base
C. Anterior ST-segment elevation
D. None of the above

Takotsubo syndrome or apical ballooning syndrome is due to sudden emotional or physiologic trauma leading to dysfunction of mid-portion & apex of LV with hyperdynamic function at ventricular base. More common in women, it presents with chest pain, anterior ST-segment elevation & mildly elevated cardiac enzymes without significant epicardial coronary artery disease. Prognosis is favorable & complete & spontaneous resolution of ventricular dysfunction occurs within weeks.

1712. Which of the following is the most common vascular deceleration injury?

Scand J Trauma Resusc Emerg Med. 2009;17:42

A. Post-pericardiotomy syndrome
B. Takotsubo syndrome
C. Commotio cordis
D. Rupture of the aorta

Rupture of aorta, usually just above aortic valve or at the site of ligamentum arteriosum, is the most common vascular deceleration injury with clinical presentation similar to that of aortic dissection.

Non-ST-Segment Elevation Acute Coronary Syndrome (Non-ST-Segment Elevation Myocardial Infarction and Unstable Angina)

1713. Acute coronary syndrome (ACS) includes?

Harrison's 20th Ed. Chapter 268 Page 1866

A. ST-segment elevation MI (STEMI)
B. Non-ST-segment elevation MI (NSTEMI)
C. Unstable angina (UA)
D. All of the above

Patients with IHD fall into two large groups — those with stable angina secondary to chronic coronary artery disease and patients with acute coronary syndromes (ACS). ACS include patients with acute myocardial infarction with ST-segment elevation (STEMI) on their presenting ECG and those with non-ST-segment elevation acute coronary syndrome (NSTE-ACS). NSTE-ACS include patients with non-ST-segment elevation myocardial infarction (NSTEMI), who have evidence of myocyte necrosis and those with unstable angina (UA), who do not have evidence of myocyte necrosis.

1714. Which of the following about non-ST-segment elevation myocardial infarction (NSTEMI) is false?

Harrison's 20th Ed. Chapter 268 Page 1866

A. Acute coronary syndrome (ACS)
B. Non-ST-segment ↑ acute coronary syndrome (NSTE-ACS)
C. Evidence of myocyte necrosis
D. None of the above

1715. Which of the following about unstable angina (UA) is false?

Harrison's 20th Ed. Chapter 268 Page 1866

A. Acute coronary syndrome (ACS)
B. Non-ST-segment ↑ acute coronary syndrome (NSTE-ACS)
C. No evidence of myocyte necrosis
D. None of the above

1716. Which of the following statements is false?

Harrison's 20th Ed. Chapter 268 Page 1866

A. Relative incidence of NSTEMI is rising
B. Relative incidence of STEMI is declining
C. Relative incidence of UA is declining
D. None of the above

The relative incidence of NSTEMI is rising due to increasing burden of diabetes & chronic kidney disease in an aging population. Relative incidence of STEMI is declining due to greater use of aspirin, statins, and less smoking. Among patients with NSTE-ACS, the proportion with NSTEMI is rising while that with UA is falling because of the wider use of troponin assays with higher sensitivity to detect myocyte necrosis, thereby reclassifying UA as NSTEMI.

1717. Which of the following is the most common pathophysiologic process in the development of UA?

Harrison's 20th Ed. Chapter 268 Page 1866

A. Plaque rupture with superimposed nonocclusive thrombus
B. Dynamic obstruction
C. Progressive mechanical obstruction
D. Increased myocardial oxygen demand &/or decreased supply

UA/NSTEMI can be caused by a reduction in oxygen supply and/or by an increase in myocardial oxygen demand (tachycardia or severe anemia) superimposed on a coronary obstruction. Pathophysiologic processes leading to UA are plaque rupture or erosion with superimposed nonocclusive thrombus (most common cause), dynamic obstruction (coronary spasm, as in Prinzmetal's variant angina), progressive mechanical obstruction [rapidly advancing coronary atherosclerosis or restenosis following percutaneous coronary intervention (PCI)] & secondary UA related to increased myocardial oxygen demand and/or decreased supply (anemia). More than one of these processes may be involved in many patients.

1718. Among patients with NSTE-ACS, what percentage would have left main stenosis coronary artery disease?

Harrison's 20th Ed. Chapter 268 Page 1866

A. 10%
B. 20%
C. 30%
D. 40%

1719. Among patients with NSTE-ACS, what percentage would have three-vessel coronary artery disease?

Harrison's 20th Ed. Chapter 268 Page 1866

A. 5%
B. 15%
C. 35%
D. 40%

1720. Among patients with NSTE-ACS, what percentage would have two-vessel coronary artery disease?

Harrison's 20th Ed. Chapter 268 Page 1866

A. 10%
B. 20%
C. 30%
D. 40%

1721. Among patients with NSTE-ACS, what percentage would have single-vessel coronary artery disease?

Harrison's 20th Ed. Chapter 268 Page 1866

A. 5%
B. 20%
C. 30%
D. 40%

1722. Among patients with UA/NSTEMI, what percentage would have no critical coronary artery stenosis?

Harrison's 20th Ed. Chapter 268 Page 1866

A. 5%
B. 15%
C. 30%
D. 40%

Among patients with NSTE-ACS studied angiographically, ~10% have stenosis of left main coronary artery, 35% have three-vessel CAD, 20% have two-vessel disease, 20% have single-vessel disease and 15% have no apparent critical epicardial coronary artery stenosis.

1723. Vulnerable plaques are composed of?

Harrison's 20th Ed. Chapter 268 Page 1866

A. Rich lipid core and thin fibrous cap
B. Rich lipid core and thick fibrous cap
C. Poor lipid core and thin fibrous cap
D. Poor lipid core and thick fibrous cap

Histologic studies indicate that the coronary plaques prone to disruption are those with a rich lipid core and a thin fibrous cap.

1724. Which of the following is true for unstable angina (UA)?
Harrison's 20th Ed. Chapter 268 Page 1868

A. Occurs at rest lasting > 10 minutes
B. Relatively recent onset angina pectoris
C. Occurs with a crescendo pattern
D. All of the above

UA is defined as angina pectoris or equivalent ischemic discomfort with at least one of three features: it occurs at rest usually lasting > 10 minutes, it is severe and of relatively recent onset (previous 2 weeks), and/or it occurs with a crescendo pattern. The diagnosis of NSTEMI is established if a patient with the clinical features of UA develops evidence of myocardial necrosis, as reflected in elevated cardiac biomarkers.

1725. The clinical hallmark of NSTE-ACS is chest pain that is?
Harrison's 20th Ed. Chapter 268 Page 1868

A. Substernal
B. Retrosternal
C. Suprasternal
D. Any of the above

Clinical hallmark of UA/NSTEMI is chest pain, typically located in the substernal region or sometimes in epigastrium, that radiates to the neck & jaw, left shoulder, and/or the left arm.

1726. Which of the following is considered as anginal equivalent?
Harrison's 20th Ed. Chapter 268 Page 1868

A. Dyspnea
B. Epigastric discomfort
C. Nausea
D. All of the above

Anginal equivalents are dyspnea, epigastric discomfort, nausea, or weakness. They may occur instead of chest discomfort.

1727. Anginal equivalents are more frequent in?
Harrison's 20th Ed. Chapter 268 Page 1868

A. Women
B. Elderly
C. Patients with diabetes mellitus
D. All of the above

Anginal equivalents are more frequent in women, the elderly, and patients with diabetes mellitus.

1728. T-wave inversions in NSTE-ACS have more specificity for myocardial ischemia if they are?
Harrison's 20th Ed. Chapter 268 Page 1868

A. ≥ 0.1 mV deep
B. ≥ 0.2 mV deep
C. ≥ 0.3 mV deep
D. ≥ 0.4 mV deep

T-wave changes in NSTE-ACS are more common but are less specific signs of ischemia, unless they are new and deep T-wave inversions (≥ 0.3 mV).

1729. Minor troponin elevations can be caused by?
Harrison's 20th Ed. Chapter 268 Page 1868

A. Heart failure
B. Myocarditis
C. Pulmonary embolism
D. All of the above

Minor troponin elevations are due to congestive heart failure, myocarditis or pulmonary embolism.

1730. Which of the following is a cause of elevated cardiac troponin?
Harrison's 20th Ed. Chapter 268 Page 1868 Table 268-1

A. Tachyarrhythmias
B. Aortic stenosis
C. Aortic dissection
D. All of the above

1731. Which of the following is a cause of elevated cardiac troponin?
Harrison's 20th Ed. Chapter 268 Page 1868 Table 268-1

A. Pericarditis
B. Takotsubo cardiomyopathy
C. Coronary spasm
D. All of the above

1732. Which of the following is a cause of elevated cardiac troponin?
Harrison's 20th Ed. Chapter 268 Page 1868 Table 268-1

A. Hypertensive emergencies
B. Amyloidosis
C. Hemochromatosis
D. All of the above

1733. Which of the following is a cause of elevated cardiac troponin?
Harrison's 20th Ed. Chapter 268 Page 1868 Table 268-1

A. Snake venom
B. Hypo or hyperthyroidism
C. Stroke
D. All of the above

1734. Which of the following improves the accuracy & speed of the diagnostic evaluation in NSTEMI-ACS?
Harrison's 20th Ed. Chapter 268 Page 1868

A. ECG
B. Cardiac biomarkers
C. Stress testing
D. Coronary computed tomographic angiography (CCTA)

1735. ECG & cardiac markers are typically obtained at what timings after presentation?
Harrison's 20th Ed. Chapter 268 Page 1868

A. Baseline, at 1 hour & at 3 hours
B. Baseline, at 3 hour & at 6 hours
C. Baseline, at 4–6 hours & at 12 hours
D. Baseline, at 6 hours & 24 hours

ECGs and cardiac markers are typically obtained at baseline and at 4-6 hours and 12 hours after presentation.

1736. What percentage of patients with documented NSTE-ACS carry a risk of early death (30 days)?
Harrison's 20th Ed. Chapter 268 Page 1868

A. 1 to 2%
B. 1 to 4%
C. 1 to 6%
D. 1 to 10%

1737. What percentage of patients with documented NSTE-ACS carry a risk of recurrent ACS?

Harrison's 20th Ed. Chapter 268 Page 1868

A. 1–4% during the first year
B. 3–8% during the first year
C. 5–15% during the first year
D. 9–35% during the first year

1 to 10% patients with documented NSTE-ACS carry a risk of early death (30 days). 5 - 15% patients with documented NSTE-ACS carry a risk of recurrent ACS during the first year.

1738. Number of independent risk factors included in clinical risk scoring system developed from Thrombolysis in Myocardial Infarction (TIMI) Trials is?

Harrison's 20th Ed. Chapter 268 Page 1868

A. 5
B. 7
C. 9
D. 11

Clinical risk scoring system developed from the Thrombolysis in Myocardial Infarction (TIMI) Trials includes seven independent risk factors. They are age ≥ 65 years, 3 or more of the traditional risk factors for coronary heart disease, known history of coronary artery disease or coronary stenosis of at least 50%, daily aspirin use in the prior week, more than one anginal episode in the past 24 hour, ST segment deviation of at least 0.5 mm, and an elevated cardiac specific biomarker above the upper limit of normal.

1739. Risk factor for CAD include?

Harrison's 20th Ed. Chapter 268 Page 1868

A. Elevated levels of creatinine
B. Brain natriuretic peptides
C. C-reactive protein
D. All of the above

Besides the seven independent risk factors in Thrombolysis in Myocardial Infarction (TIMI) Trials, other risk factors are diabetes mellitus, left ventricular dysfunction & elevated levels of creatinine, brain natriuretic peptides & C-reactive protein.

1740. B-type natriuretic peptide is a marker of?

Harrison's 20th Ed. Chapter 268 Page 1868

A. Vascular inflammation
B. Increased myocardial wall tension
C. Plaque rupture
D. All of the above

C-reactive protein is a marker of vascular inflammation and B-type natriuretic peptide is a marker of increased myocardial wall tension.

1741. According to which study, early invasive strategy conferred a 40% reduction in recurrent cardiac events in patients with an elevated cTn level?

Harrison's 20th Ed. Chapter 268 Page 1868

A. TRITON-TIMI 38 Trial
B. TACTICS-TIMI 18 Trial
C. FREEDOM Trial
D. SYNTAX Trial

TACTICS-TIMI 18 Trial, an early invasive strategy conferred a 40% reduction in recurrent cardiac events in patients with an elevated cTn level, whereas no benefit was observed in those without detectable troponin.

1742. Inhaled oxygen is given in patients of NSTE-ACS who have arterial O_2 saturation of?

Harrison's 20th Ed. Chapter 268 Page 1869

A. < 100%
B. < 96%
C. < 90%
D. < 86%

Inhaled oxygen is given in patients of NSTE-ACS who have arterial O_2 saturation of <90%, and/or in those with heart failure and rales.

1743. Instead of sublingual nitrates, intravenous nitroglycerin is recommended if ischemic pain persists after?

Harrison's 20th Ed. Chapter 268 Page 1869

A. Three doses given 5 minutes apart
B. Three doses given 15 minutes apart
C. Three doses given 30 minutes apart
D. Three doses given 60 minutes apart

Nitrates should first be given sublingually or by buccal spray (0.3-0.6 mg) if the patient is having ischemic pain. If pain persists after three doses given 5 minutes apart, intravenous nitroglycerin (5–10 μg/minute using nonabsorbing tubing) is recommended. The rate of infusion may be increased by 10 μg/minute every 3–5 minute until symptoms are relieved, systolic arterial pressure falls to <100 mm Hg or the dose reaches 200 μg/minute.

1744. Nitrates must not be administered if sildenafil (Viagra) has been used by the patient within the previous?

Harrison's 20th Ed. Chapter 268 Page 1869

A. 3 hours
B. 6 hours
C. 12 hours
D. 24 hours

Absolute contraindications to the use of nitrates are hypotension or the recent use of a phosphodiesterase type 5 (PDE-5) inhibitor, sildenafil or vardenafil (within 24 hours), or tadalafil (within 48 hours).

1745. In ACS, oral beta blockade is recommended to being heart rate to?

Harrison's 20th Ed. Chapter 268 Page 1869

A. 40 - 50 beats / minute
B. 50 - 60 beats / minute
C. 60 - 70 beats / minute
D. 70 - 80 beats / minute

In patients with acute coronary syndrome (ACS), oral beta blockade targeted to a heart rate of 50–60 beats/minute is recommended.

1746. In NSTE-ACS, verapamil or diltiazem, are recommended for patients who have?

Harrison's 20th Ed. Chapter 268 Page 1869

A. Lack of improvement after full-dose of nitrates
B. Lack of improvement after full-dose of beta blockers
C. Contraindications to nitrates or beta blockers
D. All of the above

Heart rate slowing calcium channel blockers (verapamil or diltiazem) are recommended for patients who have persistent symptoms or ECG signs of ischemia after treatment with full-dose nitrates & beta blockers and in patients with contraindications to either class of these agents.

1747. Administration of statins prior to percutaneous coronary intervention (PCI) reduces?

Harrison's 20th Ed. Chapter 268 Page 1869

A. Arrhythmias
B. Peri-procedural MI
C. Hypotension
D. All of the above

Early administration of intensive HMG-CoA reductase inhibitors (statins) prior to percutaneous coronary intervention (PCI), and continued thereafter, reduces peri-procedural MI and recurrences of ACS.

1748. Inadequate lipid lowering response to maximally tolerated statin is?

Harrison's 20th Ed. Chapter 268 Page 1869

A. < 10% decrease in LDL-C from untreated baseline
B. < 20% decrease in LDL-C from untreated baseline
C. < 40% decrease in LDL-C from untreated baseline
D. < 50% decrease in LDL-C from untreated baseline

Inadequate lipid lowering response to maximally tolerated statin is <50% decrease in LDL-C from untreated baseline or LDL-C on treatment >70 mg/dL.

1749. In patients with acute coronary syndrome (ACS), typical initial dose of aspirin is?

Harrison's 20th Ed. Chapter 268 Page 1869

A. 75 mg / day
B. 162 mg / day
C. 325 mg / day
D. 1000 mg / day

In patients with acute coronary syndrome (ACS), the typical initial dose of aspirin is 325 mg/day, with lower doses (75 - 100 mg/day) recommended thereafter.

1750. "Aspirin resistance" has been noted what percentage of patients?

Harrison's 19th Ed. Page1596

A. 0.2 - 0.8%
B. 1 - 1.6%
C. 1.6 - 2%
D. 2 - 8%

"Aspirin resistance" has been noted in 2-8% of patients.

1751. Letter "C" in CURE trial stands for?

Harrison's 19th Ed. Page 1596

A. Coronary
B. Carotid
C. Clopidogrel
D. Cardiac

CURE is CURE trial stands for Clopidogrel in Unstable Angina to Prevent Recurrent Events.

1752. Prasugrel is contraindicated in patients with?

Harrison's 20th Ed. Chapter 268 Page 1870

A. Peripheral artery disease
B. Prior stroke or transient ischemic attack
C. Tuberculosis
D. Hypertension

Thienopyridine drug prasugrel has a more rapid onset, and higher level of platelet inhibition than clopidogrel. Dose is 60 mg load followed by 10 mg/day for up to 15 months. It is contraindicated in patients with prior stroke or transient ischemic attack.

1753. With prasugrel therapy, which of the following was prone to serious bleeding?

N Engl J Med. 2009;361:941

A. Elderly
B. Underweight
C. Patients with previous stroke or transient ischemic attack
D. All of the above

With prasugrel therapy, three subgroups appeared to be particularly prone to serious bleeding—the elderly, the underweight, and patients with a previous stroke or transient ischemic attack.

1754. Which of the following is a reversible platelet P2Y12 inhibitor?

Harrison's 20th Ed. Chapter 268 Page 1870

A. Clopidogrel
B. Prasugrel
C. Ticagrelor
D. All of the above

Ticagrelor is a reversible and direct-acting oral antagonist of the adenosine diphosphate receptor P2Y12. It reduces the risk of cardiovascular death, MI, or stroke by 16% compared with clopidogrel in ACS patients without increasing the risk of total bleeding.

1755. Dual antiplatelet therapy (DAPT) should continue for how long in patients with NSTE-ACS?

Harrison's 20th Ed. Chapter 268 Page 1870

A. At least 3 months
B. At least 6 months
C. At least 1 year
D. At least 2 years

Dual antiplatelet therapy (DAPT) should continue for at least 1 year in patients with NSTE-ACS, especially those with a drug-eluting stent, to prevent stent thrombosis.

1756. Which of the following is an intravenous P2Y12 inhibitor?

Harrison's 20th Ed. Chapter 268 Page 1871

A. Cangrelor
B. Ticlopidine
C. Clopidogrel
D. Ticagrelor

Cangrelor is an intravenous, direct and rapidly acting, P2Y12 inhibitor.

1757. Besides aspirin & clopidogrel, triple antiplatelet therapy uses which of the following as the third drug?

Harrison's 20th Ed. Chapter 268 Page 1871

A. Cangrelor
B. Bivalirudin
C. Glycoprotein IIb/IIIa inhibitors
D. Prasugrel

The addition of intravenous glycoprotein IIb/IIIa inhibitors to aspirin and a P2Y12 inhibitor (triple antiplatelet therapy) should be reserved for unstable patients undergoing PCI. These include patients with recurrent rest pain, elevated cTn, and ECG changes, & those who have a coronary thrombus evident on angiography.

1758. Which of the following is a direct thrombin inhibitor?

Harrison's 20th Ed. Chapter 268 Page 1871

A. Heparin
B. Bivalirudin
C. Fondaparinux
D. Enoxaparin

Fondaparinux is a Factor Xa inhibitor. Bivalirudin is a direct thrombin inhibitor. Enoxaparin is a low molecular weight heparin (LMWH).

1759. Laboratory test used to measure the antiplatelet effects of aspirin is?
Biomark Med. 2011 Feb;5(1):31-42

A. Optical platelet aggregation
B. Skin bleeding time
C. Urinary 11-dehydrothromboxane B2
D. All of the above

The direct measurement of inhibition of thromboxane-forming capacity is the most specific pharmacological assay for aspirin. Measurement of urinary levels of the TXB(2) metabolite, 11-dehydro-thromboxane B(2), represents an index of TXA(2) biosynthesis in vivo.

1760. Which of the following is an intravenous antiplatelet agent?
Harrison's 20th Ed. Chapter 268 Page 1870 Table 268-3

A. Abciximab
B. Tirofiban
C. Cangrelor
D. All of the above

1761. The Global Registry of Acute Coronary Events (GRACE) risk score estimates probability of death within how many months of hospital discharge in patients with ACS?
Am J Cardiol. 2016;118(8):1105-1110

A. 3 months
B. 6 months
C. 1 year
D. 2 years

The Global Registry of Acute Coronary Events (GRACE) risk score provides an estimate of the probability of death within 6 months of hospital discharge in patients with acute coronary syndrome (ACS).

1762. The Global Registry of Acute Coronary Events (GRACE) risk score 2.0 estimates probability of death within how many months of hospital discharge in patients with ACS?
Am J Cardiol. 2016;118(8):1105-1110

A. 3 months
B. 6 months
C. 1 year
D. 2 years

GRACE Risk Score 2.0 simplified algorithm for predicting 1-year mortality in ACS patients.

1763. Immediate invasive strategy in patients with NSTE-ACS is recommended in all except?
Harrison's 20th Ed. Chapter 268 Page 1871 Table 268-4

A. Refractory angina
B. Hemodynamic instability
C. Temporal change in troponin
D. Sustained ventricular tachycardia or ventricular fibrillation

1764. Patients at high ischemic risk include?
Harrison's 20th Ed. Chapter 268 Page 1871

A. Prior MI
B. Diabetes mellitus
C. Congestive heart failure
D. All of the above

1765. Patients at high ischemic risk should continue DAPT for?
Harrison's 20th Ed. Chapter 268 Page 1871

A. 1 year
B. 2 years
C. 3 years
D. 5 years

Patients at high ischemic risk (those with prior MI, diabetes mellitus, vein graft stent, congestive heart failure) who are also at low risk of bleeding, continuation of DAPT for 3 years is beneficial.

1766. Prinzmetal's variant angina is due to?
Harrison's 20th Ed. Chapter 268 Page 1871

A. Focal spasm of an epicardial coronary artery
B. Focal spasm of an intramyocardial coronary artery
C. Diffuse spasm of an epicardial coronary artery
D. Diffuse spasm of an intramyocardial coronary artery

Described by Prinzmetal in 1959, Prinzmetal's variant angina is due to focal spasm of an epicardial coronary artery, leading to severe myocardial ischemia. It may be related to hypercontractility of vascular smooth muscle due to vasoconstrictor mitogens, leukotrienes, or serotonin.

1767. Prinzmetal's variant angina may be associated with?
Harrison's 20th Ed. Chapter 268 Page 1872

A. Migraine
B. Raynaud's phenomenon
C. Aspirin-induced asthma
D. All of the above

Prinzmetal's variant angina is a manifestation of a vasospastic disorder and is associated with migraine, Raynaud's phenomenon or aspirin-induced asthma.

1768. In Prinzmetal's variant angina, focal spasm is most common in?
N Engl J Med. 2017; 376:e52

A. Right coronary artery
B. Left anterior descending coronary artery
C. Left circumflex coronary artery
D. Posterior descending coronary artery

Focal spasm is most common in right coronary artery, and it may occur at one or more sites in one artery or in multiple arteries simultaneously. Atherosclerotic plaques in at least one proximal coronary artery occur in ~ half of patients & in these patients, spasm usually occurs within 1 cm of plaque.

1769. Which of the following can be used to provoke focal coronary spasm in Prinzmetal's variant angina?
Harrison's 20th Ed. Chapter 268 Page 1872

A. Ergonovine
B. Acetylcholine
C. Hyperventilation
D. All of the above

Ergonovine, acetylcholine & hyperventilation can provoke focal coronary stenosis. It is used to establish the diagnosis of Prinzmetal's variant angina.

1770. Which of the following is false regarding Prinzmetal's variant angina?
Harrison's 20th Ed. Chapter 268 Page 1872

A. Nitrates and Ca^{++} channel blockers are main treatments
B. Ca^{++} channel blockers given in maximally tolerated doses
C. Aspirin is of therapeutic value
D. Aspirin may increase the severity of ischemic episodes

Nitrates & calcium channel blockers are the main treatments for Prinzmetal's variant angina. Calcium antagonists are extremely effective in preventing coronary artery spasm of variant angina & they should be prescribed in maximally tolerated doses. Prazosin, a selective alpha adrenoreceptor blocker, has also been found to be of value in some patients, while aspirin may increase the severity of ischemic episodes. The response to beta blockers is variable.

Ischemic Heart Disease

1771. Which of the following is a determinant of myocardial oxygen demand (MVO_2)?
Harrison's 20th Ed. Chapter 267 Page 1850

A. Heart rate
B. Myocardial contractility
C. Myocardial wall tension (stress)
D. All of the above

The major determinants of myocardial oxygen demand (MVO_2) are heart rate, myocardial contractility, and myocardial wall tension (stress).

1772. Oxygen-carrying capacity of the blood is determined by?
Harrison's 20th Ed. Chapter 267 Page 1850

A. Inspired level of oxygen
B. Pulmonary function
C. Hemoglobin concentration and function
D. All of the above

An adequate supply of oxygen to the myocardium requires a satisfactory level of oxygen-carrying capacity of the blood. Apart from adequate level of coronary blood flow it is determined by inspired level of oxygen, pulmonary function and hemoglobin concentration and function.

1773. Majority of blood flow through coronary arteries is during?
Harrison's 20th Ed. Chapter 267 Page 1850

A. Systole
B. Diastole
C. Presystole
D. Prediastole

Blood flows through coronary arteries in a phasic fashion, with majority occurring during diastole.

1774. In the absence of significant flow-limiting atherosclerotic obstructions, major determinant of total coronary resistance is found in?
Harrison's 20th Ed. Chapter 267 Page 1850

A. Large epicardial arteries (R_1)
B. Prearteriolar vessels (R_2)
C. Arteriolar and intramyocardial capillary vessels (R_3)
D. R_2 & R_3

About 75% of the total coronary resistance to flow occurs across three sets of arteries: (1) large epicardial arteries (Resistance 1 = R_1), (2) prearteriolar vessels (R_2), and (3) arteriolar and intramyocardial capillary vessels (R_3). In the absence of significant flow-limiting atherosclerotic obstructions, R_1 is trivial. The major determinant of coronary resistance is found in R_2 and R_3.

1775. Which of the following statements is false?
Harrison's 20th Ed. Chapter 267 Page 1850

A. Large epicardial coronary arteries are conductance vessels
B. Intramyocardial arterioles are resistance vessels
C. Abnormal constriction of conductance vessels can cause Prinzmetal's angina
D. Abnormal constriction of resistance vessels can cause Prinzmetal's angina

Although the large epicardial coronary arteries are capable of constriction and relaxation, in healthy persons they serve as conduits and are referred to as conductance vessels, while the intramyocardial arterioles normally exhibit changes in tone and are therefore referred to as resistance vessels. Abnormal constriction of the conductance vessels can cause severe ischemia in Prinzmetal's angina. Abnormal constriction or failure of normal dilation of coronary resistance vessels causes ischemia termed as microvascular angina.

1776. What is the size of the epicardial coronary arteries?
Harrison's 20th Ed. Chapter 267 Page 1851 Figure 267-1

A. > 100 μm
B. > 200 μm
C. > 300 μm
D. > 400 μm

1777. What is the size of the arterioles in the coronary microcirculation?
Harrison's 20th Ed. Chapter 267 Page 1851 Figure 267-1

A. < 10 μm
B. < 40 μm
C. < 80 μm
D. < 100 μm

1778. Which of the following offers maximum percentage of total resistance to flow?
Harrison's 20th Ed. Chapter 267 Page 1851 Figure 267-1

A. Epicardial arteries
B. Small arteries
C. Arterioles
D. Capillaries

1779. Principal function of small arteries & arterioles is?
Harrison's 20th Ed. Chapter 267 Page 1851 Figure 267-1

A. Transport
B. Regulation
C. Exchange
D. All of the above

1780. Which of the following is part of the coronary microcirculation?
Harrison's 20th Ed. Chapter 267 Page 1851 Figure 267-1

A. Small arteries
B. Arterioles
C. Capillaries
D. All of the above

1781. Main stimulus for vasomotion in epicardial arteries is?
Harrison's 20th Ed. Chapter 267 Page 1851 Figure 267-1

A. Flow
B. Pressure
C. Metabolites
D. All of the above

1782. Coronary blood flow can be limited compromised by?
Harrison's 20th Ed. Chapter 267 Page 1850

A. Spasm
B. Arterial thrombi
C. Coronary emboli
D. All of the above

Coronary blood flow also can be limited by spasm (Prinzmetal's angina, vasoconstrictors), arterial thrombi, coronary emboli and ostial narrowing due to aortitis.

1783. Microvascular angina best relates to which of the following?
Harrison's 20th Ed. Chapter 267 Page 1851

A. Failure of normal dilation of coronary resistance vessels
B. Coronary emboli
C. Coronary ostial narrowing
D. All of the above

Abnormal constriction or failure of normal dilation of the coronary resistance vessels also can cause ischemia. When it causes angina, this condition is referred to as microvascular angina.

1784. Which of the following is a normal function of the vascular endothelium?
Harrison's 20th Ed. Chapter 267 Page 1851

A. Local control of vascular tone
B. Maintenance of an antithrombotic surface
C. Control of inflammatory cell adhesion & diapedesis
D. All of the above

Normal functions of the vascular endothelium include local control of vascular tone, maintenance of an antithrombotic surface and control of inflammatory cell adhesion and diapedesis.

1785. Which of the following define the atherosclerotic plaque?
Harrison's 20th Ed. Chapter 267 Page 1851

A. Subintimal collections of fat
B. Subintimal collections of smooth muscle cells
C. Subintimal collections of fibroblasts
D. All of the above

Subintimal collections of fat, smooth muscle cells, fibroblasts and intercellular matrix define the atherosclerotic plaque.

1786. Which of the following contribute to a state of "vulnerable blood"?
Harrison's 20th Ed. Chapter 267 Page 1851

A. Increased concentrations of platelet microparticles
B. Increased concentrations of von Willebrand factor
C. Increased concentrations of coagulation factor VII
D. All of the above

Alterations in the nature of the circulating blood like hyperglycemia, increased concentrations of LDL cholesterol, tissue factor, fibrinogen, von Willebrand factor, coagulation factor VII and platelet microparticles lead to a state of "vulnerable blood". The combination of a "vulnerable vessel" in a patient with "vulnerable blood" promotes a state of hypercoagulability and hypofibrinolysis. This is especially true in patients with diabetes mellitus.

1787. Which of the following sites has the most predilection for atherosclerotic plaques to develop?
Harrison's 20th Ed. Chapter 267 Page 1851

A. Origin of epicardial arteries
B. Branch points in epicardial arteries
C. Terminal regions of epicardial arteries
D. Any of the above

Atherosclerotic plaques have a predilection to develop at sites of increased turbulence in coronary flow like branch points in the epicardial arteries.

1788. Coronary blood flow at rest may be reduced, when the diameter is reduced by?
Harrison's 20th Ed. Chapter 267 Page 1851

A. 50%
B. 60%
C. 70%
D. 80%

When a stenosis reduces the diameter of an epicardial coronary artery by 50%, there is a limitation of the ability to increase flow to meet increased myocardial demand. When the diameter is reduced by ~80%, blood flow at rest may be reduced.

1789. Gregg effect best relates to which of the following?
Z Kardiol. 2001;90(5):319-26

A. Congenital cataracts among infants
B. Increase in myocardial oxygen consumption with increase in coronary perfusion pressure
C. Failure of aldosterone to suppress
D. Disruption of adrenal androgen secretion

In 1958, Gregg reported that myocardial oxygen consumption increased when coronary perfusion pressure was increased.

1790. Which of the following collateral vessels is false?
Harrison's 20th Ed. Chapter 267 Page 1851

A. Promoted by chronic severe coronary narrowing
B. Promoted by myocardial ischemia
C. May sustain viability of myocardium at rest but not during conditions of increased demand
D. None of the above

1791. Which of the following occur when a proximal epicardial artery is stenosed?
Harrison's 20th Ed. Chapter 267 Page 1851

A. Pressure gradient develops across the proximal stenosis
B. Poststenotic pressure falls
C. Myocardial blood flow becomes dependent on pressure in the coronary artery distal to stenosis
D. All of the above

1792. Myocardial ischemia causes disturbance in which of the following?
Harrison's 20th Ed. Chapter 267 Page 1851

A. Mechanical functions of the myocardium
B. Biochemical functions of the myocardium
C. Electrical functions of the myocardium
D. All of the above

1793. Which of the following about coronary atherosclerosis is false?
Harrison's 20th Ed. Chapter 267 Page 1852

A. Focal process
B. Causes nonuniform ischemia
C. Causes loss of endothelial control of dilation
D. None of the above

1794. Normal myocardium metabolizes which of the following?
Harrison's 20th Ed. Chapter 267 Page 1852

A. Fatty acids
B. Amino acids
C. Lactate
D. All of the above

Normal myocardium metabolizes fatty acids and glucose to carbon dioxide and water.

1795. Which of the following occurs during myocardial ischemia?
Harrison's 20th Ed. Chapter 267 Page 1852

A. Intracellular pH is reduced
B. Intracellular creatine phosphate is reduced
C. Intracellular glucose is converted to lactate
D. All of the above

With severe oxygen deprivation, fatty acids cannot be oxidized and glucose is converted to lactate. Intracellular pH and myocardial stores of high-energy phosphates (ATP, creatine phosphate) are reduced.

1796. During myocardial ischemia, impairment of cell membrane function leads to?
Harrison's 20th Ed. Chapter 267 Page 1852

A. Leakage of potassium from myocytes
B. Uptake of sodium by myocytes
C. Increase in cytosolic calcium
D. All of the above

Impaired myocyte cell membrane function due to ischemia leads to leakage of potassium and uptake of sodium by myocytes as well as an increase in cytosolic calcium.

1797. Minimum duration of total occlusion of epicardial vessel in absence of collaterals for development of myocardial necrosis is?
Harrison's 20th Ed. Chapter 267 Page 1852

A. > 20 minutes
B. > 25 minutes
C. > 30 minutes
D. > 35 minutes

Severity & duration of imbalance between myocardial oxygen supply & demand determine whether damage is reversible (≤20 minutes for total occlusion in the absence of collaterals) or whether it is permanent, with subsequent myocardial necrosis (>20 minutes).

1798. In ECG, transient ST-segment depression reflects?
Harrison's 20th Ed. Chapter 267 Page 1852

A. Subendocardial ischemia
B. Transmural ischemia
C. Epicardial ischemia
D. All of the above

1799. In ECG, transient ST-segment elevation reflects?
Harrison's 20th Ed. Chapter 267 Page 1852

A. Subendocardial ischemia
B. Transmural ischemia
C. Epicardial ischemia
D. All of the above

Ischemia also causes characteristic changes in ECG such as repolarization abnormalities in the form of inversion of T waves and, when more severe, by displacement of ST segments. Transient ST-segment depression reflects patchy subendocardial ischemia, while ST-segment elevation is caused by more severe transmural ischemia.

1800. Coronary atherosclerosis begins to develop at what age?
Harrison's 20th Ed. Chapter 267 Page 1852

A. < 20 years
B. 20 - 30 years
C. 30 - 40 years
D. > 40 years

Postmortem studies have shown that coronary atherosclerosis often begins to develop prior to age 20 and is widespread even among adults who were asymptomatic during life.

1801. Which of the following statements about angina pectoris is false?
Harrison's 20th Ed. Chapter 267 Page 1852

A. Males constitute ~70% of all patients with angina pectoris
B. Angina pectoris in women is often atypical in presentation
C. Angina pectoris only rarely presents as frank pain
D. None of the above

1802. Squeezing, central, substernal discomfort in angina pectoris is termed?
Harrison's 20th Ed. Chapter 267 Page 1853

A. Landolfi's sign
B. Levine's sign
C. Lhermitte's sign
D. Carvolo's sign

Squeezing, central, substernal discomfort indicative of angina pectoris is termed as Levine's sign.

1803. Which of the following statements about angina is false?
Harrison's 20th Ed. Chapter 267 Page 1853

A. Angina is usually crescendo-decrescendo in nature
B. Typically lasts for 10 to 15 minutes
C. Pain can radiate to both arms
D. Rarely localized below umbilicus or above mandible

Angina is usually crescendo-decrescendo in nature, typically lasts 2 to 5 minutes, and can radiate to left shoulder and to both arms, especially to the ulnar surfaces of forearm and hand. It can also arise in or radiate to the back, interscapular region, root of the neck, jaw, teeth, and epigastrium. Angina is rarely localized below the umbilicus or above the mandible.

1804. Radiation of chest pain towards which of the following is more typical of pericarditis?
Harrison's 20th Ed. Chapter 267 Page 1853

A. Interscapular region
B. Jaw
C. Epigastrium
D. Trapezius muscles

Chest discomfort due to myocardial ischemia does not radiate to the trapezius muscles; such a radiation pattern is more typical of pericarditis.

1805. "Angina decubitus" refers to anginal pain occuring when the patient is in which of the following positions?
Harrison's 20th Ed. Chapter 267 Page 1853

A. Squatting
B. Sitting with legs hanging
C. Recumbent
D. Any of the above

Episodes of angina that occur at night while the patient is recumbent is termed as angina decubitus.

1806. Nocturnal angina may be due to?
Harrison's 20th Ed. Chapter 267 Page 1853

A. Episodic tachycardia
B. Changes in respiratory pattern during sleep
C. Expansion of intrathoracic blood volume
D. All of the above

Nocturnal angina may be due to episodic tachycardia, diminished oxygenation as the respiratory pattern changes during sleep or expansion of intrathoracic blood volume that occurs with recumbency.

1807. Expansion of the intrathoracic blood volume during recumbency leads to?
Harrison's 20th Ed. Chapter 267 Page 1853

A. Increase in end-diastolic volume
B. Increase in wall tension
C. Increase in myocardial oxygen demand
D. All of the above

1808. Atypical presentations of angina pectoris are more frequent in?
Harrison's 20th Ed. Chapter 267 Page 1853, N Engl J Med. 2005;352:2524-33

A. Older patients
B. Diabetics
C. Women
D. All of the above

1809. Anginal "equivalents" are all except?
Harrison's 20th Ed. Chapter 267 Page 1853

A. Dyspnea
B. Fatigue
C. Palpitation
D. Faintness

1810. Anginal "equivalents" are more common in?
Harrison's 20th Ed. Chapter 267 Page 1853

A. Women
B. Smoker
C. Hypertension
D. Diabetes mellitus

Anginal "equivalents" are symptoms of myocardial ischemia other than angina. These include dyspnea, fatigue and faintness and are more common in the elderly and in diabetic patients.

1811. Which of the following point towards an unstable anginal syndrome?
Harrison's 20th Ed. Chapter 267 Page 1853

A. Angina occurring with less exertion than in the past
B. Angina occurring at rest
C. Angina awakening the patient from sleep
D. All of the above

1812. Coronary reactivity testing can be done by which of the following vasoactive agents?
Harrison's 20th Ed. Chapter 267 Page 1853

A. Adenosine
B. Acetylcholine
C. Nitroglycerin
D. All of the above

Coronary reactivity testing can be done by vasoactive agents such as intracoronary adenosine, acetylcholine and nitroglycerin.

1813. Abnormal cardiac nociception may be ameliorated by?
Harrison's 20th Ed. Chapter 267 Page 1853

A. Calcium antagonists
B. Statins
C. Nicorandil
D. Imipramine

Abnormal cardiac nociception is more difficult to manage and may be ameliorated in some cases by imipramine.

1814. Disorders that may cause angina in absence of coronary atherosclerosis are all except?
Harrison's 20th Ed. Chapter 267 Page 1854

A. Hypertrophic cardiomyopathy
B. Aortic regurgitation
C. Pulmonary hypertension
D. Systemic hypertension

Aortic stenosis, aortic regurgitation, pulmonary hypertension and hypertrophic cardiomyopathy may cause angina in the absence of coronary atherosclerosis.

1815. Which of the following statements is false?
Harrison's 20th Ed. Chapter 391 Page 2825

A. Angina is the commonest initial symptom of CHD in women
B. Myocardial infarction is the commonest initial symptom of CHD in men
C. Women with MI are more likely to present with cardiac arrest or cardiogenic shock
D. None of the above

In the Framingham study, angina was the most common initial symptom of CHD in women, whereas myocardial infarction (MI) was the most common initial presentation in men. Women more often have atypical symptoms such as nausea, vomiting, indigestion, and upper back pain. Women with MI are more likely to present with cardiac arrest or cardiogenic shock, whereas men are more likely to present with ventricular tachycardia. Younger women with MI are more likely to die than are men of similar age.

1816. Poor exercise tolerance is defined as?
Harrison's 20th Ed. Chapter 467 Page 3447

A. Inabi!ity to walk four blocks
B. Inabi!ity to climb two flights of stairs at normal pace
C. Meet a metabolic equivalent (MET) level of 4
D. All of the above

Poor exercise tolerance is defined as inabi!ity to walk four blocks or climb two flights of stairs at a normal pace or to meet a metabolic equivalent (MET) level of 4 because of the development of dyspnea, angina or excessive fatigue.

1817. Which of the following can closely mimic angina?
Harrison's 20th Ed. Chapter 11 Page 76

A. Esophageal reflux
B. Esophageal spasm
C. Peptic ulcer
D. Gall bladder disease

The pain of esophageal spasm is commonly an intense squeezing discomfort that is retrosternal in location and like angina may be relieved by nitroglycerin or dihydropyridine calcium channel antagonists.

1818. Cardiac cephalgia best relates to?
Harrison's 20th Ed. Chapter 422 Page 3106

A. Primary cough headache
B. Primary exercise headache
C. Primary thunderclap headache
D. Primary sex headache

Cardiac cephalgia refers exertional headache. Pain from angina may be referred to the head, probably by central connections of vagal afferents. The link to exercise is the main clinical clue that headache is of cardiac origin.

1819. Which of the following makes it unlikely that the chest pain is caused by myocardial ischemia?
Harrison's 20th Ed. Chapter 267 Page 1854

A. Tenderness of the chest wall
B. Localization of discomfort with a single fingertip on chest
C. Reproduction of the pain with palpation of chest
D. All of the above

1820. Which of the following is useful in therapeutic decision-making about the initiation of hypolipidemic treatment?
Harrison's 20th Ed. Chapter 267 Page 1854

A. Lp(a)
B. CRP
C. Homocysteine
D. All of the above

Evidence exists that ↑ level of high-sensitivity C-reactive protein (CRP) (between 0 - 3 mg/dL) is an independent risk factor for IHD and is useful in therapeutic decision-making about initiation of hypolipidemic treatment.

1821. Which of the following ECG change is more specific for the diagnosis of angina pectoris?
Harrison's 20th Ed. Chapter 267 Page 1854

A. Dynamic ST-segment and T-wave changes
B. Disturbances of cardiac rhythm
C. Intraventricular conduction defect
D. All of the above

Dynamic ST-segment and T-wave changes that accompany episodes of angina pectoris and disappear thereafter are more specific in patients with angina pectoris.

1822. All of the following are indications of discontinuing exercise stress testing except?
Harrison's 20th Ed. Chapter 267 Page 1854

A. Chest discomfort
B. Severe shortness of breath
C. Dizziness
D. Rise in systolic blood pressure > 40 mm Hg

1823. All of the following are indications of discontinuing exercise stress testing except?
Harrison's 20th Ed. Chapter 267 Page 1854

A. ST-segment depression > 0.2 mV (2 mm)
B. Fall in systolic blood pressure > 10 mm Hg
C. Development of supraventricular tachyarrhythmia
D. Development of ventricular tachyarrhythmia

Treadmill exercise stress test is discontinued upon evidence of chest discomfort, severe shortness of breath, dizziness, severe fatigue, ST-segment depression > 0.2 mV (2 mm), a fall in systolic blood pressure >10 mm Hg, or the development of a ventricular tachyarrhythmia.

1824. Which of the following represents baseline in ECG?
Harrison's 20th Ed. Chapter 267 Page 1854

A. PR segment
B. ST segment
C. QT segment
D. TP segment

The PR segment is considered as the baseline in ECG.

1825. Ischemic ST-segment response on standard exercise treadmill testing (ETT) is?
Harrison's 20th Ed. Chapter 267 Page 1854

A. Flat or downsloping depression of the ST segment
B. > 0.1 mV below baseline
C. Lasting longer than 0.08 seconds
D. All of the above

The ischemic ST-segment response on standard exercise treadmill testing (ETT) is defined as flat or downsloping depression of the ST segment >0.1 mV below baseline (PR segment) and lasting longer than 0.08 seconds.

1826. On standard exercise treadmill testing (ETT), which of the following is not considered characteristic of ischemia or is not diagnostic?
Harrison's 20th Ed. Chapter 267 Page 1854

A. Upsloping or junctional ST-segment changes
B. Conduction disturbances
C. Ventricular arrhythmias
D. All of the above

On standard exercise treadmill testing (ETT), upsloping or junctional ST-segment changes are not considered characteristic of ischemia and do not constitute a positive test. Although T-wave abnormalities, conduction disturbances, and ventricular arrhythmias that develop during exercise should be noted, they are also not diagnostic.

1827. In standard exercise treadmill testing (ETT), target heart rate (THR) is defined as?
Harrison's 20th Ed. Chapter 267 Page 1854

A. 65% of maximal predicted heart rate for age and sex
B. 75% of maximal predicted heart rate for age and sex
C. 85% of maximal predicted heart rate for age and sex
D. 95% of maximal predicted heart rate for age and sex

Negative exercise tests in which the target heart rate (85% of maximal predicted heart rate for age and sex) is not achieved are considered nondiagnostic.

1828. The standard Bruce treadmill protocol begins at what speed and gradient?
Harrison's 20th Ed. Chapter 267 Page 1857 Table 267-2

A. 1.7 miles per hour and 0% gradient
B. 1.7 miles per hour and 5% gradient
C. 1.7 miles per hour and 10% gradient
D. 1.7 miles per hour and 12% gradient

The standard Bruce treadmill protocol begins at 1.7 MPH and 10% gradient and progresses every 3 min to a higher speed and elevation.

1829. In standard Bruce treadmill protocol, what is the maximum speed and maximum gradient?
Harrison's 20th Ed. Chapter 267 Page 1857 Table 267-2

A. 5 miles per hour and 18% gradient
B. 5 miles per hour and 22% gradient
C. 6 miles per hour and 18% gradient
D. 6 miles per hour and 22% gradient

1830. The standard Bruce treadmill protocol progresses to a higher speed and elevation every?
Harrison's 20th Ed. Chapter 267 Page 1857 Table 267-2

A. 1 minute
B. 2 minutes
C. 3 minutes
D. 4 minutes

The standard Bruce treadmill protocol progresses to a higher speed and elevation every 3 minutes.

1831. Methoxyisobutyl isonitrite (MIBI) best relates to?

Harrison's 20th Ed. Chapter 267 Page 1855 Figure 267-3

A. 2D echocardiography
B. Nuclear perfusion scan
C. Cardiac MR scan
D. Cardiac PET scan

1832. False-positive or false negative results occur in what proportion of ECG stress tests?

Harrison's 20th Ed. Chapter 267 Page 1854

A. 25%
B. 33%
C. 50%
D. 75%

Pretest probability of ECG stress tests being false-positive or false negative for coronary artery disease (CAD) exists in the patient or population is 33%.

1833. Likelihood of CAD in a positive ECG stress test is increased in?

Harrison's 20th Ed. Chapter 267 Page 1854

A. Males who are > 50 years
B. History of typical angina pectoris
C. Who develop chest discomfort during the test
D. All of the above

A positive result on exercise indicates that the likelihood of CAD is 98% in males who are > 50 years with a history of typical angina pectoris and who develop chest discomfort during the test. The likelihood decreases if the patient has atypical or no chest pain by history and/or during the test.

1834. Incidence of false-positive exercise stress electrocardiography is significantly increased in?

Harrison's 20th Ed. Chapter 267 Page 1854

A. Patients taking digitalis and antiarrhythmic agents
B. Patients with ventricular hypertrophy
C. Patients with abnormal serum potassium levels
D. All of the above

Incidence of false-positive tests is significantly increased in patients with low probabilities of IHD like asymptomatic men <40 years or in premenopausal women with no risk factors for premature atherosclerosis. It is also increased in patients taking cardioactive drugs like digitalis & antiarrhythmic agents, or in those with intraventricular conduction disturbances, resting ST-segment & T-wave abnormalities, ventricular hypertrophy, or abnormal serum potassium levels.

1835. False-negative stress test is usual in obstructive disease limited to which coronary artery?

Harrison's 20th Ed. Chapter 267 Page 1854

A. Left anterior descending coronary artery
B. Left circumflex coronary artery
C. Right coronary artery
D. Posterior descending artery

Obstructive disease limited to circumflex coronary artery results in a false-negative stress test since lateral portion of heart which it supplies is not well represented on the surface 12-lead ECG.

1836. Overall sensitivity of exercise stress electrocardiography is?

Harrison's 20th Ed. Chapter 267 Page 1854

A. ~ 55%
B. ~ 65%
C. ~ 75%
D. ~ 85%

Overall sensitivity of exercise stress electrocardiography is only ~75%.

1837. Modified (heart rate limited) exercise stress tests can be earliest performed safely in patients of uncomplicated MI after how many days?

Harrison's 20th Ed. Chapter 267 Page 1854

A. 3 days
B. 6 days
C. 9 days
D. 12 days

Modified (heart rate limited rather than symptom-limited) exercise tests can be performed safely in patients as early as 6 days after uncomplicated MI.

1838. Contraindications to exercise stress testing include all except?

Harrison's 20th Ed. Chapter 267 Page 1854

A. Rest angina within 48 hours
B. Unstable rhythm
C. Severe aortic stenosis
D. Severe mitral stenosis

1839. Contraindications to exercise stress testing include all except?

Harrison's 20th Ed. Chapter 267 Page 1854

A. Acute myocarditis
B. Uncontrolled heart failure
C. Hypertension
D. Active infective endocarditis

Contraindications to exercise stress testing include rest angina within 48 hours, unstable rhythm, severe aortic stenosis, acute myocarditis, uncontrolled heart failure, severe pulmonary hypertension and active infective endocarditis.

1840. Adverse prognostic signs in exercise stress testing include all except?

Harrison's 20th Ed. Chapter 267 Page 1854

A. Failure of blood pressure to increase
B. Development of angina
C. Severe ST-segment depression at low workload
D. ST-segment depression persisting for > 3 minutes after termination of exercise

Failure of BP to increase or an actual decrease with signs of ischemia during the exercise test is an important adverse prognostic sign, since it may reflect ischemia induced global left ventricular dysfunction. Development of angina and/or severe (>0.2 mV) ST-segment depression at a low workload (before completion of stage II of Bruce protocol), and/or ST-segment depression that persists for ">5 minutes" after the termination of exercise increases the specificity of the test and suggests severe IHD and a high risk of future adverse events.

1841. Stress myocardial perfusion imaging is more informative than exercise test in all of the following conditions except?

Harrison's 20th Ed. Chapter 267 Page 1854

A. Wolff-Parkinson-White syndrome
B. Left bundle branch block
C. Right bundle branch block
D. Paced ventricular rhythm

When resting ECG is abnormal (Wolff-Parkinson-White syndrome, >1 mm of resting ST segment depression, left bundle branch block, paced ventricular rhythm), information gained from an exercise test can be enhanced by stress myocardial perfusion imaging.

1842. Which of the following drugs can be used in place of exercise for noninvasive stress testing?

Harrison's 20th Ed. Chapter 267 Page 1854

A. Intravenous nitroglycerine
B. Intravenous dopamine
C. Intravenous adenosine
D. Intravenous phenylephrine

Intravenous dipyridamole or adenosine can be used in place of exercise for noninvasive stress testing to create a coronary "steal" by temporarily increasing flow in nondiseased segments of the coronary vasculature at the expense of diseased segments. Graded incremental infusion of dobutamine may be administered to increase MVO_2.

1843. Agatston score is used for?
Harrison's 20th Ed. Chapter 267 Page 1857

A. Regional wall motion abnormalities
B. Myocardial ischemia quantification
C. Coronary calcium quantification
D. Collateral blood flow quantification

Coronary calcium detected by electron beam computed tomography (EBCT) & multidetector computed tomography (MDCT) is quantified using the Agatston score which is based on the area & density of calcification.

1844. Glagov effect, or positive remodeling refers to?
N Engl J Med. 2005;352:2524-33

A. As coronary plaque burden increases, atherosclerotic mass tends to stay external to lumen, which allows diameter of lumen to be maintained
B. Coronary plaque tends to produce different levels of coronary obstruction at different times
C. Coronary plaque is unduly unstable
D. All of the above

Coronary arteriography outlines the lumina of the coronary arteries. It provides no information about the arterial wall, and severe atherosclerosis that does not encroach on the lumen may go undetected.

1845. Which of the following is associated with coronary artery aneurysms?
Circulation. 2004;110:2747-2771

A. Kawasaki disease
B. Antiphospholipid antibody syndrome
C. Syphilis
D. Bacterial endocarditis

Vasculitis of the coronary arteries (intimal proliferation and infiltration of the vessel wall with mononuclear cells) occurs in Kawasaki disease leading to beadlike aneurysms and thromboses, myocardial ischemia and infarction. Coronary artery aneurysms or ectasia develop in ~15% to 25% of untreated children and may lead to ischemic heart disease or sudden death.

1846. Which of the following about Kawasaki disease is false?
Circulation. 2004;110:2747-2771

A. Acute, self-limited vasculitis
B. Unknown etiology
C. Occurs predominantly in infants and young children
D. None of the above

Kawasaki disease is an acute, self-limited vasculitis of unknown etiology that occurs predominantly in infants and young children. It is characterized by fever, bilateral nonexudative conjunctivitis, erythema of the lips and oral mucosa, strawberry tongue, changes in the extremities, rash, and cervical lymphadenopathy.

1847. The principal prognostic indicator in patients with IHD is?
Harrison's 20th Ed. Chapter 267 Page 1858

A. Age
B. Functional state of the left ventricle
C. Location and severity of coronary artery narrowing
D. All of the above

The principal prognostic indicators in patients with IHD are age, functional state of left ventricle, location(s) and severity of coronary artery narrowing, and the severity or activity of myocardial ischemia.

1848. Which of the following indicate an increased risk for adverse coronary events?
Harrison's 20th Ed. Chapter 267 Page 1858

A. Angina pectoris of recent onset
B. Unstable angina
C. Early postmyocardial infarction angina
D. All of the above

Angina pectoris of recent onset, unstable angina, early postmyocardial infarction angina, angina unresponsive or poorly responsive to medical therapy, and angina accompanied by symptoms of congestive heart failure all indicate an increased risk for adverse coronary events.

1849. Which of the following indicate an increased risk for adverse coronary events?
Harrison's 20th Ed. Chapter 267 Page 1858

A. Episodes of pulmonary edema
B. Mitral regurgitation
C. LVEF <0.40 by echocardiography
D. All of the above

Physical signs of heart failure, episodes of pulmonary edema, transient S3, and mitral regurgitation, cardiac enlargement and reduced (<0.40) LV ejection fraction indicate an ↑ risk for adverse coronary events.

1850. Which of the following indicates a high risk for coronary events?
Harrison's 20th Ed. Chapter 267 Page 1858

A. Inability to exercise for 6 minutes (stage II of Bruce protocol)
B. ST-segment ↓ for >5 minutes after cessation of exercise
C. A decline in systolic pressure >10 mm Hg during exercise
D. All of the above

Indicators of a high risk for coronary events are inability to exercise for 6 minutes (stage II of Bruce protocol) of ETT; onset of myocardial ischemia at low workloads (≥0.1 mV ST segment depression before completion of stage II, ≥0.2 mV ST-segment depression at any stage, ST-segment depression for >5 minutes after cessation of exercise, a decline in systolic pressure >10 mm Hg during exercise, or the development of ventricular tachyarrhythmias during exercise).

1851. On cardiac catheterization, which of the following is associated with a poor prognosis?
Harrison's 20th Ed. Chapter 267 Page 1858

A. Elevations of LV end-diastolic pressure
B. Elevations of LV end-diastolic volume
C. Reduced LV ejection fraction
D. All of the above

On cardiac catheterization, elevations of LV end-diastolic pressure and ventricular volume and reduced ejection fraction are the most important signs of LV dysfunction and are associated with a poor prognosis.

1852. Obstructive lesions of which of the following coronary artery is associated with a greater risk?
Harrison's 20th Ed. Chapter 267 Page 1858

A. Left anterior descending coronary artery
B. Right coronary artery
C. Left circumflex coronary artery
D. Posterior descending artery

Obstructive lesions of the left main (>50% luminal diameter) or left anterior descending coronary artery proximal to the origin of the first septal artery are associated with a greater risk than are lesions of the right or left circumflex coronary artery because of the greater quantity of myocardium at risk.

1853. Which of the following reflect episodes of rapid progression in coronary lesions?
Harrison's 20th Ed. Chapter 267 Page 1858

A. Recent onset of symptoms
B. Development of severe ischemia during stress testing
C. Unstable angina pectoris
D. All of the above

The recent onset of symptoms, development of severe ischemia during stress testing, and unstable angina pectoris reflect episodes of rapid progression in coronary lesions.

1854. Which of the following indicates an increased risk of coronary events?
Harrison's 20th Ed. Chapter 267 Page 1858

A. Elevated levels of plasma CRP
B. Extensive coronary calcification on electron beam CT
C. Increased carotid intimal thickening on ultrasound
D. All of the above

1855. Advanced age refers to?
Harrison's 20th Ed. Chapter 267 Page 1858

A. > 65 years
B. > 70 years
C. > 75 years
D. > 80 years

1856. Obesity often is accompanied by which of the following risk factors?
Harrison's 20th Ed. Chapter 267 Page 1859

A. Diabetes mellitus
B. Hypertension
C. Hyperlipidemia
D. All of the above

Obesity often is accompanied by three other risk factors: diabetes mellitus, hypertension, and hyperlipidemia.

1857. Target LDL cholesterol level in diabetes mellitus is?
Harrison's 20th Ed. Chapter 267 Page 1859

A. < 70 mg/dL
B. < 100 mg/dL
C. < 150 mg/dL
D. < 180 mg/dL

1858. Which of the following markedly lowers LDL-C levels?
Harrison's 20th Ed. Chapter 267 Page 1860

A. Monoclonal antibodies against PCSK9
B. Monoclonal antibodies against IL-5
C. Monoclonal antibodies against LFA-1
D. Monoclonal antibodies against CD15s

The proprotein convertase subtilisin/kexin type 9 (PCSK9) is a secreted protein that binds to LDL receptor & targets it for lysosomal degradation. Normally, after LDL binds to LDL receptor, it is internalized along with the receptor, and in the low pH of the endosome, the LDL receptor dissociates from the LDL and recycles to the cell surface. When circulating PCSK9 binds LDL receptor, the complex is internalized and the receptor is directed to lysosome, rather than to cell surface, reducing the number of active LDL receptors. Loss-of-function mutations in PCSK9 markedly lower LDL-C levels. Injectable monoclonal antibodies against PCSK9 are capable of producing dramatic lowering of LDL cholesterol beyond that achieved with a statin alone.

1859. Nitroglycerin deteriorates with exposure to?
Can Med Assoc J. 1974;110(7):788-791

A. Air
B. Moisture
C. Sunlight
D. All of the above

Nitroglycerin deteriorates with exposure to air, moisture, and sunlight.

1860. Increase in which of the following causes relaxation of vascular smooth muscle?
Harrison's 20th Ed. Chapter 267 Page 1861

A. Guanosine diphosphate (GDP)
B. Guanosine triphosphate (GTP)
C. Cyclic guanosine monophosphate
D. Platelet guanylyl cyclase

When metabolized, organic nitrates release nitric oxide (NO) that binds to guanylyl cyclase in vascular smooth muscle cells, leading to an increase in cyclic guanosine monophosphate, which causes relaxation of vascular smooth muscle. Nitroglycerin and related nitrates used to treat angina produce vasodilation by elevating cyclic GMP.

1861. To minimize nitrate tolerance, patient should be kept free of the drug for a minimum of how many hours each day?
Harrison's 20th Ed. Chapter 267 Page 1861

A. 2 hours
B. 4 hours
C. 6 hours
D. 8 hours

In order to minimize the effects of nitrate tolerance, minimum effective dose should be used and a minimum of 8 hours each day kept free of the drug.

1862. β-adrenergic blocker can be discontinued with doses tapered over?
Harrison's 20th Ed. Chapter 267 Page 1861

A. 1 week
B. 2 weeks
C. 3 weeks
D. 4 weeks

Since sudden discontinuation of β-adrenergic blockers can intensify ischemia, its doses should be tapered over 2 weeks.

1863. Asymptomatic persons with severe coronary atherosclerosis include?
Harrison's 17th Ed. 1526

A. Patients with higher pain thresholds
B. Patients with higher endorphin levels
C. Diabetics with autonomic dysfunction
D. All of the above

Asymptomatic persons with severe coronary atherosclerosis who exhibit ST-segment changes during activity include those who exhibit higher thresholds to electrically induced pain, higher endorphin levels and diabetics with autonomic dysfunction.

1864. Which of the following drug is useful in the management of angina pectoris?
Harrison's 20th Ed. Chapter 267 Page 1862, Table 267–7

A. Betaxolol
B. Ranolazine
C. Pentaerythritol tetranitrate
D. All of the above

Betaxolol is a selective beta 1 blocker. Ranolazine casts its antianginal effect through blockage of late inward sodium current. Pentaerythritol tetranitrate is used sublingually for its antianginal effect.

1865. Sildenafil was initially developed as?

Harrison's 19th Ed. Page 43

A. Mast cell stabilizer
B. Bronchodilator
C. Antianginal drug
D. Antipletelet drug

Sildenafil was initially developed as an antianginal, but its effects to alleviate erectile dysfunction not only led to a new drug indication but also to increased understanding of the role of type 5 phosphodiesterase in erectile tissue. Sildenafil leads to inhibition of phosphodiesterase type 5 isoform that inactivates cyclic guanosine monophosphate (GMP) in the vasculature.

1866. Which of the following is a second-generation dihydropyridine calcium antagonist?

Harrison's 20th Ed. Chapter 267 Page 1861

A. Nicardipine
B. Isradipine
C. Felodipine
D. All of the above

1867. Which of the following is not a dihydropyridine calcium channel blocker?

Harrison's 20th Ed. Chapter 267 Page 1860, Table 267–6

A. Amlodipine
B. Felodipine
C. Diltiazem
D. Isradipine

1868. Which of the following is a nondihydropyridine calcium channel blocker?

Harrison's 20th Ed. Chapter 267 Page 1860, Table 267–6

A. Nicardipine
B. Nifedipine
C. Nisoldipine
D. Verapamil

1869. Which of the following calcium channel blocker has the longest duration of action?

Harrison's 20th Ed. Chapter 267 Page 1860, Table 267–6

A. Amlodipine
B. Isradipine
C. Nisoldipine
D. Nicardipine

1870. Which of the following calcium channel blocker may be associated with increased risk of mortality if administered during acute myocardial infarction?

Harrison's 20th Ed. Chapter 267 Page 1860, Table 267–6

A. Amlodipine
B. Diltiazem (Immediate release)
C. Nifedipine (Immediate release)
D. Verapamil (Immediate release)

Nifedipine (Immediate release) may be associated with increased risk of mortality if administered during acute myocardial infarction. In general, short-acting dihydropyridines should be avoided because of the risk of precipitating infarction, particularly in the absence of beta blockers.

ST-Segment Elevation Myocardial Infarction

1871. Who coined the term angina pectoris?

American Journal of Clinical Medicine. 2011;8(1):15

A. Carl Weigert
B. William Heberden
C. William Osler
D. George Dock

William Heberden coined the term angina pectoris in 1768. Carl Weigert in 1880 clearly correlated myocardial infarction as a disease of the coronary arteries. In 1910, Russian clinicians, Obraztsov and Strazhesko, actually documented clinical features of myocardial infarction in a living patient. In 1918, James Herrick was one of the first to encourage electrocardiography, which had been created by Einthoven in 1902.

1872. Acute coronary syndrome refers to?

N Engl J Med. 2006; 354:1524-1527

A. Myocardial infarction with ST-segment elevation
B. Myocardial infarction without ST-segment elevation
C. Unstable angina
D. All of the above

Acute coronary syndromes is defined as myocardial infarction with ST-segment elevation, myocardial infarction without ST-segment elevation, and unstable angina. They share a common pathophysiology i.e. atherosclerotic plaque rupture, erosion, or both with superimposed intracoronary thrombosis, commonly known as atherothrombosis.

1873. What percentage of acute myocardial infarction related deaths occur before the stricken individual reaches the hospital?

Harrison's 20th Ed. Chapter 269 Page 1872

A. ~ 10%
B. ~ 20%
C. ~ 30%
D. ~ 50%

About half of acute myocardial infarction (AMI)-related deaths occur before the stricken individual reaches the hospital.

1874. The in-hospital mortality rate after admission for acute myocardial infarction (AMI) is?

Harrison's 20th Ed. Chapter 269 Page 1873

A. ~ 1%
B. ~ 5%
C. ~ 10%
D. ~ 15%

The in-hospital mortality rate after admission for AMI is ~5%.

1875. The 1-year mortality rate after AMI is?

Harrison's 20th Ed. Chapter 269 Page 1873

A. ~ 1%
B. ~ 5%
C. ~ 10%
D. ~ 15%

The 1-year mortality rate after AMI is about 15%.

1876. AMI-related mortality is how many times higher in elderly patients (>75 years) as compared with younger patients?

Harrison's 20th Ed. Chapter 269 Page 1873

A. ~ 1 x
B. ~ 2 x
C. ~ 3 x
D. ~ 4 x

AMI-related mortality is ~ 4 times higher in elderly patients (>75 years) as compared with younger patients.

1877. Which of the following statements about acute coronary syndromes is false?

Harrison's 20th Ed. Chapter 269 Page 1873 Figure 269-1

A. Majority of patients with ST-segment elevation ultimately develop Q-wave on ECG (QwMI)
B. Majority of patients without ST-segment elevation (NSTEMI) ultimately develop Q-wave on ECG (QwMI)
C. Patients without ST-segment elevation are suffering from either unstable angina or a non-ST-segment elevation MI (NSTEMI)
D. None of the above

Of patients with ST-segment elevation, the majority ultimately develop a Q-wave on the ECG (QwMI). Majority of patients presenting with NSTEMI do not develop a Q-wave on the ECG.

1878. Histologically, coronary plaques prone to disruption are those with?

Harrison's 20th Ed. Chapter 269 Page 1873

A. Rich lipid core and thin fibrous cap
B. Rich lipid core and thick fibrous cap
C. Poor lipid core and thin fibrous cap
D. Poor lipid core and thick fibrous cap

Histologic studies indicate that the coronary plaques prone to disruption are those with a rich lipid core and a thin fibrous cap.

1879. Agonists that promote platelet activation at the site of ruptured plaque include all except?

Harrison's 20th Ed. Chapter 269 Page 1873

A. Collagen
B. ATP
C. Epinephrine
D. Serotonin

After an initial platelet monolayer forms at the site of the ruptured plaque, various agonists like collagen, ADP, epinephrine and serotonin promote platelet activation.

1880. Which of the following best describes thromboxane A_2?

Harrison's 20th Ed. Chapter 269 Page 1873

A. Adhesive protein
B. Local vasoconstrictor
C. Resistance to fibrinolysis
D. Platelet aggregator

At the site of disrupted plaque, agonists like collagen, ADP, epinephrine, serotonin promote platelet activation and from them thromboxane A_2 - a potent local vasoconstrictor is released and potential resistance to fibrinolysis develops.

1881. Fibrinogen can bind to how many platelets simultaneously?
Harrison's 20th Ed. Chapter 269 Page 1873

A. 1
B. 2
C. 3
D. 4

Fibrinogen is a multivalent molecule and can bind to two different platelets simultaneously, resulting in platelet cross-linking & aggregation.

1882. Cyclooxygenase is also known as?
N Engl J Med. 2001; 345:1809-1817

A. Prostaglandin G/H synthase
B. Prostaglandin D/E synthase
C. Prostaglandin M/N synthase
D. Prostaglandin U/V synthase

Aspirin acts by irreversibly acetylating a serine residue at position 529 in platelet prostaglandin G/H synthase, an enzyme colloquially known as cyclooxygenase.

1883. Out of the following, which is the least likely condition that increases risk of developing STEMI?
Harrison's 20th Ed. Chapter 269 Page 1874

A. Collagen vascular disease
B. Unstable angina
C. Cocaine abuse
D. Alcohol abuse

Patients at increased risk of developing STEMI include those with multiple coronary risk factors and those with unstable angina or Prinzmetal's variant angina. Less common underlying medical conditions predisposing patients to STEMI include hypercoagulability, collagen vascular disease, cocaine abuse, and intracardiac thrombi or masses that can produce coronary emboli.

1884. Which of the following best relates to management of STEMI?
Harrison's 20th Ed. Chapter 269 Page 1874

A. The linking theory
B. Attention to time
C. Chain of survival
D. The weak link

Management of STEMI aims at providing expeditious implementation of a reperfusion strategy through a highly integrated system termed as "chain of survival" which involves prehospital care that extends to early hospital management.

1885. STEMI tends to occur most commonly at?
Harrison's 20th Ed. Chapter 269 Page 1874

A. Early morning, few hours before awakening
B. Morning, within a few hours after awakening
C. After meals
D. Late evening, following return from work

Although STEMI may commence at any time of the day or night, circadian variations have been reported such that clusters are seen in the morning within a few hours of awakening.

1886. Which of the following is false regarding 'pain' in STEMI?
Harrison's 20th Ed. Chapter 269 Page 1874

A. Most common presenting complaint
B. Deep and visceral
C. Different in character to discomfort of angina pectoris
D. May radiate as high as occipital area

Pain is the most common presenting complaint in STEMI. Pain is deep & visceral. It is similar in character to discomfort of angina pectoris but is more severe, lasts longer and does not usually subside with cessation of activity. Typically. pain involves central portion of chest and/or epigastrium & on occasion it radiates to arms.

1887. Which of the following is false regarding 'pain' in STEMI?
Harrison's 20th Ed. Chapter 269 Page 1874

A. Does not radiate below umbilicus
B. May radiate to trapezius
C. Pain does not subside with cessation of activity
D. Painless STEMIs is greater in diabetics

Pain of STEMI may radiate as high as occipital area but not below umbilicus. Pain does not subside with cessation of activity, in contrast to angina pectoris. Radiation of discomfort to trapezius is not seen in patients with STEMI & distinguishes it from pericarditis. Painless STEMIs is more in diabetes mellitus, and it increases with age. In elderly, STEMI may present as sudden-onset breathlessness, which may progress to pulmonary edema.

1888. Which of the following best relates to acute coronary syndrome?
Br Med J 1964;2:688

A. Crum symnoni
B. Strum preci
C. Angor animi
D. Klent groci

Angor animi (also referred to as angina animi, Gardner's disease and also angina pectoris sine dolore), in medicine, is a symptom defined as a patient's perception that they are in fact dying.

1889. Sympathetic nervous system hyperactivity is more common in?
Harrison's 20th Ed. Chapter 269 Page 1874

A. Anterior infarction
B. Inferior infarction
C. Posterior infarction
D. Lateral infarction

1890. Parasympathetic nervous system hyperactivity is more common in?
Harrison's 20th Ed. Chapter 269 Page 1874

A. Anterior infarction
B. Inferior infarction
C. Posterior infarction
D. Lateral infarction

Combination of substernal chest pain lasting >30 minutes & diaphoresis suggests STEMI. 25% patients with anterior infarction have manifestations of sympathetic nervous system hyperactivity (tachycardia and/or hypertension), and up to one-half with inferior infarction show parasympathetic hyperactivity (bradycardia and/or hypotension).

1891. Which of the following is not an auscultatory finding in myocardial infarction?
Harrison's 20th Ed. Chapter 269 Page 1874

A. Decreased intensity of S1
B. Paradoxical splitting of S2
C. Early systolic apical systolic murmur
D. Pericardial friction rub

A transient midsystolic or late systolic apical systolic murmur due to dysfunction of the mitral valve apparatus may be present in myocardial infarction.

1892. In most patients with transmural myocardial infarction, systolic pressure declines by how much from the preinfarction state?

Harrison's 20th Ed. Chapter 269 Page 1874

A. ~ 5–10 mm Hg
B. ~ 10–15 mm Hg
C. ~ 15–20 mm Hg
D. ~ 20–25 mm Hg

In most patients with transmural myocardial infarction, systolic pressure declines by ~ 10—15 mm Hg from the preinfarction state.

1893. In temporal staging of myocardial infarction, acute stage is?

Harrison's 20th Ed. Chapter 269 Page 1874

A. First few hours
B. First few hours to 3 days
C. First few hours to 5 days
D. First few hours to 7 days

1894. In temporal staging of myocardial infarction, healing stage is?

Harrison's 20th Ed. Chapter 269 Page 1874

A. 3 to 10 days
B. 7 to 15 days
C. 10 to 21 days
D. 7 to 28 days

Myocardial infarction (MI) progresses through three temporal stages—acute (first few hours to 7 days), healing (7 to 28 days) and healed (≥ 29 days).

1895. Development of a Q wave on ECG is more dependent on?

Harrison's 20th Ed. Chapter 269 Page 1874

A. Transmurality of myocardial infarction
B. Volume of infarcted myocardial tissue
C. Thickness of the opposite myocardial wall
D. All of the above

Contemporary studies using MRI suggest that the development of a Q wave on the ECG is more dependent on the volume of infarcted myocardial tissue rather than transmurality of infarction.

1896. Which of the following was earliest to be used for diagnosis of patients with suspected myocardial infarction?

Chest 1997;111(1):1-3

A. Serum glutamic-oxaloacetic transaminase (SGOT)
B. Lactic dehydrogenase (LDH)
C. Creatine kinase (CK)
D. Troponin T

Serum glutamic-oxaloacetic transaminase (SGOT) assay was used for the diagnosis & management of patients with suspected myocardial infarction in 1954, followed by lactic dehydrogenase (LDH) isoenzymes in 1957, and creatine kinase (CK) in 1966 and CK isoenzyme analysis (CK-MB) in mid 70's.

1897. "I" in troponin I stands for?

J. Biol. Chem. 1973;248:2125-2133

A. Interactive
B. Inhibitory
C. Increased
D. In-situ

The nomenclature "troponin C (TnC), troponin I, and troponin T," for the three constituents of the troponin complex was coined in 1973, based on their functional properties ("C" for calcium binding, "I" for inhibitory, and "T" for tropomyosin binding). The inhibitory element within the troponin complex is TnI, which binds to actin-tropomyosin to inhibit actomyosin Mg++-ATPase in the absence of intracellular calcium.

1898. Which of the following about cardiac biomarkers is false?

Harrison's 20th Ed. Chapter 269 Page 1874

A. Detected in serum
B. Cardiac biomarkers are proteins
C. Released from necrotic heart muscle
D. None of the above

Serum cardiac biomarkers are proteins released from necrotic heart muscle after STEMI.

1899. Which of the following statements about troponins is false?

Chest 1997;111(1):1-3

A. Troponin complex is not found in smooth muscle
B. Cardiac troponin I has smaller molecular weight than troponin T
C. Cardiac troponin T varies from skeletal troponin T by a unique set of amino acids
D. None of the above

1900. Which of the following regulates muscle contraction in smooth muscle?

J. Biol. Chem. 1973;248:2125-2133

A. Thrombomodulin
B. Uromodulin
C. Calmodulin
D. Oxyntomodulin

Troponin complex is not found in smooth muscle, where calmodulin regulates muscle contraction.

1901. Levels of cTnI and cTnT may remain elevated for how many days after STEMI?

Harrison's 20th Ed. Chapter 269 Page 1875

A. 1 to 3 days
B. 2 to 5 days
C. 7 to 10 days
D. 10 to 21 days

Levels of cardiac-specific troponin T (cTnT) and cardiac-specific troponin I (cTnI) detected by highly specific monoclonal antibodies may remain elevated for 7 to 10 days after STEMI.

1902. After disruption of cardiomyocyte sarcolemmal membrane, biomarkers are released first from?

Harrison's 20th Ed. Chapter 269 Page 1873, Figure 269-3

A. Sarcolemma
B. Cytoplasmic pool
C. Mitochondria
D. Endoplasmic reticulum

After disruption of the sarcolemmal membrane of the cardiomyocyte, the cytoplasmic pool of biomarkers is released first.

1903. Cardiac biomarkers that are released into the interstitium are first cleared by?

Harrison's 20th Ed. Chapter 269 Page 1873, Figure 269-3

A. Arterioles
B. Venules
C. Capillaries
D. Lymphatics

Cardiac biomarkers that are released into the interstitium are first cleared by lymphatics followed subsequently by spillover into the venous system.

1904. Cardiac troponin levels rise to how many times the upper reference limit in "classic" acute myocardial infarction?

Harrison's 20th Ed. Chapter 269 Page 1873, Figure 269-3

A. ~ 20-50 times
B. ~ 100-200 times
C. ~ 200-500 times
D. ~ 500-1000 times

Cardiac troponin levels rise to about 20–50 times the upper reference limit in "classic" acute myocardial infarction (MI). cTn are found as structural (bound) proteins and as a small free pool that exists in the cytosol, which is about 6–8% for cTnT and 3.5% for cTnI.

1905. Cardiac troponins are particularly valuable in distinguishing?

Harrison's 20th Ed. Chapter 269 Page 1875

A. Angina pectoris from UA
B. UA from NSTEMI
C. NSTEMI from STEMI
D. All of the above

Cardiac troponins are of particular value in distinguishing UA from NSTEMI.

1906. Which of the following can elevate serum troponin concentrations?

Cleveland Clin J Med. 2018;85(4):274-277

A. Sepsis
B. Chemotherapy
C. Stress cardiomyopathy
D. All of the above

Sepsis, stroke, chronic kidney disease, pulmonary disease, chemotherapy, heart failure, and stress cardiomyopathy can all raise serum troponin concentrations.

1907. Which of the following chemotherapeutic agents is associated with cardiotoxicity?

Cleveland Clin J Med. 2018;85(4):274-277

A. Anthracyclines
B. Trastuzumab
C. Mitomycin
D. All of the above

Chemotherapeutic agents associated with cardiotoxicity include anthracyclines, trastuzumab, chlormethine, and mitomycin.

1908. In sepsis, troponin elevations are caused by?

Cleveland Clin J Med. 2018;85(4):274-277

A. Decreased clearance of troponin fragments by kidneys
B. Cytokine-induced cardiac damage
C. Increased endogenous & exogenous catecholamines damage cardiac myocytes
D. All of the above

Patients with a troponin elevation at the time of diagnosis of sepsis had a risk of death almost twice that of patients without a troponin elevation.

1909. Macrotroponin is composed of troponin I fragments and?

Cleveland Clin J Med. 2018;85(4):274-277

A. IgM antibodies
B. IgG antibodies
C. IgA antibodies
D. IgE antibodies

Macrotroponin, a molecule found in patients with autoantibodies against troponin I, is composed of troponin I fragments and IgG antibodies and can also cause a false-positive troponin immunoassay.

1910. Which of the following is a biomarker in acute myocardial infarction?

BMC Medicine 2010;8:34

A. C-terminal-provasopressin (Copeptin)
B. Heart-Type Fatty Acid Binding Protein (H-FABP)
C. Troponin T
D. All of the above

1911. Which of the following is a biomarker of plaque instability and inflammation?

BMC Medicine 2010;8:34

A. HsCRP (High-sensitivity C-reactive Protein)
B. Myeloperoxidase (MPO)
C. Pregnancy associated Plasma Protein A (PaPPA)
D. All of the above

1912. Which of the following biomarker is associated with cardiovascular death?

BMC Medicine 2010;8:34

A. NTproBNP
B. TIMP1
C. MMP 9
D. All of the above

1913. Which of the following about creatine kinase is false?

Clin Rheumatol. 2016 ;35(6):1541-1547

A. Enzyme
B. Primarily found in muscle tissue
C. Catalyzes conversion of creatine & ATP into phosphocreatine & ADP
D. None of the above

Creatine kinase is an enzyme primarily found in muscle tissue that catalyzes the conversion of creatine and adenosine triphosphate (ATP) into phosphocreatine and adenosine diphosphate (ADP).

1914. Which of the following about creatine kinase is false?

Cleveland Clin J Med. 2000;67(11):37-843

A. Better for detecting reinfarctions soon after the first event
B. More reliable for estimating the size of myocardial infarction
C. Clearance of CK-MB is not affected by renal function
D. None of the above

1915. Which of the following is true for levels of creatine phosphokinase (CK) in STEMI?

Harrison's 20th Ed. Chapter 269 Page 1875

A. Rises within 10 to 30 minutes
B. Rises within 30 minutes to 1 hour
C. Rises within 1 to 4 hours
D. Rises within 4 to 8 hours

1916. Which of the following is true for levels of creatine phosphokinase (CK) in STEMI?

Harrison's 20th Ed. Chapter 269 Page 1875

A. Returns to normal within 24 hours
B. Returns to normal by 24 to 48 hours
C. Returns to normal by 48 to 72 hours
D. Returns to normal by 72 to 96 hours

CK rises within 4 to 8 hours and generally returns to normal by 48 to 72 hours.

1917. What ratio (relative index) of CKMB mass : CK activity suggests myocardial infarction?

Harrison's 20th Ed. Chapter 269 Page 1875

A. ≥ 1.2
B. ≥ 1.8
C. ≥ 2.2
D. ≥ 2.5

A ratio (relative index) of CKMB mass : CK activity ≥2.5 "suggests" myocardial rather than a skeletal muscle source for the CKMB elevation.

1918. When patients with STEMI undergo reperfusion, which of the following is false about cardiac biomarkers?

Harrison's 20th Ed. Chapter 269 Page 1875

A. Are detected sooner
B. Rise to a higher peak value
C. Decline more rapidly
D. None of the above

When patients with STEMI undergo reperfusion, cardiac biomarkers are detected sooner, rise to a higher peak value, but decline more rapidly.

1919. Potential sources of total CK elevation are all except?

Cleve Clin J Med. 2016 ;83(1):37-42

A. Muscular dystrophy
B. Myopathies
C. Polymyositis
D. Hyperthyroidism

Hyperthyroidism is typically associated with normal serum CK concentrations.

1920. Potential sources of total CK elevation are all except?

Cleve Clin J Med. 2016 ;83(1):37-42

A. Alcohol binge
B. Hypothyroidism
C. Stroke
D. Prolonged immobilization

Potential sources of total CK elevation are skeletal muscular diseases (muscular dystrophy, myopathies and polymyositis), electrical cardioversion, hypothyroidism, stroke, surgery, skeletal muscle damage secondary to trauma, convulsions and prolonged immobilization.

1921. Mechanism of CK elevation in response to statins is?

Cleve Clin J Med. 2016 ;83(1):37-42

A. Increased muscle membrane fragility due to decreased cholesterol content
B. Inhibition of isoprenoid production
C. Depletion of ubiquinone
D. All of the above

Mechanisms of CK elevation in response to statins include increased muscle membrane fragility due to decreased cholesterol content, inhibition of isoprenoid production (step in synthesis of membrane proteins), and depletion of ubiquinone, leading to mitochondrial dysfunction.

1922. Macro CK type 1 is associated with?

Cleve Clin J Med. 2016 ;83(1):37-42

A. Malignancies
B. Autoimmune diseases
C. Skeletal trauma
D. Renal failure

Macro CK type 1 is found in ~1.2% of the general population. The complexes are composed of CK & immunoglobulin and are associated with autoimmune diseases. Macro CK type 2 complexes consist of CK and an undetermined protein and are associated with malignancies.

1923. Which of the following is false about myoglobin in STEMI?

Harrison's 20th Ed. Chapter 269 Page 1873, Figure 269-3

A. First serum cardiac markers to rise after STEMI
B. High cardiac specificity
C. Rapidly excreted in urine
D. Blood levels return to normal within 24 hours

Myoglobin and CK isoforms are one of the first serum cardiac markers that rises after STEMI but it lacks cardiac specificity. It is rapidly excreted in urine therefore blood levels return to normal range within 24 hours of the onset of myocardial infarction.

1924. Abnormalities of wall motion on 2D echocardiography are present in?

Harrison's 20th Ed. Chapter 269 Page 1875

A. Acute STEMI
B. Acute severe ischemia
C. Old myocardial scar
D. All of the above

Abnormalities of wall motion on 2D echocardiography are almost universally present in acute STEMI. They are also found in old myocardial scar or from acute severe ischemia.

1925. MI can be detected accurately with?

Harrison's 20th Ed. Chapter 269 Page 1876

A. Myocardial perfusion imaging with [201_{T1}]
B. Myocardial perfusion imaging with [$99m_{Tc}$] -sestamibi
C. Radionuclide ventriculography with [$99m_{Tc}$] - labeled RBCs
D. High-resolution cardiac MRI

1926. Which of the following about high-resolution cardiac MRI is false?

Harrison's 20th Ed. Chapter 269 Page 1876

A. Standard imaging agent is gadolinium
B. Little gadolinium enters normal myocardium
C. Produces bright signal in areas of infarction
D. None of the above

MI can be detected accurately with high-resolution cardiac MRI using a technique referred to as late enhancement. Infarct zone appears as a bright signal in areas of infarction that appears in stark contrast to the dark areas of normal myocardium.

1927. Which of the following appears in the criteria for acute Myocardial infarction?

Harrison's 20th Ed. Chapter 269 Page 1876 Table 269-1

A. RBBB
B. LBBB
C. CHB
D. All of the above

1928. In percutaneous coronary intervention (PCI)-related MI, cTn levels (with normal baseline values) rise by?

Harrison's 20th Ed. Chapter 269 Page 1876 Table 269-1

A. 2 times
B. 3 times
C. 4 times
D. 5 times

Percutaneous coronary intervention (PCI)-related MI is arbitrarily defined by elevation of cTn values >5 x 99th percentile URL in patients with normal baseline values.

1929. In percutaneous coronary intervention (PCI)-related MI, cTn levels (with elevated baseline values) rise by?

Harrison's 20th Ed. Chapter 269 Page 1876 Table 269-1

A. > 10%
B. > 20%
C. > 30%
D. > 40%

Percutaneous coronary intervention (PCI)-related MI is arbitrarily defined by a rise of cTn values >20% if the baseline values are elevated.

1930. In myocardial infarction associated with CABG, cTn levels rise by?

Harrison's 20th Ed. Chapter 269 Page 1876 Table 269-1

A. 3 times
B. 5 times
C. 10 times
D. 15 times

In myocardial infarction associated with CABG, cTn levels rise by >10 x 99th percentile URL.

1931. Spontaneous myocardial infarction related to atherosclerotic plaque rupture is classified as?

Harrison's 20th Ed. Chapter 269 Page 1877 Table 269-2

A. Type 1
B. Type 2
C. Type 3
D. Type 4a

1932. Myocardial infarction secondary to an ischemic imbalance is classified as?

Harrison's 20th Ed. Chapter 269 Page 1877 Table 269-2

A. Type 1
B. Type 2
C. Type 3
D. Type 4a

1933. Myocardial infarction related to percutaneous coronary intervention (PCI) is classified as?

Harrison's 20th Ed. Chapter 269 Page 1877 Table 269-2

A. Type 3
B. Type 4a
C. Type 4b
D. Type 5

1934. Myocardial infarction related to stent thrombosis is classified as?

Harrison's 20th Ed. Chapter 269 Page 1877 Table 269-2

A. Type 3
B. Type 4a
C. Type 4b
D. Type 5

1935. Myocardial infarction related to coronary artery bypass grafting (CABG) is classified as?

Harrison's 20th Ed. Chapter 269 Page 1877 Table 269-2

A. Type 3
B. Type 4a
C. Type 4b
D. Type 5

1936. Most out-of-hospital deaths from STEMI are due to the sudden development of?

Harrison's 20th Ed. Chapter 269 Page 1876

A. Ventricular asystole
B. Ventricular fibrillation
C. Complete heart block
D. Torsades de pointes

Most out-of-hospital deaths from STEMI are due to the sudden development of ventricular fibrillation, mostly within the first 24 hours of the onset of symptoms, and of these, over half occur in the first hour.

1937. The greatest delay in obtaining hospital care in patients with suspected STEMI occurs in?

Harrison's 20th Ed. Chapter 269 Page 1876

A. Between onset of pain & patient's decision to call for help
B. Transportation to the hospital
C. Emergency department
D. Cardiac catheterization laboratory

The greatest delay usually occurs not during transportation to the hospital but, rather, between the onset of pain and the patient's decision to call for help. The goal is to minimize time from first medical contact (FMC) to initiation of reperfusion therapy within 120 minutes.

1938. In the Emergency department, the goals for the management of patients with suspected STEMI is?

Harrison's 20th Ed. Chapter 269 Page 1876

A. Control of cardiac discomfort
B. Identification of patients for urgent reperfusion therapy
C. Avoidance of inappropriate discharge of patients with STEMI
D. All of the above

In Emergency department, goals for management of patients with suspected STEMI include control of cardiac discomfort, rapid identification of patients who are candidates for urgent reperfusion therapy, triage of lower-risk patients to appropriate location in hospital, & avoidance of inappropriate discharge of patients with STEMI.

1939. Angiography & revascularization should not be performed within how many hours after administration of fibrinolytic therapy?

Harrison's 20th Ed. Chapter 269 Page 1878 Figure 269-4

A. First half - 1 hour
B. First 1 - 2 hours
C. First 2 - 3 hours
D. First 3 - 6 hours

Angiography and revascularization should not be performed within the first 2 - 3 hours after administration of fibrinolytic therapy.

1940. Who is credited for the concept of low doses of aspirin in myocardial infarction?

American Journal of Clinical Medicine. 2011;8(1):15

A. Carl Weigert
B. Lawrence Craven
C. William Osler
D. George Dock

In 1950, Lawrence Craven, a general practitioner in Glendale, California hypothesized that aspirin was preventive of coronary thrombosis. However, Craven's work languished in obscurity for decades.

1941. Aspirin is effective in?
Harrison's 20th Ed. Chapter 269 Page 1876

A. Unstable angina
B. NSTEMI
C. STEMI
D. All of the above

Aspirin is essential in the management of patients with suspected STEMI and is effective across the entire spectrum of acute coronary syndromes.

1942. Aspirin should be given in a dose of?
Harrison's 20th Ed. Chapter 269 Page 1876

A. 75–162 mg
B. 160–325 mg
C. 325–625 mg
D. 625–1000 mg

Aspirin must be given immediately in doses of 160-325 mg to inhibit cyclooxygenase-1 in platelets with reduction of thromboxane A2 levels. This should be followed by daily oral administration of aspirin in a dose of 75 - 162 mg.

1943. In acute MI patients with hypoxemia, O_2 is administered by nasal prongs or face mask at the rate of?
Harrison's 20th Ed. Chapter 269 Page 1877

A. 2–4 L/minute
B. 4–6 L/minute
C. 6–8 L/minute
D. 8–10 L/minute

In STEMI patients, whose arterial O_2 saturation is normal, supplemental O_2 is of limited clinical benefit. When hypoxemia is present, O_2 is given by nasal prongs or face mask @ 2 - 4 L/minute for the first 6 to 12 hours after infarction and then according to the situation.

1944. In STEMI, three doses of sublingual nitroglycerin (0.4 mg) should be administered at an interval of?
Harrison's 20th Ed. Chapter 269 Page 1877

A. 5 minutes
B. 10 minutes
C. 30 minutes
D. One hour

Sublingual nitroglycerin can be given safely to most patients with STEMI. Up to three doses of 0.4 mg should be administered at about 5 minute intervals.

1945. Therapy with nitrates in STEMI should be avoided in?
Harrison's 20th Ed. Chapter 269 Page 1877

A. Low systolic arterial pressure (< 90 mm Hg)
B. When there is clinical suspicion of RV infarction
C. Who have taken 'sildenafil' within preceding 24 hours
D. All of the above

Therapy with nitrates is avoided in MI patients who have low systolic arterial pressure (<90 mm Hg), if RV infarction is suspected, in patients who have taken phosphodiesterase-5 inhibitor sildenafil within the preceding 24 hours since it may potentiate the hypotensive effects of nitrates.

1946. Which of the following raises clinical suspicion of right ventricular (RV) infarction?
Harrison's 20th Ed. Chapter 269 Page 1877

A. Inferior infarction on ECG
B. Elevated jugular venous pressure
C. Clear lungs
D. All of the above

Clinical suspicion of RV infarction is indicated by inferior infarction on ECG, elevated jugular venous pressure, clear lungs & hypotension.

1947. Idiosyncratic hypotensive reaction to nitrates is reversed promptly by?
Harrison's 20th Ed. Chapter 269 Page 1877

A. IV Calcium gluconate
B. IV Atropine
C. IV Norepinephrine
D. IV Fluids

An idiosyncratic reaction to nitrates, consisting of sudden marked hypotension can be reversed promptly by the rapid administration of intravenous atropine.

1948. Which of the following about morphine in acute MI is false?
Harrison's 20th Ed. Chapter 269 Page 1877

A. Morphine has a vagotonic effect
B. May cause advanced heart block particularly in patients with anterior wall infarction
C. Shoule be given IV rather than subcutaneously
D. None of the above

Morphine has vagotonic effect & may cause bradycardia or advanced degrees of heart block particularly in patients with posteroinferior infarction. These side effects respond to atropine. Morphine is routinely administered by repetitive (every 5 min) intravenous injection of small doses (2–4 mg) rather than by subcutaneous administration of a larger quantity, because absorption may be unpredictable by subcutaneous route.

1949. Which of the following about IV β-blockers in acute MI is false?
Harrison's 20th Ed. Chapter 269 Page 1877

A. Useful in the control of pain of STEMI
B. Reduce the risks of reinfarction
C. Reduce the risks of ventricular fibrillation
D. None of the above

Intravenous beta blockers are useful in the control of pain of STEMI by diminishing myocardial O2 demand & ischemia. Intravenous beta blockers reduce risks of reinfarction & ventricular fibrillation.

1950. In acute MI, IV metoprolol is given as?
Harrison's 20th Ed. Chapter 269 Page 1877

A. 5 mg every 2–5 minutes for a total of three doses
B. 10 mg every 2–5 minutes for a total of five doses
C. 5 mg every 10–15 minutes for a total of three doses
D. 5 mg every 10–15 minutes for a total of five doses

A commonly employed regimen is metoprolol, 5 mg every 2-5 minutes for a total of three doses, provided the patient has a heart rate >60 beats/minute, systolic pressure > 100 mm Hg, a PR interval <0.24 seconds and rales that are no higher than 10 cm up from the diaphragm. Fifteen minutes after the last intravenous dose, an oral regimen is initiated of 50 mg every 6 hours for 48 hours, followed by 100 mg every 12 hours.

1951. Which of the following has no role in the control of chest discomfort in STEMI?
Harrison's 20th Ed. Chapter 269 Page 1877

A. Sublingual nitroglycerin
B. Morphine
C. Beta blockers
D. Calcium antagonists

Calcium antagonists are of little value in acute setting of STEMI. Short-acting dihydropyridines may be associated with an increased mortality risk.

1952. After fibrinolytic therapy, angiography & revascularization should not be performed for?

Harrison's 20th Ed. Chapter 269 Page 1878 Figure 269-4

A. 1 to 2 hours
B. 2 to 3 hours
C. 3 to 4 hours
D. 4 to 6 hours

Angiography and revascularization should not be performed within the first 2 to 3 hours after administration of fibrinolytic therapy.

1953. Reperfusion therapy is not helpful in?

Harrison's 20th Ed. Chapter 269 Page 1877

A. ST-segment ↑ of ≥ 2 mm in 2 contiguous precordial leads
B. ST-segment ↑ of ≥ 1 mm in two adjacent limb leads
C. Absence of ST-segment elevation
D. None of the above

In the absence of ST-segment elevation, fibrinolysis is not helpful, and it may be harmful.

1954. In STEMI, the goal is to keep total ischemic time within?

Harrison's 20th Ed. Chapter 269 Page 1878 Figure 269-4

A. 30 minutes
B. 60 minutes
C. 90 minutes
D. 120 minutes

In STEMI, the goal is to keep total ischemic time within 120 minutes.

1955. ECG finding in a patient of acute MI that makes a candidate suitable for reperfusion therapy is?

Harrison's 20th Ed. Chapter 269 Page 1877

A. ST-segment elevation of at least 1 mm in two contiguous precordial leads
B. ST-segment elevation of at least 2 mm in two contiguous precordial leads
C. ST-segment elevation of at least 1 mm in three contiguous precordial leads
D. ST-segment elevation of at least 2 mm in three contiguous precordial leads

The primary tool for screening patients and making triage decisions is the initial 12-lead ECG. When ST-segment elevation of at least 2 mm in two contiguous precordial leads and 1 mm in two adjacent limb leads is present, a patient should be considered candidate for reperfusion therapy. In the absence of ST-segment elevation, fibrinolysis is not helpful, in fact harmful.

1956. What proportion of patients with STEMI may achieve spontaneous reperfusion of infarct-related coronary artery within 24 hours?

Harrison's 20th Ed. Chapter 269 Page 1877

A. One - fourth
B. One - third
C. One - half
D. Two - third

Up to one–third of patients with STEMI may achieve spontaneous reperfusion of the infarct-related coronary artery within 24 hours.

1957. Which of the following extends the "window" of time for salvage of myocardium by reperfusion strategies?

Harrison's 20th Ed. Chapter 269 Page 1878

A. Treatment of congestive heart failure (CHF)
B. Minimization of tachycardia
C. Control of hypertension
D. All of the above

Protection of the ischemic myocardium by maintenance of an optimal balance between myocardial O_2 supply & demand through pain control, treatment of congestive heart failure, and minimization of tachycardia & hypertension extends the "window" of time for salvage of myocardium by reperfusion strategies.

1958. Which of the following drugs should be avoided in patients with STEMI?

Harrison's 20th Ed. Chapter 269 Page 1878

A. Glucocorticoids
B. Nonsteroidal anti-inflammatory agents
C. Short-acting dihydropyridines calcium antagonists
D. All of the above

1959. Glucocorticoids are deleterious in patients with STEMI due to?

Harrison's 20th Ed. Chapter 269 Page 1878

A. They impair infarct healing & result in a larger infarct scar
B. They increase the risk of myocardial rupture
C. They increase coronary vascular resistance
D. All of the above

Glucocorticoids & nonsteroidal anti-inflammatory agents (other than aspirin), should be avoided in STEMI as they impair infarct healing resulting in a larger infarct scar & increase the risk of myocardial rupture. They also increase coronary vascular resistance, thereby potentially reducing flow to ischemic myocardium.

1960. In STEMI, the golden hour refers to?

Am Heart J. 2010;160(6):1079-84

A. First 15 minutes
B. First 30 minutes
C. First 60 minutes
D. First 180 minutes

1961. The first description of the coronary care unit (CCU) was given by?

American Journal of Clinical Medicine. 2011;8(1):15

A. Carl Weigert
B. Lawrence Craven
C. Desmond Julian
D. George Dock

The very first description of the coronary care unit (CCU) was presented to the British Thoracic Society in July 1961 by Desmond Julian.

1962. A cardiologist is considered as an "experienced operator" if he has does how many percuteneous coronary intervention (PCI) cases per year?

Heart 2004;90:e37

A. ≥ 15
B. ≥ 25
C. ≥ 50
D. ≥ 75

A cardiologist is considered as an "experienced operator" if he does ≥75 percutaneous coronary intervention (PCI) cases per year.

1963. A cardiological unit is considered as a "dedicated medical center" if it does how many percuteneous coronary intervention (PCI) cases per year?

Heart 2004;90:e37

A. ≥ 5
B. ≥ 15
C. ≥ 25
D. ≥ 33

A cardiological unit is considered as a "dedicated medical center" if it does ≥33 percutaneous coronary intervention (PCI) cases per year.

1964. Primary PCI is preferred over fibrinolysis when?

Harrison's 20th Ed. Chapter 269 Page 1878

A. Diagnosis is in doubt
B. Cardiogenic shock is present
C. Bleeding risk is increased
D. All of the above

Primary PCI is preferred over fibrinolysis when the diagnosis is in doubt, cardiogenic shock is present, bleeding risk is increased, or symptoms have been present for at least 2 - 3 hours when the clot is more mature and less easily lysed by fibrinolytic drugs.

1965. In STEMI, fibrinolytic therapy should ideally be initiated within?

Harrison's 20th Ed. Chapter 269 Page 1878

A. 10 minutes of presentation
B. 30 minutes of presentation
C. 60 minutes of presentation
D. 90 minutes of presentation

In STEMI, fibrinolytic therapy should ideally be initiated within 30 minutes of presentation (door-to-needle time 30 minutes) with a principal goal to promptly restore full coronary arterial patency (TIMI grade 3).

1966. Value of reducing delay time between onset of symptoms and initiation of treatment was illustrated by?

American Journal of Clinical Medicine. 2011;8(1):15

A. GISSI-2
B. ISIS-3
C. GUSTO-1
D. All of the above

GISSI-2, ISIS-3, and GUSTO-1 concluded that the choice of thrombolytic therapy was much less important to ultimate survival than was the delay time between onset of symptoms and initiation of treatment.

1967. Which of the following is a characteristic of an ideal fibrinolytic agent?

American Journal of Clinical Medicine. 2011;8(1):15

A. One that would achieve 100% patency in a short time period
B. Has minimal bleeding complications
C. Improves microvascular function and flow
D. All of the above

1968. Which of the following fibrinolytic agent acts by promoting conversion of plasminogen to plasmin?

Harrison's 20th Ed. Chapter 269 Page 1878

A. Tissue plasminogen activator (tPA)
B. Streptokinase
C. Tenecteplase (TNK)
D. All of the above

Tissue plasminogen activator (tPA), streptokinase, tenecteplase (TNK) & reteplase (rPA) are fibrinolytic agents that act by promoting conversion of plasminogen to plasmin, which subsequently lyses fibrin thrombi.

1969. Which of the following is a 'bolus fibrinolytic' agent?

Harrison's 20th Ed. Chapter 269 Page 1878

A. Streptokinase
B. Tenecteplase (TNK)
C. Urokinase
D. Tissue plasminogen activator (tPA)

1970. Which of the following is a 'bolus fibrinolytic' agent?

Harrison's 20th Ed. Chapter 269 Page 1878

A. Streptokinase
B. Reteplase (rPA)
C. Urokinase
D. Tissue plasminogen activator (tPA)

Tenecteplase (TNK) & reteplase (rPA) are bolus fibrinolytics since their administration does not require a prolonged intravenous infusion.

1971. Angiographically flow in the culprit coronary artery is assessed by which of the following grading system?

Harrison's 20th Ed. Chapter 269 Page 1878

A. TIMI
B. ISIS
C. CURE
D. CAPRIE

When assessed angiographically, flow in the culprit coronary artery is described by a simple qualitative scale called the thrombolysis in myocardial infarction (TIMI) grading system.

1972. Method of angiographic assessment of the efficacy of fibrinolysis is?

Harrison's 20th Ed. Chapter 269 Page 1879

A. TIMI flow grade
B. TIMI frame count
C. TIMI myocardial perfusion grade
D. All of the above

Qualitative scale to angiographically assess flow in the culprit coronary artery is the thrombolysis in myocardial infarction (TIMI) grading system. Grade 0 - complete occlusion of infarct-related artery (IRA), grade 1 - some penetration of contrast material beyond the point of obstruction but without perfusion of distal coronary bed, grade 2 - perfusion of entire infarct vessel into distal bed, but with flow that is delayed compared with that of a normal artery and grade 3 - full perfusion of the infarct vessel with normal flow. Additional methods of angiographic assessment of efficacy of fibrinolysis include counting the number of frames on cine film required for dye to flow from the origin of the IRA to a landmark in distal vascular bed (TIMI frame count) and determining the rate of entry and exit of contrast dye from microvasculature in myocardial infarct zone (TIMI myocardial perfusion grade).

1973. Which TIMI flow grade indicates full perfusion of infarct vessel with normal flow following reperfusion therapy?

Harrison's 20th Ed. Chapter 269 Page 1879

A. TIMI 1
B. TIMI 2
C. TIMI 3
D. TIMI 4

TIMI grade 3 indicates full perfusion of the infarct vessel with normal flow which is the goal of reperfusion therapy.

1974. In STEMI, fibrinolytic therapy can reduce the relative risk of in-hospital death by up to?

N Engl J Med. 2013;368:1379-87

A. 10%
B. 25%
C. 50%
D. 75%

In STEMI, fibrinolytic therapy can reduce the relative risk of in-hospital death by up to 50% when administered within the first hour of the onset of symptoms. Benefit is maintained for at least 10 years.

1975. Which of the following is given as a "single" weight-based intravenous bolus?
Harrison's 20th Ed. Chapter 269 Page 1879

A. Tissue plasminogen activator (tPA)
B. Reteplase (rPA)
C. Tenecteplase (TNK)
D. Streptokinase (STK)

TNK is given as a "single" weight-based intravenous bolus of 0.53 mg/kg over 10 seconds.

1976. Which of the following fibrinolytic agent is administered in a double-bolus regimen?
Harrison's 20th Ed. Chapter 269 Page 1879

A. Tissue plasminogen activator (tPA)
B. Reteplase (rPA)
C. Tenecteplase (TNK)
D. Streptokinase (STK)

tPA is given as a 15 mg bolus followed by 50 mg intravenously over the first 30 minutes, followed by 35 mg over the next 60 minutes. Streptokinase is administered as 1.5 million units (MU) intravenously over 1 hour. rPA is administered in a double-bolus regimen consisting of a 10-MU bolus given over 2 - 3 minutes, followed by a second 10-MU bolus 30 minutes later.

1977. Combination reperfusion regimens involve giving a fibrinolytic agent with which of the following?
Harrison's 20th Ed. Chapter 269 Page 1879

A. Aspirin
B. Clopidogrel
C. Intravenous glycoprotein IIb/IIIa inhibitor
D. Percutaneous coronary intervention (PCI)

Combination reperfusion regimens for coronary reperfusion combine an intravenous glycoprotein IIb/IIIa inhibitor with a reduced dose of a fibrinolytic agent.

1978. Clear contraindications to the use of fibrinolytic agents are all except?
Harrison's 20th Ed. Chapter 269 Page 1879

A. Cerebrovascular hemorrhage at any time
B. Nonhemorrhagic stroke at any time
C. Suspicion of aortic dissection
D. Active internal bleeding

Clear contraindications to the use of fibrinolytic agents include a history of cerebrovascular hemorrhage at any time, a nonhemorrhagic stroke or other cerebrovascular event within the past year, marked hypertension (>180/110 mm Hg) at any time during acute presentation, suspicion of aortic dissection, and active internal bleeding (excluding menses).

1979. In STEMI, which of the following is a relative contraindication to fibrinolytic therapy?
Harrison's 20th Ed. Chapter 269 Page 1879

A. Current use of anticoagulants (INR >=2)
B. Pregnancy
C. Hemorrhagic diabetic retinopathy
D. All of the above

Relative contraindications to fibrinolytic therapy, which require clinical consideration of risk:benefit ratio include current use of anticoagulants (INR >=2), a recent (<2 weeks) invasive or surgical procedure or prolonged (>10 minute) cardiopulmonary resuscitation, known bleeding diathesis, pregnancy, a hemorrhagic ophthalmic condition (hemorrhagic diabetic retinopathy), active peptic ulcer disease, and a history of severe hypertension that is currently adequately controlled.

1980. For what period, streptokinase should not be given, if the patient has received it in past?
Harrison's 20th Ed. Chapter 269 Page 1879

A. Never in life
B. 5 days to 2 years
C. 1 to 2 years
D. 3 to 5 years

Because of the risk of an allergic reaction, patients should not receive streptokinase if that agent had been received within the preceding 5 days to 2 years.

1981. Allergic reactions to streptokinase occur in about what percentage of patients who receive it?
Harrison's 20th Ed. Chapter 269 Page 1879

A. 1%
B. 2%
C. 3%
D. 4%

Allergic reactions to streptokinase occur in ~2% of patients who receive it.

1982. Minor degree of hypotension occurs in what percentage of patients who receive streptokinase?
Harrison's 20th Ed. Chapter 269 Page 1879

A. 4–10%
B. 10–16%
C. 16–30%
D. 30–40%

Minor hypotension occurs in 4 - 10% of patients given STK, marked hypotension occurs rarely.

1983. Hemorrhagic stroke occurs in about what percentage of patients who receive streptokinase?
Harrison's 20th Ed. Chapter 269 Page 1879

A. 0.1–0.5%
B. 0.5–0.9%
C. 0.9–1.5%
D. 1.5–2.4%

Hemorrhagic stroke, the most serious complication, occurs in ~0.5 - 0.9% of patients receiving fibrinolytic agents. Rate of intracranial hemorrhage with tPA or rPA is slightly higher than with STK.

1984. Integrated approach in the management of STEMI addresses patients to receive?
Harrison's 20th Ed. Chapter 269 Page 1879

A. Fibrinolytic therapy
B. Percutaneous coronary intervention (PCI)
C. Coronary artery bypass grafting (CABG)
D. All of the above

Prior approaches that segregated pharmacologic and catheter-based approaches to reperfusion have been replaced with an integrated approach to triage & transfer of STEMI patients to receive PCI.

1985. Failure of reperfusion refers to persistent chest pain & ST-segment elevation beyond?

Harrison's 20th Ed. Chapter 269 Page 1879

A. > 30 minutes
B. > 60 minutes
C. > 90 minutes
D. > 120 minutes

Cardiac catheterization & coronary angiography should be carried out after fibrinolytic therapy if there is evidence of failure of reperfusion, which means persistent chest pain & ST-segment elevation >90 minutes. Rescue PCI should be considered in such a situation.

1986. Development of recurrent ischemia is handled by?

Harrison's 20th Ed. Chapter 269 Page 1879

A. Rescue PCI
B. Urgent PCI
C. Elective PCI
D. Any of the above

1987. Patients with confirmed STEMI and low risk may be safely transferred out of the coronary care unit within?

Harrison's 20th Ed. Chapter 269 Page 1879

A. 6 hours
B. 12 hours
C. 24 hours
D. 48 hours

Patients with confirmed STEMI & low risk (no prior MI & no persistent chest discomfort, CHF, hypotension or cardiac arrhythmias) may be safely transferred out of CCU within 24 hours.

1988. Patients with STEMI should be kept at bed rest for the first?

Harrison's 20th Ed. Chapter 269 Page 1879

A. 3–6 hours
B. 6–12 hours
C. 12–24 hours
D. 24–48 hours

Patients with STEMI should be at bed rest for the first 6–12 hours. In the absence of complications, patients should be encouraged, under supervision, to resume an upright posture by dangling their feet over the side of the bed & sitting in a chair within the first 24 hours. By day 3 after MI, patients should increase their ambulation progressively to a goal of 185 meters (600 ft) three times a day.

1989. STEMI patients should receive either nothing or only clear liquids by mouth for the first?

Harrison's 20th Ed. Chapter 269 Page 1879

A. 4-6 hours
B. 4-8 hours
C. 4-10 hours
D. 4-12 hours

STEMI patients should receive either nothing or only clear liquids by mouth for the first 4–12 hours.

1990. The typical coronary care unit diet should provide?

Harrison's 20th Ed. Chapter 269 Page 1879

A. ≤ 30% of total calories as fat
B. Cholesterol content should be ≤ 300 mg/day
C. Complex carbohydrates should be 50—55% of total calories
D. All of the above

The typical coronary care unit diet should provide ≤30% of total calories as fat and have a cholesterol content of ≤300 mg/day. Complex carbohydrates should make up 50–55% of total calories.

1991. In STEMI, diet rich in which of the following is recommended?

Harrison's 20th Ed. Chapter 269 Page 1879

A. Potassium
B. Magnesium
C. Fiber
D. All of the above

In STEMI, foods that are high in potassium, magnesium, and fiber, but low in sodium are recommended.

1992. Which of the following drugs used in coronary care unit can produce delirium, particularly in the elderly?

Harrison's 20th Ed. Chapter 269 Page 1880

A. Atropine
B. H_2 blockers
C. Narcotics
D. All of the above

Atropine, H2 blockers & narcotics can produce delirium, particularly in the elderly.

1993. In STEMI, goal of treatment with antiplatelet and anticoagulant agents is?

Harrison's 20th Ed. Chapter 269 Page 1880

A. To maintain patency of infarct-related artery (IRA)
B. To reduce likelihood of mural thrombus formation
C. To reduce likelihood of deep venous thrombosis
D. All of the above

1994. Data from Antiplatelet Trialists' Collaboration shows a relative reduction in mortality of how much in patients with MI receiving antiplatelet agents?

Harrison's 20th Ed. Chapter 269 Page 1880

A. 12%
B. 21%
C. 27%
D. 34%

Data from Antiplatelet Trialists' Collaboration patients with MI showed a relative reduction of 27% in mortality rate, from 14.2% in control patients to 10.4% in patients receiving antiplatelet agents.

1995. In STEMI, the maximum recommended dose of unfractionated heparin (UFH) given as an initial bolus is?

Harrison's 20th Ed. Chapter 269 Page 1880

A. 2500 U
B. 4000 U
C. 5000 U
D. 7500 U

1996. In STEMI, the maximum recommended dose of unfractionated heparin (UFH) given after the initial bolus is?

Harrison's 20th Ed. Chapter 269 Page 1880

A. 500 U / hour
B. 1000 U / hour
C. 1500 U / hour
D. 2000 U / hour

1997. In STEMI, with the use of UFH, activated partial thromboplastin time during maintenance therapy should be?

Harrison's 20th Ed. Chapter 269 Page 1880

A. 1.5 times the control value
B. 1.5–2 times the control value
C. 2.5–3 times the control value
D. 3–3.5 times the control value

In STEMI, the recommended dose of unfractionated heparin (UFH) is an initial bolus of 60 U/kg (maximum 4000 U) followed by an initial infusion of 12 U/kg per hour (maximum 1000 U/hour). Activated partial thromboplastin time during maintenance therapy should be 1.5 - 2 times the control value.

1998. In STEMI, which of the following can be used as an alternative to UFH for anticoagulation?
Harrison's 20th Ed. Chapter 269 Page 1880

A. Fondaparinux
B. Bivalirudin
C. Enoxaparin
D. All of the above

Advantages of low-molecular-weight heparin (LMWH) preparations include high bioavailability permitting subcutaneous administration, reliable anticoagulation without monitoring, and greater antiXa:IIa activity.

1999. Unique pentasaccharide sequence of heparin consists of?
The Journal of Biological Chemistry. 2009; 284(40):27054-27064

A. D-fructosamine and hexosamine
B. D-nitrosamine and N-acetylglucosamine
C. D-glucosamine and uronic acid
D. D-glucuronic acid and N-acetyl-D-glucosamine

2000. Which of the following is essential for heparin for binding and activating antithrombin?
The Journal of Biological Chemistry. 2009; 284(40):27054-27064

A. 1-O-sulfo group
B. 2-O-sulfo group
C. 3-O-sulfo group
D. 4-O-sulfo group

The key structural unit of heparin is a unique pentasaccharide sequence which consists of three D-glucosamine and two uronic acid residues. The central D-glucosamine residue contains a unique 3-O-sulfo moiety that is rare outside of this sequence. Removal of unique 3-O-sulfo group results in complete loss of the anticoagulant activity.

2001. Which of the following about fondaparinux is false?
N Engl J Med. 2006; 354:1524-1527

A. Synthetic pentasaccharide
B. Inhibits factor Xa within clot, prevents thrombus progression
C. Does not inhibit platelet function
D. None of the above

2002. Which of the following about fondaparinux is false?
Harrison's 20th Ed. Chapter 269 Page 1880

A. Synthetic version of the pentasaccharide sequence of heparin
B. Should not be used alone during PCI
C. Does not cause heparin-induced thrombocytopenia
D. None of the above

2003. The first LMW heparin was?
N Engl J Med. 2006; 354:1524-1527

A. Enoxaparin
B. Dalteparin
C. Parnaparin
D. Tinzaparin

2004. Which of the following about LMW heparin is false?
Harrison's 20th Ed. Chapter 269 Page 1880

A. LMWH is prepared from unfractionated heparin
B. Mean molecular weight of LMWH is about 5000
C. LMWH is cleared almost exclusively by the kidneys
D. None of the above

2005. Which of the following clinical trials evaluated fondaparinux in STEMI?
Harrison's 20th Ed. Chapter 269 Page 1880, N Engl J Med. 2006; 354:1524-1527

A. OASIS-2
B. OASIS-4
C. OASIS-6
D. OASIS-8

In Organization to Assess Strategies in Acute Ischemic Syndromes (OASIS-6) trial, fondaparinux was compared with a control group treated with UFH (N= 3221) & patients who had myocardial infarction with ST-segment elevation and who presented relatively late (N= 12,902). Primary end point of death or reinfarction at 30 days was significantly lower in the fondaparinux group.

2006. Which of the under mentioned myocardial infarction has an increased risk of systemic or pulmonary thromboembolism?
Harrison's 20th Ed. Chapter 269 Page 1880

A. Anterior
B. Inferior
C. Posterior
D. Lateral

Patients with anterior myocardial infarction, severe LV dysfunction, heart failure, history of embolism, 2D echocardiographic evidence of mural thrombus or atrial fibrillation are at increased risk of systemic or pulmonary thromboembolism.

2007. In STEMI, acute intravenous beta blockade leads to?
Harrison's 20th Ed. Chapter 269 Page 1880

A. Improvement in the myocardial O_2 supply-demand relationship
B. Decrease in chest pain
C. Reduces infarct size
D. All of the above

In STEMI, acute intravenous beta blockade improves the myocardial O2 supply-demand relationship, decreases pain, reduces infarct size, and decreases the incidence of serious ventricular arrhythmias.

2008. In STEMI patients who undergo fibrinolysis, beta blockers do not reduce?
Harrison's 20th Ed. Chapter 269 Page 1880

A. Mortality rate
B. Recurrent ischemia
C. Reinfarction
D. None of the above

In STEMI patients who undergo fibrinolysis soon after onset of chest pain, no incremental reduction in mortality rate is seen with beta blockers, but recurrent ischemia and reinfarction are reduced.

2009. STEMI patients with excellent long-term prognosis are?

Harrison's 20th Ed. Chapter 269 Page 1880

A. Patients <55 years
B. Patients with no previous MI
C. Patients with normal ventricular function
D. All of the above

STEMI patients with excellent long–term prognosis are those with an expected mortality rate of <1% per year, patients <55 years, no previous MI, with normal ventricular function, no complex ventricular ectopy, and no angina.

2010. High-risk STEMI patients are?

Harrison's 20th Ed. Chapter 269 Page 1880

A. Those who are elderly
B. Those who have an anterior infarction
C. Those who have had a prior infarction
D. All of the above

2011. ACE inhibitors should be continued indefinitely in patients who have?

Harrison's 20th Ed. Chapter 269 Page 1881

A. Clinically evident CHF
B. In patients with reduction in global LV function
C. In patients with a large regional wall motion abnormality
D. All of the above

ACE inhibitors should be continued indefinitely in patients who have clinically evident CHF, in patients with a reduction in global LV function (LV ejection fraction ≤40%) or a large regional wall motion abnormality, or in hypertensive individuals.

2012. Which of the following medication is least useful during the first 24-48 hours after the onset of myocardial infarction?

Harrison's 20th Ed. Chapter 269 Page 1881

A. Intravenous nitroglycerin
B. Angiotensin-converting enzyme (ACE) inhibitors
C. Beta blockers
D. Unfractionated heparin (UFH)

Benefits of routine use of intravenous nitroglycerin are less in contemporary era where beta-adrenoceptor blockers & ACE inhibitors are routinely prescribed for patients with STEMI.

2013. In STEMI, serum levels of which of the following should be corrected to minimize the risk of arrhythmias?

Harrison's 20th Ed. Chapter 269 Page 1881

A. Calcium
B. Potassium
C. Magnesium
D. All of the above

Serum magnesium should be measured in all patients of STEMI on admission, and any deficits should be corrected to minimize the risk of arrhythmias.

2014. After STEMI, left ventricle undergoes changes in which of the following in noninfarcted segments?

Harrison's 20th Ed. Chapter 269 Page 1881

A. Shape
B. Size
C. Thickness
D. All of the above

After STEMI, left ventricle undergoes a series of changes in shape, size & thickness in both, infarcted and noninfarcted segments, a process referred to as ventricular remodeling.

2015. Overall cardiac chamber enlargement is more following infarction of?

Harrison's 20th Ed. Chapter 269 Page 1881

A. Inferior wall
B. Posterior wall
C. Anterior wall
D. Any of the above

Overall cardiac chamber enlargement is more following infarction of anterior wall & apex of left ventricle.

2016. Which of the following is the primary cause of in-hospital death from STEMI?

Harrison's 20th Ed. Chapter 269 Page 1881

A. Pump failure
B. Arrhythmia
C. Thromboembolism
D. Sepsis

Presently, pump failure is the primary cause of in-hospital death from STEMI.

2017. Early mortality in STEMI refers to death within how many days of infarction?

Harrison's 20th Ed. Chapter 269 Page 1881

A. 3 days
B. 7 days
C. 10 days
D. 14 days

Early mortality in STEMI refers to death within 10 days of infarction.

2018. The most common clinical signs of pump failure is?

Harrison's 20th Ed. Chapter 269 Page 1881

A. Tachycardia
B. Hypotension
C. Pulmonary rales
D. Raised JVP

The most common clinical signs of pump failure are pulmonary rales and S3 / S4 gallop sounds.

2019. Which of the following is the characteristic hemodynamic finding of pump failure?

Harrison's 20th Ed. Chapter 269 Page 1881

A. Elevated LV filling volume
B. Elevated RV filling volume
C. Elevated RA pressure
D. Elevated pulmonary artery pressure

Elevated LV filling pressure & elevated pulmonary artery pressure are the characteristic hemodynamic findings of pump failure.

2020. Patients with rales at lung bases, S3 gallop, tachypnea, or signs of right heart failure belong to which Killip class?

Harrison's 20th Ed. Chapter 269 Page 1881

A. Killip class I
B. Killip class II
C. Killip class III
D. Killip class IV

Killip classification divides patients into four groups. Class I–no signs of pulmonary or venous congestion, class II–rales at lung bases, S3 gallop, tachypnea, or signs of right heart failure, class III–severe heart failure, pulmonary edema and class IV–shock with systolic pressure <90 mm Hg, peripheral vasoconstriction, peripheral cyanosis, mental confusion, and oliguria.

2021. Infarction of what percentage of left ventricle results in cardiogenic shock?

Harrison's 20th Ed. Chapter 269 Page 1881

A. About 20%
B. About 30%
C. About 35%
D. About 40%

Hemodynamic evidence of abnormal LV function appears when contraction is seriously impaired in 20 to 25% of the left ventricle. Infarction of ≥40% of left ventricle results in cardiogenic shock.

2022. After STEMI, which of the following is an ideal class of drugs for the long-term management of ventricular dysfunction?

Harrison's 20th Ed. Chapter 269 Page 1881

A. Diuretics
B. Digitalis
C. Nitrates
D. ACE inhibitors

ACE inhibitors are an ideal class of drugs for the long term management of ventricular dysfunction after STEMI.

2023. Incidence of cardiogenic shock is?

Harrison's 20th Ed. Chapter 269 Page 1882

A. ~ 1%
B. ~ 3%
C. ~ 5%
D. ~ 7%

The incidence of cardiogenic shock is ~7%. In recent years, practice of prompt reperfusion, efforts to reduce infarct size and treatment of ongoing ischemia and other complications of MI contributed to the reduction.

2024. In STEMI, what proportion of patients present with cardiogenic shock on admission?

Harrison's 20th Ed. Chapter 269 Page 1882

A. 1%
B. 5%
C. 10%
D. 20%

Only 10% of patients with STEMI present with cardiogenic shock on admission. 90% develop it during hospitalization.

2025. Which of the following is not true for cardiogenic shock?

Harrison's 20th Ed. Chapter 269 Page 1882

A. Sustained systolic arterial pressure of <60 mm Hg
B. Cardiac index < 2.2 L/(min/m_2)
C. Elevated pulmonary capillary wedge pressure (>18 mm Hg)
D. Generally associated with mortality rate of >50%

Cardiogenic shock (CS) is characterized by systemic hypoperfusion due to severe depression of cardiac index [<2.2 (L/min)/m2] & sustained systolic arterial hypotension (<90 mm Hg), despite an elevated filling pressure (PCWP > 18 mm Hg). In-hospital mortality rate is >50%.

2026. Clinically significant RV infarction can cause?

Harrison's 20th Ed. Chapter 269 Page 1882

A. Jugular venous distention
B. Kussmaul's sign
C. Hepatomegaly
D. All of the above

Approximately one-third of patients with inferior infarction demonstrate at least a minor degree of RV necrosis. Clinically significant RV infarction causes signs of severe RV failure i.e. jugular venous distention, Kussmaul's sign, hepatomegaly with or without hypotension.

2027. Which of the following ECG lead is most helpful in diagnosing right ventricular myocardial infarction?

Harrison's 20th Ed. Chapter 269 Page 1882

A. V_1R
B. V_2R
C. V_3R
D. V_4R

ST-segment elevations of right-sided precordial ECG leads, particularly lead V_4R, are frequently present in the first 24 hours in patients with RV infarction.

2028. What is true for right ventricular myocardial infarction?

Harrison's 20th Ed. Chapter 269 Page 1882

A. Associated with occlusion of proximal RCA
B. ST-segment elevation of >1 mm in lead V_4R
C. Upright T wave in lead V_4R during initial hours
D. All of the above

2029. Catheterization study in a patient with right ventricular myocardial infarction resembles?

Harrison's 20th Ed. Chapter 269 Page 1882

A. Constrictive pericarditis
B. Pericardial effusion
C. Cardiac tamponade
D. Any of the above

In RV infarction, catheterization study of the right side of heart resembles constrictive pericarditis i.e. steep right atrial "y" descent and an early diastolic dip & plateau in RV waveforms.

2030. Objective of therapy for RV infarction is?

Harrison's 20th Ed. Chapter 269 Page 1882

A. To maintain adequate RV preload
B. To reduce pulmonary capillary wedge
C. To reduce pulmonary arterial pressures
D. All of the above

Therapy for RV infarction consists of volume expansion to maintain adequate RV preload, efforts to improve LV performance with attendant reduction in pulmonary capillary wedge & pulmonary arterial pressures.

2031. Mechanisms responsible for infarction-related arrhythmias is?

Harrison's 20th Ed. Chapter 269 Page 1882

A. Autonomic nervous system imbalance
B. Electrolyte disturbances
C. Slowed conduction in zones of ischemic myocardium
D. All of the above

The mechanisms responsible for infarction-related arrhythmias include autonomic nervous system imbalance, electrolyte disturbances, ischemia and slowed conduction in zones of ischemic myocardium.

2032. Warning arrhythmia refers to?

Harrison's 20th Ed. Chapter 269 Page 1882

A. Early systolic ventricular extrasystoles
B. Early diastolic ventricular extrasystoles
C. Late systolic ventricular extrasystoles
D. Late diastolic ventricular extrasystoles

2033. Which of the following is effective in abolishing ventricular ectopic activity in patients with STEMI?

Harrison's 20th Ed. Chapter 269 Page 1882

A. Nitrates
B. Beta-adrenoceptor blocking agents
C. Inhibitors of the $P2Y_{12}$ ADP receptor
D. Digitalis

Beta-adrenoceptor blocking agents are effective in abolishing ventricular ectopic activity in patients with STEMI and in the prevention of ventricular fibrillation.

2034. In patients with STEMI, serum magnesium should be adjusted to?
Harrison's 20th Ed. Chapter 269 Page 1882

A. ~ 1.0 mmol / L
B. ~ 2.0 mmol / L
C. ~ 3.0 mmol / L
D. ~ 4.0 mmol / L

Hypokalemia and hypomagnesemia are risk factors for ventricular fibrillation in patients with STEMI. To reduce the risk, serum potassium concentration should be adjusted to ~4.5 mmol/L and magnesium to ~2.0 mmol/L.

2035. Prophylactic use of lidocaine in STEMI increases?
Harrison's 20th Ed. Chapter 269 Page 1882

A. Overall mortality
B. Risk of bradycardia
C. Risk of asystole
D. All of the above

2036. Ventricular tachycardia or fibrillation refractory to electroshock is more responsive after patient is treated with?
Harrison's 20th Ed. Chapter 269 Page 1882

A. Epinephrine
B. Bretylium
C. Amiodarone
D. All of the above

Ventricular tachycardia or fibrillation that is refractory to electroshock may be more responsive after patient is treated with epinephrine (1 mg intravenously or 10 mL of a 1:10,000 solution via the intracardiac route), bretylium (5 mg/kg bolus) or amiodarone (75 to 150 mg bolus).

2037. Torsades des pointes may occur in patients with STEMI with the use of?
Harrison's 20th Ed. Chapter 269 Page 1882

A. Amiodarone
B. Lidocaine
C. Quinidine
D. All of the above

Torsades des pointes may occur in patients with STEMI as a consequence of hypoxia, hypokalemia, or co-administration of digoxin or quinidine.

2038. Which of the following about accelerated idioventricular rhythm (AIVR) is false?
Harrison's 20th Ed. Chapter 269 Page 1882

A. Benign
B. Occurs transiently during fibrinolytic therapy
C. Ventricular rate is 60–100 beats/minute
D. None of the above

Accelerated idioventricular rhythm (AIVR) or "slow ventricular tachycardia" is a ventricular rhythm with a rate of 60- 100 beats/minute. It often occurs transiently during fibrinolytic therapy at the time of reperfusion. AIVR is benign and does not presage the development of classic ventricular tachycardia. Most episodes of AIVR do not require treatment.

2039. Synchronized electroshock is recommended if supraventricular abnormal rhythm persists for?
Harrison's 20th Ed. Chapter 269 Page 1882

A. > 2 hours
B. > 6 hours
C. > 12 hours
D. > 24 hours

If supraventricular abnormal rhythm persists for >2 hours with a ventricular rate > 120 beats/minute, or if tachycardia induces heart failure, shock, or ischemia, a synchronized electroshock (100-200 J monophasic waveform) should be used.

2040. Which of the following about accelerated junctional rhythms is false?
Harrison's 20th Ed. Chapter 269 Page 1882

A. Occur in patients with inferoposterior infarction
B. Occur in patients with digitalis excess
C. Right atrial or coronary sinus pacing is indicated
D. None of the above

2041. Heart block in inferior infarction results from the release of?
Harrison's 20th Ed. Chapter 269 Page 1882

A. Adenosine
B. Bradykinin
C. Natriuretic peptide
D. All of the above

Heart block in inferior infarction results from increased vagal tone and/or the release of adenosine and therefore is transient.

2042. Implantable cardioverter/defibrillator (ICD) is recommended for which of the following?
Harrison's 19th Ed. 1609, Figure 295-5

A. LVEF is <30-40% and NYHA class II
B. LVEF is <30-40% and NYHA class III
C. LVEF is <30-35% and NYHA class I
D. All of the above

Patients with depressed left ventricular function at least 40 days post-STEMI are referred for insertion of an implantable cardioverter/defibrillator (ICD) if the LVEF is <30–40% with NYHA class II-III or if LVEF is <30–35% with NYHA class I functional status. Patients with preserved left ventricular function (LVEF >40%) do not receive an ICD regardless of NYHA functional class.

2043. Which of the following is false about recurrent post STEMI angina?
Harrison's 20th Ed. Chapter 269 Page 1884

A. Develops in ~25% of patients hospitalized for STEMI
B. More frequent in those who have successful fibrinolysis
C. Repeat fibrinolysis is an alternative
D. None of the above

Recurrent angina develops in ~25% of patients hospitalized for STEMI. It is even higher in patients who undergo successful fibrinolysis. Repeat administration of a fibrinolytic agent is an alternative to early mechanical revascularization.

2044. Pain of pericarditis radiates to?
Harrison's 20th Ed. Chapter 269 Page 1884

A. Right trapezius muscle
B. Left trapezius muscle
C. Both trapezius muscles
D. Any of the above

Pain radiating to either trapezius muscle is typical of pericarditis.

2045. Complication of LV aneurysm is?

Harrison's 20th Ed. Chapter 269 Page 1882

A. CHF
B. Arterial embolism
C. Ventricular arrhythmias
D. All of the above

Complications of LV aneurysm do not usually occur for weeks to months after STEMI. They include CHF, arterial embolism and ventricular arrhythmias. Apical aneurysms are the most common.

2046. Maximal (symptom limited) exercise stress test may be carried out how many weeks after myocardial infarction?

Harrison's 20th Ed. Chapter 269 Page 1882

A. 2-4 weeks
B. 4-6 weeks
C. 6-10 weeks
D. 10-12 weeks

Maximal (symptom limited) exercise stress test may be carried out 4-6 weeks after myocardial infarction to detect residual ischemia and ventricular ectopy.

2047. Usual duration of hospitalization for an uncomplicated STEMI is about?

Harrison's 20th Ed. Chapter 269 Page 1882

A. 3 days
B. 5 days
C. 7 days
D. 10 days

Usual duration of hospitalization for an uncomplicated STEMI is about 5 days.

2048. Intravenous antiplatelet drugs include?

Journal of Blood Medicine 2012:3:33-42

A. Abciximab
B. Eptifibatide
C. Tirofiban
D. All of the above

Three potent parenteral GpIIb/IIIa inhibitors are Abciximab (chimeric monoclonal Fab fragment of human & murine protein that binds to GpIIb/IIIa), Eptifibatide (synthetic cyclic heptapeptide with a KGD sequence) and Tirofiban (synthetic peptidomimetic based on the RGD sequence).

2049. ATP in "National Cholesterol Education Project ATP III" stands for?

N Engl J Med. 2014; 370:1422-1431

A. Adult Treatment Panel
B. Advanced Treatment Panel
C. Aggressive Treatment Panel
D. Angina Treatment Panel

Adult Treatment Panel III (ATP III).

2050. The technique "Percutaneous transluminal coronary angioplasty" (PTCA) was first introduced by?

N Engl J Med. 2001; 344:144-145

A. Andreas Gruentzig
B. Denton Cooley
C. Michael DeBakey
D. Christian Bernard

In 1977, Andreas Gruentzig introduced percutaneous transluminal coronary angioplasty (PTCA).

2051. During percutaneous coronary intervention (PCI), steerable guidewire put into coronary artery lumen has a diameter of?

BMJ. 2003;326(7399):1137-1140

A. < 0.4 mm
B. < 0.6 mm
C. < 0.8 mm
D. < 1 mm

During PCI, steerable guidewire put into coronary artery lumen has a diameter of < 0.4 mm.

2052. What suggests involvement of right coronary artery rather than left circumflex artery as the culprit vessel in inferior MI?

N Engl J Med. 2003;348:933-40

A. Greater ST-segment elevation in lead II than in lead III & ST-segment depression of >1 mm in leads I & aVL
B. Greater ST-segment elevation in lead III than in lead II & ST-segment depression of >1 mm in leads I & aVL
C. Greater ST-segment elevation in lead aVF than in lead II or III & ST-segment depression of >1 mm in leads I & aVL
D. Greater ST-segment elevation in lead II & III than in lead aVF & ST-segment depression of >1 mm in leads I & aVL

2053. In inferior MI, ST-segment depression in leads V1 and V2 suggest concomitant infarction of?

N Engl J Med. 2003;348:933-40

A. Lateral wall of left ventricle
B. Posterior wall of left ventricle
C. Anterior wall of left ventricle
D. Atrial infarction

2054. Most sensitive electrocardiographic sign of right ventricular infarction is?

N Engl J Med. 2003;348:933-40

A. ST-segment elevation of >1 mm in V_4R with upright T wave during first 12 hours
B. ST-segment elevation of >1 mm in V_4R with inverted T wave during first 12 hours
C. ST-segment elevation of >1 mm in V_4R with upright T wave after first 12 hours
D. ST-segment elevation of >1 mm in V_4R with inverted T wave after first 12 hours

2055. Proximal occlusion of the left anterior descending artery is indicated by?

N Engl J Med. 2003;348:933-40

A. Anterior wall MI, ST elevation in V_1, V_2, and V_3
B. Anterior wall MI, ST elevation in V_1, V_2, and V_3 & aVL
C. Anterior wall MI, ST elevation in V_1, V_2, V_3 & aVL with ST depression of >1 mm in lead aVF
D. Anterior wall MI, ST elevation in V_1, V_2, V_3 & aVL with ST depression of >1 mm in lead II, III and aVF

2056. Which of the following statements about blood supply of sinus node is true?

N Engl J Med. 2003;348:933-40

A. Supplied by RCA in 60% of people and by the left circumflex artery in 40%
B. Supplied by RCA in 40% of people and by left circumflex artery in 60%
C. Supplied by RCA in 80% of people and by left circumflex artery in 20%
D. Supplied by RCA in 60% of people and by left anterior descending artery in 40%

2057. Which of the following statements about blood supply of atrioventricular node is true?

N Engl J Med. 2003;348:933-40

A. Supplied by RCA in 50% of people and by left circumflex artery in 50%
B. Supplied by RCA in 60% of people and by left circumflex artery in 40%
C. Supplied by RCA in 75% of people and by left circumflex artery in 25%
D. Supplied by RCA in 90% of people and by left circumflex artery in 10%

2058. Which of the following statements about blood supply of bundle of His is true?

N Engl J Med. 2003;348:933-40

A. Supplied by atrioventricular nodal branch of LAD
B. Supplied by atrioventricular nodal branch of RCA + septal perforators of LAD
C. Supplied by atrioventricular nodal branch of left circumflex artery + septal perforators of LAD
D. Supplied by septal branch of left circumflex artery

2059. Which of the following statements about blood supply of right bundle branch is true?

N Engl J Med. 2003;348:933-40

A. Supplied by septal perforators of LAD
B. Supplied by septal perforators of RCA
C. Supplied by septal perforators of left circumflex artery
D. None of the above

2060. Which of the following is an electrocardiographic predictor of myocardial reperfusion following thrombolysis?

N Engl J Med. 2003;348:933-40

A. T-wave inversion in < 4 hours after MI
B. ST-segment resolution during first 90 minutes
C. Accelerated idioventricular rhythm
D. All of the above

Hypertensive Vascular Disease

2061. According to JNC 7, stage 2 hypertension is?
N Engl J Med. 2006;355:385-92

A. 120/80 mm Hg
B. 140-159/90-99
C. ≥ 160/100 mm Hg
D. 180/110 mm Hg

2062. Isolated systolic hypertension is defined as a systolic pressure of >=140 mm Hg and a diastolic pressure below?
N Engl J Med. 2006;355:385-92

A. 70 mm Hg
B. 80 mm Hg
C. 90 mm Hg
D. 100 mm Hg

2063. Among adults, diastolic blood pressure increases progressively until what age, after which it tends to decrease?
Harrison's 20th Ed. Chapter 271 Page 1891

A. ~ 45 years
B. ~ 55 years
C. ~ 65 years
D. ~ 75 years

Among adults, diastolic blood pressure increases progressively with age until ~55 years, after which it tends to decrease.

2064. The probability that a middle-aged or elderly individual will develop hypertension in his or her lifetime is?
Harrison's 20th Ed. Chapter 271 Page 1891

A. 10%
B. 30%
C. 60%
D. 90%

Probability that a middle-aged / elderly individual will develop hypertension in lifetime is 90%.

2065. Which of the following statements about age-related increase of blood pressure is false?
Harrison's 20th Ed. Chapter 271 Page 1891

A. Augmented by high NaCl intake
B. Augmented by low dietary intakes of calcium
C. Augmented by low dietary intakes of potassium
D. None of the above

Hypertension prevalence is related to dietary NaCl intake, & age-related increase of BP is augmented by high NaCl intake. Low dietary intakes of calcium & potassium contribute to risk of hypertension.

2066. Which of the following is a stronger correlate of blood pressure?
Harrison's 20th Ed. Chapter 271 Page 1891

A. Urine sodium
B. Urine potassium
C. Urine sodium-to-potassium ratio
D. All of the above

The urine sodium-to-potassium ratio is a stronger correlate of blood pressure than is either sodium or potassium alone.

2067. High BP before age 55 occurs how many times more frequently among persons with a positive family history of hypertension?
Harrison's 19th Ed. 1612

A. 1.8 times
B. 2.8 times
C. 3.8 times
D. 4.8 times

High blood pressure before age 55 occurs 3.8 times more frequently among persons with a positive family history of hypertension.

2068. Which of the following is considered as a hypertension-related gene?
Harrison's 20th Ed. Chapter 271 Page 1891

A. Alpha-adducin gene
B. MDR1 gene
C. NAT2 gene
D. All of the above

Alpha adducin gene encodes a cytoskeletal protein important for renal tubular sodium absorption. It is thought to be associated with increased renal tubular absorption of sodium, and variants of this gene may be associated with hypertension and salt sensitivity of blood pressure.

2069. Which of the following best relate to the genetics of hypertension?
Harrison's 20th Ed. Chapter 271 Page 1891

A. Epigenetic signature
B. Epigenetic reset
C. Epigenetic dysregulation
D. Epigenetic imprint

2070. Hypertension-related genes relate to?
Harrison's 20th Ed. Chapter 271 Page 1891

A. Renin-angiotensin aldosterone system
B. Atrial natriuretic peptide
C. Beta-2 adrenoreceptor
D. All of the above

2071. Which of the following genes is possibly related to hypertension?
Harrison's 20th Ed. Chapter 271 Page 1891

A. Gene encoding AT_1 receptor
B. Gene encoding aldosterone synthase
C. Gene encoding β_2 adrenoreceptor
D. All of the above

Genes possibly related to hypertension include genes encoding the AT1 receptor, aldosterone synthase, atrial natriuretic peptide and the b2 adrenoreceptor.

2072. Which of the following statements about genesis of hypertension is false?
Harrison's 20th Ed. Chapter 271 Page 1892

A. Vascular volume is a primary determinant of arterial pressure over the long term
B. Nonchloride salts of sodium have little or no effect on blood pressure
C. Salt-wasting disorders are associated with low blood pressure levels
D. None of the above

2073. Which of the following modulate blood pressure over the short term?
Harrison's 20th Ed. Chapter 271 Page 1892

A. Adrenergic reflexes
B. Hormonal factors
C. Volume-related factors
D. All of the above

Adrenergic reflexes modulate blood pressure over the short term. Adrenergic function, in concert with hormonal & volume-related factors contributes to long-term regulation of arterial pressure.

2074. Which of the following is an endogenous catecholamine?
Harrison's 20th Ed. Chapter 271 Page 1892, British J of Pharmacology. 2012;165:2015-2033

A. Norepinephrine
B. Epinephrine
C. Dopamine
D. All of the above

The three endogenous catecholamines are norepinephrine, epinephrine, and dopamine. They play important roles in tonic and phasic cardiovascular regulation.

2075. The activities of the adrenergic receptors are mediated by?
Harrison's 20th Ed. Chapter 271 Page 1892

A. Receptor Tyrosine Kinase
B. Cytokine Receptor–Linked Kinase
C. Guanosine nucleotide-binding regulatory proteins
D. Serine Kinase

The activities of adrenergic receptors are mediated by guanosine nucleotide-binding regulatory proteins (G proteins) & by intracellular concentrations of downstream second messengers.

2076. Physiologic responsiveness to catecholamines depends on?
Harrison's 20th Ed. Chapter 271 Page 1892

A. Receptor affinity
B. Receptor density
C. Receptor-effector coupling efficiency
D. All of the above

2077. When activated by catecholamines, which of the following receptors act as negative feedback controllers, inhibiting further norepinephrine release?
Harrison's 20th Ed. Chapter 271 Page 1892

A. α_1
B. α_2
C. β_1
D. β_2

When activated by catecholamines, α_2 receptors act as negative feedback controllers, inhibiting further norepinephrine release.

2078. In the kidney, activation of which of the following increases renal tubular reabsorption of sodium?
Harrison's 20th Ed. Chapter 271 Page 1892

A. α_1-adrenergic receptors
B. α_2-adrenergic receptors
C. β_1-adrenergic receptors
D. β_2-adrenergic receptors

In kidney, activation of a_1-adrenergic receptors increases renal tubular reabsorption of sodium.

2079. Activation of which of the following receptors by epinephrine relaxes vascular smooth muscle leading to vasodilation?
Harrison's 20th Ed. Chapter 271 Page 1892

A. α_1
B. α_2
C. β_1
D. β_2

Activation of b_2 receptors by epinephrine relaxes vascular smooth muscle & results in vasodilation.

2080. Antihypertensive agents act as?
Harrison's 20th Ed. Chapter 271 Page 1892

A. α_1 receptor inhibitors
B. α_2 receptor agonists
C. β_1 receptor inhibitors
D. Any of the above

2081. Which of the following about clonidine is false?
Harrison's 20th Ed. Chapter 271 Page 1892

A. Antihypertensive agent
B. Centrally acting α_1 agonist
C. Inhibits sympathetic outflow
D. Abrupt cessation of therapy leads to rebound hypertension due to upregulation of α_1 receptors

Clonidine is a centrally acting α2 agonist.

2082. The autonomic nervous system maintains cardiovascular homeostasis via which of the following signals?
Harrison's 20th Ed. Chapter 271 Page 1892

A. Pressure signals
B. Volume signals
C. Chemoreceptor signals
D. All of the above

The autonomic nervous system maintains cardiovascular homeostasis via pressure, volume, and chemoreceptor signals.

2083. Which of the following is false about Renin?
Harrison's 20th Ed. Chapter 271 Page 1892

A. Prorenin is an enzymatically inactive precursor
B. Synthesized in renal afferent renal arteriole
C. Plasma contains 2–5 times more prorenin than renin
D. None of the above

2084. Which of the following is not a primary stimuli for renin secretion?
Harrison's 20th Ed. Chapter 271 Page 1892

A. Decreased NaCl transport in thick ascending limb of loop of Henle
B. Increased NaCl transport in thick ascending limb of loop of Henle
C. Decreased pressure or stretch within renal afferent arteriole
D. Sympathetic nervous system stimulation of renin-secreting cells via beta$_1$ adrenoreceptors

Three primary stimuli for renin secretion are decreased NaCl transport in thick ascending limb of loop of Henle (macula densa mechanism), decreased pressure or stretch within renal afferent arteriole (baroreceptor mechanism), and sympathetic nervous system stimulation of renin-secreting cells via beta1 adrenoreceptors. Renin secretion is inhibited by increased NaCl transport in thick ascending limb of loop of Henle.

2085. Renin is best related to which of the following?
Harrison's 20th Ed. Chapter 271 Page 1892

A. Metallo-protease
B. Aspartyl protease
C. Cysteine protease
D. Serine protease

Renin is an aspartyl protease that is synthesized as an enzymatically inactive precursor called prorenin.

2086. Most renin in the circulation is synthesized in?
Harrison's 20th Ed. Chapter 271 Page 1892

A. Renal afferent renal arteriole
B. Renal efferent renal arteriole
C. Glomeruli
D. All of the above

Most renin in the circulation is synthesized in the renal afferent renal arteriole.

2087. Which of the following directly inhibits renin secretion?
Harrison's 20th Ed. Chapter 271 Page 1892

A. Angiotensin I
B. Angiotensin II
C. Angiotensinogen
D. Prorenin

Angiotensin II directly inhibits renin secretion due to angiotensin II type 1 receptors on juxtaglomerular cells. Renin secretion increases in response to pharmacologic blockade of ACE or angiotensin II receptors.

2088. Which of the following statements is false?
Harrison's 20th Ed. Chapter 271 Page 1893

A. Angiotensin I is an inactive decapeptide
B. Angiotensin II is an active octapeptide
C. ACE-kininase II is located in pulmonary circulation
D. ACE-kininase II activates bradykinin

In circulation, active renin cleaves angiotensinogen to form an inactive decapeptide, angiotensin I. ACE-kininase II is a converting enzyme, located primarily in pulmonary circulation, converts angiotensin I to active octapeptide, angiotensin II. It also inactivates vasodilator bradykinin.

2089. Which of the following statements is false about angiotensin II?
Harrison's 20th Ed. Chapter 271 Page 1893

A. Acts on angiotensin II type 1 receptors on cell membranes
B. Potent pressor substance
C. Stimulates secretion of aldosterone
D. None of the above

2090. Which of the following is a functional effect of angiotensin II type 2 receptor (AT_2)?
Harrison's 20th Ed. Chapter 271 Page 1893

A. Vasodilation
B. Sodium excretion
C. Inhibition of cell growth & matrix formation
D. All of the above

Angiotensin II type 2 (AT_2) receptor is widely distributed in kidneys and has the opposite functional effects of AT_1 receptor. AT_2 receptor induces vasodilation, sodium excretion and inhibition of cell growth and matrix formation.

2091. Which of the following is a renin-secreting tumor?
Harrison's 20th Ed. Chapter 271 Page 1893

A. Germinoma
B. Benign hemangiopericytoma
C. Choriocarcinoma
D. Osteoblastoma

Renin-secreting tumors include benign hemangiopericytomas of the juxtaglomerular apparatus, renal carcinomas & Wilms tumors.

2092. Renin-producing carcinomas may be found in?
Harrison's 20th Ed. Chapter 271 Page 1893

A. Lung
B. Liver
C. Pancreas
D. All of the above

Renin-producing carcinomas have been described in lung, liver, pancreas, colon and adrenals.

2093. Angiotensinogen, renin, and angiotensin II are also synthesized locally in?
Harrison's 20th Ed. Chapter 271 Page 1893

A. Uterus
B. Brain
C. Spleen
D. All of the above

Angiotensinogen, renin, and angiotensin II are also synthesized locally in brain, pituitary, aorta, arteries, heart, adrenal glands, kidneys, adipocytes, leukocytes, ovaries, testes, uterus, spleen, and skin.

2094. Angiotensin II in tissues may be formed by the enzymatic activity of?
Harrison's 20th Ed. Chapter 271 Page 1893

A. Tonin
B. Chymase
C. Cathepsins
D. All of the above

Angiotensin II in tissues may be formed by the enzymatic activity of renin or by other proteases like tonin, chymase, and cathepsins.

2095. Which of the following is the primary trophic factor regulating synthesis & secretion of aldosterone by zona glomerulosa of adrenal cortex?
Harrison's 20th Ed. Chapter 271 Page 1893

A. Potassium
B. Adrenocorticotropic hormone (ACTH)

C. Angiotensin II
D. All of the above

Angiotensin II is the primary trophic factor regulating synthesis & secretion of aldosterone by zona glomerulosa of adrenal cortex. Aldosterone synthesis is also dependent on potassium and acute elevations of adrenocorticotropic hormone (ACTH).

2096. Excess tissue angiotensin II contributes to?
Harrison's 20th Ed. Chapter 271 Page 1893

A. Atherosclerosis
B. Cardiac hypertrophy
C. Renal failure
D. All of the above

Excess tissue angiotensin II contributes to atherosclerosis, cardiac hypertrophy & renal failure.

2097. Which of the following best relates to angiotensin II?
Harrison's 20th Ed. Chapter 271 Page 1893

A. Anaphylactoid reaction
B. Mitogen
C. Thrombocytopenia
D. Hyperlipidemia

Tissue angiotensin II is a mitogen that stimulates growth and contributes to modeling and repair.

2098. Which of the following influence the synthesis & secretion of aldosterone by zona glomerulosa of adrenal cortex?
Harrison's 20th Ed. Chapter 271 Page 1893

A. Angiotensin II
B. Potassium
C. Adrenocorticotropic hormone (ACTH)
D. All of the above

2099. Which of the following is the primary tropic factor regulating synthesis & secretion of aldosterone by zona glomerulosa?
Harrison's 20th Ed. Chapter 271 Page 1893

A. Angiotensin II
B. Potassium
C. Adrenocorticotropic hormone (ACTH)
D. All of the above

Angiotensin II is the primary tropic factor regulating synthesis & secretion of aldosterone by zona glomerulosa of adrenal cortex. Aldosterone secretion may be decreased in potassium-depleted individuals. Acute elevations of adrenocorticotropic hormone (ACTH) increase aldosterone secretion.

2100. Aldosterone increases sodium reabsorption by?
Harrison's 20th Ed. Chapter 271 Page 1893

A. ATP-sensitive potassium channel
B. Voltage-sensitive sodium channel
C. Amiloride-sensitive Na^+ channel
D. All of the above

2101. Increased aldosterone secretion may result in?
Harrison's 20th Ed. Chapter 271 Page 1893

A. Hypokalemia
B. Alkalosis
C. Endothelial dysfunction
D. All of the above

Aldosterone is a potent mineralocorticoid that increases sodium reabsorption by amiloride-sensitive epithelial sodium channels (ENaC) on apical surface of principal cells of renal cortical collecting duct. Increased aldosterone secretion may result in hypokalemia, alkalosis, fibrosis, endothelial dysfunction, inflammation, and oxidative stress, as well as an overall increase in cardiovascular morbidity & mortality.

2102. Mineralocorticoid receptors are expressed in which of the following?
Harrison's 19th Ed. 1614

A. Colon
B. Salivary glands
C. Sweat glands
D. All of the above

Mineralocorticoid receptors also are expressed in the colon, salivary glands, and sweat glands.

2103. Which of the following has no affinity for the mineralocorticoid receptor?
Harrison's 20th Ed. Chapter 271 Page 1893

A. Aldosterone
B. Cortisol
C. Cortisone
D. All of the above

Cortisol binds to mineralocorticoid receptors but is a less potent mineralocorticoid than aldosterone because cortisol is converted to cortisone by enzyme 11 β-hydroxysteroid dehydrogenase type 2. Cortisone has no affinity for the mineralocorticoid receptor.

2104. Myocardial fibrosis, nephrosclerosis, vascular inflammation and remodeling are the effects of which of the following?
Harrison's 20th Ed. Chapter 271 Page 1893

A. Aldosterone
B. Cortisol
C. Cortisone
D. All of the above

Aldosterone and/or mineralocorticoid receptor activation induces structural & functional alterations in heart, kidney & blood vessels, leading to myocardial fibrosis, nephrosclerosis & vascular inflammation and remodeling, as a consequence of oxidative stress. These effects are amplified by a high salt intake.

2105. In CHF, low-dose spironolactone reduces the risk of progressive heart failure & sudden death from cardiac causes by?
Harrison's 20th Ed. Chapter 271 Page 1893

A. 10%
B. 20%
C. 30%
D. 40%

In CHF, low-dose spironolactone reduces the risk of progressive heart failure and sudden death from cardiac causes by 30%.

2106. Resistance to blood flow varies inversely with?
Harrison's 20th Ed. Chapter 271 Page 1893

A. Second power of the radius
B. Third power of the radius
C. Fourth power of the radius
D. Fifth power of the radius

Vascular radius & compliance of resistance arteries are important determinants of arterial pressure. Resistance to flow varies inversely with the fourth power of the radius.

2107. Which of the following contribute to vascular remodeling?
Harrison's 20th Ed. Chapter 271 Page 1893

A. Apoptosis
B. Low-grade inflammation
C. Vascular fibrosis
D. All of the above

2108. Which of the following is related to the functional properties of large arteries?
Harrison's 20th Ed. Chapter 271 Page 1893

A. Cardiac output
B. Peripheral resistance
C. Pulse pressure
D. All of the above

Pulse pressure is related to the functional properties of large arteries.

2109. Aortic augmentation index is calculated as the ratio of?
Harrison's 20th Ed. Chapter 271 Page 1894

A. Central arterial pressure - to - pulse pressure
B. Pulse pressure - to - central arterial pressure
C. Central arterial pressure - to - mean blood pressure
D. Mean blood pressure - to - central arterial pressure

The aortic augmentation index is a surrogate index of arterial stiffening. It is calculated as the ratio of central arterial pressure-to-pulse pressure. Central blood pressure and the aortic augmentation index are strong, independent predictors of cardiovascular disease and all-cause mortality.

2110. Intracellular pH (pHi) is regulated by?
Harrison's 20th Ed. Chapter 271 Page 1894

A. Na^+ - H^+ exchange
B. Na^+ - dependent HCO_3^- - Cl^- exchange
C. Cation-independent HCO_3 - Cl^- exchange
D. All of the above

Intracellular pH (pHi) of vascular smooth muscle cells determine vascular tone and vascular growth. Ion transport mechanisms that regulate pHi include Na+-H+ exchange, Na+-dependent HCO_3^--Cl^- exchange and cation-independent HCO_3^-–Cl^- exchange.

2111. Which of the following is increased in hypertension?
Harrison's 20th Ed. Chapter 271 Page 1894

A. Sympathetic outflow
B. Activity of the Na^+ - H^+ exchanger
C. Atrial natriuretic factor
D. All of the above

2112. Which of the following is a vasoconstrictor?
Harrison's 20th Ed. Chapter 271 Page 1894

A. Nitric oxide
B. Acetylcholine
C. Endothelin
D. All of the above

Vascular endothelium synthesizes & releases nitric oxide, a potent vasodilator. Acetylcholine is an endothelium-dependent vasodilator. Endothelin is a vasoconstrictor peptide produced by endothelium.

2113. Which of the following occurs in hypertension?
Harrison's 20th Ed. Chapter 271 Page 1894

A. Impaired endothelium-dependent vasodilation
B. Increased circulating levels of autoantibodies
C. Disruption of renal pressure-natriuresis curve
D. All of the above

2114. Which of the following is an early consequence of hypertension-related heart disease?
Harrison's 20th Ed. Chapter 271 Page 1894

A. Systolic dysfunction
B. Diastolic dysfunction
C. Left ventricular hypertrophy
D. All of the above

Diastolic dysfunction is an early consequence of hypertension-related heart disease.

2115. Cerebral blood flow remains unchanged when mean arterial pressure is between?
Harrison's 20th Ed. Chapter 271 Page 1894

A. 50–100 mm Hg
B. 50–150 mm Hg
C. 50–200 mm Hg
D. 50–250 mm Hg

Cerebral blood flow remains unchanged over mean arterial pressure of 50–150 mm Hg.

2116. Differential diagnosis of hypertensive encephalopathy includes?
Harrison's 20th Ed. Chapter 271 Page 1895

A. Pseudotumor cerebri
B. Acute intermittent porphyria
C. Uremic encephalopathy
D. All of the above

2117. Mechanisms of kidney-related hypertension is?
Harrison's 20th Ed. Chapter 271 Page 1895

A. Diminished capacity to excrete sodium
B. Excessive renin secretion in relation to volume status
C. Sympathetic nervous system overactivity
D. All of the above

2118. Which of the following is synthesized in adrenal medulla and released into circulation upon adrenal stimulation?
Harrison's 19th Ed. 1615

A. Epinephrine
B. Norepinephrine
C. Dopamine
D. All of the above

Adrenergic neurons synthesize norepinephrine & dopamine, which are stored in vesicles within neuron. When neuron is stimulated, these neurotransmitters are released into synaptic cleft. Epinephrine is synthesized in adrenal medulla & released into circulation upon adrenal stimulation.

2119. Atherosclerotic, hypertension-related vascular lesions in the kidney primarily affect?
Harrison's 20th Ed. Chapter 271 Page 1895

A. Preglomerular arterioles
B. Glomerular capillaries
C. Postglomerular arterioles
D. All of the above

Atherosclerotic, hypertension-related vascular lesions in the kidney primarily affect preglomerular arterioles, resulting in ischemic changes in the glomeruli and postglomerular structures.

2120. Renal lesion associated with malignant hypertension is?
Harrison's 20th Ed. Chapter 271 Page 1895

A. Fibrinoid necrosis of afferent arterioles
B. Fibrinoid necrosis of glomerular capillaries
C. Fibrinoid necrosis of efferent arterioles
D. All of the above

Renal lesion associated with malignant hypertension consists of fibrinoid necrosis of the afferent arterioles.

2121. For every 20 mm Hg increase in SBP & 10 mm Hg increase in DBP, cardiovascular disease risk increases by?
Harrison's 20th Ed. Chapter 271 Page 1895

A. 1.5 times
B. 2 times
C. 2.5 times
D. 3 times

Cardiovascular disease risk doubles for every 20 mm Hg increase in systolic and 10 mm Hg increase in diastolic pressure.

2122. Among older individuals, which of the following is the least powerful predictor of cardiovascular disease?
Harrison's 20th Ed. Chapter 271 Page 1895

A. Systolic blood pressure
B. Diastolic blood pressure
C. Pulse pressure
D. None of the above

Among older individuals, systolic blood pressure & pulse pressure are more powerful predictors of cardiovascular disease than diastolic blood pressure.

2123. Blood pressure tends to be higher during which of the following times?
Harrison's 20th Ed. Chapter 271 Page 1895

A. Early morning hours soon after waking
B. Following meals
C. Evenings
D. Night

Blood pressure tends to be higher in the early morning hours, soon after waking, than at other times of day. Myocardial infarction and stroke are more frequent in the early morning hours.

2124. Generally, night time blood pressures are lower than day time blood pressures by?
Harrison's 20th Ed. Chapter 271 Page 1895

A. 5–10%
B. 10–20%
C. 20–30%
D. 30–40%

Nighttime blood pressures are generally 10–20% lower than daytime blood pressures.

2125. Which of the following about hypertension is false?
Harrison's 20th Ed. Chapter 271 Page 1895

A. More severe in glomerular than in interstitial diseases
B. Low-renin patients have volume-dependent hypertension
C. White coat hypertension does not develop into sustained hypertension
D. ~80–95% of hypertensive patients have essential hypertension

Individuals with white coat hypertension are at increased risk for developing sustained hypertension.

2126. Which of the following is a secondary cause of systolic & diastolic hypertension?
Harrison's 20th Ed. Chapter 271 Page 1896 Table 271-3

A. 17α-hydroxylase deficiency
B. 11β-hydroxylase deficiency
C. 11-hydroxysteroid dehydrogenase deficiency
D. All of the above

2127. Which of the following is a secondary cause of systolic & diastolic hypertension?
Harrison's 20th Ed. Chapter 271 Page 1896 Table 271-3

A. Hypothyroidism
B. Hyperthyroidism
C. Hypercalcemia
D. All of the above

2128. Which of the following is a secondary cause of systolic & diastolic hypertension?
Harrison's 20th Ed. Chapter 271 Page 1896 Table 271-3

A. Cyclosporine
B. High-dose estrogens
C. Erythropoietin
D. All of the above

2129. Which of the following about primary hypertension is false?
Harrison's 20th Ed. Chapter 271 Page 1896

A. Tends to be familial
B. High-renin patients have vasoconstrictor form of hypertension
C. Low-renin patients have volume-dependent hypertension
D. None of the above

2130. Association between aldosterone & blood pressure is striking in?
Harrison's 20th Ed. Chapter 271 Page 1896

A. Native American
B. Polynesian
C. African Americans
D. Maori population

Association between aldosterone & blood pressure is more striking in African Americans. Aldosterone antagonist Spironolactone may be an effective antihypertensive agent.

2131. Metabolic syndrome consists of all except?
Harrison's 20th Ed. Chapter 271 Page 1896

A. Diabetes mellitus
B. Abdominal obesity
C. Hypertension
D. Dyslipidemia

Constellation of insulin resistance, abdominal obesity, hypertension & dyslipidemia is called metabolic syndrome.

2132. Which of the following is the most common cause of secondary hypertension?
Harrison's 20th Ed. Chapter 271 Page 1896

A. Obesity & metabolic syndrome
B. Renal disease
C. Obstructive sleep apnea
D. Psychogenic

Virtually all disorders of kidney may cause hypertension and renal disease is the most common cause of secondary hypertension.

2133. Which of the following about patients with fibromuscular dysplasia is false?
Harrison's 20th Ed. Chapter 271 Page 1896

A. Lesions are frequently bilateral
B. Strong predilection for young black women
C. Have more favorable outcomes with vascular repair
D. Potentially curable form of hypertension

Fibromuscular dysplasia may occur at any age and it has a strong predilection for young white women.

2134. Which is the most common histologic variant of fibromuscular dysplasia?
Harrison's 19th Ed. 1617

A. Medial fibroplasia
B. Perimedial fibroplasia
C. Medial hyperplasia
D. Intimal fibroplasia

Histologic variants of fibromuscular dysplasia include medial fibroplasia, perimedial fibroplasia, medial hyperplasia & intimal fibroplasia. Medial fibroplasia is the most common variant (66%).

2135. Lesions of fibromuscular dysplasia mostly affect which portion of renal artery?
Harrison's 20th Ed. Chapter 271 Page 1897

A. Proximal
B. Mid
C. Distal
D. Any of the above

Lesions of fibromuscular dysplasia are frequently bilateral and in contrast to atherosclerotic renovascular disease tend to affect more distal portions of renal artery.

2136. Which of the following raises the possibility of renovascular hypertension?
Harrison's 20th Ed. Chapter 271 Page 1897

A. Severe or refractory hypertension
B. Recent loss of hypertension control
C. Deterioration of renal function with ACE inhibitor use
D. All of the above

2137. What percentage of patients with renovascular hypertension have an abdominal or flank bruit?
Harrison's 20th Ed. Chapter 271 Page 1897

A. ~ 10%
B. ~ 25%
C. ~ 50%
D. ~ 75%

~50% of patients with renovascular hypertension have an abdominal or flank bruit. Bruit is more likely to be hemodynamically significant if it lateralizes or extends throughout systole into diastole.

2138. Which of the following serves as "gold standard" for evaluation and identification of renal artery lesions?
Harrison's 20th Ed. Chapter 271 Page 1897

A. DTPA scan
B. Gadolinium-contrast magnetic resonance angiography
C. Contrast arteriography
D. Doppler ultrasound of the renal arteries

Contrast arteriography remains the "gold standard" for evaluation and identification of renal artery lesions.

2139. Renal blood flow may be evaluated with?
Harrison's 20th Ed. Chapter 271 Page 1897

A. 2-[^{18}F]fluoro-2-deoxy-D-glucose (FDG) scan
B. [^{131}I]-orthoiodohippurate (OIH) scan
C. ^{99}mTc scan
D. ^{90}Yttrium scan

As a screening test, renal blood flow is evaluated with a radionuclide [^{131}I]-orthoiodohippurate (OIH) scan.

2140. [^{99}mTc]-diethylenetriamine pentaacetic acid (DTPA) scan estimates which of the following?
Harrison's 20th Ed. Chapter 271 Page 1897

A. Renal blood flow
B. Renal blood flow velocity
C. Glomerular filtration rate
D. All of the above

Glomerular filtration rate (GFR) is evaluated with a [^{99}mTc]-diethylenetriamine pentaacetic acid (DTPA) scan before and after a single dose of captopril.

2141. Which of the following test is sufficiently reliable for a causal relationship between a renal artery lesion & hypertension?
Harrison's 20th Ed. Chapter 271 Page 1897

A. DTPA scan
B. Gadolinium-contrast magnetic resonance angiography
C. Doppler ultrasound of the renal arteries
D. None of the above

No single test is sufficiently reliable to determine a causal relationship between a renal artery lesion and hypertension.

2142. In renal artery obstruction, functionally significant lesions occlude?
Harrison's 20th Ed. Chapter 271 Page 1897

A. > 30% of the lumen
B. > 50% of the lumen
C. > 70% of the lumen
D. > 90% of the lumen

Functionally significant renal artery lesions generally occlude more than 70% of the lumen of the affected renal artery.

2143. Which of the following predict a functionally significant renal artery and response to vascular repair?
Harrison's 20th Ed. Chapter 271 Page 1897

A. Occlusion of >70% of lumen of the affected renal artery
B. Presence of collateral vessels to the ischemic kidney

C. Lateralizing renal vein renin ratio

D. All of the above

Renin secretion is increased in the ischemic kidney but is suppressed in the contralateral kidney. The ratio of the measurement from ischemic kidney to the measurement from contralateral kidney is the renal vein renin ratio. A ratio higher than 1.5 constitutes a positive test result and is suggestive of functionally important renovascular disease.

2144. Which of the following is false about primary aldosteronism?

Harrison's 20th Ed. Chapter 271 Page 1897

A. Potentially curable form of hypertension

B. Aldosterone production is independent of RAS

C. Patients rarely have edema

D. None of the above

2145. Which of the following is not a feature of primary aldosteronism?

Harrison's 20th Ed. Chapter 271 Page 1897

A. Sodium retention

B. Mild to moderate hypertension

C. Unprovoked hypokalemia

D. High PRA

Excess aldosterone production in primary aldosteronism is independent of the renin-angiotensin system (RAS) and leads to sodium retention, hypertension, hypokalemia, and low PRA. In patients on diuretics, serum potassium <3.1 mEq/L also raises the possibility of primary aldosteronism.

2146. Hypokalemic hypertension is seen in?

Harrison's 20th Ed. Chapter 271 Page 1897

A. Primary aldosteronism

B. Glucocorticoid-induced hypertension

C. Pheochromocytoma

D. All of the above

Besides primary aldosteronism, hypokalemic hypertension may be a consequence of secondary aldosteronism, other mineralocorticoid- and glucocorticoid-induced hypertensive disorders, and pheochromocytoma.

2147. Plasma aldosterone (adult) level in supine position with patient on normal sodium diet normally is?

Harrison's 18th Ed., Appendix: Laboratory Values of Clinical Importance, Table 2

A. < 16 ng/dL

B. < 32 ng/dL

C. < 48 ng/dL

D. < 72 ng/dL

2148. What ratio of plasma aldosterone to plasma renin activity is indicative of aldosterone-producing adenoma?

Harrison's 20th Ed. Chapter 271 Page 1897

A. > 10 : 1

B. > 20 : 1

C. > 30 : 1

D. > 40 : 1

A ratio of >30 : 1 of plasma aldosterone to plasma renin activity (PA / PRA) is indicative of aldosterone-producing adenoma provided plasma aldosterone concentration is >555 pmol/L (>20 ng/dL). It can be confirmed by demonstrating failure to suppress plasma aldosterone to <277 pmol/L (<10 ng/dL) after IV infusion of 2 liters of isotonic saline over 4 hours.

2149. Plasma aldosterone is suppressed by all except?

Harrison's 20th Ed. Chapter 271 Page 1897

A. Oral NaCl load

B. Fludrocortisone

C. Captopril

D. Spironolactone

Aldosterone antagonists, angiotensin receptor antagonists, and ACE inhibitors may increase renin. Aldosterone antagonists may increase aldosterone. IV infusion of isotonic saline, oral NaCl load, fludrocortisone, or captopril suppress aldosterone.

2150. Which of the following is the most common cause of sporadic primary aldosteronism?

Harrison's 20th Ed. Chapter 271 Page 1898

A. Glucocorticoid-remediable primary aldosteronism

B. Bilateral adrenal hyperplasia

C. Familial aldosteronism type II

D. Familial aldosteronism type III

The two most common causes of sporadic primary aldosteronism are an aldosterone-producing adenoma and bilateral adrenal hyperplasia. Together, they account for >90% of all patients with primary aldosteronism.

2151. Which of the following is false about aldosterone-producing adrenal adenoma?

Harrison's 20th Ed. Chapter 271 Page 1898

A. Tumor is almost always unilateral

B. Measures < 3 cm in diameter

C. Aldosterone biosynthesis more responsive to ACTH

D. None of the above

2152. Glucocorticoid-remediable hyperaldosteronism (GRA) best relates to?

Harrison's 20th Ed. Chapter 271 Page 1898

A. Mutations in KCNJ5 gene

B. Chimeric karyotype

C. Chimeric gene duplication

D. All of the above

Glucocorticoid-remediable hyperaldosteronism is a monogenic autosomal dominant disorder characterized by moderate to severe early age hypertension. Hypokalemia is usually mild or absent. Normally, angiotensin II stimulates aldosterone production by adrenal zona glomerulosa, whereas ACTH stimulates cortisol production in zona fasciculata. Due to a chimeric gene on chromosome 8, ACTH also regulates aldosterone secretion by zona fasciculata in glucocorticoid-remediable hyperaldosteronism. Consequently, there is overproduction in zona fasciculata of both aldosterone & hybrid steroids (18-hydroxycortisol & 18-oxocortisol). Suppression of ACTH with low-dose glucocorticoids corrects hyperaldosteronism, hypertension & hypokalemia.

2153. Glucocorticoid-remediable hyperaldosteronism is also called?

Harrison's 20th Ed. Chapter 49 Page 305

A. Familial hyperaldosteronism type I (FH-I)

B. Familial hyperaldosteronism type II (FH-II)

C. Familial hyperaldosteronism type III (FH-III)

D. Familial hyperaldosteronism type IV (FH-IV)

Familial hyperaldosteronism type I (FH-I) is also known as glucocorticoid-remediable hyperaldosteronism. FH-I is caused by a chimeric gene duplication between the homologous 11β-hydroxylase (CYP11B1) and aldosterone synthase (CYP11B2) genes, fusing the adrenocorticotropic hormone (ACTH) responsive 11β-hydroxylase promoter to the coding region of aldosterone synthase. This chimeric gene is under the control of ACTH and thus repressible by glucocorticoids.

2154. Which of the following is caused by mutations in the KCNJ5 gene?

Harrison's 20th Ed. Chapter 49 Page 305

A. Familial hyperaldosteronism type I (FH-I)

B. Familial hyperaldosteronism type II (FH-II)

C. Familial hyperaldosteronism type III (FH-III)

D. Familial hyperaldosteronism type IV (FH-IV)

Familial hyperaldosteronism type III (FH-III) is caused by mutations in the KCNJ5 gene, which encodes G-protein-activated inward rectifier K^+ channel 4 (GIRK4).

2155. Surgery is not indicated in which of the following?
Harrison's 20th Ed. Chapter 271 Page 1898

A. Bilateral adrenal hyperplasia
B. Glucocorticoid-remediable primary aldosteronism
C. Familial aldosteronism type II
D. All of the above

2156. Laboratory screening for Cushing's syndrome is done by?
Harrison's 20th Ed. Chapter 271 Page 1898

A. 24-hour excretion rates of urine-free cortisol
B. Overnight dexamethasone-suppression test
C. Late night salivary cortisol
D. All of the above

2157. In pheochromocytoma, hypotension rather than hypertension is the presentation, the hormone secreted is?
Harrison's 20th Ed. Chapter 271 Page 1898

A. Epinephrine
B. Norepinephrine
C. Corticosterone
D. Cortisol

When epinephrine is the predominant catecholamine secreted in pheochromocytoma, the patients may present with hypotension rather than hypertension.

2158. Inherited pheochromocytomas may be associated with?
Harrison's 20th Ed. Chapter 271 Page 1898

A. Multiple endocrine neoplasia (MEN) type 2A & type 2B
B. von Hippel-Lindau disease
C. Neurofibromatosis
D. All of the above

~20% of pheochromocytomas are familial with autosomal dominant inheritance. Inherited pheochromocytomas may be associated with multiple endocrine neoplasia (MEN) type 2A and type 2B, von Hippel-Lindau disease and neurofibromatosis.

2159. Mutations of which of the following genes are associated with paraganglioma syndromes?
Harrison's 20th Ed. Chapter 271 Page 1898

A. Activin receptor–like kinase gene
B. Succinate dehydrogenase genes
C. Tyrosinase gene
D. Serine threonine kinase gene

Mutations of succinate dehydrogenase genes are associated with paraganglioma syndromes, characterized by head and neck paragangliomas.

2160. Which of the following is the most common congenital cardiovascular cause of hypertension?
Harrison's 20th Ed. Chapter 271 Page 1899

A. Patent ductus arteriosus
B. Venrticular septal defect
C. Coarctation of the aorta
D. Atrial septal defect

2161. Coarctation of the aorta is associated with which of the following syndromes?
Harrison's 20th Ed. Chapter 271 Page 1899

A. Klinefelter's syndrome
B. Parkes Weber syndrome
C. Hennekam's syndrome
D. Turner's syndrome

Coarctation of the aorta is the most common congenital cardiovascular cause of hypertension. The incidence is 1–8 per 1000 live births. It is usually sporadic but occurs in 35% of children with Turner's syndrome.

2162. Which of the following is a complication of coarctation of the aorta?
Harrison's 20th Ed. Chapter 271 Page 1899

A. Ischemic heart disease
B. Cerebral hemorrhage
C. Aortic aneurysm
D. All of the above

2163. In which of the following conditions, males may present with pseudohermaphroditism and hypertension?
Harrison's 20th Ed. Chapter 271 Page 1899 Table 271-4

A. Glucocorticoid-remediable hyperaldosteronism
B. 11β-hydroxylase deficiency
C. 17α-hydroxylase deficiency
D. 11β-hydroxysteroid dehydrogenase deficiency

With 17α-hydroxylase deficiency, synthesis of sex hormones & cortisol is decreased. Consequently, these individuals do not mature sexually. Males may present with pseudohermaphroditism and females with primary amenorrhea and absent secondary sexual characteristics. Because cortisol-induced negative feedback on pituitary ACTH production is diminished, ACTH-stimulated adrenal steroid synthesis proximal to the enzymatic block is increased. Hypertension and hypokalemia are consequences of increased synthesis of mineralocorticoids proximal to the enzymatic block, particularly desoxycorticosterone. Increased steroid production and, hence, hypertension may be treated with low-dose glucocorticoids.

2164. Which of the following conditions may result in hypertension?
Harrison's 20th Ed. Chapter 271 Page 1899

A. Hypercalcemia
B. Acromegaly
C. Hypothyroidism, hyperthyroidism
D. All of the above

2165. Which of the following is a form of monogenic hypertension?
Harrison's 20th Ed. Chapter 271 Page 1899

A. Liddle's syndrome
B. Hypertension exacerbated in pregnancy
C. Glucocorticoid-remediable primary aldosteronism
D. All of the above

2166. Supplementation of which of the following may be associated with reduced stroke mortality?
Harrison's 20th Ed. Chapter 271 Page 1901

A. Potassium
B. Calcium
C. Sodium
D. Alcohol

Potassium supplementation may be associated with reduced stroke mortality.

2167. "Hypertensive headache" occurs during?
Harrison's 19th Ed. 1621

A. Morning
B. Afternoon
C. Evening
D. Night

2168. "Hypertensive headache" is localized to?
Harrison's 19th Ed. 1621

A. Occipital region
B. Frontal region
C. Temporal region
D. Any of the above

Characteristically, hypertensive headache occurs in morning & is localized to occipital region.

2169. Width of the blood pressure bladder cuff should equal at least what percentage of the arm circumference?
Harrison's 19th Ed. 1445

A. 10%
B. 20%
C. 30%
D. 40%

2170. Length of blood pressure bladder cuff bladder should encircle at least what percentage of the arm circumference?
Harrison's 19th Ed. 1445

A. 20%
B. 40%
C. 60%
D. 80%

Width of the blood pressure bladder cuff should equal at least 40% of the arm circumference; the length of the cuff bladder should encircle at least 80% of the arm circumference.

2171. Optical funduscopic changes in hypertension include?
Harrison's 19th Ed. 1622

A. Increased arteriolar light reflex
B. Arteriovenous crossing defects
C. Hemorrhages and exudates
D. All of the above

With increasing severity of hypertension and atherosclerotic disease, progressive funduscopic changes include increased arteriolar light reflex, arteriovenous crossing defects, hemorrhages and exudates and in patients with malignant hypertension — papilledema.

2172. Blunting of the day-night blood pressure pattern occurs in?
Harrison's 19th Ed. 1627

A. Sleep apnea
B. Autonomic neuropathy
C. African Americans populations
D. All of the above

Attenuated nighttime blood pressure "dip" is associated with increased cardiovascular disease risk. Blunting of day-night blood pressure pattern occurs in sleep apnea, autonomic neuropathy & in African Americans.

2173. One standard drink contains how many grams of ethanol?
Harrison's 20th Ed. Chapter 271 Page 1901

A. ~ 10 grams
B. ~ 14 grams
C. ~ 18 grams
D. ~ 24 grams

One standard drink contains ~14 grams of ethanol.

2174. DASH trial stands for?
Harrison's 20th Ed. Chapter 271 Page 1901

A. Death and survival in hypertension
B. Diastolic and systolic hypertension
C. Dietary approaches to stop hypertension
D. Duration and severity of hypertension

DASH stands for Dietary Approaches to Stop Hypertension.

2175. Which of the following about lowering of SBP & DBP is false?
Harrison's 20th Ed. Chapter 271 Page 1901

A. Risk reductions of 35–40% for stroke
B. Risk reductions of 12–16% for CHD
C. Risk reductions of > 50% for heart failure
D. Risk reductions of > 75% for renal failure

Lowering SBP by 10-12 mm Hg & DBP by 5-6 mm Hg reduces relative risk by 35-40% for stroke, 12-16% for CHD within 5 years of initiation of treatment and >50% risk reduction of heart failure.Benefit of BP lowering on progression of renal failure is less apparent.

2176. Additive blood pressure lowering effect of thiazide diuretics is least when combined with?
Harrison's 20th Ed. Chapter 271 Page 1901

A. Beta blockers
B. Calcium channel blocker
C. Angiotensin-converting enzyme inhibitors (ACEIs)
D. Angiotensin receptor blockers (ARBs)

2177. Which of the following is a side effect of thiazide diuretic?
Harrison's 20th Ed. Chapter 271 Page 1901

A. Hypokalemia
B. Insulin resistance
C. Increased cholesterol
D. All of the above

2178. Which of the following act by inhibiting epithelial sodium channels in the distal nephron?
Harrison's 20th Ed. Chapter 271 Page 1901

A. Thiazides
B. Furosemide
C. Eplerenone
D. Amiloride

Potassium-sparing diuretics, amiloride and triamterene, act by inhibiting epithelial sodium channels in the distal nephron. Thiazides inhibit the Na^+/Cl^- pump in the distal convoluted tubule and hence increase sodium excretion. Loop diuretics inhibit the Na^+-K^+-$2Cl^-$ cotransporter in the thick ascending limb of the loop of Henle. Eplerenone is an aldosterone antagonist.

2179. Angiotensin-converting enzyme inhibitors act by which of the following mechanism?

Harrison's 20th Ed. Chapter 271 Page 1901

A. Decrease production of angiotensin II
B. Increase bradykinin levels
C. Reduce sympathetic nervous system activity
D. All of the above

ACEIs decrease the production of angiotensin II, increase bradykinin levels, and reduce sympathetic nervous system activity.

2180. Angiotensin receptor blockers (ARB) provide selective blockade of?

Harrison's 20th Ed. Chapter 271 Page 1901

A. AT_1 receptors
B. AT_2 receptors
C. AT_3 receptors
D. AT_4 receptors

ARBs provide selective blockade of AT_1 receptors, and the effect of angiotensin II on unblocked AT_2 receptors may augment their hypotensive effect.

2181. Which of the following diminishes the adverse effects of diuretics on glucose metabolism?

Harrison's 20th Ed. Chapter 271 Page 1902

A. ACEIs and ARBs
B. Beta blockers
C. Calcium antagonists
D. Alpha antagonists

ACEIs & ARBs improve insulin action & ameliorate the adverse effects of diuretics on glucose metabolism.

2182. Which of the following reduces the risk of developing diabetes in high-risk hypertensive patients?

Harrison's 20th Ed. Chapter 271 Page 1902

A. Valsartan
B. Lisinopril
C. Captopril
D. Ramipril

Valsartan (an ARB) reduces the risk of developing diabetes in high-risk hypertensive patients.

2183. Combining angiotensin-converting enzyme inhibitors with which of the following is associated with more adverse events?

Harrison's 20th Ed. Chapter 271 Page 1902

A. Angiotensin receptor blockers
B. Beta blockers
C. Calcium channel blocker
D. Alpha blocking agents

ACEI/ARB combination therapy is associated with more adverse events like cardiovascular death, myocardial infarction, stroke, and hospitalization for heart failure, without increases in benefit.

2184. Which of the following predisposes to renal insufficiency induced by ACEIs and ARBs?

Harrison's 20th Ed. Chapter 271 Page 1902

A. Dehydration
B. CHF
C. Use of nonsteroidal anti-inflammatory drugs
D. All of the above

2185. Dry cough occurs in what percentage of patients taking ACEIs?

Harrison's 20th Ed. Chapter 271 Page 1902

A. ~ 5%
B. ~ 10%
C. ~ 15%
D. ~ 20%

Dry cough occurs in ~15% of patients, and angioedema occurs in <1% of patients taking ACEIs.

2186. Which of the following is a direct renin inhibitor?

Harrison's 20th Ed. Chapter 271 Page 1902

A. Guanfacine
B. Doxazosin
C. Aliskiren
D. Terazosin

Aliskiren is an oral, nonpeptide competitive inhibitors of the enzymatic activity of renin.

2187. Which of the following trials studied Aliskiren in Type 2 Diabetes?

N Engl J Med. 2012; 367:2204-2213

A. ALTITUDE
B. ATMOSPHERE
C. CHARM-Added
D. Val-HeFT

ALTITUDE Clinical Trial studied the addition of aliskiren to standard therapy with renin–angiotensin system blockade in patients with type 2 diabetes who are at high risk for cardiovascular & renal events. It concluded that addition may be harmful.

2188. Which of the following about spironolactone is false?

Harrison's 20th Ed. Chapter 271 Page 1903

A. Nonselective aldosterone antagonist
B. Binds to progesterone
C. Binds to androgen receptors
D. None of the above

2189. Spironolactone is effective in patients with?

Harrison's 20th Ed. Chapter 271 Page 1903

A. Low-renin essential hypertension
B. Resistant hypertension
C. Primary aldosteronism
D. All of the above

Spironolactone is a nonselective aldosterone antagonist that may be used alone or in combination with a thiazide diuretic. It is particularly effective agent in patients with low-renin essential hypertension, resistant hypertension, and primary aldosteronism. Because spironolactone binds to progesterone and androgen receptors, side effects may include gynecomastia, impotence, and menstrual abnormalities.

2190. Which of the following is a selective aldosterone antagonist?

Harrison's 20th Ed. Chapter 271 Page 1903

A. Aliskiren
B. Eplerenone
C. Candesartan
D. Minoxidil

Eplerenone is a selective aldosterone antagonist.

2191. Which of the following clinical trials evaluated eplerenone?
N Engl J Med. 2011; 364:11-21

A. SHIFT trial
B. CHARM-Added trial
C. RALES trial
D. EPHESUS trial

Eplerenone Post–Acute Myocardial Infarction Heart Failure Efficacy and Survival Study (EPHESUS).

2192. β-Adrenergic receptor blockers lower blood pressure by?
Harrison's 20th Ed. Chapter 271 Page 1903

A. Decreasing cardiac output
B. Central nervous system effect
C. Inhibition of renin release
D. All of the above

β-Adrenergic receptor blockers lower blood pressure by decreasing cardiac output (reduction of heart rate & contractility). Other mechanisms include a central nervous system effect & inhibition of renin release.

2193. Which of the following blocks both β receptors and peripheral a-adrenergic receptors?
Harrison's 20th Ed. Chapter 271 Page 1903

A. Carvedilol
B. Aliskiren
C. Eplerenone
D. Minoxidil

Carvedilol and labetalol block both β receptors and peripheral α-adrenergic receptors.

2194. Which of the following about Nebivolol is false?
Harrison's 20th Ed. Chapter 271 Page 1903

A. Beta blocker
B. Cardioselective
C. Enhances nitric oxide activity
D. None of the above

Nebivolol is a cardioselective β blocker with vasodilator action due to enhancement of nitric oxide activity.

2195. Selective alpha antagonists include all except?
Harrison's 20th Ed. Chapter 271 Page 1902 Table 271-8

A. Prazosin
B. Doxazosin
C. Terazosin
D. Phenoxybenzamine

Phenoxybenzamine is a nonselective alpha antagonist.

2196. Which of the following antihypertensive drugs is contraindicated in pregnancy?
Harrison's 20th Ed. Chapter 271 Page 1902 Table 271-8

A. Aliskiren
B. Minoxidil
C. Clonidine
D. All of the above

2197. Which of the following drug is contraindicated in pregnancy?
Harrison's 20th Ed. Chapter 271 Page 1902 Table 271-8

A. Captopril
B. Losartan
C. Aliskiren
D. All of the above

2198. Which of the following is false about α-Adrenergic Blockers?
Harrison's 20th Ed. Chapter 271 Page 1903

A. Do not reduce cardiovascular morbidity / mortality & CHF
B. Effective in treating men with prostatic hypertrophy
C. Useful in management of patients with pheochromocytoma
D. None of the above

2199. Peripheral sympatholytics act by depleting nerve terminal?
Harrison's 20th Ed. Chapter 271 Page 1903

A. Epinephrine
B. Norepinephrine
C. Acethylcholine
D. All of the above

Peripheral sympatholytics decrease peripheral resistance and venous constriction by depleting nerve terminal norepinephrine.

2200. Calcium antagonists reduce vascular resistance through?
Harrison's 20th Ed. Chapter 271 Page 1903

A. K - channel blockade
B. L - channel blockade
C. M - channel blockade
D. N - channel blockade

Calcium antagonists reduce vascular resistance through L-channel blockade, which reduces intracellular calcium and blunts vasoconstriction.

2201. Which of the following is not a class of calcium antagonists?
Harrison's 20th Ed. Chapter 271 Page 1903

A. Phenylalkylamines
B. Phenylpyridines
C. Benzothiazepines
D. Dihydropyridines

Calcium antagonists are of three classes — phenylalkylamines (verapamil), benzothiazepines (diltiazem), and 1,4-dihydropyridines (amlodipine, felodipine, isradipine, nicardipine, nifedipine and nisoldipine).

2202. Edema with dihydropyridine calcium channel blockers is due to?
Harrison's 20th Ed. Chapter 271 Page 1903

A. Net salt retention
B. Net water retention
C. Increase in transcapillary pressure gradients
D. All of the above

Edema with dihydropyridine use are related to their potencies as arteriolar dilators. Edema is due to an increase in transcapillary pressure gradients, not to net salt and water retention.

2203. Which of the following is a direct vasodilator?
Harrison's 20th Ed. Chapter 271 Page 1903

A. Hydralazine
B. Minoxidil
C. Sodium nitroprusside
D. All of the above

2204. Which of the following is true about Hydralazine?
Harrison's 20th Ed. Chapter 271 Page 1903

A. Direct vasodilator
B. Antioxidant
C. Nitric-oxide enhancer
D. All of the above

Hydralazine is a potent direct vasodilator that has antioxidant and nitric-oxide enhancing actions.

2205. Which of the following drug is used in patients with renal insufficiency who are refractory to all other drugs?

Harrison's 20th Ed. Chapter 271 Page 1903

A. Minoxidil
B. Aliskiren
C. Hydralazine
D. Methyldopa

Minoxidil is used most frequently in patients with renal insufficiency who are refractory to all other drugs.

2206. Patients with high-renin hypertension may be more responsive to which of the following?

Harrison's 20th Ed. Chapter 271 Page 1903

A. ACE inhibitors
B. Beta blockers
C. Calcium antagonists
D. Diuretics

2207. Patients with low-renin hypertension are more responsive to which of the following?

Harrison's 20th Ed. Chapter 271 Page 1903

A. ACE inhibitors
B. Beta blockers
C. Calcium antagonists
D. Direct vasodilators

Younger patients may be more responsive to beta blockers & ACE inhibitors, whereas patients over age 50 may be more responsive to diuretics & calcium antagonists. Patients with high-renin hypertension may be more responsive to ACE inhibitors & angiotensin receptor blockers, whereas patients with low-renin hypertension are more responsive to diuretics and calcium antagonists.

2208. Which of the following influences the selection of antihypertensive agents?

Harrison's 20th Ed. Chapter 271 Page 1903

A. Age
B. Ethnicity
C. Comorbid conditions
D. All of the above

2209. In HOPE (Heart Outcomes Prevention Evaluation) trial, which of the following ACE inhibitors was studied?

The American Journal of Medicine 2005;118, 695-705

A. Lisinopril
B. Ramipril
C. Enalapril
D. Perindopril

2210. In ALLHAT (Antihypertensive and Lipid-Lowering Treatment to Prevent Heart Attack Trial), which of the following ACE inhibitors was studied?

The American Journal of Medicine 2005;118, 695-705

A. Lisinopril
B. Ramipril
C. Enalapril
D. Perindopril

2211. Which of the following antihypertensives is inferior to other agents in reducing all-cause mortality?

Harrison's 20th Ed. Chapter 271 Page 1904

A. ACE Inhibitors
B. Diuretics
C. Calcium antagonists
D. Beta blockers

Antihypertensive and Lipid-Lowering Treatment to Prevent Heart Attack Trial (ALLHAT) concluded that occurrence of CHD, nonfatal MI & overall mortality was virtually identical in hypertensive patients treated with either ACEI (lisinopril), a diuretic (chlorthalidone), or a calcium antagonist (amlodipine). However, Beta blockers are inferior to other classes of agents for prevention of cardiovascular events, stroke, renal failure, and all-cause mortality.

2212. Which of the following drug has renal protective effects?

Harrison's 20th Ed. Chapter 271 Page 1904

A. Aliskiren
B. ACE Inhibitors
C. ARBs
D. All of the above

In hypertension & diabetes, renal protection with aliskiren is comparable to that with ACEIs & ARBs.

2213. Better stroke protection is provided by?

Harrison's 20th Ed. Chapter 271 Page 1904

A. ACE inhibitors
B. Beta blockers
C. Calcium channel blockers
D. All of the above

ACE inhibitors provide better coronary protection than calcium channel blockers, whereas calcium channel blockers provide more stroke protection than either ACE inhibitors or beta blockers.

2214. Resistant hypertension refers to BP persistently above what level despite taking 3 or more antihypertensives, including a diuretic, in reasonable combination and at full doses?

Harrison's 20th Ed. Chapter 271 Page 1905

A. >130/90 mm Hg
B. >140/90 mm Hg
C. >150/90 mm Hg
D. >160/90 mm Hg

Resistant hypertension refers to patients with BP persistently >140/90 mm Hg despite taking three or more antihypertensive agents, including a diuretic, in reasonable combination & at full doses.

2215. "Pseudoresistance" refers to?

Harrison's 20th Ed. Chapter 271 Page 1905

A. Lower office and high home blood pressures
B. High office and lower home blood pressures
C. Higher office and high home blood pressures
D. Lower office and low home blood pressures

"Pseudoresistance" refers to high office blood pressures & lower home blood pressures.

2216. If the radial pulse remains palpable despite occlusion of the brachial artery by the cuff, the maneuver is called?

Harrison's 20th Ed. Chapter 271 Page 1905

A. Roger maneuver
B. Osler maneuver
C. Happit maneuver
D. Weber maneuver

Osler maneuver refers to the radial pulse that remains palpable despite occlusion of brachial artery by cuff.

2217. Which of the following is most important in malignant hypertension?

Harrison's 20th Ed. Chapter 271 Page 1905

A. Underlying hypertension
B. Absolute level of blood pressure
C. Rate of rise of blood pressure
D. Response to treatment

In malignant hypertension, absolute level of blood pressure is not as important as its rate of rise.

2218. Which of the following occurs pathologically in malignant hypertension?

Harrison's 20th Ed. Chapter 271 Page 1905

A. Diffuse necrotizing vasculitis
B. Arteriolar thrombi
C. Fibrin deposition in arteriolar walls
D. All of the above

Pathologically, malignant hypertension is associated with diffuse necrotizing vasculitis, arteriolar thrombi, and fibrin deposition in arteriolar walls.

2219. Malignant hypertension is associated with?

Harrison's 20th Ed. Chapter 271 Page 1905

A. Progressive retinopathy
B. Microangiopathic hemolytic anemia
C. Encephalopathy
D. All of the above

Clinically, in malignant hypertension, there occurs progressive retinopathy (arteriolar spasm, hemorrhages, exudates, and papilledema), deteriorating renal function with proteinuria, microangiopathic hemolytic anemia, and encephalopathy.

2220. Which of the following can contribute to the development of malignant hypertension?

Harrison's 20th Ed. Chapter 271 Page 1905

A. Monoamine oxidase inhibitors
B. Cocaine
C. Amphetamines
D. All of the above

2221. In malignant hypertension, the initial goal of therapy is to reduce mean arterial blood pressure by no more than?

Harrison's 20th Ed. Chapter 271 Page 1905

A. 10%
B. 25%
C. 40%
D. 60%

In malignant hypertension, the initial goal of therapy is to reduce mean arterial blood pressure by no more than 25% within minutes to 2 hours or to a blood pressure in the range of 160/100 - 110 mm Hg.

2222. Which of the following drugs is used in the treatment of hypertensive encephalopathy?

Harrison's 20th Ed. Chapter 271 Page 1905

A. Nitroprusside
B. Labetalol
C. Nicardipine
D. All of the above

2223. Which of the following is a short-acting oral antihypertensive useful in the management of malignant hypertension without encephalopathy?

Harrison's 20th Ed. Chapter 271 Page 1905

A. Captopril
B. Clonidine
C. Labetalol
D. All of the above

2224. SBP above what level should be lowered in patients with cerebral infarction who are not candidates for thrombolytic therapy?

Harrison's 20th Ed. Chapter 271 Page 1905

A. > 180 mm Hg
B. > 200 mm Hg
C. > 220 mm Hg
D. > 240 mm Hg

2225. DBP above what level should be lowered in patients with cerebral infarction who are not candidates for thrombolytic therapy?

Harrison's 20th Ed. Chapter 271 Page 1905

A. > 100 mm Hg
B. > 110 mm Hg
C. > 120 mm Hg
D. > 130 mm Hg

For patients with cerebral infarction who are not candidates for thrombolytic therapy, antihypertensive therapy is given only for those with a systolic blood pressure >220 mm Hg or a diastolic blood pressure >130 mm Hg.

2226. Recommended BP goal for patients with cerebral infarction who are undergoing thrombolytic therapy is?

Harrison's 20th Ed. Chapter 271 Page 1905

A. SBP < 200 mm Hg and DBP < 110 mm Hg
B. SBP < 185 mm Hg and DBP < 110 mm Hg
C. SBP < 200 mm Hg and DBP < 100 mm Hg
D. SBP < 185 mm Hg and DBP < 100 mm Hg

If thrombolytic therapy is to be used in patients with cerebral infarction, the recommended goal blood pressure is <185 mm Hg systolic pressure and <110 mm Hg diastolic pressure.

2227. Adrenergic crisis due to catecholamine excess is due to?

Harrison's 20th Ed. Chapter 271 Page 1905

A. Cocaine or amphetamine overdose
B. Acute spinal cord injuries
C. Interaction of tyramine-containing compounds with monoamine oxidase inhibitors
D. All of the above

2228. Adrenergic crisis is treated with?

Harrison's 20th Ed. Chapter 271 Page 1905

A. Labetalol
B. Esmolol
C. Phentolamine
D. Hydralazine

Besides pheochromocytoma, adrenergic crisis due to catecholamine excess may be due to cocaine or amphetamine overdose, clonidine withdrawal, acute spinal cord injuries and an interaction of tyramine-containing compounds with monoamine oxidase inhibitors. These patients may be treated with phentolamine or nitroprusside.

2229. Esmolol is the preferred parenteral drug for?
Harrison's 20th Ed. Chapter 271 Page 1905 Table 271-9

A. Aortic dissection
B. Preeclampsia/eclampsia of pregnancy
C. Stroke
D. Adrenergic crisis

2230. Preferred parenteral drug for hypertensive emergency during preeclampsia / eclampsia of pregnancy is?
Harrison's 20th Ed. Chapter 271 Page 1905 Table 271-9

A. Hydralazine
B. Labetalol
C. Nicardipine
D. All of the above

2231. Which of the following antihypertensive agents is given as "IV bolus" in hypertensive emergencies?
Harrison's 20th Ed. Chapter 271 Page 1905 Table 271-10

A. Hydralazine
B. Esmolol
C. Phentolamine
D. Labetalol

2232. Risk factors for preeclampsia include all except?
Harrison's 20th Ed. Chapter 466 Page 3440

A. Nulliparity
B. Diabetes mellitus
C. Anemia
D. Obesity

Risk factors for the development of preeclampsia include nulliparity, diabetes mellitus, a history of renal disease or chronic hypertension, a prior history of preeclampsia, extremes of maternal age (>35 years or <15 years), obesity, antiphospholipid antibody syndrome and multiple gestation.

2233. Risk factors for preeclampsia include all except?
Harrison's 20th Ed. Chapter 466 Page 3440

A. Factor V Leiden mutation
B. Angiotensinogen gene T235
C. Antiphospholipid antibody syndrome
D. Smoking

2234. Medications or substances that can raise blood pressure or antagonize effects of antihypertensive drugs include all except?
N Engl J Med. 2006;355:385-92

A. Ginseng
B. Anabolic steroids
C. Erythropoietin
D. Chloroquine

2235. Medications or substances that can raise blood pressure or antagonize effects of antihypertensive drugs include all except?
N Engl J Med. 2006;355:385-92

A. Nonsteroidal antiinflammatory drugs
B. Excessive alcohol use
C. High sodium intake
D. Appetite stimulants

2236. High sodium intake is defined by?
N Engl J Med. 2006;355:385-92

A. Urinary sodium excretion of >50 mmol per day
B. Urinary sodium excretion of >100 mmol per day
C. Urinary sodium excretion of >150 mmol per day
D. None of the above

2237. Frequency of salt sensitivity is increased among?
N Engl J Med. 2006;355:385-92

A. > 60 years of age
B. Black or obese
C. Renal impairment
D. All of the above

2238. Which of the following suggest a diagnosis of atherosclerotic renovascular disease?
N Engl J Med. 2006;355:385-92

A. Abdominal bruit
B. Hypokalemia
C. Recent increase in severity of hypertension
D. All of the above

2239. Which of the following suggest aldosteronism as cause of secondary hypertension?
N Engl J Med. 2006;355:385-92

A. Abnormal ratio of aldosterone to renin
B. Abnormal response to sodium loading
C. Adrenal adenoma on CT or MRI
D. All of the above

2240. Which of the following suggest pheochromocytoma as cause of secondary hypertension?
N Engl J Med. 2006;355:385-92

A. Norepinephrine >80 μg/24 hours
B. VMA >5 mg/24 hours
C. Elevated plasma metanephrines
D. All of the above

2241. To prevent hypertensive crisis, patients taking MAOIs must avoid?
N Engl J Med. 2005;353:1819-34

A. Phenylalanine diet
B. Tryptophan diet
C. Tyramine diet
D. All of the above

2242. Which of the following is amino acid derived hormone?
N Engl J Med. 2005;353:1819-34

A. Dopamine
B. Catecholamines
C. Thyroid hormone
D. All of the above

2243. In hypertension during pregnancy, which of the following drugs would be safest?

N Engl J Med. 1998;338:1131

A. Labetalol
B. Beta-adrenergic–receptor antagonists
C. Prazosin
D. Calcium channel blocker

2244. If ACE inhibitors are given during pregnancy, what teratogenic effects can happen?

N Engl J Med. 1998;338:1131

A. Prolonged renal failure in neonates
B. Decreased skull ossification
C. Renal tubular dysgenesis
D. All of the above

2245. If Warfarin is given during pregnancy, what teratogenic effect can happen?

N Engl J Med. 1998;338:1131

A. Neonatal meconium ileus
B. Anomalies of teeth and bone
C. Ebstein's anomaly
D. Dandy–Walker syndrome

2246. Mothers who took warfarin during 1st trimester could have all of the following congenital malformations in infants except?

Harrison's 20th Ed. Chapter 114 Page 854, N Engl J Med. 2002;347:110

A. Severe nasal hypoplasia
B. Stippled epiphyseal calcifications
C. Chondrodysplasia punctata
D. Chiari type I malformation

Warfarin crosses the placenta and can cause fetal abnormalities that include a characteristic embryopathy, which consists of nasal hypoplasia and stippled epiphyses. The risk of embryopathy is highest if warfarin is given in the first trimester of pregnancy.

2247. Which of the following anticoagulants does not cross placenta?

Harrison's 20th Ed. Chapter 114 Page 854

A. Warfarin
B. Anisindione
C. Heparin
D. None of the above

Heparin, LMWH, or fondaparinux can be given during pregnancy for prevention or treatment of thrombosis.

2248. Which of the following is a vasoconstrictor?

Lancet 2005:365:417-430

A. Norepinephrine
B. Endothelin
C. Angiotensin II
D. All of the above

2249. Hypertensive retinopathy was first described by?

N Engl J Med. 2004;351:2310-7

A. Marcus Gunn
B. William Osler
C. Keith Wegener
D. Alexender Fleming

2250. Which of the following is called "Age pigment"?

Heart Lung and Circulation 2005;14:107-114

A. Calpains
B. Melanin
C. Lipofuscin
D. Bilirubin

Renovascular Disease

2251. Which of the following regions of kidney have blood circulation excess of its metabolic requirements?

Harrison's 20th Ed. Chapter 272 Page 1906

A. Renal cortex
B. Superficial medullary segments
C. Deeper medullary segments
D. Renal papilla

Renal vasculature is complex with rich arteriolar flow to cortex in excess of metabolic requirements, consistent with its primary function as a filtering organ.

2252. Vascular disorders that commonly threaten the blood supply of the kidney include?

Harrison's 20th Ed. Chapter 272 Page 1906

A. Large vessel atherosclerosis
B. Fibromuscular diseases
C. Embolic disorders
D. All of the above

2253. Which of the following is predictive of systemic atherosclerotic disease events?

Harrison's 20th Ed. Chapter 272 Page 1906

A. Microalbuminuria
B. Urinary albumin excretion (UAE)
C. Urine albumin / creatinine ratio
D. All of the above

2254. Large-vessel renal artery occlusive disease most commonly results from?

Harrison's 20th Ed. Chapter 272 Page 1906

A. Intimal dissection
B. Fibromuscular dysplasia (FMD)
C. Atherosclerotic disease
D. Extrinsic compression of the vessel

Large-vessel renal artery occlusive disease results most commonly from atherosclerotic disease. Also from extrinsic compression of the vessel, intimal dissection & fibromuscular dysplasia (FMD).

2255. Which of the following about systemic hypertension due to renal artery stenosis is false?

Harrison's 20th Ed. Chapter 272 Page 1906

A. Angiotensin dependence in the early stages
B. Loss of circadian blood pressure (BP) rhythms
C. Accelerated target organ injury
D. Revascularization lowers BP to normal

Revascularization (endovascular or surgical) alone rarely lowers BP to normal in renal artery stenosis.

2256. Minimum renal artery velocity that predicts hemodynamically significant lesion is?

Harrison's 20th Ed. Chapter 272 Page 1906

A. > 100 cm per second
B. > 200 cm per second
C. > 300 cm per second
D. > 400 cm per second

Minimum renal artery velocity (by Doppler ultrasound) that predicts hemodynamically significant (>60% vessel lumen occlusion) lesion is >200 cm per second.

2257. Normal study of which of the following investigations excludes renovascular hypertension?

Harrison's 20th Ed. Chapter 272 Page 1907 Table 272-1

A. Captopril renography with ^{99}mTc MAG3
B. Duplex ultrasonography
C. Computed tomographic angiography
D. Magnetic resonance angiography

Captopril-enhanced renography has a strong negative predictive value when normal.

2258. Which of the following is considered as "gold standard" for diagnosis of large-vessel renal disease?

Harrison's 20th Ed. Chapter 272 Page 1907 Table 272-1

A. Intraarterial angiography
B. Duplex ultrasonography
C. Computed tomographic angiography
D. Magnetic resonance angiography

2259. Vascular lesions in malignant hypertension best relate to?

Harrison's 20th Ed. Chapter 272 Page 1909

A. Avascular necrosis
B. Cystic medial necrosis
C. Fibrinoid necrosis
D. Subintimal foam cells

The hemodynamic stress of malignant hypertension leads to fibrinoid necrosis of small blood vessels, thrombotic microangiography, a nephritic urinalysis, and acute renal failure. The renal lesion associated with malignant hypertension consists of fibrinoid necrosis of the afferent arterioles, extending into glomerulus, and may result in focal necrosis of glomerular tuft.

2260. Which of the following predispose to subtle focal sclerosing glomerular disease, with severe hypertension?

Harrison's 20th Ed. Chapter 272 Page 1909

A. SERPINA1
B. APOL1
C. TCR-α
D. DRB1

2261. Vascular lesions of hypertensive nephrosclerosis are also seen in?

Harrison's 20th Ed. Chapter 272 Page 1909

A. Aging
B. Dyslipidemia
C. Glucose intolerance
D. All of the above

Deep Venous Thrombosis and Pulmonary Thromboembolism

2262. Which is the most common preventable cause of death among hospitalized patients?
Harrison's 20th Ed. Chapter 273 Page 1910

A. Deep venous thrombosis (DVT)
B. Pulmonary embolism (PE)
C. Postthrombotic syndrome
D. All of the above

PE is the most common preventable cause of death among hospitalized patients.

2263. Postthrombotic syndrome is also known as?
Harrison's 20th Ed. Chapter 273 Page 1910

A. Chronic thromboembolic pulmonary hypertension
B. Chronic venous insufficiency
C. Deep venous thrombosis
D. Pulmonary embolism

Postthrombotic syndrome is also known as chronic venous insufficiency.

2264. Virchow's triad consists of all except?
Harrison's 20th Ed. Chapter 273 Page 1910

A. Inflammation
B. Venous stasis
C. Hypercoagulability
D. Endothelial injury

Virchow's triad of venous stasis, hypercoagulability and endothelial injury leads to recruitment of activated platelets, which release microparticles.

2265. Wells Clinical Prediction Rule is used for?
Harrison's 20th Ed. Chapter 3 Page 19

A. ILD
B. COPD
C. Pulmonary embolism
D. Cystic fibrosis

Wells Clinical Prediction Rule is a semi-quantitative clinical scoring system for suspected pulmonary embolism (PE). The Wells Scoring System has a maximum of 12.5 points. If the score is <= 4 points, the likelihood of PE is only 8%.

2266. Microparticles contain proinflammatory mediators that bind?
Harrison's 20th Ed. Chapter 273 Page 1910

A. Platelets
B. Neutrophils
C. Eosinophils
D. Basophils

2267. Which of the following about neutrophil extracellular traps is false?
Harrison's 20th Ed. Chapter 273 Page 1910

A. Nuclear material of neutrophils
B. Web-like extracellular networks
C. Prothrombotic
D. None of the above

Microparticles contain proinflammatory mediators that bind neutrophils, stimulating them to release their nuclear material and form web-like extracellular prothrombotic networks called neutrophil extracellular traps which contain histones that stimulate platelet aggregation and promote platelet-dependent thrombin generation.

2268. Which of the following intracellular components has antimicrobial properties?
Harrison's 20th Ed. Chapter 116 Page 871

A. Histones
B. Myeloperoxidase
C. Elastase
D. All of the above

Neutrophil extracellular traps (NETs) are composed of DNA and other intracellular components with antimicrobial properties, such as histones, myeloperoxidase, and elastase.

2269. Venous thrombi form and flourish in an environment of?
Harrison's 20th Ed. Chapter 273 Page 1910

A. Stasis
B. Low oxygen tension
C. Upregulation of proinflammatory genes
D. All of the above

Venous thrombi form and flourish in an environment of stasis, low oxygen tension and upregulation of proinflammatory genes.

2270. Which of the following is the most common autosomal dominant genetic mutation that leads to a prothrombotic state?
Harrison's 20th Ed. Chapter 273 Page 1910

A. Prothrombin gene mutation
B. Thrombin gene mutation
C. Fibrinogen gene mutation
D. Fibrin gene mutation

Factor V Leiden and prothrombin gene mutation are the two most common autosomal dominant genetic mutation that lead to a prothrombotic state. Presence of genetic mutations such as heterozygous factor V Leiden and prothrombin gene mutation does not appear to increase the risk of recurrent VTE.

2271. Leiden is the name of a city in?
Cleveland Clinic J of Medicine 2000;67(11):825

A. Austria
B. Netherland
C. France
D. Germany

2272. Factor V Leiden best relates to which of the following?
Cleveland Clinic J of Medicine 2000;67(11):825

A. G1691A
B. G1691B
C. G1691C
D. G1691D

Factor V Leiden is a single point mutation. A G-to-A substitution at nucleotide 1691 (G1691A) of the gene that codes for factor V occurs. Inherited in an autosomal-dominant fashion, it has the effect of rendering factors V and Va resistant to degradation by activated protein C.

2273. Factor V Leiden results in a condition known as?
Circulation. 2003;107:e94-e97

A. Activated protein S resistance
B. Activated antithrombin resistance

C. Activated protein C resistance

D. All of the above

Activated protein C, a natural anticoagulant, breaks down factor Va and factor Villa, resulting in less thrombin generation and less fibrin. Activated protein C resistance was first described in 1993. >90% of cases are due to factor V Leiden mutation. Remaining 10% being due to pregnancy, OCP use, select antiphospholipid antibodies, and other factor V point mutations such as factor V Hong Kong and factor V Cambridge.

2274. Heterozygous Factor V Leiden increases the lifetime risk of having a venous thromboembolic event by?

Cleveland Clinic J of Medicine 2000;67(11):825

A. ~ 3 fold

B. ~ 5 fold

C. ~ 7 fold

D. ~ 9 fold

Factor V Leiden increases the risk of developing a DVT during pregnancy by about 7-fold. Persons homozygous for the mutation (who have two abnormal copies) have an astounding 80-fold increased risk.

2275. A woman who has factor V Leiden and takes oral contraceptive pills (OCP) has an increased risk of developing a DVT by?

Circulation. 2003;107:e94-e97

A. ~ 15 fold

B. ~ 25 fold

C. ~ 35 fold

D. ~ 45 fold

A woman who has factor V Leiden and takes oral contraceptive pills (OCP) has a 35-fold increased risk of developing a DVT.

2276. Factor V Leiden causes resistance to?

Harrison's 20th Ed. Chapter 273 Page 1910

A. Antithrombin

B. Protein C

C. Protein S

D. All of the above

Factor V Leiden causes resistance to the endogenous anticoagulant - activated protein C. Activated protein C inactivates clotting factors V and VIII.

2277. Which of the following is a naturally occurring coagulation inhibitor?

Harrison's 20th Ed. Chapter 273 Page 1910

A. Antithrombin

B. Protein C

C. Protein S

D. All of the above

Antithrombin, protein C and protein S are naturally occurring coagulation inhibitors.

2278. Which of the following is the most common acquired cause of thrombophilia?

Harrison's 20th Ed. Chapter 273 Page 1910

A. Antiphospholipid antibody syndrome

B. Cigarette smoking

C. Chronic obstructive pulmonary disease

D. Oral contraceptives

Antiphospholipid antibody syndrome is the most common acquired cause of thrombophilia and is associated with venous or arterial thrombosis.

2279. Which of the following is a predisposing factor of thrombophilia?

Harrison's 20th Ed. Chapter 273 Page 1910

A. Air pollution

B. Systemic arterial hypertension

C. Obesity

D. All of the above

Common predisposing factors of thrombophilia include cancer, obesity, cigarette smoking, systemic arterial hypertension, chronic obstructive pulmonary disease, chronic kidney disease, blood transfusion, long-haul air travel, air pollution, oral contraceptives, pregnancy, postmenopausal hormone replacement, surgery and trauma.

2280. Which of the following medical conditions contribute to the likelihood of VTE?

Harrison's 20th Ed. Chapter 273 Page 1910

A. Antiphospholipid antibody syndrome

B. Systemic arterial hypertension

C. Chronic obstructive pulmonary disease

D. All of the above

Acquired predispositions to VTE include long-haul air travel, obesity, cigarette smoking, oral contraceptives, pregnancy, postmenopausal hormone replacement, surgery, trauma. Medical conditions include APLA syndrome, cancer, systemic arterial hypertension & COPD.

2281. Increased pulmonary vascular resistance leads to increase in?

Harrison's 20th Ed. Chapter 273 Page 1910

A. Serotonin

B. Brain natriuretic peptide

C. Cardiac troponin

D. All of the above

2282. Which of the following is not a pathophysiologic abnormality in pulmonary embolism?

Harrison's 20th Ed. Chapter 273 Page 1911

A. Impaired gas exchange

B. Alveolar hypoventilation

C. Increased airway resistance

D. Decreased pulmonary compliance

2283. Massive pulmonary embolism is characterized by extensive thrombosis affecting how much of the pulmonary vasculature?

Harrison's 20th Ed. Chapter 273 Page 1911

A. At least 10%

B. At least 25%

C. At least 33%

D. At least 50%

Massive pulmonary embolism is characterized by extensive thrombosis affecting at least half of the pulmonary vasculature.

2284. Which of the following is the hallmark of massive PE?

Harrison's 20th Ed. Chapter 273 Page 1911

A. Dyspnea

B. Cyanosis

C. Hypotension

D. All of the above

Dyspnea, syncope, hypotension and cyanosis are hallmarks of massive PE.

2285. Which of the following is normal in submassive PE?
Harrison's 20th Ed. Chapter 273 Page 1911

A. Pulmonary artery pressure
B. Right ventricular diastolic function
C. Right ventricular systolic function
D. Systemic arterial pressure

Submassive PE is characterized by RV dysfunction despite normal systemic arterial pressure. The combination of right heart failure & release of cardiac biomarkers indicates a high risk of clinical deterioration.

2286. Lower extremity DVT usually begins in?
Harrison's 20th Ed. Chapter 273 Page 1911

A. Calf
B. Thigh
C. Pelvis
D. Any of the above

Lower extremity DVT usually begins in the calf and propagates proximally to the popliteal vein, femoral vein and iliac veins.

2287. Which of the following signs is related to DVT?
N Engl J Med. 1946; 234:288-291, J Am Med Assoc. 1949;140(5):476

A. Peabody's sign
B. Pratt's test
C. Lisker's sign
D. All of the above

2288. "LEFT" rule used in the diagnosis of deep-vein thrombosis in pregnancy consists of all except?
N Engl J Med. 2015;373:540-7

A. Left calf circumference ≥2 cm more than right calf
B. Edema
C. First-trimester presentation
D. Tachycardia

The "LEFT" rule is used to assess three variables to predict the likelihood of a diagnosis of deep-vein thrombosis in pregnancy: left (L) calf circumference (a difference of ≥2 cm or more from the right calf is positive), edema (E), and first-trimester presentation (FT).

2289. Which of the following is false for gestational deep-vein thrombosis?
N Engl J Med. 2015;373:540-7

A. Usually occurs in the left leg
B. Proximal rather than distal
C. Associated with increased risk of embolic complications
D. None of the above

2290. Which of the following signs is related to DVT?
JAPI. 2007;55:5-30

A. Louvel's sign
B. Lowenberg's sign
C. Bancroft's sign
D. All of the above

Peabody's sign - calf muscle spasm occurs on raising the affected leg with the foot extended. Pratt's test - pain elicited by compression on the popliteal vein in the proximal calf. Lisker's sign - tenderness when anteromedial part of tibia is percussed. Louvel's sign - pain in the distribution of affected vein which occurs during coughing or sneezing (Valsalva maneuver), and which disappears when the vein is compressed proximally. Lowenberg's sign - pain is elicited rapidly when a blood pressure cuff is placed around calf and inflated to ~80mm Hg. Bancroft's sign (Also known as Moses' sign) - pain is elicited when calf muscle is compressed forwards against tibia, but not when the calf muscle is compressed from side to side.

2291. Which of the following is also called dorsiflexion sign of DVT?
JAPI. 2007;55:5-30

A. Louvel's sign
B. Lowenberg's sign
C. Bancroft's sign
D. Homans' sign

Homans' sign or the dorsiflexion sign refers to discomfort behind the knee on forced dorsiflexion of the foot.

2292. Which of the following is a part of the classification of pulmonary embolism?
Harrison's 20th Ed. Chapter 273 Page 1911

A. Massive PE
B. Submassive PE
C. Low-risk PE
D. All of the above

2293. Eponym "The Great Masquerader" is used for?
Harrison's 20th Ed. Chapter 273 Page 1911

A. Deep venous thrombosis (DVT)
B. Pulmonary embolism (PE)
C. Venous thromboembolism (VTE)
D. All of the above

2294. "The Great Masquerader" eponym applies to?
Harrison's 20th Ed. Chapter 273 Page 1911 (2616, 2740)

A. Fibromyalgia
B. Pulmonary embolism (PE)
C. Pheochromocytoma
D. All of the above

Apart from PE, term masquerader has been used for fibromyalgia & pheochromocytoma. Historically, syphilis and tuberculosis were labeled as the "great masqueraders"

2295. The most common symptom of pulmonary embolism is?
Harrison's 20th Ed. Chapter 273 Page 1911

A. Unexplained breathlessness
B. Unexplained syncope
C. Unexplained hypotension
D. Unexplained cyanosis

The most common symptom of pulmonary embolism is unexplained breathlessness.

2296. Clinical improvement often fails to occur in which of the following when occult PE occurs concomitantly?
Harrison's 20th Ed. Chapter 273 Page 1911

A. Asthma
B. Pneumonia
C. Sarcoidosis
D. All of the above

When occult PE occurs concomitantly with overt congestive heart failure or pneumonia, clinical improvement often fails to occur despite standard medical treatment of the concomitant illness. This scenario presents a clinical clue to the possible coexistence of PE.

2297. Which of the following eponyms is used to describe presentation of DVT?
Harrison's 20th Ed. Chapter 273 Page 1911

A. Creepy ant
B. Blueberry muffin
C. Charley horse
D. Goose bump

With DVT, the most common symptom is a cramp or "charley horse" in the lower calf that persists and intensifies over several days.

2298. DVT is likely if?

Harrison's 20th Ed. Chapter 273 Page 1911

A. Sudden, severe calf discomfort
B. Fever and chills
C. Marked thigh swelling, tenderness and erythema
D. Leg is diffusely edematous

2299. Which of the following is likely in massive DVT?

Harrison's 20th Ed. Chapter 273 Page 1911

A. Sudden, severe calf discomfort
B. Severe thigh swelling
C. Diffusely edematous leg
D. Any of the above

Sudden, severe calf discomfort suggests a ruptured Baker's cyst. Severe thigh swelling & marked tenderness in inguinal area & common femoral vein occurs in massive DVT. If leg is diffusely edematous, DVT is unlikely, rather acute exacerbation of venous insufficiency due to postphlebitic syndrome is likely.

2300. Upper extremity venous thrombosis may present with?

Harrison's 20th Ed. Chapter 273 Page 1911

A. Numbness in fingers
B. Asymmetry in supraclavicular fossa
C. Pain in nail beds of fingers
D. All of the above

Upper extremity venous thrombosis may present with asymmetry in the supraclavicular fossa or in the circumference of the upper arms.

2301. May-Thurner Syndrome best relates to?

Proc (Bayl Univ Med Cent) 2012;25(3):231–233

A. Right Iliofemoral deep venous thrombosis
B. Left Iliofemoral deep venous thrombosis
C. Bilateral Iliofemoral deep venous thrombosis
D. Any of the above

First described in 1957, May-Thurner syndrome (MTS) is also known as the iliac vein compression syndrome. In this anatomical variant an overriding right common iliac artery causes compression of the left common iliac vein against the lumbar spine (L5). The anatomical defect occurs high in the pelvis, an area that is not easily visualized by ultrasound.

2302. Which of the following suggests a small pulmonary embolism?

Harrison's 20th Ed. Chapter 273 Page 1912

A. Dyspnea
B. Pleuritic pain
C. Syncope
D. Hypotension

2303. Which of the following suggests a massive pulmonary embolism?

Harrison's 19th Ed. 1632

A. Cough
B. Pleuritic pain
C. Dyspnea
D. Hemoptysis

Dyspnea is the most frequent symptom of PE, and tachypnea is its most frequent sign. Dyspnea, syncope, hypotension or cyanosis indicates a massive PE. Pleuritic pain, cough or hemoptysis suggests a small embolism located distally near the pleura. This condition is exquisitely painful because the thrombus lodges peripherally, near the innervation of pleural nerves.

2304. Which of the following nonthrombotic PE can occur after total hip or knee replacement?

Harrison's 20th Ed. Chapter 273 Page 1912

A. Fat
B. Bone marrow
C. Cotton
D. Bony fragment

Nonthrombotic PE etiologies include fat embolism after pelvic or long bone fracture, tumor embolism, bone marrow and air embolism. Cement embolism and bony fragment embolism can occur after total hip or knee replacement. Intravenous drug users may inject themselves with substances that can embolize such as hair, talc and cotton. Amniotic fluid embolism occurs when fetal membranes leak or tear at placental margin.

2305. The sensitivity of the D-dimer for DVT is?

Harrison's 20th Ed. Chapter 273 Page 1912

A. > 60%
B. > 70%
C. > 80%
D. > 90%

2306. The sensitivity of the D-dimer for PE is?

Harrison's 20th Ed. Chapter 273 Page 1912

A. > 65%
B. > 75%
C. > 85%
D. > 95%

The sensitivity of the D-dimer is >80% for DVT (including isolated calf DVT) and >95% for PE.

2307. Levels of D-dimer increase in?

Harrison's 20th Ed. Chapter 273 Page 1912

A. Myocardial infarction
B. Sepsis
C. Second or third trimester of pregnancy
D. All of the above

Levels of D-dimer increase in myocardial infarction, pneumonia, sepsis, cancer, postoperative state, and second or third trimester of pregnancy.

2308. All are true for pulmonary embolism except?

Harrison's 20th Ed. Chapter 273 Page 1912

A. Plasma D-dimer ELISA assay has high (-) predictive value
B. ABG lacks diagnostic utility
C. Westermark's sign in chest X-ray is focal oligemia
D. Palla's sign is enlarged (L) descending pulmonary artery

Quantitative ELISA plasma D-dimer level is elevated (>500 ng/mL) in more than 90% of patients with PE, reflecting plasmin's breakdown of fibrin and indicating endogenous thrombolysis. D-dimer assay is not specific and levels increase in patients with MI, sepsis etc. Plasma D-dimer ELISA has a high negative predictive value (99.6%) and can be used to help exclude PE. It has a sensitivity of 96.4%. Arterial blood gases lack diagnostic utility for PE.

2309. Which of the following biomarkers increase in PE?

Harrison's 20th Ed. Chapter 273 Page 1912

A. Serum troponin
B. Plasma heart-type fatty acid-binding protein
C. NT-pro-brain natriuretic peptide
D. All of the above

Serum troponin and plasma heart-type fatty acid-binding protein levels increase because of RV microinfarction. Myocardial stretch causes release of brain natriuretic peptide or NT-pro-brain natriuretic peptide.

2310. ECG change in pulmonary embolism include?

Harrison's 20th Ed. Chapter 273 Page 1912

A. T wave inversion in $V_{1\text{-}4}$
B. Sinus tachycardia
C. $S_1Q_3T_3$ pattern
D. All of the above

ECG abnormalities in PE include sinus tachycardia and $S_1Q_3T_3$ sign (S wave in lead I, Q wave in lead III & an inverted T wave in lead III).

2311. Most frequent ECG finding in pulmonary embolism is?

Harrison's 20th Ed. Chapter 273 Page 1912

A. New-onset atrial fibrillation
B. $S_1Q_3T_3$ pattern
C. QRS axis greater than 90º
D. T-wave inversion in leads V_1 to V_4

In PE, T-wave inversion in leads V_1 to V_4 is the most frequent change (right ventricular strain).

2312. Which of the following parameter is looked at in venous ultrasonography for DVT?

Harrison's 20th Ed. Chapter 273 Page 1912

A. Intima-media thickness
B. Diameter of the vein
C. Vein compressibility
D. All of the above

Venous ultrasonography of deep-venous system relies on loss of vein compressibility as the primary diagnostic criterion for DVT.

2313. Which of the following is found in venous ultrasonography for the diagnosis of acute DVT?

Harrison's 20th Ed. Chapter 273 Page 1912

A. Homogeneous and low echogenicity thrombus
B. Hetrogeneous and low echogenicity thrombus
C. Homogeneous and high echogenicity thrombus
D. Hetrogeneous and high echogenicity thrombus

The diagnosis of acute DVT is more reliable when thrombus is directly visualized which is homogeneous & with low echogenicity.

2314. Which of the following is found in venous ultrasonography for the diagnosis of acute DVT?

Harrison's 20th Ed. Chapter 273 Page 1912

A. Dilated vein
B. Loss of vein compressibility
C. Absent collateral channels
D. All of the above

Venous flow dynamics can be examined with Doppler imaging.

2315. Augmentation of Doppler flow pattern in venous Doppler imaging is done by?

Harrison's 20th Ed. Chapter 273 Page 1912

A. Valsalva maneuver
B. Passive leg raising
C. Manual calf compression
D. All of the above

Loss of normal respiratory variation is caused by an obstructing DVT in venous flow dynamics study with Doppler imaging. Normally, manual calf compression causes augmentation of the Doppler flow pattern.

2316. Which of the following is a feature of pulmonary embolism on chest X-ray?

Harrison's 20th Ed. Chapter 273 Page 1912

A. Westermark's sign
B. Hampton's hump
C. Palla's sign
D. All of the above

2317. Palla's sign refers to?

Harrison's 20th Ed. Chapter 273 Page 1912

A. Focal oligemia
B. Peripheral wedged-shaped density above diaphragm
C. Enlarged right descending pulmonary artery
D. Enlarged left descending pulmonary artery

2318. Westermark's sign refers to?

Harrison's 20th Ed. Chapter 273 Page 1912

A. Focal oligemia
B. Peripheral wedged-shaped density above diaphragm
C. Enlarged right descending pulmonary artery
D. Enlarged left descending pulmonary artery

2319. Hampton's hump refers to?

Harrison's 20th Ed. Chapter 273 Page 1912

A. Focal oligemia
B. Peripheral wedged-shaped density above diaphragm
C. Enlarged right descending pulmonary artery
D. Enlarged left descending pulmonary artery

In a dyspneic patient, a normal or near-normal chest X-ray suggests PE. Other abnormalities include focal oligemia (Westermark's sign), a peripheral wedged-shaped density above the diaphragm (Hampton's hump), or an enlarged right descending pulmonary artery (Palla's sign).

2320. Which of the following is the principal imaging test for the diagnosis of PE?

Harrison's 20th Ed. Chapter 273 Page 1912

A. Lung Scanning
B. Chest X-ray
C. Chest CT with intravenous contrast
D. Echocardiography

Computed tomography of chest with intravenous contrast is the principal imaging test for diagnosis of PE. Multidetector-row spiral CT scanners can image small peripheral emboli. Sixth-order branches can be visualized with resolution superior to that of conventional invasive contrast pulmonary angiography.

2321. "Triple rule-out CT" helps in the diagnosis of?
Harrison's 20th Ed. Chapter 273 Page 1912

A. Pulmonary embolism
B. Acute aortic syndrome
C. Acute coronary syndrome
D. All of the above

2322. "Triple rule-out CT" best relates to?
Harrison's 20th Ed. Chapter 273 Page 1912

A. Ultrasonography
B. ECG
C. Echocardiography
D. All of the above

"Triple rule-out CT" utilizes ECG synchronized acquisition, adjusts contrast material timing & opacifies both thoracic aorta & pulmonary artery circulation to exclude PE, acute aortic & acute coronary syndrome.

2323. Which of the following is false?
Harrison's 20th Ed. Chapter 273 Page 1913

A. Normal or nearly normal chest X-ray often occurs in PE
B. Normal venous ultrasound does not exclude PE
C. Lung scanning is the second-line diagnostic test for PE
D. None of the above

PE is unlikely in normal/nearly normal lung scan. Echocardiography is not a reliable diagnostic tool for acute PE.

2324. Pulmonary perfusion scan that has a high probability for PE should have how many segmental perfusion defects in the presence of normal ventilation scan?
Harrison's 20th Ed. Chapter 273 Page 1913

A. One or more
B. Two or more
C. Three or more
D. Four or more

A high probability pulmonary perfusion scan for PE is defined as having two or more segmental perfusion defects in the presence of normal ventilation scan.

2325. Which of the following radiolabeled inhaled gas is used in ventilation scan?
Harrison's 20th Ed. Chapter 273 Page 1912

A. Helium (He)
B. Neon (Ne)
C. Krypton (Kr)
D. Argon (Ar)

Xenon-133, Krypton-81m, or Technetium-99m DTPA are the radiolabeled inhaled gases used in ventilation scan which improves the specificity of the perfusion scan.

2326. Which of the following about perfusion scan is false?
Harrison's 20th Ed. Chapter 273 Page 1912

A. Agent used is macro aggregated albumin labeled with a gamma-emitting radionuclide like technetium^{99}m (^{99}mTc-MAA).
B. Injected intravenously
C. Gamma camera acquires the images
D. None of the above

2327. Echocardiography is the least useful diagnostic tool for?
Harrison's 20th Ed. Chapter 273 Page 1913

A. Acute myocardial infarction
B. Pulmonary embolism
C. Pericardial tamponade
D. Aortic dissection

Echocardiography is not a reliable diagnostic imaging tool for acute PE because most patients with PE have normal echocardiograms.

2328. In echocadiography, McConnell's sign is specific for which of the following?
Harrison's 20th Ed. Chapter 273 Page 1913

A. HOCM
B. Pulmonary embolism
C. Acute rheumatic fever
D. Infective endocarditis

Echocardiographic McConnell's sign refers to right ventricular free wall hypokinesis with normal or hyperkinetic right ventricular apical motion and is specific for PE.

2329. Transesophageal echocardiography can identify which of the following?
Harrison's 20th Ed. Chapter 273 Page 1913

A. Saddle PE
B. Right main PE
C. Left main PE
D. All of the above

Transesophageal echocardiography can identify saddle, right main or left main PE.

2330. Definitive diagnostic test for pulmonary embolism is?
Harrison's 20th Ed. Chapter 273 Page 1913

A. V/Q scan
B. MR Angiography
C. CT Chest
D. Selective pulmonary angiography

Selective pulmonary angiography demonstrating intraluminal filling defect in more than one projection is the most specific examination available for establishing the definitive diagnosis of PE. Although chest CT with contrast has replaced invasive pulmonary angiography as a diagnostic test, invasive catheter-based diagnostic testing is reserved for patients with technically unsatisfactory chest CTs and those in whom an interventional procedure such as catheter-directed thrombolysis or embolectomy is planned.

2331. Secondary signs of PE on pulmonary angiography include?
Harrison's 20th Ed. Chapter 273 Page 1913

A. Prolonged arterial phase with slow filling
B. Tortuous, tapering peripheral vessels
C. Segmental oligemia or avascularity
D. All of the above

Secondary signs of PE on pulmonary angiography include abrupt occlusion ("cutoff") of vessels, segmental oligemia or avascularity, prolonged arterial phase with slow filling & tortuous, tapering peripheral vessels.

2332. In pulmonary embolism, which of the following identify high-risk patients?
Harrison's 20th Ed. Chapter 273 Page 1914

A. Hemodynamic instability
B. Right ventricular dysfunction on echocardiography

C. Elevation of troponin level
D. All of the above

Hemodynamic instability, right ventricular dysfunction on echocardiography, or elevation of the troponin level due to right ventricular microinfarction identify high-risk PE. RV enlargement on chest CT indicates a 5x increased likelihood of death within next 30 days compared with PE patients with normal RV size on chest CT.

2333. In PE, which of the following is the most widely used approach to risk stratification?
Harrison's 20th Ed. Chapter 273 Page 1914

A. Elevation of troponin level
B. $S_1Q_3T_3$ pattern in ECG
C. Detection of RV hypokinesis by echocardiography
D. Increased levels of D-dimer

In PE, detection of RV hypokinesis on echocardiography is most widely used for risk stratification.

2334. Which of the following is a heparin-based parenteral anticoagulant?
Harrison's 20th Ed. Chapter 273 Page 1914

A. Argatroban
B. Rivaroxaban
C. Fondaparinux
D. Bivalirudin

The three heparin-based parenteral anticoagulants are unfractionated heparin (UFH), low-molecular-weight heparin (LMWH) and fondaparinux.

2335. Which of the following is a direct thrombin inhibitor?
Harrison's 20th Ed. Chapter 273 Page 1914

A. Argatroban
B. Dabigatran
C. Bivalirudin
D. All of the above

Direct thrombin inhibitors are argatroban, dabigatran, or bivalirudin and should be used in patients with proven or suspected heparin-induced thrombocytopenia.

2336. Primary therapy of PE is?
Harrison's 20th Ed. Chapter 273 Page 1914

A. Anticoagulation with heparin
B. Anticoagulation with warfarin
C. Thrombolysis
D. Placement of inferior vena cava filter

Primary therapy consists of clot dissolution with thrombolysis or removal of PE by embolectomy. Anticoagulation with heparin and warfarin or placement of an inferior vena cava filter constitutes secondary prevention of recurrent PE.

2337. Which of the following prevents postphlebitic syndrome?
Harrison's 20th Ed. Chapter 273 Page 1914

A. Vascular compression stockings
B. Aspirin
C. Warfarin
D. Clopidogrel

Only therapy to prevent postphlebitic syndrome is daily use of below-knee 30 - 40 mm Hg vascular compression stockings.

2338. In massive pulmonary embolism, immediately effective anticoagulation is initiated with?
Harrison's 20th Ed. Chapter 273 Page 1914

A. Unfractionated heparin (UFH)
B. Low molecular weight heparin (LMWH)
C. Fondaparinux
D. Any of the above

In massive PE, immediately effective anticoagulation is initiated with a parenteral drug - UFH, LMWH (Enoxaparin, Tinzaparin), fondaparinux, argatroban, bivalirudin, rivaroxaban or apixaban.

2339. A typical initial intravenous bolus of unfractionated heparin in PE is?
Harrison's 20th Ed. Chapter 273 Page 1914

A. 60 U / kg
B. 80 U / kg
C. 100 U / kg
D. 120 U / kg

UFH is dosed to achieve a target activated partial thromboplastin time (aPTT) that is 2 - 3 times the upper limit of laboratory normal. This is usually equivalent to an aPTT of 60 - 80 seconds. For UFH, a typical initial intravenous bolus is 80 U/kg, followed by an initial infusion rate of 18/kg per hour.

2340. What is the dose of Fondaparinux in patients weighing between 50 - 100 kg?
Harrison's 20th Ed. Chapter 114 Page 851

A. 2.5 mg
B. 5 mg
C. 7.5 mg
D. 10 mg

Fondaparinux is an anti-Xa pentasaccharide. It is administered by once-daily subcutaneous injection. Patients weighing <50 kg receive 5 mg, 50-100 kg patients receive 7.5 mg, and patients weighing >100 kg receive 10 mg. 2.5 mg of Fondaparinux is used to prevent VTE.

2341. Warfarin inhibits which of the following?
Harrison's 20th Ed. Chapter 114 Page 853

A. Vitamin K epoxide reductase
B. Vitamin K epoxide oxidase
C. Vitamin K epoxide hydrolase
D. All of the above

Warfarin inhibits vitamin K epoxide reductase (VKOR) thereby blocking the γ-carboxylation process. This results in the synthesis of vitamin K-dependent clotting proteins (factors II, VII, IX and X) that are only partially γ-carboxylated. Warfarin acts as an anticoagulant because these partially γ-carboxylated proteins have reduced or absent biologic activity.

2342. Which of the following about warfarin is false?
Harrison's 20th Ed. Chapter 114 Page 853

A. Initially developed as a rodenticide
B. Warfarin is a racemic mixture of R and S isomers
C. S-warfarin is most active
D. None of the above

2343. Warfarin acts by preventing carboxylation activation of which coagulation factor?
Harrison's 20th Ed. Chapter 273 Page 1914

A. II
B. VII
C. X
D. All of the above

Warfarin is a vitamin K antagonist that prevents carboxylation activation of coagulation factors II, VII, IX, and X.

2344. Heparin should be overlapped with oral anticoagulation for at least how many days?

Harrison's 20th Ed. Chapter 273 Page 1914

A. 2 to 3 days
B. 3 to 4 days
C. 4 to 5 days
D. 5 to 6 days

Warfarin requires 5-7 days to achieve a therapeutic effect. During that period, the parenteral and oral agents are overlapped. If warfarin is initiated as monotherapy during an acute thrombotic illness, a paradoxical exacerbation of hypercoagulability increases the likelihood of thrombosis. Overlapping UFH, LMWH, fondaparinux or parenteral direct thrombin inhibitors with warfarin for at least 5 days will nullify the early procoagulant effect of warfarin.

2345. Which of the following affect warfarin metabolism?

Harrison's 20th Ed. Chapter 273 Page 1914

A. Drug-drug and drug-food interactions
B. Age, sex, weight
C. Concomitant drugs
D. All of the above

2346. Antidote for bleeding from fondaparinux is?

Harrison's 20th Ed. Chapter 273 Page 1914

A. Protamine sulfate
B. Vitamin K
C. Recombinant factor VIIa
D. None of the above

There is no specific antidote for bleeding from fondaparinux, direct thrombin inhibitors or factor Xa inhibitors.

2347. Which of the following is an oral anticoagulant?

Harrison's 20th Ed. Chapter 114 Page 848

A. Dabigatran etexilate
B. Rivaroxaban
C. Apixaban
D. All of the above

2348. Which of the following is an oral anticoagulant?

Harrison's 20th Ed. Chapter 114 Page 848

A. Lepirudin
B. Bivalirudin
C. Argatroban
D. None of the above

Currently available oral anticoagulants include warfarin; dabigatran etexilate, an oral thrombin inhibitor; and rivaroxaban, apixaban, and edoxaban, which are oral factor Xa inhibitors. Parenteral anticoagulants include heparin, low molecular-weight heparin (LMWH), fondaparinux (a synthetic pentasaccharide), lepirudin, desirudin, bivalirudin, and argatroban.

2349. Catastrophic bleeding associated with warfarin administration is best treated by?

Harrison's 20th Ed. Chapter 112 Page 837

A. Fresh-frozen plasma
B. Recombinant factor VIIa therapy (rFVIIa)
C. Vitamin K
D. All of the above

For life-threatening or intracranial hemorrhage due to heparin or LMWH, protamine sulfate can be administered. Major bleeding from warfarin is best managed with prothrombin complex concentrate. With non-life threatening bleeding, fresh-frozen plasma can be used. Recombinant human coagulation factor VIIa (rFVIIa) is used to manage catastrophic bleeding from warfarin. For minor bleeding or to manage an excessively high INR in the absence of bleeding, oral vitamin K may be administered.

2350. Individuals with loss-of-function alleles in which of the following are at increased risk for bleeding with warfarin?

Harrison's 20th Ed. Chapter 63 Page 423

A. CYP2C8
B. CYP2C9
C. CYP2C19
D. CYP2C21

CYP2C9 mediates elimination of warfarin. Individuals with loss-of-function alleles in CYP2C9, responsible for metabolism of the active S-enantiomer of warfarin are at increased risk for bleeding.

2351. Risk of upper gastrointestinal bleeding is increased by how much in those taking warfarin and an NSAID?

Harrison's 20th Ed. Chapter 63 Page 426

A. Twice
B. Thrice
C. Four times
D. Five times

In patients treated with warfarin, risk of upper gastrointestinal bleeding is increased almost threefold by concomitant use of an NSAID.

2352. Most common nonbleeding side effect of warfarin is?

Harrison's 19th Ed. 354

A. Alopecia
B. Skin necrosis
C. Seizure
D. Osteoporosis

Most common nonbleeding side effect of warfarin is alopecia. Warfarin-induced skin necrosis is rare.

2353. Warfarin embryopathy occurs with warfarin exposure during?

Harrison's 20th Ed. Chapter 114 Page 854

A. Second to sixth weeks of gestation
B. Sixth to twelfth weeks of gestation
C. Twelfth to sixteen weeks of gestation
D. Twenty to twenty four weeks of gestation

Warfarin is teratogenic. Warfarin embryopathy is most common with exposure during 6th to 12th weeks of gestation. Warfarin therapy is contraindicated in first trimester due to its association with fetal chondrodysplasia punctata. In the second and third trimesters, warfarin may cause fetal optic atrophy and mental retardation.

2354. Warfarin can be administered safely during?

Harrison's 20th Ed. Chapter 114 Page 854

A. Second trimester of pregnancy
B. Postpartum period
C. Breast feeding
D. All of the above

Warfarin is safe during second trimester, postpartum and breast feeding period.

2355. Warfarin use during pregnancy can cause?

N Engl J Med. 2015;373:540-7

A. Central nervous system abnormalities
B. Pregnancy loss
C. Fetal anticoagulation
D. All of the above

Warfarin is contraindicated in pregnancy as it crosses placenta and is associated with embryopathy, central nervous system abnormalities, pregnancy loss, and fetal anticoagulation with possible bleeding.

2356. Which of the following about Novel oral anticoagulants (NOACs) is false?
Harrison's 20th Ed. Chapter 273 Page 1915

A. Administered in a fixed dose
B. Establish effective anticoagulation within hours of ingestion
C. Require no laboratory coagulation monitoring
D. None of the above

Novel oral anticoagulants (NOACs) are administered in a fixed dose, result in effective anticoagulation within hours of ingestion, require no laboratory coagulation monitoring, and have few drug-drug or drug-food interactions.

2357. "Bridging" with a parenteral anticoagulant is required when which of the following is used?
Harrison's 20th Ed. Chapter 273 Page 1915

A. Betrixaban
B. Warfarin
C. Rivaroxaban
D. All of the above

Rivaroxaban is a factor Xa inhibitor, and dabigatran is a direct thrombin inhibitor. Because of these drugs' rapid onset of action & relatively short half-life compared with warfarin, "bridging" with a parenteral anticoagulant is not required.

2358. "Bridging" with a parenteral anticoagulant is required when which of the following is used?
Harrison's 20th Ed. Chapter 273 Page 1915

A. Betrixaban
B. Rivaroxaban
C. Apixaban
D. None of the above

Betrixaban, rivaroxaban and apixaban are direct factor Xa inhibitors, and are approved as monotherapy for acute and extended treatment of DVT and PE, without a parenteral "bridging" anticoagulant.

2359. Which of the following is a dabigatran antibody?
Harrison's 20th Ed. Chapter 273 Page 1915

A. Mepolizumab
B. Reslizumab
C. Idarucizumab
D. Benralizumab

The dabigatran antibody, idarucizumab, is an effective & rapidly acting antidote for dabigatran.

2360. Andexanet is an antidote for?
Harrison's 20th Ed. Chapter 273 Page 1915

A. Betrixaban
B. Rivaroxaban
C. Apixaban
D. All of the above

Andexanet is a universal anti-Xa antidote for betrixaban, rivaroxaban, apixaban & edoxaban.

2361. Bleeding from warfarin is managed with?
Harrison's 20th Ed. Chapter 273 Page 1915

A. Prothrombin complex concentrate
B. Fresh-frozen plasma
C. Intravenous vitamin K
D. All of the above

Major bleeding from warfarin is best managed with prothrombin complex concentrate. With less serious bleeding, fresh-frozen plasma or IV vitamin K can be used. Oral vitamin K is effective for managing minor bleeding or an excessively high INR in the absence of bleeding.

2362. Duration of anticoagulation for PE following surgery or trauma is?
Harrison's 20th Ed. Chapter 273 Page 1915

A. 3 - 6 months
B. 6 - 12 months
C. 12 - 18 months
D. Indefinite

Duration of anticoagulation for PE following surgery or trauma is 3 - 6 months.

2363. Duration of anticoagulation for PE with moderate or high levels of anticardiolipin antibodies is?
Harrison's 20th Ed. Chapter 273 Page 1915

A. 3 - 6 months
B. 6 - 12 months
C. 12 - 18 months
D. Indefinite

Duration of anticoagulation for PE with moderate or high levels of anticardiolipin antibodies is indefinite, even if initial VTE was provoked by trauma or surgery.

2364. Indefinite-duration anticoagulation is recommended for?
Harrison's 20th Ed. Chapter 273 Page 1915

A. Patients with high levels of anticardiolipin antibodies
B. Patients with idiopathic VTE
C. Patients with cancer and VTE
D. All of the above

2365. Which of the following is considered unprovoked VTE?
Harrison's 20th Ed. Chapter 273 Page 1915

A. That occurs following surgery, trauma
B. That occurs during long-haul air travel
C. That occurs following estrogen therapy
D. That occurs following indwelling central venous catheter

VTE that occurs during long-haul air travel is considered unprovoked. Among patients with idiopathic, unprovoked VTE, recurrence rate is high after cessation of anticoagulation.

2366. First-line inotropic agent for treatment of PE-related shock is?
Harrison's 20th Ed. Chapter 273 Page 1915

A. Dopamine / dobutamine
B. Phenylephrine
C. Vasopressin
D. Norepinephrine

Dopamine and dobutamine are first-line inotropic agents for treatment of PE-related shock. Other agents that may be effective include norepinephrine, vasopressin or phenylephrine.

2367. Successful fibrinolytic therapy in PE leads to?
Harrison's 20th Ed. Chapter 273 Page 1915

A. Rapidly reversal of right heart failure
B. Lowers rate of death
C. Prevention of recurrent PE
D. All of the above

The only FDA approved indication for PE fibrinolysis is massive PE. Successful fibrinolytic therapy in PE rapidly reverses right heart failure and leads to a lower rate of death and recurrent PE.

2368. The preferred fibrinolytic regimen in PE is?

Harrison's 20th Ed. Chapter 273 Page 1915

A. Recombinant tissue plasminogen activator (tPA)

B. Streptokinase

C. Urokinase

D. Alteplase

Preferred fibrinolytic regimen is 100 mg of tPA administered as a continuous peripheral intravenous infusion over 2 hours. Lower dose i.e. 50 mg of TPA is associated with fewer bleeding complications.

2369. PE patients respond to fibrinolysis for up to how many days after the PE has occurred?

Harrison's 20th Ed. Chapter 273 Page 1915

A. 1 day

B. 3 days

C. 7 days

D. 14 days

PE patients respond to fibrinolysis for up to 14 days after the PE has occurred.

2370. What is the risk of intracranial hemorrhage following fibrinolysis in PE?

Harrison's 20th Ed. Chapter 273 Page 1915

A. 0.1 - 0.3%

B. 0.3 - 0.9%

C. 0.9 - 1.9%

D. 2 - 3%

The overall major bleeding rate is about 10%, including a 2 - 3% risk of intracranial hemorrhage.

Diseases of the Aorta

2371. In adults, aortic diameter at the origin is approximately?
Harrison's 20th Ed. Chapter 274 Page 1917

A. 2 cm
B. 3 cm
C. 4 cm
D. 5 cm

In adults, aortic diameter at the origin is ~3 cm, 2.5 cm in descending portion in thorax, and 1.8 to 2 cm in abdomen.

2372. Aortic wall intima is composed of all except?
Harrison's 20th Ed. Chapter 274 Page 1917

A. Endothelium
B. Subendothelial connective tissue
C. Internal elastic lamina
D. Smooth muscle cells

Aortic wall thin intima is composed of endothelium, subendothelial connective tissue, and an internal elastic lamina.

2373. Vasa vasorum and nervi vascularis are located in which of the following structures of aorta?
Harrison's 20th Ed. Chapter 274 Page 1917

A. Endothelium
B. Tunica media
C. Adventitia
D. All of the above

Vasa vasorum & nervi vascularis are located in adventitia composed of connective tissue.

2374. Kommerell's diverticulum is an anatomic remnant of?
Harrison's 20th Ed. Chapter 274 Page 1917

A. Left umblical artery
B. Right aortic arch
C. Ductus arteriosus
D. Left atrial appendage

Kommerell's diverticulum is an anatomic remnant of a right aortic arch.

2375. Coarctation of the aorta may be associated with?
Harrison's 20th Ed. Chapter 274 Page 1917

A. Bicuspid aortic valve
B. Aortic arch hypoplasia
C. Intracranial aneurysms
D. All of the above

2376. Which of the following about coarctation of the aorta is false?
Harrison's 20th Ed. Chapter 274 Page 1917

A. Occurs near the insertion of ligamentum arteriosum
B. Occurs adjacent to the right subclavian artery
C. Associated with congenital heart defects
D. None of the above

2377. In a pseudoaneurysm, which of the following layers is not disrupted?
Harrison's 20th Ed. Chapter 274 Page 1917

A. Intima
B. Media
C. Adventitia
D. None of the above

In pseudoaneurysm, intimal & medial layers are disrupted & dilatation is lined by adventitia only. A true aneurysm involves all three layers of the vessel wall.

2378. A fusiform aneurysm affects what proportion of the circumference of a segment of the vessel?
Harrison's 20th Ed. Chapter 274 Page 1917

A. 25%
B. 50%
C. 75%
D. 100%

A fusiform aneurysm affects the entire circumference of a segment of the vessel, resulting in a diffusely dilated artery. A saccular aneurysm involves only a portion of circumference, resulting in an outpouching of the vessel wall.

2379. Which of the following factors is not associated with degenerative aortic aneurysms?
Harrison's 20th Ed. Chapter 274 Page 1917

A. Aging
B. Alcohol
C. Cigarette smoking
D. Hypercholesterolemia

Factors associated with degenerative aortic aneurysms include aging, cigarette smoking, hypercholesterolemia, male sex, and a family history of aortic aneurysms.

2380. The most common pathologic condition associated with degenerative aortic aneurysms is?
Harrison's 20th Ed. Chapter 274 Page 1917

A. Atherosclerosis
B. Genetic or developmental
C. Vasculitis
D. Infection

Most common pathologic condition associated with degenerative aortic aneurysms is atherosclerosis.

2381. Cystic medial necrosis affects which component of the aortic wall?
Harrison's 20th Ed. Chapter 274 Page 1918

A. Intima
B. Media
C. Adventitia
D. All of the above

Cystic medial necrosis is a histopathologic term used to describe degeneration of collagen & elastic fibers in tunica media of aorta.

2382. Most common pathological condition for ascending aortic aneurysm is?

Harrison's 20th Ed. Chapter 274 Page 1918

A. Hypertension
B. Atherosclerosis
C. Cystic medial necrosis
D. Tuberculosis

Cystic medial necrosis characteristically affects the proximal aorta, leading to circumferential weakness, dilatation and development of fusiform aneurysm.

2383. Cystic medial necrosis is prevalent in patients with?

Harrison's 20th Ed. Chapter 274 Page 1918

A. Marfan syndrome
B. Ehlers-Danlos syndrome type IV
C. Loeys-Dietz syndrome
D. All of the above

Cystic medial necrosis is particularly prevalent in patients with Marfan syndrome, Loeys-Dietz syndrome, Ehlers-Danlos syndrome type IV, hypertension, congenital bicuspid aortic valves, and familial thoracic aortic aneurysm syndromes.

2384. Mutations of the gene that encodes fibrillin-1 are present in patients with?

Harrison's 20th Ed. Chapter 274 Page 1918

A. Marfan syndrome
B. Ehlers-Danlos syndrome type IV
C. Loeys-Dietz syndrome
D. Osteogenesis Imperfecta (OI)

Mutations of the gene that encodes fibrillin-1 are present in patients with Marfan syndrome.

2385. Loeys-Dietz syndrome is caused by mutations in the genes that encode?

Harrison's 20th Ed. Chapter 274 Page 1918

A. COL5A1
B. TNXB
C. TGF-β receptors 1 (TGFBR1)
D. PLOD1

Loeys-Dietz syndrome is due to mutations in genes that encode TGF-β 1 (TGFBR1) & 2 (TGFBR2).

2386. Loeys-Dietz syndrome (LDS) is characterized by all except?

Harrison's 20th Ed. Chapter 274 Page 1918

A. Aortic aneurysms
B. Hearing loss
C. Cleft palate
D. Hypertelorism

Loeys-Dietz syndrome (LDS) is characterized by aortic aneurysms, cleft palate & hypertelorism. LDS is related to Marfan Syndrome.

2387. Mutations of type III procollagen results in?

Harrison's 20th Ed. Chapter 274 Page 1918

A. Ehlers-Danlos type I syndrome
B. Ehlers-Danlos type II syndrome
C. Ehlers-Danlos type III syndrome
D. Ehlers-Danlos type IV syndrome

Mutations of type III procollagen have been implicated in Ehlers-Danlos type IV syndrome.

2388. Syphilitic aneurysms are mostly located in?

Harrison's 20th Ed. Chapter 274 Page 1918

A. Ascending aorta
B. Thoracic aorta
C. Abdominal aorta
D. All of the above

Approximately 90% of syphilitic aneurysms are located in ascending aorta or aortic arch. Syphilis is a relatively uncommon cause of aortic aneurysm.

2389. Tuberculous aneurysms are mostly located in?

Harrison's 20th Ed. Chapter 274 Page 1918

A. Ascending aorta
B. Thoracic aorta
C. Abdominal aorta
D. All of the above

Tuberculous aneurysms typically affect thoracic aorta. Direct extension of tubercular infection from hilar lymph nodes or contiguous abscesses or from bacterial seeding resulting granulomatous destruction of medial layer is the pathogenetic mechanism.

2390. All of the following conditions can lead to dilatation of the ascending aorta except?

Harrison's 20th Ed. Chapter 274 Page 1918

A. Ankylosing spondylitis
B. Rheumatoid arthritis
C. Reiter's syndrome
D. Behcet's disease

Spondyloarthropathies like ankylosing spondylitis, rheumatoid arthritis, psoriatic arthritis, relapsing polychondritis and Reiter's syndrome are associated with dilatation of the ascending aorta while Behcet's disease, IgG4-related systemic disease and Cogan's syndrome cause thoracic & abdominal aortic aneurysms.

2391. Most common pathological condition associated with aneurysms of aortic arch & descending thoracic aorta is?

Harrison's 20th Ed. Chapter 274 Page 1918

A. Hypertension
B. Atherosclerosis
C. Cystic medial necrosis
D. Tuberculosis

Atherosclerosis is the most frequent cause of aneurysms of aortic arch & descending thoracic aorta.

2392. Most common pathological condition for distal abdominal aortic aneurysm below renal arteries is?

Harrison's 20th Ed. Chapter 274 Page 1919

A. Hypertension
B. Atherosclerosis
C. Cystic medial necrosis
D. Tuberculosis

At least 90% of all abdominal aortic aneurysms >4.0 cm are affected by atherosclerosis, and most of these aneurysms are below the level of the renal arteries.

2393. What percentage of atherosclerotic aneurysms are located in distal abdominal aorta, below the renal arteries?

Harrison's 20th Ed. Chapter 274 Page 1919

A. 25%
B. 33%
C. 50%
D. 75%

75% of atherosclerotic aneurysms are located in distal abdominal aorta, below the renal arteries.

2394. For descending thoracic aneurysms, risk of rupture increases substantially beyond?

Harrison's 20th Ed. Chapter 274 Page 1918

A. > 4 cm
B. > 5 cm
C. > 6 cm
D. > 7 cm

The average growth rate of thoracic aneurysms is 0.1 - 0.2 cm per year. Risk of rupture increases substantially for ascending aortic aneurysms >6 cm and descending thoracic aneurysms >7 cm.

2395. The annual risk of aneurysmal rupture of thoracic aortic aneurysms that are > 6 cm in diameter is?

Harrison's 20th Ed. Chapter 274 Page 1918

A. 3%
B. 5%
C. 7%
D. 9%

The risk of aneurysmal rupture is ~2 - 3% per year for thoracic aortic aneurysms <4.0 cm in diameter to 7% per year for those >6 cm in diameter.

2396. Aneurysmal dilation of ascending aorta causes congestive heart failure as a consequence of?

Harrison's 20th Ed. Chapter 274 Page 1918

A. Aortic stenosis
B. Aortic regurgitation
C. Hypertension
D. All of the above

Aneurysmal dilation of ascending aorta causes CHF as a consequence of aortic regurgitation.

2397. Chest X-ray finding that suggests thoracic aortic aneurysm is?

Harrison's 20th Ed. Chapter 274 Page 1918

A. Widening of the mediastinal shadow
B. Displacement or compression of trachea
C. Displacement or compression of left main stem bronchus
D. All of the above

2398. Which of the following reduce rate of aortic dilation in Marfan's syndrome by blocking TGF-β signaling?

Harrison's 20th Ed. Chapter 274 Page 1918

A. β-Adrenergic blockers
B. Angiotensin receptor antagonists
C. Diuretics
D. All of the above

Angiotensin receptor antagonists reduce the rate of aortic dilation in patients with Marfan's syndrome by blocking TGF-β signaling.

2399. Operative repair is indicated in asymptomatic aneurysms when aortic root or ascending aortic diameter is?

Harrison's 20th Ed. Chapter 274 Page 1919

A. ≥ 3.5 cm
B. ≥ 4.5 cm
C. ≥ 5.5 cm
D. ≥ 6.5 cm

2400. Operative repair is indicated in asymptomatic aneurysms when growth rate is?

Harrison's 20th Ed. Chapter 274 Page 1919

A. > 0.1 cm per year
B. > 0.3 cm per year
C. > 0.5 cm per year
D. > 0.7 cm per year

Operative repair with placement of a prosthetic graft is indicated in patients with symptomatic ascending thoracic aortic aneurysms and for most asymptomatic aneurysms, including those associated with bicuspid aortic valves, when aortic root or ascending aortic diameter is ≥5.5 cm, or when the growth rate is >0.5 cm per year.

2401. As abdominal aortic aneurysms expand, patients complain of pain in?

Harrison's 20th Ed. Chapter 274 Page 1919

A. Chest
B. Lower back
C. Scrotum
D. Any of the above

2402. Which of the following is effective in managing abdominal aortic aneurysm?

Harrison's 20th Ed. Chapter 274 Page 1919

A. Statins
B. β-adrenergic blockers
C. Renin-angiotensin inhibitors
D. All of the above

2403. Which of the following is an acute aortic syndrome?

Harrison's 20th Ed. Chapter 274 Page 1919

A. Aortic dissection
B. Intramural hematoma
C. Penetrating atherosclerotic ulcer
D. All of the above

The four major acute aortic syndromes are aortic rupture, aortic dissection, intramural hematoma and penetrating atherosclerotic ulcer.

2404. Which of the following acute aortic syndromes is least aggressive?

Harrison's 20th Ed. Chapter 274 Page 1919

A. Aortic dissection
B. Intramural hematoma
C. Penetrating atherosclerotic ulcer
D. Aortic rupture

Penetrating atherosclerotic ulcers are caused by erosion of a plaque into aortic media. They are usually localized and are not associated with extensive propagation.

2405. Aortic dissection commonly occurs at?

Harrison's 20th Ed. Chapter 274 Page 1919

A. Right lateral wall of ascending aorta
B. Left lateral wall of ascending aorta
C. Right lateral wall of thoracic descending aorta
D. Right lateral wall of thoracic descending aorta

Aortic dissection is caused by a circumferential or, less frequently, transverse tear of the intima. It often occurs along the right lateral wall of the ascending aorta where the hydraulic shear stress is high. Another common site is the descending thoracic aorta just below the ligamentum arteriosum.

2406. Acute intramural hematoma result from rupture of?
Harrison's 20th Ed. Chapter 274 Page 1920

A. Intima
B. Vasa vasorum
C. Collateral artery
D. Any of the above

Acute intramural hematoma results from rupture of vasa vasorum with hemorrhage into wall of the aorta.

2407. Acute intramural hematoma most commonly occurs in?
Harrison's 20th Ed. Chapter 274 Page 1920

A. Ascending aorta
B. Arch of aorta
C. Descending thoracic aorta
D. Descending abdominal aorta

Most of acute intramural hematomas occur in descending thoracic aorta.

2408. Stanford & DeBakey classifications are used to classify?
Harrison's 20th Ed. Chapter 274 Page 1920

A. Peripheral vascular disease
B. Aortic dissection
C. Renal artery stenosis
D. Internal carotid artery lesions

2409. Aortic dissection is the major cause of morbidity and mortality in patients with?
Harrison's 20th Ed. Chapter 274 Page 1920

A. Marfan's syndrome
B. Loeys-Dietz syndrome
C. Ehlers-Danlos syndrome
D. All of the above

2410. Incidence of aortic dissection is increased in patients with?
Harrison's 20th Ed. Chapter 274 Page 1920

A. Takayasu's arteritis
B. Bicuspid aortic valve
C. Coarctation of aorta
D. All of the above

2411. Incidence of aortic dissection is increased during which of the following period of pregnancy?
Harrison's 20th Ed. Chapter 274 Page 1920

A. Second trimester of pregnancy
B. Third trimester of pregnancy
C. Intrapartum period
D. Post partum period

Incidence of aortic dissection is increased in normal women during 3rd trimester of pregnancy.

2412. Which of the following about aortic dissection is false?
Harrison's 20th Ed. Chapter 274 Page 1921

A. Peak incidence is in sixth & seventh decades
B. Men are more affected than women (2:1)
C. Acute aortic regurgitation is common
D. None of the above

2413. Which of the following drugs should be avoided while managing hypertension in acute aortic dissection?
Harrison's 20th Ed. Chapter 274 Page 1921

A. Beta adrenergic blockers
B. Sodium nitroprusside
C. Diazoxide
D. Diltiazem

2414. Which of the following drugs should be avoided while managing hypertension in acute aortic dissection?
Harrison's 20th Ed. Chapter 274 Page 1921

A. Labetalol
B. Sodium nitroprusside
C. Hydralazine
D. Verapamil

For acute dissection, parenteral beta-adrenergic blockers (IV propranolol, metoprolol, labetalol or esmolol) should be administered to achieve a heart rate of ~60 beats/min. Sodium nitroprusside infusion is used to lower SBP to <120 mm Hg. Verapamil, diltiazem or enalaprilat may be used parenterally. Isolated use of direct vasodilators like diazoxide and hydralazine is contraindicated because these agents can increase hydraulic shear and may propagate dissection.

2415. Acute occlusion in distal abdominal aorta usually results from?
Harrison's 20th Ed. Chapter 274 Page 1922

A. Saddle embolus from the heart
B. In situ thrombosis
C. Extramural compression
D. Accidently during pelvic surgery

2416. Aortitis may be caused by?
Harrison's 20th Ed. Chapter 274 Page 1922

A. Cogan's syndrome
B. Erdheim-Chester disease
C. IgG4-related systemic disease
D. All of the above

2417. Infection that may cause aortitis is?
Harrison's 20th Ed. Chapter 274 Page 1922

A. Syphilis
B. Tuberculosis
C. Salmonella
D. All of the above

2418. Which of the following is termed pulseless disease?
Harrison's 20th Ed. Chapter 274 Page 1922

A. Infective aortitis
B. Giant cell arteritis
C. Takayasu's arteritis
D. Syphilitic aortitis

Takayasu' s arteritis is also termed pulseless disease because of the frequent occlusion of the large arteries originating from the aorta.

2419. Takayasu's arteritis predominantly involves which of the following?
Harrison's 20th Ed. Chapter 274 Page 1922

A. Ascending aorta
B. Descending thoracic aorta
C. Descending abdominal aorta
D. All of the above

Takayasu's arteritis is an inflammatory disease that involves the ascending aorta and aortic arch causing obstruction of the aorta and its major arteries.

2420. Which of the following about Takayasu's arteritis is false?
Harrison's 20th Ed. Chapter 274 Page 1922

A. Panarteritis
B. Affects young females of Asian descent
C. Progressive course with no definitive therapy
D. None of the above

2421. Which of the following may be associated with polymyalgia rheumatica?
Harrison's 20th Ed. Chapter 274 Page 1922

A. Infective aortitis
B. Giant cell arteritis
C. Takayasu's arteritis
D. Syphilitic aortitis

Giant cell arteritis is a disease of the old with focal granulomatous lesions involving the entire arterial wall. It may be associated with polymyalgia rheumatica.

2422. Which of the following disorders associated with aortitis involve the ascending aorta?
Harrison's 20th Ed. Chapter 274 Page 1922

A. Rheumatoid arthritis
B. Ankylosing spondylitis
C. Psoriatic arthritis
D. All of the above

Rheumatoid arthritis, ankylosing spondylitis, psoriatic arthritis, reactive arthritis (Reiter's syndrome), relapsing polychondritis and inflammatory bowel disorders may all be associated with aortitis involve the ascending aorta.

2423. Which of the following bacteria cause aortitis by infecting the aorta at sites of atherosclerotic plaque?
Harrison's 20th Ed. Chapter 274 Page 1922

A. Staphylococcus
B. Streptococcus
C. Salmonella
D. All of the above

2424. The initial lesion in syphilitic aortitis is in?
Harrison's 20th Ed. Chapter 274 Page 1922

A. Intima
B. Media
C. Adventitia
D. All of the above

The initial lesion in syphilitic aortitis is an obliterative endarteritis of the vasa vasorum, especially in the adventitia.

2425. Linear calcification of the ascending aorta is a feature of?
Harrison's 20th Ed. Chapter 274 Page 1922

A. Infective aortitis
B. Giant cell arteritis
C. Takayasu's arteritis
D. Syphilitic aortitis

Arterial Diseases of the Extremities

2426. Which of the following is a cause of peripheral artery disease (PAD)?

Harrison's 20th Ed. Chapter 275 Page 1923

A. Vasculitis
B. Entrapment
C. Cystic adventitial disease
D. All of the above

Atherosclerosis is the leading cause of PAD in patients >40 years old. Other causes include thrombosis, embolism, vasculitis, fibromuscular dysplasia, entrapment, cystic adventitial disease and trauma.

2427. Out of the following vessels, which is the most often involved in PAD?

Harrison's 20th Ed. Chapter 275 Page 1923

A. Abdominal aorta
B. Iliac arteries
C. Femoral and popliteal arteries
D. Tibial and peroneal arteries

The primary sites of involvement are the abdominal aorta and iliac arteries (30% of symptomatic patients), the femoral and popliteal arteries (80-90% of patients) and the more distal vessels including the tibial and peroneal arteries (40-50% of patients).

2428. Which of the following about intermittent claudication is false?

Harrison's 20th Ed. Chapter 275 Page 1923

A. Occurs during exercise & is relieved by rest
B. More common in lower than in upper extremities
C. Worse at night
D. None of the above

2429. Which of the following is a physical finding of PAD?

Harrison's 20th Ed. Chapter 275 Page 1923

A. Hair loss
B. Thickened nails
C. Smooth and shiny skin
D. All of the above

Important physical findings of PAD include decreased or absent pulses distal to the obstruction, the presence of bruits over the narrowed artery and muscle atrophy. With more severe disease, hair loss, thickened nails, smooth and shiny skin, reduced skin temperature and pallor or cyanosis are common physical signs. In patients with critical limb ischemia, ulcers or gangrene may occur.

2430. In patients with peripheral arterial disease, the ankle:brachial index (ABI) is?

Harrison's 20th Ed. Chapter 275 Page 1923

A. < 0.4
B. < 0.6
C. < 0.8
D. < 1

In hemodynamically significant arterial stenoses, systolic blood pressure in leg is decreased. Ratio of ankle and brachial artery pressures (ankle:brachial index or ABI) is 1.00 to 1.40 in normal individuals. ABI <0.90 is abnormal and diagnostic of PAD. A ratio of <0.5 is consistent with severe ischemia.

2431. ABI > 1.40 indicates?

Harrison's 20th Ed. Chapter 275 Page 1923

A. Hyperplastic artery
B. Noncompressible artery secondary to vascular calcification
C. Arteriovenous communication
D. None of the above

ABIs > 1.40 indicates noncompressible arteries secondary to vascular calcification.

2432. Which of the following is false about PAD?

Harrison's 20th Ed. Chapter 275 Page 1923

A. Decline of the ABI immediately after exercise
B. Blunting of amplitude of pulse volume contour
C. ABI values of 0.91 - 0.99 are considered borderline
D. None of the above

2433. Which of the following drugs is effective in patients with PAD?

Harrison's 20th Ed. Chapter 275 Page 1924

A. Cilostazol
B. Pentoxifylline
C. Angiotensin converting enzyme inhibitors
D. All of the above

Cilostazol is a phosphodiesterase inhibitor with vasodilator and antiplatelet properties. Pentoxifylline is a substituted xanthine derivative and increases blood flow to the microcirculation and enhances tissue oxygenation.

2434. Which of the following about fibromuscular dysplasia is false?

Harrison's 20th Ed. Chapter 275 Page 1925

A. Affects medium size and small arteries
B. Occurs predominantly in females
C. Usually involves renal and carotid arteries
D. None of the above

2435. In fibromuscular dysplasia, which of the following is the most common histologic type?

Harrison's 20th Ed. Chapter 275 Page 1925

A. Medial fibroplasia
B. Perimedial fibroplasia
C. Medial hyperplasia
D. Intimal fibroplasia

The histologic classification of fibromuscular dysplasia includes intimal fibroplasia, medial dysplasia and adventitial hyperplasia. Medial dysplasia is subdivided into medial fibroplasia, perimedial fibroplasia and medial hyperplasia. Medial fibroplasia is the most common type and is characterized by alternating areas of thinned media and fibromuscular ridges. The internal elastic lamina usually is preserved.

2436. "String of beads" appearance on angiography is typical of?

Harrison's 20th Ed. Chapter 275 Page 1925

A. Fibromuscular dysplasia
B. Thromboangiitis obliterans
C. Takayasu's arteritis
D. Giant cell (temporal) arteritis

"String of beads" appearance on angiography is characteristic of fibromuscular dysplasia caused by thickened fibromuscular ridges contiguous with thin, less-involved portions of the arterial wall.

2437. Clinical features of thromboangiitis obliterans include?
Harrison's 20th Ed. Chapter 275 Page 1925

A. Claudication of affected extremity
B. Raynaud's phenomenon
C. Migratory superficial vein thrombophlebitis
D. All of the above

Clinical features of thromboangiitis obliterans include a triad of claudication of the affected extremity, Raynaud's phenomenon, and migratory superficial vein thrombophlebitis.

2438. Which out of the following is false about thromboangiitis obliterans?
Harrison's 20th Ed. Chapter 275 Page 1925

A. Most frequently in men < 40 years of age
B. Definite relationship to cigarette smoking
C. Involves small & medium-size arteries & veins of extremities
D. None of the above

2439. Which out of the following is false about thromboangiitis obliterans?
Harrison's 20th Ed. Chapter 275 Page 1925

A. Smooth tapering segmental lesions in distal vessels
B. Collateral vessels at sites of vascular occlusion
C. Proximal atherosclerotic disease is usually absent
D. None of the above

2440. Which of the following is a cause of acute arterial occlusion?
Harrison's 20th Ed. Chapter 275 Page 1926

A. Embolism
B. Thrombus in situ
C. Arterial dissection
D. All of the above

Principal causes of acute arterial occlusion include embolism, thrombus in situ, arterial dissection and trauma.

2441. In lower extremities, emboli lodge most frequently in?
Harrison's 20th Ed. Chapter 275 Page 1926

A. Femoral artery
B. Iliac artery
C. Popliteal artery
D. Tibioperoneal arteries

In lower extremities, emboli lodge most frequently in femoral artery, followed by iliac artery, aorta, and popliteal and tibioperoneal arteries.

2442. "Blue toe" syndrome is best related to?
Harrison's 20th Ed. Chapter 275 Page 1927 Figure 275-2

A. Frostbite
B. Raynaud's phenomenon
C. Atheroembolism
D. Arteriovenous Fistula

Atheroembolism causes cyanotic discoloration & impending necrosis of the toes termed as "blue toe syndrome".

2443. Paget-Schroetter syndrome is best related to?
Harrison's 20th Ed. Chapter 275 Page 1927

A. Frostbite
B. Thoracic Outlet Compression Syndrome
C. Atheroembolism
D. Arteriovenous Fistula

Thoracic outlet compression syndrome may be divided into arterial, venous & neurogenic forms. Patients with neurogenic thoracic outlet compression may develop shoulder & arm pain, weakness, & paresthesias. Patients with arterial compression experience claudication, Raynaud's phenomenon, ischemic tissue loss & gangrene. Venous compression causes thrombosis of subclavian & axillary veins, often associated with effort & is referred to as Paget-Schroetter syndrome.

2444. Which of the following maneuvers is useful in diagnosis of thoracic outlet compression syndrome?
Harrison's 20th Ed. Chapter 275 Page 1927

A. Hyperabduction maneuver
B. Scalene maneuver
C. Costoclavicular maneuver
D. All of the above

Maneuvers used for diagnosis of thoracic outlet compression syndrome include abduction & external rotation test, in which affected arm is abducted by 90° & shoulder is externally rotated. Scalene maneuver (extension of neck & rotation of head to side of symptoms). Costoclavicular maneuver (posterior rotation of shoulders) & hyperabduction maneuver (raising arm to 180°).

2445. Which of the following is the most common peripheral artery aneurysm?
Harrison's 20th Ed. Chapter 275 Page 1927

A. Femoral artery
B. Popliteal artery
C. Tibial artery
D. Dorsalis pedis artery

Popliteal artery aneurysms are the most common peripheral artery aneurysms.

2446. Nicoladoni-Branham sign refers to?
Harrison's 20th Ed. Chapter 275 Page 1927

A. Tenderness in supraclavicular fossa
B. Compression of large arteriovenous fistula causing reflex slowing of heart rate
C. Hyperabduction maneuver causing subclavian bruits
D. Hyperabduction maneuver causing loss of pulses in arm

Compression of a large arteriovenous fistula may cause reflex slowing of the heart rate. This is called Nicoladoni-Branham sign.

2447. On cold exposure, which of the following is the first to occur in Raynaud's phenomenon?
Harrison's 20th Ed. Chapter 275 Page 1928

A. Pallor
B. Cyanosis
C. Rubor
D. None of the above

Raynaud's phenomenon is characterized by episodic digital ischemia, manifested clinically by sequential development of digital blanching or pallor, cyanosis, & rubor of fingers or toes following cold exposure & subsequent rewarming.

2448. In Raynaud's phenomenon, patients experience throbbing pain during which phase?
Harrison's 20th Ed. Chapter 275 Page 1928

A. Pallor
B. Cyanosis
C. Rubor
D. None of the above

Blanching or pallor represents the ischemic phase of Raynaud's phenomenon and results from vasospasm of digital arteries. During ischemic phase, capillaries & venules dilate and cyanosis results from deoxygenated blood that is present in these vessels. A sensation of cold or numbness or paresthesia of the digits often accompanies the phases of pallor and cyanosis. With rewarming, the digital vasospasm resolves, and blood flow into the dilated arterioles and capillaries increases dramatically. This "reactive hyperemia" imparts a bright red color to the digits. In addition to rubor and warmth, patients often experience a throbbing, painful sensation during the hyperemic phase.

2449. Which of the following about Raynaud's disease is false?
Harrison's 20th Ed. Chapter 275 Page 1928

A. 50% with Raynaud's phenomenon have Raynaud's disease
B. Women are affected 5 times more than men
C. Age of presentation is between 20 and 40 years
D. Toes are involved more frequently than fingers

Over 50% of patients with Raynaud's phenomenon have Raynaud's disease. Women are affected about five times more often than men, and the age of presentation is usually between 20 and 40 years. Fingers are involved more frequently than the toes.

2450. Which of the following may be involved in Raynaud's phenomenon?
Harrison's 20th Ed. Chapter 275 Page 1929

A. Earlobes
B. Tip of the nose
C. Penis
D. All of the above

Rarely, the earlobes, the tip of the nose and the penis are involved in Raynaud's phenomenon.

2451. Which of the following about Raynaud's phenomenon is false?
Harrison's 20th Ed. Chapter 275 Page 1929

A. Occurs frequently in patients who also have migraine
B. Occurs frequently in patients who also have variant angina
C. Radial, ulnar and pedal pulses are abnormal
D. Fingers and toes perspire excessively between attacks

Raynaud's phenomenon occurs frequently in patients who also have migraine headaches or variant angina. Radial, ulnar, and pedal pulses are normal. The fingers and toes may be cool between attacks and may perspire excessively.

2452. Which of the following drugs does not cause Raynaud's phenomenon?
Harrison's 20th Ed. Chapter 275 Page 1929

A. Methysergide
B. α-adrenergic receptor antagonists
C. β-adrenergic receptor antagonists
D. None of the above

2453. Which of the following drugs cause Raynaud's phenomenon?
Harrison's 20th Ed. Chapter 275 Page 1928 Table 275-1

A. Bleomycin
B. Vinblastine
C. Cisplatin
D. All of the above

Drugs that can cause Raynaud's phenomenon include ergot derivatives, methysergide, beta-adrenergic receptor blockers, bleomycin, vinblastine and cisplatin.

2454. Which of the following diseases can present as Raynaud's phenomenon?
Harrison's 20th Ed. Chapter 275 Page 1929

A. Scleroderma
B. Systemic lupus erythematosus
C. Dermatomyositis or polymyositis
D. All of the above

Raynaud's phenomenon occurs in patients with systemic sclerosis (scleroderma), systemic lupus erythematosus (SLE), dermatomyositis or polymyositis, rheumatoid arthritis, atherosclerosis of extremities, thromboangiitis obliterans, acute occlusion of large and medium-sized arteries by a thrombus or embolus, thoracic outlet compression syndrome, primary pulmonary hypertension, blood dyscrasias, use of vibrating hand tools, pianists and keyboard operators. Electric shock injury to the hands or frostbite may lead to the later development of Raynaud's phenomenon.

2455. Which of the following drug is useful in Raynaud's phenomenon?
Harrison's 20th Ed. Chapter 275 Page 1929

A. Nifedipine
B. Prazosin
C. Methyldopa
D. All of the above

2456. Which of the following drug is useful in Raynaud's phenomenon?
Harrison's 20th Ed. Chapter 275 Page 1929

A. Amlodipine
B. Terazosin
C. Phenoxybenzamine
D. All of the above

Dihydropyridine calcium channel antagonists (nifedipine, isradipine, felodipine & amlodipine) are useful. Postsynaptic alpha 1-adrenergic antagonist prazosin, doxazosin & terazosin may be effective. Sympatholytic agents methyldopa, guanethidine & phenoxybenzamine may be useful. Digital sympathectomy is helpful in those who are unresponsive to medical therapy.

2457. Which of the following is false about acrocyanosis?
Harrison's 20th Ed. Chapter 275 Page 1929

A. Persistent cyanosis of the hands
B. Normal pulses
C. Trophic skin changes and ulcerations do not occur
D. None of the above

In acrocyanosis, there is arterial vasoconstriction & secondary dilation of capillaries & venules with resulting persistent cyanosis of hands & feet. Pain, ulcers & gangrene do not occur. Pulses are normal & blanching does not occur.

2458. Secondary acrocyanosis is associated with?
Harrison's 20th Ed. Chapter 275 Page 1929

A. Brain tumour
B. Lung cancer
C. Infective hepatitis
D. Anorexia nervosa

Secondary acrocyanosis may result from hypoxemia, connective tissue diseases, atheroembolism, antiphospholipid antibodies, cold agglutinins, or cryoglobulins, and is associated with anorexia nervosa and orthostatic tachycardia syndrome.

2459. "Atrophie blanche en plaque" is the term given to?
Harrison's 20th Ed. Chapter 275 Page 1929

A. Myxoedema dermopathy
B. Thyroid acropachy
C. Primary livedo reticularis with ulceration
D. Secondary livedo reticularis

Primary livedo reticularis with ulceration is called atrophie blanche en plaque.

2460. Secondary livedo reticularis can occur with?
Harrison's 20th Ed. Chapter 275 Page 1929

A. Atheroembolism
B. SLE
C. Anticardiolipin antibodies
D. All of the above

Secondary livedo reticularis can occur with atheroembolism, SLE, anticardiolipin antibodies, hyperviscosity, cryoglobulinemia & Sneddon's syndrome (ischemic stroke & livedo reticularis).

2461. The other name of 'Pernio' is?
Harrison's 20th Ed. Chapter 275 Page 1930

A. Acrocyanosis
B. Erythromelalgia
C. Chilblains
D. Frostbite

2462. Which of the following best relates to Pernio (Chilblains)?
Harrison's 20th Ed. Chapter 275 Page 1930

A. Atheroembolism
B. Mechanical trauma
C. Vasculitic disorder
D. All of the above

Pernio (Chilblains) is a vasculitic disorder associated with exposure to cold. Raised erythematous lesions develop on lower part of legs & feet in cold weather. These are associated with pruritus and a burning sensation, and they may blister and ulcerate.

2463. Which of the following is false about erythromelalgia?
Harrison's 20th Ed. Chapter 275 Page 1930

A. Characterized by burning pain and erythema of extremities
B. Feet involved more frequently than hands
C. Males affected more frequently than females
D. None of the above

Erythromelalgia is characterized by burning pain and erythema of the extremities. The feet are involved more frequently than hands, and males are affected more frequently than females.

2464. Which of the following is false about erythromelalgia?
Harrison's 20th Ed. Chapter 275 Page 1930

A. May be secondary to myeloproliferative disorders
B. May occur as an adverse effect of nifedipine
C. May occur as an adverse effect of bromocriptine
D. Burning sensation is precipitated by exposure to cold environment

Secondary erythromelalgia occurs with myeloproliferative disorders such as polycythemia vera and essential thrombocytosis. Less-common causes include drugs, such as calcium channel blockers, bromocriptine, and pergolide; neuropathies; connective tissue diseases, such as SLE and paraneoplastic syndromes. Patients complain of burning in the extremities that is precipitated by exposure to a warm environment and aggravated by a dependent position. The symptoms are relieved by exposing the affected area to cool air or water or by elevation.

2465. Frostbite usually affects which of the following?
Harrison's 20th Ed. Chapter 275 Page 1930

A. Nose
B. Chin
C. Cheeks
D. All of the above

Frostbite affects distal aspects of extremities or exposed parts of face like ears, nose, chin & cheeks.

2466. In superficial frostbite, after rewarming, which of the following occurs?
Harrison's 20th Ed. Chapter 275 Page 1930

A. Cyanosis and erythema
B. Wheal-and-flare formation
C. Edema and superficial blisters
D. All of the above

2467. In frostbite, the temperature of the water bath used for rewarming should be?
Harrison's 20th Ed. Chapter 275 Page 1930

A. 32° – 36°C
B. 36° – 40°C
C. 40° – 44°C
D. 44° – 48°C

Initial treatment is rewarming, which is accomplished by immersion of the affected part in a water bath at temperatures of 40°–44°C (104°–111°F).

Chronic Venous Disease and Lymphedema

2468. Chronic venous diseases include?
Harrison's 20th Ed. Chapter 276 Page 1930

A. Telangiectasias & reticular veins
B. Varicose veins
C. Chronic venous insufficiency
D. All of the above

Chronic venous diseases include telangiectasias & reticular veins, varicose veins, chronic venous insufficiency with edema, skin changes, and ulceration.

2469. Which of the following is the longest vein in the body?
Harrison's 20th Ed. Chapter 276 Page 1930

A. Popliteal vein
B. Common iliac vein
C. Great saphenous vein
D. Common femoral vein

2470. Which of the following about varicose veins is false?
Harrison's 20th Ed. Chapter 276 Page 1930

A. Deep veins
B. Dilated, bulging, tortuous veins
C. Measure at least 3 mm in diameter
D. Due to defective structure & function of the valves

Varicose veins are dilated, bulging, tortuous superficial veins, measuring at least 3 mm in diameter.

2471. Primary varicose veins result from?
Harrison's 20th Ed. Chapter 276 Page 1931

A. Defective structure & function of valves of saphenous veins
B. Intrinsic weakness of the vein wall
C. High intraluminal pressure
D. All of the above

2472. Secondary varicose veins result from?
Harrison's 20th Ed. Chapter 276 Page 1931

A. Deep-venous insufficiency
B. Deep venous obstruction
C. Incompetent perforating veins
D. All of the above

Secondary varicose veins result from venous hypertension.

2473. The Klippel-Trenaunay syndrome is characterized by?
J Cardiovasc Ultrasound. 2015;23(4):266-270

A. Vascular nevus
B. Varicose veins
C. Soft tissue and bony hypertrophy of limb
D. All of the above

The Klippel-Trenaunay syndrome is characterized by a triad of vascular nevus, varicose veins, and soft tissue and bony hypertrophy of limb. The venous stasis in vascular malformations of lower limbs increases the chance of thrombus formation and PTE.

2474. Venulitis is a feature of?
Harrison's 20th Ed. Chapter 276 Page 1930

A. Thromboangiitis obliterans
B. Behçet's syndrome
C. Homocystinuria
D. All of the above

Venulitis occurring in thromboangiitis obliterans, Behçet's syndrome and homocystinuria may cause venous thrombosis.

2475. 'Phlegmasia cerulea dolens' refers to?
N Engl J Med. 2007; 356:e3

A. Deoxygenated hemoglobin in stagnant veins giving cyanotic hue to limb
B. Pain on antigravity movement of DVT affected limb
C. DVT affected veins that are likely to embolize
D. Chronic venous insufficiency

Phlegmasia cerulea dolens or blue, painful leg, is an uncommon manifestation of deep-vein thrombosis and results from massive thrombosis compromising venous outflow, which causes ischemia.

2476. 'Phlegmasia alba dolens' refers to?
Damar Cer Derg 2017;26(3):111-115

A. Deoxygenated hemoglobin in stagnant veins giving cyanotic hue to limb
B. Pain on antigravity movement of DVT affected limb
C. DVT affected veins that are likely to embolize
D. Pallor in markedly edematous DVT affected legs

Phlegmasia alba dolens is a condition characterized by limb swelling (edema), tenderness, pain, lividity, and bullous lesions followed by whitening of the limb due to venous stasis caused by femoral vein thrombosis. The collateral vessels are either not affected or affected less extensively than phlegmasia cerulea dolens.

2477. Dermatologic findings associated with venous stasis include?
Harrison's 20th Ed. Chapter 276 Page 1931

A. Lipodermatosclerosis
B. Atrophie blanche
C. Phlebectasia corona
D. All of the above

Dermatologic findings associated with venous stasis include hyperpigmentation, erythema, eczema, lipodermatosclerosis, atrophie blanche, and a phlebectasia corona.

2478. Lipodermatosclerosis is best related to?
Harrison's 20th Ed. Chapter 276 Page 1931

A. Fat deposition
B. Thrombin deposition
C. Collagen deposition
D. Hemosiderin deposition

Lipodermatosclerosis is the combination of induration, hemosiderin deposition, and inflammation, and typically occurs in the lower part of the leg just above the ankle.

2479. Lipodermatosclerosis is a form of?
Harrison's 20th Ed. Chapter 54 Page 352

A. Dermatitis
B. Vasculitis
C. Panniculitis
D. Cellulitis

Panniculitis, an inflammation of the fat. Various forms of panniculitis, are erythema nodosum, erythema induratum/nodular vasculitis, lupus panniculitis, lipodermatosclerosis, α1-antitrypsin deficiency, factitial, and fat necrosis secondary to pancreatic disease.

2480. Which of the following is a feature of Atrophie blanche?
Harrison's 20th Ed. Chapter 276 Page 1931

A. White patch of scar tissue
B. Focal telangiectasias and hyperpigmented border
C. Develops near medial malleolus
D. All of the above

Atrophie blanche is a white patch of scar tissue, often with focal telangiectasias and a hyperpigmented border that usually develops near medial malleolus.

2481. Which of the following is the characteristic pattern of phlebectasia corona?
Harrison's 20th Ed. Chapter 276 Page 1931

A. Crown-shaped
B. Fan-shaped
C. Tear drop-shaped
D. Dome-shaped

Phlebectasia corona is a fan-shaped pattern of intradermal veins near the ankle or on the foot.

2482. Which of the following tests is used to diagnose varicose veins?
Harrison's 20th Ed. Chapter 276 Page 1932, Ann R Coll Surg Engl. 2006;88(3):309-312

A. Brodie–Trendelenburg test
B. Perthes test
C. Schwarts test
D. All of the above

Brodie–Trendelenburg test is used to determine whether varicose veins are secondary to deep-venous insufficiency. As the patient is lying supine, the leg is elevated and the veins allowed to empty. Then, a tourniquet is placed on the proximal part of the thigh and the patient is asked to stand. Filling of the varicose veins within 30 s indicates that the varicose veins are caused by deep-venous insufficiency and incompetent perforating veins. Primary varicose veins with superficial venous insufficiency are the likely diagnosis if venous refilling occurs promptly after tourniquet removal. The Perthes test assesses the possibility of deep venous obstruction. A tourniquet is placed on the mid thigh after the patient has stood, and the varicose veins are filled. The patient is then instructed to walk for 5 min. A patent deep-venous system and competent perforating veins enable the superficial veins below the tourniquet to collapse. Deep venous obstruction is likely to be present if the superficial veins distend further with walking.

Brodie-Trendelenburg (tourniquet) test, cough impulse and tap test (Ann R Coll Surg Engl. 2006;88(3):309-312).

Brodie-Trendeleburg test, Schwarts test, Morrissey's cough impulse test, Parthe's test, multiple tourniquet test

2483. Persistent lymphedema leads to infiltration of?
Harrison's 20th Ed. Chapter 276 Page 1933

A. Mononuclear cells
B. Fibroblasts
C. Adipocytes
D. All of the above

Persistent lymphedema leads to inflammatory & immune responses characterized by infiltration of mononuclear cells, fibroblasts & adipocytes, leading to adipose & collagen deposition in skin & subcutaneous tissues.

2484. Smooth muscle cells first appear in which of the following?
Harrison's 20th Ed. Chapter 276 Page 1933

A. Lymphatic capillaries
B. Microlymphatic precollector vessels
C. Collecting lymphatic vessels
D. Larger lymphatic conduits

2485. Bileaflet valves first appear in which of the following?
Harrison's 20th Ed. Chapter 276 Page 1933

A. Lymphatic capillaries
B. Microlymphatic precollector vessels
C. Collecting lymphatic vessels
D. Larger lymphatic conduits

2486. Superficial & deep lymphatic vessels in legs communicate at?
Harrison's 20th Ed. Chapter 276 Page 1933

A. Popliteal lymph nodes
B. Pelvic lymph nodes
C. Para aortic lymph nodes
D. All of the above

Superficial & deep lymphatic vessels in legs communicate at the popliteal & inguinal lymph nodes.

2487. Thoracic duct connects with?
Harrison's 20th Ed. Chapter 276 Page 1933

A. Right brachiocephalic vein
B. Left brachiocephalic vein
C. Inferior vena cava
D. Superior vena cava

Pelvic lymphatic vessels drain into the thoracic duct, which connects with the left brachiocephalic vein.

2488. Which of the following is a clinical subtype of primary lymphedema?
Harrison's 20th Ed. Chapter 276 Page 1933

A. Congenital lymphedema
B. Lymphedema praecox
C. Lymphedema tarda
D. All of the above

2489. Lymphedema tarda usually begins after the age of?
Harrison's 20th Ed. Chapter 276 Page 1933

A. 1 year
B. 14 years
C. 25 years
D. 35 years

Congenital lymphedema appears shortly after birth, lymphedema praecox has its onset at the time of puberty and lymphedema tarda usually begins after age 35.

2490. Which of the following genes is involved in the development of lymphatic valves?
Harrison's 20th Ed. Chapter 276 Page 1933

A. KIF11
B. GATA2
C. CCBE1
D. FOXC2

Mutations of the GATA2 gene, which is involved in the development of lymphatic valves, cause lymphedema and predisposes to acute myeloid leukemia.

2491. Milroy's disease is best described as?
Harrison's 20th Ed. Chapter 276 Page 1933

A. Congenital lymphedema
B. Lymphedema praecox
C. Lymphedema tarda
D. Bacterial lymphangitis

Familial forms of congenital lymphedema (Milroy's disease) and lymphedema praecox (Meige's disease) may be inherited in an autosomal dominant manner with variable penetrance.

2492. Mutations in which of the following genes causes Milroy's disease?
Harrison's 20th Ed. Chapter 276 Page 1933

A. LSC1
B. VEGFR3
C. CCBE1
D. FOXC2

Milroy's disease is caused by mutations in genes expressing vascular endothelial growth factor receptor 3 (VEGFR3) which determines lymphangiogenesis.

2493. Mutations in which of the following genes causes cholestasis-lymphedema syndrome?
Harrison's 20th Ed. Chapter 276 Page 1933

A. LSC1
B. VEGFR3
C. CCBE1
D. FOXC2

2494. Mutations in which of the following genes causes lymphedema-distichiasis syndrome?
Harrison's 20th Ed. Chapter 276 Page 1933

A. LSC1
B. VEGFR3
C. CCBE1
D. FOXC2

2495. Mutations in which of the following genes causes hypotrichosis, lymphedema, telangiectasia syndrome?
Harrison's 20th Ed. Chapter 276 Page 1933

A. LSC1
B. VEGFR3
C. SOX18
D. FOXC2

2496. Double row of eyelashes relates to which of the following genes?
Harrison's 20th Ed. Chapter 276 Page 1933

A. LSC1
B. VEGFR3
C. SOX18
D. FOXC2

2497. Mutations in which of the following genes causes microcephaly-lymphedema syndrome?
Harrison's 20th Ed. Chapter 276 Page 1933

A. KIF11
B. GATA2
C. CCBE1
D. FOXC2

2498. Primary lymphedema may be associated with?
Harrison's 20th Ed. Chapter 276 Page 1934

A. Turner syndrome
B. Klinefelter syndrome
C. Noonan syndrome
D. All of the above

2499. Primary lymphedema may be associated with?
Harrison's 20th Ed. Chapter 276 Page 1934

A. Yellow nail syndrome
B. Intestinal lymphangiectasia syndrome
C. Lymphangiomyomatosis
D. All of the above

Primary lymphedema may be associated with Turner's syndrome, Klinefelter's syndrome, Noonan's syndrome, yellow nail syndrome, intestinal lymphangiectasia syndrome, and lymphangiomyomatosis.

2500. Lymphedema is found in which of the following?
Harrison's 20th Ed. Chapter 276 Page 1934

A. Noonan's syndrome
B. Yellow nail syndrome
C. Klippel-Trenaunay syndrome
D. All of the above

Patients with a chromosomal aneuploidy (Turner's syndrome, Klinefelter's syndrome) or trisomy 18, 13 or 21 may develop lymphedema. Other disorders include Klippel-Trenaunay syndrome, Parkes-Weber syndrome, Hennekam's syndrome, Noonan's syndrome, yellow nail syndrome, intestinal lymphangiectasia syndrome, lymphangiomyomatosis and neurofibromatosis type 1.

2501. Most common cause of secondary lymphedema worldwide is?
Harrison's 20th Ed. Chapter 276 Page 1934

A. Bacterial lymphangitis
B. Filariasis
C. Radiation therapy for breast carcinoma
D. Pregnancy

Most common cause of secondary lymphedema worldwide is filariasis.

2502. Filariasis is caused by?
Harrison's 20th Ed. Chapter 276 Page 1934 Table 276-2

A. Wucheria bancrofti
B. Brugia malayi
C. B. timori
D. Any of the above

2503. Infectious causes of secondary lymphedema include?
Harrison's 20th Ed. Chapter 276 Page 1934

A. Streptococcal infection
B. Lymphogranuloma venereum
C. Tuberculosis
D. All of the above

2504. Podoconiosis best relates to?
Harrison's 20th Ed. Chapter 276 Page 1934

A. Surgical excision of axillary and inguinal lymph nodes
B. Irradiation of axillary and inguinal lymph nodes
C. Silicate particles in soil
D. Self-induced or factitious lymphedema

Podoconiosis refers to absorption of silicate particles in soil derived from volcanic rock following barefoot exposure.

2505. Inability to tent the skin at the base of the toes is called?
Harrison's 20th Ed. Chapter 276 Page 1934

A. Stemmer's sign
B. Signet-ring sign
C. Hoover's sign
D. Atoll sign

2506. Which of the following is related to lymphedema?
Harrison's 20th Ed. Chapter 276 Page 1934

A. Squaring of the toes
B. Peau d'orange
C. Acanthosis and verrucous overgrowths
D. All of the above

2507. Which of the following disorders cause unilateral leg swelling?
Harrison's 20th Ed. Chapter 276 Page 1934

A. Deep-vein thrombosis
B. Chronic venous insufficiency
C. Lymphedema
D. All of the above

2508. Sparing of the feet is observed in which of the following?
Harrison's 20th Ed. Chapter 276 Page 1934

A. Myxedema
B. Lipedema
C. Lymphedema
D. All of the above

Lipedema is usually seen in women and is caused by accumulation of adipose tissue in leg from thigh to the ankle, with sparing of the feet.

2509. Which of the following is characteristic of lymphedema on magnetic resonance imaging (MRI)?
Harrison's 20th Ed. Chapter 276 Page 1935

A. Honeycomb pattern in the epifascial compartment
B. Mosaic pattern in the epifascial compartment
C. Crazy paving in the epifascial compartment
D. Eggshell pattern in the epifascial compartment

2510. In primary lymphedema, lymphatic channels are?
Harrison's 20th Ed. Chapter 276 Page 1934

A. Absent
B. Hypoplastic
C. Ectatic
D. Any of the above

Pulmonary Hypertension

2511. In Pulmonary hypertension (PH), mean pulmonary artery pressure is?

Harrison's 20th Ed. Chapter 277 Page 1935

A. > 16 mm Hg
B. > 18 mm Hg
C. > 20 mm Hg
D. > 22 mm Hg

Pulmonary hypertension (PH) is a spectrum of diseases involving the pulmonary vasculature and is defined as an elevation in pulmonary arterial pressures (mean pulmonary artery pressure >22 mm Hg).

2512. In Pulmonary hypertension (PH), the estimated systolic PAP is?

Harrison's 20th Ed. Chapter 277 Page 1935

A. > 28 mm Hg
B. > 32 mm Hg
C. > 36 mm Hg
D. > 40 mm Hg

In pulmonary hypertension (PH), the estimated systolic PAP is >36 mm Hg.

2513. Pulmonary arterial hypertension (PAH) is characterized by symptoms of?

Harrison's 20th Ed. Chapter 277 Page 1935

A. Dyspnea
B. Chest pain
C. Syncope
D. All of the above

Pulmonary arterial hypertension (PAH) is characterized by dyspnea, chest pain and syncope.

2514. Which of the following is the most common symptom attributable to pulmonary hypertension?

Harrison's 20th Ed. Chapter 277 Page 1936

A. Edema
B. Exertional dyspnea
C. Syncope
D. Peripheral edema

Most common symptom attributable to pulmonary hypertension is exertional dyspnea. Other symptoms are fatigue, angina pectoris (RV ischemia), syncope, near syncope & peripheral edema.

2515. Which of the following underlie the development of PAH?

Harrison's 20th Ed. Chapter 277 Page 1936

A. Vascular proliferation
B. Thrombosis
C. Inflammation
D. All of the above

Vasoconstriction, vascular proliferation, thrombosis, and inflammation underlie the development of PAH.

2516. In PH, which of the following characterize the pathological findings in the pulmonary vasculature?

Harrison's 20th Ed. Chapter 277 Page 1936

A. Intimal proliferation & fibrosis
B. Medial hypertrophy
C. In situ thrombosis
D. All of the above

Intimal proliferation & fibrosis, medial hypertrophy, and in situ thrombosis characterize the pathological findings in the pulmonary vasculature.

2517. In PH, with decreased compliance of pulmonary vasculature, the compensatory response is?

Harrison's 20th Ed. Chapter 277 Page 1936

A. Tachypnea
B. Tachycardia
C. Hypertension
D. All of the above

2518. Which of the following occurs in plexogenic pulmonary arteriopathy?

Harrison's 20th Ed. Chapter 277 Page 1936 Figure 277-1

A. Medial hypertrophy of muscular pulmonary arteries
B. Obstructive lesions of small muscular pulmonary arteries
C. Proliferative lesions of small muscular pulmonary arteries
D. All of the above

2519. Pathobiologic process that result in pulmonary arterial hypertension is?

Harrison's 20th Ed. Chapter 277 Page 1936

A. Inhibition of voltage-regulated potassium channel
B. Increased serotonin uptake in smooth-muscle cells
C. Hypoxia-induced activation of hypoxia-inducible factor-1α
D. All of the above

In PAH, abnormalities in molecular pathways regulating the pulmonary vascular endothelial and smooth-muscle cells include inhibition of voltage-regulated potassium channel, mutations in the bone morphogenetic protein-2 receptor, increased serotonin uptake in smooth-muscle cells due to overactivation of the serotonin transporter, hypoxia-induced activation of hypoxia-inducible factor-1α, activation of nuclear factor of activated T cells and excessive thrombin deposition related to a procoagulant state. There is a loss of apoptosis of smooth-muscle cells allowing their proliferation, and emergence of apoptosis-resistant endothelial cells which can obliterate the vascular lumen.

2520. Which of the following is the most important initial screening test for the diagnosis of PH?

Harrison's 20th Ed. Chapter 277 Page 1937

A. Doppler echocardiography
B. Echocardiogram with bubble study
C. Cardiopulmonary exercise test (CPET)
D. High-resolution computed tomography (HRCT)

An echocardiogram with bubble study is the most important initial screening test for the diagnosis of PH.

2521. Which of the following can cause PH?

Harrison's 20th Ed. Chapter 277 Page 1937

A. Valvular heart disease
B. Left ventricular systolic & diastolic function
C. Intra-cardiac shunts
D. All of the above

All forms of PH demonstrate a hypertrophied & dilated right ventricle with elevated estimated pulmonary artery systolic pressure.

2522. Which of the following is the gold standard for diagnosis & assessment of disease severity?

Harrison's 20th Ed. Chapter 277 Page 1937

A. Doppler echocardiography
B. CT angiograms
C. Ventilation-perfusion (V/Q) scanning
D. Right heart catheterization (RHC) with pulmonary vasodilator testing

Invasive hemodynamic monitoring (right heart catheterization) is the gold standard for diagnosis & assessment of disease severity.

2523. Classic findings of PH on high-resolution computed tomography include?

Harrison's 20th Ed. Chapter 277 Page 1937

A. Enlarged pulmonary arteries
B. Peripheral pruning of small vessels
C. Enlarged right ventricle & right atrium
D. All of the above

2524. Centrilobular ground glass infiltrate & thickened septal lines seen in the absence of left heart disease on high-resolution CT suggest?

Harrison's 20th Ed. Chapter 277 Page 1937

A. Emphysema
B. Asthma
C. Pulmonary venous disease
D. Interstitial lung disease

2525. Which of the following is the classic finding in PAH?

Harrison's 20th Ed. Chapter 277 Page 1938

A. Abnormal Ventilation-perfusion (V/Q) scanning
B. Abnormal CT angiogram
C. Isolated reduction in DLCO
D. All of the above

An isolated reduction in diffusing capacity of lungs for carbon monoxide (DLCO) is a classic finding in PAH.

2526. Which of the finding in right heart catheterization study define precapillary PH or PAH?

Harrison's 20th Ed. Chapter 277 Page 1938

A. Increased mean PAP (mPAP >25 mm Hg)
B. Pulmonary capillary wedge pressure (PCWP) ≤15 mm Hg
C. PVR >3 Wood units
D. All of the above

An increased mean PAP (mPAP >25 mm Hg), pulmonary capillary wedge pressure (PCWP), left atrial pressure, or left ventricular enddiastolic pressure (LVEDP) ≤15 mm Hg and PVR >3 Wood units define precapillary PH or PAH in right heart catheterization (RHC) study. Post capillary PH is differentiated from precapillary PH by the PCWP being ≥15 mm Hg.

2527. In vasodilator testing, decrease in mPAP by how much is considered as a positive pulmonary vasodilator response?

Harrison's 20th Ed. Chapter 277 Page 1938

A. ≥ 3 mm Hg
B. ≥ 5 mm Hg
C. ≥ 10 mm Hg
D. ≥ 15 mm Hg

2528. Positive responders to vasodilator testing are considered for long-term treatment with?

Harrison's 20th Ed. Chapter 277 Page 1938

A. Angiotensin converting enzyme inhibitors
B. Calcium channel blockers
C. Tadalafil
D. All of the above

Short acting vasodilators like inhaled nitric oxide (NO) or inhaled epoprostenol are used for vasodilator testing. A decrease in mPAP by ≥10 mm Hg to an absolute level ≤40 mm Hg without a decrease in CO is considered as a positive pulmonary vasodilator response. Positive responders are considered for long-term treatment with calcium channel blockers (CCB).

2529. PH due to left heart disease is classified by WHO as?

Harrison's 20th Ed. Chapter 277 Page 1939

A. WHO Group I PH
B. WHO Group II PH
C. WHO Group III PH
D. WHO Group IV PH

WHO recognizes five categories of PH (I to V), including PAH, PH due to left heart disease, PH due to chronic lung disease, PH associated with chronic thromboemboli, and a group of miscellaneous diseases that only rarely cause PH.

2530. Based on RHC, PAH is defined as?

Harrison's 20th Ed. Chapter 277 Page 1939

A. Pulmonary arterial pressure (mPAP) ≥25 mm Hg
B. PVR > 240 dyne-s/cm^5
C. PCWP or LVEDP of ≤15 mm Hg
D. All of the above

Based on RHC, PAH is defined as a sustained elevation in resting mean pulmonary arterial pressure (mPAP) ≥25 mm Hg, PVR > 240 dyne-s/cm^5, and PCWP or LVEDP of ≤15 mm Hg.

2531. PAH may be associated with?

Harrison's 20th Ed. Chapter 277 Page 1939

A. HIV
B. Connective tissue disease
C. Portal hypertension
D. All of the above

PAH may be associated with HIV, connective tissue disease, and portal hypertension.

2532. Prevalence of PAH is increased in which of the following connective tissue diseases?

Harrison's 20th Ed. Chapter 277 Page 1939

A. Polymyositis
B. Systemic sclerosis
C. Sjögren's syndrome
D. All of the above

2533. Of the following collagen vascular diseases, PAH is commonest in?

Harrison's 20th Ed. Chapter 277 Page 1939

A. Systemic lupus erythematosus
B. Scleroderma
C. Rheumatoid arthritis
D. Dermatomyositis

All collagen vascular diseases may be associated with PAH. It is common with CREST syndrome & scleroderma. It is less frequent in SLE, Sjögren's syndrome, dermatomyositis, polymyositis & RA.

2534. Prevalence of PAH is increased in?
Harrison's 20th Ed. Chapter 277 Page 1939

A. Scleroderma renal crisis
B. Limited cutaneous scleroderma
C. Diffuse cutaneous scleroderma
D. Scleromyxedema

2535. CREST syndrome includes all except?
Harrison's 20th Ed. Chapter 363 Page 2621

A. Calcinosis
B. Raynaud's phenomenon
C. Sclerodactyly
D. Thrombosis

CREST syndrome includes Calcinosis, Raynaud's phenomenon, Esophageal involvement, Sclerodactyly, and Telangiectasia.

2536. Portopulmonary hypertension is observed in?
Harrison's 20th Ed. Chapter 277 Page 1939

A. Primary biliary cholangitis
B. Autoimmune hepatitis
C. Hepatocellular carcinoma
D. None of the above

Portopulmonary hypertension occurs in 2 - 10% of patients with established portal hypertension. Its occurrence is independent of the cause of liver disease & is seen in patients with non-hepatic causes of portal hypertension.

2537. Which of the following is the characteristic event in portopulmonary hypertension?
Harrison's 20th Ed. Chapter 277 Page 1939

A. Medial hyperplasia
B. Intrapulmonary shunting
C. Intimal fibrosis
D. Pulmonary venous obliteration

In portopulmonary hypertension, there occurs an abnormal vasodilation of pulmonary vasculature leading to intrapulmonary shunting.

2538. WHO Group II PH includes patients with?
Harrison's 20th Ed. Chapter 277 Page 1939

A. Left heart systolic dysfunction
B. Aortic and mitral valve disease
C. Heart failure with preserved ejection fraction (HFpEF)
D. All of the above

2539. The hallmark of Group II PH is?
Harrison's 20th Ed. Chapter 277 Page 1939

A. Intrinsic pulmonary arterial disease
B. Pulmonary venous hypertension
C. Obstruction of the pulmonary vasculature
D. All of the above

The hallmark of Group II PH is elevated left atrial pressure with resulting pulmonary venous hypertension, although transpulmonary gradient and PVR remain normal.

2540. Which of the following carry a higher overall risk of PH?
Harrison's 20th Ed. Chapter 277 Page 1939

A. Left heart systolic dysfunction
B. Aortic and mitral valve disease
C. Heart failure with preserved ejection fraction (HFpEF)
D. All of the above

Studies suggest that HFpEF may carry a higher overall risk of PH.

2541. Which of the following can produce pulmonary hypertension?
Harrison's 20th Ed. Chapter 277 Page 1939

A. Portal Hypertension
B. Obstructive sleep apnea (OSA)
C. Sickle cell disease
D. All of the above

2542. Sleep-disordered breathing is classified by WHO as?
Harrison's 20th Ed. Chapter 277 Page 1939

A. WHO Group I PH
B. WHO Group II PH
C. WHO Group III PH
D. WHO Group IV PH

Sleep-disordered breathing is included in Group III PH.

2543. Globally, which of the following is one of the most common causes of PH?
Harrison's 20th Ed. Chapter 277 Page 1939

A. Schistosomiasis
B. Chronic thromboembolic disease
C. Left heart systolic dysfunction
D. Pulmonary arterial hypertension

Globally, schistosomiasis is one of the most common causes of PH.

2544. Which of the following is the action of Prostacyclin (PGI_2)?
Harrison's 20th Ed. Chapter 277 Page 1940

A. Vasodilation
B. Antiproliferative effects on vascular smooth muscle
C. Inhibits platelet aggregation
D. All of the above

2545. Which of the following reduces pulmonary artery pressure acutely with little effect on systemic vascular bed?
Harrison's 19th Ed. 1660

A. Inhaled nitric oxide
B. Intravenous adenosine
C. Intravenous epoprostenol
D. All of the above

Inhaled nitric oxide, IV adenosine & IV epoprostenol reduce pulmonary artery pressure acutely which is a fall in mean pulmonary artery pressure (MPAP) >=10 mm Hg & a final MPAP <40 mm Hg.

2546. Conventional therapy for pulmonary arterial hypertension includes?
Harrison's 19th Ed. Page 1660

A. Anticoagulation
B. Diuretics

Cardiology

C. Calcium channel blockers

D. All of the above

Anticoagulant therapy is advocated for all patients with PAH as warfarin increases survival of patients with PAH. Diuretic therapy relieves peripheral edema & reduces RV volume overload in presence of tricuspid regurgitation. Patients who have substantial reductions in pulmonary arterial pressure in response to short-acting vasodilators at the time of cardiac catheterization should be treated initially with calcium channel blockers.

2547. Phosphodiesterase-5 is responsible for the hydrolysis of which of the following in pulmonary vascular smooth muscle?

Harrison's 20th Ed. Chapter 277 Page 1940

A. Cyclic GMP

B. Cyclic AMP

C. Endothelin-1

D. Inositol 1,4,5-trisphosphate (IP_3)

Phosphodiesterase-5 (PDE-5) is responsible for the hydrolysis of cyclic 3',5'-guanosine monophosphate (cyclic GMP) in pulmonary vascular smooth muscle which induces relaxation of smooth muscle. Inhibitors of PDE-5 such as sildenafil, vardenafil, and tadalafil reduce the breakdown of cyclic GMP. Nitric oxide increases the production of cyclic GMP.

2548. Which of the following prostacyclins is used for treatment of PAH?

Harrison's 20th Ed. Chapter 277 Page 1940

A. Iloprost

B. Epoprostenol

C. Treprostinil

D. All of the above

2549. Which of the following is an 'Endothelin Receptor Antagonist' used in the treatment of pulmonary arterial hypertension?

Harrison's 20th Ed. Chapter 277 Page 1940

A. Epoprostenol

B. Treprostinil

C. Bosentan

D. Sildenafil

Endothelin receptor antagonists bosentan and ambrisentan are approved for treatment of PAH. Liver functions must be monitored monthly throughout the duration of use. Bosentan is contraindicated in patients who are on cyclosporine or glyburide concurrently. Sildenafil is a phosphodiesterase-5 inhibitor. Treprostinil is an analogue of epoprostenol.

2550. Which of the following is an ET receptor antagonist?

Harrison's 20th Ed. Chapter 277 Page 1940

A. Ambrisentan

B. Bosentan

C. Macitentan

D. All of the above

Ambrisentan is a selective ET-A receptor antagonist while Bosentan and Macitentan are non-selective ET receptor antagonists.

2551. Selexipag best relates to?

Harrison's 20th Ed. Chapter 277 Page 1940

A. Prostaglandin I_2 (IP) receptor

B. Endothelin-1 (ET-1) receptor

C. β2-receptor

D. Adenosine A_1-receptor

Selexipag is an oral nonprostanoid diphenylpyrazine derived selective IP prostacyclin receptor agonist that binds the prostaglandin I2 (IP) receptor.

2552. Which of the following about Nitric oxide (NO) is false?

Harrison's 20th Ed. Chapter 277 Page 1940

A. Derives from endothelial cells

B. Activate guanylyl cyclase to generates cGMP

C. Induces vasodilation, inhibits platelet activation

D. None of the above

2553. Phosphodiesterase type 5 enzymes metabolize?

Harrison's 20th Ed. Chapter 277 Page 1940

A. cGMP

B. cAMP

C. CREB

D. All of the above

Nitric oxide (NO) derived from endothelial cells activate guanylyl cyclase that generates cGMP in vascular smooth muscle cells & platelets. cGMP induces vasodilation through relaxation of arterial smooth muscle cells & inhibits platelet activation. Phosphodiesterase-5 (PDE5) inhibitors increase cyclic guanosine monophosphate (cGMP) levels.

2554. Riociguate increases the production of?

Harrison's 20th Ed. Chapter 277 Page 1940

A. Prostacyclin (PGI_2)

B. Nitric oxide

C. Endothelin

D. All of the above

Riociguat is a soluble guanylyl cyclase stimulator acting synergistically with endogenous NO, and also directly stimulating soluble guanylyl cyclase independent of NO availability. Riociugat acts by increasing the production of nitric oxide.

2555. Which of the following best relates to familial pulmonary arterial hypertension?

Harrison's 20th Ed. Chapter 476 Page 3517

A. Tumor necrosis factor (TNF) receptor superfamily

B. Serine protease inhibitor (serpin) superfamily

C. Transforming growth factor β (TGF-β) superfamily

D. GPCR superfamily

2556. Which of the following is a member of transforming growth factor β (TGF-β) superfamily?

Harrison's 20th Ed. Chapter 476 Page 3517-8

A. Bone morphogenetic protein receptor-2 (BMPR-2)

B. Activin receptor-like kinase-1 (Alk-1)

C. Endoglin

D. All of the above

ANSWERS

1. D
2. D
3. D
4. D
5. B
6. A
7. D
8. D
9. C
10. D
11. C
12. B
13. C
14. D
15. D
16. C
17. C
18. A
19. C
20. C
21. D
22. D
23. A
24. A
25. D
26. D
27. A
28. A
29. B
30. C
31. A
32. D
33. D
34. B
35. C
36. D
37. B
38. A
39. D
40. D
41. D
42. D
43. B
44. C
45. D
46. D
47. A
48. D
49. D
50. B
51. B
52. C
53. A
54. A
55. A
56. B
57. C
58. D
59. A
60. D
61. C
62. B
63. D
64. D
65. D
66. D
67. C
68. D
69. C
70. B
71. A
72. B
73. C
74. D
75. C
76. D
77. A
78. D
79. C
80. D
81. D
82. C
83. D
84. C
85. A
86. D
87. A
88. B
89. D
90. B
91. A
92. C
93. C
94. D
95. D
96. D
97. A
98. C
99. B
100. D
101. B
102. A
103. A
104. D
105. D
106. D
107. C
108. A
109. B
110. B
111. C
112. D
113. D
114. C
115. B
116. D
117. D
118. D
119. B
120. A
121. C
122. D
123. A
124. D
125. D
126. D
127. B
128. C
129. D
130. D
131. D
132. B
133. A
134. A
135. D
136. D
137. D
138. A
139. D
140. C
141. D
142. B
143. B
144. D
145. D
146. D
147. C
148. B
149. D
150. D
151. D
152. C
153. C
154. D
155. A
156. B
157. A
158. C
159. A
160. A
161. B
162. B
163. B
164. C
165. B
166. C
167. B
168. D
169. B
170. A
171. C
172. B
173. B
174. B
175. C
176. A
177. C
178. A
179. D
180. D
181. B
182. D
183. A
184. B
185. C
186. C
187. B
188. D
189. B
190. D
191. A
192. C
193. D
194. D
195. B
196. B
197. A
198. D
199. B
200. D
201. B
202. A
203. D
204. D
205. A
206. C
207. B
208. D
209. D
210. A
211. D
212. D
213. B
214. A
215. B
216. D
217. C
218. A
219. C
220. D
221. A
222. B
223. C
224. B
225. C
226. B
227. A
228. A
229. B
230. C
231. B
232. B
233. A
234. D

ANSWERS

235. A	274. D	313. A	352. C	391. B	430. C
236. C	275. D	314. D	353. C	392. D	431. D
237. C	276. D	315. C	354. D	393. D	432. D
238. D	277. D	316. D	355. C	394. A	433. C
239. D	278. B	317. D	356. C	395. A	434. D
240. D	279. D	318. D	357. D	396. B	435. D
241. D	280. D	319. C	358. D	397. C	436. D
242. C	281. D	320. C	359. D	398. D	437. D
243. A	282. B	321. C	360. D	399. D	438. D
244. D	283. D	322. A	361. D	400. C	439. D
245. B	284. A	323. D	362. D	401. D	440. D
246. C	285. B	324. D	363. D	402. D	441. C
247. A	286. B	325. B	364. D	403. B	442. D
248. A	287. D	326. D	365. D	404. D	443. A
249. B	288. B	327. C	366. D	405. D	444. B
250. B	289. A	328. D	367. D	406. D	445. A
251. B	290. D	329. A	368. C	407. D	446. D
252. C	291. C	330. D	369. C	408. C	447. D
253. B	292. C	331. B	370. A	409. A	448. A
254. C	293. D	332. D	371. A	410. B	449. A
255. B	294. C	333. D	372. B	411. C	450. B
256. B	295. B	334. D	373. D	412. D	451. D
257. D	296. D	335. B	374. D	413. C	452. B
258. A	297. A	336. B	375. C	414. A	453. C
259. D	298. C	337. A	376. D	415. D	454. D
260. A	299. C	338. B	377. D	416. B	455. D
261. D	300. C	339. C	378. D	417. C	456. C
262. D	301. A	340. D	379. B	418. B	457. C
263. B	302. C	341. C	380. D	419. D	458. D
264. D	303. B	342. B	381. B	420. D	459. A
265. D	304. C	343. D	382. B	421. A	460. D
266. D	305. D	344. D	383. A	422. D	461. B
267. D	306. B	345. D	384. D	423. D	462. A
268. B	307. D	346. D	385. B	424. C	463. C
269. A	308. C	347. C	386. A	425. D	464. D
270. D	309. D	348. A	387. D	426. D	465. D
271. D	310. D	349. A	388. C	427. A	466. B
272. A	311. A	350. C	389. D	428. B	467. C
273. B	312. A	351. D	390. A	429. A	468. D

ANSWERS

469. D
470. B
471. B
472. A
473. C
474. C
475. C
476. D
477. A
478. B
479. C
480. A
481. D
482. C
483. D
484. D
485. D
486. A
487. C
488. B
489. D
490. A
491. C
492. C
493. D
494. A
495. A
496. C
497. D
498. A
499. A
500. D
501. D
502. A
503. B
504. B
505. B
506. D
507. D
508. D
509. D
510. D
511. C
512. C
513. C
514. D
515. D
516. D
517. D
518. D
519. C
520. D
521. D
522. A
523. A
524. B
525. D
526. D
527. D
528. D
529. D
530. A
531. D
532. B
533. C
534. D
535. B
536. B
537. A
538. D
539. D
540. D
541. D
542. B
543. B
544. B
545. D
546. A
547. B
548. C
549. D
550. D
551. A
552. D
553. B
554. A
555. C
556. A
557. D
558. B
559. D
560. D
561. D
562. C
563. B
564. D
565. D
566. D
567. D
568. A
569. A
570. D
571. C
572. D
573. D
574. C
575. C
576. D
577. D
578. D
579. D
580. D
581. C
582. D
583. D
584. D
585. B
586. C
587. B
588. D
589. A
590. C
591. B
592. D
593. A
594. D
595. D
596. C
597. C
598. D
599. D
600. B
601. B
602. D
603. D
604. D
605. D
606. A
607. D
608. D
609. D
610. D
611. D
612. D
613. A
614. D
615. A
616. A
617. B
618. A
619. B
620. D
621. D
622. B
623. A
624. D
625. D
626. C
627. D
628. C
629. D
630. D
631. A
632. B
633. D
634. D
635. D
636. D
637. C
638. D
639. C
640. B
641. D
642. D
643. C
644. D
645. D
646. D
647. D
648. C
649. A
650. D
651. A
652. D
653. C
654. D
655. B
656. D
657. B
658. C
659. B
660. B
661. B
662. D
663. B
664. D
665. D
666. D
667. D
668. D
669. D
670. B
671. D
672. A
673. D
674. D
675. D
676. A
677. D
678. B
679. A
680. B
681. C
682. D
683. D
684. A
685. C
686. D
687. D
688. D
689. C
690. D
691. A
692. D
693. D
694. D
695. D
696. D
697. A
698. A
699. D
700. D
701. D
702. D

ANSWERS

703. D
704. D
705. D
706. A
707. D
708. A
709. B
710. B
711. B
712. D
713. D
714. B
715. D
716. D
717. D
718. B
719. D
720. D
721. D
722. B
723. D
724. C
725. D
726. D
727. B
728. D
729. D
730. D
731. A
732. D
733. D
734. D
735. D
736. D
737. B
738. C
739. D
740. A
741. D
742. D
743. D
744. D
745. D
746. D
747. D
748. A
749. D
750. D
751. D
752. D
753. D
754. D
755. D
756. D
757. D
758. D
759. D
760. D
761. D
762. D
763. B
764. D
765. C
766. A
767. B
768. A
769. C
770. D
771. D
772. B
773. D
774. A
775. A
776. D
777. C
778. D
779. B
780. B
781. D
782. D
783. D
784. C
785. D
786. D
787. D
788. D
789. B
790. C
791. B
792. D
793. C
794. D
795. D
796. D
797. C
798. C
799. D
800. A
801. D
802. A
803. D
804. D
805. D
806. D
807. D
808. D
809. D
810. A
811. D
812. C
813. D
814. D
815. D
816. D
817. A
818. D
819. B
820. D
821. A
822. D
823. D
824. D
825. B
826. B
827. C
828. D
829. C
830. D
831. B
832. A
833. B
834. C
835. D
836. D
837. B
838. D
839. B
840. C
841. D
842. D
843. A
844. A
845. A
846. D
847. D
848. D
849. A
850. D
851. D
852. B
853. A
854. B
855. A
856. A
857. A
858. D
859. D
860. B
861. B
862. B
863. A
864. A
865. D
866. A
867. C
868. B
869. C
870. D
871. A
872. C
873. D
874. D
875. D
876. A
877. D
878. D
879. D
880. D
881. D
882. D
883. C
884. A
885. C
886. C
887. D
888. D
889. B
890. B
891. B
892. D
893. B
894. C
895. D
896. D
897. C
898. D
899. D
900. C
901. D
902. D
903. D
904. D
905. B
906. C
907. B
908. D
909. D
910. D
911. C
912. A
913. D
914. D
915. A
916. B
917. A
918. B
919. D
920. D
921. D
922. D
923. D
924. D
925. B
926. D
927. D
928. D
929. D
930. D
931. A
932. D
933. B
934. D
935. C
936. D

ANSWERS

937. D	976. A	1015. C	1054. C	1093. A	1132. C
938. B	977. D	1016. A	1055. C	1094. D	1133. B
939. D	978. D	1017. C	1056. B	1095. A	1134. A
940. D	979. C	1018. D	1057. A	1096. D	1135. C
941. D	980. B	1019. C	1058. D	1097. D	1136. D
942. A	981. B	1020. C	1059. B	1098. C	1137. D
943. B	982. D	1021. D	1060. D	1099. D	1138. D
944. D	983. D	1022. A	1061. D	1100. D	1139. D
945. A	984. C	1023. D	1062. D	1101. C	1140. C
946. D	985. B	1024. B	1063. C	1102. C	1141. C
947. D	986. C	1025. C	1064. D	1103. D	1142. D
948. C	987. B	1026. A	1065. C	1104. D	1143. D
949. B	988. D	1027. A	1066. B	1105. B	1144. D
950. D	989. D	1028. D	1067. D	1106. C	1145. A
951. D	990. A	1029. D	1068. A	1107. D	1146. B
952. C	991. B	1030. B	1069. D	1108. D	1147. D
953. B	992. A	1031. B	1070. A	1109. A	1148. D
954. D	993. C	1032. C	1071. B	1110. D	1149. A
955. D	994. D	1033. D	1072. B	1111. A	1150. D
956. B	995. D	1034. D	1073. C	1112. A	1151. D
957. C	996. D	1035. D	1074. D	1113. D	1152. B
958. C	997. D	1036. D	1075. D	1114. B	1153. A
959. C	998. D	1037. D	1076. C	1115. D	1154. D
960. C	999. C	1038. C	1077. B	1116. C	1155. A
961. C	1000. D	1039. D	1078. B	1117. C	1156. D
962. D	1001. C	1040. C	1079. B	1118. D	1157. D
963. D	1002. C	1041. D	1080. D	1119. A	1158. D
964. A	1003. D	1042. B	1081. C	1120. D	1159. D
965. D	1004. D	1043. D	1082. B	1121. D	1160. B
966. A	1005. D	1044. C	1083. A	1122. A	1161. C
967. D	1006. B	1045. C	1084. D	1123. C	1162. D
968. C	1007. D	1046. D	1085. C	1124. B	1163. D
969. D	1008. C	1047. B	1086. D	1125. B	1164. D
970. B	1009. A	1048. D	1087. D	1126. D	1165. D
971. D	1010. D	1049. C	1088. D	1127. C	1166. D
972. D	1011. A	1050. D	1089. A	1128. D	1167. D
973. D	1012. D	1051. B	1090. D	1129. D	1168. D
974. D	1013. D	1052. B	1091. B	1130. B	1169. C
975. D	1014. B	1053. D	1092. D	1131. D	1170. C

ANSWERS

1171. B	1210. B	1249. B	1288. A	1327. C	1366. B
1172. B	1211. B	1250. D	1289. D	1328. B	1367. D
1173. C	1212. A	1251. C	1290. C	1329. A	1368. D
1174. C	1213. C	1252. B	1291. D	1330. D	1369. D
1175. B	1214. D	1253. C	1292. D	1331. D	1370. B
1176. D	1215. A	1254. D	1293. C	1332. D	1371. D
1177. A	1216. B	1255. C	1294. D	1333. C	1372. B
1178. D	1217. C	1256. B	1295. D	1334. B	1373. B
1179. D	1218. D	1257. A	1296. D	1335. D	1374. A
1180. A	1219. B	1258. D	1297. D	1336. C	1375. B
1181. D	1220. A	1259. D	1298. D	1337. D	1376. B
1182. D	1221. D	1260. B	1299. D	1338. D	1377. C
1183. D	1222. B	1261. B	1300. D	1339. D	1378. A
1184. C	1223. C	1262. B	1301. A	1340. D	1379. D
1185. D	1224. C	1263. D	1302. C	1341. D	1380. B
1186. B	1225. C	1264. D	1303. B	1342. C	1381. D
1187. D	1226. C	1265. D	1304. B	1343. C	1382. B
1188. C	1227. D	1266. D	1305. D	1344. D	1383. D
1189. D	1228. A	1267. B	1306. C	1345. C	1384. D
1190. B	1229. A	1268. C	1307. C	1346. D	1385. D
1191. A	1230. A	1269. B	1308. B	1347. C	1386. A
1192. A	1231. D	1270. D	1309. A	1348. D	1387. B
1193. D	1232. D	1271. D	1310. D	1349. A	1388. B
1194. C	1233. D	1272. B	1311. D	1350. C	1389. D
1195. C	1234. A	1273. C	1312. D	1351. D	1390. D
1196. C	1235. A	1274. C	1313. B	1352. B	1391. D
1197. D	1236. C	1275. A	1314. D	1353. C	1392. B
1198. C	1237. B	1276. D	1315. D	1354. D	1393. C
1199. D	1238. B	1277. B	1316. C	1355. C	1394. A
1200. A	1239. A	1278. D	1317. C	1356. C	1395. D
1201. A	1240. B	1279. D	1318. D	1357. D	1396. D
1202. B	1241. A	1280. B	1319. D	1358. C	1397. D
1203. D	1242. C	1281. D	1320. D	1359. C	1398. D
1204. C	1243. C	1282. D	1321. D	1360. D	1399. C
1205. D	1244. C	1283. D	1322. D	1361. A	1400. D
1206. D	1245. D	1284. D	1323. D	1362. D	1401. D
1207. D	1246. D	1285. C	1324. D	1363. A	1402. A
1208. A	1247. C	1286. D	1325. D	1364. D	1403. D
1209. A	1248. C	1287. D	1326. C	1365. D	1404. D

ANSWERS

1405. D	1444. C	1483. D	1522. D	1561. D	1600. B
1406. A	1445. C	1484. C	1523. D	1562. D	1601. D
1407. C	1446. D	1485. D	1524. D	1563. D	1602. D
1408. D	1447. D	1486. D	1525. A	1564. D	1603. C
1409. C	1448. D	1487. D	1526. D	1565. D	1604. B
1410. B	1449. C	1488. D	1527. D	1566. D	1605. C
1411. D	1450. D	1489. B	1528. D	1567. D	1606. D
1412. D	1451. D	1490. B	1529. C	1568. C	1607. A
1413. B	1452. D	1491. B	1530. C	1569. D	1608. A
1414. D	1453. B	1492. D	1531. D	1570. D	1609. C
1415. D	1454. D	1493. D	1532. D	1571. D	1610. A
1416. B	1455. A	1494. B	1533. A	1572. D	1611. C
1417. C	1456. C	1495. D	1534. D	1573. B	1612. D
1418. B	1457. D	1496. D	1535. D	1574. D	1613. B
1419. B	1458. A	1497. D	1536. D	1575. D	1614. B
1420. B	1459. D	1498. D	1537. D	1576. D	1615. D
1421. D	1460. A	1499. D	1538. B	1577. D	1616. B
1422. C	1461. B	1500. D	1539. D	1578. D	1617. C
1423. C	1462. C	1501. D	1540. C	1579. D	1618. A
1424. A	1463. B	1502. D	1541. C	1580. C	1619. A
1425. D	1464. C	1503. C	1542. B	1581. D	1620. A
1426. D	1465. C	1504. D	1543. B	1582. D	1621. D
1427. D	1466. C	1505. B	1544. D	1583. D	1622. B
1428. B	1467. D	1506. A	1545. D	1584. D	1623. C
1429. B	1468. C	1507. A	1546. B	1585. D	1624. D
1430. D	1469. D	1508. D	1547. D	1586. A	1625. A
1431. A	1470. C	1509. D	1548. C	1587. D	1626. A
1432. D	1471. D	1510. C	1549. C	1588. B	1627. A
1433. D	1472. A	1511. D	1550. D	1589. C	1628. A
1434. D	1473. B	1512. D	1551. C	1590. C	1629. B
1435. D	1474. A	1513. D	1552. D	1591. D	1630. D
1436. D	1475. A	1514. C	1553. D	1592. B	1631. B
1437. D	1476. B	1515. B	1554. D	1593. B	1632. A
1438. C	1477. B	1516. B	1555. D	1594. D	1633. A
1439. B	1478. D	1517. D	1556. D	1595. C	1634. D
1440. B	1479. D	1518. D	1557. D	1596. A	1635. C
1441. D	1480. B	1519. D	1558. A	1597. A	1636. D
1442. C	1481. A	1520. D	1559. A	1598. C	1637. D
1443. A	1482. D	1521. D	1560. D	1599. B	1638. A

ANSWERS

1639. D
1640. D
1641. B
1642. B
1643. C
1644. D
1645. D
1646. A
1647. D
1648. D
1649. B
1650. D
1651. B
1652. B
1653. D
1654. A
1655. D
1656. D
1657. D
1658. D
1659. D
1660. B
1661. D
1662. D
1663. D
1664. C
1665. C
1666. B
1667. B
1668. D
1669. B
1670. D
1671. D
1672. D
1673. B
1674. C
1675. D
1676. A
1677. C
1678. D
1679. D
1680. A
1681. C
1682. D
1683. C
1684. C
1685. C
1686. D
1687. C
1688. D
1689. D
1690. A
1691. D
1692. B
1693. C
1694. B
1695. D
1696. A
1697. D
1698. D
1699. D
1700. B
1701. C
1702. A
1703. C
1704. C
1705. B
1706. A
1707. D
1708. A
1709. D
1710. B
1711. D
1712. D
1713. D
1714. D
1715. D
1716. D
1717. A
1718. A
1719. C
1720. B
1721. B
1722. B
1723. A
1724. D
1725. A
1726. D
1727. D
1728. C
1729. D
1730. D
1731. D
1732. D
1733. D
1734. D
1735. C
1736. D
1737. C
1738. B
1739. D
1740. B
1741. B
1742. C
1743. A
1744. D
1745. B
1746. D
1747. B
1748. D
1749. B
1750. D
1751. C
1752. B
1753. D
1754. C
1755. C
1756. A
1757. C
1758. B
1759. D
1760. D
1761. B
1762. C
1763. C
1764. D
1765. C
1766. A
1767. D
1768. A
1769. D
1770. C
1771. D
1772. D
1773. B
1774. D
1775. D
1776. D
1777. D
1778. C
1779. B
1780. D
1781. A
1782. D
1783. A
1784. D
1785. D
1786. D
1787. B
1788. D
1789. B
1790. D
1791. D
1792. D
1793. D
1794. A
1795. D
1796. D
1797. A
1798. A
1799. B
1800. A
1801. D
1802. B
1803. B
1804. D
1805. C
1806. D
1807. D
1808. D
1809. C
1810. D
1811. D
1812. D
1813. D
1814. D
1815. D
1816. D
1817. B
1818. B
1819. D
1820. B
1821. A
1822. D
1823. C
1824. A
1825. D
1826. D
1827. C
1828. C
1829. D
1830. C
1831. B
1832. B
1833. D
1834. D
1835. B
1836. C
1837. B
1838. D
1839. C
1840. D
1841. C
1842. C
1843. C
1844. A
1845. A
1846. D
1847. D
1848. D
1849. D
1850. D
1851. D
1852. A
1853. D
1854. D
1855. C
1856. D
1857. A
1858. A
1859. D
1860. C
1861. D
1862. B
1863. D
1864. D
1865. C
1866. D
1867. C
1868. D
1869. A
1870. C
1871. B
1872. D

ANSWERS

1873. D
1874. B
1875. D
1876. D
1877. B
1878. A
1879. B
1880. B
1881. B
1882. A
1883. D
1884. C
1885. B
1886. C
1887. B
1888. C
1889. A
1890. B
1891. C
1892. B
1893. D
1894. D
1895. B
1896. A
1897. B
1898. D
1899. D
1900. C
1901. C
1902. B
1903. D
1904. A
1905. B
1906. D
1907. D
1908. D
1909. B
1910. D
1911. D
1912. D
1913. D
1914. D
1915. D
1916. C
1917. D
1918. D
1919. D
1920. A
1921. D
1922. B
1923. B
1924. D
1925. D
1926. D
1927. B
1928. D
1929. B
1930. C
1931. A
1932. B
1933. B
1934. C
1935. D
1936. B
1937. A
1938. D
1939. C
1940. B
1941. D
1942. B
1943. A
1944. A
1945. D
1946. D
1947. B
1948. B
1949. D
1950. A
1951. D
1952. B
1953. C
1954. D
1955. B
1956. B
1957. D
1958. D
1959. D
1960. C
1961. C
1962. D
1963. D
1964. D
1965. B
1966. D
1967. D
1968. D
1969. B
1970. B
1971. A
1972. D
1973. C
1974. C
1975. C
1976. B
1977. C
1978. B
1979. D
1980. B
1981. B
1982. A
1983. B
1984. B
1985. C
1986. B
1987. C
1988. B
1989. D
1990. D
1991. D
1992. D
1993. D
1994. C
1995. B
1996. B
1997. B
1998. D
1999. C
2000. C
2001. D
2002. D
2003. A
2004. D
2005. C
2006. A
2007. D
2008. A
2009. D
2010. D
2011. D
2012. A
2013. C
2014. D
2015. C
2016. A
2017. C
2018. C
2019. D
2020. B
2021. D
2022. D
2023. D
2024. C
2025. A
2026. D
2027. D
2028. D
2029. A
2030. D
2031. D
2032. B
2033. B
2034. B
2035. D
2036. D
2037. C
2038. D
2039. A
2040. D
2041. A
2042. D
2043. D
2044. D
2045. D
2046. B
2047. B
2048. D
2049. A
2050. A
2051. A
2052. B
2053. B
2054. A
2055. C
2056. A
2057. D
2058. B
2059. A
2060. D
2061. C
2062. C
2063. B
2064. D
2065. D
2066. C
2067. C
2068. A
2069. C
2070. D
2071. D
2072. D
2073. A
2074. D
2075. C
2076. D
2077. B
2078. A
2079. D
2080. D
2081. B
2082. D
2083. D
2084. B
2085. B
2086. A
2087. B
2088. D
2089. D
2090. D
2091. B
2092. D
2093. D
2094. D
2095. C
2096. D
2097. B
2098. D
2099. A
2100. C
2101. D
2102. D
2103. C
2104. A
2105. C
2106. C

ANSWERS

2107. D
2108. C
2109. A
2110. D
2111. D
2112. C
2113. D
2114. B
2115. B
2116. D
2117. D
2118. A
2119. A
2120. A
2121. B
2122. B
2123. A
2124. B
2125. C
2126. D
2127. D
2128. D
2129. D
2130. C
2131. A
2132. B
2133. B
2134. A
2135. C
2136. D
2137. C
2138. C
2139. B
2140. C
2141. D
2142. C
2143. D
2144. D
2145. D
2146. D
2147. A
2148. C
2149. D
2150. B
2151. D
2152. C
2153. A
2154. C
2155. D
2156. D
2157. A
2158. D
2159. B
2160. C
2161. D
2162. D
2163. C
2164. D
2165. D
2166. A
2167. A
2168. A
2169. D
2170. D
2171. D
2172. D
2173. B
2174. C
2175. D
2176. B
2177. D
2178. D
2179. D
2180. A
2181. A
2182. A
2183. A
2184. D
2185. C
2186. C
2187. A
2188. D
2189. D
2190. B
2191. D
2192. D
2193. A
2194. D
2195. D
2196. A
2197. D
2198. D
2199. B
2200. B
2201. B
2202. C
2203. D
2204. D
2205. A
2206. A
2207. C
2208. D
2209. B
2210. A
2211. D
2212. D
2213. C
2214. B
2215. B
2216. B
2217. C
2218. D
2219. D
2220. D
2221. B
2222. D
2223. D
2224. C
2225. D
2226. B
2227. D
2228. C
2229. A
2230. D
2231. C
2232. C
2233. D
2234. D
2235. D
2236. C
2237. D
2238. D
2239. D
2240. D
2241. C
2242. D
2243. A
2244. D
2245. D
2246. D
2247. C
2248. D
2249. A
2250. C
2251. A
2252. D
2253. B
2254. C
2255. D
2256. B
2257. A
2258. A
2259. C
2260. B
2261. D
2262. B
2263. B
2264. A
2265. C
2266. B
2267. D
2268. D
2269. D
2270. A
2271. B
2272. A
2273. C
2274. C
2275. C
2276. B
2277. D
2278. A
2279. D
2280. D
2281. D
2282. B
2283. D
2284. D
2285. D
2286. A
2287. D
2288. D
2289. D
2290. D
2291. D
2292. D
2293. B
2294. D
2295. A
2296. B
2297. C
2298. C
2299. B
2300. B
2301. B
2302. B
2303. C
2304. D
2305. C
2306. D
2307. D
2308. D
2309. D
2310. D
2311. D
2312. C
2313. A
2314. D
2315. C
2316. D
2317. C
2318. A
2319. B
2320. C
2321. D
2322. B
2323. D
2324. B
2325. C
2326. D
2327. B
2328. B
2329. D
2330. D
2331. D
2332. D
2333. C
2334. C
2335. D
2336. C
2337. A
2338. D
2339. B
2340. C

ANSWERS

2341. A	2377. C	2413. C	2449. D	2485. B	2521. D
2342. D	2378. D	2414. C	2450. D	2486. A	2522. D
2343. D	2379. B	2415. A	2451. C	2487. B	2523. D
2344. D	2380. A	2416. D	2452. B	2488. D	2524. C
2345. D	2381. B	2417. D	2453. D	2489. D	2525. C
2346. D	2382. C	2418. C	2454. D	2490. B	2526. D
2347. D	2383. D	2419. A	2455. D	2491. A	2527. C
2348. D	2384. A	2420. D	2456. D	2492. B	2528. B
2349. B	2385. C	2421. B	2457. D	2493. A	2529. B
2350. B	2386. B	2422. D	2458. D	2494. D	2530. D
2351. B	2387. D	2423. D	2459. C	2495. C	2531. D
2352. A	2388. A	2424. C	2460. D	2496. D	2532. B
2353. B	2389. B	2425. D	2461. C	2497. A	2533. B
2354. D	2390. D	2426. D	2462. C	2498. D	2534. B
2355. D	2391. B	2427. C	2463. D	2499. D	2535. D
2356. D	2392. B	2428. D	2464. D	2500. D	2536. D
2357. B	2393. D	2429. D	2465. D	2501. B	2537. B
2358. D	2394. D	2430. D	2466. D	2502. D	2538. D
2359. C	2395. C	2431. B	2467. C	2503. D	2539. B
2360. D	2396. B	2432. D	2468. D	2504. C	2540. C
2361. D	2397. D	2433. D	2469. C	2505. A	2541. D
2362. A	2398. B	2434. D	2470. A	2506. D	2542. C
2363. D	2399. C	2435. A	2471. D	2507. D	2543. A
2364. D	2400. C	2436. A	2472. D	2508. B	2544. D
2365. B	2401. D	2437. D	2473. D	2509. A	2545. D
2366. A	2402. A	2438. D	2474. D	2510. D	2546. D
2367. D	2403. D	2439. D	2475. A	2511. D	2547. A
2368. A	2404. C	2440. D	2476. D	2512. C	2548. D
2369. D	2405. A	2441. A	2477. D	2513. D	2549. C.
2370. D	2406. B	2442. C	2478. D	2514. B	2550. D
2371. B	2407. C	2443. B	2479. C	2515. D	2551. A
2372. D	2408. B	2444. D	2480. D	2516. D	2552. D
2373. C	2409. D	2445. B	2481. B	2517. B	2553. A
2374. B	2410. D	2446. B	2482. D	2518. D	2554. D
2375. D	2411. B	2447. A	2483. D	2519. D	2555. C
2376. B	2412. D	2448. C	2484. B	2520. B	2556. D

Respiratory 3

Approach to the Patient with Disease of the Respiratory System

1. Stethoscope was invented by René Laënnec in which year?
N Engl J Med 2014;370:744-51

A. 1780
B. 1802
C. 1816
D. 1860

Stethoscope was invented by René Laënnec in year 1816.

2. Tracheal Sounds are produced by turbulent airflow in?
N Engl J Med 2014;370:744-51

A. Pharynx
B. Glottis
C. Subglottic region
D. All of the above

Tracheal Sounds are produced by turbulent airflow in the pharynx, glottis, and subglottic region.

3. Which of the following is related to Velcro?
N Engl J Med 2014;370:744-51

A. Fine crackles
B. Coarse crackles
C. Pleural friction rub
D. Stridor

Fine crackles have a distinctive sound similar to the sound heard when joined strips of Velcro are gently separated, they have been called Velcro rales.

4. Fine crackles tend to be minimal or even absent in?
N Engl J Med 2014;370:744-51

A. Idiopathic pulmonary fibrosis
B. Sarcoidosis
C. Asbestosis
D. Nonspecific interstitial pneumonitis

Though not pathognomonic, fine crackles are prominent in idiopathic pulmonary fibrosis, appearing first in basal areas of lungs and progressing to upper zones with disease progression. Fine crackles are also found in asbestosis, nonspecific interstitial pneumonitis, and interstitial fibrosis associated with connective-tissue disorders. Fine crackles tend to be minimal or even absent in sarcoidosis, because sarcoidosis primarily affects central lung zones not abutting pleura.

5. Squawks are heard in patients with?
N Engl J Med 2014;370:744-51

A. Hypersensitivity pneumonitis
B. Bronchiectasis
C. Pneumonia
D. All of the above

Squawks are typically heard from middle to the end of inspiration in patients with interstitial diseases, especially hypersensitivity pneumonitis. Also heard in bronchiectasis and pneumonia.

6. Which of the following is the most common of diseases of the respiratory system?
Harrison's 20th Ed. Chapter 278 Page 1943

A. Obstructive lung diseases
B. Restrictive disorders
C. Pulmonary vascular diseases
D. Neoplastic diseases of lung

Diseases of respiratory system are obstructive lung diseases, restrictive disorders and abnormalities of pulmonary vasculature. Obstructive lung diseases are most common.

7. Which of the following is included in the category of obstructive lung diseases?
Harrison's 20th Ed. Chapter 278 Page 1943 Table 278–1

A. Asthma
B. Bronchiectasis
C. Bronchiolitis
D. All of the above

Obstructive lung diseases include disorders of the airways such as asthma, chronic obstructive pulmonary disease (COPD), bronchiectasis, and bronchiolitis. Bronchitis and Tracheitis is included under the infectious pathology.

8. Which of the following is a type of restrictive lung disease?
Harrison's 20th Ed. Chapter 278 Page 1943

A. Parenchymal lung diseases
B. Abnormalities of chest wall and pleura
C. Neuromuscular disease
D. All of the above

9. Which of the following is a disorder of pulmonary vasculature?
Harrison's 20th Ed. Chapter 278 Page 1943

A. Pulmonary embolism
B. Pulmonary hypertension
C. Pulmonary veno-occlusive disease
D. All of the above

10. Acute shortness of breath is usually associated with?
Harrison's 20th Ed. Chapter 278 Page 1943

A. Myocardial infarction
B. Pulmonary embolism
C. Pneumothorax
D. All of the above

Acute shortness of breath is usually associated with laryngeal edema, bronchospasm, myocardial infarction, pulmonary embolism, or pneumothorax.

11. Cough that persists for more than how many weeks is defined as chronic cough?
Harrison's 20th Ed. Chapter 278 Page 1943

A. 2 weeks
B. 4 weeks
C. 6 weeks
D. 8 weeks

Cough that persists for more than eight weeks is defined as chronic cough.

12. Chest pain caused by diseases of respiratory system usually originates from involvement of?

Harrison's 20th Ed. Chapter 278 Page 1943

A. Parietal pleura
B. Visceral pleura
C. Pulmonary parenchyma
D. Bronchial airways

Lung parenchyma is not innervated with pain fibers. Chest pain from respiratory disorders results from either diseases of parietal pleura (pneumothorax) or pulmonary vascular diseases (pulmonary hypertension).

13. Which of the following is associated with smoking?

Harrison's 20th Ed. Chapter 278 Page 1944

A. Bronchogenic lung cancer
B. Desquamative interstitial pneumonitis
C. Pulmonary Langerhans cell histiocytosis
D. All of the above

COPD, neoplasia, spontaneous pneumothorax, respiratory bronchiolitis–interstitial lung disease, desquamative interstitial pneumonitis (DIP), pulmonary Langerhans cell histiocytosis & pulmonary hemorrhage with Goodpasture's syndrome are associated with smoking.

14. Asymmetric expansion of the chest is due to?

Harrison's 20th Ed. Chapter 278 Page 1944

A. Endobronchial obstruction of a large airway
B. Unilateral parenchymal or pleural disease
C. Unilateral phrenic nerve paralysis
D. All of the above

15. Which of the following about lung auscultation is false?

Harrison's 20th Ed. Chapter 278 Page 1944

A. Wheeze & rhonchi have same meaning
B. Crackles are typically inspiratory sounds
C. Wheezes are more prominent during expiration
D. Stridor occurs primarily during inspiration

16. Which of the following about lung auscultation is false?

Harrison's 20th Ed. Chapter 278 Page 1944

A. Crackles are created when alveoli & small airways open & close with respiration
B. Wheezes reflect oscillation of airway walls with airflow limitation
C. Rhonchi is the sound created when there is free liquid in the airway lumen
D. None of the above

17. Which of the following about stridor is false?

Harrison's 20th Ed. Chapter 278 Page 1944

A. High-pitched
B. Focal inspiratory wheeze
C. Heard over the neck
D. Manifestation of upper airway obstruction

Stridor or a low-pitched, focal inspiratory wheeze heard over the neck. It is a manifestation of upper airway obstruction.

18. Crackles sounding like Velcro being ripped apart is a feature of?

Harrison's 20th Ed. Chapter 278 Page 1944

A. Bronchiectasis
B. Pleuritis
C. IPF
D. Pulmonary edema

Crackles, or rales are a sign of alveolar disease. Diseases that result in fibrosis of the interstitium (IPF) result in crackles sounding like Velcro being ripped apart.

19. Which of the following is useful in distinguishing crackles due to alveolar fluid and those due to interstitial fibrosis?

Harrison's 20th Ed. Chapter 278 Page 1944

A. Air entry
B. Percussion note
C. Tactile fremitus
D. Egophony

Egophony helps to distinguish between crackles associated with alveolar fluid and those associated with interstitial fibrosis. Egophony is auscultation of sound "AH" instead of "EEE" when a patient phonates "EEE." This change in note is due to abnormal sound transmission through consolidated lung and will be present in pneumonia but not in IPF.

20. Chest hyperresonance in pneumothorax is best appreciated at?

Harrison's 20th Ed. Chapter 278 Page 1944

A. Apex
B. Axillary region
C. Interscapular region
D. Bases of lung

Chest hyperresonance, particularly at apex, indicates air in pleural space (pneumothorax).

21. All of the following can cause clubbing except?

Harrison's 20th Ed. Chapter 278 Page 1944

A. Lung cancer
B. ILD
C. Empyema
D. Wegener's granulomatosis

22. Schamroth's sign is seen in?

Hutchison's Hunter

A. Koilonychia
B. Platynychia
C. Clubbing
D. None of the above

23. Clubbing of the digits is not a sign of?

Harrison's 20th Ed. Chapter 278 Page 1944

A. COPD
B. Crohn's disease
C. Bacterial endocarditis
D. Interstitial lung disease

Clubbing of the digits is not a sign of COPD, and its presence should alert clinician to initiate an investigation for causes of clubbing. Even cyanosis is a late finding in cor pulmonale & is secondary to a low cardiac output with systemic vasoconstriction & ventilation-perfusion mismatches in lung.

24. Which of the following is a feature of hypertrophic osteoarthropathy (HOA)?

Harrison's 20th Ed. Chapter 367 Page 2643

A. Clubbing of digits
B. Periosteal new bone formation
C. Synovial effusions
D. All of the above

HOA is characterized by clubbing of digits and, in more advanced stages, by periosteal new bone formation and synovial effusions.

25. Which of the following about primary hypertrophic osteoarthropathy is false?

Harrison's 20th Ed. Chapter 367 Page 2643

A. Autosomal dominant disorder
B. Periosteal new bone formation
C. Smooth & undulating periosteal surface
D. Hyperhydrosis

*Primary or idiopathic hypertrophic osteoarthropathy is an autosomal dominant disorder characterized by periosteal new bone formation of distal extremities with **irregular** periosteal surface, clubbing, hyperhydrosis, thickening of skin of face & forehead, progressive enlargement of hands & feet, and arthralgias. In secondary hypertrophic osteopathy due to pulmonary disorders, exuberant periosteal new bone formation occurs with smooth and undulating periosteal surface.*

26. Role of which of the following explains acquired HOA?

Harrison's 20th Ed. Chapter 367 Page 2643

A. RBC
B. Platelets
C. WBC
D. All of the above

Recent studies have suggested a role for platelets in the development of HOA. Megakaryocytes & large platelet particles, present in venous circulation, get fragmented in their passage through normal lung. In patients with cyanotic congenital heart disease and in right-to-left shunts, these large platelet particles bypass lung and reach distal extremities, where they interact with endothelial cells. Platelet-endothelial activation in distal portion of extremities results in release of platelet-derived growth factor (PDGF) leading to proliferation of connective tissue & periosteum. Stimulation of fibroblasts by PDGF & transforming growth factor results in cell growth and collagen synthesis.

27. Levels of which of the following are elevated in HOA?

Harrison's 20th Ed. Chapter 367 Page 2643

A. Factor IX
B. Factor X
C. von Willebrand factor
D. All of the above

Elevated plasma levels of von Willebrand factor antigen have been found in patients with both primary and secondary forms of HOA, indicating endothelial activation or damage.

28. Touraine-Solente-Golé syndrome refers to?

Harrison's 20th Ed. Chapter 367 Page 2643

A. Primary or familial hypertrophic osteoarthropathy
B. Hemophilic arthropathy
C. Arthropathy of acromegaly
D. Arthropathy of hemochromatosis

Primary or familial HOA is called pachydermoperiostitis or Touraine-Solente-Golé syndrome. Usually begins insidiously at puberty, this autosomal dominant trait with variable expression and is nine times more common in boys than in girls.

29. Which of the following is not a feature of primary hypertrophic osteoarthropathy (HOA)?

Harrison's 19th Ed. 2244

A. Clubbing
B. Periostitis
C. Ptosis
D. Anhidrosis

Primary HOA is characterized by clubbing, periostitis, and unusual skin features. The skin becomes thickened and coarse. Deep nasolabial folds develop, and the forehead may become furrowed. Patients may have heavy-appearing eyelids and ptosis. The skin is often greasy, and there may be excessive sweating of the hands and feet.

30. Cutis verticis gyrata is a feature of?

Harrison's 20th Ed. Chapter 367 Page 2643

A. Scleroderma
B. Primary HOA
C. Diabetes mellitus
D. Syphilis

In primary HOA, skin over scalp becomes very thick & corrugated (cutis verticis gyrata).

31. Associated abnormalities observed in primary HOA include all except?

Harrison's 20th Ed. Chapter 367 Page 2643

A. Hypertrophic gastropathy
B. Synovial hypertrophy
C. Bone marrow failure
D. Female escutcheon

Associated abnormalities in primary HOA include hypertrophic gastropathy, bone marrow failure, female escutcheon, gynecomastia, and cranial suture defects. Noninflammatory effusions occur in wrists, knees & ankles. Synovial hypertrophy is not found.

32. The sensation experienced by patient in clubbed fingers is?

Harrison's 20th Ed. Chapter 367 Page 2643

A. Burning
B. Itching
C. Tingling
D. All of the above

Patients with clubbing may experience a burning sensation in their fingertips.

33. Fishman's classification is used for?

Circulation 1966;33:145

A. Cyanosis
B. Anemia
C. Clubbing
D. Jaundice

An objective measurement of finger clubbing can be made by determining the diameter at the base of the nail and at the distal interphalangeal joint of all 10 digits. Clubbing is present when the sum of the individual digit ratios is >10.

34. Which of the following is present in clubbing?

Harrison's 20th Ed. Chapter 367 Page 2643

A. Periungual erythema
B. Drumstick appearance
C. Hyperextended distal interphalangeal joint
D. All of the above

Marked periungual erythema is usually present. When clubbing is advanced, the finger may have a drumstick appearance, and the distal interphalangeal joint can be hyperextended. Periosteal involvement in the distal extremities may produce a burning or deep-seated aching pain. The pain can be quite incapacitating and is aggravated by dependency and relieved by elevation of the affected limbs. The overlying soft tissue may be swollen, and the skin slightly erythematous. Pressure applied over the distal forearms and legs may be quite painful.

35. In a patient with clubbing, pain may be present in all of the following joints except?

Harrison's 20th Ed. Chapter 367 Page 2643

A. Ankles
B. Knees
C. Hip
D. Wrists

With clubbing, pain & symmetric arthritis-like changes in shoulders, knees, ankles, wrists & elbows is observed.

36. Which of the following is uncommon in secondary HOA?

Harrison's 20th Ed. Chapter 367 Page 2644

A. Excessive sweating
B. Oiliness of the skin
C. Thickening of facial skin
D. All of the above

Unlike primary HOA, excessive sweating and oiliness of the skin and thickening of the facial skin are uncommon in secondary HOA.

37. Out of the following malignancies, HOA is most common in?

Harrison's 20th Ed. Chapter 367 Page 2644

A. Carcinoma of esophagus
B. Lung metastases
C. Pleural tumors
D. Thymoma

HOA is most common in bronchogenic carcinoma and pleural tumors. Lung metastases infrequently cause HOA.

38. Unilateral clubbing may be found in which of the following?

Harrison's 20th Ed. Chapter 367 Page 2644 Table 367-3

A. Aneurysms of major extremity arteries
B. Infected arterial grafts
C. Arteriovenous fistulas of brachial vessels
D. All of the above

Unilateral clubbing is seen in association with aneurysms of major extremity arteries, with infected arterial grafts & with arteriovenous fistulas of brachial vessels.

39. Clubbing of toes but not fingers is found in?

Harrison's 20th Ed. Chapter 367 Page 2644 Table 367-3

A. Infected abdominal aortic aneurysm
B. Coarctation of aorta
C. Budd-Chiari syndrome
D. Tetralogy of Fallot

40. Clubbing of toes but not fingers is found in?

Harrison's 20th Ed. Chapter 367 Page 2644 Table 367-3

A. VSD
B. Patent ductus arteriosus
C. Budd-Chiari syndrome
D. Tetralogy of Fallot

Clubbing of the toes but not fingers is seen in an infected abdominal aortic aneurysm & PDA. Differential cyanosis refers to cyanotic and clubbed toes but not the fingers.

41. Clubbing of a single digit may be found in all except?

Harrison's 20th Ed. Chapter 367 Page 2644

A. Trauma
B. Tophaceous gout
C. Cystic fibrosis
D. Sarcoidosis

Clubbing of a single digit may follow trauma, in tophaceous gout and sarcoidosis. With advanced lung disease, clubbing of digits appears in virtually all patients with CF.

42. Which of the following is not a feature of thyroid acropachy?

Harrison's 20th Ed. Chapter 367 Page 2644

A. Hypothyroidism
B. Clubbing
C. Periostitis of hand bones
D. Periostitis of feet bones

Hyperthyroidism (Graves' disease) associated with clubbing & periostitis of bones of hands & feet is called thyroid acropachy. It is strongly associated with thyroid dermopathy.

43. Clubbing without cyanosis is frequent in?

Harrison's 20th Ed. Chapter 36 Page 237

A. Infective endocarditis
B. Inflammatory bowel disease
C. Jackhammer operators
D. All of the above

Disturbances of Respiratory Function

44. What is the approximate lung surface area?

Harrison's 20th Ed. Chapter 279 Page 1945

A. 50 m^2
B. 60 m^2
C. 70 m^2
D. 80 m^2

Alveolar surface area is ~70 m^2 and volume of thoracic cavity is 7 liters.

45. The respiratory system includes?

Harrison's 20th Ed. Chapter 279 Page 1945

A. Lungs
B. Neuromuscular system
C. Chest wall (diaphragm & intercostal muscles)
D. All of the above

Respiratory system includes lungs, neuromuscular system, chest wall (diaphragm & intercostal muscles) & pulmonary circulation.

46. In pulmonary circulation, how many capillaries are present per alveolus?

Harrison's 20th Ed. Chapter 60 Page 395

A. ~ 100
B. ~ 1000
C. ~ 10000
D. ~ 100000

In pulmonary circulation, extensive capillary bed with ~1000 capillaries per alveolus exists.

47. What portion of the fresh air inspired with each breath does not reach alveoli but remains in conducting airways of lung?

Respir Care 2008;53(7):885– 89

A. ~ 10%
B. ~ 20%
C. ~ 30%
D. ~ 40%

~30% of inspired fresh air of each breath does not reach alveoli but remains in the conducting airways of lung (anatomic dead space) or ~1 mL of dead space for every pound of body weight..

48. Total ventilation each minute is approximately?

A. 5 Liters
B. 7 Liters
C. 9 Liters
D. 11 Liters

Total ventilation each minute is ~7 liters (2 liters/minute of dead space ventilation and 5 liters/minute of alveolar ventilation).

49. Each breath has a tidal volume of approximately?

A. 200 mL
B. 300 mL
C. 400 mL
D. 500 mL

Normal individual at rest inspires ~12 to 16 times per minute, each breath has a tidal volume of ~500 mL.

50. The volume of gas that is exhaled from lungs in going from TLC to RV is?

Harrison's 20th Ed. Chapter 279 Page 1946 Figure 279-2

A. Expiratory reserve volume (ERV)
B. Functional residual capacity (FRC)
C. Vital capacity (VC)
D. Tidal volume (VT)

Volume of gas exhaled from lungs in going from TLC to RV is vital capacity.

51. $FEF_{25-75\%}$ is also called?

A. Maximal early expiratory flow rate
B. Maximal mid expiratory flow rate
C. Maximal late expiratory flow rate
D. Maximal pan expiratory flow rate

Average expiratory flow rate during the middle 50% of VC [forced expiratory flow (FEF) between 25 & 75% of VC, or $FEF_{25-75\%}$ is also called maximal midexpiratory flow rate (MMFR)].

52. Total lung capacity (TLC) is a sum of?

Harrison's 20th Ed. Chapter 279 Page 1946 Figure 279-2

A. VC + RV
B. VC + FRC
C. VC + ERV
D. VC + IC

Spirographic tracings consist of 4 lung capacities (TLC, VC, IC & FRC) & 3 lung volumes (RV, ERV & V_T).

53. Total lung capacity (TLC) is a sum of?

Harrison's 20th Ed. Chapter 279 Page 1946 Figure 279-2

A. VC + ERV
B. VC + FRC
C. FRC + Tidal volume (V_T)
D. FRC + IC

54. Total lung capacity (TLC) is a sum of?

Harrison's 20th Ed. Chapter 279 Page 1946 Figure 279-2

A. VC + ERV
B. VC + FRC
C. IC + ERV + RV
D. FRC + V_T

55. Vital capacity (VC) is a sum of?

Harrison's 20th Ed. Chapter 279 Page 1946 Figure 279-2

A. IC - VT
B. IC + VT
C. IC + ERV
D. IC - ERV

56. Transpulmonary pressure (P_{TP}) refers to?

A. Alveolar pressure-pleural pressure
B. Pleural pressure-alveolar pressure
C. Endexpiratory-endinspiratory pleural pressure
D. Endinspiratory-endexpiratory pleural pressure

Transpulmonary pressure or P_{TP} is defined as alveolar pressure minus pleural pressure.

57. Volume of gas in the lungs at the end of a normal exhalation is denoted by?
Harrison's 20th Ed. Chapter 279 Page 1946 Figure 279-2

A. Tidal volume (V_T)
B. Residual volume (RV)
C. Expiratory reserve volume (ERV)
D. Functional residual capacity (FRC)

FRC is defined as the volume of gas in the lungs at the end of a normal exhalation.

58. Which of the following respiratory functions can be measured by a spirometer?
Harrison's 20th Ed. Chapter 279 Page 1946

A. Vital Capacity (VC)
B. Expiratory reserve volume (ERV)
C. Inspiratory capacity (IC)
D. All of the above

59. Which of the following respiratory functions cannot be measured by a spirometer?
Harrison's 20th Ed. Chapter 279 Page 1946

A. VC
B. ERV
C. IC
D. Residual Volume (RV)

60. Which of the following respiratory functions cannot be measured by a spirometer?
Harrison's 20th Ed. Chapter 279 Page 1946

A. VC
B. ERV
C. IC
D. Functional Residual Capacity (FRC)

61. Which of the following respiratory functions cannot be measured by a spirometer?
Harrison's 20th Ed. Chapter 279 Page 1946

A. VC
B. ERV
C. IC
D. Total Lung Capacity (TLC)

VC, expiratory reserve volume (ERV), and inspiratory capacity (IC) are measured by having the patient breathe into and out of a spirometer. RV, FRC, and TLC cannot be measured by a spirometer because they include the volume of gas present in the lungs even after a maximal expiration.

62. The excursion between full and minimal lung inflation is called?
Harrison's 20th Ed. Chapter 279 Page 1946

A. Tidal volume
B. FRC
C. Vital capacity
D. Inspiratory capacity

The excursion between full and minimal lung inflation is called vital capacity (VC). VC provides little information about the intrinsic properties of the respiratory system.

63. Most distal generation of airways is?
Harrison's 20th Ed. Chapter 279 Page 1946

A. Respiratory bronchiole
B. Terminal bronchiole
C. Alveolar duct
D. Alveolus

Most distal generation of airways is respiratory bronchioles.

64. Maximal expiratory flow at any lung volume is determined by?
Harrison's 20th Ed. Chapter 279 Page 1947

A. Gas density
B. Airway cross-section and distensibility
C. Elastic recoil pressure of lung
D. All of the above

Maximal expiratory flow at any lung volume is determined by gas density, airway cross-section & distensibility, elastic recoil pressure of lung and frictional pressure loss to flow-limiting airway site.

65. Maximal expiratory flow is elevated in?
Harrison's 20th Ed. Chapter 279 Page 1947

A. Asthma
B. Chronic bronchitis
C. Pulmonary fibrosis
D. Emphysema

Under normal conditions, maximal expiratory flow falls with lung volume due mainly to the dependence of lung recoil pressure on lung volume. In pulmonary fibrosis, lung recoil pressure is increased at any lung volume and thus the maximal expiratory flow is elevated.

66. Pulmonary function values are expressed as a percentage of normal predicted values except for?
Harrison's 20th Ed. Chapter 279 Page 1949 Figure 279-6

A. RV
B. FEV1
C. DLCO
D. R_{aw}

Pulmonary function values are expressed as a percentage of normal predicted values except for airways resistance - R_{aw} which is expressed as cmH_2O/L per second. (normal <2 cm H_2O/L per second).

67. Residual volume is minimum is which of the following?
Harrison's 20th Ed. Chapter 279 Page 1949 Figure 279-6

A. Pulmonary fibrosis
B. Myasthenia gravis
C. Acute asthma
D. Severe emphysema

68. Residual volume is maximum is which of the following?
Harrison's 20th Ed. Chapter 279 Page 1949 Figure 279-6

A. Pulmonary fibrosis
B. Myasthenia gravis
C. Acute asthma
D. Severe emphysema

69. DL_{CO} is minimum is which of the following?
Harrison's 20th Ed. Chapter 279 Page 1949 Figure 279-6

A. Pulmonary fibrosis
B. Myasthenia gravis
C. Acute asthma
D. Severe emphysema

70. FRC is maximum is which of the following?
Harrison's 20th Ed. Chapter 279 Page 1949 Figure 279-6

A. Pulmonary fibrosis
B. Myasthenia gravis
C. Acute asthma
D. Severe emphysema

71. Airways resistance - R_{aw} is maximum is which of the following?
Harrison's 20th Ed. Chapter 279 Page 1949 Figure 279-6

A. Pulmonary fibrosis
B. Myasthenia gravis
C. Acute asthma
D. Severe emphysema

72. Normal value for the ratio FEV_1/FVC is?
Harrison's 20th Ed. Chapter 279 Page 1949

A. 0.25 to 0.50
B. 0.50 to 0.75
C. 0.75 to 0.80
D. 0.80 to 1.00

73. During maximal inspiration from RV to TLC, inspiratory flow is most rapid at?
Harrison's 19th Ed. 306e-5

A. Beginning of inspiration
B. Midpoint of inspiration
C. Terminal point of inspiration
D. None of the above

During maximal inspiration from RV to TLC, inspiratory flow is most rapid at midpoint of inspiration.

74. Maximal inspiratory pressure (MIP) and maximal expiratory pressure (MEP) are useful in assessing?
Harrison's 20th Ed. Chapter 290 Page 2012

A. Strength of respiratory muscles
B. Lung recoil
C. Airway obstruction
D. All of the above

Strength of respiratory muscles is determined by estimating the maximal inspiratory pressure (MIP) and the maximal expiratory pressure (MEP).

75. Abnormality noted on routine testing of pulmonary function in early obstructive disease is?
Harrison's 19th Ed. 306e-5

A. Increased FEV1/VC
B. Depression in FEF25–75%
C. Coved early portion of flow-volume curve
D. All of the above

With early obstructive disease, FEV_1/VC may be normal. Only abnormalities noted may be depression in $FEF_{25-75\%}$ & coved terminal portion of forced expiratory flow-volume curve.

76. Which of the following is true in obstructive lung disease?
Harrison's 19th Ed. 306e-5

A. Decreased TLC
B. Ratio RV/TLC increased
C. Increased VC
D. None of the above

In obstructive disease, TLC is normal or increased, residual volume is elevated and RV/TLC is increased. VC is frequently decreased.

77. Which of the following is decreased in pulmonary parenchymal restrictive lung disease?
Harrison's 19th Ed. 306e-5

A. TLC
B. VC
C. RV
D. All of the above

In pulmonary parenchymal restrictive disease, total lung capacity (TLC), forced vital capacity (FVC), functional residual capacity (FRC) & residual volume (RV) are decreased. FEF rates are preserved.

78. Which of the following is decreased in neuromuscular weakness causing pulmonary extraparenchymal restrictive lung disease?
Harrison's 19th Ed. 306e-5

A. TLC
B. VC
C. MIP
D. All of the above

With extraparenchymal pulmonary disease due to neuromuscular disease (respiratory muscle weakness), TLC is decreased, RV is not significantly affected & MIP is decreased. Expiratory flow rates are preserved.

79. Helium dilution & body plethysmography are used for estimating?
Harrison's 20th Ed. Chapter 279 Page 1950

A. VC
B. ERV
C. IC
D. RV

80. Helium dilution & body plethysmography are used for estimating?
Harrison's 20th Ed. Chapter 279 Page 1950

A. VC
B. ERV
C. IC
D. TLC

81. Helium dilution & body plethysmography are used for estimating?

Harrison's 20th Ed. Chapter 279 Page 1950

A. VC
B. ERV
C. IC
D. FRC

Helium dilution and body plethysmography are used to measure RV, FRC & TLC.

82. Normal spirometry, normal lung volumes, and a low DL_{CO} suggests the diagnosis of?

Harrison's 20th Ed. Chapter 279 Page 1951

A. Myasthenia gravis
B. Pulmonary fibrosis
C. Pulmonary vascular disease
D. Emphysema

Isolated reduction in DL_{co} is the classic finding in PAH. Normal spirometry, normal lung volumes, and a low DLCO should prompt further evaluation for pulmonary vascular disease.

83. Normal mean pulmonary artery pressure is?

Harrison's 20th Ed. Chapter 252 Page 1768

A. 15 mm Hg
B. 18 mm Hg
C. 22 mm Hg
D. 28 mm Hg

Normal mean pulmonary artery pressure is 15 mm Hg, as compared to ~95 mm Hg for the normal mean aortic pressure.

84. In an upright person, pulmonary arterial pressure (PAP) is lowest at?

Am J Respir Crit Care Med. 2013;187(6):576–583

A. Apex of lung
B. Lung base
C. Right middle lobe
D. Apical segment of lower lobe

85. In an upright person, pulmonary arterial pressure (PAP) is highest at?

Am J Respir Crit Care Med. 2013;187(6):576–583

A. Apex of lung
B. Lung base
C. Right middle lobe
D. Apical segment of lower lobe

In an upright person, perfusion is least at apex of lung & greatest at base. Ventilation-perfusion ratios are higher at lung apices than at the lung bases.

86. In upright position, pulmonary perfusion is least at?

Am J Respir Crit Care Med. 2013;187(6):576–583

A. Apex
B. Lung base
C. Right middle lobe
D. Apical segment of lower lobe

87. Pulmonary vascular resistance (PVR) is calculated by?

Harrison's 20th Ed. Chapter 237 Page 1712

A. $PVR = 60(PAP_m - PCW)/CO$
B. $PVR = 70(PAP_m - PCW)/CO$
C. $PVR = 80(PAP_m - PCW)/CO$
D. $PVR = 90(PAP_m - PCW)/CO$

Pulmonary vascular resistance (PVR) = 80[Mean pulmonary arterial pressure (PAP_m) - pulmonary capillary wedge pressure (PCW)]/cardiac output (CO). PAP & PCW are measured directly ith flow-directed Swan-Ganz catheter in pulmonary artery. CO is obtained by thermodilution method.

88. Normal value for pulmonary vascular resistance is?

Harrison's 20th Ed. Chapter 237 Page 1712

A. 5 to 20 $dyn{\cdot}s/cm^5$
B. 20 to 150 $dyn{\cdot}s/cm^5$
C. 150 to 250 $dyn{\cdot}s/cm^5$
D. 250 to 500 $dyn{\cdot}s/cm^5$

Normal value for pulmonary vascular resistance is ~50–150 $dyn \cdot s/cm^5$.

89. Normally, O_2 & CO_2 diffusion equilibration is complete in what time of RBCs transit through pulmonary capillary bed?

BJA Education, 2016;16(10):341–348

A. 1/3
B. 1/2
C. 3/4
D. Throughout transit time

Normally, O_2 & CO_2 diffusion is rapid. Equilibration is complete within one-third of transit time of RBC's through pulmonary capillary bed.

90. Hemoglobin is almost fully (~90%) saturated at a PO_2 of?

BJA Education, 2016;16(10):341–348

A. 60 mm Hg
B. 70 mm Hg
C. 80 mm Hg
D. 90 mm Hg

Hemoglobin is almost fully (~90%) saturated at a P_{O2} of 60 mm Hg.

91. When fully saturated, each gram of hemoglobin is capable of carrying?

BJA Education, 2016;16(10):341–348

A. 0.34 mL of O_2
B. 1.34 mL of O_2
C. 2.34 mL of O_2
D. 3.34 mL of O_2

When fully saturated, each gram of Hb is capable of carrying 1.34 mL O_2

92. Amount of O_2 transported bound to hemoglobin is?

BJA Education, 2016;16(10):341–348

A. ~ 10 mL per deciliter of blood
B. ~ 20 mL per deciliter of blood
C. ~ 30 mL per deciliter of blood
D. ~ 40 mL per deciliter of blood

Amount of O_2 transported bound to hemoglobin is ~20 mL per deciliter of blood.

93. Amount of O_2 transported dissolved in plasma is?
BJA Education, 2016;16(10):341–348

A. ~ 0.3 mL O_2 per deciliter of blood
B. ~ 1.3 mL O_2 per deciliter of blood
C. ~ 2.3 mL O_2 per deciliter of blood
D. ~ 3.3 mL O_2 per deciliter of blood

Amount of O_2 transported dissolved in plasma is ~0.3 mL per deciliter of blood.

94. In mixed venous blood, the P_{O2} is normally about?
BJA Education, 2016;16(10):341–348

A. 40 mm Hg
B. 60 mm Hg
C. 80 mm Hg
D. 100 mm Hg

In mixed venous blood, the P_{O2} is normally ~40 mmHg

95. In a healthy young person breathing room air, the PA_{O2}–Pa_{O2} is normally?
BJA Education, 2016;16(10):341–348

A. < 15 mm Hg
B. < 30 mm Hg
C. < 45 mm Hg
D. < 60 mm Hg

In healthy person breathing room air, PA_{O2} – Pa_{O2} is normally <15 mmHg for subjects <=30 years and increases by ~3 mmHg per decade after age 30.

96. Pulse oximeter calculates O_2 saturation by measuring absorption of how many wavelengths of light?
Harrison's 20th Ed. Chapter 293 Page 2028

A. 2
B. 5
C. 8
D. 12

Pulse oximeter calculates O_2 saturation by measuring absorption of two wavelengths of light by oxygenated & nonoxygenated Hb. Percentage of Hb saturated with oxygen - Sa_{O2} is displayed.

97. Which of the following wavelengths are utilized in pulse oximetry?
Harrison's 20th Ed. Chapter 293 Page 2028

A. 460 nm and 740 nm
B. 560 nm and 840 nm
C. 660 nm and 940 nm
D. 760 nm and 1040 nm

Pulse oximetry works on the basis of differences in absorptive properties of oxygenated & deoxygenated hemoglobin. At wavelengths of 660 nm, oxyhemoglobin reflects light more effectively than does deoxyhemoglobin, whereas the reverse is true in infrared spectrum (940 nm). Pulse oximeter passes both wavelengths of light & relative intensity of light transmission at these two wavelengths is recorded. From this information, relative percentage of oxyhemoglobin is derived.

98. Specific relationship between Pa_{O2} & Sa_{O2} depends on?
BJA Education, 2016;16(10):341–348

A. Temperature
B. pH
C. Erythrocyte concentration of 2,3-diphosphoglycerate
D. All of the above

Arterial P_{O2} of 60 mm Hg corresponds to Sa_{O2} of 90%. Specific relationship between Pa_{O2} & Sa_{O2} depends on temperature, pH & RBC concentration of 2,3-DPG.

99. CO-oximeter can distinguish which of the following?
BJA Education, 2016;16(10):341–348

A. Oxyhemoglobin
B. Carboxyhemoglobin
C. Methemoglobin
D. All of the above

CO-oximeter uses at least four wavelengths of light and is capable of distinguishing oxyhemoglobin, deoxygenated hemoglobin, carboxyhemoglobin & methemoglobin.

100. What concentration of carbon monoxide is inhaled to assess DL_{CO}?
BJA Education, 2016;16(10):341–348

A. 0.3%
B. 0.5%
C. 0.75%
D. 0.1%

To assess the diffusing capacity of lung for carbon monoxide (DL_{CO}), 0.3% of carbon monoxide is inhaled in a single breath & held for ~10 seconds.

101. The hallmark of hypoventilation as a cause of hypoxemia is?
Harrison's 20th Ed. Chapter 290 Page 2011

A. Decrease in Pa_{CO2}
B. Elevation in Pa_{CO2}
C. Decrease in Pa_{O2}
D. Elevation in Pa_{O2}

Hallmark of hypoventilation as a cause of hypoxemia is an elevation in Pa_{CO2}.

102. Which of the following is rarely responsible for hypoxemia?
Harrison's 20th Ed. Chapter 279 Page 1948

A. Abnormalities in diffusion
B. Decrease in inspired P_{O2}
C. Hypoventilation
D. Shunting

Abnormalities in diffusion are rarely responsible for hypoxemia.

103. Disease associated with lowered DL_{CO} is?
Harrison's 20th Ed. Chapter 279 Page 1951

A. Interstitial lung disease
B. Emphysema
C. Pulmonary vascular disease
D. All of the above

Lowered DL_{CO} is found in interstitial lung disease, emphysema & pulmonary vascular disease.

104. Diffusing capacity (DL_{CO}) may be elevated in?
Harrison's 20th Ed. Chapter 279 Page 1951

A. Goodpasture syndrome
B. Interstitial lung disease
C. Emphysema
D. All of the above

Diffusing capacity may be elevated in congestive heart failure and in alveolar hemorrhage as in Goodpasture syndrome. Hb in RBCs in alveolar lumen binds CO leading to increased DL_{CO}.

105. For cyanosis to occur, hemoglobin concentration should be more than?

Harrison's 20th Ed. Chapter 36 Page 236

A. 3 gm%
B. 4 gm%
C. 5 gm%
D. 6 gm%

Cyanosis becomes apparent when the concentration of reduced hemoglobin in capillary blood exceeds 4 gm/dL. It is the absolute, rather than the relative, quantity of reduced hemoglobin that is important in producing cyanosis.

106. In peripheral cyanosis, the extremities are?

Harrison's 20th Ed. Chapter 36 Page 237

A. Hypothermic
B. Hyperthermic
C. Normothermic
D. Any of the above

107. In which condition, cyanosis does not occur?

Harrison's 20th Ed. Chapter 36 Page 236

A. Peripheral circulatory failure
B. Cyanotic congenital heart disease
C. Carbon monoxide poisoning
D. All of the above

108. Which of the following site is best for detecting central cyanosis?

Harrison's 20th Ed. Chapter 36 Page 236

A. Skin
B. Nails
C. Oral mucous membranes
D. Ear lobule

Examination of mucous membranes in oral cavity & conjunctivae rather than skin is more helpful in the detection of cyanosis.

109. Cyanosis usually becomes manifest at an altitude of?

Harrison's 20th Ed. Chapter 36 Page 236

A. 1000 meters
B. 2000 meters
C. 4000 meters
D. 6000 meters

Cyanosis usually becomes manifest at an altitude of 4000 meters (13,000 ft).

110. Which of the following comes first in clinical manifestation of Raynaud's phenomenon?

Harrison's 20th Ed. Chapter 36 Page 237

A. Blanching or pallor
B. Cyanosis
C. Rubor or erythema
D. Edema

Raynaud's phenomenon is characterized by episodic digital ischemia & a triphasic color response manifested clinically by sequential development of digital blanching (vasoconstriction), cyanosis (ischemia) & rubor (reperfusion) of fingers or toes following cold exposure & subsequent rewarming.

111. Which of the following is false about acrocyanosis?

Harrison's 20th Ed. Chapter 275 Page 1929

A. Episodic peripheral cyanosis of the hands
B. Cyanosis intensified by cold
C. Trophic skin changes & ulcerations do not occur
D. Normal pulses

In acrocyanosis, there is arterial vasoconstriction & secondary dilation of capillaries & venules with resulting persistent peripheral cyanosis of the hands & feet, intensified by cold exposure, normal pulses, moist palms, no trophic skin changes & ulcerations.

112. In frostbite, after rewarming, which of the following occurs?

Harrison's 20th Ed. Chapter 275 Page 1930

A. Cyanosis & erythema
B. Wheal-and-flare formation
C. Edema & superficial blisters
D. All of the above

In frostbite, after rewarming there is cyanosis & erythema, wheal-and-flare formation, edema, and superficial blisters.

113. Differential cyanosis in patent ductus arteriosus means?

Harrison's 20th Ed. Chapter 234 Page 1667

A. Cyanosis in fingers but not toes
B. Cyanosis in toes but not fingers
C. Cyanosis in lips & cheek but not fingers & toes
D. None of the above

In PDA with severe pulmonary vascular disease, reversal of flow through ductus results in shunting of unoxygenated blood to descending aorta. Toes, but not fingers become cyanotic and clubbed - differential cyanosis.

114. Which of the following is false about hemoptysis?

Harrison's 20th Ed. Chapter 35 Page 233

A. Bright red color
B. Alkaline pH
C. Massive hemoptysis is > 400 mL/day
D. None of the above

Massive hemoptysis is defined as >400 mL of blood produced in 24 hours or 100–150 mL expectorated at one time.

115. Hemoptysis can originate from disease of?

Harrison's 20th Ed. Chapter 35 Page 233

A. Airways
B. Pulmonary parenchyma
C. Pulmonary vasculature
D. All of the above

Hemoptysis can originate from disease of airways (acute or chronic bronchitis, bronchiectasis, cystic fibrosis, bronchogenic carcinoma or bronchial carcinoid tumors), pulmonary parenchyma (pneumonia, lung abscess, tuberculosis, Aspergillosis, Goodpasture's syndrome, idiopathic pulmonary hemosiderosis), or pulmonary vasculature (pulmonary thromboembolic disease, pulmonary arteriovenous malformations).

116. A dilated vessel in a pulmonary tuberculosis cavity is called?

Harrison's 20th Ed. Chapter 35 Page 233

A. Rasmussen's aneurysm
B. Bouchart's aneurysm
C. Charcot's aneurysm
D. Beyer's aneurysm

In pulmonary tuberculosis, massive hemoptysis may occur from rupture of a dilated vessel in a cavity (Rasmussen's aneurysm).

117. Kussmaul breathing is seen in?
Harrison's 20th Ed. Chapter 300 Page 2072

A. Metabolic acidosis
B. Hypoglycemia
C. Superior vena cava syndrome
D. Pneumothorax

118. Kussmaul breathing may also occur with?
Harrison's 20th Ed. Chapter 300 Page 2072

A. Bacterial meningitis
B. Pontomesencephalic lesions
C. Herpes zoster
D. All of the above

Kussmaul breathing is a rapid, deep usually implies metabolic acidosis but may also occur with pontomesencephalic lesions.

119. Which of the following statements about stridor is false?
Harrison's 20th Ed. Chapter 300 Page 2072

A. Occurs primarily during inspiration
B. Represents flow through a narrowed lower airway
C. Occurs in an infant with croup
D. Occurs in a patient with retropharyngeal growth

120. Radiographic "thumbprint sign" is seen in?
Harrison's 20th Ed. Chapter 31 Page 217

A. Laryngitis
B. Croup syndrome
C. Acute epiglottitis
D. All of the above

Neck radiographs in acute epiglottitis (supraglottitis) typically reveal an enlarged edematous epiglottis referred to as the thumbprint sign.

121. "Hot potato" voice is a feature of?
Harrison's 20th Ed. Chapter 31 Page 214

A. Oropharyngeal candidiasis (thrush)
B. Lemierre's disease
C. Vincent's angina
D. Ludwig's angina

Ludwig's angina is a rapidly progressive cellulitis of sublingual & submandibular spaces following infected or recently extracted tooth (lower II & III molars). Patients speak in a "hot potato" voice.

122. "Trench mouth" is related to?
Harrison's 20th Ed. Chapter 31 Page 214

A. Oropharyngeal candidiasis (thrush)
B. Lemierre's disease
C. Vincent's angina
D. Ludwig's angina

Vincent's angina (acute necrotizing ulcerative gingivitis or trench mouth) is a form of gingivitis characterized by painful, inflamed gingiva with ulcerations of interdental papillae that bleed easily.

123. Harrison's groove is characteristic of?
Pediatr Radiol. 2010;40(7):1184-9

A. Emphysema
B. Pneumothorax
C. Rickets
D. Pleural effusion

124. Tietze syndrome refers to painful swelling of?
Harrison's 20th Ed. Chapter 367 Page 2644

A. Ribs
B. Costochondral articulations
C. Intercostal muscles
D. All of the above

Tietze syndrome is manifested by painful swelling of one or more costochondral articulations, usually II or III costochondral joint presenting as anterior chest pain radiating to arms or shoulders, aggravated by sneezing, coughing, deep inspirations or twisting motions of chest.

125. Which of the following is false about costochondritis?
Harrison's 20th Ed. Chapter 367 Page 2644

A. Pain of costochondral articulations without swelling
B. Observed mostly in women over age 40 years
C. Affects III, IV and V costochondral joints
D. None of the above

Costochondritis is pain of costochondral articulations without swelling, observed mostly in women over age 40 years and tends to affect the III, IV and V costochondral joints.

126. Xiphoidalgia & slipping rib syndrome usually involve which rib?
Harrison's 20th Ed. Chapter 367 Page 2644

A. Second
B. Fifth
C. Seventh
D. Tenth

Xiphoidalgia & slipping rib syndrome usually involve the tenth rib.

127. Pectus carinatum is also called?
Harrison's 20th Ed. Chapter 234 Page 1667

A. Rachitic rosaries
B. Kyphoscoliosis
C. Pigeon-breast
D. Barrel chest

Pectus carinatum is also called Pigeon-breast. It is the reverse of pectus excavatum with the sternum protruding anteriorly. It is associated with congenital ASD or VSD & severe prolonged childhood asthma.

128. Which of the following is false about "Pectus excavatum"?
Harrison's 20th Ed. Chapter 234 Page 1667

A. Also called Funnel chest
B. Pulmonary function tests are nearly normal
C. Lower sternum commonly involved
D. None of the above

In Pectus excavatum, lower portion of sternum is displaced posteriorly and the anterior ribs are markedly bowed, which results in a depressed panel in the anterior chest. Respiratory symptoms are uncommon & pulmonary function tests are nearly normal.

129. Straight back syndrome occurs in patients with?
Harrison's 20th Ed. Chapter 234 Page 1667

A. Aortic stenosis (AS)
B. Aortic regurgitation (AR)
C. Hypertrophic obstructive cardiomyopathy (HOCM)
D. Mitral valve prolapse (MVP)

Straight back syndrome refers to loss of normal kyphosis of thoracic spine and occurs in patients with mitral valve prolapse (MVP) and its variants.

130. 'Sulfur granule pus' is seen in infection with?

Harrison's 20th Ed. Chapter 170 Page 1220

A. Tuberculosis
B. Mycoplasma
C. Actinomycosis
D. Hodgkin's disease

Sulfur granules are characteristic of actinomycosis.

131. Mondor's disease refers to?

J Med Case Rep. 2018;12:4

A. Subcutaneous anterior thoracic phlebitis
B. Herpes zoster infection of thoracic nerve roots
C. Angina inversa
D. Xiphoidalgia

132. Which of the following is false about Da Costa's syndrome?

Lancet 2001;358(9290):1376

A. Chronic anxiety
B. Often, pain occurs after excercise
C. Pain is usually left submammary
D. None of the above

133. Which of the following is false about Bornholm disease?

Harrison's 20th Ed. Chapter 199 Page 1470

A. Also called epidemic pleurodynia
B. Pain is like that of pleurisy
C. Due to Coxsackie B virus
D. None of the above

Pleurodynia presents with acute onset of fever & spasms of pleuritic chest or upper abdominal pain. Most cases are due to coxsackievirus B and occur during epidemics.

134. Hamman's sign is characteristic of?

Harrison's 20th Ed. Chapter 289 Page 2010

A. Diaphragmatic paralysis
B. Pneumomediastinum
C. Kyphoscoliosis
D. Tension pneumothorax

In pneumomediastinum, there is gas in the interstices of mediastinum. Subcutaneous emphysema in suprasternal notch and Hamman's sign (crunching or clicking noise synchronous with heartbeat & best heard in left lateral decubitus position) are characteristic features.

135. All of the following can cause diffuse nodular opacities in chest X-Ray except?

N Engl J Med 2005;353:2042-55

A. Metastatic neoplasm
B. Pneumoconiosis
C. Eosinophilic granuloma
D. Sarcoidosis

136. Specialized tissues that sense the local oxygen tension include all except?

N Engl J Med 2005;353:2042-55

A. Glomus cells of carotid body
B. Neuroepithelial bodies in lungs
C. Systemic veins
D. Chromaffin cells of fetal adrenal medulla

137. Specialized tissues that sense the local oxygen tension include all except?

N Engl J Med 2005;353:2042-55

A. Smooth-muscle cells of resistance pulmonary arteries
B. Hepatic vein
C. Fetoplacental arteries
D. Ductus arteriosus

138. Vasodilators produced by endothelium are all except?

N Engl J Med 2005;353:2042-55

A. Nitric oxide
B. Prostacyclin
C. Both of the above
D. None of the above

139. Vasoconstrictors produced by endothelium are all except?

N Engl J Med 2005;353:2042-55

A. Endothelin
B. Thromboxane A_2
C. Both of the above
D. None of the above

140. Angiotensin-converting enzyme (ACE) is present in?

N Engl J Med 2005;353:2042-55

A. Pulmonary vascular endothelium
B. Liver
C. Kidneys
D. Intestines

141. Which of the following is related to asterixis?

Harrison's 20th Ed. Chapter 428 Page 3138

A. Tic
B. Myoclonus
C. Chorea
D. Hemiballismus

Asterixis in hepatic failure is a negative myoclonus consisting of a brief loss of muscle activity.

142. Most specific sign of a metabolic encephalopathy is?

Harrison's 20th Ed. Chapter 300 Page 2071

A. Bilateral Asterixis
B. Confusion
C. Seizure
D. Vomiting

In a drowsy and confused patient, bilateral asterixis is a sign of metabolic encephalopathy or drug intoxication.

143. Asterixis can be found in?

Harrison's 20th Ed. Chapter 337 Page 2413

A. Any tonically held posture
B. Tonically held tongue
C. Voluntary limb motion
D. All of the above

Asthma

144. Which of the following statements about asthma is false?
Harrison's 20th Ed. Chapter 281 Page 1957

A. 10–12% adults and 15% children affected by asthma
B. Peak age of presentation is 3 years
C. Sex ratio in adults is equal
D. None of the above

In childhood asthma, male:female ratio is 2:1, but in adulthood the sex ratio is equalized.

145. Which of the following about asthma is false?
Harrison's 20th Ed. Chapter 281 Page 1957

A. Most patients with asthma in affluent countries are atopic
B. Severity of asthma varies significantly within a patient
C. Onset of asthma in adulthood rarely become permanently asymptomatic
D. Inflammatory disease of airways

Severity of asthma does not vary significantly within a given patient.

146. Asthma is a disease of?
Harrison's 20th Ed. Chapter 281 Page 1957

A. Large airway
B. Medium airway
C. Terminal bronchiole
D. Respiratory bronchiole

147. The term "atopy" in Greek means?
N Engl J Med 2001;344:30

A. Inert
B. Out of place
C. Explosive
D. Mischief

148. Allergic rhinitis is found in what percentage of asthmatic patients?
Harrison's 20th Ed. Chapter 281 Page 1957

A. ~ 40%
B. ~ 60%
C. ~ 80%
D. ~ 100%

Allergic rhinitis is found in over 80% of asthmatic patients.

149. Which of the following is false about difficult-to-treat asthma?
N Engl J Med 2017;377:965-76

A. That remains uncontrolled despite high-dose of inhaled glucocorticoids
B. That remains uncontrolled despite high-dose of other controllers
C. That requires high-dose of inhaled glucocorticoids to remain well controlled
D. None of the above

Difficult-to-treat asthma is asthma that remains uncontrolled despite treatment with high-dose inhaled glucocorticoids or other controllers, or that requires such treatment to remain well controlled. Severe asthma is a subset of difficult-to-control asthma; the term is used to describe patients with asthma that remains uncontrolled despite treatment with high-dose inhaled glucocorticoids combined with a long acting β2-agonist (LABA), a leukotriene modifier, or theophylline for the previous year or treatment with systemic glucocorticoids for at least half the previous year. The term is also used to describe asthma that requires such treatment in order to remain well controlled; it excludes patients in whom asthma is vastly improved with optimization of adherence, inhaler technique, and treatment of coexisting conditions. The criteria for uncontrolled asthma include exacerbations, poor symptom control, lung-function impairment, or a combination of these.

150. Which of the following is called 'house-dust mite'?
Harrison's 20th Ed. Chapter 281 Page 1957

A. Dermatophagoides pteronyssinus
B. Betula verrucosa
C. Phleum pratense
D. Ambrosia artemisiifolia

Dermatophagoides pteronyssinus is called house dust mite.

151. Atopy is due to the genetically determined production of?
Harrison's 20th Ed. Chapter 281 Page 1958

A. IgA antibody
B. IgE antibody
C. IgG antibody
D. IgM antibody

Atopy is due to the genetically determined production of specific IgE antibody

152. Which of the following statements about nonatopic or intrinsic asthma is false?
Harrison's 20th Ed. Chapter 281 Page 1958

A. Negative skin test to common inhalant allergens
B. Normal serum IgE levels
C. Have mild asthma
D. Commonly have nasal polyps

Patients with nonatopic or intrinsic asthma usually have more severe, later onset and persistent asthma.

153. Polymorphism of genes for which of the following is associated with atopy?
Harrison's 20th Ed. Chapter 281 Page 1958

A. IL-5
B. IL-9
C. IL-13
D. All of the above

Asthma is polygenic. Interaction of many genes is important and these may differ in different populations. The most consistent findings have been associations with polymorphisms of genes on chromosome 5q, including the T helper 2 (TH2) cells interleukin (IL)-4, IL-5, IL-9 and IL-13 which are associated with atopy.

154. Novel gene associated with asthma is?
Harrison's 20th Ed. Chapter 281 Page 1958

A. ADAM–33
B. DPP–10
C. ORMDL3
D. All of the above

Asthma is polygenic. Novel genes associated with asthma include ADAM–33, DPP–10 and ORMDL3.

155. ORMDL3 best relates to?

Harrison's 20th Ed. Chapter 281 Page 1958

A. Mitochondria
B. Golgi apparatus
C. Endoplasmic reticulum
D. All of the above

XBP1, ORMDL3, OCTN are genes that are associated with fundamental cell biologic processes such as endoplasmic reticulum (ER) and metabolic stress to regulate the secretory activity of cells.

156. Which of the following is strongly linked with asthma in genetic association studies?

Harrison's 20th Ed. Chapter 281 Page 1958

A. TNFAIP3
B. ORMDL3
C. PTPN2
D. IL23R

Asthma is caused by a combination of poorly understood genetic & environmental factors. Orosomucoid like 3 (ORMDL3) has been strongly linked with asthma in genetic association studies. ORMDL3 is a member of a gene family that encodes transmembrane proteins anchored in the endoplasmic reticulum and asthma patients have elevated expression levels of this gene.

157. Thunderstorm asthma is due to?

Harrison's 20th Ed. Chapter 281 Page 1959

A. Fungal spores
B. Domestic pets
C. Pollen grains
D. Cockroaches

Pollens cause allergic rhinitis rather than asthma. In thunderstorms, pollen grains are disrupted & particles that are released can trigger severe asthma exacerbations (thunderstorm asthma).

158. Which of the following upper respiratory tract virus is the most common trigger of acute severe asthma exacerbation?

Harrison's 20th Ed. Chapter 281 Page 1959

A. Rhinovirus
B. Respiratory syncytial virus
C. Coronavirus
D. All of the above

Rhinovirus, respiratory syncytial virus, and coronavirus are the most common triggers of acute severe asthma exacerbations.

159. Cough associated with angiotensin-converting enzyme inhibitors best relates to?

Harrison's 20th Ed. Chapter 281 Page 1959

A. Type I interferons
B. Kinins
C. Cysteinyl leukotrienes
D. All of the above

Angiotensin-converting enzyme inhibitors inhibit breakdown of kinins, which are bronchoconstrictors and produce the characteristic cough.

160. Severity of exercise induced asthma depends on?

Harrison's 20th Ed. Chapter 281 Page 1959

A. Level of ventilation achieved
B. Temperature of environment
C. Humidity of inspired air
D. All of the above

EIA is worse in cold, dry climates than in hot, humid conditions.

161. Which of the following is false about exercise induced asthma (EIA)?

Harrison's 20th Ed. Chapter 281 Page 1959

A. No long-term sequelae
B. Does not increase airway reactivity
C. Attacks follow exertion
D. None of the above

162. Which of the following is false about exercise induced asthma (EIA)?

Harrison's 20th Ed. Chapter 281 Page 1959

A. Begins after exercise has ended
B. Recovers spontaneously within ~30 minutes
C. Best prevented by inhaled glucocorticoids
D. None of the above

163. Which of the following may also be a trigger of asthma?

Harrison's 20th Ed. Chapter 281 Page 1959

A. Anger
B. Orgasm
C. Laughter
D. All of the above

Laughter may also be a trigger of asthma.

164. Patients with aspirin-induced asthma may benefit from?

Harrison's 20th Ed. Chapter 281 Page 1960

A. Salt free diet
B. Pepper free diet
C. Salicylate free diet
D. Sulphar free diet

Patients with aspirin-induced asthma may benefit from a salicylate-free diet.

165. After what length of time, aspirin-induced asthma develops after drug administration?

Harrison's 20th Ed. Chapter 281 Page 1960

A. Within 1 hour
B. Within 6 hours
C. Within 12 hours
D. Within 24 hours

Most NSAIDs, including aspirin, cause immediate, allergy-like symptoms in susceptible individuals. Urticaria/angioedema may be delayed up to 24 hours. The rhinosinusitis-asthma syndrome generally develops within 1 hour of drug administration.

166. Which of the following is supposedly protective for the occurrence of childhood-onset asthma?

Harrison's 20th Ed. Chapter 281 Page 1960

A. M. tuberculosis
B. Chlamydia trachomatis
C. H. pylori
D. All of the above

Recent studies have shown an inverse association of $cagA^+$ H. pylori with childhood-onset asthma, hay fever, and atopic disorders.

167. Infection with which of the following may be associated with a reduced risk of asthma?

Harrison's 20th Ed. Chapter 281 Page 1960

A. Mycoplasma
B. Chlamydophila
C. Hookworm
D. All of the above

Infection with hookworm may be associated with a reduced risk of asthma.

168. Which of the following diet is associated with an increased risk of asthma?

Harrison's 20th Ed. Chapter 281 Page 1960

A. Diet low in magnesium
B. Diet low in omega-3 polyunsaturated fats
C. Diet high in omega-6 polyunsaturated fats
D. All of the above

Diets low in vitamin C and vitamin A, magnesium, selenium and omega-3 polyunsaturated fats (fish oil) or high in sodium and omega-6 polyunsaturated fats are associated with an increased risk of asthma. Vitamin D deficiency may also predispose to the development of asthma.

169. Airway mucosa in asthma is infiltrated with?

Harrison's 20th Ed. Chapter 281 Page 1960

A. Activated eosinophils
B. T lymphocytes
C. Activated mucosal mast cells
D. All of the above

Autopsy results from patients of established asthma show airway mucosa infiltrated with activated eosinophils and T lymphocytes, and activation of mucosal mast cells. Degree of inflammation is poorly related to disease severity.

170. In asthma, characteristic histologic finding in airways is?

Harrison's 20th Ed. Chapter 281 Page 1960

A. Normal parenchymal attachments
B. Thickened airway smooth muscle
C. Goblet cell metaplasia
D. Thickening of basement membrane

In asthma, characteristic finding is thickening of basement membrane due to subepithelial types III and V collagen deposition.

171. Type 2 inflammation in airway is characterized by presence of which of the following cytokines?

N Engl J Med 2017;377:965-76

A. Interleukin–4
B. Interleukin–5
C. Interleukin–13
D. All of the above

Type 2 inflammation in respiratory airway is characterized by presence of interleukin-4, interleukin-5, and interleukin-13 cytokines produced by type 2 helper T (Th2) cells. Interleukin-4 and interleukin-5 promote the production of IgE and eosinophils, respectively. Most of the recently approved biologic interventions target type 2 inflammation.

172. Sputum eosinophilia, defined as what percentage of leukocytes in a sample?

N Engl J Med 2017;377:965-76

A. 2% or more
B. 3% or more
C. 4% or more
D. 5% or more

Sputum eosinophilia, defined as 2% or more of leukocytes in a sample.

173. Which of the following about thymic stromal lymphopoietin (TSLP) is false?

N Engl J Med 2017;377:965-76

A. Stimulates type 2 helper T (Th2) cells
B. Stimulates innate lymphoid cells of group 2 (ILC2)
C. Helps produce type 2 cytokines interleukin (IL) 4, IL-5 & IL-13
D. None of the above

Type 2 inflammation is initiated by adaptive immune system on recognition of allergens through the actions of thymic stromal lymphopoietin (TSLP). TSLP stimulates type 2 helper T (Th2) cells & innate lymphoid cells of group 2 (ILC2) to differentiate & produce type 2 cytokines interleukin (IL) 4, IL-5, and IL-13.

174. Type 2 cytokine interleukin production is best related to?

N Engl J Med 2017;377:965-76

A. GATA1 transcription factor
B. GATA2 transcription factor
C. GATA3 transcription factor
D. GATA4 transcription factor

Type 2 helper T (Th2) cells & innate lymphoid cells of group 2 (ILC2) differentiation depends on activation of the GATA3 transcription factor.

175. Cytokines result in the production of IgE through the action of?

N Engl J Med 2017;377:965-76

A. IL–4
B. IL–5
C. IL–13
D. All of the above

Cytokines result in the production of IgE through the action of IL-4 & subsequent activation of mast cells, which depend on stem cell factor & its receptor, KIT, for normal development and survival.

176. Activation and recruitment of eosinophils is through?

N Engl J Med 2017;377:965-76

A. IL–4
B. IL–5
C. IL–13
D. All of the above

Activation and recruitment of eosinophils is through IL-5.

177. Which of the following is an action of IL-13?

N Engl J Med 2017;377:965-76

A. Acts on smooth muscle to induce hyperresponsiveness & remodeling
B. Stimulates epithelium to increase cytokine production
C. Stimulates mucus production
D. All of the above

IL-13 acts on smooth muscle to induce hyperresponsiveness and remodeling; it also stimulates the epithelium to increase cytokine production and stimulates mucus production.

178. Prostaglandin D2 (PGD2) is synthesized by?
N Engl J Med 2017;377:965-76

A. Eosinophils
B. Mast cells
C. Neutrophils
D. All of the above

Mast cells synthesize prostaglandin D2 (PGD2), which stimulates upstream cells & eosinophils through its actions at the receptor known as CRTH2.

179. Which of the following produces non type 2 inflammation?
N Engl J Med 2017;377:965-76

A. Irritants
B. Pollutants
C, Microbes, viruses
D. All of the above

The type 2 pathway can be activated by infectious agents & irritants that stimulate innate immune system through production of cytokines like IL-33 (through its receptor ST2) & IL-25 (through its receptor IL-17RB), which in turn stimulate ILC2 and Th2 cells.

180. Which of the following have a role in down-regulating neutrophilic inflammation & antagonizing effects of leukotrienes?
N Engl J Med 2017;377:965-76

A. Hepoxilin
B. Lipoxin
C. Eoxins
D. All of the above

lipoxins is a synthesize pro-resolving compound, which down-regulates neutrophilic inflammation and antagonizes effects of leukotrienes.

181. Which of the following plays a major role in attracting and stimulating neutrophils?
N Engl J Med 2017;377:965-76

A. IL–4
B. IL–5
C. IL–13
D. IL–17

Type 17 helper T (Th17) cells and their products play a major role in attracting & stimulating neutrophils.

182. Which of the following is false about "Paucigranulocytic" asthma?
N Engl J Med 2017;377:965-76

A. No cellular evidence of activation
B. Poor cellular evidence of activation
C. Increased cellular evidence of activation
D. Any of the above

Some patients with severe asthma may not have cellular evidence of activation of the pathways and are considered to have "paucigranulocytic" asthma.

183. Which of the following is a peripheral biomarker of severe asthma?
N Engl J Med 2017;377:965-76

A. Blood eosinophil count
B. FeNO
C. IgE levels
D. All of the above

184. Which of the following is a marker of eosinophilic inflammation in the airway?
Harrison's 20th Ed. Chapter 281 Page 1960

A. Fragmented parenchymal attachments
B. Thickened airway smooth muscle
C. Goblet cell metaplasia
D. Thickening of basement membrane

In the pathology of asthma, a characteristic finding is thickening of basement membrane due to subepithelial collagen deposition. This feature is also found in eosinophilic bronchitis presenting as cough who do not have asthma. It is a marker of eosinophilic inflammation in airway as eosinophils release fibrogenic mediators.

185. Thickening of basement membrane in airway mucosa due to subepithelial collagen deposition is a feature of?
Harrison's 20th Ed. Chapter 281 Page 1960

A. Atopic asthma
B. Nonatopic asthma
C. Aspirin-sensitive asthma
D. All of the above

Pathology of asthma is remarkably uniform in different types of asthma, including atopic, nonatopic, occupational, aspirin-sensitive, and pediatric asthma.

186. Which of the following is a histopathologic feature of a small airway in fatal asthma?
Harrison's 20th Ed. Chapter 281 Page 1960 Figure 281-1

A. Goblet cell aplasia
B. Goblet cell dysplasia
C. Goblet cell metaplasia
D. Any of the above

Histopathologic feature in a small airway in fatal asthma include shed or friable epithelium, lumen occlusion with a mucous plug, goblet cell metaplasia, thickened airway wall due to subepithelial collagen deposition, increase in basement membrane thickness and airway smooth muscle, vasodilation and increased numbers of blood vessels (angiogenesis). Involvement of airways may be patchy.

187. Physiologic abnormality of asthma is?
Harrison's 20th Ed. Chapter 281 Page 1960

A. Increased physiological dead space
B. Increased anatomic dead space
C. Airway hyperresponsiveness (AHR)
D. All of the above

188. Mast cell is the key effector cell of the biologic response in?
Harrison's 20th Ed. Chapter 281 Page 1961

A. Allergic rhinitis
B. Urticaria
C. Anaphylaxis
D. All of the above

Mast cell is the key effector cell of the biologic response in allergic rhinitis, urticaria, anaphylaxis, and systemic mastocytosis.

189. In asthmatic patients, mast cells are localized to airway?
Harrison's 20th Ed. Chapter 281 Page 1961

A. Epithelial cells
B. Fibroblasts
C. Smooth muscle
D. Parenchyma

In asthmatic patients, mast cells are localized to airway smooth muscle layer.

190. Activated mast cells are found at the airway surface in?
Harrison's 20th Ed. Chapter 281 Page 1961

A. Asthma patients
B. Normal subjects
C. Patients with eosinophilic bronchitis
D. All of the above

Activated mast cells are found at the airway surface and also in the airway smooth-muscle layer in asthma patients, but not in normal subjects or patients with eosinophilic bronchitis.

191. Mast cells release which of the following bronchoconstrictor mediators?
Harrison's 20th Ed. Chapter 281 Page 1961

A. Histamine
B. Prostaglandin D2
C. Cysteinyl-leukotrienes
D. All of the above

Mast cells release bronchoconstrictor mediators like histamine, prostaglandin D_2, and cysteinyl-leukotrienes besides several cytokines, chemokines, growth factors, and neurotrophins.

192. Which of the following is an action of inflammatory mediators?
Harrison's 20th Ed. Chapter 281 Page 1961

A. Contract airway smooth muscle
B. Increase microvascular leakage
C. Increase airway mucus secretion
D. All of the above

Inflammatory mediators like histamine, prostaglandin D_2, and cysteinyl-leukotrienes contract airway smooth muscle, increase microvascular leakage, increase airway mucus secretion and attract other inflammatory cells.

193. In "sensitization", IgE gets attached to human mast cells and?
Harrison's 20th Ed. Chapter 281 Page 1961

A. Basophils
B. Eosinophils
C. Monocytes
D. Lymphocytes

The fixation of IgE to human mast cells and basophils, a process termed sensitization, prepares these cells for subsequent antigen-specific activation.

194. Which chain of FcεR1 is solely responsible for IgE binding?
Harrison's 20th Ed. Chapter 281 Page 1961

A. α chain
B. β chain
C. γ chain
D. All of the above

FcεR1 is composed of one α, one β, and two disulfide-linked γ chains, which together cross the plasma membrane seven times. The α chain is responsible for IgE binding, and the β and γ chains provide signal transduction.

195. Bronchial asthma is associated with increased levels of?
Harrison's 20th Ed. Chapter 281 Page 1961

A. Leukotrienes
B. PGI_1
C. PGI_2
D. Thromboxane

196. Mechanism by which aspirin produces bronchospasm is?
Harrison's 20th Ed. Chapter 281 Page 1961

A. Induction of Haptines
B. Chronic overexcretion of cysteinyl leukotrienes
C. Production of T cell derived cytokines
D. All of the above

Aspirin-sensitive asthma is a well defined subtype of asthma that is usually preceded by perennial rhinitis and nasal polyps in nonatopic patients with a late onset of the disease. Aspirin, even in small doses, characteristically provokes rhinorrhea, conjunctival irritation, facial flushing, and wheezing. There is a genetic predisposition to increased production of cysteinyl-leukotrienes with functional polymorphism of cys-leukotriene C synthase. Asthma is triggered by COX inhibitors, but is persistent even in their absence. All nonselective COX inhibitors should be avoided, but selective COX2 inhibitors are safe to use when an anti-inflammatory analgesic is needed. Aspirin-sensitive asthma responds to usual therapy with ICS. Although antileukotrienes should be effective in these patients, they are no more effective than in allergic asthma. Occasionally, aspirin desensitization is necessary, but this should only be undertaken in specialized centers.

197. Which of the following is a cysteinyl leukotriene?
N Engl J Med 2007;357:1841-54

A. LTC_4
B. LTD_4
C. LTE_4
D. All of the above

198. Cysteinyl leukotrienes were earlier known as?
N Engl J Med 2007;357:1841-54

A. Structural inflammatory cell
B. Slow-reacting substance of anaphylaxis
C. Crystal structure molecule
D. Exacerbation molecule

Cysteinyl leukotrienes C4, D4 & E4 were previously termed "slow-reacting substance of anaphylaxis".

199. "Trienes" in word leukotriene stand for?
N Engl J Med 2007;357:1841-54

A. Three conjugated double bonds
B. Three cysteinyl molecules
C. Three metabolic pathways
D. Three sulphar molecules

Leukotrienes ("leuko"-WBCs & "trienes"-3 conjugated double bonds) is a family of products of 5-lipoxygenase pathway of arachidonic acid metabolism. Capacity to form leukotrienes from arachidonate is confined to leukocytes.

200. Synthesis of leukotrienes from arachidonic acid is initiated by 5-lipoxygenase in concert with?
N Engl J Med 2007;357:1841-54

A. 5-lipoxygenase-activating protein (FLAP)
B. 5-lipoxygenase-associated protein (FLAP)
C. 5-lipoxygenase-augmenting protein (FLAP)
D. 5-lipoxygenase-assisted protein (FLAP)

Synthesis of leukotrienes from substrate arachidonic acid is initiated by 5-lipoxygenase enhanced by 5-lipoxygenase - activating protein (FLAP).

201. Products of 5-lipoxygenase pathway besides leukotrienes are?
N Engl J Med 2007;357:1841-54

A. 5-hydroxyeicosatetraenoic acid
B. 5-oxo-eicosatetraenoic acid
C. Lipoxins
D. All of the above

Products of the 5-lipoxygenase pathway besides leukotrienes are 5-hydroxyeicosatetraenoic acid, 5-oxo-eicosatetraenoic acid, and lipoxins.

202. FcεRI-α is intracellular in which of the following?
N Engl J Med 2001;344:30

A. Mast cells
B. Basophils
C. Eosinophils
D. All of the above

Fc portion of circulating IgE binds to high-affinity receptors (FcεRI) present on the surfaces of mast cells and basophils. Chemokines are involved in attracting inflammatory cells from the bronchial circulation into the airways. Eotaxin (CCL11) is selectively attractant to eosinophils via CCR3 and is expressed by epithelial cells of asthmatics, whereas CCL17 (TARC) and CCL22 (MDC) from epithelial cells attract T_H2 cells via CCR4.

203. Macrophages are derived from?
Harrison's 20th Ed. Chapter 281 Page 1961

A. Eosinophils
B. Basophils
C. Monocytes
D. Any of the above

Macrophages are derived from blood monocytes.

204. Dendritic cells are?
Harrison's 20th Ed. Chapter 281 Page 1961

A. Specialized eosinophil-like cells
B. Specialized basophil-like cells
C. Specialized macrophage-like cells
D. All of the above

Dendritic cells are specialized macrophage-like cells in airway epithelium, which are the major antigen-presenting cells.

205. Which of the following about macrophages is false?
Harrison's 20th Ed. Chapter 281 Page 1961

A. Activated by allergens
B. Initiate inflammatory response
C. Release anti-inflammatory mediators
D. None of the above

Macrophages are activated by allergens via low affinity IgE receptors (FcεRII). Macrophages initiate inflammatory response via release of certain cytokines. They also release anti-inflammatory mediators (IL-10).

206. In asthmatic patients, which of the following instructs dendritic cells to release chemokines that attract T_H2 cells into airways?
Harrison's 20th Ed. Chapter 281 Page 1961

A. IL-12
B. Tumor necrosis factor (TNF-α)
C. Thymic stromal lymphopoietin (TSLP)
D. All of the above

Dendritic cells take up allergens, process them to peptides, and migrate to local lymph nodes to present allergenic peptides to uncommitted T-lymphocytes for programming to allergen-specific T cells. Cytokine thymic stromal lymphopoietin (TSLP) released from epithelial cells in asthmatic patients instructs dendritic cells to release chemokines that attract T_H2 cells into airways.

207. Blocking antibodies to which of the following causes a profound and prolonged reduction in circulating and sputum eosinophils?
Harrison's 20th Ed. Chapter 281 Page 1961

A. Interleukin-2
B. Interleukin-4
C. Interleukin-5
D. Interleukin-13

Blocking antibodies to IL-5 causes a profound & prolonged reduction in circulating & sputum eosinophils, but is not associated with reduced AHR or asthma symptoms.

208. Which of the following is a feature of asthma with neutrophil predominance?
Harrison's 20th Ed. Chapter 281 Page 1961

A. Silent chest
B. Resistant to anti-inflammatory effects of corticosteroids
C. Frequent fungal infections
D. Acanthosis nigricans

209. Which of the following cells predominate in normal airways?
Harrison's 20th Ed. Chapter 281 Page 1961

A. T_H1
B. T_H2
C. T_H3
D. T_H4

210. Which of the following cells predominate in asthmatics?
Harrison's 20th Ed. Chapter 281 Page 1961

A. T_H1
B. T_H2
C. T_H3
D. T_H4

211. Which of the following leads to eosinophilic inflammation in asthmatics?
Harrison's 20th Ed. Chapter 281 Page 1961

A. IL–5
B. IL–4
C. IL–13
D. All of the above

The naïve immune system and immune system of asthmatics express T_H2 phenotype, whereas in normal airways T_H1 cells predominate. T_H2 cells, through the release of IL-5, are associated with eosinophilic inflammation and, through the release of IL-4 and IL-13, are associated with increased IgE formation.

212. Differentiation of Th1 cells depends on?
N Engl J Med 2002;346:857

A. Interleukin-12
B. Interleukin-4
C. Interferon-γ
D. All of the above

IL-10 & IL-12 are anti-inflammatory and may be deficient in asthma.

213. Differentiation of Th2 cells depends on?

N Engl J Med 2002;346:857

A. Interleukin-12
B. Interleukin-4
C. Interferon-γ
D. All of the above

214. Which of the following is not produced by Th2 cells?

N Engl J Med 2001;344:30

A. Interleukin-2
B. Interleukin-4
C. Interleukin-5
D. Interleukin-13

T_H2 cytokines IL-4, IL-5 & IL-13 mediate allergic inflammation, whereas proinflammatory cytokines tumor necrosis factor alpha and IL-1beta amplify the inflammatory response.

215. Which of the following in bronchial asthma is false?

N Engl J Med 2002;346:857

A. Interferon-γ from Th1 cells inhibits Th2 cells
B. Interleukin-4 from Th2 cells inhibits Th1 cells
C. Bronchial lymphocytes in asthma lack T-bet transcription factor
D. None of the above

216. Which of the following cytokines may be deficient in asthma?

Harrison's 20th Ed. Chapter 281 Page 1962

A. IL-4
B. IL-5
C. IL-12
D. IL-13

Cytokines IL-10 & IL-12 are anti-inflammatory and may be deficient in asthma.

217. Type 2 innate lymphoid cells (ILC2) are activated by?

Harrison's 20th Ed. Chapter 281 Page 1962 Figure 281-5

A. IL-5
B. IL-25, IL-33
C. CCL17, CCL22
D. Thymus stimulated lymphopoietin (TSLP)

Allergen interacts with dendritic cells and releases thymus stimulated lymphopoeitin (TSLP) which stimulates activated dendritic cells to release the chemokines CCL17 and CCL22, which attract T helper 2 (T_H2) lymphocytes. Allergens and viral infection may release interleukin (IL)-25 and -33, which recruit and activate type 2 innate lymphoid cells (ILC2). Both T_H2 and ILC2 cells release IL-5 and epithelial cells release CCL11 (eotaxim), which together lead to recruitment of eosinophils into the airways.

218. Stimulating factor for eosinophils is?

Harrison's 20th Ed. Chapter 281 Page 1962

A. Interleukin 3
B. Interleukin 4
C. Interleukin 5
D. Interleukin 8

Interleukin 5 stimulates the release of eosinophils into the circulation & extends their survival.

219. Which of the following is a T_H2 cytokine?

Harrison's 20th Ed. Chapter 281 Page 1962

A. IL-4
B. IL-5
C. IL-13
D. All of the above

T_H2 cytokines are IL-4, IL-5 and IL-13. They mediate allergic inflammation.

220. Which of the following is a proinflammatory cytokine?

Harrison's 20th Ed. Chapter 281 Page 1962

A. IL-1β
B. TSLP
C. IL-10
D. IL-12

221. Which of the following has a proinflammatory effect?

Harrison's 20th Ed. Chapter 281 Page 1962

A. IL-1β
B. TNF-α
C. Substance P
D. All of the above

Proinflammatory cytokines are TNF-α and IL-1β. They amplify the inflammatory response and play a role in more severe disease. Neurotransmitter - substance P have inflammatory effect.

222. Cytokine TSLP is released from?

Harrison's 20th Ed. Chapter 281 Page 1962

A. Dendritic cells
B. T_H2 cells
C. Epithelial cells
D. All of the above

TSLP is an upstream cytokine released from epithelial cells of asthmatics that orchestrates the release of chemokines that selectively attract T_H2 cells.

223. Which of the following is an anti-inflammatory cytokine?

Harrison's 20th Ed. Chapter 281 Page 1962

A. IL-8
B. IL-9
C. IL-10
D. IL-11

IL-10 and IL-12 are anti-inflammatory cytokines and may be deficient in asthma.

224. Which of the following is selectively attractant to eosinophils in asthmatics?

Harrison's 20th Ed. Chapter 281 Page 1962

A. Eotaxin
B. Chemotaxin
C. Bronchotaxin
D. Pulmotaxin

Chemokine Eotaxin (CCL11), expressed by epithelial cells of asthmatics, is attractant to eosinophils via CCR3, whereas CCL17 (TARC) and CCL22 (MDC) from epithelial cells attract T_H2 cells via CCR4.

225. Evidence for increased oxidative stress in asthma is provided by increased concentrations of which of the following in exhaled breath condensates?

Harrison's 20th Ed. Chapter 281 Page 1962

A. 6-isoprostane
B. 7-isoprostane
C. 8-isoprostane
D. 9-isoprostane

Evidence for increased oxidative stress in asthma is provided by increased concentrations of 8-isoprostane (product of oxidized arachidonic acid) in exhaled breath condensates and increased ethane (product of lipid peroxidation) in the expired air of asthmatic patients.

226. In airways, Nitric Oxide (NO) is produced mainly by?

Harrison's 20th Ed. Chapter 281 Page 1962

A. Epithelial cells
B. Fibroblasts
C. Smooth muscle
D. All of the above

Nitric oxide (NO) is produced by airway epithelial cells & macrophages in the airway by NO synthases. Its level in expired air of asthma patients is higher than normal due to eosinophilic inflammation.

227. Level of NO in expired air in asthma is related to?

Harrison's 20th Ed. Chapter 281 Page 1962

A. Bronchoconstriction
B. Mucus hypersecretion
C. Eosinophilic inflammation
D. Airway hyperresponsiveness (AHR)

Nitric oxide (NO) is produced particularly by airway epithelial cells and macrophages. Its level NO in expired air (Fractional exhaled NO or F_ENO) in asthmatics is higher than normal and is related to eosinophilic inflammation.

228. Which of the following favours Th2 phenotype?

Harrison's 20th Ed. Chapter 281 Page 1962

A. Transcription factor GATA-3
B. c-maf
C. Prostaglandin E2
D. All of the above

Proinflammatory transcription factors like nuclear factor κB & activator protein 1 (AP-1) are activated in asthmatic airways leading to expression of multiple inflammatory genes. Specific transcription factor GATA-3 regulates expression of T_H2 cytokines in T cells.

229. Which of the following contribute to the airway smooth muscle abnormality in asthma?

Harrison's 20th Ed. Chapter 281 Page 1963

A. Endothelin-1
B. Endothelin-2
C. Endothelin-3
D. Endothelin-4

In asthmatic airways there is a characteristic hypertrophy & hyperplasia of airway smooth muscle due to stimulation by growth factors such as platelet-derived growth factor (PDGF) or endothelin-1 released from inflammatory or epithelial cells. In vitro airway smooth muscle from asthmatic patients usually shows no increased responsiveness to constrictors.

230. Which of the following induces mucus hypersecretion in experimental models of asthma?

Harrison's 20th Ed. Chapter 281 Page 1963

A. IL-13
B. IL-14
C. IL-15
D. IL-16

IL-13 induces mucus hypersecretion in experimental models of asthma.

231. The characteristic structural change in asthma is?

Harrison's 20th Ed. Chapter 281 Page 1963

A. Fibrosis
B. Angiogenesis
C. Mucus hyperplasia
D. All of the above

The characteristic structural changes in asthma are increased airway smooth muscle, fibrosis, angiogenesis and mucus hyperplasia.

232. Airflow limitation is represented by?

Harrison's 20th Ed. Chapter 281 Page 1963

A. Reduced FEV_1
B. Reduced FEV_1/FVC ratio
C. Reduced peak expiratory flow (PEF)
D. All of the above

Airflow limitation is confirmed by reduced FEV_1, FEV_1/FVC ratio, and PEF.

233. Which of the following is false about asthma?

Harrison's 20th Ed. Chapter 281 Page 1963

A. Bronchial hyperemia
B. Ventilatory failure is very uncommon
C. Low PCO_2
D. None of the above

234. Which of the following does not trigger asthma via mast cell activation?

Harrison's 20th Ed. Chapter 281 Page 1963

A. Exercise
B. Hyperventilation
C. Fog
D. Irritant dusts

235. Sulfur dioxide triggers asthma symptoms by?

Harrison's 20th Ed. Chapter 281 Page 1963

A. Mast cell activation
B. Adrenergic reflex
C. Cholinergic reflex
D. All of the above

Most of the triggers for asthma symptoms act indirectly. Allergens, exercise, hyperventilation and fog via mast cell activation. Irritant dusts and sulfur dioxide via a cholinergic reflex. Direct bronchoconstrictors are histamine & methacholine.

Respiratory

236. The characteristic symptom of asthma is?
Harrison's 20th Ed. Chapter 281 Page 1963

A. Wheezing
B. Dyspnea
C. Coughing
D. All of the above

The characteristic symptoms of asthma are wheezing, dyspnea & coughing.

237. Prodromal symptom that may precede an asthma attack is?
Harrison's 20th Ed. Chapter 281 Page 1963

A. Itching under the axilla
B. Itching over epigastrium
C. Itching under the chin
D. Itching behind the ears

Prodromal symptoms that may precede an asthma attack are itching under the chin, discomfort between scapulae or inexplicable fear (impending doom).

238. Which of the following symptoms is considered 'sine qua non' for asthma?
Harrison's 20th Ed. Chapter 281 Page 1963

A. Dyspnea
B. Cough
C. Wheezing
D. All of the above

239. Which of the following is most common & characteristic feature of asthma?
Harrison's 20th Ed. Chapter 281 Page 1963

A. Cough
B. Nocturnal awakening with dyspnea and/or wheeze
C. Constriction feeling in chest
D. Perspiration

240. Bronchial reactivity reaches its peak around?

A. 3 AM
B. 6 AM
C. 12 Noon
D. 12 Midnight

241. Cough-variant asthma is seen in?
Harrison's 20th Ed. Chapter 281 Page 1963

A. Children
B. Adolescents
C. Adults
D. Elderly

Cough due to asthma in the absence of wheezing, shortness of breath, and chest tightness is referred to as "cough-variant asthma." Children particularly may present with a predominant nonproductive cough or cough-variant asthma that ties the onset of cough to typical triggers for asthma and resolution of cough upon withdrawal from exposure to them. Cough-variant asthma typically responds well to inhaled glucocorticoids and intermittent use of inhaled beta-agonist bronchodilators.

242. Reversibility of asthma is defined as an increase in FEV_1 15 minutes after inhaled short-acting $beta_2$-agonist of?
Harrison's 20th Ed. Chapter 281 Page 1963

A. > 12% or 50 mL
B. > 12% or 100 mL
C. > 12% or 150 mL
D. > 12% or 200 mL

Reversibility of asthma means a >12% or 200 mL increase in FEV_1 15 minutes after inhaled short-acting $beta_2$-agonist or, by a 2- to 4-week trial of oral glucocorticoids (prednisolone 30-40 mg daily).

243. In asthma, increased airway responsiveness (AHR) is measured by?
Harrison's 20th Ed. Chapter 281 Page 1963

A. Carbon dioxide
B. Nitric Oxide (NO)
C. Methacholine
D. All of the above

Increased airway responsiveness (AHR) is measured by methacholine or histamine challenge with calculation of provocative concentration that reduces FEV_1 by 20% (PC_{20}).

244. Aim of asthma therapy is to reduce peak expiratory flow (PEF) circadian variation to?
Harrison's 20th Ed. Chapter 281 Page 1964 Table 281-2

A. < 5%
B. < 10%
C. < 15%
D. < 20%

Aim of asthma therapy is to reduce PEF circadian variation to < 20%.

245. Which of the following test can be used to measure airway inflammation?
Harrison's 20th Ed. Chapter 281 Page 1964

A. Skin prick tests
B. Spirometry and flow-volume loop
C. Exhaled nitric oxide (F_ENO)
D. Serum IgE

F_ENO is used as a noninvasive test to measure airway inflammation, for compliance with therapy and demonstrating effectiveness of anti-inflammatory therapy with ICS.

246. Asthma is a feature of which of the following?
Harrison's 20th Ed. Chapter 281 Page 1964

A. Cogan's syndrome
B. Churg-strauss syndrome
C. Henoch-Schönlein purpura
D. All of the above

247. Which of the following may be associated with wheezing?
Harrison's 20th Ed. Chapter 281 Page 1964

A. Eosinophilic pneumonias
B. Polyarteritis nodosa
C. Churg-Strauss syndrome
D. All of the above

Eosinophilic pneumonias and systemic vasculitis, including Churg-Strauss syndrome and polyarteritis nodosa, may be associated with wheezing. Churg-Strauss syndrome (allergic angiitis & granulomatosis) is characterized by asthma, peripheral & tissue eosinophilia, extravascular granuloma formation, and vasculitis of multiple organ systems.

248. Asthma is related to which of the following?
Harrison's 20th Ed. Chapter 281 Page 1964

A. Atopic dermatitis (AD)
B. Allergic contact dermatitis (ACD)
C. Seborrheic Dermatitis
D. All of the above

Atopic dermatitis (AD) is the cutaneous expression of the atopic state, characterized by a family history of asthma, allergic rhinitis, or eczema. ~80% coexpress allergic rhinitis or asthma.

249. Asthma is a feature of which of the following?
Harrison's 20th Ed. Chapter 281 Page 1964

A. Zollinger-Ellison syndrome
B. Verner-Morrison syndrome
C. Carcinoid syndrome
D. All of the above

Apart from flushing, diarrhea & cardiac manifestations, wheezing or asthma-like symptoms (8–18%) and pellagra-like skin lesions (2–25%) are also seen.

250. Which of the following is not a bronchodilator drug?
Harrison's 20th Ed. Chapter 281 Page 1964

A. Beta2-adrenergic agonists
B. Anticholinergics
C. Inhaled corticosteroids (ICSs)
D. Theophylline

Three classes of bronchodilators are Beta$_2$-adrenergic agonists, anticholinergics & theophylline.

251. Major side effect of β_2 adrenergic agonists is?
Harrison's 20th Ed. Chapter 281 Page 1964

A. Tachycardia
B. Hyperglycemia
C. Tremors
D. Hypertension

252. Which of the following is related to beta$_2$-agonists?
Harrison's 20th Ed. Chapter 281 Page 1965

A. G protein
B. Adenylyl cyclase
C. Cyclic adenosine monophosphate (AMP)
D. All of the above

Beta$_2$-agonists activate beta$_2$-adrenergic receptors which are coupled through a stimulatory G protein to adenylyl cyclase, resulting in increased intracellular cyclic adenosine monophosphate (AMP), which relaxes smooth muscle cells.

253. Actions of Beta$_2$-agonists include all except?
Harrison's 20th Ed. Chapter 281 Page 1965

A. Reduction in airway hyperresponsiveness (AHR)
B. Inhibition of mast cell mediator release
C. Reduction in plasma exudation
D. Inhibition of sensory nerve activation

In contrast to corticosteroids, beta$_2$-agonist have no effects on inflammatory cells in airways and there is no reduction in AHR.

254. Which of the following is used in the prevention of EIA?
Harrison's 20th Ed. Chapter 281 Page 1965

A. Short-acting Beta2-agonists (SABAs)
B. Inhaled Corticosteroids (ICSs)
C. Cromolyn sodium
D. All of the above

255. Which of the following LABAs is given once daily?
Harrison's 20th Ed. Chapter 281 Page 1965

A. Salmeterol
B. Formoterol
C. Indacaterol
D. All of the above

Long-acting β2-agonists (LABAs) include salmeterol and formoterol, both of which have a duration of action over 12 hours and are given twice daily by inhalation. Indacaterol is given once daily.

256. MART stands for?
N Engl J Med 2017;377:965-76

A. Maintenance and radical therapy
B. Maintenance and rapid therapy
C. Maintenance and random therapy
D. Maintenance and quick-relief therapy

MART stands for maintenance and quick-relief therapy. It involves a low-dose inhaled glucocorticoid and formoterol as the patient's regular therapy and as quick-relief therapy.

257. Which of the following is false about asthma–COPD overlap?
N Engl J Med 2017;377:965-76

A. Severe asthma
B. Clinical features of both asthma and COPD
C. High morbidity
D. None of the above

Patients with severe asthma, especially those with a history of smoking, may have clinical features of both asthma and COPD (often called asthma–COPD overlap); these patients have high morbidity and a high rate of health care use.

258. Which of the following about beta$_2$-agonists is false?
Harrison's 20th Ed. Chapter 281 Page 1965

A. SABAs are useful in preventing EIA
B. LABAs should not be given without ICSs
C. Mast cell tolerance prevented by concomitant ICSs
D. None of the above

259. Non-bronchodilator effect of beta-2 agonists is?
Harrison's 20th Ed. Chapter 281 Page 1965

A. Inhibition of mast cell mediator release
B. Reduction in plasma exudation
C. Inhibition of sensory nerve activation
D. All of the above

Non-bronchodilator effects of beta-2 agonists are inhibition of mast cell mediator release, reduction in plasma exudation & inhibition of sensory nerve activation.

260. Which of the following about asthma treatment is false?
Harrison's 20th Ed. Chapter 281 Page 1965

A. Increased use of SABAs means asthma is not controlled
B. LABAs do not control underlying inflammation
C. LABAs should not be given without ICS therapy
D. None of the above

261. Which of the following is a bronchodilator?
Harrison's 20th Ed. Chapter 281 Page 1965

A. β_2-adrenergic agonists
B. Anticholinergics
C. Theophylline
D. All of the above

Three classes of bronchodilator are β_2-adrenergic agonists, anticholinergics & theophylline.

262. Theophylline activates which of the following?
Harrison's 20th Ed. Chapter 281 Page 1965

A. Growth factor - related receptor tyrosine kinase
B. Histone deacetylase-2
C. DNA methyltransferase
D. All-trans-retinoic acid (ATRA)

Theophylline activates key nuclear enzyme histone deacetylase-2, which is a critical mechanism for switching off activated inflammatory genes.

263. Nausea, vomiting & headaches produced by theophylline are due to?
Harrison's 20th Ed. Chapter 281 Page 1965

A. Adenosine receptor antagonism
B. Phosphodiesterase inhibition
C. Muscarinic receptor antagonis
D. All of the above

Nausea, vomiting & headaches produced by theophylline are due to phosphodiesterase inhibition.

264. Cardiac arrhythmias produced by theophylline is due to?
Harrison's 20th Ed. Chapter 281 Page 1965

A. Adenosine A1 receptor antagonism
B. Phosphodiesterase inhibition
C. Muscarinic receptor antagonis
D. All of the above

Theophylline side effects like cardiac arrhythmias & epileptic seizures occur due to adenosine A1 receptor antagonism.

265. Theophylline side effects are rare at plasma concentrations below?
Harrison's 20th Ed. Chapter 281 Page 1965

A. 10 mg/L
B. 20 mg/L
C. 30 mg/L
D. 40 mg/L

Theophylline side effects are rare at plasma concentrations <10 mg/L.

266. Therapeutic plasma concentration of theophylline is?
Harrison's 20th Ed. Chapter 281 Page 1965

A. 5–15 μg/mL
B. 20–40 μg/mL
C. 5–15 μg/mL
D. 20–40 μg/mL

267. Plasma concentrations of theophylline may be elevated by?
Harrison's 20th Ed. Chapter 281 Page 1966 Table 281-3

A. Erythromycin
B. Ciprofloxacin
C. Zafirlukast
D. All of the above

Theophylline is metabolized by CYP450 in liver. Its plasma concentrations may be elevated by drugs like erythromycin, allopurinol, cimetidine, ciprofloxacin, zileuton, zafirlukast.

268. All of the following drugs increase theophylline level except?
Harrison's 20th Ed. Chapter 281 Page 1966 Table 281-3

A. Rifampin
B. Erythromycin
C. Ciprofloxacin
D. Cimetidine

269. All of the following drugs increase theophylline level except?
Harrison's 20th Ed. Chapter 281 Page 1965

A. Allopurinol
B. Propranolol
C. Cephalosporins
D. Phenytoin

270. Which of the following does not belong to the controller therapy of asthma?
Harrison's 20th Ed. Chapter 281 Page 1965

A. Long-acting beta2-agonists (LABAs)
B. Inhaled corticosteroids (ICSs)
C. Cromolyn sodium
D. Antileukotrienes

Drugs for asthma are divided into bronchodilators & controllers. Bronchodilators provide rapid relief of symptoms through relaxation of airway smooth muscle, while controllers inhibit inflammatory process.

271. Which of the following is an action of corticosteroids in asthma?
Harrison's 20th Ed. Chapter 281 Page 1965

A. Inhibition of transcription factor NF-kB
B. Inhibition of transcription factor activator protein (AP)-1
C. Recruitment of histone deacetylase-2 (HDAC2) to inflammatory gene complex
D. All of the above

Corticosteroids also activate anti-inflammatory gene mitogen-activated protein (MAP) kinase phosphatase-1 and increase the expression of β2-receptors.

272. Metabolic & endocrine side effects of corticosteroids are mediated through?

Harrison's 20th Ed. Chapter 281 Page 1966

A. Anti-inflammatory proteins
B. Anti-inflammatory enzymes
C. Transcriptional activation
D. Adhesion molecules

Metabolic and endocrine side effects of corticosteroids are also mediated through transcriptional activation.

273. First-line therapy for patients with persistent asthma is?

Harrison's 20th Ed. Chapter 281 Page 1966

A. Long acting beta2-adrenergic agonists
B. Anticholinergics
C. Inhaled Corticosteroids (ICSs)
D. Theophylline

ICSs are the first-line therapy for persistent asthma. If symptoms are not controled, LABA is added.

274. Which of the following is a major problem in therapy with intramuscular triamcinolone acetonide?

Harrison's 20th Ed. Chapter 281 Page 1966

A. Osteoporosis
B. Depression
C. Cataracts
D. Proximal myopathy

Proximal myopathy is a major problem with intramuscular triamcinolone acetonide therapy.

275. In asthma, cysteinyl-leukotrienes are produced mainly by?

Harrison's 20th Ed. Chapter 281 Page 1966

A. Mast cells
B. Neutrophils
C. Macrophages
D. Basophils

Cysteinyl-leukotrienes are produced predominantly by mast cells in asthma.

276. Antileukotrienes (montelukast & zafirlukast) block which of the following?

Harrison's 20th Ed. Chapter 281 Page 1966

A. cys-LT_1-receptors
B. cys-LT_2-receptors
C. cys-LT_3-receptors
D. All of the above

Cysteinyl-leukotrienes are potent bronchoconstrictors, cause microvascular leakage, and increase eosinophilic inflammation through activation of cys-LT_1-receptors. Antileukotrienes (montelukast & zafirlukast) block cys-LT_1-receptors.

277. Which of the following medicine is used as steroid-sparing therapy?

Harrison's 20th Ed. Chapter 281 Page 1966

A. Methotrexate
B. Cyclosporin A
C. IV gamma globulin
D. All of the above

Immunomodulators have been used to reduce requirement for OCS in patients with severe asthma. Methotrexate, cyclosporin A, azathioprine, gold, and IV gamma globulin are used as steroid-sparing therapies, but none of these treatments has any long-term benefit and each is associated with a relatively high risk of side effects.

278. What proportion of inhaled corticosteroids by MDI goes to the lungs?

Harrison's 20th Ed. Chapter 281 Page 1966

A. 5–10%
B. 10–20%
C. 20–30%
D. 30–50%

279. Which of the following is an Anti-IgE antibody?

N Engl J Med 2017;377:965-76

A. Mepolizumab
B. Reslizumab
C. Omalizumab
D. All of the above

280. Which of the following about Omalizumab is false?

N Engl J Med 2017;377:965-76

A. It is a monoclonal antibody
B. Binds to free IgE
C. Prevents activation of mast cells, basophils & dendritic cells
D. None of the above

Omalizumab is a monoclonal antibody that binds to free IgE. It prevents activation of mast cells, basophils, & dendritic cells. It down-regulates the high-affinity receptor for the Fc region of IgE (FcεRI).

281. Which of the following binds to interleukin-5 receptor, producing eosinophil apoptosis?

N Engl J Med 2017;377:965-76

A. Mepolizumab
B. Reslizumab
C. Benralizumab
D. All of the above

Benralizumab binds to the interleukin-5 receptor, producing eosinophil apoptosis.

282. Which of the following block Interleukin-4 or Interleukin-13 signaling?

N Engl J Med 2017;377:965-76

A. Lebrikizumab
B. Tralokinumab
C. Dupilumab
D. All of the above

283. Which of the following is an anti-CRTH2 drug?

N Engl J Med 2017;377:965-76

A. Lebrikizumab
B. Tralokinumab
C. Dupilumab
D. Fevipiprant

Fevipiprant is an anti-CRTH2 oral pill. It blocks signaling at CRTH2 - the PGD2 receptor. CRTH2 denotes chemoattractant receptor homologue expressed by type 2 helper T cells.

284. Anti IgE monoclonal antibody used in bronchial asthma is?
Harrison's 20th Ed. Chapter 281 Page 1966, N Engl J Med 2006;354:2689-95

A. Mepolizumab
B. Omalizumab
C. Keliximab
D. Altrakincept

Humanized anti-IgE monoclonal antibody omalizumab blocks circulating IgE without binding to cell-bound IgE and inhibits IgE-mediated reactions. Approved for persistent allergic asthma not controlled by inhaled glucocorticoid therapy.

285. Omalizumab is given in bronchial asthma by which route?
Harrison's 20th Ed. Chapter 281 Page 1966, N Engl J Med 2006;354:2689-95

A. Subcutaneous
B. Intravenous
C. Intramuscular
D. Aerosol

Omalizumab is usually given as a subcutaneous injection every 2 - 4 weeks.

286. Which of the following about Omalizumab is false?
N Engl J Med 2006;354:2689-95

A. Recombinant humanized IgG1 monoclonal anti-IgE antibody
B. Not anaphylactogenic
C. Total serum IgE levels will increase during treatment
D. None of the above

Omalizumab is a recombinant humanized IgG1 monoclonal anti-IgE antibody that binds to IgE molecule at the same epitope on Fc that binds to FcεRI. It is not anaphylactogenic since it cannot interact with IgE that is already bound to cell surfaces and cannot induce degranulation of mast cells or basophils. Omalizumab binds to circulating IgE forming small, biologically inert IgE - anti-IgE complexes without activating complement cascade.

287. Omalizumab cannot be given if the total IgE is?
BMJ 2009;338:b494

A. > 100 IU/L
B. > 300 IU/L
C. > 500 IU/L
D. > 700 IU/L

Omalizumab cannot be given if the total IgE is >700 IU/L, which effectively excludes highly atopic patients. Recommended dose is 0.016 mg /per kg body weight per international unit of IgE every four weeks, administered subcutaneously at either two-week or four-week intervals. Dose is based on estimated amount of drug that is required to reduce circulating free IgE levels to <10 IU/mL.

288. Speleotherapy is best related to?
The European Journal of General Practice. 2019;25(2):1-12

A. Mountain
B. Lagoon
C. Cave
D. Iceberg

Speleotherapy comes from a Greek word meaning cave. Speleotherapy was first formulated by Polish physician F. Bochkowsky who noticed that salt miners had a very low incident of respiratory diseases.

289. How frequent use of a reliever medication indicates the need for regular controller therapy?
Harrison's 20th Ed. Chapter 281 Page 1967 Table 281-4

A. > once a week
B. > twice times a week
C. > thrice times a week
D. > four times a week

Use of a reliever medication > twice a week indicates need for regular controller therapy.

290. The mainstay of treatment in acute severe asthma is?
Harrison's 20th Ed. Chapter 281 Page 1968

A. High dose short-acting inhaled $beta_2$-agonists
B. High dose inhaled corticosteroids (ICSs)
C. Intravenous $beta_2$-agonists
D. Intravenous corticosteroids

The mainstay of treatment is high doses of short-acting inhaled $Beta_2$-agonists.

291. Treatment of choice in severely ill asthma patients with impending respiratory failure is?
Harrison's 20th Ed. Chapter 281 Page 1968

A. High dose short-acting inhaled $beta_2$-agonists
B. High dose inhaled corticosteroids (ICSs)
C. Intravenous $beta_2$-agonists
D. Intravenous corticosteroids

In severely ill patients with impending respiratory failure, intravenous $Beta_2$-agonists may be given.

292. Which of the following have a role in acute severe asthma patients who are refractory to inhaled therapies?
Harrison's 20th Ed. Chapter 281 Page 1968

A. Magnesium sulfate
B. Halothane
C. Aminophylline
D. All of the above

293. Which of the following is a nonstandard bronchodilator?
Harrison's 20th Ed. Chapter 281 Page 1968

A. Magnesium sulfate
B. Methotrexate
C. Gold salts
D. Colchicine

294. Refractory asthma is defined as difficult to control asthma despite?
Harrison's 20th Ed. Chapter 281 Page 1968

A. Maximal inhaled therapy
B. Maximal inhaled + oral therapy
C. Maximal inhaled + oral + IV therapy
D. All of the above

Approximately 5% of asthmatics are difficult to control despite maximal inhaled therapy.

295. The most common reason for poor control of asthma is?
Harrison's 20th Ed. Chapter 281 Page 1968

A. Continued exposure to allergens
B. Use of cyclooxygenase (COX) inhibitors
C. Noncompliance with medication
D. Gastroesophageal reflux

Most common reason for poor control of asthma is noncompliance with medication (ICS).

296. Premenstrual worsening of asthma is treated by?

Harrison's 20th Ed. Chapter 281 Page 1968

A. Corticosteroids
B. Progesterone
C. Oestrogen
D. Anticholinergics

Severe premenstrual worsening of asthma, unresponsive to corticosteroids requires treatment with progesterone or gonadotropin-releasing factors.

297. Corticosteroid resistant asthma is defined as failure to respond to what dose & duration of oral prednisolone?

Harrison's 20th Ed. Chapter 281 Page 1968

A. 40 mg OD for 2 weeks
B. 60 mg OD for 2 weeks
C. 80 mg OD for 2 weeks
D. 100 mg OD for 2 weeks

Corticosteroid resistant asthma is defined as failure to respond to 40 mg OD for 2 weeks of oral prednisolone.

298. Mechanism of corticosteroid resistant asthma may be?

Harrison's 20th Ed. Chapter 281 Page 1968

A. Excess of transcription factor AP-1
B. Increase in glucocorticoid receptor (GR)-β
C. Reduction in histone deacetylase activity
D. All of the above

Mechanism of corticosteroid resistant asthma may be excess of transcription factor AP-1, increase in glucocorticoid receptor-β, abnormal pattern of histone acetylation in response to corticosteroids, defect in IL-10 production and reduction in histone deacetylase activity.

299. Oral and intravenous administration produces the same effect in case of?

Harrison's 20th Ed. Chapter 281 Page 1968

A. Methylprednisolone
B. Prednisolone
C. Prednisone
D. Hydrocortisone

300. The most potent anti-inflammatory agent available for bronchial asthma is?

Harrison's 20th Ed. Chapter 281 Page 1968

A. Glucocorticoids
B. Nedocromil
C. Ketotifen
D. Zafirlucast

301. Treatment of choice in type 2 brittle asthma is?

Harrison's 20th Ed. Chapter 281 Page 1968

A. Oral corticosteroids
B. Continuous infusion of beta$_2$-agonists
C. Continuous infusion of corticosteroids
D. Subcutaneous epinephrine

Type I brittle asthma-chaotic variations in lung function despite appropriate therapy. Some show a persistent pattern of variability and may require oral corticosteroids or, at times, continuous infusion of Beta$_2$-agonists. Type II brittle asthma—normal or near-normal lung function but precipitous, unpredictable falls in lung function that may result in death, do not respond well to corticosteroids and inhaled bronchodilators, most effective therapy is subcutaneous epinephrine.

302. Which of the following therapy is not effective in severe asthma?

Harrison's 20th Ed. Chapter 281 Page 1968

A. Anti TNF therapy
B. Omalizumab
C. Infusions of β2-agonists
D. Low doses of theophylline

303. Aspirin sensitive asthma is associated with?

Harrison's 20th Ed. Chapter 281 Page 1968

A. Extrinsic asthma
B. Urticaria
C. Nasal polyp
D. Obesity

Aspirin-sensitive asthma is a well-defined subtype of late onset asthma that is preceded by perennial rhinitis & nasal polyps in nonatopic patients.

304. Which of the following happens in aspirin sensitive asthma?

Harrison's 20th Ed. Chapter 281 Page 1969

A. Rhinorrhea
B. Conjunctival injection
C. Facial flushing
D. All of the above

Aspirin characteristically provokes rhinorrhea, conjunctival injection, facial flushing and wheezing.

305. Functional polymorphism of which of the following is observed in aspirin sensitive asthma?

Harrison's 20th Ed. Chapter 281 Page 1969

A. cys-leukotriene C1 synthase
B. cys-leukotriene C2 synthase
C. cys-leukotriene C3 synthase
D. cys-leukotriene C4 synthase

306. Drugs for asthma that are safe and without teratogenic potential include all except?

Harrison's 20th Ed. Chapter 281 Page 1969

A. Short-acting beta$_2$-agonists
B. Long-acting beta$_2$-agonists
C. ICSs
D. Theophylline

Drugs for asthma that are safe and without teratogenic potential include SABAs, ICSs & theophylline. There is less safety information about LABAs, antileukotrienes & anti-IgE.

307. Which of the following about asthma and pregnancy is false?

Harrison's 20th Ed. Chapter 281 Page 1969

A. ~ one-third improve during pregnancy
B. ~ one-third deteriorate during pregnancy
C. ~ one-third remain unchanged during pregnancy
D. None of the above

~ one-third of asthmatic patients who are pregnant improve during the course of a pregnancy, one-third deteriorate, and one-third are unchanged.

308. Early onset bronchial asthma is associated with all except?
Harrison's 20th Ed. Chapter 281 Page 1969

A. Rhinitis
B. Family history of urticaria
C. Personal history of eczema
D. Normal levels of IgE in serum

309. Heightened airway responsiveness in bronchial asthma can be demonstrated by the use of?
Harrison's 20th Ed. Chapter 281 Page 1969

A. Histamine
B. Methacholine
C. Isocapnic hyperventilation of cold air
D. All of the above

310. When sleep disruption is a prominent side effect of asthma treatment, which drug is preferred?
Harrison's 20th Ed. Chapter 281 Page 1969

A. Theophylline sustained release preparations
B. Inhaled beclomethasone
C. Inhaled Adrenergic agonists
D. Oral glucocorticoids

Prominent daily variation in airway resistance in asthmatics results in marked increases in asthmatic symptoms at night, especially during sleep. Treatment with theophylline, adrenergic agonists or glucocorticoids can independently disrupt sleep. When sleep disruption is a side effect of asthma treatment, inhaled glucocorticoids (beclomethasone) that do not disrupt sleep may be useful.

311. Most successful means of bronchial asthma management is?
Harrison's 20th Ed. Chapter 281 Page 1969

A. Glucocorticoids
B. Glucocorticoids + β_2 agonists
C. Desensitization/Immunotherapy
D. Elimination of provocative agent

312. Bronchial asthma occuring in women at specific predictable time during menstrual cycle is called?
Clin Surg. 2019; 4: 2516

A. Functional asthma
B. Periodic asthma
C. Mittelschmerz asthma
D. Catamenial asthma

313. All are "quick relief medications" for bronchial asthma except?
Am J Respir Crit Care Med 2019; 199, P7-P8

A. β adrenergic agonists
B. Methylxanthines
C. Anticholinergics
D. Glucocorticoids

"Quick relief medications" for bronchial asthma are β-adrenergic agonists, methylxanthines and anticholinergics.

314. All are "long-term control medications" for bronchial asthma except?
Am Fam Physician. 2016;94(6):454-462

A. Glucocorticoids
B. All β adrenergic agonists
C. Mast cell stabilizing agents
D. Leukotriene modifiers

"Long-term control medications" for bronchial asthma are glucocorticoids, long-acting β2-agonists, combined medications, mast cell stabilizing agents, leukotriene modifiers and methylxanthines.

315. In patients of bronchial asthma with coexistent heart disease, which of the following drugs is preferred?
Am Fam Physician. 2016;94(6):454-462

A. Anticholinergic drugs
B. Methylxanthines
C. β adrenergic stimulants
D. None of the above

316. Which of the traditional medicine was used in the treatment of asthma?
Harrison's 20th Ed. Chapter 469 Page 3465

A. Ginkgo biloba
B. Ma huang
C. Hypericum perforatum
D. All of the above

Ephedra sinica, or ma huang, a product used in traditional Chinese medicine was used for short-term treatment of asthma and bronchial congestion.

317. Which of the following promotes histamine release from tissue mast cells & may worsen bronchospasm in patients with asthma?
Harrison's 20th Ed. Chapter 295 Page 2035

A. Ketamine
B. Morphine
C. Fentanyl
D. Propofol

Morphine can promote histamine release from tissue mast cells and may worsen bronchospasm in patients with asthma.

318. The 5-lipoxygenase inhibitor used in asthma is?
Oxidative Medicine and Cellular Longevity 2019

A. Bupropion
B. Zolpidem
C. Zileuton
D. Zafirlucast

319. "Balance oxygen" used for treatment of severe airway obstruction is?
Crit Care. 2001; 5(4): 179–181

A. 70–80% Hydrogen
B. 70–80% Nitrogen
C. 70–80% Oxygen
D. 70–80% Helium

Treatment with 70 to 80% helium (balance oxygen) may be beneficial in severe airway obstruction.

320. Intranasal glucocorticoids include?

Harrison's 20th Ed. Chapter 281 Page 1969

A. Fluticasone furoate
B. Ciclesonide
C. Mometasone furoate
D. All of the above

Intranasal glucocorticoids include beclomethasone, flunisolide, triamcinolone, budesonide, fluticasone propionate, fluticasone furoate, ciclesonide and mometasone furoate.

321. Which is a "Soft steroid" used in bronchial asthma?

Pulm Pharmacol Ther. 2003;16(6):321-5

A. Budesonide
B. Flunisolide
C. Ciclesonide
D. Dexamethasone

322. Potassium channel opener used in bronchial asthma is?

The Journal of Headache and Pain 2017;18:90

A. Levcromakalim
B. Nicorandil
C. Minoxidil
D. All of the above

323. Renal Natriuretic Peptide (ANP) analogue used in bronchial asthma is?

Clin Sci (Lond). 2016; 130(2): 57–77

A. Urodilatin
B. Nesiritide
C. Ariflo
D. Roflumilast

324. Phosphodiesterase inhibitors used in bronchial asthma are all except?

Harrison's 20th Ed. Chapter 286 Page 1997

A. Ariflo
B. Roflumilast
C. Urodilatin
D. Cilostazol

325. Monoclonal antibody to IL-5 is?

Harrison's 20th Ed. Chapter 106 Page 1967

A. Mepolizumab
B. Omalizumab
C. Keliximab
D. Altrakincept

IL-5 is the dominant eosinophil growth factor and can be specifically inhibited with the monoclonal antibody mepolizumab. Mepolizumab & reslizumab blocks IL-5, benralizumab blocks its receptor.

326. Which of the following is a monoclonal antibody directed against alpha subunit of interleukin-4 receptor?

N Engl J Med 2018;378:2533

A. Mepolizumab
B. Reslizumab
C. Dupilumab
D. Benralizumab

Dupilumab is a monoclonal antibody directed against alpha subunit of interleukin-4 receptor that inhibits interleukin-4 & interleukin-13 signaling. It has a salutary treatment effect in severe asthma. Mepolizumab & reslizumab are directed against interleukin-5, whereas benralizumab is directed against interleukin-5 receptor.

327. Which of the following targets the CD52 antigen?

Harrison's 20th Ed. Chapter 138 Page 1032

A. Alemtuzumab
B. Adalimumab
C. Certolizumab
D. Etanercept

Alemtuzumab targets CD52 antigen, which is expressed by eosinophils but not by neutrophils.

328. Which of the following statements is false?

Harrison's 20th Ed. Chapter 106 Page 1967

A. IL-5 is a survival factor for eosinophils
B. IL-5 is the dominant eosinophil growth factor
C. Mepolizumab is an anti-IL-5 agent
D. None of the above

329. Anti CD 4 monoclonal antibody used in bronchial asthma is?

BMJ 2009;338:b494

A. Mepolizumab
B. Omalizumab
C. Gomilumab
D. Altrakincept

Gomilumab is a humanised monoclonal antibody against tumour necrosis factor.

330. Immunomodulators used in bronchial asthma are?

Allergy Asthma Immunol Res. 2010; 2(4): 228–234

A. Mycophenolate mofetil
B. Leflunomide
C. Brequinar sodium
D. All of the above

331. Which oral β agonist is administered once daily in bronchial asthma?

Allergy Asthma Immunol Res. 2010; 2(4): 228–234

A. Albuterol
B. Bambuterol
C. Formoterol
D. Salmeterol

332. Pneumococcal polysaccharide (PPSV) vaccination is indicated for patients with?

Harrison's 20th Ed. Chapter 141 Page 1071

A. Severe asthma
B. Nephrotic syndrome
C. Cirrhosis
D. All of the above

Pneumococcal polysaccharide (PPSV) vaccination is indicated for patients with chronic lung disease (including asthma), chronic cardiovascular diseases, diabetes mellitus, chronic liver diseases; cirrhosis, chronic alcoholism, sickle cell disease, splenectomy, chronic renal failure, nephrotic syndrome) and cochlear implants and cerebrospinal fluid leaks.

333. Flushing is a feature of which of the following?

Harrison's 20th Ed. Chapter 80 Page 605

A. Systemic mastocytosis
B. Chronic myeloid leukemia
C. Menopause
D. All of the above

Flushing occurs in systemic mastocytosis, chronic myeloid leukemia with increased histamine release, menopause, reactions to alcohol or glutamate, side effects of chlorpropamide, calcium channel blockers, and nicotinic acid. None of these conditions cause increased urinary 5-HIAA.

334. Creola bodies are made up of?

Pediatr Allergy Immunol. 2004;15(2):159-62

A. Airway epithelium
B. Airway smooth muscle
C. Thick and stringy mucus
D. All of the above

Airway epithelium which is sloughed into bronchial lumen appears in the form of Creola bodies.

335. Curschmann's spirals in sputum is seen in?

Pediatr Allergy Immunol. 2004;15(2):159-62

A. Tubercular cavity
B. Bronchial Asthma
C. Bronchiectasis
D. All of the above

336. At necropsy, in a case of acute asthma, feature not found is?

Pediatr Allergy Immunol. 2004;15(2):159-62

A. Gross overdistension of lungs
B. Failure of lungs to collapse when pleural cavities are opened
C. Gelatinous plugs of exudate in terminal bronchioles
D. Destructive emphysema

Most conspicuous feature of lungs of asthma patients at necropsy is their gross overdistension, failure to collapse when pleural cavities are opened and numerous gelatinous plugs of exudate in most of the bronchial branches down to the terminal bronchioles.

337. In acutely ill asthmatic patient, residual volume is about?

Am J Respir Crit Care Med 2003;168:740–759

A. 100% of normal
B. 250% of normal
C. 300% of normal
D. 400% of normal

In acutely ill asthmatic patients, residual volume approaches 400% of normal, while functional residual capacity doubles.

338. Which of the following is found during acute exacerbation of asthma?

Am J Respir Crit Care Med 2003;168:740–759

A. Hypoxia
B. Hypocapnia
C. Respiratory alkalosis
D. All of the above

339. Ominous finding during acute exacerbation of asthma is?

Am J Respir Crit Care Med 2003;168:740–759

A. Normal arterial carbon dioxide tension
B. Metabolic acidosis
C. Cyanosis
D. All of the above

340. Which of the following indicate severe and prolonged bronchial obstruction in asthma?

Am J Respir Crit Care Med 2003;168:740–759

A. High pitched wheezing
B. Visibly active accessory muscles of respiration
C. Paradoxical pulse
D. All of the above

341. All of the following have relation with severity of asthma except?

Am J Respir Crit Care Med 2003;168:740–759

A. Respiratory rate
B. Pulsus paradoxus
C. Inability to speak
D. Use of accessory muscles of respiration

Hypersensitivity Pneumonitis and Pulmonary Infiltrates with Eosinophilia

342. Hypersensitivity pneumonitis (HP) is also called?
Harrison's 20th Ed. Chapter 282 Page 1970

A. Extrinsic allergic alveolitis
B. Intrinsic allergic alveolitis
C. Immunologic alveolitis
D. Decaying alveolitis

Hypersensitivity pneumonitis (HP) is also called extrinsic allergic alveolitis. Eosinophilia is not a feature of HP.

343. Hypersensitivity pneumonitis (HP) is also called?
Harrison's 20th Ed. Chapter 282 Page 1970

A. Gardener's lung
B. Mountain lung
C. Farmer's lung
D. Pollen lung

Term "Farmer's lung" is used for HP due to inhalation of antigens present in moldy hay, such as thermophilic actinomyces, Micropolyspora faeni, and Aspergillus species.

344. Hot tub lung best related to?
Harrison's 20th Ed. Chapter 282 Page 1970

A. Molds in air conditioners or humidifiers
B. Isocyanates
C. Mycobacterium avium complex
D. Cigarette smoking

Hot tub lung refers to a hypersensitivity reaction to Mycobacterium avium complex, which is present in hot tubs or whirlpools and is differentiated from actual infection.

345. The clinical presentation of HP can be?
Harrison's 20th Ed. Chapter 282 Page 1971

A. Acute
B. Subacute
C. Chronic
D. Any of the above

The clinical presentation of HP can be acute, subacute, or chronic.

346. In acute HP, symptoms occur within how many hours after exposure to antigen?
Harrison's 20th Ed. Chapter 282 Page 1971

A. 4 to 8 hours
B. 12 to 24 hours
C. 24 to 48 hours
D. 48 to 72 hours

In acute HP, symptoms (cough, fever, chills, malaise, dyspnea) occur 4 to 8 hours after exposure to antigen and usually clear within a few days if there is no further exposure to antigen.

347. Which of the following is false about acute hypersensitivity pneumonitis (HP)?
Harrison's 20th Ed. Chapter 282 Page 1971

A. Neutrophilia
B. Eosinophilia
C. Lymphopenia
D. Presence of rheumatoid factor

Following acute exposure to antigen, neutrophilia & lymphopenia are present. Eosinophilia is not a feature. Raised ESR, C-reactive protein, rheumatoid factor, and serum immunoglobulins also occur.

348. Which of the following can be found in BAL of HP patients?
Harrison's 20th Ed. Chapter 282 Page 1971

A. Lymphocytosis
B. CD4+/CD8+ lymphocyte ratio < 1
C. Bronchoalveolar mastocytosis
D. All of the above

BAL in HP patients shows marked lymphocytic alveolitis, alveolar neutrophilia in acute cases and bronchoalveolar mastocytosis.

349. Which of the following is false in lung biopsy of HP patients?
Harrison's 20th Ed. Chapter 282 Page 1971

A. Mononuclear bronchiolitis
B. Interstitial infiltrates of lymphocytes & plasma cells
C. Necrotizing granulomas
D. Thickened interstitium

Granulomas in HP are noncaseating in the vicinity of small airways and nonnecrotizing.

350. The most important tool in diagnosing HP is?
Harrison's 20th Ed. Chapter 282 Page 1971

A. Pulmonary function tests
B. Radiographic tests
C. BAL
D. High index of suspicion

Most important tool in diagnosing HP is high index of suspicion.

351. Strongest predictor among clinical prediction rule for HP is?
Harrison's 20th Ed. Chapter 282 Page 1971

A. Exposure to an antigen known to cause HP
B. Presence of serum precipitins
C. Symptoms occurring 4-8 hours after antigen exposure
D. Recurrent symptoms

Clinical prediction rule for predicting the presence of HP includes six statistically significant predictors, the strongest of which is exposure to an antigen known to cause HP. Other predictive criteria were the presence of serum precipitins, recurrent symptoms, symptoms occurring 4-8 hours after antigen exposure, crackles on inspiration and weight loss.

352. Which of the following is included in the differential diagnosis of HP?
Harrison's 20th Ed. Chapter 282 Page 1971

A. IPF
B. Nonspecific interstitial pneumonitis (NSIP)
C. Sarcoidosis
D. All of the above

353. Which of the following about organic dust toxic syndrome is false?

Harrison's 20th Ed. Chapter 282 Page 1972

A. More common than HP
B. Follows heavy exposure to organic dusts
C. Transient fever & muscle aches
D. None of the above

354. Which of the following about organic dust toxic syndrome is false?

Harrison's 20th Ed. Chapter 282 Page 1972

A. Serum precipitins are absent
B. Chest X-ray is usually normal
C. Self-limited disorder without long-term sequelae
D. None of the above

Organic dust toxic syndrome (ODTS) is more common than HP. It follows heavy exposure to organic dusts. Transient fever & muscle aches, with or without dyspnea & cough occur. Serum precipitins are absent, CxR is normal. ODTS is a self-limited disorder without significant long-term sequelae.

355. Which of the following is not a feature of acute eosinophilic pneumonia?

Harrison's 20th Ed. Chapter 282 Page 1972

A. Acute respiratory failure
B. Peripheral eosinophilia
C. Pulmonary eosinophilia
D. Diffuse pulmonary infiltrates

Acute eosinophilic pneumonia is a syndrome characterized by fevers, acute respiratory failure that often requires mechanical ventilation, diffuse pulmonary infiltrates and pulmonary eosinophilia in a previously healthy individual. In contrast to other pulmonary eosinophilic syndromes, acute eosinophilic pneumonia is often not associated with peripheral eosinophilia upon presentation. However, between 7 and 30 days of disease onset, peripheral eosinophilia often occurs with mean eosinophil counts of 1700.

356. Which of the following is false about acute eosinophilic pneumonia?

Harrison's 20th Ed. Chapter 282 Page 1972

A. Multisystem organ failure absent
B. > 25% eosinophilia on BAL fluid
C. IgE levels are normal
D. HRCT is always abnormal

Erythrocyte sedimentation rate, C-reactive protein and IgE levels are high.

357. Which of the following is false about acute eosinophilic pneumonia?

Harrison's 20th Ed. Chapter 282 Page 1972

A. Affects males with no history of asthma
B. High degree of corticosteroid responsiveness
C. Excellent prognosis
D. None of the above

In acute eosinophilic pneumonia, complete clinical and radiographic recovery without recurrence or residual sequelae occurs in almost all patients within several weeks of initiation of therapy.

358. Which of the following is seen in HRCT of HP patients?

Harrison's 20th Ed. Chapter 282 Page 1972

A. Abnormality is bilateral
B. Patchy ground-glass or reticular opacities
C. Pleural effusions
D. All of the above

HRCT is always abnormal with bilateral random patchy ground-glass or reticular opacities and small pleural effusions in as many as two-thirds of patients. Pleural fluid is characterized by a high pH with marked eosinophilia.

359. Which of the following is false about chronic eosinophilic pneumonia?

Harrison's 20th Ed. Chapter 282 Page 1973

A. Affects females
B. Majority of patients have asthma
C. Eosinophilia in both tissue and blood
D. None of the above

360. "Photographic negative pulmonary edema" appearance on chest X-ray and chest CT is pathognomonic of?

Harrison's 20th Ed. Chapter 282 Page 1973

A. Acute eosinophilic pneumonia
B. Chronic eosinophilic pneumonia
C. Eosinophilic granulomatosis with polyangiitis (EGPA)
D. Allergic bronchopulmonary aspergillosis (ABPA)

361. Which of the following is false about chronic eosinophilic pneumonia?

Harrison's 20th Ed. Chapter 282 Page 1973

A. Peripheral eosinophilia (> 30%of TLC)
B. BAL eosinophil count ~ 60%
C. Nonrespiratory manifestations are common
D. Relapse common following treatment

Unlike EGPA or hypereosinophilic syndrome, nonrespiratory manifestations (arthralgias, neuropathy, skin lesions and GI symptoms) are uncommon.

362. Besides lung, which other organ is involved in allergic angiitis granulomatosis or Churg-Strauss syndrome?

Harrison's 20th Ed. Chapter 282 Page 1973

A. Skin
B. Kidney
C. Nervous system
D. All of the above

In eosinophilic granulomatosis with polyangiitis (EGPA), previously known as allergic angiitis granulomatosis or Churg-Strauss syndrome, lungs, heart, skin, GI tract and nervous system are involved.

363. Which of the following is false about eosinophilic granulomatosis with polyangiitis (EGPA)?

Harrison's 20th Ed. Chapter 282 Page 1974

A. Asthma
B. Eosinophilic vasculitis
C. Involvement of multiple end organs
D. None of the above

364. The primary feature of EGPA is?

Harrison's 20th Ed. Chapter 282 Page 1974

A. Neuropathy
B. Paranasal sinus abnormality
C. Asthma
D. All of the above

The primary features of EGPA include asthma, peripheral eosinophilia, neuropathy, pulmonary infiltrates, paranasal sinus abnormality and presence of eosinophilic vasculitis.

365. Prodromal phase of EGPA is characterized by?
Harrison's 20th Ed. Chapter 282 Page 1974

A. Asthma
B. Fever
C. Weight loss
D. Fatigue

366. Neurologic manifestation of EGPA is?
Harrison's 20th Ed. Chapter 282 Page 1974

A. Mononeuritis multiplex (mostly of peroneal nerve)
B. Cerebral hemorrhage
C. Cerebral infarction
D. All of the above

367. Which of the following is a primary target organ in EGPA?
Harrison's 20th Ed. Chapter 282 Page 1974

A. Heart
B. Skin
C. GI tract
D. Nervous system

The heart is a primary target organ in EGPA and cardiac involvement has a worse prognosis.

368. Which of the following is elevated in EGPA?
Harrison's 20th Ed. Chapter 282 Page 1974

A. Systemic eosinophils
B. ANCAs
C. IgE
D. All of the above

369. Which of the following is a chest X-ray abnormality in EGPA?
Harrison's 20th Ed. Chapter 282 Page 1974

A. Bilateral, nonsegmental patchy infiltrates
B. Reticulonodular and nodular disease without cavitation
C. Pleural effusions
D. All of the above

Chest X-ray abnormalities are extremely common in EGPA and consist of bilateral, nonsegmental, patchy infiltrates that may migrate and may be interstitial or alveolar in appearance. Reticulonodular and nodular disease without cavitation, pleural effusions and hilar adenopathy.

370. The most common CT finding in EGPA is?
Harrison's 20th Ed. Chapter 282 Page 1974

A. Airspace consolidation
B. Hyperinflation
C. Interlobular septal thickening
D. Lymph node enlargement

The most common CT findings include bilateral ground-glass opacity and airspace consolidation that is predominantly subpleural. Other CT findings include bronchial wall thickening, hyperinflation, interlobular septal thickening, lymph node enlargement and pericardial and pleural effusions.

371. Which of the following does not have a role in the treatment of EGPA?
Harrison's 20th Ed. Chapter 282 Page 1974

A. Cyclophosphamide
B. Intravenous gamma globulin
C. Interferon α
D. Plasma exchange

372. In diagnosis of hypereosinophilic syndrome (HES), eosinophil count should be over?
Harrison's 20th Ed. Chapter 282 Page 1975

A. 500/μL of peripheral blood with end organ damage
B. 1000/μL of peripheral blood with end organ damage
C. 1250/μL of peripheral blood with end organ damage
D. 1500/μL of peripheral blood with end organ damage

Hypereosinophilic syndrome (HES) is characterized by persistent presence of >1500 eosinophils per microliter of peripheral blood with end organ damage or dysfunction and with no secondary cause of eosinophilia.

373. Which of the following variant of HES is responsive to imatinib?
Harrison's 20th Ed. Chapter 282 Page 1975

A. Chronic eosinophilic leukemia
B. PDGFRα-associated HES
C. FIP1-negative variant associated with clonal eosinophilia
D. All of the above

374. In hypereosinophilic syndrome, the cardiac abnormality is?
Harrison's 20th Ed. Chapter 282 Page 1975

A. Tricuspid valve abnormalities
B. Endomyocardial fibrosis
C. Restrictive, biventricular cardiomyopathy
D. All of the above

375. Which of the following is false about HES?
Harrison's 20th Ed. Chapter 282 Page 1975

A. High levels of blood, BAL and tissue eosinophilia
B. Elevated IgE
C. Ground-glass lung opacities on HRCT
D. None of the above

HES are typically not associated with ANCA or elevated IgE.

376. Tropical eosinophilia is usually caused by?
Harrison's 20th Ed. Chapter 282 Page 1975

A. Wuchereria bancrofti
B. Ascaris
C. Ancylostoma
D. Strongyloides stercoralis

Tropical eosinophilia is caused by filarial infection (Wuchereria bancrofti or W. malayi). It is treated successfully with diethylcarbamazine. Eosinophilic pneumonias also occur with Ascaris, Ancyclostoma sp., Toxocara sp. & Strongyloides stercoralis.

377. Drug-induced eosinophilic pneumonias can be caused by?
Harrison's 20th Ed. Chapter 282 Page 1975

A. Nitrofurantoin
B. Sulfonamides
C. Penicillin
D. All of the above

378. Drug-induced eosinophilic pneumonias can be caused by?

Harrison's 20th Ed. Chapter 282 Page 1975

A. Thiazides
B. Tricyclic antidepressants
C. Isoniazid
D. All of the above

Drug-induced eosinophilic pneumonias can be caused by nitrofurantoin, sulfonamides, penicillin, chlorpropamide, thiazides, tricyclic antidepressants, hydralazine, gold salts, isoniazid, indomethacin.

379. BAL fluid of normal nonsmoker individual, percentage of eosinophils is?

N Engl J Med 2009;360:1870-84

A. < 2%
B. < 4%
C. < 6%
D. < 8%

BAL fluid of normal nonsmoker individual, percentage of eosinophils is less than 2%.

380. Most common route of entry of aspergillus spores is?

N Engl J Med 2009;360:1870-84

A. Inhalation
B. Ingestion
C. Urinary tract
D. Skin

Invasive aspergillosis principally involves sinopulmonary tract. Inhalation is the most common route of entry of aspergillus spores.

381. Invasive aspergillosis of lung tissue is found in?

N Engl J Med 2009;360:1870-84

A. Granulocyte count in peripheral blood of <500/uL
B. Treatment with supraphysiologic doses of glucocorticoids
C. History of treatment with cytotoxic drugs
D. All of the above

382. Aspergillus infection in a neutropenic patient is characterized by?

N Engl J Med 2009;360:1870-84

A. Hyphal invasion of blood vessels
B. Thrombosis, necrosis
C. Hemorrhagic infarction
D. All of the above

383. Term allergic bronchopulmonary aspergillosis (ABPA) denotes the condition of patients with preexisting asthma who have?

N Engl J Med 2009;360:1870-84

A. Eosinophilia
B. IgE antibody to Aspergillus
C. Fleeting pulmonary infiltrates from bronchial plugging
D. All of the above

Main diagnostic criteria of Allergic Bronchopulmonary Aspergillosis (ABPA) include bronchial asthma, pulmonary infiltrates, peripheral eosinophilia (>1000/μL), immediate wheal-and-flare response to A fumigatus, serum precipitins to A. fumigatus, elevated serum IgE and central bronchiectasis.

384. Endobronchial saprophytic pulmonary aspergillosis presents in a patient with prior?

N Engl J Med 2009;360:1870-84

A. Pulmonary tuberculosis
B. Sarcoidosis
C. Histoplasmosis
D. All of the above

385. In allergic bronchopulmonary aspergillosis (ABPA), fleeting eosinophilic infiltrates involve which lobes of lung?

N Engl J Med 2009;360:1870-84

A. Upper lobes
B. Middle lobes
C. Lower lobes
D. Any of the above

In ABPA, fleeting eosinophilic infiltrates typically involve upper lobes of lungs.

386. The earliest CT finding in invasive aspergillosis is?

N Engl J Med 2009;360:1870-84

A. Pulmonary nodules
B. Pulmonary infiltrate
C. Pleural effusion
D. Pneumothorax

387. Halo sign & crescent sign are radiological findings in?

N Engl J Med 2009;360:1870-84

A. Invasive aspergillosis of the lung
B. Bronchiectasis
C. Bronchogenic carcinoma
D. Atelectasis

Earliest radiologic sign of invasive aspergillosis is a nodule. "Halo sign" is defined as a macronodule surrounded by a perimeter of ground-glass opacity corresponding to alveolar hemorrhage.

388. Detection of galactomannan antigen in serum suggests the diagnosis of?

N Engl J Med 2009;360:1870-84

A. Invasive aspergillosis of the lung
B. Bronchiectasis
C. Bronchogenic carcinoma
D. Atelectasis

Antigen-based diagnosis relies on serum detection of either galactomannan or beta-D-glucan, two constituents of fungal-cell walls.

389. Which of the following can give false positive results for galactomannan antigen?

N Engl J Med 2009;360:1870-84

A. Concomitant use of piperacillin–tazobactam antibiotic
B. Concomitant use of beta-lactam antibiotic
C. Gluconate containing IV fluids
D. All of the above

False positive results for galactomannan antigen are due to concomitant use of piperacillin–tazobactam, other beta-lactam antibiotics, and gluconate containing IV fluids.

390. Drug of choice as primary therapy for invasive aspergillosis is?
N Engl J Med 2009;360:1870-84

A. Posaconazole
B. Itraconazole
C. Voriconazole
D. Amphotericin B

Drug of choice as primary therapy for invasive aspergillosis is Voriconazole. 6 mg/kg IV BD for 2 doses, then 4 mg/kg BD as initial therapy. Oral therapy for adults - 200 mg BD or 4 mg/kg BD.

391. Which of the following is an "Echinocandin"?
N Engl J Med 2009;360:1870-84

A. Caspofungin
B. Micafungin
C. Anidulafungin
D. All of the above

Fungal beta-glucans are ubiquitous cell-wall constituents of fungi and trigger inflammatory responses in macrophages through their exposure on surface of germinating aspergillus conidia. Dectin-1 and TLR2 recognize distinct beta-glucan motifs and stimulate proinflammatory cytokine production. Echinocandins are antifungal agents acting on the cell wall by inhibiting beta-glucan synthesis.

392. Drugs for treatment of aspergillosis include?
N Engl J Med 2009;360:1870-84

A. IV amphotericin B
B. Liposomal amphotericin B
C. Itraconazole
D. All of the above

393. Drugs for treatment of aspergillosis include?
N Engl J Med 2009;360:1870-84

A. Intravenous voriconazole
B. Intravenous caspofungin
C. Itraconazole
D. All of the above

394. Which of the following is not effective in treatment of aspergillosis?
N Engl J Med 2009;360:1870-84

A. Fluconazole
B. Voriconazole
C. Caspofungin
D. Itraconazole

Fluconazole is not effective for the treatment of aspergillosis.

395. Triad of presentation of disseminated candidiasis includes all except?
Harrison's 20th Ed. Chapter 16 Page 114

A. Fever
B. Thrush
C. Myalgias
D. Eruptive nodules

Disseminated candidiasis (often due to Candida tropicalis) may have a triad of fever, myalgias and eruptive nodules.

396. Which of the following conditions presents with exquisitely tender nodules on lower extremities?
Harrison's 20th Ed. Chapter 16 Page 114

A. Aspergillosis
B. Erythema nodosum
C. Sweet syndrome
D. All of the above

397. Invasive infection occurs with those species of Aspergillus that grow at?
Harrison's 20th Ed. Chapter 212 Page 1532

A. 34°C
B. 35°C
C. 36°C
D. 37°C

Only those Aspergillus species that grow at 37°C can cause invasive infection.

398. Which of the following causes most cases of invasive aspergillosis?
Harrison's 20th Ed. Chapter 212 Page 1532

A. A. fumigatus
B. A. flavus
C. A. jumigatus
D. A. niger

A. fumigatus is responsible for most cases of invasive aspergillosis, almost all cases of chronic aspergillosis and most allergic syndromes.

399. Risk factor for invasive aspergillosis is?
Harrison's 20th Ed. Chapter 212 Page 1533

A. Neutropenia
B. Glucocorticoid use
C. Neutrophil and/or phagocyte dysfunction
D. All of the above

400. Which of the following drugs carries an increased risk of invasive aspergillosis?
Harrison's 20th Ed. Chapter 212 Page 1533

A. Infliximab
B. Adalimumab
C. Rituximab
D. All of the above

Therapy with infliximab, adalimumab, alemtuzumab, daclizumab, rituximab and possibly bevacizumab therapy also carries an increased risk of invasive aspergillosis and also severe liver disease and high levels of stored iron in bone marrow.

401. Underlying pulmonary disease in patients with chronic pulmonary aspergillosis is?
Harrison's 20th Ed. Chapter 212 Page 1533

A. Tuberculosis
B. Prior pneumothorax
C. Chronic obstructive pulmonary disease
D. All of the above

Patients with chronic pulmonary aspergillosis have a wide spectrum of underlying pulmonary disease, including tuberculosis, atypical mycobacterial infection, sarcoidosis, rheumatoid lung disease, prior pneumothorax, chronic obstructive pulmonary disease or lung surgery.

402. Most cases of invasive aspergillosis involve?
Harrison's 20th Ed. Chapter 212 Page 1533

A. Lungs
B. Maxillary sinus
C. Bronchial airways
D. External ear

More than 80% of cases of invasive aspergillosis involve the lungs. Sinuses are involved in 5 - 10% of cases of invasive aspergillosis.

403. Which of the following is most typical in acute cerebral aspergillosis?
Harrison's 20th Ed. Chapter 212 Page 1534

A. Cerebral abscess
B. Hemorrhagic infarction
C. Meningitis
D. Mycotic aneurysm

Hematogenous dissemination to the brain is a devastating complication of invasive aspergillosis. In acute disease, hemorrhagic infarction is most typical and cerebral abscess is common. Rarer manifestations include meningitis, mycotic aneurysm, and cerebral granuloma.

404. Chronic cavitary pulmonary aspergillosis is also called?
Harrison's 20th Ed. Chapter 212 Page 1534

A. Chronic necrotizing aspergillosis
B. Complex aspergilloma
C. Semi-invasive aspergillosis
D. Any of the above

Chronic cavitary pulmonary aspergillosis is also called semi-invasive aspergillosis, chronic necrotizing aspergillosis, or complex aspergilloma.

405. Which of the following is typical of cavitary pulmonary aspergillosis?
Harrison's 20th Ed. Chapter 212 Page 1534

A. Subpleural nodules
B. Bullae
C. Pericavitary infiltrates
D. Atelectasis

Cavities may have a fluid level or a well-formed fungal ball, but pericavitary infiltrates and multiple cavities, with or without pleural thickening, are typical. An irregular internal cavity surface and thickened cavity walls are indicative of disease activity. Radiologic features of invasive pulmonary aspergillosis include nodules and pleural-based infarction or cavitation, with pleural fluid apparent in 10% of patients. Chest CT may reveal a characteristic halo consisting of a mass-like infiltrate surrounded by an area of low attenuation. The presence of a "crescent sign" on chest X-ray or chest CT, in which the mass progresses to central cavitation is characteristic of invasive Aspergillus infection but may develop as the lesions are resolving. The earliest radiologic sign of invasive aspergillosis is a nodule. A "halo sign," defined as a macronodule surrounded by a perimeter of ground-glass opacity corresponding to alveolar hemorrhage, is suggestive of invasive aspergillosis in patients with compatible host factors.

406. In diabetic patients, vast majority of fungal balls are caused by?
Harrison's 20th Ed. Chapter 212 Page 1534

A. A. fumigatus
B. A. flavus
C. A. jumigatus
D. A. niger

The vast majority of fungal balls are caused by A. fumigates, but A. niger has been implicated, particularly in diabetic patients; aspergillomas due to A. niger can lead to oxalosis with renal dysfunction.

407. The most significant complication of aspergilloma (fungal ball) is?
Harrison's 20th Ed. Chapter 212 Page 1534

A. Wheezing
B. Weight loss
C. Nondescript chest discomfort
D. Hemoptysis

The most significant complication of aspergilloma is life-threatening hemoptysis, which may be the presenting manifestation. Bronchial artery embolization is preferred for problematic hemoptysis.

408. Almost all cases of allergic bronchopulmonary aspergillosis represents a hypersensitivity reaction to?
Harrison's 20th Ed. Chapter 212 Page 1535

A. A. fumigatus
B. A. flavus
C. A. jumigatus
D. A. niger

409. Allergic bronchopulmonary aspergillosis occurs in what percentage of patients with asthma?
Harrison's 20th Ed. Chapter 212 Page 1535

A. 1%
B. 1.5%
C. 2%
D. 2.5%

ABPA occurs in ~2.5% of patients with asthma and in up to 15% of adults with cystic fibrosis.

410. All of the following is true for allergic bronchopulmonary aspergillosis except?
Harrison's 20th Ed. Chapter 212 Page 1535

A. Serum total IgE > 100 IU/mL
B. Halo sign on HRCT scan
C. Central bronchiectasis
D. Eosinophilia

The cardinal diagnostic test for ABPA is an elevated serum level of total IgE, usually > 1000 IU/mL). Halo sign on HRCT scan is a localized ground-glass appearance representing hemorrhagic infarction surrounding a nodule.

411. Predominant involvement of the central airways is seen in?
Harrison's 20th Ed. Chapter 284 Page 1984

A. Allergic bronchopulmonary aspergillosis (ABPA)
B. Mounier-Kuhn syndrome
C. Williams-Campbell syndrome
D. All of the above

Predominant involvement of central airways is seen in allergic bronchopulmonary aspergillosis (ABPA), in which an immune-mediated reaction to Aspergillus damages the bronchial wall. Congenital causes of central airway-predominant bronchiectasis resulting from cartilage deficiency include tracheobronchomegaly (Mounier-Kuhn syndrome) and Williams-Campbell syndrome.

412. Aspergillus hyphae are hyaline, narrow and septate with branching at?
Harrison's 20th Ed. Chapter 212 Page 1535

A. 30°
B. 45°
C. 60°
D. 90°

Aspergillus hyphae are hyaline, narrow and septate with branching at 45°.

413. Aspergillus antigen test relies on detection of?

Harrison's 20th Ed. Chapter 212 Page 1535, N Engl J Med 2009;360:1870-84

A. Aflatoxin B1

B. Tannic acid

C. Galactomannan

D. Safrole

The Aspergillus antigen test relies on detection of galactomannan release from Aspergillus organisms during growth. Antigen-based diagnosis relies on serum detection of either galactomannan or beta-D-glucan, two constituents of fungal-cell walls. The galactomannan assay is relatively specific for invasive aspergillosis, whereas the beta-d-glucan assay also detects other invasive fungal diseases, including candidiasis, other mold pathogens (excluding zygomycetes), and Pneumocystis jiroveci (formerly called P. carinii).

414. Which of the antifungal drug is active against Aspergillus?

Harrison's 20th Ed. Chapter 212 Page 1536

A. Voriconazole

B. Amphotericin B

C. Caspofungin

D. All of the above

Antifungal drugs active against Aspergillus include voriconazole, itraconazole, posaconazole, caspofungin, micafungin and amphotericin B (AmB).

415. Which of the following is the preferred agent for invasive aspergillosis?

Harrison's 20th Ed. Chapter 212 Page 1536

A. Voriconazole

B. Amphotericin B

C. Caspofungin

D. Posaconazole

Voriconazole is the preferred agent for invasive aspergillosis. Caspofungin, posaconazole, and lipid-associated AmB are second line agents. The duration of therapy for invasive aspergillosis varies from ~3 months to several years, depending on the patient's immune status and response to therapy.

416. Which of the following is the preferred oral agent for chronic & allergic forms of aspergillosis?

Harrison's 20th Ed. Chapter 212 Page 1536

A. Voriconazole

B. Itraconazole

C. Caspofungin

D. Posaconazole

Itraconazole is currently the preferred oral agent for chronic and allergic forms of aspergillosis. Chronic cavitary pulmonary aspergillosis probably requires lifelong therapy. Glucocorticoids should be used in chronic cavitary pulmonary aspergillosis only if covered by adequate antifungal therapy.

417. Which of the following may produce mass lesions of the brain?

Harrison's 20th Ed. Chapter 70 Page 506

A. Nocardia

B. Aspergillus

C. Toxoplasma

D. All of the above

Infections associated with mass lesions of the brain may be caused by bacteria (particularly Nocardia), fungi (particularly Cryptococcus or Aspergillus) or parasites (Toxoplasma) .

418. Starting in the second month post solid organ transplant, which of the following is the more common opportunistic infections of the CNS?

Harrison's 20th Ed. Chapter 301 Page 2082

A. Nocardia

B. Toxoplasma

C. Aspergillosis

D. All of the above

Starting in the second month post solid organ transplant, opportunistic infections of the CNS become more common, including Nocardia and Toxoplasma species as well as fungal infections such as aspergillosis.

Occupational and Environmental Lung Disease

419. "Pneumoconiosis" is the term used for diseases associated with inhaling?

Prim Care Respir J. 2013;22(2):249–252

A. Mineral dusts
B. Chemicals
C. Proteins
D. All of the above

Occupational lung diseases are a broad group of diagnoses caused by the inhalation of dusts, chemicals, or proteins. "Pneumoconiosis" is the term used for the diseases associated with inhaling mineral dusts.

420. "Fugitive dust" includes?

Circulation. 2010;121:2331-2378

A. Pollens
B. Windblown dust
C. Dust from mechanical industrial processes
D. All of the above

421. What percentage of burden of adult asthma & COPD is due to occupational factors?

Harrison's 20th Ed. Chapter 283 Page 1976

A. 5 – 10%
B. 15 – 20%
C. 25 – 30%
D. 30 – 40%

15–20% of the burden of adult asthma & chronic obstructive pulmonary disease (COPD) is estimated to be due to occupational factors.

422. OSHA stands for?

Harrison's 20th Ed. Chapter 283 Page 1976

A. Occupational Safety and Health Administration
B. Occupational Safety and Health Authority
C. Occupational surveillance and Health Administration
D. Occupational surveillance and Health Authority

Workers in United States have the right to know about potential hazards in their workplaces under federal Occupational Safety and Health Administration (OSHA) regulations.

423. Particles below what size can be carried to lower airways?

Harrison's 20th Ed. Chapter 283 Page 1977

A. 10 μm
B. 7.5 μm
C. 5 μm
D. 2.5 μm

Particles >10–15 μm in diameter do not penetrate beyond nose & throat. Particles <10 μm in size are deposited below larynx.

424. Coarse-mode fraction contains particles of what size?

Harrison's 20th Ed. Chapter 283 Page 1977

A. ~ 2.5–10 μm
B. ~ 10–19.9 μm
C. ~ 20–20.9 μm
D. ~ 30–30.9 μm

Particles of silica, aluminum and iron are of the size of ~2.5–10 μm and represent coarse-mode fraction. They mostly deposit in tracheobronchial tree. Respirable particles that can deposit & be carried to lower airways, is of the size <2.5 μm (fine-mode fraction). Particulate matter (PM) is broadly categorized by aerodynamic diameter: All particles <10 μm (thoracic particles [PM10]), all particles <2.5 μm (fine particles [PM2.5]), all particles <0.1 μm (UFP), and particles between 2.5 and 10 μm (coarse particles [PM10–2.5]). Hence, PM10 contains within it the coarse and $PM_{2.5}$ fractions, and $PM_{2.5}$ includes ultrafine particles (UFP) particles.

425. Asbestos includes?

Harrison's 20th Ed. Chapter 283 Page 1977

A. Chrysolite
B. Amosite
C. Crocidolite
D. All of the above

Asbestos is a generic term for mineral silicates like chrysolite, amosite, anthophyllite & crocidolite (blue asbestos).

426. Major health effect from exposure to asbestos is?

Harrison's 20th Ed. Chapter 283 Page 1977

A. Pleural fibrosis
B. Diffuse interstitial pulmonary fibrosis
C. Cancers of respiratory tract, pleura & peritoneum
D. All of the above

Major health effects from asbestos exposure are pleural & diffuse interstitial pulmonary fibrosis & cancers of respiratory tract, pleura and rarely peritoneum.

427. Exposure for what duration is required before asbestosis becomes manifest?

Harrison's 20th Ed. Chapter 283 Page 1978

A. 6 months
B. 3 years
C. 5 years
D. 10 years

Usually, exposure has taken place for at least 10 years before asbestosis becomes manifest.

428. In chest radiography, which of the following is suggestive of asbestosis?

Harrison's 20th Ed. Chapter 283 Page 1978

A. Irregular or linear opacities in lower lung fields
B. "Ground-glass" appearance in lung fields
C. Subpleural curvilinear lines parallel to pleural surface
D. All of the above

429. In chest radiography, which of the following is suggestive of asbestosis?

Harrison's 20th Ed. Chapter 283 Page 1978 Figure 283-1

A. Bilateral calcified pleural plaques
B. Bilateral subpleural reticulation
C. Subpleural lines
D. All of the above

Diffuse pleural thickening is defined as >3 mm in thickness & extending >5 cm in transverse dimension and >8 cm in craniocaudad extent.

430. Pleural plaques most commonly develop along?
J Thorac Imaging 2009;24:310-320

A. Posterolateral chest wall between sixth & tenth ribs
B. Along peripheral diaphragm
C. Along cardiac border
D. Any of the above

Pleural plaques most commonly develop along posterolateral chest wall between sixth & tenth ribs and along the central diaphragm.

431. "Comet tail sign" best relates to?
J Thorac Imaging 2009;24:310-320

A. Asbestosis
B. Silicosis
C. Berylliosis
D. Coal worker's pneumoconiosis (CWP)

On HRCT, in asbestos-related pleural disease, rounded atelectasis (asbestos pseudotumor) manifests as a peripheral mass abutting pleura with or without lung distortion & with a curving tail of bronchovascular structures spiraling into the mass ("comet tail sign").

432. The clinical & pathological features of acute silicosis are similar to those of?
Harrison's 20th Ed. Chapter 283 Page 1978

A. ABPA
B. Asthma
C. Acute pneumonitis
D. Pulmonary alveolar proteinosis

Clinical & pathological features of acute silicosis are similar to those of pulmonary alveolar proteinosis.

433. "Crazy paving" HRCT pattern is characteristic of?
Harrison's 20th Ed. Chapter 283 Page 1979 Figure 283-2

A. Asbestosis
B. Berylliosis
C. Silicosis
D. Coal worker's pneumoconiosis (CWP)

Silicosis chest radiograph shows profuse miliary infiltration or consolidation and "crazy paving" is a characteristic HRCT pattern (diffuse ground-glass densities with thickened intralobular & interlobular septa, producing polygonal shapes).

434. "Eggshell" pattern of hilar node calcification is seen in?
Harrison's 20th Ed. Chapter 283 Page 1979

A. Asbestosis
B. Berylliosis
C. Silicosis
D. Coal worker's pneumoconiosis (CWP)

Calcification of hilar nodes produces a characteristic "eggshell" pattern in simple silicosis.

435. Potential clinical complication of silicosis is?
Harrison's 20th Ed. Chapter 283 Page 1979

A. Mycobacterium tuberculosis infection
B. Rheumatoid arthritis
C. Scleroderma
D. All of the above

Silica is cytotoxic to alveolar macrophages. Lung infections (Mycobacterium tuberculosis, atypical mycobacteria & fungi) are therefore common. Autoimmune connective tissue disorders like rheumatoid arthritis or scleroderma also occur.

436. Caplan's syndrome is?
Harrison's 20th Ed. Chapter 283 Page 1979

A. Seronegative Rheumatoid arthritis + Neutropenia
B. Seropositive Rheumatoid arthritis + splenomegaly
C. Seropositive Rheumatoid arthritis + progressive massive fibrosis (PMF)
D. Seronegative Rheumatoid arthritis + bronchial asthma

Caplan's syndrome occurs in patients with silicosis includes seropositive rheumatoid arthritis with characteristic pneumoconiotic nodules leading to progressive massive fibrosis (PMF).

437. Caplan syndrome was first described in?
Harrison's 20th Ed. Chapter 283 Page 1979

A. Coal miners
B. Stone cutters
C. Sand blasters
D. Cement workers

Caplan syndrome was first described in coal miners but subsequently in patients with silicosis.

438. Which of the following is called black lung disease?
J Commun Disord. 1975;8(2):129-40

A. Berylliosis
B. Byssinosis
C. Coal worker's pneumoconiosis
D. Farmer's lung

439. Coughing up of a black sputum is called?
J Thorac Imaging 2009;24:310-320

A. Melanoptisis
B. Melanoptosis
C. Melanoptysis
D. Melanopthysis

Coughing up of a black sputum is called melanoptysis.

440. Which of the following about Coal worker's pneumoconiosis is false?
Harrison's 20th Ed. Chapter 283 Page 1979

A. Occurs after 15–20 years of exposure to coal dust
B. Effects of coal dust are additive to those of cigarette smoking
C. Nodules are confined to upper half of lungs
D. None of the above

441. Histopathological lesion of which of the following environment-associated disease is similar to sarcoidosis?
Harrison's 20th Ed. Chapter 283 Page 1980

A. Asbestosis
B. Berylliosis
C. Coal worker's pneumoconiosis (CWP)
D. Silicosis

Beryllium is commonly associated with a chronic granulomatous inflammatory disease that is similar to sarcoidosis. In CBD, there is evidence of a specific cell-mediated immune response (delayed hypersensitivity) to beryllium. Hilar adenopathy is less common though.

442. Which of the following test provides evidence of occupational exposures to beryllium?

Harrison's 20th Ed. Chapter 283 Page 1980

A. Beryllium neutrophil proliferation test
B. Beryllium lymphocyte proliferation test
C. Beryllium eosinophil proliferation test
D. Beryllium monocyte proliferation test

Beryllium lymphocyte proliferation test (BeLPT) provides evidence of occupational exposures to beryllium. BeLPT compares the in vitro proliferation of lymphocytes from blood or BAL in presence of beryllium salts with that of unstimulated cells. Proliferation is measured by lymphocyte uptake of radiolabeled thymidine.

443. Which of the following CxR features of sarcoidosis is seen in Berylliosis?

Harrison's 20th Ed. Chapter 283 Page 1980

A. Ground glass infiltrates
B. Nodules along septal lines
C. Mosaic attenuation
D. Central nodular opacities

444. Which of the following confers increased risk of chronic beryllium disease (CBD)?

Harrison's 20th Ed. Chapter 283 Page 1980

A. Glu69 polymorphism of HLA–DP chain
B. Glu79 polymorphism of HLA–DP chain
C. Glu89 polymorphism of HLA–DP chain
D. Glu99 polymorphism of HLA–DP chain

Glu69 polymorphism of the HLA-DP chain confers increased risk of CBD.

445. In lung biopsy, which of the following finding is required to make the diagnosis of CBD?

Harrison's 20th Ed. Chapter 283 Page 1980

A. Noncaseating granulomas in lung tissue
B. Monocytic infiltration in lung tissue
C. Accumulation of beryllium-specific CD4+ T cells
D. All of the above

446. When sarcoidosis appears to be the diagnosis, one should always consider?

Harrison's 20th Ed. Chapter 283 Page 1980

A. Chronic beryllium disease (CBD)
B. Farmer's lung
C. Byssinosis
D. Mushroom worker's disease

447. Giant cell interstitial pneumonia best relates to?

Harrison's 20th Ed. Chapter 283 Page 1980

A. Polymer fume fever
B. Metal fume fever
C. Hard metal pneumoconiosis
D. Building-associated illness

Hard metal pneumoconiosis, formerly classified as giant cell interstitial pneumonia, results from exposure to tungsten carbide, cobalt, and diamond dust produced in hard-metal industry.

448. Which of the following best relates to byssinosis?

Harrison's 20th Ed. Chapter 283 Page 1980

A. Smoke inhalation
B. Hypersensitivity pneumonitis
C. Asthma-like syndrome
D. Hard metal

449. Other names for byssinosis include?

Chest. 1953;24(6):674-678

A. Monday fever
B. Brown lung disease
C. Mill fever
D. All of the above

450. "Monday chest tightness" is seen in?

Harrison's 20th Ed. Chapter 283 Page 1980

A. Bagassosis
B. Byssinosis
C. Berylliosis
D. Asbestosis

Cotton dust exposure (Byssinosis) is characterized clinically by chest tightness toward the end of first day of workweek ("Monday chest tightness").

451. "Monday chest tightness" responds best to?

Harrison's 20th Ed. Chapter 283 Page 1980

A. Bronchodilators
B. Antihistamines
C. Oxygen therapy
D. All of the above

452. Which of the following about Byssinosis is false?

Harrison's 20th Ed. Chapter 283 Page 1980

A. Occurs >10 years of exposure
B. Obstructive pattern on pulmonary function testing
C. Endotoxin levels play a role
D. None of the above

453. Findings in which of the following are virtually identical to the characteristic findings in cigarette smokers?

Harrison's 20th Ed. Chapter 283 Page 1980

A. Acute farmer's lung
B. Firefighters and fire victims
C. Radiation-related workers
D. Grain dust - exposed workers

Presentation of obstructive airway disease in grain dust-exposed workers is virtually identical to characteristic findings in cigarette smokers.

454. Thermophilic actinomycetes can cause all except?

Harrison's 20th Ed. Chapter 283 Page 1970 Table 282-1

A. Bagassosis
B. Farmer's lung
C. Mushroom worker's lung
D. Tobacco worker's lung

455. Which of the following is not a feature of acute farmer's lung?
Harrison's 20th Ed. Chapter 283 Page 1980

A. Onset 4–8 hour after exposure
B. Fever with chills
C. Cough and dyspnea
D. Wheezing

Acute farmer's lung presents 4–8 hours after exposure with fever, chills, malaise, cough & dyspnea without wheezing.

456. Exposure to which of the following can cause nasopharyngeal cancer?
Harrison's 20th Ed. Chapter 283 Page 1981 Table 283-2

A. Ammonia
B. Ozone
C. Sulfur dioxide
D. Formaldehyde

457. Exposure to which of the following can cause acute respiratory distress syndrome (ARDS)?
Harrison's 20th Ed. Chapter 283 Page 1981 Table 283-2

A. Ammonia
B. Acid fumes
C. Cadmium fumes
D. Formaldehyde

458. Exposure to which of the following can cause respiratory arrest & lactic acidosis?
Harrison's 20th Ed. Chapter 283 Page 1981 Table 283-2

A. Phosgene
B. Isocyanates
C. Hydrogen sulfide
D. Nitrogen dioxide

459. All can cause chronic bronchitis except?
Harrison's 20th Ed. Chapter 283 Page 1981 Table 283-2

A. Phosgene
B. Hydrogen sulphide
C. Ozone
D. Ammonia

460. Exposure to which of the following can cause occupational asthma?
Harrison's 20th Ed. Chapter 283 Page 1981

A. Diisocyanates
B. Aromatic amines
C. Acid anhydrides
D. All of the above

461. Polymer fume fever and metal fume fever present as?
Harrison's 20th Ed. Chapter 283 Page 1981

A. Influenza-like syndrome
B. Malaria
C. Pel Ebstein fever
D. Heat stroke

462. Which of the following provides "butter" flavor in the manufacture of microwave popcorn?
Harrison's 20th Ed. Chapter 283 Page 1981

A. Aromatic amines
B. Fluoropolymers
C. Zinc oxide
D. Diacetyl

Flavor worker's lung is a newly recognized occupational lung disease characterized by development of obliterative bronchiolitis after exposure to diacetyl (2,3-butanedione), a ketone used in butter flavoring of microwave popcorn.

463. Which of the following agent from diesel exhaust is a respiratory carcinogen?
Harrison's 20th Ed. Chapter 283 Page 1981

A. Acrylonitrile
B. Isopropanol
C. Polycyclic aromatic hydrocarbons
D. Vinyl chloride

In addition to asbestos, other agents either proven or suspected to be respiratory carcinogens include acrylonitrile, arsenic compounds, beryllium, bis(chloromethyl) ether, chromium (hexavalent), formaldehyde (nasal), isopropanol (nasal sinuses), mustard gas, nickel carbonyl (nickel smelting), polycyclic aromatic hydrocarbons (coke oven emissions and diesel exhaust), secondhand tobacco smoke, silica (both mining and processing), talc (possible asbestos contamination in both mining and milling), vinyl chloride (sarcomas), wood (nasal cancer only) and uranium.

464. Photochemically derived pollution ("smog") was originally thought to be confined to?
Harrison's 20th Ed. Chapter 283 Page 1981

A. Barcelona
B. Dhaka
C. New Delhi
D. Los Angeles

Photochemically derived pollution ("smog") was originally thought to be confined to Los Angeles.

465. Which of the following agent has been implicated in "Tight-building syndrome"?
Harrison's 20th Ed. Chapter 283 Page 1982

A. Dust mites
B. Perfumes
C. Latex particles
D. None of the above

Nonspecific responses occur in "tight-building syndrome" or better termed "building-associated illness". No particular agent has been implicated in its causation.

466. Which of the following is false about "nuisance dusts"?
Am J Public Health. 2013;103(2):238-249

A. Do not affect architecture of terminal bronchioles/acini
B. Clinical effects are reversible
C. Pulmonary function tests are usually normal
D. None of the above

467. Siderosis is due to?

J Med Case Reports. 2008;2:257

A. Iron & iron oxides
B. Tin oxide
C. Barium sulfate
D. Antimony salts

Siderosis, also referred to as welder's lung or silver polisher's lung, is a lung disease caused by inhalation of iron particles, whether through dust or fumes.

468. Baritosis is due to?

Thorax. 1976;31(1):30-9

A. Iron & iron oxides
B. Tin oxide
C. Barium sulfate
D. Antimony salts

Baritosis is a benign type of pneumoconiosis, which is caused by long-term exposure to barium dust.

469. Stannosis is due to?

Lancet. 1961;1:1089–93

A. Iron & iron oxides
B. Tin oxide
C. Barium sulfate
D. Antimony salts

470. Flock worker's lung is best related to?

Ann Intern Med. 1998;129(4):261-272

A. Nylon
B. Bauxite
C. Mercury
D. Radiation

471. Mad hatter syndrome is best related to?

The British Journal of Psychiatry 1995;167(1):95-8

A. Nylon
B. Phosphorus
C. Mercury
D. Radiation

472. Phossy jaw is best related to?

JAMA. 2010;303(22):2303

A. Nylon
B. Phosphorus
C. Mercury
D. Radiation

Bronchiectasis

473. Patterns of bronchiectasis were described by?
Harrison's 20th Ed. Chapter 284 Page 1983

A. RTH Laënnec
B. Lynne Reid
C. Jean Athanase Sicard
D. PJ Cole

Different patterns of bronchiectasis were described by Reid in 1950.

474. Which of the following is false about bronchiectasis?
Harrison's 20th Ed. Chapter 284 Page 1983

A. Abnormal & permanent dilatation of bronchi
B. Affects older individuals
C. Affects women more than men
D. None of the above

475. Which of the following forms of bronchiectasis is due to an underlying systemic or infectious disease process?
Harrison's 20th Ed. Chapter 284 Page 1983

A. Cylindrical or tubular bronchiectasis
B. Varicose bronchiectasis
C. Focal bronchiectasis
D. Diffuse

Diffuse bronchiectasis is characterized by widespread bronchiectatic changes throughout the lung and often arises from an underlying systemic or infectious disease process.

476. Bronchiectasis more pronounced in upper lung fields is most common in?
Harrison's 20th Ed. Chapter 284 Page 1984

A. Cystic fibrosis (CF)
B. Scleroderma
C. Idiopathic pulmonary fibrosis
D. Due to Mycobacterium avium-intracellulare complex (MAC)

More pronounced bronchoectatic involvement of the upper lung fields is most common in cystic fibrosis (CF), in postradiation fibrosis, corresponding to the lung region radiated.

477. Bronchiectasis more pronounced in lower lung fields is most common in?
Harrison's 20th Ed. Chapter 284 Page 1984

A. Cystic fibrosis (CF)
B. Scleroderma
C. Idiopathic pulmonary fibrosis
D. Due to Mycobacterium avium-intracellulare complex (MAC)

478. Bronchiectasis more pronounced in lower lung fields is most common in?
Harrison's 20th Ed. Chapter 284 Page 1984

A. Scleroderma
B. Idiopathic pulmonary fibrosis
C. Hypogammaglobulinemia
D. All of the above

Bronchiectasis with predominant involvement of the lower lung fields is due to chronic recurrent aspiration (due to esophageal motility disorders like scleroderma), end-stage fibrotic lung disease (traction bronchiectasis from idiopathic pulmonary fibrosis), or recurrent immunodeficiency-associated infections (hypogammaglobulinemia).

479. Bronchiectasis more pronounced in mid lung fields is most common in?
Harrison's 20th Ed. Chapter 284 Page 1984

A. Cystic fibrosis (CF)
B. Scleroderma
C. Idiopathic pulmonary fibrosis
D. Due to Mycobacterium avium-intracellulare complex (MAC)

Bronchiectasis due to infection by nontuberculous mycobacteria (NTM), mostly Mycobacterium avium-intracellulare complex (MAC) preferentially affects midlung fields. Congenital causes of bronchiectasis with predominant midlung field involvement include the dyskinetic/immotile cilia syndrome.

480. Bronchiectasis of relatively proximal airways suggests?
Harrison's 20th Ed. Chapter 284 Page 1984

A. Infection with M. avium complex
B. ABPA
C. Tuberculosis
D. Cystic fibrosis

Bronchiectasis accompanying ABPA involves proximal airways & is associated with mucoid impaction. An immune-mediated reaction to Aspergillus damages the bronchial wall.

481. Which of the following is a congenital cause of bronchiectasis?
Harrison's 20th Ed. Chapter 284 Page 1984

A. McCune-Albright syndrome
B. Laurence-Moon-Biedl syndrome
C. Kallmann syndrome
D. Mounier-Kuhn syndrome

482. Which of the following is a congenital cause of bronchiectasis?
Harrison's 20th Ed. Chapter 284 Page 1984

A. Pallister-Hall syndrome
B. Prader-Willi syndrome
C. Laron syndrome
D. Williams-Campbell syndrome

Congenital causes of central airway predominant bronchiectasis resulting from cartilage deficiency include tracheobronchomegaly (Mounier-Kuhn syndrome) and Williams-Campbell syndrome.

483. Mechanism of infectious bronchiectasis is?
Harrison's 20th Ed. Chapter 284 Page 1984

A. British hypothesis
B. Elastase : antielastase hypothesis
C. Vicious cycle hypothesis
D. Dutch hypothesis

Mechanism of infectious bronchiectasis is the "vicious cycle hypothesis" in which susceptibility to infection and poor mucociliary clearance result in microbial colonization of the bronchial tree.

484. In bronchiectasis, which of the following components of the wall of airways is destroyed?
Harrison's 20th Ed. Chapter 284 Page 1984

A. Cartilage
B. Muscle
C. Elastic tissue
D. All of the above

Normal structural components of larger-airway wall-cartilage, smooth muscle & elastic tissue are destroyed and may be replaced by fibrous tissue due to significant small-airway wall inflammation.

485. Which of the following is an action of α_1 antitrypsin?
Harrison's 20th Ed. Chapter 284 Page 1984

A. Antiprotease
B. Neutralizes damaging effects of neutrophil elastase
C. Enhances bacterial killing
D. All of the above

486. Bronchiectasis may occur with which of the following?
Harrison's 20th Ed. Chapter 284 Page 1984

A. Ulcerative colitis
B. Rheumatoid arthritis
C. Sjogren's syndrome
D. All of the above

Bronchiectasis occurs rarely in ulcerative colitis, rheumatoid arthritis & Sjogren's syndrome. Bronchiectasis due to noninfectious causes may occur in immune-mediated reactions that damage the bronchial wall (Sjögren's syndrome & rheumatoid arthritis).

487. Which of the following is false about bronchiectasis?
Harrison's 20th Ed. Chapter 284 Page 1984

A. Parenchyma supplied by affected airways is abnormal
B. Vascularity of bronchial wall is increased
C. Broncho-pulmonary arterial anastomoses
D. None of the above

488. In which pattern of bronchiectasis, bronchi end in blind sacs without recognizable distal bronchial structures?
Harrison's 20th Ed. Chapter 284 Page 1984

A. Cylindrical or tubular
B. Varicose
C. Saccular
D. All of the above

In saccular (cystic) bronchiectasis, bronchi end in blind sacs without recognizable bronchial structures distal to the sacs.

489. Which of the following is the most severe form of bronchiectasis?
N Engl J Med 2002;346:1383

A. Cylindrical or tubular
B. Varicose bronchiectasis
C. Saccular or cystic
D. None of the above

490. Traction bronchiectasis as seen in HRCT is a feature of?
N Engl J Med 2002;346:1383

A. Asthma
B. Chronic bronchitis
C. Pulmonary fibrosis
D. Allergic bronchopulmonary aspergillosis

491. Which of the following is the least common cause of bronchiectasis?
Harrison's 20th Ed. Chapter 284 Page 1984

A. Adenovirus
B. Staphylococcus aureus
C. Tuberculosis
D. Mycoplasma

Adenovirus, influenza virus, Staph. aureus, Klebsiella, anaerobes, Bordetella pertussis, M. tuberculosis are important causes of bronchiectasis.

492. Which of the following is not a feature of Kartagener's syndrome?
Harrison's 20th Ed. Chapter 284 Page 1984

A. Situs inversus
B. Colonic diverticula
C. Bronchiectasis
D. Sinusitis

Kartagener's syndrome includes situs inversus, bronchiectasis and sinusitis.

493. Which of the following is related to bronchiectasis?
Harrison's 20th Ed. Chapter 284 Page 1984

A. Tram tracks
B. Signet-ring sign
C. "Tree-in-bud" pattern
D. All of the above

In chest radiographs, presence of "tram tracks" indicates dilated airways and is consistent with bronchiectasis. Chest CT findings include airway dilation that is detected as parallel "tram tracks" or as "signet-ring sign" i.e. a cross-sectional area of the airway with a diameter at least 1.5 times that of the adjacent vessel, lack of bronchial tapering (including the presence of tubular structures within 1 cm from the pleural surface), bronchial wall thickening in dilated airways, inspissated secretions (e.g., the "tree-in-bud" pattern), or cysts emanating from the bronchial wall (especially pronounced in cystic bronchiectasis.

494. "Tram tracks" and "ring shadows" are chest radiological signs seen in?
Harrison's 20th Ed. Chapter 284 Page 1984

A. Bronchopneumonia
B. Bronchiectasis
C. Bronchogenic carcinoma
D. Aspergillosis

Dilated airways with thickened walls due to peribronchial inflammation are often crowded together in parallel. When seen longitudinally, they appear as "tram tracks", when seen in cross-section, they produce "ring shadows".

495. Nodular bronchiectasis is suggestive of?
Harrison's 20th Ed. Chapter 284 Page 1984

A. Infection with Mycobacterium avium complex
B. ABPA
C. Cystic fibrosis
D. P. aeruginosa infection

Presence of multiple small pulmonary nodules (nodular bronchiectasis) suggests infection with M. avium complex.

496. FEV_1 declines by how much per year in healthy individuals?

Harrison's 20th Ed. Chapter 284 Page 1984

A. 10–20 mL

B. 20–30 mL

C. 30–40 mL

D. 40–50 mL

Forced expiratory volume in 1 second (FEV_1) declines by 20 - 30 mL per year in healthy subjects.

497. Phrase "clean-outs" best relates to?

Harrison's 20th Ed. Chapter 284 Page 1984

A. Administration of an oral antibiotic

B. Use of a rotating schedule of oral antibiotics

C. Inhalation of aerosolized antibiotics

D. Intermittent administration of IV antibiotics

498. Which of the following is not a feature of 'Yellow nail syndrome'?

Harrison's 20th Ed. Chapter 284 Page 1984

A. Lymphedema

B. Pleural effusion

C. Mediastinal lymphadenopathy

D. Yellow discoloration of nails

Yellow nail syndrome is due to hypoplastic lymphatics. The triad of lymphedema, pleural effusion and yellow discoloration of nails is accompanied by bronchiectasis in ~40% of patients.

499. Which of the following causes 'Green nail syndrome'?

Harrison's 20th Ed. Chapter 159 Page 1171

A. Stenotrophomonas maltophilia

B. Acinetobacter baumannii

C. Pseudomonas aeruginosa

D. All of the above

"Green nail syndrome" is caused by P. aeruginosa paronychia. It is due to frequent submersion of hands in water. The green discoloration results from diffusion of pyocyanin into nail bed.

500. Which lobe of lung is involved in "Dry" bronchiectasis?

doi: 10.1183/13993003.01899-2015

A. Upper lobe

B. Middle lobe

C. Lower lobe

D. Any of the above

Bronchiectasis with upper lobe involvement may be suggestive of either tuberculosis or ABPA.

Cystic Fibrosis

501. The median survival for patients with CF is about?
Harrison's 20th Ed. Chapter 285 Page 1986

A. 27 years
B. 37 years
C. 47 years
D. 57 years

Due to improvements in therapy, the median survival is >37.4 years for patients with CF.

502. CF is characterized by?
Harrison's 20th Ed. Chapter 285 Page 1986

A. Bronchiolectasis
B. Exocrine pancreatic insufficiency
C. Intestinal dysfunction
D. All of the above

CF is characterized by chronic bacterial infection of airways that leads to bronchiectasis and bronchiolectasis, exocrine pancreatic insufficiency and intestinal dysfunction, abnormal sweat gland function, and urogenital dysfunction.

503. Cystic fibrosis (CF) is characterized by all except?
Harrison's 20th Ed. Chapter 285 Page 1986

A. Polygenic disorder
B. Autosomal recessive
C. Bronchiolectasis
D. Exocrine pancreatic insufficiency

Cystic fibrosis (CF) is a monogenic autosomal recessive disorder.

504. If both parents are carriers of disease-causing CFTR mutations, what is the chance of a fetus being affected?
Harrison's 20th Ed. Chapter 285 Page 1986

A. 1 : 2
B. 1 : 3
C. 1 : 4
D. 1 : 8

Because CF is an autosomal recessive disorder, a fetus has a 1 : 4 chance of being affected if both parents are carriers of disease-causing CFTR mutations.

505. CFTR stands for?
Harrison's 20th Ed. Chapter 285 Page 1986

A. CF transmembrane resistance regulator
B. CF transmembrane conductance regulator
C. CF transport regulator
D. CF transcription regulator

CFTR stands for CF transmembrane conductance regulator.

506. Which of the following bacteria is routinely cultured from CF sputum?
Harrison's 20th Ed. Chapter 285 Page 1986

A. Staphylococcus aureus
B. Haemophilus influenzae
C. Pseudomonas aeruginosa
D. All of the above

A complex bacterial flora that includes Staphylococcus aureus, Haemophilus influenzae and Pseudomonas aeruginosa (among other pathogens) is routinely cultured from CF sputum.

507. Concretions refer to?
Harrison's 20th Ed. Chapter 285 Page 1986

A. Broncolithiasis
B. Inhaled foreign body
C. Tenacious exocrine secretions
D. All of the above

Tenacious exocrine secretions (concretions) obstruct pancreatic ducts & impair production and flow of digestive enzymes to the duodenum.

508. Which of the following is a sequelae of exocrine pancreatic insufficiency?
Harrison's 20th Ed. Chapter 285 Page 1986

A. Fat-soluble vitamin insufficiency
B. High levels of serum immunoreactive trypsinogen
C. Loss of pancreatic islet cell mass
D. All of the above

509. Which of the following is observed in CF?
Harrison's 20th Ed. Chapter 285 Page 1986

A. Multilobular cirrhosis
B. Meconium ileus
C. Complete involution of the vas deferens
D. All of the above

510. The CFTR protein contains how many amino acids?
Harrison's 20th Ed. Chapter 285 Page 1986

A. 1280
B. 1380
C. 1480
D. 1580

CFTR protein is a single polypeptide chain with 1480 amino acids. It functions as a cyclic AMP - regulated Cl^- channel and as a regulator of other ion channels.

511. Fully processed form of CFTR is found in?
Harrison's 20th Ed. Chapter 285 Page 1986

A. Plasma membrane
B. Nuclear membrane
C. Cytoplasm
D. Rough endoplasmic reticulum

Fully processed CFTR is found in the plasma membrane in normal epithelia.

512. In a normal cell, CFTR is synthesized in?

Harrison's 20th Ed. Chapter 285 Page 1986

A. Golgi apparatus
B. Rough endoplasmic reticulum
C. Mitochondria
D. Nucleus

CFTR is synthesized in rough endoplasmic reticulum (RER), glycosylated in Golgi apparatus & functions as a Cl⁻ channel & regulator of other ion channels when located in plasma membrane.

513. CFTR gene is located on chromosome?

Harrison's 20th Ed. Chapter 456 Page 3351 Figure 456-3

A. 4
B. 7
C. 12
D. 13

CF is due to mutations in the gene located on the long arm of chromosome 7 that encodes CF transmembrane conductance regulator (CFTR) protein.

514. CFTR gene contains how many exons?

Harrison's 20th Ed. Chapter 456 Page 3351 Figure 456-3

A. 22
B. 25
C. 27
D. 29

CFTR gene contains 27 exons. There are currently 1963 reported mutations in the CFTR gene. CFTR is protein missing or nonfunctional in most severe cases of cystic fibrosis.

515. CFTR mutation along with which other mutation increases the risk of pancreatitis?

Harrison's 20th Ed. Chapter 341 Page 2445

A. Cationic trypsinogen (PRSS1)
B. Chymotrypsin C gene (CTRC)
C. Pancreatic secretory trypsin inhibitor gene (SPINK1)
D. All of the above

A combination of two CFTR mutations and an N34S SPINK1 mutation increased the risk of pancreatitis 900-fold.

516. Absence of CFTR synthesis is labeled as which class of defects in the CFTR gene?

Harrison's 20th Ed. Chapter 285 Page 1988 Figure 285-2

A. I
B. II
C. III
D. IV

517. Which of the following is abnormal in Class IV CFTR gene mutation?

Harrison's 20th Ed. Chapter 285 Page 1988 Figure 285-2

A. Defective protein synthesis
B. Defective protein maturation & premature degradation
C. Defective gating/regulation
D. Defective conductance through ion channel pore

Classes of defects in the CFTR gene include the absence of synthesis (class 1); defective protein maturation and premature degradation (class II); disordered gating/regulation, such as diminished adenosine triphosphate (ATP) binding and hydrolysis (class III); defective conductance through the ion channel pore (class IV); a reduced number of CFTR transcripts due to a promoter or splicing abnormality (class V); and accelerated turnover from the cell surface (class VI).

518. Adenosine triphosphate (ATP) in CFTR epithelial anion channel is utilized for?

Harrison's 20th Ed. Chapter 285 Page 1987

A. Chloride transport
B. Bicarbonate transport
C. Ion channel mechanochemistry and gating
D. All of the above

Cystic Fibrosis Transmembrane Conductance Regulator (CFTR) is an integral membrane protein that functions as an epithelial anion channel or a passive conduit for chloride & bicarbonate transport across plasma membranes of epithelial tissues, with direction of ion flow dependent on the electrochemical driving force. Gating of CFTR involves conformational cycling between an open & closed configuration & is augmented by hydrolysis of adenosine triphosphate (ATP). Anion flux mediated by CFTR "does not involve active transport" against a concentration gradient but utilizes energy provided from ATP hydrolysis for ion channel mechanochemistry and gating.

519. In respiratory airways, CFTR is necessary to provide?

Harrison's 20th Ed. Chapter 285 Page 1987

A. Depth of periciliary fluid layer (PCL)
B. Formation of mucus
C. Extrusion of glandular secretion onto airway surface
D. All of the above

In respiratory mucosa, CFTR is necessary to provide sufficient depth of the periciliary fluid layer (PCL), allowing normal ciliary extension and mucociliary transport. CFTR-deficient airway cells exhibit depleted PCL, causing ciliary collapse & failure to clear overlying mucus.

520. Airway remodeling and bronchiectasis in CF is due to?

Harrison's 20th Ed. Chapter 285 Page 1987

A. Aggressive, unrelenting neutrophilic inflammation
B. Aggressive, unrelenting eosinophilic inflammation
C. Aggressive, unrelenting basophilic inflammation
D. All of the above

The CF airway is characterized by an aggressive, unrelenting, neutrophilic inflammatory response with release of proteases & oxidants leading to airway remodeling & bronchiectasis.

521. In CF, most common genetic abnormalities are in class?

Harrison's 20th Ed. Chapter 285 Page 1987

A. I
B. II
C. III
D. IV

CFTR mutations that disrupt protein maturation are termed class II defects and are by far the most common genetic abnormalities.

522. The most common mutation in CF is termed as?

Harrison's 20th Ed. Chapter 285 Page 1987, N Engl J Med 2005;352:1992-2001

A. ΔF_{508}
B. N1303K
C. G85E
D. G91R

Most common mutation in CF is termed ΔF508 or F508del. CFTR with ΔF508 mutation lacks a phenylalanine (F) residue at CFTR position 508. CFTR encoding F508del retains partial ion channel function but protein maturation is arrested in endoplasmic reticulum and CFTR fails to arrive at the plasma membrane. Instead, F508del CFTR is misrouted & undergoes endoplasmic reticulum-associated degradation via the proteasome. Other clinically important mutations - N1303K, G85E, and G91R lead to misfolded CFTR protein that is prematurely degraded.

523. In CF, defective gating/regulation best relates to?

Harrison's 20th Ed. Chapter 285 Page 1987

A. G542X
B. R553X
C. G551D
D. W1282X

CFTR ion channels when properly trafficked to apical cell surface but are unable to open and/or gate leads to an inability to transport Cl^- or HCO_3^- in the presence of ATP (a class III abnormality). Such channel proteins include G551D (a glycine to aspartic acid replacement at CFTR position 551).

524. In CF, which of the following is a class I defect?

Harrison's 20th Ed. Chapter 285 Page 1987

A. G542X
B. R553X
C. W1282X
D. All of the above

CFTR nonsense alleles such as G542X, R553X and W1282X (premature termination codon replaces glycine, arginine or tryptophan at positions 542, 553 or 1282 respectively) are among the common class I defects, in addition to large deletions or other major disruptions of the gene.

525. CF patients homozygous for ρF508 have normal sweat electrolytes in the presence of which second mutation?

N Engl J Med 1997;336:487

A. R553X
B. R554X
C. R555X
D. R556X

Patients homozygous for ΔF508 mutation have normal sweat electrolyte concentrations if a second mutation - R553X is also present.

526. Cellular function ascribed to CFTR is?

N Engl J Med 2005;352:1992-2001

A. Conducts chloride across cell membrane
B. Down-regulates transepithelial sodium transport
C. Regulates Ca^{++} activated chloride & K^+ channels
D. All of the above

CFTR conducts chloride across the cell membrane & is regulated by protein kinase A (PKA) in a cAMP-dependent fashion. Other cellular functions of CFTR are down-regulation of transepithelial sodium transport, regulation of calcium-activated chloride & potassium channels.

527. Diagnostic biophysical hallmark of CF airway epithelia is?

Harrison's 20th Ed. Chapter 285 Page 1987

A. Lowered transepithelial electric potential difference
B. Raised transepithelial electric potential difference
C. Plasma membrane fenestration
D. Plasma membrane rigidity

Diagnostic biophysical hallmark of CF airway epithelia is raised transepithelial electric potential difference which reflects both the rate of active ion transport and epithelial resistance to ion flow.

528. Cystic fibrosis (CF) is characterized by all except?

Harrison's 20th Ed. Chapter 285 Page 1987

A. Increased airway Na^+ absorption
B. Increased airway Cl^- secretion
C. Reduced salt & water content of mucus
D. Decreased volume of periciliary liquid

Capacity to initiate cyclic AMP mediated Cl^- secretion is diminished in CF airway epithelia due to absence/dysfunction of CFTR Cl^- channel. Accelerated Na^+ absorption in CF reflects absence of CFTR inhibitory effects on Na^+ channels.

529. Which of the following is best related to airway surfaces in CF?

Harrison's 20th Ed. Chapter 285 Page 1987

A. Edematous
B. Atrophic
C. Hypertrophic
D. Dehydrated

Due to faulty regulation of Na^+ absorption and inability to secrete Cl^- via CFTR reduce the volume of liquid on airway surfaces and appear "dehydrated".

530. Which of the following is mostly infected in CF?

Harrison's 20th Ed. Chapter 285 Page 1988

A. Mucus layer
B. Epithelia
C. Airway wall
D. All of the above

Infection in CF airways involves mucus layer rather than epithelial or airway wall.

531. Which of the following is false about mucus layer in CF airways?

Harrison's 20th Ed. Chapter 285 Page 1988

A. Mucus stasis
B. Mucus hypoxemia
C. Mucus dehydration
D. None of the above

O_2 tension is very low in CF mucus (mucus hypoxemia). Mucus stasis is due to dehydration of mucus and periciliary liquid layers. It produces adhesion of mucus to airway surface causing failure to clear mucus from airways by ciliary and cough-dependent mechanisms.

532. CF airways are predisposed to chronic infection by?

Harrison's 20th Ed. Chapter 285 Page 1988

A. Staphylococcus aureus
B. Pseudomonas aeruginosa
C. Strict anaerobes
D. All of the above

533. CF patients fail to secrete which of the following in pancreatic duct?

Harrison's 20th Ed. Chapter 285 Page 1988

A. Na^+
B. HCO_3^-
C. Water
D. All of the above

In CF, failure to secrete Na^+, HCO_3^- and water leads to retention of enzymes in pancreas & destruction of virtually all pancreatic tissue.

534. Cholelithiasis occurs with increased frequency in?

Harrison's 20th Ed. Chapter 285 Page 1988

A. Cystic fibrosis (CF)
B. Crohn's disease (CD)
C. Wilson Disease
D. All of the above

In addition to the above three illnesses, cholelithiasis occurs with increased frequency in polyglandular autoimmune syndrome Type I.

535. Which of the following can occur in CF?
Harrison's 20th Ed. Chapter 285 Page 1988

A. Thickened biliary secretions
B. Focal biliary cirrhosis
C. Bile-duct proliferation
D. All of the above

In CF, defective hepatic ductal salt (Cl^-) & water secretion causes thickened biliary secretions, focal biliary cirrhosis, and bile-duct proliferation in ~ 25–30% of patients. Chronic cholecystitis and cholelithiasis also occur.

536. In CF, sweat emerging on the skin surface contains?
N Engl J Med 2005;352:1992-2001

A. High level of salt
B. Low level of salt
C. Normal level of salt
D. Any of the above

In CF, sweat emerging on the skin surface contains a high level of salt.

537. Elevated electrolyte levels in sweat can be due to?
N Engl J Med 1997;336:487

A. Cystic fibrosis
B. Fucosidosis
C. Glycogen storage disease type 1
D. All of the above

538. Elevated electrolyte levels in sweat can be due to?
N Engl J Med 1997;336:487

A. Mucopolysaccharidosis
B. Hypothyroidism
C. Vasopressin-resistant diabetes insipidus
D. All of the above

539. Elevated electrolyte levels in sweat can be due to?
N Engl J Med 1997;336:487

A. Adrenal insufficiency
B. Familial cholestasis
C. Familial hypoparathyroidism
D. All of the above

540. Recovery of which bacteria in bronchoalveolar lavage fluid supports the diagnosis of CF?
N Engl J Med 1997;336:487

A. Klebsiella pneumoniae
B. Proteus mirabilis
C. Escherichia coli
D. Pseudomonas aeruginosa

Recovery of Pseudomonas aeruginosa in BAL fluid supports the diagnosis of CF.

541. In lower respiratory tract, the first symptom of CF is?
Harrison's 20th Ed. Chapter 285 Page 1988

A. Cough
B. Dyspnea
C. Pain chest
D. Hemoptysis

In the lower respiratory tract, the first symptom of CF is cough.

542. Which of the following is often the first organism recovered from lung secretions in newly diagnosed CF patients?
Harrison's 20th Ed. Chapter 285 Page 1988

A. P. aeruginosa
B. Haemophilus influenzae
C. Aspergillus fumigatus
D. Klebsiella

Haemophilus influenzae and S. aureus are often the first organisms recovered from lung secretions in newly diagnosed CF patients.

543. Infection with which of the following is rare in CF?
Harrison's 20th Ed. Chapter 285 Page 1988

A. Haemophilus influenzae
B. Mycobacterium tuberculosis
C. P. aeruginosa
D. Aspergillus fumigatus

Mycobacterium tuberculosis is rare in patients with CF.

544. Which of the following is a significant cause of infection in patients with cystic fibrosis?
Harrison's 20th Ed. Chapter 285 Page 1988

A. Pseudomonas aeruginosa
B. Burkholderia cepacia
C. Aspergillus
D. All of the above

P. aeruginosa remains the most common contributing factor to respiratory failure in CF and is responsible for the majority of deaths among CF patients.

545. Chronic infection due to P. aeruginosa is seen in?
Harrison's 20th Ed. Chapter 285 Page 1988

A. Bronchiectasis
B. Chronic relapsing panbronchiolitis
C. Cystic fibrosis
D. All of the above

546. Distal intestinal obstruction syndrome (DIOS) consists of all except?
J Cyst Fibros. 2011;10 Suppl 2:S24-8

A. Left lower quadrant pain
B. Loss of appetite
C. Emesis
D. Palpable mass

In children & young adults, meconium ileus equivalent or distal intestinal obstruction syndrome (DIOS) occurs consisting of right lower quadrant pain, loss of appetite, emesis & often a palpable mass.

547. Which of the following can also cause pulmonary disease and azoospermia?

N Engl J Med 1997;336:487

A. Chédiak-Higashi syndrome
B. Young's syndrome
C. Felty's syndrome
D. Job's Syndrome

Young's syndrome can cause pulmonary disease and azoospermia. > 95% of male patients with CF are azoospermic, reflecting obliteration of the vas deferens due to defective liquid secretion.

548. All of the following are useful tests for CF except?

Harrison's 20th Ed. Chapter 285 Page 1988

A. Sweat chloride concentration
B. Semen Analysis
C. Serum lipids
D. Nasal Potential-Difference Measurements

A combination of clinical criteria & abnormal CFTR function (sweat tests, nasal PD measurements, and CFTR mutation analysis) are required for diagnosis of CF.

549. What value of sweat Cl^- concentration is typical in CF adults?

N Engl J Med 1997;336:487

A. > 40 mEq/L
B. > 50 mEq/L
C. > 60 mEq/L
D. > 70 mEq/L

Typically in adults a sweat Cl^- concentration of >70 mEq/L is pathognomonic for CF.

550. Normal mean nasal potential-difference is?

N Engl J Med 1997;336:487

A. – 4.7 mV
B. – 24.7 mV
C. – 44.7 mV
D. – 64.7 mV

Normal mean nasal potential-difference is – 24.7 mV. In CF, nasal transepithelial PD is raised

551. In CF, information of nasal potential-difference measurements can be augmented by the use of?

N Engl J Med 1997;336:487

A. Amiloride
B. Chloride-free solution
C. Isoproterenol
D. All of the above

Nasal potential-difference measurements (including responses to amiloride, chloride-free solution, and isoproterenol) may demonstrate abnormal CFTR function more reliably than the sweat test.

Pneumonia

552. Pneumonia is an infection of?

Harrison's 20th Ed. Chapter 121 Page 908

A. Pulmonary parenchyma
B. Terminal bronchiole
C. Respiratory bronchiole
D. All of the above

Pneumonia is an infection of the pulmonary parenchyma.

553. HCAP stands for?

Harrison's 20th Ed. Chapter 121 Page 908

A. Hospital-community acquired pneumonia
B. Hospital-community associated pneumonia
C. Healthcare-associated pneumonia
D. Healthcare-acquired pneumonia

Pneumonia is categorized as either community-acquired pneumonia (CAP) or healthcare-associated pneumonia (HCAP). HCAP includes hospital-acquired pneumonia (HAP) & ventilator-associated pneumonia (VAP).

554. Which of the following is the most common route for bacterial pneumonia?

Harrison's 20th Ed. Chapter 121 Page 909

A. Aerosolization
B. Contiguous extension
C. Microaspiration of oropharyngeal secretions
D. Hematogenous spread

Most common mechanism by which microorganisms gain access to lower respiratory tract is by aspiration from the oropharynx.

555. Which of the following is instrumental in clearing and killing pathogens at the alveolar level?

Harrison's 20th Ed. Chapter 121 Page 909

A. Resident alveolar macrophages
B. Surfactant protein A
C. Surfactant protein D
D. All of the above

Resident alveolar macrophages are assisted by local proteins (surfactant proteins A and D) in clearing and killing pathogens at the alveolar level.

556. Which of the following triggers the clinical syndrome of pneumonia?

Harrison's 20th Ed. Chapter 121 Page 909

A. Host inflammatory response
B. Proliferation of microorganisms
C. Alveolar capillary leak
D. All of the above

Alveolar macrophages initiate the inflammatory response. The host inflammatory response, rather than the proliferation of microorganisms, triggers the clinical syndrome of pneumonia.

557. Release of which of the following results in fever?

Harrison's 20th Ed. Chapter 121 Page 909

A. Interleukin (IL) 1
B. Interleukin (IL) 8
C. Granulocyte colony-stimulating factor
D. All of the above

558. Which of the following stimulates release of neutrophils & their attraction to lung?

Harrison's 20th Ed. Chapter 121 Page 909

A. Interleukin (IL) 1
B. Interleukin (IL) 8
C. Interleukin (IL) 12
D. Interleukin (IL) 14

Release of inflammatory mediators interleukin (IL) 1 & tumor necrosis factor (TNF) results in fever. Chemokines IL-8 & granulocyte colony-stimulating factor stimulate release of neutrophils & their attraction to lung.

559. Which of the following leads to dyspnea in pneumonia?

Harrison's 20th Ed. Chapter 121 Page 909

A. Decreased compliance due to capillary leak
B. Hypoxemia
C. Increased secretions
D. All of the above

Decreased compliance due to capillary leak, hypoxemia, increased respiratory drive, increased secretions and infection-related bronchospasm all lead to dyspnea.

560. Macrophage is the dominant cell type in alveolar space in which of the following pathological phase of pneumonia?

Harrison's 20th Ed. Chapter 121 Page 909

A. Edema
B. Red hepatization
C. Gray hepatization
D. Resolution

In the resolution phase, macrophage is the dominant cell type in alveolar space.

561. Neutrophil is the dominant cell type in alveolar space in which of the following pathological phases of pneumonia?

Harrison's 20th Ed. Chapter 121 Page 909

A. Edema
B. Red hepatization
C. Gray hepatization
D. Resolution

In the third phase i.e. gray hepatization, neutrophil is the predominant cell, fibrin deposition is abundant, and bacteria have disappeared.

562. Successful containment of infection & improvement in gas exchange occurs in which of the following pathological phases of pneumonia?

Harrison's 20th Ed. Chapter 121 Page 909

A. Edema
B. Red hepatization
C. Gray hepatization
D. Resolution

Phase of gray hepatization corresponds with successful containment of the infection and improvement in gas exchange.

563. Four pathological phases of pneumonia are best described for?

Harrison's 20th Ed. Chapter 121 Page 909

A. Pneumococcal pneumonia
B. Viral pneumonia
C. Pneumocystis pneumonia
D. All of the above

Four pathological phases of pneumonia are described best for lobar pneumococcal pneumonia and may not apply to pneumonias of all etiologies, especially viral or Pneumocystis pneumonia.

564. Bronchopneumonia pattern is most common in?

Harrison's 20th Ed. Chapter 121 Page 909

A. Bacterial CAP
B. Nosocomial pneumonia
C. Viral pneumonia
D. Pneumocystis pneumonia

Due to microaspiration mechanism, bronchopneumonia pattern is most common in nosocomial pneumonias. Lobar pattern is more common in bacterial CAP.

565. Which of the following is the most common cause of CAP in OPD, Non-ICU and ICU?

Harrison's 20th Ed. Chapter 121 Page 910 Table 121-2

A. Streptococcus pneumoniae
B. Haemophilus influenzae
C. Mycoplasma pneumoniae
D. Chlamydia pneumoniae

Streptococcus pneumoniae is most common of CAP in OPD, Non-ICU and ICU.

566. Which of the following is the least common cause of CAP in OPD patients?

Harrison's 20th Ed. Chapter 121 Page 910 Table 121-2

A. Legionella spp.
B. Haemophilus influenzae
C. Mycoplasma pneumoniae
D. C. pneumoniae

567. Which of the following is the least common cause of CAP in ICU patients?

Harrison's 20th Ed. Chapter 121 Page 910 Table 121-2

A. Influenza A and B viruses
B. Legionella spp.
C. H. influenzae
D. Mycoplasma pneumoniae

568. Community-acquired pneumonia (CAP) is caused by?

Harrison's 20th Ed. Chapter 121 Page 910

A. Metapneumoviruses
B. Coronaviruses
C. Community-acquired strains of MRSA
D. All of the above

Newly identified pathogens that cause CAP include metapneumoviruses, the coronaviruses responsible for severe acute respiratory syndrome (SARS) and Middle East respiratory syndrome and community-acquired strains of methicillin-resistant Staphylococcus aureus (MRSA).

569. Which of the following is not a "typical" bacterial pathogen causing CAP?

Harrison's 20th Ed. Chapter 121 Page 910

A. S. aureus
B. Klebsiella pneumoniae
C. Pseudomonas aeruginosa
D. Mycoplasma pneumoniae

CAP can be caused by "typical" bacterial pathogens or "atypical" organisms. Typical category includes S. pneumoniae, Haemophilus influenzae, S. aureus, Klebsiella pneumoniae and Pseudomonas aeruginosa. The "atypical" organisms include Mycoplasma pneumoniae, Chlamydia pneumoniae, Legionella species, respiratory viruses like influenza viruses, adenoviruses, human metapneumovirus and respiratory syncytial viruses.

570. Which of the following is false about "atypical" pathogens causing CAP?

Harrison's 20th Ed. Chapter 121 Page 910

A. Cannot be cultured on standard media
B. Cannot be seen on Gram's stain
C. Are intrinsically resistant to all b-lactam agents
D. None of the above

571. "Atypical" pathogens causing CAP must be treated with?

Harrison's 20th Ed. Chapter 121 Page 910

A. Macrolide
B. Fluoroquinolone
C. Tetracycline
D. Any of the above

572. Which of the following complicates influenza infection?

Harrison's 20th Ed. Chapter 121 Page 910

A. Streptococcus pneumoniae
B. Haemophilus influenzae
C. Staphylococcus aureus
D. H. influenzae

S. aureus pneumonia is well known to complicate influenza infection.

573. Which of the following is not an independent risk factor for community-acquired pneumonia?

Harrison's 20th Ed. Chapter 121 Page 910

A. Alcoholism
B. Asthma
C. Immunosuppression
D. Age > 50 years

Risk factors for CAP include alcoholism, asthma, immunosuppression, institutionalization, and an age of ≥70 years.

574. Which of the following is the strongest independent predictor of invasive pneumococcal disease in immunocompetent young adults?

Harrison's 20th Ed. Chapter 121 Page 910

A. Alcoholism
B. Cigarette smoking
C. Chronic obstructive pulmonary disease
D. Male gender

Risk factors for pneumococcal pneumonia include dementia, seizure disorders, heart failure, cerebrovascular disease, alcoholism, tobacco smoking, chronic obstructive pulmonary disease, and HIV infection. Cigarette smoking is the strongest independent predictor of invasive pneumococcal disease among immunocompetent young adults.

575. A recent hotel stay or ship cruise predisposes a person to pneumonia due to?

Harrison's 20th Ed. Chapter 121 Page 910

A. Legionella
B. Enterobacteriaceae
C. CA-MRSA
D. P. aeruginosa

Risk factors for Legionella infection include diabetes, hematologic malignancy, cancer, renal disease, HIV, smoking, male, and a recent hotel stay or ship cruise.

576. In CAP, gross hemoptysis is suggestive of infection with?

Harrison's 20th Ed. Chapter 121 Page 911

A. P. aeruginosa
B. Legionella
C. CA-MRSA
D. S. aureus

Gross hemoptysis is suggestive of CA-MRSA pneumonia.

577. Pneumatoceles on chest radiography suggest infection with?

Harrison's 20th Ed. Chapter 121 Page 911

A. Enterobacteriaceae
B. P. aeruginosa
C. M. tuberculosis
D. S. aureus

In CAP, pneumatoceles suggest infection with S. aureus.

578. To be adequate for culture, sputum sample should have?

Harrison's 20th Ed. Chapter 121 Page 911

A. >25 PMN and <10 squamous cells per low power field
B. >25 PMN and <20 squamous cells per low power field
C. >50 PMN and <10 squamous cells per low power field
D. >50 PMN and <20 squamous cells per low power field

To be adequate for culture, a sputum sample must have >25 neutrophils (PMN) and <10 squamous epithelial cells per low-power field.

579. Urinary antigen detection by ELISA is done for which of the following lung infections?

Harrison's 20th Ed. Chapter 121 Page 911

A. Legionella pneumophila serogroup 1
B. C. burnetii
C. Histoplasma capsulatum
D. Neisseria meningitidis

580. Urinary antigen detection by ELISA is done for which of the following lung infections?

Harrison's 20th Ed. Chapter 121 Page 911

A. S. pneumoniae
B. Mycobacterium tuberculosis
C. Histoplasma capsulatum
D. Neisseria meningitidis

Pneumococcal & Legionella pneumophila serogroup 1 antigens can be detected in urine.

581. In pneumonia, following etiologic agents can be diagnosed serologically except?

Harrison's 20th Ed. Chapter 121 Page 911

A. Mycoplasma pneumoniae
B. Chlamydia pneumoniae
C. Chlamydia psittaci
D. Histoplasma capsulatum

582. In pneumonia, following etiologic agents can be diagnosed serologically except?

Harrison's 20th Ed. Chapter 121 Page 911

A. Legionella spp.
B. Coxiella burnetii
C. Adenovirus
D. Coccidioides immitis

583. Number of variables included in the Pneumonia Severity Index (PSI) is?

Harrison's 20th Ed. Chapter 121 Page 912

A. 8
B. 15
C. 20
D. 26

To determine the PSI, points are given for 20 variables and patients are assigned to one of five classes. PSI a prognostic model used to identify patients at low risk of dying.

584. Number of variables included in the CURB-65 criteria is?

Harrison's 20th Ed. Chapter 121 Page 912

A. 3
B. 4
C. 5
D. 6

CURB-65 criteria is a severity-of-illness score. CURB-65 criteria include five variables - confusion (C), urea >7 mmol/L (U), respiratory rate 30/minute (R), blood pressure, systolic 90 mm Hg or diastolic 60 mm Hg (B) and age 65 years (65).

585. Patients should be admitted to the hospital when the CURB-65 score is more than?

Harrison's 20th Ed. Chapter 121 Page 912

A. 0
B. 1
C. 2
D. 3

With a CURB-65 score of 2, 30-day mortality rate is 9.2% & patients should be admitted in hospital.

586. Methicillin resistance in S. aureus is determined by?

Harrison's 20th Ed. Chapter 121 Page 913

A. ermB gene
B. mecA gene
C. gyrA gene
D. parC gene

Methicillin resistance in S. aureus is determined by the mecA gene, which encodes for resistance to all β-lactam drugs.

587. CA-MRSA has which type of SCCmec element?

Harrison's 20th Ed. Chapter 121 Page 913

A. Type I
B. Type II
C. Type III
D. Type IV

Out of the five staphylococcal chromosomal cassette mec (SCCmec) types described, typical hospital-acquired strains have type II or III, whereas CA-MRSA has a type IV SCCmec element.

588. Which of the following is a superantigen in CA-MRSA strains?

Harrison's 20th Ed. Chapter 121 Page 913

A. Enterotoxins B
B. Enterotoxins C
C. Panton-Valentine leukocidin
D. All of the above

CA-MRSA strains also carry genes for superantigens, such as enterotoxins B and C and Panton-Valentine leukocidin that can create cytolytic pores in polymorphonuclear neutrophils, monocytes, and macrophages.

589. Which of the following bacteria is typically resistant to cephalosporins?

Harrison's 20th Ed. Chapter 121 Page 913

A. Escherichia coli
B. Enterobacter spp.
C. CA-MRSA
D. All of the above

Enterobacter spp. are typically resistant to cephalosporins. Drugs of choice for these are usually fluoroquinolones or carbapenems.

590. If CA-MRSA pneumonia infection is suspected, which of the following should be added to initial empirical regimen?

Harrison's 20th Ed. Chapter 121 Page 914

A. Tobramycin
B. Meropenem
C. Linezolid
D. Piperacillin/tazobactam

If CA-MRSA infection is suspected, either linezolid or vancomycin should be added to the initial empirical regimen.

591. In treatment of CAP, which of the following is an alternative to the macrolide?

Harrison's 20th Ed. Chapter 121 Page 914

A. Aztreonam
B. Linezolid
C. Levofloxacin
D. Doxycycline

Doxycycline is an alternative to the macrolide.

592. In empirical treatment of community-acquired pneumonia, which of the following has significantly higher mortality rate?

Harrison's 20th Ed. Chapter 121 Page 914

A. Macrolide + second-generation cephalosporin
B. Second- or third-generation cephalosporin alone
C. Fluoroquinolone
D. Aminoglycoside + any other antibiotic

Combination of an aminoglycoside & any other antibiotic has a significantly higher mortality rate.

593. Therapy of longer duration is recommended for all of the following pathogens causing community-acquired pneumonia except?

Harrison's 20th Ed. Chapter 121 Page 914

A. Legionella spp.
B. P. aeruginosa
C. S. pneumoniae
D. Enterobacteriaceae

Pneumonia due to Legionella spp., P. aeruginosa, or Enterobacteriaceae usually requires therapy of longer duration (often up to 21 days).

594. Which of the following is intrinsically resistant to many of the empirical antibiotic regimens?

Harrison's 20th Ed. Chapter 121 Page 915

A. Acinetobacter
B. Stenotrophomonas maltophilia
C. Burkholderia cepacia
D. All of the above

Acinetobacter, Stenotrophomonas maltophilia, and Burkholderia cepacia are intrinsically resistant to many of the empirical antibiotic regimens.

595. Drotrecogin alfa (activated) should be considered for CAP patients if?

Crit Care. 2007;11(Suppl 5):S7

A. Persistent septic shock
B. APACHE II scores of ≥25
C. Infection by S. pneumoniae
D. All of the above

Immunomodulatory therapy with drotrecogin alfa (activated) should be considered for CAP patients with persistent septic shock & APACHE II scores of ≥25, particularly if infection is by S. pneumoniae.

596. In community-acquired pneumonia, complicating pleural effusion should be drained for all the following reasons except?

Harrison's 20th Ed. Chapter 121 Page 914

A. If the fluid has a pH of <7
B. If the fluid has a glucose level of < 2.2 mmol/L
C. If the fluid has a LDH content of > 500 units
D. If the fluid has is positive on Gram's staining or culture

A significant pleural effusion in pneumonia should be tapped if fluid has a pH of <7, glucose <2.2 mmol/L and LDH >1000 U/L or if bacteria are seen or cultured.

597. "Round pneumonia" is due to infection with?

Harrison's 20th Ed. Chapter 141 Page 1068

A. P. aeruginosa
B. S. pneumoniae
C. CA-MRSA
D. Mycoplasma pneumoniae

"Round pneumonia" is a distinctly spherical consolidation on chest radiography, is associated with a pneumococcal etiology. Round pneumonia is seen In children and is uncommon in adults.

598. In treated pneumonia, a follow-up radiograph is done after how many weeks?

Harrison's 20th Ed. Chapter 121 Page 914

A. One week
B. 3 weeks
C. 4–6 weeks
D. 8–12 weeks

Chest radiographic abnormalities are slowest to resolve & may require 4–12 weeks to clear. A follow-up radiograph can be done ~4–6 weeks later.

599. Which of the following is an MDR pathogen in the causation of VAP?

Harrison's 20th Ed. Chapter 121 Page 915 Table 121-6

A. Acinetobacter spp.
B. Legionella pneumophila
C. Enterobacter spp.
D. All of the above

600. Which of the following is an MDR pathogen in the causation of VAP?

Harrison's 20th Ed. Chapter 121 Page 915 Table 121-6

A. Pseudomonas aeruginosa
B. Streptococcus pneumoniae
C. Haemophilus influenzae
D. Proteus spp.

601. Which of the following is a critical factor in the pathogenesis of VAP?

Harrison's 20th Ed. Chapter 121 Page 915

A. Colonization of oropharynx with pathogenic microorganisms
B. Aspiration of organisms from oropharynx into lower respiratory tract
C. Compromise of normal host defense mechanisms
D. All of the above

Three factors are critical in the pathogenesis of VAP: colonization of oropharynx with pathogenic microorganisms, aspiration of these organisms from oropharynx into lower respiratory tract and compromise of normal host defense mechanisms.

602. Which of the following is best related to causation of VAP endotracheal tube?

Harrison's 20th Ed. Chapter 121 Page 915

A. Matrix biofilm on endotracheal tube's surface
B. Pseudomembrane biofilm on endotracheal tube's surface
C. Glycocalyx biofilm on endotracheal tube's surface
D. Proteinaceous biofilm on endotracheal tube's surface

Pathogenic bacteria form a glycocalyx biofilm on the endotracheal tube's surface that protects them from antibiotics and host defenses.

603. Which of the following statements about VAP is false?

Harrison's 20th Ed. Chapter 121 Page 915

A. P. aeruginosa almost never cause infection in patients without prior exposure to antibiotics
B. State of immunoparalysis corresponds to the greatest risk of developing VAP
C. Hyperglycemia affects neutrophil function
D. None of the above

604. Which of the following is included in the differential diagnosis of VAP?

Harrison's 20th Ed. Chapter 121 Page 916

A. Atypical pulmonary edema
B. Hypersensitivity pneumonitis
C. Pulmonary embolism
D. All of the above

Differential diagnosis of VAP includes atypical pulmonary edema, pulmonary contusion, alveolar hemorrhage, hypersensitivity pneumonitis, acute respiratory distress syndrome & pulmonary embolism.

605. Clinical Pulmonary Infection Score (CPIS) was developed for the diagnosis of?

Clinical Infectious Diseases. 1988; 51(1),:S131–S135

A. CAP
B. HAP
C. HCAP
D. VAP

Clinical Pulmonary Infection Score (CPIS) was developed for the diagnosis of VAP.

606. Which of the following statements about VAP is false?

Harrison's 20th Ed. Chapter 121 Page 916

A. Higher mortality rates with initially inappropriate empirical antibiotic therapy
B. The major difference from CAP is the markedly lower incidence of atypical pathogens in VAP
C. For patients with risk factors for MDR infection is for three antibiotics
D. None of the above

607. The most sensitive component of the CPIS is improvement in?

Clinical Infectious Diseases. 1988; 51(1),:S131–S135

A. Oxygenation
B. Body temperature
C. Leucocytosis
D. Tracheal aspirate culture

The most sensitive component of the CPIS is improvement in oxygenation.

608. In VAP, clinical improvement, if it occurs, is usually evident within how many hours of initiation of antimicrobial treatment?

Clinical Infectious Diseases. 1988; 51(1),:S131–S135

A. 6–12 hours
B. 12–24 hours
C. 24–48 hours
D. 48–72 hours

In VAP, clinical improvement, if it occurs, is usually evident within 48–72 h of the initiation of antimicrobial treatment.

609. Pneumonia caused by which pathogen signifies that patients immune system is so compromised that death is almost inevitable?

Harrison's 20th Ed. Chapter 121 Page 918

A. P. aeruginosa
B. S. maltophilia
C. Acinetobacter spp.
D. Klebsiella pneumoniae

Pneumonia caused by S. maltophilia is a marker for a patient whose immune system is so compromised that death is almost inevitable.

Lung Abscess

610. Which of the following is false about primary lung abscesses?
Harrison's 20th Ed. Chapter 122 Page 919

A. Major risk factor is aspiration
B. Caused by anaerobic bacteria
C. Absence of underlying pulmonary or systemic condition
D. None of the above

~80% of lung abscesses are primary.

611. Lemierre's disease best relates to?
Harrison's 20th Ed. Chapter 122 Page 919 Table 122-1

A. Strongyloides stercoralis
B. Blastomyces
C. Fusobacterium necrophorum
D. Gemella

Anaerobe Fusobacterium necrophorum is the organism involved in the causation of life-threatening Lemierre's disease, also called postanginal septicemia. Typical clinical triad of Lemierre's disease includes pharyngitis, tender/swollen neck and noncavitating pulmonary infiltrates.

612. Of the following, which is the most common pulmonary site of primary lung abscess?
Harrison's 20th Ed. Chapter 122 Page 920

A. Anterior segments of upper lobes
B. Posterior segments of lower lobes
C. Right middle lobe
D. None of the above

Dependent areas of lung, particularly posterior upper lobes & posterior segments of lower lobes are the most common pulmonary site of lung abscess.

613. Which of the following is false about primary lung abscesses?
Harrison's 20th Ed. Chapter 122 Page 920

A. Mostly affects middle-aged men
B. Right lung is affected more commonly than the left
C. Microbiology is often polymicrobial
D. None of the above

614. Which of the following in lung abscess indicates anaerobic infection?
Harrison's 20th Ed. Chapter 122 Page 920

A. Putrid breath
B. Sputum
C. Empyema fluid
D. All of the above

In lung abscess, putrid breath, sputum, or empyema fluid indicates anaerobic infection.

615. Which of the following can be a finding on physical examination in a case of lung abscess?
Harrison's 20th Ed. Chapter 122 Page 920

A. Tenderness over mastoid
B. Absence of a gag reflex
C. Carotid artery bruit
D. Goiter

616. Cavitary lung lesions can be produced by?
Harrison's 20th Ed. Chapter 122 Page 920

A. Granulomatosis with polyangiitis
B. Septic emboli
C. Lung infarction
D. All of the above

The differential diagnosis of lung abscesses includes other noninfectious processes that result in cavitary lung lesions including lung infarction, malignancy, sequestration, vasculitides (granulomatosis with polyangiitis), lung cysts or bullae containing fluid and septic emboli (from tricuspid valve endocarditis).

617. An abscess of what diameter is less likely to respond to antibiotic therapy without additional interventions?
Harrison's 20th Ed. Chapter 122 Page 921

A. > 2 – 3 cm
B. > 3 – 4 cm
C. > 5 – 6 cm
D. > 6 – 8 cm

An abscess >6–8 cm in diameter is less likely to respond to antibiotic therapy without additional interventions.

618. Poor prognostic factor for primary lung abscesses is?
Harrison's 20th Ed. Chapter 122 Page 921

A. Presence of aerobic bacteria
B. Sepsis at presentation
C. Symptom duration of >8 weeks
D. All of the above

Poor prognostic factors for primary abscesses include an age >60, the presence of aerobic bacteria, sepsis at presentation, symptom duration of >8 weeks and abscess size >6 cm.

619. Multiple small pulmonary abscesses in contiguous areas of lung is called?
Ann Thorac Surg 2009;87:310–1

A. Lung chancre
B. Lung carbuncle
C. Lung gangrene
D. Lung pemphigus

Lung abscess refers to microbial infection of lung resulting in necrosis of pulmonary parenchyma. Necrotizing pneumonia or lung gangrene refers to multiple small pulmonary abscesses in contiguous areas of the lung, usually resulting from a more virulent infection.

620. Lung abscess may occur in association with?
Harrison's 20th Ed. Chapter 122 Page 920

A. Aspiration
B. CA-MRSA infection
C. P. aeruginosa infection
D. All of the above

Lung abscess may occur in association with aspiration or with infection caused by a single CAP pathogen, such CA-MRSA, P. aeruginosa, or S. pneumoniae.

621. Most common cause of primary lung abscess is?

Harrison's 20th Ed. Chapter 122 Page 920

A. Aspiration
B. Periodontal disease
C. Alcoholism
D. Immunoglobulin deficiency

Aspiration is the most common cause of lung abscess.

622. Most common causative organisms for primary lung abscess is?

Harrison's 20th Ed. Chapter 122 Page 920

A. Anaerobic bacteria
B. S. aureus
C. Klebsiella pneumoniae
D. M. tuberculosis

Anaerobic bacteria are the most common causative organisms for lung abscess.

623. Acute lung abscess in a healthy young patient, along with influenza, is likely to be due to?

Harrison's 20th Ed. Chapter 122 Page 920

A. Klebsiella pneumoniae
B. Staphylococcus aureus
C. M. tuberculosis
D. All of the above

Acute lung abscess in a healthy young patient, especially in conjunction with influenza, is likely to be due to Staphylococcus aureus. Other bacteria include S. milleri, K. pneumoniae, Group A Streptococcus, Gemella, Legionella, and Actinomyces spp. Parasites include Entamoeba histolytica, Paragonimus westermani, Strongyloides stercoralis.

624. Which of the following about primary lung abscess is false?

Harrison's 20th Ed. Chapter 122 Page 920

A. Right lung is affected more often than left
B. Posterior upper lobes are the most common location
C. Superior lower lobes are the most common location
D. None of the above

625. Which of the following agent is found almost exclusively in patients with defective cell-mediated immunity?

Harrison's 20th Ed. Chapter 122 Page 919 Table 122-1

A. Nocardia asteroides
B. Burkholderia pseudomallei
C. Paragonimus westermani
D. S. milleri

Agents that are found almost exclusively in patients with defective cell-mediated immunity are Nocardia asteroides and Rhodococcus equi. Other agents include M. tuberculosis, Legionella spp., P. aeruginosa, Enterobacteriaceae (Klebsiella pneumoniae), Aspergillus spp., Cryptococcus spp.

626. Which of the following clinical features of nonspecific lung abscess is uncommon?

Harrison's 20th Ed. Chapter 122 Page 920

A. Fatigue
B. Cough
C. Sputum production
D. Fever with chills

Chills are uncommon.

627. Foul odor of sputum is due to the organisms' production of?

Harrison's 20th Ed. Chapter 122 Page 920

A. Short-chain fatty acids
B. Medium-chain fatty acids
C. Long-chain fatty acids
D. All of the above

Foul odor of sputum is due to the organisms' production of short-chain fatty acids, such as butyric or succinic acid.

628. Which of the following is uncommon in lung abscess?

Harrison's 20th Ed. Chapter 122 Page 920

A. Fever with chills
B. Lymphadenopathy
C. Anaerobic bacteria in expectorated sputum cultures
D. All of the above

Lymphadenopathy is not associated with bacterial lung abscess and suggests an alternative diagnosis. Anaerobic bacteria, the most common causes of primary lung abscess, are not detected in expectorated sputum cultures.

629. Which of the following drugs is now standard therapy for lung abscess?

Harrison's 20th Ed. Chapter 122 Page 920

A. Penicillin
B. Clindamycin
C. Metronidazole
D. TMP-SMZ

Penicillin "was" the mainstay of empiric antibiotic therapy for lung abscess. Due to frequent β-lactamase producing organisms, clindamycin is now standard therapy.

630. Which of the following should not be used for pulmonary infections?

Harrison's 20th Ed. Chapter 115 Page 865 Table 115-5

A. Linezolid
B. Daptomycin
C. Aerosolized colistin
D. Aminoglycosides

Daptomycin should not be used for pulmonary infections.

631. Poor prognostic factor in lung abscess is?

Harrison's 20th Ed. Chapter 122 Page 921

A. Presence of aerobic bacteria
B. Symptom duration of >8 weeks
C. Abscess size >6 cm
D. All of the above

Poor prognostic factors in lung abscess include an age >60 years, presence of aerobic bacteria, sepsis at presentation, symptom duration of >8 weeks and abscess size >6 cm.

632. Virulence factor 'pneumolysin' interacts with any cell whose membrane contains?

Harrison's 20th Ed. Chapter 146 Page 1100

A. Peptides
B. Cholesterol
C. Triglyceride
D. Amino acids

All pneumococci produce pneumolysin that interacts with any cell whose membrane contains cholesterol. Pneumococci also produce neuraminidase, hyaluronidase, and IgA1 protease.

633. Which of the following is a cytolysin?

Harrison's 20th Ed. Chapter 146 Page 1100

A. Streptolysin O
B. Pneumolysin
C. Perfringolysin O
D. All of the above

Cholesterol-dependent cytolysins streptolysin O, pneumolysin, perfringolysin O and listeriolysin O are produced by extracellular pathogens.

634. In the clinical entity designated ALPS, 'S' stands for?

Avicenna J Med. 2013;3(2):53–55

A. Smoking
B. Sepsis
C. Sedantry
D. Supine

Clinical entity designated ALPS (alcoholism, leukopenia, pneumococcal sepsis) is associated with a mortality rate of 80%.

635. 'PORT risk score' is used to classify?

Harrison's 20th Ed. Chapter 121 Page 914

A. Community-acquired pneumonia
B. Bronchiectasis
C. Interstitial lung disease
D. Pulmonary thromboembolism

PORT stands for Pneumonia Patient Outcomes Research Team. PORT risk class stratifies mortality rate in Community-Acquired Pneumonia.

636. The single most useful clinical sign of severity of pneumonia in a person without underlying lung disease is?

Dtsch Arztebl Int. 2014;111(29-30):503–508

A. Respiratory rate >30/minute
B. Pulse rate > 100/minute
C. Hypothermia
D. Postural fall of SBP > 10 mm Hg

The single most useful clinical sign of the severity of pneumonia is a respiratory rate of >30/minute in a person without underlying lung disease.

637. Which of the following bacterial pneumonia has the highest mortality rate?

PLoS Med. 2009; 6(5): e1000081

A. P. aeruginosa
B. Klebsiella spp.
C. E. coli
D. S. aureus

Mortality rate is highest (>50%) for pneumonia due to P. aeruginosa, followed by Klebsiella spp., E. coli, S. aureus, and Acinetobacter spp. (30 to 35%).

638. Microorganisms isolated from sputum that should always be considered pathogens include?

Mater Sociomed. 2013; 25(4): 226–229

A. Mycobacterium tuberculosis
B. Legionella spp.
C. Blastomyces dermatitidis
D. All of the above

639. Microorganisms isolated from sputum that should always be considered pathogens include?

Mater Sociomed. 2013; 25(4): 226–229

A. Blastomyces dermatitidis
B. Histoplasma capsulatum
C. Coccidioides immitis
D. All of the above

Certain microorganisms, if isolated from sputum, should always be considered pathogens. These include M. tuberculosis, Legionella spp., B. dermatitidis, H. capsulatum, and C. immitis.

640. Aerobic pathogen most often implicated in causation of aspiration-associated lung abscesses is?

Harrison's 20th Ed. Chapter 172 Page 1231

A. Streptococcus milleri
B. Bacteroides fragilis
C. Prevotella oralis
D. Fusobacterium nucleatum

Most aspiration-associated lung abscesses are due to a combination of aerobic and anaerobic bacteria, with an average of six or seven bacterial species identified in an individual case. Streptococcus milleri is one of the principal aerobic pathogens.

641. Gastric acid aspiration leading to aspiration pneumonitis requires following characteristics of gastric aspirate?

N Engl J Med. 2001;344(9):665-71

A. pH < 2.5 & gastric aspirate volume of > 0.3 mL/kg
B. pH < 5 & gastric aspirate volume of > 0.3 mL/kg
C. pH < 2.5 & gastric aspirate volume of > 0.6 mL/kg
D. pH < 5 & gastric aspirate volume of > 0.6 mL/kg

Gastric aspirate pH of <2.5 & volume >0.3 mL/kg (20 to 25 mL in adults) is required for the development of aspiration pneumonitis.

642. Which of the following is a respiratory fluoroquinolone?

Harrison's 20th Ed. Chapter 115 Page

A. Moxifloxacin
B. Gemifloxacin
C. Levofloxacin
D. All of the above

Respiratory fluoroquinolones include moxifloxacin, gemifloxacin and levofloxacin.

643. Hospital-acquired pneumonia (HAP) is defined as pneumonia occurring how many hours after hospital admission?

Can J Infect Dis Med Microbiol. 2008;19(1):19–53

A. At least 12 hours
B. At least 24 hours
C. At least 36 hours
D. At least 48 hours

HAP is defined as pneumonia occurring at least 48 hours after hospital admission and not incubating at the time of admission.

644. Cefoxitin, Cefotetan, and Cefmetazole belong to which generation of cephalosporins?

Antimicrob Agents Chemother. 1973;3(2):254–261

A. First
B. Second
C. Third
D. None of the above

Cephamycins (cefoxitin, cefotetan, & cefmetazole) are structurally different from true cephalosporins & display enhanced stability in the presence of ESBLs. Some consider cephamycins to be subset of second-generation cephalosporins.

645. ESBL-producing isolates should be considered resistant to?

J of Clinical Microbiology, 2010:1019–1025

A. All penicillins
B. Cephalosporins
C. Aztreonam
D. All of the above

ESBL-producing isolates should be considered resistant to all penicillins, cephalosporins & aztreonam.

Chronic Obstructive Pulmonary Disease

646. COPD includes?

Harrison's 20th Ed. Chapter 286 Page 1990

A. Emphysema
B. Chronic bronchitis
C. Small airways disease
D. All of the above

COPD includes emphysema, chronic bronchitis and small airways disease all characterized by airflow limitation that is not fully reversible. Chronic bronchitis without chronic airflow obstruction is not included within COPD.

647. Obstructive lung disease is diagnosed if?

Harrison's 20th Ed. Chapter 286 Page 1990

A. FEV1/FVC < 0.7
B. FEV1/FVC > 0·7
C. FVC/FEV1 < 0·7
D. FVC/FEV1 > 0·7

COPD is characterized by an FEV1 value that is <80% of the predicted normal value and an FEV1/FVC ratio of <0.70.

648. Which of the following is responsible for physiologic alterations that occur with COPD?

Harrison's 20th Ed. Chapter 286 Page 1990

A. Large airways
B. Medium airways
C. Small airways and alveolar space
D. All of the above

Changes in large airways cause cough and sputum, while changes in small airways and alveoli are responsible for physiologic alterations.

649. Which of the following is responsible for increased resistance in most individuals with COPD?

Harrison's 20th Ed. Chapter 286 Page 1990

A. Large airways
B. Medium airways
C. Small airways
D. All of the above

Major site of increased resistance in COPD is in airways ≤2 mm diameter.

650. Cells secreting surfactant are called?

Harrison's 20th Ed. Chapter 286 Page 1990

A. Kulchitsky cell
B. Clara cell
C. Langerhans cell
D. C cell

In COPD, characteristic cellular changes include goblet cell metaplasia, with these mucus-secreting cells replacing surfactant-secreting Clara cells. Reduced surfactant may increase surface tension at the air-tissue interface, predisposing to airway narrowing or collapse.

651. Gas exchanging airspaces include?

Harrison's 20th Ed. Chapter 286 Page 1990

A. Respiratory bronchiole
B. Alveolar duct
C. Alveoli
D. All of the above

Gas-exchanging airspaces are respiratory bronchioles, alveolar ducts and alveoli. Emphysema is characterized by destruction of all these three.

652. Which of the following is false in smokers?

Harrison's 20th Ed. Chapter 286 Page 1990

A. In BAL fluid, macrophages are > 95% of total cell count
B. Neutrophils account for 1 to 2% of cells
C. CD8+ T lymphocytes are increased in alveolar space
D. None of the above

In smokers' BAL fluid, macrophages comprise >95% of the total cell count, and neutrophils, nearly absent in nonsmokers' lavage, account for 1–2% of the cells. $CD8^+$ lymphocytes are also increased in alveolar space of smokers.

653. Which of the following is false?

Harrison's 20th Ed. Chapter 286 Page 1990

A. Panacinar emphysema is seen in α_1 AT deficiency
B. Centriacinar emphysema is seen in cigarette smokers
C. Panacinar emphysema has predilection for upper lobes
D. Centriacinar emphysema is most prominent in the upper lobes and superior segments of lower lobes

Panacinar emphysema is usually observed in patients with alpha$_1$AT deficiency, and has a predilection for the lower lobes.

654. Which of the following is the most typical finding in COPD?

Harrison's 20th Ed. Chapter 286 Page 1991

A. Increase in the residual volume
B. Persistent reduction in forced expiratory flow rates
C. Increase in residual volume/total lung capacity ratio
D. Nonuniform distribution of ventilation

Persistent reduction in forced expiratory flow rates is the most typical finding in COPD. Increases in residual volume & RV/TLC ratio, nonuniform distribution of ventilation & ventilation-perfusion mismatching also occur.

655. In COPD, at rest, PaO_2 usually remains near normal until the FEV_1 is decreased to?

Harrison's 20th Ed. Chapter 286 Page 1991

A. ~ 25% of predicted
B. ~ 33% of predicted
C. ~ 50% of predicted
D. ~ 75% of predicted

PaO_2 usually remains near normal until the FEV_1 is decreased to ~50% of predicted at rest.

656. In COPD, $PaCO_2$ usually remains near normal until the FEV_1 is decreased to?

Harrison's 20th Ed. Chapter 286 Page 1991

A. ~ 25% of predicted
B. ~ 33% of predicted
C. ~ 50% of predicted
D. ~ 75% of predicted

In COPD, elevation of P_aCO_2 is not expected until FEV_1 is <25% of predicted.

657. Pulmonary hypertension leading to cor pulmonale & CHF due to COPD occurs in those with FEV_1 (<25% of predicted) and?

Harrison's 20th Ed. Chapter 286 Page 1991

A. Chronic hypoxemia (PaO_2 <75 mm Hg)
B. Chronic hypoxemia (PaO_2 <65 mm Hg)
C. Chronic hypoxemia (PaO_2 <55 mm Hg)
D. Chronic hypoxemia (PaO_2 <45 mm Hg)

PHT severe enough to cause cor pulmonale & RVF due to COPD occurs only in those who have marked decreases in FEV_1 (<25% of predicted) together with chronic hypoxemia (P_aO_2<55 mm Hg).

658. Which of the following accounts most for the reduction in PaO_2 that occurs in COPD?

Harrison's 20th Ed. Chapter 286 Page 1991

A. Bronchospasm
B. Shunting
C. Ventilation/perfusion mismatching
D. Bronchial tree plugging

Ventilation/perfusion mismatching accounts for all of the reduction in PaO_2 that occurs in COPD. Shunting is minimal.

659. Asthma, chronic bronchitis and emphysema are variations of the same basic disease is hypothesised by?

J Allergy Clin Immunol. 2015;136(3):521-9

A. American hypothesis
B. British hypothesis
C. Canadian hypothesis
D. Dutch hypothesis

Dutch hypothesis suggests that asthma, chronic bronchitis & emphysema are variations of the same basic disease which is modulated by environmental & genetic factors to produce these pathologically distinct entities. British hypothesis states that asthma & COPD are fundamentally different diseases.

660. Which of the following is a risk factor for COPD?

Harrison's 20th Ed. Chapter 286 Page 1994

A. Severe a1AT deficiency
B. Airway hyperresponsiveness
C. Cigarette smoking
D. All of the above

661. Which allele is associated with normal α1antitrypsin levels?

Harrison's 20th Ed. Chapter 286 Page 1994

A. S
B. M
C. Z
D. Null

Protease inhibitor (PI or SERPINA1) locus encodes α_1AT. M allele is associated with normal α_1AT levels. S allele is associated with slightly reduced α_1AT levels.

662. Which allele is associated with markedly reduced α1antitrypsin levels?

Harrison's 20th Ed. Chapter 286 Page 1994

A. S
B. M
C. Z
D. Null

Z allele is associated with markedly reduced α_1AT levels. Null alleles lead to absence of any α_1AT. Individuals with two Z alleles or one Z and one null allele are referred to as Pi^Z, which is the most common form of severe α_1AT deficiency.

663. α1- antitrypsin is mainly produced in?

Lancet 2005;365:2225-36

A. Lung
B. Liver
C. Kidney
D. Spleen

α1-antitrypsin deficiency is a genetic disorder, clinically characterised by liver disease & early-onset emphysema. α1 AT is mainly produced in liver. Its main function is to protect lung against proteolytic damage from neutrophil elastase.

664. α1- antitrypsin is the prototypic member of which superfamily of proteins?

Lancet 2005;365:2225-36

A. Glutamine protease inhibitor
B. Methionine protease inhibitor
C. Threonine protease inhibitor
D. Serine protease inhibitor

665. Mutation that causes severe α1 antitrypsin deficiency arises in which gene?

Lancet 2005;365:2225-36

A. SERPINA 1
B. SERPINA 2
C. SERPINA 3
D. SERPINA 4

Most frequent mutation that causes severe α1-AT deficiency arises in SERPINA1 gene & gives rise to Z allele. This mutation reduces concentrations in serum of α1 AT by retaining polymerised molecules within hepatocytes.

666. Risk for emphysema increases when level of serum α1-AT is?

Lancet 2005;365:2225-36

A. < 11 µmol/L
B. < 21 µmol/L
C. < 31 µmol/L
D. < 41 µmol/L

An amount of α1-AT below the serum protective threshold of 11 µmol/L increases risk for emphysema.

667. SERPINA1 gene was formerly known as?

Lancet 2005;365:2225-36

A. PR
B. PI
C. PX
D. PZ

SERPINA1 gene was formerly known as protease inhibitor (PI).

668. α1 antitrypsin deficiency is inherited as?
Lancet 2005;365:2225-36

A. Autosomal co-dominant
B. Autosomal recessive
C. X linked
D. None of the above

α1-antitrypsin deficiency is inherited as an autosomal co-dominant disorder, for which more than 100 alleles have been identified.

669. SERPINA1 gene is located on?
Lancet 2005;365:2225-36

A. Long arm of chromosome 12
B. Long arm of chromosome 13
C. Long arm of chromosome 14
D. Long arm of chromosome 15

SERPINA1 gene is located on long arm of chromosome 14. It spans 12·2 kb & is organized into four coding (2, 3, 4, 5) & three non-coding (1a, 1b, 1c) exons.

670. Normal α1 antitrypsin concentrations in serum is?
Lancet 2005;365:2225-36

A. 5 – 13 mol/L
B. 13 – 20 mol/L
C. 20 – 53 mol/L
D. 65 – 90 mol/L

671. Normal α1 antitrypsin concentrations in serum is?
Lancet 2005;365:2225-36 Table 2

A. 15 – 50 mg/dL
B. 50 – 150 mg/dL
C. 150 – 350 mg/dL
D. 350 – 550 mg/dL

Normal alleles are typified by α1-antitrypsin concentrations in serum of 20 - 53 μmol/L. Typically, deficient alleles lead to α1 AT levels <20 μmol/L.

672. Dysfunctional variants leading to abnormal function of α1 antitrypsin can cause?
Lancet 2005;365:2225-36

A. Emphysema
B. Cirrhosis liver
C. Bleeding diathesis
D. All of the above

673. Dysfunctional variants leading to abnormal function of α1 antitrypsin can cause?
Lancet 2005;365:2225-36

A. c-ANCA-positive vasculitis
B. Cirrhosis liver
C. Bleeding diathesis
D. All of the above

Dysfunctional variants lead to abnormal function of α1 antitrypsin with reduced binding to neutrophil elastase (as in the F variant) or, as with Pittsburgh, structural abnormality that causes the protein to serve as a thrombin inhibitor rather than as an antielastolytic protein, causing a bleeding diathesis.

674. Testing for α1 antitrypsin concentration in serum is done by?
Lancet 2005;365:2225-36

A. Nephelometry
B. Rocket immunoelectrophoresis
C. Radial immunodiffusion
D. All of the above

Testing for α1-AT deficiency in serum is done by nephelometry, rocket immunoelectrophoresis or radial immunodiffusion. Clinical laboratory test used most frequently to screen for α_1AT deficiency is measurement of the immunologic level of α_1AT in serum

675. α1 antitrypsin plays a major role in inactivating?
Lancet 2005;365:2225-36

A. Macrophage elastase
B. Neutrophil elastase
C. Lymphocyte elastase
D. Eosinophil elastase

α1 AT is the prototypic member of serine protease inhibitor (serpin) superfamily of proteins, which have a major role in inactivating neutrophil elastase to maintain protease-antiprotease balance.

676. α1 antitrypsin deficiency, conformational instability of which structure of serpins leads to mutations and polymerization?
Lancet 2005;365:2225-36

A. α-sheet
B. β-sheet
C. γ-sheet
D. δ-sheet

Conformational instability of the β-sheet structure of the serpins underlies their susceptibility to mutations and polymerisation.

677. α1 antitrypsin deficiency can predispose to which of the following liver disorders?
Lancet 2005;365:2225-36

A. Chronic hepatitis
B. Cirrhosis
C. Hepatoma
D. All of the above

678. α1 antitrypsin deficiency can predispose to which of the following skin disorders?
Lancet 2005;365:2225-36

A. Pemphigus
B. Panniculitis
C. Psoriasis
D. All of the above

α1-AT deficiency can predispose to lung disease (emphysema, bronchiectasis), liver disorders (chronic hepatitis, cirrhosis, hepatoma), skin disease (panniculitis), and vasculitis (anticytoplasmic antibody-positive vasculitis - Wegener's granulomatosis).

679. Emphysema associated with α_1 antitrypsin deficiency, distinctive features include?
Lancet 2005;365:2225-36

A. Early onset (fourth and fifth decade)
B. Panacinar pathology
C. Disproportionate involvement of lung bases
D. All of the above

Emphysema associated with α1-AT deficiency is early onset (IV & V decades), panacinar pathology, & disproportionate emphysematous involvement of lung bases (compared with more apical distribution seen in α1 AT replete COPD).

680. In α_1 antitrypsin deficiency, retained α_1 antitrypsin aggregates are found in which orgenelle of hepatocytes as inclusions?
Lancet 2005;365:2225-36

A. Endoplasmic reticulum
B. Mitochondria
C. Golgi apparatus
D. All of the above

681. Which amino acid is essential in the reactive center of α_1-antitrypsin to inhibits neutrophil elastase?
N Engl J Med 2002;346:45

A. Serine
B. Methionine
C. Threonine
D. Lysine

Inhibition is initiated by docking of protease with serpin. Alpha1-antitrypsin with a methionine at its reactive center inhibits neutrophil elastase.

682. Which of the following increase the risk of COPD in Pi^Z subjects?
Harrison's 20th Ed. Chapter 286 Page 1994

A. Asthma
B. Male gender
C. Cigarette smoking
D. All of the above

683. Which of the following is used to assess a patient of COPD?
Cleveland Clinic Journal of Medicine 2014;81(6):373

A. BODE index
B. Modified British Medical Research Council dyspnea scale
C. COPD Assessment Test (CAT)
D. All of the above

The BODE index (body mass index, obstruction, dyspnea score, and exercise oximetry). The modified British Medical Research Council (mMRC) dyspnea scale has five grades, numbered 0 through 4. The COPD Assessment Test (CAT) is a proprietary questionnaire. Patients use a 6-point scale (numbered 0 through 5) to rate eight symptoms (cough, mucus production, chest tightness, shortness of breath on exertion, limitations in home activities, lack of confidence leaving the home, poor sleep, and lack of energy). A total score of 10 or higher is abnormal.

684. "Fewer symptoms, high risk" patients belong to which group of GOLD guidelines?
Cleveland Clinic Journal of Medicine 2014;81(6):373

A. Group A
B. Group B
C. Group C
D. Group D

Four GOLD groups according to new GOLD guidelines are Group A (fewer symptoms, low risk), Group B (more symptoms, low risk), Group C (fewer symptoms, high risk) and Group D (more symptoms, high risk).

685. Patient who has an FEV1 of 40%, no history of exacerbations, and a CAT score of 20 would be in which GOLD group?
Cleveland Clinic Journal of Medicine 2014;81(6):373

A. Group A
B. Group B
C. Group C
D. Group D

Patient who has an FEV1 of 40% (severe airflow limitation), no history of exacerbations, and a CAT score of 20 would be in group D.

686. COTE index best relates to?
Cleveland Clinic Journal of Medicine 2014;81(6):373

A. Overall health status
B. Frequent exacerbations
C. Comorbidities in COPD patients
D. All of the above

Doctors must be aware of comorbidities in COPD patients. COTE index (COPD-Specific Comorbidity Test) awards points as follows: 6 points for cancer of the lung, esophagus, pancreas, or breast, or for anxiety, 2 points for all other cancers, liver cirrhosis, atrial fibrillation or flutter, diabetes with neuropathy, or pulmonary fibrosis, 1 point for congestive heart failure, gastric or duodenal ulcer, or coronary artery disease. COTE index score of 4 or higher was associated with a risk of death 2.2 times higher in each quartile of BODE index.

687. Which of the following is not included in the three cardinal symptoms of COPD exacerbation?
Cleveland Clinic Journal of Medicine 2014;81(6):373

A. Shortness of breath
B. Fever
C. Increase in sputum volume
D. Sputum purulence

The three cardinal symptoms of COPD exacerbation are shortness of breath, increase in sputum volume, and sputum purulence.

688. Which of the following is a disease-specific instrument designed to measure impact on overall health, daily life, and perceived well-being in patients with obstructive airways disease?
Cleveland Clinic Journal of Medicine 2014;81(6):373

A. Juniper Respiratory Questionnaire
B. St. George's Respiratory Questionnaire
C. Bouchet Respiratory Questionnaire
D. Andersson Respiratory Questionnaire

Chronic Respiratory Questionnaire (CRQ) and the St George's Respiratory Questionnaire (SGRQ) are the two most widely used quality of life questionnaires in chronic obstructive pulmonary disease (COPD).

689. Which of the following about "Roflumilast" is false?
Cleveland Clinic Journal of Medicine 2014;81(6):373

A. Oral phosphodiesterase 4 inhibitor
B. Anti-inflammatory properties
C. No acute bronchodilatory effect
D. None of the above

Roflumilast is an oral phosphodiesterase 4 inhibitor approved for treating exacerbations & symptoms of chronic bronchitis in patients with severe COPD. Phosphodiesterase 4, one of the 11 isoforms of the enzyme, is found in immune & inflammatory cells and promotes inflammatory responses. Roflumilast has anti-inflammatory properties but no acute bronchodilatory effect.

690. Which of the following is a side effect of Roflumilast?
Cleveland Clinic Journal of Medicine 2014;81(6):373

A. Alopecia
B. Photosensitivity
C. Cataract
D. Depression

Apart from diarrhea, weight loss, decreased appetite, and nausea, clinicians should be aware of psychiatric side effects of roflumilast, which include depression and, possibly, suicide.

691. Which of the following is a novel long-acting muscarinic M3 antagonist for the treatment of COPD?
Cleveland Clinic Journal of Medicine 2014;81(6):373

A. Aclidinium
B. Hypedinium
C. Clidinium
D. Geranium

Aclidinium bromide is a long-acting antimuscarinic recently approved by FDA. Its dosage is 400 μg twice daily by inhalation. Aclidinium has an advantage over tiotropium in patients who have nocturnal symptoms.

692. Which of the following is a long-acting beta-2 agonist?
Cleveland Clinic Journal of Medicine 2014;81(6):373

A. Salmeterol
B. Formoterol
C. Arformoterol
D. All of the above

Salmeterol, formoterol, and arformoterol are long-acting beta-2 agonists in clinical use that are taken twice daily.

693. Which of the following is an "ultra-long-acting" beta agonist?
Cleveland Clinic Journal of Medicine 2014;81(6):373

A. Solucaterol
B. Minicaterol
C. Indacaterol
D. Flucaterol

Indacaterol is the first once-daily beta agonist or "ultra-long-acting" beta agonist (75 to 300 μg once daily) because it has a high affinity for the lipid raft domain of the cell membrane where beta-2 receptors are coupled to second messengers. The drug has a 24-hour duration of action and provides adequate pharmacologic stenting of airways.

694. Which of the following is a common symptoms in COPD?
Harrison's 20th Ed. Chapter 286 Page 1995

A. Cough
B. Sputum production
C. Exertional dyspnea
D. All of the above

695. Principal feature of advancing COPD is?
Harrison's 20th Ed. Chapter 286 Page 1995

A. Worsening dyspnea on exertion
B. Cough
C. Sputum production
D. All of the above

Three most common symptoms in COPD are cough, sputum production & exertional dyspnea. As COPD advances, the principal feature is worsening dyspnea on exertion.

696. Sitting in "tripod" position, facilitates action of which of the following muscles?
Harrison's 20th Ed. Chapter 286 Page 1995

A. Sternocleidomastoid muscle
B. Scalene muscle
C. Intercostal muscles
D. All of the above

Use of accessory muscles of respiration is done by sitting in characteristic "tripod" position that facilitates the actions of sternocleidomastoid, scalene, and intercostal muscles.

697. Which of the following is false for patients with predominant emphysema?
Harrison's 20th Ed. Chapter 286 Page 1995

A. "Pink puffers"
B. Thin and noncyanotic at rest
C. Prominent use of accessory muscles
D. None of the above

Patients with chronic bronchitis are more likely to be heavy and cyanotic— "blue bloaters".

698. Which of the following is a poor prognostic factor in COPD?
Harrison's 20th Ed. Chapter 286 Page 1995

A. Diffuse loss of subcutaneous adipose tissue
B. Significant weight loss
C. Bitemporal wasting
D. All of the above

Independent poor prognostic factors in advanced COPD are systemic wasting, significant weight loss, bitemporal wasting & diffuse loss of subcutaneous adipose tissue.

699. Systemic wasting in advanced COPD is related to?
Harrison's 20th Ed. Chapter 286 Page 1995

A. Neutrophil elastase
B. Matrix metalloproteinase-12 (MMP-12)
C. TNF-α
D. Transforming growth factor β (TGF-b)

Systemic wasting in advanced COPD is related to both inadequate oral intake and elevated levels of inflammatory cytokines (TNF-α).

700. In COPD, Hoover's sign refers to?
Harrison's 20th Ed. Chapter 286 Page 1995

A. Use of accessory muscles
B. Pursed-lip breathing
C. Diffuse loss of subcutaneous adipose tissue
D. Paradoxical inward movement of rib cage with inspiration

Hoover's sign refers to paradoxical inward movement of rib cage with inspiration.

701. Which of the following is not a sign of COPD?
Harrison's 20th Ed. Chapter 286 Page 1995

A. Expiratory wheezing
B. Bitemporal wasting
C. Clubbing of the digits
D. Right heart failure

Clubbing of the digits is not a sign of COPD, and its presence should alert the clinician to rule out lung cancer or else.

702. Which of the following is the basis for Gold criteria for COPD severity?
Harrison's 20th Ed. Chapter 286 Page 1995

A. Airflow obstruction
B. Exercise performance
C. Arterial blood gases and oximetry
D. Body mass index

The hallmark and important prognostic factor of COPD is airflow obstruction and is the basis for the Global Initiative for Lung Disease (GOLD) classification for COPD severity.

703. Which of the following influence the natural history of patients with COPD?

Harrison's 20th Ed. Chapter 286 Page 1995

A. Smoking cessation
B. Oxygen therapy in chronically hypoxemic patients
C. Lung volume reduction surgery
D. All of the above

704. Which of the following interventions does not influence the natural history of patients with COPD?

Harrison's 20th Ed. Chapter 286 Page 1995

A. Antibiotics
B. Smoking cessation
C. Oxygen therapy in chronically hypoxemic patients
D. Lung volume reduction surgery

Only three interventions i.e.smoking cessation, oxygen therapy in chronically hypoxemic patients, and lung volume reduction surgery in selected patients with emphysema influence the natural history of patients with COPD.

705. Cigarette smoking increases risk for which of the following?

Lancet 2004;364:791-802

A. Atherosclerotic vascular disease
B. Osteoporosis
C. Peptic ulcer disease
D. All of the above

Cigarette smoking increases atherosclerotic vascular disease risk, osteoporosis & peptic ulcer disease.

706. The other action of 'Bupropion' used in nicotine replacement therapy is?

Lancet 2004;364:791-802

A. Antihypertensive
B. Antidepressant
C. Anticholinergic
D. Analgesic

Antidepressant bupropion is shown to be effective in smoking cessation.

707. Bupropion use is contraindicated in patients of?

Lancet 2004;364:791-802

A. Diabetes mellitus
B. Hypertension
C. Seizure
D. Hypothryoidism

Bupropion is contraindicated in those with increased risk of seizures.

708. Which of the following drugs have been found useful in smoking cessation?

Lancet 2004;364:791-802

A. Clonidine
B. Nortriptyline
C. Varenicline
D. All of the above

Clonidine & tricyclic antidepressant nortriptyline have been found useful in smoking cessation as second-line treatments. Varenicline is an $\alpha_4\beta_2$ nicotinic acetylcholine receptor partial agonist.

709. Adverse effect of Varenicline is?

Harrison's 20th Ed. Chapter 286 Page 1996

A. Dysphagia
B. Suicidal ideation
C. Hemoptysis
D. Seizure

Therapy with an antidepressant bupropion or nicotine replacement therapy with varenicline are approved by USFDA as first-line treatments for nicotine dependence. Both drugs increase suicidal ideation and must be used with caution. Varenicline is more efficacious than bupropion or placebo.

710. Nicotine replacement therapy can be carried out by all routes except?

Harrison's 20th Ed. Chapter 286 Page 1996

A. Per rectal
B. Transdermal patches
C. Inhaler
D. Nasal spray

Nicotine replacement therapy is available as gum, transdermal patches, inhaler & nasal spray.

711. Bronchodilator effect of anticholinergics is due to blocking the action of acetylcholine on?

Lancet 2004;364:791-802

A. M1 muscarinic receptors
B. M2 muscarinic receptors
C. M3 muscarinic receptors
D. M4 muscarinic receptors

Anticholinergics are effective bronchodilators because they block the action of acetylcholine on M3 muscarinic receptors that induce contraction on airway smooth muscle.

712. Which of the following is a long-acting β_2 adrenergic receptor agonist?

Lancet 2004;364:791-802

A. Formoterol fumarate
B. Albuterol sulfate
C. Tiotropium bromide
D. None of the above

713. Besides bronchodilator action, theophylline also has which of the following therapeutic effects?

Lancet 2004;364:791-802

A. Anti-inflammatory effects
B. Inotropoic & diuretic effects
C. Augmenting skeletal muscle strength
D. All of the above

Besides the bronchodilator effects of theophylline in COPD, it has anti-inflammatory, inotropoic and diuretic effects and has effects in augmenting skeletal muscle strength.

714. Only therapy demonstrated to decrease mortality in COPD patients is?

Harrison's 20th Ed. Chapter 286 Page 1996

A. Supplemental oxygen
B. Beta agonists
C. Theophylline
D. Glucocorticoids

Supplemental O_2 is the only pharmacologic therapy demonstrated to decrease mortality in COPD. Supplemental O_2 should be supplied to keep arterial saturations ≥ 90%.

715. Which of the following is an action of N-acetyl cysteine?

Harrison's 20th Ed. Chapter 286 Page 1997

A. Antioxidant
B. Anti-inflammtory
C. Bronchodilator
D. Mast cell stabilizer

N-acetyl cysteine is used in COPD patients for its mucolytic and antioxidant properties.

716. Eligibility for α_1 antitrypsin augmentation therapy requires a serum α_1 antitrypsin level of?

Harrison's 20th Ed. Chapter 286 Page 1997

A. < 6 μM
B. < 8 μM
C. < 10 μM
D. < 11 μM

Eligibility for α_1 antitrypsin augmentation therapy requires a serum α_1 antitrypsin level < 11 μM (~ 50 mg/dL) PI^Z & null-null individuals and not in those with normal pulmonary function and a normal chest CT scan.

717. Which of the following vaccines is recommended before administering α_1 antitrypsin augmentation therapy?

Harrison's 20th Ed. Chapter 286 Page 1997

A. Influenza vaccine
B. Polyvalent pneumococcal vaccine
C. Hepatitis B vaccination
D. All of the above

Despite sterilization procedures for blood-derived products and the absence of reported cases of viral infection from α_1 antitrypsin augmentation therapy, some physicians recommend hepatitis B vaccination prior to starting augmentation therapy.

718. Which of the following vaccines are recommended in COPD patients?

Harrison's 20th Ed. Chapter 286 Page 1997

A. Polyvalent pneumococcal vaccine
B. Influenza vaccine
C. Vaccination for Bordetella pertussis
D. All of the above

719. LVRS is used in the management of?

Harrison's 20th Ed. Chapter 286 Page 1997

A. Bronchial asthma
B. ILD
C. Chronic bronchitis
D. Emphysema

Lung volume reduction surgery (LVRS) reduce volume of lung in emphysema.

720. Lung volume reduction surgery (LVRS) is not recommended if pulmonary artery systolic pressure is?

Harrison's 20th Ed. Chapter 286 Page 1997

A. > 15 mm Hg
B. > 25 mm Hg
C. > 35 mm Hg
D. > 45 mm Hg

LVRS is not recommended if patients of emphysema have significant pleural disease, a pulmonary artery systolic pressure >45 mm Hg, extreme deconditioning, congestive heart failure, or other severe comorbid conditions.

721. Patients with which of the following are not candidates for LVRS?

Harrison's 20th Ed. Chapter 286 Page 1997

A. FEV1 < 20% of predicted
B. Diffusely distributed emphysema on CT scan
C. DLCO < 20% of predicted
D. All of the above

722. Patients with which of the following are most likely to benefit from LVRS?

Harrison's 20th Ed. Chapter 286 Page 1997

A. Upper lobe predominant emphysema
B. Middle lobe predominant emphysema
C. Lower lobe predominant emphysema
D. Any of the above

Patients with upper lobe predominant emphysema and a low postrehabilitation exercise capacity are most likely to benefit from LVRS.

723. Which of the following reduce exacerbation rates in patients with COPD?

Harrison's 20th Ed. Chapter 286 Page 1997

A. Influenza vaccine
B. Inhaled glucocorticoids
C. Azithromycin
D. All of the above

724. Bacteria frequently implicated in COPD exacerbations include all except?

Harrison's 20th Ed. Chapter 286 Page 1997

A. Streptococcus pneumoniae
B. Haemophilus influenzae
C. Staphylococcus aureus
D. Moraxella catarrhalis

Bacteria frequently implicated in COPD exacerbations include S. pneumoniae, H. influenzae, Moraxella catarrhalis, M. pneumoniae or Chlamydia pneumoniae.

725. Which of the following is not a parameter in 'BODE score' used as a predictor for COPD mortality?

Lancet 2004;364:985-996

A. Breathing rate
B. Airflow obstruction
C. Dyspnea
D. Exercise capacity

726. Which of the following drugs is not included in the "not recommended or contraindicated" list in GOLD guidelines?

Lancet 2004; 364: 791–802 Table 2

A. Mucolytics
B. Narcotics
C. Antitussives
D. Vasodilators

Use of mucolytic, antioxidant, immunoregulators, respiratory stimulants is not recommended in pharmacological treatments of COPD. Antitussives & vasodilators are contraindicated. Narcotics can relieve dyspnoea (potentially dangerous due to ventilatory suppression) & is used to manage symptoms in terminal situations.

727. Which of the following is true as "Lung regeneration agent"?
Lancet 2004;364:985-996

A. Retinoic acid (all-trans)
B. Retinoic acid receptor g agonists
C. Stem cells
D. All of the above

Lung regeneration agents include Retinoic acid (all-trans), Retinoic acid receptor γ agonists & Stem cells.

728. Which of the following is used in the "Augmentation therapy" of COPD?
Lancet 2005;365:2225-36

A. Smoking cessation
B. Vaccines
C. Human plasma a1 antitrypsin
D. Supplemental oxygen

In COPD, specific treatment of α1-AT deficiency consists of infusion of purified pooled human plasma α1 antitrypsin - known as augmentation therapy.

729. Pooled human plasma is the source of which of the following preparations of purified α1 antitrypsin?
Lancet 2005;365:2225-36

A. Prolastin
B. Aralast
C. Zemaira
D. All of the above

730. Which season is appropriate for giving influenza vaccination yearly in patients of COPD?
Lancet 2004;364:791-802

A. Autumn
B. Winter
C. Spring
D. Summer

Influenza vaccination reduces serious illness & death in COPD patients by 50%. Vaccination should be given once in autumn.

731. Etiological factor in acute exacerbations of COPD includes?
Lancet 2004;364:883-895

A. Viral infections
B. Bacterial infections
C. Particulate air pollutants
D. All of the above

Main etiological factors in acute exacerbations of COPD are viral & bacterial infections & air pollutants.

732. Risk factors predicting increased hospital admission for acute exacerbations in COPD include all except?
Lancet 2004;364:883-895

A. Low body-mass index
B. High arterial carbon dioxide tension ($PaCO_2$)
C. Degree of hypoxaemia
D. High mean pulmonary arterial pressure

733. Risk factors predicting increased hospital admission for acute exacerbations in COPD include all except?
Lancet 2004;364:883-895

A. Gas-exchange impairment
B. Severity of airflow obstruction
C. High arterial carbon dioxide tension ($PaCO_2$)
D. High mean pulmonary arterial pressure

Neither the severity of airflow obstruction nor the degree of hypoxaemia are predictive of hospital admission in COPD

734. Which of the following is an effective respiratory stimulant?
Lancet 2004;364:883-895

A. Doxapram
B. Cilomilast
C. Gefitinib
D. Batimastat

Doxapram is an effective respiratory stimulant and can provide only minor short-term improvement in blood gas tensions in COPD.

Respiratory

Interstitial Lung Diseases

735. Interstitial lung diseases are characterized by?

N Engl J Med 2018;378:1811-23

A. Cellular proliferation
B. Interstitial inflammation
C. Interstitial fibrosis
D. All of the above

The family of interstitial lung diseases is characterized by cellular proliferation, interstitial inflammation, fibrosis, or a combination of such findings within the alveolar wall that is not due to infection or cancer.

736. Which of the following is the predominant phenotype in most cases of interstitial lung diseases?

N Engl J Med 2018;378:1811-23

A. Cellular proliferation
B. Interstitial inflammation
C. Interstitial fibrosis
D. All of the above

Interstitial fibrosis is the predominant phenotype in most cases of interstitial lung diseases.

737. Which of the following contribute to the development of dyspnea in ILD?

Harrison's 20th Ed. Chapter 287 Page 1999

A. Increased work of breathing
B. Increased drive to breathe
C. Stimulation of pulmonary receptors
D. All of the above

In ILD, there is no stimulation of vascular receptors or metaboreceptors.

738. Which of the following initial features is most frequent in ILD patients?

Harrison's 20th Ed. Chapter 287 Page 1999

A. Wheezing
B. Chest pain
C. Progressive exertional dyspnea
D. Hemoptysis

Patients with ILDs seek medical attention mainly due to progressive exertional dyspnea or a persistent, nonproductive cough. Hemoptysis, wheezing, and chest pain may be present.

739. Which of the following is central to the diagnosis of ILDs?

Harrison's 20th Ed. Chapter 287 Page 1999

A. Pulmonary function tests
B. Imaging findings
C. Histopathology
D. None of the above

No single piece of data confers a diagnosis alone in ILDs. Diagnosis is based on combined information obtained from a patient's clinical presentation, measures of pulmonary function, imaging, immune serologies, and histopathology. A multidisciplinary approach is required for diagnosis.

740. ILDs involve which of the following in lung parenchyma?

Harrison's 20th Ed. Chapter 287 Page 1999

A. Capillary endothelium
B. Perivascular tissues
C. Lymphatic tissues
D. All of the above

ILDs involve parenchyma of lung-alveoli, alveolar epithelium, capillary endothelium, & spaces between these structures, as well as perivascular & lymphatic tissues.

741. Which of the following conditions has a strong association with smoking?

Harrison's 20th Ed. Chapter 287 Page 1999 Table 287-1

A. Idiopathic pulmonary fibrosis (IPF)
B. Nonspecific interstitial pneumonia
C. Respiratory bronchiolitis associated ILD
D. Systemic sclerosis associated ILD

742. Digital clubbing is common in which of the following conditions?

Harrison's 20th Ed. Chapter 287 Page 1999 Table 287-1

A. Idiopathic pulmonary fibrosis (IPF)
B. Nonspecific interstitial pneumonia
C. Sarcoidosis
D. Systemic sclerosis associated ILD

743. Lung response is alveolitis, interstitial inflammation and fibrosis in all of the following ILDs except?

Harrison's 19th Ed. 1708, Table 315-1

A. Hypersensitivity pneumonitis
B. Goodpasture's syndrome
C. Idiopathic pulmonary hemosiderosis
D. Asbestosis

ILDs are groups in two based on the major underlying histopathology i.e. they are either associated with predominant inflammation and fibrosis or they have predominantly granulomatous reaction in interstitial or vascular areas. Hypersensitivity pneumonitis belongs to the later group.

744. Etiology of which of the following interstitial lung diseases is known?

Harrison's 20th Ed. Chapter 287 Page 2000

A. Sarcoidosis
B. Idiopathic pulmonary fibrosis (IPF)
C. Pulmonary fibrosis associated with CTDs
D. None of the above

Sarcoidosis, IPF and pulmonary fibrosis associated with connective tissue diseases (CTD) are the most common ILDs of unknown etiology. Among the ILDs of known cause, the largest group includes occupational & environmental exposures.

745. Which of the following is quite rare among patients < 50 years?
Harrison's 20th Ed. Chapter 287 Page 2000

A. Sarcoidosis
B. Idiopathic pulmonary fibrosis (IPF)
C. Pulmonary Langerhans cell histiocytosis (PLCH)
D. Lymphangioleiomyomatosis (LAM)

IPF occurs most commonly in patients >60 years and is quite rare among patients <50 years.

746. Which of the following is a pathologic hallmark of IPF?
Harrison's 20th Ed. Chapter 287 Page 2000

A. Usual interstitial pneumonia (UIP)
B. Non-specific interstitial pneumonia (NSIP)
C. Cryptogenic organizing pneumonia (COP)
D. Desquamative interstitial pneumonia (DIP)

On HRCT chest, classic UIP pattern is considered diagnostic of IPF.

747. Which of the following ILD tends to present between the ages of 20 and 40 years?
Harrison's 20th Ed. Chapter 287 Page 2000

A. Sarcoidosis
B. Lymphangioleiomyomatosis (LAM)
C. Pulmonary Langerhans cell histiocytosis (PLCH)
D. All of the above

ILDs like sarcoidosis, CTD associated ILD, LAM, pulmonary Langerhans cell histiocytosis (PLCH) tend to present between 20 and 40 years of age.

748. ILDs that present at age < 50 years include all except?
Harrison's 20th Ed. Chapter 287 Page 2000

A. IPF
B. Lymphangioleiomyomatosis (LAM)
C. PLCH
D. Sarcoidosis

Most patients with sarcoidosis, ILD associated with CTD, lymphangio-leiomyomatosis (LAM), PLCH, and inherited forms of ILD (familial IPF, Gaucher's disease, Hermansky-Pudlak syndrome) present between the ages of 20 and 40 years. Most patients with IPF are older than 50 years.

749. Interstitial lung disease in which of these conditions is more common in men?
Harrison's 20th Ed. Chapter 287 Page 2000

A. Lymphangioleiomyomatosis (LAM)
B. Tuberous sclerosis
C. Hermansky-Pudlak syndrome
D. Rheumatoid arthritis

LAM & pulmonary involvement in tuberous sclerosis occur exclusively in premenopausal women. ILD in Hermansky-Pudlak syndrome & in CTDs is more common in women. ILD in rheumatoid arthritis (RA) is more common in men. IPF and pneumoconioses is more common in men.

750. Which of the following ILDs relate to tuberous sclerosis?
Harrison's 20th Ed. Chapter 287 Page 2000

A. Sarcoidosis
B. Lymphangioleiomyomatosis (LAM)
C. Pulmonary Langerhans cell histiocytosis (PLCH)
D. Idiopathic pulmonary fibrosis (IPF)

751. ILDs with symptoms and signs form a chronic presentation include all except?
Harrison's 20th Ed. Chapter 287 Page 2000

A. Sarcoidosis
B. Pulmonary Langerhans cell histiocytosis (PLCH)
C. Churg-Strauss syndrome
D. IPF

ILDs with s/s as a chronic presentation (months to years) include IPF, sarcoidosis, pulmonary Langerhans cell histiocytosis (PLCH), pneumoconioses, and CTDs.

752. ILDs with acute presentation include all except?
Harrison's 20th Ed. Chapter 287 Page 2000

A. Sarcoidosis
B. Eosinophilic pneumonia
C. Hypersensitivity pneumonitis
D. Churg-Strauss syndrome

Acute presentation (days to weeks) occurs with allergy (drugs, fungi, helminths), acute interstitial pneumonia (AIP), eosinophilic pneumonia, hypersensitivity pneumonitis & granulomatosis with polyangiitis (GPA). Episodic presentations include eosinophilic pneumonia, hypersensitivity pneumonitis, COP, vasculitides, pulmonary hemorrhage, and Churg-Strauss syndrome.

753. ILDs with acute presentation include?
Harrison's 20th Ed. Chapter 287 Page 2000

A. Sarcoidosis
B. Drug-induced ILDs
C. Cryptogenic organizing pneumonia (COP)
D. All of the above

Subacute presentations (weeks to months) can occur in most of the ILDs (sarcoidosis, CTD associated ILD, drug-induced ILD, or COP).

754. Which of the following features is most frequent in ILD patients?
Harrison's 20th Ed. Chapter 287 Page 2000

A. Wheezing
B. Chest pain
C. Progressive exertional dyspnea
D. Hemoptysis

Patients with ILDs seek medical attention mainly due to progressive exertional dyspnea or a persistent, nonproductive cough. Hemoptysis, wheezing, and chest pain may be present.

755. Patients with idiopathic pulmonary fibrosis typically have all the following features except?
Harrison's 20th Ed. Chapter 287 Page 2000

A. Exertional dyspnea
B. Productive cough
C. Fine bibasilar inspiratory crackles
D. An abnormal chest radiograph on presentation

Cough, particularly a dry cough can be the most prominent symptom in patients with IPF.

756. In ILD, cough with hemoptysis suggests?
Harrison's 20th Ed. Chapter 287 Page 2000

A. Goodpasture's syndrome
B. GPA
C. LAM
D. Any of the above

In ILD, cough with hemoptysis is rare. However it could suggest an ILD associated with diffuse alveolar hemorrhage (DAH) (Goodpasture's syndrome), GPA, or LAM.

757. Which of the following anti-neoplastic agent can cause ILD?
Harrison's 20th Ed. Chapter 287 Page 2001

A. Cyclophosphamide
B. Bleomycin
C. Cyclosporine
D. All of the above

758. Which of the following medicines can cause ILD?
Harrison's 20th Ed. Chapter 287 Page 2001

A. Nitrofurantoin
B. Amiodarone
C. Bleomycin
D. All of the above

Nitrofurantoin, amiodarone and bleomycin are known to cause ILD.

759. Gene involved in the maintenance of telomere length is?
N Engl J Med 2018;378:1811-23

A. TERT
B. TERC
C. PARN
D. All of the above

Mutations in TERT, TERC, PARN, and RTEL1 are the genes involved in the maintenance of telomere length. They are associated with an increased risk of IPF.

760. Which of the following gene is associated with both familial and idiopathic forms of pulmonary fibrosis?
Harrison's 20th Ed. Chapter 287 Page 2001

A. APOL1
B. GANAB
C. TERT
D. TSC2

761. Which of the following gene is associated with both familial and idiopathic forms of pulmonary fibrosis?
Harrison's 20th Ed. Chapter 287 Page 2001

A. MUC5B
B. MUC1
C. UMOD
D. REN

Replicated genetic factors for pulmonary fibrosis (both familial & idiopathic forms) include a mucin gene (MUC5B) and telomerase reverse transcriptase gene (TERT).

762. Which of the following is called smoking related ILD?
Harrison's 20th Ed. Chapter 287 Page 2001

A. Desquamative interstitial pneumonia (DIP)
B. Sarcoidosis
C. Usual interstitial pneumonia (UIP)
D. Non-specific interstitial pneumonia (NSIP)

763. Patients with all of the following are almost always current or former smokers except?
Harrison's 20th Ed. Chapter 287 Page 2001

A. Pulmonary Langerhans cell histiocytosis (PLCH)
B. Lymphangioleiomyomatosis (LAM)
C. Desquamative interstitial pneumonia (DIP)
D. Goodpasture's syndrome

Patients with PLCH, desquamative interstitial pneumonia (DIP), Goodpasture's syndrome, respiratory bronchiolitis, and pulmonary alveolar proteinosis are almost always current or former smokers. 75% of patients with IPF have a history of smoking.

764. Which of the following may be one of the earliest signs of the ILD?
Harrison's 20th Ed. Chapter 287 Page 2001

A. End-inspiratory fine crackles
B. End-expiratory fine crackles
C. End-inspiratory coarse crackles
D. End-expiratory coarse crackles

End-inspiratory fine crackles at lung bases are found in most patients with IPF and may be one of the earliest signs of the disease.

765. Wheezing can be found in which of the following forms of ILD?
Harrison's 20th Ed. Chapter 287 Page 2001

A. Sarcoidosis
B. Hypersensitivity pneumonitis (HP)
C. Eosinophilic GPA
D. All of the above

Wheezing is uncommon in most forms of ILD but can be present in sarcoidosis, HP, and eosinophilic GPA.

766. Which of the following is a sign of advanced ILD?
Harrison's 20th Ed. Chapter 287 Page 2001

A. Cyanosis
B. Digital clubbing
C. Cor pulmonale
D. All of the above

Signs of advanced ILD include cyanosis, digital clubbing, cor pulmonale & honeycombing on HRCT.

767. Pulmonary-function test in patients with idiopathic pulmonary fibrosis will show?
Harrison's 20th Ed. Chapter 287 Page 2001

A. Reduction in total lung capacity
B. Reduction in functional residual capacity
C. Reduction in residual volume
D. All of the above

Most forms of ILD produce a restrictive defect with reduced total lung capacity (TLC), functional residual capacity, and residual volume. FEV_1 and FVC are reduced, but these changes are related to the decreased TLC. FEV_1/FVC ratio is usually normal or increased. Lung volumes decrease as lung stiffness worsens with disease progression.

768. Which of the following is typical of interstitial lung diseases?
N Engl J Med 2018;378:1811-23

A. Reduced forced vital capacity (FVC)
B. Reduced total lung capacity
C. Reduction in DLco
D. All of the above

A reduced forced vital capacity (FVC), a reduced total lung capacity, and a reduction in DLco are typical of interstitial lung diseases.

769. Spirometric results and lung volumes can be normal in early ILD or when which of the following is also present?

N Engl J Med 2018;378:1811-23

A. Chronic bronchitis
B. Emphysema
C. Asthma
D. Pulmonary embolism

Spirometric results and lung volumes can be normal during the early stages of interstitial lung disease or when emphysema is also present.

770. Which of the following about decreased DI_{CO} in most ILDs is false?

Harrison's 20th Ed. Chapter 287 Page 2001

A. Common nonspecific finding in most ILDs
B. Due to mismatching of ventilation & perfusion (V/Q)
C. Does not correlate with disease stage
D. None of the above

771. Secondary interstitial pneumonia best relates to?

Harrison's 20th Ed. Chapter 287 Page 2001

A. Idiopathic pulmonary fibrosis (IPF)
B. Non-specific interstitial pneumonia (NSIP)
C. Desquamative interstitial pneumonia (DIP)
D. Connective tissue disease-associated ILDs

772. Which of the following chest X-ray findings is indicative of a poor prognosis in a case of ILD?

Harrison's 20th Ed. Chapter 287 Page 2002

A. Bibasilar reticular pattern
B. Honeycombing
C. Nodular pattern of alveolar filling
D. Mixed pattern of alveolar filling

Most common chest radiograph abnormality in ILD is a bibasilar reticular pattern. Radiographic finding of honeycombing suggests small cystic spaces & progressive fibrosis which carry a poor prognosis.

773. Chest CT findings in IPF include?

Harrison's 20th Ed. Chapter 287 Page 2002

A. Subpleural reticulation with a posterior basal predominance
B. Honeycombing
C. Traction bronchiectasis
D. All of the above

774. Which of the following is included to describe a UIP pattern?

Harrison's 20th Ed. Chapter 287 Page 2002

A. Subpleural reticulation with a posterior basal predominance
B. Honeycombing
C. Traction bronchiectasis
D. All of the above

775. Which of the following finding on HRCT goes against the diagnosis of IPF?

Harrison's 20th Ed. Chapter 287 Page 2002

A. Extensive ground glass opacities
B. Mosaic attenuation
C. Upper lung predominance
D. All of the above

Chest CT findings of subpleural reticulation with posterior basal predominance, honeycombing and traction bronchiectasis collectively are referred to as a UIP pattern - diagnostic of IPF. Presence of extensive ground glass opacities, bronchovascular changes, micronodules, mosaic attenuation, or an upper lung predominance raises suspicion for an alternative diagnosis.

776. Honeycombing best relates to?

Harrison's 20th Ed. Chapter 287 Page 2002

A. Necrosis
B. Fibrosis
C. Apoptosis
D. All of the above

777. Pathologic changes that characterize idiopathic pulmonary fibrosis are all except?

N Engl J Med. 2001; 345:517

A. Predilection for peripheral subpleural parenchyma
B. Fibrotic zones with associated honeycombing alternate with areas of relatively unaffected lung tissue
C. Fibrotic areas vary in age and activity
D. "Fibroblast foci" occur at sites of chronic lung injury

"Fibroblast foci" occur at sites of acute lung injury.

778. HRCT in idiopathic pulmonary fibrosis shows all except?

Harrison's 20th Ed. Chapter 287 Page 2002 Figure 287-2

A. Bibasal peripheral lower lobe reticular opacities
B. Peripheral "honeycombing"
C. Traction bronchiectasis
D. Pleural thickening

HRCT lung scans in IPF show patchy, predominantly basilar, subpleural reticular opacities, with traction bronchiectasis and honeycombing.

779. HRCT finding that goes against the diagnosis of idiopathic pulmonary fibrosis is?

Harrison's 20th Ed. Chapter 287 Page 2002

A. Extensive ground-glass abnormality
B. Nodular opacities with upper or mid-zone predominance
C. Prominent hilar or mediastinal lymphadenopathy
D. All of the above

HRCT findings that suggest an alternative diagnosis to IPF include extensive ground-glass abnormality, nodular opacities, upper or mid-zone predominance & prominent hilar or mediastinal lymphadenopathy.

780. Reversed halo or atoll sign best relates to?

Harrison's 20th Ed. Chapter 287 Page 2002 Figure 287-2

A. Idiopathic pulmonary fibrosis (IPF)
B. Non-specific interstitial pneumonia (NSIP)
C. Cryptogenic organizing pneumonia (COP)
D. Sarcoidosis

Reversed halo or atoll sign refers to peribronchiolar, or perilobar opacities with a rim of subpleural sparing - diagnostic of cryptogenic organizing pneumonia (COP).

781. Mosaic attenuation best relates to?
Harrison's 20th Ed. Chapter 287 Page 2002 Figure 287-2

A. Large airways involvement
B. Small airways involvement
C. Bronchovascular bundles
D. Ground glass infiltrates

782. Which of the following statements about ILDs is false?
Harrison's 20th Ed. Chapter 287 Page 1999

A. Non-malignant disorders
B. Not caused by identified infectious agents
C. May have granulomatous or inflammatory/fibrosis pattern
D. None of the above

ILDs are nonmalignant disorders not caused by identified infectious agents. Two major histopathologic patterns are granulomatous or inflammation & fibrosis.

783. Granulomas in granulomatous lung disease consists of?
Harrison's 20th Ed. Chapter 287 Page 1999

A. T lymphocytes
B. Macrophages
C. Epithelioid cells
D. All of the above

Granulomas in granulomatous lung disease consist of T lymphocytes, macrophages, and epithelioid cells organized into discrete structures in the lung parenchyma. Granulomatous lesions can progress to fibrosis. Sarcoidosis and hypersensitivity pneumonitis are prime examples.

784. The initial insult leading to inflammation and fibrosis in ILD is to?
Harrison's 20th Ed. Chapter 287 Page 1999

A. Vascular endothelium
B. Epithelial surface
C. Perivascular tissues
D. Lymphatic tissues

The initial insult is an injury to the epithelial surface that causes inflammation in the air spaces and alveolar walls. Inflammation spreads to adjacent portions of interstitium and vasculature and eventually causes interstitial fibrosis.

785. Which of the following is usually not a clinical feature of sarcoidosis?
Harrison's 20th Ed. Chapter 287 Page 1999

A. Dyspnea
B. Wheezing
C. Hemoptysis
D. Substernal chest pain

Dyspnea is a common and prominent complaint in patients with ILD, especially sarcoidosis. Wheezing and clinically significant chest pain, though uncommon in ILD, is noted in patients with sarcoidosis. Frank hemoptysis rarely a presenting manifestations of sarcoidosis.

786. Frank hemoptysis in ILD suggests the possibility which of the following ILDs?
Harrison's 20th Ed. Chapter 287 Page 2000

A. Diffuse alveolar hemorrhage (DAH) syndromes
B. Lymphangioleiomyomatosis (LAM)
C. GPA
D. Any of the above

Frank hemoptysis and blood-streaked sputum are rarely presenting manifestations of ILD but can be seen in the diffuse alveolar hemorrhage (DAH) syndromes, LAM, tuberous sclerosis, and the granulomatous vasculitides.

787. Which of the following is an unusual manifestation in ILDs?
Harrison's 20th Ed. Chapter 287 Page 2000

A. Wheezing
B. Clinically significant chest pain
C. Frank hemoptysis
D. All of the above

788. Which of the following laboratory abnormality is common in sarcoidosis?
Harrison's 20th Ed. Chapter 287 Page 2000

A. Elevated serum angiotensin-converting enzyme level
B. Presence of serum precipitins
C. Antineutrophil cytoplasmic antibodies
D. Anti-basement membrane antibodies

Elevation of serum ACE level is common in sarcoidosis.

789. In which of the following ILDs, nodular opacities in upper lung zones is frequent?
Harrison's 20th Ed. Chapter 287 Page 2001

A. Sarcoidosis
B. PLCH
C. Chronic hypersensitivity pneumonitis
D. All of the above

ILDs that show nodular opacities with a predilection for the upper lung zones include sarcoidosis, PLCH, chronic hypersensitivity pneumonitis, silicosis, berylliosis, RA (necrobiotic nodular form), and ankylosing spondylitis.

790. Which of the following is a bronchoalveolar lavage (BAL) finding in sarcoidosis?
Harrison's 20th Ed. Chapter 260 Page 2605

A. Eosinophils >25%
B. Hemosiderin-laden macrophages
C. CD4 : CD8 ratio > 3.5
D. Atypical hyperplastic type II pneumocytes

791. Birbeck granule best relates with?
Harrison's 20th Ed. Chapter 106 Page 792

A. Eosinophilic lung disease
B. Pulmonary Langerhans cell histiocytosis
C. Hypersensitivity pneumonitis
D. Berylliosis

792. Marked lymphocytosis (>50%) in bronchoalveolar lavage (BAL) is a feature of?
Harrison's 20th Ed. Chapter 282 Page 1971

A. Organizing pneumonia
B. Eosinophilic lung disease
C. Hypersensitivity pneumonitis
D. Pulmonary Langerhans cell histiocytosis

793. Which of the following is false about idiopathic pulmonary fibrosis?

Harrison's 20th Ed. Chapter 287 Page 1999

A. Most common form of idiopathic interstitial pneumonia
B. Has a distinctly poor response to therapy
C. Has a bad prognosis
D. None of the above

794. Usual interstitial pneumonia (UIP), nonspecific interstitial pneumonia, organizing pneumonia etc are categories of ILD based on?

Harrison's 20th Ed. Chapter 287 Page 2004

A. Clinical presentation
B. Radiological findings
C. Histopathologic patterns
D. Response to treatment

Important histopathologic patterns found in ILDs include usual interstitial pneumonia (UIP), nonspecific interstitial pneumonia, respiratory bronchiolitis/desquamative interstitial pneumonia, organizing pneumonia, diffuse alveolar damage (acute or organizing), and lymphocytic interstitial pneumonia.

795. Histologic hallmark of Usual interstitial pneumonia (UIP) is?

Harrison's 20th Ed. Chapter 287 Page 2003 Figure 287-3

A. Alternating areas of normal lung & interstitial inflammation
B. Foci of proliferating fibroblasts
C. Dense collagen fibrosis
D. All of the above

The histologic hallmark and chief diagnostic criterion of UIP is a heterogeneous appearance at low magnification with alternating areas of normal lung, interstitial inflammation, foci of proliferating fibroblasts, dense collagen fibrosis, and honeycomb changes affecting peripheral, subpleural parenchyma most severely. Lesion is idiopathic and not associated with another condition.

796. Which of the following drug improves cough in patients with IPF?

N Engl J Med 2018;378:1811-23

A. N-acetylcysteine (NAC)
B. Warfarin
C. Thalidomide
D. Glucocorticoids

There is no effective therapy for IPF. Thalidomide appears to improve cough in patients with IPF.

797. In patients with idiopathic pulmonary fibrosis, which of the following antifibrotic agent slows loss of lung function?

N Engl J Med 2018;378:1811-23

A. Dapsone
B. Pirfenidone
C. Statins
D. Triamcinolone

Recent clinical trials show benefit of pirfenidone and of nintedanib in patients with idiopathic pulmonary fibrosis, with significant slowing of the loss of lung function.

798. Which of the following drug is effective in acute exacerbations of IPF?

N Engl J Med 2018;378:1811-23

A. Glucocorticoids
B. Azathioprine
C. Interferon gamma-1b
D. None of the above

No therapy has been found to be effective in the management of acute exacerbations of IPF.

799. Which of the following drug is safe and effective in the treatment of IPF?

N Engl J Med 2018;378:1811-23

A. Nintedanib
B. Vandetanib
C. Cabozantinib
D. Axitinib

Nintedanib is a tyrosine kinase inhibitor that targets growth factor pathways, including those downstream from vascular endothelial growth factor receptors 1, 2, and 3, fibroblast growth factor receptors 1, 2, and 3, and platelet-derived growth factor receptor.

800. Patients with IPF are at increased risk for?

N Engl J Med 2018;378:1811-23

A. Venous thromboembolism
B. Lung cancer
C. Pulmonary hypertension
D. All of the above

Patients with IPF are at increased risk for venous thromboembolism, lung cancer, and pulmonary hypertension.

801. Which of the following about Idiopathic Nonspecific Interstitial Pneumonia (NSIP) is false?

Harrison's 20th Ed. Chapter 287 Page 2003

A. Good prognosis
B. Presents at a younger age
C. Occurs in women who have never smoked
D. None of the above

Idiopathic NSIP is a subacute restrictive process with presentation similar to IPF, most common in women of younger age who have never smoked.

802. Typical feature of NSIP is?

Harrison's 20th Ed. Chapter 287 Page 2003

A. Honeycombing
B. Uniformity of interstitial involvement
C. Nodular lesions
D. Pleural calcification

HRCT of NSIP shows bilateral, subpleural ground-glass opacities. Honeycombing is unusual. Key histopathologic features are uniformity of interstitial involvement across biopsy section.

803. Which of the following is a feature of idiopathic NSIP?

Harrison's 20th Ed. Chapter 287 Page 2003

A. Honeycombing is unusual
B. Uniformity of interstitial involvement across biopsy section
C. Improvement after treatment with glucocorticoids
D. All of the above

804. Hamman Rich Syndrome is the name given to?

Harrison's 20th Ed. Chapter 287 Page 2004

A. Acute interstitial pneumonia (AIP)
B. Hypersensitivity pneumonitis
C. Desquamative interstitial pneumonia (DIP)
D. Respiratory bronchiolitis

Hamman Rich Syndrome refers to acute interstitial pneumonia (AIP).

805. Which of the following is a fulminant form of ILD?

Harrison's 20th Ed. Chapter 287 Page 2004

A. Acute interstitial pneumonia (AIP)
B. Hypersensitivity pneumonitis
C. Desquamative interstitial pneumonia (DIP)
D. Respiratory bronchiolitis

AIP is a fulminant form of lung injury characterized histologically by diffuse alveolar damage on lung biopsy. Onset of drug-Induced ILD may be abrupt and fulminant, or insidious.

806. AIP is similar in presentation to?

Harrison's 20th Ed. Chapter 287 Page 2004

A. Spontaneous pneumothorax
B. Acute respiratory distress syndrome (ARDS)
C. Bronchial asthma
D. CHF

AIP is similar in presentation to acute respiratory distress syndrome (ARDS).

807. Which of the following is known as idiopathic BOOP?

Harrison's 20th Ed. Chapter 287 Page 2004

A. Cryptogenic organizing pneumonia
B. Desquamative interstitial pneumonia
C. Respiratory bronchiolitis
D. Lymphocytic interstitial pneumonia

Cryptogenic Organizing Pneumonia (COP) is also known as idiopathic BOOP (bronchiolitis obliterans with organizing pneumonia).

808. Which of the following ILD is associated with cigarette smoking?

Harrison's 20th Ed. Chapter 287 Page 2003

A. Desquamative interstitial pneumonia (DIP)
B. Respiratory bronchiolitis - associated ILD (RB-ILD)
C. Pulmonary Langerhans cell histiocytosis (PLCH)
D. All of the above

809. Which of the following is false about desquamative interstitial pneumonia (DIP)?

Harrison's 20th Ed. Chapter 287 Page 2000

A. Found exclusively in cigarette smokers
B. Macrophages in intraalveolar spaces
C. Minimal interstitial fibrosis
D. Has a worse prognosis than IPF

DIP occurs exclusively in cigarette smokers. Histologic hallmark is diffuse and uniform accumulation of macrophages in intraalveolar spaces with minimal interstitial fibrosis. DIP has a better prognosis than IPF.

810. Which of the following about Pulmonary Langerhans Cell Histiocytosis (PLCH) is false?

Harrison's 20th Ed. Chapter 287 Page 2000

A. Smoking-related
B. HRCT shows nodules & thin-walled cysts
C. Increased DLCO
D. Persistent/progressive disease

Most frequent pulmonary function abnormality is a markedly reduced DL_{CO} along with restrictive disease pattern, airflow limitation & diminished exercise capacity.

811. Radiographic features of PLCH include all except?

Harrison's 20th Ed. Chapter 287 Page 2000

A. Reticular or nodular opacities
B. Bizarre-shaped, thin-walled upper zone cysts
C. Honeycombing
D. Sparing of the costophrenic angles

CxR of PLCH include a ill-defined or stellate nodules, reticular or nodular opacities, bizarre-shaped upper zone thin-walled cysts & sparing of costophrenic angles. Honeycombing is a feature of IPF.

812. Most common form of pulmonary involvement in connective tissue disorders is?

Harrison's 20th Ed. Chapter 287 Page 2003

A. Respiratory bronchiolitis
B. Desquamative interstitial pneumonia
C. Cryptogenic organizing pneumonia
D. Nonspecific interstitial pneumonia

Commonest form of pulmonary involvement in connective tissue disorders is nonspecific interstitial pneumonia.

813. NSIP histopathologic pattern means?

Harrison's 20th Ed. Chapter 287 Page 2003

A. Uniformity of interstitial involvement
B. Less temporal and spatial heterogeneity
C. Little or no honeycombing
D. All of the above

814. UIP histopathologic pattern means?

Harrison's 20th Ed. Chapter 287 Page 2002

A. Affect peripheral, subpleural parenchyma mostly
B. Alternating areas of normal lung & interstitial inflammation
C. Honeycombing common
D. All of the above

815. Rheumatoid pneumoconiosis is also called?

Harrison's 20th Ed. Chapter 283 Page 1979

A. Hermansky-Pudlak syndrome
B. Churg-Strauss syndrome
C. Caplan's syndrome
D. Goodpasture's syndrome

Caplan's syndrome is the term given to rheumatoid pneumoconiosis. Caplan's syndrome is a rare subset of pulmonary nodulosis characterized by the development of nodules and pneumoconiosis following silica exposure.

816. Pulmonary manifestations of RA include?

Harrison's 20th Ed. Chapter 351 Page 2529

A. Pleurisy with or without effusion
B. Nonpneumoconiotic intrapulmonary rheumatoid nodules
C. Organized pneumonia
D. All of the above

Pulmonary manifestations of RA include pleurisy with or without effusion, ILD, necrobiotic nodules (nonpneumoconiotic intrapulmonary rheumatoid nodules) with or without cavities, Caplan syndrome (rheumatoid pneumoconiosis), pulmonary hypertension secondary to rheumatoid pulmonary vasculitis, organized pneumonia and upper airway obstruction due to cricoarytenoid arthritis.

817. Which of the following is the most common pulmonary manifestation of RA?

Harrison's 20th Ed. Chapter 351 Page 2529

A. Pleuritis
B. Interstitial lung disease (ILD)
C. Respiratory bronchiolitis
D. Bronchiectasis

Pleuritis, the most common pulmonary manifestation of RA, may produce pleuritic chest pain and dyspnea, as well as a pleural friction rub and effusion. Pleural effusions tend to be exudative with increased numbers of monocytes and neutrophils.

818. Most common pulmonary manifestation in Systemic Lupus Erythematosus (SLE) is?

Harrison's 20th Ed. Chapter 351 Page 2520

A. Atelectasis
B. Pleuritis
C. Pulmonary vascular disease
D. Infectious pneumonia

Pleuritis with or without effusion is the most common pulmonary manifestation in SLE.

819. Which of the following diseases is associated with ILD?

Harrison's 20th Ed. Chapter 287 Page 2005

A. Systemic sclerosis (SSc)
B. Sjogren's syndrome
C. Ankylosing spondylitis (AS)
D. All of the above

820. ILD occurs more commonly in the subgroup of polymyositis & dermatomyositis patients having which antibody?

Harrison's 20th Ed. Chapter 287 Page 2005

A. Anti-Smith antibody
B. Anti-Ro antibody
C. Anti-Jo-1 antibody
D. Anti-La antibody

80% of patients of PM/DM with anti-Jo-1 antibodies (directed to histidyl tRNA synthetase) have interstitial lung disease.

821. Which of the following about pulmonary alveolar proteinosis (PAP) is false?

Can Respir J 2012;19(4):243-245

A. Impaired ability to process surfactant
B. Accumulation of PAS positive lipoproteinaceous material in distal air spaces
C. Extensive lung inflammation
D. Preserved lung architecture

There is a defect in macrophage function with impaired ability to process surfactant. Amorphous, PAS-positive lipoproteinaceous material accumulates in distal air spaces. There is little or no lung inflammation, and the underlying lung architecture is preserved.

822. In pulmonary alveolar proteinosis (PAP), the neutralizing IgG antibody is against which of the following?

Can Respir J 2012;19(4):243-245

A. Surfactant
B. GM-CSF
C. PAS positive lipoproteinaceous material
D. All of the above

PAP is an autoimmune disease with neutralizing antibody of IgG isotype against granulocyte-macrophage colony-stimulating factor (GM-CSF). Neutralization of GM-CSF bioactivity by the antibody causes dysfunction of alveolar macrophages, which results in reduced surfactant clearance. Elevated serum anti-GM-CSF titer is highly sensitive & specific for diagnosis of acquired PAP.

823. Which of the following is the most common class of Pulmonary Alveolar Proteinosis (PAP)?

Can Respir J 2012;19(4):243-245

A. Acquired
B. Congenital
C. Secondary
D. None of the above

There are three distinct classes of PAP. Acquired (>90%), congenital, and secondary.

824. Secondary pulmonary alveolar proteinosis (PAP) is caused by which of the following malignancies?

Can Respir J 2012;19(4):243-245

A. Lung
B. Pleural
C. Hematopoietic
D. Hepatic

825. Secondary PAP is caused by?

Can Respir J 2012;19(4):243-245

A. Lysinuric protein intolerance
B. Acute silicosis
C. Hematopoietic malignancies
D. All of the above

Secondary PAP is caused by lysinuric protein intolerance, acute silicosis, immuno-deficiency disorders, hematopoietic malignancies and hematopoietic disorders.

826. Congenital PAP is caused by mutation in?

Can Respir J 2012;19(4):243-245

A. SP-A gene
B. SP-B gene
C. SP-C gene
D. SP-D gene

Congenital PAP is transmitted in autosomal recessive manner & is caused by mutation in SP-B gene.

827. In PAP, which of the following is frequent?

Can Respir J 2012;19(4):243-245

A. Polycythemia
B. Hypergammaglobulinemia
C. Increased LDH
D. All of the above

Apart from elevated serum levels of lung surfactant proteins A & D, polycythemia, hypergammaglobulinemia and increased LDH levels are frequent in PAP.

828. Radiographically, 'bat-wing' distribution of lung opacities is suggestive of which of the following?

Can Respir J 2012;19(4):243-245

A. Churg-Strauss syndrome
B. Pulmonary lymphangioleiomyomatosis (LAM)
C. Pulmonary alveolar proteinosis (PAP)
D. Goodpasture's syndrome

Radiographically, bilateral symmetric alveolar opacities located centrally in mid and lower lung zones result in a 'bat-wing' distribution in PAP.

829. Pulmonary lymphangioleiomyomatosis (LAM) is seen in?

Harrison's 20th Ed. Chapter 287 Page 2000

A. Female child
B. Premenopausal women
C. Postmenopausal women
D. Any of the above

Pulmonary LAM afflicts premenopausal women and should be suspected in young women with emphysema, recurrent pneumothorax, or chylous pleural effusion. The disease accelerates during pregnancy and abates after oopherectomy.

830. In pulmonary lymphangioleiomyomatosis (LAM), there occurs proliferation of which of the following?

Lung India 2018;35:154-6

A. Type 1 pneumocytes
B. Type 2 pneumocytes
C. Pulmonary lymphatic vessels
D. Atypical pulmonary interstitial smooth muscle

Pathologically, pulmonary LAM is characterized by the proliferation of atypical pulmonary interstitial smooth muscle and cyst formation.

831. Atypical smooth-muscle cells that proliferate in pulmonary lymphangioleiomyomatosis (LAM) react with which of the following monoclonal antibody?

Lung India 2018;35:154-6

A. HMB42
B. HMB43
C. HMB44
D. HMB45

Immature-appearing smooth-muscle cells react with monoclonal antibody HMB45, which recognizes gp100 originally found in human melanoma cells.

832. Which of the following modalities of treatment is useful in pulmonary lymphangioleiomyomatosis (LAM)?

Eur Respir J 2006; 27: 1056–1065

A. Oophorectomy
B. Progesterone
C. Tamoxifen
D. All of the above

Oophorectomy, progesterone, sirolimus, tamoxifen & luteinizing hormone-releasing hormone analogues have been used in pulmonary LAM. Lung transplantation offers the only hope for cure.

833. Inherited diseases that produce interstitial lung disease include?

Clin Chest Med 33:95, 2012

A. Tuberous sclerosis
B. Neurofibromatosis
C. Niemann-Pick disease
D. All of the above

834. Inherited diseases that produce interstitial lung disease include?

Clin Chest Med 33:95, 2012

A. Gaucher's disease
B. Hermansky-Pudlak syndrome
C. Niemann-Pick disease
D. All of the above

Inherited disorders associated with ILD include phakomatoses, tuberous sclerosis, neurofibromatosis, Niemann-Pick disease, Gaucher's disease and Hermansky-Pudlak syndrome.

835. Which of the following may cause interstitial lung disease (ILD)?

Harrison's 20th Ed. Chapter 71 Page 521

A. Imatinib
B. Erlotinib
C. Gefitinib
D. All of the above

Molecular targeted agents like imatinib, erlotinib and gefitinib are potent inhibitors of tyrosine kinases and may cause interstitial lung disease (ILD).

Disorders of the Pleura

836. Parietal pleura covers which of the following?
N Engl J Med 2018;378:740-51

A. Chest wall
B. Diaphragm
C. Mediastinum
D. All of the above

Pleural space is between the visceral and parietal pleura. Visceral pleura cover the lungs while parietal pleura covers the chest wall, diaphragm, and mediastinum. In humans, parietal & visceral pleura merge at the hilum of lungs. Elephants do not have a pleural space.

837. Pressure in the pleural space is?
N Engl J Med 2018;378:740-51

A. 3 to 5 mm of water
B. (-) 3 to (-) 5 mm of water
C. 3 to 5 cm of water
D. (-) 3 to (-) 5 cm of water

Pressure in the pleural space is negative, approximately −3 to −5 cm of water.

838. Which of the following is produced by pleurae?
N Engl J Med 2018;378:740-51

A. Hyaluronic acid rich glycoproteins
B. Nitric oxide
C. Transforming growth factor β
D. All of the above

The pleurae are covered by metabolically active mesothelial cells which produce hyaluronic acid rich glycoproteins, nitric oxide and transforming growth factor β.

839. In normal humans, what volume of fluid is contained within each pleural cavity?
N Engl J Med 2018;378:740-51

A. ~ 0.16 mL per kilogram body weight
B. ~ 0.26 mL per kilogram body weight
C. ~ 0.36 mL per kilogram body weight
D. ~ 0.46 mL per kilogram body weight

In normal humans, approximately 0.26 ml of fluid per kilogram of body weight is contained within each pleural cavity.

840. In healthy adults, pleural space contains how much of pleural fluid?
Cleveland Clinic Journal Of Medicine 2008;75:303

A. 5 to 10 mL
B. 25 to 50 mL
C. 50 to 100 mL
D. 100 to 150 mL

In healthy adults, pleural space contains ~ 5 to 10 mL of pleural fluid (0.1 mg/kg body weight).

841. Which of the following is not related to pleural effusion?
Cleveland Clinic Journal Of Medicine 2008;75:303

A. Skodaic resonance
B. Calot's triangle
C. Grocco triangle
D. Garland triangle

Skodaic resonance (area of hyperresonance above a pleural effusion), Succussion splash (splashing sound produced by violently shaking patients with hydropneumothorax), Grocco triangle (right-angle triangle of dullness found over posterior region of chest opposite a large pleural effusion), Garland triangle (small area of resonance next to spine in patients with large unilateral pleural effusions).

842. Contralateral tracheal or mediastinal shift occurs when the size of pleural effusion is?
Cleveland Clinic Journal Of Medicine 2008;75:303

A. 300 – 500 mL
B. 500 – 750 mL
C. 750 – 1000 mL
D. > 1,500 mL

Physical findings are normal if <300 mL of fluid is present. Large effusions (>1500 mL) is associated with significant asymmetry of chest expansion, contralateral tracheal or mediastinal shift and bulging of intercostal spaces.

843. What quantity of pleural fluid must be present to be detected by physical examination?
Cleveland Clinic Journal Of Medicine 2008;75:303

A. 100 mL
B. 150 mL
C. 350 mL
D. 500 mL

At least 500 mL of fluid must be present to be detected an effusion by physical examination.

844. Which of the following statements is false?
Harrison's 20th Ed. Chapter 288 Page 2006

A. Normally, fluid enters pleural space from capillaries in parietal pleura
B. Normally, fluid is removed via lymphatics situated in parietal pleura
C. Fluid can enter pleural space from peritoneal cavity
D. Lymphatics have the capacity to absorb 2 times more fluid than is normally formed in pleural spaces

Lymphatics have a capacity to absorb 20 times more fluid than is normally formed.

845. Which of the following is true for exudative pleural effusions?
Harrison's 20th Ed. Chapter 288 Page 2006

A. Pleural fluid protein/serum protein >0.5
B. Pleural fluid LDH/serum LDH >0.6
C. Pleural fluid LDH > two-thirds normal upper limit for serum
D. All of the above

846. Which of the following is true for transudative pleural effusions?

Harrison's 20th Ed. Chapter 288 Page 2006

A. Pleural fluid protein/serum protein >0.5

B. Pleural fluid LDH/serum LDH >0.6

C. Pleural fluid LDH > two-thirds normal upper limit for serum

D. None of the above

Light's criteria - Out of the following, exudative pleural effusions meet at least one, whereas transudative pleural effusions meet none. Pleural fluid protein/serum protein >0.5, pleural fluid LDH/serum LDH >0.6 and pleural fluid LDH more than two-thirds normal upper limit for serum. Still, if clinically transudative effusion is strongly suspected, difference between albumin levels in serum and pleural fluid is estimated. If this difference is >3.1 g/dL, pleural effusion is transudative.

847. According to Light's criteria, a patient is considered to have an exudative effusion when?

N Engl J Med 2018;378:740-51

A. Ratio of pleural fluid protein to serum protein higher than 0.5

B. Ratio of pleural fluid LDH to serum LDH higher than 0.6

C. Pleural fluid LDH higher than 200 IU per liter

D. Any of the above

According to Light's criteria, a patient is considered to have an exudative effusion when any one of the following findings is present - ratio of pleural fluid protein to serum protein higher than 0.5, ratio of pleural fluid lactate dehydrogenase (LDH) level to serum LDH level higher than 0.6, or a pleural fluid LDH level higher than 200 IU per liter (or >67% of the upper limit of the normal range for serum LDH level).

848. Which of the following statements about pleural effusions is false?

N Engl J Med 2018;378:740-51

A. Light's criteria correctly identify nearly all exudates

B. With Light's criteria, 25% of transudates are misclassified as exudates

C. The error is frequent in patients with congestive heart failure who are receiving diuretic therapy

D. None of the above

Light's criteria correctly identify nearly all exudates, ~25% of transudates are misclassified as exudates, especially in patients who have underlying congestive heart failure and have received diuretics. In patients with suspected CHF who are receiving diuretic therapy, serum protein level that is >3.1 g/dL higher than that in pleural fluid or a serum albumin level that is >1.2 g/dL higher than that in pleural fluid helps in identify transudates that were misclassified as exudates with the use of Light's criteria.

849. Which of the following statements about pleural effusions is false?

N Engl J Med 2018;378:740-51

A. Pleural fluid is primarily produced from the parietal pleura

B. Hydrostatic pressures are higher on parietal pleura than on visceral pleura

C. Oncotic pressures are equivalent on parietal pleura & visceral pleura

D. None of the above

The amount of fluid in the pleural space is dependent on the balance of hydrostatic and oncotic pressures between parietal & visceral pleura and pleural space. Because hydrostatic pressures are higher on the parietal pleura than on the visceral pleura and oncotic pressures are equivalent, pleural fluid is primarily produced from the parietal pleura. Lymphatic vessels on the parietal pleura are responsible for the majority of pleural fluid resorption.

850. Estimation of which of the following helps differentiate exudative effusion from transudative effusion?

N Engl J Med 2018;378:740-51

A. Uric acid

B. CPK

C. Cholesterol

D. All of the above

A pleural fluid protein level >3 gram/dL or a pleural fluid cholesterol level >45 mg/dL has been shown to indicate the presence of an exudative effusion as accurately as Light's criteria.

851. Which of the following test is virtually diagnostic of pleural effusion secondary to congestive heart failure?

Harrison's 20th Ed. Chapter 288 Page 2007, N Engl J Med 2018;378:740-51

A. Pleural fluid LDH

B. Pleural fluid N-terminal pro-brain natriuretic peptide

C. Pleural fluid sodium

D. Pleural fluid osmolality

Pleural fluid NT-pro BNP >1500 pg/mL is virtually diagnostic of an effusion secondary to CHF.

852. Who said "Persons who become affected with empyema after pleurisy, if they get clear of it in forty days from the breaking of it, escape the disease; but if not, it passes into phthisis"?

N Engl J Med 2018;378:740-51

A. Hippocrates

B. William Osler

C. Aristotle

D. Light

853. Most common cause of pleural effusion is?

Harrison's 20th Ed. Chapter 288 Page 2007

A. Left ventricular failure

B. Bacterial pneumonia

C. Cirrhosis liver

D. Viral infection

Most common cause of pleural effusion is LVF. Isolated right-sided pleural effusions are more common than left-sided effusions in heart failure.

854. Which of the following is a cause of transudative effusion?

N Engl J Med 2018;378:740-51

A. Superior vena cava obstruction

B. Myxedema

C. Glomerulonephritis

D. All of the above

855. In the scoring system "RAPID", R stands for?

N Engl J Med 2018;378:740-51

A. Race

B. Renal function

C. Respiratory rate

D. Roentgenographic finding

Rahman developed a scoring system called RAPID (renal function, age, purulence, infection source, and dietary factors) to help identify parapneumonic effusion patients who are at risk for a poor outcome at the time of their presentation.

856. Which of the following is false for 'Hepatic Hydrothorax'?
Harrison's 20th Ed. Chapter 288 Page 2007

A. Occur in ~5% of patients with cirrhosis & ascites
B. Due to direct movement of peritoneal fluid through small holes in diaphragm into pleural space
C. Effusion is usually left-sided
D. Transjugular intrahepatic portal systemic shunt helpful

Hepatic Hydrothorax is usually "right-sided".

857. Parapneumonic effusions are associated with?
Harrison's 20th Ed. Chapter 288 Page 2007

A. Bacterial pneumonia
B. Lung abscess
C. Bronchiectasis
D. All of the above

Parapneumonic effusions are associated with bacterial pneumonia, lung abscess, or bronchiectasis. Grossly purulent effusion is termed empyema.

858. Which of the following is the likely pathogen in pneumonia presenting with a subacute illness, weight loss, brisk leukocytosis and possibility of aspiration?
Harrison's 20th Ed. Chapter 288 Page 2007

A. Bacterial infection
B. Anaerobic infection
C. Fungal infection
D. Viral infection

Patients with "anaerobic infections" present with a subacute illness, weight loss, brisk leukocytosis, mild anemia, & predisposition for aspiration.

859. Therapeutic thoracentesis is indicated if pleural free fluid separates lung from chest wall by?
Harrison's 20th Ed. Chapter 288 Page 2007

A. > 5 mm
B. > 10 mm
C. > 15 mm
D. > 20 mm

If pleural free fluid separates lung from the chest wall by >10 mm, a therapeutic thoracentesis should be performed.

860. Factors indicating the likely need for a procedure more invasive than a thoracentesis are all except?
Harrison's 20th Ed. Chapter 288 Page 2007

A. Loculated pleural fluid
B. Pleural fluid pH < 7.40
C. Pleural fluid glucose <60 mg/dL
D. Positive Gram stain or culture of pleural fluid

Factors indicating the likely need for a procedure more invasive than a thoracentesis include loculated pleural fluid, pleural fluid pH < 7.20, pleural fluid glucose <60 mg/dL, (+) Gram stain or culture, gross pus in pleural space.

861. Which out of the following is the commonest cause of malignant pleural effusion?
Harrison's 20th Ed. Chapter 288 Page 2007

A. Hepatoma
B. Ca. Pancreas
C. Ca. Thyroid
D. Lymphoma

862. Which out of the following is the commonest cause of malignant pleural effusion?
Harrison's 20th Ed. Chapter 288 Page 2007

A. Hepatoma
B. Leukemia
C. Mesotheliomas
D. Ca. Breast

Lung carcinoma, breast carcinoma & lymphoma are the cause of ~75% of all malignant pleural effusions.

863. The only symptom that can be attributed to the malignant pleural effusion itself is?
Harrison's 20th Ed. Chapter 288 Page 2007

A. Dyspnea
B. Pain
C. Cough
D. Hemoptysis

Only symptom that can be attributed to pleural effusion itself is dyspnea. Dyspnea is frequently out of proportion to the size of pleural effusion.

864. Which of the following about malignant pleural effusion is false?
Harrison's 20th Ed. Chapter 288 Page 2007

A. To be treated symptomatically
B. Indicates disseminated disease
C. Most malignancies associated with PE are not curable
D. None of the above

Patients with malignant pleural effusion are treated symptomatically as presence of effusion indicates disseminated disease & most malignancies associated with pleural effusion are not curable with chemotherapy.

865. Most malignant mesotheliomas are related to exposure to?
Harrison's 20th Ed. Chapter 288 Page 2007

A. Silica
B. Asbestos
C. Benzene
D. Carbon

Malignant mesotheliomas are primary tumors that arise from the mesothelial cells that line the pleural cavities. Most are related to asbestos exposure.

866. Chest radiograph of patients with mesothelioma reveals?
Harrison's 20th Ed. Chapter 288 Page 2007

A. Pleural effusion
B. Generalized pleural thickening
C. Shrunken hemithorax
D. All of the above

Chest radiograph in patients with mesothelioma reveals a pleural effusion, generalized pleural thickening, and a shrunken hemithorax.

867. Shortness of breath in mesothelioma should be treated with?
Harrison's 20th Ed. Chapter 288 Page 2007

A. Bronchodilators
B. Glucocorticoids
C. Opiates
D. ACE inhibitors

Shortness of breath in mesothelioma is treated with oxygen and/or opiates.

868. The diagnosis most commonly overlooked in differential diagnosis of an undiagnosed pleural effusion is?
Harrison's 20th Ed. Chapter 288 Page 2007

A. Pulmonary embolism
B. Left ventricular failure
C. Malignancy
D. AIDS

Diagnosis most commonly overlooked in differential diagnosis of an undiagnosed pleural effusion is pulmonary embolism.

869. Which is the most common symptom in cases of pleural effusion secondary to pulmonary embolization?
Harrison's 20th Ed. Chapter 288 Page 2007

A. Dyspnea
B. Pain
C. Cough
D. Hemoptysis

Dyspnea is the most common symptom in with pleural effusion due to PE.

870. In pleural effusion secondary to pulmonary embolization, if pleural effusion increases in size after anticoagulation, the possibility is?
Harrison's 20th Ed. Chapter 288 Page 2007

A. Recurrent emboli
B. Hemothorax
C. Pleural infection
D. Any of the above

If pleural effusion secondary to PE increases in size after anticoagulation, probability is of recurrent emboli or a hemothorax or a pleural infection.

871. Tuberculous pleural effusions are due to?
Harrison's 20th Ed. Chapter 288 Page 2007

A. Hematogenous spread of tubercular bacilli
B. Contiguous spread of tubercular bacilli
C. Hypersensitivity reaction to tuberculous protein in pleural space
D. All of the above

Tuberculous pleural effusions are due to a hypersensitivity reaction to tuberculous protein in pleural space.

872. Which of the following is false about tuberculous pleural effusion?
Harrison's 20th Ed. Chapter 288 Page 2008

A. Contains predominantly small lymphocytes
B. Adenosine deaminase level > 40 IU/L
C. Interferon g level >140 pg/mL
D. Recommended treatment of pleural & pulmonary tuberculosis is not identical

Tuberculous pleural fluid is an exudate with predominantly small lymphocytes. TB markers in pleural fluid like ADA is > 40 IU/L, interferon γ is > 140 pg/mL, or positive PCR for tuberculous DNA. The recommended treatment of pleural and pulmonary tuberculosis is "identical".

873. Pleural effusion that produces no shift of mediastinal structures to opposite side is suggestive of?
Harrison's 20th Ed. Chapter 288 Page 2008

A. Tuberculosis
B. Mesothelioma
C. Pulmonary adenocarcinoma
D. Metastasis to pleura

874. Which of the following is false about AIDS & pleural effusions?
Harrison's 20th Ed. Chapter 288 Page 2008

A. Pleural effusions are uncommon
B. Most common cause is Kaposi's sarcoma
C. Pleural effusions very uncommon with P. carinii infection
D. None of the above

Pleural effusions are uncommon in AIDS patients. The most common cause is Kaposi's sarcoma. Other common causes are TB, cryptococcosis, and primary effusion lymphoma. Pleural effusions are very uncommon with Pneumocystis carinii infection.

875. The most common cause of chylothorax is?
Harrison's 20th Ed. Chapter 288 Page 2008

A. Malignancy
B. Trauma
C. Developmental anomaly
D. Necrotizing infection

Chylothorax occurs when thoracic duct is disrupted and chyle accumulates in pleural space. The most common cause of chylothorax is trauma.

876. Which of the following is characteristic of pleural fluid biochemical analysis in a case of chylothorax?
Harrison's 20th Ed. Chapter 288 Page 2008

A. LDL > 120 mg/dL
B. Triglyceride > 110 mg/dL
C. HDL < 40 mg/dL
D. Total cholesterol > 300 mg/dL

In chylothorax, thoracentesis reveals milky fluid and biochemical analysis reveals a triglyceride level of > 110 mg/dL.

877. The treatment of choice for most chylothoraces is?
Harrison's 20th Ed. Chapter 288 Page 2008

A. Tube thoracostomy with chest tube drainage
B. Pleurodesis
C. Implantation of a pleuroperitoneal shunt
D. Ligation of thoracic duct

Treatment of choice for most chylothoraces is insertion of a chest tube plus administration of octreotide. If these fail, a pleuroperitoneal shunt is placed unless patient has chylous ascites.

878. Hemothorax is diagnosed when hematocrit of pleural fluid is how much of the peripheral blood hematocrit?
Harrison's 20th Ed. Chapter 288 Page 2008

A. > 25%
B. > 33%
C. > 50%
D. > 75%

If hematocrit of bloody pleural fluid is >50% that of the peripheral blood, patient has a hemothorax.

879. Most hemothoraces are the result of?
Harrison's 20th Ed. Chapter 288 Page 2008

A. Trauma
B. Rupture of a blood vessel
C. Tumor
D. Tuberculosis

Most hemothoraces are due to trauma. Other causes include rupture of a blood vessel or tumor.

880. The treatment of choice for most hemothorax is?
Harrison's 20th Ed. Chapter 288 Page 2008

A. Tube thoracostomy with chest tube drainage
B. Pleurodesis
C. Thoracotomy
D. Blood transfusion

Most patients with hemothorax are treated with tube thoracostomy, which allows continuous quantification of bleeding. If pleural hemorrhage exceeds 200 mL/hour, thoracotomy is considered.

881. Which WBC predominates in drug-induced pleural effusion?
Harrison's 20th Ed. Chapter 288 Page 2008

A. Neutrophil
B. Lymphocyte
C. Monocyte
D. Eosinophil

Several drugs can cause pleural effusion. Associated fluid is usually eosinophilic.

882. Drug-induced pleural disease can be due to all except?
Harrison's 20th Ed. Chapter 288 Page 2008, Table 288-1

A. Nitrofurantoin
B. Dantrolene
C. Chloroquine
D. Methysergide

883. Drug-induced pleural disease can be due to all except?
Harrison's 20th Ed. Chapter 288 Page 2008, Table 288-1

A. Cephalosporins
B. Bromocriptine
C. Procarbazine
D. Amiodarone

Drug-induced Exudative pleural disease can be due to Nitrofurantoin, Dantrolene, Methysergide, Bromocriptine, Procarbazine, Amiodarone.

884. Pleural effusions that occur following coronary artery bypass surgery within the first weeks are which sided?
Harrison's 20th Ed. Chapter 288 Page 2008

A. Right-sided
B. Left-sided
C. Bilateral
D. Any of the above

Pleural effusions commonly occur within weeks following CABG surgery are left-sided & bloody, with large numbers of eosinophils & respond to therapeutic thoracenteses. Effusions occurring after first few weeks are left-sided & clear yellow with more of small lymphocytes & tend to recur.

885. Which of the following medical manipulations can cause pleural effusion?
Harrison's 20th Ed. Chapter 288 Page 2008

A. Endoscopic variceal sclerotherapy
B. Radiation therapy
C. Intravascular insertion of central lines
D. All of the above

Medical manipulations that induce pleural effusions include abdominal surgery, endoscopic variceal sclerotherapy, radiation therapy, liver or lung transplantation, or intravascular insertion of central lines.

886. Which of the following about pneumothorax is false?
Harrison's 20th Ed. Chapter 288 Page 2009

A. Spontaneous pneumothorax occurs without antecedent trauma to thorax
B. Primary spontaneous pneumothorax occurs in the absence of underlying lung disease
C. Secondary spontaneous pneumothorax occurs in presence of underlying lung disease
D. In tension pneumothorax, pressure in pleural space is positive at the end of inspiration

In tension pneumothorax, pressure in pleural space is positive throughout the respiratory cycle.

887. Which of the following is false about primary spontaneous pneumothorax?
Harrison's 20th Ed. Chapter 288 Page 2009

A. Usually due to rupture of apical pleural blebs
B. Occur almost exclusively in smokers
C. 50% of patients with an initial primary spontaneous pneumothorax will have a recurrence
D. None of the above

Primary spontaneous pneumothoraces are due to rupture of apical pleural blebs that lie within or immediately under the visceral pleura. They occur almost exclusively in smokers. Approximately one-half of patients with an initial primary spontaneous pneumothorax will have a recurrence.

888. Which of the following treatments for primary spontaneous pneumothorax surely prevents recurrences?
Harrison's 20th Ed. Chapter 288 Page 2009

A. Simple aspiration
B. Stapling of blebs
C. Pleural abrasion
D. All of the above

Initial recommended treatment for primary spontaneous pneumothorax is simple aspiration. If the lung does not expand or if patient has recurrent pneumothorax, thoracoscopy with stapling of blebs and pleural abrasion is indicated. Thoracoscopy or thoracotomy with pleural abrasion is ~100% successful in preventing recurrences.

889. Secondary spontaneous pneumothoraces are most frequently found in?

Harrison's 20th Ed. Chapter 288 Page 2009

A. During mechanical ventilation or resuscitative efforts
B. Asthma
C. COPD
D. Lung malignancy

Most secondary spontaneous pneumothoraces are due to COPD, but pneumothoraces have been reported with virtually every lung disease.

890. Patients with secondary spontaneous pneumothorax should be treated in the first instance with?

Harrison's 20th Ed. Chapter 288 Page 2009

A. Tube thoracostomy
B. Bleb resection
C. Pleural abrasion
D. Simple aspiration

Nearly all patients with secondary pneumothorax should be treated with tube thoracostomy.

891. Which of the following is a cause of iatrogenic pneumothorax?

Harrison's 20th Ed. Chapter 288 Page 2009

A. Transthoracic needle aspiration
B. Thoracentesis
C. Insertion of central intravenous catheters
D. All of the above

Leading causes of iatrogenic pneumothorax are transthoracic needle aspiration, thoracentesis and insertion of central intravenous catheters.

892. Tension pneumothorax is most frequently found in?

Harrison's 20th Ed. Chapter 288 Page 2009

A. During mechanical ventilation/resuscitative efforts
B. Asthma
C. COPD
D. Lung malignancy

Tension Pneumothorax usually occurs during mechanical ventilation or resuscitative efforts.

893. In treating 'Tension pneumothorax', a large-bore needle is inserted into pleural space through?

Harrison's 20th Ed. Chapter 288 Page 2009

A. Second anterior intercostal space
B. Third anterior intercostal space
C. Fourth anterior intercostal space
D. Fifth anterior intercostal space

Tension pneumothorax is a medical emergency. A large-bore needle is inserted into pleural space through 2nd anterior intercostal space. Needle is left in place until a thoracostomy tube can be inserted.

Disorders of the Mediastinum

894. Mediastinum is separated into how many compartments?
Harrison's 20th Ed. Chapter 289 Page 2009

A. 2
B. 3
C. 4
D. 5

Mediastinum is the region between pleural sacs, separated in 3 compartments.

895. Thoracic duct is present in which compartment of mediastinum?
Harrison's 20th Ed. Chapter 289 Page 2009

A. Anterior
B. Middle
C. Posterior
D. None of the above

896. Azygos and hemiazygos veins are present in which compartment of mediastinum?
Harrison's 20th Ed. Chapter 289 Page 2009

A. Anterior
B. Middle
C. Posterior
D. None of the above

Anterior mediastinum extends from the sternum anteriorly to pericardium & brachiocephalic vessels posteriorly. It contains thymus gland, anterior mediastinal lymph nodes & internal mammary arteries & veins. Middle mediastinum lies between anterior & posterior mediastina & contains heart, ascending & transverse arches of aorta, venae cavae, brachiocephalic arteries & veins, phrenic nerves, trachea, main bronchi & their contiguous lymph nodes & pulmonary arteries & veins. Posterior mediastinum is bounded by pericardium & trachea anteriorly & vertebral column posteriorly. It contains descending thoracic aorta, esophagus, thoracic duct, azygos & hemiazygos veins & posterior group of mediastinal lymph nodes.

897. Lymphomas are most common lesion in which mediastinal compartment?
Harrison's 20th Ed. Chapter 289 Page 2009

A. Anterior
B. Middle
C. Posterior
D. Any of the above

898. Lymph node enlargement from metastases are most common lesion in which mediastinal compartment?
Harrison's 20th Ed. Chapter 289 Page 2009

A. Anterior
B. Middle
C. Posterior
D. Any of the above

The most common lesions in the anterior mediastinum are thymomas, lymphomas, teratomatous neoplasms, and thyroid masses. The most common masses in the middle mediastinum are vascular masses, lymph node enlargement from metastases or granulomatous disease, and pleuropericardial and bronchogenic cysts. In the posterior mediastinum, neurogenic tumors, meningoceles, meningomyeloceles, gastroenteric cysts, and esophageal diverticula are commonly found.

899. Hamman 's sign is characteristic of?
Harrison's 20th Ed. Chapter 289 Page 2010

A. Pneumomediastinum
B. Chronic mediastinitis
C. Tension pneumothorax
D. Traumatic pneumothorax

900. Hamman's sign is best elicited in which position?
Harrison's 20th Ed. Chapter 289 Page 2010

A. Upright
B. Supine
C. Left lateral
D. Prone

Physical examination in pneumomediastinum reveals subcutaneous emphysema in suprasternal notch & Hamman's sign, which is a crunching or clicking noise synchronous with heartbeat & best heard in left lateral decubitus position.

901. In pneumomediastinum, mediastinal air is absorbed faster if the patient is given?
Harrison's 20th Ed. Chapter 289 Page 2010

A. High concentrations of oxygen
B. CO_2 inhalation
C. IV Hypertonic saline
D. High doses of IV glucocorticoids

In pneumomediastinum, the mediastinal air will be absorbed faster if the patient inspires high concentrations of oxygen.

902. Word egophony comes from Greek "ego" which means?
Cleveland Clinic Journal Of Medicine 2008;75:303

A. Temper
B. Silence
C. Cat
D. Goat

Word egophony comes from Greek "ego" meaning goat. It describes change in pronounced sound of E to A. Mechanism in massive pleural effusions is upward displacement & compression or consolidation of lung at the top of effusion.

Disorders of Ventilation

903. In health and at sea level, arterial level of carbon dioxide (Pa_{CO2}) is maintained between?

Harrison's 20th Ed. Chapter 290 Page 2010

A. 35 & 41 mm Hg

B. 36 & 42 mm Hg

C. 37 & 43 mm Hg

D. 38 & 44 mm Hg

In health the arterial level of carbon dioxide (Pa_{CO2}) is maintained between 37 and 43 mm Hg at sea level.

904. In the equation Pa_{CO2}= (k)($V._{CO2}$)/V. A, V. $_{CO2}$ represents?

Harrison's 20th Ed. Chapter 290 Page 2010

A. Carbon dioxide excretion

B. Carbon dioxide production

C. Carbon dioxide excess

D. Carbon dioxide retention

V. $_{CO2}$ represents the carbon dioxide production, k is a constant and V. A is fresh gas alveolar ventilation.

905. V. A is calculated by which of the following formula?

Harrison's 20th Ed. Chapter 290 Page 2010

A. Minute ventilation x (1-Vd/Vt)

B. Minute ventilation/(1-Vd/Vt)

C. Minute ventilation + (1-Vd/Vt)

D. Minute ventilation - (1-Vd/Vt)

V. A can be calculated as minute ventilation x(1-Vd/Vt) where Vd/Vt represents dead space fraction.

906. Disturbances of Pa_{CO2} reflect which of the following?

Harrison's 20th Ed. Chapter 290 Page 2010

A. Altered CO_2 production

B. Minute ventilation

C. Dead space fraction

D. All of the above

All disorders of ventilation result in abnormal measurements of Pa_{CO2}. All disturbances of Pa_{CO2} must reflect altered CO_2 production, minute ventilation, or dead space fraction.

907. Dorsal respiratory group (DRG) & ventral respiratory column (VRC) are located in?

Harrison's 20th Ed. Chapter 290 Page 2010

A. Pleura

B. Lung parenchyma

C. Bronchial airways

D. Medulla oblongata

The spontaneous cycle of inspiration & expiration is automatically generated in medulla through dorsal respiratory group (DRG) and ventral respiratory column (VRC).

908. DRG acts as the initial integration site for which of the following?

Harrison's 20th Ed. Chapter 290 Page 2010

A. P_{aO2}

B. Pa_{CO2}

C. pH

D. All of the above

DRG acts as the initial integration site for afferent nerves bringing in information about partial pressure of arterial oxygen (Pa_{O2}), Pa_{CO2}, pH, and blood pressure from carotid and aortic chemoreceptors and baroreceptors to the central nervous system (CNS).

909. Which of the following nerves relay information from stretch receptors & juxtapulmonary-capillary receptors in lung parenchyma & chest wall to DRG?

Harrison's 20th Ed. Chapter 290 Page 2010

A. Vagus nerve

B. Phrenic nerve

C. Intercostal nerves

D. All of the above

Vagus nerve relays information from stretch receptors and juxtapulmonary-capillary receptors in the lung parenchyma and chest wall to the DRG.

910. Pre-Bötzinger complex is a part of?

Harrison's 20th Ed. Chapter 290 Page 2010

A. DRG

B. VRC

C. Parafacial respiratory group (pFRG)

D. All of the above

911. Which of the following is responsible for the generation of inspiratory activity?

Harrison's 20th Ed. Chapter 290 Page 2010

A. DRG

B. Parafacial respiratory group (pFRG)

C. Pre-Bötzinger complex

D. All of the above

912. Which of the following is responsible for the generation of expiratory activity?

Harrison's 20th Ed. Chapter 290 Page 2010

A. DRG

B. Parafacial respiratory group (pFRG)

C. Pre-Bötzinger complex

D. All of the above

The respiratory rhythm is generated within the VRC, as well as the more rostrally located parafacial respiratory group (pFRG), which is particularly important for the generation of active expiration. One particularly important area within the VRC is the so-called pre-Bötzinger complex. This area is responsible for the generation of various forms of inspiratory activity, and lesioning of the pre-Bötzinger complex leads to the complete cessation of breathing. The neural output of these medullary respiratory networks can be voluntarily suppressed or augmented by input from higher brain centers and the autonomic nervous system. During normal sleep there is an attenuated response to hypercapnia and hypoxemia resulting in mild nocturnal hypoventilation that corrects upon awakening.

913. Which of the following confirms chronic alveolar hypoventilation?

Harrison's 20th Ed. Chapter 290 Page 2011

A. Elevated plasma bicarbonate
B. Elevated Pa_{CO_2}
C. Normal pH
D. All of the above

Elevated plasma bicarbonate in the absence of volume depletion is suggestive of hypoventilation. An arterial blood gas demonstrating elevated Pa_{CO2} with a normal pH confirms chronic alveolar hypoventilation.

914. Which of the following is used to identify patients of alveolar hypoventilation?

Harrison's 20th Ed. Chapter 290 Page 2011

A. Berlin questionnaire
B. Epworth sleepiness scale (ESS)
C. STOP-Bang questionnaire
D. All of the above

915. Which out of the following measures daytime sleepiness?

Harrison's 20th Ed. Chapter 290 Page 2011

A. Berlin questionnaire
B. Epworth sleepiness scale (ESS)
C. STOP-Bang questionnaire
D. All of the above

Berlin questionnaire has been validated in a primary care setting and identifies patients likely to have OSA. ESS measures daytime sleepiness. STOP-Bang survey is used in preoperative clinics to identify patients at risk of having OSA.

916. Sleepiness score is named after?

Harrison's 20th Ed. Chapter 290 Page 2011

A. Dereck
B. Epworth
C. Hall
D. Garcia

Epworth Sleepiness Score helps to detect troublesome sleepiness.

917. Which of the following parameter in PFT is used to monitor for respiratory muscle involvement in diseases with progressive muscle weakness?

Harrison's 20th Ed. Chapter 290 Page 2012

A. Maximum inspiratory pressure
B. Maximum expiratory pressure
C. Forced vital capacity (FVC)
D. All of the above

Respiratory muscle weakness has to be profound before lung volumes are compromised and hypercapnia develops. Measurement of maximum inspiratory and expiratory pressures or forced vital capacity (FVC) can be used to monitor for respiratory muscle involvement in diseases with progressive muscle weakness.

918. Which of the following stimulates respiration?

Harrison's 20th Ed. Chapter 290 Page 2012

A. Acetazolamide
B. Estrogen
C. Testosterone
D. Norepinephrine

Pharmacologic agents that stimulate respiration are medroxyprogesterone and acetazolamide.

919. Which of the following is false about diagnosis of Obesity Hypoventilation Syndrome?

Harrison's 20th Ed. Chapter 290 Page 2012

A. Body mass index (BMI) ≥ 30 kg/m^2
B. Pa_{CO_2} ≥ 45 mm Hg
C. Pa_{O_2} < 80 mm Hg
D. Chronic daytime alveolar hypoventilation

Diagnosis of obesity hypoventilation syndrome (OHS) requires body mass index (BMI) ≥30 kg/m^2, sleep-disordered breathing and chronic daytime alveolar hypoventilation, defined as Pa_{CO_2}≥45 mm Hg, and Pa_{O_2} <70 mm Hg in the absence of other known causes of hypercapnia.

920. Ondine's curse is best related to?

Harrison's 20th Ed. Chapter 290 Page 2012

A. Hyperventilation
B. Obstructive sleep apnea syndrome
C. Central hypoventilation syndrome (CCHS)
D. Obesity hypoventilation syndrome

Central Hypoventilation Syndrome can present later in life or in the neonatal period where it is often called Ondine's curse or congenital central hypoventilation syndrome (CCHS).

921. Which of the following gene has been implicated in the pathogenesis of congenital central hypoventilation syndrome?

Harrison's 20th Ed. Chapter 290 Page 2012

A. PHOX1b
B. PHOX2b
C. PHOX3b
D. PHOX4b

Abnormalities in the gene encoding PHOX2b, a transcription factor with a role in neuronal development, have been implicated in the pathogenesis of congenital central hypoventilation syndrome.

Sleep Apnea

922. Obstructive sleep apnea/hypopnea syndrome (OSAHS) relates to?
Harrison's 20th Ed. Chapter 291 Page 2013

A. Unexplained excessive daytime sleepiness
B. Five obstructed apneas per hour of sleep
C. Five obstructed hypopneas per hour of sleep
D. All of the above

OSAHS may be defined as coexistence of unexplained excessive daytime sleepiness with at least five obstructed breathing events (apnea or hypopnea) per hour of sleep.

923. Apnea-hypopnea index [AHI] is calculated as?
Harrison's 20th Ed. Chapter 291 Page 2013

A. Number of episodes/number of hours of sleep
B. (Number of episodes x number of hours of sleep)/12
C. (Number of episodes x number of hours of sleep)/24
D. (Number of episodes/number of hours of sleep)/24

Apnea-hypopnea index [AHI] is calculated as the number of episodes divided by the number of hours of sleep.

924. OSAHS is diagnosed if the AHI is above?
Harrison's 20th Ed. Chapter 291 Page 2013

A. 5
B. 10
C. 15
D. 20

OSAHS is diagnosed in the absence of symptoms if the AHI is above 15.

925. Apneas of what duration are considered significant?
Harrison's 20th Ed. Chapter 291 Page 2013

A. At least 6 second
B. At least 7 second
C. At least 9 second
D. At least 10 second

Apneas are defined in adults as breathing pauses lasting 10 seconds or when there is ≥3% drop in oxygen saturation and/or a brain cortical arousal.

926. AHI represents which of the following?
Harrison's 20th Ed. Chapter 291 Page 2013

A. Frequency of breathing disturbances
B. Duration of apneas & hypopneas
C. Degree of sleep fragmentation
D. Level of daytime sleepiness

OSAHS severity is based on the frequency of breathing disturbances (AHI), the amount of oxygen desaturation with respiratory events, duration of apneas & hypopneas, degree of sleep fragmentation and the level of daytime sleepiness.

927. In hypopnea, ventilation is reduced from the previous baseline during sleep by at least?
Harrison's 20th Ed. Chapter 291 Page 2015 Table 291-1

A. 20%
B. 30%
C. 40%
D. 50%

Hypopnea is defined as a ≥30% reduction in airflow for at least 10 seconds during sleep that is accompanied by either ≥3% desaturation or an arousal.

928. How many obstructive events & arousals per hour of sleep define severe OSA?
Harrison's 20th Ed. Chapter 291 Page 2015 Table 291-2

A. > 5
B. > 10
C. > 20
D. > 30

In severe OSA (significant daytime sleepiness or >30 obstructive events and arousals per hour of sleep), nasal continuous positive airway pressure (CPAP) is the treatment of choice. Mild OSAHS: AHI of 5–14 events/hour, Moderate OSAHS: AHI of 15–29 events/hour and Severe OSAHS: AHI of ≥ 30 events/hour.

929. Sleep apnea is defined as an intermittent cessation of airflow most commonly at the level of?
Harrison's 20th Ed. Chapter 291 Page 2014

A. Soft palate
B. Tongue base
C. Lateral pharyngeal walls
D. Epiglottis

The airway may collapse at various levels. Most common is soft palate. Others include tongue base, lateral pharyngeal walls and/or epiglottis.

930. OSAHS is most severe?
Harrison's 20th Ed. Chapter 291 Page 2014

A. During REM (rapid eye movement) sleep
B. In supine position
C. In individuals with small pharyngeal lumen
D. All of the above

OSAHS may be most severe during REM (rapid eye movement) sleep, when neuromuscular output to the skeletal muscles is particularly low and in the supine position due to gravitational forces. Individuals with a small pharyngeal lumen require relatively high levels of neuromuscular innervation to maintain patency during wakefulness and are thus predisposed to excessive airway collapsibility during sleep.

931. Which of the following statements is false?
Harrison's 20th Ed. Chapter 291 Page 2014

A. Sleep apneas can be central or obstructive
B. In CSA, neural drive to respiratory muscles is transiently abolished
C. In OSA, airflow ceases despite respiratory drive
D. None of the above

Sleep apneas can be central or obstructive. In CSA, neural drive to all respiratory muscles is transiently abolished. In OSA airflow ceases despite continuing respiratory drive because of occlusion of oropharyngeal airway.

932. The definitive event in obstructive sleep apnea is occlusion of upper airway usually at the level of?
Harrison's 20th Ed. Chapter 291 Page 2015

A. Nasopharynx
B. Oropharynx
C. Laryngopharynx
D. All of the above

In obstructive sleep apnea (OSA), airflow ceases despite continuing respiratory drive because of occlusion of oropharyngeal airway.

933. Main factor leading to collapse of upper airway in OSA is?
Harrison's 20th Ed. Chapter 291 Page 2015

A. Critical sub-atmospheric pressure in inspiration
B. Critical supra-atmospheric pressure in inspiration
C. Spasm of airway adductor muscles
D. All of the above

The immediate factor leading to collapse of upper airway in OSA is generation of a critical subatmospheric pressure during inspiration that exceeds the ability of airway dilator and abductor muscles to maintain airway stability.

934. Which of the following predispose to the development of OSA?
Harrison's 20th Ed. Chapter 291 Page 2014

A. Acromegaly
B. Adenotonsillar hypertrophy
C. Retrognathia
D. All of the above

935. Which of the following predispose to the development of OSA?
Harrison's 20th Ed. Chapter 291 Page 2014

A. Macroglossia
B. Obesity
C. Menopause
D. All of the above

Alcohol depresses activity of upper airway muscles & arousal response that terminates each apnea. Structural compromise due to adenotonsillar hypertrophy, retrognathia & macroglossia aggravate OSA. Obesity reduces size of upper airways by increasing fat deposition in soft tissues of pharynx or by compressing the pharynx by superficial fat masses in neck.

936. Factors that predispose to OSAHS include all except?
Harrison's 20th Ed. Chapter 291 Page 2014

A. Male gender
B. Shortening of mandible
C. Shortening of maxilla
D. Elderly

937. Factors that predispose to OSAHS include all except?
Harrison's 20th Ed. Chapter 291 Page 2014

A. Smoking
B. Myotonic dystrophy
C. Lambert-Eaton myasthenic syndrome
D. Ehlers Danlos syndrome

Factors predisposing to OSAHS include obesity, shortening of mandible &/or maxilla, male gender, middle age (40–65 years), hypothyroidism, acromegaly, myotonic dystrophy, Ehlers Danlos syndrome & smoking.

938. Risk factors for sleep apnea include all except?
N Engl J Med 2002;347:498

A. Obesity
B. Increased neck circumference
C. Short neck
D. Craniofacial abnormalities

939. Risk factors for sleep apnea include all except?
N Engl J Med 2002;347:498

A. Hypothyroidism
B. Acromegaly
C. Mental retardation
D. Obesity

940. Which of the following can cause day time sleepiness?
N Engl J Med 2002;347:498

A. Circadian-rhythm abnormality
B. Narcolepsy
C. Periodic limb movement disorder
D. All of the above

941. Which of the following contribute to the pathogenesis of OSAHS?
Harrison's 20th Ed. Chapter 291 Page 2014

A. Ventilatory sensitivity
B. Arousal threshold
C. Neuromuscular responses to CO2
D. All of the above

942. Which of the following genetic syndrome is best related to OSAHS?
Harrison's 20th Ed. Chapter 291 Page 2014

A. Pendred's syndrome
B. Usher's syndrome
C. Treacher-Collins syndrome
D. Waardenburg's syndrome

Genetic syndromes that reduce upper airway patency are Down syndrome and Treacher-Collins syndrome.

943. A 10% weight gain is associated with?
Harrison's 20th Ed. Chapter 291 Page 2014

A. > 10% increase in AHI
B. > 20% increase in AHI
C. > 30% increase in AHI
D. > 40% increase in AHI

A 10% weight gain is associated with a >30% increase in AHI.

944. Obesity predisposes to OSAHS through?
Harrison's 20th Ed. Chapter 291 Page 2014

A. Narrowing effects of upper airway fat on pharyngeal lumen
B. Reduction in chest wall compliance
C. Decrease in lung volumes
D. All of the above

Obesity predisposes to OSAHS through the narrowing effects of upper airway fat on the pharyngeal lumen, reduction in chest wall compliance and decrease in lung volumes, resulting in a loss of caudal traction on upper airway structures.

945. Which of the following statements is false?

Harrison's 20th Ed. Chapter 291 Page 2014

A. Majority of snoring individuals do not have OSA disorder

B. Snoring is not associated with long-term health risks

C. Dyspnea is unusual

D. Patients with OSA are equally prone to motor vehicle accidents as normal individuals

Most pervasive manifestation of OSA is excessive daytime sleepiness. Motor vehicle accidents in OSA are 7 times more as compared with normal.

946. Electrographic variable studied in polysomnography for OSA is?

N Engl J Med 2002;347:498

A. Electroencephalogram

B. Electrooculogram

C. Submental or chin electromyogram

D. All of the above

Definitive investigation for suspected OSA is overnight polysomnography (PSG). It includes recording of electroencephalography, chin electromyography and electro-oculography, limb movements by leg sensors and snoring intensity.

947. Respiratory disturbance index (RDI) includes which of the following?

Harrison's 20th Ed. Chapter 291 Page 2015 Table 291-2

A. Number of respiratory effort related arousals (RERA)

B. Number of apneas

C. Number of hypopneas

D. All of the above

Respiratory disturbance index (RDI) includes the number of respiratory effort related arousals (RERA) in addition to the number of apneas plus hypopneas.

948. Which out of the following drug is useful in OSA?

N Engl J Med 2002;347:498

A. Codeine

B. Fluoxetine

C. Theophylline

D. Domperidone

949. Which out of the following drug is useful in OSA?

N Engl J Med 2002;347:498

A. Acetazolamide

B. Ipratropium bromide

C. Theophylline

D. Protriptyline

Medications are generally ineffective in management of OSA, except in patients with predominantly rapid eye movement sleep related events in whom protriptyline or fluoxetine may be beneficial.

950. Uvulopalatopharyngoplasty in OSA involves?

N Engl J Med 2002;347:498

A. Resection of tonsils

B. Resection of Uvula & Posterior palate

C. Reorientation of tonsillar pillars

D. All of the above

951. Which of the following is central in the pathogenesis of CSA disorders?

Harrison's 20th Ed. Chapter 291 Page 2017

A. PCO_2 level

B. PO_2 level

C. pH level

D. All of the above

PCO_2 level of wakefulness is lower than that required for rhythm generation in sleep. Common to all CSA disorders is a PCO_2 level during sleep that falls transiently below the critical PCO_2 required for respiratory rhythm generation.

Approach to the Patient with Critical Illness

952. Which of the following is the most commonly used severity-of-illness (SOI) scoring system in North America?
Harrison's 20th Ed. Chapter 293 Page 2023

A. APACHE I system
B. APACHE II system
C. APACHE III system1
D. APACHE IV system

APACHE II scoring system is the most commonly used severity-of-illness (SOI) scoring system in North America.

953. About 50% mortality is expected when APACHE II score in nonoperative cases is?
Harrison's 20th Ed. Chapter 293 Page 2025 Figure 293-1

A. 15 – 19
B. 20 – 24
C. 25 – 29
D. 30 – 34

954. Mean arterial pressure (MAP) is the product of cardiac output and?
Harrison's 20th Ed. Chapter 293 Page 2024

A. Heart rate
B. Stroke volume
C. Pulse pressure
D. Systemic vascular resistance (SVR)

Mean arterial pressure (MAP) is the product of cardiac output & systemic vascular resistance (SVR).

955. Clinical evidence of diminished cardiac output includes?
Harrison's 20th Ed. Chapter 293 Page 2024

A. Narrow pulse pressure
B. Cool extremities
C. Delayed capillary refill
D. All of the above

Clinical evidence of diminished cardiac output includes a narrow pulse pressure, cool extremities and delayed capillary refill. If a hypotensive patient has clinical signs of increased cardiac output, it can be inferred that the reduced blood pressure is from decreased SVR.

956. Most common cause of high cardiac output hypotension is?
Harrison's 20th Ed. Chapter 293 Page 2025

A. Sepsis
B. Thyrotoxicosis
C. Anaphylaxis
D. Peripheral arteriovenous shunts

The most common cause of high cardiac output hypotension is sepsis. Other causes include liver failure, severe pancreatitis, burns and other trauma that elicit the systemic inflammatory response syndrome (SIRS), anaphylaxis, thyrotoxicosis, and peripheral arteriovenous shunts.

957. Respiratory failure can be?
Harrison's 20th Ed. Chapter 293 Page 2025

A. Hypoxemic
B. Hypercarbic
C. Combined
D. Any of the above

958. Alveolar unit consists of all except?
Harrison's 20th Ed. Chapter 293 Page 2025

A. Respiratory bronchiole
B. Terminal bronchiole
C. Alveolar duct
D. Alveoli

959. CO_2 challenge test is used to test which component of respiratory system?
Harrison's 20th Ed. Chapter 293 Page 2010

A. Nervous system
B. Muscles of breathing
C. Airways
D. Pulmonary vasculature

960. $P_{0.1}$ test is used to test which component of respiratory system?
Ann. Intensive Care 2019;9:104

A. Nervous system
B. Muscles of breathing
C. Airways
D. Pulmonary vasculature

Occlusion pressure at 100 ms (P0.1), defined as the negative pressure measured 100 ms after the initiation of an inspiratory effort performed against a closed respiratory circuit, has been shown to be well correlated with central respiratory drive and respiratory effort.

961. Rapid-shallow-breathing index (RSBI) is calculated by?
Tanaffos 2012; 11(3): 28-31

A. Respiratory rate/FVC
B. Respiratory rate/IC
C. Respiratory rate/tidal volume
D. Respiratory rate/minute volume

962. Type I respiratory failure best relates to which of the following?
Harrison's 20th Ed. Chapter 293 Page 2026

A. Alveolar hypoventilation
B. Alveolar flooding
C. Hypoperfusion of respiratory muscles
D. Lung atelectasis

963. Type 1 respiratory failure occurs in?
Harrison's 20th Ed. Chapter 293 Page 2026

A. Near-drowning
B. Multiple blood transfusions
C. Pancreatitis
D. All of the above

Type 1 respiratory failure occurs in clinical settings such as sepsis, gastric aspiration, pneumonia, near-drowning, multiple blood transfusions and pancreatitis.

964. Type II respiratory failure best relates to which of the following?
Harrison's 20th Ed. Chapter 293 Page 2026

A. Alveolar hypoventilation
B. Alveolar flooding
C. Hypoperfusion of respiratory muscles
D. Lung atelectasis

965. Type III respiratory failure best relates to which of the following?
Harrison's 20th Ed. Chapter 293 Page 2026

A. Alveolar hypoventilation
B. Alveolar flooding
C. Hypoperfusion of respiratory muscles
D. Lung atelectasis

966. Type IV respiratory failure best relates to which of the following?
Harrison's 20th Ed. Chapter 293 Page 2027

A. Alveolar hypoventilation
B. Alveolar flooding
C. Hypoperfusion of respiratory muscles
D. Lung atelectasis

967. Under normal conditions, respiratory muscles consume what proportion of total cardiac output?
Harrison's 20th Ed. Chapter 293 Page 2027

A. 3%
B. 4%
C. 5%
D. 6%

Under normal conditions, respiratory muscles consume <5% of total cardiac output and oxygen delivery.

968. All are true about Type I respiratory failure except?
Harrison's 20th Ed. Chapter 293 Page 2027

A. Decreased PaO_2
B. Decreased $PaCO_2$
C. Normal $PaCO_2$
D. Normal A-a gradient

969. Type I respiratory failure consists of?
Harrison's 20th Ed. Chapter 293 Page 2027

A. Decreased PaO_2, Normal or decreased $PaCO_2$
B. Decreased PaO_2, increased $PaCO_2$
C. Decreased PaO_2, decreased $PaCO_2$
D. Increased PaO_2, increased $PaCO_2$

970. In type II respiratory failure, there is?
Harrison's 20th Ed. Chapter 293 Page 2027

A. Decreased PaO_2, decreased $PaCO_2$
B. Decreased PaO_2, increased $PaCO_2$
C. Normal PaO_2, normal $PaCO_2$
D. Increased PaO_2, decreased $PaCO_2$

971. Type II respiratory failure is seen in?
Harrison's 20th Ed. Chapter 293 Page 2027

A. COPD with cor pulmonale
B. CRF
C. ARDS
D. Pulmonary fibrosing alveolitis

972. In hypothyroidism, which type of respiratory failure occurs?
Harrison's 20th Ed. Chapter 293 Page 2026

A. Type I
B. Type II
C. Type III
D. Type IV

973. In Guillain-Barre syndrome, which type of respiratory failure occurs?
Harrison's 20th Ed. Chapter 293 Page 2026

A. Type I
B. Type II
C. Type III
D. Type IV

974. In multiple blood transfusions, which type of respiratory failure occurs?
Harrison's 20th Ed. Chapter 293 Page 2026

A. Type I
B. Type II
C. Type III
D. Type IV

975. In ARDS, which type of respiratory failure occurs?
Harrison's 20th Ed. Chapter 293 Page 2026

A. Type I
B. Type II
C. Type III
D. Type IV

976. Perioperative respiratory failure is also called?
Harrison's 20th Ed. Chapter 293 Page 2026

A. Type I
B. Type II
C. Type III
D. Type IV

977. Respiratory failure type IV is seen in?
Harrison's 20th Ed. Chapter 293 Page 2027

A. ARDS
B. COPD
C. CRF
D. Shock

978. The ratio of partial pressure arterial oxygen and fraction of inspired oxygen is called?
Rom J Anaesth Intensive Care. 2018;(1):49-54

A. Carrico index
B. Girard index
C. Abraham index
D. Pronovost index

The ratio of partial pressure arterial oxygen and fraction of inspired oxygen, called P/F ratio or Carrico index, is a comparison between the oxygen level in the blood and the oxygen concentration that is breathed. PaO_2/FiO_2 ratio ≤ 200 mm Hg gets diagnosis of ARDS.

979. Intubated patients having which of the following should undergo spontaneous breathing trial?
Harrison's 20th Ed. Chapter 293 Page 2027

A. PaO_2/FiO_2 >200
B. PEEP ≤ 5 cm H_2O
C. Cough & airway reflexes intact
D. All of the above

Intubated patients having the following should undergo spontaneous breathing trial for 30–120 minutes: stable oxygenation (PaO_2/FiO_2 >200 & PEEP ≤5 cmH_2O), cough & airway reflexes intact, and no vasopressor agents or sedatives.

980. Spontaneous breathing trial is declared a failure and must be stopped if?
Harrison's 20th Ed. Chapter 293 Page 2027

A. Respiratory rate > 35/minute for >5 minutes
B. O2 saturation < 90%
C. HR >140/min or 20% increase or decrease from baseline
D. Any of the above

Spontaneous breathing trial is declared a failure and stopped if any of the following occur. Respiratory rate >35/minute for >5 minutes, O_2 saturation <90%, heart rate >140/min or a 20% increase or decrease from baseline, systolic blood pressure <90 mm Hg or >180 mm Hg and increased anxiety or diaphoresis.

981. Successful spontaneous breathing trial means that the ratio of respiratory rate & tidal volume in liters (f/V_T) is?
Harrison's 20th Ed. Chapter 293 Page 2027

A. < 55
B. < 105
C. < 135
D. < 165

If, at the end of the spontaneous breathing trial, the ratio of the respiratory rate and tidal volume in liters (f/V_T) is <105, patient can be extubated.

982. Postparalytic syndrome refers to?
Harrison's 20th Ed. Chapter 293 Page 2027

A. Neuropathy
B. Pneumothorax
C. Myopathy
D. Pneumonia

Use of neuromuscular blocking agents to facilitate mechanical ventilation may result in prolonged weakness - a myopathy known as the postparalytic syndrome.

983. Multiorgan system failure is defined by the simultaneous presence of physiologic dysfunction and/or failure of?
Harrison's 20th Ed. Chapter 293 Page 2027

A. Two or more organs
B. Three or more organs
C. Four or more organs
D. Five or more organs

Syndrome of multiorgan system failure is defined by the simultaneous presence of physiologic dysfunction and/or failure of two or more organs. Organ failure must persist beyond 24 hours. SIRS is a common basis for multiorgan system failure.

984. The "gold standard" for monitoring in the ICU is?
Harrison's 20th Ed. Chapter 293 Page 2027

A. Pulse oximetry
B. Arterial blood-gas analysis
C. Circulatory status
D. Respiratory system mechanics

For monitoring in the ICU, evaluation of respiratory gas exchange is done by arterial blood-gas analysis which is the "gold standard".

985. Oxyhemoglobin reflects light more effectively than deoxyhemoglobin at wavelengths of?
Harrison's 20th Ed. Chapter 293 Page 2028

A. 660 nm
B. 720 nm
C. 860 nm
D. 940 nm

In pulse oximetry, at wavelengths of 660 nm, oxyhemoglobin reflects light more effectively than does deoxyhemoglobin, whereas the reverse is true in the infrared spectrum (940 nm). A pulse oximeter passes both wavelengths of light through a finger, and the relative intensity of light transmission at these two wavelengths is analyzed to derive relative percentage of oxyhemoglobin.

986. Normally, respiratory system compliance is about?
Harrison's 20th Ed. Chapter 293 Page 2028

A. 10 mL per cmH_2O
B. 50 mL per cmH_2O
C. 100 mL per cmH_2O
D. 150 mL per cmH_2O

End-inspiratory pause (plateau pressure) is a static measurement, affected only by respiratory system compliance, not airway resistance. Normally, respiratory system compliance is ~100 mL per cmH_2O.

987. Normally, the content of O_2 in mixed venous blood (CO_2) is?
Harrison's 20th Ed. Chapter 293 Page 2028

A. 12.76 mL O_2 per dL blood
B. 13.76 mL O_2 per dL blood
C. 14.76 mL O_2 per dL blood
D. 15.76 mL O_2 per dL blood

Oxygen delivery (Q_{O2}) is a function of cardiac output and content of O_2 in arterial blood (Ca_{O2}). Normally, content of O_2 in mixed venous blood (C_{O2}) is 15.76 mL O_2 per dL blood, since the mixed venous blood is 75% saturated.

988. Normal tissue extraction ratio for O_2 is?
Harrison's 20th Ed. Chapter 293 Page 2028

A. 8%
B. 15%
C. 25%
D. 33%

The normal tissue extraction ratio for O_2 is $Ca_{O2} - C_{O2}/Ca_{O2}$ ([21.16–15.76]/21.16) or 25%.

Acute Respiratory Distress Syndrome

989. Which of the following is not a part of definition of acute respiratory distress syndrome (ARDS)?
Harrison's 20th Ed. Chapter 294 Page 2030

A. Severe dyspnea of rapid onset
B. Hypercapnia
C. Hypoxemia
D. Diffuse pulmonary infiltrates leading to respiratory failure

Acute respiratory distress syndrome (ARDS) is a clinical syndrome of severe dyspnea of rapid onset, hypoxemia and diffuse pulmonary infiltrates leading to respiratory failure. Increased pulmonary vascular permeability leading to interstitial and alveolar edema fluid rich in protein is a central feature of ARDS.

990. Diagnostic criteria for mild ARDS is?
Harrison's 20th Ed. Chapter 294 Page 2031 Table 294-2

A. $PaO_2/FiO_2 \leq 300$ mm Hg
B. Acute onset
C. Pulmonary capillary wedge pressure ≤ 18 mm Hg
D. All of the above

991. Diagnostic criteria for moderate ARDS include all except?
Harrison's 20th Ed. Chapter 294 Page 2031 Table 294-2

A. $PaO_2/FiO_2 \leq 200$ mm Hg
B. $PaO_2/FiO_2 \leq 100$ mm Hg
C. Acute onset
D. Pulmonary capillary wedge pressure ≤ 18 mm Hg

992. Diagnostic criteria for severe ARDS include all except?
Harrison's 20th Ed. Chapter 294 Page 2031 Table 294-2

A. $PaO_2/FiO_2 \leq 200$ mm Hg
B. $PaO_2/FiO_2 \leq 100$ mm Hg
C. Acute onset
D. Pulmonary capillary wedge pressure ≤ 18 mm Hg

$PaO_2/FiO_2 \leq 300$ mm Hg is typical of Acute lung injury (ALI). Acute onset and PCWP ≤ 18 mm Hg being the same as in ARDS.

993. Which of the following is the most common situation leading to ARDS?
Harrison's 20th Ed. Chapter 294 Page 2010

A. Multiple bone fractures
B. Head trauma
C. Burns
D. Near drowning

994. All are predisposing factors of ARDS except?
Harrison's 20th Ed. Chapter 294 Page 2031

A. Fat embolism
B. Sepsis
C. Multiple blood transfusions
D. Status asthmaticus

Among patients with trauma, pulmonary contusion, multiple bone fractures, and chest wall trauma/flail chest are the most frequently reported surgical conditions in ARDS, whereas head trauma, near drowning, toxic inhalation, and burns are rare causes.

995. Secondary factors that increases the risk for ARDS include?
N Engl J Med 2000 ;342 :1335

A. Chronic alcohol abuse
B. Chronic lung disease
C. Low serum pH
D. All of the above

996. Secondary factors that increases risk for ARDS include except?
N Engl J Med 2000;342:1335

A. Chronic alcohol abuse
B. Chronic lung disease
C. Low serum pH
D. High serum pH

997. Scores for Acute Physiology, Age, and Chronic Health Evaluation (APACHE II) can range from?
N Engl J Med 2003;348:683-93, Harrison's 20th Ed. Chapter 294 Page 2031

A. 0 to 61
B. 0 to 71
C. 0 to 81
D. 0 to 91

Trauma patients with APACHE II score ≥16 have a 2.5-fold increase in risk of ARDS. Those with a score >20 have an incidence of ARDS that is 3 fold greater than those with APACHE II scores ≤9.

998. Cause of pulmonary oedema in ARDS is?
Harrison's 20th Ed. Chapter 294 Page 2031

A. Increased vascular permeability
B. Increased hydrostatic pressure
C. Lymphatic obstruction
D. Physiological

999. Usually, pulmonary capillary wedge pressure in ARDS is?
Harrison's 20th Ed. Chapter 294 Page 2031

A. Markedly increased
B. Moderately increased
C. Normal
D. Decreased

ARDS is also called "low-pressure pulmonary edema".

1000. All are true about ARDS except?
Harrison's 20th Ed. Chapter 294 Page 2031

A. Widespread atelectasis
B. Increased surfactant
C. Ground glass mottling in X-Ray chest
D. Cyanosis

1001. All are true about ARDS except?
Harrison's 20th Ed. Chapter 294 Page 2031

A. Pulmonary hypertension
B. Normal PCWP
C. Hypoxemia
D. Low protein pulmonary edema

1002. Phases of ARDS are all except?
Harrison's 20th Ed. Chapter 294 Page 2031

A. Exudative
B. Serofibrinous
C. Proliferative
D. Fibrotic

Natural history of ARDS, each having its own characteristic clinico-pathologic features is marked by three phases, i.e. exudative, proliferative, and fibrotic.

1003. Which of the following is a lipid mediator?
Harrison's 20th Ed. Chapter 294 Page 2031

A. Interleukin 1
B. Interleukin 8
C. Tumor necrosis factor α
D. Leukotriene B4

1004. Which of the following cytokine is present in lung in early exudative phase of ARDS?
Harrison's 20th Ed. Chapter 294 Page 2031

A. Interleukin 1
B. Interleukin 8
C. Tumor necrosis factor a
D. All of the above

Significant concentrations of cytokines (interleukin 1, interleukin 8, and tumor necrosis factor α) and lipid mediators (leukotriene B4) are present in the lung in early exudative phase of ARDS.

1005. Which of the following is not a feature of exudative phase of ARDS?
Harrison's 20th Ed. Chapter 294 Page 2031 Figure 294-1

A. Alveolar edema
B. Neutrophil-rich leukocytic infiltration
C. Prominent interstitial inflammation
D. Formation of hyaline membrane whorls

Exudative phase is notable for early alveolar edema and neutrophil-rich leukocytic infiltration of the lungs with subsequent formation of hyaline membranes from diffuse alveolar damage.

1006. Which of the following is not a feature of exudative phase of ARDS?
Harrison's 20th Ed. Chapter 294 Page 2031

A. Injury to alveolar capillary endothelial cells
B. Injury to type I pneumocytes
C. Proliferation of type II pneumocytes
D. Vascular obliteration by microthrombi & fibrocellular proliferation

1007. Which of the following is false about early ARDS?
Harrison's 20th Ed. Chapter 294 Page 2031

A. Alveolar edema involves dependent portions of lung
B. Hypercapnia is prominent in early ARDS
C. Chest X-ray in ARDS rarely shows cardiomegaly
D. None of the above

In exudative phase of ARDS, alveolar edema involves "dependent" portions of lung, leading to diminished aeration & atelectasis. With severe hypoxemia, hypercapnia secondary to an increase in pulmonary dead space is prominent. C × R rarely shows cardiomegaly, pleural effusions or pulmonary vascular redistribution.

1008. After exposure to a precipitating ARDS risk factor, exudative phase encompasses how many days?
Harrison's 20th Ed. Chapter 294 Page 2031

A. First 1 day
B. First 3 days
C. First 5 days
D. First 7 days

Exudative phase encompasses first 7 days of illness after exposure to a precipitating ARDS risk factor.

1009. Chest radiograph in exudative phase of ARDS shows alveolar & interstitial opacities involving?
Harrison's 20th Ed. Chapter 294 Page 2031

A. One-third of lung fields
B. One half of lung fields
C. Two-thirds of lung fields
D. Three-quarters of lung fields

CxR in exudative phase of ARDS reveals alveolar & interstitial opacities involving at least three-quarters of the lung fields.

1010. Chest X-ray in exudative phase of ARDS rarely shows?
Harrison's 20th Ed. Chapter 294 Page 2031

A. Cardiomegaly
B. Pleural effusions
C. Pulmonary vascular redistribution
D. All of the above

Chest X-ray in exudative phase of ARDS rarely shows cardiomegaly, pleural effusions or pulmonary vascular redistribution.

1011. In D/D of ARDS, which one of the following is least likely?
Harrison's 20th Ed. Chapter 294 Page 2031

A. Cardiogenic pulmonary edema
B. Hypersensitivity pneumonitis
C. Diffuse pneumonia
D. Alveolar hemorrhage

In D/D of ARDS, most common disorders are cardiogenic pulmonary edema, diffuse pneumonia, and alveolar hemorrhage. Less frequent diagnoses include acute interstitial lung diseases, hypersensitivity pneumonitis, radiation pneumonitis and neurogenic pulmonary edema.

1012. Proliferative phase of ARDS usually lasts from?
Harrison's 20th Ed. Chapter 294 Page 2031

A. Day 7 to 10
B. Day 7 to 14
C. Day 7 to 18
D. Day 7 to 21

Proliferative phase of ARDS usually lasts from day 7 to day 21.

1013. Histologically, in proliferative phase of ARDS, pulmonary infiltrate is?

Harrison's 20th Ed. Chapter 294 Page 2032

A. Neutrophil predominant
B. Lymphocyte predominant
C. Eosinophil predominant
D. Basophil predominant

In proliferative phase of ARDS, first signs of resolution are evident with initiation of lung repair, organization of alveolar exudates & a shift from a neutrophil to a lymphocyte-predominant pulmonary infiltrate.

1014. Which of the following represents a reparative process in proliferative phase of ARDS?

Harrison's 20th Ed. Chapter 294 Page 2032

A. Organization of alveolar exudates
B. Lymphocyte-predominant pulmonary infiltrate
C. Proliferation of type II pneumocytes
D. All of the above

As part of the reparative process, there is a proliferation of type II pneumocytes along alveolar basement membranes.

1015. Increased risk of pneumothorax is present in which phase of ARDS?

Harrison's 20th Ed. Chapter 294 Page 2033

A. Exudative phase
B. Proliferative phase
C. Fibrotic phase
D. All of the above

Increased risk of pneumothorax is present in fibrotic phase of ARDS.

1016. Histologically, in fibrotic phase of ARDS, which of the following occurs?

Harrison's 20th Ed. Chapter 294 Page 2033

A. Extensive alveolar duct fibrosis
B. Extensive interstitial fibrosis
C. Large bullae
D. All of the above

Histologically, alveolar edema & inflammatory exudates of earlier phases convert to extensive alveolar duct & interstitial fibrosis. Acinar architecture is markedly disrupted, leading to emphysema-like changes with large bullae.

1017. Which of the following is false about normal alveolar epithelium?

N Engl J Med 2002;342:1335

A. Flat type I cells make up 90% of alveolar surface area and are easily injured
B. Cuboidal type II cells make up 10% of alveolar surface area and are more resistant to injury
C. Type II cell functions include surfactant production, ion transport, and proliferation & differentiation to type I cells after injury
D. None of the above

1018. In ARDS, what measure of tidal volume is preferred?

Harrison's 20th Ed. Chapter 294 Page 2033

A. 6 mL/kg predicted body weight
B. 8 mL/kg predicted body weight
C. 10 mL/kg predicted body weight
D. 12 mL/kg predicted body weight

Significantly lower mortality was observed in large-scale, randomized controlled trials in the low tidal volume patients (6 mL/kg predicted body weight) as compared to conventional tidal volume patients (12 mL/kg).

1019. In ARDS, which of the following is a theoretical "optimal PEEP" for alveolar recruitment?

Harrison's 20th Ed. Chapter 294 Page 2033

A. 0 – 5 mm Hg
B. 5 – 12 mm Hg
C. 12 – 15 mm Hg
D. 15 – 18 mm Hg

In ARDS, 12–15 mm Hg is a theoretical "optimal PEEP" for alveolar recruitment.

1020. Inverse ratio ventilation refers to?

Harrison's 20th Ed. Chapter 295 Page 2037

A. Prone-position ventilation
B. Inspiratory time is longer than expiratory time
C. Expiratory time is longer than inspiratory time
D. Ventilating at extremely high respiratory rates

In inverse ratio ventilation technique, inspiratory time is lengthened so that it is longer than expiratory time. With diminished time to exhale, dynamic hyperinflation leads to increased end-expiratory pressure, similar to ventilator-prescribed PEEP.

1021. Mechanical ventilation strategies used for ARDS are?

Harrison's 20th Ed. Chapter 295 Page 2033

A. Partial liquid ventilation (PLV)
B. High-frequency ventilation (HFV)
C. Extracorporeal membrane oxygenation (ECMO)
D. All of the above

1022. Which of the following belongs to recommendation category "A" in management of ARDS?

Harrison's 20th Ed. Chapter 295 Page 2034 Table 294-3

A. Glucocorticoid treatment
B. Low tidal volume
C. Prone position
D. Minimized left atrial filling pressures

1023. Which of the following belongs to recommendation category "B" in management of ARDS?

Harrison's 20th Ed. Chapter 295 Page 2034 Table 294-3

A. Glucocorticoid treatment
B. Surfactant replacement
C. High-frequency ventilation
D. Minimized left atrial filling pressures

1024. Which of the following belongs to recommendation category "C" in management of ARDS?

Harrison's 20th Ed. Chapter 294 Page 2034 Table 294-3

A. Low tidal volume mechanical ventilation

B. Early neuromuscular blockade

C. Inhaled vasodilators

D. Minimized left atrial filling pressures

Recommendation category A includes low tidal volume mechanical ventilation and early neuromuscular blockade (with cisatracurium besylate). Category B includes minimized left atrial filling pressures. Category C includes high-PEEP or "open lung", prone position, recruitment maneuvers and ECMO. Category D includes high-frequency ventilation, glucocorticoid treatment, surfactant replacement, inhaled NO, inhaled epoprostenol and other anti-inflammatory therapy (ketoconazole, PGE1, NSAIDs).

1025. Which of the following is similar in presentation to acute respiratory distress syndrome (ARDS)?

Harrison's 20th Ed. Chapter 294 Page 2034

A. Acute interstitial pneumonia

B. Pulmonary Langerhans cell histiocytosis

C. Cryptogenic organizing pneumonia

D. Desquamative interstitial pneumonia

Acute Interstitial Pneumonia (Hamman-Rich Syndrome) is similar in presentation to acute respiratory distress syndrome (ARDS). AIP probably corresponds to the subset of cases of idiopathic ARDS. AIP is a fulminant form of lung injury characterized histologically by diffuse alveolar damage. Most patients are >40 years of age.

1026. Adult respiratory distress syndrome (ARDS) can be caused by which of the following?

Harrison's 20th Ed. Chapter 294 Page 2031

A. Carbon monoxide

B. Opioid

C. Prolonged anoxia

D. All of the above

ARDS can be caused by poisoning with carbon monoxide, cyanide, an opioid, paraquat, phencyclidine, a sedative-hypnotic, or salicylate; by inhalation of irritant gases, fumes, or vapors (acids and alkali, ammonia, aldehydes, chlorine, hydrogen sulfide, isocyanates, metal oxides, mercury, phosgene, polymers); or by prolonged anoxia, hyperthermia, or shock.

ANSWERS

1. C
2. D
3. A
4. B
5. D
6. A
7. D
8. D
9. D
10. D
11. D
12. A
13. D
14. D
15. A
16. D
17. A
18. C
19. D
20. A
21. D
22. C
23. A
24. D
25. C
26. B
27. C
28. A
29. D
30. B
31. B
32. A
33. C
34. D
35. C
36. D
37. C
38. D
39. A
40. B
41. C
42. A
43. D
44. C
45. D
46. B
47. C
48. B
49. D
50. C
51. B
52. A
53. D
54. C
55. C
56. A
57. D
58. D
59. D
60. D
61. D
62. C
63. A
64. D
65. C
66. D
67. A
68. D
69. D
70. D
71. C
72. C
73. B
74. A
75. B
76. B
77. D
78. D
79. D
80. D
81. D
82. C
83. A
84. A
85. B
86. A
87. C
88. B
89. A
90. A
91. B
92. B
93. A
94. A
95. A
96. A
97. C
98. D
99. D
100. A
101. B
102. A
103. D
104. A
105. B
106. A
107. C
108. C
109. C
110. A
111. A
112. D
113. B
114. D
115. D
116. A
117. A
118. B
119. B
120. C
121. D
122. C
123. C
124. B
125. D
126. D
127. C
128. D
129. D
130. C
131. A
132. D
133. D
134. B
135. D
136. C
137. B
138. C
139. C
140. A
141. B
142. A
143. D
144. D
145. B
146. C
147. B
148. C
149. D
150. A
151. B
152. C
153. D
154. D
155. C
156. B
157. C
158. D
159. B
160. D
161. D
162. D
163. C
164. C
165. A
166. C
167. C
168. D
169. D
170. D
171. D
172. A
173. D
174. C
175. A
176. B
177. D
178. B
179. D
180. B
181. D
182. A
183. D
184. D
185. D
186. C
187. C
188. D
189. C
190. A
191. D
192. D
193. A
194. A
195. A
196. B
197. D
198. B
199. A
200. A
201. D
202. C
203. C
204. C
205. D
206. C
207. C
208. B
209. A
210. B
211. A
212. A
213. B
214. A
215. D
216. C
217. B
218. C
219. D
220. A
221. D
222. C
223. C
224. A
225. C
226. A
227. C
228. A
229. A
230. A
231. D
232. D
233. D
234. D
235. C
236. D
237. C
238. C
239. B
240. A
241. A
242. D
243. C
244. D
245. C
246. B
247. D
248. A
249. C
250. C
251. C
252. D
253. A
254. D
255. C
256. D
257. D
258. D

ANSWERS

259.	D	302.	A	345.	D	388.	A	431.	A	474.	D
260.	D	303.	C	346.	A	389.	D	432.	D	475.	D
261.	D	304.	D	347.	B	390.	C	433.	C	476.	A
262.	B	305.	D	348.	D	391.	D	434.	C	477.	B
263.	B	306.	B	349.	C	392.	D	435.	D	478.	D
264.	A	307.	D	350.	D	393.	D	436.	C	479.	D
265.	A	308.	D	351.	A	394.	A	437.	A	480.	B
266.	A	309.	D	352.	D	395.	B	438.	C	481.	D
267.	D	310.	B	353.	D	396.	B	439.	C	482.	D
268.	A	311.	D	354.	D	397.	D	440.	D	483.	C
269.	C	312.	D	355.	B	398.	A	441.	B	484.	D
270.	A	313.	D	356.	C	399.	D	442.	B	485.	D
271.	D	314.	B	357.	D	400.	D	443.	B	486.	D
272.	C	315.	A	358.	D	401.	D	444.	A	487.	D
273.	C	316.	B	359.	D	402.	A	445.	D	488.	C
274.	D	317.	B	360.	B	403.	B	446.	A	489.	C
275.	A	318.	C	361.	C	404.	D	447.	C	490.	C
276.	A	319.	D	362.	D	405.	C	448.	C	491.	D
277.	D	320.	D	363.	D	406.	D	449.	D	492.	B
278.	B	321.	C	364.	D	407.	D	450.	B	493.	D
279.	C	322.	A	365.	A	408.	A	451.	B	494.	B
280.	D	323.	A	366.	D	409.	D	452.	D	495.	A
281.	C	324.	C	367.	A	410.	A	453.	D	496.	B
282.	D	325.	A	368.	D	411.	D	454.	D	497.	D
283.	D	326.	C	369.	D	412.	B	455.	D	498.	C
284.	B	327.	A	370.	A	413.	C	456.	D	499.	C
285.	A	328.	D	371.	D	414.	D	457.	C	500.	A
286.	D	329.	C	372.	D	415.	A	458.	C	501.	B
287.	D	330.	D	373.	B	416.	B	459.	C	502.	D
288.	C	331.	B	374.	D	417.	D	460.	D	503.	A
289.	B	332.	D	375.	B	418.	D	461.	A	504.	C
290.	A	333.	D	376.	A	419.	A	462.	D	505.	B
291.	C	334.	A	377.	D	420.	D	463.	C	506.	D
292.	D	335.	B	378.	D	421.	B	464.	D	507.	C
293.	A	336.	D	379.	A	422.	A	465.	D	508.	D
294.	A	337.	D	380.	A	423.	D	466.	D	509.	D
295.	C	338.	D	381.	D	424.	A	467.	A	510.	C
296.	B	339.	D	382.	D	425.	D	468.	C	511.	A
297.	A	340.	D	383.	D	426.	D	469.	B	512.	B
298.	D	341.	A	384.	D	427.	D	470.	A	513.	B
299.	C	342.	A	385.	A	428.	D	471.	C	514.	C
300.	A	343.	C	386.	A	429.	D	472.	B	515.	C
301.	D	344.	C	387.	A	430.	A	473.	B	516.	A

ANSWERS

517. D
518. C
519. D
520. A
521. B
522. A
523. C
524. D
525. A
526. D
527. B
528. B
529. D
530. A
531. D
532. D
533. D
534. D
535. D
536. A
537. D
538. D
539. D
540. D
541. A
542. B
543. B
544. D
545. D
546. A
547. B
548. C
549. D
550. B
551. D
552. A
553. C
554. C
555. D
556. A
557. A
558. B
559. D
560. D
561. C
562. C
563. A
564. B
565. A
566. A
567. D
568. D
569. D
570. D
571. D
572. C
573. D
574. B
575. A
576. C
577. D
578. A
579. A
580. A
581. D
582. D
583. C
584. C
585. C
586. B
587. D
588. D
589. B
590. C
591. D
592. D
593. C
594. D
595. D
596. C
597. B
598. C
599. D
600. A
601. D
602. C
603. D
604. D
605. D
606. D
607. A
608. D
609. B
610. D
611. C
612. B
613. D
614. D
615. B
616. D
617. D
618. D
619. C
620. D
621. A
622. A
623. D
624. D
625. A
626. D
627. A
628. D
629. B
630. B
631. D
632. B
633. D
634. B
635. A
636. A
637. A
638. D
639. D
640. A
641. A
642. D
643. D
644. D
645. D
646. D
647. A
648. C
649. C
650. B
651. D
652. D
653. C
654. B
655. C
656. A
657. C
658. C
659. D
660. D
661. B
662. C
663. B
664. D
665. A
666. A
667. B
668. A
669. C
670. C
671. C
672. D
673. D
674. D
675. B
676. B
677. D
678. B
679. D
680. A
681. B
682. D
683. D
684. C
685. D
686. C
687. B
688. B
689. D
690. D
691. A
692. D
693. C
694. D
695. A
696. D
697. D
698. D
699. C
700. D
701. C
702. A
703. D
704. A
705. D
706. B
707. C
708. D
709. B
710. A
711. C
712. A
713. D
714. A
715. A
716. D
717. C
718. D
719. D
720. D
721. D
722. A
723. D
724. C
725. A
726. B
727. D
728. C
729. D
730. A
731. D
732. C
733. B
734. A
735. D
736. C
737. D
738. C
739. D
740. D
741. C
742. A
743. A
744. D
745. B
746. A
747. D
748. A
749. D
750. B
751. C
752. A
753. D
754. C
755. B
756. D
757. B
758. D
759. D
760. C
761. A
762. A
763. B
764. A
765. D
766. D
767. D
768. D
769. B
770. D
771. D
772. B
773. D
774. D

ANSWERS

775. D
776. B
777. D
778. D
779. D
780. C
781. B
782. D
783. D
784. B
785. C
786. D
787. D
788. A
789. D
790. C
791. B
792. C
793. D
794. C
795. D
796. C
797. B
798. D
799. A
800. D
801. D
802. B
803. D
804. A
805. A
806. B
807. A
808. D
809. D
810. C
811. C
812. D
813. D
814. D
815. C
816. D
817. A
818. B
819. A
820. C
821. C
822. B
823. A
824. C
825. D
826. B
827. D
828. C
829. B
830. D
831. D
832. D
833. D
834. D
835. D
836. D
837. D
838. D
839. B
840. A
841. B
842. D
843. D
844. D
845. D
846. D
847. D
848. D
849. D
850. C
851. B
852. A
853. A
854. D
855. B
856. C
857. D
858. B
859. B
860. B
861. D
862. D
863. A
864. D
865. B
866. D
867. C
868. A
869. A
870. D
871. C
872. D
873. B
874. D
875. B
876. B
877. A
878. C
879. A
880. A
881. D
882. C
883. A
884. B
885. D
886. D
887. D
888. C
889. C
890. A
891. D
892. A
893. A
894. B
895. C
896. C
897. A
898. B
899. A
900. C
901. A
902. D
903. C
904. B
905. A
906. D
907. D
908. D
909. A
910. B
911. C
912. B
913. D
914. D
915. B
916. B
917. D
918. A
919. C
920. C
921. B
922. D
923. A
924. C
925. D
926. A
927. B
928. D
929. A
930. D
931. D
932. B
933. A
934. D
935. D
936. D
937. C
938. C
939. C
940. D
941. D
942. C
943. C
944. D
945. D
946. D
947. D
948. B
949. D
950. D
951. A
952. B
953. C
954. D
955. D
956. A
957. D
958. B
959. A
960. A
961. C
962. B
963. D
964. A
965. D
966. C
967. C
968. D
969. A
970. B
971. A
972. B
973. B
974. A
975. A
976. C
977. D
978. A
979. D
980. D
981. B
982. C
983. A
984. B
985. A
986. C
987. D
988. C
989. B
990. D
991. B
992. A
993. A
994. D
995. D
996. D
997. B
998. A
999. C
1000. B
1001. D
1002. B
1003. D
1004. D
1005. C
1006. C
1007. D
1008. D
1009. D
1010. D
1011. B
1012. D
1013. B
1014. C
1015. C
1016. D
1017. D
1018. A
1019. C
1020. B
1021. D
1022. B
1023. D
1024. C
1025. A
1026. D

Nephrology 4

NEPHROLOGY

Azotemia and Urinary Abnormalities

1. Broad casts in urinary sediment is a diagnostic clue for which of the major nephrology syndromes?
Harrison's 20th Ed. Chapter 48 Page 289 Table 48-1

A. Acute nephritis
B. Nephrotic syndrome
C. Chronic renal failure
D. All of the above

2. Nocturia is a diagnostic clue for which of the major nephrology syndromes?
Harrison's 20th Ed. Chapter 48 Page 289 Table 48-1

A. Urinary tract obstruction
B. Renal tubule defects
C. Chronic renal failure
D. All of the above

3. Lipiduria is a diagnostic clue for which of the major nephrology syndromes?
Harrison's 20th Ed. Chapter 48 Page 289 Table 48-1

A. Acute nephritis
B. Nephrotic syndrome
C. Chronic renal failure
D. Renal tubular defects

4. Which of the following is a common finding in chronic renal failure?
Harrison's 20th Ed. Chapter 48 Page 289 Table 48-1

A. Hypocalcemia
B. Hyperphosphatemia
C. Hyperparathyroidism
D. All of the above

5. Azotemia for more than how many months is labeled as chronic renal failure?
Harrison's 20th Ed. Chapter 48 Page 289 Table 48-1

A. > 1 month
B. > 3 months
C. > 6 months
D. > 12 months

Azotemia for > 3 months is labeled as chronic renal failure.

6. Which of the following is a typical finding in chronic renal failure?
Harrison's 20th Ed. Chapter 48 Page 289 Table 48-1

A. Kidneys reduced in size bilaterally
B. Broad casts in urinary sediment
C. Azotemia for >3 months
D. All of the above

7. Renal osteodystrophy is a finding in?
Harrison's 20th Ed. Chapter 48 Page 289 Table 48-1

A. Acute nephritis
B. Nephrotic syndrome
C. Chronic renal failure
D. Renal tubular defects

8. Hypercoagulable state is a finding in?
Harrison's 20th Ed. Chapter 48 Page 289 Table 48-1

A. Acute nephritis
B. Nephrotic syndrome
C. Chronic renal failure
D. Renal tubular defects

9. Flank tenderness is a finding in?
Harrison's 20th Ed. Chapter 48 Page 289 Table 48-1

A. Acute nephritis
B. Nephrolithiasis
C. Urinary tract obstruction
D. All of the above

10. Large kidneys are a finding in?
Harrison's 20th Ed. Chapter 48 Page 289 Table 48-1

A. Acute nephritis
B. Nephrolithiasis
C. Urinary tract obstruction
D. Renal tubular defects

11. Renal calcification is a finding in?
Harrison's 20th Ed. Chapter 48 Page 289 Table 48-1

A. Acute nephritis
B. Chronic renal failure
C. Urinary tract obstruction
D. Renal tubular defects

12. "Tubular" proteinuria (<1 gram/24 hours) is a finding in?
Harrison's 20th Ed. Chapter 48 Page 289 Table 48-1

A. Urinary tract obstruction
B. Renal tubule defects
C. Chronic renal failure
D. All of the above

13. Which of the following is not a finding in renal tubule defects?
Harrison's 20th Ed. Chapter 48 Page 289 Table 48-1

A. Renal calcification
B. Electrolyte disorders
C. Hypoalbuminemia
D. Large kidneys

14. Circulatory congestion is a typical finding in?

Harrison's 20th Ed. Chapter 48 Page 289 Table 48-1

A. Acute nephritis
B. Chronic renal failure
C. Nephrotic syndrome
D. All of the above

15. Normal combined kidney volume is about?

Can J Kidney Health Dis. 2017;4:1-6

A. 100 to 150 cm^3
B. 150 to 200 cm^3
C. 200 to 300 cm^3
D. 250 to 400 cm^3

Normal combined kidney volume is about 250 to 400 cm^3.

16. Formula for calculation of total kidney volume (TKV) is?

Can J Kidney Health Dis. 2017;4:1-6

A. Length × width × thickness × (π/2)
B. Length × width × thickness × (π/4)
C. Length × width × thickness × (π/6)
D. Length × width × thickness × (π/8)

Ellipsoid formula to calculate TKV is length × width × thickness × (π/6).

17. Which of the following is the primary metric for kidney "function"?

Harrison's 20th Ed. Chapter 48 Page 288

A. Creatinine clearance
B. Glomerular filtration rate
C. Fractional excretion of sodium
D. Albumin-to-creatinine ratio

GFR is the primary metric for kidney "function".

18. Which of the following is used as a surrogate to estimate GFR?

Harrison's 20th Ed. Chapter 48 Page 289

A. Blood urea
B. Plasma creatinine
C. Urine creatinine
D. Creatinine clearance

As direct GFR measurement is not feasible, plasma creatinine is used as a surrogate to estimate GFR.

19. Value of GFR is expressed in?

Harrison's 20th Ed. Chapter 48 Page 289

A. mL/minute
B. mL/hour
C. mL/day
D. mL/kg/minute

20. Value of creatinine clearance is expressed in?

Harrison's 20th Ed. Chapter 48 Page 289

A. mL/minute
B. mL/hour
C. mL/day
D. mL/kg/minute

Creatinine clearance & GFR is calculated for a defined time period (24 hours) & is expressed in mL/minute.

21. In general, patients do not develop symptomatic uremia until GFR is?

Harrison's 20th Ed. Chapter 48 Page 289

A. < 15 mL/minute
B. < 45 mL/minute
C. < 60 mL/minute
D. < 90 mL/minute

In general, patients do not develop symptomatic uremia until renal insufficiency is usually quite severe (GFR < 15 mL/minute).

22. Azotemia best relates to?

Harrison's 20th Ed. Chapter 48 Page 289

A. Retention of nitrogenous waste products
B. Decreased urine output
C. Circulatory overload
D. All of the above

Azotemia is defined as retention of nitrogenous waste products.

23. Azotemia may result from?

Harrison's 20th Ed. Chapter 48 Page 289

A. Reduced renal perfusion
B. Intrinsic renal disease
C. Postrenal processes
D. All of the above

Azotemia may result from reduced renal perfusion (40-80% of cases of acute renal failure), intrinsic renal disease or postrenal processes (ureteral obstruction).

24. In a patient of azotemia due to chronic renal failure, which of the following is false?

Harrison's 20th Ed. Chapter 48 Page 290 Figure 48-1

A. Small kidneys, thin cortex
B. Bland sediment
C. Isosthenuria
D. None of the above

25. In patient of prerenal azotemia, which of the following is false?

Harrison's 20th Ed. Chapter 48 Page 290 Figure 48-1

A. Normal urinalysis with oliguria
B. FeNa < 1%
C. Urine osmolality > 500 mOsmol
D. None of the above

26. In a patient of acute tubular necrosis, which of the following is false?

Harrison's 20th Ed. Chapter 48 Page 290 Figure 48-1

A. Normal urinalysis with oliguria
B. FeNa > 1%
C. Urine osmolality < 350 mOsmol
D. None of the above

27. Which of the following is the first observation in investigations that helps in arriving at the cause of azotemia?

Harrison's 20th Ed. Chapter 48 Page 290 Figure 48-1

A. Renal size
B. Hydronephrosis
C. Cortical thickness
D. Urinary sediment

28. In azotemia, RBC cast with proteinuria point towards the diagnosis of?

Harrison's 20th Ed. Chapter 48 Page 290 Figure 48-1

A. Glomerulonephritis
B. Renal artery occlusion
C. Interstitial nephritis
D. All of the above

29. In azotemia, muddy brown cast with proteinuria point towards the diagnosis of?

Harrison's 20th Ed. Chapter 48 Page 290 Figure 48-1

A. Glomerulonephritis
B. Prerenal azotemia
C. Interstitial nephritis
D. Acute tubular necrosis

30. In azotemia, WBC cast with eosinophilia point towards the diagnosis of?

Harrison's 20th Ed. Chapter 48 Page 290 Figure 48-1

A. Glomerulonephritis
B. Prerenal azotemia
C. Interstitial nephritis
D. Acute tubular necrosis

31. Which of the following is false about creatinine?

Harrison's 20th Ed. Chapter 48 Page 290

A. Small, freely filtered solute, not reabsorbed by tubules
B. Produced from muscle
C. Excreted at a relatively constant rate
D. None of the above

32. For a 20- to 50-year-old man, creatinine excretion should be?

Harrison's 20th Ed. Chapter 48 Page 290

A. 6.5–15.0 mg/kg body weight
B. 18.5–25.0 mg/kg body weight
C. 28.5–35.0 mg/kg body weight
D. 36.5–44.0 mg/kg body weight

For a 20 to 50 year old man, creatinine excretion should be 18.5–25.0 mg/kg body weight. For a woman of the same age, it should be 16.5–22.4 mg/kg body weight.

33. Creatinine clearance (CrCl) is calculated by?

Harrison's 20th Ed. Chapter 48 Page 290

A. $(P_{cr} X T_{min})/(U_{vol} X U_{cr})$
B. $(U_{vol} X U_{cr})/(P_{cr} X T_{min})$
C. $(U_{vol} X P_{cr})/(U_{cr} X T_{min})$
D. $(P_{cr} X U_{cr})/(U_{vol} X T_{min})$

Creatinine clearance (CrCl) is calculated by $(U_{vol} X U_{cr})/(P_{cr} X T_{min})$

34. Which of the following variable is not included in the Cockcroft-Gault formula?

Harrison's 20th Ed. Chapter 48 Page 290

A. Age
B. Weight
C. Plasma creatinine
D. Blood urea

Cockcroft-Gault formula is as follows : CrCl (mL/min) = (140 – age (years) × weight (kg) × [0.85 if female])/(72 × PCr (mg/dL).

35. For calculating GFR by Cockcroft-Gault formula, the value is multiplied by what factor for women?

Harrison's 20th Ed. Chapter 48 Page 290

A. 0.55
B. 0.65
C. 0.75
D. 0.85

For calculating GFR by Cockcroft-Gault formula, the value is multiplied by 0.85 for women a lower fraction of the body weight is composed of muscle.

36. Which of the following variable is not included in the Modification of Diet in Renal Disease (MDRD) formula?

Harrison's 20th Ed. Chapter 48 Page 290

A. Age
B. Gender
C. Ethnicity
D. Height

MDRD formula is as follows : eGFR (mL/min per 1.73 m^2) = 186.3 × PCr ($e^{-1.154}$) × age ($e^{-0.203}$) × (0.742 if female) × (1.21 if black).

37. Which of the following is not used to estimate GFR?

Harrison's 20th Ed. Chapter 48 Page 290

A. Insulin clearance
B. MDRD (modification of diet in renal disease)
C. Cockcroft-Gault formula
D. CKD-EPI

38. MDRD equation better correlates with true GFR when GFR is?

Harrison's 20th Ed. Chapter 48 Page 290

A. < 90 mL/min per 1.73 m^2
B. < 60 mL/min per 1.73 m^2
C. < 30 mL/min per 1.73 m^2
D. < 15 mL/min per 1.73 m^2

The MDRD equation is better correlated with true GFR when the GFR is < 60 mL/min per 1.73 m^2.

39. Cystatin C estimation is a renal function equivalent of?

N Engl J Med. 2006;354:2473-83

A. Urea
B. Creatinine
C. Ammonium
D. Inulin

40. Which of the following is false about Cystatin C?

Harrison's 20th Ed. Chapter 48 Page 290

A. Member of cysteine protease inhibitors
B. Produced from all nucleated cells
C. Production not affected by diet or nutritional status
D. None of the above

Cystatin C is a member of cystatin superfamily of cysteine protease inhibitors, produced at a relatively constant rate from all nucleated cells. Cystatin C production is not affected by diet or nutritional status. It provides a more sensitive indicator of GFR than the plasma creatinine concentration.

41. Laboratory abnormalities characteristic of chronic renal failure include?

Harrison's 20th Ed. Chapter 48 Page 291

A. Anemia
B. Hypocalcemia
C. Hyperphosphatemia
D. All of the above

42. Abnormalities characteristic of chronic renal failure include?

Harrison's 20th Ed. Chapter 48 Page 291

A. Isosthenuria
B. Small kidneys on ultrasound
C. Cortical thinning
D. All of the above

Laboratory abnormalities characteristic of chronic renal failure include anemia, hypocalcemia and hyperphosphatemia. Radiographic evidence of renal osteodystrophy is also characteristic of chronic renal failure but is a very late finding. Other typical findings include proteinuria, nonconcentrated urine (isosthenuria; isosmotic with plasma) and small kidneys on ultrasound with increased echogenicity and cortical thinning.

43. Decreased circulating blood volume due to volume sequestration occurs in?

Harrison's 20th Ed. Chapter 48 Page 291

A. Pancreatitis
B. Peritonitis
C. Rhabdomyolysis
D. All of the above

44. Profound renal vasoconstriction occurs in?

Harrison's 20th Ed. Chapter 48 Page 291

A. Severe heart failure
B. Hepatorenal syndrome
C. Nonsteroidal antiinflammatory drugs (NSAIDs) use
D. All of the above

45. There occurs a steep decline in GFR when mean arterial pressure falls below?

Harrison's 20th Ed. Chapter 48 Page 291

A. 80 mm Hg
B. 90 mm Hg
C. 100 mm Hg
D. 110 mm Hg

Once the mean arterial pressure falls below 80 mm Hg, there is a steep decline in GFR.

46. Which of the following statements is false?

Harrison's 20th Ed. Chapter 48 Page 291

A. Prostaglandin dilate afferent arterioles of glomerulus
B. Angiotensin II constricts efferent arterioles of glomerulus
C. Arterial hypovolemia leads to release of vasopressin (AVP)
D. None of the above

47. Patients are most susceptible to hemodynamically mediated acute renal failure from which drug combinations?

Harrison's 20th Ed. Chapter 48 Page 291

A. NSAIDs + aminoglycosides
B. NSAIDs + ACE inhibitors/ARBs
C. NSAIDs + Azithromycin
D. NSAIDs + Alcohol

Patients taking NSAIDs and/or ACE inhibitors/ARBs are most susceptible to hemodynamically mediated acute renal failure when blood volume is reduced for any reason.

48. The BUN/P_{Cr} ratio in prerenal azotemia is?

Harrison's 20th Ed. Chapter 48 Page 291 Table 48-2

A. > 5:1
B. > 10:1
C. > 15:1
D. > 20:1

BUN/P_{Cr} ratio in prerenal azotemia is > 20:1. It is 10–15:1 in oliguric acute renal failure.

49. Which of the following is false in prerenal azotemia?

Harrison's 20th Ed. Chapter 48 Page 291 Table 48-2

A. Urine sodium (U_{Na}) <20 mEq/L
B. Urine osmolality >500 mOsmol/L H_2O
C. Fractional excretion of sodium (FE_{Na}) >2%
D. Urine/plasma creatinine (U_{Cr}/P_{Cr}) >40

In prerenal azotemia, Fractional excretion of sodium (FE_{Na}) is <1%. In prerenal conditions, renal tubules are intact capable of concentrating urine (>500 mOsmol), avid Na retention (urine Na concentration <20 mmolfL, fractional excretion of Na < 1%) and U_{cr}/P_{cr} >40. The prerenal urine sediment is usually normal or has hyaline and granular casts whereas the sediment of ATN usually is filled with cellular debris, tubular epithelial casts and dark (muddy brown) granular casts.

50. Which of the following formula is correct to calculate fractional excretion of sodium (FE_{Na})?

Harrison's 20th Ed. Chapter 48 Page 291 Table 48-2

A. $U_{Na} + U_{cr} \times 100 \div (P_{Na} + P_{cr})$
B. $U_{Na} \times P_{cr} \times 100 \div (P_{Na} \times U_{cr})$
C. $U_{Na} \times P_{cr} \times 100 - (P_{Na} \times U_{cr})$
D. $U_{Na} \times P_{cr} \times 100 + (P_{Na} \times U_{cr})$

51. Which of the following is a radiopharmaceutical used for evaluation of the kidneys?

J Nucl Med 1996; 37:1883-1890

A. Technetium-99m mercaptoacetyl triglycine (MAG3)
B. Technetium-99m diethylene triamine penta-acetic acid (DTPA)
C. Technetium-99m dimercaptosuccinic acid (DMSA)
D. All of the above

52. Intrinsic renal disease can arise from processes involving which of the following?

Harrison's 20th Ed. Chapter 48 Page 291

A. Large renal vessels
B. Intrarenal microvasculature
C. Glomeruli or the tubulo-interstitium
D. All of the above

Intrinsic renal disease can arise from processes involving large renal vessels, intrarenal microvasculature and glomeruli or the tubulointerstitium.

53. Enhanced reabsorption of Na^+ by collecting duct occurs due to?

Harrison's 20th Ed. Chapter 48 Page 291

A. Increased aldosterone
B. Increased AVP secretion
C. Suppressed atrial natriuretic peptide secretion
D. All of the above

Enhanced reabsorption of Na^+ by collecting duct is in response to increased aldosterone, increased AVP secretion & suppressed atrial natriuretic peptide secretion.

54. Ischemic and toxic ATN account for what percentage of cases of acute intrinsic renal failure?

Harrison's 20th Ed. Chapter 48 Page 291

A. ~ 10%
B. ~ 40%
C. ~ 60%
D. ~ 90%

Ischemic and toxic ATN account for -90% of cases of acute intrinsic renal failure.

55. Evidence of which of the following is present in ATN?

Harrison's 20th Ed. Chapter 48 Page 291

A. Structural collecting duct injury
B. Structural glomerular injury
C. Structural tubule injury
D. All of the above

Prerenal azotemia and ATN are part of a spectrum of renal hypoperfusion. Prolonged renal hypoperfusion can lead to acute tubular necrosis (ATN) and evidence of structural tubule injury is present in ATN.

56. Renal blood flow constitutes what percentage of cardiac output?

Harrison's 20th Ed. Chapter 48 Page 291

A. 5%
B. 10%
C. 15%
D. 25%

Renal blood flow is approximately 25% of cardiac output, or 1000 mL/minute.

57. Medications cause nephrotoxic ATN by?

Harrison's 20th Ed. Chapter 48 Page 292

A. Intrarenal vasoconstriction
B. Direct tubule toxicity
C. Tubular obstruction
D. All of the above

Medications cause nephrotoxic ATN by inducing a combination of intrarenal vasoconstriction, direct tubule toxicity, and/or tubular obstruction.

58. Process that can cause acute kidney injury (AKI) is?

Harrison's 20th Ed. Chapter 48 Page 292

A. Drug-induced interstitial nephritis
B. Infections
C. Systemic diseases
D. All of the above

Acute kidney injury (AKI) is a subtype of acute renal failure due to involvement of tubules & interstitium. These processes include drug-induced interstitial nephritis (antibiotics, NSAIDs, diuretics), severe infections (bacterial and viral), systemic diseases (systemic lupus erythematosus) and infiltrative disorders (sarcoidosis, lymphoma or leukemia).

59. To demonstrate urinary eosinophils, which of the following stains is used?

Harrison's 20th Ed. Chapter 48 Page 292

A. Periodic acid–Schiff (PAS) stain
B. Hansel's stain
C. Warthin-Starry stain
D. Gram stain

To demonstrate urinary eosinophils, Wright's or Hansel's stain is used. The classic sediment finding in allergic interstitial nephritis is a predominance (>10%) of urinary eosinophils.

60. Renal arteries can be occluded due to?

Harrison's 20th Ed. Chapter 48 Page 292

A. Atheroemboli
B. Thromboemboli
C. In situ thrombosis
D. All of the above

Renal arteries can be occluded with atheroemboli, thromboemboli, in situ thrombosis, aortic dissection or vasculitis.

61. Atheroembolic renal failure most often is associated with?

Harrison's 20th Ed. Chapter 48 Page 292

A. Blunt abdominal trauma
B. Recent aortic instrumentation
C. Acute pancreatitis
D. All of the above

Atheroembolic renal failure can occur spontaneously but most often is associated with recent aortic instrumentation.

62. Stigmata of atheroemboli is?

Harrison's 20th Ed. Chapter 48 Page 292

A. Livedo reticularis
B. Distal peripheral infarcts
C. Eosinophilia
D. All of the above

Stigmata of atheroemboli are livedo reticularis, distal peripheral infarcts, eosinophilia.

63. Which of the following statements is false?

Harrison's 20th Ed. Chapter 48 Page 292

A. Renal artery thrombosis leads to mild proteinuria & hematuria
B. Renal vein thrombosis leads to heavy proteinuria & hematuria
C. Eosinophils in urine suggest atheroembolic renal disease
D. None of the above

Eosinophils in urine suggest allergic interstitial nephritis or atheroembolic renal disease.

64. Diseases of the renal microvasculature include?

Harrison's 20th Ed. Chapter 48 Page 292

A. Hemolytic-uremic syndromes
B. Thrombotic thrombocytopenic purpura
C. Malignant hypertension
D. All of the above

Diseases of the renal microvasculature include hemolytic-uremic syndromes, thrombotic thrombocytopenic purpura and malignant hypertension.

65. Oliguria refers to a 24-hour urine output of?

Harrison's 20th Ed. Chapter 48 Page 292

A. < 200 mL
B. < 300 mL
C. < 400 mL
D. < 500 mL

Oliguria refers to a 24-hour urine output of < 400 mL.

66. Anuria refers to a 24-hour urine output of?

Harrison's 20th Ed. Chapter 48 Page 292

A. < 300 mL
B. < 200 mL
C. < 100 mL
D. < 50 mL

Anuria is the complete absence of urine formation (< 100 mL).

67. Urine output of > 400 mL/day in acute or chronic azotemia is called?

Harrison's 20th Ed. Chapter 48 Page 292

A. False anuria
B. Nonanuria
C. Nonoliguria
D. False azotemia

Nonoliguria refers to urine output >400 mL/day in patients with acute or chronic azotemia.

68. Which of the following statements is false?

Harrison's 20th Ed. Chapter 48 Page 292

A. Oliguria is never normal
B. RBC casts are highly specific for glomerulonephritis
C. Hematuria without RBC casts can be an indication of glomerular disease
D. None of the above

69. Which of the following is false about dipstick measurement of proteinuria?

Harrison's 20th Ed. Chapter 48 Page 293

A. False-positive when urine pH is > 7.0
B. False-positive when urine is very concentrated
C. False-positive when urine is contaminated with blood
D. None of the above

Dipstick measurement detects albumin and gives false-positive results when urine pH > 7.0, urine is very concentrated or contaminated with blood.

70. Unit of expression of albumin-to-creatinine ratio (ACR) is?

Harrison's 20th Ed. Chapter 48 Page 293

A. mg/mg
B. mg/dL
C. mg/gram
D. mg%

Albumin-to-creatinine ratio (ACR) is expressed in mg/gram. 24-hour albumin excretion rate (AER) is expressed as mg/24 hour.

71. Proteins of what size are freely filtered by the kidneys?

Harrison's 20th Ed. Chapter 48 Page 293

A. < 20 kDa
B. < 30 kDa
C. < 40 kDa
D. < 50 kDa

Smaller proteins (<20 kDa) are freely filtered but are readily reabsorbed by the proximal tubule.

72. Normal individuals excrete what amount of total protein in urine?

Harrison's 20th Ed. Chapter 48 Page 293

A. < 150 mg/day
B. < 200 mg/day
C. < 250 mg/day
D. < 300 mg/day

73. Normal individuals excrete what amount of albumin in urine?

Harrison's 20th Ed. Chapter 48 Page 293

A. < 30 mg/day
B. < 100 mg/day
C. < 200 mg/day
D. < 300 mg/day

Normal individuals excrete <150 mg/day of total protein and <30 mg/day of albumin.

74. Which of the following is secreted by renal tubules?

Harrison's 20th Ed. Chapter 48 Page 293

A. Tamm-Horsfall protein
B. IgA
C. Urokinase
D. All of the above

75. Which of the following is not secreted by renal tubules?

Harrison's 20th Ed. Chapter 48 Page 293

A. Tamm-Horsfall protein
B. IgA
C. Urokinase
D. β_2-microglobulin

Tamm-Horsfall, IgA, and urokinase in urine is secreted by the tubules. Small amounts of β_2-microglobulin, apoproteins, enzymes, and peptide hormones are filtered.

76. Size of pores of normal glomerular endothelial cell is?

Harrison's 20th Ed. Chapter 48 Page 293

A. ~50 nm
B. ~100 nm
C. ~150 nm
D. ~200 nm

Normal glomerular endothelial cell forms a barrier composed of pores of ~100 nm that hold back blood cells but allow passage of most proteins.

77. Disease that allows "selective" loss of albumin is?

Harrison's 20th Ed. Chapter 48 Page 293

A. Diabetes
B. Focal segmental glomerulosclerosis (FSGS)
C. Minimal change disease
D. Hypertension

"Selective" loss of albumin is seen in minimal change disease. Diabetes & FSGS lead to "nonselective" loss of all plasma proteins. Hypertension, CRF cause increased tubular protein loss.

78. Urinary protein excretion of >3.5 grams/day can occur without the features of nephrotic syndrome in?
Harrison's 20th Ed. Chapter 48 Page 293

A. Diabetes
B. Amyloidosis
C. Minimal change disease
D. All of the above

79. Urinary protein excretion of >3.5 grams/day can occur without the features of nephrotic syndrome in?
Harrison's 20th Ed. Chapter 48 Page 293

A. Focal segmental glomerulosclerosis (FSGS)
B. Membranous glomerulopathy
C. Membranoproliferative glomerulonephritis (MPGN)
D. All of the above

80. Mechanism of renal failure due to plasma cell dyscrasias is?
Harrison's 20th Ed. Chapter 48 Page 293

A. Fusion of glomerular epithelial cell foot processes
B. Disruption of basement membrane & slit diaphragms
C. Tubule obstruction (cast nephropathy)
D. All of the above

Renal failure from plasma cell dyscrasias (multiple myeloma) occurs due to tubule obstruction (cast nephropathy) and light chain deposition.

81. Mechanisms of edema formation in hypoalbuminemia is the activation of?
Harrison's 20th Ed. Chapter 48 Page 293

A. Renin-angiotensin system
B. Antidiuretic hormone
C. Sympathetic nervous system
D. All of the above

Hypoalbuminemia in nephrotic syndrome is due to excessive urinary losses & increased proximal tubule catabolism of filtered albumin. Edema forms from renal sodium retention & reduced plasma oncotic pressure. Mechanisms include activation of renin-angiotensin system, antidiuretic hormone, & sympathetic nervous system, all of which promote excessive renal salt & water reabsorption.

82. In nephrotic syndrome, which of the following protein is lost?
Harrison's 20th Ed. Chapter 48 Page 293

A. Thyroxine-binding globulin
B. Cholecalciferol-binding protein
C. Transferrin
D. All of the above

In nephrotic syndrome, thyroxine-binding globulin, cholecalciferol-binding protein, transferrin, metal-binding proteins, antithrombin III, proteins S & C, fibrinogen and IgG are lost.

83. Hypercoagulable state in nephrotic syndrome is due?
Harrison's 20th Ed. Chapter 48 Page 293

A. Urinary loss of Antithrombin III
B. Urinary loss of Proteins S & C
C. Hyperfibrinogenemia
D. All of the above

Hypercoagulable state in severe nephrotic syndrome is due to urinary losses of antithrombin III, proteins S & C, hyperfibrinogenemia and enhanced platelet aggregation.

84. Normal red blood cell excretion in urine is?
Harrison's 20th Ed. Chapter 48 Page 294

A. ~ 2 million RBCs per day
B. ~ 3 million RBCs per day
C. ~ 4 million RBCs per day
D. ~ 5 million RBCs per day

Normal red blood cell excretion is up to 2 million RBCs per day.

85. Hematuria is defined as how many RBCs per high-power field?
Harrison's 20th Ed. Chapter 48 Page 294

A. 2–5
B. 5–8
C. 8–12
D. 12–15

Hematuria is defined as 2 to 5 RBCs per high-power field (HPF) & can be detected by dipstick.

86. Persistent or significant hematuria means?
Harrison's 20th Ed. Chapter 48 Page 294

A. > 3 RBCs/HPF on three urinalyses
B. Single urinalysis with > 100 RBCs
C. Gross hematuria
D. All of the above

Persistent or significant hematuria means >3 RBCs/HPF on three urinalyses, or a single urinalysis with >100 RBCs, or gross hematuria.

87. Isolated hematuria may be a feature of all except?
Harrison's 20th Ed. Chapter 48 Page 294

A. Urogenital neoplasms
B. Hypercalciuria
C. Hyperoxaluria
D. Hyperuricosuria

Urogenital neoplasms present as isolated painless hematuria with nondysmorphic RBCs. Hypercalciuria & hyperuricosuria are risk factors for unexplained isolated hematuria in children & adults.

88. Isolated glomerular hematuria can occur in?
Harrison's 20th Ed. Chapter 48 Page 294

A. IgA nephropathy
B. Hereditary nephritis
C. Thin basement membrane disease
D. All of the above

Common etiologies of isolated glomerular hematuria are IgA nephropathy, hereditary nephritis, and thin basement membrane disease.

89. Which of the following urinary feature is diagnostic of glomerulonephritis?
Harrison's 20th Ed. Chapter 48 Page 294

A. Hematuria with dysmorphic RBCs
B. RBC casts
C. Protein excretion >500 mg/day
D. All of the above

Hematuria with dysmorphic RBCs, RBC casts, and protein excretion >500 mg/day is virtually diagnostic of glomerulonephritis. RBC casts form as RBCs that enter tubule fluid become trapped in a cylindrical mold of gelled Tamm-Horsfall protein.

90. In urine, WBCs and/or WBC casts are seen in?
Harrison's 20th Ed. Chapter 48 Page 294

A. Interstitial nephritis
B. Systemic lupus erythematosus
C. Transplant rejection
D. All of the above

WBCs and/or WBC casts in urine are seen in tubulointerstitial diseases like interstitial nephritis, SLE and transplant rejection.

91. Urinary sediment of ATN has which of the following?
Harrison's 20th Ed. Chapter 48 Page 294

A. Cellular debris
B. RBC cast
C. Waxy cast
D. Broad cast

Urinary sediment of ATN is filled with cellular debris & dark (muddy brown) granular casts.

92. Waxy casts refer to?
Harrison's 20th Ed. Chapter 48 Page 294

A. Lipid bodies
B. Oval fat bodies
C. Degenerated cellular casts
D. All of the above

In chronic renal diseases, degenerated cellular casts called waxy casts can be seen in the urine.

93. Broad casts are diagnostic of?
Harrison's 20th Ed. Chapter 48 Page 294

A. Pyelonephritis
B. Chronic renal failure
C. Membranoproliferative glomerulonephritis (MPGN)
D. All of the above

Broad casts arise in dilated tubules of enlarged nephrons that have undergone compensatory hypertrophy in response to reduced renal mass as in chronic renal failure.

94. Which of the following statements is false?
Harrison's 20th Ed. Chapter 48 Page 294

A. Normal individuals excrete < 150 mg/day of total protein
B. Normal individuals excrete ~ 30 mg/day of albumin
C. Polyuria is defined as urine output of > 3 L/day
D. None of the above

95. Polyuria is defined as a 24-hour urine output of?
Harrison's 20th Ed. Chapter 48 Page 294

A. > 2 L/day
B. > 3 L/day
C. > 4 L/day
D. > 5 L/day

Polyuria is defined as a 24-hour urine output of >3 L/day.

96. Polyuria results from which of the following mechanisms?
Harrison's 20th Ed. Chapter 48 Page 294

A. Excretion of nonabsorbable solutes
B. Defect in AVP production
C. Defect in AVP renal responsiveness
D. All of the above

Polyuria results from excretion of nonabsorbable solutes (glucose) or excretion of water due to a defect in AVP production or defect in AVP renal responsiveness. Estimation of urine osmolality distinguishes them.

97. An average person excretes how much of solutes per day?
Harrison's 20th Ed. Chapter 48 Page 294

A. 200–600 mOsmol/day
B. 600–800 mOsmol/day
C. 800–1400 mOsmol/day
D. 1400–1800 mOsmol/day

Average person excretes 600 - 800 mOsmol of solutes per day, primarily as urea & electrolytes.

98. In polyuria (>3 L/day) with dilute urine (<250 mOsmol/L), the cause is?
Harrison's 20th Ed. Chapter 48 Page 294

A. Polydipsia
B. Central diabetes insipidus
C. Nephrogenic diabetes insipidus
D. All of the above

99. In polyuria (>3 L/day) with urine osmolality >300 mOsmol/L, the cause is?
Harrison's 20th Ed. Chapter 48 Page 294

A. Polydipsia
B. Central diabetes insipidus
C. Nephrogenic diabetes insipidus
D. Solute diuresis

In polyuria (>3 L/day) with dilute urine (<250 mOsmol/L), the cause can be polydipsia, central diabetes insipidus, or nephrogenic diabetes insipidus. If the urine volume is >3 L/day and urine osmolality is >300 mOsmol/L, a solute diuresis is present.

100. Which of the following is a poorly reabsorbed solute?
Harrison's 20th Ed. Chapter 48 Page 294

A. Glucose
B. Mannitol
C. Urea
D. All of the above

Poorly reabsorbed solutes are glucose, mannitol or urea.

101. Which of the following is a "salt-wasting disorder"?
Harrison's 20th Ed. Chapter 48 Page 294

A. Cystic renal diseases
B. Bartter's syndrome
C. Resolving ATN
D. All of the above

Cystic renal diseases, Bartter's syndrome, or a resolving ATN are salt-wasting disorders.

102. Which of the following drugs can cause primary polydipsia?
Harrison's 20th Ed. Chapter 48 Page 294 Figure 48-4

A. Thioridazine
B. Chlorpromazine
C. Anticholinergic agents
D. All of the above

103. Which of the following can cause solute diuresis?

Harrison's 20th Ed. Chapter 48 Page 294 Figure 48-4

A. Lithium
B. Demeclocycline
C. Diuretics
D. Ethanol

104. Which of the following can cause central diabetes insipidus (vasopressin-sensitive)?

Harrison's 20th Ed. Chapter 48 Page 294 Figure 48-4

A. Sheehan's syndrome
B. Guillain-Barre syndrome
C. Empty sella syndrome
D. All of the above

105. In psychogenic polydipsia, which of the following is false?

Harrison's 20th Ed. Chapter 48 Page 294 Figure 48-4

A. Polyuria
B. Urine osmolality < 250 mOsmol
C. Low serum sodium
D. None of the above

Urine osmolality is maximally dilute at 50 mOsmol/L.

106. Which of the following is the best method to distinguish between central & nephrogenic diabetes insipidus?

Harrison's 20th Ed. Chapter 48 Page 294

A. Urine osmolality
B. Plasma AVP level
C. Water deprivation test
D. All of the above

Estimation of plasma AVP level is the best method for distinguishing between central & nephrogenic diabetes insipidus. Water deprivation test along with exogenous vasopressin may distinguish primary polydipsia from central & nephrogenic diabetes insipidus.

Fluid and Electrolyte Disturbances

107. Water comprises what percentage of body weight in women?
Harrison's 20th Ed. Chapter 49 Page 295

A. ~ 50%
B. ~ 60%
C. ~ 70%
D. ~ 80%

108. Water comprises what percentage of body weight in men?
Harrison's 20th Ed. Chapter 49 Page 295

A. ~ 50%
B. ~ 60%
C. ~ 70%
D. ~ 80%

Water comprises ~50% of body weight in women and ~60% in men.

109. What percentage of total body water is found as intracellular fluid (ICF)?
Harrison's 20th Ed. Chapter 49 Page 295

A. 15–35%
B. 35–55%
C. 55–75%
D. 75–95%

110. What percentage of total body water is found as extracellular fluid (ECF)?
Harrison's 20th Ed. Chapter 49 Page 295

A. 15–25%
B. 25–45%
C. 45–55%
D. 55–75%

55–75% of body water is present as intracellular fluid (ICF) & 25–45% as extracellular fluid (ECF).

111. Ratio of water in intravascular and extravascular spaces is?
Harrison's 20th Ed. Chapter 49 Page 295

A. 1:2
B. 2:1
C. 1:3
D. 3:1

Ratio of intravascular (plasma water) & extravascular (interstitial) ECF water is 1:3.

112. Which of the following is true for Osmolality?
Harrison's 20th Ed. Chapter 49 Page 295

A. Osmoles of solute per milligram of water (Osm/mg)
B. Osmoles of solute per milliliter of water (Osm/mL)
C. Osmoles of solute per kilogram of water (Osm/kg)
D. Osmoles of solute per liter of water (Osm/L)

Osmolality is defined as the concentration of all solutes in a given weight of water and is expressed as milliosmoles or osmoles of solute per kilogram of water (mOsm/kg H_2O). Osmolarity is the measure of osmoles of solute per liter of water (mOsm/L H_2O). Osmolarity = Osmolality × 0.995

113. Plasma osmolality (mOsm/kg H_2O) is calculated by?
Harrison's 20th Ed. Chapter 49 Page 295

A. 2 × plasma [Na^+ + K^+] + glucose/18 + BUN/1.8
B. 2 × plasma [Na^+ + K^+] + glucose/18 + BUN/2.8
C. 2 × plasma [Na^+ + K^+] + glucose/18 + BUN/3.8
D. 2 × plasma [Na^+ + K^+] + glucose/18 + BUN/4.8

Plasma osmolality (mOsm/kg H_2O) is calculated as 2 × plasma [Na^++K^+](mEq/L) + glucose(mg/dL)/18 + BUN(mg/dL)/2.8.

114. Which of the following is correct?
Harrison's 20th Ed. Chapter 49 Page 295

A. ECF osmolality = ICF osmolality
B. ECF osmolality < ICF osmolality
C. ECF osmolality > ICF osmolality
D. All of the above

Osmotic equilibrium refers to ECF osmolality = ICF osmolality.

115. Which of the following is a reflection of ECF volume?
Harrison's 20th Ed. Chapter 49 Page 296

A. Total body Na^+
B. Total body K^+
C. Total body Cl^-
D. Total body HCO_3^-

Total body Na^+ content reflects ECF volume as it is restricted to extracellular compartment.

116. Difference between ICF and ECF composition is due to?
Harrison's 20th Ed. Chapter 49 Page 295

A. Transporters
B. Channels
C. ATP-driven membrane pumps
D. All of the above

117. Which of the following is an organic phosphate ester?
Harrison's 20th Ed. Chapter 49 Page 295

A. ATP
B. Creatine phosphate
C. Phospholipids
D. All of the above

Apart from potassium, the predominant ICF osmoles are organic phosphate esters like ATP, creatine phosphate, and phospholipids.

118. A change in ICF osmolality is due to a change in?
Harrison's 20th Ed. Chapter 49 Page 295

A. ICF water content
B. ICF Na^+ content
C. ICF K^+ content
D. ICF Cl^- content

A change in ICF osmolality is usually due to a change in ICF water content.

119. Which of the following is known as "ineffective osmole"?
Harrison's 20th Ed. Chapter 49 Page 295

A. Inositol
B. Phospholipids
C. Urea
D. All of the above

An osmole is the number of moles that a solute contributes to the osmotic pressure of a solution. Water travels from a low solute concentration to a high solute concentration in order to establish equilibrium. Osmotic pressure is what drives osmosis. It's the force that pulls water from areas of low solute concentration to high solute concentration. Solutes like urea do not contribute to water shift across cell membranes and are known as ineffective osmoles. Ineffective osmoles like urea & glucose do not play a role in stimulating thirst.

120. Regulation of water balance is governed by a high-gain feedback mechanism involving?
N Engl J Med. 2015;372:1349-58

A. Hypothalamus
B. Neurohypophysis
C. Kidneys
D. All of the above

121. AVP gene codes for?
N Engl J Med. 2015;372:1349-58

A. 9–amino acid peptide arginine vasopressin
B. Carrier protein neurophysin-2
C. Glycoprotein copeptin
D. All of the above

AVP gene codes for three peptides — the 9–amino acid peptide arginine vasopressin, a carrier protein called neurophysin-2, and a small glycoprotein called copeptin.

122. Which of the following is considered as a second "antidiuretic hormone"?
N Engl J Med. 2015;372:1349-58

A. Copeptin
B. Oxytocin
C. Neurophysin-2
D. All of the above

Oxytocin gene has a structure that is very similar to that of the arginine vasopressin gene expressed in oxytocinergic cells in the supraoptic & paraventricular nuclei of hypothalamus. Vasopressin secretion is increased by osmotic stimuli. It binds to vasopressin receptors in kidney and produces similar, although weaker, responses than AVP. Consequently, oxytocin is considered to be a second "antidiuretic hormone".

123. Transient vasopressin-resistant diabetes insipidus of pregnancy is due to?
N Engl J Med. 2015;372:1349-58

A. Aquanase
B. Nephrinase
C. Vasopressinase
D. Vasopressinine

Rarely, in III trimester of pregnancy, a syndrome called transient vasopressin-resistant diabetes insipidus of pregnancy occurs as a result of placental secretion of vasopressinase (also called oxytocinase), which hydrolyzes circulating vasopressin and oxytocin. Affected patients have a response to desmopressin acetate, which is resistant to this enzyme.

124. Which of the following collaborate to maintain human body fluid osmolality?
Harrison's 20th Ed. Chapter 49 Page 295

A. Water ingestion
B. Vasopressin secretion
C. Renal water transport
D. All of the above

Vasopressin secretion, water ingestion & renal water transport collaborate to maintain human body fluid osmolality between 280 & 295 mOsm/kg.

125. Osmotic threshold for AVP release is?
Harrison's 20th Ed. Chapter 49 Page 295 Figure 49-1

A. 275 mOsmol/kg
B. 285 mOsmol/kg
C. 295 mOsmol/kg
D. 305 mOsmol/kg

AVP secretion is stimulated as systemic osmolality increases above a threshold level of ~285 mOsm/kg. It maintains plasma osmolality within a 1–2% range. Plasma AVP becomes detectable in euvolemic, healthy individuals at a threshold of ~285 mOsm/kg, above which there is a linear relationship between osmolality and circulating AVP.

126. In hypothalamus, vasopressin (AVP) is synthesized in?
Harrison's 20th Ed. Chapter 49 Page 295

A. Neuroendocrine cells of the periventricular nucleus
B. Neuroendocrine cells of the preoptic area
C. Magnocellular neurons
D. Parvocellular neurosecretory cells of paraventricular nucleus

Vasopressin (AVP) is synthesized in magnocellular neurons within the hypothalamus.

127. Thirst is mediated by?
Harrison's 20th Ed. Chapter 49 Page 295

A. Increase in effective osmolality
B. Decrease in ECF volume
C. Decrease in blood pressure
D. All of the above

Primary stimulus for water ingestion is thirst mediated either by an increase in effective osmolality or a decrease in ECF volume or blood pressure.

128. 'Osmoreceptors' are located in?
Harrison's 20th Ed. Chapter 49 Page 295

A. Posterior pituitary
B. Anterolateral hypothalamus
C. Posteromedial hypothalamus
D. All of the above

Osmoreceptors, located in the anterolateral hypothalamus, are stimulated by a rise in tonicity.

129. Arginine vasopressin is synthesized in?
Harrison's 20th Ed. Chapter 49 Page 295

A. Hypothalamus
B. Anterior pituitary gland
C. Posterior pituitary gland
D. All of the above

130. Arginine vasopressin (AVP) is secreted by?
Harrison's 20th Ed. Chapter 49 Page 295

A. Hypothalamus
B. Anterior pituitary gland
C. Posterior pituitary gland
D. All of the above

Arginine vasopressin (AVP) or antidiuretic hormone (ADH) is a polypeptide synthesized in supraoptic & paraventricular nuclei of hypothalamus & secreted by posterior pituitary gland.

131. Thirst is mediated by?

Harrison's 20th Ed. Chapter 49 Page 295

A. Increase in effective osmolality
B. Decrease in ECF volume
C. Decrease in blood pressure
D. All of the above

Primary stimulus for water ingestion is thirst mediated either by an increase in effective osmolality or a decrease in ECF volume or blood pressure.

132. Half-life of AVP in the circulation is?

Harrison's 20th Ed. Chapter 49 Page 295

A. 1–2 minutes
B. 2–4 minutes
C. 4–8 minutes
D. 10–20 minutes

AVP has a half-life in the circulation of only 10–20 minutes.

133. Nonosmotic factors that regulate AVP secretion include?

Harrison's 20th Ed. Chapter 49 Page 295

A. Nausea
B. Serotonin
C. Intracerebral angiotensin II
D. All of the above

Nonosmotic factors that regulate AVP secretion include effective circulating (arterial) volume, nausea, pain, stress, hypoglycemia, pregnancy, intracerebral angiotensin II, serotonin and multiple drugs.

134. Receptor to which AVP binds in renal collecting ducts is?

Harrison's 20th Ed. Chapter 49 Page 295

A. U_2 receptor
B. V_2 receptor
C. W_2 receptor
D. X_2 receptor

AVP acts on renal V2 type receptors in the thick ascending limb of Henle and principal cells of the collecting duct (CD), increasing intracellular levels of cyclic AMP and activating protein kinase A (PKA) - dependent phosphorylation of multiple transport proteins.

135. Which of the following about V2 vasopressin receptor is false?

N Engl J Med. 2015;372:1349-58

A. G protein–coupled receptor
B. Functions mediated by the heterotrimeric G-protein G_s
C. Located chiefly in renal epithelia
D. None of the above

136. V2 receptor acts chiefly in?

N Engl J Med. 2015;372:1349-58

A. Principal cells of renal collecting duct
B. Distal convoluted tubule cells
C. Cells of the thick ascending limb of Henle
D. All of the above

V2 receptor acts chiefly in the principal cells of the renal collecting duct, the connecting tubule cells, the distal convoluted tubule cells, and the cells of the thick ascending limb of Henle.

137. Which of the following aquaporin is present in renal proximal tubule & thin descending limb of the loop of Henle?

N Engl J Med. 2015;372:1349-58

A. Aquaporin-1 gene
B. Aquaporin-2 gene
C. Aquaporin-3 gene
D. Aquaporin-4 gene

138. Which of the following aquaporin is present in renal connecting tubule & collecting duct?

N Engl J Med. 2015;372:1349-58

A. Aquaporin-2 gene
B. Aquaporin-3 gene
C. Aquaporin-4 gene
D. All of the above

139. Water channels in collecting ducts activated by AVP are encoded by?

Harrison's 20th Ed. Chapter 49 Page 295

A. Aquaporin-1 gene
B. Aquaporin-2 gene
C. Aquaporin-3 gene
D. Aquaporin-4 gene

AVP binds to V_2 receptors on basolateral membrane of principal cells in the collecting duct activating the water channels which are encoded by aquaporin-2 gene.

140. Loss or gain of approximately how much water will change plasma Na^+ concentration by ~1 mmol per liter?

N Engl J Med. 2015;372:55-65

A. 1 mL per kilogram of body weight
B. 2 mL per kilogram of body weight
C. 3 mL per kilogram of body weight
D. 4 mL per kilogram of body weight

Loss or gain of approximately 3 mL of water per kilogram of body weight will change the plasma sodium concentration by approximately 1 mmol per liter.

141. Site where AVP exerts its principal effect is?

Lancet 2005;365:417-430

A. Proximal convoluted tubule
B. Loop of Henle
C. Distal convoluted tubule
D. Cortical & papillary portions of collecting duct

142. Site of action of loop diuretics is?

Lancet 2005;365:417-430

A. Proximal convoluted tubule
B. Thin ascending limb of Henle's loop
C. Medullary thick ascending limb of Henle
D. All of the above

Na:K:2Cl cotransporter is the site of action of the powerful loop diuretics in the medullary thick ascending limb of Henle, and its mutations give rise to Bartter's syndrome.

143. Normally, major quantity of phosphate is reabsorbed in?
Lancet 2005;365:417-430

A. Proximal convoluted tubule
B. Loop of Henle
C. Distal convoluted tubule
D. Collecting duct

144. The principle site of action of parathyroid hormone (PTH) is?
Lancet 2005;365:417-430

A. Proximal convoluted tubule
B. Loop of Henle
C. Distal convoluted tubule
D. Collecting duct

145. Fluid that enters the distal convoluted tubule is always?
N Engl J Med. 2015;372:55-65

A. Isoosmotic
B. Hypoosmotic
C. Hyperosmotic
D. None of the above

146. The terminal segment of the distal nephron is?
N Engl J Med. 2015;372:55-65

A. Cortical collecting tubule
B. Papillary collecting duct
C. Terminal duct
D. None of the above

147. Calcium reabsorption in cortical thick ascending limb of Henle's loop (cTAL) requires which of the following?
N Engl J Med. 2015;372:55-65

A. PTH
B. $1,25(OH)_2D$
C. Paracellin-1
D. Calbindin-D28k

Mutations in CLDN16 encoding paracellin-1, a transmembrane protein located within the tight junction complex, leads to familial hypomagnesemia with hypercalciuria & nephrocalcinosis, suggesting that the ion conductance of the paracellular pathway in thick limb is regulated.

148. In cells & in ECF, phosphorus exists in which form?
N Engl J Med. 2015;372:55-65

A. $H_2PO_4^-$
B. $NaHPO_4^-$
C. HPO_4^{2-}
D. All of the above

149. In adults, above what level of fasting serum phosphate concentration is called hyperphosphatemia?
N Engl J Med. 2015;372:55-65

A. 2.5 mg/dL
B. 3.5 mg/dL
C. 4.5 mg/dL
D. 5.5 mg/dL

Hyperphosphatemia is defined in adults as a fasting serum phosphate concentration > 1.8 mmol/L or 5.5 mg/dL. It results from impaired glomerular filtration, hypoparathyroidism, excessive delivery of phosphate into the ECF from bone, gut, or parenteral phosphate therapy. Upper limit of normal serum phosphate concentrations is higher in children & neonates (2.4 mmol/L or 7 mg/dL).

150. Normally, the concentration of magnesium in serum is?
N Engl J Med. 2015;372:55-65

A. 0.7 to 1.2 mg/dL
B. 1.2 to 1.6 mg/dL
C. 1.5 to 2.0 mg/dL
D. 2.4 to 2.9 mg/dL

The concentration of magnesium in serum is closely regulated within the range of 0.7 - 1 mmol!L or 1.5 - 2 mEq/L. One-half of the 25 gram (1000 mmol) of total body magnesium is located in bone and only 1% of body magnesium resides in the ECF. Almost all extraskeletal magnesium is present within cells, where the total concentration is 5 mM.

151. Which of the following should be supplemented in patients with hypomagnesemia?
N Engl J Med. 2015;372:55-65

A. Calcium
B. Potassium
C. Phosphate
D. All of the above

152. Maximal urine osmolality can be?
Harrison's 20th Ed. Chapter 49 Page 296, N Engl J Med. 2015;372:55-65

A. 500 mOsmol/kg
B. 800 mOsmol/kg
C. 1000 mOsmol/kg
D. 1200 mOsmol/kg

Under "antidiuretic" conditions, with increased circulating AVP, kidneys reabsorbs water filtered at glomerulus, equilibrating the osmolality across CD epithelium to excrete a hypertonic or concentrated urine (osmolality of up to 1200).

153. Minimum urine osmolality in humans can be?
Harrison's 20th Ed. Chapter 49 Page 296, N Engl J Med. 2015;372:55-65

A. 50 mOsmol/kg
B. 100 mOsmol/kg
C. 150 mOsmol/kg
D. 200 mOsmol/kg

In the absence of circulating AVP, insertion of aquaporin-2 channels & water absorption across CD is essentially abolished, resulting in secretion of a hypotonic, dilute urine (osmolality as low as 30-50 mOsm/kg).

154. Maximally dilute urine occurs in which of the following?
N Engl J Med. 2015;372:55-65

A. Untreated diabetes insipidus
B. Spontaneous recovery from hyponatremia
C. Administration of a vasopressin antagonist
D. All of the above

155. Individuals eating a typical western diet consume what amount of NaCl daily?
N Engl J Med. 2015;372:55-65

A. ~ 50 mmol
B. ~ 150 mmol
C. ~ 250 mmol
D. ~ 500 mmol

Individuals eating a typical western diet consume ~150 mmol of NaCl daily.

156. Major regulatory mechanism controlling sodium excretion is?
Harrison's 20th Ed. Chapter 49 Page 296

A. GFR
B. Tubule Na^+ reabsorption
C. Tubule water reabsorption
D. All of the above

Tubule Na^+ reabsorption, and not GFR, is the major regulatory mechanism controlling Na^+ excretion.

157. Kidneys filter how many millimoles of Na^+ per day?
Harrison's 20th Ed. Chapter 49 Page 296

A. 20,200
B. 25,200
C. 30,200
D. 35,200

Kidneys filter ~25,200 mmol of Na^+ per day. This is equivalent to ~1.5 kg of salt.

158. How many millimoles of Na^+ is excreted per day?
Harrison's 20th Ed. Chapter 49 Page 296

A. 100 mM
B. 400 mM
C. 800 mM
D. 1000 mM

99.6% of filtered Na^+-Cl^- is reabsorbed to excrete 100 mM per day.

159. Which of the following play a role in the renal absorption of sodium?
Harrison's 20th Ed. Chapter 49 Page 296

A. Na^+-K^+-$2Cl^-$ cotransporter (NKCC2)
B. Na^+-Cl^- cotransporter (NCC)
C. Epithelial Na^+ channels (ENaC)
D. All of the above

160. Majority of filtered sodium is reabsorbed in?
Harrison's 20th Ed. Chapter 49 Page 296

A. Proximal convoluted tubule
B. Thick ascending limb of loop of Henle
C. Distal convoluted tubule
D. Cortical and medullary collecting ducts

161. Reabsorption of filtered sodium mediated by 'Na^+ - K^+ - $2Cl^-$ cotransporter' occurs in?
Harrison's 20th Ed. Chapter 49 Page 296

A. Proximal convoluted tubule
B. Thick ascending limb of the loop of Henle (TALH)
C. Distal convoluted tubule
D. Cortical and medullary collecting ducts

162. Reabsorption of filtered sodium mediated by 'thiazide - sensitive Na^+ - Cl^- cotransporter' occurs in?
Harrison's 20th Ed. Chapter 49 Page 296

A. Proximal convoluted tubule
B. Thick ascending limb of loop of Henle (TALH)
C. Distal convoluted tubule
D. Cortical & medullary collecting ducts

Almost two-thirds of filtered Na^+ is reabsorbed in the proximal convoluted tubule. 25-30% occurs in TALH via apical furosemide-sensitive Na^+-K^+-$2Cl^-$ co-transporter. 5% occurs in DCT mediated by thiazide-sensitive Na^+-Cl^- co-transporter. Na^+ reabsorption also occurs in cortical and medullary collecting ducts.

163. Distal nephron comprises of?
Harrison's 20th Ed. Chapter 49 Page 296

A. Distal convoluted tubule (DCT)
B. Connecting tubule (CNT)
C. Collecting ducts (CD)
D. All of the above

164. Amiloride-sensitive epithelial Na^+ channels (ENaC) are located in?
Harrison's 20th Ed. Chapter 49 Page 296

A. Proximal convoluted tubule
B. Thin descending limb of loop of Henle
C. Thick ascending limb of loop of Henle (TALH)
D. Collecting ducts (CD)

165. Chloride ions are primarily reabsorbed by?
Harrison's 20th Ed. Chapter 49 Page 296

A. Principal cells
B. β–intercalated cells
C. Macula densa
D. All of the above

Cl^- ions are primarily reabsorbed by intercalated cells, via apical Cl^- exchange (Cl^--OH^- and Cl^--HCO_3^- exchange, mediated by the SLC26A4 anion exchanger.

166. Angiotensin II acts at which of the following?
Harrison's 20th Ed. Chapter 49 Page 296

A. Proximal convoluted tubule
B. Thick ascending limb of loop of Henle (TALH)
C. Distal convoluted tubule
D. Cortical & medullary collecting ducts

Angiotensin II activates proximal Na^+ - Cl^- reabsorption like adrenergic receptors under the influence of renal sympathetic innervation. Locally generated dopamine has a natriuretic effect.

167. Aldosterone-sensitive distal nephron comprises of?
Harrison's 20th Ed. Chapter 49 Page 296

A. Distal convoluted tubule (DCT)
B. Connecting tubule (CNT)
C. Collecting duct (CD)
D. All of the above

Aldosterone-sensitive distal nephron comprises of distal convoluted tubule (DCT), Connecting tubule (CNT) and collecting duct (CD). Aldosterone primarily activates Na-Cl reabsorption within the aldosterone-sensitive distal nephron.

168. Na^+ absorption and promoting K^+ excretion is a function of?
Harrison's 20th Ed. Chapter 49 Page 296

A. Na^+–K^+–$2Cl^-$ cotransporter
B. Thiazide–sensitive Na^+–Cl^- cotransporter
C. Epithelial Na^+ channels (ENaC)
D. All of the above

Aldosterone activates ENaC channel in principal cells inducing Na^+ absorption & promoting K^+ excretion.

169. AVP maintains circulatory integrity by?
Harrison's 20th Ed. Chapter 49 Page 297

A. Inducing vasoconstriction
B. Increasing sympathetic nervous system tone
C. Increasing renal retention of water and $Na^+–Cl^-$
D. All of the above

AVP maintains circulatory integrity by inducing vasoconstriction, increasing sympathetic nervous system tone, increasing renal retention of both water and Na - Cl and modulating the arterial baroreceptor reflex. Most of these responses involve activation of systemic V_{1A} AVP receptors but concomitant activation of V2 receptors in the kidney can result in renal water retention and hyponatremia.

170. Aquaporin-2 dysregulation occurs in?
N Engl J Med. 2015;372:1349-58

A. Congestive heart failure
B. Hepatic cirrhosis
C. Syndrome of inappropriate antidiuretic hormone secretion
D. All of the above

Aquaporin-2 dysregulation occurs in syndromes associated with renal water retention & dilutional hyponatremia, mainly severe congestive heart failure, hepatic cirrhosis, and the syndrome of inappropriate antidiuretic hormone secretion (SIADH).

171. Type I Bartter's syndrome is associated with?
N Engl J Med. 2015;372:1349-58

A. Bumetanide-sensitive sodium-potassium-chloride cotransporter
B. Thiazide-sensitive sodium-chloride cotransporter
C. Vasopressin receptor V2
D. Vasopressin-regulated urea channel

In the thick ascending limbs of Henle, transport of sodium & chloride from lumen is mediated by the bumetanide-sensitive sodium–potassium–chloride cotransporter. Vasopressin upregulates this cotransporter by increasing the expression of SLC12A1, which codes for the cotransporter protein. Up-regulation of sodium–potassium–chloride cotransporter does not affect salt excretion, primarily because thick ascending limb is upstream from macula densa, which compensates for changes in salt delivery by adjusting glomerular filtration rate. This compensatory process is called glomerulotubular feedback. Bumetanide and other loop diuretics increase salt excretion because they inhibit sodium–potassium–chloride cotransporter in macula densa, thereby blocking the feedback to the glomerulus. Type I Bartter's syndrome is due to loss-of-function mutations in SLC12A1 and is manifested by a salt-losing syndrome rather than by a simple defect in water balance.

172. Gitelman's syndrome is associated with?
N Engl J Med. 2015;372:1349-58

A. Bumetanide-sensitive sodium-potassium-chloride cotransporter
B. Thiazide-sensitive sodium-chloride cotransporter
C. Vasopressin receptor V2
D. Vasopressin-regulated urea channel

Vasopressin also regulates salt transport in distal convoluted tubule by upregulating apical thiazide-sensitive sodium–chloride cotransporter,. It transports salt at a high rate but is impermeable to water and thereby contributes to dilution of the tubular fluid. This cotransporter is also regulated by aldosterone. Inactivating mutations in thiazide-sensitive sodium–chloride cotransporter cause Gitelman's syndrome, which is manifested by hypotension, hypokalemia, hypomagnesemia, hypocalciuria, and metabolic alkalosis.

173. Deafness is invariably associated with which type of Bartter's syndrome?
N Engl J Med. 2015;372:1349-58

A. Type 1
B. Type 2
C. Type 3
D. Type 4

Bartter type 4 is due to mutations in barttin which is also expressed in inner ear. Deafness is invariably associated with Bartter type 4.

174. Which of the following is false for Bartter's syndrome?
N Engl J Med. 2015;372:1349-58

A. Inherited as autosomal recessive trait
B. Due to abnormality in renal tubule transport proteins
C. Prostaglandin E production is low
D. Metabolic abnormalities similar to diuretic abuse

In Bartter's syndrome, RAS activation causes increased levels of cyclooxygenase 2 (COX-2) & marked overproduction of renal prostaglandins (PGE2).

175. Hyperprostaglandin E syndrome is related to?
N Engl J Med. 2015;372:1349-58

A. Bartter's syndrome
B. Gitelman's syndrome
C. Liddle's syndrome
D. All of the above

Hyperprostaglandin E syndrome is a severe form of Bartter's syndrome. Neonates present with pronounced volume depletion, fever, vomiting and diarrhea from PGE_2 overproduction.

176. Protein affected in Bartter's syndrome is?
N Engl J Med. 2015;372:1349-58

A. NKCC2
B. ROMK
C. Barttin
D. All of the above

Bartter's syndrome is the result of mutations in ion transport proteins in TAL. Type 1 is due to apical loop-diuretic sensitive sodium-potassium-chloride co-transporter protein NKCC2, type 2 is due to apical potassium channel ROMK, type 3 is due to basolateral chloride channel ClC-Kb and Bartter type 4 results from mutations in barttin, an essential subunit of ClC-Ka and ClC-Kb that enables transport of the chloride channels to the cell surface.

177. Which of the following electrical situations occur in Bartter's syndrome?
N Engl J Med. 2015;372:1349-58

A. Loss of lumen-positive electrical transport potential
B. Loss of lumen-negative electrical transport potential
C. Loss of cell-positive electrical transport potential
D. Loss of cell-negative electrical transport potential

In Bartter's syndrome, loss of lumen-positive electrical transport potential that normally drives paracellular reabsorption of sodium, calcium & magnesium causes NaCl wasting, hypercalciuria & mild hypomagnesemia.

178. Gitelman's syndrome is due to mutations in?
N Engl J Med. 2015;372:1349-58

A. Apical loop-diuretic sensitive Na-K-Cl co-transporter
B. Apical potassium channel
C. Thiazide-sensitive Na-Cl co-transporter (NCCT)
D. Basolateral chloride channel ClC-Kb

Gitelman's syndrome is due to mutations in thiazide-sensitive Na-Cl co-transporter (NCCT) in DCT.

179. Gitelman's syndrome is distinguished from Bartter's syndrome by?
N Engl J Med. 2015;372:1349-58

A. Hypokalemia
B. Metabolic alkalosis
C. Elevated renin and aldosterone levels
D. Hypomagnesemia

Severe magnesium wasting occurs in Gitelman's syndrome.

180. Gitelman's syndrome is distinguished from Bartter's syndrome by?

N Engl J Med. 2015;372:1349-58

A. Hypokalemia
B. Metabolic alkalosis
C. Elevated renin and aldosterone levels
D. Hypocalciuria

Gitelman's syndrome is distinguished from Bartter's syndrome by presence of severe hypomagnesemia & hypocalciuria. Hypercalciuria marked overproduction of renal prostaglandins (PGE2) occurs in Bartter's syndrome.

181. Carpopedal spasm, cramps & tetany are clinical features of?

N Engl J Med. 2015;372:1349-58

A. Bartter's syndrome
B. Gitelman's syndrome
C. Liddle's syndrome
D. Von Hippel-Lindau disease

Gitelman's syndrome is characterized by hypocalciuria, severe hypomagnesemia resulting in carpopedal spasm, cramps and tetany. Autosomal recessive familial hypomagnesemia with hypercalciuria and nephrocalcinosis (FHHNC), autosomal recessive hypomagnesemia with secondary hypocalcemia (HSH), autosomal dominant hypomagnesemia, and autosomal dominant hypoparathyroidism can also produce such presentation.

182. Which of the following best relate to Liddle's syndrome?

N Engl J Med. 2015;372:1349-58

A. Unregulated sodium reabsorption
B. Overactive ENaC in cortical collecting duct
C. Chloride-independent sodium reabsorption
D. All of the above

183. Which of the following is false for Liddle's syndrome?

N Engl J Med. 2015;372:1349-58

A. Hypertension
B. Hypokalemia
C. High aldosterone levels
D. Metabolic alkalosis

Liddle's syndrome mimics a state of aldosterone excess. Features include early and severe hypertension, hypokalemia & metabolic alkalosis. Plasma aldosterone & renin levels are low.

184. Which of the following drug is ineffective in treatment of Liddle's syndrome?

N Engl J Med. 2015;372:1349-58

A. Spironolactone
B. Amiloride
C. Triamterene
D. All of the above

Amiloride or triamterene block ENaC and, combined with salt restriction, provide effective therapy for hypertension and hypokalemia.

185. Polyuria is a prominent feature of all except?

N Engl J Med. 2015;372:1349-58

A. ADPKD
B. Medullary cystic kidney disease (MCKD)
C. Bartter's syndrome
D. Gitelman's syndrome

186. During antenatal period, fetal polyuria causes maternal polyhydramnios and premature labor in?

N Engl J Med. 2015;372:1349-58

A. ADPKD
B. Medullary cystic kidney disease (MCKD)
C. Bartter's syndrome
D. Gitelman's syndrome

In antenatal period, fetal polyuria may cause maternal polyhydramnios & premature labor in Bartter's syndrome.

187. ENaC best relates to?

N Engl J Med. 2015;372:1349-58

A. Amiloride-sensitive epithelial sodium channel
B. Thiazide-sensitive Na-Cl co-transporter
C. Na-K-2Cl co-transporter
D. Sodium-bicarbonate co-transporter

ENaC is an amiloride-sensitive epithelial sodium channel.

188. Which of the following about aquaporin-1 is false?

N Engl J Med. 2015;372:1349-58

A. Expressed in proximal tubule
B. Expressed in thin descending limb of the loop of Henle
C. Not regulated by vasopressin
D. None of the above

189. Which of the following about aquaporin-2 is false?

N Engl J Med. 2015;372:1349-58

A. Expressed throughout the collecting-duct system
B. Regulated by vasopressin
C. Half-life of aquaporin-2 protein is increased by vasopressin
D. None of the above

Aquaporin-2 is expressed throughout collecting-duct system i.e., in the region of renal tubule where vasopressin regulates osmotic transport of water. Aquaporin-2 mediates "apical" component of transepithelial water transport, and its regulation by vasopressin controls the overall rate of water permeation across the collecting-duct epithelium.

190. Which of the following about aquaporin-3 is false?

N Engl J Med. 2015;372:1349-58

A. Localized to the basolateral plasma membrane
B. Present in collecting-duct principal cells, connecting-tubule cells, and inner medullary collecting-duct cells
C. Conducts glycerol in addition to water
D. None of the above

Like aquaporin-2, aquaporin-3 is regulated by vasopressin.

191. Which of the following about aquaporin-4 is false?

N Engl J Med. 2015;372:1349-58

A. Localized to the basolateral plasma membrane
B. Present in the collecting-duct system
C. Not regulated by vasopressin
D. None of the above

192. In erythrocytes, aquaporin-3 is responsible for which of the following blood-group antigen?

N Engl J Med. 2015;372:1349-58

A. KEL
B. GIL
C. MNS
D. LU

Aquaporin-3 is widely expressed throughout body. In RBCs, it is responsible for GIL blood-group antigen.

193. Urea-channel proteins (UT-A1 & UT-A3) are produced from which of the following gene?

N Engl J Med. 2015;372:1349-58

A. SLC12A2
B. SLC13A2
C. SLC14A2
D. SLC15A2

Urea-channel proteins (UT-A1 & UT-A3) are produced from the same gene, SLC14A2. In the inner medullary collecting duct, vasopressin rapidly & reversibly increases transepithelial urea permeability, allowing urea to exit and become trapped within countercurrent exchange system. Accumulation of urea in the medullary interstitium by this mechanism contributes to the high osmolality in the inner medulla.

194. Amiloride-sensitive epithelial Na^+ channel (ENaC) best relates to?

N Engl J Med. 2015;372:1349-58

A. Nedd4-1
B. Nedd4-2
C. Nedd4-3
D. Nedd4-4

The activity of ENaC is increased by SGK1-mediated phosphorylation of Nedd4-2, a protein that promotes recycling of the Na+ channel from the plasma membrane.

195. Which of the following channels is regulated by vasopressin?

N Engl J Med. 2015;372:1349-58

A. Epithelial Sodium Channel
B. Urea Channel
C. Aquaporin-2
D. All of the above

196. X-linked nephrogenic diabetes insipidus is associated with?

N Engl J Med. 2015;372:1349-58

A. Bumetanide-sensitive sodium-potassium-chloride cotransporter
B. Thiazide-sensitive sodium-chloride cotransporter
C. Vasopressin receptor V2
D. Vasopressin-regulated urea channel

Most patients with non–X-linked nephrogenic diabetes insipidus have mutations in AQP2.

197. Autosomal nephrogenic diabetes insipidus is associated with?

N Engl J Med. 2015;372:1349-58

A. Epithelial sodium channel Beta subunit
B. Epithelial sodium channel Gamma subunit
C. Vasopressin receptor V2
D. Aquaporin-2

198. Which of the following is false about hereditary nephrogenic diabetes insipidus (NDI)?

N Engl J Med. 2015;372:1349-58

A. High plasma levels of vasopressin
B. Hyponatremia
C. Polyuria
D. Seizures & mental retardation

Hereditary nephrogenic diabetes insipidus (NDI) presents in infancy with severe vasopressin-resistant polyuria, dehydration, failure to thrive, and dilute urine despite the presence of hypernatremia.

Hypovolemia

199. True volume depletion or hypovolemia refers to?

Harrison's 20th Ed. Chapter 49 Page 297

A. Salt loss
B. Water loss
C. Contraction of ECFV
D. All of the above

True volume depletion, or hypovolemia, refers to a state of combined salt & water loss, leading to contraction of the ECFV. The loss of salt & water may be renal or nonrenal in origin.

200. Which of the following can cause osmotic diuresis?

Harrison's 20th Ed. Chapter 49 Page 297

A. Glucose
B. Urea
C. Mannitol
D. All of the above

201. Which of the following causes natriuresis by inhibiting proximal tubular Na^+ - Cl^- absorption?

Harrison's 20th Ed. Chapter 49 Page 297

A. Acetazolamide
B. Trimethoprim
C. Pentamidine
D. All of the above

Acetazolamide induces natriuresis as a side effect by inhibiting proximal tubular Na^+ - Cl^- absorption.

202. Which of the following causes natriuresis by inhibiting distal tubular amiloride-sensitive ENaC channel?

Harrison's 20th Ed. Chapter 49 Page 297

A. Acetazolamide
B. Trimethoprim
C. Doxycycline
D. All of the above

Trimethoprim & pentamidine inhibit distal tubular Na^+ reabsorption through amiloride-sensitive ENaC channel leading to urinary Na^+-Cl^- loss.

203. Which of the following reduce Na^+-Cl^- reabsorption by the aldosterone-sensitive distal nephron?

Harrison's 20th Ed. Chapter 49 Page 297

A. Mineralocorticoid deficiency
B. Mineralocorticoid resistance
C. Inhibition of mineralocorticoid receptor (MLR)
D. All of the above

204. What quantity of fluid enters gastrointestinal tract daily as secretions?

Harrison's 20th Ed. Chapter 49 Page 297

A. ~ 3 liters
B. ~ 5 liters
C. ~ 7 liters
D. ~ 9 liters

~ 9 liters of fluid enters GI tract daily, 2 by ingestion & 7 liters by secretion.

205. Fecal fluid loss is?

Harrison's 20th Ed. Chapter 49 Page 297

A. 100–200 mL/day
B. 200–300 mL/day
C. 300–400 mL/day
D. 400–500 mL/day

Fecal fluid loss is 100 - 200 mL/day.

206. Which of the following secretions is alkaline?

Harrison's 20th Ed. Chapter 49 Page 297

A. Biliary
B. Pancreatic
C. Intestinal
D. All of the above

Biliary, pancreatic and intestinal secretions are alkaline.

207. What is the magnitude of "insensible losses" in healthy adults?

Harrison's 20th Ed. Chapter 49 Page 297

A. 250–500 mL/day
B. 500–650 mL/day
C. 750–1000 mL/day
D. 1000–1500 mL/day

"Insensible losses" refers to the evaporation of water from skin and respiratory tract. They are a major route for loss of solute-free water. It is typically 500-650 mL/day in healthy adults.

208. Reliable sign of hypovolemia is?

Harrison's 20th Ed. Chapter 49 Page 297

A. Decreased jugular venous pressure (JVP)
B. Orthostatic tachycardia
C. Orthostatic hypotension
D. All of the above

Diminished skin turgor & dry oral mucous membranes are less reliable markers of a decreased ECFV in adult patients. More reliable signs of hypovolemia include a decreased jugular venous pressure (JVP), orthostatic tachycardia (increase of >15-20 beats/minute upon standing) and orthostatic hypotension (>10-20 mm Hg drop in blood pressure on standing).

209. In nonrenal hypovolemia, which of the following is true?

Harrison's 20th Ed. Chapter 49 Page 298

A. Urine Na^+ <20 mM, Urine osmolality >450 mOsm/kg
B. Urine Na^+ >20 mM, Urine osmolality <450 mOsm/kg
C. Urine Na^+ <20 mM, Urine osmolality <450 mOsm/kg
D. Urine Na^+ >20 mM, Urine osmolality >450 mOsm/kg

In nonrenal hypovolemiaurine, urine Na^+ concentration is typically <20 mM with a urine osmolality of >450 mOsm/kg. This is because neurohumoral response to hypovolemia stimulates an increase in renal tubular Na^+ and water reabsorption.

210. In hypovolemia and hypochloremic alkalosis, which of the following is true?

Harrison's 20th Ed. Chapter 49 Page 298

A. Urine Na^+ <20 mM, urine pH <7.0
B. Urine Na^+ >20 mM, urine pH >7.0
C. Urine Na^+ >20 mM, urine pH <7.0
D. Urine Na^+ <20 mM, urine pH >7.0

Patients with hypovolemia and hypochloremic alkalosis due to vomiting, diarrhea or diuretics will typically have a urine Na^+ concentration >20 mM and urine pH of >7.0, due to the increase in filtered HCO_3^-. Urine Cl^- concentration in therefore a more accurate indicator of volume status, with a level <25 mM suggestive of hypovolemia.

211. Isotonic, "normal" saline (0.9% NaCl) contains what amount of sodium?

Harrison's 20th Ed. Chapter 49 Page 298

A. 134 mM
B. 144 mM
C. 154 mM
D. 164 mM

212. Red cell transfusion is given to hypovolemic patients due to severe hemorrhage/anemia keeping hematocrit levels below?

Harrison's 20th Ed. Chapter 49 Page 298

A. 25%
B. 35%
C. 45%
D. 55%

Hypovolemic patients due to severe hemorrhage or anemia should receive red cell transfusions, without increasing the hematocrit beyond 35%.

213. Plasma osmolality is calculated by?

Harrison's 20th Ed. Chapter 49 Page 297

A. Na^+ + (Glucose/18) + (BUN/2.8)
B. $2Na^+$ + (Glucose/18) + (BUN/2.8)
C. $3Na^+$ + (Glucose/18) + (BUN/2.8)
D. $4Na^+$ + (Glucose/18) + (BUN/2.8)

BUN are expressed in milligrams per deciliter: Posm = $2Na^+$ + Glucose/18 + BUN/2.8.

214. What level of BUN : creatinine ratio distinguishes pre-renal azotemia (PRA) from acute tubular necrosis (ATN)?

Clin Kidney J. 2012;5(2):187-191

A. 5:1
B. 10:1
C. 15:1
D. 20:1

The blood urea nitrogen (BUN)/creatinine ratio (BCR) is used to distinguish pre-renal azotemia (PRA) and acute tubular necrosis (ATN), with a typical threshold of 20 (0.081 in international units).

215. An increased BUN : creatinine ratio may be due to?

Clin Kidney J. 2012;5(2):187-191

A. Prerenal azotemia
B. GI bleeding
C. Glucocorticoid therapy
D. All of the above

Increased BUN (relative to creatinine) may be due to prerenal azotemia, increased urea production as in hyperalimentation (high-protein), glucocorticoid therapy, and gastrointestinal bleeding.

216. Which of the following statements is false?
Clin Kidney J. 2012;5(2):187-191

A. A 70 gram protein diet produces about 12 gram of urea/day
B. BUN is roughly one-half of the blood urea
C. >99% of urea synthesis occurs in liver
D. None of the above

Hyponatremia

217. Much of the sodium in the body is bound to?
N Engl J Med. 2015;372:55-65

A. Bone
B. Cartilage
C. Connective tissue
D. All of the above

A substantial amount of sodium is bound to large polyanionic macromolecules called proteoglycans, which make up the ground substance of bone, connective tissue, cartilage and skin. These tissues could serve as sodium reservoirs, taking up or releasing sodium in response to the needs of the body.

218. Hyponatremia is defined as a plasma Na^+ concentration of?
Harrison's 20th Ed. Chapter 49 Page 298

A. < 115 mM
B. < 125 mM
C. < 135 mM
D. < 145 mM

Hyponatremia is defined as a plasma Na^+ concentration <135 mM. This is almost always the result of an increase in circulating AVP and/or increased renal sensitivity to AVP, combined with an intake of free water.

219. Hyponatremia can be?
Harrison's 20th Ed. Chapter 49 Page 298

A. Hypovolemic
B. Euvolemic
C. Hypervolemic
D. All of the above

Hyponatremia is subdivided diagnostically into three groups, depending on clinical history and volume status—hypovolemic, euvolemic & hypervolemic.

220. Which of the following is the cause of hypovolemic hyponatremia with U_{Na} > 20?
Harrison's 20th Ed. Chapter 49 Page 298 Figure 49-5

A. Diuretic excess
B. Mineral corticoid deficiency
C. Salt losing deficiency
D. All of the above

221. Which of the following is the cause of hypovolemic hyponatremia with U_{Na} > 20?
Harrison's 20th Ed. Chapter 49 Page 298 Figure 49-5

A. Ketonuria
B. Osmotic diuresis
C. Cerebral salt wasting syndrome
D. All of the above

222. Which of the following is the cause of euvolemic hyponatremia with U_{Na} > 20?
Harrison's 20th Ed. Chapter 49 Page 298 Figure 49-5

A. Glucocorticoid deficiency
B. Hypothyroidism
C. SIADH
D. All of the above

223. Which of the following is the cause of hypervolemic hyponatremia with U_{Na} > 20?
Harrison's 20th Ed. Chapter 49 Page 298 Figure 49-5

A. Hyperthyroidism
B. Cushing's syndrome
C. Acromegaly
D. Acute or chronic renal failure

224. Which of the following is the cause of hypervolemic hyponatremia with U_{Na} < 20?
Harrison's 20th Ed. Chapter 49 Page 298 Figure 49-5

A. Nephrotic syndrome
B. Cirrhosis
C. Cardiac failure
D. All of the above

225. In hypovolemic hyponatremia, AVP helps preserve blood pressure via?
Harrison's 20th Ed. Chapter 49 Page 299

A. V1A receptors
B. V1B receptors
C. V1C receptors
D. V1D receptors

In hypovolemic hyponatremia, increase in circulating AVP helps preserve blood pressure via vascular & baroreceptor V1A receptors and increases water reabsorption via renal V2 receptors.

226. In nonrenal hypovolemic hyponatremia, without adequate oral replacement, urine Na^+ concentration is typically?
Harrison's 20th Ed. Chapter 49 Page 299

A. < 10 mM
B. < 20 mM
C. < 30 mM
D. < 40 mM

227. In renal hypovolemic hyponatremia, urine Na^+ concentration is typically?
Harrison's 20th Ed. Chapter 49 Page 299

A. > 10 mM
B. > 20 mM
C. > 30 mM
D. > 40 mM

228. Hyperkalemia & hyponatremia in a hypotensive and/or hypovolemic patient with high urine Na^+ strongly suggests?
Harrison's 20th Ed. Chapter 49 Page 299

A. Alcoholic ketoacidosis
B. Medullary cystic disease
C. Thiazide diuretics use
D. Primary adrenal insufficiency

229. Which of the following is a salt-losing nephropathy?
Harrison's 20th Ed. Chapter 49 Page 299

A. Interstitial nephropathies
B. Medullary cystic disease
C. Recovery phase of acute tubular necrosis
D. All of the above

Typical causes of salt-losing nephropathies include reflux nephropathy, interstitial nephropathies, postobstructive uropathy, medullary cystic disease and the recovery phase of acute tubular necrosis.

230. 'Diuretic-induced hyponatremia' is almost always due to?
Harrison's 20th Ed. Chapter 49 Page 299

A. Thiazide diuretics
B. Loop diuretics
C. Aldosterone antagonists
D. All of the above

Diuretic-induced hyponatremia is almost always due to thiazide diuretics which lead to Na^+ & K^+ depletion & AVP-mediated water retention. Thiazides do not inhibit the renal concentrating mechanism. Loop diuretics decrease tonicity of medullary interstitium & impair maximal urinary concentrating capacity which limits ability of AVP to promote water retention.

231. Which of the following can cause hypovolemic hyponatremia?
Harrison's 20th Ed. Chapter 49 Page 299

A. Glycosuria
B. Ketonuria
C. Bicarbonaturia
D. All of the above

232. Syndrome of "cerebral salt wasting" is due to?
Harrison's 20th Ed. Chapter 49 Page 299

A. Subarachnoid hemorrhage
B. Traumatic brain injury
C. Meningitis
D. All of the above

Syndrome of "cerebral salt wasting" is due to subarachnoid hemorrhage, traumatic brain injury, craniotomy, encephalitis and meningitis. Unlike SIADH, it typically responds to aggressive Na^+-Cl^- repletion.

233. Which of the following is false in hypervolemic hyponatremia?
Harrison's 20th Ed. Chapter 49 Page 299

A. Reduced plasma Na^+ concentration
B. Increase in total body Na^+-Cl^-
C. Increase in total body water
D. None of the above

Patients with hypervolemic hyponatremia develop an increase in total-body Na^+-Cl^- that is accompanied by a "proportionately greater" increase in total body water, leading to a reduced plasma Na^+ concentration.

234. Which of the following is an 'osmolyte'?
Harrison's 20th Ed. Chapter 49 Page 300, N Engl J Med. 2015;372:55-65

A. Myo-inositol
B. Betaine
C. Creatine
D. All of the above

Organic solutes, also called osmolytes are creatine, betaine, glutamate, myo-inositol & taurine. These are small intracellular molecules regulated through osmolyte-accumulating transporters (taurine transporter TauT and the myo-inositol transporter SMIT).

235. Which of the following is not a secretory diarrhea?
Harrison's 20th Ed. Chapter 49 Page 299

A. Cholera
B. Carcinoid
C. Lactulose induced
D. VIPoma

236. Which of the following conditions can cause hyponatremia?
Harrison's 20th Ed. Chapter 49 Page 299

A. Hypothyroidism
B. Hyperthyroidism
C. Cushing's disease
D. Pheochromocytoma

Adrenal insufficiency & hypothyroidism may cause hyponatremia. Hypothyroidism decreases cardiac output and GFR and thus increased AVP secretion leading to hyponatremia.

237. Which of the following statements is false?
Harrison's 20th Ed. Chapter 49 Page 299

A. Glucocorticoids exert a negative feedback on AVP release
B. Thiazides do not inhibit renal concentrating mechanism
C. SIAD is the most frequent cause of euvolemic hyponatremia
D. None of the above

238. Which of the following is the most common pattern of AVP secretion recognized in patients with SIAD?
Harrison's 20th Ed. Chapter 49 Page 300

A. Unregulated, erratic AVP secretion
B. Failure to suppress AVP secretion at lower serum osmolalities
C. "Reset osmostat," with a lower threshold osmolality
D. No detectable circulating AVP

Four distinct patterns of AVP secretion have been recognized in patients with SIAD, independent of the underlying cause. First, unregulated, erratic AVP secretion seen in about a third of patients, with no obvious correlation between serum osmolality & circulating AVP levels. Second, patients fail to suppress AVP secretion at lower serum osmolalities, with a normal response curve to hyperosmolar conditions. Third, a "reset osmostat" with a lower threshold osmolality and a left-shifted osmotic response curve. Fourth, patients with essentially no detectable circulating AVP, suggesting either a gain in function in renal water reabsorption or a circulating antidiuretic substance that is distinct from AVP.

239. Drugs that stimulate release of AVP or enhance its action include?
Harrison's 20th Ed. Chapter 49 Page 299 Table 49-1

A. SSRIs
B. Tricyclic antidepressants
C. Antipsychotic drugs
D. All of the above

240. Drugs that stimulate release of AVP or enhance its action include?
Harrison's 20th Ed. Chapter 49 Page 299 Table 49-1

A. Nicotine
B. Nonsteroidal antiinflammatory drugs
C. Narcotics
D. All of the above

241. Drugs that stimulate release of AVP or enhance its action include?

Harrison's 20th Ed. Chapter 49 Page 299 Table 49-1

A. Vincristine
B. Cyclophosphamide
C. Ifosfamide
D. All of the above

242. Drugs that either stimulate AVP secretion or enhance its action on the kidney includes all except ?

Harrison's 20th Ed. Chapter 49 Page 299 Table 49-1

A. Chlorpropamide
B. Clofibrate
C. Carbamazepine
D. Phenytoin

Drugs that either stimulate AVP secretion or enhance its action on kidney are chlorpropamide, clofibrate, carbamazepine and NSAIDs.

243. Which of the following can cause syndrome of inappropriate antidiuresis (SIAD)?

Harrison's 20th Ed. Chapter 49 Page 299 Table 49-1

A. Endurance exercise
B. General anesthesia
C. Nausea, pain
D. All of the above

244. Which of the following can cause syndrome of inappropriate antidiuresis (SIAD)?

Harrison's 20th Ed. Chapter 49 Page 299 Table 49-1

A. Guillain-Barré syndrome
B. Acute intermittent porphyria
C. Meningitis
D. All of the above

245. Which of the following can cause syndrome of inappropriate antidiuresis (SIAD)?

Harrison's 20th Ed. Chapter 49 Page 299 Table 49-1

A. Asthma
B. Bacterial pneumonia
C. Respiratory failure associated with positive-pressure breathing
D. All of the above

246. Which of the following can cause syndrome of inappropriate antidiuresis (SIAD)?

Harrison's 20th Ed. Chapter 49 Page 299 Table 49-1

A. Aspergillosis
B. Cystic fibrosis
C. Tuberculosis
D. All of the above

247. Syndrome of inappropriate antidiuresis (SIAD) is most common with which of the following malignancies?

Harrison's 20th Ed. Chapter 49 Page 300

A. Small-cell lung carcinoma
B. Lymphoma
C. Pancreatic cancer
D. Prostate cancer

248. Syndrome of inappropriate antidiuresis (SIAD) is most common with which of the following drugs?

Harrison's 20th Ed. Chapter 49 Page 300

A. SSRIs
B. Narcotics
C. Nonsteroidal antiinflammatory drugs
D. Carbamazepine

249. Which of the following is useful in distinguishing between hypervolemic & euvolemic hyponatremia?

Harrison's 20th Ed. Chapter 49 Page 300

A. Serum triglyceride
B. Serum uric acid
C. Serum lipase
D. Serum amylase

Serum uric acid is low (<4 mg/dL) in patients with SIAD, consistent with suppressed proximal tubular transport in the setting of increased distal tubular Na-Cl and water transport. In contrast, patients with hypovolemic hyponatremia will be hyperuricemic, due to a shared activation of proximal tubular Na-Cl and urate transport.

250. Phenomenon of 'hyponatremia' in beer drinkers is called?

Harrison's 20th Ed. Chapter 49 Page 300

A. Beer syndrome
B. Beer flush
C. Beer potomania
D. Beer psychosis

Beer is very low in protein and salt content, containing only 1-2 mM of Na^+. Beer drinkers who consume large volumes of beer, which may exceed renal excretory capacity and result in hyponatremia. This is referred to as beer potomania. Saline hydration corrects causative plasma Na^+ concentration deficit.

251. Which of the following statements about hyponatremia is false?

Harrison's 20th Ed. Chapter 49 Page 300

A. Hyponatremia induces generalized cellular swelling
B. Symptoms of hyponatremia are primarily neurologic
C. Normocapneic or hypercapneic respiratory failure
D. None of the above

252. Urine osmolality is calculated with which of the following formula?

Am J Nephrol. 1990;10(2):89-102

A. $2 \times (U_{Na}) + U_K$ + (urinary urea nitrogen/2.8) + (urine glucose/18)
B. $3 \times (U_{Na}) + U_K$ + (urinary urea nitrogen/2.8) + (urine glucose/18)
C. $4 \times (U_{Na}) + U_K$ + (urinary urea nitrogen/2.8) + (urine glucose/18)
D. $5 \times (U_{Na}) + U_K$ + (urinary urea nitrogen/2.8) + (urine glucose/18)

Urine Osmolality = 2 x (urine Na) + Urine K + (urinary urea nitrogen/2.8) + (urine glucose/18)

253. Which of the following statements is false?

Am J Nephrol. 1990;10(2):89-102

A. Osmolarity refers to concentration per liter of solution
B. Osmolality refers to concentration per kilogram of solution
C. Osmolarity is affected by temperature & pressure, whereas osmolality is not
D. None of the above

Osmolality measures only the number of particles present in a solution, while specific gravity determines not only the number but also weight of the particles in a solution.

254. Urine tonicity is calculated by?

Am J Nephrol. 1990;10(2):89-102

A. $[Na^+] + [K^+] - [Cl^-]$
B. $[Na^+] \times [K^+]$
C. $[Na^+] \times [K^+] \div [Cl^-]$
D. $[Na^+] + [K^+]$

Urine tonicity is calculated as the sum of concentrations of Na^+ and K^+. The normal 24-hour urine osmolality is 500 - 800 mOsm/kg of water. Random urine osmolality should average 300—900 mOsm/kg of water. After 12–14 hours of fluid intake restriction, the urine osmolality should exceed 850 mOsm/kg of water.

255. 'Syndrome of inappropriate antidiuretic hormone secretion' (SIADH) causes?

Harrison's 20th Ed. Chapter 49 Page 300

A. Normovolemic hyponatremia
B. Hypovolemic hyponatremia
C. Hypervolemic hyponatremia
D. All of the above

Syndrome of inappropriate antidiuretic hormone secretion (SIADH) is the most common cause of normovolemic or euvolemic hyponatremia. The urine sodium value of 50 mEq/L conferred the best accuracy in separating SIADH from hypovolemic hyponatremia.

256. 'Osmotic diuresis' is defined as a solute excretion rate of more than?

Harrison's 20th Ed. Chapter 49 Page 300

A. ~ 250 mOsmol/day
B. ~ 450 mOsmol/day
C. ~ 550 mOsmol/day
D. ~ 750 mOsmol/day

Osmotic diuresis refers to a solute excretion rate of > ~750 mOsmol/day.

257. Organic osmolytes include which of the following?

Harrison's 20th Ed. Chapter 49 Page 300

A. Creatine
B. Betaine
C. Glutamate
D. All of the above

Organic osmolytes include creatine, betaine, glutamate, myoinositol and taurine.

258. Hyponatremia lasting for how many hours is termed as chronic hyponatremia?

Harrison's 20th Ed. Chapter 49 Page 300

A. 24 Hours
B. 48 Hours
C. 60 Hours
D. 72 Hours

259. Stupor, seizures, and coma occur when plasma sodium concentration falls below?

Harrison's 20th Ed. Chapter 49 Page 300

A. 125 mM
B. 127 mM
C. 129 mM
D. 131 mM

Stupor, seizures & coma occur when plasma Na^+ concentration falls below 125 mM.

260. In hyponatremia, plasma Na^+ concentration during the first 24 hours should not be more than?

Harrison's 20th Ed. Chapter 49 Page 300

A. 2–3 mM
B. 4–6 mM
C. 6–8 mM
D. 8–10 mM

Overly rapid correction of hyponatremia (>8–10 mM in 24 hours or 18 mM in 48 hours) is associated with a disruption in integrity of the blood-brain barrier, allowing the entry of immune mediators that may contribute to demyelination.

261. In a 70 kg man, to raise plasma Na^+ concentration from 110 to 120 mmol/L, what is the amount of Na^+ required?

Harrison's 20th Ed. Chapter 49 Page 300

A. 420 mmol
B. 440 mmol
C. 460 mmol
D. 480 mmol

To raise plasma Na^+ concentration from 110 to 120 mmol/L in a 70-kg man requires 420 mmol [(120 – 110)x70x0.6] of Na^+. Total body water is 50 & 60% of lean body weight in women or men respectively.

262. Osmotic demyelination syndrome (ODS) includes?

Harrison's 20th Ed. Chapter 49 Page 300

A. Flaccid paralysis
B. Dysarthria
C. Dysphagia
D. All of the above

If hyponatremia is corrected too rapidly, osmotic demyelination syndrome (ODS) develops which is characterized by paraparesis or quadriparesis, dysphagia, dysarthria, diplopia, a "locked-in syndrome," and/or loss of consciousness (central pontine myelinolysis). Patients with chronic hyponatremia are most susceptible to development of ODS.

263. The lesions of ODS classically affects which of the following?

Harrison's 20th Ed. Chapter 49 Page 301

A. Pons
B. Cerebellum
C. Thalamus
D. Cerebral cortex

The lesions of ODS classically affect the pons. Clinically, patients with central pontine myelinolysis present 1 or more days after overcorrection of hyponatremia with paraparesis or quadriparesis, dysphagia, dysarthria, diplopia, a "locked-in syndrome" and/or loss of consciousness. Other regions of the brain can also be involved in ODS, most commonly in association with lesions of the pons but occasionally in isolation. In order of frequency, the lesions of extrapontine myelinolysis can occur in the cerebellum, lateral geniculate body, thalamus, putamen and cerebral cortex or subcortex.

264. Risk factors for ODS include?

Harrison's 20th Ed. Chapter 49 Page 301

A. Rapid or overcorrection of hyponatremia
B. Prior cerebral anoxic injury
C. Hypokalemia
D. All of the above

Besides, rapid or overcorrection of hyponatremia, risk factors for ODS include prior cerebral anoxic injury, menstruating women, prepubescent children, hypokalemia, and malnutrition.

265. Which of the following is related to central pontine myelinolysis?
Harrison's 20th Ed. Chapter 49 Page 301

A. Cerebral oedema
B. Cerebral dehydration
C. Cerebral atrophy
D. None of the above

Acute brain dehydration produced by rapid correction disrupts the tight junctions of blood-brain barrier. Disruption of BBB results in an influx of activated complement into brain which is toxic to oligodendrocytes that produce and maintain myelin in CNS. Clinical symptoms of central pontine myelinolysis do not occur until a few days after rapid Na^+ correction. The classic presentation is pseudobulbar palsy & spastic quadriparesis.

266. Rapid correction of hyponatremia leads to?
N Engl J Med. 2015;372:55-65

A. Triggering apoptosis
B. Disrupts blood–brain barrier
C. Brain demyelination
D. All of the above

Rapid correction of hyponatremia is a hypertonic stress to astrocytes that are depleted of osmolytes, triggering apoptosis, disruption of the blood–brain barrier, and, eventually, brain demyelination.

267. Pseudohyponatremia is defined as the coexistence of?
Harrison's 20th Ed. Chapter 49 Page 301

A. Hyponatremia with increased plasma tonicity
B. Hyponatremia with decreased plasma tonicity
C. Normonatremia with increased plasma tonicity
D. Normonatremia with decreased plasma tonicity

Pseudohyponatremia is defined as the coexistence of hyponatremia with a normal or increased plasma tonicity.

268. Which of the following about pseudohyponatremia is false?
Harrison's 20th Ed. Chapter 49 Page 301

A. Iso-osmolar & isotonic hyponatremia
B. Severe hypertriglyceridemia or paraproteinemia
C. Increase in solid phase of plasma
D. None of the above

Pseudohyponatremia is a spurious form of iso-osmolar & isotonic hyponatremia when severe hypertriglyceridemia or paraproteinemia increases substantially the solid phase of plasma.

269. Patients with hyponatremia have an effective osmolality of?
Harrison's 20th Ed. Chapter 49 Page 301

A. < 295 mOsm/kg
B. < 285 mOsm/kg
C. < 275 mOsm/kg
D. < 265 mOsm/kg

Patients with hyponatremia have an effective osmolality of < 275 mOsm/kg.

270. Plasma sodium concentration falls by how much for every 100 mg/dL rise in plasma glucose concentration?
Harrison's 20th Ed. Chapter 49 Page 301

A. 1.1–1.6 mM
B. 1.6–2.4 mM
C. 2.4–3.2 mM
D. 3.2–4.4 mM

Plasma Na^+ concentration falls by ~ 1.6 - 2.4 mM for every 100 mg/dL increase in glucose due to glucose-induced water efflux from cells. This "true" hyponatremia resolves after correction of hyperglycemia.

271. Which of the following is a cause of hypovolemic hyponatremia?
Harrison's 20th Ed. Chapter 49 Page 301

A. Hypothyroidism
B. Secondary adrenal failure due to pituitary insufficiency
C. Primary adrenal failure
D. All of the above

272. "Gold standard" for diagnosis of hypovolemic hyponatremia is plasma Na^+ correction after?
Harrison's 20th Ed. Chapter 49 Page 301

A. Hydration with normal saline
B. Intake of oral salt
C. Restriction of water intake
D. All of the above

Ultimate "gold standard" for the diagnosis of hypovolemic hyponatremia is the demonstration that plasma Na^+ concentration corrects after hydration with normal saline.

273. Which of the following statements is false?
Harrison's 20th Ed. Chapter 49 Page 301

A. Urine osmolality <100 mOsm/kg is suggestive of polydipsia
B. Urine osmolality >400 mOsm/kg indicates AVP excess
C. Urine Na^+ is <20 mM in beer potomania
D. None of the above

274. Which of the following is a cause of euvolemic hyponatremia?
Harrison's 20th Ed. Chapter 49 Page 301

A. Hypothyroidism
B. Secondary adrenal failure due to pituitary insufficiency
C. SIAD
D. All of the above

275. Syndrome of inappropriate antidiuretic hormone secretion (SIADH) is also called?
Ther Adv Endocrinol Metab. 2012;3(2):61-73

A. Achard-Thiers syndrome
B. Liebenberg syndrome
C. Schwartz-Bartter syndrome
D. Donnai-Barrow syndrome

Schwartz-Bartter described SIADH as hyponatremia with corresponding hypo-osmolality, continued renal excretion of sodium, urine less than maximally dilute, absence of clinical evidence of volume depletion, absence of other causes of hyponatremia and correction of hyponatremia by fluid restriction.

276. Patients with which of the following conditions have a very high risk of developing ODS?
Harrison's 20th Ed. Chapter 49 Page 301

A. Beer potomania
B. CHF
C. Hypothyroidism
D. Secondary adrenal failure

Patients with beer potomania have a very high risk of developing ODS due to the associated hypokalemia, alcoholism, malnutrition and high risk of overcorrecting plasma Na^+ concentration.

277. Which of the following are modalities to correct plasma Na^+ concentration?

Harrison's 20th Ed. Chapter 49 Page 301

A. Fluid restriction
B. Potassium replacement
C. Increased solute intake
D. All of the above

Modalities to correct plasma Na^+ concentration include fluid restriction, potassium replacement, oral urea and/or increased solute intake.

278. Which of the following are modalities to correct plasma Na^+ concentration in patients with SIAD?

Harrison's 20th Ed. Chapter 49 Page 301

A. Oral furosemide
B. Demeclocycline
C. Oral urea
D. All of the above

279. Which of the following statements about SIADH is false?

Harrison's 20th Ed. Chapter 49 Page 301

A. Hypoosmotic hyponatremia
B. Urine osmolality >100 mOsmol/kg
C. Hypervolemia
D. Normal sodium balance

Patients with SIADH are usually euvolemic.

280. Which of the following statements about SIADH is false?

Harrison's 20th Ed. Chapter 49 Page 301

A. Normal renal, adrenal, and thyroid function
B. Normal potassium and acid-base balance
C. Hypouricemia
D. None of the above

SIADH is characterized by hypoosmotic hyponatremia in the setting of an inappropriately concentrated urine (urine osmolality >100 mOsmol/kg). Patients are typically normovolemic & have normal Na^+ balance. They tend to be mildly volume-expanded secondary to water retention & have a urine Na^+ excretion rate equal to intake (urine Na^+ concentration usually >40 mmol/L). By definition, they have normal renal, adrenal & thyroid function & usually have normal K^+ & acid-base balance. Hypouricemia in SIADH is due to uricosuric state induced by volume expansion. In contrast, hypovolemic patients tend to be hyperuricemic secondary to increased proximal urate reabsorption.

281. What percentage of increase in brain volume can be fatal?

Cleveland clinic J of Medicine 2007;74(5):377-383

A. 2% to 4%
B. 4% to 6%
C. 6% to 8%
D. 8% to 10%

If plasma is dilute, water diffuses into brain by osmosis causing dilution of extracellular fluid in brain & swelling of brain cells. An increase in brain volume of 8% to 10% can be fatal. By cerebral osmoregulatory (adaptive) mechanism brain cells pump out myoinositol, glutamine, glycerophosphoryl-choline, betaine, creatine & taurine to restore osmolality of cerebral ECF & limiting swelling of brain cells. Acute hyponatremia may cause cerebral edema due to underlying osmotic interactions between brain cells and the extracellular fluid compartment.

282. Sodium required to correct hyponatremia can be estimated by multiplying the deficit in plasma sodium concentration by?

Ther Adv Endocrinol Metab. 2012;3(2):61-73

A. Weight
B. Height
C. Total body water
D. Urine output in liters

Quantity of Na^+ required to increase plasma Na^+ concentration by a given amount can be estimated by multiplying the deficit in plasma Na^+ concentration by total body water.

283. Which of the following formula is used to calculate the change in serum sodium expected from a saline infusion?

Ther Adv Endocrinol Metab. 2012;3(2):61-73

A. Holliday-Segar formula
B. Adrogué-Madias formula
C. Schmidt formula
D. Buckley-Leblanc formula

284. Quantity of sodium in 0.9% (normal, isotonic) saline is?

Ther Adv Endocrinol Metab. 2012;3(2):61-73

A. 77 mM
B. 154 mM
C. 256 mM
D. 513 mM

285. Quantity of sodium in 3% (hypertonic) saline is?

Ther Adv Endocrinol Metab. 2012;3(2):61-73

A. 77 mM
B. 154 mM
C. 256 mM
D. 513 mM

286. Physiologic functions of AVP include?

Lancet 2008;371:1624-32

A. Contraction of vascular smooth muscle
B. Stimulation of liver glycogenolysis
C. Regulation of corticotropin release
D. All of the above

Physiologic functions of AVP or antidiuretic hormone include contraction of vascular smooth muscle, stimulation of liver glycogenolysis, regulation of corticotropin release and renal antidiuresis.

287. Inappropriately elevated levels of AVP are found in?

Drugs. 2007;67(6):847-58

A. Congestive heart failure
B. Cirrhosis of liver
C. SIADH
D. All of the above

Inappropriately elevated levels of AVP occur in CHF, cirrhosis liver, treatment with diuretics & SIADH.

288. Which of the following is a arginine-vasopressin-receptor subtype?

Lancet 2008;371:1624-32

A. V1a
B. V1b
C. V2
D. All of the above

Arginine vasopressin (AVP) is a neuropeptide hormone. Three arginine-vasopressin-receptor subtypes V1a, V1b, and V2 belong to the large rhodopsin-like G-protein-coupled receptor family. V1A & V1B receptors are linked to phosphoinositol signaling pathway, with intracellular calcium acting as the second messenger, whereas V2 receptors are linked to adenylate cyclase signaling pathway, with intracellular cyclic adenosine monophosphate (cAMP) acting as second messenger.

289. V(1A) receptors located in?
Lancet 2008;371:1624-32

A. Vascular smooth muscle cells & myocardium
B. Collecting tubules
C. Anterior pituitary
D. All of the above

290. V(2) receptors located in?
Lancet 2008;371:1624-32

A. Vascular smooth muscle cells & myocardium
B. Collecting tubules
C. Anterior pituitary
D. All of the above

291. V(1B) receptors located in?
Lancet 2008;371:1624-32

A. Vascular smooth muscle cells & myocardium
B. Collecting tubules
C. Anterior pituitary
D. All of the above

Activation of V(1A) receptors located in vascular smooth muscle cells & myocardium results in vasoconstriction & increased afterload & hypertrophy. V(2) receptors located in principal cells of renal-collecting-duct system & mediate free water absorption. V(1B) receptors are located in anterior pituitary & mediate adrenocorticotropin hormone release. Cardiovascular & renal effects of AVP are mediated primarily by V(1A) and V(2) receptors.

292. Which of the following is a combined V(1A)/V(2)-receptor antagonist?
Lancet 2008;371:1624-32

A. Mozavaptan
B. Tolvaptan
C. Conivaptan
D. Lixivaptan

Conivaptan is a combined V(1A)/V(2)-receptor antagonist (non-selective) that induces diuresis as well as haemodynamic improvement.

293. Which of the following is a selective V(1A) receptor antagonist?
Lancet 2008;371:1624-32

A. Mozavaptan
B. Tolvaptan
C. Relcovaptan
D. Lixivaptan

Relcovaptan is a selective V1a-receptor antagonist used in the treatment of Raynaud's disease, dysmenorrhoea, and tocolysis.

294. Which of the following is a V2-receptor antagonist?
Lancet 2008;371:1624-32

A. Mozavaptan
B. Satavaptan
C. Tolvaptan
D. All of the above

V2-receptor antagonists—mozavaptan, lixivaptan, satavaptan & tolvaptan, induce a highly hypotonic diuresis without substantially affecting excretion of electrolytes (by contrast with effects of diuretics). These are effective in the treatment of euvolaemic & hypervolaemic hyponatraemia.

295. Which of the following is administered intravenously?
Lancet 2008;371:1624-32

A. Mozavaptan
B. Tolvaptan
C. Conivaptan
D. Lixivaptan

Conivaptan is available for intravenous (IV) administration, whereas the other three agents are for oral administration.

296. Which of the following is a Benzodiazepine derivative?
Lancet 2008;371:1624-32

A. Mozavaptan
B. Tolvaptan
C. Conivaptan
D. Lixivaptan

Tolvaptan, Mozavaptan & Conivaptan are benzazepine derivative, Satavaptan is N-arylsulfonyl oxindole derivative, Lixivaptan is a Benzodiazepine derivative.

297. Vaptans are metabolised by which of the following hepatic cytochrome enzymes?
Lancet 2008;371:1624-32

A. CYP2D6
B. CYP2C9
C. CYP3A4
D. CYP2C19

298. Vaptans are excreted through?
Lancet 2008;371:1624-32

A. Urine
B. Faeces
C. Lungs
D. All of the above

299. V2-receptor antagonists are contraindicated in which of the following conditions?
Lancet 2008;371:1624-32

A. Hypovolaemic hyponatraemia
B. Euvolaemic hyponatraemia
C. Hypervolaemic hyponatraemia
D. None of the above

Conivaptan & other V2-receptor antagonists are contraindicated in patients with hypovolaemic hyponatraemia, since it is an aquaretic.

300. Non-peptide vasopressin receptor antagonists are called?
Lancet 2008;371:1624-32

A. Captans
B. Vaptans
C. Naptans
D. Saptans

Vaptans are orally & intravenously active non-peptide vasopressin receptor antagonists. AVP receptor antagonists induces free water diuresis without natriuresis or kaliuresis, an effect termed aquaresis.

301. Na^+ deficit is calculated by?

Lancet 2008;371:1624-32

A. 0.3 × body weight × (target plasma Na^+–starting plasma Na^+ concentration)
B. 0.4 × body weight × (target plasma Na^+–starting plasma Na^+ concentration)
C. 0.5 × body weight × (target plasma Na^+–starting plasma Na^+ concentration)
D. 0.6 × body weight × (target plasma Na^+–starting plasma Na^+ concentration)

Na^+ deficit = 0.6 x body weight x (target plasma Na^+ concentration - starting plasma Na^+ concentration.

302. AVP antagonists do not have an approved role in the management of?

Lancet 2008;371:1624-32

A. Acute hyponatremia
B. Heart failure
C. Cirrhosis
D. SIAD

AVP antagonists do not have an approved role in the management of acute hyponatremia. AVP antagonists (vaptans) are highly effective in SIAD and in hypervolemic hyponatremia due to heart failure or cirrhosis.

Hypernatremia

303. Hypernatremia is defined as a plasma sodium concentration more than?

Harrison's 20th Ed. Chapter 49 Page 302

A. 135 mmol/L
B. 140 mmol/L
C. 145 mmol/L
D. 150 mmol/L

Hypernatremia is defined as a plasma Na^+ concentration >145 mmol/L.

304. Which of the following about hypernatremia is false?

Harrison's 20th Ed. Chapter 49 Page 302

A. Associated with mortality rates of 40–60%
B. Result due to losses of H_2O in excess of Na^+
C. Diarrhea is the most common gastrointestinal cause
D. None of the above

305. Which of the following about hypernatremia is false?

Harrison's 20th Ed. Chapter 49 Page 302

A. State of iso-osmolality
B. Results in ICF volume contraction
C. Stimulates thirst
D. Excretion of minimum volume of maximally concentrated urine

Hypernatremia is a state of hyperosmolality.

306. Which of the following is a cause of adipsic diabetes insipidus?

Harrison's 20th Ed. Chapter 49 Page 302

A. Primary or metastatic tumor
B. Occlusion or ligation of the anterior communicating artery
C. Hydrocephalus
D. All of the above

Causes of adipsic DI include primary or metastatic tumor, occlusion or ligation of the anterior communicating artery, trauma, hydrocephalus & inflammation.

307. Which of the following causes osmotic diuresis?

Harrison's 20th Ed. Chapter 49 Page 303

A. Hyperglycemia
B. Excess urea
C. Mannitol
D. All of the above

308. Which of the following can cause nephrogenic diabetes insipidus (NDI)?

Harrison's 20th Ed. Chapter 49 Page 303

A. Loss of function mutations in X-linked V2 receptor
B. Mutations in AVP-responsive aquaporin-2 water channel
C. Recessive deficiency of aquaporin-1 water channel
D. All of the above

309. Which of the following can cause polyuria and NDI?

Harrison's 20th Ed. Chapter 49 Page 303

A. Hypercalcemia
B. Hypokalemia
C. Lithium
D. All of the above

In hypercalcemia, calcium signals directly through calcium-sensing receptor to downregulate Na^+, K^+ & Cl^- transport by TALH & water transport in principal cells, thus reducing renal concentrating ability. In hypokalemia, the renal response to AVP are inhibited and aquaporin-2 expression is downregulated.

310. Which of the following best relates to lithium therapy?

Harrison's 20th Ed. Chapter 49 Page 303

A. (Lif)/Stat3
B. Mapk1/3
C. Glycogen synthase kinase-3 (GSK3)
D. All of the above

311. Which of the following when used with lithium can mitigate lithium associated NDI?

Harrison's 20th Ed. Chapter 49 Page 303

A. Triamterene
B. Amiloride
C. Spironolactone
D. All of the above

Lithium causes NDI by direct inhibition of renal glycogen synthase kinase-3 (GSK3). GSK3 is required for the response of principal cells to A VP. Entry of lithium through amiloride-sensitive Na^+ channel ENaC is required for the effect of the drug on principal cells, such that combined therapy of lithium and amiloride can mitigate lithium associated NDI.

312. Which of the following about glycogen synthase kinase-3 (GSK3) is false?

Curr Opin Nephrol Hypertens. 2012;21(5):541-546

A. Serine/threonine protein kinase
B. Inhibits glycogen synthase
C. Exists in two isoforms–GSK3α and GSK3β
D. None of the above

Lithium is a reversible & highly specific inhibitor of GSK3. Glycogen synthase kinase-3 (GSK3) inhibition by LiCl increases cyclooxygenase 2 expression and reduces aquaporin 2 expression.

313. Which of the following about nephrogenic diabetes insipidus is false?

Harrison's 20th Ed. Chapter 49 Page 303

A. Congenital Nephrogenic diabetes insipidus (NDI) is X-linked recessive trait due to mutations in V2 receptor gene
B. Congenital Nephrogenic diabetes insipidus (NDI) may be due to mutation in autosomal aquaporin-2 gene
C. Lithium, hypercalcemia & hyperkalemia cause sporadic NDI
D. Pregnant women, in II or III trimester, may develop NDI due to excessive vasopressinase from placenta

Lithium, hypercalcemia and hypokalemia can cause sporadic NDI.

314. Gestational DI best relates to?

Harrison's 20th Ed. Chapter 49 Page 303

A. Leucine-rich proteins
B. Vasopressinase
C. Carnitine
D. Cryoglobulin

Gestational DI is a complication of late-term pregnancy in which there is increased activity of a circulating placental protease with "vasopressinase" activity leading to reduced circulating AVP & polyuria, often accompanied by hypernatremia. DDAVP is an effective therapy, given its resistance to the vasopressinase enzyme.

315. Major symptoms of hypernatremia are?

Harrison's 20th Ed. Chapter 49 Page 303

A. Cardiac
B. Neurologic
C. Respiratory
D. Gastroenterological

Major symptoms of hypernatremia are neurologic like altered mental status, weakness, neuromuscular irritability, focal neurologic deficits & coma or seizures.

316. Which of the following can occur in acute hypernatremia?

Harrison's 20th Ed. Chapter 49 Page 303

A. Parenchymal or subarachnoid hemorrhage
B. Subdural hematoma
C. Rhabdomyolysis
D. All of the above

317. Increasing plasma Na^+ by how much is considered as overcorrection?

Harrison's 20th Ed. Chapter 49 Page 303

A. > 2 mM/day
B. > 5 mM/day
C. > 8 mM/day
D. > 10 mM/day

318. Which of the following laboratory investigation is useful in a case of hypernatremia?

Harrison's 20th Ed. Chapter 49 Page 303

A. Serum osmolality
B. Urine osmolality
C. Urine electrolytes
D. All of the above

319. Which of the following indicate to an extrarenal source of water loss primarily responsible for hypernatremia?

Harrison's 20th Ed. Chapter 49 Page 303

A. Serum osmolality >295 mOsm/kg
B. Excretion of low volumes (<500 mL/day) of urine
C. Urine osmolality >800 mOsm/kg
D. All of the above

320. Which of the following is false about patients with baseline hypernatremia?

Harrison's 20th Ed. Chapter 49 Page 303

A. Hypertonicity
B. Adequate stimulus for AVP by posterior pituitary
C. Water deprivation test is unnecessary
D. None of the above

321. Which of the following is false about patients with nephrogenic diabetes insipidus (NDI)?

Harrison's 20th Ed. Chapter 49 Page 303

A. Will not to respond to DDAVP
B. DDAVP will not ↑ urine osmolality by <50% or <150 mOsm/kg
C. Normal or high circulating AVP level
D. None of the above

322. Which of the following is false about patients with central diabetes insipidus (CDI)?

Harrison's 20th Ed. Chapter 49 Page 303

A. Will respond to DDAVP
B. DDAVP will not ↑ urine osmolality by >50% but <800 mOsm/kg
C. Reduced circulating AVP
D. None of the above

323. After administering 'desmopressin', urine osmolality should increase by how much in CDI?

Harrison's 20th Ed. Chapter 49 Page 303

A. At least 10%
B. At least 25%
C. At least 35%
D. At least 50%

324. After administering 'desmopressin', urine osmolality should increase by how much in NDI?

Harrison's 20th Ed. Chapter 49 Page 303

A. At least 10%
B. At least 25%
C. At least 35%
D. None of the above

CDI & NDI can be distinguished by administering AVP analogue desmopressin (10 μg intranasally) after careful water restriction. Urine osmolality should increase by at least 50% in CDI & will not change in NDI.

325. Which of the following prevents degradation of placental vasopressinase?

Harrison's 20th Ed. Chapter 49 Page 303

A. Hydroxyproline
B. Tyrosinase
C. 1,10-phenanthroline
D. All of the above

In pregnant women, AVP assays should be drawn in tubes containing protease inhibitor 1,10-phenanthroline, to prevent in vitro degradation of AVP by placental vasopressinase.

326. In women, what percentage of body weight is total-body water (TBW)?

Harrison's 20th Ed. Chapter 49 Page 302 Table 49-3

A. 40%
B. 50%
C. 60%
D. 70%

327. In men, what percentage of body weight is total-body water (TBW)?

Harrison's 20th Ed. Chapter 49 Page 302 Table 49-3

A. 40%
B. 50%
C. 60%
D. 70%

50% of body weight in women and 60% in men is the estimated total-body water (TBW).

328. Which of the following is the correct formula to calculate free-water deficit?

Harrison's 20th Ed. Chapter 49 Page 302 Table 49-3

A. $[(Na^+ - 120)/140] \times TBW$
B. $[(Na^+ - 130)/140] \times TBW$
C. $[(Na^+ - 140)/140] \times TBW$
D. $[(Na^+ - 150)/140] \times TBW$

Free-water deficit is calculated by the formula $[(Na^+ - 140)/140] \times TBW$.

329. Which of the following variable is not included in the formula to calculate free-water clearance (C_eH_2O)?

Harrison's 20th Ed. Chapter 49 Page 302 Table 49-3

A. Urinary $[Na^+]$
B. Urinary $[K^+]$
C. Plasma $[Na^+]$
D. Plasma $[K^+]$

Formula to calculate free-water clearance (C_eH_2O) is Urinary volume × [1 - (urinary [Na+] + urinary [K+])/plasma [Na+]].

330. Normal insensible water loss is?

Harrison's 20th Ed. Chapter 49 Page 302 Table 49-3

A. ~ 2 mL/kg per day
B. ~ 5 mL/kg per day
C. ~ 10 mL/kg per day
D. ~ 15 mL/kg per day

331. It is imperative to correct hypernatremia 'slowly' to avoid?

Harrison's 20th Ed. Chapter 49 Page 304

A. Acute renal failure
B. Heart failure
C. Cerebral edema
D. All of the above

It is imperative to correct hypernatremia slowly to avoid cerebral edema.

332. In hypernatremia due to water loss, water deficit should be corrected in which of the following ways?

Harrison's 20th Ed. Chapter 49 Page 304

A. Rapidly
B. Over 12 to 24 hours
C. Over 24 to 36 hours
D. Slowly over at least 48 to 72 hours

In hypernatremia due to water loss, water deficit should be corrected slowly over 48–72 hours, raising plasma Na^+ concentration by no more than 10 mM/day except in patients with acute hypernatremia (<48 hours) due to sodium loading, who can safely be corrected rapidly at a rate of 1 mM/hour.

333. DDAVP can be administered through which of the following routes?

Harrison's 20th Ed. Chapter 49 Page 304

A. Intravenous
B. Intranasal
C. Oral
D. All of the above

Patients with central DI should respond to the administration of intravenous, intranasal or oral DDAVP.

334. Which of the following drugs is useful in NDI patients who have to take lithium?

Harrison's 20th Ed. Chapter 49 Page 304

A. Amiloride
B. Chlorpropamide
C. Clofibrate
D. Carbamazepine

Amiloride is useful NDI patients who have to take lithium. Nephrotoxicity of lithium requires it to be taken up into collecting duct cells via amiloride-sensitive Na^+ channel.

335. Which of the following is useful for 'chronic' management of polyuria from NDI?

Harrison's 20th Ed. Chapter 49 Page 304

A. Thiazides
B. Amiloride
C. NSAIDs
D. All of the above

336. Which of the following about diabetes insipidus is false?

Harrison's 20th Ed. Chapter 49 Page 303

A. CDI is characterized by impaired AVP secretion
B. NDI results from renal resistance to actions of AVP
C. Familial CDI is inherited as autosomal recessive
D. Familial CDI is due to mutation in propressophysin gene

Familial form of CDI is inherited as autosomal dominant and is attributed to mutations in propressophysin (AVP precursor) gene.

337. 'Solute excretion rate' is?

N Engl J Med. 2015; 372:2207-2216

A. Urine volume × Osmolality
B. Urine volume × Urine sodium
C. Urine volume × Urine potassium
D. Urine volume × Urine bicarbonate

The product of urine volume & osmolality is called solute excretion rate. Or, urinary volume in liters per day = Solute excretion in mOsm per day/urinary osmolality in mOsm per liter.

Hypokalemia

338. Potassium delivery to distal nephron approximates?

Harrison's 20th Ed. Chapter 49 Page 304

A. Dietary excess
B. Dietary intake
C. Dietary deficiency
D. Daily requirement

339. What percentage of daily intake of potassium is excreted in stool?

Harrison's 20th Ed. Chapter 49 Page 304

A. 1%
B. 5%
C. 10%
D. 15%

Entire daily intake of potassium is excreted, approximately 90% in urine & 10% in the stool. K^+ delivery to distal nephron [DCT + cortical collecting duct (CCD)] approximates dietary intake.

340. 98% of total-body potassium is intracellular, chiefly in?

Harrison's 20th Ed. Chapter 49 Page 304

A. Fat cells
B. Skin cells
C. Muscle cells
D. Liver cells

98% of total-body potassium is intracellular, chiefly in muscle. Most of the cellular K^+ in the body resides in the intracellular fluid (ICF) (~50 mEq/kg, 98%), largely in the skeletal muscles (3,000 mEq), red blood cells (300 mEq), and liver (200 mEq). Total K^+ content in the extracellular fluid (ECF) is very low (<1 mEq/kg, ~2%) and similar to the daily dietary intake and renal excretion of K^+.

341. All regulation of renal potassium excretion & total body potassium balance occurs in?

Harrison's 20th Ed. Chapter 49 Page 304

A. Proximal convoluted tubule
B. Loop of Henle
C. Distal nephron
D. All of the above

Virtually all regulation of renal K^+ excretion & total body K^+ balance occurs in distal nephron.

342. Normal plasma potassium concentration inside cells is about?

Pediatr Nephrol. 2011;26:377-384

A. 50 mmol/L
B. 100 mmol/L
C. 150 mmol/L
D. 200 mmol/L

Normal plasma K^+ concentration is 3.5 - 5.0 mmol/L, whereas that inside cells is about 150 mmol/L. <2% of total body K^+ content (2500–4500 mmol) is in ECF.

343. Normally, ratio of ICF to ECF K^+ concentration is about?

Electrolyte Blood Press. 2010;8(1):38-50

A. 28:1
B. 35:1
C. 48:1
D. 58:1

Normally, ratio of ICF to ECF K^+ concentration is ~ 35:1 due to resting membrane potential and is crucial for normal neuromuscular function.

344. What percentage of filtered potassium is reabsorbed in proximal tubule by diffusion and solvent drag?

Pediatr Nephrol. 2011;26:377-384

A. ~ 15–25%
B. ~ 25–45%
C. ~ 45–60%
D. ~ 60–75%

Approximately 60–75% of the filtered potassium is reabsorbed in the proximal tubule (PT) by diffusion and solvent drag, mainly coupled to Na^+ transport, mainly by the Na^+/H^+ antiporter.

345. What percentage of filtered potassium is reabsorbed in the thick ascending limb of the Loop of Henle (TALH)?

Pediatr Nephrol. 2011;26:377-384

A. ~ 15–20%
B. ~ 20–45%
C. ~ 45–60%
D. ~ 60–75%

~15-20% of the filtered potassium is reabsorbed in the thick ascending limb of the Loop of Henle (TALH), mainly by the Na-K-2Cl cotransporter (NKCC2). This cotransporter is inhibited by loop diuretics (furosemide).

346. Distal convoluted tubule (DCT) is the site of excretion of?

Pediatr Nephrol. 2011;26:377-384

A. Potassium
B. Calcium
C. Magnesium
D. All of the above

Distal convoluted tubule (DCT) is the site of the apical sodium chloride cotransporter (NCCT), which is blocked by thiazides. It modulates excretion of not only potassium but also calcium and magnesium.

347. The basolateral Na-K ATPase pump actively transports potassium in & sodium out of the cell in a ratio of?

Harrison's 20th Ed. Chapter 49 Page 304

A. 1:2
B. 2:3
C. 3:4
D. 4:5

The basolateral Na^+, K^+-ATPase pump actively transports K^+ in and Na^+ out of the cell in a 2:3 ratio, and the passive outward diffusion of K^+ is quantitatively the most important factor that generates the resting membrane potential. The main hormones that increase the activity of Na^+,K^+-ATPase include β2-adrenergic agonists, insulin, and thyroid hormone.

348. Renal adaptive mechanisms allow the kidneys to maintain potassium homeostasis until the GFR drops to?

Pediatr Nephrol. 2011;26:377-384

A. < 60 ml/min/1.73 m^2
B. < 45 ml/min/1.73 m^2
C. < 30 ml/min/1.73 m^2
D. < 15 ml/min/1.73 m^2

Renal adaptive mechanisms allow the kidneys to maintain potassium homeostasis until the glomerular filtration rate (GFR) drops to less than 15 ml/min/1.73 m^2.

349. K^+ intake in an average western diet is?

Pediatr Nephrol. 2011;26:377-384

A. 10–40 mmol/day
B. 40–120 mmol/day
C. 120–350 mmol/day
D. 350–550 mmol/day

K^+ intake in an average western diet is 40–120 mmol/day, or approximately 1 mmol/kg per day, 90% of which is absorbed by the gastrointestinal tract.

350. Which is the most important site of K^+ secretion in the kidney?

Harrison's 20th Ed. Chapter 49 Page 304

A. Proximal tubule
B. Thick ascending limb of loop of Henle
C. Distal tubule convolute
D. Cortical collecting duct

Although, K^+ is transported along the entire nephron, it is the principal cells of the connecting segment (CNT) and cortical collecting duct (CD) that play a dominant role in renal K^+ secretion.

351. Which of the following is a flow-sensitive channel for potassium secretion?

Harrison's 20th Ed. Chapter 49 Page 304

A. Renal outer medullary K^+ channel (ROMK)
B. "Big potassium" (BK) or maxi-K K^+ channel
C. ENaC channel
D. All of the above

The maxi-K^+ channel (also known as the large-conductance K^+ (BK) channel) is characterized by a large single channel conductance and quiescence in the basal state and activation under conditions of increased flow. In addition to increased delivery of Na^+ and dilution of luminal K^+ concentration, recruitment of maxi-K^+ channels contributes to flow-dependent increased K^+ secretion.

352. Which of the following mediates bulk of constitutive K^+ secretion?

Harrison's 20th Ed. Chapter 49 Page 304

A. Renal outer medullary K^+ channel (ROMK)
B. "Big potassium" (BK) or maxi-K K^+ channel
C. ENaC channel
D. All of the above

Two major K^+ channels mediate distal tubular K^+ secretion. They are secretory K^+ channel ROMK (renal outer medullary K^+ channel, also known as Kir1.1 or KcnJ1) and the flow-sensitive "big potassium" (BK) or maxi-K K^+ channel. ROMK mediates bulk of constitutive K^+ secretion.

353. Which of the following hormones has a major influence on potassium excretion?

Harrison's 20th Ed. Chapter 49 Page 304

A. Aldosterone
B. Renin
C. Angiotensin II
D. All of the above

Aldosterone has a major influence on potassium excretion. It increases the activity of ENaC channels to amplify the driving force for K^+ secretion across the luminal membrane of principal cells. Aldosterone as key regulator of renal potassium homeostasis binds to the nuclear mineralocorticoid receptor (MR) within the distal tubule and the principal cells in the CCD. It activates the basolateral Na^+/K^+-ATPase, thereby increasing Na^+ and water reabsorption into the blood and secretion of K^+ into the urine. Aldosterone also upregulates the amiloride sensitive sodium channels (ENaCs) in the apical membrane of CCD and stimulates H^+ secretion by intercalated CCD cells, thereby influencing acid/base balance.

354. Hypokalemia is defined as a plasma potassium concentration of?

Harrison's 20th Ed. Chapter 49 Page 304

A. < 3.5 mM
B. < 3.6 mM
C. < 3.7 mM
D. < 3.8 mM

Hypokalemia is defined as a plasma K^+ concentration <3.5 mM.

355. Which of the following can cause treatment-resistant hypokalemia?

Harrison's 20th Ed. Chapter 49 Page 304

A. Hypomagnesemia
B. Hypocalcemia
C. Hyponatremia
D. All of the above

Systemic hypomagnesemia can also cause treatment-resistant hypokalemia, due to a combination of reduced cellular uptake of K^+ and exaggerated renal secretion.

356. Spurious hypokalemia or "pseudohypokalemia" best relates to?

Harrison's 20th Ed. Chapter 49 Page 304

A. Erythrocytosis
B. Leukocytosis
C. Thrombocytosis
D. All of the above

Spurious hypokalemia or "pseudohypokalemia" can occasionally result from in vitro cellular uptake of K^+ after venipuncture due to profound leukocytosis in acute leukemia.

357. Which of the following promote Na^+/K^+-ATPase-mediated cellular uptake of K^+?

Harrison's 20th Ed. Chapter 49 Page 304

A. Insulin
B. β-adrenergic activity
C. Alkalosis
D. All of the above

Insulin, β-adrenergic activity, thyroid hormone and alkalosis promote Na^+/K^+-ATPase-mediated cellular uptake of K^+ leading to hypokalemia.

358. Inhibition of the passive efflux of K^+ occurs with?

Harrison's 20th Ed. Chapter 49 Page 304

A. Arsenic
B. Barium
C. Cobalt
D. All of the above

Inhibition of the passive efflux of K^+ can also cause hypokalemia. This typically occurs due to systemic inhibition of K^+ channels by toxic barium ions.

359. In malnourished patients given a carbohydrate load, stimulation of endogenous insulin can lead to?

Harrison's 20th Ed. Chapter 49 Page 304

A. Hypokalemia
B. Hypomagnesemia
C. Hypophosphatemia
D. All of the above

In malnourished patients given a carbohydrate load, stimulation of endogenous insulin can provoke hypokalemia, hypomagnesemia and/or hypophosphatemia.

360. Which of the following can cause hypokalemia?

Harrison's 20th Ed. Chapter 49 Page 304

A. Pseudoephedrine and ephedrine
B. Ritodrine
C. Theophylline
D. All of the above

β2 agonists, bronchodilators (salmeterol), tocolytics (ritodrine) and "hidden" sympathomimetics (pseudoephedrine & ephedrine), are powerful activators of cellular K^+ uptake may cause unexpected hypokalemia.

361. Thyrotoxic periodic paralysis (TPP) best relates to?
Harrison's 20th Ed. Chapter 49 Page 305

A. Kir1.6
B. Kir2.6
C. Kir3.6
D. Kir4.6

TPP is linked to genetic variation in Kir2.6, a muscle-specific, thyroid hormone responsive K^+ channel.

362. Patients with TPP typically develop paralytic episodes most frequently between?
Harrison's 20th Ed. Chapter 49 Page 305

A. 1 AM and 6 AM
B. 6 AM and 12 Noon
C. 12 Noon and 6 PM
D. 6 PM and 12 Midnight

Patients with TPP typically present with weakness of extremities & limb girdles, with paralytic episodes that occur most frequently between 1 & 6 AM. Signs & symptoms of hyperthyroidism are not invariably present.

363. Which of the following occurs in thyrotoxic periodic paralysis?
Harrison's 20th Ed. Chapter 49 Page 305

A. Hypokalemia
B. Hypophosphatemia
C. Hypomagnesemia
D. All of the above

In TPP, hypokalemia is usually profound and almost invariably accompanied by hypophosphatemia and hypomagnesemia.

364. Which of the following reverses hypokalemia, hypophosphatemia and paralysis in TPP?
Harrison's 20th Ed. Chapter 49 Page 305

A. Glucagon
B. Adrenaline
C. Propranolol
D. Amiodarone

Hypokalemia in TPP is attributed to both direct & indirect activation of the Na^+/ K^+-ATPase, resulting in increased uptake of K^+ by muscle and other tissues. High-dose propranolol (3 mg/kg) rapidly reverses the associated hypokalemia, hypophosphatemia and paralysis.

365. Which of the following is the least likely cause of hypokalemia?
Harrison's 20th Ed. Chapter 49 Page 305

A. Ileostomy
B. Loss of gastric secretions
C. Chronic laxative abuse
D. Colonic pseudo-obstruction

K^+ concentration of gastric fluid is only 5–10 mmol/L and is a less likely cause of hypokalemia. Loss of gastric contents results in volume depletion & metabolic alkalosis, both promote kaliuresis. Celiac disease, ileostomy, villous adenomas, inflammatory bowel disease, colonic pseudo-obstruction (Ogilvie's syndrome), VIPomas and chronic laxative abuse can also cause significant hypokalemia.

366. Which of the following is false about acute colonic pseudo-obstruction (ACPO)?
World J Gastroenterol. 2017;23(30):5634-5644

A. Acute colonic dilatation
B. Absence of intrinsic mechanical obstruction
C. Absence of extrinsic inflammatory process
D. All of the above

Acute colonic pseudo-obstruction (ACPO) is characterised by acute colonic dilatation in the absence of intrinsic mechanical obstruction or extrinsic inflammatory process. "Sympathetic deprivation" of the colon as its mechanism was first postulated by Ogilvie. "Ogilvie's syndrome" has also been used to refer to ACPO, though this term is now discouraged due to ambiguity regarding its meaning.

367. Which of the following is a cause of decreased potassium intake?
Harrison's 20th Ed. Chapter 49 Page 305 Table 49-4

A. Ingestion of excess carbohydrates
B. Ingestion of excess proteins
C. Ingestion of excess fats
D. Ingestion of clay (geophagia)

Ingestion of clay (geophagia) is a cause of decreased K^+ intake as it binds dietary K^+ & iron.

368. Which of the following statements is false?
Harrison's 20th Ed. Chapter 49 Page 305

A. Thiazides cause more hypokalemia than loop diuretics
B. Thiazides cause hypocalciuria
C. Loop diuretics cause hypercalciuria
D. None of the above

Thiazides cause more hypokalemia than loop diuretics although they have lesser natriuretic effect. Diuretic effect of thiazides is due to inhibition of the Na^+-Cl^- cotransporter NCC in DCT cells that leads to increased delivery of luminal Na^+ to principal cells immediately downstream in CNT & cortical CD. This augments Na^+ entry via ENaC, increases lumen-negative potential difference and amplifies K^+ secretion. Thiazides cause hypokalemia also secondary to thiazide-associated hypocalciuria, versus hypercalciuria seen with loop diuretics. The increases in downstream luminal calcium in response to loop diuretics inhibit ENaC in principal cells, thus reducing the lumen-negative potential difference and attenuating distal K^+ excretion.

369. Which of the following drugs increase K^+ excretion by acting as nonreabsorbable anions in distal nephron?
Harrison's 20th Ed. Chapter 49 Page 305

A. Aminoglycosides
B. Amphotericin
C. Carbenicillin
D. Foscarnet

370. Which of the following drugs cause hypokalemia and hypomagnesemia?
Harrison's 20th Ed. Chapter 49 Page 305

A. Aminoglycosides
B. Amphotericin
C. Foscarnet
D. All of the above

High doses of penicillin-related antibiotics (nafcillin, dicloxacillin, ticarcillin, oxacillin and carbenicillin) can increase obligatory K^+ excretion by acting as nonreabsorbable anions in the distal nephron. Renal tubular toxins cause renal K^+ and magnesium wasting, leading to hypokalemia and hypomagnesemia. These include aminoglycosides, amphotericin, foscarnet, cisplatin & ifosfamide.

371. In congenital adrenal hyperplasia, hypertension & hypokalemia is due to increase in circulating?
Harrison's 20th Ed. Chapter 49 Page 305

A. 11-deoxycorticosterone
B. 12-deoxycorticosterone
C. 13-deoxycorticosterone
D. 14-deoxycorticosterone

Congenital adrenal hyperplasia is caused by defects in either steroid 11β-hydroxylase or steroid 17α-hydroxylase. Increase in circulating 11-deoxycorticosterone causes hypertension and hypokalemia.

372. Aldosterone is secreted by zona glomerulosa cells of adrenal cortex in response to?
Harrison's 20th Ed. Chapter 49 Page 305

A. High renin
B. High angiotensin II
C. Hyperkalemia
D. All of the above

Aldosterone is secreted by the zona glomerulosa cells of the adrenal cortex in response to high renin and angiotensin II or hyperkalemia.

373. Glucocorticoid-remediable hyperaldosteronism (GRA) is also called?

Harrison's 20th Ed. Chapter 49 Page 305

A. Familial hyperaldosteronism type I (FH-I)

B. Familial hyperaldosteronism type II (FH-II)

C. Familial hyperaldosteronism type III (FH-III)

D. Familial hyperaldosteronism type IV (FH-IV)

Familial hyperaldosteronism type I (FH-I) is also known as glucocorticoid-remediable hyperaldosteronism (GRA). FH-II and FH-III are forms of isolated primary genetic hyperaldosteronism in which aldosterone production is not repressible by exogenous glucocorticoids.

374. FH-I is caused by a chimeric gene duplication between?

Harrison's 20th Ed. Chapter 49 Page 305

A. CYP11B1 and CYP11B2

B. CYP11B1 and CYP11B3

C. CYP11B1 and CYP11B4

D. CYP11B1 and CYP11B5

FH-I is caused by a chimeric gene duplication between homologous 11β-hydroxylase (CYP11B1) and aldosterone synthase (CYP11B2) genes, fusing the adrenocorticotropic hormone (ACTH) responsive 11β-hydroxylase promoter to the coding region of aldosterone synthase. This chimeric gene is under the control of ACTH and thus repressible by glucocorticoids.

375. FH-III is caused by mutations in which of the following gene?

Harrison's 20th Ed. Chapter 49 Page 305

A. ABCB11

B. ATP8B1

C. UDPGT

D. KCNJ5

FH-III is caused by mutations in KCNJ5 gene, which encodes G-protein-activated inward rectifier K^+ channel 4 (GIRK4). These mutations lead to acquisition of sodium permeability in the mutant GIRK4 channels causing an exaggerated membrane depolarization in adrenal glomerulosa cells and activation of voltage-gated calcium channels. The resulting calcium influx is sufficient to produce aldosterone secretion & cell proliferation, leading to adrenal adenomas & hyper-aldosteronism.

376. Acquired causes of primary hyperaldosteronism include?

Harrison's 20th Ed. Chapter 49 Page 306

A. Aldosterone producing adenomas (APAs)

B. Primary or unilateral adrenal hyperplasia (PAH)

C. Idiopathic hyperaldosteronism (IHA)

D. All of the above

Acquired causes of primary hyperaldosteronism include aldosterone producing adenomas (APAs), primary or unilateral adrenal hyperplasia (PAH), idiopathic hyperaldosteronism (IHA) due to bilateral adrenal hyperplasia and adrenal carcinoma.

377. What value of plasma aldosterone : PRA ratio is suggestive of primary hyperaldosteronism?

Harrison's 20th Ed. Chapter 49 Page 306

A. > 20

B. > 30

C. > 40

D. > 50

Plasma aldosterone : PRA ratio of >50, due to suppression of circulating renin and an elevation of circulating aldosterone, is suggestive of primary hyperaldosteronism. However, hypokalemia and multiple antihypertensive drugs may alter aldosterone:PRA ratio.

378. Which of the following converts cortisol to cortisone?

Harrison's 20th Ed. Chapter 49 Page 306

A. 11β-hydroxysteroid dehydrogenase-1 (11βHSD-1)

B. 11β-hydroxysteroid dehydrogenase-2 (11βHSD-2)

C. 17α-hydroxylase

D. 11β-hydroxylase

The glucocorticoid cortisol has equal affinity for the mineralocorticoid receptor (MLR) to that of aldosterone, with resultant "mineralocorticoid-like" activity. However, cells in the aldosterone-sensitive distal nephron are protected from this "illicit" activation by the enzyme 11β-hydroxysteroid dehydrogenase-2 (11βHSD-2), which converts cortisol to cortisone; cortisone has minimal affinity for the MLR.

379. 'Syndrome of apparent mineralocorticoid excess' is due to deficiency of?

Harrison's 20th Ed. Chapter 49 Page 306

A. 11α-HSDH-2

B. 11β-HSDH-2

C. 12α-HSDH-2

D. 12β-HSDH-2

Cortisol is converted to cortisone by 11β-hydroxysteroid dehydrogenase 2 (11β-HSDH-2). 11β-HSDH-2 deficiency or suppression allows cortisol to bind to the aldosterone receptor & leads to syndrome of apparent mineralocorticoid excess (SAME).

380. Syndrome of apparent mineralocorticoid excess (SAME) is characterized by?

Harrison's 20th Ed. Chapter 49 Page 306

A. Hypertension

B. Hypokalemia

C. Hypercalciuria

D. All of the above

381. Syndrome of apparent mineralocorticoid excess (SAME) is characterized by?

Harrison's 20th Ed. Chapter 49 Page 306

A. Metabolic alkalosis

B. Suppressed PRA

C. Suppressed aldosterone

D. All of the above

Syndrome of apparent mineralocorticoid excess (SAME) is characterized by hypertension, hypokalemia, hypercalciuria and metabolic alkalosis with suppressed PRA and suppressed aldosterone.

382. Conditions that inhibit the activity of '11βHSD-2' include?

Harrison's 20th Ed. Chapter 49 Page 306

A. Glycyrrhetinic/glycyrrhizinic acid

B. Chewing tobacco

C. Carbenoxolone

D. All of the above

Glycyrrhetinic acid (in licorice), chewing tobacco & carbenoxolone inhibit activity of 11βHSD-2.

383. Which of the following is a cause of hypokalemia?

Harrison's 20th Ed. Chapter 49 Page 306

A. Metabolic alkalosis

B. Treatment of DKA with insulin

C. Uncontrolled hyperglycemia

D. All of the above

384. Which of the following is a cause of hypokalemia?

A. Patients of pernicious anemia treated with vitamin B12
B. Patients of neutropenia treated with GM-CSF
C. Massive transfusion with thawed washed RBCs
D. All of the above

Treatment of DKA with insulin causes hypokalemia due movement of K^+ inside the cells with glucose like anabolic states. Uncontrolled hyperglycemia causes K^+ depletion due to osmotic diuresis.

385. Primary hyperaldosteronism is due to dysregulated aldosterone secretion by?

A. Adrenal adenoma
B. Adrenal carcinoma
C. Adrenocortical hyperplasia
D. All of the above

Primary hyperaldosteronism is due to dysregulated aldosterone secretion by an adrenal adenoma (Conn's syndrome) or carcinoma or to adrenocortical hyperplasia.

386. Tumor that produce renin include?

A. Renal cell carcinoma
B. Ovarian carcinoma
C. Wilms' tumor
D. All of the above

Renin-secreting tumors of juxtaglomerular apparatus, renal cell carcinoma, ovarian carcinoma, and Wilms' tumor produce renin.

387. Which of the following is false about 'Liddle's syndrome'?
Harrison's 20th Ed. Chapter 49 Page 306

A. Autosomal dominant
B. Hypertension
C. Hypokalemic metabolic alkalosis
D. Excess renin and aldosterone secretion

Liddle's syndrome is an autosomal dominant gain-in-function mutations of ENaC subunits. The result is increased expression of activated ENaC channels at the plasma membrane of principal cells. It is characterized by hypertension, hypokalemic metabolic alkalosis, renal K^+ wasting & suppressed renin & aldosterone secretion.

388. Which of the following is false about 'Liddle's syndrome'?
Harrison's 20th Ed. Chapter 49 Page 306

A. Blunted aldosterone response to ACTH
B. Reduced urinary aldosterone excretion
C. Unresponsive to spironolactone yet sensitive to amiloride
D. None of the above

Patients with Liddle's syndrome classically manifest severe hypertension with hypokalemia, unresponsive to spironolactone yet sensitive to amiloride. Hypertension and hypokalemia are variable aspects of the Liddle's phenotype; more consistent features include a blunted aldosterone response to ACTH and reduced urinary aldosterone excretion.

389. Loss of transport functions of which nephron segment causes Bartter's syndrome (BS)?
Harrison's 20th Ed. Chapter 49 Page 306

A. PCT
B. TALH
C. DCT
D. All of the above

Loss of the transport functions of TALH nephron segment with reduction in renal concentrating ability causes Bartter's syndrome, a hereditary hypokalemic alkalosis.

390. Loss of transport functions of which nephron segment causes Gitelman's syndrome (GS)?
Harrison's 20th Ed. Chapter 49 Page 306

A. PCT
B. TALH
C. DCT
D. All of the above

Loss of the transport functions of in the thiazide-sensitive Na-Cl cotransporter of DCT nephron segment reduction in renal concentrating ability causes Gitelman's syndrome, a hereditary hypokalemic alkalosis.

391. Which of the following statements is false?
Harrison's 20th Ed. Chapter 49 Page 306

A. Bartter's syndrome relates to Na^+, K^+ & Cl^- transport of TALH
B. Gitelman's syndrome relates to thiazide-sensitive Na^+-Cl^- cotransporter of DCT
C. Urinary calcium excretion is a critical diagnostic test in BS/GS
D. None of the above

392. Bartter's syndrome is characterized by?
Harrison's 20th Ed. Chapter 49 Page 306

A. Hypokalemia
B. Metabolic alkalosis
C. Hyperreninemic hyperaldosteronism
D. All of the above

Bartter's syndrome is characterized by hypokalemia, metabolic alkalosis, hyperreninemic hyperaldosteronism secondary to ECF volume contraction, increase in urinary calcium excretion & juxtaglomerular apparatus hyperplasia.

393. Systemic symptoms of Bartter's syndrome are due to?
Harrison's 20th Ed. Chapter 49 Page 306

A. Increase in plasma renin
B. Increase in plasma aldosterone
C. Increase in renal prostaglandin
D. All of the above

In Bartter's syndrome, renal prostaglandin synthesis & excretion are significantly increased, accounting for much of the systemic symptoms.

394. Which of the following is a critical diagnostic test in Gitelman's syndrome (GS)?
Harrison's 20th Ed. Chapter 49 Page 306

A. Plasma renin activity (PRA)
B. Aldosterone
C. Urinary calcium excretion
D. Urinary magnesium excretion

395. Which of the following is a feature of Gitelman's syndrome?
Harrison's 20th Ed. Chapter 49 Page 306

A. Hypomagnesemia
B. Hypocalciuria
C. Chondrocalcinosis
D. All of the above

396. Which of the following statements is false?

Harrison's 20th Ed. Chapter 49 Page 306

A. GS is genetically homogeneous
B. Patients with GS are uniformly hypomagnesemic
C. Patients with GS exhibit marked hypocalciuria
D. None of the above

Hypomagnesemic patients are clinically refractory to K^+ replacement in the absence of Mg^{++} repletion.

397. Which of the following laboratory abnormalities is seen only in chronic renal failure?

Harrison's 20th Ed. Chapter 49 Page 306

A. Anemia
B. Hypocalcemia
C. Hyperphosphatemia
D. Radiographic evidence of renal osteodystrophy

398. Hypokalemia has prominent effects on which of the following?

Harrison's 20th Ed. Chapter 49 Page 306

A. Cardiac
B. Skeletal muscle cells
C. Intestinal muscle cells
D. All of the above

Hypokalemia has prominent effects on cardiac (precipitant of arrhythmia), skeletal (weakness, paralysis, skeletal myopathy, rhabdomyolysis) and intestinal muscle cells (intestinal ileus).

399. Electrocardiographic changes in hypokalemia include?

Harrison's 20th Ed. Chapter 49 Page 306

A. Broad flat T waves
B. ST depression
C. QT prolongation
D. All of the above

Electrocardiographic changes in hypokalemia include broad flat T waves, ST depression and QT prolongation.

400. Electrocardiographic changes in hypokalemia are most marked when serum K^+ is?

Harrison's 20th Ed. Chapter 49 Page 306

A. < 3.5 mmol/L
B. < 3.2 mmol/L
C. < 3.0 mmol/L
D. < 2.7 mmol/L

Electrocardiographic changes in hypokalemia are most marked when serum K^+ is <2.7 mmol/L.

401. Which of the following is false regarding ECG changes of hypokalemia?

Harrison's 20th Ed. Chapter 49 Page 306

A. Delayed ventricular repolarization
B. Do not correlate well with plasma K^+ levels
C. Prominent U wave
D. Shortened QU interval

ECG changes of hypokalemia are due to delayed ventricular repolarization and do not correlate well with the plasma K^+ concentration. Early changes include flattening or inversion of T wave, prominent U wave, ST-segment depression, and prolonged QU interval.

402. Which of the following ECG changes denote severe potassium depletion?

Harrison's 20th Ed. Chapter 49 Page 306

A. Prominent U wave
B. Inversion of T wave
C. Prolonged PR interval
D. Prolonged QU interval

Severe K^+ depletion may result in a prolonged PR interval, decreased voltage and widening of the QRS complex and ventricular arrhythmias.

403. Which of the following occurs in hypokalemia?

Harrison's 20th Ed. Chapter 49 Page 306

A. Phosphaturia
B. Hypocitraturia
C. Activation of renal ammoniagenesis
D. All of the above

The functional effects of hypokalemia on the kidney can include Na-Cl and HCO_3 retention, polyuria, phosphaturia, hypocitraturia and an activation of renal ammoniagenesis. Bicarbonate retention and other acid-base effects of hypokalemia can contribute to the generation of metabolic alkalosis.

404. Hypokalemia is associated frequently with?

Harrison's 20th Ed. Chapter 49 Page 306

A. Metabolic alkalosis
B. Respiratory acidosis
C. Respiratory alkalosis
D. All of the above

Metabolic alkalosis is associated with hypokalemia due to K^+ redistribution and excessive renal K^+ loss.

405. What value of a 24-h K^+ excretion is indicative of an extrarenal cause of hypokalemia?

Harrison's 20th Ed. Chapter 49 Page 307

A. < 15 mmol
B. < 30 mmol
C. < 45 mmol
D. < 60 mmol

A 24 hour K^+ excretion of <15 mmol is indicative of an extrarenal cause of hypokalemia. The etiology of hypokalemia can simply be divided into two groups: those with a low K^+ excretion rate and those with a high K^+ excretion rate.

406. Which of the following is a feature of hypokalemia due to renal K^+ wasting?

Electrolyte Blood Press. 2010;8(1):38-50

A. Chronic
B. Related to disorders with increased flow rate to the CCD
C. Related to disorders with increased K^+ in the CCD
D. None of the above

Hypokalemia due to renal K^+ wasting is chronic and usually related to disorders with either increased flow rate to the CCD or increased K^+ in the CCD (fast Na^+ or slow Cl^-).

407. Which of the following suggests hypokalemia due to gastrointestinal potassium loss?

Harrison's 20th Ed. Chapter 49 Page 307 Figure 49-7

A. Serum K^+ < 3.5 mmol/L
B. Urine K^+ < 15 mmol/day
C. Metabolic acidosis
D. All of the above

408. Which of the following suggests hypokalemia due to profuse sweating?

Harrison's 20th Ed. Chapter 49 Page 307 Figure 49-7

A. Serum K^+ < 3.5 mmol/L
B. Urine K^+ < 15 mmol/day
C. Normal acid-base status
D. All of the above

409. Which of the following suggests hypokalemia due to remote diuretic use?

Harrison's 20th Ed. Chapter 49 Page 307 Figure 49-7

A. Serum K^+ < 3.5 mmol/L
B. Urine K^+ < 15 mmol/day
C. Metabolic alkalosis
D. All of the above

410. Hypokalemia with minimal renal potassium excretion suggests that potassium loss is through?

Harrison's 20th Ed. Chapter 49 Page 307

A. Skin
B. Gastrointestinal tract
C. Diuretic use
D. All of the above

Hypokalemia with minimal renal K^+ excretion (<15 mmol/day of K^+ in urine) suggests that K^+ was lost via the skin or gastrointestinal tract or that there is a remote history of vomiting or diuretic use.

411. Plasma renin activity and aldosterone levels are high in patients with?

Electrolyte Blood Press. 2010;8(1):38-50

A. Renin-secreting tumor
B. Renal vascular stenosis
C. Malignant hypertension
D. All of the above

Plasma renin activity and aldosterone levels are high in patients with renin-secreting tumor, renal vascular stenosis, malignant hypertension, and pheochromocytoma.

412. High plasma aldosterone levels but low plasma renin activity indicates?

Harrison's 20th Ed. Chapter 49 Page 307 Figure 49-7

A. Cushing's syndrome
B. Malignant hypertension
C. Renal artery stenosis
D. Primary hyperaldosteronism

413. Primary hyperaldosteronism can be caused by?

Electrolyte Blood Press. 2010;8(1):38-50

A. Bilateral adrenal hyperplasia
B. Adrenal adenoma/carcinoma
C. Glucocorticoid-remediable aldosteronism (GRA)
D. All of the above

High plasma aldosterone levels but low plasma renin activity indicates primary hyperaldosteronism which can be caused by bilateral adrenal hyperplasia, adrenal adenoma/carcinoma, and glucocorticoid-remediable aldosteronism (GRA).

414. High plasma aldosterone levels but low plasma renin activity indicates?

Harrison's 20th Ed. Chapter 49 Page 307 Figure 49-7

A. Familial hyperaldosteronism type I (FH-I)
B. Familial hyperaldosteronism type II (FH-II)
C. Familial hyperaldosteronism type III (FH-III)
D. All of the above

415. Which of the following is false about Cushing's syndrome?

Harrison's 20th Ed. Chapter 49 Page 307 Figure 49-7

A. Urine K^+ > 15 mmol/day
B. TTKG < 2
C. Low aldosterone
D. High cortisol

416. Which of the following is false about Liddle's syndrome?

Harrison's 20th Ed. Chapter 49 Page 307 Figure 49-7

A. Urine K^+ < 15 mmol/day
B. TTKG > 4
C. Low aldosterone
D. Normal cortisol

417. Which of the following is false about renal artery stenosis?

Harrison's 20th Ed. Chapter 49 Page 307 Figure 49-7

A. Urine K^+ < 15 mmol/day
B. TTKG > 4
C. High aldosterone
D. High renin

418. Hypokalemia with acidosis is seen in?

Harrison's 20th Ed. Chapter 49 Page 307

A. Lower gastrointestinal losses
B. Diabetic ketoacidosis
C. Renal tubular acidosis
D. All of the above

419. Hypokalemia with alkalosis is seen in?

Harrison's 20th Ed. Chapter 49 Page 307

A. Diuretic use
B. Gitelman syndrome
C. Bartter syndrome
D. All of the above

420. Hypokalemia with potassium wasting is seen in?

Harrison's 20th Ed. Chapter 49 Page 307

A. Diabetic ketoacidosis
B. Renal tubular acidosis
C. Diuretic use
D. All of the above

421. Hypokalemia with potassium wasting is seen in all except ?

Harrison's 20th Ed. Chapter 49 Page 307

A. Vomiting
B. Gitelman syndrome
C. Bartter syndrome
D. Surreptitious vomiting (bulimia)

422. Secretion of K^+ in cortical & outer medullary collecting ducts is influenced by?

Indian J Pediatr. 2007;74(7):679-686

A. Aldosterone
B. Plasma K^+ concentration
C. Anion composition of the luminal fluid
D. All of the above

Secretion of K^+ in cortical & outer medullary collecting ducts accounts for the majority of its excretion in urine that is influenced by aldosterone, plasma K^+ concentration and anion composition of the luminal fluid.

423. Which of the following is a spot urine index of renal response to hypokalemia?

Electrolyte Blood Press. 2010;8(1):38-50

A. Fractional excretion of K^+
B. Urine K^+/creatinine ratio
C. Urine osmolality/creatinine
D. All of the above

Four spot urine indices of renal response to hypokalemia have been used: fractional excretion of K+, TTKG, urine K+/creatinine ratio and urine osmolality/creatinine.

424. Which of the following is the formula for calculating transtubular potassium gradient (TTKG)?

Harrison's 20th Ed. Chapter 49 Page 310

A. (Urine K^+ × serum osmolality) ÷ (Serum K^+ × urine osmolality)
B. (Serum K^+ × urine osmolality) ÷ (Urine K^+ × serum osmolality)
C. (Urine K^+ × urine osmolality) ÷ (Serum K^+ × serum osmolality)
D. (Serum K^+ × serum osmolality) ÷ (Urine K^+ × urine osmolality)

Formula to calculate TTKG is (urine/plasma $[K^+]$) ÷ (urine/plasma osmolality). The TTKG is an index of the gradient of K^+ in the distal tubular lumen and interstitial blood capillaries, independent of urine flow rate. TTKG provides an accurate estimate of aldosterone effect on late distal and cortical collecting tubules.

425. What value of transtubular K^+ concentration gradient (TTKG) is indicative of hypokalemia?

Harrison's 20th Ed. Chapter 49 Page 307

A. < 1
B. < 2
C. < 3
D. < 4

TTKG should be <3 in the presence of hypokaleemia. TTKG is the ratio of K^+ concentration in lumen of CCD ($[K^+]_{CCD}$) to that in peritubular capillaries or plasma ($[K^+]_P$). The TTKG in normal persons varies but is generally within the range of 6–12.

426. What value of urinary K^+ to creatinine ratio is compatible with excessive renal K^+ excretion?

Harrison's 20th Ed. Chapter 49 Page 307

A. > l0 mmol/gram creatinine
B. > l1 mmol/gram creatinine
C. > l2 mmol/gram creatinine
D. > l3 mmol/gram creatinine

Urinary K^+ to creatinine ratio of > l3 mmol/g creatinine (>1.5 mmol/mmol creatinine) is compatible with excessive renal K^+ excretion.

427. Hypokalemic patients with vomiting due to bulimia typically have a urinary Cl^- of?

Harrison's 20th Ed. Chapter 49 Page 307

A. < 10 mmol/L
B. < 20 mmol/L
C. < 30 mmol/L
D. < 40 mmol/L

Hypokalemic patients with vomiting due to bulimia typically have a urinary Cl^- <10 mmol/L.

428. Urine Na^+, K^+, and Cl^- Which of the following is persistently elevated in Gitelman's syndrome (GS)?

Harrison's 20th Ed. Chapter 49 Page 307

A. Urine Na^+
B. Urine K^+
C. Urine Cl^-
D. All of the above

Urine Na^+, K^+, and Cl^- are persistently elevated in Gitelman's syndrome (GS), due to loss of function in the thiazide-sensitive Na^+-Cl^- cotransporter.

429. Which of the following statements is false?

Harrison's 20th Ed. Chapter 49 Page 308

A. Patients with Liddle's syndrome respond to amiloride
B. Patients with Liddle's syndrome do not respond to spironolactone
C. Patients with SAME respond to spironolactone
D. None of the above

430. High-dose propranolol (3 mg/kg) should be considered in which of the following redistributive hypokalemia conditions?

Harrison's 20th Ed. Chapter 49 Page 308

A. Thyrotoxic periodic paralysis (TPP)
B. Theophylline overdose
C. Acute head injury
D. All of the above

In redistributive hypokalemia, as in TPP, theophylline overdose, and acute head injury, excessive activity of sympathetic nervous system plays a dominant role. High-dose propranolol (3 mg/kg) will correct hypokalemia without the risk of rebound hyperkalemia.

431. It is generally safer to correct hypokalemia via which route?

Harrison's 20th Ed. Chapter 49 Page 308

A. Oral
B. Peripheral vein
C. Central vein
D. Per rectum

It is generally safer to correct hypokalemia via the oral route.

432. Which is the preparation of choice for correction of hypokalemia with metabolic alkalosis?

Harrison's 20th Ed. Chapter 49 Page 308

A. Potassium chloride
B. Potassium bicarbonate
C. Potassium citrate
D. None of the above

Potassium chloride is preferred for more rapid correction of hypokalemia. Potassium phosphate, oral or IV, may be appropriate in patients with combined hypokalemia and hypophosphatemia. Potassium bicarbonate and citrate (metabolized to HCO_3^-) tend to alkalinize and is more appropriate for hypokalemia associated with chronic diarrhea or RTA. Hypomagnesemic patients are refractory to K^+ replacement alone.

433. Serum K^+ drops by about how much for every 100-mmol reduction in total-body stores?

Harrison's 20th Ed. Chapter 49 Page 308

A. 0.17 mM
B. 0.27 mM
C. 0.37 mM
D. 0.47 mM

In the absence of abnormal K^+ redistribution, the total deficit correlates with serum K^+, such that serum K^+ drops by approximately 0.27 mM for every 100-mmol reduction in total-body stores. Loss of 400-800 mmol of total-body K^+ results in a reduction in serum K^+ by approximately 2.0 mM.

434. A decrement of 1 mmol/L in plasma potassium concentration may represent a total body potassium deficit of?

Harrison's 20th Ed. Chapter 49 Page 308

A. 20 to 40 mmol
B. 50 to 100 mmol
C. 100 to 200 mmol
D. 200 to 400 mmol

A decrement of 1 mmol/L in plasma K^+ concentration reflects total body K^+ deficit of 200–400 mmol.

435. Plasma potassium levels of < 3 mmol/L require how much potassium to correct the deficit?

Harrison's 20th Ed. Chapter 49 Page 308

A. 100 mmol
B. 200 mmol
C. 400 mmol
D. 600 mmol

Patients with plasma levels <3.0 mmol/L require >600 mmol of K^+ to correct the deficit.

436. Rate of IV infusion of potassium in severe hypokalemia should not exceed?

Harrison's 20th Ed. Chapter 49 Page 308

A. 20 mmol/hour
B. 40 mmol/hour
C. 60 mmol/hour
D. 80 mmol/hour

Rate of K^+ infusion should not exceed 20 mmol/hour unless paralysis or malignant ventricular arrhythmias are present.

437. Through a peripheral vein, maximum concentration of administered K^+ should be no more than?

Harrison's 20th Ed. Chapter 49 Page 308

A. 20 mmol/L
B. 40 mmol/L
C. 60 mmol/L
D. 80 mmol/L

The maximum concentration of administered K^+ should be no more than 40 mmol/L via a peripheral vein or 60 mmol/L via a central vein.

438. Ideally, for infusion KCl should be mixed in?

Harrison's 20th Ed. Chapter 49 Page 308

A. Normal saline
B. Dextrose solutions
C. Ringer solutions
D. All of the above

Ideally, KCl is mixed in normal saline as dextrose solutions may initially exacerbate hypokalemia due to insulin-mediated movement of K^+ into cells.

Hyperkalemia

439. Hyperkalemia is defined as a plasma K^+ concentration of?

Harrison's 20th Ed. Chapter 49 Page 308

A. > 4.5 mM
B. > 5.0 mM
C. > 5.5 mM
D. > 6.0 mM

Hyperkalemia is defined as a plasma K^+ concentration of 5.5 mM. Levels >6.0 mM are called as severe hyperkalemia.

440. Which of the following is the most frequent underlying cause of hyperkalemia?

Harrison's 20th Ed. Chapter 49 Page 308

A. Redistribution
B. Reduced tissue uptake
C. Decrease in renal K^+ excretion
D. Excessive intake of K^+

A decrease in renal K^+ excretion is the most frequent underlying cause of hyperkalemia. Excessive intake of K^+ is a rare cause.

441. ↑ed dietary intake of K^+ can cause hyperkalemia in?

Harrison's 20th Ed. Chapter 49 Page 308

A. Diabetics with hyporeninemic hypoaldosteronism
B. Chronic kidney disease
C. Drugs that impact the renin-angiotensin-aldosterone axis
D. All of the above

Dietary intake can have a mäjor effect in susceptible patients like diabetics with hyporeninemic hypoaldosteronism and chronic kidney disease. Drugs that impact on the renin-angiotensin-aldosterone axis are also a major cause of hyperkalemia.

442. Pseudohyperkalemia or factitious hyperkalemia results from?

Harrison's 20th Ed. Chapter 49 Page 308

A. Prolonged use of tourniquet
B. Hemolysis
C. Marked leukocytosis
D. All of the above

Pseudohyperkalemia refers to an artificially elevated "plasma" K^+ concentration due to movement of K^+ out of cells on venipuncture in asymptomatic patient with no obvious underlying cause. Serum K^+ concentration is normal. Prolonged tourniquet use, cooling of blood following venipuncture, hemolysis & marked leukocytosis, erythrocytosis or thrombocytosis, acute anxiety with respiratory alkalosis contribute to its occurrence.

443. Hereditary pseudohyperkalemia is caused by increases in?

Harrison's 20th Ed. Chapter 49 Page 308

A. Passive K^+ permeability of erythrocytes
B. Active K^+ permeability of erythrocytes
C. Passive K^+ permeability of leucocytes
D. Active K^+ permeability of leucocytes

Hereditary pseudohyperkalemia is caused by increases in the passive K^+ permeability of erythrocytes. Causative mutations have been described in red cell anion exchanger (AE1, encoded by the SLC4A1 gene), leading to reduced red cell anion transport, hemolytic anemia, the acquisition of a novel AE1-mediated K^+ leak and pseudohyperkalemia.

444. Acidosis leading to hyperkalemia is seen in?

Harrison's 20th Ed. Chapter 49 Page 308

A. Non-anion gap causes of metabolic acidosis
B. Lactic acidosis
C. Ketoacidosis
D. All of the above

Acidosis leading to hyperkalemia is limited to non-anion gap causes of metabolic acidosis. Hyperkalemia due to an acidosis induced shift of potassium from the cells into ECF does not occur in the anion gap acidoses-lactic acidosis and ketoacidosis.

445. Hyperkalemia can occur due to?

Harrison's 20th Ed. Chapter 49 Page 308

A. Hypertonic mannitol
B. Hypertonic saline
C. Intravenous immune globulin
D. All of the above

Hyperkalemia due to hypertonic mannitol, hypertonic saline & intravenous immune globulin is attributed to a "solvent drag" effect as water moves out of cells along the osmotic gradient.

446. Hyperkalemia can occur due to?

Harrison's 20th Ed. Chapter 49 Page 308

A. Lysine
B. Arginine
C. Epsilon-aminocaproic acid
D. All of the above

Cationic amino acids like lysine, arginine and the structurally related drug epsilon-aminocaproic acid, cause efflux of K^+ and hyperkalemia through an effective cation-K^+ exchange.

447. Which of the following poisoning is typically associated with hyperkalemia?

Harrison's 20th Ed. Chapter 49 Page 308

A. Arsenic
B. Benzene
C. Fluoride
D. Mangnese

Fluoride poisoning is typically associated with hyperkalemia because fluoride ions inhibit Na^+/K^+-ATPase.

448. Which of the following drug can cause acute hyperkalemia?

Harrison's 20th Ed. Chapter 49 Page 308

A. Ethanol
B. Succinylcholine
C. Ketamine
D. Lidocaine

Succinylcholine depolarizes muscle cells, causing an efflux of K^+ through acetylcholine receptors (AChRs).

449. Hyperkalemia can result from?

Harrison's 20th Ed. Chapter 49 Page 308

A. Intravascular hemolysis
B. Tumor lysis syndrome
C. Rhabdomyolysis
D. All of the above

Intravascular hemolysis, tumor lysis syndrome, and rhabdomyolysis lead to K^+ release from cells as a result of tissue breakdown. Red cell transfusion is a well described cause of hyperkalemia, typically in the setting of massive transfusions.

450. Which of the following foods is rich in potassium?

Harrison's 20th Ed. Chapter 49 Page 308

A. Tomatoes
B. Bananas
C. Citrus fruits
D. All of the above

Foods rich in potassium include tomatoes, bananas and citrus fruits.

451. Which of the following is false about hyporeninemic hypoaldosteronism?

Harrison's 20th Ed. Chapter 49 Page 308

A. Suppressed PRA & aldosterone
B. Reduced renal excretion of NH_4^+
C. Positive urinary anion gap and urine pH <5.5
D. None of the above

Hyporeninemic hypoaldosteronism is a very common predisposing factor in several overlapping subsets of hyperkalemic patients: diabetics, the elderly and patients with renal insufficiency. Classically, patients should have suppressed PRA and aldosterone. About 50% have an associated acidosis, with a reduced renal excretion of NH_4^+, a positive urinary anion gap & urine pH <5.5. Most patients have secondary increases in circulating atrial natriuretic peptide (ANP) that inhibit both renal renin release and adrenal aldosterone release.

452. Hyporeninemic hypoaldosteronism is seen in?

Harrison's 20th Ed. Chapter 49 Page 308

A. Mild renal insufficiency
B. Diabetic nephropathy
C. Chronic tubulointerstitial disease
D. All of the above

Hyporeninemic hypoaldosteronism is seen in mild renal insufficiency, diabetic nephropathy or chronic tubulointerstitial disease.

453. Hyperkalemia out of proportion to GFR can also be seen in?

Harrison's 20th Ed. Chapter 49 Page 308

A. Sickle cell anemia
B. Interstitial nephritis
C. Obstructive uropathy
D. All of the above

Hyperkalemia out of proportion to GFR is seen in tubulointerstitial disease that affects the distal nephron like amyloidosis, sickle cell anemia, interstitial nephritis and obstructive uropathy.

454. Which of the following is also known as hereditary hypertension with hyperkalemia?

Harrison's 20th Ed. Chapter 49 Page 308

A. Autosomal recessive pseudohypoaldosteronism type 1
B. Autosomal dominant pseudohypoaldosteronism type 1
C. Pseudohypoaldosteronism type II
D. All of the above

Hereditary renal causes of hyperkalemia have overlapping clinical features with hypoaldosteronism are labeled as pseudohypoaldosteronism (PHA). PHA type II (PHA-II) is also known as hereditary hypertension with hyperkalemia.

455. Pseudohypoaldosteronism type II is also called?

Harrison's 20th Ed. Chapter 271 Page 1899 Table 271-4

A. Spragg's syndrome
B. Leopold's syndrome
C. Marcelo's syndrome
D. Gordon's syndrome

Gordon's syndrome is characterized by hyperkalemia, metabolic acidosis, normal GFR, volume-expansion with suppressed renin & aldosterone levels. It is refractory to kaliuretic effect of exogenous mineralocorticoids.

456. Autosomal dominant form of PHA type 1 is due to loss-of-function mutations in?

Harrison's 20th Ed. Chapter 49 Page 308

A. NCC
B. ENaC
C. MLR
D. WNKI

457. Autosomal recessive form of PHA type 1 is due to mutation in?

Harrison's 20th Ed. Chapter 49 Page 308

A. NCC
B. ENaC
C. MLR
D. WNKI

PHA type 1 (PHA-I) has both an autosomal recessive and an autosomal dominant form. Autosomal dominant form is due to loss-of-function mutations in MLR. Recessive form is caused by various combinations of mutations in the three subunits of ENaC, resulting in impaired Na^+ channel activity in principal cells and other tissues.

458. Autosomal recessive form of PHA type II is due to mutation in?

Harrison's 20th Ed. Chapter 49 Page 308

A. ENaC
B. MLR
C. WNK1
D. All of the above

459. Patients with recessive PHA-I present as?

Harrison's 20th Ed. Chapter 49 Page 308

A. Lifelong salt wasting
B. Hypotension
C. Hyperkalemia
D. All of the above

Patients with recessive PHA-I suffer from lifelong salt wasting, hypotension and hyperkalemia, whereas the phenotype of autosomal dominant PHA-1 due to MLR dysfunction improves in adulthood.

460. PHA type II is in every respect the mirror image of?

Harrison's 20th Ed. Chapter 49 Page 308

A. Liddle's syndrome
B. Bartter's syndrome
C. Gitelman's syndrome
D. Gordon's syndrome

PHA type II is in every respect the mirror image of GS. PHA-II behaves like a gain of function in NCC and treatment with thiazides results in resolution of the entire clinical phenotype. However, the NCC gene is not directly involved in PHA-II, which is caused by mutations in WNK1 & WNK4 serine-threonine kinases or the upstream Kelch-like 3 (KLHL3) and Cullin 3 (CUL3), two components of an E3 ubiquitin ligase complex that regulates these kinases. These proteins collectively regulate NCC activity, with PHA-II associated activation of the transporter.

461. Clinical features of PHA type II include?

Harrison's 20th Ed. Chapter 49 Page 308

A. Hypertension
B. Hyperkalemia
C. Hyperchloremic metabolic acidosis
D. All of the above

Clinical features of PHA type II include hypertension, hyperkalemia, hyperchloremic metabolic acidosis, suppressed PRA and aldosterone, hypercalciuria and reduced bone density.

462. Pseudohypoaldosteronism is characterized by all except?

Harrison's 20th Ed. Chapter 49 Page 308

A. High renin & aldosterone levels
B. End-organ resistance to aldosterone
C. Renal sodium wasting
D. Hypertension

463. Pseudohypoaldosteronism is characterized by all except ?

Harrison's 20th Ed. Chapter 49 Page 308

A. Hyperkalemia
B. Metabolic alkalosis
C. Renal sodium wasting
D. Hypotension

Pseudohypoaldosteronism (PHA) is characterized by hyperkalemia, metabolic acidosis, renal Na^+ wasting, hypotension, high renin and aldosterone levels, and end-organ resistance to aldosterone.

464. Which of the following cause hyperkalemia?

Harrison's 20th Ed. Chapter 49 Page 308

A. Renin inhibitors
B. MLRs
C. ACE inhibitors & angiotensin receptor blockers
D. All of the above

ACE inhibitors, angiotensin receptor blockers, renin inhibitors and MLRs are predictable and common causes of hyperkalemia.

465. Which of the following cause hyperkalemia?

Harrison's 20th Ed. Chapter 49 Page 308

A. Yasmin-28
B. Nafamostat
C. Pentamidine
D. All of the above

Yasmin-28 is an oral contraceptive agent that contains progestin drospirenon which inhibits the MLR and can cause hyperkalemia. Nafamostat is a protease inhibitor used for pancreatitis. It inhibits aldosterone induced renal proteases that activate ENaC by proteolytic cleavage.

466. Which of the following cause hyperkalemia?

Harrison's 20th Ed. Chapter 49 Page 308

A. Theophylline
B. Chloroquine
C. Tacrolimus
D. Licorice

Cyclosporine, tacrolimus, NSAIDs and cyclooxygenase 2 (COX2) inhibitors cause hyperkalemia by their the ability to cause hyporeninemic hypoaldosteronism.

467. Which of the following blocks the apical ENaC activity in the distal nephron?

Harrison's 20th Ed. Chapter 49 Page 308

A. Amiloride
B. Trimethoprim
C. Pentamidine
D. All of the above

Trimethoprim & pentamidine impair K^+ secretion by blocking distal nephron Na^+ reabsorption.

468. Which of the following medications affect aldosterone secretion?

Harrison's 20th Ed. Chapter 49 Page 308

A. Angiotensin-converting enzyme (ACE) inhibitors
B. Angiotensin II receptor blockers (ARBs)
C. Heparin
D. All of the above

469. Which of the following medications cause tubular resistance to the action of aldosterone?

Harrison's 20th Ed. Chapter 49 Page 308

A. Trimethoprim
B. Spironolactone
C. Pentamidine
D. Digoxin

Trimethoprim, an antibiotic similar to potassium-sparing diuretic amiloride, competitively inhibits luminal sodium transport channels, causing a reduction in negative luminal charge and decreased potassium secretion.

470. Which of the following medications cause transmembrane shifting of potassium?

Harrison's 20th Ed. Chapter 49 Page 308

A. Spironolactone
B. Nonsteroidal anti-inflammatory drugs
C. Nonselective beta blockers
D. Heparin

Catecholamine-stimulated renin release is inhibited by beta blockade and causes a decrease in the amount of aldosterone synthesis. To a greater extent, however, beta blockers decrease the function of Na+/K+-ATPase by decreasing the amount of cyclic adenosine monophosphate (cAMP) in the cells.

471. Cardiac arrhythmias associated with hyperkalemia include?

Harrison's 20th Ed. Chapter 49 Page 310

A. Slow idioventricular rhythms
B. Ventricular tachycardia
C. Ventricular fibrillation
D. All of the above

Cardiac arrhythmias associated with hyperkalemia include sinus bradycardia, sinus arrest, slow idioventricular rhythms, ventricular tachycardia, ventricular fibrillation and asystole.

472. The earliest ECG change in hyperkalemia is?

Harrison's 20th Ed. Chapter 49 Page 310

A. Increased T-wave amplitude
B. Prolonged PR interval
C. Prolonged QRS duration
D. Loss of P waves

473. sine wave pattern in ECG in hyperkalemia is seen when serum K^+ levels are more than?

Harrison's 20th Ed. Chapter 49 Page 310

A. 5.5 mM
B. 6.5 mM
C. 7.0 mM
D. 8.0 mM

Electrocardiographic manifestations in hyperkalemia progress from tall peaked T waves (5.5-6.5 mM), to a loss of P waves (6.5-7.5 mM) to a widened QRS complex (7.0-8.0 mM) and ultimately a sine wave pattern (>8.0 mM).

474. In ECG, hyperkalemia can cause which of the following?

Harrison's 20th Ed. Chapter 49 Page 310

A. Long QT syndrome
B. Torsade de pointis
C. Type 1 Brugada pattern
D. All of the above

475. Hyperkalemic Brugada's sign can be differentiated from genetic Brugada's syndrome by?

Harrison's 20th Ed. Chapter 49 Page 310

A. Absence of P waves
B. Marked QRS widening
C. Abnormal QRS axis
D. All of the above

Hyperkalemia can cause a type 1 Brugada pattern in the electrocardiogram (ECG), with a pseudo-right bundle branch block and persistent coved ST segment elevation in at least two precordial leads. Hyperkalemic Brugada's sign occurs in critically ill patients with severe hyperkalemia and can be differentiated from genetic Brugada's syndrome by an absence of P waves, marked QRS widening and an abnormal QRS axis. Most patients are male, and many are critically ill. There is absence of congenital sodium channel anomaly. This change is reversible and typically resolves with resolution of hyperkalemia.

476. Sine wave pattern seen in severe hyperkalemia is due to merging of?

Harrison's 20th Ed. Chapter 49 Page 310

A. P + QRS
B. QRS + T
C. P + QRS + T
D. All of the above

The earliest ECG changes in hyperkalemia include increased T-wave amplitude. More severe degrees result in prolonged PR interval and QRS duration, AV conduction delay and loss of P waves. Progressive widening of QRS complex and merging with T wave produces a sine wave pattern. The terminal event is ventricular fibrillation or asystole.

477. Which of the following cardiac structure is most sensitive to hyperkalemia?

Emergency Medicine Practice 2016;18(11):1-24

A. Atrial myocardium
B. Ventricular myocardium
C. SA node
D. HIS bundle

↑ed extracellular K^+ causes an increase in transmembrane permeability & influx of K^+ into cells leading to a decrease in magnitude of the resting potential, a decrease in velocity of phase 0 of action potential & delayed conduction between myocytes. Effects of these changes are dependent upon tissue affected, with atrial myocardium being the most sensitive & specialized tissue (SA node & HIS bundle) being the least sensitive.

478. Which of the following regarding secondary hyperkalemic paralysis is false?

Harrison's 20th Ed. Chapter 49 Page 310

A. Autosomal dominant disorder
B. Episodic weakness/paralysis precipitated by exercise
C. Due to mutation in gene for skeletal muscle Na^+ channel
D. None of the above

Secondary hyperkalemic paralysis is an autosomal dominant disorder characterized by episodic weakness or paralysis, precipitated by stimuli that normally lead to mild hyperkalemia (exercise). Genetic defect is due to mutation in gene for skeletal muscle Na^+ channel.

479. Which of the following parameter is not required in calculating TTKG?

Harrison's 20th Ed. Chapter 49 Page 310

A. Serum Osmolality
B. Urine Osmolality
C. pH
D. Serum K

To calculate following parameters are required : Serum Osmolality (mOsm/kg), Urine Osmolality (mOsm/kg), Serum K (mEq/L) and Urine K (mEq/L).

480. Formula for calculating Transtubular Potassium Gradient (TTKG) is?

Harrison's 20th Ed. Chapter 49 Page 310

A. $(K^+_{serum} \times K^+_{Urine})/(Osm_{serum} \times Osm_{Urine})$
B. $(Osm_{serum} \times K^+_{serum})/(K^+_{Urine} \times Osm_{Urine})$
C. $(K^+_{Urine} \times Osm_{serum})/(K^+_{serum} \times Osm_{Urine})$
D. $(K^+_{serum} \times Osm_{Urine})/(Osm_{serum} \times K^+_{Urine})$

Correct formula for TTKG is $(P_{Osm} \times U_{Potassium})/(P_{Potassium} \times U_{Osm})$. It is valid only when Uosm >300 & UNa >25.

481. TTKG in a normal person on a normal diet is?

Indian J Pediatr 2007;74(7):679-686

A. 2–6
B. 6–12
C. 12–20
D. 20–29

The TTKG in normal persons varies but is generally within 6–12 range. Hypokalemia from extrarenal causes results in renal K⁺ conservation and a TTKG <2. A higher value suggests renal K⁺ losses, as in hyperaldosteronism. During hyperkalemia, the expected TTKG is >10. An inappropriately low TTKG (< 8) in hyperkalemia suggests hypoaldosteronism or renal tubular resistance to aldosterone. Administration of mineralocorticoid fludrocortisone (0.05 mg) enables TTKG to rise to >7 in patients with hypoaldosteronism. When it does not increase after mineralocorticoid challenge, tubular resistance to aldosterone is suspected.

482. Which of the following statements is false?

Indian J Pediatr 2007;74(7):679-686

A. Hypokalemia should result in a TTKG < 3
B. Hyperkalemia should result in a TTKG > 7–8
C. Hypokalemia not resulting in a TTKG<2 suggests renal K^+ loss
D. Hyperkalemia not resulting in a TTKG>10 suggests type I renal tubular acidosis

Hyperkalemia not resulting in a TTKG>10 suggests type IV renal tubular acidosis.

483. Renal excretion of potassium is dependent on?

Emergency Medicine Practice 2016;18(11):1-24

A. Rate of flow in the distal nephron
B. Aldosterone
C. Secretory pathways of potassium
D. All of the above

Renal excretion of potassium is dependent upon the rate of flow in the distal nephron, aldosterone, and the secretory pathways of potassium.

484. Which of the following suggests tubular resistance as a cause of hyperkalemia?

Harrison's 20th Ed. Chapter 49 Page 311 Figure 49-8

A. ↓ed urinary K^+ excretion
B. TTKG < 5
C. TTKG < 8 after 9α Fludrocortisone challenge
D. All of the above

485. Which of the following suggests ACE inhibitors as a cause of hyperkalemia?

Harrison's 20th Ed. Chapter 49 Page 311 Figure 49-8

A. TTKG ≥ 8 after 9α Fludrocortisone challenge
B. Low aldosterone
C. High renin
D. All of the above

486. Which of the following suggests primary adrenal insufficiency as a cause of hyperkalemia?

Harrison's 20th Ed. Chapter 49 Page 311 Figure 49-8

A. TTKG ≥ 8 after 9α Fludrocortisone challenge
B. Low aldosterone
C. High renin
D. All of the above

487. Which of the following suggests advanced kidney failure as a cause of hyperkalemia?

Harrison's 20th Ed. Chapter 49 Page 311 Figure 49-8

A. ↓ed urinary K^+ excretion (< 40 mmol/day)
B. TTKG > 8
C. Reduced tubular flow
D. All of the above

488. Significant hyperkalemia is considered when plasma K^+ concentration is?

Harrison's 20th Ed. Chapter 49 Page 310

A. ≥ 4.5 mM
B. ≥ 5.5 mM
C. ≥ 6.5 mM
D. ≥ 7.5 mM

489. In hyperkalemia, calcium administration acts by?

Harrison's 20th Ed. Chapter 49 Page 310

A. Raising the action potential threshold
B. Reducing excitability
C. No change in the resting membrane potential
D. All of the above

Calcium raises the action potential threshold & reduces excitability, without changing the resting membrane potential. Thus, calcium reverses the depolarization blockade due to hyperkalemia.

490. In severe hyperkalemia, 10 mL of 10% calcium gluconate should be infused over?

Harrison's 20th Ed. Chapter 49 Page 310

A. Half to 1 minute
B. 1 to 2 minutes
C. 2 to 3 minutes
D. 5 to 10 minutes

IV Calcium gluconate decreases membrane excitability. Usual dose is 10 mL of a 10% solution infused over 2–3 minutes with cardiac monitoring. Its effect is short-lived (30-60 min). Dose can be repeated if no change in ECG is seen after 5–10 minutes.

491. Hypercalcemia potentiates the cardiac toxicity of?

Harrison's 20th Ed. Chapter 49 Page 310

A. Amiodarone
B. Beta blockers
C. Theophylline
D. Digoxin

Hypercalcemia potentiates the cardiac toxicity of digoxin.

492. Which of the following is true for insulin-glucose treatment in hyperkalemia?

Harrison's 20th Ed. Chapter 49 Page 310

A. 5 units of IV regular insulin + 25 grams of IV glucose
B. 10 units of IV regular insulin + 25 grams of IV glucose
C. 15 units of IV regular insulin + 25 grams of IV glucose
D. 20 units of IV regular insulin + 25 grams of IV glucose

In hyperkalemia, the recommended dose is 10 units of intravenous regular insulin followed immediately by 50 mL of 50% dextrose (D50W, 25 g of glucose total) with avoidance of hypoglycemia. The effect begins in 10-20 minutes, peaks at 30-60 minutes, and lasts for 4-6 hours. In hyperkalemic patients with glucose concentrations of ≥200-250 mg/dL, insulin should be administered without glucose.

493. In hyperkalemia, inhaled Albuterol should not be used without?

Harrison's 20th Ed. Chapter 49 Page 310

A. IV Calcium
B. IV Insulin
C. IV Bicarbonate
D. All of the above

Inhaled Albuterol and insulin with glucose have an additive effect on plasma K^+ concentration.

494. Which of the following has no role in the acute treatment of hyperkalemia?

Harrison's 20th Ed. Chapter 49 Page 311

A. Intravenous calcium
B. Insulin
C. Albuterol
D. Intravenous bicarbonate

495. Severity of hyperkalemia is determined by?

Harrison's 20th Ed. Chapter 49 Page 311

A. Symptoms
B. Plasma K^+ concentration
C. ECG abnormalities
D. All of the above

Severity of hyperkalemia is determined by symptoms, plasma K^+ & ECG abnormalities.

496. The appropriate renal response to hyperkalemia is to excrete how much of K^+ daily?

Harrison's 20th Ed. Chapter 49 Page 311

A. At least 50 mmol
B. At least 100 mmol
C. At least 200 mmol
D. At least 300 mmol

The appropriate renal response to hyperkalemia is to excrete at least 200 mmol of K^+ daily.

497. Potentially fatal hyperkalemia occurs when plasma potassium concentration exceeds?

Harrison's 20th Ed. Chapter 49 Page 311

A. 5.5 mmol/L
B. 6.5 mmol/L
C. 7.5 mmol/L
D. 8.5 mmol/L

Potentially fatal hyperkalemia rarely occurs unless plasma K^+ concentration exceeds 7.5 mmol/L.

498. Which of the following is used for lowering potassium levels in severe hyperkalemia?

Harrison's 20th Ed. Chapter 49 Page 311

A. Insulin-glucose infusion
B. Alkali therapy with IV $NaHCO_3$
C. β_2 adrenergic agonists
D. All of the above

499. Which of the following reduce plasma K^+ levels by shifting K^+ into cells?

Harrison's 20th Ed. Chapter 49 Page 311

A. Glucose–insulin therapy
B. Alkali therapy with IV $NaHCO_3$
C. β_2-adrenergic agonists
D. All of the above

Alkali therapy with IV $NaHCO_3$ shifts K^+ into cells. β_2-adrenergic agonists promote cellular uptake of K^+.

500. Which of the following is false regarding sodium polystyrene sulfonate (SPS)?

Harrison's 20th Ed. Chapter 49 Page 311

A. Exchanges Na^+ for K^+ in gastrointestinal tract
B. Increases fecal excretion of K^+
C. Always given in a premade suspension with 33% sorbitol
D. None of the above

501. Which of the following is false regarding sodium polystyrene sulfonate (SPS)?

Harrison's 20th Ed. Chapter 49 Page 311

A. Anion-exchange resin
B. One gram binds 1 mmol of K^+ & releases 2-3 mmol of Na^+
C. Usual dose is 25–50 gram orally
D. Can be administered as retention enema

Sodium polystyrene sulfonate is a cation-exchange resin that promotes the exchange of Na^+ for K^+ in the gastrointestinal tract. Each gram binds 1 mmol of K^+ and releases 2–3 mmol of Na^+. Usual dose is 25-50 grams in 100 mL of 20% sorbitol orally to prevent constipation. It can also be administered as a retention enema.

502. Which of the following is a complication of SPS?

Harrison's 20th Ed. Chapter 49 Page 311

A. Anaphylaxis
B. Hepatitis
C. Intestinal obstruction
D. Intestinal necrosis

Intestinal necrosis typically of the colon or ileum is a rare but usually fatal complication of SPS. Coadministration of SPS with sorbitol increases the risk of intestinal necrosis.

503. Patiromer binds K^+ in exchange for?

Harrison's 20th Ed. Chapter 49 Page 312

A. Na^+
B. Ca^{++}
C. H^+
D. NH_4^+

Patiromer (Veltassa®) is a nonabsorbed polymer which binds K^+ in exchange for Ca++ in the intestine. Its side-effect is hypomagnesemia.

504. Which of the following is used in the treatment of hyperkalemia?

Harrison's 20th Ed. Chapter 49 Page 312

A. ZS-8

B. ZS-9

C. ZS-10

D. ZS-11

ZS-9 (Sodium zirconium cyclosilicate) is an inorganic, nonabsorbable crystalline compound that exchanges both Na^+ and H^+ ions in exchange for K^+ and $NH4^+$ in the intestine.

505. The most rapid & effective way of lowering plasma potassium concentration is?

Harrison's 20th Ed. Chapter 49 Page 312

A. Insulin-glucose infusion

B. Calcium gluconate infusion

C. Peritoneal dialysis

D. Hemodialysis

The most rapid and effective way of lowering the plasma K^+ concentration is hemodialysis. Although dialysis removes 1 mmol/L of serum potassium in the first hour and 2 mmol/L by 3 hours, a rebound of serum potassium can be seen post dialysis. The magnitude of postdialysis serum K^+ rebound is proportional to the predialysis serum K^+ level, with 35% of the reduction equated by 1 hour post treatment. Peritoneal dialysis is only 15-20% as effective as hemodialysis.

Hypercalcemia and Hypocalcemia

506. What is the normal range of serum parathyroid hormone (intact)?

Harrison's 20th Ed. Chapter 50 Page 309

A. 1–8 pg/mL
B. 8–51 pg/mL
C. 51–95 pg/mL
D. 95–135 pg/mL

Normal range of serum parathyroid hormone (intact) is 8–51 pg/mL or 8–51 ng/L.

507. What is the normal range of serum phosphatase, alkaline?

Harrison's 19th Ed 2762

A. 1-33 U/L
B. 33-96 U/L
C. 96-146 U/L
D. 146-216 U/L

508. What is the normal range of serum magnesium?

Harrison's 19th Ed 2761

A. 0.5-1.2 mg/dL
B. 1.5-2.3 mg/dL
C. 2.8-4.3 mg/dL
D. 4.5-6.3 mg/dL

Normal range of serum magnesium is 1.5–2.3 mg/dL or 0.62–0.95 mmol/L.

509. What is the normal range of serum calcium?

Harrison's 19th Ed 2758

A. 5.7-8.2 mg/dL
B. 8.7-10.2 mg/dL
C. 10.7-13.2 mg/dL
D. 13.7-18.2 mg/dL

Normal range of serum calcium is 8.7–10.2 mg/dL or 2.2–2.6 mmol/L.

510. What is the normal range of serum vitamin D 1,25-dihydroxy, total?

Harrison's 19th Ed 2766

A. 5-15 pg/mL
B. 15-75 pg/mL
C. 75-125 pg/mL
D. 125-175 pg/mL

Normal range of serum calcium is 15–75 pg/mL or 36–180 pmol/L.

511. What is the normal range of plasma vitamin D 25-dihydroxy, total?

Harrison's 19th Ed 2766

A. 5-30 ng/mL
B. 30-100 ng/mL
C. 100-200 ng/mL
D. 230-400 ng/mL

Normal range of serum calcium is 30–100 ng/mL or 75–250 nmol/L.

512. Calcium ion regulates which of the following physiologic processes?

Harrison's 20th Ed. Chapter 50 Page 312

A. Neuromuscular signaling
B. Hormone secretion
C. Blood coagulation
D. All of the above

The calcium ion plays a critical role in normal cellular function and signaling, regulating neuromuscular signaling, cardiac contractility, hormone secretion and blood coagulation.

513. Feedback mechanisms for maintenance of extracellular calcium concentrations involve?

Harrison's 20th Ed. Chapter 50 Page 312

A. Parathyroid glands
B. Kidney
C. Intestine
D. All of the above

Extracellular calcium concentrations are maintained through feedback mechanisms involving parathyroid hormone (PTH) and active vitamin D metabolite 1,25-dihydroxyvitamin D [1,25(OH)$_2$D]. Feedback mechanisms are orchestrated by integrating signals between parathyroid glands, kidney, intestine & bone.

514. Decrease in serum calcium leads to?

Harrison's 20th Ed. Chapter 50 Page 312 Figure 50-1

A. Increase in parathyroid hormone (PTH)
B. Resorption of calcium from bone
C. Stimulates renal 1,25(OH)$_2$D production
D. All of the above

515. Which of the following is the action of PTH?

Harrison's 20th Ed. Chapter 50 Page 312 Figure 50-1

A. Increased tubular reabsorption of calcium by kidney
B. Resorption of calcium from bone
C. Stimulates renal 1,25(OH)$_2$D production
D. All of the above

A decrease in extracellular (ECF) calcium (Ca^+) triggers an increase in parathyroid hormone (PTH) secretion via the calcium sensor receptor on parathyroid cells. PTH causes increased tubular reabsorption of calcium by kidney and resorption of calcium from bone. PTH also stimulates renal 1,25(OH)$_2$D production. 1,25(OH)$_2$D then acts principally on intestine to increase calcium absorption.

516. Which of the following statements is false?

Harrison's 20th Ed. Chapter 50 Page 312 Figure 50-1

A. Normal serum calcium is 8.9-10.1 mg/dL (2.2-2.5 mM)
B. Ectopic PTH secretion by tumors is extremely rare
C. Hypercalcemia invariably leads to dehydration
D. None of the above

Normally, plasma PTH level varies inversely with plasma calcium level. Ectopic secretion of authentic PTH is a rare cause of hypercalcemia, having been well documented in only eight patients to date.

517. Excess PTH production not appropriately suppressed by increased serum calcium concentrations occurs in?

Harrison's 20th Ed. Chapter 50 Page 313

A. Hypercalcemia of malignancy
B. Parathyroid adenoma
C. Sarcoidosis
D. Hyperthyroidism

Excess PTH production not appropriately suppressed by increased serum calcium concentrations occurs in primary neoplastic disorders of parathyroid glands like parathyroid adenomas, hyperplasia, or carcinoma.

518. Which of the following is related to familial hypocalciuric hypercalcemia (FHH)?

Harrison's 20th Ed. Chapter 50 Page 313

A. PTH-related peptide (PTHrP)
B. $1,25(OH)_2D$
C. Calcium sensor receptor (CaSR) mutations
D. Exogenous calcium overload

Inappropriate PTH secretion for existing level of serum calcium occurs with heterozygous inactivating calcium sensor receptor (CaSR) mutations, which impair extracellular calcium sensing by parathyroid glands and kidneys, resulting in familial hypocalciuric hypercalcemia (FHH). Hypercalcemia is typically not treated in patients with familial hypocalciuric hypercalcemia, because the elevation in serum calcium is typically mild and produces few if any symptoms.

519. Calcium-sensing receptor (CaSR) is expressed in?

Am J Physiol Renal Physiol. 2010;298(3):F485-F499

A. Parathyroid hormone (PTH)-secreting parathyroid glands
B. Calcitonin (CT)-secreting thyroidal C cells
C. Kidney
D. All of the above

520. Which of the following determine how much Ca^{++} moves into or out of the body?

Am J Physiol Renal Physiol. 2010;298(3):F485-F499

A. Intestines
B. Bone
C. Kidney
D. All of the above

521. Ca^{++} fluxes are regulated by?

Am J Physiol Renal Physiol. 2010;298(3):F485-F499

A. Parathyroid hormone (PTH)
B. Calcitonin (CT)
C. 1,25-dihydroxyvitamin D3 [$1,25(OH)_2D3$]
D. All of the above

Key CaSR-expressing, homeostatic tissues include parathyroid hormone (PTH)-secreting parathyroid glands, calcitonin (CT)-secreting thyroidal C cells, intestines, bone, and kidney. The last three determine how much Ca^{++} moves into or out of the body (intestine and kidney, respectively) or how Ca^{++} moves between the extracellular fluids (ECF) and bone. These Ca^{++} fluxes are regulated by PTH and CT, PTHrP as well as by 1,25-dihydroxyvitamin D3 [$1,25(OH)_2D3$], whose renal synthesis is homeostatically regulated.

522. The CaSR belongs to?

Am J Physiol Renal Physiol. 2010;298(3):F485-F499

A. Family A of the G protein-coupled receptors
B. Family B of the G protein-coupled receptors
C. Family C of the G protein-coupled receptors
D. Family D of the G protein-coupled receptors

The CaSR belongs to family C of the G protein-coupled receptors. Family C also includes metabotropic glutamate receptors, $GABA_B$ receptors, receptors for taste and pheromones, and an amino acid- and divalent cation-sensing receptor called GPRC6A.

523. The biologically active cell surface CaSR, upon binding Ca^{++}, activates which of the following G proteins?

Am J Physiol Renal Physiol. 2010;298(3):F485-F499

A. Gq/11
B. Gi
C. G12/13
D. All of the above

The biologically active cell surface CaSR, upon binding Ca^{++}, activates G proteins Gq/11, Gi, and G12/13, which stimulate phospholipase C (PLC), thereby producing diacylglycerol & inositol 1,4,5-trisphosphate (IP3). The latter releases Ca^{++} from intracellular stores, inhibit adenylate cyclase, and activate Rho kinase, respectively.

524. CaSR controls which of the following parathyroid functions?

Am J Physiol Renal Physiol. 2010;298(3):F485-F499

A. PTH secretion
B. PTH synthesis
C. Parathyroid cellular proliferation
D. All of the above

The CaSR controls three important aspects of parathyroid function relevant to the kidney: PTH secretion, PTH synthesis, and parathyroid cellular proliferation. CaSR also controls expression of the PTH gene.

525. Which of the following is related to PTH-related peptide (PTHrP)?

Harrison's 20th Ed. Chapter 50 Page 313

A. Hypercalcemia of malignancy
B. Milk-alkali syndrome
C. Familial hypocalciuric hypercalcemia (FHH)
D. Sarcoidosis

Many solid tumors produce PTH-related peptide (PTHrP) which binds PTH receptor & mimicks effects of PTH on bone & kidney like PTHrP-mediated hypercalcemia of malignancy & suppression of PTH.

526. Enhanced conversion of 25(OH)D to $1,25(OH)_2D$ leading to hypercalcemia is related to?

Harrison's 20th Ed. Chapter 50 Page 313

A. Hypercalcemia of malignancy
B. Milk-alkali syndrome
C. Familial hypocalciuric hypercalcemia (FHH)
D. Sarcoidosis

Hypercalcemia in sarcoidosis or lymphomas is caused by enhanced conversion of 25(OH)D to potent $1,25(OH)_2D$ that enhances intestinal calcium absorption resulting in hypercalcemia & suppressed PTH.

527. Hypercalcemia with suppressed PTH secretion in hyperthyroidism is due to?

Harrison's 20th Ed. Chapter 50 Page 313

A. Enhanced intestinal calcium absorption
B. Increased calcium mobilization from bone
C. PTHrP-mediated hypercalcemia
D. Increased parathyroid cell mass

Hyperthyroidism or osteolytic metastases directly increase calcium mobilization from bone leading to hypercalcemia with suppressed PTH secretion.

528. Granulomatous disease that cause excessive $1,25(OH)_2D$ production is?

Harrison's 20th Ed. Chapter 50 Page 313 Table 50-1

A. Sarcoidosis
B. Tuberculosis
C. Silicosis
D. All of the above

Granulomatous diseases that cause excessive $1,25(OH)_2D$ production are Sarcoidosis, Tuberculosis and Silicosis.

529. Hypercalcemia due to excess secretion of 1,25(OH)$_2$ D occurs in which of the following?

N Engl J Med. 2005;352:373-9

A. Astrocytoma
B. Squamous-cell lung cancer
C. Ovarian cancer
D. Lymphoma

Some lymphomas secrete the active form of vitamin D, 1,25-dihydroxyvitamin D (1,25(OH)$_2$D), causing hypercalcemia as a result of the combination of enhanced osteoclastic bone resorption and enhanced intestinal absorption of calcium.

530. Endocrine disorder that causes hypercalcemia is?

Harrison's 20th Ed. Chapter 50 Page 313 Table 50-1

A. Adrenal insufficiency
B. Pheochromocytoma
C. VIPoma
D. All of the above

Endocrine disorders that can cause hypercalcemia are adrenal insufficiency, pheochromocytoma, VIPoma.

531. Medication that causes hypercalcemia is?

Harrison's 20th Ed. Chapter 50 Page 313 Table 50-1

A. Thiazides
B. Vitamin A
C. Antiestrogens
D. All of the above

532. Medication that may independently lead to hypercalcemia is?

N Engl J Med. 2005;352:373-9

A. Lithium
B. Vitamin D
C. Thiazides
D. All of the above

Medications that independently lead to hypercalcemia are lithium, calcitriol, vitamin D & thiazides.

533. Tertiary hyperparathyroidism refers to?

Harrison's 20th Ed. Chapter 50 Page 313 Table 50-1

A. Inactivating mutations in the CaSR or in G proteins
B. Long-term stimulation of PTH secretion in renal insufficiency
C. Overproduction of PTHrP
D. Lytic skeletal metastases

Tertiary hyperparathyroidism refers to long-term stimulation of PTH secretion in renal insufficiency.

534. Primary increase in bone resorptlon occurs in which of the following?

Harrison's 20th Ed. Chapter 50 Page 313 Table 50-1

A. Overproduction of PTHrP
B. Lytic skeletal metastases
C. Hyperthyroidism
D. All of the above

Primary increase in bone resorptlon occurs in hyperthyroidism and immobilization.

535. Type of hypercalcemia associated with cancer is?

N Engl J Med. 2005;352:373-9

A. Local osteolytic hypercalcemia
B. Humoral hypercalcemia of malignancy
C. 1,25(OH)$_2$D-secreting lymphomas
D. All of the above

In addition to the above three, ectopic hyperparathyroidism due to ectopic secretion of authentic PTH is a rare cause of hypercalcemia.

536. True hypercalcemia refers to?

N Engl J Med. 2005;352:373-9

A. Elevated serum level of total calcium
B. Elevated serum level of nonionized calcium
C. Elevated serum level of ionized calcium
D. All of the above

Elevated serum level of ionized calcium is true hypercalcemia.

537. Basic mechanism of true hypercalcemia is?

N Engl J Med. 2005;352:373-9

A. Enhanced osteoclastic bone resorption
B. Enhanced renal tubular reabsorption of calcium
C. Enhanced intestinal absorption of calcium
D. All of the above

True hypercalcemia is due to enhanced osteoclastic bone resorption (in local osteolytic hypercalcemia, humoral hypercalcemia of malignancy (HHM), 1,25(OH)$_2$D secreting lymphomas, & ectopic hyperparathyroidism), enhanced renal tubular reabsorption of calcium (in HHM & ectopic hyperparathyroidism), and enhanced intestinal absorption of calcium (in 1,25(OH)$_2$D-secreting lymphomas & ectopic hyperparathyroidism).

538. While treating hypercalcemia, serum phosphorus level should be kept in the range of?

N Engl J Med. 2005;352:373-9

A. 0.5–1.0 mg/dL
B. 1.0–2.0 mg/dL
C. 2.0–2.5 mg/dL
D. 2.5–3.0 mg/dL

539. While treating hypercalcemia, calcium - phosphorus product should be kept ideally below?

N Engl J Med. 2005;352:373-9

A. 5
B. 10
C. 20
D. 30

While treating hypercalcemia, serum phosphorus level should be kept in the range of 2.5–3.0 mg/dL and the calcium - phosphorus product below 40, ideally in the range of 30.

540. Serum levels of calcium in mild hypercalcemia are up to?

Harrison's 20th Ed. Chapter 50 Page 313

A. 7–8.5 mg/dL
B. 8–9.5 mg/dL
C. 9–10.5 mg/dL
D. 11–11.5 mg/dL

Serum levels of calcium in mild hypercalcemia is upto 11–11.5 mg/dL and is usually asymptomatic.

541. Serum levels of calcium in severe hypercalcemia is more than?
Harrison's 20th Ed. Chapter 50 Page 313

A. 11 mg/dL
B. 12 mg/dL
C. 13 mg/dL
D. 14 mg/dL

Serum levels of calcium in severe hypercalcemia is > 14.0 mg/dL. Patients with a serum calcium concentration >14 mg/dL (3.5 mmol/L) require treatment, regardless of symptoms.

542. Which of the following occurs in acute severe hypercalcemia (>12–13 mg/dL)?
Harrison's 20th Ed. Chapter 50 Page 313

A. Pancreatitis
B. Peptic ulcer disease
C. Nephrolithiasis
D. All of the above

Severe acute hypercalcemia (>12–13 mg/dL) may result in lethargy, stupor, coma or pancreatitis.

543. ECG changes in hypercalcemia include all except?
Harrison's 20th Ed. Chapter 50 Page 313

A. Bradycardia
B. AV block
C. Short QT interval
D. Prolonged PR interval

ECG changes in hypercalcemia include bradycardia, AV block & short QT interval.

544. Changes in serum calcium is preferably monitored by which of the following in ECG?
Harrison's 20th Ed. Chapter 50 Page 313

A. Heart rate
B. QRS amplitude
C. QT interval
D. ST segment

Changes in serum calcium can be monitored by following the QT interval.

545. What percentage of serum total calcium is ionized?
Harrison's 20th Ed. Chapter 50 Page 313

A. 10%
B. 25%
C. 50%
D. 80%

~50% of total calcium is ionized & rest is bound principally to albumin.

546. With a decrease in serum albumin of 1.0 g/dL, what quantity should be added to serum total calcium?
Harrison's 19th Ed 314

A. 0.2 mg/dL
B. 0.4 mg/dL
C. 0.6 mg/dL
D. 0.8 mg/dL

Serum albumin levels are determined to obtain "correct serum calcium". 0.8 mg/dL should be aded to total calcium for every decrement in serum albumin of 1.0 g/dL below the reference value of 4.1 g/dL for albumin, and conversely for elevations in serum albumin. In patients with hyperalbuminemia due to severe volume depletion and multiple myeloma, who have a calcium-binding paraprotein, have increased protein binding of calcium. This can cause an elevation in serum total calcium concentration without any rise in serum ionized calcium concentration. This phenomenon is called pseudohypercalcemia (or factitious hypercalcemia) since the patient has a normal ionized serum calcium concentration.

547. Chronic hypercalcemia is most commonly caused by?
Harrison's 20th Ed. Chapter 50 Page 313

A. Medication use
B. Primary hyperparathyroidism
C. Underlying malignancy
D. Sarcoidosis

Primary hyperparathyroidism is the most common cause of chronic hypercalcemia, followed by hypercalcemia due to an underlying malignancy.

548. Increases in PTH are often accompanied by?
Harrison's 20th Ed. Chapter 50 Page 313

A. Hypokalemia
B. Hyperphosphatemia
C. Hypophosphatemia
D. Hypernatremia

Increases in PTH are often accompanied by hypophosphatemia.

549. Lab findings in primary hyperparathyroidism include?
Harrison's 20th Ed. Chapter 50 Page 313

A. Elevated serum calcium
B. Low serum phosphorus
C. Increased PTH level
D. All of the above

If the PTH level is increased (or "inappropriately normal") in the setting of elevated calcium and low phosphorus, the diagnosis is almost always primary hyperparathyroidism.

550. Lab findings in hypercalcemia due to underlying malignancy include?
Harrison's 20th Ed. Chapter 50 Page 313

A. Hypercalcemia
B. Suppressed PTH level
C. Elevated PTHrP level
D. All of the above

551. In familial hypocalciuric hypercalcemia (FHH), calcium/creatinine clearance ratio is?
Harrison's 20th Ed. Chapter 50 Page 313

A. < 0.01
B. < 0.05
C. < 0.1
D. < 0.2

Calcium/creatinine clearance ratio (urine calcium/serum calcium divided by urine creatinine/serum creatinine) of <0.01 is suggestive of FHH.

552. Classic laboratory finding in milk alkali syndrome is?
N Engl J Med. 2008;358:1952-6

A. Hypercalcemia
B. Metabolic alkalosis
C. Impaired renal function
D. All of the above

Hypercalcemia, metabolic alkalosis & impaired renal function are classic laboratory findings in patients with milk alkali syndrome in those with excess oral intake of calcium and milk.

553. Effective treatments to reduce serum calcium is by?
Harrison's 20th Ed. Chapter 50 Page 313

A. Inhibiting bone resorption
B. Increasing urinary calcium excretion
C. Decreasing intestinal calcium absorption
D. All of the above

Effective treatments reduce serum calcium by inhibiting bone resorption, increasing urinary calcium excretion, or decreasing intestinal calcium absorption.

554. Initial therapy of significant hypercalcemia begins with?
Harrison's 20th Ed. Chapter 50 Page 313

A. Volume expansion with IV saline
B. Zoledronic acid
C. Calcitonin
D. Glucocorticoids

Initial therapy of significant hypercalcemia begins with volume expansion with saline (200–500 mL/hour, depending on patient's cardiovascular status & renal function) as hypercalcemia invariably leads to dehydration. Saline itself is calciuretic. Loop diuretics should not be administered until after full hydration has been achieved. Thiazide diuretics should not be used as they stimulate renal calcium reabsorption.

555. Bisphosphonate that is used for the treatment of hypercalcemia of malignancy in adults is?
Harrison's 20th Ed. Chapter 50 Page 313

A. Zoledronic acid
B. Pamidronate
C. Ibandronate
D. All of the above

Bisphosphonates that are commonly used for the treatment of hypercalcemia of malignancy in adults are Zoledronic acid, Pamidronate, clodronate, etidronate and Ibandronate. The bisphosphonates are nonhydrolyzable analogs of inorganic pyrophosphate that adsorb to the surface of bone hydroxyapatite and inhibit calcium release by interfering with osteoclast-mediated bone resorption.

556. Drug that inhibits bone resorption is?
Harrison's 20th Ed. Chapter 50 Page 314

A. Zoledronic acid
B. Pamidronate
C. Etidronate
D. All of the above

Intravenous bisphosphonates are the best studied, safest and most effective agents for use in patients with hypercalcemia associated with cancer. They work by blocking osteoclastic bone resorption. Ibandronate and Clodronate are the other two besides the above three.

557. Which of the following is an alternative to bisphosphonates in hypercalcemia?
Harrison's 20th Ed. Chapter 50 Page 314

A. Glucocorticoids
B. Gallium nitrate
C. Intravenous phosphate
D. Ketoconazole

An alternative to bisphosphonates is gallium nitrate (200 mg/m^2 IV daily for 5 days). It is effective, but has potential nephrotoxicity.

558. Which of the following is an alternative to bisphosphonates in hypercalcemia?
Harrison's 20th Ed. Chapter 50 Page 314

A. Glucocorticoids
B. Denosumab
C. Hydroxychloroquine
D. Ketoconazole

Denosumab (an antibody to RANKL) is a potent inhibitor of bone resorption, effective in treating hypercalcemia refractory to bisphosphonates. Its dose is 120 mg SC on days 1, 8, 15, and 29, and then every 4 weeks.

559. Salmon calcitonin is approved for the treatment of?
Harrison's 20th Ed. Chapter 405 Page 21962

A. Multiple myeloma
B. Paget's disease
C. Osteopetrosis
D. All of the above

The subcutaneous injectable form of salmon calcitonin is approved for the treatment of Paget's disease but is rarely used due to its low potency and should be reserved for patients who either do not tolerate bisphosphonates or have a contraindication to their use.

560. Which of the following is the preferred treatment in patients with $1,25(OH)_2D$-mediated hypercalcemia?
Harrison's 20th Ed. Chapter 50 Page 314

A. Zoledronic acid
B. Glucocorticoids
C. Gallium nitrate
D. All of the above

561. Glucocorticoids are the preferred therapy in hypercalcemia due to?
Harrison's 20th Ed. Chapter 50 Page 314

A. Malignancy
B. Severe hyperparathyroidism
C. Sarcoidosis
D. Familial hypocalciuric hypercalcemia (FHH)

In patients with $1,25(OH)_2D$-mediated hypercalcemia, glucocorticoids are the preferred therapy, as they decrease $1,25(OH)_2D$ production.

562. Pharmacologic therapy for hypercalcemia associated with cancer include?
N Engl J Med. 2005;352:373-9

A. Mithramycin
B. Calcitonin
C. Gallium nitrate
D. All of the above

563. Dose of Zoledronic acid is?
Harrison's 20th Ed. Chapter 50 Page 314

A. 2 mg IV infusion over 30-minutes
B. 4 mg IV infusion over 30-minutes
C. 6 mg IV infusion over 30-minutes
D. 8 mg IV infusion over 30-minutes

564. Drugs that decreases $1,25(OH)_2D$ production is?
Harrison's 20th Ed. Chapter 50 Page 314

A. Ketoconazole
B. Chloroquine
C. Hydroxychloroquine
D. All of the above

Other drugs, such as ketoconazole, chloroquine, and hydroxychloroquine, may decrease $1,25(OH)_2D$ production and are used occasionally.

565. Which of the following is the skeletal complication of severe form of primary hyperparathyroidism?
Harrison's 20th Ed. Chapter 50 Page 314

A. Osteomalacia
B. Osteitis fibrosa cystica
C. Hyperostosis
D. All of the above

Primary hyperparathyroidism often presents in its severe form with skeletal complications like osteitis fibrosa cystica. It is the distinctive bone manifestation of hyperparathyroidism.

566. Which of the following is a calcimimetic?
Harrison's 20th Ed. Chapter 381 Page 2748

A. Cinacalpet
B. Cinacalcet
C. Cinacalnet
D. Cinacalvet

Cinacalcet is a calcimimetic, which act via calcium-sensing receptor. It is used to treat primary hyperparathyroidism, in some patients when surgery is unsuccessful or contraindicated. Calcimimetics lower PTH secretion lower calcium but do not affect bone mass density (BMD).

Hypocalcemia

567. Main defense against hypocalcemia is?
Harrison's 20th Ed. Chapter 50 Page 314

A. Calcium
B. Vitamin D
C. PTH
D. PTH-related peptide (PTHrP)

PTH is the main defense against hypocalcemia.

568. Hypoparathyroidism is a cardinal feature of?
Harrison's 20th Ed. Chapter 50 Page 314

A. Autoimmune endocrinopathies
B. Hereditary endocrinopathies
C. Inflammatory endocrinopathies
D. All of the above

Hypoparathyroidism is a cardinal feature of autoimmune endocrinopathies (Isolated or part of APS-1, autoimmune polyendocrinopathy syndrome).

569. Which of the following syndromes is associated with hypoparathyroidism?
Harrison's 20th Ed. Chapter 50 Page 314

A. Sjogren's syndrome
B. Syndrome of apparent mineralocorticoid excess (SAME)
C. Immunodysregulation polyendocrinopathy enteropathy X-linked syndrome (IPEX)
D. DiGeorge's syndrome (CATCH-22)

A form of hypoparathyroidism associated with defective development of both the thymus and the parathyroid glands is termed the DiGeorge syndrome or the velocardiofacial syndrome. The chromosome 22 defect is now termed DSG1. A defect in chromosome 10p is also now recognized-and is called DSG2.

570. Which of the following syndromes is associated with hypoparathyroidism?
Harrison's 20th Ed. Chapter 403 Page 2937

A. Kenney-Caffey syndrome Type I
B. Sanjad-Sakati syndrome
C. Kearns-Sayre syndrome (KSS)
D. All of the above

571. Which of the following leads to reduced parathyroid function?
Harrison's 20th Ed. Chapter 50 Page 314

A. Iron deficiency
B. Hypomagnesemia
C. Hypokalemia
D. VIPoma

572. Pseudohypoparathyroidism best relates to?
Harrison's 20th Ed. Chapter 50 Page 314 Table 50-2

A. Vitamin D resistance
B. G protein mutations
C. Calcium chelators
D. PTH receptor mutations

573. Which of the following can lead to secondary hyperparathyroidism?
Harrison's 20th Ed. Chapter 50 Page 314 Table 50-2

A. Hungry bone syndrome
B. Osteoblastic metastasis of prostate cancer
C. Acute pancreatitis
D. All of the above

574. Which of the following drug can lead to secondary hyperparathyroidism?
Harrison's 20th Ed. Chapter 50 Page 314 Table 50-2

A. Plicamycin
B. Phenytoin
C. Ketoconazole
D. All of the above

575. Degree of hypocalcemia is most in which of these disorders?
Harrison's 20th Ed. Chapter 50 Page 314

A. Hypoparathyroidism
B. Vitamin D deficiency
C. Impaired 1,25$(OH)_2$D production
D. Vitamin D resistance

Degree of hypocalcemia is most in hypoparathyroidism.

576. Hypocalcemia may occur in?
Harrison's 20th Ed. Chapter 50 Page 314

A. Rhabdomyolysis
B. Tumor lysis
C. Pancreatitis
D. All of the above

Hypocalcemia may occur in severe tissue injury like burns, rhabdomyolysis, tumor lysis, or pancreatitis.

577. Paresthesias in moderate to severe hypocalcemia involve?
Harrison's 20th Ed. Chapter 50 Page 314

A. Fingers
B. Toes
C. Circumoral regions
D. All of the above

Moderate to severe hypocalcemia is associated with paresthesias, usually of the fingers, toes, and circumoral regions, and is caused by increased neuromuscular irritability.

578. Chvostek's sign is present in what percentage of normal individuals?
Harrison's 20th Ed. Chapter 50 Page 314

A. ~ 4%
B. ~ 6%
C. ~ 8%
D. ~ 10%

Chvostek's sign i.e. twitching of circumoral muscles in response to tapping of facial nerve just anterior to the ear is present in ~10% of normal individuals.

579. For eliciting Trousseau's sign, BP cuff is inflated how much above patient's systolic blood pressure?
Harrison's 20th Ed. Chapter 50 Page 314

A. 5 mm Hg
B. 10 mm Hg
C. 15 mm Hg
D. 20 mm Hg

Trousseau's sign refers to carpal spasm in hypocalcemia induced by inflation of a BP cuff to 20 mm Hg above patient's SBP for 3 minutes.

580. Which of the following is false about severe hypocalcemia?
Harrison's 20th Ed. Chapter 50 Page 314

A. Seizures
B. Bronchospasm
C. Laryngospasm
D. Short QT interval

Severe hypocalcemia can induce seizures, carpopedal spasm, bronchospasm, laryngospasm, and prolongation of the QT interval.

581. Nutritional vitamin D deficiency is best assessed by?
Harrison's 20th Ed. Chapter 50 Page 314

A. Serum 25-hydroxyvitamin D levels
B. Serum 1,25$(OH)_2$D levels
C. Serum calcium levels
D. Serum PTH levels

582. Vitamin D resistance is best assessed by?
Harrison's 20th Ed. Chapter 50 Page 314

A. Serum 25-hydroxyvitamin D levels
B. Serum 1,25$(OH)_2$D levels
C. Serum calcium levels
D. Serum PTH levels

Nutritional vitamin D deficiency is best assessed by obtaining serum 25-hydroxyvitamin D levels, which reflect vitamin D stores. In renal insufficiency or suspected vitamin D resistance, serum 1,25$(OH)_2$D levels are informative.

583. Acute, symptomatic hypocalcemia is initially managed with?
Harrison's 20th Ed. Chapter 50 Page 314

A. Vitamin D_2 or D_3
B. Magnesium sulphate
C. Calcium gluconate
D. All of the above

Acute, symptomatic hypocalcemia is initially managed with calcium gluconate, 10 mL of 10% (90 mg or 2.2 mmol) intravenously, diluted in 50 mL of 5% dextrose or 0.9% sodium chloride, given intravenously over 5 minutes.

584. Which of the following is used for the treatment of refractory hypoparathyroidism?
Harrison's 20th Ed. Chapter 50 Page 315

A. PTH (1-82)
B. PTH (1-83)
C. PTH (1-84)
D. PTH (1-85)

Recombinant parathyroid hormone rhPTH (1-84) has recently been approved by the FDA for the treatment of refractory hypoparathyroidism. N-terminal fragment of PTH is rhPTH (1-34).

Acidosis and Alkalosis

585. Systemic arterial pH is maintained between 7.35 & 7.45 by?
Harrison's 20th Ed. Chapter 51 Page 315

A. Central nervous system
B. Respiratory system
C. Kidney
D. All of the above

Control of arterial CO_2 tension ($PaCO_2$) by central nervous and respiratory systems & control of plasma bicarbonate by kidneys stabilize arterial pH by excretion or retention of acid or alkali maintains systemic arterial pH between 7.35 & 7.45.

586. Henderson-Hasselbalch equation is used to determine?
Harrison's 20th Ed. Chapter 51 Page 315

A. $PaCO_2$
B. PaO_2
C. Systemic pH
D. Anion gap

587. Which of the following is not a parameter in Henderson-Hasselbalch equation?
Harrison's 20th Ed. Chapter 51 Page 315

A. $PaCO_2$
B. PaO_2
C. pH
D. HCO_3^-

588. Henderson-Hasselbalch equation for systemic pH is?
Harrison's 20th Ed. Chapter 51 Page 315

A. $4.1 + \log (HCO_3^-/(PaCO_2 \times 0.0301))$
B. $5.1 + \log (HCO_3^-/(PaCO_2 \times 0.0301))$
C. $6.1 + \log (HCO_3^-/(PaCO_2 \times 0.0301))$
D. $7.1 + \log (HCO_3^-/(PaCO_2 \times 0.0301))$

Henderson-Hasselbalch equation includes metabolic & respiratory components that regulate systemic pH.

589. Increases or decreases in $PaCO_2$ represent derangements of?
Harrison's 20th Ed. Chapter 51 Page 315

A. Neural respiratory control
B. Compensatory response to alteration in plasma $[HCO_3^-]$
C. Both A and B
D. None of the above

590. Which of the following statements is false?
Harrison's 20th Ed. Chapter 51 Page 315

A. Usual steady-state $PaCO_2$ is 60 mm Hg
B. CO_2 underexcretion produces hypercapnia
C. CO_2 overexcretion causes hypocapnia
D. $PaCO_2$ regulated primarily by neural respiratory factors

Usual steady-state $PaCO_2$ is maintained at 40 mm Hg.

591. Which of the following statements is false?
Harrison's 20th Ed. Chapter 51 Page 315

A. Hypercapnia is the result of hypoventilation
B. Primary alteration of $PaCO_2$ evokes renal adaptation
C. $PaCO_2$ changes result from alteration in plasma $[HCO_3^-]$
D. None of the above

592. Which of the following conditions returns the pH to a normal value?
Harrison's 20th Ed. Chapter 51 Page 315

A. Metabolic acidosis
B. Metabolic alkalosis
C. Chronic respiratory alkalosis
D. Chronic metabolic alkalosis

Compensatory responses return pH toward, but not to, the normal value. Chronic respiratory alkalosis when prolonged is an exception to this rule and often returns the pH to a normal value.

593. Which of the following formula (Winter's) is correct?
Harrison's 20th Ed. Chapter 51 Page 315

A. $PaCO_2 = (1.3 \times [HCO_3^-]) + 8 \pm 2$
B $PaCO_2 = (1.4 \times [HCO_3^-]) + 8 \pm 2$
C. $PaCO_2 = (1.5 \times [HCO_3^-]) + 8 \pm 2$
D. $PaCO_2 = (1.6 \times [HCO_3^-]) + 8 \pm 2$

Winter's formula for expected CO_2 is (1.5 × Bicarbonate) + 8 ± 2

594. In simple metabolic acidosis, $PaCO_2$ would decrease by how much for each mmol/L decrease in $[HCO_3^-]$?
Harrison's 20th Ed. Chapter 51 Page 315 Table 51-1

A. 1.25 mm Hg
B. 1.50 mm Hg
C. 1.75 mm Hg
D. 2.00 mm Hg

Degree of respiratory compensation in simple metabolic acidosis is predicted by $PaCO_2 = (1.5 \times [HCO_3^-]) + 8 \pm 2$. Thus, $PaCO_2$ decreases by 1.25 mm Hg for each mmol/L decrease in $[HCO_3^-]$ or $PaCO_2 = [HCO_3^-] + 15$. Values for $PaCO_2$ <24 or >28 mm Hg define a mixed disturbance (metabolic acidosis and respiratory alkalosis or metabolic alkalosis and respiratory acidosis, respectively).

595. In simple metabolic alkalosis, $PaCO_2$ would increase by how much for each mmol/L increase in $[HCO_3^-]$?
Harrison's 20th Ed. Chapter 51 Page 315 Table 51-1

A. 0.25 mm Hg
B. 0.50 mm Hg
C. 0.75 mm Hg
D. 1.00 mm Hg

$PaCO_2$ increases by 0.75 mm Hg for each mmol/L increase in $[HCO_3^-]$ or $PaCO_2$ will increase by 6 mm Hg per 10 mmol/L increase in $[HCO_3^-]$.

596. In acute respiratory alkalosis, $[HCO_3^-]$ would decrease by how much for each mm Hg decrease in $PaCO_2$?
Harrison's 20th Ed. Chapter 51 Page 315 Table 51-1

A. 0.1 mmol/L
B. 0.2 mmol/L
C. 0.3 mmol/L
D. 0.4 mmol/L

597. In chronic respiratory alkalosis, [HCO_3^-] would decrease by how much for each mm Hg decrease in $PaCO_2$?

Harrison's 20th Ed. Chapter 51 Page 315 Table 51-1

A. 0.1 mmol/L
B. 0.2 mmol/L
C. 0.3 mmol/L
D. 0.4 mmol/L

598. In acute respiratory acidosis, [HCO_3^-] would increase by how much for each mm Hg increase in $PaCO_2$?

Harrison's 20th Ed. Chapter 51 Page 315 Table 51-1

A. 0.1 mmol/L
B. 0.2 mmol/L
C. 0.3 mmol/L
D. 0.4 mmol/L

599. In chronic respiratory acidosis, [HCO_3^-] would increase by how much for each mm Hg increase in $PaCO_2$?

Harrison's 20th Ed. Chapter 51 Page 315 Table 51-1

A. 0.1 mmol/L
B. 0.2 mmol/L
C. 0.3 mmol/L
D. 0.4 mmol/L

600. Acid-base nomogram is drawn between arterial blood pH and?

Harrison's 20th Ed. Chapter 51 Page 315 Table 51-1

A. Arterial plasma [HCO_3^-]
B. Arterial plasma $PaCO_2$
C. Arterial plasma PaO_2
D. Arterial blood [H^+]

601. Which of the following statements about mixed acid-base disorders is false?

Harrison's 20th Ed. Chapter 51 Page 316

A. Due to independently coexisting disorders
B. Relationship is not as compensatory responses
C. Can lead to dangerous extremes of pH
D. None of the above

Mixed acid-base disorders are due to independently coexisting disorders and not merely as compensatory responses. They can lead to dangerous extremes of pH.

602. Which of the following indicate metabolic acidosis - respiratory acidosis?

Harrison's 20th Ed. Chapter 51 Page 316 Table 51-2

A. Na^+ 140; K^+ 4.0; Cl^- 106; HCO_3^- 14; AG 20; $PaCO_2$ 24; pH 7.39
B. Na^+ 140; K^+ 4.0; Cl^- 102; HCO_3^- 18; AG 20; $PaCO_2$ 38; pH 7.30
C. Na^+ 140; K^+ 4.0; Cl^- 91; HCO_3^- 33; AG 16; $PaCO_2$ 38; pH 7.55
D. Na^+ 140; K^+ 3.5; Cl^- 88; HCO_3^- 42; AG 10; $PaCO_2$ 67; pH 7.42

603. Which of the following indicate metabolic acidosis - respiratory alkalosis?

Harrison's 20th Ed. Chapter 51 Page 316 Table 51-2

A. Na^+ 140; K^+ 4.0; Cl^- 106; HCO_3^- 14; AG 20; $PaCO_2$ 24; pH 7.39
B. Na^+ 140; K^+ 4.0; Cl^- 102; HCO_3^- 18; AG 20; $PaCO_2$ 38; pH 7.30
C. Na^+ 140; K^+ 4.0; Cl^- 91; HCO_3^- 33; AG 16; $PaCO_2$ 38; pH 7.55
D. Na^+ 140; K^+ 3.5; Cl^- 88; HCO_3^- 42; AG 10; $PaCO_2$ 67; pH 7.42

604. Which of the following indicate metabolic alkalosis - respiratory alkalosis?

Harrison's 20th Ed. Chapter 51 Page 316 Table 51-2

A. Na^+ 140; K^+ 4.0; Cl^- 106; HCO_3^- 14; AG 20; $PaCO_2$ 24; pH 7.39
B. Na^+ 140; K^+ 4.0; Cl^- 102; HCO_3^- 18; AG 20; $PaCO_2$ 38; pH 7.30
C. Na^+ 140; K^+ 4.0; Cl^- 91; HCO_3^- 33; AG 16; $PaCO_2$ 38; pH 7.55
D. Na^+ 140; K^+ 3.5; Cl^- 88; HCO_3^- 42; AG 10; $PaCO_2$ 67; pH 7.42

605. Which of the following indicate metabolic alkalosis - respiratory acidosis?

Harrison's 20th Ed. Chapter 51 Page 316 Table 51-2

A. Na^+ 140; K^+ 4.0; Cl^- 106; HCO_3^- 14; AG 20; $PaCO_2$ 24; pH 7.39
B. Na^+ 140; K^+ 4.0; Cl^- 102; HCO_3^- 18; AG 20; $PaCO_2$ 38; pH 7.30
C. Na^+ 140; K^+ 4.0; Cl^- 91; HCO_3^- 33; AG 16; $PaCO_2$ 38; pH 7.55
D. Na^+ 140; K^+ 3.5; Cl^- 88; HCO_3^- 42; AG 10; $PaCO_2$ 67; pH 7.42

606. Which of the following indicate metabolic acidosis - metabolic alkalosis?

Harrison's 20th Ed. Chapter 51 Page 316 Table 51-2

A. Na^+ 140; K^+ 4.0; Cl^- 106; HCO_3^- 14; AG 20; $PaCO_2$ 24; pH 7.39
B. Na^+ 140; K^+ 3.0; Cl^- 95; HCO_3^- 25; AG 20; $PaCO_2$ 40; pH 7.42
C. Na^+ 140; K^+ 4.0; Cl^- 91; HCO_3^- 33; AG 16; $PaCO_2$ 38; pH 7.55
D. Na^+ 140; K^+ 3.5; Cl^- 88; HCO_3^- 42; AG 10; $PaCO_2$ 67; pH 7.42

607. Which of the following indicate metabolic acidosis - metabolic acidosis?

Harrison's 20th Ed. Chapter 51 Page 316 Table 51-2

A. Na^+ 140; K^+ 4.0; Cl^- 106; HCO_3^- 14; AG 20; $PaCO_2$ 24; pH 7.39
B. Na^+ 140; K^+ 3.0; Cl^- 95; HCO_3^- 25; AG 20; $PaCO_2$ 40; pH 7.42
C. Na^+ 135; K^+ 3.0; Cl^- 110; HCO_3^- 10; AG 15; $PaCO_2$ 25; pH 7.20
D. Na^+ 140; K^+ 3.5; Cl^- 88; HCO_3^- 42; AG 10; $PaCO_2$ 67; pH 7.42

608. Which acid-base disorder is expected in lactic acidosis or sepsis in ICU?

Harrison's 20th Ed. Chapter 51 Page 316 Table 51-2

A. Metabolic acidosis–respiratory alkalosis
B. Metabolic acidosis–respiratory acidosis
C. Metabolic acidosis–metabolic alkalosis
D. Metabolic acidosis–metabolic acidosis

609. Which acid-base disorder is expected in severe pneumonia or pulmonary edema?

Harrison's 20th Ed. Chapter 51 Page 316 Table 51-2

A. Metabolic acidosis–respiratory alkalosis
B. Metabolic acidosis–respiratory acidosis
C. Metabolic acidosis–metabolic alkalosis
D. Metabolic acidosis–metabolic acidosis

610. Which acid-base disorder is expected in liver disease and diuretics?

Harrison's 20th Ed. Chapter 51 Page 316 Table 51-2

A. Metabolic acidosis–respiratory alkalosis
B. Metabolic acidosis–respiratory acidosis
C. Metabolic alkalosis–respiratory alkalosis
D. Metabolic acidosis–metabolic acidosis

611. Which acid-base disorder is expected in COPD on diuretics?
Harrison's 20th Ed. Chapter 51 Page 316 Table 51-2

A. Metabolic acidosis–respiratory alkalosis
B. Metabolic acidosis–respiratory acidosis
C. Metabolic alkalosis–respiratory alkalosis
D. Metabolic alkalosis–respiratory acidosis

612. Which acid-base disorder is expected in uremia with vomiting?
Harrison's 20th Ed. Chapter 51 Page 316 Table 51-2

A. Metabolic acidosis–respiratory alkalosis
B. Metabolic acidosis–respiratory acidosis
C. Metabolic acidosis–metabolic alkalosis
D. Metabolic acidosis–metabolic acidosis

613. Which acid-base disorder is expected in treatment of diabetic ketoacidosis?
Harrison's 20th Ed. Chapter 51 Page 316 Table 51-2

A. Metabolic acidosis–respiratory alkalosis
B. Metabolic acidosis–respiratory acidosis
C. Metabolic acidosis–metabolic alkalosis
D. Metabolic acidosis–metabolic acidosis

614. In clinical laboratory, which of the following is calculated from the Henderson-Hasselbalch equation?
Harrison's 20th Ed. Chapter 51 Page 316

A. pH
B. $PaCO_2$
C. $[HCO_3^-]$
D. All of the above

In clinical laboratory, pH and $PaCO_2$ are measured and $[HCO_3^-]$ is calculated from Henderson-Hasselbalch equation.

615. Which of the following is not used in the calculation of AG?
Harrison's 20th Ed. Chapter 51 Page 317

A. Na^+
B. K^+
C. Cl^-
D. HCO_3^-

616. Anionic gap (AG) is calculated by?
Harrison's 20th Ed. Chapter 51 Page 317

A. $AG = Na^+ + (Cl^- – HCO_3^-)$
B. $AG = Na^+ – (Cl^- – HCO_3^-)$
C. $AG = Na^+ + (Cl^- + HCO_3^-)$
D. $AG = Na^+ – (Cl^- + HCO_3^-)$

AG represents unmeasured anions in plasma (normal range is from 6 to 12 mmol/L, with an average of ~10 mmol/L) and is calculated as $AG = Na^+ – (Cl^- + HCO_3^-)$.

617. Anion gap represents "unmeasured" anions like?
Harrison's 20th Ed. Chapter 51 Page 317

A. Anionic proteins (Albumin)
B. Phosphate
C. Sulfate
D. All of the above

Unmeasured anions include anionic proteins, phosphate, sulfate, and organic anions. Unmeasured cations include calcium, magnesium & potassium.

618. Increase in AG is most often due to?
Harrison's 20th Ed. Chapter 51 Page 317

A. Increase in unmeasured anions
B. Increase in measured anions
C. Decrease in unmeasured cations
D. Decrease in measured cations

Increase in AG is most often due to increase in unmeasured anions and less commonly due to decrease in unmeasured cations (Ca^{++}, Mg^{++}, K^+).

619. Increase in AG is due to?
Harrison's 20th Ed. Chapter 51 Page 317

A. Increase in unmeasured anions
B. Increase in acid anions
C. Decrease in unmeasured cations
D. All of the above

Acetoacetate and lactate are acid anions. Lithium is an abnormal cation. Plasma cell dyscrasias produce cationic immunoglobulins.

620. A fall in serum albumin by 1 g/dL from the normal value (4.5 g/dL) decreases the anion gap by?
Harrison's 20th Ed. Chapter 51 Page 317

A. 1.5 mEq/L
B. 2.0 mEq/L
C. 2.5 mEq/L
D. 3.0 mEq/L

A fall in serum albumin by 1 g/dL from normal value (4.5 g/dL) decreases anion gap by 2.5 mEq/L.

621. Normal values of which of the following ensures the absence of an acid-base disturbance?
Harrison's 20th Ed. Chapter 51 Page 317

A. HCO_3^-
B. $PaCO_2$
C. pH
D. None of the above

Normal values for $[HCO_3^-]$, $PaCO_2$ and pH do not ensure the absence of an acid-base disturbance.

622. In cases of high-AG metabolic acidosis, increase in the AG (ΔAG) must be compared to?
Harrison's 20th Ed. Chapter 51 Page 317

A. Decline in $[HCO_3^-]$ (ΔHCO_3^-)
B. Decline in [pH] (ΔpH)
C. Rise in PCO_2
D. All of the above

In cases of high-AG metabolic acidosis it is valuable to compare the decline in $[HCO_3^-]$ (ΔHCO_3^- i.e. 25 – patient's $[HCO_3^-]$) with the increase in the AG (ΔAG: patient's AG – 10).

623. In acid-base disturbances, changes in $[Cl^-]$ must be compared to?
Harrison's 20th Ed. Chapter 51 Page 317 Table 51-3

A. $[Na^+]$
B. $[K^+]$
C. $[HCO_3^-]$
D. All of the above

624. Metabolic acidosis can occur because of?
Harrison's 20th Ed. Chapter 51 Page 317

A. Increase in endogenous acid production
B. Loss of bicarbonate
C. Accumulation of endogenous acids
D. All of the above

Metabolic acidosis occurs due to an increase in endogenous acid production (lactate & ketoacids), loss of bicarbonate (diarrhea), or accumulation of endogenous acids (renal failure).

625. Metabolic acidosis has profound effect on which of the following systems?
Harrison's 20th Ed. Chapter 51 Page 317

A. Respiratory
B. Cardiac
C. Nervous
D. All of the above

Metabolic acidosis has profound effects on the respiratory, cardiac, and nervous systems.

626. Fall in blood pH is accompanied by?
Harrison's 20th Ed. Chapter 51 Page 317

A. Increase in ventilation
B. Peripheral arterial vasodilation
C. Central venoconstriction
D. All of the above

Fall in blood pH is accompanied by increase in tidal volume (Kussmaul respiration), peripheral arterial vasodilation & central venoconstriction.

627. Non-AG metabolic acidosis is also called?
Harrison's 20th Ed. Chapter 51 Page 317

A. Hyperchloremic acidosis
B. Hypochloremic acidosis
C. Hyperkalemic acidosis
D. Hypokalemic acidosis

Clinical metabolic acidosis is of two types - high-AG and non-AG or hyperchloremic acidosis.

628. Increment (Δ) in AG (ΔAG) is estimated by?
Harrison's 20th Ed. Chapter 51 Page 317

A. Patient's AG × 10
B. Patient's AG + 10
C. Patient's AG – 10
D. Patient's AG ÷ 10

Potential [HCO_3^-] can be estimated from the increment (Δ) in the AG (ΔAG = patient's AG – 10).

629. Which of the following acid anion in plasma is metabolizable?
Harrison's 20th Ed. Chapter 51 Page 317

A. β-hydroxybutyrate
B. Acetoacetate
C. Lactate
D. All of the above

Metabolizable acid anion in plasma are β-hydroxybutyrate, acetoacetate & lactate.

630. Which of the following can cause ketoacidosis?
Harrison's 20th Ed. Chapter 51 Page 317 Table 51-4

A. Diabetes mellitus
B. Alcohol
C. Starvation
D. All of the above

631. Which of the following toxins can cause high-anion gap metabolic acidosis?
Harrison's 20th Ed. Chapter 51 Page 317 Table 51-4

A. Ethylene glycol
B. Methanol
C. Salicylates
D. All of the above

632. Which of the following toxins can cause high-anion gap metabolic acidosis?
Harrison's 20th Ed. Chapter 51 Page 317 Table 51-4

A. Propylene glycol
B. Pyroglutamic acid (5-oxoproline)
C. Salicylates
D. All of the above

633. Shohl's solution is?
Harrison's 20th Ed. Chapter 51 Page 317

A. Neutral
B. Acidic
C. Alkaline
D. All of the above

634. Sodium salt in Shohl's solution is?
Harrison's 20th Ed. Chapter 51 Page 320

A. Chloride
B. Citrate
C. Bicarbonate
D. Sulphate

635. In a pure AG severe metabolic acidosis, goal is to increase the [HCO_3^-] to?
Harrison's 20th Ed. Chapter 51 Page 317

A. 10 mEq/L
B. 15 mEq/L
C. 20 mEq/L
D. 25 mEq/L

636. In a pure AG severe metabolic acidosis, goal is to increase the pH to?
Harrison's 20th Ed. Chapter 51 Page 317

A. 7.20
B. 7.25
C. 7.35
D. 7.45

In severe acidosis i.e. pH < 7.20, goal is to increase [HCO_3^-] to 10 mEq/L and pH to 7.20 and not to increase these values to normal.

637. Which of the following can cause high anion-gap metabolic acidosis?
Harrison's 20th Ed. Chapter 51 Page 317

A. Lactic acidosis, ketoacidosis
B. Acute and chronic renal failure
C. Ingested toxins & their metabolites
D. All of the above

638. Which of the following 'toxins' can cause high-anion-gap metabolic acidosis?
Harrison's 20th Ed. Chapter 51 Page 318

A. Ethylene glycol
B. Methanol
C. Salicylates
D. All of the above

639. Which of the following 'ketoacidosis' producing states can cause high-anion-gap metabolic acidosis?
Harrison's 20th Ed. Chapter 51 Page 318

A. Diabetic ketoacidosis
B. Alcoholic ketoacidosis
C. Starvation ketoacidosis
D. All of the above

640. Normal serum lactate level is?
Harrison's 20th Ed. Chapter 51 Page 318

A. 0.5–1.7 mmol/L
B. 1.7–2.3 mmol/L
C. 2.5–3.7 mmol/L
D. 3.5–4.7 mmol/L

Normal serum lactate level is 0.5–1.7 mmol/L.

641. Type A lactic acidosis is due to all except?
Harrison's 20th Ed. Chapter 51 Page 318

A. Severe anemia
B. Mitochondrial enzyme defects
C. Diabetes mellitus
D. Shock

642. Type B lactic acidosis is due to all except?
Harrison's 20th Ed. Chapter 51 Page 318

A. Renal failure
B. Hepatic failure
C. Circulatory failure
D. Carbon monoxide poisoning

643. Which of the following can cause Type B lactic acidosis?
Harrison's 20th Ed. Chapter 51 Page 318

A. Biguanides
B. Ethanol
C. Methanol
D. All of the above

644. Which of the following can cause Type B lactic acidosis?
Harrison's 20th Ed. Chapter 51 Page 318

A. Isoniazid
B. AZT analogues
C. Fructose
D. All of the above

Increase in plasma L-lactate may be secondary to poor tissue perfusion (type A) - circulatory insufficiency (shock, cardiac failure), severe anemia, mitochondrial enzyme defects, and inhibitors (carbon monoxide, cyanide) or to aerobic disorders (type B) - malignancies, NRTI drugs, DM, renal or hepatic failure, thiamine deficiency, infections, seizures, or drugs/toxins (biguanides, ethanol, methanol, propylene glycol, isoniazid, and fructose).

645. Pyroglutamic acidemia best relates to?
Harrison's 20th Ed. Chapter 51 Page 318

A. Isoniazid
B. AZT analogues
C. Biguanides
D. Acetaminophen

Pyroglutamic acidemia is seen in critically ill patients receiving acetaminophen, which is associated with depletion of glutathione.

646. D-Lactic acid acidosis may be associated with?
Harrison's 20th Ed. Chapter 51 Page 318

A. Jejunoileal bypass
B. Short bowel syndrome
C. Intestinal obstruction
D. All of the above

D-Lactic acid acidosis, which may be associated with jejunoileal bypass, short bowel syndrome or intestinal obstruction, is due to formation of D-lactate by gut bacteria.

647. HCO_3^- stimulates which of the following?
Harrison's 20th Ed. Chapter 51 Page 318

A. Fructose-1,6-biphosphatase
B. Fructose-2,6-biphosphatase
C. Phosphofructokinase
D. Phosphoglycerate kinase

HCO_3^- stimulates phosphofructokinase. Therefore, $NaHCO_3$ therapy in L-lactic acid acidosis may paradoxically depress cardiac performance and exacerbate acidosis by enhancing lactate production.

648. In DKA, the relationship between ΔAG and ΔHCO_3^- is typically?
Harrison's 20th Ed. Chapter 51 Page 318

A. ~1:1
B. ~1:2
C. ~1:3
D. ~1:4

In DKA, the relationship between ΔAG and ΔHCO_3^- is typically ~1:1.

649. Which of the following develops during treatment of DKA?
Harrison's 20th Ed. Chapter 51 Page 318

A. Hyperchloremic acidosis
B. Hyperchloremic alkalosis
C. Hypochloremic acidosis
D. Hypochloremic alkalosis

Volume overexpansion with IV fluid administration contributes to the development of a hyperchloremic acidosis during treatment of DKA.

650. Which of the following is false about alcoholic ketoacidosis (AKA)?

Harrison's 20th Ed. Chapter 51 Page 318

A. Occurs when alcohol consumption is abruptly curtailed
B. Elevated ketones are predominantly β-hydroxybutyrate
C. Mixed acid-base disorders are common
D. None of the above

651. The nitroprusside ketone reaction can detect?

Harrison's 20th Ed. Chapter 51 Page 318

A. Acetoacetic acid
B. β-hydroxybutyrate
C. Both A and B
D. None of the above

Nitroprusside ketone reaction can detect acetoacetic acid but not β-hydroxybutyrate, so the degree of ketosis and ketonuria can be underestimated.

652. Which of the following about alcoholic ketoacidosis is false?

Harrison's 20th Ed. Chapter 51 Page 318

A. Occurs in chronic alcoholics when alcohol consumption is abruptly curtailed
B. Associated with binge drinking, vomiting, starvation and volume depletion
C. Glucagon levels are decreased
D. Increasingly (+) nitroprusside reaction as patient improves

653. Which of the following about alcoholic ketoacidosis is false?

Harrison's 20th Ed. Chapter 51 Page 318

A. Acidosis is because of elevated β-hydroxybutyrate
B. Nitroprusside ketone reaction does not detect β-hydroxybutyrate
C. Insulin levels are high
D. Triglyceride levels are increased

Chronic alcoholics can develop ketoacidosis when alcohol consumption is abruptly curtailed and nutrition is poor. AKA is usually associated with binge drinking, vomiting, abdominal pain, starvation and volume depletion. Typically, insulin levels are low, and triglyceride, cortisol, glucagon and growth hormone levels are increased.

654. Which of the following is exacerbated by glucose infusion for treatment of alcoholic ketoacidosis (AKA)?

Harrison's 20th Ed. Chapter 51 Page 318

A. Hypophosphatemia
B. Hypokalemia
C. Hypomagnesemia
D. All of the above

Hypophosphatemia usually emerges 12–24 hours after admission and may be exacerbated by glucose infusion. If severe, may induce rhabdomyolysis. Hypophosphatemia, hypokalemia and hypomagnesemia may coexist in AKA.

655. Which of the following is used in the treatment of salicylate induced acidosis?

Harrison's 20th Ed. Chapter 51 Page 318

A. Activated charcoal
B. Acetazolamide
C. Sodium bicarbonate
D. All of the above

656. Which of the following should be anticipated with vigorous bicarbonate therapy?

Harrison's 20th Ed. Chapter 51 Page 319

A. Hyperkalemia
B. Hypokalemia
C. Hypernatremia
D. Hyponatremia

Hypokalemia should be anticipated with vigorous bicarbonate therapy.

657. Kidneys regulate plasma [HCO_3^-] by?

Harrison's 20th Ed. Chapter 51 Page 319

A. Reabsorption of filtered HCO_3^-
B. Formation of titratable acid
C. Excretion of NH_4^+ in urine
D. All of the above

658. Kidneys excrete how much HCO_3^- ions per day?

Harrison's 20th Ed. Chapter 51 Page 319

A. About 2000 mmol
B. About 3000 mmol
C. About 4000 mmol
D. About 5000 mmol

659. Kidneys excrete how much H^+ ions per day?

Harrison's 20th Ed. Chapter 51 Page 319

A. About 2000 mmol
B. About 3000 mmol
C. About 4000 mmol
D. About 5000 mmol

Kidney filters ~4000 mmol of HCO_3^- per day and to reabsorb this filtered load of HCO_3^-, renal tubules must secrete 4000 mmol of hydrogen ions.

660. Which part of nephron reabsorbs most of HCO_3^- ions?

Harrison's 20th Ed. Chapter 51 Page 319

A. Proximal convoluted tubule
B. Loop of Henle
C. Distal convoluted tubule
D. Collecting ducts

80–90% of HCO_3^- is reabsorbed in the proximal convoluted tubule of kidney.

661. NH_4^+ production & excretion are impaired in?

Harrison's 20th Ed. Chapter 51 Page 319

A. Chronic renal failure
B. Hyperkalemia
C. Renal tubular acidosis
D. All of the above

NH_4^+ production & excretion are impaired in chronic renal failure, hyperkalemia & renal tubular acidosis.

662. Normally, what quantity of H^+ is secreted daily by distal nephron?

Harrison's 20th Ed. Chapter 51 Page 319

A. 40–60 mmol
B. 60–80 mmol
C. 80–100 mmol
D. 100–120 mmol

Distal nephron reabsorbs remainder of filtered HCO_3^- and secretes 40–60 mmol/day of H^+.

663. Secreted H^+ is represented in the urine as?
Harrison's 20th Ed. Chapter 51 Page 319

A. NH_4^+
B. Titratable acid
C. Titratable acid & NH_4^+
D. All of the above

Secreted H^+ is represented in urine as titratable acid and NH_4^+.

664. Under most physiologic conditions, osmotic pressure of blood is generated by?
Harrison's 20th Ed. Chapter 51 Page 319

A. Sodium
B. Urea
C. Glucose
D. All of the above

Under most physiologic conditions, sodium, urea and glucose generate osmotic pressure of blood.

665. Plasma osmolality (P_{osm}) is calculated by?
Harrison's 20th Ed. Chapter 51 Page 319

A. P_{osm} = 2Na⁺ + Glucose (mmol/L) + Urea (mmol/L)
B. P_{osm} = 2Na⁺ + Glucose (mmol/L) + BUN (mmol/L)
C. P_{osm} = 2Na⁺ + Glucose (mmol/L) + (3 × Albumin)
D. P_{osm} = 2Na⁺ + 3Glucose (mmol/L)

Plasma osmolality (P_{osm}) = $2Na^+$ + Glucose (mmol/L) + BUN (mmol/L), or P_{osm} = $2Na^+$ + Glucose (mg/dL)/18 + BUN (mg/dL)/2.8.

666. Osmolar gap is calculated by?
Harrison's 20th Ed. Chapter 51 Page 319

A. Calculated osmolality–measured osmolality
B. $2Na^+$ + Glucose (mmol/L) + (3 × Albumin)
C. $2Na^+$ + 3Glucose (mmol/L)
D. $2Na^+$ + Glucose (mmol/L) + Urea (mmol/L)

Difference between calculated osmolality and measured osmolality is called osmolar gap and is proportional to concentration of unmeasured solute.

667. Unit of osmolality is?
Harrison's 20th Ed. Chapter 51 Page 319

A. mOsm/kg/H_2O
B. mOsm/kg/Plasma
C. mOsm/kg/Serum
D. mOsm/kg/Blood

Unit of osmolality is mOsm/kg/H_2O.

668. Which of the following is an osmolyte?
Harrison's 20th Ed. Chapter 51 Page 319

A. Mannitol
B. Methanol
C. Acetone
D. All of the above

Osmolytes include mannitol, radiocontrast media, ethanol, isopropyl alcohol, ethylene glycol, propylene glycol, methanol and acetone.

669. Which of the following can cause an elevated osmolal gap?
Harrison's 20th Ed. Chapter 51 Page 319

A. Ethylene glycol
B. Methanol
C. Isopropyl alcohol
D. All of the above

Ethylene glycol, methanol and isopropyl alcohol cause an elevated osmolal gap. Ethylene glycol and methanol cause a high-AG acidosis.

670. Which of the following is a metabolite of ethylene glycol?
Harrison's 20th Ed. Chapter 51 Page 319

A. Lactic acid
B. Tricarboxylic acid
C. Oxalic acid
D. Hydrochloric acid

Ethylene glycol (used in antifreeze) causes metabolic acidosis and damage to CNS, heart, lungs and kidneys. Its metabolites are oxalic acid, glycolic acid, and other organic acids.

671. Which of the following is false about ethylene glycol toxicity?
Harrison's 20th Ed. Chapter 51 Page 319

A. Oxalate crystals in urine
B. Presence of an osmolar gap in serum
C. High-AG acidosis
D. None of the above

672. Which of the following is useful in the treatment of ethylene glycol toxicity?
Harrison's 20th Ed. Chapter 51 Page 319

A. Thiamine supplements
B. Pyridoxine supplements
C. Fomepizole
D. All of the above

673. The chemical name of Fomepizole is?
Harrison's 20th Ed. Chapter 51 Page 319

A. 2-methylpyrazole
B. 3-methylpyrazole
C. 4-methylpyrazole
D. 5-methylpyrazole

674. Fomepizole is a?
Harrison's 20th Ed. Chapter 51 Page 319

A. Aldehyde dehydrogenase inhibitor
B. Alcohol dehydrogenase inhibitor
C. Ketone dehydrogenase inhibitor
D. None of the above

Fomepizole or 4-methylpyrazole is an alcohol dehydrogenase inhibitor. It is used to treat ethylene glycol induced acidosis in an IV loading dose of 15 mg/kg.

675. In ethylene glycol intoxication, ethanol IV should be infused to achieve a blood level of?
Harrison's 20th Ed. Chapter 51 Page 319

A. 10 mg/dL
B. 50 mg/dL
C. 100 mg/dL
D. 150 mg/dL

Ethanol IV should be infused to achieve a blood level of 100 mg/dL (22 mmol/L).

676. In ethylene glycol intoxication, hemodialysis is indicated when osmolar gap exceeds?

Harrison's 20th Ed. Chapter 51 Page 319

A. 10 mOsm/kg
B. 20 mOsm/kg
C. 30 mOsm/kg
D. 40 mOsm/kg

Hemodialysis is indicated when the arterial pH is < 7.3 or the osmolar gap exceeds 20 mOsm/kg.

677. Which of the following about methanol is false?

Harrison's 20th Ed. Chapter 51 Page 319

A. Also called 'wood alcohol'
B. Has high molecular weight
C. Metabolites include formaldehyde and formic acid
D. Intoxication cause severe optic nerve & CNS damage

Methanol or wood alcohol causes metabolic acidosis. Its metabolites formaldehyde & formic acid cause optic nerve & CNS damage. It has a low molecular weight (32 Da).

678. Which of the following is metabolized by alcohol dehydrogenase?

Harrison's 20th Ed. Chapter 51 Page 319

A. Propylene glycol
B. Ethylene glycol
C. Methanol
D. All of the above

Propylene glycol, ethylene glycol and methanol are metabolized by alcohol dehydrogenase.

679. AG acidosis is not present in which of the following?

Harrison's 20th Ed. Chapter 51 Page 319

A. Ethylene glycol ingestion
B. Isopropyl alcohol ingestion
C. Methanol ingestion
D. Acetaminophen

680. Isopropyl alcohol is metabolized by alcohol dehydrogenase to?

Harrison's 20th Ed. Chapter 51 Page 319

A. Acetone
B. Acetoacetic acid
C. β-hydroxybutyric acid
D. All of the above

Isopropyl alcohol is metabolized by alcohol dehydrogenase to acetone. In Isopropyl alcohol ingestion, acidosis is not present because acetone is rapidly excreted.

681. Which of the following about acetaminophen-induced acidosis is false?

Harrison's 20th Ed. Chapter 51 Page 319

A. High-AG metabolic acidosis
B. 5-Oxoproline accumulation
C. No elevation of osmolar gap
D. None of the above

682. Which of the following about uremic acidosis is false?

Harrison's 20th Ed. Chapter 51 Page 319

A. Reduced rate of NH_4^+ production and excretion
B. $[HCO_3^-]$ levels rarely < 15 mmol/L
C. Anion gap (AG) rarely > 20 mmol/L
D. None of the above

Uremic acidosis is characterized by reduced rate of NH_4^+ production & excretion due to decreased renal mass. $[HCO_3^-]$ rarely falls to <15 mmol/L and AG is rarely >20 mmol/L.

683. Urine anion gap (UAG) is calculated by the formula?

Harrison's 20th Ed. Chapter 51 Page 320

A. $[Na^+ + K^+]_u/[Cl^-]_u$
B. $[Na^+ + K^+]_u \times [Cl^-]_u$
C. $[Na^+ + K^+]_u - [Cl^-]_u$
D. $[Na^+ + K^+]_u + [Cl^-]_u$

Urinary NH_4^+ levels are estimated by urine anion gap (UAG) i.e. $[Na^+ + K^+]_u - [Cl^-]_u$. Under normal circumstances, the UAG is positive due to the presence of dissolved anions. When $[Cl^-]_u > [Na^+ + K^+]$, the UAG is negative which indicates that urine ammonium level is appropriately increased, suggesting an extrarenal cause of the acidosis. When urine anion gap is positive, urine ammonium level is low, suggesting a renal cause of acidosis. Because urinary ammonia is not directly measured by the clinical laboratory, it is estimated by measuring UAG or urine osmolar gap. Both calculations only give a qualitative and not a quantitative measure of urinary ammonia. The usual UAG ranges from 20–90 mEq/L and NH_4^+ = 80 – UAG.

684. Which of the following is the correct Winter's formula for expected CO_2?

Clin J Am Soc Nephrol. 2012;7:1-8

A. (Bicarbonate × 1.3) + 8 ± 2
B. (Bicarbonate × 1.4) + 8 ± 2
C. (Bicarbonate × 1.5) + 8 ± 2
D. (Bicarbonate × 1.6) + 8 ± 2

Winter's formula for calculating expected CO_2 is (Bicarbonate × 1.5) + 8 ± 2.

685. Which of the following statements is false?

Clin J Am Soc Nephrol. 2012;7:1-8

A. Anion gaps of 25 or greater deserve a thorough evaluation
B. Winter's equation helps for appropriate respiratory response
C. Delta gap used to diagnose a "double" metabolic abnormality
D. None of the above

686. Which of the following about Delta gap is false?

Clin J Am Soc Nephrol. 2012;7:1-8

A. Delta gap is defined as rise in AG minus fall in bicarbonate
B. Delta gap = (change in anion gap)–(change in bicarbonate)
C. Delta gap = $(Na^+–Cl^-)–36$
D. None of the above

687. Which of the following interpretations of generated delta ratio is false?

Clin J Am Soc Nephrol. 2012;7:1-8

A. –6 = Mixed high and normal anion gap acidosis
B. –6 to 6 = Only a high anion gap acidosis exists
C. > 6 = Mixed high anion gap acidosis and metabolic alkalosis
D. None of the above

Delta gap = Delta AG – Delta HCO_3 = (AG-12) – (24-bicarbonate) Or Delta Gap = Anion Gap - Baseline Gap. Delta HCO_3 = 25 - HCO_3. Delta Gradient = Delta Gap - Delta HCO_3. If Delta gap is < -6, then a NAGMA is present. If the gap is > 6, then an underlying metabolic alkalosis is present. If the gap is between -6 & 6, then only an anion gap acidosis exists.

Nephrology

688. Which of the following about Delta gap is false?
Clin J Am Soc Nephrol. 2012;7:1-8

A. Delta ratio = (Decrease in Anion Gap/Increase in bicarbonate)
B. Delta ratio = (change in anion gap)/(change in bicarbonate)
C. Delta gap is defined as rise in AG minus the fall in bicarbonate
D. The normal value for delta gap is zero

Delta ratio = (Increase in Anion Gap/Decrease in bicarbonate). The normal value for delta gap is zero, and it should remain zero as anion gap and bicarbonate change together (mole for mole, in opposite directions). If the bicarbonate is changing significantly less than the anion gap, the delta gap will become more and more positive, reflecting that an alkalosis is present. If the change in bicarbonate is significantly greater than the change in anion gap, there is clearly some acidosis present which is unrelated to the anion gap rise, and the delta gap will be very negative.

689. Which of the following values of delta ratio indicates purely due to a high anion gap metabolic acidosis?
Clin J Am Soc Nephrol. 2012;7:1-8

A. 0.4
B. 0.4–0.8
C. 0.8–1.0
D. > 2.0

Interpretation of the generated delta ratio is : 0.4 = normal anion gap metabolic acidosis, 0.4–0.8 = mixed high and normal anion gap acidosis exists, 0.8–1.0 = purely due to a high anion gap metabolic acidosis, 1.0–2.0 = still purely a high anion gap metabolic acidosis, Over 2.0 = high anion gap acidosis with pre-existing metabolic alkalosis.

690. Delta Gradient significantly > 0 usually indicates?
Clin J Am Soc Nephrol. 2012;7:1-8

A. A mixed high anion gap metabolic acidosis plus a primary metabolic alkalosis
B. A mixed high anion gap metabolic acidosis plus a chronic respiratory acidosis
C. A non-acidotic high anion gap state (excess penicillin)
D. All of the above

691. Delta Gradient significantly < 0 may result from?
Clin J Am Soc Nephrol. 2012;7:1-8

A. A mixed high anion gap metabolic acidosis plus a normal anion gap metabolic acidosis
B. A mixture of high anion gap metabolic acidosis plus chronic respiratory alkalosis plus hyperchloremia acidosis
C. A high anion gap acidosis with a pre-existing low anion gap state (hypoalbuminemia, para-proteinemia)
D. All of the above

A simple high anion gap metabolic acidosis produces a Delta Gradient around 0.

692. Which of the following statements is false?
Harrison's 20th Ed. Chapter 51 Page 320

A. Kidneys acidify urine by secreting NH_4^+
B. NH_4^+ is usually secreted coupled to Cl^-
C. Urinary Cl provides an indirect measurement of NH_4^+ secretion
D. None of the above

The kidneys acidify urine by secreting NH_4^+, which is usually secreted coupled to Cl^-. Therefore, urinary Cl^- provides an indirect measurement of NH_4^+ secretion.

693. Vomiting is a clue to which of the following acid-base disorder?
Harrison's 20th Ed. Chapter 51 Page 320

A. Metabolic acidosis
B. Metabolic alkalosis
C. Respiratory acidosis
D. Respiratory alkalosis

694. History of smoking/COPD is a clue to which of the following acid-base disorder?
Harrison's 20th Ed. Chapter 51 Page 320

A. Metabolic acidosis
B. Metabolic alkalosis
C. Respiratory acidosis
D. Respiratory alkalosis

695. History of liver disease is a clue to which of the following acid-base disorder?
Harrison's 20th Ed. Chapter 51 Page 320

A. Metabolic acidosis
B. Metabolic alkalosis
C. Respiratory acidosis
D. Respiratory alkalosis

696. Tachypnea is a clue to which of the following acid-base disorder?
Harrison's 20th Ed. Chapter 51 Page 320

A. Metabolic acidosis
B. Metabolic alkalosis
C. Respiratory acidosis
D. Respiratory alkalosis

697. In acidemia, which of the following looks like a laboratory error?
Harrison's 20th Ed. Chapter 51 Page 320

A. Low HCO_3^-, High PCO_2
B. Low HCO_3^-, Low PCO_2
C. High HCO_3^-, High PCO_2
D. High HCO_3^-, Low PCO_2

698. In acidemia, which of the following suggests predominant respiratory acidosis?
Harrison's 20th Ed. Chapter 51 Page 320

A. Low HCO_3^-, High PCO_2
B. Low HCO_3^-, Low PCO_2
C. High HCO_3^-, High PCO_2
D. High HCO_3^-, Low PCO_2

699. In acidemia, which of the following suggests predominant metabolic acidosis?
Harrison's 20th Ed. Chapter 51 Page 320

A. Low HCO_3^-, High PCO_2
B. Low HCO_3^-, Low PCO_2
C. High HCO_3^-, High PCO_2
D. High HCO_3^-, Low PCO_2

700. In acidemia, which of the following suggests mixed metabolic acidosis and respiratory acidosis?

Harrison's 20th Ed. Chapter 51 Page 320

A. Low HCO_3^-, High PCO_2
B. Low HCO_3^-, Low PCO_2
C. High HCO_3^-, High PCO_2
D. High HCO_3^-, Low PCO_2

701. In alkalemia, which of the following looks like a laboratory error?

Harrison's 20th Ed. Chapter 51 Page 320

A. Low HCO_3^-, High PCO_2
B. Low HCO_3^-, Low PCO_2
C. High HCO_3^-, High PCO_2
D. High HCO_3^-, Low PCO_2

702. In alkalemia, which of the following suggests predominant respiratory alkalosis?

Harrison's 20th Ed. Chapter 51 Page 320

A. Low HCO_3^-, High PCO_2
B. Low HCO_3^-, Low PCO_2
C. High HCO_3^-, High PCO_2
D. High HCO_3^-, Low PCO_2

703. In alkalemia, which of the following suggests predominant metabolic alkalosis?

Harrison's 20th Ed. Chapter 51 Page 320

A. Low HCO_3^-, High PCO_2
B. Low HCO_3^-, Low PCO_2
C. High HCO_3^-, High PCO_2
D. High HCO_3^-, Low PCO_2

704. In alkalemia, which of the following suggests mixed metabolic alkalosis and respiratory alkalosis?

Harrison's 20th Ed. Chapter 51 Page 320

A. Low HCO_3^-, High PCO_2
B. Low HCO_3^-, Low PCO_2
C. High HCO_3^-, High PCO_2
D. High HCO_3^-, Low PCO_2

705. Under normal conditions in individuals with a normal acid-base status, the average urinary pH is?

Harrison's 20th Ed. Chapter 51 Page 320

A. 3–4
B. 4–5
C. 5–6
D. 6–7

Under normal conditions in individuals with a normal acid-base status, the average urinary pH is 5–6. In patients with hyperchloremic metabolic acidosis & alkaline urine, considered as urine pH >5.5, RTA of some type is strongly suggested.

706. 'Extrarenal cause' of acidosis is suggested by?

Harrison's 20th Ed. Chapter 51 Page 320

A. Negative urine anion gap (UAG)
B. Positive urine anion gap
C. Zero urine anion gap
D. All of the above

707. Which of the following about renal tubular acidosis is false?

Harrison's 20th Ed. Chapter 51 Page 320

A. Can be inherited or acquired
B. Kidney's ability to reabsorb HCO_3^- or excreted NH_3 affected
C. Normal anionic gap (Hyperchloremic)
D. None of the above

In RTA, the capacity for normal urinary acidification is impaired, resulting in net acid retention and hyperchloremic metabolic acidosis. The defining feature of most cases of RTA is impaired renal acid-base buffering and the development of non-anion gap metabolic acidosis, renal performance is otherwise satisfactory.

708. Which of the following about renal tubular acidosis is false?

Harrison's 20th Ed. Chapter 51 Page 320

A. Limited urinary acid secretion is feature of Distal RTA
B. Restricted urinary HCO_3^- reabsorption is a feature of proximal RTA
C. Hypoaldosteronism hyperkalemic is feature of Type 4 RTA
D. None of the above

The 3 major forms of RTA are classified by their respective tubular transport defects, each of which produces persistent hyperchloremic metabolic acidosis. Distal RTA is characterized by limited urinary acid secretion, proximal RTA by restricted urinary bicarbonate reabsorption, and hyperkalemic RTA by hypoaldosteronism.

709. Fanconi syndrome is characterized by?

Harrison's 20th Ed. Chapter 51 Page 320

A. Glycosuria
B. Generalized aminoaciduria
C. Phosphaturia
D. All of the above

Fanconi syndrome refers to glycosuria, generalized aminoaciduria, and phosphaturia due to generalized proximal tubular dysfunction (type 2 RTA). Fanconi syndrome is a malabsorptive state of the proximal convoluted tubules, while proximal RTA refers only to the deficiency in HCO_3^- retention. Nutritional deficiencies typical of Fanconi syndrome include hypophosphatemia, hyponatremia, and rarely, hypoglycemia or hypoproteinemia.

710. Disorder associated with proximal RTA and Fanconi syndrome is?

Harrison's 20th Ed. Chapter 51 Page 320

A. Cystinosis
B. Lowe's syndrome
C. Wilson's disease
D. All of the above

Disorders that are associated with proximal RTA and Fanconi syndrome should be specifically screened for, including cystinosis, Lowe's syndrome, galactosemia and Wilson's disease.

711. Which of the following syndrome is associated with distal RTA?

Harrison's 20th Ed. Chapter 51 Page 320

A. Restless leg syndrome
B. Sjögren's syndrome
C. Hungry bone syndrome
D. Alport's syndrome

712. Which of the following about distal RTA (type 1 RTA) is false?

Harrison's 20th Ed. Chapter 51 Page 320

A. Lifelong disease
B. Frequent manifestation is nephrolithiasis during adolescence
C. Inability of kidneys to excrete hydrogen (H^+)
D. None of the above

713. Typical findings in classic distal RTA (type 1 RTA) include?

Harrison's 20th Ed. Chapter 51 Page 320

A. Hypokalemia
B. Low urinary NH_4^+ excretion
C. Urine pH > 5.5
D. All of the above

714. The typical findings in classic distal RTA (type 1 RTA) include all except?

Harrison's 20th Ed. Chapter 51 Page 320

A. Hyperkalemia
B. Non-AG metabolic acidosis
C. Low urinary NH_4^+ excretion
D. High urine pH

Typical findings of classic distal RTA (type 1 RTA) include hypokalemia, hyperchloremic acidosis or non-AG metabolic acidosis, low urinary NH_4^+ excretion (positive UAG, low urine $[NH_4^+]$), and high urine pH (pH > 5.5).

715. Hyperkalemia is indicative of which of the following RTA?

Harrison's 20th Ed. Chapter 51 Page 320

A. Distal RTA
B. Proximal RTA
C. Mixed RTA
D. Hypoaldosteronism RTA

Hypokalemia is characteristic of distal RTA & proximal RTA, while hyperkalemia is indicative of hyperkalemic RTA. The acidosis is thought to be induced by hyperkalemia that retards urinary NH_4^+ excretion.

716. Findings in classic distal RTA (type 1 RTA) include?

Harrison's 20th Ed. Chapter 51 Page 320

A. Nephrolithiasis
B. Nephrocalcinosis
C. Bone disease
D. All of the above

Most patients have hypocitraturia and hypercalciuria, so nephrolithiasis, nephrocalcinosis and bone disease are common.

717. Type 1 RTA may be associated with?

Harrison's 20th Ed. Chapter 51 Page 320

A. Systemic lupus erythematosus
B. Sjogren syndrome
C. Chronic hepatitis
D. All of the above

Type 1 RTA in older children may be associated with systemic lupus erythematosus, Sjogren syndrome or chronic hepatitis.

718. Which of the following renal tubular acidosis type is rare?

Harrison's 20th Ed. Chapter 51 Page 320

A. 1
B. 2
C. 3
D. 4

719. Serum anion gap is normal in which of the following renal tubular acidosis (RTA) type?

Harrison's 20th Ed. Chapter 51 Page 320

A. 1
B. 2
C. 4
D. All of the above

Inherited renal tubular acidosis presents as nonanion gap (hyperchloremic) metabolic acidosis from proximal tubular bicarbonate wasting or impaired distal net acid excretion.

720. Hereditary diseases that cause type 1 RTA include?

Harrison's 20th Ed. Chapter 51 Page 320

A. Ehler-Danlos syndrome
B. Fabry's disease
C. Wilson's disease
D. All of the above

721. Systemic disorder that cause type 1 RTA include?

Harrison's 20th Ed. Chapter 51 Page 320

A. Sjogren's syndrome
B. Chronic active hepatitis
C. Lupus
D. All of the above

722. Which of the following inherited disorders produce Type 2 (Proximal) RTA?

Harrison's 20th Ed. Chapter 51 Page 320

A. Wilson's disease
B. Cystinosis
C. Glycogen storage disease type I
D. All of the above

Inherited disorders that produce Type 2 (Proximal) RTA are Wilson's disease, cystinosis, tyrosinemia, galactosemia, hereditary fructose intolerance, glycogen storage disease type I, and Lowe's syndrome.

723. Serum potassium is high in which of the following RTA?

Harrison's 20th Ed. Chapter 51 Page 320

A. 1
B. 2
C. 4
D. All of the above

Type 4 RTA is acquired in association with moderate renal dysfunction & is characterized by hyperkalemia.

724. Drug-induced type 4 RTA is due to which of the following drugs?

Harrison's 20th Ed. Chapter 51 Page 320

A. NSAIDs
B. ACE inhibitors
C. Heparin
D. All of the above

725. Which of the following statements is false?

Harrison's 20th Ed. Chapter 51 Page 320

A. Type 1 RTA is due to impaired H^+ ion secretion or HCO_3^- reabsorption in distal nephron
B. Type 2 RTA is due to impaired HCO_3^- reabsorption in proximal tubule
C. Type 1 RTA may present as "marble-brain disease"
D. None of the above

726. Marble-brain disease consists of?
Journal of Molecular Biology 2004;342(2):619-633

A. Osteopetrosis
B. Short stature
C. Mental retardation
D. All of the above

727. Marble-brain disease is due to mutations in?
Journal of Molecular Biology 2004;342(2):619-633

A. CA2
B. SLC3A1
C. SLC6A19
D. CLCN5

Marble-brain disease consists of osteopetrosis, short stature, and mental retardation with dRTA. It is due to mutations in CA2 (carbonic anhydrase II).

728. Which of the following is not a feature of Type 1 (Distal) RTA?
Harrison's 20th Ed. Chapter 51 Page 320

A. Hypokalemia
B. Hypocitraturia
C. Hypocalciuria
D. Rickets or osteomalacia

Type 1 (Distal) RTA presents as hypokalemia, hypocitraturia, hypercalciuria, nephrocalcinosis, nephrolithiasis. Chronic untreated acidosis may lead to rickets or osteomalacia.

729. In Type 1 (Distal) RTA, patients fail to acidify urine to pH?
Harrison's 20th Ed. Chapter 51 Page 320

A. < 5.5
B. < 6.5
C. < 7.0
D. < 7.5

In Type 1 (Distal) RTA, patients fail to acidify urine to pH <5.5 even after acid loading with oral ammonium chloride or calcium chloride.

730. Which of the following stone is formed in Type 1 (Distal) RTA?
Harrison's 20th Ed. Chapter 51 Page 320

A. Uric acid
B. Cystine
C. Calcium oxalate
D. Calcium phosphate

Increased proximal citrate absorption leads to hypocitraturia and together with hypercalciuria predisposes to nephrocalcinosis & calcium phosphate stone formation.

731. Bicarbonate replacement dose in Type 1 (Distal) RTA is?
Harrison's 20th Ed. Chapter 51 Page 320

A. 0.2–1 mmol/kg/day
B. 1–3 mmol/kg/day
C. 3–5 mmol/kg/day
D. 5–10 mmol/kg/day

In Type 1 (Distal) RTA, bicarbonate replacement dose is 1–3 mmol/kg/day in divided doses. While, in Type 2 (proximal) RTA the dose is 5–15 mmol/kg/day along with supplemental potassium & vitamin D.

732. Renal glucosuria is due to mutations in which gene?
Harrison's 20th Ed. Chapter 51 Page 320

A. SLC6A19
B. SLC5A2
C. SLC3A1
D. SLC7A9

Renal isolated glucosuria with normal blood glucose concentration is due to mutations in SLC5A2 gene that encodes sodium-glucose co-transporter SGLT2 in the proximal renal tubule.

733. Low-molecular-weight proteinuria is a feature of?
Harrison's 20th Ed. Chapter 303 Page 2095

A. Renal glucosuria
B. Hartnup disease
C. Cystinuria
D. Dent's disease

Low-molecular-weight proteinuria, hypercalciuria, nephrocalcinosis and nephrolithiasis are features of Dent's disease.

734. Cerebellar ataxia & pellagra-like skin lesions are a feature of?
Harrison's 20th Ed. Chapter 414 Page 3023

A. Renal glucosuria
B. Hartnup disease
C. Cystinuria
D. Dent's disease

In Hartnup disease, tryptophan is retained in intestinal lumen & converted to indole compounds that are toxic to CNS. Consequent niacin deficiency leads to skin manifestations.

735. Inherited systemic disorders associated with Fanconi syndrome include?
Harrison's 20th Ed. Chapter 410 Page 3001

A. Wilson's disease
B. Galactosemia
C. Tyrosinemia
D. All of the above

736. Acquired disorders associated with Fanconi syndrome include?
Harrison's 20th Ed. Chapter 410 Page 3001

A. Multiple myeloma
B. Heavy metal toxicity
C. Chemotherapeutic drugs
D. All of the above

737. Which of the following RTA is principally associated with carbonic anhydrase II deficiency?
Harrison's 20th Ed. Chapter 51 Page 320

A. Distal RTA
B. Proximal RTA
C. Mixed RTA
D. Hypoaldosteronism RTA

Type 3 RTA is a mixed syndrome that has diagnostic findings characteristic of both distal & proximal RTA. Type 3 RTA manifests with debilitating congenital syndromes in children and is principally associated with carbonic anhydrase II deficiency.

738. Which of the following is type 4 renal tubular acidosis?
Harrison's 20th Ed. Chapter 51 Page 320

A. Distal RTA
B. Proximal RTA
C. Mixed RTA
D. Hypoaldosteronism RTA

Distal RTA is Type 1, Proximal RTA is Type 2, Mixed RTA is Type 3 (combined pRTA & dRTA), & Hypoaldosteronism RTA is Type 4.

739. Which of the following is false about hyperkalemic RTA?
Harrison's 20th Ed. Chapter 51 Page 320

A. Consequence of aldosterone deficiency or insensitivity
B. Occurs more frequently in adults than children
C. Usually an acquired rather than a heritable defect
D. None of the above

740. Clinical features that suggest RTA include all except?
Harrison's 20th Ed. Chapter 51 Page 320

A. Mental retardation
B. Polyuria
C. Polydipsia
D. Refractory rickets

Clinical features that suggest RTA include growth retardation, failure to thrive, polyuria, polydipsia, preference for savory foods and refractory rickets.

741. Mnemonic "MUDPILES" is to remember causes of?
Lancet. 2008;327 Issue 9642:892

A. Metabolic acidosis
B. Metabolic alkalosis
C. Respiratory acidosis
D. Respiratory alkalosis

Useful to memorize causes of anion gap metabolic acidemias. Letters in MUDPILES represent methanol, uremia, diabetic & alcoholic ketoacidosis, paraldehyde, iron or isoniazid (INH), lactic acidemia, ethylene glycol toxicity, and salicylates. Paraldehyde can be replaced with propylene glycol.

742. In mnemonic "KUSMALE" for metabolic acidosis, "M" stands for?
Lancet. 2008;327 Issue 9642:892

A. Methanol
B. Medication
C. Male
D. None of the above

Mnemonic KUSMALE for metabolic acidosis represents Ketoacidosis, Uremia, Salicylate poisoning, Methanol, Aldehyde (paraldehyde), Lactate, and Ethylene glycol.

743. In mnemonic "GOLD MARK" for metabolic acidosis, "O" stands for?
Lancet. 2008;327 Issue 9642:892

A. Oxyphenbutazone
B. Ofloxacin
C. Oxoproline
D. Omega 3 fatty acids

GOLD MARK mnemonic for anion-gap metabolic acidoses represents Glycols (ethylene and propylene), Oxoproline, L-lactate, D-lactate, Methanol, Aspirin, Renal failure, and Ketoacidosis.

744. In mnemonic "CAT MUDPILES" for anion gap metabolic acidosis differential, "C" stands for?
Lancet. 2008;327 Issue 9642:892

A. Carbon monoxide
B. Calcium
C. Cholesterol
D. Cancer

Mnemonic "CAT MUDPILES" for anion gap metabolic acidosis differential is Cyanide and carbon monoxide poisoning, Arsenic, Toluene, Methanol, Metformin, Uremia, DKA, Paraldehyde, Iron, INH, Lactate, Ethylene glycol, Salicylates.

745. In mnemonic "KULT IMPACT" for anion gap metabolic acidosis differential, "K" stands for?
Lancet. 2008;327 Issue 9642:892

A. Ketones
B. Kidney failure
C. Potassium
D. KIM-1

"KULT IMPACT", provides a practical and organized way of remembering the differential of metabolic acidosis. Ketones: diabetic ketoacidosis (DKA), alcoholic ketoacidosis, starvation ketoacidosis, Uremia, Lactate, Toxins, Iron, Isoniazid, Metformin, Phenformin, Paraldehyde, Aspirin, Acetaminophen, Alcohols (toxic), Cyanide, Carbon, Toluene

746. In mnemonic "KARMEL" for anion gap metabolic acidosis differential, "A" stands for?
Lancet. 2008;327 Issue 9642:892

A. Aspirin
B. Alcohol
C. Aldehyde
D. Acidoses

Mnemonic KARMEL stands for Ketoacidosis, Aspirin, Renal failure, Methanol, Ethylene glycol, Lactic acidosis.

747. In mnemonic "KUPIN" for anion gap metabolic acidosis differential, "I" stands for?
Lancet. 2008;327 Issue 9642:892

A. Iron
B. Isoniazid
C. Ingestion
D. Inhalation

Mnemonic KUPIN stands for Ketoacidosis (DKA, AKA), Uremia, Production (Lactic acidosis), Ingestion (Ethylene glycol, methanol), Need to Remember Drugs (aspirin, Metformin).

748. In mnemonic "DUMPSALE" for anion gap metabolic acidosis differential, "S" stands for?
Lancet. 2008;327 Issue 9642:892

A. Starvation
B. Salicylates
C. Salt
D. All of the above

Mnemonic DUMPSALE was proposed by of D. Robert Dufour. "I" of MUDPILES was omitted as "I" are exceedingly rare in clinical practice. DUMPSALE stands for Diabetic ketoacidosis, Uremia, Methanol, Paraldehyde, Salicylates, Alcoholic ketoacidosis, Lactic acidosis, Ethylene Glycol.

749. In mnemonic "ACE GIFT" for anion gap metabolic acidosis differential, "C" stands for?
Lancet. 2008;327 Issue 9642:892

A. Chronic renal failure
B. Cystatin C
C. Cyanide
D. Chloroform

Mnemonic for the toxins is ACE GIFTs: Aspirin, Cyanide, Ethanolic ketosis, Glycols (ethylene & propylene), Isoniazid, Ferrous iron, Toluene. Most of these cause a lactic acidosis.

750. Mnemonic "HARD POPS" is to remember causes of?

Lancet. 2008;327 Issue 9642:892

A. Anion gap metabolic acidosis
B. Non-anion gap metabolic acidosis
C. Respiratory acidosis
D. Respiratory alkalosis

Mnemonic "HARD POPS" stands for hyperalimentation (resulting from amino acid load in TPN), Amphotericin, Acetazolamide, Renal failure, RTA (type I, II, IV), diarrhea, Pancreatic fistula, Obstructive uropathy (RTA IV), PEE (ureteroenteric drain/ileal conduit), Saline.

751. Which condition does not cause anion gap acidosis?

Harrison's 20th Ed. Chapter 51 Page 320

A. Alcohol
B. Diabetic ketoacidosis
C. Lactic acid
D. Acetazolamide

Anion gap acidosis can be due to alcohol, methanol, diabetic ketoacidosis, iron, isoniazid, lactic acid, ethylene glycol, carbamazepine, aspirin, and toluene. Acetazolamide causes non-anion gap acidosis. Other causes of non-anion gap acidosis are hyperalimentation, renal tubular acidosis, diarrhea, spironolactone, and pancreatic fistula. Lactic acid is the most common cause of metabolic acidosis.

752. Which of the following does not cause a non-anion gap acidosis?

Harrison's 20th Ed. Chapter 51 Page 320

A. Total parenteral nutrition
B. Intense exercise
C. Acetazolamide
D. Pancreatic fistula

Diarrhea is the most common cause of non-anion gap acidosis. During exercise, there is a build up of lactate and the acidosis is that of anion gap. Other causes of non-anion gap acidosis include total parenteral nutrition, acetazolamide, and renal tubular acidosis. Enteric fistulas and pancreatico-duodenal fistulas are abdominal causes of non-anion gap acidosis.

753. Which of the following pairs is not correctly associated?

Harrison's 20th Ed. Chapter 51 Page 320

A. Metabolic alkalosis with mild dehydration
B. Non-anion gap metabolic acidosis and hypokalemia with hyperalimentation solutions
C. Hypokalemia and metabolic alkalosis with urinary chloride > 20 mEq/L
D. Metabolic alkalosis and urinary chloride < 20 mEq/L with infusion of normal saline

There are two types of non-anion gap metabolic acidosis. The first is due to a bicarbonate deficit and usually is associated with low serum potassium. This can occur with pancreatic fistulas, renal tubular acidosis, or diarrhea. The second is caused by an excess of chloride anion but serum potassium usually is normal. Common causes of this second type of non-anion gap metabolic acidosis include large volumes of normal saline for resuscitation and excess chloride salts in hyperalimentation solutions.

754. What type of metabolic acidosis is associated with diarrhea?

Harrison's 20th Ed. Chapter 51 Page 320

A. Normal anion gap
B. Anion gap of 20
C. Anion gap of 15
D. Anion gap of 25

A normal anion gap is usually seen with diarrhea causing metabolic acidosis. The anion gap is elevated if it is greater than 16. To calculate the anion gap the formula [Na]-[Cl]+[HCO$_3$] is used. The anions that aren't measure and create the gap are calcium, magnesium, gamma globulins, and potassium.

755. Which of the following electrolyte abnormalities is associated with metabolic acidosis?

Harrison's 20th Ed. Chapter 51 Page 320

A. Hypokalemia
B. Hyperkalemia
C. Hypercalcemia
D. Hypocalcemia

Acidosis results in the shift of potassium into the extracellular space. This results in hyperkalemia. This is seen in diabetic ketoacidosis. Administration of insulin to treat DKA causes the potassium to shift back into the cells and can create a state of hypokalemia.

756. Which of the following laboratory results is not consistent with a metabolic acidosis with respiratory compensation?

Harrison's 20th Ed. Chapter 51 Page 320

A. Arterial pH of 7.32
B. PCO_2 of 33 mm Hg
C. PO_2 of 110 mm Hg
D. Serum bicarbonate concentration of 20 mEq/L

An arterial pH of 7.32 indicates mild acidosis. A PCO_2 of 33 mm Hg indicates hypocapnia. The combination of acidosis with hypocapnia indicates that the hypocapnia is most likely compensatory and one would expect a lower PO_2. Serum bicarbonate of 20 is mildly elevated.

757. Which of the following findings is not present in metabolic acidosis?

Harrison's 20th Ed. Chapter 51 Page 320

A. pH of 7.25
B. PCO_2 of 30 mm Hg
C. PO_2 of 70 mm Hg
D. PCO_2 of 60 mm Hg

Metabolic acidosis is primarily noticed by reduced pH and increased HCO_3. This leads to compensatory hyperventilation and loss of PCO_2. A PCO_2 of 60 is not seen in such cases. The level of PCO_2 is actually expected to be lower.

758. A patient with pH=7.34, PCO_2 = 31, HCO_3 = 20 has what type of acid-base imbalance?

Harrison's 20th Ed. Chapter 51 Page 320

A. Compensated metabolic alkalosis
B. Compensated respiratory acidosis
C. Compensated respiratory alkalosis
D. Compensated metabolic acidosis

The correct interpretation is compensated metabolic acidosis. Normal PCO_2 is 35–45. The PCO_2 is decreased because the patient is compensating for the acidosis by breathing more quickly and reducing the amount of CO_2. Normal HCO_3 is 22–26. Bicarbonate is lost in the urine as a buffer during metabolic acidosis. Since the pH is normal, the acid-base balance is compensated.

759. Which of the following would explain an arterial blood gas with a pH of 7.36, PO_2 of 105, PCO_2 of 32 mm Hg, and bicarbonate of 17 mEq/L?

Harrison's 20th Ed. Chapter 51 Page 320

A. Respiratory and metabolic acidosis
B. Metabolic acidosis with respiratory compensation
C. Respiratory acidosis with metabolic compensation
D. Respiratory alkalosis with metabolic compensation

The low bicarbonate indicates metabolic acidosis. Bicarbonate is lost in the urine as a buffer during metabolic acidosis. The patient has been hyperventilating to reduce the PCO_2. Since the pH is a normal value, there is respiratory compensation.

760. A patient has the following laboratory values: sodium 135 mEq/L, potassium 2.7 mEq/L, HCO_3 9 mEq/L, chloride 116 mEq/L, BUN 18 mg/dL, creatinine 1.0 mg/dL. The arterial blood gas shows PO_2 = 80 mm Hg, PCO_2 = 24 mm Hg, pH = 7.29. The possibility is?

A. Non-anion gap metabolic acidosis
B. Respiratory acidosis with compensatory metabolic alkalosis
C. Anion gap metabolic acidosis
D. Metabolic alkalosis

The patient is acidotic with low PCO_2 ruling out respiratory acidosis. The anion gap is normal. There is a reduction in PCO_2 showing respiratory compensation.

761. A febrile patient presents to the emergency room with hypotension. Preliminary laboratory analysis reveals elevated lactic acid levels and evidence of metabolic acidosis. What is the major blood buffer which will help the patient counteract the acidosis?

A. Calcium carbonate
B. Water
C. Citric acid
D. Bicarbonate

The buffer present in blood plasma is composed of bicarbonate and carbonic acid. A buffer solution is composed of a weak acid and its conjugate base. Although a mixture of citric acid and sodium citrate can act as a buffer in the urine, it is not a major blood buffer. Bicarbonate combines with hydrogen ions forming carbonic acid. This becomes carbon dioxide and water. The carbon dioxide is removed by the lungs. This is called compensatory respiratory alkalosis.

762. What metabolic derangement is associated with shock?
Harrison's 20th Ed. Chapter 51 Page 320

A. Metabolic acidosis
B. Metabolic alkalosis
C. Respiratory acidosis
D. Respiratory alkalosis

Shock is associated with metabolic acidosis. Increasing lactate levels due to lack of tissue perfusion accounts for the metabolic acidosis. Other causes of metabolic acidosis include aspirin poisoning, diarrhea, diabetic ketoacidosis, and methanol poisoning.

763. Which chemical is increased in metabolic acidosis?
Harrison's 20th Ed. Chapter 51 Page 320

A. Sodium
B. BUN
C. Potassium
D. Albumin

Shock is the most common cause of metabolic acidosis. It results in an increase of lactic acid levels. There will be concern for hyperkalemia in acidotic states.

764. What electrolyte abnormality is most likely to be found in a patient with severe diarrhea?
Harrison's 20th Ed. Chapter 51 Page 320

A. Hyperkalemia
B. Hypercalcemia
C. Acidosis
D. Hypermagnesemia

Gastrointestinal tract secretions below the stomach are alkaline. Therefore, diarrhea tends to cause a metabolic acidosis. It is also usually associated with hypokalemia.

765. Which is consistent with metabolic acidosis?
Harrison's 20th Ed. Chapter 51 Page 320

A. High extracellular hydrogen ions
B. Low extracellular hydrogen ions
C. High extracellular sodium ions
D. Low extracellular sodium ions

Metabolic acidosis is associated with high extracellular hydrogen ions. Metabolic alkalosis is associated with low extracellular hydrogen ions. Hypernatremia is associated with high extracellular hydrogen ions. Hyponatremia is associated with low extracellular hydrogen ions.

766. A homeless patient presents with nausea, vomiting, and blurry vision. Laboratory results show serum pH 7.30, Na 145 mmol/L, Cl 100 mmol/L, and HCO_3 19 mmol/L. What is the likely diagnosis?

A. Methanol intoxication
B. Isopropyl alcohol intoxication
C. Ethylene glycol intoxication
D. Ethanol intoxication

The pH is < 7.35 and HCO_3 is less than normal range, therefore a metabolic acidosis is present. Anion gap is 21. An anion gap metabolic acidosis is present. Methanol is an alcohol found in windshield washer fluid. Classic findings are an anion gap metabolic acidosis in the setting of vision loss.

767. Hyporeninemic hypoaldosteronism can be seen in?
Harrison's 20th Ed. Chapter 51 Page 320

A. Diabetes mellitus
B. Tubulointerstitial disease
C. CKD
D. All of the above

Hyporeninemic hypoaldosteronism causes hyperchloremic or non-AG metabolic acidosis, in older adults with diabetes mellitus or tubulointerstitial disease and renal insufficiency (CKD).

768. Which of the following drugs can cause non-anionic gap acidosis?
Harrison's 20th Ed. Chapter 51 Page 320 Table 51-5

A. Cholestyramine
B. Acetazolamide
C. Topiramate
D. All of the above

769. Which of the following drugs can cause non-anionic gap acidosis?
Harrison's 20th Ed. Chapter 51 Page 320 Table 51-5

A. Amphotericin B
B. Ifosfamide
C. Calcium chloride
D. All of the above

Metabolic Alkalosis

770. Which of the following can induce metabolic alkalosis?
Harrison's 20th Ed. Chapter 51 Page 321

A. Intracellular shift, excessive GI/renal H^+ ion loss
B. Retention or addition of HCO_3^- ions
C. Volume contraction
D. All of the above

Metabolic alkalosis is a primary increase in serum HCO_3^- concentration as a result of loss of H^+ from body or a gain in HCO_3^- manifests as alkalemia (pH >7.40), usually compensated by alveolar hypoventilation with a rise in arterial carbon dioxide tension ($PaCO_2$) to decrease change in pH. Processes that drive hydrogen intracellularly include hypokalemia. HCO_3^- concentration >35 mEq/L is almost always caused by primary metabolic alkalosis. The serum HCO_3^- usually does not increase above 38 mmol/L.

771. Ability to eliminate bicarbonate is impaired due to?
Harrison's 20th Ed. Chapter 51 Page 321

A. Chloride depletion
B. Hypokalemia
C. Hyperaldosteronism
D. All of the above

Ability to eliminate bicarbonate is impaired due to hypovolemia, reduced effective arterial blood volume, chloride depletion, hypokalemia, reduced glomerular filtration rate, and/or hyperaldosteronism.

772. Metabolic alkalosis is manifested by all except?
Harrison's 20th Ed. Chapter 51 Page 321

A. Elevated arterial pH
B. Increase in serum [HCO_3^-]
C. Hyperchloremia
D. Increase in $PaCO_2$

773. Which of the following statements about metabolic alkalosis is false?
Harrison's 20th Ed. Chapter 51 Page 321

A. Loss of nonvolatile acid
B. Due to net gain of [HCO_3^-]
C. Kidneys retain, rather than excrete excess alkali
D. None of the above

Metabolic alkalosis manifests as elevated arterial pH, increased serum [HCO_3^-] & increased $PaCO_2$ due to compensatory alveolar hypoventilation. It is often accompanied by hypochloremia & hypokalemia.

774. Metabolic alkalosis frequently occurs in association with?
Harrison's 20th Ed. Chapter 51 Page 321

A. Respiratory acidosis
B. Respiratory alkalosis
C. Metabolic acidosis
D. All of the above

Metabolic alkalosis frequently occurs as a mixed acid base disorder in association with other disorders such as respiratory acidosis or alkalosis or metabolic acidosis.

775. The $PaCO_2$ increases how much for each mmol/L increase in [HCO_3^-] above normal?
Harrison's 20th Ed. Chapter 51 Page 315 Table 51-1

A. 0.25 mm Hg
B. 0.50 mm Hg
C. 0.75 mm Hg
D. 1.00 mm Hg

776. The $PaCO_2$ increases how much for each 10 mmol/L increase in [HCO_3^-] above normal?
Harrison's 20th Ed. Chapter 51 Page 315 Table 51-1

A. 2 mm Hg
B. 4 mm Hg
C. 6 mm Hg
D. 8 mm Hg

777. Which of the following is high in metabolic alkalosis?
Harrison's 20th Ed. Chapter 51 Page 315 Table 51-1

A. pH
B. HCO_3^-
C. $PaCO_2$
D. All of the above

778. Which of the following formula is correct?
Harrison's 20th Ed. Chapter 51 Page 315 Table 51-1

A. $PaCO_2$ = [HCO_3^-] + 12
B. $PaCO_2$ = [HCO_3^-] + 13
C. $PaCO_2$ = [HCO_3^-] + 14
D. $PaCO_2$ = [HCO_3^-] + 15

779. In reduced GFR, kidneys will retain excess alkali and maintain alkalosis if there is?
Harrison's 20th Ed. Chapter 51 Page 321

A. Volume deficiency
B. Chloride deficiency
C. K^+ deficiency
D. All of the above

Kidneys will retain, rather than excrete, excess alkali & maintain alkalosis if volume deficiency, chloride deficiency, and K^+ deficiency exist in combination with a reduced GFR or hypokalemia exists because of autonomous hyperaldosteronism.

780. Assessment of which of the following is necessary to establish the cause of metabolic alkalosis?
Harrison's 20th Ed. Chapter 51 Page 321

A. Status of the extracellular fluid volume (ECFV)
B. Recumbent & upright blood pressure
C. Serum [K^+]
D. All of the above

781. Which of the following suggests primary mineralocorticoid excess?
Harrison's 20th Ed. Chapter 51 Page 321

A. Metabolic alkalosis
B. Low plasma renin activity
C. Normal values for urine [Na^+] & [Cl^-]
D. All of the above

Metabolic alkalosis, low plasma renin activity and normal values for urine [Na^+] and [Cl^-], in a patient who is not taking diuretics, suggest primary mineralocorticoid excess.

782. Hypokalemia and alkalosis in a normotensive, nonedematous patient suggests?
Harrison's 20th Ed. Chapter 51 Page 321

A. Magnesium deficiency
B. Vomiting
C. Diuretic ingestion
D. All of the above

783. Hypokalemia and alkalosis in a normotensive, nonedematous patient suggests?
Harrison's 20th Ed. Chapter 51 Page 321

A. Bartter's syndrome
B. Gitelman's syndrome
C. Exogenous alkali
D. All of the above

Combination of hypokalemia & alkalosis in a normotensive, nonedematous patient can be due to Bartter's or Gitelman's syndrome, magnesium deficiency, vomiting, exogenous alkali, or diuretic ingestion.

784. Which of the following findings favor the diagnosis of metabolic alkalosis due to vomiting or alkali ingestion?
Harrison's 20th Ed. Chapter 51 Page 321

A. Alkaline urine
B. Elevated urine [Na^+] & [K^+]
C. Low urine [Cl^-]
D. All of the above

785. In metabolic alkalosis, acidic urine with low urine Na^+, K^+, and Cl^-, point towards the diagnosis of?
Harrison's 20th Ed. Chapter 51 Page 321

A. Prior vomiting
B. Posthypercapnic state
C. Prior diuretic ingestion
D. All of the above

786. In metabolic alkalosis, acidic urine with normal urine Na^+, K^+, and Cl^-, point towards the diagnosis of?
Harrison's 20th Ed. Chapter 51 Page 321

A. Magnesium deficiency
B. Bartter's or Gitelman's syndrome
C. Current diuretic ingestion
D. All of the above

787. In metabolic alkalosis, Bartter's or Gitelman's syndrome are mainly differentiated by?
Harrison's 20th Ed. Chapter 51 Page 321

A. Urine potassium
B. Urine magnesium
C. Urine calcium
D. Urine sodium

Hypocalciuria is a feature of Gitelman's syndrome.

788. Acetate load is increased resulting in alkalosis in patients receiving?
Harrison's 20th Ed. Chapter 51 Page 321

A. Parenteral hyperalimentation solutions
B. Transfusions
C. Antacids
D. All of the above

789. Citrate load is increased resulting in alkalosis in patients receiving?
Harrison's 20th Ed. Chapter 51 Page 321

A. Parenteral hyperalimentation solutions
B. Transfusions
C. Antacids
D. All of the above

790. Which of the following is true for urine in patients who are vomiting?
Harrison's 20th Ed. Chapter 51 Page 321

A. Acidic urine, elevated $[Na]_u$ and $[K]_u$, low $[Cl]_u$
B. Alkaline urine, low $[Na]_u$ and $[K]_u$, low $[Cl]_u$
C. Acidic urine, low $[Na]_u$ and $[K]_u$, low $[Cl]_u$
D. Alkaline urine, elevated $[Na]_u$ and $[K]_u$, low $[Cl]_u$

If urine is alkaline, with elevated [Na^+] & [K^+] but low [Cl^-], diagnosis is either vomiting or alkali ingestion.

791. High urine chloride metabolic alkalemia includes?
Disease-a-Month 2004;50:122-162

A. Bartter syndrome
B. Gitleman syndrome
C. Liddle's syndrome
D. All of the above

792. High urine chloride metabolic alkalemia with hypertension includes all except?
Disease-a-Month 2004;50:122-162

A. Conn's Syndrome
B. Cushing disease
C. Bartter's syndrome
D. Liddle's syndrome

793. High urine chloride metabolic alkalemia without hypertension includes all except?
Disease-a-Month 2004;50:122-162

A. Excess bicarbonate administration
B. Gitelman syndrome
C. Bartter's syndrome
D. Liddle's syndrome

794. Conn syndrome lead to?
Disease-a-Month 2004;50:122-162

A. Hypernatremia
B. Hypokalemia
C. Hydrogen ion loss in urine
D. All of the above

Metabolic alkalosis is split into 2 categories: Chloride responsive with urine chloride <10 mEq/L and chloride resistant with urine chloride >20 mEq/L. Chloride responsive etiologies include loss of H^+ via GI tract, congenital chloride diarrhea syndrome, contraction alkalosis, diuretic therapy, post-hypercapnia syndrome, cystic fibrosis, & exogenous alkalotic agent use. Chloride-resistant etiologies include retention of bicarbonate, shift of H^+ into intracellular spaces, hyperaldosteronism, Bartter syndrome, & Gitelman syndrome.

795. "Contraction alkalosis" best relates to?
Harrison's 20th Ed. Chapter 51 Page 322

A. Vomiting
B. Gastric aspiration
C. Diuretic use
D. All of the above

Diuretics or chloride diarrhea increase excretion of salt & acutely diminish ECFV without altering total body [HCO_3^-] content. Serum [HCO_3^-] increases because reduced ECFV "contracts" around [HCO_3^-] in plasma. This is called contraction alkalosis. Or, volume contraction around a constant amount of extracellular [HCO_3^-].

796. In chronic use of diuretics, metabolic alkalosis is maintained by persistence of?
Harrison's 20th Ed. Chapter 51 Page 322

A. Contraction of the ECFV
B. Secondary hyperaldosteronism
C. K^+ deficiency
D. All of the above

797. Which of the following statements is false?
Harrison's 20th Ed. Chapter 51 Page 322

A. Hypokalemia upregulates renal ammoniagenesis
B. Hypokalemia upregulates renal H^+, K^+-ATPase
C. Alkalosis due to severe K^+ depletion is salt resistant
D. None of the above

798. K^+ depletion occurs concomitant with Mg^{++} deficiency in?
Harrison's 20th Ed. Chapter 51 Page 322

A. Chronic administration of diuretics
B. Alcoholics with malnutrition
C. Transfusions of whole blood
D. Parenteral hyperalimentation

Potassium depletion often occurs concomitant with magnesium deficiency in alcoholics with malnutrition.

799. Lactate or ketones are metabolized to yield?
Harrison's 20th Ed. Chapter 51 Page 322

A. H^+
B. HCO_3^-
C. Cl^-
D. All of the above

Lactate or ketones are metabolized to yield an equivalent amount of HCO_3^-.

800. Which of the following is false about Liddle's syndrome?
Harrison's 20th Ed. Chapter 51 Page 322

A. Increased activity of collecting duct sodium channel
B. Hypertension due to volume expansion
C. Hypokalemic alkalosis
D. Elevated aldosterone levels

Liddle's syndrome results from increased activity of collecting duct Na^+ channel (ENaC) manifests as hypertension due to volume expansion leading to hypokalemic alkalosis & normal aldosterone levels.

801. Presentation of metabolic alkalosis is similar to?
Harrison's 20th Ed. Chapter 51 Page 322

A. Hypercalcemia
B. Hypocalcemia
C. Hyperkalemia
D. All of the above

Changes in central and peripheral nervous system function with metabolic alkalosis are similar to those of hypocalcemia.

802. Renal HCO_3^- loss can be accelerated by administration of?
Harrison's 20th Ed. Chapter 51 Page 322

A. Acetazolamide
B. Thiazide diuretics
C. Furosemide
D. Aluminum hydroxide

Renal HCO_3^- loss can be accelerated by administration of acetazolamide, a carbonic anhydrase inhibitor which is usually effective in patients with adequate renal function but can worsen K^+ losses.

Respiratory Acidosis

803. In acute respiratory acidosis, $[HCO_3^-]$ levels increase by how much for every 10 mm Hg increase in $PaCO_2$?
Harrison's 20th Ed. Chapter 51 Page 322

A. 1 mmol/L
B. 2 mmol/L
C. 3 mmol/L
D. 4 mmol/L

Carbon dioxide is the "respiratory acid" and is the only acid which can be controlled by respiration. When the PCO_2 is high, respiratory acidosis occurs.

804. In chronic respiratory acidosis, $[HCO_3^-]$ levels increase by how much for every 10 mm Hg increase in $PaCO_2$?
Harrison's 20th Ed. Chapter 51 Page 322

A. 1 mmol/L
B. 2 mmol/L
C. 3 mmol/L
D. 4 mmol/L

In acute respiratory acidosis, there is an increase of 1 mmol/L of HCO_3^- for every 10-mm Hg increase in $PaCO_2$. In chronic respiratory acidosis (>24 hours), the $[HCO_3^-]$ increases by 4 mmol/L for every 10-mmHg increase in $PaCO_2$.

805. In respiratory acidosis, serum HCO_3^- usually does not increase above?
Harrison's 20th Ed. Chapter 51 Page 322

A. 28 mmol/L
B. 38 mmol/L
C. 48 mmol/L
D. 58 mmol/L

In respiratory acidosis, serum HCO_3^- usually does not increase above 38 mmol/L.

806. In respiratory acidosis, papilledema is due to?
Harrison's 20th Ed. Chapter 51 Page 322

A. Vasoconstriction
B. Vasodilatation
C. Hyperviscosity
D. Renal failure

In respiratory acidosis, papilledema, abnormal reflexes and focal muscle weakness is due to vasoconstriction secondary to loss of the vasodilator effects of CO_2.

807. Diagnosis of respiratory acidosis requires measurement of?
Harrison's 20th Ed. Chapter 51 Page 323

A. $PaCO_2$
B. PaO_2
C. $[HCO_3^-]$
D. All of the above

Diagnosis of respiratory acidosis requires, by definition, measurement of $PaCO_2$ & arterial pH.

Respiratory Alkalosis

808. In chronic respiratory alkalosis a 1-mm Hg fall in $PaCO_2$ causes a drop in $[HCO_3^-]$ of?
Harrison's 20th Ed. Chapter 51 Page 324

A. 0.1–0.2 mmol/L
B. 0.2–0.3 mmol/L
C. 0.3–0.4 mmol/L
D. 0.4–0.5 mmol/L

In chronic respiratory alkalosis a 1 mm Hg fall in $PaCO_2$ causes a 0.4 to 0.5 mmol/L drop in $[HCO_3^-]$ and a 0.003 rise in pH.

809. $[HCO_3^-]$ falls by how much for each 10-mm Hg decrease in $PaCO_2$ in acute hypocapnia?
Harrison's 20th Ed. Chapter 51 Page 324

A. 2 mmol/L
B. 3 mmol/L
C. 4 mmol/L
D. 5 mmol/L

810. $[HCO_3^-]$ falls by how much for each 10-mm Hg decrease in $PaCO_2$ in chronic hypocapnia?

Harrison's 20th Ed. Chapter 51 Page 324

A. 2 mmol/L
B. 3 mmol/L
C. 4 mmol/L
D. 5 mmol/L

In acute hypocapnia, $[HCO_3^-]$ falls by 2 mmol/L and 4 mmol/L for each 10-mmHg decrease in $PaCO_2$ in acute and chronic hypocapnia respectively.

811. In pure respiratory alkalosis, plasma HCO_3^- is usually more than?

Harrison's 20th Ed. Chapter 51 Page 324

A. 12 mmol/L
B. 14 mmol/L
C. 16 mmol/L
D. 18 mmol/L

It is unusual to see a plasma HCO_3^- < 12 mmol/L due to pure respiratory alkalosis.

812. Which of the following shift inside the cell in acute respiratory alkalosis?

Harrison's 20th Ed. Chapter 51 Page 324

A. Na^+
B. K^+
C. PO_4^-
D. All of the above

Acute respiratory alkalosis causes intracellular shifts of Na^+, K^+, and PO_4^-. Hypocapnia-induced hypokalemia is usually minor.

813. Most common acid-base disturbance in critically ill patients is?

Harrison's 20th Ed. Chapter 51 Page 324

A. Acute respiratory acidosis
B. Acute respiratory alkalosis
C. Chronic respiratory acidosis
D. Chronic respiratory alkalosis

Chronic respiratory alkalosis is the most common acid-base disturbance in critically ill patients.

814. Most common cause of drug-induced respiratory alkalosis is by?

Harrison's 20th Ed. Chapter 51 Page 324

A. Salicylates
B. Theophylline
C. Progesterone
D. Aminophylline

Salicylates are the most common cause of drug-induced respiratory alkalosis as a result of direct stimulation of the medullary chemoreceptor. Methylxanthines, theophylline and aminophylline stimulate ventilation & increase ventilatory response to CO_2. Progesterone increases ventilation & lowers arterial $PaCO_2$. Chronic respiratory alkalosis is a common feature of pregnancy.

815. Which of the following is an early finding in gram-negative septicemia?

Harrison's 20th Ed. Chapter 51 Page 324

A. Fever
B. Hypoxemia
C. Respiratory alkalosis
D. Hypotension

Respiratory alkalosis is often an early finding in gram-negative septicemia, before fever, hypoxemia, or hypotension develops.

816. What is the anion gap in a patient if albumin is 2 g/dL, Na^+ is 140 mEq/L, Cl^- is 100 mEq/L, and HCO_3 is 20 mEq/L?

Harrison's 20th Ed. Chapter 51 Page 324

A. 15
B. 20
C. 25
D. 30

817. Which of the following is an ineffective osmole?

Harrison's 20th Ed. Chapter 51 Page 324

A. Inositol
B. Urea
C. Betaine
D. Glutamine

818. For each decrease in blood pH of 0.10, the plasma potassium rises by?

Harrison's 20th Ed. Chapter 51 Page 324

A. 0.5 mmol/L
B. 0.6 mmol/L
C. 0.7 mmol/L
D. 0.8 mmol/L

819. Normal range of urine ammonia is?

Harrison's 19th Ed. 2768

A. 10–30 mEq/day
B. 30–50 mEq/day
C. 50–100 mEq/day
D. 100–150 mEq/day

820. Normal range of urine creatinine is?

Harrison's 19th Ed. 2768

A. 1.0–1.6 g/day
B. 1.6–2.2 g/day
C. 2.2–2.6 g/day
D. 2.6–3.0 g/day

821. Normal range of urine potassium is?

Harrison's 19th Ed. 2769

A. 5–25 mEq/day
B. 25–100 mEq/day
C. 100–200 mEq/day
D. 200–300 mEq/day

822. Normal range of urine sodium is?

Harrison's 19th Ed. 2769

A. 10–60 mEq/day
B. 60–100 mEq/day
C. 100–260 mEq/day
D. 260–460 mEq/day

823. Normal range of urine uric acid is?

Harrison's 19th Ed. 2769

A. 50–250 mg/day
B. 250–800 mg/day
C. 800–1800 mg/day
D. 1800–3000 mg/day

824. Normal range of urine urea nitrogen is?

Harrison's 19th Ed. 2769

A. 6–17 g/day
B. 17–37 g/day
C. 37–57 g/day
D. 57–87 g/day

825. Normal range of urine osmolality is?

Harrison's 19th Ed. 2769

A. 50–100 mOsmol/kg
B. 100–800 mOsmol/kg
C. 800–1000 mOsmol/kg
D. 1000–1500 mOsmol/kg

Cellular and Molecular Biology of the Kidney

826. In kidneys, number of different cell types found is about?
Harrison's 20th Ed. Chapter 303 Page 2089

A. 10
B. 30
C. 50
D. 80

Kidney is one of the highly differentiated organs in body containing nearly 30 different cell types.

827. Which of the following is a function of kidneys?
Harrison's 20th Ed. Chapter 303 Page 2089

A. Endocrine function
B. Regulation of blood pressure
C. Solute and water transport
D. All of the above

Endocrine functions, the regulation of blood pressure and intraglomerular hemodynamics, solute and water transport, acid-base balance, and removal of drug metabolites are all accomplished by intricate mechanisms of renal response.

828. How many glomeruli does each kidney contain in a normal-birth-weight adult?
Harrison's 20th Ed. Chapter 303 Page 2089

A. ~ 100,000
B. ~ 400,000
C. ~ 900,000
D. ~ 1200,000

There are ~900,000 glomeruli in each kidney in normal-birth-weight adults. It is estimated that each kilogram in birth weight confers on average 260,000 more nephrons. Barker hypothesis proposes that adult disease has fetal origins and is based on epidemiologic studies showing a correlation between birth weight and the incidence of cardiovascular disease.

829. Which of the following is the first step in renal nephrogenesis?
Harrison's 20th Ed. Chapter 303 Page 2089 Figure 303-1

A. Comma-shaped bodies
B. Pretubular aggregation
C. S-shaped bodies
D. Ureteric bud induction and condensation

The various steps in renal nephrogenesis are : Ureteric bud induction and condensation, pretubular aggregation, Comma-shaped bodies, S-shaped bodies, Capillary loop and mature glomerulus. Human kidney development initiates around 4 weeks of gestation and ends around 34–37 weeks of gestation.

830. VEGF-A and angiopoietin-1 are secreted by?
Harrison's 20th Ed. Chapter 303 Page 2089

A. Bowman capsule
B. Podocytes
C. Mesangial cells
D. Juxtaglomerular cells

Glomeruli evolve as complex capillary filters with fenestrated endothelia under the guiding influence of VEGF-A & angiopoietin-1 secreted by adjacently developing podocytes. VEGF-A is a potent angiogenic factor related to normal and pathological angiogenesis. It is secreted by podocytes. Hypoxia is a key regulator of VEGF gene expression. It acts through tyrosine-kinase receptors, which are known as VEGF receptor 1 and 2 (VEGFR1 and 2), predominantly expressed in the glomerular capillaries. Two co-receptors called neuropilins 1 and 2 amplify the VEGFR2 signal. Angiopoietin is a growth factor.

831. Which of the following gene is involved in glomerulotubular development?
Harrison's 20th Ed. Chapter 303 Page 2089 Figure 303-1, Development. 2005;132(24):5437-49

A. Gdnf
B. Wt1
C. Flk1
D. All of the above

Kidney development is considered as the interaction of metanephric mesenchyme and ureteric bud to be the major inductive event that maintains tubular differentiation and branching morphogenesis. The mesenchyme produces Gdnf, which stimulates branching, and the ureteric bud stimulates continued growth of the mesenchyme and differentiation of nephrons from the induced mesenchyme. Null mutation of the Wt1 gene eliminates outgrowth of the ureteric bud, but Gdnf has been identified as a target of Pax2, but not of Wt1. Vegfa expression in mesenchyme is regulated by Wt1. Signaling through Flk1 is required to maintain expression of Pax2 in the mesenchyme of the early kidney, and for Pax2 to stimulate expression of Gdnf.

832. Contractile actin-myosin fibers are found in which of the following tissues of kidney?
Harrison's 20th Ed. Chapter 303 Page 2089

A. Glomeruli
B. Mesangial cells
C. Renal interstitium
D. All of the above

Glomerular capillaries are in the midst of a mesangial matrix and together form the Bowman's capsule. Mesangial cells contain contractile actin-myosin fibers to maintain structural integrity.

833. Vasa recta best relates to?
Harrison's 20th Ed. Chapter 303 Page 2089

A. Cortical nephrons
B. Juxtamedullary nephrons
C. Renal interstitium
D. Epithelial podocytes

Juxtamedullary nephrons have individual capillaries called vasa recta that run alongside the long loops of Henle. The peritubular capillaries surrounding cortical nephrons are shared among adjacent nephrons. Juxtamedullary nephron contains large glomeruli located near the corticomedullary border and a large network of vasa recta, more than cortical nephron. Consequently they have a high glomerular filtration rate. Afferent arterioles of cortical nephrons are larger than their respective efferent arterioles, while they are equal in juxtamedullary nephrons.

834. Pars Recta best relates to?
Harrison's 20th Ed. Chapter 303 Page 2089

A. Proximal tubule
B. Loop of Henle
C. Distal tubule
D. Collecting duct

Pars recta is the straight portion of the proximal tubule of the juxtamedullary nephron located in the outer stripe of the medulla (medullary rays).

835. Which of the following about kidney structure is false?
Harrison's 20th Ed. Chapter 303 Page 2089

A. Majority of nephrons are cortical
B. Majority of glomeruli located in mid-to-outer cortex
C. Cortical nephrons perform most of glomerular filtration
D. None of the above

836. Which of the following about kidney structure is false?

Harrison's 20th Ed. Chapter 303 Page 2089

A. Cortical nephrons have short loops of Henle
B. Juxtamedullary nephrons have long loops of Henle
C. Peritubular capillaries surrounding cortical nephrons are shared among adjacent nephrons
D. None of the above

Majority of nephrons are cortical, with glomeruli located in mid-to-outer cortex. Cortical nephrons have short loops of Henle, whereas juxtamedullary nephrons have long loops of Henle. Peritubular capillaries surrounding cortical nephrons are shared among adjacent nephrons. Juxtamedullary nephrons use separate capillaries called vasa recta. Cortical nephrons perform most of the glomerular filtration & their afferent arterioles are larger than their respective efferent arterioles. Juxtamedullary nephrons create a hyperosmolar gradient that allows for production of concentrated urine.

837. Juxtamedullary nephrons represent what percentage of the total number of nephrons?

Harrison's 20th Ed. Chapter 303 Page 2089

A. ~ 5%
B. ~ 10%
C. ~ 15%
D. ~ 20%

Juxtamedullary nephrons represent ~15% of the total number of nephrons. The main difference between cortical nephron & juxtamedullary nephron is that cortical nephron contains a short loop of Henle which only extends into outer region of renal medulla whereas juxtamedullary nephron have a large glomerulus, increasing the glomerular filtration rate of the nephron. longer loop of Henle which extends deeper into the inner medulla. Juxtamedullary nephrons have a vital role in concentrating urine or water conservation.

838. Slit-pore membrane formation is related to?

Harrison's 20th Ed. Chapter 303 Page 2089

A. Annexin-4
B. Podocin
C. Neph 1-3 proteins
D. All of the above

Podocytes attach to the basement membrane by special foot processes and share a slit-pore membrane with their neighbor. Slit-pore membrane forms a filter for plasma water & solute by synthetic interaction of nephrin, annexin-4, CD2AP, FAT, ZO-1, P-cadherin, podocin, TRPC6, PLCE1, and Neph 1-3 proteins.

839. Renal interstitium contains all of the following cells except?

Harrison's 20th Ed. Chapter 303 Page 2089

A. Fibroblasts
B. Osteoblasts
C. Dendritic cells
D. Lipid-laden macrophages

Renal interstitium is the functional space surrounding glomeruli & their downstream tubules. It is home to resident & trafficking cells like fibroblasts, dendritic cells, lymphocytes, and lipid-laden macrophages.

840. Renal blood flow normally drains what percentage of the cardiac output?

Harrison's 20th Ed. Chapter 303 Page 2090

A. ~ 5%
B. ~ 10%
C. ~ 15%
D. ~ 20%

Renal blood flow normally drains approximately 20% of the cardiac output or 1000 mL/minute.

841. Cortical nephron has how many capillary beds arranged in series?

Harrison's 20th Ed. Chapter 303 Page 2090

A. 1
B. 2
C. 3
D. 4

Cortical nephron has two capillary beds arranged in series separated by efferent arteriole that regulates hydrostatic pressure in both capillary beds.

842. Driving force for glomerular filtration at efferent arteriole is?

Harrison's 20th Ed. Chapter 303 Page 2090

A. Zero
B. 10
C. 20
D. 30

As the oncotic pressure rises along the length of the glomerular capillary, the driving force for filtration falls to zero before reaching the efferent arteriole.

843. What percentage of renal plasma flow is filtered into Bowman's space?

Harrison's 20th Ed. Chapter 303 Page 2090

A. ~ 20%
B. ~ 45%
C. ~ 60%
D. ~ 80%

~20% of the renal plasma flow is filtered into Bowman's space.

844. Autoregulation of glomerular filtration is the result of?

Harrison's 20th Ed. Chapter 303 Page 2090

A. Autonomous vasoreactive reflex in afferent arteriole
B. Tubuloglomerular feedback
C. Angiotensin II mediated vasoconstriction of efferent arteriole
D. All of the above

Autoregulation of glomerular filtration is the result of an autonomous vasoreactive (myogenic) reflex in the afferent arteriole, tubuloglomerular feedback, and angiotensin II mediated vasoconstriction of the efferent arteriole.

845. Which of the following is the first line of defense against fluctuations in renal blood flow in autoregulation of glomerular filtration?

Harrison's 20th Ed. Chapter 303 Page 2090

A. Myogenic reflex in afferent arteriole
B. Tubuloglomerular feedback
C. Angiotensin II mediated vasoconstriction of efferent arteriole
D. None of the above

Myogenic reflex is a first line of defense against fluctuations in renal blood flow.

846. Tubuloglomerular feedback changes the rate of filtration & tubular flow by reflex vasoconstriction or dilatation of?

Harrison's 20th Ed. Chapter 303 Page 2090

A. Afferent arteriole
B. Efferent arteriole
C. Vasa recta
D. All of the above

847. Tubuloglomerular feedback is mediated by?
Harrison's 20th Ed. Chapter 303 Page 2090

A. Juxtaglomerular apparatus
B. Macula densa
C. Granular cells in the wall of afferent arteriole
D. All of the above

848. Macula densa is located in which of the following?
Harrison's 20th Ed. Chapter 303 Page 2090

A. Proximal tubule
B. Thick ascending limb of the loop of Henle
C. Distal tubule
D. Collecting duct

Tubuloglomerular feedback is mediated by specialized cells in thick ascending limb of the loop of Henle called macula densa that act as sensors of solute concentration & flow of tubular fluid.

849. Which of the following blunts tubuloglomerular feedback?
Harrison's 20th Ed. Chapter 303 Page 2090

A. Angiotensin II
B. Reactive oxygen species
C. Nitric oxide
D. Adenosine

Angiotensin II & reactive oxygen species enhance, while nitric oxide blunts tubuloglomerular feedback.

850. Juxtaglomerular apparatus is located in?
Harrison's 20th Ed. Chapter 303 Page 2090

A. Afferent arteriole
B. Efferent arteriole
C. Distal tubule
D. Collecting duct

Juxtaglomerular apparatus is located within the wall of afferent arteriole near macula densa and its granular cells release renin.

851. Which of the following is a potent vasoconstrictor of the afferent arteriole?
Harrison's 20th Ed. Chapter 303 Page 2090

A. Adenosine
B. ATP
C. Angiotensin II
D. Nitric oxide (NO)

ATP is metabolized in the extracellular space to generate adenosine, a potent vasoconstrictor of the afferent arteriole.

852. Renin catalyzes the conversion of?
Harrison's 20th Ed. Chapter 303 Page 2090

A. Angiotensinogen to angiotensin I
B. Angiotensin I to angiotensin II
C. Angiotensin II to angiotensin III
D. All of the above

Renin is a proteolytic enzyme released from juxtaglomerular apparatus. It catalyzes conversion of angiotensinogen to angiotensin I.

853. Angiotensin-converting enzyme catalyzes conversion of?
Harrison's 20th Ed. Chapter 303 Page 2090

A. Angiotensinogen to angiotensin I
B. Angiotensin I to angiotensin II
C. Angiotensin II to angiotensin III
D. All of the above

Angiotensin I is converted to angiotensin II by angiotensin-converting enzyme (ACE).

854. Which of the following is false about angiotensin II?
Harrison's 20th Ed. Chapter 303 Page 2090

A. Enhances tubuloglomerular feedback
B. Evokes vasoconstriction of efferent arteriole
C. Inhibits renin secretion through a negative feedback loop
D. None of the above

855. Which of the following is false about angiotensin II?
Harrison's 20th Ed. Chapter 303 Page 2090

A. Renin & ACE activity eventually produce angiotensin II
B. Stimulation of proximal tubular Na^+/H^+ exchange by angiotensin II directly increases Na^+ reabsorption
C. Angiotensin II also promotes Na+ reabsorption along the collecting duct by stimulating aldosterone secretion
D. None of the above

856. Angiotensin II causes constriction of?
Harrison's 20th Ed. Chapter 303 Page 2090

A. Afferent glomerular arteriole
B. Efferent glomerular arteriole
C. Renal artery
D. All of the above

Constriction of the efferent glomerular arteriole by angiotensin II indirectly increases the filtration fraction and raises peritubular capillary oncotic pressure to promote tubular Na^+ reabsorption. Angiotensin II inhibits renin secretion through a negative feedback loop.

857. Which of the following about cells lining the various tubular segments is false?
Harrison's 20th Ed. Chapter 303 Page 2090

A. Apical membrane faces the tubular lumen
B. Basolateral membrane faces the interstitium
C. Renal epithelial cells are polarized
D. Membrane proteins have symmetric assignment

Membrane proteins of renal epithelial cells mediating transport processes have asymmetric assignment of proteins. This provides the machinery for directional movement of fluid & solutes by the nephron.

858. Which of the following is not a major tubular segment of the nephron?
Harrison's 20th Ed. Chapter 303 Page 2091 Figure 303-3

A. Proximal tubular cells
B. Thick ascending limb of the loop of Henle cells
C. Distal convoluted tubular & cortical collecting duct cells
D. Typical cell in the outer medullary collecting duct

The five major tubular segments are proximal tubular cells, typical cell in the thick ascending limb of the loop of Henle, distal convoluted tubular cell, cortical collecting duct cells and typical cell in the inner medullary collecting duct.

859. Epithelial cellular transport is mediated by?
Harrison's 20th Ed. Chapter 303 Page 2091

A. Transporters
B. Channels
C. Pumps
D. All of the above

Cell membranes are composed of hydrophobic lipids that repel water and aqueous solutes. Epithelial cellular transport i.e. movement of fluid & solutes "sequentially" across apical & basolateral cell membranes (or vice versa) is mediated by transporters, channels, or pumps.

860. Paracellular transport occurs through?
Harrison's 20th Ed. Chapter 303 Page 2091

A. Leaky junctions
B. Tight junctions
C. Perforated junctions
D. Slit junctions

Paracellular transport occurs through tight junctions.

861. Leaky epithelia is present in?
Harrison's 20th Ed. Chapter 303 Page 2091

A. Proximal convoluted tubule
B. Distal convoluted tubule
C. Collecting duct
D. All of the above

Proximal tubule contains leaky epithelia which are best suited for bulk fluid reabsorption. Distal nephron segments (distal convoluted tubule & collecting duct) contain tight epithelia with little water permeability and provide refined control & regulation of transport.

862. Facilitated diffusion occurs through which of the following?
Harrison's 20th Ed. Chapter 303 Page 2093

A. Pumps
B. Channels
C. Transporters
D. Co-transporters

863. Secondary active transport occurs through which of the following?
Harrison's 20th Ed. Chapter 303 Page 2093

A. Pumps
B. Channels
C. Transporters
D. Co-transporters

864. Passive transport occurs through which of the following?
Harrison's 20th Ed. Chapter 303 Page 2093

A. Pumps
B. Channels
C. Transporters
D. Co-transporters

865. Active transport occurs through which of the following?
Harrison's 20th Ed. Chapter 303 Page 2093

A. Pumps
B. Channels
C. Transporters
D. Co-transporters

Movement of solutes & water across cell membranes is made possible by pumps (active transport), channels (passive transport), transporters (facilitated diffusion), and co-transporters (secondary active transport).

866. Ion-translocating ATPases include?
Harrison's 20th Ed. Chapter 303 Page 2093

A. Na^+/K^+-ATPase
B. H^+-ATPase
C. Ca^{++}-ATPase
D. All of the above

Ion-translocating ATPases that mediate active transport ("pumps") are the ubiquitous Na^+/K^+-ATPase, the H^+-ATPases, and Ca^{++}-ATPases.

867. Which of the following is false about active transport pumps?
Harrison's 20th Ed. Chapter 303 Page 2094

A. Electrogenic
B. Ion-translocating ATPases
C. Establish a voltage or membrane potential
D. None of the above

868. Which of the following solute moves by simple diffusion or passive transport?
Harrison's 20th Ed. Chapter 303 Page 2094

A. K^+
B. Na^+
C. Cl^-
D. All of the above

In kidney, movement by simple diffusion or passive transport occurs of water, K^+, Na^+, and Cl^-.

869. Which of the following is a transporter?
Harrison's 20th Ed. Chapter 303 Page 2094

A. Carrier
B. Symporter
C. Antiporter
D. All of the above

870. GLUT2 is a?
Harrison's 20th Ed. Chapter 303 Page 2094

A. Pump
B. Channel
C. Transporter
D. Co-transporter

GLUT2 is a hexose transporter that mediates glucose transport by tubular cells.

871. Carriers or uniporters are related to?
Harrison's 20th Ed. Chapter 303 Page 2094

A. Active transport
B. Passive transport
C. Facilitated diffusion
D. Secondary active transport

872. Symporters or co-transporters, antiporters or exchangers are related to?
Harrison's 20th Ed. Chapter 303 Page 2094

A. Active transport
B. Passive transport
C. Facilitated diffusion
D. Secondary active transport

Facilitated diffusion is a specialized type of passive transport mediated by simple transporters called carriers or uniporters. Many transporters operate by translocating two or more ions/solutes either in the same direction (symporters or co-transporters) or in opposite directions (antiporters or exchangers) across the cell membrane.

873. Proximal tubule reabsorbs which of the following?

Harrison's 20th Ed. Chapter 303 Page 2095

A. NaCl and water
B. Bicarbonate
C. Glucose & amino acids
D. All of the above

874. Which of the following is "most" absorbed in proximal tubule?

Harrison's 20th Ed. Chapter 303 Page 2095

A. NaCl
B. Water
C. Bicarbonate
D. Glucose & amino acids

Proximal tubule is responsible for reabsorbing ~60% of filtered NaCl and water as well as ~90% of filtered bicarbonate, phosphate & most critical nutrients (glucose & amino acids) through cellular & paracellular transport mechanisms. Proximal tubular cells reclaim nearly all filtered bicarbonate by a mechanism dependent on carbonic anhydrases.

875. Which of the following is false about peritubular capillaries?

Harrison's 20th Ed. Chapter 303 Page 2095

A. Have high oncotic pressure
B. Have low hydrostatic pressure
C. Vasa recta are medullary peritubular capillaries
D. None of the above

876. Which of the following statements is false?

Harrison's 20th Ed. Chapter 303 Page 2095

A. Aquaporin-1 present on apical & basolateral membranes
B. Na^+/K^+-ATPase pump is on basolateral membranes
C. Filtered bicarbonate first titrated by protons
D. Carbonic acid diffuses into the cell

Carbonic acid is metabolized by brush border carbonic anhydrase to water and carbon dioxide. Dissolved CO_2 diffuses into the cell, whereby cytoplasmic carbonic anhydrase reforms carbonic acid which dissociates into H^+ and bicarbonate anions. Bicarbonate exits the cell through a basolateral Na^+/HCO_3^- co-transporter.

877. Which of the following about acetazolamide is false?

Harrison's 20th Ed. Chapter 303 Page 2095

A. Carbonic anhydrase inhibitor
B. Blocks proximal tubule bicarbonate reabsorption
C. Diuretic
D. Acidifies urine

Acetazolamide is a carbonic anhydrase inhibitor, a weak diuretic, blocks proximal tubule bicarbonate reabsorption and alkalinizes urine. Dorzolamide, methazolamide, brinzolamide and dichlorphenamide are also carbonic anhydrase inhibitors. The increased distal nephron sodium delivery caused by acetazolamide results in increased potassium secretion and thus carbonic anhydrase inhibitors typically result in moderate increases of urinary potassium excretion.

878. Renal NH_3 is produced in the proximal tubule by?

Harrison's 20th Ed. Chapter 303 Page 2095

A. Inositol metabolism
B. Glutamine metabolism
C. Taurine metabolism
D. Arginine metabolism

Renal NH_3 is produced by glutamine metabolism in the proximal tubule (ammoniagenesis), diffuses out of the proximal tubular cell and traps H^+, which is secreted by Na^+/H^+ exchange, to form ammonium ion ($NH4^+$).

879. Glutamine is synthesized in?

Harrison's 20th Ed. Chapter 303 Page 2095

A. Kidneys
B. Liver
C. Intestines
D. Cartilage

Glutamine is synthesized in the liver and transported via circulation to kidney proximal tubule, where it is taken up by specific transporters.

880. Which of the following is a urinary buffer?

Harrison's 20th Ed. Chapter 303 Page 2095

A. Phosphate buffer
B. Bicarbonate buffer
C. Ammonia buffer
D. All of the above

881. Which of the following about urinary buffer is false?

Harrison's 20th Ed. Chapter 303 Page 2095

A. Increases urine pH
B. Ammonia (NH_3) and phosphate are urinary buffers
C. Cellular K^+ levels inversely modulate proximal tubular ammoniagenesis
D. None of the above

For every H^+ which enters urine, one sodium ion is reabsorbed from urine into the blood and is conserved. For every H^+ ion excreted & every Na^+ ion conserved, one bicarbonate ion is also reabsorbed into the blood.

882. Which of the following about carbonic anhydrase is false?

Harrison's 20th Ed. Chapter 303 Page 2095

A. Carbonic anhydrase is present at brush border
B. Carbonic anhydrase is present in cytoplasm
C. Carbonic anhydrase inhibitors alkalinize the urine
D. None of the above

883. The kidneys regulate hydrogen ion concentration by?

Harrison's 20th Ed. Chapter 303 Page 2095

A. Reabsorption of filtered bicarbonate
B. Secretion of titratable acid
C. Secretion of ammonia
D. All of the above

The kidneys regulate hydrogen ion concentration by three mechanisms: reabsorption of filtered bicarbonate, secretion of titratable acid, and secretion of ammonia. The renal excretion of acid (H^+) is achieved by titratable acidity and ammonium (NH_4^+) excretion.

884. The urine has a physiological pH of?

Harrison's 20th Ed. Chapter 303 Page 2095

A. 2.8–5.5
B. 3.8–6.5
C. 4.8–7.5
D. 5.8–8.5

The urine has a physiological pH of 4.8–7.5 with a mean of ~6.

885. Titratable acid is defined as the amount of strong base needed to titrate the pH of the urine back to pH?

Harrison's 20th Ed. Chapter 303 Page 2095

A. 7.1
B. 7.2
C. 7.3
D. 7.4

Titratable acid is defined as the amount of strong base needed to titrate the pH of the urine back to pH 7.4. Titratable acid refers to the excretion of protons with urinary buffers. Under normal conditions, ~one-third to one-half of net acid excretion by the kidneys is in the form of titratable acid. The other one-half to two-thirds is the excretion of NH_4^+. ($H^+ + NH_3 \leftrightarrow NH_4^+$). Therefore, net acid excretion = titratable acid + ammonium - urinary HCO_3^-

886. The major titratable acid in the urine is?

Harrison's 20th Ed. Chapter 303 Page 2095

A. HPO_4^{--}
B. $H_2PO_4^-$
C. HCl
D. HNO_3

Filtered hydrogen phosphate ion (HPO_4^{--}) is titrated in proximal tubule by secreted H^+ to form $H_2PO_4^-$, and this reaction constitutes a major component of the urinary buffer referred to as titratable acid. Thus, the major titratable acid in the urine is the monovalent organic phosphate ($H_2PO_4^-$). Buffering by phosphate and, to a lesser extent, other buffers such as urate and creatinine is called titratable acidity.

887. Reabsorption of filtered phosphate ion is regulated by?

Harrison's 20th Ed. Chapter 303 Page 2095

A. Calcium
B. Calcitonin
C. Parathyroid hormone
D. All of the above

Most filtered phosphate ion (HPO_4^{--}) is reabsorbed by the proximal tubule through a sodium-coupled cotransport process that is regulated by parathyroid hormone (PTH).

888. Which of the following statements is false?

Harrison's 20th Ed. Chapter 303 Page 2095

A. H^+ requires combination with buffers for excretion
B. H^+ requires formation of ammonium for excretion
C. For each H^+ excreted as titratable acid, there is one new HCO_3^- transferred to blood
D. None of the above

For each H^+ excreted as titratable acid, there is one new HCO_3^- transferred to blood. For each H^+ excreted as NH_4^+, there is also one new HCO_3^- transferred to blood.

889. Which of the following statements is false?

Harrison's 20th Ed. Chapter 303 Page 2095

A. Renal tubular cells synthesize ammonia by enzymatic deamination of amino acids
B. Ammonia acts as an acceptor of hydrogen ions, forming $NH4^+$
C. Ammonium ion is lipid insoluble
D. None of the above

Renal tubular cells synthesize ammonia by enzymatic deamination of amino acids. Ammonia diffuses down its concentration gradient into the tubular fluid where it acts as an acceptor of hydrogen ions, forming ammonium ions. The ammonium ion is lipid insoluble; thus it is trapped in the tubule lumen and excreted in the urine.

890. Which of the following is relevant in the renal control of plasma HCO_3^-?

Harrison's 20th Ed. Chapter 303 Page 2095

A. Sodium-hydrogen exchanger NHE_3
B. Basolateral Na^+/K^+-ATPase
C. Apical H^+-ATPase
D. All of the above

The kidneys regulate the [HCO_3^-] by conserving or excreting the HCO_3^- present in the glomerular ultrafiltrate and by producing new HCO_3^- which enters the body fluids as the kidneys excrete ammonium salts and titratable acids (this sum is called net acid) in the urine.

891. H^+ secretion from cells across the luminal membrane is mostly in exchange for?

Harrison's 20th Ed. Chapter 303 Page 2095

A. Na^+ ions
B. K^+ ions
C. HCO_3^- ions
D. All of the above

892. Soluble carbonic anhydrase is also called?

Harrison's 20th Ed. Chapter 303 Page 2095

A. Type I
B. Type II
C. Type III
D. Type IV

H^+ secretion from cells across the luminal membrane is mostly in exchange for Na^+ ions. Secreted H^+ reacts with filtered HCO_3^- to form H_2CO_3. In the presence of carbonic anhydrase (type IV), luminal H_2CO_3 rapidly dehydrates to $CO_2 + H_2O$. Inside the cell, dissociation of H_2O into OH^- and H^+ is promoted by hydroxylation of CO_2 ($OH^- + CO_2 => HCO_3^-$) to generate bicarbonate, catalyzed by soluble (type II) carbonic anhydrase.

893. Bicarbonate exits the cell through the basolateral membrane in a cotransport ratio with Na^+ of?

Harrison's 20th Ed. Chapter 303 Page 2095

A. 1:1
B. 2:1
C. 3:1
D. 4:1

Bicarbonate exits the cell through the basolateral membrane in a 3:1 cotransport with Na^+. The net result is that $NaHCO_3$ disappears from the lumen and appears in the blood-side of the proximal tubule cells.

894. Proximal reabsorption HCO_3^- is stimulated by?

Harrison's 20th Ed. Chapter 303 Page 2095

A. Respiratory acidosis
B. Decreases in cellular K^+
C. High levels of Angiotensin II
D. All of the above

Proximal reabsorption HCO_3^- is stimulated by decreases in cell pH (due to metabolic acidosis, respiratory acidosis or to decreases in cell K^+) and high levels of Angiotensin II which stimulate Na-H exchange. The most potent stimulator of NH_4^+ generation and excretion is metabolic acidosis.

895. Which of the following inherited disorders involve the proximal tubule?

Harrison's 20th Ed. Chapter 303 Page 2095 Table 303-1

A. Fanconi-Bickel syndrome
B. Dent disease
C. Hartnup disorder
D. All of the above

Inherited disorders involving the proximal tubule are proximal renal tubular acidosis, Fanconi-Bickel syndrome, isolated renal glycosuria, cystinuria (type I and non type I), Lysinuric protein intolerance, Hartnup disorder, Hereditary hypophosphatemic rickets with hypercalcemia, renal hypouricemia (type 1 & 2), Dent disease, X-linked-recessive nephrolithiasis with renal failure, X-linked-recessive hypophosphatemic rickets.

896. Which of the following inherited disorders involve the loop of Henle?

Harrison's 20th Ed. Chapter 303 Page 2095 Table 303-1

A. Familial hypocalciuric hypercalcemia
B. Bartter syndrome
C. Primary hypomagnesemia
D. All of the above

Inherited disorders involving the loop of Henle are Bartter syndrome (type 1, 2 & 3), autosomal dominant hypocalcemia with Bartter-like syndrome, Familial hypocalciuric hypercalcemia, Primary hypomagnesemia and isolated renal magnesium loss.

897. Which of the following inherited disorders involve the distal tubule and collecting duct?

Harrison's 20th Ed. Chapter 303 Page 2095 Table 303-1

A. Gitelman syndrome
B. Pseudoaldosteronism (Liddle's syndrome)
C. Gordon's syndrome
D. All of the above

Inherited disorders involving the distal tubule and collecting duct are Gitelman syndrome, primary hypomagnesemia with secondary hypocalcemia, pseudoaldosteronism (Liddle's syndrome), recessive pseudohypoaldosteronism type 1, pseudohypoaldosteronism type 2 (Gordon's hyperkalemia-hypertension syndrome), X-linked nephrogenic diabetes insipidus, nephrogenic diabetes insipidus (autosomal), Distal renal tubular acidosis.

898. Which of the following is related to Glucose transporter, GLUT2 gene?

Harrison's 20th Ed. Chapter 303 Page 2095 Table 303-1

A. Hartnup disorder
B. Bartter's syndrome
C. Fanconi-Bickel syndrome
D. Liddle's syndrome

899. Chloride channel gene is affected in which of the following Bartter's syndrome?

Harrison's 20th Ed. Chapter 303 Page 2095 Table 303-1

A. Type I
B. Type II
C. Type III
D. All of the above

900. Which of the following gene is affected in autosomal dominant distal renal tubular acidosis?

Harrison's 20th Ed. Chapter 303 Page 2095 Table 303-1

A. Anion exchanger-1
B. Vasopressin V2 receptor
C. Sodium chloride cotransporter
D. Calcium-sensing receptor

901. Which of the following gene is affected in Hartnup disorder?

Harrison's 20th Ed. Chapter 303 Page 2095 Table 303-1

A. Urate-anion exchanger
B. Neutral amino acid transporter
C. Amino acid transporter
D. Sodium bicarbonate cotransporter

902. Which of the following drugs is not filtered at the glomerulus?

Harrison's 20th Ed. Chapter 303 Page 2095

A. Penicillins
B. Cephalosporins
C. Salicylates
D. All of the above

Protein-bound drugs like penicillins, cephalosporins, and salicylates are not filtered at the glomerulus and are secreted by proximal tubule by specific transporters.

903. Which of the following is a biogenic amine neurotransmitter?

Harrison's 20th Ed. Chapter 303 Page 2095

A. Dopamine
B. Acetylcholine
C. Epinephrine
D. All of the above

Organic cations secreted by the proximal tubule include various biogenic amine neurotransmitters (dopamine, acetylcholine, epinephrine, norepinephrine, and histamine) and creatinine.

904. Which of the following drugs is secreted by ATP-dependent transporter P-glycoprotein?

Harrison's 20th Ed. Chapter 303 Page 2095

A. Cyclosporine
B. Digoxin
C. Tacrolimus
D. All of the above

The ATP-dependent transporter P-glycoprotein is highly expressed in brush border membranes and secretes cyclosporine, digoxin, tacrolimus, and various cancer chemotherapeutic agents. P-glycoprotein (P-gp) is a plasma membrane ATP-binding cassette transporter, responsible for multidrug resistance in tumor cells.

905. Which of the following present in proximal tubular cell bioactivates circulating 25-hydroxy vitamin D?

Harrison's 20th Ed. Chapter 303 Page 2095

A. 1α-hydroxylase
B. 7α-hydroxylase
C. 17-α-hydroxylase
D. 21-hydroxylase

Circulating 25-hydroxy vitamin D (calcidiol) is bioactivated by proximal tubular 1α-hydroxylase to produce 1,25-di-hydroxy vitamin D (calcitriol) which is the most active form of the hormone, that acts on the small intestine to promote calcium absorption.

906. Which of the following statements about fibroblast growth factor (FGF) is false?

Harrison's 20th Ed. Chapter 303 Page 2095

A. Fibroblast growth factor 23 (FGF23) is produced in osteoblasts and osteocytes
B. Parathyroid hormone (PTH) and active vitamin D regulate FGF23 production
C. Klotho is the required co-factor of FGF23
D. None of the above

FGF23 requires Klotho protein as a coreceptor for high affinity binding to cognate FGF receptors (FGFRs).

907. Fibroblast growth factor 23 (FGF23) belongs to which of the following class of phosphate-regulating factors?

Kidney Int. 2004;65(1):1-14

A. Phosphataxin
B. Phosphatonin
C. Phosphatorin
D. Phosphatine

Phosphorus balance is primarily regulated by PTH but may also respond to fibroblast growth factor 23 (FGF-23) and its cofactor, klotho, which together and separately promote renal excretion of phosphorus.

908. Which of the following is a phosphatonin?

Clin Cases Miner Bone Metab. 2012;9(1):9-12

A. FGF-23
B. sFRP-4
C. MEPE
D. All of the above

FGF23, sFRP-4, MEPE, and FGF7 are phosphatonins.

909. Which of the following diseases has a high fibroblast growth factor (FGF)-23 level?

Kidney Int. 2004;65(1):1-14

A. X-linked hypophosphatemia (XLH)
B. Autosomal dominant hypophosphatemic rickets (ADHR)
C. Oncogenic osteomalacia (OOM)
D. All of the above

910. Which of the following is a feature of secondary hyperparathyroidism?

doi:10.4061/2011/364890 Kidney Int. 2004;65(1):1-14

A. Elevated serum phosphate
B. Low calcitriol
C. High PTH levels
D. All of the above

911. Proteins encoded by SLC3A1 and SLC7A9 genes transport which of the following amino acids?

Harrison's 20th Ed. Chapter 303 Page 2095

A. Cystine
B. Lysine
C. Arginine
D. All of the above

Cystine, lysine, arginine and ornithine are transported by a system comprising two proteins encoded by the SLC3A1 and SLC7A9 genes. Mutations in either of them impair reabsorption of these amino acids and cause cystinuria.

912. Absorptive endocytosis relates to the transport of?

Harrison's 20th Ed. Chapter 303 Page 2095

A. Amino acids
B. Peptide hormones
C. Biogenic amine neurotransmitters
D. Protein-bound drugs

Peptide hormones like insulin and growth hormone, β_2-microglobulin, albumin are taken up by the proximal tubule through a process of absorptive endocytosis and are degraded in acidified endocytic lysosomes.

913. Which of the following is not a major segment of loop of Henle?

Harrison's 20th Ed. Chapter 303 Page 2095

A. Descending thin limb
B. Descending thick limb
C. Ascending thin limb
D. Ascending thick limb

Loop of Henle consists of 3 major segments - descending & ascending thin limb & ascending thick limb.

914. Major segments of Loop of Henle are based on?

Harrison's 20th Ed. Chapter 303 Page 2095

A. Cellular morphology
B. Anatomic location
C. Specialization of function
D. All of the above

915. Site of action of loop diuretics is?

Harrison's 20th Ed. Chapter 303 Page 2095

A. Proximal convoluted tubule
B. Loop of Henle
C. Distal convoluted tubule
D. Collecting duct

Site of action of loop diuretics is loop of Henle.

916. Water-permeability is highest in?

Harrison's 20th Ed. Chapter 303 Page 2095

A. Descending thin limb
B. Ascending thin limb
C. Ascending thick limb
D. Proximal convoluted tubule

Descending thin limb of loop of Henle is highly water-permeable due to dense expression of aquaporin-1 water channels. Water permeability is negligible in the ascending limb.

917. Which of the following is false about countercurrent multiplication?

Harrison's 20th Ed. Chapter 303 Page 2095

A. Uses Na^+ transporters in TALH
B. Descending thin limb of LOH is permeable to water
C. TALH is not permeable to water
D. None of the above

Epithelium of the ascending thin and thick limb of Henle's loop is impermeable to water and there are no lymphatics in the inner medulla and few in the outer medulla. Any water added to the interstitium must be removed by ascending vasa recta (AVR).

918. "Countercurrent multiplication" leads to?

Harrison's 20th Ed. Chapter 303 Page 2095

A. Hypotonic medullary interstitium
B. Hypertonic medullary interstitium
C. Isotonic medullary interstitium
D. All of the above

Loop of Henle and vasa recta establishes a hypertonic medullary interstitium by phenomenon called countercurrent multiplication.

919. Which of the following is a capillary network in a nephron?

Harrison's 20th Ed. Chapter 303 Page 2095

A. Glomerular capillaries
B. Peritubular capillaries
C. Vasa recta
D. All of the above

920. Which of the following statements is false?

Am J Physiol Regul Integr Comp Physiol. 2003;284:R1153-R1175

A. Ratio of ascending to descending vasa recta is 2:1
B. Endothelium of ascending vasa recta (AVR) is fenestrated
C. Endothelium of descending vasa recta (DVR) is continuous
D. None of the above

921. Which of the following occurs in medullary interstitium as blood flows from corticomedullary junction toward the papillary tip?

Am J Physiol Regul Integr Comp Physiol. 2003;284:R1153-R1175

A. Rising interstitial concentrations of NaCl from PCT
B. Rising interstitial concentrations of urea from collecting duct
C. Water flows via AQP1 channels from DVR lumen to medullary interstitium
D. All of the above

922. Water is supplied to the medullary interstitium by reabsorption from?

Harrison's 20th Ed. Chapter 303 Page 2095

A. Pars recta of proximal tubule in outer medulla
B. Descending thin limb of Henle's loop in the inner medulla
C. Collecting duct
D. All of the above

A small difference in osmotic pressure (the single effect) is multiplied by countercurrent flow in adjacent channels of the limbs of Henle's loop to produce a large axial difference in osmotic pressure between the renal cortex and the tip of the renal papilla. This multiplier generates a hypertonic renal medulla. Countercurrent exchange preserves medullary hypertonicity rather than create it.

923. Which of the following about countercurrent multiplication (CCM) is false?

Harrison's 20th Ed. Chapter 303 Page 2095

A. Exchange occurs between capillary & interstitium of the medulla rather than between two adjacent capillary loops
B. Solute diffuses from medullary interstitium to blood flowing down the descending vas rectum
C. As blood returns in the ascending vas rectum, solute diffuses into the interstitium
D. None of the above

Exchange occurs between capillary and interstitium of the medulla rather than between two adjacent capillary loops. Solute diffuses from the medullary interstitium to the blood flowing down the descending vas rectum. As blood returns in the ascending vas rectum, the solute concentration difference is reversed and solute diffuses into the interstitium. This effectively "traps" solute in the interstitium by recycling between ascending and descending capillary. In this way, blood circulates through the renal medulla without "washing out" its hypertonicity. The greater the solute permeability of the capillary, the more complete the exchange.

924. Which of the following is false about loop of Henle?

Harrison's 20th Ed. Chapter 303 Page 2095

A. Site of action for loop diuretics
B. Contributes to reabsorption of calcium ions
C. Contributes to reabsorption of magnesium ions
D. None of the above

925. Which of the following is the primary target for loop diuretics?

Harrison's 20th Ed. Chapter 303 Page 2095

A. Na^+/Cl^- co-transporter
B. $Na^+/K^+/2Cl^-$ co-transporter
C. Na^+/K^+-ATPase
D. Apical Ca^{++}-selective channels (TRPV5)

In the thick ascending limb, high level of secondary active NaCl transport is enabled by $Na^+/K^+/2Cl^-$ cotransporter on the apical membrane in series with basolateral Cl^- channels & Na^+/K^+-ATPase The $Na^+/K^+/2Cl^-$ co-transporter is the primary target for loop diuretics.

926. Tubular concentration of K^+ is?

Harrison's 20th Ed. Chapter 303 Page 2096

A. ~ 2 mEq/L
B. ~ 4 mEq/L
C. ~ 6 mEq/L
D. ~ 8 mEq/L

Tubular concentration of K^+ is similar to plasma i.e. about 4 mEq/L.

927. Which of the following is an inherited disorder of the thick ascending limb?

Harrison's 20th Ed. Chapter 303 Page 2096

A. Gitelman's syndrome
B. Bartter's syndrome
C. Gordon's syndrome
D. Liddle's syndrome

Bartter's syndrome is an inherited disorder of thick ascending limb. It leads to a salt-wasting renal disease with hypokalemia & metabolic alkalosis.

928. Loss-of-function mutations in which of the following can cause Bartter's syndrome?

Harrison's 20th Ed. Chapter 303 Page 2096

A. NKCC2
B. KCNJ1
C. CLCNKB
D. All of the above

Loss-of-function mutations in one of five distinct genes encoding components of the $Na^+/K^+/2Cl^-$ cotransporter (NKCC2), apical K^+ channel (KCNJ1), basolateral Cl^- channel (CLCNKB, BSND), or calcium-sensing receptor (CASR) can cause Bartter's syndrome.

929. Positive electrostatic charge in the lumen relative to interstitium is caused by?

Harrison's 20th Ed. Chapter 303 Page 2096

A. Mg^{2+} reabsorption
B. Ca^{2+} reabsorption
C. Potassium recycling
D. All of the above

Potassium recycling contributes to a positive electrostatic charge in lumen relative to the interstitium.

930. Which of the following is a transmembrane protein located within the tight junction complex?

Harrison's 20th Ed. Chapter 303 Page 2096

A. Hensin
B. Paracellin-1
C. Nedd4-2
D. All of the above

Mutations in CLDN16 encoding paracellin-1, a transmembrane protein located within the tight junction complex, leads to familial hypomagnesemia with hypercalcuria and nephrocalcinosis.

931. Which of the following about TRPV5 is true?

Harrison's 20th Ed. Chapter 303 Page 2096

A. Basolateral Na^+/K^+-ATPase and Cl^- channels
B. Apical K^+ channels
C. Ca^+ selective channel
D. Thiazide-sensitive Na^+/Cl^- cotransporter

TRPV5 stands for Transient Receptor Potential Cation Channel Subfamily V Member 5. Diseases associated with TRPV5 include Hypervitaminosis D and Idiopathic Hypercalciuria.

932. Which of the following about TRPV5 is false?

Harrison's 20th Ed. Chapter 303 Page 2096

A. Apical Ca^{++}-selective channel
B. Promotes active renal calcium reabsorption
C. Localized to distal convoluted tubule and collecting tubule
D. None of the above

TRPV5 is a transient receptor potential channel involved in calcium reabsorption. The renal handling of calcium is similar to active intestinal absorption, but uses TRPV5 instead of TRPV6. Phosphatidylinositol 4,5-bisphosphate (PI(4,5)P2) and calmodulin (CaM) directly bind to TRPV5 and activate or inactivate the channel, respectively. PI(4,5)P2 is found in the inner leaflet of the plasma membrane.

933. Which of the following about calmodulin (CaM) is false?
N Engl J Med. 1986; 314:1164-1170

A. Calcium sensing protein
B. Endogenous inactivator of TRPV5
C. Calmodulin's structure is similar to that of troponin C
D. None of the above

Calmodulin (CaM) is an abbreviation for calcium-modulated protein.

934. A molecular complex of which of the following proteins is critical for Mg^{2+} reabsorption in thick ascending limb of Henle?
Harrison's 20th Ed. Chapter 303 Page 2096

A. TRPM1 and TRPM2
B. TRPM3 and TRPM4
C. TRPM5 and TRPM6
D. TRPM6 and TRPM7

A molecular complex of TRPM6 and TRPM7 proteins is critical for Mg^{2+} reabsorption in the thick ascending limb of Henle.

935. Loss-of-function mutations of SLC12A3 encoding the apical Na^+/Cl^- co-transporter cause?
Harrison's 20th Ed. Chapter 303 Page 2096

A. Gitelman's syndrome
B. Bartter's syndrome
C. Gordon's syndrome
D. Liddle's syndrome

Loss-of-function mutations of SLC12A3 encoding the apical Na^+/Cl^- co-transporter cause Gitelman's syndrome - a salt-wasting disorder associated with hypokalemic alkalosis and hypocalciuria.

936. Mutations in genes encoding WNK kinases, WNK-1 & WNK-4 cause?
Harrison's 20th Ed. Chapter 303 Page 2096

A. Gitelman's syndrome
B. Bartter's syndrome
C. Gordon's syndrome
D. Liddle's syndrome

Mutations in genes encoding WNK kinases, WNK-1 and WNK-4 cause pseudohypoaldosteronism type II or Gordon's syndrome characterized by familial hypertension with hyperkalemia.

937. Which of the following modulates the final composition of the urine?
Harrison's 20th Ed. Chapter 303 Page 2096

A. Proximal convoluted tubule
B. Loop of Henle
C. Distal convoluted tubule
D. Collecting duct

The collecting duct modulates the final composition of urine. Its two major divisions are cortical collecting duct and inner medullary collecting duct.

938. Which of the following about principal cells of cortical collecting duct is false?
Harrison's 20th Ed. Chapter 303 Page 2096

A. Main Na^+ reabsorbing cells
B. Site of action of aldosterone
C. Site of action of K^+-sparing diuretics
D. None of the above

Principal cells are the main water and Na^+ reabsorbing & K^+ secreting cells and the site of action of aldosterone, K^+-sparing diuretics, and mineralocorticoid receptor antagonists such as spironolactone and eplerenone.

939. Which of the following is true for type A intercalated cells of cortical collecting duct?
Harrison's 20th Ed. Chapter 303 Page 2096

A. Acid secretion & bicarbonate reabsorption
B. Bicarbonate secretion & acid reabsorption
C. Acid & bicarbonate secretion
D. Acid & bicarbonate reabsorption

940. Which of the following is true for type B intercalated cells of cortical collecting duct?
Harrison's 20th Ed. Chapter 303 Page 2096

A. Acid secretion & bicarbonate reabsorption
B. Bicarbonate secretion & acid reabsorption
C. Acid & bicarbonate secretion
D. Acid & bicarbonate reabsorption

Type A intercalated cells of cortical collecting duct mediate acid secretion and bicarbonate reabsorption. Type B intercalated cells mediate bicarbonate secretion and acid reabsorption.

941. Activating mutations occur in which of the following channels in Liddle's syndrome?
Harrison's 20th Ed. Chapter 303 Page 2096

A. Na^+
B. K^+
C. Cl^-
D. HCO_3^-

942. Epithelial Na^+ channel (ENaC) are sensitive to?
Harrison's 20th Ed. Chapter 303 Page 2096

A. Amiloride
B. Aldosterone
C. Spironolactone
D. Eplerenone

In principal cells, passive apical Na^+ entry occurs through an amiloride-sensitive, epithelial Na^+ channel (ENaC) with basolateral exit mediated by the Na^+/K^+-ATPase.

943. In principal cells of cortical collecting ducts, sodium reabsorptive process is tightly regulated by?
Harrison's 20th Ed. Chapter 303 Page 2096

A. Renin
B. Angiotensin II
C. Aldosterone
D. All of the above

In principal cells of cortical collecting ducts, sodium reabsorptive process is tightly regulated by aldosterone which enters the cell across basolateral membrane, binds to cytoplasmic mineralocorticoid receptor, and translocates into nucleus, where it modulates gene transcription, resulting in increased Na^+ reabsorption and K^+ secretion.

944. All of the following are features of Liddle's syndrome except?
Harrison's 20th Ed. Chapter 303 Page 2096

A. Hypokalemia
B. Hypernatremia
C. Hypertension
D. Metabolic alkalosis

In Liddle's syndrome, activating mutations occur in epithelial Na^+ channel (ENaC) causing increase in Na^+ reclamation that produces hypokalemia, hypertension, and metabolic alkalosis.

945. Which of the following block ENaC?
Harrison's 20th Ed. Chapter 303 Page 2096

A. Trimethoprim
B. Pentamidine
C. Triamterene
D. All of the above

K^+-sparing diuretics amiloride & triamterene block ENaC, causing reduced Na^+ reabsorption. Trimethoprim & pentamidine, block ENaCs and predispose to hyperkalemia.

946. Which of the following statements about intercalated cells is false?
Harrison's 20th Ed. Chapter 303 Page 2097

A. Intercalated cells do not participate in Na^+ reabsorption
B. Intercalated cells mediate acid-base secretion
C. Type A intercalated cells have Cl^-/HCO_3^- exchanger on the apical membrane
D. Type B intercalated cells have Cl^-/HCO_3^- exchanger on the apical membrane

Type A intercalated cells have an apical proton pump (H^+-ATPase) that mediates acid secretion and a basolateral Cl^-/HCO_3^- anion exchanger for bicarbonate reabsorption. Type B intercalated cells have the Cl^-/HCO_3^- exchanger on the apical membrane to mediate bicarbonate secretion while the proton pump resides on the basolateral membrane to enable acid reabsorption.

947. Extracellular protein hensin is best related to?
Harrison's 20th Ed. Chapter 303 Page 2097

A. Principal cells
B. Intercalated cells
C. Podocytes
D. Mesangial cells

In acidemia, kidneys uses type A intercalated cells to secrete excess H^+ & generate more HCO_3^-. In bicarbonate excess with alkalemia type B intercalated cells predominate. Extracellular protein 'hensin' mediates this adaptation.

948. Atrial natriuretic peptide or renal natriuretic peptide (urodilatin) acts on?
Harrison's 20th Ed. Chapter 303 Page 2097

A. Cortical collecting duct
B. Inner medullary collecting duct
C. Distal convoluted tubule
D. All of the above

The two major divisions of collecting duct are the cortical collecting duct and inner medullary collecting duct. Natriuretic peptides like atrial natriuretic peptide or renal natriuretic peptide (urodilatin) interact with either apical (urodilatin) or basolateral (atrial natriuretic peptides) receptors on inner medullary collecting duct cells.

949. Which of the following is false about renal natriuretic peptide (urodilatin)?
Harrison's 20th Ed. Chapter 303 Page 2097

A. Secreted by renal tubular epithelia
B. Interacts with apical receptors on inner medullary collecting duct cells
C. Attenuates net Na^+ reabsorption
D. None of the above

950. Urodilatin resembles which of the following?
Harrison's 20th Ed. Chapter 303 Page 2097

A. Atrial natriuretic peptide
B. Aldosterone
C. Renin
D. PGE_2

951. Routine surrogate marker for assessing clinical tonicity is the concentration of?
Harrison's 20th Ed. Chapter 303 Page 2098 Figure 303-4

A. Na^+
B. K^+
C. Cl^-
D. All of the above

Routine surrogate marker for assessing clinical tonicity is the concentration of serum Na^+.

952. Which of the following water channels "aquaporin" is not present in inner medullary collecting duct cells?
Harrison's 20th Ed. Chapter 303 Page 2098

A. Aquaporin-1
B. Aquaporin-2
C. Aquaporin-3
D. Aquaporin-4

Inner medullary collecting duct cells have vasopressin-regulated water channels (aquaporin-2 on apical & aquaporin-3 & 4 on basolateral membrane). Aquaporin-1 water channels are densely expressed in descending thin limb of loop of Henle.

953. Which of the following aquaporin is not regulated by vasopressin in the collecting duct?
Harrison's 20th Ed. Chapter 303 Page 2098

A. Aquaporin 1
B. Aquaporin 2
C. Aquaporin 3
D. Aquaporin 4

Aquaporin 1 is active in all water-permeable segments of proximal & distal tubules, while aquaporins 2, 3, and 4 are regulated by vasopressin in the collecting duct.

954. Which of the following TRPV channels is osmoreceptive?
Harrison's 20th Ed. Chapter 303 Page 2098

A. $TRPV1^+$
B. $TRPV2^+$
C. $TRPV3^+$
D. $TRPV4^+$

Vanilloid receptors Transient receptor potential (TRPV) channels respond to changes in tonicity. $TRPV4^+$ neuronal cells connected to supraoptic and paraventricular nuclei in hypothalamus are osmoreceptive. They modulate release of vasopressin by posterior lobe of the pituitary gland.

955. Aldosterone leads to which of the following in principal cells of the collecting duct?
Harrison's 20th Ed. Chapter 303 Page 2098

A. Increase activity of apical membrane Na^+ channel
B. Increase activity of apical membrane K^+ channel
C. Increase activity of basolateral Na^+/K^+-ATPase
D. All of the above

Aldosterone binds to cytoplasmic mineralocorticoid receptors in principal cells of collecting duct & increases activity of apical membrane Na^+ channel, apical membrane K^+ channel & basolateral Na^+/K^+-ATPase.

956. Aldosterone mediates its effects by which of the following genes?

Harrison's 20th Ed. Chapter 303 Page 2098

A. SLC2A2
B. CLCN5
C. SGK1
D. CASR

Aldosterone mediates its effects in part by serum/glucocorticoid-induced kinase 1 (SGK1).

957. Which of the following is false about aldosterone escape?

Harrison's 20th Ed. Chapter 303 Page 2098

A. Chronic exposure to aldosterone
B. Decreased proximal tubular Na^+ reabsorption
C. Facilitated by atrial natriuretic peptides
D. None of the above

958. Who proposed the "Hyperfiltration hypothesis"?

Kidney International. 1996; 49:1774-1777

A. JL Olson
B. Timothy W. Meyer
C. HG Rennke
D. Barry Brenner

Barry Brenner in his hyperfiltration hypothesis in 1982 demonstrated that alterations in glomerular hemodynamics associated with renal ablation are accompanied by structural lesions and suggest that sustained single nephron hyperfiltration (SNGFR) may have maladaptive consequences by damaging remnant glomeruli.

959. Nephrons are not generated after how many weeks of gestation?

Mol Cell Pediatr. 2017;4:12

A. 30–32
B. 32–34
C. 34–36
D. 36–40

Nephrons are not generated after 34–36 weeks of gestation or after birth.

960. Reduced nephron numbers at birth may be due to?

Mol Cell Pediatr. 2017;4:12

A. Developmental abnormalities
B. Genetic predisposition
C. Malnutrition
D. All of the above

Reduced nephron numbers at birth may be due to developmental abnormalities, genetic predisposition and environmental factors such as malnutrition.

961. Which of the following is a CAKUT disorder?

Harrison's 20th Ed. Chapter 309 Page 2156

A. Kidney agenesis
B. Ureteropelvic junction obstruction
C. Vesicoureteral reflux
D. All of the above

Congenital abnormalities of the kidney and urinary tract (CAKUT) disorders include kidney hypoplasia, kidney agenesis, ureteropelvic junction obstruction, and vesicoureteral reflux.

962. Which of the following can be caused by prenatal exposure of ACE inhibitors or angiotensin receptor blockers?

Harrison's 20th Ed. Chapter 309 Page 2156

A. Kidney dysgenesis
B. Ureteropelvic junction obstruction
C. Vesicoureteral reflux
D. All of the above

963. Which of the following is a syndromic forms of CAKUT?

Harrison's 20th Ed. Chapter 309 Page 2156

A. Hepatorenal syndrome
B. Branchio-oto-renal syndrome
C. Pulmonary-renal syndrome
D. All of the above

Branchio-oto-renal (BOR) syndrome and autosomal dominant renal coloboma syndrome are syndromic forms of CAKUT. BOR is characterized by developmental abnormalities in neck, ears, and kidney, and is caused by mutations in EYA1 & SIX1 genes. Mutations in the PAX2 transcription factor gene causes the autosomal dominant renal coloboma syndrome.

964. Time of most rapid nephrogenesis is?

Mol Cell Pediatr. 2017;4:12

A. Early gestation
B. Mid gestation
C. Late gestation
D. All of the above

Mid gestation is the time of most rapid nephrogenesis.

965. Deficiency of which of the following predisposes to abnormal kidney development?

Mol Cell Pediatr. 2017;4:12

A. Vitamin A
B. Sodium
C. Zinc
D. All of the above

966. Which of the following medications taken by mother influences kidney development?

Mol Cell Pediatr. 2017;4:12

A. Dexamethasone
B. Angiotensin converting enzyme inhibitors
C. Gentamicin
D. All of the above

Factors implicated as predisposing to abnormal kidney development include deficiency in vitamin A, sodium, zinc or iron, and medications like dexamethasone, Gentamicin, Nonsteroidal anti-inflammatory drugs, angiotensin converting enzyme inhibitors and angiotensin receptor antagonists.

967. Who was the first to describe association between low birth weight & later cardiovascular death?

Indian Pediatrics 2009;46:S48-S54

A. Barry Brenner
B. Timothy W. Meyer
C. David Barker
D. Neal Bricker

Barker fetal origins hypothesis proposed that intrauterine growth retardation, low birth weight, and premature birth have a causal relationship to the origins of hypertension, coronary heart disease, and non-insulin-dependent diabetes, in middle age.

968. Nephrons of which of the followng can regenerate?

J Am Soc Nephrol. 2006;17:2390-2401

A. Duck
B. Bat
C. Fish
D. Dog

Nephrons of mammals, in contrast to those of fish, cannot regenerate.

969. Which of the following participates in compensatory renal growth after nephron loss?

Pediatr Endocrinol Rev. 2012;10(1):152-63

A. Hepatocyte growth factor
B. Glucose transporters
C. Insulin-like growth factor
D. All of the above

970. Whose name is associated with intact nephron hypothesis?

Nephrol Dial Transplant 2015;30:1602–1604

A. Herbert Lubowitz
B. Neil Bricker
C. Doris Rolf
D. Fred Weisser

An exposition of the Intact Nephron Hypothesis was published by Bricker et. al. in American Journal of Medicine (1960). Dr. Bricker defined the "intact nephron hypothesis" that the number of functioning nephrons is reduced in chronic renal disease and that the remaining nephrons undergo adaptations that maintain renal homeostasis.

971. Bricker's trade-off hypothesis best relates to?

Nutrients. 2017;9(5):427

A. Calcium
B. Phosphorus
C. PTH
D. All of the above

Slatopolsky and Bricker's trade-off hypothesis in 1972 is based on the effects of uremia on the balance between calcium, phosphorus & PTH levels. Elevations in PTH that occur in CKD restore calcium & phosphorus levels but lead to hyperplasia of parathyroid gland & secondary hyperparathyroidism (trade-off).

972. Urine specific gravity of 1.010 equals how many mOsmol/L of urine osmolality?

Harrison's 18th Ed 2291

A. 300
B. 325
C. 350
D. 375

Urine specific gravity of 1.010 equals ~350 mOsmol/L of urine osmolality.

973. Delta metabolic acidosis occurs when GFR falls below?

Harrison's 18th Ed 2292

A. 25 mL/minute
B. 40 mL/minute
C. 60 mL/minute
D. 75 mL/minute

When GFR falls below 25 mL/minute, organic acids accumulate producing a delta metabolic acidosis.

Acute Kidney Injury

974. Which of the following about acute kidney injury (AKI) is false?
Harrison's 20th Ed. Chapter 304 Page 2099

A. Clinical rather than a structural diagnosis
B. Increase in serum creatinine (SCr) concentration
C. Often associated with a reduction in urine volume
D. None of the above

975. Which of the following is not a cause of community-acquired acute kidney injury (AKI)?
Harrison's 20th Ed. Chapter 304 Page 2099

A. Volume depletion
B. Nephrotoxic medication administration
C. Obstruction of the urinary tract
D. Malignancy

AKI may be community-acquired or hospital-acquired. Common causes of community-acquired AKI include volume depletion, heart failure, adverse effects of medications, obstruction of the urinary tract, or malignancy. Most common clinical settings for hospital-acquired AKI are sepsis, major surgical procedures, critical illness involving heart or liver failure, and nephrotoxic medication administration.

976. Which of the following is the cause of AKI?
Harrison's 20th Ed. Chapter 304 Page 2099

A. Prerenal azotemia
B. Intrinsic renal parenchymal disease
C. Postrenal obstruction
D. All of the above

Causes of AKI have traditionally been divided into three broad categories : prerenal azotemia, intrinsic renal parenchymal disease and postrenal obstruction. Prerenal azotemia is the most common form of AKI.

977. Which of the following is a cause of prerenal AKI?
Harrison's 20th Ed. Chapter 304 Page 2099 Figure 304-1

A. Congestive heart failure
B. Liver failure
C. Hypovolemia
D. All of the above

978. Which of the following is not a cause of intrinsic AKI?
Harrison's 20th Ed. Chapter 304 Page 2099 Figure 304-1

A. Sepsis
B. Ischemia
C. Hemolysis
D. Congestive heart failure

979. Which of the following is a cause of intrinsic AKI?
Harrison's 20th Ed. Chapter 304 Page 2099 Figure 304-1

A. Malignant hypertension
B. TTP-HUS
C. Acute glomerulonephritis
D. All of the above

980. Which of the following is an endogenous nephrotoxin?
Harrison's 20th Ed. Chapter 304 Page 2099 Figure 304-1

A. Rhabdomyolysis
B. Myeloma
C. Hemolysis
D. All of the above

981. "Azo" means?
Harrison's 20th Ed. Chapter 304 Page 2099

A. Urea
B. Ammonia
C. Nitrogen
D. Waste

Word azotemia is derived from "azo" meaning nitrogen.

982. Term azotemia is used mostly for?
Harrison's 20th Ed. Chapter 304 Page 2099

A. Prerenal ARF
B. Intrinsic ARF
C. Postrenal ARF
D. All of the above

Prerenal acute renal failure is also called azotemia.

983. Acute tubular necrosis (ATN) best relates to?
Harrison's 20th Ed. Chapter 304 Page 2099

A. Sepsis
B. Ischemic injury
C. Vasculitis
D. Nephrotoxin

Prolonged periods of prerenal azotemia may lead to ischemic injury. This is termed as acute tubular necrosis (ATN).

984. Which of the following about acute renal failure is false?
Lancet 2005;365:417-430

A. Abrupt & sustained decrease in renal function with retention of nitrogenous and non-nitrogenous waste products
B. Acute & sustained increase in serum creatinine of 0.5 mg/dL, if the baseline is < 2.5 mg/dL
C. Increase in serum creatinine of > 20% if the baseline is > 2.5 mg/dL
D. None of the above

985. RIFLE system is used to classify?
Lancet 2005;365:417-430

A. Acute renal failure
B. Chronic renal failure
C. Glomerulonephritis
D. Nephrotic syndrome

RIFLE = Risk-Injury-Failure-Loss-End-stage kidney disease (ESKD). RIFLE classification was established by the Acute Dialysis Quality Initiative (ADQI) group in order to supply the obligation for uniform definition, early detection, and grading of AKI. After this, the AKIN criteria were created by the Acute Kidney Injury Network (AKIN) for further refinement of the definition of AKI.

986. Which of the following about prerenal azotemia is false?
Lancet 2005;365:417-430

A Integrity of renal tissue is disturbed
B. Appropriate physiological response to renal hypoperfusion
C. Certain drugs can provoke acute prerenal failure
D. Persistent renal hypoperfusion leads to ischemic ATN

By definition, no parenchymal damage to the kidney occurs in prerenal azotemia. It is rapidly reversible once parenchymal blood flow and intraglomerular hemodynamics are restored.

987. Typical histological features of human acute tubular necrosis include?
Lancet 2005;365:417-430

A. Loss of brush border in proximal tubular cells
B. Sloughing of tubular cells into the lumen
C. Interstitial oedema
D. All of the above

988. In kidneys, most of the blood supply is directed to?
Lancet 2005;365:417-430

A. Renal cortex
B. Outer medulla
C. Medullary rays
D. None of the above

989. In established acute tubular necrosis, selective reduction in blood supply occurs in?
Lancet 2005;365:417-430

A. Renal cortex
B. Outer medulla
C. Medullary rays
D. None of the above

990. Vasoconstrictors implicated in reduced renal blood flow in acute tubular necrosis are?
Lancet 2005;365:417-430

A. Angiotensin II
B. Thromboxane A_2
C. Prostaglandin H_2
D. All of the above

991. Vasoconstrictors implicated in the reduced renal blood flow in acute tubular necrosis are?
Lancet 2005;365:417-430

A. Leukotrienes C4 and D4
B. Endothelin 1
C. Adenosine
D. All of the above

992. Which of the following about urine findings in pre-renal ARF is false?
Lancet 2005;365:417-430

A. Specific gravity about 1.020
B. Urine osmolality > 500
C. Fractional excretion of sodium (%) < 1
D. Fractional excretion of urea (%) > 35

993. Which of the following about urine findings in pre-renal ARF is false?
Lancet 2005;365:417-430

A. Urine sodium < 10 mmol/L
B. Urine osmolality > 500
C. Fractional excretion of sodium (%) > 2
D. Fractional excretion of urea (%) < 35

994. Which of the following about urine findings in pre-renal ARF is false?
Lancet 2005;365:417-430

A. Fractional excretion of uric acid (%) < 7
B. Fractional excretion of Lithium (%) < 7
C. Low brush border enzyme levels
D. None of the above

995. Which of the following about urine findings in renal ARF is false?
Lancet 2005;365:417-430

A. Specific gravity about 1.010
B. Urine osmolality > 300
C. Fractional excretion of sodium (%) > 2
D. Fractional excretion of urea (%) < 35

996. Which of the following about urine findings in renal ARF is false?
Lancet 2005;365:417-430

A. Urine sodium > 20 mmol/kg
B. Urine osmolality > 300
C. Fractional excretion of sodium (%) < 1
D. Fractional excretion of urea (%) > 35

997. Which of the following about urine findings in renal ARF is false?
Lancet 2005;365:417-430

A. Fractional excretion of uric acid (%) > 15
B. Fractional excretion of Lithium (%) > 20
C. High brush border enzyme levels
D. None of the above

998. Biomarkers proposed for the early diagnosis of acute renal failure include?
Lancet 2005;365:417-430

A. Urinary interleukin 18
B. Intestinal form of alkaline phosphatase
C. N-acetyl-β-glucosaminidase & alanine aminopeptidase
D. All of the above

999. Biomarkers specifically higher in ischaemic ATN is?
Lancet 2005;365:417-430

A. Urinary interleukin 18
B. Kidney injury molecule 1
C. N-acetyl-β-glucosaminidase
D. Alanine aminopeptidase

1000. Normal GFR is maintained by?

Harrison's 20th Ed. Chapter 304 Page 2099

A. Renal blood flow
B. Afferent renal arteriole resistance
C. Efferent renal arteriole resistance
D. All of the above

Normal GFR is maintained by renal blood flow and the relative resistances of afferent and efferent renal arterioles, which determine the glomerular plasma flow rate and the transcapillary hydraulic pressure gradient that drive glomerular ultrafiltration.

1001. Which of the following is a mediator of homeostatic response to decreased effective circulating volume or cardiac output?

Harrison's 20th Ed. Chapter 304 Page 2099

A. Angiotensin II
B. Norepinephrine
C. Vasopressin (antidiuretic hormone)
D. All of the above

1002. Glomerular filtration is maintained despite reduced renal blood flow by?

Harrison's 20th Ed. Chapter 304 Page 2099

A. Angiotensin II
B. Norepinephrine
C. Vasopressin (antidiuretic hormone)
D. All of the above

Glomerular filtration is maintained despite reduced renal blood flow by angiotensin II–mediated renal efferent vasoconstriction, which maintains glomerular capillary hydrostatic pressure closer to normal, if renal blood flow reduction is not excessive.

1003. Which of the following occur in response to low renal perfusion pressure?

Harrison's 20th Ed. Chapter 304 Page 2100

A. Increased intrarenal biosynthesis of prostaglandins
B. Increased intrarenal biosynthesis of kallikrein and kinins
C. Increased intrarenal biosynthesis of nitric oxide (NO)
D. All of the above

1004. Myogenic reflex relates best to?

Harrison's 20th Ed. Chapter 304 Page 2100

A. Afferent arteriole
B. Efferent arteriole
C. Glomerular capillaries
D. All of the above

In a low perfusion pressure situation, a myogenic reflex within the afferent arteriole leads to dilation, thereby maintaining glomerular perfusion.

1005. Agents that impair autoregulation of renal blood flow include?

Lancet 2005;365:417-430

A. NSAIDs
B. ACE inhibitors
C. Angiotensin-II-receptor blockers
D. All of the above

1006. Which of the following about prerenal azotemia is false?

Harrison's 20th Ed. Chapter 304 Page 2099

A. Related to intraglomerular hemodynamics
B. No parenchymal damage to the kidney
C. May lead to ischemic injury–acute tubular necrosis (ATN)
D. None of the above

1007. Acute tubular necrosis (ATN) relates best with?

Harrison's 20th Ed. Chapter 304 Page 2099

A. Prerenal ARF
B. Intrinsic ARF
C. Postrenal ARF
D. All of the above

More severe or prolonged prerenal ARF (renal hypoperfusion) may lead to ischemic injury of kidneys leading to acute tubular necrosis (ATN).

1008. Prerenal ARF can result from which of the following?

Harrison's 20th Ed. Chapter 304 Page 2099

A. Low cardiac output
B. Systemic vasodilatation
C. Selective intrarenal vasoconstriction
D. All of the above

Prerenal ARF can complicate any disease that induces hypovolemia, low cardiac output, systemic vasodilatation or selective intrarenal vasoconstriction.

1009. Which of the following is an action of Angiotensin II?

Harrison's 20th Ed. Chapter 304 Page 2099

A. Increased biosynthesis of Prostaglandin E_2
B. Increased biosynthesis of prostacyclin
C. Preferential constriction of efferent arterioles
D. All of the above

Angiotensin II increases biosynthesis of vasodilator prostaglandins (Pg E_2 & prostacyclin) resulting in afferent arteriolar vasodilation. Angiotensin II also induces preferential constriction of efferent arterioles.

1010. Which of the following drugs cause impairment of renal autoregulatory responses?

Harrison's 20th Ed. Chapter 304 Page 2099

A. Nonsteroidal anti-inflammatory drugs
B. Angiotensin-converting enzyme inhibitors
C. Angiotensin II receptor blockers
D. All of the above

Impairment of renal autoregulatory responses is caused by COX inhibitors (NSAID's), ACE inhibitors & angiotensin II receptor blockers. The combined use of NSAIDs with ACE inhibitors or ARBs poses a higher risk for developing prerenal azotemia.

1011. Autoregulation by tubuloglomerular feedback mechanism is mediated by?

Harrison's 20th Ed. Chapter 304 Page 2100

A. Prostaglandins
B. Kallikrein
C. Nitric oxide (NO)
D. All of the above

Autoregulation by tubuloglomerular feedback mechanism, in which decreases in solute delivery to macula densa elicit dilation of juxtaposed afferent arteriole in order to maintain glomerular perfusion, is mediated, in part, by nitric oxide (NO).

1012. Renal autoregulation fails when systolic blood pressure falls below?

Harrison's 20th Ed. Chapter 304 Page 2100

A. 100 mm Hg
B. 90 mm Hg
C. 80 mm Hg
D. 70 mm Hg

Even in healthy adults, renal autoregulation usually fails once the systolic blood pressure falls below 80 mm Hg.

1013. Hepatorenal syndrome (HRS) is a form of?

Harrison's 20th Ed. Chapter 304 Page 2101

A. Prerenal ARF
B. Intrinsic ARF
C. Intratubular obstruction
D. Postrenal ARF

Hepatorenal syndrome (HRS) is a unique form of prerenal ARF.

1014. Which of the following is false about hepatorenal syndrome?

Harrison's 20th Ed. Chapter 304 Page 2101

A. Kidneys are structurally normal
B. Kidneys fail due to intense renal vasoconstriction
C. Type I HRS is the more aggressive form
D. None of the above

1015. Which of the following is a cause of intrinsic AKI?

Harrison's 20th Ed. Chapter 304 Page 2101

A. Sepsis
B. Ischemia
C. Endogenous and exogenous nephrotoxins
D. All of the above

1016. Which of the following leads to intrinsic ARF?

Harrison's 20th Ed. Chapter 304 Page 2101

A. Ischemic or nephrotoxic tubular injury
B. Tubulointerstitial diseases
C. Diseases of renal microcirculation & glomeruli
D. All of the above

Intrinsic causes of ARF can be ischemic or nephrotoxic tubular injury, tubulointerstitial diseases, diseases of renal microcirculation & glomeruli and diseases of larger renal vessels. Prerenal azotemia and ischemia-associated AKI represent a continuum of manifestations of renal hypoperfusion.

1017. In AKI associated with sepsis, which of the following is most affected?

Harrison's 20th Ed. Chapter 304 Page 2102

A. Glomeruli
B. Tubulointerstitium
C. Vessels
D. All of the above

1018. Which of the following play a role in the pathophysiology of sepsis-induced AKI?

Harrison's 20th Ed. Chapter 304 Page 2102

A. Inflammation
B. Mitochondrial dysfunction
C. Interstitial edema
D. All of the above

1019. Activation of which of the following leads to renal vasoconstriction?

Harrison's 20th Ed. Chapter 304 Page 2102

A. Renin-angiotensin-aldosterone system
B. Vasopressin
C. Endothelin
D. All of the above

Renal vasoconstriction occurs from activation of sympathetic nervous system, renin-angiotensin-aldosterone system, vasopressin, and endothelin.

1020. Hypovolemia leads to activation of?

Harrison's 20th Ed. Chapter 304 Page 2102

A. Sympathetic nervous system
B. Renin-angiotensin-aldosterone system
C. Release of arginine vasopressin
D. All of the above

Hypovolemia triggers neurohormonal responses that include activation of the sympathetic nervous system and renin-angiotensin-aldosterone system, and release of arginine vasopressin.

1021. Which of the following about healthy human kidneys is false?

Harrison's 20th Ed. Chapter 304 Page 2102

A. Receive 20% of the cardiac output
B. Consume 10% of resting oxygen
C. Constitute 0.5% of the human body mass
D. None of the above

Healthy kidneys receive 20% of the cardiac output and consume 10% of resting oxygen, despite constituting only 0.5% of the human body mass.

1022. Which of the following is the site of the most hypoxic region in the body?

Harrison's 20th Ed. Chapter 304 Page 2102

A. Pituitary
B. Hypothalamus
C. Renal medulla
D. Retina

Kidneys are the site of most hypoxic regions in the body, the renal medulla, outer medulla is particular.

1023. Ischemic renal injury is most prominent in?

Harrison's 20th Ed. Chapter 304 Page 2102

A. S_1 segment of proximal tubule
B. S_2 segment of proximal tubule
C. S_3 segment of proximal tubule
D. Cortical thick ascending limb of loop of Henle

Ischemic renal injury is most prominent in metabolically very active S_3 segment of PCT and in medullary portion of the thick ascending limb of the loop of Henle.

1024. Which of the following cause vasoconstriction of glomerular and medullary microvasculature?

Harrison's 20th Ed. Chapter 304 Page 2102 Figure 304-4

A. Endothelin
B. Thromboxane A2
C. Adenosine
D. All of the above

1025. Which of the following cause vasodilation of glomerular and medullary microvasculature?
Harrison's 20th Ed. Chapter 304 Page 2102 Figure 304-4

A. PGE_2
B. Acetylcholine
C. Bradykinin
D. All of the above

1026. AKI from atheroembolic disease following percutaneous catheterization of aorta, or spontaneously, is due to?
Harrison's 20th Ed. Chapter 304 Page 2102

A. Air embolization
B. Fat embolization
C. Cholesterol crystal embolization
D. All of the above

AKI from atheroembolic disease following percutaneous catheterization of aorta, or spontaneously, is due to cholesterol crystal embolization.

1027. Intra-abdominal pressure that causes abdominal compartment syndrome is?
Harrison's 20th Ed. Chapter 304 Page 2102

A. > 20 mm Hg
B. > 30 mm Hg
C. > 40 mm Hg
D. > 50 mm Hg

Intra-abdominal pressure that causes abdominal compartment syndrome is usually >20 mm Hg.

1028. Microvascular causes of AKI include which of the following?
Harrison's 20th Ed. Chapter 304 Page 2103

A. Antiphospholipid antibody syndrome
B. Malignant nephrosclerosis
C. Scleroderma
D. All of the above

Microvascular causes of AKI include the thrombotic microangiopathies (antiphospholipid antibody syndrome, radiation nephritis, malignant nephrosclerosis and thrombotic thrombocytopenic purpura/hemolytic-uremic syndrome [TTP-HUS]), scleroderma and atheroembolic disease.

1029. Which of the following structures of the kidney are vulnerable to nephrotoxin associated injury?
Harrison's 20th Ed. Chapter 304 Page 2103

A. Tubules
B. Vasculature
C. Collecting system
D. All of the above

All structures of the kidney are vulnerable to nephrotoxin associated injury, including the tubules, interstitium, vasculature, and collecting system.

1030. Risk factor for nephrotoxin associated AKI is?
Harrison's 20th Ed. Chapter 304 Page 2103

A. Older age
B. CKD
C. Prerenal azotemia
D. All of the above

1031. Which of the following is false about the clinical course (serum creatinine) of contrast nephropathy?
Harrison's 20th Ed. Chapter 304 Page 2103

A. Begins to rise 24–48 hours after exposure
B. Peaks within 3–5 days
C. Resolves within 1 week
D. None of the above

Clinical course of contrast nephropathy is characterized by a rise in serum creatinine (SCr) beginning 24–48 hours after exposure, peaking within 3–5 days and resolving within 1 week.

1032. Which of the following diagnostic agents can cause AKI?
Harrison's 20th Ed. Chapter 304 Page 2103

A. Iodinated contrast agents
B. High-dose gadolinium
C. Oral sodium phosphate solution
D. All of the above

Iodinated contrast agents are used for cardiovascular and computed tomography (CT) imaging, high-dose gadolinium is used for magnetic resonance imaging (MRI) and oral sodium phosphate solutions is used as bowel purgative.

1033. Contrast nephropathy is due to?
Harrison's 20th Ed. Chapter 304 Page 2103

A. Hypoxia in renal outer medulla
B. Cytotoxic damage to tubules
C. Tubule obstruction with precipitated contrast material
D. All of the above

1034. Which of the following drugs binds to tubular membrane cholesterol and introduces pores?
Harrison's 20th Ed. Chapter 304 Page 2103

A. Aminoglycosides
B. Amphotericin B
C. Vancomycin
D. Acyclovir

Amphotericin B binds to tubular membrane cholesterol and introduces pores.

1035. Clinical features of amphotericin B nephrotoxicity include?
Harrison's 20th Ed. Chapter 304 Page 2103

A. Hypomagnesemia
B. Hypocalcemia
C. Nongap metabolic acidosis
D. All of the above

Clinical features of amphotericin B nephrotoxicity include polyuria, hypomagnesemia, hypocalcemia and nongap metabolic acidosis.

1036. AKI typically manifests after how many days of aminoglycoside therapy?
Harrison's 20th Ed. Chapter 304 Page 2103

A. 1–3 days
B. 3–5 days
C. 5–7 days
D. 7–10 days

AKI typically manifests after 5–7 days of aminoglycoside therapy and can present even after the drug has been discontinued. Hypomagnesemia is a common finding.

1037. Which of the following drugs precipitate in tubules and cause AKI by tubular obstruction?

Harrison's 20th Ed. Chapter 304 Page 2103

A. Aminoglycosides
B. Amphotericin B
C. Vancomycin
D. Acyclovir

Acyclovir precipitates in tubules and causes AKI by tubular obstruction, particularly when given as an intravenous bolus at high doses (500 mg/m^2) or in the setting of hypovolemia.

1038. Which of the following drugs is associated with AKI due to tubular toxicity?

Harrison's 20th Ed. Chapter 304 Page 2103

A. Foscarnet
B. Pentamidine
C. Tenofovír
D. All of the above

1039. Which of the following drugs is associated with AKI due to acute interstitial nephritis?

Harrison's 20th Ed. Chapter 304 Page 2103

A. Cephalosporins
B. Quinolones
C. Rifampin
D. All of the above

Foscarnet, pentamidine, tenofovír and cidofovir are associated with AKI due to tubular toxicity. AKI secondary to acute interstitial nephritis can occur as a consequence of exposure to many antibiotics, including penicillins, cephalosporins, quinolones, sulphonamides and rifampin.

1040. Which of the following drugs can cause injury to the glomerular microvasculature (thrombotic microangiopathy)?

Harrison's 20th Ed. Chapter 304 Page 2103

A. Cisplatin
B. Carboplatin
C. Ifosfamide
D. Bevacizumab

Antiangiogenesis agent bevacizumab can cause proteinuria and hypertension via injury to the glomerular microvasculature (thrombotic microangiopathy) as do mitomycin C and gemcitabine.

1041. Which of the following is a metabolic product of ethylene glycol?

Harrison's 20th Ed. Chapter 304 Page 2103

A. Oxalic acid
B. Glycolaldehyde
C. Glyoxylate
D. All of the above

Ethylene glycol, present in automobile antifreeze, is metabolized to oxalic acid, glycolaldehyde & glyoxylate, which may cause AKI through direct tubular injury & tubular obstruction.

1042. Which of the following is the cause of "Chinese herb nephropathy" and "Balkan nephropathy"?

Harrison's 20th Ed. Chapter 304 Page 2103

A. Aristolochic acid
B. Ethylene glycol
C. 2-hydroxyethoxyacetic acid (HEAA)
D. Melamine

Aristolochic acid was found to be the cause of "Chinese herb nephropathy" and "Balkan nephropathy" due to contamination of medicinal herbs or farming.

1043. Which of the following is an environmental toxin?

Harrison's 20th Ed. Chapter 304 Page 2103

A. Melamine
B. Diethylene glycol
C. Ethylene glycol
D. All of the above

1044. Which of the following is an endogenous nephrotoxin?

Harrison's 20th Ed. Chapter 304 Page 2103

A. Myoglobin
B. Hemoglobin
C. Myeloma light chains
D. All of the above

Endogenous nephrotoxins include calcium, myoglobin, hemoglobin, uric acid, oxalate & myeloma light chains.

1045. Endogenous nephrotoxins include all except?

Harrison's 20th Ed. Chapter 304 Page 2103

A. Calcium
B. Magnesium
C. Urate
D. Oxalate

1046. Presence of which of the following suggests a diagnosis of acute renal failure due to rhabdomyolysis?

Harrison's 20th Ed. Chapter 304 Page 2103

A. Hyperkalemia
B. Hyperphosphatemia
C. Hypocalcemia
D. All of the above

Hyperkalemia, hyperphosphatemia, hypocalcemia, hyperuricemia and raised creatine kinase (MM isoenzyme) suggest a diagnosis of rhabdomyolysis.

1047. Uromodulin is also called?

Harrison's 20th Ed. Chapter 304 Page 2103

A. Bence Jones protein
B. Tamm-Horsfall protein
C. C-reactive protein
D. Heat shock protein

Uromodulin, also known as Tamm-Horsfall protein, encoded by UMOD gene on chromosome 16, is exclusively produced in the kidney and is the most abundant protein in normal urine under physiological conditions.

1048. Tamm-Horsfall protein (uromodulin) is secreted by epithelial cells of?

Harrison's 20th Ed. Chapter 304 Page 2103

A. Proximal convoluted tubule
B. Loop of Henle
C. Distal convoluted tubule
D. All of the above

Tamm-Horsfall protein (uromodulin) is secreted by epithelial cells of the thick ascending limb of the loop of Henle.

1049. Which of the following is the pathophysiological hallmark of postrenal AKI?

Harrison's 20th Ed. Chapter 304 Page 2104

A. Abrupt increase in intratubular pressures
B. Compromised filtration barrier and blood flow
C. Damage to glomerular podocytes
D. Precipitation of proteins in renal tubules

The pathophysiology of postrenal AKI involves hemodynamic alterations triggered by an abrupt increase in intratubular pressures or increased retrograde hydrostatic pressure & interference with glomerular filtration.

1050. Which of the following point towards the presence of AKI?

Harrison's 20th Ed. Chapter 304 Page 2104

A. Rise in SCr from baseline of 0.3 mg/dL within 48 hours
B. At least 50% higher SCr than baseline within 1 week
C. Reduction in urine output to <0.5 mL/kg/hour for > 6 hours
D. All of the above

Presence of AKI is usually inferred by an elevation in SCr concentration. AKI is defined by a rise from baseline of at least 0.3 mg/dL within 48 hours or 50% higher than baseline within 1 week or a reduction in urine output to less than 0.5 mL/kg per hour for longer than 6 hours. Serial blood tests showing continued substantial rise of SCr represents clear evidence of AKI.

1051. Clue suggestive of CKD is?

Harrison's 20th Ed. Chapter 304 Page 2104

A. Small, shrunken kidneys with cortical thinning in USG
B. Evidence of renal osteodystrophy
C. Hyperphosphatemia and hypocalcemia
D. All of the above

Clues suggestive of CKD can come from radiologic studies (small, shrunken kidneys with cortical thinning on renal ultrasound or evidence of renal osteodystrophy) or laboratory tests such as normocytic anemia in the absence of blood loss or secondary hyperparathyroidism with hyperphosphatemia and hypocalcemia consistent with CKD.

1052. In AKI, presence of livedo reticularis points to the diagnosis of?

Harrison's 20th Ed. Chapter 304 Page 2104

A. Systemic vasculitis
B. Atheroembolic disease
C. Acute abdominal compartment syndrome
D. Rhabdomyolysis

Atheroembolic disease can be associated with livedo reticularis & other signs of emboli to legs.

1053. Which of the following is false about prerenal azotemia?

Harrison's 20th Ed. Chapter 304 Page 2105 Table 304-1

A. BUN/creatinine ratio > 20
B. FeNa < 1%
C. Urine osmolality > 500 mOsm/kg
D. None of the above

Response to restoration of hemodynamics is most diagnostic.

1054. Urine heme positive with few red blood cells is suggestive of?

Harrison's 20th Ed. Chapter 304 Page 2105 Table 304-1

A. Rhabdomyolysis
B. Hemolysis
C. Tumor lysis
D. Multiple myeloma

1055. Hyperphosphatemia, hypocalcemia, hyperuricemia are suggestive of?

Harrison's 20th Ed. Chapter 304 Page 2105 Table 304-1

A. Rhabdomyolysis
B. Hemolysis
C. Tumor lysis
D. Multiple myeloma

1056. Schistocytes on peripheral blood smear are suggestive of?

Harrison's 20th Ed. Chapter 304 Page 2105 Table 304-1

A. Atheroembolic disease
B. TTP/HUS
C. Glomerulonephritis/vasculitis
D. Hemolysis

"Typical HUS" refers to AKI with a diarrheal prodrome, due to Shiga toxin released from Escherichia coli. "Atypical HUS" constitutes the majority of adult cases of HUS and is due to inherited or acquired complement dysregulation. "TTP-HUS" refers to sporadic cases in adults.

1057. Eosinophilia & sterile pyuria is suggestive of?

Harrison's 20th Ed. Chapter 304 Page 2105 Table 304-1

A. Interstitial nephritis
B. Tubular injury
C. Glomerulonephritis/vasculitis
D. All of the above

1058. Hypocomplementemia & eosinophiluria is suggestive of?

Harrison's 20th Ed. Chapter 304 Page 2105 Table 304-1

A. Atheroembolic disease
B. TTP/HUS
C. Glomerulonephritis/vasculitis
D. Hemolysis

1059. Which of the following is a calcineurin inhibitor?

Harrison's 20th Ed. Chapter 304 Page 2105

A. Tacrolimus
B. Sirolimus
C. Everolimus
D. All of the above

CNI or calcineurin inhibitors include cyclosporine and tacrolimus. They have an afferent arteriolar constrictor effect on the kidney. They may cause TTP/HUS.

1060. Which of the following is a cause of complete anuria?

Harrison's 20th Ed. Chapter 304 Page 2106

A. Renal artery occlusion
B. Overwhelming septic shock
C. Severe proliferative glomerulonephritis
D. All of the above

Complete anuria early in the course of AKI is uncommon. It may however be seen in complete urinary tract obstruction, renal artery occlusion, overwhelming septic shock, severe ischemia (with cortical necrosis), or severe proliferative glomerulonephritis or vasculitis.

1061. Oliguria is defined as?

Harrison's 20th Ed. Chapter 304 Page 2106

A. Urine output < 100 mL/day
B. Urine output < 200 mL/day
C. Urine output < 300 mL/day
D. Urine output < 400 mL/day

Oliguria is defined as urine output of <400 mL/day contributing to extracellular fluid overload.

1062. Nephrogenic diabetes insipidus is characteristic of?
Harrison's 20th Ed. Chapter 304 Page 2106

A. Long-standing urinary tract obstruction
B. Tubulointerstitial disease
C. Nephrotoxicity from cisplatin or aminoglycosides
D. All of the above

Nephrogenic diabetes insipidus is characteristic of long-standing urinary tract obstruction, tubulointerstitial disease, or nephrotoxicity from cisplatin or aminoglycosides.

1063. Urine is strongly positive for heme by dipstick in?
Harrison's 20th Ed. Chapter 304 Page 2106

A. Hemoglobinuria
B. Hematuria
C. Myoglobinuria
D. All of the above

Urine is strongly positive for heme by dipstick in hemoglobinuria, hematuria & myoglobinuria. If the dipstick is positive for hemoglobin but few red blood cells are evident in the urine sediment, then rhabdomyolysis or hemolysis should be suspected.

1064. Pigmented "muddy brown" granular cast is characteristic of?
Harrison's 20th Ed. Chapter 304 Page 2106

A. Prerenal ARF
B. Ischemic or nephrotoxic ATN
C. Postrenal ARF
D. All of the above

Pigmented "muddy brown" granular cast is characteristic of ATN due to ischemic or nephrotoxic etiology. AKI from ATN due to ischemic injury, sepsis or certain nephrotoxins has characteristic urine sediment findings: pigmented "muddy brown" granular casts and tubular epithelial cell casts.

1065. Broad granular casts are characteristic of?
Harrison's 20th Ed. Chapter 304 Page 2106

A. Glomerular injury
B. Acute tubulointerstitial nephritis
C. Ischemic or nephrotoxic ATN
D. Chronic kidney disease

Broad granular casts are characteristic of chronic kidney disease.

1066. Oxalate crystal is best related with?
Harrison's 20th Ed. Chapter 304 Page 2106

A. Envelope-shaped
B. Needle-shaped
C. Round-shaped
D. Elliptical-shaped

The finding of oxalate crystals in AKI should prompt an evaluation for ethylene glycol toxicity.

1067. Hippurate crystal is best related with?
Harrison's 20th Ed. Chapter 304 Page 2106

A. Envelope-shaped
B. Needle-shaped
C. Round-shaped
D. Elliptical-shaped

Ethylene glycol toxicity causes oxalate (envelope-shaped) & hippurate (needle-shaped) crystals.

1068. Abundant uric acid crystals may be seen in?
Harrison's 20th Ed. Chapter 304 Page 2106

A. Atheroembolic disease
B. Cystitis
C. Tumor lysis syndrome
D. Ethylene glycol toxicity

Abundant uric acid crystals may be seen in the tumor lysis syndrome.

1069. In AKI, the rise in SCr is characteristically delayed in?
Harrison's 20th Ed. Chapter 304 Page 2107

A. Contrast nephropathy
B. Atheroembolic disease
C. Aminoglycoside antibiotics and cisplatin toxicity
D. All of the above

In aminoglycoside antibiotics and cisplatin toxicity, the rise in SCr is characteristically delayed for 3–5 days to 2 weeks after initial exposure.

1070. Which of the following cause kidney injury through intrarenal vasoconstriction?
Harrison's 20th Ed. Chapter 304 Page 2107

A. Radiocontrast agents
B. Cyclosporine
C. Tacrolimus
D. All of the above

Radiocontrast agents, cyclosporine & tacrolimus cause kidney injury through intrarenal vasoconstriction.

1071. In acute renal failure, systemic eosinophilia suggests?
Harrison's 20th Ed. Chapter 304 Page 2107

A. Allergic interstitial nephritis
B. Atheroembolic disease
C. Polyarteritis nodosa
D. All of the above

In acute renal failure, systemic eosinophilia suggests allergic interstitial nephritis, atheroembolic disease, polyarteritis nodosa and Churg-Strauss vasculitis. .

1072. Eosinophilia is found in which of the following causes of acute renal failure?
Harrison's 20th Ed. Chapter 304 Page 2107

A. Renal artery thrombosis
B. HUS/TTP
C. Hemolysis
D. Atheroembolic disease

Peripheral eosinophilia can accompany interstitial nephritis, atheroembolic disease, polyarteritis nodosa and Churg-Strauss vasculitis.

1073. Acute renal failure impairs which of the following?
Harrison's 20th Ed. Chapter 304 Page 2107

A. Renal excretion of sodium, potassium & water
B. Divalent cation homeostasis
C. Urinary acidification mechanisms
D. All of the above

ARF impairs renal excretion of sodium, potassium, and water and perturbs divalent cation homeostasis and urinary acidification mechanisms.

1074. In acute renal failure, severe anemia in the absence of hemorrhage suggests?

Harrison's 20th Ed. Chapter 304 Page 2107

A. Hemolysis
B. Multiple myeloma
C. Thrombotic microangiopathy
D. All of the above

In acute renal failure, severe anemia in the absence of hemorrhage suggests hemolysis, multiple myeloma, or thrombotic microangiopathy (HUS or TTP).

1075. Laboratory finding of thrombotic microangiopathy is?

Harrison's 20th Ed. Chapter 304 Page 2107

A. Schistocytes on peripheral blood smear
B. Elevated lactate dehydrogenase level
C. Low haptoglobin content
D. All of the above

Laboratory findings of thrombotic microangiopathy include thrombocytopenia, schistocytes on peripheral blood smear, elevated lactate dehydrogenase level and low haptoglobin content.

1076. Increased serum LDH is found in which of the following causes of acute renal failure?

Harrison's 20th Ed. Chapter 304 Page 2107

A. Renal artery thrombosis
B. HUS/TTP
C. Hemolysis
D. All of the above

Increased serum LDH is found in acute renal failure due to renal artery, HUS/TTP, thrombosis, hemolysis, acute urate nephropathy & tumor lysis syndrome.

1077. AKI leads to which of the following?

Harrison's 20th Ed. Chapter 304 Page 2107

A. Hyperkalemia
B. Hyperphosphatemia
C. Hypocalcemia
D. All of the above

AKI leads to hyperkalemia, hyperphosphatemia, and hypocalcemia.

1078. Which of the following occur in tumor lysis syndrome?

Harrison's 20th Ed. Chapter 304 Page 2107

A. Marked hyperphosphatemia
B. Normal or marginally elevated creatine kinase
C. Markedly elevated serum uric acid
D. All of the above

AKI causes hyperkalemia, hyperphosphatemia and hypocalcemia. Marked hyperphosphatemia with accompanying hypocalcemia suggests rhabdomyolysis or tumor lysis syndrome. Creatine phosphokinase levels & serum uric acid are elevated in rhabdomyolysis, while tumor lysis syndrome shows normal or marginally elevated creatine kinase and markedly elevated serum uric acid.

1079. High titers of which of the following is seen in glomerulonephritis and vasculitis?

Harrison's 20th Ed. Chapter 304 Page 2107

A. Antineutrophil cytoplasmic antibodies (ANCAs)
B. Antiglomerular basement membrane (Anti-GBM) antibodies
C. Cryoglobulins
D. All of the above

Findings in glomerulonephritis and vasculitis include depressed complement levels and high titers of antinuclear antibodies (ANAs), antineutrophil cytoplasmic antibodies (ANCAs), antiglomerular basement membrane (Anti-GBM) antibodies, and cryoglobulins.

1080. Disproportionate BUN elevation is seen in?

Harrison's 20th Ed. Chapter 304 Page 2107

A. Upper gastrointestinal bleeding
B. Hyperalimentation
C. Glucocorticoid use
D. All of the above

Disproportionate BUN elevation is seen in upper gastrointestinal bleeding, hyperalimentation, increased tissue catabolism and glucocorticoid use. This is due to low tubular flow rate and increased renal medullary recycling of urea seen in prerenal azotemia.

1081. Hypocomplementemia is found in which of the following causes of acute renal failure?

Harrison's 20th Ed. Chapter 304 Page 2107

A. Renal artery thrombosis
B. Ethylene glycol ingestion
C. Multiple myeloma
D. Atheroembolic disease

1082. Fractional excretion of sodium (FE_{Na}) is calculated as?

Lancet 2005;365:417-430

A. [(Urine sodium × Plasma sodium)÷ (Plasma creatinine × urine creatinine)] × 100
B. [(Urine creatinine × Plasma creatinine)÷ (Plasma sodium × Urine sodium)] × 100
C. [(Urine sodium × Urine creatinine)÷ (Plasma sodium × Plasma creatinine)] × 100
D. [(Urine sodium × Plasma creatinine)÷ (Plasma sodium × Urine creatinine)] × 100

The fractional excretion of sodium (FeNa) is the fraction of the filtered sodium load that is reabsorbed by the tubules and is a measure of both the kidney's ability to reabsorb sodium as well as endogenously and exogenously administered factors that affect tubular reabsorption. FE_{Na} relates sodium clearance to creatinine clearance. Patients with prerenal ARF typically have a FE_{Na} of <1.0%. FE_{Na} may be >1.0% in prerenal ARF if patients are on diuretics or with preexisting CKD, salt-wasting syndromes or adrenal insufficiency. In ischemic AKI, the FeNa is above 1% because of tubular injury and resultant inability to reabsorb sodium.

1083. FeNa depends on?

Harrison's 20th Ed. Chapter 304 Page 2107

A. Sodium intake
B. Effective intravascular volume
C. GFR
D. All of the above

FeNa depends on sodium intake, effective intravascular volume, GFR, diuretic intake and intact tubular reabsorptive mechanisms. Low FeNa is suggestive, but not synonymous, with effective intravascular volume depletion.

1084. FeNa below 1% may be present in?

Harrison's 20th Ed. Chapter 304 Page 2107

A. Early sepsis
B. Rhabdomyolysis
C. Contrast nephropathy
D. All of the above

FeNa below 1% may be present in sepsis (often early in the course), rhabdomyolysis and contrast nephropathy.

1085. Kidney size may be increased in which of the following chronic renal diseases?

Harrison's 20th Ed. Chapter 304 Page 2107

A. Diabetic nephropathy
B. Amyloidosis
C. HIV associated nephropathy
D. All of the above

Kidney size may be normal or increased in diabetic nephropathy, amyloidosis, polycystic kidney disease and HIV associated nephropathy.

1086. Enlarged kidneys in a patient with AKI suggests?

Harrison's 20th Ed. Chapter 304 Page 2107

A. Acute interstitial nephritis
B. Multiple myeloma
C. HIV -associated nephropathy
D. Rhabdomyolysis

Enlarged kidneys in a patient with AKI suggests acute interstitial nephritis.

1087. Nephrogenic system fibrosis (NSF) is best related to?

Harrison's 20th Ed. Chapter 304 Page 2107

A. Renal artery thrombosis
B. Ethylene glycol ingestion
C. Gadolinium-based contrast agent
D. Multiple myeloma

MRI with gadolinium-based contrast agents should be avoided in severe AKI due to the possibility of inducing nephrogenic system fibrosis.

1088. Kidney biopsy is avoided when the probable diagnosis is?

Harrison's 20th Ed. Chapter 304 Page 2107

A. Prerenal azotemia
B. Postrenal AKI
C. Ischemic or nephrotoxic AKI
D. All of the above

1089. In oliguric AKI, what urinary flow rate after IV furosemide identifies patients at higher risk of progression to severe AKI?

Harrison's 20th Ed. Chapter 304 Page 2107

A. < 100 mL over 1 hour
B. < 200 mL over 1 hour
C. < 100 mL over 2 hour
D. < 200 mL over 2 hour

In cases of oliguric AKI, in response to bolus intravenous furosemide (1.0 - 1.5 mg/kg), urine output of < 200 mL over 2 hour may identify patients at higher risk of progression to more severe AKI, and the need for renal replacement therapy.

1090. Which of the following observation is associated with severity and worsening of AKI?

Harrison's 20th Ed. Chapter 304 Page 2107

A. Inadequate response to bolus intravenous furosemide
B. ↑ed renal tubular epithelial cells in urine sediment
C. ↑ed granular casts in urine sediment
D. All of the above

1091. Which of the following about kidney injury molecule-1 (KIM-1) is false?

Harrison's 20th Ed. Chapter 304 Page 2108

A. Type 1 transmembrane protein with two extracellular domains
B. Expressed in injured proximal tubular cells
C. Not expressed in extrarenal tissues
D. None of the above

Kidney injury molecule-1 (KIM-1) is a type 1 transmembrane protein that is abundantly expressed in proximal tubular cells (S3 segment) injured by ischemia or nephrotoxins. KIM-1 is not expressed in the absence of tubular injury or in extrarenal tissues. Its role is to confer phagocytic properties to tubular cells, enabling them to clear debris from tubular lumen after kidney injury. KIM-1 can be detected shortly after ischemic or nephrotoxic injury in urine. Urinary KIM-1 can be used as a specific biomarker for early diagnosis of AKI.

1092. Which of the following about Neutrophil gelatinase associated lipocalin (NGAL) is false?

Harrison's 20th Ed. Chapter 304 Page 2108

A. Also known as lipocalin-2 or siderocalin
B. Binds to iron siderophore complexes & protects proximal tubule
C. Upregulated after inflammation and kidney injury
D. None of the above

Neutrophil gelatinase associated lipocalin (NGAL, also known as lipocalin-2 or siderocalin) is another novel biomarker of AKI. It was first discovered as a protein in granules of human neutrophils. NGAL can bind to iron siderophore complexes and may have tissue-protective effects in the proximal tubule. NGAL is highly upregulated after inflammation and kidney injury and can be detected in the plasma and urine within 2 hours of cardiopulmonary bypass-associated AKI.

1093. Which of the following is a biomarker of AKI?

Harrison's 20th Ed. Chapter 304 Page 2108

A. Neutrophil gelatinase associated lipocalin (NGAL)
B. Insulin-like growth factor binding protein 7 (IGFBP7)
C. Tissue inhibitor of metalloproteinase-2 (TIMP-2)
D. All of the above

1094. Which of the following is a biomarker of AKI?

Harrison's 20th Ed. Chapter 304 Page 2108

A. Neutrophil gelatinase associated lipocalin (NGAL)
B. Interleukin (IL) 18
C. Kidney injury molecule-1 (KIM-1)
D. All of the above

Other biomarkers of AKI include interleukin (IL) 18, a proinflammatory cytokine of the IL-1 superfamily that may mediate ischemic proximal tubular injury and L-type fatty acid binding protein, which is expressed in ischemic proximal tubule cells and may be renoprotective by binding free fatty acids and lipid peroxidation products.

1095. Which of the following is the hallmark of AKI?

Harrison's 20th Ed. Chapter 304 Page 2108

A. Elevated BUN concentration
B. Elevated creatine concentration
C. Oliguria
D. Impaired salt and water excretion

Buildup of nitrogenous waste products, manifested as an elevated BUN concentration, is a hallmark of AKI.

1096. BUN itself poses little direct toxicity at levels below?
Harrison's 20th Ed. Chapter 304 Page 2108

A. 10 mg/dL
B. 30 mg/dL
C. 70 mg/dL
D. 100 mg/dL

BUN itself poses little direct toxicity at levels below 100 mg/dL. At higher concentrations, mental status changes and bleeding complications arise. Other toxins normally cleared by the kidney may be responsible for the symptom complex known as uremia.

1097. Urine output is lowest in which of the following phases of ischemic ATN?
Harrison's 20th Ed. Chapter 304 Page 2109

A. Initiation
B. Extension
C. Maintenance
D. Recovery

During maintenance phase that lasts for 1–2 weeks, urine output is lowest due to reduced GFR and uremic complications may appear.

1098. Diuresis occurs in which of the following phases of ischemic ATN?
Harrison's 20th Ed. Chapter 304 Page 2109

A. Initiation
B. Extension
C. Maintenance
D. Recovery

Diuresis occurs in the recovery phase. Recovery from AKI can be accompanied by polyuria which if untreated can lead to significant volume depletion. The polyuric phase of recovery may be due to an osmotic diuresis from retained urea and other waste products as well as delayed recovery of tubular reabsorptive functions.

1099. Which of the following can occur during recovery phase of ARF?
Harrison's 20th Ed. Chapter 304 Page 2109

A. Hypernatremia
B. Hypokalemia
C. Hypophosphatemia
D. All of the above

Vigorous diuresis during recovery phase of ARF may lead to intravascular volume depletion causing hypernatremia, hypokalemia, hypomagnesemia, hypophosphatemia and hypocalcemia.

1100. Which of the following is not a feature of AKI?
Harrison's 20th Ed. Chapter 304 Page 2109

A. Hyperphosphatemia
B. Hypocalcemia
C. Hypomagnesemia
D. Metabolic acidosis

ARF is complicated by hyponatremia, hyperkalemia, hyperphosphatemia, hypocalcemia, hypermagnesemia and metabolic acidosis.

1101. Hyperkalemia in AKI is severe in?
Harrison's 20th Ed. Chapter 304 Page 2109

A. Rhabdomyolysis
B. Hemolysis
C. Tumor lysis syndrome
D. All of the above

Hyperkalemia in acute renal failure may be severe in patients with rhabdomyolysis, hemolysis, and tumor lysis syndrome due to release of intracellular potassium from damaged cells.

1102. Hyperphosphatemia in AKI is severe in?
Harrison's 20th Ed. Chapter 304 Page 2109

A. Rhabdomyolysis
B. Hemolysis
C. Tumor lysis syndrome
D. All of the above

AKI can lead to hyperphosphatemia, particularly in highly catabolic patients or those with AKI from rhabdomyolysis, hemolysis and tumor lysis syndrome. Metastatic deposition of calcium phosphate leads to hypocalcemia apart from derangements in vitamin D-parathyroid hormone-fibroblast growth factor-23 axis.

1103. Which of the following is a major complication of AKI?
Harrison's 20th Ed. Chapter 304 Page 2109

A. Anemia and bleeding
B. Arrhythmias, pericarditis and pericardial effusion
C. Infections
D. All of the above

Direct hematologic effects from AKI-related uremia include decreased erythropoiesis and platelet dysfunction. Major cardiac complications of AKI are arrhythmias, pericarditis and pericardial effusion. Infections are a dreaded complication of AKI. Direct hematologic effects from AKI-related uremia include decreased erythropoiesis and platelet dysfunction.

1104. AKI due to scleroderma (scleroderma renal crisis) should be treated with?
Harrison's 20th Ed. Chapter 304 Page 2109

A. Terlipressin
B. Octreotide
C. Midodrine
D. ACE inhibitors

AKI due to scleroderma (scleroderma renal crisis) should be treated with ACE inhibitors.

1105. Which of the following is a phosphate binder?
Harrison's 20th Ed. Chapter 304 Page 2110

A. Lanthanum
B. Sevelamer
C. Aluminum hydroxide
D. All of the above

1106. Which of the following is an oral phosphate binder?
Harrison's 20th Ed. Chapter 304 Page 2110

A. Calcium carbonate
B. Calcium acetate
C. Aluminum hydroxide
D. All of the above

Hyperphosphatemia is common in AKI and can usually be treated by limiting intestinal absorption of phosphate using phosphate binders (calcium carbonate, calcium acetate, lanthanum, sevelamer, or aluminum hydroxide).

1107. Absolute indication for dialysis in ARF is?
Harrison's 20th Ed. Chapter 304 Page 2110

A. Uremic syndrome
B. Hyperkalemia
C. Acidosis
D. All of the above

Absolute indications for dialysis are symptoms or signs of uremic syndrome, refractory hypervolemia, hyperkalemia, or acidosis.

1108. In patients of AKI on dialysis, what is the recommended protein intake?

Harrison's 20th Ed. Chapter 304 Page 2110

A. 0.1–0.4 gram/kg per day
B. 0.4–0.8 gram/kg per day
C. 0.8–1.0 gram/kg per day
D. 1.0–1.5 gram/kg per day

According to the Kidney Disease Improving Global Outcomes (KDIGO) guidelines, patients with AKI should get a total energy intake of 20–30 kcal/kg per day. Protein intake should vary depending on the severity of AKI : 0.8–1.0 g/kg per day in noncatabolic AKI without the need for dialysis; 1.0–1.5 g/kg per day in patients on dialysis; and up to a maximum of 1.7 g/kg per day if hypercatabolic and receiving continuous renal replacement therapy.

1109. Uremic bleeding may respond to administration of?

Harrison's 20th Ed. Chapter 304 Page 2110

A. Desmopressin
B. Estrogens
C. Dialysis
D. All of the above

Uremic bleeding may respond to desmopressin, estrogens or dialysis.

1110. Severe complications of uremia include?

Harrison's 20th Ed. Chapter 304 Page 2110

A. Pericardial rub or effusion
B. Encephalopathy
C. Uremic bleeding
D. All of the above

Severe complications of uremia include asterixis, pericardial rub or effusion, encephalopathy and uremic bleeding. The initiation of dialysis should not await the development of a life-threatening complication of renal failure.

1111. Continuous renal replacement therapy (CRRT) is preferred in patients with?

Harrison's 20th Ed. Chapter 304 Page 2110

A. Severe hemodynamic instability
B. Cerebral edema
C. Significant volume overload
D. All of the above

CRRT is preferred in patients with severe hemodynamic instability, cerebral edema or significant volume overload.

1112. Which of the following prolong QT interval?

Harrison's 20th Ed. Chapter 304 Page 2110

A. Quinidine
B. Subarachnoid hemorrhage
C. Hypocalcemia
D. All of the above

1113. "Sine-wave" pattern in ECG is seen in?

Harrison's 20th Ed. Chapter 304 Page 2110

A. Hypokalemia
B. Hyperkalemia
C. Hypercalcemia
D. Hypothermia

1114. Which of the following may prevent or attenuate ARF?

Lancet 2005;365:417-430

A. Allopurinol
B. Forced alkaline diuresis
C. Rasburicase
D. All of the above

Allopurinol, forced alkaline diuresis, Rasburicase, N-acetylcysteine help in preventing development of ARF due to various causes.

1115. In acute renal failure, mortality is high when there is?

Lancet 2005;365:417-430

A. Multiorgan failure
B. High concentration of TNF-α
C. Low production of interleukin 10
D. All of the above

1116. Which of the following is a "salt-wasting nephropathy"?

Lancet 2005;365:417-430

A. Chronic pyelonephritis
B. Polycystic disease
C. Medullary cystic disease
D. All of the above

1117. To convert the values for urea nitrogen to millimoles/liter, multiply by?

A. 0.157
B. 0.257
C. 0.357
D. 0.457

1118. To convert the values for creatinine to micromoles/liter, multiply by?

A. 68.4
B. 78.4
C. 88.4
D. 98.4

1119. To convert the values for glucose to millimoles per liter, multiply by?

A. 0.4551
B. 0.5551
C. 0.6551
D. 0.7551

1120. To convert the values for calcium to millimoles per liter, multiply by?

A. 0.150
B. 0.250
C. 0.350
D. 0.450

1121. To convert the values for phosphorus to millimoles per liter, multiply by?

A. 0.1229
B. 0.2229
C. 0.3229
D. 0.4229

1122. To convert the values for magnesium to millimoles per liter, multiply by?

A. 0.200
B. 0.300
C. 0.400
D. 0.500

Chronic Kidney Disease

1123. The risk of CKD progression is closely linked to?
Harrison's 20th Ed. Chapter 305 Page 2111

A. Albuminuria
B. Urine output
C. Age
D. All of the above

The risk of CKD progression is closely linked to both - GFR and amount of albuminuria.

1124. Chronic kidney disease (CKD) is defined as?
Kidney International Supplements. 2018;8:91-165

A. Abnormalities of kidney structure or function
B. Present for >3 months
C. Implications for health
D. All of the above

1125. CKD is classified based on?
Kidney International Supplements. 2018;8:91-165

A. Cause
B. GFR
C. Albuminuria
D. All of the above

CKD is defined as abnormalities of kidney structure or function, present for >3 months, with implications for health. CKD is classified based on cause, GFR category (G1–G5), and albuminuria category (A1–A3), abbreviated as CGA.

1126. Chronic kidney disease (CKD) is divided into how many stages by Kidney Disease Improving Global Outcome (KDIGO)?
Harrison's 20th Ed. Chapter 305 Page 2111

A. 3
B. 4
C. 5
D. 6

CKD is divided into six stages by Kidney Disease Improving Global Outcome (KDIGO 2012) which CKD stratified by both estimated GFR and the degree of albuminuria, in order to predict risk of progression of CKD.

1127. Chronic renal failure typically corresponds to which of the following CKD stages?
Harrison's 20th Ed. Chapter 305 Page 2111

A. 1–3
B. 2–4
C. 3–5
D. 4–5

Term CRF applies to the process of continuing significant irreversible reduction in nephron number and typically corresponds to CKD stages 3–5.

1128. End-stage renal disease denotes which stage of CKD?
Harrison's 20th Ed. Chapter 305 Page 2111

A. 2
B. 3
C. 4
D. 5

End-stage renal disease denotes stage 5 of CKD.

1129. Factors that increase the risk for CKD include?
Harrison's 20th Ed. Chapter 305 Page 2111

A. Small for gestation birth weight
B. Childhood obesity
C. Family history of kidney disease
D. All of the above

Factors that increase the risk for CKD include small for gestation birth weight, childhood obesity, hypertension, diabetes mellitus, autoimmune disease, advanced age, African ancestry, family history of kidney disease, previous episode of acute kidney injury and the presence of proteinuria, abnormal urinary sediment or structural abnormalities of the urinary tract.

1130. Which of the following genes is associated with CKD?
Harrison's 20th Ed. Chapter 305 Page 2111

A. APOL1
B. APOE
C. ROSA26
D. MTHFR

1131. Normal annual mean decline in GFR with age is?
Harrison's 20th Ed. Chapter 305 Page 2111

A. ~1 mL/min per year per 1.73 m^2
B. ~1.5 mL/min per year per 1.73 m^2
C. ~2 mL/min per year per 1.73 m^2
D. ~2.5 mL/min per year per 1.73 m^2

1132. Mean value of GFR at the age of 70 years is?
Harrison's 20th Ed. Chapter 305 Page 2111

A. 70 mL/min per 1.73 m^2
B. 80 mL/min per 1.73 m^2
C. 90 mL/min per 1.73 m^2
D. 100 mL/min per 1.73 m^2

Normal annual mean decline in GFR with age is ~1 mL/min per year per 1.73 m^2, reaching a mean value of 70 mL/min per 1.73 m^2 at the age of 70 years.

1133. What is the GFR value (mL/min per 1.73 m^2) in stage 5 of chronic kidney disease (CKD)?
Harrison's 20th Ed. Chapter 305 Page 2112 Figure 305-1

A. < 15
B. 15–29
C. 30–59
D. 60–89

GFR in CKD (mL/min per 1.73 m^2) - Stage G1 = >90, stage G2 = 60–89, stage G3a = 45–59, stage G3b = 30–44, stage G4 = 15–29 and stage G5 = <15.

1134. Modification of Diet in Renal Disease (MDRD) formula for estimating GFR (mL/min per 1.73 m^2) is?
Harrison's 20th Ed. Chapter 305 Page 2113 Table 305-1

A. $1.56 \times (S_{Cr})^{-1.154} \times (age)^{-0.203}$
B. $1.66 \times (S_{Cr})^{-1.154} \times (age)^{-0.203}$
C. $1.76 \times (S_{Cr})^{-1.154} \times (age)^{-0.203}$
D. $1.86 \times (S_{Cr})^{-1.154} \times (age)^{-0.203}$

1135. Cockcroft-Gault equation for estimating creatinine clearance (ml/minute) is?

Harrison's 19th Ed. 1813 Table 335-1

A. (120-age × body weight in kg)/(72 × plasma creatinine)

B. (130-age × body weight in kg)/(72 × plasma creatinine)

C. (140-age × body weight in kg)/(72 × plasma creatinine)

D. (150-age × body weight in kg)/(72 × plasma creatinine)

1136. In the Chronic Kidney Disease Epidemiology Collaboration (CKD-EPI) equation, what is the value of constant K for males?

Harrison's 20th Ed. Chapter 305 Page 2113 Table 305-1

A. 0.3

B. 0.5

C. 0.7

D. 0.9

CKD-EPI Equation for GFR = $141 \times \min(S_{Cr}/\kappa, 1)^{\alpha} \times \max(S_{Cr}/\kappa, 1)^{-1.209} \times 0.993^{Age}$. Constant κ is 0.7 for females and 0.9 for males. α is –0.329 for females and –0.411 for males.

1137. Cockcroft - Gault equation is used for estimation of?

Harrison's 19th Ed. 1813

A. Urinary anion gap

B. Serum anion gap

C. Glomeruler filtration rate (GFR)

D. Fractional excretion of sodium

1138. Modification of Diet in Renal Disease (MDRD) equation is used for estimation of?

Harrison's 20th Ed. Chapter 305 Page 2113 Table 305-1

A. Urinary anion gap

B. Serum anion gap

C. Glomeruler filtration rate (GFR)

D. Fractional excretion of sodium

1139. Which of the following is a biomarker for prediction of first major cardiovascular events and death?

N Engl J Med. 2006; 355:2631-2639

A. C-reactive protein

B. B-type natriuretic peptide

C. Aldosterone

D. All of the above

1140. Which of the following is a biomarker for prediction of first major cardiovascular events and death?

N Engl J Med. 2006; 355:2631-2639

A. Renin

B. D-dimer

C. Urinary albumin-to-creatinine ratio

D. All of the above

Biomarkers for prediction of first major cardiovascular events and death include C-reactive protein, B-type natriuretic peptide, N-terminal pro–atrial natriuretic peptide, aldosterone, renin, fibrinogen, D-dimer, plasminogen-activator inhibitor type 1, lipoprotein-associated phospholipase A_2, homocysteine and urinary albumin-to-creatinine ratio.

1141. Which of the following is a biomarker of neurohormonal activity?

N Engl J Med. 2006; 355:2631-2639

A. B-type natriuretic peptide

B. Serum aldosterone

C. Plasma renin

D. All of the above

C-reactive protein is a marker of inflammation. B-type natriuretic peptide, N-terminal pro–atrial natriuretic peptide, serum aldosterone, and plasma renin are markers of neurohormonal activity. Fibrinogen is a marker of thrombosis & inflammation. Plasminogen-activator inhibitor type 1 is a marker of fibrinolytic potential & endothelial function. D-dimer is a marker of thrombosis. Homocysteine is a marker of endothelial function and oxidant stress. Urinary albumin-to-creatinine ratio is a marker of glomerular endothelial function.

1142. Which of the following about urinary albumin & creatinine excretion in healthy individuals is false?

N Engl J Med. 2006; 355:2631-2639

A. Average daily urinary protein excretion in adults is 80 mg/day

B. Albumin represents ~15% of daily urinary protein excretion

C. Creatinine excretion is ~ 1 gram per 1.73 m^2 BSA

D. None of the above

Average daily urinary protein excretion in adults is 80 mg/day, with normal excretion considered to be <150 mg/day. Albumin represents ~15% of daily urinary protein excretion in healthy people, with other plasma proteins (e.g., immunoglobulins, beta-2-microglobulin) and Tamm-Horsfall protein constituting the remaining 85%. Urinary excretion of abnormal quantities of protein for ≥3 months, with or without a decrease in glomerular filtration rate (GFR), is diagnostic of chronic kidney disease.

1143. Which of the following hypothesis relates diabetes and cardiovascular disease?

Diabetes. 1995 Apr;44(4):369-74

A. Knudson two-hit hypothesis

B. The "common soil" hypothesis

C. Threshold hypothesis

D. Grandmother hypothesis

Unlike classical microvascular complications, large-vessel atherosclerosis can precede development of diabetes, suggesting that rather than atherosclerosis being a complication of diabetes, both conditions have common genetic & environmental antecedents, i.e., they spring from a "common soil." (Stern, 1995).

1144. Which of the following about urinary albumin excretion (UAE) is false?

J Am Heart Assoc. 2016;5:e003245

A. Normoalbuminuria is <30 mg/day or UACR <30 mg/g

B. Microalbuminuria is 30–300 mg/day or UACR 30–300 mg/g

C. Macroalbuminuria is >300 mg/day or UACR >300 mg/g

D. None of the above

Urinary albumin excretion is classified as normoalbuminuria (<30 mg/day or UACR <30 mg/g), microalbuminuria (30–300 mg/day or UACR 30–300 mg/g), and macroalbuminuria (>300 mg/day or UACR >300 mg/g).

1145. In men, what value of urinary albumin to creatinine ratio (UACR) is indicative of primary kidney disease?

Harrison's 20th Ed. Chapter 305 Page 2111

A. > 4 mg albumin/gram creatinine

B. > 7 mg albumin/gram creatinine

C. > 12 mg albumin/gram creatinine

D. > 17 mg albumin/gram creatinine

1146. In women, what value of urinary albumin to creatinine ratio (UACR) is indicative of primary kidney disease?

Harrison's 20th Ed. Chapter 305 Page 2111

A. > 14 mg albumin/gram creatinine
B. > 20 mg albumin/gram creatinine
C. > 25 mg albumin/gram creatinine
D. > 33 mg albumin/gram creatinine

UACR above 17 mg albumin/gram creatinine in men and 25 mg albumin/gram creatinine in women serves as a marker for early detection of primary kidney disease, systemic microvascular disease & endothelial dysfunction.

1147. Out of the following, which is the most common cause of chronic kidney disease?

Harrison's 20th Ed. Chapter 305 Page 2113

A. Diabetes mellitus
B. Hypertension
C. Glomerulonephritis
D. Cystic kidney disease

Most frequent cause of CKD is diabetic nephropathy, secondary to type 2 diabetes mellitus. Hypertensive nephropathy is a common cause of CKD in the elderly.

1148. Uremic "Toxins" include?

Harrison's 20th Ed. Chapter 305 Page 2113

A. By-products of protein & amino acid metabolism
B. End products of aliphatic amine metabolism
C. End products of aromatic amino acid metabolism
D. All of the above

1149. Uremic "Toxins" include?

Harrison's 20th Ed. Chapter 305 Page 2113

A. Urea
B. Creatine
C. Urates and hippurates
D. All of the above

Apart from the above ones, PTH is also a uremic toxin.

1150. Which of the following is a nitrogenous excretory product?

Harrison's 20th Ed. Chapter 305 Page 2113

A. Polyamines
B. Myoinositol
C. Phenols
D. All of the above

1151. Which of the following is a nitrogenous excretory product?

Harrison's 20th Ed. Chapter 305 Page 2113

A. Benzoates
B. Indoles
C. Phenols
D. All of the above

Hundreds of toxins that accumulate in renal failure have been implicated in the uremic syndrome. These include water-soluble, hydrophobic, protein-bound, charged and uncharged compounds. Additional categories of nitrogenous excretory products include guanidino compounds, urates and hippurates, products of nucleic acid metabolism, polyamines, myoinositol, phenols, benzoates and indoles.

1152. Which of the following dysfunctions occur in uremic syndrome?

Harrison's 20th Ed. Chapter 305 Page 2113

A. Renal excretory failure
B. Progressive systemic inflammation
C. Loss of hormone regulation
D. All of the above

Uremic syndrome manifests as accumulation of toxins due to renal excretory failure, loss of fluid & electrolyte homeostasis & hormone regulation and progressive systemic inflammation with vascular & nutritional consequences.

1153. Plasma levels of which of the following hormones rise with renal failure?

Harrison's 20th Ed. Chapter 305 Page 2113

A. Parathyroid hormone (PTH)
B. Prolactin
C. Luteinizing hormone
D. All of the above

Plasma levels of many hormones like PTH, FGF-23, insulin, glucagon, steroid hormones including vitamin D and sex hormones and prolactin change in CKD as a result of reduced excretion, decreased degradation or abnormal regulation.

1154. Which of the following is not a negative acute-phase reactant?

Harrison's 20th Ed. Chapter 305 Page 2113

A. Transthyretin
B. Fetuin (AHSG)
C. Albumin
D. Fibrinogen

Fetuin (AHSG), a glycoprotein is synthesized by hepatocytes & is present in the circulation. It has the highest capacity of inhibiting soft tissue calcification.

1155. Which of the following is an acute-phase reactant?

Harrison's 20th Ed. Chapter 305 Page 2113

A. Thrombocytosis
B. Serum amyloid A (SAA)
C. Ferritin
D. All of the above

1156. Which of the following is a loop diuretic?

Harrison's 20th Ed. Chapter 305 Page 2114

A. Furosemide
B. Bumetanide
C. Torsemide
D. All of the above

1157. Combination with which of the following provides a synergistic effect in patients receiving long-term therapy with loop diuretic agents?

Harrison's 20th Ed. Chapter 305 Page 2114

A. Metolazone
B. Chlorthalidone
C. Spironolactone
D. Acetazolamide

Metolazone in combination provides a synergistic effect and is often required in patients receiving long-term therapy with loop diuretic agents. Resistance to loop diuretics in CKD often mandates use of higher doses than those used in patients with higher GFR. The combination of loop diuretics with metolazone may be helpful.

1158. In CKD, hyperkalemia may be precipitated by?
Harrison's 20th Ed. Chapter 305 Page 2114

A. Hemolysis
B. Transfusion of stored red blood cells
C. Metabolic acidosis
D. All of the above

1159. Which of the following is a potassium-sparing diuretic?
Harrison's 20th Ed. Chapter 305 Page 2114

A. Amiloride
B. Eplerenone
C. Triamterene
D. All of the above

1160. Which of the following inhibits sodium chloride co-transporter of the distal convoluted tubule?
Harrison's 20th Ed. Chapter 305 Page 2114

A. Amiloride
B. Eplerenone
C. Metolazone
D. All of the above

Metolazone inhibits the sodium chloride co-transporter of the distal convoluted tubule. It promotes renal salt excretion.

1161. Which of the following is involved in CKD with earlier & more severe disruption of K^+-secretory mechanisms?
Harrison's 20th Ed. Chapter 305 Page 2114

A. Glomerulus
B. Proximal tubule
C. Loop of Henle
D. Distal tubule

CKD can be associated with earlier & more severe disruption of K^+-secretory mechanisms in distal nephron, out of proportion to the decline in GFR.

1162. Which of the following preferentially affects distal nephron?
Harrison's 20th Ed. Chapter 305 Page 2114

A. Diabetic nephropathy
B. Sickle cell nephropathy
C. HIV nephropathy
D. Polycystic kidney disease

Obstructive uropathy & sickle cell nephropathy preferentially affect the distal nephron.

1163. Which of the following leads to hyporeninemic hypoaldosteronism?
Harrison's 20th Ed. Chapter 305 Page 2114

A. Diabetes mellitus
B. Obstructive uropathy
C. Sickle cell nephropathy
D. All of the above

In CKD, potassium levels may rise out of proportion to decline in GFR in conditions that lead to hyporeninemic hypoaldosteronism like diabetes, obstructive uropathy & sickle cell nephropathy.

1164. Which of the following promotes potassium loss through the GI tract?
Harrison's 20th Ed. Chapter 305 Page 2114

A. Calcium resonium
B. Sodium polystyrene
C. Patiromer
D. All of the above

Potassium-binding resins like calcium resonium, sodium polystyrene or patiromer promote potassium loss through the GI tract and may reduce the incidence of hyperkalemia in CKD.

1165. In adult males, persistence in urine of how much albumin per gram of creatinine signifies chronic renal damage?
Harrison's 20th Ed. Chapter 305 Page 2111

A. > 11 mg
B. > 13 mg
C. > 15 mg
D. > 17 mg

1166. In adult females, persistence in urine of how much albumin per gram of creatinine signifies chronic renal damage?
Harrison's 20th Ed. Chapter 305 Page 2111

A. > 18 mg
B. > 21 mg
C. > 23 mg
D. > 25 mg

Persistence in urine of >17 mg of albumin per gram of creatinine in adult males and 25 mg albumin per gram of creatinine in adult females signifies CKD.

1167. Which of the following suggests chronic kidney disease?

A. Anemia
B. Evidence of renal osteodystrophy
C. Small scarred kidneys
D. All of the above

Findings that suggest chronic kidney disease include anemia, evidence of renal osteodystrophy (radiologic or laboratory) and small scarred kidneys.

1168. A persistent reduction in GFR to less than what level per minute per 1.73 m² is defined as chronic kidney disease?
Lancet 2005;365:417-430

A. 60 mL
B. 70 mL
C. 80 mL
D. 90 mL

1169. In a case of CRF, oral acetylcysteine with hydration significantly lowers the risk of?
Lancet 2005;365:417-430

A. Contrast nephropathy
B. Uremic pericarditis
C. Uremic encephalopathy
D. All of the above

1170. Most rapid way to remove potassium in severe hyperkalemia is?
Lancet 2005;365:417-430

A. Intravenous calcium
B. Infusion of glucose & insulin
C. Na–K exchange resin (sodium polystyrene sulfonate)
D. Hemodialysis

Nephrology

1171. Decreased GFR occurs due to?

Lancet 2005;365:417-430

A. Reduced glomerular hydraulic pressure
B. Elevated Bowman's space hydraulic pressure
C. Rise in plasma colloid osmotic pressure
D. All of the above

1172. Decreased GFR occurs due to?

Lancet 2005;365:417-430

A. Reduced glomerular blood flow
B. Reduced glomerular permeability
C. Diminished filtration surface area
D. All of the above

1173. The molecular weight of inulin is about?

Lancet 2005;365:417-430

A. 4800
B. 5000
C. 5200
D. 5400

Molecular weight of inulin is ~5200. It pass freely across glomerular filtration barrier, appearing at approximately the same concentration in Bowman's space as in plasma.

1174. Which of the following is curve A-type solute?

Lancet 2005;365:417-430

A. Sodium
B. Urate
C. Urea
D. All of the above

Curve A-type solutes include urea and creatinine. These depend largely on glomerular filtration for urinary excretion. Their secretion contributes little to overall excretion. The clinical course of CRF usually also approximates curve A.

1175. Which of the following are curve B-type solutes?

Lancet 2005;365:417-430

A. Phosphate (PO_4^{3-})
B. Urate
C. Potassium & Hydrogen ions
D. All of the above

1176. Which of the following is not a curve B-type solute?

Lancet 2005;365:417-430

A. Sodium
B. Potassium
C. Hydrogen
D. None of the above

1177. Which of the following is a curve C-type solute?

Lancet 2005;365:417-430

A. Sodium
B. Potassium
C. Hydrogen
D. Urate

In contrast to solutes of the curve A type, plasma levels of phosphate, urate, and potassium and hydrogen ions usually do not rise until the GFR falls to a small percentage of normal. With progressive renal failure this pattern of response (curve B) reflects the participation of tubule transport mechanisms in the excretion of these substances.

1178. In CKD, principal complications of abnormalities of calcium and phosphate metabolism occur in?

Harrison's 20th Ed. Chapter 305 Page 2114

A. Skeleton
B. Vascular bed
C. Soft tissues
D. All of the above

Principal complications of abnormalities of calcium & phosphate metabolism in CKD occur in skeleton and the vascular bed, with occasional severe involvement of soft tissues.

1179. In CKD, which of the following bone disease is associated with high bone turnover?

Harrison's 20th Ed. Chapter 305 Page 2114

A. Adynamic bone disease
B. Osteomalacia
C. Osteitis fibrosa cystica
D. All of the above

1180. Which of the following is the classic lesion of secondary hyperparathyroidism?

Harrison's 20th Ed. Chapter 305 Page 2114

A. Adynamic bone disease
B. Osteomalacia
C. Osteitis fibrosa cystica
D. All of the above

In CKD, the major disorders of bone disease can be classified into those associated with high bone turnover with increased PTH levels (osteitis fibrosa cystica, classic lesion of secondary hyperparathyroidism), osteomalacia due to reduced action of the active forms of vitamin D, and low bone turnover with low or normal PTH levels (adynamic bone disease) or their combinations.

1181. Plasma concentration of which of the following remains normal throughout the course of CRF?

Harrison's 20th Ed. Chapter 305 Page 2114

A. Potassium
B. Sodium
C. Calcium
D. Hydrogen

For sodium chloride (NaCl), plasma concentrations remain normal throughout the course of CRF, despite unrestricted intake of these substances (curve C). Hyponatremia is not commonly seen in CKD patients but, when present, often responds to water restriction.

1182. Clinical manifestations of severe hyperparathyroidism include?

Harrison's 20th Ed. Chapter 305 Page 2115

A. Bone pain and fragility
B. Brown tumors
C. Erythropoietin (EPO) resistance
D. All of the above

Clinical manifestations of severe hyperparathyroidism include bone pain and fragility, brown tumors, compression syndromes, and erythropoietin (EPO) resistance related to bone marrow fibrosis.

1183. Which of the following about PTH is false?

Harrison's 20th Ed. Chapter 305 Page 2115

A. Uremic toxin
B. Stimulates Ca^{++} reabsorption in the distal convoluted tubule
C. Stimulates proximal tubular 1α-hydroxylation of vitamin D
D. None of the above

Most filtered phosphate ion is reabsorbed by the proximal tubule through a sodium-coupled cotransport process that is regulated by parathyroid hormone (PTH). FGF-23 stimulation of PTH also increases renal phosphate excretion.

1184. Which of the following growth patterns is seen when cell mass of parathyroid glands increases with CKD?

Harrison's 20th Ed. Chapter 305 Page 2115

A. Diffuse hyperplasia (polyclonal)
B. Nodular growth (monoclonal) within diffuse hyperplasia
C. Diffuse monoclonal hyperplasia ("adenoma" or tertiary autonomous hyperparathyroidism)
D. All of the above

Owing to increased PTH production from parathyroid cells, its cell mass increases progressively with CKD. Growth patterns may be diffuse hyperplasia (polyclonal), nodular growth (monoclonal) within diffuse hyperplasia or diffuse monoclonal hyperplasia ("adenoma" or tertiary autonomous hyperparathyroidism).

1185. Which of the following about FGF-23 is false?

Harrison's 20th Ed. Chapter 305 Page 2115

A. Secreted by osteocytes
B. Is part of a family of phosphatonins
C. Promotes renal phosphate excretion
D. None of the above

FGF-23 is a phosphaturic hormone relevant in pathophysiological scheme of secondary hyperparathyroidism.

1186. FGF-23 is a member of which of the following subfamily?

Harrison's 20th Ed. Chapter 305 Page 2115

A. FGF-19
B. FGF-21
C. FGF-23
D. All of the above

The FGF-19 subfamily is composed of three proteins - FGF-19, FGF-21, and FGF-23. FGF-23 is a central regulator of phosphate homeostasis and calcitriol blood levels. FGF-19 inhibits expression of enzyme cholesterol 7-α hydroxylase (CYP7A1), which is the first & rate-limiting step in bile acid synthesis. FGF-21 stimulates insulin independent glucose uptake in adipocytes & lowers triglycerides.

1187. Which of the following about FGF-23 is false?

Harrison's 20th Ed. Chapter 305 Page 2115

A. Increases renal phosphate excretion (phosphaturic hormone)
B. Stimulates PTH
C. Suppresses formation of $1,25(OH)_2D_3$
D. None of the above

FGF-23 increases renal phosphate excretion, stimulates PTH, which also increases renal phosphate excretion and suppresses formation of $1,25(OH)_2D_3$ leading to diminished phosphorus absorption from the GI tract. FGF23 forms a ternary complex with klotho protein and renal FGF receptors to reduce renal phosphate reabsorption.

1188. High levels of FGF-23 is an independent risk factor for?

Harrison's 20th Ed. Chapter 305 Page 2115

A. Coronary artery disease
B. Left ventricular hypertrophy
C. Acute pancreatitis
D. Cirrhosis liver

High levels of FGF-23 are also an independent risk factor for left ventricular hypertrophy and mortality in CKD, dialysis and renal transplant patients with a lower eGFR despite normal phosphate levels.. Higher FGF-23 level is associated with higher atherosclerosis score.

1189. FGF23 is associated with?

Harrison's 20th Ed. Chapter 305 Page 2115

A. Vascular dysfunction
B. Atherosclerosis
C. Left ventricular hypertrophy
D. All of the above

1190. Which of the following about FGF23 is false?

Harrison's 20th Ed. Chapter 305 Page 2115

A. Its increase occurs well before an elevation in PTH in CKD
B. Potent inhibitor of renal 1-alpha hydroxylase
C. Reduces $1,25(OH)_2$ vitamin D
D. None of the above

1191. Which of the following about FGF23 is false?

Harrison's 20th Ed. Chapter 305 Page 2115

A. Regulator of calcium-phosphate metabolism
B. Responsible for inception of secondary hyperparathyroidism
C. Responsible for cardiovascular morbidity & mortality in CKD
D. None of the above

In CKD, FGF-23 is a stronger predictor of mortality than serum phosphate level.

1192. Brown tumor relates best with?

Harrison's 20th Ed. Chapter 305 Page 2115

A. Subcuteneous tissue
B. Bone
C. Brain
D. Liver

Bone histology in hyperparathyroidism may show bone cysts, at times with hemorrhagic elements giving it brown color, hence the term brown tumor.

1193. Clinical clues indicating the imminent development of uremic complications are?

Harrison's 20th Ed. Chapter 305 Page 2115

A. Muscle twitching & cramps
B. Asterixis
C. Non-compliance of treatment
D. All of the above

1194. Adynamic bone disease best relates to?

Harrison's 20th Ed. Chapter 305 Page 2115

A. Aluminium-containing phosphate binders
B. Excessive PTH suppression
C. Low calcium exposure
D. All of the above

1195. Adynamic bone disease can result from?

Harrison's 20th Ed. Chapter 305 Page 2115

A. Use of vitamin D preparations
B. Excessive calcium-containing phosphate binders
C. High-calcium dialysis solutions
D. All of the above

Adynamic bone disease is a state of reduced bone volume & mineralization. It results from excessive PTH suppression from the use of vitamin D preparations or from excessive calcium exposure in the form of calcium-containing phosphate binders or high-calcium dialysis solutions.

1196. Complications of adynamic bone disease include?

Harrison's 20th Ed. Chapter 305 Page 2115

A. Increased incidence of fracture & bone pain
B. Increased vascular & cardiac calcification
C. Tumoral calcinosis
D. All of the above

Complications of adynamic bone disease include an increased incidence of fracture and bone pain and an association with increased vascular and cardiac calcification. Occasionally, the calcium will precipitate in the soft tissues into large concretions termed "tumoral calcinosis". Very low PTH levels are associated with adynamic bone disease and possible consequences of fracture and ectopic calcification.

1197. Metastatic calcification is seen in?

Harrison's 20th Ed. Chapter 405 Page 2966

A. Sarcoidosis
B. Vitamin D intoxication
C. Milk-alkali syndrome
D. All of the above

Metastatic calcification is seen in conditions associated with hypercalcemia, such as in sarcoidosis, vitamin D intoxication, milk-alkali syndrome, and primary hyperparathyroidism.

1198. Which of the following contributes to soft tissue calcifications in CKD?

Harrison's 20th Ed. Chapter 405 Page 2966

A. Increased production of parathyroid hormone (PTH)
B. Increased production of fibroblast growth factor-23
C. Klotho deficiency
D. All of the above

1199. Which of the following is a phosphaturic agent?

Harrison's 20th Ed. Chapter 405 Page 2966

A. Thyroxine
B. Vitamin D
C. Acetazolamide
D. All of the above

Acetazolamide is a phosphaturic agent.

1200. Osteomalacia best relates to?

Harrison's 20th Ed. Chapter 305 Page 2115

A. Calcium
B. PTH
C. $1,25(OH)_2D_3$
D. FGF-23

Osteomalacia in CKD is consequent to reduced production and action of $1,25(OH)_2D_3$, leading to non-mineralized osteoid.

1201. Calciphylaxis best relates to?

Harrison's 20th Ed. Chapter 305 Page 2115

A. Metastatic calcification
B. Calcific uremic arteriolopathy
C. Calcific chronic pancreatitis
D. Calcific tendinitis

1202. Which of the following about calciphylaxis is false?

Harrison's 20th Ed. Chapter 305 Page 2115

A. Seen almost exclusively in patients with advanced CKD
B. Preceded by livedo reticularis
C. Patches of ischemic necrosis
D. None of the above

Calciphylaxis or calcific uremic arteriolopathy is a devastating condition seen almost exclusively in patients with advanced CKD. It is heralded by livedo reticularis and advances to patches of ischemic necrosis, especially on the legs, thighs, abdomen and breasts.

1203. Which of the following about vascular calcification is false?

Harrison's 20th Ed. Chapter 305 Page 2115

A. Matrix GLA protein prevents vascular calcification
B. Low levels of fetuin permit more rapid vascular calcification
C. Diffuse vascular calcifications associated with Paget's disease
D. None of the above

1204. Which of the following about vascular calcification is false?

Harrison's 20th Ed. Chapter 305 Page 2115

A. Warfarin can cause arterial vascular calcification
B. Hyperphosphatemia & hypercalcemia increase vascular calcification
C. Ankle:brachial index >1.40 indicates vascular calcification
D. None of the above

1205. Which of the following is a phosphate binder?

Harrison's 20th Ed. Chapter 305 Page 2115

A. Calcium chloride
B. Calcium acetate
C. Calcium gluconate
D. Calcium hydroxide

Examples of phosphate binders are calcium acetate and calcium carbonate.

1206. Which of the following is a phosphate binder?

Harrison's 20th Ed. Chapter 305 Page 2115

A. Sevelamer
B. Lanthanum
C. Calcium carbonate
D. All of the above

Sevelamer & lanthanum are non-calcium-containing polymers that bind phosphates and do not predispose CKD patients to hypercalcemia. They also attenuate calcium deposition in the vascular bed. Low serum phosphate stimulates renal proximal tubular synthesis of $1,25(OH)_2D$, by suppressing blood levels of FGF23.

1207. Which of the following is a phosphate binding agent?

Harrison's 20th Ed. Chapter 305 Page 2115

A. Calcium acetate
B. Sevelamer hydrochloride
C. Aluminum hydroxide
D. All of the above

Agents limiting intestinal absorption of phosphate (phosphate binders) are calcium carbonate, calcium acetate, lanthanum, sevelamer, & aluminum hydroxide.

1208. In CKD, increased cardiovascular mortality has a strong association with?

Harrison's 20th Ed. Chapter 305 Page 2115

A. Hypercalcemia
B. Hyperphosphatemia
C. Chronic inflammation
D. Soft tissue calcification

Epidemiologic evidence shows a strong association between hyperphosphatemia & increased cardiovascular mortality in patients with CKD.

1209. Which of the following drugs is a risk factor for Calciphylaxis?
Harrison's 20th Ed. Chapter 305 Page 2115

A. Aspirin
B. Statins
C. Warfarin
D. All of the above

Warfarin therapy decreases vitamin K–dependent regeneration of matrix GLA protein which prevents vascular calcification.

1210. Calcimimetic agents that enhance the sensitivity of the parathyroid cell to the suppressive effect of calcium is?
Harrison's 20th Ed. Chapter 305 Page 2116

A. Sevelamer
B. Calcitriol
C. Cinacalcet
D. Lanthanum

1211. Which of the following about cinacalcet is false?
Harrison's 20th Ed. Chapter 305 Page 2116

A. Oral calcimimetic agent
B. Directly lowers PTH levels
C. Increases calcium-sensing receptor to extracellular calcium
D. None of the above

Calcimimetic agents that enhance the sensitivity of the parathyroid cell to the suppressive effect of calcium. Cinacalcet, a calcimimetic agent that acts by allosteric activation of the calcium-sensing receptor on parathyroid tissue. Sevelamer and lanthanum are non-calcium-containing polymers that function as phosphate binders. They do not predispose CKD patients to hypercalcemia and may attenuate calcium deposition in the vascular bed.

1212. Which of the following trials is related to Cinacalcet therapy?
N Engl J Med. 2012; 367:2482-2494

A. HEMO Study
B. EVOLVE trial
C. AURORA Study
D. SHARP Study

Evaluation of Cinacalcet Hydrochloride Therapy to Lower Cardiovascular Events (EVOLVE) trial tested the hypothesis that treatment with cinacalcet reduces the risks of death & nonfatal cardiovascular events among patients with secondary hyperparathyroidism, who were undergoing dialysis.

1213. In CKD, target PTH level should be between?
Harrison's 20th Ed. Chapter 305 Page 2116

A. 25–100 pg/mL
B. 75–200 pg/mL
C. 150–300 pg/mL
D. 350–500 pg/mL

1214. Which of the following is a consequence of very low PTH level?
Harrison's 20th Ed. Chapter 305 Page 2116

A. Adynamic bone disease
B. Fracture
C. Ectopic calcification
D. All of the above

In CKD, target PTH level should be between 150 and 300 pg/mL. Very low PTH levels cause adynamic bone disease, fracture and ectopic calcification.

1215. The CKD-related risk factor of vascular disease is?
Harrison's 20th Ed. Chapter 305 Page 2116

A. Increased FGF-23
B. Sleep apnea
C. Generalized inflammation
D. All of the above

1216. The CKD-related risk factor of vascular disease is?
Harrison's 20th Ed. Chapter 305 Page 2116

A. Anemia
B. Hyperphosphatemia
C. Hyperparathyroidism
D. All of the above

The CKD-related risk factors comprise anemia, hyperphosphatemia, hyperparathyroidism, increased FGF-23, sleep apnea and generalized inflammation.

1217. Fetuin best relates to which of the following?
Harrison's 20th Ed. Chapter 305 Page 2113

A. Angiogenesis
B. Negative acute-phase reactant
C. NK cell function
D. B cell activation

"Negative acute-phase reactants" include serum albumin and fetuin. Serum fetuin-A concentrations are inversely associated with CAC severity independent of traditional CVD risk factors and kidney function in community-living individuals free of clinically apparent CVD.

1218. Which of the following statements about fetuin-A is false?
J Am Soc Nephrol. 2009;20:1264-1274

A. Calcification inhibitor (inhibits ectopic calcification)
B. Also called α_2-Heremans-Schmid glycoprotein
C. Synthesized and secreted by the liver
D. None of the above

1219. Which of the following statements is false?
Harrison's 20th Ed. Chapter 305 Page 2116

A. Cardiac troponin levels are elevated in CKD
B. LVH & dCMP are the strongest risk factors for CV morbidity & mortality in CKD
C. In dialysis patients, low blood pressure carries a worse prognosis than does high blood pressure
D. All of the above

1220. Which of the following is associated with poor prognosis in late-stage CKD patients?
Harrison's 20th Ed. Chapter 305 Page 2116

A. Low blood pressure
B. Reduced body mass index
C. Hypolipidemia
D. All of the above

In late-stage CKD, low BP, reduced BMI & hypolipidemia indicate the presence of a malnutrition-inflammation state, with poor prognosis.

1221. Which of the following should be the first line of therapy in CKD?
Harrison's 20th Ed. Chapter 305 Page 2117

A. Salt restriction
B. Volume management
C. Antihypertensive agent
D. Dialysis

Salt restriction should be the first line of therapy. When volume management alone is not sufficient, the choice of antihypertensive agent is similar to that in the general population.

1222. In CKD patients with diabetes or proteinuria > 1 gram/day, blood pressure should be reduced to?

Harrison's 20th Ed. Chapter 305 Page 2117

A. < 110/70 mm Hg
B. < 125/75 mm Hg
C. < 130/80 mm Hg
D. < 140/90 mm Hg

In CKD patients with diabetes or proteinuria > 1 gram/day, BP should be reduced to <130/80 mm Hg. Renoprotective effect of antihypertensive medications is gauged by consequent reduction of proteinuria.

1223. Which of the following about potassium is false?

The American Journal of Medicine. 2018;131(5):459-460

A. K^+ is absorbed in small intestine via paracellular pathway
B. K^+ is secreted in proximal colon
C. K^+ is absorbed in distal colon
D. None of the above

Majority of potassium is absorbed in small intestine via paracellular pathway, which is driven by the K^+ concentration & positive charge. Fine tuning of K^+ absorption occurs in colon. K^+ is secreted in proximal colon, mainly mediated by calcium-dependent, large-conductance potassium channel (BK or Big Potassium channel), and absorbed in distal colon, mediated by hydrogen potassium ATPase.

1224. Which of the following is a potassium-binding agent for treatment of patients with hyperkalemia?

Harrison's 20th Ed. Chapter 305 Page 2117

A. Sodium polystyrene sulfonate (SPS)
B. Sodium zirconium cyclosilicate
C. Patiromer
D. All of the above

Sodium polystyrene sulfonate (SPS) is a nonspecific sodium-cation exchange resin sometimes associated with colonic necrosis. Sodium zirconium cyclosilicate is a selective potassium cation trapping agent while Patiromer is a calcium-potassium cation exchange resin.

1225. Which of the following about sodium polystyrene sulfonate (SPS) is false?

Harrison's 20th Ed. Chapter 305 Page 2117

A. Oral synthetic cation-exchange resin
B. Binds potassium, calcium and magnesium
C. Not absorbed into the systemic circulation
D. None of the above

Sodium polystyrene sulfonate and calcium polystyrene sulfonate may cause ischemic colitis, related to coadministration with sorbitol.

1226. Nonabsorbed polymer of Patiromer binds potassium in exchange for?

N Engl J Med. 2015;372:211-21

A. Sodium
B. Calcium
C. Magnesium
D. All of the above

The active moiety of patiromer for oral suspension is a nonabsorbed polymer that binds potassium in exchange for calcium predominantly in the distal colon, where the concentration of free potassium is highest, thus increasing fecal potassium excretion and lowering serum potassium levels. Patiromer cannot be used as an emergency treatment for life-threatening hyperkalemia because of its delayed onset of action (7 hours).

1227. Which of the following is a potential side effect of Patiromer acetate?

N Engl J Med. 2015;372:211-21

A. Hypercalcemia
B. Hypomagnesemia
C. Hypokalemia
D. All of the above

Calcium released from patiromer in exchange for potassium can have multiple fates: it can bind to phosphorous and/or oxalate forming insoluble calcium phosphate and/or calcium oxalate salts and be excreted in the stool; it can rebind with patiromer; or it can be systematically absorbed leading to hypercalcemia, although it has not been reported in any major clinical trials. Patiromer also has the ability to bind to magnesium in the colon, which can result in hypomagnesemia.

1228. Which of the following about uremic pericarditis is false?

Harrison's 20th Ed. Chapter 305 Page 2117

A. Absolute indication for urgent initiation of dialysis
B. Propensity to hemorrhage in pericardial fluid
C. Hemodialysis should be performed without heparin
D. None of the above

1229. Pericardial effusion is a side effect of?

Harrison's 20th Ed. Chapter 305 Page 2117

A. Prazosin
B. Minoxidil
C. Eplerenone
D. Labetalol

Side effects of minoxidil include hypertrichosis and pericardial effusion.

1230. Normocytic, normochromic anemia is almost always present by which stage of CKD?

Harrison's 20th Ed. Chapter 305 Page 2117

A. Stage 1
B. Stage 2
C. Stage 3
D. Stage 4

Normocytic, normochromic anemia is almost always present by stage 4 of CKD.

1231. Primary cause of anemia in patients with CKD is?

Harrison's 20th Ed. Chapter 305 Page 2117

A. Insufficient erythropoietin (EPO)
B. Iron deficiency
C. Anemia of chronic disease
D. All of the above

Primary cause of anemia in patients with CKD is insufficient production of erythropoietin (EPO) by the diseased kidneys.

1232. Anemia resistant to erythropoietic-stimulating agents (ESA) when iron stores are adequate may be due to?

Harrison's 20th Ed. Chapter 305 Page 2118

A. Inadequate dialysis
B. Severe hyperparathyroidism
C. Chronic hemolysis
D. All of the above

Anemia resistant to recommended doses of ESA in the face of adequate iron stores may be due to some combination of the following: acute or chronic inflammation, inadequate dialysis, severe hyperparathyroidism, chronic blood loss or hemolysis, chronic infection or malignancy.

1233. Use of erythropoietic-stimulating agents (ESA) in CKD may be associated with?

Harrison's 20th Ed. Chapter 305 Page 2118

A. Increased risk of stroke in patients with type 2 diabetes
B. Increase in thromboembolic events
C. Faster progression of renal decline
D. All of the above

Use of ESA in CKD may be associated with an increased risk of stroke in those with type 2 diabetes, an increase in thromboembolic events, and a faster progression of renal decline.

1234. In CKD, blood transfusions increase the risk of?

Harrison's 20th Ed. Chapter 305 Page 2118

A. Hepatitis
B. Iron overload
C. Transplant sensitization
D. All of the above

Blood transfusions increase the risk of hepatitis, iron overload and transplant sensitization.

1235. In CKD, current practice is to target a hemoglobin concentration of?

Harrison's 20th Ed. Chapter 305 Page 2118

A. 9–10.5 gram/dL
B. 10–11.5 gram/dL
C. 11–12.5 gram/dL
D. 12–13.5 gram/dL

In CKD, current practice is to target a hemoglobin concentration of 10–11.5 gram/dL.

1236. Patients with later stages of CKD may have?

Harrison's 20th Ed. Chapter 305 Page 2118

A. Decreased activity of platelet factor III
B. Abnormal platelet aggregation & adhesiveness
C. Impaired prothrombin consumption
D. All of the above

Patients with later stages of CKD may have a prolonged bleeding time, decreased activity of platelet factor III, abnormal platelet aggregation and adhesiveness and impaired prothrombin consumption.

1237. Abnormal bleeding time and coagulopathy in renal failure may be reversed temporarily with?

Harrison's 20th Ed. Chapter 305 Page 2118

A. Desmopressin (DDAVP)
B. IV conjugated estrogens
C. Erythropoietin (EPO) therapy
D. All of the above

Abnormal BT & coagulopathy in renal failure may be reversed temporarily with desmopressin (DDAVP), cryoprecipitate, IV conjugated estrogens, blood transfusions and ESA therapy.

1238. Which of the following will usually correct a prolonged bleeding time in CKD patients?

Harrison's 20th Ed. Chapter 305 Page 2118

A. Desmopressin (DDAVP)
B. IV conjugated estrogens
C. Erythropoietin (EPO) therapy
D. Optimal dialysis

Optimal dialysis will usually correct a prolonged bleeding time. A brief run of hemodialysis (without heparin) may also be considered prior to renal biopsy to normalize the bleeding time.

1239. Peripheral neuropathy of CKD becomes clinically evident after which stage of CKD?

Harrison's 20th Ed. Chapter 305 Page 2118

A. Stage 1
B. Stage 2
C. Stage 3
D. Stage 4

Peripheral neuropathy usually becomes clinically evident after stage 4 of CKD.

1240. Which of the following is true for peripheral neuropathy of CKD?

Harrison's 20th Ed. Chapter 305 Page 2118

A. Sensory nerves involved more than motor
B. Lower extremities involved more than upper
C. Distal parts of extremities involved more than proximal
D. All of the above

1241. Uremic fetor is due to breakdown of urea to ammonia in?

Harrison's 20th Ed. Chapter 305 Page 2118

A. Saliva
B. Lung
C. Mucous membranes of mouth
D. All of the above

Uremic fetor (urine-like odor on breath) is due to breakdown of urea to ammonia in saliva.

1242. Which active variant of sodium glucose co-transporter (SGLT) is responsible for 90% of glucose reabsorption in kidneys?

Int J Appl Basic Med Res. 2015;5(3):161–163

A. SGLT-1
B. SGLT-2
C. SGLT-3
D. SGLT-4

Reabsorption of glucose in kidney is mediated by insulin independent sodium glucose co-transporter (SGLT), which has six active variants SGLT-1 to SGLT-6. SGLT-2 is responsible for 90% of renal proximal tubule glucose reabsorption, whereas SGLT-1 is responsible for remaining 10% reabsorption in kidneys.

1243. SGLT1 transporter is expressed in which of the following organs?

Am J Physiol Renal Physiol. 2015;309(11):F889-F900

A. Gut
B. Heart
C. Lungs
D. All of the above

SGLT1 transporter is expressed in gut, heart, and lungs. In gut, it transports glucose & galactose. SGLT2 is highly localized to the kidney.

1244. The maximum glucose transport capacity (Tm) of proximal tubule is?

Am J Physiol Renal Physiol. 2015;309(11):F889-F900

A. ~ 175 mg/minute
B. ~ 275 mg/minute
C. ~ 375 mg/minute
D. ~ 475 mg/minute

The maximum glucose transport capacity (Tm) of the proximal tubule, on average, is ~375 mg/minute. In normal individuals with a mean day-long plasma glucose concentration of ~100 mg/dL, the filtered glucose load (~125 mg/minute or 180 gram/day) is less than the maximal renal glucose transport capacity. In poorly controlled diabetic individuals, filtered glucose load may exceed 375 mg/minute, and all of the filtered glucose in excess of the Tm is excreted in the urine. In healthy individuals, plasma glucose threshold at which glucosuria begins is ~180 mg/dL due to nonlinear transition in the reabsorption and excretion curves (splay).

1245. Prototype compound of SGLT inhibitors is?
Int J Appl Basic Med Res. 2015;5(3):161–163

A. Arborizin
B. Phlorizin
C. Temporizin
D. Cetirizin

Prototype compound of SGLT inhibitors is a bitter white glycoside Phlorizin (O-glucoside phlorizin dihydrochalcones, a type of flavonoid). Phlorizin, isolated from the bark of apple trees, was the first renal sodium-glucose cotransport inhibitor to be identified.

1246. Which class of drugs approved for the treatment of T2DM reduces kidney function decline and cardiovascular events?
Harrison's 20th Ed. Chapter 305 Page 2119

A. Biguanides
B. Glucagon-like peptide 1 (GLP-1)
C. DPP-4 inhibitors
D. SGLT inhibitors

By inhibiting sodium, along with glucose, transport in proximal tubule and increasing sodium delivery to juxtaglomerular apparatus, SGLT2 inhibitors cause afferent renal arteriolar vasoconstriction, decreased intraglomerular pressure, and reduction in GFR hyperfiltration.

1247. Pregnancy is associated with high rate of spontaneous abortion, when GFR is?
Harrison's 20th Ed. Chapter 305 Page 2119

A. ~ 90 mL/minute
B. ~ 70 mL/minute
C. ~ 40 mL/minute
D. ~ 30 mL/minute

Pregnancy is associated with high rate of spontaneous abortion, when GFR is ~ 40 mL/minute. At this stage, only ~ 20% of pregnancies lead to live births.

1248. Skin pigmentation in advanced CKD is due to?
Harrison's 20th Ed. Chapter 305 Page 2119

A. Chromogens
B. Chromolytes
C. Urochromes
D. Renochromes

Patients become more pigmented in advanced CKD, even on dialysis due to deposition of retained pigmented metabolites called urochromes.

1249. Disorders associated with ESRD include?
Harrison's 20th Ed. Chapter 305 Page 2119

A. Calciphylaxis
B. Uremic frost
C. Nephrogenic fibrosing dermopathy
D. All of the above

Uremic frost is infrequently seen because of early dialytic intervention. When BUN level is high, concentration of urea in sweat is increased greatly. Evaporation results in the deposition of urea crystals on skin as fine white-to-yellow crystals that dissolve readily when challenged by a drop of water.

1250. Nephrogenic fibrosing dermopathy is similar to?
Harrison's 20th Ed. Chapter 305 Page 2119

A. Guttate morphea
B. Scleromyxedema
C. Linear scleroderma
D. Diffuse fasciitis with eosinophilia

Nephrogenic fibrosing dermopathy, seen in CKD, is a progressive subcutaneous induration on arms & legs similar to scleromyxedema.

1251. Which of the following can precipitate nephrogenic fibrosing dermopathy?
Harrison's 20th Ed. Chapter 305 Page 2119

A. Vitamin D
B. Metformin
C. Aluminum
D. Gadolinium

Exposure to magnetic resonance contrast agent, gadolinium may precipitate nephrogenic fibrosing dermopathy or nephrogenic systemic fibrosis (NSF) between 5 & 75 days following exposure.

1252. Rapid removal of gadolinium can be done by?
Harrison's 20th Ed. Chapter 305 Page 2119

A. Forced diuresis
B. IV calcium
C. Hemodialysis
D. All of the above

Rapid removal of gadolinium can be done by hemodialysis.

1253. Which of the following test must be done in all unexplained anemic with normal serum calcium CKD patients >35 years?
Harrison's 20th Ed. Chapter 305 Page 2119

A. Hepatitis B
B. Serum and urine protein electrophoresis
C. Serum concentrations of PTH
D. Serum vitamin B_{12} and folate

Serum and urine protein electrophoresis for multiple myeloma must be done in all patients >35 years with unexplained CKD, especially if there is associated anemia and elevated or even inappropriately normal serum calcium concentration.

1254. In which of the following conditions, kidney size may be normal in the face of CKD?
Harrison's 20th Ed. Chapter 305 Page 2119

A. Diabetic nephropathy
B. HIV nephropathy
C. Amyloidosis
D. All of the above

1255. Which of the following measures attenuate contrast-induced worsening of renal function?
Harrison's 20th Ed. Chapter 305 Page 2119

A. Sodium bicarbonate containing solutions
B. N acetylcysteine
C. Use of least nephrotoxic potential radiographic contrast agent
D. All of the above

1256. Contraindications to renal biopsy include?
Harrison's 20th Ed. Chapter 305 Page 2120

A. Bilaterally small kidneys
B. Uncontrolled hypertension
C. Active urinary tract infection
D. All of the above

1257. Contraindications to renal biopsy include?
Harrison's 20th Ed. Chapter 305 Page 2120

A. Bleeding diathesis
B. Ongoing anticoagulation
C. Severe obesity
D. All of the above

1258. If bleeding time is ↑ed at the time of renal biopsy, which of the following is administered immediately prior to the procedure?
Harrison's 20th Ed. Chapter 305 Page 2120

A. Protamine
B. Desmopressin
C. N acetylcysteine
D. IV calcium

If bleeding time is increased at the time of renal biopsy, desmopressin should be administered immediately prior to the procedure. A brief run of hemodialysis, without heparin, also helps.

1259. Which of the following can be a superimposed acute process in CKD?
Harrison's 20th Ed. Chapter 305 Page 2120

A. ECFV depletion
B. Urinary infection or obstruction
C. Nephrotoxin exposure
D. All of the above

Potentially reversible uper imposed acute or subacute processes like ECFV depletion, uncontrolled hypertension, urinary tract infection, new obstructive uropathy, exposure to nephrotoxic agents (NSAIDs or radiographic dye), and reactivation or flare of the original disease, such as lupus or vasculitis, may complicate CKD.

1260. Which of the following have an antiproteinuric and renoprotective effect?
Harrison's 20th Ed. Chapter 305 Page 2120

A. ACE inhibitors and ARBs
B. Diltiazem
C. Verapamil
D. All of the above

1261. CKD is likely if bilateral kidney size is?
Harrison's 20th Ed. Chapter 305 Page 2120

A. < 8.5 cm
B. < 9.0 cm
C. < 9.5 cm
D. < 10 cm

Finding of bilaterally reduced kidney size (<8.5 cm) favors CKD.

1262. Dose adjustment is not needed, if the medication's excretion by nonrenal route is?
Harrison's 20th Ed. Chapter 305 Page 2120

A. > 60%
B. > 70%
C. > 80%
D. > 90%

For those medication in which >70% excretion is by a nonrenal route (hepatic elimination), dose adjustment may not be needed.

1263. Which of the following drugs that should be avoided in CKD?
Harrison's 20th Ed. Chapter 305 Page 2120

A. Metformin
B. Meperidine
C. Gadolinium
D. All of the above

Drugs that should be avoided in CKD include metformin, meperidine & gadolinium.

1264. Clear indications for initiation of renal replacement therapy include?
Harrison's 20th Ed. Chapter 305 Page 2121

A. Pericarditis
B. Progressive neuropathy due to uremia
C. Encephalopathy
D. All of the above

1265. Clear indications for initiation of renal replacement therapy include?
Harrison's 20th Ed. Chapter 305 Page 2121

A. Muscle irritability
B. Anorexia & nausea not relieved by protein restriction
C. Refractory fluid & electrolyte abnormalities
D. All of the above

1266. Clear indications for initiation of renal replacement therapy include?
Harrison's 20th Ed. Chapter 305 Page 2121

A. Unresponsive volume overload
B. Unresponsive hyperkalemia
C. Progressive metabolic acidosis
D. All of the above

Clear indications for initiation of renal replacement therapy in CKD include pericarditis, encephalopathy, intractable muscle cramping, anorexia, nausea, malnutrition, & refractory fluid & electrolyte abnormalities (hyperkalemia).

1267. Clinical clues indicating the imminent development of uremic complications are?
Harrison's 20th Ed. Chapter 305 Page 2121

A. History of hiccoughing
B. Intractable pruritus
C. Morning nausea & vomiting
D. All of the above

Dialysis in the Treatment of Renal Failure

1268. Which of the following dialysis process is specific to the management of acute renal failure?

Harrison's 20th Ed. Chapter 306 Page 2121

A. Continuous renal replacement therapies (CRRT)
B. Prolonged intermittent renal replacement therapy (PIRRT)
C. Slow low-efficiency dialysis (SLED)
D. All of the above

1269. Which of the following is the leading cause of ESRD?

Harrison's 20th Ed. Chapter 306 Page 2122

A. Hypertension
B. Diabetes mellitus
C. Glomerulonephritis
D. Obstructive uropathy

The leading cause of ESRD is diabetes mellitus (~45% of newly diagnosed cases of ESRD). Other include hypertension (~30%), glomerulonephritis, polycystic kidney disease and obstructive uropathy.

1270. Mortality rates for patients with ESRD are lowest in?

Harrison's 20th Ed. Chapter 306 Page 2122

A. Japan
B. USA
C. Australia
D. UAE

Mortality rates for patients with ESRD are lowest in Europe and Japan.

1271. Which of the following is an accepted criteria for initiating patients on maintenance dialysis?

Harrison's 20th Ed. Chapter 306 Page 2122

A. Presence of uremic symptoms
B. Acidosis refractory to medical therapy
C. Bleeding diathesis
D. All of the above

Accepted criteria for initiating patients on maintenance dialysis include presence of uremic symptoms, presence of hyperkalemia unresponsive to conservative measures, persistent extracellular volume expansion despite diuretic therapy, acidosis refractory to medical therapy, bleeding diathesis and creatinine clearance or estimated glomerular filtration rate (GFR) below 10 mL/minute per 1.73 m^2. There is no benefit to initiating dialysis preemptively at a GFR of 10–14 mL/minute per 1.73 m^2 compared to initiating dialysis for symptoms of uremia.

1272. Complications of advanced chronic kidney disease (CKD) include?

Harrison's 20th Ed. Chapter 306 Page 2122

A. Anemia
B. Acidosis
C. Secondary hyperparathyroidism
D. All of the above

Complications of advanced chronic kidney disease (CKD) include hypertension, anemia, acidosis, and secondary hyperparathyroidism.

1273. Which of the following is the most common therapeutic modality for ESRD?

Harrison's 20th Ed. Chapter 306 Page 2122

A. Hemodialysis
B. Continuous ambulatory peritoneal dialysis (CAPD)
C. Continuous cyclic peritoneal dialysis (CCPD)
D. Reanl transplantation

In ESRD, treatment options include hemodialysis (institutional or domiciliary), peritoneal dialysis as either continuous ambulatory peritoneal dialysis (CAPD) or continuous cyclic peritoneal dialysis (CCPD) or transplantation. Hemodialysis remains the most common therapeutic modality for ESRD.

1274. What is the size of urea molecule?

Harrison's 20th Ed. Chapter 306 Page 2122

A. 50 Da
B. 60 Da
C. 70 Da
D. 80 Da

1275. What is the size of creatinine molecule?

Harrison's 20th Ed. Chapter 306 Page 2122

A. 100 Da
B. 113 Da
C. 123 Da
D. 132 Da

Size of urea molecule is 60 Da, while that of creatinine is 113 Da. According to laws of diffusion, the larger the molecule, the slower is its rate of transfer across the membrane.

1276. Middle molecules have a molecular mass between?

Harrison's 20th Ed. Chapter 306 Page 2122

A. 500 & 1500 Da
B. 1500 & 3000 Da
C. 3000 & 5000 Da
D. 5000 & 8000 Da

Compounds with a molecular mass between 500 & 1500 Da are middle molecules.

1277. Which of the following processes occur in hemodialysis?

Harrison's 20th Ed. Chapter 306 Page 2122

A. Diffusive clearance
B. Ultrafiltration
C. Convective clearance
D. All of the above

1278. The rate of diffusive transport across a semipermeable membrane depends on?

Harrison's 20th Ed. Chapter 306 Page 2122

A. Magnitude of the concentration gradient
B. Membrane surface area
C. Mass transfer coefficient of the membrane
D. All of the above

1279. Mass transfer coefficient of the semipermeable membrane depends on?

Harrison's 20th Ed. Chapter 306 Page 2122

A. Porosity and thickness of the membrane
B. Size of the solute molecule
C. Conditions of flow on two sides of the membrane
D. All of the above

1280. Convective clearance best relates to?

Harrison's 20th Ed. Chapter 306 Page 2122

A. Supersaturation
B. Solvent drag
C. Ultrafiltration
D. All of the above

Convective clearance occurs because of solvent drag, with solutes being swept along with water across the semipermeable dialysis membrane.

1281. Which of the following is a component to hemodialysis?

Harrison's 20th Ed. Chapter 306 Page 2122

A. Dialyzer
B. Composition and delivery of the dialysate
C. Blood delivery system
D. All of the above

The three essential components to hemodialysis are the dialyzer, the composition and delivery of the dialysate, and the blood delivery system.

1282. Which of the following is a category of dialysis membrane?

Harrison's 20th Ed. Chapter 306 Page 2122

A. Cellulose
B. Cellulosynthetic
C. Synthetic
D. All of the above

Categories of dialysis membranes are cellulose, substituted cellulose, cellulosynthetic and synthetic.

1283. Reprocessing agent used in a hemodialyzer include?

Harrison's 20th Ed. Chapter 306 Page 2122

A. Formaldehyde
B. Peracetic acid–hydrogen peroxide
C. Glutaraldehyde
D. All of the above

Formaldehyde, peracetic acid–hydrogen peroxide, glutaraldehyde and bleach are used as reprocessing agents.

1284. Surface area of modern dialysis membranes in adult patients is?

Harrison's 20th Ed. Chapter 306 Page 2122

A. 0.5–1.0 m^2
B. 1.5–2.0 m^2
C. 2.5–3.0 m^2
D. 3.5–4.0 m^2

Surface area of modern dialysis membranes in adult patients is ~1.5–2.0 m^2.

1285. Which of the following improve the 'Biocompatibility' of a dialysis membrane?

Harrison's 20th Ed. Chapter 306 Page 2122

A. More free hydroxyl groups on membrane surface
B. Less free hydroxyl groups on membrane surface
C. More free sulphydral groups on membrane surface
D. Less free sulphydral groups on membrane surface

Bioincompatibility is defined as the ability of dialysis membrane to activate complement cascade. Cellulosic membranes are bioincompatible because of the presence of free hydroxyl groups on membrane surface.

1286. Which of the following is a form of synthetic membrane?

Harrison's 20th Ed. Chapter 306 Page 2122

A. Polysulfone
B. Poly methyl methacrylate
C. Polyacrylonitrile
D. All of the above

Examples of synthetic membranes are polysulfone, poly methyl methacrylate, and polyacrylonitrile membranes. These are more biocompatible because of the absence of free hydroxyl groups.

1287. Which of the following is false about ion concentration of dialysate?

Harrison's 20th Ed. Chapter 306 Page 2122

A. K^+ concentration of dialysate varies from 0 to 4 mmol/L
B. Ca^+ is 1.25 mmol/L or 2.5 mEq/L
C. Na^+ concentration is 136–140 mmol/L
D. None of the above

1288. During each hemodialysis session, patient is exposed to approximately how much water as dialysate?

Harrison's 20th Ed. Chapter 306 Page 2122

A. 80 L
B. 120 L
C. 180 L
D. 250 L

Patients are exposed to ~120 liters of water during each dialysis treatment.

1289. Blood flow rate in the extracorporeal circuit in hemodialysis machine ranges from?

Harrison's 20th Ed. Chapter 306 Page 2122

A. 50 to 100 mL/minute
B. 100 to 200 mL/minute
C. 250 to 450 mL/minute
D. 500 to 750 mL/minute

Blood flow rate in extracorporeal circuit in hemodialysis machine ranges from 250–450 mL/minute.

1290. 'Breschia-Cimino fistula' is used for?

Harrison's 20th Ed. Chapter 306 Page 2123

A. Dialysis access
B. Ventriculo-atrial shunt
C. Peritono-caval shunt
D. Peripheral arterial bypass

In Brescia-Cimino fistula, cephalic vein is anastomosed end-to-side to radial artery for dialysis access (arterialization of the vein).

1291. Prosthetic material for arteriovenous graft is?

Harrison's 20th Ed. Chapter 306 Page 2123

A. Polytetrafluoroethylene (PTFE)
B. Polyethylene (PE)
C. Polyvinylidene fluoride (PVDF)
D. Polytrifluoroethylene

Polytetrafluoroethylene (PTFE) is one of the most stable polymers known.

1292. Most common dialysis access-related complication is?
Harrison's 20th Ed. Chapter 306 Page 2123

A. Infection
B. Thrombosis
C. Embolism
D. Perforation

Most important complication of AV grafts is thrombosis of the graft & graft failure, due to intimal hyperplasia at anastomosis between graft & recipient vein.

1293. Most tunneled catheters are placed in?
Harrison's 20th Ed. Chapter 306 Page 2123

A. Internal jugular vein
B. External jugular vein
C. Femoral vein
D. Subclavian vein

Most tunneled catheters are placed in the internal jugular veins. External jugular, femoral, and subclavian veins may also be used.

1294. In hemodialysis, dialysate flows in an opposite counter-current direction at the rate of?
Harrison's 20th Ed. Chapter 306 Page 2123

A. 100 to 300 mL/minute
B. 300 to 500 mL/minute
C. 500 to 800 mL/minute
D. 800 to 1000 mL/minute

Dialysate flows in an opposite counter-current direction at 500–800 mL/minute while heparinized blood is pumped through the dialyzer at a flow rate of 300–450 mL/minute.

1295. The dose of dialysis is governed by?
Harrison's 20th Ed. Chapter 306 Page 2123

A. Patient size
B. Residual kidney function
C. Dietary protein intake
D. All of the above

The dose of dialysis, which is defined as a derivation of fractional urea clearance during a single treatment, is governed by patient size, residual kidney function, dietary protein intake, the degree of anabolism or catabolism, and the presence of comorbid conditions.

1296. What level of urea reduction ratio (URR) per treatment, defines minimal standards for adequacy among ESRD patients?
Harrison's 20th Ed. Chapter 306 Page 2123

A. 35%
B. 45%
C. 55%
D. 65%

Current target is a urea reduction ratio (fractional reduction in BUN per hemodialysis session) of >65– 70% (dose of dialysis).

1297. What level of KT/V per treatment, defines minimal standards for adequacy among ESRD patients?
Harrison's 20th Ed. Chapter 306 Page 2123

A. 0.8
B. 1.0
C. 1.2
D. 1.4

Current target is body water–indexed clearance x time product (KT/V) above 1.2.

1298. For the majority of patients with ESRD, how many hours of dialysis is required each week?
Harrison's 20th Ed. Chapter 306 Page 2124

A. 3 to 9 hours
B. 9 to 12 hours
C. 12 to 24 hours
D. 24 to 36 hours

For the majority of patients with ESRD, between 9 and 12 hours of dialysis are required each week, usually divided into three equal sessions.

1299. Most common acute complication of hemodialysis is?
Harrison's 20th Ed. Chapter 306 Page 2124

A. Infection
B. Hypotension
C. Anemia
D. Muscle cramps

1300. Hypotension as the most common acute complication of hemodialysis is particularly seen in?
Harrison's 20th Ed. Chapter 306 Page 2124

A. Hypertensives
B. Diabetics
C. Heart failure
D. All of the above

Hypotension is the most common acute complication of hemodialysis, particularly among diabetics. Other complications of ESRD include a high incidence of infection, progressive debility and frailty, protein-energy malnutrition and impaired cognitive function.

1301. In dialysate, presence of which of the following is a common cause of hypotension?
Harrison's 20th Ed. Chapter 306 Page 2124

A. Acetate
B. Bicarbonate
C. Calcium
D. Aluminium

Because of the vasodilatory & cardiodepressive effects of acetate, its use as buffer in dialysate is a common cause of hypotension. Since the introduction of bicarbonate-containing dialysate, dialysis-associated hypotension has become less common.

1302. In the management of hypotension during dialysis, administration of which of the following is useful?
Harrison's 20th Ed. Chapter 306 Page 2124

A. 100 to 250 mL of isotonic saline
B. 10 mL of 23% saturated hypertonic saline
C. Salt-poor albumin
D. All of the above

Hypotension during dialysis is managed with discontinuing ultrafiltration, 100–250 mL of isotonic saline or 10 mL of 23% saturated hypertonic saline, and administration of salt-poor albumin.

1303. Hypotension during dialysis can be prevented by?
Harrison's 20th Ed. Chapter 306 Page 2124

A. Careful evaluation of dry weight
B. Withholding of antihypertensive medications
C. Avoiding heavy meals during dialysis
D. All of the above

1304. Hypotension during dialysis can be prevented by?
Harrison's 20th Ed. Chapter 306 Page 2124

A. Ultrafiltration modeling
B. Midodrine
C. Cooling of dialysate during dialysis treatment
D. All of the above

1305. Excessively rapid fluid removal during hemodialysis refers to?
Harrison's 20th Ed. Chapter 306 Page 2124

A. > 8 mL/kg per hour
B. > 13 mL/kg per hour
C. > 18 mL/kg per hour
D. > 23 mL/kg per hour

Hypotension during dialysis can be prevented by by ultrafiltration modeling, such that more fluid is removed at the beginning rather than the end of dialysis procedure. Excessively rapid fluid removal i.e. >13 mL/kg per hour should be avoided.

1306. Which of the following may prevent muscle cramps during hemodialysis?
Harrison's 20th Ed. Chapter 306 Page 2124

A. Reducing volume removal during dialysis
B. Use of sodium modeling
C. Ultrafiltration profiling
D. All of the above

1307. Which of the following is false about anaphylactoid reactions to the dialyzer?
Harrison's 20th Ed. Chapter 306 Page 2124

A. Occur with bioincompatible cellulosic-containing membranes
B. Type A reactions are hypersensitivity reaction to ethylene oxide
C. Type B reaction activate complement & release of cytokine
D. None of the above

Anaphylactoid reactions to dialyzer, particularly on its first use, occur mostly with bioincompatible cellulosic-containing membranes. Dialyzer reactions can be divided into two types, A and B. Type A reactions are attributed to an IgE mediated intermediate hypersensitivity reaction to ethylene oxide used in the sterilization of new dialyzers. This reaction typically occurs soon after initiation & can progress to full-blown anaphylaxis if the therapy is not promptly discontinued. Treatment with steroids or epinephrine may be needed. Type B reaction consists of a symptom complex of nonspecific chest & back pain, which results from complement activation & cytokine release occurring several minutes into the dialysis run & typically resolve with continued dialysis.

1308. In peritoneal dialysis, how much dextrose-containing solution is infused in the peritoneal cavity?
Harrison's 20th Ed. Chapter 306 Page 2124

A. 1.5 to 3 Liters
B. 4 to 6 Liters
C. 6 to 8 Liters
D. 10 to 12 Liters

1309. In peritoneal dialysis, for how many hours dextrose-containing solution is allowed to remain in the peritoneal cavity?
Harrison's 20th Ed. Chapter 306 Page 2124

A. 1 to 2 hours
B. 2 to 4 hours
C. 4 to 6 hours
D. 6 to 8 hours

In peritoneal dialysis, 1.5–3 liters of a dextrose-containing solution is infused into peritoneal cavity & allowed for 2–4 hours.

1310. Which of the following about peritoneal dialysis is false?
Harrison's 20th Ed. Chapter 306 Page 2124

A. Metabolic byproducts removed through convective clearance
B. Metabolic byproducts removed through diffusive clearance
C. Absorption of solutes & water occurs via peritoneal lymphatics into lymphatic circulation
D. None of the above

In PD, metabolic byproducts are removed through a combination of convective clearance generated through ultrafiltration and diffusive clearance down a concentration gradient. Absorption of solutes and water from the peritoneal cavity occurs across peritoneal membrane into peritoneal capillary circulation and via peritoneal lymphatics into lymphatic circulation.

1311. Which of the following can be used in place of dextrose in peritoneal dialysis solution?
Harrison's 20th Ed. Chapter 306 Page 2124

A. Maltodextrin
B. Cyclodextrin
C. Icodextrin
D. All of the above

Icodextrin is a nonabsorbable carbohydrate that can be used in place of dextrose.

1312. Additive to peritoneal dialysis solutions may be?
Harrison's 20th Ed. Chapter 306 Page 2124

A. Heparin
B. Antibiotics
C. Insulin
D. All of the above

Additives to peritoneal dialysis solutions are heparin, antibiotics and insulin.

1313. Advantage of continuous renal replacement therapy (CRRT) over intermittent hemodialysis in ARF is?
Harrison's 20th Ed. Chapter 306 Page 2125

A. Better tolerated hemodynamically
B. Gradual correction of biochemical abnormalities
C. Highly effective in removing fluid
D. All of the above

1314. Continuous renal replacement therapy (CRRT) techniques include?
Harrison's 20th Ed. Chapter 306 Page 2125

A. Continuous arteriovenous hemodiafiltration with dialysis
B. Continuous arteriovenous hemodiafiltration without dialysis
C. Continuous veno-venous hemodiafiltration with dialysis
D. All of the above

1315. Which of the following is a type of 'Peritoneal dialysis'?
Harrison's 20th Ed. Chapter 306 Page 2125

A. Continuous ambulatory peritoneal dialysis (CAPD)
B. Continuous cyclic peritoneal dialysis (CCPD)
C. Nocturnal intermittent peritoneal dialysis (NIPD)
D. All of the above

1316. Which of the following is false for CAPD?
Harrison's 20th Ed. Chapter 306 Page 2125

A. Dialysis solution is manually infused into peritoneal cavity
B. Dialysis solution remains in peritoneal cavity through night
C. Drainage of spent dialysate is performed manually
D. None of the above

1317. Which of the following statements is false?
Harrison's 20th Ed. Chapter 306 Page 2125

A. In CCPD, exchanges are performed in automated fashion
B. In CCPD, the last exchange remains in abdomen
C. In NIPD, the abdomen is left dry during the day
D. None of the above

1318. Preferred buffer in peritoneal dialysis solution is?
Harrison's 20th Ed. Chapter 306 Page 2125

A. Lactate
B. Bicarbonate
C. Acetate
D. All of the above

Lactate is the preferred buffer in peritoneal dialysis solutions.

1319. Which of the following is a complication of peritoneal dialysis?
Harrison's 20th Ed. Chapter 306 Page 2125

A. Peritonitis
B. Weight gain
C. Residual uremia
D. All of the above

Complications of PD are peritonitis, catheter-associated nonperitonitis infections, weight gain, metabolic disturbances and residual uremia.

1320. What value of peritoneal fluid leukocyte count denotes peritonitis?
Harrison's 20th Ed. Chapter 306 Page 2125

A. $10/mm^3$
B. $40/mm^3$
C. $80/mm^3$
D. $100/mm^3$

Peritonitis is defined by a raised peritoneal fluid leukocyte count ($100/mm^3$, 50% are PMN).

1321. Most common culprit organism in peritonitis as a complication of peritoneal dialysis is?
Harrison's 20th Ed. Chapter 306 Page 2125

A. Gram-positive cocci
B. Gram-positive bacilli
C. Gram-negative cocci
D. Gram-negative bacilli

Most common culprit organisms in peritonitis as a complication of peritoneal dialysis are gram-positive cocci including Staphylococcus, reflecting the origin from skin.

1322. Nonperitonitis catheter-associated infections are termed as?
Harrison's 20th Ed. Chapter 306 Page 2125

A. Funnel infections
B. Tunnel infections
C. Channel infections
D. Chamber infections

Nonperitonitis catheter-associated infections are often termed tunnel infections.

1323. Which of the following statements is false?
Harrison's 20th Ed. Chapter 306 Page 2125

A. Acetate in PD solution can accelerate peritoneal sclerosis
B. Bicarbonate in PD solution can precipitate calcium
C. Bicarbonate in PD solution can caramelize glucose
D. None of the above

1324. Which of the following study evaluated cardiovascular risk reduction in ESRD patients?
Harrison's 20th Ed. Chapter 306 Page 2125

A. 4D
B. AURORA
C. SHARP
D. All of the above

1325. Clinical abnormalities in uremia that develop only after initiation of dialysis therapy are all except?

A. Adynamic osteomalacia
B. Dialysis disequilibrium syndrome
C. Hypotension & arrhythmias
D. Hypothermia

1326. Clinical abnormalities in uremia that develop only after initiation of dialysis therapy are all except?

A. Hepatitis
B. Idiopathic ascites
C. Peritonitis
D. Muscular irritability

1327. Clinical abnormalities in uremia that develop only after initiation of dialysis therapy are all except?

A. Leukopenia
B. Hypocomplementemia
C. Muscle cramps
D. Hypernatremia & hyponatremia

1328. Clinical abnormalities in uremia that improve with dialysis and erythropoietin therapy are all except?

A. Fatigue
B. Impaired mentation
C. Lethargy
D. Sleep disorders

1329. Clinical abnormalities in uremia that improve with dialysis and erythropoietin therapy are all except?

A. Pallor
B. Anemia
C. Bleeding diathesis
D. Leukopenia

1330. Gastrointestinal disturbances in uremia that usually improve with optimal dialysis & related therapy are all except?

A. Anorexia, nausea and vomiting
B. Uremic fetor
C. Gastroenteritis
D. Idiopathic ascites

1331. Gastrointestinal disturbances in uremia that develop only after initiation of dialysis therapy are all except?

A. Hepatitis
B. Idiopathic ascites
C. Peritonitis
D. Uremic fetor

1332. Endocrine-metabolic disturbances in uremia that develop only after initiation of dialysis therapy are all except?

A. Carbohydrate intolerance
B. Adynamic osteomalacia
C. Secondary hyperparathyroidism
D. Vitamin D-deficient osteomalacia

1333. Endocrine-metabolic disturbances in uremia that improve with optimal dialysis & related therapy are all except?

A. Carbohydrate intolerance
B. Vitamin D-deficient osteomalacia
C. Hypothermia
D. All of the above

1334. Endocrine-metabolic disturbances in uremia that tends to persist or even progress, despite optimal dialysis & related therapy are all except?

A. Increased Lp(a) level
B. Decreased high-density lipoprotein level
C. Infertility and sexual dysfunction
D. None of the above

1335. Endocrine-metabolic disturbances in uremia that tends to persist or even progress, despite optimal dialysis & related therapy are all except?

A. Amenorrhea
B. Impaired growth & development
C. Infertility & sexual dysfunction
D. None of the above

1336. Neuromuscular disturbances in uremia that usually improve with optimal dialysis & related therapy are all except?

A. Asterixis
B. Muscular irritability
C. Coma
D. Sleep disorder

1337. Neuromuscular disturbances in uremia that develops only after initiation of dialysis therapy are all except?

A. Muscle cramps
B. Myoclonus
C. Dialysis disequilibrium syndrome
D. Myopathy

1338. Neuromuscular disturbances in uremia that improve with dialysis and erythropoietin therapy are all except?

A. Fatigue
B. Impaired mentation
C. Lethargy
D. Asterixis

1339. Cardiovascular & pulmonary disturbances in uremia that usually improve with optimal dialysis & related therapy are all except?

A. CHF/pulmonary edema
B. Pericarditis
C. Uremic lung
D. Hypotension & arrhythmias

1340. Dermatologic disturbances in uremia that usually improve with optimal dialysis & related therapy are all except?

A. Ecchymoses
B. Uremic frost
C. Pallor
D. Pruritus

Transplantation in the Treatment of Renal Failure

1341. 1-year survival in deceased-donor kidney transplants is?
Harrison's 20th Ed. Chapter 307 Page 2126

A. 76%
B. 84%
C. 92%
D. 97%

1342. 1-year survival in living-donor kidney transplants is?
Harrison's 20th Ed. Chapter 307 Page 2126

A. 76%
B. 84%
C. 92%
D. 97%

Deceased-donor kidney transplants have a 92% 1-year survival and living-donor kidney transplants have a 97% 1-year survival.

1343. Currently, the "average" (t½) life expectancy of a deceased-donor kidney transplants is around?
Harrison's 20th Ed. Chapter 307 Page 2126

A. 10 years
B. 15 years
C. 20 years
D. 25 years

1344. Currently, the "average" (t½) life expectancy of a living-donor kidney transplants is around?
Harrison's 20th Ed. Chapter 307 Page 2126

A. 7 years
B. 14 years
C. 21 years
D. 28 years

Currently, the "average" (t½) life expectancy of a living-donor kidney transplants is around 14 years and that of a deceased-donor kidney transplants is ~10 years.

1345. Mortality rates after kidney transplantation are highest in?
Harrison's 20th Ed. Chapter 307 Page 2126

A. First day
B. First week
C. First month
D. First year

Mortality rates after transplantation are highest in the first year.

1346. Most kidney transplantation patients succumb at varying rates to a chronic process consisting of?
Harrison's 20th Ed. Chapter 307 Page 2126

A. Interstitial fibrosis
B. Tubular atrophy
C. Glomerulopathy
D. All of the above

Most kidney transplantation patients succumb at varying rates to a chronic process consisting of interstitial fibrosis, tubular atrophy, vasculopathy, and glomerulopathy.

1347. Potential kidney recipients with the highest expected postransplant survival are provided with kidney donor profile index (KDPI) score of?
Harrison's 20th Ed. Chapter 307 Page 2126

A. < 10%
B. < 20%
C. < 30%
D. < 40%

Kidney donor profile Index (KDPI) score from 0 to 100% quantifies potential risk of graft failure after kidney transplant based on 10 donor factors. Lower KDPI values are associated with higher expected post-transplant survival. Kidneys with KDPI <20% are allocated to the 20% of the potential recipients with highest expected post-transplant survival.

1348. Kidneys from which of the following categories is least preferred for transplantation?
Harrison's 20th Ed. Chapter 307 Page 2126 Table 307-1

A. Brought in dead
B. Unsuccessful resuscitation
C. Awaiting cardiac arrest
D. Cardiac arrest after brainstem death

1349. Kidneys from which of the following categories is preferred for transplantation?
Harrison's 20th Ed. Chapter 307 Page 2126 Table 307-1

A. Brought in dead
B. Unsuccessful resuscitation
C. Awaiting cardiac arrest
D. Cardiac arrest in a hospital patient

The five categories of non-heart-beating donor (donation after cardiac death (DCD) are I: Brought in dead, II: Unsuccessful resuscitation, III: Awaiting cardiac arrest, IV: Cardiac arrest after brainstem death and V: Cardiac arrest in a hospital patient.

1350. Which of the following statements is false?
Harrison's 20th Ed. Chapter 307 Page 2126

A. High KDPI kidneys have a poorer survival
B. Graft survival is higher for living-donor recipients
C. Transplanted kidney is placed in the inguinal fossa
D. None of the above

1351. Which of the following is relevant for selection of donors for renal allografts is?
Harrison's 20th Ed. Chapter 307 Page 2127

A. HLA antigens
B. ABH(O) blood groups
C. Endothelial antigens
D. All of the above

1352. Which of the following statements is false?
Harrison's 20th Ed. Chapter 307 Page 2127

A. The Rh system is not expressed on graft tissue
B. T lymphocytes express class I antigens
C. B lymphocytes express both class I & class II antigens
D. None of the above

1353. Which of the following statements is false?
Harrison's 20th Ed. Chapter 307 Page 2127

A. CD4+ lymphocyte respond to class II (HLA-DR) incompatibility
B. CD8+ cytotoxic lymphocyte precursors respond to class I (HLA-A, -B) antigens
C. Graft rejection is initiated by CD4 helper T lymphocytes (TH)
D. None of the above

1354. Which of the following corresponds to complete HLA mismatch?
Harrison's 20th Ed. Chapter 307 Page 2127

A. 0/6
B. 2/6
C. 4/6
D. 6/6

1355. Which of the following assays is most sensitive for recipient - donor matching?
Harrison's 20th Ed. Chapter 307 Page 2127

A. Cytotoxic cross-match of recipient serum & donor T lymphocytes
B. Flow cytometric-based crossmatch assay
C. ABO compatibility
D. All of the above

1356. Anti-thymocyte globulin (ATG) comes under which of the following categories of induction therapy?
Harrison's 20th Ed. Chapter 307 Page 2128

A. Monoclonal antibody
B. Polyclonal antibody
C. Depletional agents
D. Nondepletional agents

1357. Alemtuzumab is directed to?
Harrison's 20th Ed. Chapter 307 Page 2128

A. CD28 protein
B. CD42 protein
C. CD52 protein
D. CD68 protein

Alemtuzumab is directed to the CD52 protein, widely distributed on immune cells such as B and T cells, natural killer cells, macrophages, and some granulocytes.

1358. In kidney transplantation patients, most frequently used combination for maintenance immunosuppressive therapy is?
Harrison's 20th Ed. Chapter 307 Page 2128

A. Prednisone + mTOR inhibitors
B. Prednisone + Calcineurin inhibitor
C. Prednisone + antimetabolite
D. Prednisone + calcineurin inhibitor + antimetabolite

All kidney transplant recipients should receive maintenance immunosuppressive therapies except identical twins. The most frequently used combination is triple therapy with prednisone, a calcineurin inhibitor, and an antimetabolite.

1359. Which of the following is used as prophylaxis for acute rejection in the immediate post renal transplant period?
Harrison's 20th Ed. Chapter 307 Page 2128, Biologics. 2009;3:319-336

A. Eculizumab
B. Daclizumab
C. Bevacizumab
D. Certolizumab pegol

Anti-interleukin-2 receptor antibodies, basiliximab and daclizumab are used for the prevention of acute rejection in renal transplantation.

1360. All kidney transplant recipients should receive maintenance immunosuppressive therapies except?
Harrison's 20th Ed. Chapter 307 Page 2129

A. Father–child
B. Mother–child
C. Identical twins
D. All of the above

All kidney transplant recipients must receive maintenance immunosuppressive therapies except identical twins.

1361. Which of the following is FDA-approved for kidney transplant recipients?
Harrison's 20th Ed. Chapter 307 Page 2129

A. Abatacept
B. Belatacept
C. Rilonacept
D. All of the above

Belatacept is a fusion protein that binds costimulatory ligands (CD80 and CD86) present on antigen presenting cells, interrupting their binding to CD28 on T cells. This inhibition leads to T cell anergy and apoptosis.

1362. Which of the following antimetabolite is used for maintenance therapy in kidney transplant recipients?
Harrison's 20th Ed. Chapter 307 Page 2129

A. Azathioprine
B. Methotrexate
C. 5-flucytosine
D. All of the above

Azathioprine and Mycophenolate mofetil are used for maintenance therapy in kidney transplant recipients.

1363. Which of the following about steroids in kidney transplant recipients is false?
Harrison's 20th Ed. Chapter 307 Page 2129

A. Prevents release of IL-6 & IL-1 by monocytes-macrophages
B. Methylprednisolone used in treatment of acute rejection
C. Methylprednisolone not effective in chronic rejection
D. None of the above

1364. Which of the following side effect is more common with tacrolimus as compared to cyclosporine?
Harrison's 20th Ed. Chapter 307 Page 2129

A. Nephrotoxicity
B. Hepatotoxicity
C. Diabetes mellitus
D. Tremor

Tacrolimus has a similar side-effect profile as cyclosporine ((nephrotoxicity, hepatotoxicity, hirsutism, tremor, gingival hyperplasia, and diabetes). Tacrolimus does not produce hirsutism or gingival hyperplasia. De novo diabetes mellitus is more common with tacrolimus.

1365. Clinical evidence of rejection is characterized by?

Harrison's 20th Ed. Chapter 307 Page 2129

A. Fever
B. Swelling
C. Tenderness over the allograft
D. None of the above

Clinical evidence of rejection is rarely characterized by fever, swelling, and tenderness over the allograft. Rejection may present only with a rise in serum creatinine, with or without a reduction in urine volume. A rise in the serum creatinine level is a late marker of rejection, but it may be the only sign.

1366. Which of the following is suggestive of cyclosporine side effect on renal biopsy?

Harrison's 20th Ed. Chapter 307 Page 2129

A. Interstitial fibrosis
B. Isometric tubular vacuolization
C. Thickening of arteriolar walls
D. All of the above

In renal biopsy, interstitial fibrosis, isometric tubular vacuolization, and thickening of arteriolar walls are suggestive of cyclosporine side effect, but not diagnostic.

1367. Which of the following is relevant to acute kidney graft rejection?

Harrison's 20th Ed. Chapter 307 Page 2130

A. Component c3
B. Component c4d
C. Component c5
D. Component c5b-9

Evidence of antibody-mediated injury is present when endothelial injury and deposition of complement component c4d is detected by fluorescence labeling.

1368. Which of the following is not an infection during early (1–6 months) period in kidney transplant recipients?

Harrison's 20th Ed. Chapter 307 Page 2130 Table 307-4

A. Herpes zoster
B. Pneumocystis carinii
C. Cytomegalovirus
D. Legionella

1369. Which of the following is an infection during late (> 6 months) period in kidney transplant recipients?

Harrison's 20th Ed. Chapter 307 Page 2130 Table 307-4

A. BK virus (polyoma)
B. Aspergillus
C. Nocardia
D. All of the above

1370. Use of which of the following drugs increase catabolism of calcineurin inhibitors resulting in low blood levels?

Harrison's 20th Ed. Chapter 307 Page 2130

A. Erythromycin
B. Phenytoin
C. Ketoconazole
D. Diltiazem

Ketoconazole, erythromycin, diltiazem & verapamil compete with calcineurin inhibitors for P450 catabolism and cause their elevated levels. Phenytoin & carbamazepine increase their catabolism to result in low levels.

1371. Which of the following about OKT3 is false?

Immunotherapy 2016;8(8):889-906

A. Stands for ortho kung T3
B. Monoclonal antibody for CD3 surface antigen on human T cells
C. Potent mitogen
D. None of the above

1372. Which of the following viruses does not belong to polyoma group?

Harrison's 20th Ed. Chapter 307 Page 2131

A. BK
B. JC
C. CMV
D. SV40

The polyoma group (BK, JC, SV40) is a class of DNA viruses that become dormant in kidneys and can be activated by immunosuppression.

1373. Which of the following tumor occurs in patients on immunosuppressive therapy?

Harrison's 20th Ed. Chapter 307 Page 2131

A. Cancer of skin and lips
B. Carcinoma in situ of cervix
C. Non-Hodgkin's lymphoma
D. All of the above

The incidence of tumors in patients on immunosuppressive therapy is 5–6%, or ~100 times greater than that in the general population in the same age range. The most common cancers are cancer of the skin and lips and carcinoma in situ of the cervix, and non-Hodgkin's lymphoma.

1374. Many renal transplant patients have creatinine clearances of?

Harrison's 20th Ed. Chapter 307 Page 2131

A. 15–30 mL/minute
B. 30–50 mL/minute
C. 50–70 mL/minute
D. 70–90 mL/minute

Many transplant patients have creatinine clearances of 30–50 mL/minute.

Glomerular Diseases

1375. Number of glomerular capillary tufts in the two human kidneys is about?

Harrison's 20th Ed. Chapter 308 Page 2132

A. 0.6 million
B. 1.2 million
C. 1.8 million
D. 2.4 million

About 1.8 million glomerular capillary tufts are found in the two human kidneys.

1376. Each kidney contains how many glomeruli in the renal cortex?

N Engl J Med. 2006;354:1387-401

A. About 1 million
B. About 2 million
C. About 3 million
D. About 4 million

1377. Which of the following about glomerulus is false?

Harrison's 20th Ed. Chapter 308 Page 2132

A. Arteriolar portal system
B. Glomerular capillaries have fenestrated endothelial cells
C. Podocytes line the outer surface of the glomerular capillaries
D. None of the above

1378. Which of the following about glomerulus is false?

Harrison's 20th Ed. Chapter 308 Page 2132

A. Parietal epithelial cells of Bowman's capsule transition into tubular epithelia of proximal nephron
B. Parietal epithelial cells of Bowman's capsule migrate into glomerular tuft to replenish podocytes
C. Adjacent podocytes interconnect by slit-pore membranes
D. None of the above

1379. Which of the following about glomerular filtration is false?

Harrison's 20th Ed. Chapter 308 Page 2132

A. Slit-pore membrane forming a selective filtration barrier
B. Physicochemical barrier
C. Positive electrostatic charge
D. Pores in GBM & slit-pore membranes have a radius of 4 nm

Glomerular filtration takes place across a physicochemical barrier governed by pore size and negative electrostatic charge.

1380. Which of the following about albumin filtration is false?

Harrison's 20th Ed. Chapter 308 Page 2132

A. Albumin has a negative charge
B. Albumin has a physical radius of 3.6 nm
C. Albumin is reclaimed by megalin & cubilin receptors of PCT
D. None of the above

1381. Pores in the glomerular basement membrane (GBM) and slit-pore membranes have a radius of?

Harrison's 20th Ed. Chapter 308 Page 2132

A. 2 nm
B. 4 nm
C. 6 nm
D. 8 nm

Pores in GBM & slit-pore membranes have a radius of 4 nm. Albumin has a physical radius of 3.6 nm.

1382. Filtration barrier of capillary wall in glomerulus contains?

N Engl J Med. 2006;354:1387-401

A. Fenestrated endothelium
B. Glomerular basement membrane
C. Interdigitating podocyte foot processes
D. All of the above

1383. Glomerular basement membrane has a thickness of?

N Engl J Med. 2006;354:1387-401

A. 200 to 250 nm
B. 300 to 350 nm
C. 400 to 450 nm
D. 500 to 550 nm

1384. Humans with normal nephrons excrete how much albumin in daily voided urine?

Harrison's 20th Ed. Chapter 308 Page 2132

A. 1–5 mg
B. 8–10 mg
C. 15–30 mg
D. 40–60 mg

1385. Main components of glomerular basement membrane are?

N Engl J Med. 2003;348:2543-56

A. Type IV collagen
B. Laminin
C. Nidogen
D. All of the above

1386. Which of the following is instrumental in reclaiming filtered albumin along the proximal tubule?

Harrison's 20th Ed. Chapter 308 Page 2132

A. Crucin
B. Optimin
C. Megalin
D. Reglin

4000 to 9000 mg/day of albumin is filtered and is reclaimed by megalin and cubilin receptors along the proximal tubule. Humans with normal nephrons excretion average 8–10 mg of albumin in daily voided urine, approximately 20–60% of total excreted protein.

1387. Founder effect best relates to?

Harrison's 20th Ed. Chapter 308 Page 2132

A. Laplace's law
B. Hardy-Weinberg law
C. Hy's Law
D. Inverse-care law

The Hardy-Weinberg law, which is the basis of population genetics, states, in part, that in a large randommating population at equilibrium (i.e. no selection, migration or genetic drift), genotype frequencies are functions of allele frequencies and the former can be predicted from the latter.

1388. What proportion of glomerular ultrafiltrate is reabsorbed in the proximal tubules?

Lancet 2005;365:417-430

A. One-third
B. One-half
C. Two-third
D. Three-fourth

~ Two-thirds of glomerular ultrafiltrate is reabsorbed isosmotically in proximal tubule with little change in osmolality or sodium concentration of unreabsorbed fraction. With water absorption, sodium along with chloride & bicarbonate are absorbed actively to keep ultrafiltrate iso-osmotic.

1389. In earliest portion of proximal tubule, which of the following is the principal ion that accompanies reabsorption of sodium?

Lancet 2005;365:417-430

A. Chloride
B. Bicarbonate
C. Hydrogen
D. Phosphate

In the earliest portion of PCT, bicarbonate is the principal anion that accompanies reabsorption of sodium. This process occurs via a Na/H exchanger at the luminal brush border and is dependent on the activity of carbonic anhydrase.

1390. Early proximal convoluted tubule is the major site of reabsorption of?

Lancet 2005;365:417-430

A. Lactate
B. Amino acids
C. Glucose
D. All of the above

Glucose, amino acids, and organic solutes like lactate are extensively reabsorbed in the proximal tubule by cotransport mechanisms.

1391. Normally, in glomerulus, which of the following is true?

Lancet 2005;365:417-430

A. Hydraulic pressure exceeds oncotic pressure
B. Oncotic pressure exceeds hydraulic pressure
C. Oncotic pressure equals hydraulic pressure
D. All of the above

At glomerulus, hydraulic pressure exceeds oncotic pressure favoring filtration.

1392. Congenital nephrotic syndrome occurs due to mutations in?

Harrison's 20th Ed. Chapter 308 Page 2132

A. PROP-1
B. NPHS1
C. PAX-8
D. PIT-1

Congenital nephrotic syndrome occurs due to mutations in NPHS1 (nephrin) and NPHS2 (podocin).

1393. Pierson's syndrome is a form of?

N Engl J Med. 2006;354:1387-401

A. Congenital nephrotic syndrome
B. Congenital heart disease
C. Congenital bone disease
D. Congenital eye disease

1394. Focal segmental glomerulosclerosis (FSGS) occurs due to mutations in?

Harrison's 20th Ed. Chapter 308 Page 2132

A. NPHS2
B. TRPC6
C. APOL1
D. SGK1

TRPC6 cation channel mutations produce focal segmental glomerulosclerosis (FSGS) in adulthood.

1395. Polymorphisms in which of the following gene is a major risk for nondiabetic ESRD, particularly FSGS?

Harrison's 20th Ed. Chapter 308 Page 2132

A. APOL1
B. COL4A5
C. ACTN4
D. All of the above

Polymorphisms in the gene encoding apolipoprotein L1, APOL1, are a major risk for African Americans with nondiabetic end stage renal disease, particularly FSGS.

1396. Which of the following statements is false?

Harrison's 20th Ed. Chapter 308 Page 2132

A. Mutations in complement factor H cause membranoproliferative glomerulonephritis (MPGN)
B. Mutations in genes encoding for $\alpha3$, $\alpha4$, or $\alpha5$ chains of type IV collagen cause Alport's syndrome
C. α-galactosidase A deficiency causes Fabry's disease
D. None of the above

1397. Nephrosialidosis is caused by?

Harrison's 20th Ed. Chapter 308 Page 2132

A. S-Adenosylhomocysteine hydrolase deficiency
B. N acetylneuraminic acid hydrolase deficiency
C. Glycine N-methyltransferase deficiency
D. Adenosine kinase deficiency

Nephrosialidosis is an ultra-rare disorder and lacks comprehensive information about the clinical course (<20 cases in the literature). It presents as childhood-onset, steroid resistant nephrotic syndrome and is due to a mutation in NEU1 causing N acetylneuraminic acid hydrolase deficiency.

1398. Chronic glomerulosclerosis in systemic hypertension & atherosclerosis is due to?

Harrison's 20th Ed. Chapter 308 Page 2133

A. Pressure stress
B. Ischemia
C. Lipid oxidants
D. All of the above

1399. Thickening of GBM in diabetic nephropathy is secondary to the long-standing effects of?

Harrison's 20th Ed. Chapter 308 Page 2133

A. Hyperglycemia
B. Advanced glycosylation end products
C. Reactive oxygen species
D. All of the above

Diabetic nephropathy is an acquired sclerotic injury associated with thickening of GBM secondary to long-standing effects of hyperglycemia, advanced glycosylation end products and reactive oxygen species.

1400. Glomerulonephritis refers to inflammation of?

Harrison's 20th Ed. Chapter 308 Page 2133

A. Glomerular capillaries
B. Glomerular arterioles
C. Glomerular basement membrane (GBM)
D. All of the above

Inflammation of the glomerular capillaries is called glomerulonephritis.

1401. In glomerulonephritis, cytokines & proteases damage which of the following?

Harrison's 20th Ed. Chapter 308 Page 2133

A. Mesangium
B. Capillaries
C. GBM
D. All of the above

Chemokines attract neutrophils, macrophages & T cells into glomerular tuft. These react with antigens & epitopes producing more cytokines & proteases that damage mesangium, capillaries, and/or GBM.

1402. Which of the following is an antiglomerular basement membrane disease?

Harrison's 20th Ed. Chapter 308 Page 2133

A. Membranous glomerulonephritis (MGN)
B. Goodpasture's syndrome
C. Lupus nephritis
D. Granulomatosis with polyangiitis (Wegener's)

Antiglomerular basement membrane disease producing Goodpasture's syndrome. It primarily injures both lung & kidney because of the narrow distribution of the a3 NC1 domain of type IV collagen that is the target antigen.

1403. Which of the following plays an important role in the mechanism of glomerulonephritis?

Harrison's 20th Ed. Chapter 308 Page 2133

A. Deposition of immune complexes
B. Early T cell activation
C. Complement injury
D. Systemic inflammation

While the adaptive immune response is similar to that of other tissues, early T cell activation plays an important role in the mechanism of glomerulonephritis.

1404. Which of the following is associated with immune deposits along the GBM?

Harrison's 20th Ed. Chapter 308 Page 2134

A. Poststreptococcal glomerulonephritis
B. Lupus nephritis
C. Idiopathic membranous nephritis
D. All of the above

Poststreptococcal glomerulonephritis, lupus nephritis, and idiopathic membranous nephritis typically are associated with immune deposits along the GBM.

1405. Preformed circulating immune complexes precipitate along which side of the GBM?

Harrison's 20th Ed. Chapter 308 Page 2134

A. Subendothelial side
B. Subepithelial side
C. In lumen
D. All of the above

Preformed circulating immune complexes precipitate along the subendothelial side of the GBM, while immune deposits formed in situ precipitate on the subepithelial side.

1406. Complement membrane attack complex (MAC) best relates to?

Harrison's 20th Ed. Chapter 308 Page 2134

A. C3a
B. C3b
C. C5a
D. C5b-9

The five glycoproteins C5b to C9 form a complex which is responsible for the final lytic action on cells. This membrane attack complex (MAC) is formed by successive assembly of its components. The complex C5bC6C7C8(C9)$_n$ is included as an integral membrane protein complex (membrane attack complex). The free flow of small molecules and ions through the formed pores causes osmotic cell lysis. The C5 convertase (C4b2a3b of classical pathway & C3bBbC3b of alternative pathway) cleaves C5 into C5a and C5b fragments. C5a is the most potent anaphylatoxin in the complement cascade. The C5b binds to the cell surface and serves as a platform for the membrane attack complex (MAC), which consists of C5bC6789.

1407. Which of the following is the "pore-forming molecule" of complement?

Harrison's 20th Ed. Chapter 308 Page 2134

A. C3
B. C5
C. C6
D. C9

C9, a pore-forming molecule with homology to perforin, a protein used by cytotoxic T cells and natural killer cells for killing virus-infected targets. The complex of C5b678 forms a nidus for C9 binding and polymerization.

1408. Persistent glomerulonephritis that worsens renal function is always accompanied by?

Harrison's 20th Ed. Chapter 308 Page 2134

A. Interstitial nephritis
B. Renal fibrosis
C. Tubular atrophy
D. All of the above

Persistent glomerulonephritis that worsens renal function is always accompanied by interstitial nephritis, renal fibrosis, and tubular atrophy.

1409. Renal failure in glomerulonephritis best correlates histologically with the appearance of?

Harrison's 20th Ed. Chapter 308 Page 2134

A. Tubulointerstitial nephritis
B. Papillary necrosis
C. Cystic kidney disease
D. All of the above

Renal failure in glomerulonephritis best correlates histologically with the appearance of tubulointerstitial nephritis. Early acute tubulointerstitial nephritis suggests potentially recoverable renal function whereas the development of chronic interstitial fibrosis prognosticates permanent loss.

1410. Renal fibroblasts increase through which of the following mechanisms?
Harrison's 20th Ed. Chapter 308 Page 2134

A. Epithelial or endothelial mesenchymal transitions
B. Bone marrow-derived fibrocytes
C. Proliferation of resident fibroblasts
D. All of the above

At the site of injury, interstitial fibroblasts increase in number & fibrosis occurs. Renal fibroblasts increase by epithelial or endothelial mesenchymal transitions (15%), bone marrow-derived fibrocytes (35%), and the proliferation of resident fibroblasts (50%).

1411. Which of the following is active in fibrotic damage to kidneys?
Harrison's 20th Ed. Chapter 308 Page 2134

A. Transforming growth factor-β (TGF-β)
B. Fibroblast growth factor 2 (FGF-2)
C. Hypoxemia-inducible factor 1α (HIF-1α)
D. All of the above

Transforming growth factor-β (TGF-β), fibroblast growth factor 2 (FGF-2), hypoxemia-inducible factor 1α (HIF-1α), and platelet-derived growth factor (PDGF) are active in fibrosis at the site of kidney injury.

1412. Which of the following can reverse early fibrogenesis and preserve tubular architecture?
Harrison's 20th Ed. Chapter 308 Page 2134

A. Bone morphogenetic protein 2
B. Bone morphogenetic protein 7
C. Transforming growth factor β (TGF-β)
D. All of the above

In experimental studies, bone morphogenetic protein 7 and hepatocyte growth factor can reverse early fibrogenesis and preserve tubular architecture.

1413. Cause of microscopic hematuria is?
Harrison's 20th Ed. Chapter 308 Page 2134

A. Interstitial nephritis
B. Papillary necrosis
C. Cystic kidney diseases
D. All of the above

Microscopic hematuria may appear with the onset of benign prostatic hypertrophy, interstitial nephritis, papillary necrosis, hypercalciuria, renal stones, cystic kidney diseases, or renal vascular injury.

1414. Which of the following are indicative of a glomerular disease?
Harrison's 20th Ed. Chapter 308 Page 2134

A. Microscopic hematuria
B. Urinary red blood cell casts
C. Urinary dysmorphic red blood cells
D. All of the above

Sustained proteinuria >1–2 g/24 hours is also commonly associated with glomerular disease.

1415. Normal 24-hour urine protein is?
Harrison's 20th Ed. Chapter 308 Page 2134 Table 308-1

A. < 30 mg/day
B. < 100 mg/day
C. < 150 mg/day
D. < 300 mg/day

Normal 24-hour urine protein is < 150 mg/day.

1416. Albumin comprises what percentage of total proteins excreted in the urine?
Harrison's 20th Ed. Chapter 308 Page 2134 Table 308-1

A. 10–30%
B. 20–60%
C. 30–70%
D. 40–90%

Albumin represents 20–60% of the total protein excreted in the urine.

1417. Sustained isolated proteinuria is found in?
Harrison's 20th Ed. Chapter 308 Page 2135

A. Diabetic nephropathy
B. Mesangioproliferative glomerulonephritis
C. FSGS
D. All of the above

Sustained isolated proteinuria is found in diabetic nephropathy, nil lesion, mesangioproliferative glomerulonephritis, and FSGS.

1418. Orthostatic proteinuria is evident only in?
Harrison's 20th Ed. Chapter 308 Page 2135

A. Upright position
B. Recumbent position
C. Sitting position
D. Lateral position

Proteinuria only seen with upright posture is called orthostatic proteinuria.

1419. Functional proteinuria refers to?
Harrison's 20th Ed. Chapter 308 Page 2135

A. Proteinuria in females
B. Proteinuria during fever, emotional stress
C. Proteinuria in UTI
D. Proteinuria in upright posture

Benign, functional or transient proteinuria occurs in normal population. It is nonsustained and proteinuria is <1 gram/day. Fever, exercise, obesity, sleep apnea, emotional stress & congestive heart failure cause transient proteinuria.

1420. In which of the following conditions, proteinuria is selective & composed largely of albumin?
Harrison's 20th Ed. Chapter 308 Page 2135

A. Henoch-Schönlein purpura
B. Minimal change disease
C. Churg-Strauss syndrome
D. Goodpasture's syndrome

In children with minimal change disease, proteinuria is selective & composed largely of albumin.

1421. Which of the following glomerular disease can present with gross hematuria?
Harrison's 20th Ed. Chapter 308 Page 2135

A. Focal segmental glomerulosclerosis
B. Mesangioproliferative glomerulonephritis
C. IgA nephropathy
D. Subacute bacterial endocarditis

1422. Which of the following glomerular disease can present with gross hematuria?

Harrison's 20th Ed. Chapter 308 Page 2135

A. Henoch-Schönlein purpura
B. Antiphospholipid syndrome
C. Sickle cell disease
D. Nail-patella syndrome

In IgA nephropathy & sickle cell disease, gross hematuria is present.

1423. Asymptomatic hematuria is due to?

Harrison's 20th Ed. Chapter 308 Page 2135

A. IgA nephropathy (Berger's disease)
B. Thin basement membrane (TBM) disease
C. Alport's syndrome
D. All of the above

1424. Which of the following clinical syndromes is most important according to global perspective?

Harrison's 20th Ed. Chapter 308 Page 2135

A. Acute nephritic syndrome
B. Nephrotic syndrome
C. Basement membrane syndrome
D. Infectious disease–associated syndrome

Infectious disease-associated syndrome is most important if one has a global perspective. Malaria, and schistosomiasis may be the most common causes of glomerulonephritis throughout the world, closely followed by HIV and chronic hepatitis B & C. Other syndromes include acute nephritic syndromes, pulmonary-renal syndromes, nephrotic syndromes, basement membrane syndromes, glomerular vascular syndromes.

1425. Which of the following is false about a 'crescent'?

Lancet 1999;353:1509

A. Half-moon-shaped collection of cells in Bowman's space
B. Composed of proliferating parietal epithelial cells and infiltrating macrophages
C. Crescentic glomerulonephritis is also called rapidly progressive glomerulonephritis
D. None of the above

1426. Which of the following does not present as rapidly progressive glomerulonephritis (RPGN)?

Harrison's 20th Ed. Chapter 308 Page 2135 Table 308-2

A. Poststreptococcal glomerulonephritis
B. Subacute bacterial endocarditis
C. Wegener's granulomatosis
D. Henoch-Schönlein purpura

1427. Which of the following does not present as rapidly progressive glomerulonephritis (RPGN)?

Harrison's 20th Ed. Chapter 308 Page 2135 Table 308-2

A. Poststreptococcal glomerulonephritis
B. Mesangioproliferative glomerulonephritis
C. Membranoproliferative glomerulonephritis
D. Lupus nephritis

1428. Henoch-Schönlein purpura has which of the following patterns of clinical glomerulonephritis?

Harrison's 20th Ed. Chapter 308 Page 2135 Table 308-2

A. Acute nephritic syndrome
B. Pulmonary-renal syndrome
C. Glomerular vascular syndrome
D. All of the above

1429. Wegener's granulomatosis has which of the following patterns of clinical glomerulonephritis?

Harrison's 20th Ed. Chapter 308 Page 2135 Table 308-2

A. Acute nephritic syndrome
B. Pulmonary-renal syndrome
C. Glomerular vascular syndrome
D. All of the above

1430. Cryoglobulinemia has which of the following patterns of clinical glomerulonephritis?

Harrison's 20th Ed. Chapter 308 Page 2135 Table 308-2

A. Acute Nephritic syndrome
B. Pulmonary-renal syndrome
C. Glomerular vascular syndrome
D. All of the above

1431. Churg-Strauss syndrome has which of the following patterns of clinical glomerulonephritis?

Harrison's 20th Ed. Chapter 308 Page 2135 Table 308-2

A. Acute nephritic syndrome
B. Pulmonary-renal syndrome
C. Glomerular vascular syndrome
D. All of the above

1432. Which of the following can cause pulmonary-renal syndrome?

Harrison's 20th Ed. Chapter 308 Page 2135 Table 308-2

A. Henoch-Schönlein purpura
B. Microscopic polyangiitis
C. Cryoglobulinemia
D. All of the above

1433. Which of the following can cause basement membrane syndrome?

Harrison's 20th Ed. Chapter 308 Page 2135 Table 308-2

A. Alport's syndrome
B. Nail-patella syndrome
C. Thin basement membrane disease
D. All of the above

Patients with a basement membrane syndrome either have genetically abnormal basement membranes (Alport's syndrome) or an autoimmune response to basement membrane collagen IV (Goodpasture's syndrome) associated with microscopic hematuria, mild to heavy proteinuria & hypertension with variable elevations in serum creatinine.

1434. Which of the following is the most common cause of glomerulonephritis throughout the world?

Harrison's 20th Ed. Chapter 308 Page 2135

A. HIV
B. Chronic hepatitis B
C. Chronic hepatitis C
D. Malaria

Malaria and schistosomiasis may be the most common causes of glomerulonephritis throughout the world, closely followed by HIV and chronic hepatitis B and C.

1435. Which of the following stains is used to enhance basement membrane structure in renal biopsy?
Harrison's 20th Ed. Chapter 308 Page 2136

A. Hematoxylin and eosin
B. Periodic acid-Schiff (PAS)
C. Jones-methenamine silver
D. Masson's trichrome

1436. Which of the following stains is used to stain carbohydrate moieties in the membranes of the glomerular tuft & tubules?
Harrison's 20th Ed. Chapter 308 Page 2136

A. Hematoxylin and eosin
B. Periodic acid-Schiff (PAS)
C. Jones-methenamine silver
D. Masson's trichrome

1437. Which of the following stains is used to stain amyloid deposits?
Harrison's 20th Ed. Chapter 308 Page 2136

A. Congo red
B. Periodic acid-Schiff (PAS)
C. Jones-methenamine silver
D. Masson's trichrome

1438. Which of the following stains is used to stain collagen deposition and assess the degree of glomerulosclerosis & interstitial fibrosis?
Harrison's 20th Ed. Chapter 308 Page 2136

A. Congo red
B. Periodic acid-Schiff (PAS)
C. Jones-methenamine silver
D. Masson's trichrome

Renal biopsy specimen are stained with H&E for cellularity & architecture, PAS for carbohydrate moieties in glomerular tuft & tubule membranes, Jones-methenamine silver to enhance basement membrane structure, Congo red for amyloid deposits, & Masson's trichrome to identify collagen deposition to assess degree of glomerulosclerosis & interstitial fibrosis.

1439. By light microscopy, ideally how many glomeruli should be reviewed individually for discrete lesions?
Harrison's 20th Ed. Chapter 308 Page 2137

A. 1
B. 5
C. 10
D. 20

By light microscopy, ideally 20 glomeruli should be reviewed individually for discrete lesions.

1440. When cellular proliferation extends into Bowman's space, it is called?
Harrison's 20th Ed. Chapter 308 Page 2137

A. Endocapillary proliferation
B. Extracapillary proliferation
C. Synechiae
D. Crescents

Glomeruli with increased cellularity are termed as proliferative. When cells in capillary tuft proliferate, it is called endocapillary and when cellular proliferation extends into Bowman's space, it is called extracapillary.

1441. When epithelial podocytes attach to Bowman's capsule in the setting of glomerular injury, it is called?
Harrison's 20th Ed. Chapter 308 Page 2137

A. Endocapillary proliferation
B. Extracapillary proliferation
C. Synechiae
D. Crescents

When epithelial podocytes attach to Bowman's capsule in glomerular injury, it is termed synechiae.

1442. Crescents best relate to?
Harrison's 20th Ed. Chapter 308 Page 2137

A. Endocapillary proliferation
B. Extracapillary proliferation
C. Synechiae
D. All of the above

Crescents may be extension of synechiae, develop when fibrocellular/fibrin collections fill all or part of Bowman's space.

1443. Which of the following about sclerotic glomeruli is false?
Harrison's 20th Ed. Chapter 308 Page 2137

A. Acellular
B. Amorphous accumulations of proteinaceous material
C. Loss of functional capillaries & normal mesangium
D. None of the above

1444. How can background percentage of sclerosis in age-related glomerulosclerosis be estimated?
Harrison's 20th Ed. Chapter 308 Page 2137

A. (Patient's age/10) × 2
B. (Patient's age/2) – 10
C. (Patient's age/10) + 2
D. (Patient's age/2) + 10

Background percentage of sclerosis in age-related glomerulosclerosis can be estimated by dividing the patient's age in half and subtracting 10.

1445. Which of the following occurs in interstitial fibrosis?
Harrison's 20th Ed. Chapter 308 Page 2137

A. Loss of adjacency
B. Tubular dropout
C. Collagen deposition
D. All of the above

1446. 'Focal glomeulonephritis' is said to occur when lesion involves what proportion of glomeruli?
Harrison's 20th Ed. Chapter 308 Page 2137

A. < 50%
B. < 60%
C. < 70%
D. < 80%

If <50% glomeruli are involved, lesion is considered focal, else diffuse.

1447. In renal biopsy, which of the following is an ominous sign of irreversibility and progression to renal failure?
Harrison's 20th Ed. Chapter 308 Page 2137

A. Synechiae
B. Interstitial fibrosis
C. Crescents
D. All of the above

Interstitial fibrosis is an ominous sign of irreversibility & progression to renal failure.

1448. Acute nephritic syndromes classically present with?

Harrison's 20th Ed. Chapter 308 Page 2137

A. Hypertension
B. Hematuria
C. Pyuria
D. All of the above

Acute nephritic syndromes classically present with hypertension, hematuria, red blood cell casts, pyuria, and mild to moderate proteinuria.

1449. Which of the following is prototypical for acute endocapillary proliferative glomerulonephritis?

Harrison's 20th Ed. Chapter 308 Page 2137

A. Poststreptococcal glomerulonephritis
B. Endocarditis-associated glomerulonephritis
C. Lupus nephritis
D. All of the above

1450. Circulating immune-complex formation and deposition within the glomerulus is seen in?

Harrison's 20th Ed. Chapter 308 Page 2137+

A. Subacute bacterial endocarditis (SABE)
B. Lupus nephritis
C. Hepatitis-C-related cryoglobulinemia
D. All of the above

Circulating immune-complex formation and deposition within the glomerulus is seen with SABE, lupus nephritis, & hepatitis-C-related cryoglobulinemia.

1451. Poststreptococcal glomerulonephritis is prototypical for?

Harrison's 20th Ed. Chapter 308 Page 2137

A. Acute endocapillary proliferative glomerulonephritis
B. Mesangiocapillary glomerulonephritis
C. Lobar glomerulonephritis
D. Segmental necrotizing glomerulonephritis

Poststreptococcal glomerulonephritis is prototypical for acute endocapillary proliferative glomerulonephritis.

1452. Poststreptococcal glomerulonephritis develops how many weeks after streptococcal pharyngitis?

Harrison's 20th Ed. Chapter 308 Page 2137

A. 1–3 weeks
B. 2–6 weeks
C. 3–6 weeks
D. 4–8 weeks

Acute poststreptococcal glomerulonephritis (APSGN) develops after streptococcal infection with a latent period of around 1 - 3 weeks (10 days).

1453. Poststreptococcal glomerulonephritis due to impetigo develops how many weeks after the skin infection?

Harrison's 20th Ed. Chapter 308 Page 2137

A. 1–3 weeks
B. 2–6 weeks
C. 3–6 weeks
D. 4–8 weeks

Poststreptococcal glomerulonephritis due to impetigo develops 2–6 weeks after skin infection and 1–3 weeks after streptococcal pharyngitis.

1454. Which strain of streptococci is nephritogenic?

Harrison's 20th Ed. Chapter 308 Page 2137

A. H
B. O
C. M
C. N

Skin & throat infections with particular M types strains of streptococci are nephritogenic and antedate glomerular disease.

1455. Which of the following M type strain of streptococci are seen following impetigo?

Harrison's 20th Ed. Chapter 308 Page 2137

A. 47
B. 49
C. 55
D. All of the above

1456. Which of the following M type strain of streptococci are seen with pharyngitis?

Harrison's 20th Ed. Chapter 308 Page 2137

A. 1
B. 2
C. 4
D. All of the above

1457. Which of the following M type strain of streptococci are common with both impetigo & pharyngitis?

Harrison's 20th Ed. Chapter 308 Page 2137

A. 2
B. 47
C. 55
D. 60

M types 47, 49, 55, 2, 60 & 57 are seen following impetigo and M types 1, 2, 4, 3, 25, 49 & 12 with pharyngitis.

1458. The 'humps' seen in renal biopsy in poststreptococcal glomerulonephritis best relate to?

Harrison's 20th Ed. Chapter 308 Page 2137

A. Mesangium
B. Subendothelium
C. Subepithelium
D. All of the above

In APSGN, accumulation of immune complexes, complements, and plasma proteins, forming 'humps' on the outer side of glomerular tufts (subepithelium).

1459. Which of the following is an antigen from nephritogenic streptococci?

Harrison's 20th Ed. Chapter 308 Page 2137

A. Streptococcal pyrogenic exotoxin B (SPEB)
B. Streptococcal pyrogenic endotoxin B (SPEB)
C. Streptococcal plasmin exotoxin B (SPEB)
D. Streptococcal plasmin endotoxin B (SPEB)

1460. Deposition of which of the following antigens is seen in essentially all patients with early-phase APSGN?

Harrison's 20th Ed. Chapter 308 Page 2137

A. PLA2R
B. NAPlr
C. Thomsen-Friedenreich antigen
D. All of the above

Immunofluorescence staining of the renal biopsy tissues with anti-NAPlr antibody shows glomerular NAPlr deposition in essentially all patients with early-phase acute poststreptococcal glomerulonephritis (APSGN).

1461. Which of the following about NAPlr is false?

Harrison's 20th Ed. Chapter 308 Page 2137

A. Have an affinity to plasmin and glomerular proteins
B. Activates the alternative complement pathway
C. Does not co-localize with C3 in glomerular deposits
D. None of the above

A cationic cysteine proteinase known as streptococcal pyrogenic exotoxin B (SPEB) is an antigen from nephritogenic streptococci. It is generated by proteolysis of a zymogen precursor (zSPEB) and NAPlr, the nephritis-associated plasmin receptor. These two antigens have biochemical affinity for plasmin, bind as complexes and activate the alternate complement pathway. The nephritogenic antigen, SPEB, has been demonstrated inside the subepithelial 'humps' on biopsy.

1462. Deposits of IgG, IgM, C3, C4, and C5-9 in APSGN are found in?

Harrison's 20th Ed. Chapter 308 Page 2137

A. Mesangium
B. Subendothelium
C. Subepithelium
D. All of the above

1463. Deposits of nephritogenic antigen SPEB in APSGN are found in?

Harrison's 20th Ed. Chapter 308 Page 2137

A. Mesangium
B. Subendothelium
C. Subepithelium
D. All of the above

Nephritogenic antigen, SPEB, is demonstrated inside the subepithelial 'humps' on biopsy. NAPlr is localized on the inner side of glomerular tufts (endocapillary) is consistent with the predominantly endocapillary glomerular inflammation in APSGN.

1464. Nephritogenic antigens on streptococci SPEB and NAPlr have biochemical affinity for?

Harrison's 20th Ed. Chapter 308 Page 2137

A. Platelets
B. Plasmin
C. Collagen
D. Elastin

Nephritogenic antigens on streptococci SPEB and NAPlr have biochemical affinity for plasmin. NAPlr and SPEB, both bind plasmin. They protect plasmin from physiological inhibitors (Aprotinin) and thus might cause chemotaxis of inflammatory cells and degradation of glomerular basement membranes, due to the activity of plasmin. Plasmin activity may be a common final pathway in APSGN.

1465. NAPlr deposition and plasmin activity is found in which of the following glomerular disease?

Clinical Nephrology. 2006;65(2):124 -128,

A. Dense deposit disease (DDD)
B. Henoch-Schönlein Purpura nephritis (HSPN)
C. Membranoproliferative glomerulonephritis (MPGN)
D. All of the above

1466. Which of the following is a plasmin inhibitor?

Harrison's 20th Ed. Chapter 308 Page 2137

A. Renin
B. Aprotinin
C. Kallikrein
D. All of the above

Aprotinin, also known as bovine pancreatic trypsin inhibitor or BPTI, is a polypeptide extracted from bovine lung that inhibits the action of serine proteases, including plasmin and kallikrein. Aprotinin slows down fibrinolysis. It is associated with AKI and this drug was withdrawn from the market.

1467. In the immune complex theory of APSGN, which of the following is false?

Harrison's 20th Ed. Chapter 308 Page 2137

A. Glomerular deposition of nephritogenic streptococcal antigen and subsequent formation of immune complexes in situ
B. Deposition of circulating antigen-antibody complexes
C. Immune complex is localized to outer side of glomerular tufts (subepithelial site)
D. None of the above

1468. In the first week of poststreptococcal glomerulonephritis, which of the following lab. findings is false?

Harrison's 20th Ed. Chapter 308 Page 2137

A. Depressed total hemolytic complement (CH50)
B. Decreased levels of C3
C. Normal levels of C4
D. None of the above

90% patients of poststreptococcal glomerulonephritis will have depressed CH50 & decreased levels of C3 with normal levels of C4 in first week of symptoms. Positive rheumatoid factor (30–40%), cryoglobulins and circulating immune complexes (60–70%), ANCA against myeloperoxidase (10%), increased titers of ASO (30%), anti-DNAse (70%) or anti-hyaluronidase antibodies (40%) can help confirm the diagnosis.

1469. Which of the following has no role in treatment of poststreptococcal glomerulonephritis?

Harrison's 20th Ed. Chapter 308 Page 2137

A. Antibiotics
B. Antihypertensives
C. Immunosuppressive therapy
D. Dialysis

There is no role for immunosuppressive therapy in poststreptococcal glomerulonephritis even in the setting of crescents.

1470. In APSGN, complete resolution of hematuria & proteinuria occurs within what time after the onset of nephritis?

Harrison's 20th Ed. Chapter 308 Page 2137

A. 1–3 weeks
B. 3–6 weeks
C. 6–9 weeks
D. 9–12 weeks

Complete resolution of the hematuria and proteinuria in the majority of children occurs within 3–6 weeks of the onset of nephritis.

1471. 'Starry sky' appearance on immunofluorescence microscopy of renal biopsy is seen in?

Am J Kidney Dis. 2015;66(4):e31-e32

A. Acute poststreptococcal glomerulonephritis
B. Lupus nephritis
C. Glomerulonephritis in SLE
D. Goodpasture's syndrome

Post-streptococcal GN has prominent PMN infiltrate in glomerular tuft, with 'garland' or 'starry sky' appearance of IgG+C3 deposits by (immunofluorescence microscopy), & hump-shaped subepithelial deposits by EM.

1472. Which of the following is a common comorbidity of endocarditis-associated glomerulonephritis?

Harrison's 20th Ed. Chapter 308 Page 2137

A. Intravenous drug use
B. Hepatitis C
C. Diabetes mellitus
D. All of the above

Common comorbidities of endocarditis-associated glomerulonephritis are valvular heart disease, intravenous drug use, hepatitis C, and diabetes mellitus.

1473. 'Flea-bitten' kidney refers to?

Harrison's 20th Ed. Chapter 308 Page 2137

A. Subcapsular necrosis
B. Subcapsular hemorrhages
C. Subcapsular oedema
D. Subcapsular fibrosis

1474. In endocarditis-associated glomerulonephritis, immune deposits of which of the following are found in kidney?

Harrison's 20th Ed. Chapter 308 Page 2137

A. IgG
B. IgM
C. C3
D. All of the above

C3 deposition is prominent in most cases.

1475. In endocarditis-associated glomerulonephritis, immune deposits of IgG, IgM and C3 are found in?

Harrison's 20th Ed. Chapter 308 Page 2137

A. Mesangium
B. Subendothelium
C. Subepithelium
D. All of the above

Kidneys in subacute bacterial endocarditis have subcapsular hemorrhages with a 'flea-bitten' appearance. Renal biopsy reveals focal proliferation around foci of necrosis associated with abundant mesangial, subendothelial and subepithelial immune deposits of IgG, IgM and C3.

1476. Which of the following is false about endocarditis-associated glomerulonephritis?

Harrison's 20th Ed. Chapter 308 Page 2138

A. Renal deposition of circulating immune complexes in kidney
B. Complement activation
C. Circulating immune complexes
D. None of the above

1477. Which of the following may be present in endocarditis-associated glomerulonephritis?

Harrison's 20th Ed. Chapter 308 Page 2138

A. Hypocomplementemia
B. High titers of rheumatoid factor
C. High titers of type III cryoglobulins
D. All of the above

The pathogenesis of endocarditis-associated glomerulonephritis is renal deposition of circulating immune complexes in kidney with complement activation. Normocytic anemia, ↑ ESR, hypocomplementemia, high titers of rheumatoid factor, type III cryoglobulins, circulating immune complexes and ANCAs may be present.

1478. Which of the following is false about endocarditis-associated glomerulonephritis?

Harrison's 20th Ed. Chapter 308 Page 2138

A. Most commonly presents with AKI
B. Complicates staphylococcal tricuspid valve infection
C. Necrotizing and crescentic glomerulonephritis
D. None of the above

Glomerulonephritis is unusual in acute bacterial endocarditis. The most common organism in IE-associated GN is S. aureus. Streptococcus species are the next most common. Less common organisms include Bartonella henselae, Coxiella burnetii, Cardiobacterium hominis, and Gemella. The most common cardiac valve infected is tricuspid followed by mitral, aortic, pulmonic and chordae tendinae. Acute kidney injury is the most common clinical presentation and almost all patients have hematuria. Crescentic GN is the most common pattern seen on kidney biopsy specimens by light microscopy, followed by diffuse proliferative GN. Subepithelial "humps" which are classically seen in infection-related GN are infrequent.

1479. In endocarditis-associated glomerulonephritis, antibiotics are given for a period of?

Harrison's 20th Ed. Chapter 308 Page 2138

A. 1–2 weeks
B. 2–4 weeks
C. 4–6 weeks
D. 6–8 weeks

1480. Which of the following sometimes accompanies or is confused with SBE?

Harrison's 20th Ed. Chapter 308 Page 2138

A. Hepatitis B virus–associated vasculitis
B. ANCA-associated vasculitis
C. Cancer-associated vasculitis
D. Drug-induced vasculitis

ANCA-associated vasculitis sometimes accompanies or is confused with SBE and should be ruled out, as the treatment is different.

1481. Postinfectious glomerulonephritis can occur in?

Harrison's 20th Ed. Chapter 308 Page 2138

A. Ventriculoatrial shunt
B. Ventriculoperitoneal shunt
C. Infected vascular prostheses
D. All of the above

Postinfectious glomerulonephritis can occur in patients with ventriculoatrial & ventriculoperitoneal shunts, pulmonary, intraabdominal, pelvic or cutaneous infections and infected vascular prostheses.

1482. Lupus nephritis is most severe in?

Harrison's 20th Ed. Chapter 308 Page 2138

A. African-American female adolescents
B. White elderly
C. Australian aboriginals
D. Chinese young male

Lupus nephritis is most severe in African-American female adolescents as a complication of SLE.

1483. Which of the following glomerulonephritis is more common in female than in male population?
Harrison's 20th Ed. Chapter 308 Page 2138

A. Alport's syndrome
B. Goodpasture's syndrome
C. Lupus nephritis
D. Nail-patella syndrome

Lupus nephritis is two + times more in female than among male population.

1484. In lupus nephritis, the most common clinical sign of renal disease is?
Harrison's 20th Ed. Chapter 308 Page 2138

A. Hypertension
B. Active urine sediment with red blood cell casts
C. Varying degrees of renal failure
D. Proteinuria

In lupus nephritis, the most common clinical sign of renal disease is proteinuria, but hematuria, hypertension, varying degrees of renal failure and active urine sediment with red blood cell casts can be present.

1485. Remission achieved with treatment is defined as a return to near-normal renal function and proteinuria ≤?
Harrison's 20th Ed. Chapter 308 Page 2138

A. 300 mg/dL per day
B. 310 mg/dL per day
C. 320 mg/dL per day
D. 330 mg/dL per day

Remission achieved with treatment is defined as a return to near-normal renal function and proteinuria ≤ 330 mg/dL per day.

1486. Which of the following about lupus nephritis is false?
Harrison's 20th Ed. Chapter 308 Page 2138

A. Lesions limited to renal mesangium have excellent prognosis
B. Systemic lupus becomes quiescent once there is renal failure
C. Lupus nephritis class V patients are predisposed to renal-vein thrombosis
D. None of the above

1487. In lupus nephritis, which of the following antibodies correlate best with the presence of renal disease?
Harrison's 20th Ed. Chapter 308 Page 2138

A. Antiendomysial antibody
B. Anti-dsDNA antibodies
C. Anticentromere antibody
D. Anti-U3-RNP

In lupus nephritis, anti-dsDNA antibodies that fix complement correlate best with the presence of renal disease.

1488. In lupus nephritis, which of the following serves as a urinary biomarker?
J. Proteome Res. 2019; 18: 1264–1277

A. α-2-macroglobulin
B. Haptoglobin
C. α-1-antitrypsin
D. All of the above

1489. In lupus nephritis, which of the following serves as a urinary biomarker?
J. Proteome Res. 2019; 18: 1264–1277

A. Ceruloplasmin
B. Transferrin
C. Afamin
D. All of the above

Seven proteins - transferrin, α-2-macroglobulin, haptoglobin, afamin, α-1-antitrypsin, vimentin, and ceruloplasmin were confirmed to be elevated in lupus nephritis urine compared to healthy controls.

1490. Lupus nephritis is categorized in to how many classes?
Harrison's 20th Ed. Chapter 308 Page 2138 Table 308-3

A. 3
B. 4
C. 5
D. 6

1491. Which class of lupus nephritis is labeled as diffuse nephritis?
Harrison's 20th Ed. Chapter 308 Page 2138 Table 308-3

A. 3
B. 4
C. 5
D, 6

Global, diffuse proliferative lesions involving the vast majority of glomeruli are labeled as class IV. They have high anti-DNA antibody titers, low serum complement, hematuria, red blood cell casts, proteinuria, hypertension, and decreased renal function. 50% of patients have nephrotic-range proteinuria. Without treatment, this aggressive lesion has the worst renal prognosis.

1492. Which class of lupus nephritis is labeled as membranous nephritis?
Harrison's 20th Ed. Chapter 308 Page 2138 Table 308-3

A. 3
B. 4
C. 5
D. 6

1493. In lupus nephritis, lesions of which class have the most varied course?
Harrison's 20th Ed. Chapter 308 Page 2138

A. 3
B. 4
C. 5
D. 6

Class III lesions have the most varied course.

1494. Which of the following drugs is not used in the treatment of lupus nephritis?
Harrison's 20th Ed. Chapter 308 Page 2138

A. Cyclophosphamide
B. Mycophenolate mofetil
C. Ipilimumab
D. Prednisone

For lupus nephritis class 3 or 4, induction phase of treatment (high-dose corticosteroids and cyclophosphamide or MMF) generally lasts 2–6 months and is followed by a prolonged, but less intense maintenance phase (steroids and mycophenolate mofetil or azathioprine), often lasting years. It is not clear when maintenance therapy can be withdrawn.

1495. Which of the following monoclonal antibody is used in the treatment of lupus nephritis?

Harrison's 20th Ed. Chapter 308 Page 2138

A. Adalimumab
B. Belimumab
C. Certolizumab
D. Golimumab

Belimumab, a monoclonal antibody directed against the B cell survival factor BLyS, trials in nonrenal lupus showed a dose-dependent trend toward a decreased rate of renal flares in patients who had received belimumab.

1496. First name of Goodpasture was?

N Engl J Med. 2003;348:2543-56

A. Albert
B. Ellis
C. Ernest
D. Eric

Ernest Goodpasture published his observation as 'The pathology of pneumonia accompanying influenza. US Naval Med Bull 1919;13:177-97'. Stanton and Tange described the pulmonary-renal syndrome almost 40 years later, and it was they who suggested that Goodpasture's name be linked to the condition.

1497. Which of the following is not a basement membrane syndrome?

Harrison's 20th Ed. Chapter 308 Page 2139

A. Alport's syndrome
B. Goodpasture's syndrome
C. Churg-Strauss syndrome
D. Nail-patella syndrome

1498. Which of the following is true for 'anti-GBM disease'?

Harrison's 20th Ed. Chapter 308 Page 2139

A. Detectable circulating anti-GBM autoantibodies
B. Normal serum complement levels
C. Absent ANCA
D. All of the above

1499. The triad in Goodpasture's syndrome consists of all except?

Harrison's 20th Ed. Chapter 308 Page 2139

A. Lung hemorrhage
B. Renal failure
C. Proteinuria
D. Anti-GBM antibodies

Term 'Goodpasture's syndrome' is used for the triad of lung hemorrhage, renal failure and anti-GBM antibodies. 'Goodpasture's disease' or anti-GBM disease refers to glomerulonephritis caused by antibodies directed against the α3-chain of type IV collagen, with or without lung hemorrhage. Etiology is unknown.

1500. Which of the following is true for Goodpasture's syndrome?

Harrison's 20th Ed. Chapter 308 Page 2139

A. Anti-GBM nephritis
B. Lung hemorrhage
C. Autoimmune disease
D. All of the above

1501. Which of the following is a protomer of collagen IV?

N Engl J Med. 2003;348:2543-56

A. α1.α1.α2(IV)
B. α3.α4.α5(IV)
C. α5.α5.α6(IV)
D. All of the above

The six chains of collagen IV form only three sets of triple helical molecules called protomers designated as α1.α1.α2(IV), α3.α4.α5(IV), and α5.α5.α6(IV).

1502. Which chain of type IV collagen is the target antigen in Goodpasture's syndrome?

Harrison's 20th Ed. Chapter 308 Page 2139

A. α1
B. α2
C. α3
D. α4

1503. Which chain of type IV collagen is called 'Goodpasture antigen'?

Harrison's 20th Ed. Chapter 308 Page 2139

A. α3
B. α4
C. α5
D. α6

1504. Which of the following is known as 'Goodpasture protomer'?

N Engl J Med. 2003;348:2543-56

A. α3(IV) NC1
B. α5.a5.α6(IV)
C. α3.a4.α5(IV)
D. α1.a1.α2(IV)

a3.a4.a5(IV) protomer is a basement-membrane molecule of family of type IV collagens in epithelial tissues and is called the "Goodpasture protomer".

1505. α3 (IV) NC1 peptides are produced by?

N Engl J Med. 2003;348:2543-56

A. Lymph node
B. Bone marrow
C. Spleen
D. Thymus

Thymus expresses α3 (IV) NC1 peptides that can cause elimination of autoreactive CD4+ helper T cells. A few such T cells escape deletion and can engage in the production of anti–glomerular basement membrane antibodies. Linear deposits of IgG antibody along the glomerular basement membrane are seen. Autoantibodies directed against glomerular basement membrane cross-react with basement membrane of alveolar walls.

1506. Which of the following is false about Goodpasture's syndrome?

Harrison's 20th Ed. Chapter 308 Page 2139

A. Occurs in young men in late 20s
B. Occurs in men & women in 60–70s
C. Hemoptysis is largely confined to smokers
D. None of the above

1507. Exposure to which of the following can cause Goodpasture's syndrome?

Harrison's 20th Ed. Chapter 308 Page 2139

A. Infection
B. Cocaine
C. Hydrocarbon
D. All of the above

1508. Antibodies against the α1(IV) NC1 domain is seen in patients with?

Harrison's 20th Ed. Chapter 308 Page 2139

A. Leukemia
B. Paraneoplastic syndrome
C. SLE
D. All of the above

Antibodies against the α1(IV) NC1 domain is seen in patients with paraneoplastic syndrome.

1509. In Goodpasture's syndrome, which of the following indicate worse prognosis at presentation?

Harrison's 20th Ed. Chapter 308 Page 2139

A. Oliguria
B. >50% crescents on renal biopsy
C. Serum creatinine >5–6 mg/dL
D. All of the above

In Goodpasture's syndrome, prognosis at presentation is worse if there is oliguria, advanced fibrosis or >50% crescents on renal biopsy, serum creatinine >5–7 mg/dL or a need for dialysis.

1510. Patients of Goodpasture's syndrome respond to which of the following treatments?

Harrison's 20th Ed. Chapter 308 Page 2139

A. Plasmapheresis
B. Oral prednisone
C. Cyclophosphamide
D. All of the above

Patients of Goodpasture's syndrome respond to plasmapheresis, accompanied by oral prednisone and cyclophosphamide therapy.

1511. Which of the following about Goodpasture's syndrome is false?

Harrison's 20th Ed. Chapter 308 Page 2139

A. Hemoptysis is largely confined to smokers
B. Presentation with oliguria has bad outcome
C. Disease in young is usually explosive
D. None of the above

1512. Out of the following, which is the most common form of glomerulonephritis?

Harrison's 20th Ed. Chapter 308 Page 2139

A. IgA nephropathy
B. Focal sclerosing glomerulonephritis
C. Rapidly progressive/crescentic glomerulonephritis
D. Membranous glomerulonephritis

IgA nephropathy is the most common form of glomerulonephritis worldwide.

1513. IgA nephropathy is also called?

Harrison's 20th Ed. Chapter 308 Page 2139

A. Barratt disease
B. Berger disease
C. Tomino disease
D. Glassock disease

IgA nephropathy (Berger disease) is a primary glomerular disease. Berger first described it in 1968.

1514. Which of the following is false about IgA nephropathy?

Harrison's 20th Ed. Chapter 308 Page 2139

A. Female preponderance
B. Peak incidence in II & III decades of life
C. Recurrent episodes of macroscopic hematuria
D. Between episodes, urinalysis is normal

In IgA nephropathy, there is a male preponderance.

1515. IgA nephropathy resembles which of the following diseases?

Harrison's 20th Ed. Chapter 308 Page 2139

A. Wegener's granulomatosis
B. Goodpasture's syndrome
C. Henoch-Schönlein purpura
D. All of the above

Clinical and laboratory evidence suggests close similarities between Henoch-Schönlein purpura and IgA nephropathy.

1516. IgA nephropathy is differentiated from Henoch-Schönlein purpura by?

Harrison's 20th Ed. Chapter 308 Page 2139

A. Prominent systemic symptoms at a younger age (<20 years)
B. Preceding infection
C. Abdominal complaints
D. All of the above

HSP is distinguished clinically from IgA nephropathy by prominent systemic symptoms, a younger age (<20 years), preceding infection & abdominal complaints.

1517. Essentials of IgA nephropathy include?

Harrison's 20th Ed. Chapter 308 Page 2139

A. Diffuse mesangial IgA deposits
B. Clinically significant glomerular inflammation
C. Renal dysfunction
D. All of the above

1518. Deposits of IgA in glomerular mesangium are found in?

Harrison's 20th Ed. Chapter 308 Page 2139

A. Chronic liver disease
B. Crohn's disease
C. Gastrointestinal adenocarcinoma
D. All of the above

1519. Deposits of IgA in glomerular mesangium are found in?

Harrison's 20th Ed. Chapter 308 Page 2139

A. Chronic bronchiectasis
B. Idiopathic interstitial pneumonia
C. Dermatitis herpetiformis
D. All of the above

1520. Deposits of IgA in glomerular mesangium are found in?

Harrison's 20th Ed. Chapter 308 Page 2139

A. Leprosy
B. Ankylosing spondylitis
C. Sjögren's syndrome
D. All of the above

Deposits of IgA in glomerular mesangium are found in chronic liver disease, Crohn's disease, gastrointestinal adenocarcinoma, chronic obstructive bronchiectasis, idiopathic interstitial pneumonia, dermatitis herpetiformis, mycosis fungoides, leprosy, ankylosing spondylitis, relapsing polychondritis, and Sjögren's syndrome. However, IgA deposition does not produce clinically significant glomerular inflammation or renal dysfunction and therefore not called IgA nephropathy.

1521. Most IgA deposited in the kidney are derived from?
Harrison's 20th Ed. Chapter 308 Page 2139

A. Lymph node
B. Bone marrow
C. Spleen
D. Liver

IgA, particularly secretory IgA, production is done by plasma cells in bone marrow.

1522. Most IgA is cleared by?
Harrison's 20th Ed. Chapter 308 Page 2139

A. Kidney
B. Bone marrow
C. Intestines
D. Liver

IgA clearance occurs predominately in the liver.

1523. In IgA nephropathy, deposition of IgA occurs in?
Harrison's 20th Ed. Chapter 308 Page 2139

A. Glomerular capillaries
B. Glomerular mesangium
C. Glomerular basement membrane
D. All of the above

Morphologically, IgA nephropathy is characterized by diffuse deposition of IgA in glomerular mesangium. IgA deposited in the mesangium is typically polymeric and of the IgA1 subclass.

1524. Which of the following is false about IgA nephropathy?
Harrison's 20th Ed. Chapter 308 Page 2139

A. Mesangial hypercellularity
B. IgA1 subclass IgA deposits in the mesangium
C. IgM, IgG, C3 codistributed with IgA deposits
D. None of the above

1525. Which of the following is abnormal in IgA nephropathy?
Harrison's 20th Ed. Chapter 308 Page 2139

A. IgA production by plasma cells
B. IgA clearance by liver
C. Receptors for IgA
D. All of the above

1526. Which of the following is key to the pathogenesis of IgA nephropathy?
Harrison's 20th Ed. Chapter 308 Page 2139

A. Glucose-deficient IgA1
B. Galactose-deficient IgA1
C. Glucose-deficient IgA2
D. Galactose-deficient IgA2

The IgA1 produced in patients with IgA nephropathy is underglycosylated (Gd-IgA1). The galactose-deficient IgA1 may evade liver catabolism and preferentially deposit in mesangium. Susceptible individuals (second hit, such as a viral or other antigen exposure) will also produce anti–Gd-IgA1 autoantibodies (auto-Ab). The Gd-IgA1 - auto-Ab immune complexes activate the alternative pathway of complement. The immune complexes are nephritogenic, contributing to local inflammation, cellular proliferation, and ultimately fibrosis.

1527. Which of the following is a finding in patients with IgA nephropathy?
Clinical Journal of the American Society of Nephrology. 2017;12:1-10

A. Galactose-deficient IgA1
B. IgG autoantibody directed against the hinge region O-glycans
C. C3
D. All of the above

A central finding in patients with IgAN A central finding in patients with IgAN is the presence of circulating and glomerular immune complexes comprised of galactose-deficient IgA1, an IgG autoantibody directed against the hinge region O-glycans, and C3.

1528. A polymorphism which of the following gene confers susceptibility to IgA nephropathy?
Clinical Journal of the American Society of Nephrology. 2017;12:1-10

A. APOL1 gene
B. APRIL gene
C. Complement factor H regulatory proteins (CFHR's) gene
D. PKD1 gene

A polymorphism in the APRIL gene confers susceptibility to IgA nephropathy.

1529. In IgA nephropathy, histologic lesion seen on light microscopy is?
Harrison's 20th Ed. Chapter 308 Page 2139

A. DPGN
B. Segmental sclerosis
C. Segmental necrosis with cellular crescent formation
D. All of the above

Immunofluorescent pattern of IgA on renal biopsy defines IgA nephropathy, but other patterns may be seen.

1530. Which of the following about IgA nephropathy is false?
Harrison's 20th Ed. Chapter 308 Page 2140

A. Recurrent episodes of macroscopic hematuria during or immediately following an upper respiratory infection
B. Accompanied by proteinuria
C. Persistent asymptomatic microscopic hematuria
D. Nephrotic syndrome is common

Nephrotic syndrome is uncommon in IgA nephropathy.

1531. Which of the following about IgA nephropathy is false?
Harrison's 20th Ed. Chapter 308 Page 2140

A. Benign disease for the majority of patients
B. Renal function well preserved
C. Slow progression
D. Use of angiotensin-converting enzyme (ACE) inhibitors harmful

Use of angiotensin-converting enzyme (ACE) inhibitors in patients of IgA nephropathy with proteinuria or declining renal function is helpful.

1532. Which of the following is a risk factor for the loss of renal function in IgA nephropathy?
Harrison's 20th Ed. Chapter 308 Page 2140

A. Presence of hypertension
B. Presence of proteinuria
C. Absence of episodes of macroscopic hematuria
D. All of the above

In IgA nephropathy, risk factors for loss of renal function include presence of hypertension or proteinuria, absence of episodes of macroscopic hematuria, male sex, older age of onset, and extensive glomerulosclerosis or interstitial fibrosis on renal biopsy.

1533. Which out of the following has the greatest predictive power for adverse renal outcomes in IgA nephropathy?
Harrison's 20th Ed. Chapter 308 Page 2140

A. Persistent proteinuria for 6 months
B. Persistent hypertension for 6 months
C. Persistent macroscopic hematuria for 6 months
D. All of the above

Analyses of IgA nephropathy patients found persistent proteinuria for 6 months or longer to have the greatest predictive power for adverse renal outcomes.

1534. Which of the following procedures benefit select patients of IgA nephropathy?
Harrison's 20th Ed. Chapter 308 Page 2140

A. Tonsillectomy
B. Appendicectomy
C. Orchidectomy
D. None of the above

Tonsillectomy & fish oil have been suggested in small studies to benefit select patients of IgA nephropathy.

1535. When IgA nephropathy presents as RPGN, which of the following is helpful?
Harrison's 20th Ed. Chapter 308 Page 2140, N Engl J Med. 2015;373:2225-36

A. Steroids
B. Cytotoxic agents
C. Plasmapheresis
D. All of the above

Addition of immunosuppression to comprehensive supportive care was not beneficial in patients with IgA nephropathy that was characterized by moderate proteinuria & chronic kidney disease stages 1 through 3.

1536. In IgA nephropathy, which of the following is helpful?
Clinical Journal of the American Society of Nephrology. 2017;12:1-10

A. Salmeterol
B. Budesonide
C. Nifedipine
D. Tadalafil

A novel potential therapy for IgAN is a modified formulation of oral budesonide (Nefecon). This agent is proposed to act locally at the mucosal lymphoid tissue in the distal ileum and proximal large intestine to modulate IgA production.

1537. Small-vessel vasculitis rarely involves which of the following?
Harrison's 20th Ed. Chapter 308 Page 2140

A. Arterioles
B. Capillaries
C. Venules
D. Small arteries

Small-vessel vasculitis involves arterioles, capillaries, venules and rarely small arteries.

1538. ANCA stands for?
Harrison's 20th Ed. Chapter 308 Page 2140

A. Anti-neutrophilic cytoplasmic antibody
B. Anti-neutrophilic cytoplasmic autoantibody
C. Anti-neutrophilic centromeric antibody
D. Anti-neutrophilic centromeric autoantibody

1539. ANCA activates which of the following?
Harrison's 20th Ed. Chapter 308 Page 2140

A. Eosinophil
B. Basophil
C. Monocyte
D. Macrophage

ANCA, in the the pathogenesis of these small-vessel vasculitides, activates cytokine (TNFα) primed neutrophils and monocytes, which express ANCA antigens, proteinase 3 and myeloperoxidase, on their surface. B cells produce ANCAs.

1540. Which of the following is a type of ANCA?
Harrison's 20th Ed. Chapter 308 Page 2140

A. Cytoplasmic (cANCA)
B. Perinuclear (pANCA)
C. Atypical (aANCA)
D. All of the above

Cytoplasmic ANCA (C-ANCA) with specificity for PR3 are usually found in patients with GPA (Wegener granulomatosis) whereas perinuclear ANCA (P-ANCA) in patients with MPA and EGPA (Churg-Strauss syndrome). aANCA is associated with levamisole-contaminated cocaine exposure in abusers. Proteinase-3 (PR3-ANCA) is also called cANCA. Myeloperoxidase (MPO-ANCA) is also called pANCA.

1541. Which of the following about ANCA is false?
Harrison's 20th Ed. Chapter 308 Page 2140

A. P-ANCA targets & attaches to myeloperoxidase in neutrophils
B. C-ANCA targets & attaches to proteinase 3 in neutrophils
C. C-ANCA is associated with GPA, P-ANCA with MPA
D. None of the above

cANCA pattern is mostly due to the presence of anti-PR3 autoantibodies while pANCA pattern is usually due to the presence of anti-myeloperoxidase (anti-MPO) antibodies. The target proteins PR3 and MPO are both localised in the azurophile (primary) granules of polymorphonuclear cells and monocytes, from where they can be exposed on the cellular surface as a result of various inflammatory stimuli.

1542. Which of the following is false about proteinase 3 (PR3)?
Harrison's 20th Ed. Chapter 308 Page 2140

A. PR3 is GPA's main autoantigen
B. The main inhibitor of PR3 is alpha-1-antitrypsin (α1-AT)
C. PR3 allows destruction of phagocytosed bacteria in activated neutrophils favours diapedesis
D. None of the above

1543. Which of the following is a ANCA associated vasculitis?
Harrison's 20th Ed. Chapter 308 Page 2140

A. Microscopic polyangiitis (MPA)
B. Granulomatosis with polyangiitis (GPA)
C. Eosinophilic granulomatosis with polyangiitis (EGPA)
D. All of the above

Anti-neutrophil cytoplasmic antibody (ANCA)-associated vasculitis (AAV) includes microscopic polyangiitis (MPA), granulomatosis with polyangiitis (GPA, also known as Wegener's granulomatosis), eosinophilic granulomatosis with polyangiitis (EGPA, also known as Churg-Strauss syndrome) and drug-induced AAV. ANCAs have a central role in the pathogenesis of AAV because they induce excessive activation of neutrophils, which results in injury to small vessels.

1544. Which of the following antibodies play a role in the pathogenesis of AAV?

Harrison's 20th Ed. Chapter 308 Page 2140

A. Anti-GBM antibodies
B. Lysosomal-associated membrane protein 2 (LAMP-2)
C. Antibodies to ADAMTS13
D. Anti-La (SS-B) antibodies

Anti-LAMP-2 antibodies play important role in the pathogenesis of AAV. These antibodies are only found in patients with active vasculitis even those who were lacking PR3 or MPO.

1545. Which of the following is an ANCA-positive, pauci-immune glomerulonephritis?

Harrison's 20th Ed. Chapter 308 Page 2140

A. Granulomatosis with polyangiitis
B. Microscopic polyangiitis
C. Churg-Strauss syndrome
D. All of the above

1546. Anti-PR3 antibodies are more common in?

Harrison's 20th Ed. Chapter 308 Page 2140

A. Granulomatosis with polyangiitis
B. Microscopic polyangiitis
C. Churg-Strauss syndrome
D. All of the above

Anti-PR3 antibodies are more common in Wegener's granulomatosis & anti-MPO antibodies are more common in microscopic polyangiitis or Churg-Strauss syndrome.

1547. Which of the following is a classical presentation in patients with granulomatosis with polyangiitis?

Harrison's 20th Ed. Chapter 308 Page 2140

A. Significant lung disease
B. Destructive sinusitis
C. Microscopic hematuria
D. All of the above

Patients with granulomatosis with polyangiitis classically present with fever, purulent rhinorrhea, nasal ulcers, sinus pain, polyarthralgias/arthritis, cough, hemoptysis, shortness of breath, microscopic hematuria, and 0.5–1 gram/day of proteinuria. Occasionally there may be cutaneous purpura and mononeuritis multiplex.

1548. Granulomatosis with polyangiitis presenting without renal involvement is termed?

Harrison's 20th Ed. Chapter 308 Page 2140

A. Wegener's disease
B. Wegener's syndrome
C. Isolated Wegener's granulomatosis
D. Limited granulomatosis with polyangiitis

Presentation without renal involvement is termed limited granulomatosis with polyangiitis.

1549. Granulomatosis with polyangiitis is more common in?

Harrison's 20th Ed. Chapter 308 Page 2140

A. Patients exposed to epoxy resins
B. Patients exposed to silica dust
C. Patients exposed to welding fumes
D. Patients exposed to aromatic hydrocarbons

1550. Granulomatosis with polyangiitis is more common in?

Harrison's 20th Ed. Chapter 308 Page 2140

A. Folate and vitamin B12 deficiency
B. α1-antitrypsin deficiency
C. Glucose-6-phosphate dehydrogenase (G6PD) deficiency
D. Vitamin D deficiency

Granulomatosis with polyangiitis is more common in patients exposed to silica dust and those with α1-antitrypsin deficiency, which is an inhibitor of PR3.

1551. Relapse after achieving remission is more common in patients with?

Harrison's 20th Ed. Chapter 308 Page 2140

A. Microscopic polyangiitis
B. Granulomatosis with polyangiitis
C. Churg-Strauss syndrome
D. C3 Glomerulopathies

1552. In microscopic polyangiitis, which of the following is uncommon?

Harrison's 20th Ed. Chapter 308 Page 2140

A. Hematuria
B. Proteinuria
C. Significant lung disease or destructive sinusitis
D. Renal involvement

Patients of microscopic polyangiitis are similar to those with Wegener's granulomatosis, except that they rarely have significant lung disease or destructive sinusitis.

1553. Which of the following distinguishes Churg-Strauss syndrome from other small-vessel vasculitis?

Harrison's 20th Ed. Chapter 308 Page 2140

A. Pulmonary infiltrates
B. Peripheral eosinophilia
C. Glomerulonephritis
D. All of the above

Churg-Strauss syndrome is a small-vessel vasculitis associated with peripheral eosinophilia, cutaneous purpura, mononeuritis, asthma, allergic rhinitis, hypergammaglobulinemia, elevated serum IgE, and rheumatoid factor.

1554. Which of the following is a type of C3 glomerulopathy?

Harrison's 20th Ed. Chapter 308 Page 2141

A. Membranous glomerulonephritis
B. Minimal change disease
C. Dense deposit disease
D. Focal segmental glomerular sclerosis

1555. Which of the following about dense deposit disease is false?

Harrison's 20th Ed. Chapter 308 Page 2141

A. Occurs in young
B. More likely to have low serum C3 levels
C. More likely to have crescentic GN
D. None of the above

Patients with C3GN are older & have more severe arteriolar sclerosis, glomerular sclerosis & interstitial scarring on renal biopsy than patients with DDD. Older age, crescentic GN & DDD subtype were independent predictors of ESRD. Both DDD and C3GN recur after renal transplantation, often resulting in allograft loss.

1556. Mutations in which of the following complement factor regulatory protein gene causes C3 glomerulopathy?

Harrison's 20th Ed. Chapter 308 Page 2141

A. G
B. H
C. J
D. P

Factor H cleaves the active form of C3, C3b, to the inactive iC3b. Mutations in the complement factor H regulatory proteins (CFHR's) genes causes C3 glomerulopathy. The major inhibitor of the alternative pathway in the circulation is factor H which acts to block the formation of alternative pathway convertases, promotes their spontaneous dissociation and also acts as a co-factor for the cleavage of C3b to its inactive form iC3b by factor I. Properdin is the only positive regulator of the alternative pathway and acts to stabilise the alternative pathway C3 convertase.

1557. Which of the following is a principal regulator of the complement system?

Harrison's 20th Ed. Chapter 308 Page 2141

A. Complement C3
B. Membrane cofactor protein (MCP)
C. Complement factor B (CFB)
D. Complement factor H (CFH)

CFH, CFHR1–5, CFI, MCP and Thrombomodulin (THBD) inhibit or regulate the complement pathway in the fluid-phase or on the surface of host cells. C3b, CFB, CFD and properdin stabilize and activate the C3 convertase.

1558. Deficiency of complement factor H (CFH) is associated with?

Harrison's 20th Ed. Chapter 308 Page 2141

A. Focal segmental glomerular sclerosis (FSGS)
B. Atypical hemolytic uremic syndrome (aHUS)
C. Minimal change disease (MCD)
D. All of the above

Deficiency of CFH is commonly associated with aHUS.

1559. Atypical hemolytic uremic syndrome is characterized by?

Harrison's 20th Ed. Chapter 308 Page 2141

A. Microangiopathic hemolysis
B. Thrombocytopenia
C. Renal failure
D. All of the above

1560. 'Ribbons in the GBM' best relates to?

Harrison's 20th Ed. Chapter 308 Page 2141

A. Microscopic polyangiitis
B. Granulomatosis with polyangiitis
C. Dense deposit disease
D. Churg-Strauss syndrome

Dense deposit disease (DDD), formerly MPGN type II, is defined morphologically with dense deposits forming ribbons in the GBM. In its absence, the entity is categorized as C3 glomerulonephritis.

1561. Which of the following about C3 nephritic factors (C3nefs) is false?

Harrison's 20th Ed. Chapter 308 Page 2141

A. Autoantibodies
B. Stabilize the alternative pathway C3 convertase
C. Prevents C3 convertase inactivation by factor H
D. None of the above

C3 nephritic factors (C3nefs), which are autoantibodies that bind to and stabilise the alternative pathway C3 convertase by preventing its inactivation by factor H.

1562. Which of the following about C3 glomerulopathy is false?

Harrison's 20th Ed. Chapter 308 Page 2141

A. Presence of glomerular deposits composed of C3
B. Absence of significant amounts of Ig in glomerular deposits
C. Low serum C3 levels with preserved serum C4 levels
D. None of the above

1563. Histopathological & laboratory features of which of the following are indistinguishable from C3 glomerulopathy?

Harrison's 20th Ed. Chapter 308 Page 2141

A. Membranous glomerulonephritis
B. Minimal change disease
C. Post-infectious glomerulonephritis
D. Focal segmental glomerular sclerosis

Post infectious glomerulonephritis may be considered a self-limiting form of C3 glomerulopathy. Renal biopsy in post infectious GN typically shows a diffuse endocapillary glomerulonephritis with subepithelial hump-like deposits on EM. On immunofluorescence, there may be glomerular staining for IgG & C3 but some cases may show C3 deposition only. Patients usually have low levels of circulating C3.

1564. Which of the following monoclonal antibody is of use in C3 glomerulopathy?

Harrison's 20th Ed. Chapter 308 Page 2141

A. Bevacizumab
B. Eculizumab
C. Certolizumab
D. Natalizumab

Eculizumab is a monoclonal antibody directed at C5 which is activated by C3. Rational treatment of C3 glomerulopathy would involve inhibition of C3 activation.

1565. Mesangiocapillary glomerulonephritis or lobar glomerulonephritis is also called?

Harrison's 20th Ed. Chapter 308 Page 2141

A. Focal segmental glomerulosclerosis
B. Membranous glomerulonephritis
C. Membranoproliferative glomerulonephritis (MPGN)
D. Mesangioproliferative glomerulonephritis

Membranoproliferative glomerulonephritis (MPGN) is also called mesangiocapillary glomerulonephritis or lobar glomerulonephritis.

1566. Which of the following about membranoproliferative glomerulonephritis (MPGN) is false?

Harrison's 20th Ed. Chapter 308 Page 2141

A. Immune-mediated glomerulonephritis
B. Thickening of the GBM
C. Mesangioproliferative changes
D. None of the above

1567. Which of the following about membranoproliferative glomerulonephritis (MPGN) is false?

Harrison's 20th Ed. Chapter 308 Page 2141

A. Most patients have hypocomplementemia
B. Rare in African Americans
C. Usually presents in childhood or young adulthood
D. None of the above

1568. Type I membranoproliferative glomerulonephritis (MPGN) is associated with?

Harrison's 20th Ed. Chapter 308 Page 2141

A. Persistent hepatitis C infections
B. Lupus
C. Neoplastic diseases
D. All of the above

Type I MPGN is commonly associated with persistent hepatitis C infections, autoimmune diseases like lupus or cryoglobulinemia, or neoplastic diseases.

1569. Which of the following is the most proliferative type of MPGN?

Harrison's 20th Ed. Chapter 308 Page 2141

A. Type I
B. Type II
C. Type III
D. All of the above

MPGN is subdivided 'pathologically' into type I, type II, and type III disease. Type I MPGN is the most proliferative type. MPGN type I has subendothelial electron-dense deposits, type II [also called dense deposit disease DDD], with intramembranous highly electron-dense deposits and type III, with both subendothelial and subepithelial deposits.

1570. Which of the following is called 'dense deposit disease'?

Harrison's 20th Ed. Chapter 308 Page 2141

A. Type I membranoproliferative glomerulonephritis
B. Type II membranoproliferative glomerulonephritis
C. Type III membranoproliferative glomerulonephritis
D. None of the above

Low serum C3 & dense thickening of GBM containing ribbons of dense deposits and C3 characterize Type II MPGN, also called dense deposit disease.

1571. Which of the following best relates to Type I membranoproliferative glomerulonephritis?

Harrison's 20th Ed. Chapter 308 Page 2141

A. Split basement membrane
B. Tram-tracking
C. Sentinel clot
D. B ring

Renal biopsy finding in Type I MPGN shows mesangial proliferation with lobular segmentation. Mesangial interposition between the capillary basement membrane and endothelial cells, produces a double contour sometimes called 'tram-tracking'.

1572. Which of the following is false about dense deposit disease or Type II membranoproliferative glomerulonephritis?

Harrison's 20th Ed. Chapter 308 Page 2141

A. Low serum C3
B. Dense thickening of the GBM
C. Ribbons of dense deposits and C3 in GBM
D. None of the above

1573. Mesangioproliferative glomerulonephritis is seen in?

Harrison's 20th Ed. Chapter 308 Page 2142

A. IgA nephropathy
B. P. falciparum malaria
C. Resolving postinfectious glomerulonephritis
D. All of the above

Mesangioproliferative glomerulonephritis is seen in IgA nephropathy, P. falciparum malaria, resolving postinfectious glomerulonephritis, and class II lupus nephritis.

1574. Minimal change disease (MCD) is also called?

Harrison's 20th Ed. Chapter 308 Page 2142

A. Nil disease
B. Lipoid nephrosis
C. Foot process disease
D. All of the above

Minimal change disease is also called lipoid nephrosis, visceral epithelial cell disease, foot process disease, nil disease or minimal change glomerulopathy.

1575. Minimal change Disease (MCD) is associated with?

Harrison's 20th Ed. Chapter 308 Page 2142

A. Hodgkin's disease
B. Allergies
C. Use of nonsteroidal anti-inflammatory agents
D. All of the above

MCD usually presents as a primary renal disease but can be associated with Hodgkin's disease, allergies, or use of NSAID agents (secondary form). Because of the association of MCD with atopy, alimentary allergies and hypersensitivity reactions, Kark (1958), referred MCD as 'asthma of the nephron'.

1576. Minimal change disease (MCD) on electron microscopy of renal biopsy consistently shows?

Harrison's 20th Ed. Chapter 308 Page 2142

A. Mesangial proliferation
B. Mesangial interposition
C. Effacement of the foot process
D. All of the above

MCD on electron microscopy of renal biopsy consistently shows an effacement of the foot process supporting epithelial podocytes, weakening of slit-pore membranes with formation of villi on the external surface of the epithelial cells (villous transformation). There are no electron-dense deposits. This is noted along virtually the entire distribution of every capillary loop.

1577. Which of the following is false about minimal change disease?

Harrison's 20th Ed. Chapter 308 Page 2142

A. Abrupt onset of edema
B. Nephrotic syndrome (average urine protein excretion 10 g/day)
C. Severe hypoalbuminemia
D. None of the above

1578. Which of the following is false about minimal change disease?

Harrison's 20th Ed. Chapter 308 Page 2142

A. Known as nil lesion
B. Commonest cause of nephrotic syndrome in adults
C. Acellular urinary sediment
D. Selective proteinuria

80% of the MCD children are < 6 years of age. MCD is more frequent in boys than in girls.

1579. Selective proteinuria in minimal change disease is for?

Harrison's 20th Ed. Chapter 308 Page 2142

A. Albumin
B. Light chain
C. Globulin
D. All of the above

MCD causes 70–90% of nephrotic syndrome in childhood but only 10–15% of nephrotic syndrome in adults. In MCD, proteinuria is selective and largely composed of albumin. The presence of high molecular weight proteins suggests another diagnosis.

1580. Which of the following is uncommon in minimal change disease?

Harrison's 20th Ed. Chapter 308 Page 2142

A. Hematuria
B. Hypertension
C. Renal failure
D. All of the above

Hematuria, hypertension, and renal failure are uncommon.

1581. Which of the following is false about minimal change disease?

Harrison's 20th Ed. Chapter 308 Page 2142

A. No glomerular histologic changes
B. No tubulointerstitial alterations
C. No immunoglobulin or complement deposition in renal tissue
D. None of the above

1582. MCD patients with steroid resistance can develop?

Harrison's 20th Ed. Chapter 308 Page 2142

A. Focal segmental glomerulosclerosis (FSGS)
B. Mesangioproliferative glomerulonephritis
C. Microscopic polyangiitis
D. All of the above

MCD patients with steroid resistance can develop FSGS on repeat biopsy.

1583. Adults are considered steroid-resistant when there is no response after how many of therapy?

Harrison's 20th Ed. Chapter 308 Page 2142

A. 1 months
B. 2 months
C. 3 months
D. 4 months

Adults are not considered steroid-resistant until after 4 months of therapy. 80–85% of adults will achieve complete remission, but only after a longer course of 20–24 weeks.

1584. 90 to 95% of children will develop a complete remission after how many weeks of steroid therapy?

Harrison's 20th Ed. Chapter 308 Page 2142

A. 1 week
B. 4 weeks
C. 6 weeks
D. 8 weeks

90 to 95% of children will develop a complete remission after 8 weeks of steroid therapy. Primary responders are patients who have a complete remission (<0.2 mg/day of proteinuria) after a single course of prednisone.

1585. In MCD, relapses occur in what proportion of children after the first remission?

Harrison's 20th Ed. Chapter 308 Page 2142

A. 10–20%
B. 30–40%
C. 50–60%
D. 70–75%

Relapses occur in 70–75% of children after first remission. Early relapse predicts multiple subsequent relapses.

1586. Which of the following is false about minimal change disease?

Harrison's 20th Ed. Chapter 308 Page 2142

A. High levels of basal proteinuria predicts relapse
B. Frequency of relapses decreases after puberty
C. Increased risk of relapse following rapid tapering of steroids
D. None of the above

1587. Which of the following immunosuppressive drugs is used for frequent relapsers, steroid-dependent, or steroid-resistant patients?

Harrison's 20th Ed. Chapter 308 Page 2142

A. Cyclophosphamide
B. Chlorambucil
C. Mycophenolate mofetil
D. All of the above

1588. Nephrosarca best relates to?

Harrison's 20th Ed. Chapter 308 Page 2142

A. Perirenal collection of fluid
B. Intrarenal edema
C. Polyuria
D. All of the above

Nephrosarca best relates to intrarenal edema.

1589. Which of the following is common between MCD and FSGS?

Harrison's 20th Ed. Chapter 308 Page 2142

A. Proteinuria
B. Podocyte injury
C. Minimal immune deposits
D. All of the above

Distinction between MCD and FSGS is critical, because both present with proteinuria, podocyte injury, and minimal immune deposits. Light microscopy, electron microscopy, and staining for Ig and complement are critical in making the distinction between MCD and FSGS. Extensive podocyte injury with adequate numbers of normal-appearing glomeruli and nonscarred tubulointerstitium by light microscopy suggests MCD.

1590. Pathologic changes of focal segmental glomerulosclerosis (FSGS) are most prominent in glomeruli located at?

Harrison's 20th Ed. Chapter 308 Page 2142

A. Corticomedullary junction
B. Outer cortex
C. Middle cortex
D. All of the above

Pathologic changes of FSGS are most prominent in glomeruli located at corticomedullary junction.

1591. Which of the following about FSGS is false?

Harrison's 20th Ed. Chapter 308 Page 2142

A. Sclerotic lesions in glomeruli that are focal (<50%)
B. Segmental (<50% of the glomerular tuft affected)
C. Podocyte injury
D. None of the above

Podocyte injury is the earliest feature of FSGS. It is exemplified by cell body attenuation, foot process effacement, pseudocyst formation and microvillous transformation. If podocytes do not recover from initial injury, there occurs a reduction in podocyte number & a mismatch between podocyte coverage & the underlying glomerular basement membrane (GBM) surface area, leading to 'uncovered' bare areas of GBM. The glomerular parietal epithelial cells (PECs) forming the cell bridge can deposit matrix between these bridging cells to form a fibrous attachment (tuft adhesion) between the glomerular tuft and Bowman's capsule.

1592. Which of the following is considered the earliest feature of FSGS seen on light microscopy?

Harrison's 20th Ed. Chapter 308 Page 2143

A. Tubular atrophy
B. Tuft adhesion
C. Hyalinosis
D. Lipid-laden macrophages

The tuft adhesion is considered the earliest feature of FSGS seen on light microscopy in human biopsies.

1593. Which of the following gene is essential for the integrity of slit diaphragm?

Adv Chronic Kidney Dis. 2014 ;21(5):408-416

A. Nephrin
B. Podocin
C. CD2AP
D. All of the above

Nephrin, podocin, CD2AP, TRPC6, GLEPP1, MYO1E are essential for the integrity of slit diaphragm.

1594. Which of the following gene is essential for foot process-GBM interaction?

Adv Chronic Kidney Dis. 2014 ;21(5):408-416

A. α-actinin 4
B. LAMB2
C. Formin
D. TRPC6

LAMB2 and ITGA3 are essential for foot process-GBM interaction.

1595. Human conditions associated with glomerulomegaly include?

Adv Chronic Kidney Dis. 2014 ;21(5):408-416

A. Obesity
B. Hypertension
C. Oligonephronia seen in low birth weight subjects
D. All of the above

Human conditions typically associated with glomerulomegaly include obesity, hypertension and the reduced nephron number (oligonephronia) seen in low birth weight subjects.

1596. In the adult human kidney, how many podocytes are present per glomerular tuft?

Adv Chronic Kidney Dis. 2014 ;21(5):408-416

A. ~ 50–60
B. ~ 100–200
C. ~ 300–500
D. ~ 500–600

In the adult human kidney, there are ~500–600 podocytes per glomerular tuft, and turnover of adult podocytes has never been demonstrated under physiological conditions. As adult podocytes are terminally differentiated epithelial cells with a very limited ability to proliferate, podocyte loss following injury can result in a reduction in podocyte number. With the loss of <20% of podocytes, glomerulus could recover, however, > 20% podocyte loss results in FSGS.

1597. The podocyte foot processes wrap around and attach to the GBM predominantly through?

Adv Chronic Kidney Dis. 2014 ;21(5):408-416

A. α3β1 integrin
B. αvβ3 integrin
C. α-dystroglycan/β-dystroglycan
D. All of the above

The podocyte foot processes wrap around and attach to the GBM predominantly through α3β1 and αvβ3 integrins, and α-dystroglycan/β-dystroglycan.

1598. Podocytes adhere tightly to the glomerular basement membrane (GBM) via interactions between?

Adv Chronic Kidney Dis. 2014 ;21(5):408-416

A. Actin cytoskeleton
B. Integrins α3β1 and αvβ3
C. GBM components laminin 521 and type IV collagen
D. All of the above

Podocytes adhere tightly to the glomerular basement membrane (GBM) via interactions between the actin cytoskeleton, integrins α3β1 and αvβ3, and the GBM components laminin 521 and type IV collagen.

1599. Which of the following is relevant in the pathogenesis of FSGS?

Harrison's 20th Ed. Chapter 308 Page 2142

A. T cell–mediated circulating permeability factor
B. Increased soluble urokinase receptor levels
C. TGF-β–mediated cellular proliferation & matrix synthesis
D. All of the above

Possible mechanisms in FSGS include a T cell–mediated circulating permeability factor, increased soluble urokinase receptor levels, TGF-β–mediated cellular proliferation and matrix synthesis, and podocyte abnormalities associated with genetic mutations. Risk polymorphisms at the APOL1 locus encoding apolipoprotein L1 expressed in podocytes substantially explain the increased burden of FSGS among African-Americans with or without HIV-associated disease.

1600. Which of the following about APOL1 FSGS is false?

Harrison's 20th Ed. Chapter 308 Page 2143

A. Most common form in African descent populations
B. More rapid progression to ESRD
C. Strongly associated with collapsing glomerulopathy
D. None of the above

1601. Histologically, FSGS may manifest as?

Harrison's 20th Ed. Chapter 308 Page 2143, Clin J Am Soc Nephrol. 2018;13(12):1889

A. Tip variant
B. Collapsing variant
C. NOS variant
D. All of the above

1602. Which of the following variant of FSGS has better prognosis?

Harrison's 20th Ed. Chapter 308 Page 2143

A. Collapsing glomerulopathy
B. Hilar stalk lesion
C. Glomerular tip lesion
D. Endocapillary hypercellularity

1603. The clinical findings of FSGS largely manifest as?

Harrison's 20th Ed. Chapter 308 Page 2143

A. Hematuria
B. Proteinuria
C. Renal failure
D. All of the above

The clinical findings of FSGS largely manifest as proteinuria.

1604. Which of the following agents is useful in primary FSGS?
Harrison's 20th Ed. Chapter 308 Page 2143

A. Steroids over 6–9 months
B. Cyclosporine
C. Plasmapheresis
D. All of the above

Calcineurin inhibitors, including cyclosporin and tacrolimus, are mainstays of FSGS therapy for both steroid-sensitive individuals who cannot tolerate continued steroid therapy and steroid-resistant FSGS.

1605. Which of the following agents is useful in secondary FSGS?
Harrison's 20th Ed. Chapter 308 Page 2144

A. Steroids
B. Cyclosporine
C. Rituximab
D. None of the above

The treatment of secondary FSGS rests on treating the underlying cause and controlling proteinuria. There is no role for steroids or other immunosuppressive agents in secondary FSGS.

1606. What value of protein:creatinine ratio indicates nephrotic range proteinuria?
Clin J Am Soc Nephrol. 2018;13(12):1889

A. > 100–150 mg/mmol
B. > 200–250 mg/mmol
C. > 250–300 mg/mmol
D. > 300–350 mg/mmol

A protein:creatinine ratio value > 300–350 mg/mmol indicates nephrotic range proteinuria.

1607. What value of urine protein-to-creatinine ratio (uPCR) is considered as nephrotic range?
Clin J Am Soc Nephrol. 2018;13(12):1889

A. ≥ 0.8 gram/gram
B. ≥ 1.2 gram/gram
C. ≥ 1.6 gram/gram
D. ≥ 2 gram/gram

Nephrotic range proteinuria is urine protein-to-creatinine ratio (uPCR) ≥2 gram/gram.

1608. Complete remission (CR) is defined as uPCR of?
Clin J Am Soc Nephrol. 2018;13(12):1889

A. < 0.8 gram/gram
B. < 1.2 gram/gram
C. < 1.6 gram/gram
D. < 2 gram/gram

Complete remission (CR) is defined as uPCR < 0.2 g/g, and partial remission (PR) is defined as having 50% reduction from baseline proteinuria and uPCR < 2 g/g.

1609. Majority of children with nephrotic syndrome are due to?
Harrison's 20th Ed. Chapter 308 Page 2144

A. Minimal change disease (MCD)
B. Focal and segmental glomerulosclerosis (FSGS)
C. Membranous glomerulopathy
D. Membranoproliferative glomerulonephritis (MPGN)

1610. Most common cause of nephrotic syndrome in the elderly is?
Harrison's 20th Ed. Chapter 308 Page 2144

A. Minimal change disease (MCD)
B. Focal segmental glomerulosclerosis (FSGS)
C. Membranous glomerulonephritis (MGN)
D. Mesangioproliferative glomerulonephritis

Membranous glomerulonephritis (MGN) is the most common cause of nephrotic syndrome in the elderly. Idiopathic membranous nephropathy (IMN) is rare in childhood.

1611. Most common cause of nephrotic syndrome in black patients is?
Am J Kidney Dis 1996;27:647-51

A. Minimal change disease (MCD)
B. Focal segmental glomerulosclerosis (FSGS)
C. Membranous glomerulonephritis (MGN)
D. Mesangioproliferative glomerulonephritis

Membranous nephropathy is the most common cause of nephrotic syndrome in white, while FSGS is the most common cause in black patients.

1612. Experimental model of membranous glomerulonephritis (MGN) in rat is called?
Clin J Am Soc Nephrol. 2017;12:983-997

A. Lewis nephritis
B. Kupin nephritis
C. Heymann nephritis
D. Pickering nephritis

1613. Which of the following podocyte antigen is involved in neonatal membranous glomerulonephritis?
Clin J Am Soc Nephrol. 2017;12:983-997

A. Neutral endopeptidase (NEP)
B. Aryl sulfatase
C. M-type phospholipase A2 receptor type 1 (PLA2R1)
D. Thrombospondin type 1 domain containing 7A (THSD7A)

Antigens expressed by podocytes are neutral endopeptidase NEP, also called CD10 or common acute lymphoblastic leukemia antigen (CALLA) in newborns, cationic bovine serum albumin (BSA) and aryl sulfatase in childhood, the M-type phospholipase A2 receptor type 1 (PLA2R1) and thrombospondin type 1 domain containing 7A (THSD7A) in adults.

1614. Membranous glomerulonephritis (MGN) can be secondary to?
Harrison's 20th Ed. Chapter 308 Page 2144

A. Solid tumors of breast, lung, colon
B. Hepatitis B
C. Malaria
D. All of the above

MGN can be secondary to solid tumors of breast, lung, colon, hepatitis B, syphilis, malaria, schistosomiasis, & lupus, rheumatoid arthritis, IgG4 diseases or drug exposure. Worldwide, malaria and schistosomiasis are the most common causes of secondary MGN. In US, the most important causes of secondary MGN are systemic lupus erythematosus (SLE), neoplasia, hepatitis B infection, and drugs.

1615. Which of the following is false about idiopathic membranous nephropathy (IMN)?
Harrison's 20th Ed. Chapter 308 Page 2144

A. Uniform thickening of BM along peripheral capillary loops
B. Diffuse granular subepithelial deposits of IgG and C3
C. Autoantibodies against M-type phospholipase A2 receptor
D. None of the above

Membranous glomerulonephritis (MGN) is the most common primary cause of the nephrotic syndrome, accounting for ~ 20% of cases. It is characterized by basement membrane thickening and subepithelial immune deposits without cellular proliferation or infiltration. Idiopathic disease has a male and adult predominance. The peak incidence is between 30 and 50 year, and MGN is particularly likely in patients over 50 years of age who present with nephrotic syndrome.

1616. Most cases of idiopathic membranous nephropathy (IMN) have circulating IgG4 autoantibody against?

Harrison's 20th Ed. Chapter 308 Page 2144

A. IL28B
B. PLA2R
C. RIG-1
D. PNPLA3

The detection of anti-PLA2R1 antibodies in patients with nephrotic syndrome is considered as a biomarker for the diagnosis of primary/idiopathic membranous nephropathy (IMN). significant sensitivity, Specifcity of anti-PLA2R1 antibodies for IMN has been proposed close to 100%.

1617. Patients of idiopathic membranous nephropathy (IMN) have circulating IgG4 autoantibody against?

Harrison's 20th Ed. Chapter 308 Page 2144

A. α3 NC1 domain of collagen IV
B. Thrombospondin type-1 domain containing 7A (THSD7A)
C. LIM domain region of LMX1B
D. X linked inhibitor of apoptosis protein (XIAP)

Most cases of idiopathic membranous nephropathy (IMN) have circulating IgG4 autoantibody to the podocyte membrane antigen PLA2R. In 70% of cases of IMN, autoantibodies against M-type phospholipase A2 receptor (PLA2R) circulate and bind to a conformational epitope present in PLA2R on human podocytes, producing characteristic in situ deposits. 5–10% of IMN patients have autoantibodies to thrombospondin type-1 domain containing 7A (anti-THSD7A). Both antigens co-localize within glomerular subepithelial deposits with IgG4. Low or absent levels of autoantibodies to PLA2R assist in predicting both spontaneous and treatment associated remissions.

1618. Anti-PLA2R & anti-THSD7A autoantibodies are absent in membranous glomerulopathy due to?

Harrison's 20th Ed. Chapter 308 Page 2144

A. Hepatitis A
B. Hepatitis B
C. Hepatitis C
D. All of the above

Anti-PLA2R & anti-THSD7A autoantibodies are absent in membranous glomerulopathy due to Hepatitis B and sarcoidosis.

1619. In idiopathic membranous nephropathy (IMN), presence of anti-THSD7A antibodies is associated with increased risk of?

Harrison's 20th Ed. Chapter 308 Page 2144

A. Connective tissue disorders
B. Malignancy
C. Alzheimer's disease
D. All of the above

Anti-PLAR1 antibodies are very rare or absent in patients with malignancy.

1620. Which of the following associated with worse prognosis in membranous glomerulonephritis?

Harrison's 20th Ed. Chapter 308 Page 2144

A. Male gender
B. Older age
C. Hypertension
D. All of the above

Male gender, older age, hypertension, and the persistence of proteinuria are associated with worse prognosis in membranous glomerulonephritis.

1621. Which of the following is predictive of progression of membranous glomerulonephritis?

Harrison's 20th Ed. Chapter 308 Page 2144

A. Degree of tubular atrophy
B. Interstitial fibrosis
C. Levels of autoantibodies to PLA2R
D. All of the above

Degree of tubular atrophy or interstitial fibrosis is more predictive of progression of MGN than is the stage of glomerular disease. Increasing or persistently elevated anti-PLA2R levels suggest that development of spontaneous remission is unlikely and support early initiation of immunosuppressive treatment.

1622. Which of the following causes of nephrotic syndrome has the highest incidences of renal vein thrombosis, pulmonary embolism, and deep vein thrombosis?

Harrison's 20th Ed. Chapter 308 Page 2144

A. Minimal change disease (MCD)
B. Focal segmental glomerulosclerosis (FSGS)
C. Membranous glomerulonephritis (MGN)
D. Diabetic nephropathy

Thrombotic complications occur in nephrotic syndrome. MGN has the highest incidence of renal vein thrombosis, pulmonary embolism & deep vein thrombosis. Risk of venous thrombosis is higher when serum albumin is <2–2.5 gram/dL.

1623. Immunosuppressive therapy is indicated in membranous glomerulonephritis in?

Clin J Am Soc Nephrol. 2017;12:983-997

A. Those with elevated anti-PLA2R/THSD7A levels
B. Those with proteinuria >3.5 g/d at diagnosis
C. Those who fail to reduce proteinuria to <3.5 g after 6 months of supportive care or have complications of nephrotic syndrome
D. All of the above

1624. In primary MGN, immunosuppressive drugs recommended include all except?

Harrison's 20th Ed. Chapter 308 Page 2144

A. Methotrexate
B. Chlorambucil
C. Mycophenolate mofetil
D. Cyclosporine

1625. Which of the following is useful in the treatment of primary MGN?

Am J Nephrol 2018;47(suppl 1):30-42

A. Adrenocorticotropic hormone (corticotropin)
B. Bortezomib
C. Belimumab
D. All of the above

1626. Which of the following is an anti-CD20 antibody?

Am J Nephrol 2018;47(suppl 1):30-42

A. Rituximab
B. Obinutuzumab
C. Ofatumumab
D. All of the above

1627. Which of the following is a proteasome inhibitor?

Am J Nephrol 2018;47(suppl 1):30-42

A. Bortezomib
B. Delanzomib
C. Carfilzomib
D. All of the above

1628. Risk factors for the development of diabetic nephropathy include?

Harrison's 20th Ed. Chapter 308 Page 2144

A. Smoking
B. Family history of diabetic nephropathy
C. Gene polymorphisms affecting activity of RAAS axis
D. All of the above

Risk factors for the development of diabetic nephropathy include hyperglycemia, hypertension, dyslipidemia, smoking, family history of diabetic nephropathy, and gene polymorphisms affecting activity of renin angiotensin-aldosterone axis.

1629. How many years after the onset of clinical diabetes, morphologic changes appear in kidneys?

Harrison's 20th Ed. Chapter 308 Page 2144

A. 1–2 years
B. 3–4 years
C. 5–7 years
D. 7–9 years

Within 1–2 years after the onset of clinical diabetes, morphologic changes appear in the kidney.

1630. In Types 1 or 2 diabetes, microalbuminuria appears how many years after the onset of diabetes?

Harrison's 20th Ed. Chapter 308 Page 2145

A. 2–5
B. 5–10
C. 10–15
D. 15–20

In types 1 or 2 diabetes, microalbuminuria appears 5–10 years after its onset.

1631. The glomerular filtration barrier is composed of?

Harrison's 20th Ed. Chapter 308 Page 2145

A. Fenestrated endothelium
B. GBM
C. Podocyte foot processes and slit diaphragms
D. All of the above

Glomerular filtration barrier is composed of fenestrated endothelium, GBM, podocyte foot processes and slit diaphragms.

1632. Podocytes are injured in?

Harrison's 20th Ed. Chapter 308 Page 2145

A. Minimal-change disease
B. FSGS
C. Collapsing glomerulopathy
D. All of the above

Podocytes are injured in minimal-change disease, FSGS, collapsing glomerulopathy, lupus nephritis & DN.

1633. Morphologic changes in diabetic nephropathy affect which of the following renal compartments?

Arch Pathol Lab Med. 2013;137:351-359

A. Glomeruli
B. Tubules
C. Interstitium
D. All of the above

Morphologic changes in diabetic nephropathy affect all 4 renal compartments: glomeruli, tubules, interstitium, and vessels.

1634. The morphologic renal lesions in type 1 diabetes (T1DM) predominantly affect which of the following?

Semin Nephrol. 2007 ;27(2):195-207

A. Glomeruli
B. Renal tubules
C. Interstitium
D. Arterioles

The morphologic lesions in type 1 diabetes (T1DM), predominantly affect the glomeruli, with thickening of glomerular basement membrane (GBM) and mesangial expansion, although also the podocytes, renal tubules, interstitium and arterioles undergo substantial changes, especially at later stages of disease.

1635. Which of the following is first to appear in type 1 diabetes (T1DM)?

Semin Nephrol. 2007 ;27(2):195-207

A. Thickening of glomerular basement membrane (GBM)
B. Thickening of tubular basement membrane (TBM)
C. Mesangial expansion due to increase in mesangial matrix
D. Afferent and efferent arteriolar hyalinosis

GBM thickening, the first measurable change, has been detected as early as 1.5 to 2.5 years after the onset of T1DM.

1636. Which of the following is a late manifestation in type 1 diabetes (T1DM)?

Semin Nephrol. 2007 ;27(2):195-207

A. Mesangial expansion due to increase in mesangial matrix
B. Afferent and efferent arteriolar hyalinosis
C. Abnormalities of the glomerular-tubular junction (GTJA)
D. Thickening of tubular basement membrane (TBM)

Abnormalities of the glomerular-tubular junction (GTJA) as late manifestations of the disease predominantly in patients with proteinuria. GTJA were almost entirely restricted to proteinuric patients, being rare in normoalbuminuric (NA) or microalbuminuric patients (MA).

1637. In diabetes, there is loss of which of the following in the GBM?

Harrison's 20th Ed. Chapter 308 Page 2144

A. Leucine-rich proteins
B. Heparan sulfate moieties
C. Collagenases
D. All of the above

The composition of the GBM is altered in diabetes, particularly the loss of heparan sulfate moieties that form the negatively charged filtration barrier. This results in increased filtration of serum proteins into the urine, predominately negatively charged albumin.

1638. Which of the following histopathological findings occur in diabetic kidneys?

Harrison's 20th Ed. Chapter 308 Page 2144

A. Thickening of GBM
B. Expansion of mesangial matrix
C. Nodular glomerulosclerosis
D. All of the above

Diffuse thickening of GBMs is usually the earliest structural change in diabetes. Tubular basement membranes of nonatrophic tubules are also thickened. Mesangial regions are expanded, predominantly due to accumulation of mesangial matrix. There are no immune complexes. Podocytes show variable foot process effacement, especially in advanced stages.

1639. Key diagnostic feature of diabetic nephropathy is?
Am J Kidney Dis. 2015;66(5):e37-e38

A. Increased mesangial matrix
B. Nodular glomerulosclerosis with diffuse GBM thickening
C. Concomitant hyalinosis of afferent & efferent arterioles
D. All of the above

The pathologic hallmark of diabetic nephropathy is diabetic glomerulosclerosis that results from a progressive increase in extracellular matrix in the glomerular mesangium and glomerular basement membranes.

1640. Diabetic nephropathy is most commonly complicated by which of the following kidney disease?
Arch Pathol Lab Med. 2013;137:351-359

A. Membranous nephropathy
B. Acute postinfectious glomerulonephritis
C. IgA nephropathy
D. Lupus nephritis

Hyperglycaemia may cause different patterns of renal injury in T1DM compared to T2DM patients. T2DM diabetic nephropathy is probably the most common renal disease to be complicated by another distinct identifiable kidney disease, membranous nephropathy is by far the most common. Other non-diabetic renal diseases with DN include acute post-infectious glomerulonephritis, IgA nephropathy, crescentic glomerulonephritis, membranoproliferative glomerulonephritis (types I and II), lupus nephritis, nonspecific immune complex disease, and amyloid.

1641. Light microscopy characteristic features of diabetic nephropathy include?
Arch Pathol Lab Med. 2013;137:351-359

A. Glomerular hypertrophy
B. Uniform thickening of glomerular basement membrane (GBM)
C. Increase of mesangial matrix – diffuse
D. All of the above

1642. Light microscopy characteristic features of diabetic nephropathy include?
Arch Pathol Lab Med. 2013;137:351-359

A. Kimmelstiel–Wilson nodules
B. Podocyte hypertrophy & foot process broadening & effacement
C. Hyalinosis of glomerular peripheral capillaries (plasmatic insudation)
D. All of the above

1643. Light microscopy characteristic features of diabetic nephropathy include?
Arch Pathol Lab Med. 2013;137:351-359

A. Aneurysmal peripheral glomerular capillaries
B. Capsular drops
C. Extracapillary proliferation (fibro-cellular crescents)
D. All of the above

1644. Light microscopy characteristic features of diabetic nephropathy include?
Arch Pathol Lab Med. 2013;137:351-359

A. Hyalinosis of afferent and efferent arterioles
B. Thickening of the tubular basement membrane (TBM)
C. Chronic interstitial inflammation and fibrosis
D. All of the above

1645. Ultrastructural characteristic features of diabetic nephropathy include?
Arch Pathol Lab Med. 2013;137:351-359

A. Typical uniform thickening of GBM & TBM
B. Capsular drops
C. Plasmatic insudation of glomerular capillaries
D. All of the above

Glomerular insudative lesions are one of the characteristic histological features of diabetic nephropathy (DN). They are commonly known as capsular drops and fibrin caps, which are located between the parietal epithelium and Bowman's capsule or within the glomerular capillary lumen, respectively.

1646. Which of the following is pathognomic of diabetic nephropathy?
Arch Pathol Lab Med. 2013;137:351-359

A. Well-formed, intercapillary, nodular mesangial lesions
B. Thickened glomerular and tubular basement membranes
C. Hyaline arteriolosclerosis
D. All of the above

The well-formed, intercapillary, nodular mesangial lesions, along with thickened glomerular basement membranes and tubular basement membranes, and hyaline arteriolosclerosis are virtually pathognomic of diabetic nephropathy.

1647. Kimmelstiel-Wilson lesion relates best with which of the following histopathological findings in diabetic kidney?
Harrison's 20th Ed. Chapter 308 Page 2144

A. Thickening of GBM
B. Expansion of mesangial matrix
C. Nodular glomerulosclerosis
D. Hyaline arteriosclerosis

Kimmelstiel-Wilson (1936) nodules or nodular glomerulosclerosis are eosinophilic, PAS+ & Jones silver stain+ nodules. Nodular lesions are the pathological hallmark of human diabetic nephropathy (DN). The classic Kimmelstiel Wilson nodules are postulated to be the consequence of repeated mesangiolysis, with an exuberant repair response.

1648. Which of the following about Kimmelstiel-Wilson nodules is false?
Arch Pathol Lab Med. 2013;137:351-359

A. Measure 40 to 100 μm in diameter
B. Acellular
C. PAS^+ and $silver^+$
D. None of the above

The characteristic KW nodules measure 40 to 100 μm in diameter. These nodules are PAS^+ and $silver^+$ and are usually acellular, although nuclei may be present in the periphery in a circumferential manner.

1649. Which of the following lesions can be seen in diabetic nephropathy?
Arch Pathol Lab Med. 2013;137:351-359

A. Fibrin cap
B. Capsular drop
C. Tubular atrophy, tubular apoptosis, thickened tubular BM
D. All of the above

1650. Which of the following is false about hyalinotic/exudative lesion/fibrin cap in diabetic nephropathy?
Arch Pathol Lab Med. 2013;137:351-359

A. Accumulation of hyaline, eosinophilic, homogeneous material between endothelial cells & GBM of capillary loops
B. Made up of trapped plasma proteins (IgM & C1q)
C. May occlude capillary lumen
D. None of the above

Term insudative lesion is preferable over 'exudative lesion' because these lesions are localized 'inside' the lumen. The term fibrin cap is poorly chosen because these lesions actually consist of plasma proteins with a homogeneous, glassy, and hyaline appearance, as well as lipid droplets, but do not contain fibrin.

1651. Which of the following lesion is associated with the renal prognosis of DN patients?

Harrison's 20th Ed. Chapter 308 Page 2145

A. Glomerular and arteriolar insudative lesions
B. Interstitial fibrosis
C. Tubular atrophy
D. All of the above

Recent studies of biopsy-proven DN have demonstrated that glomerular and arteriolar insudative lesions are associated with the renal prognosis of DN patients, although the association is not as strong as interstitial fibrosis and tubular atrophy (IFTA) or nodular lesions.

1652. The Armanni-Ebstein lesion is associated with?

Forensic Sci Med Pathol. 2012;8(1):19-22

A. Membranous nephropathy
B. Diabetic ketoacidosis
C. Renal amyloidosis
D. Fabry's disease

The Armanni-Ebstein lesion is a histological change in the kidney consisting of sub-nuclear vacuolation of the proximal tubules. It has been most associated with diabetic ketoacidosis.

1653. Nodular glomerulosclerosis can also be seen in?

Am J Kidney Dis. 2015;66(5):e37-e38

A. Monoclonal immunoglobulin deposition disease (MIDD)
B. Amyloidosis
C. Membranoproliferative glomerulonephritides
D. All of the above

Nodular glomerulosclerosis can also be seen in monoclonal immunoglobulin deposition disease (MIDD), amyloidosis, idiopathic nodular glomerulosclerosis, membranoproliferative glomerulonephritides.

1654. Which of the following renal morphological lesion stain positive by silver stain?

Arch Pathol Lab Med. 2013;137:351-359

A. Diabetic Nephropathy
B. Monoclonal Immunoglobulin Deposition Disease
C. Amyloidosis
D. Immunotactoid Glomerulonephritis

1655. Which of the following renal morphological lesion does not stain positive by periodic acid–Schiff (PAS)?

Arch Pathol Lab Med. 2013;137:351-359

A. Diabetic Nephropathy
B. Monoclonal Immunoglobulin Deposition Disease
C. Amyloidosis
D. Immunotactoid Glomerulonephritis

1656. Which of the following renal morphological lesion does not stain positive by Congo red?

Arch Pathol Lab Med. 2013;137:351-359

A. Diabetic Nephropathy
B. Monoclonal Immunoglobulin Deposition Disease
C. Amyloidosis
D. Immunotactoid Glomerulonephritis

1657. Which of the following is different between type 1 & type 2 diabetes?

Harrison's 20th Ed. Chapter 308 Page 2145

A. Natural history of diabetic nephropathy
B. Renal biopsy findings
C. Onset of microalbuminuria
D. Presence of diabetic retinopathy

Renal biopsies from patients with Types 1 and 2 diabetes are largely indistinguishable. Natural history of diabetic nephropathy in patients with Types 1 and 2 diabetes is similar. >90% of Type 1 diabetics with nephropathy have diabetic retinopathy while only 60% of Type 2 diabetics with nephropathy have diabetic retinopathy.

1658. The pathologic changes in diabetic nephropathy are the result of?

Harrison's 20th Ed. Chapter 308 Page 2145

A. Intraglomerular hypertension
B. Direct effects of hyperglycemia on actin cytoskeleton of renal mesangial & vascular smooth-muscle cells
C. Diabetes-associated changes in circulating factors
D. All of the above

1659. Diabetes-associated changes occur in which of the following circulating factors?

Harrison's 20th Ed. Chapter 308 Page 2145

A. Atrial natriuretic factor
B. Angiotensin II
C. Insulin-like growth factor (IGF)
D. All of the above

1660. Sustained glomerular hypertension leads to?

Harrison's 20th Ed. Chapter 308 Page 2145

A. Increased mesangial matrix production
B. Alterations in GBM with disruption in filtration barrier
C. Glomerulosclerosis
D. All of the above

1661. In diabetic nephropathy, mesangial matrix production is altered by?

Harrison's 20th Ed. Chapter 308 Page 2145

A. Accumulation of advanced glycosylation end products (AGE)
B. Growth hormone
C. IGF-I
D. All of the above

1662. In diabetic nephropathy, mesangial matrix production is altered by?

Harrison's 20th Ed. Chapter 308 Page 2145

A. Angiotensin II
B. Connective tissue growth factor
C. TGF-β
D. All of the above

1663. In microalbuminuria, the range of albuminuria is?

Harrison's 20th Ed. Chapter 308 Page 2145

A. <150 mg/day
B. 20–200 mg/day
C. 30–300 mg/day
D. 40–400 mg/day

Albuminuria in the range of 30 - 300 mg/day is called microalbuminuria. Or, microalbuminuria is defined as urinary albumin excretion ≥30 and <300 mg/gCr.

1664. Dipstick positive level of albuminuria is?

Harrison's 20th Ed. Chapter 308 Page 2145

A. >30 mg
B. >150 mg
C. >300 mg
D. >500 mg

Dipstick positive level of proteinuria is >300 mg albuminuria. Macroalbuminuria is urinary albumin excretion ≥300 mg/gCr and overt proteinuria is macroalbuminuria exceeding 1 g/day.

1665. In diabetes, renal functions unrelentingly decline after what level of proteinuria?

Harrison's 20th Ed. Chapter 308 Page 2145

A. >500 mg/day
B. >1000 mg/day
C. >1500 mg/day
D. >2500 mg/day

1666. From the earliest stages of microalbuminuria, it takes how many years to reach end-stage renal disease (ESRD)?

Harrison's 20th Ed. Chapter 308 Page 2145

A. 5–10 years
B. 10–20 years
C. 20–30 years
D. >30 years

After proteinuria level of >500 mg/day, renal function decline relentlessly. From the stage of microalbuminuria, it usually takes 10–20 years to reach ESRD.

1667. Which of the following statements is false?

Harrison's 20th Ed. Chapter 308 Page 2145

A. >90% patients with type 1 diabetes & nephropathy have diabetic retinopathy
B. 60% patients with type 2 diabetes with nephropathy have diabetic retinopathy
C. Significant correlation between presence of retinopathy & presence of Kimmelstiel-Wilson nodules
D. None of the above

1668. Which of the following class of drugs may be of benefit in diabetic nephropathy?

Harrison's 20th Ed. Chapter 308 Page 2145

A. Sodium glucose transport 2 inhibitors
B. Endothelin antagonists
C. Aldosterone antagonists
D. All of the above

1669. Which of the following is a renin inhibitor?

Harrison's 20th Ed. Chapter 308 Page 2145

A. Bosentan
B. Aliskiren
C. Empagliflozin
D. Eplerenone

1670. Which of the following is an endothelin antagonist?

Harrison's 20th Ed. Chapter 308 Page 2145

A. Bosentan
B. Aliskiren
C. Empagliflozin
D. Eplerenone

1671. Which of the following is a SGLT2 inhibitor?

Harrison's 20th Ed. Chapter 308 Page 2145

A. Bosentan
B. Aliskiren
C. Empagliflozin
D. Eplerenone

1672. Which of the following is an aldosterone antagonist?

Harrison's 20th Ed. Chapter 308 Page 2145

A. Bosentan
B. Aliskiren
C. Empagliflozin
D. Eplerenone

Aliskiren is an oral, nonpeptide competitive inhibitors of the enzymatic activity of renin. Bosentan is an endothelin antagonist. Spironolactone & eplerenone are aldosterone antagonists. Empagliflozin, canagliflozin & dapagliflozin are SGLT2 inhibitors.

1673. Which of the following about Light Chain Deposition Disease (LCDD) is false?

Harrison's 20th Ed. Chapter 308 Page 2145

A. Produce kappa light chains
B. Light-chain deposits are not fibrillar
C. Light-chain deposits do not stain with Congo red
D. None of the above

Light Chain Deposition Disease (LCDD) produces nephrotic syndrome with renal failure. Congo red negative nodular deposition of nonamyloid immunoglobulin light chains is the most common pathologic finding in light chain deposition disease in light microscopy. Immunoflurescent microscopy usually demonstrates the presence of monotypic kappa light chain. Nodular glomerulosclerosis of LCDD resembles diabetic Kimmelstiel-Wilson.

1674. Which of the following about Light Chain Deposition Disease (LCDD) is false?

J Renal Inj Prev. 2013; 2(4): 127–128

A. Clinical picture is like rapidly progressive glomerulonephritis
B. Proteinuria is a combination of light chain and albumin
C. Nodular glomerulosclerosis resembles diabetic KW lesion
D. None of the above

1675. Which of the following causes renal failure but not heavy proteinuria?

Harrison's 20th Ed. Chapter 308 Page 2145

A. Amyloidosis
B. Light chain deposition disease
C. Cast nephropathy (myeloma kidney)
D. All of the above

1676. Renal vein thrombosis is common in patients with nephrotic syndrome due to?

Harrison's 20th Ed. Chapter 308 Page 2145

A. Membranous glomerulopathy
B. Membranoproliferative glomerulonephritis
C. Amyloidosis
D. All of the above

1677. Clinical features that suggest acute renal vein thrombosis include all except?

Harrison's 19th Ed. 1845

A. Sudden onset of flank or abdominal pain
B. Gross hematuria
C. Right-sided varicocele
D. Acute decline in GFR

Clinical features that suggest acute renal vein thrombosis include light-sided varicocele.

1678. Congo red stains are positive in?

Harrison's 20th Ed. Chapter 308 Page 2145

A. AA & AL amyloidosis
B. Fibrillary-Immunotactoid Glomerulopathy
C. Light chain deposition disease
D. All of the above

AA and AL amyloid fibrils are detectable with Congo red.

1679. Organs that amyloid infiltrates include?

Harrison's 20th Ed. Chapter 308 Page 2145

A. Peripheral nerves
B. Upper pharynx
C. Kidney
D. All of the above

Amyloid infiltrates the liver, heart, peripheral nerves, carpal tunnel, upper pharynx, and kidney.

1680. In systemic AL amyloidosis (primary amyloidosis), excess light chain are made into fragments by?

Harrison's 20th Ed. Chapter 308 Page 2145

A. Lymphocytes
B. Eosinophils
C. Macrophages
D. All of the above

In systemic AL amyloidosis, also called primary amyloidosis, light chains produced in excess by clonal plasma cell dyscrasias are made into fragments by macrophages leading to self-aggregation at an acid pH.

1681. Which of the following statements about primary amyloidosis is false?

Harrison's 20th Ed. Chapter 308 Page 2145

A. Excess light chains produced by clonal plasma cell dyscrasias
B. Predominant light chains are of lambda class
C. Light chain fragments self-aggregate at acid pH
D. None of the above

1682. AL amyloidosis occurs in the setting of?

Harrison's 20th Ed. Chapter 308 Page 2145

A. Multiple myeloma (MM)
B. Waldenström's macroglobulinemia
C. Lymphoma
D. All of the above

AL amyloidosis occurs in the setting of multiple myeloma (MM), Waldenström's macroglobulinemia, lymphoma, other plasmacytomas, or lymphoproliferative disorders, or without any other identifiable disease.

1683. Which of the following is true about AA amyloidosis or secondary amyloidosis?

Harrison's 20th Ed. Chapter 308 Page 2145

A. Deposition of α-pleated sheets of serum amyloid A protein
B. Deposition of β-pleated sheets of serum amyloid A protein
C. Deposition of γ-pleated sheets of serum amyloid A protein
D. Deposition of δ-pleated sheets of serum amyloid A protein

AA amyloidosis (secondary amyloidosis) is due to deposition of β-pleated sheets of serum amyloid A protein.

1684. Which of the following is true about serum amyloid A protein?

Harrison's 20th Ed. Chapter 308 Page 2145

A. Acute phase reactant
B. Membrane cofactor protein
C. Complement-regulatory protein
D. Lithogenic factor

Serum amyloid A (SAA) protein is an apolipoprotein of high-density lipoproteins that serves as a dynamic acute phase reactant. It is synthesized as a precursor by hepatocytes in response to transcriptional stimuli from various proinflammatory cytokines, such as interleukin (IL)-1, IL-6, and tumor necrosis factor (TNF) alpha.

1685. Which of the following is a positive acute-phase reactant?

Harrison's 20th Ed. Chapter 308 Page 2145

A. Ceruloplasmin
B. C-reactive protein
C. Transferrin
D. All of the above

1686. Which of the following is not a positive acute-phase reactant?

Harrison's 20th Ed. Chapter 308 Page 2145

A. Ferritin
B. Thrombocytosis
C. Serum amyloid A (SAA)
D. Albumin

Negative acute-phase reactants are albumin and fetuin. Serum amyloid A protein (SAA), a hepatic acute phase reactant.

1687. Which of the following is the function of serum amyloid A protein?

Harrison's 20th Ed. Chapter 308 Page 2146

A. Cholesterol transport
B. Immune cell attraction
C. Metalloproteases activation
D. All of the above

Serum amyloid A protein, an acute phase reactant whose physiologic functions include cholesterol transport, immune cell attraction and metalloproteases activation.

1688. Which of the following is the most common type of amyloidosis worldwide?

Clin Epidemiol. 2014;6:369-377

A. Primary AL amyloidosis
B. Secondary amyloid A (AA) amyloidosis
C. Familial amyloidosis
D. β2-microglobulin related amyloidosis

AA amyloidosis is the most common type of amyloidosis worldwide.

1689. Familial amyloidosis best relates to?

Clin Epidemiol. 2014;6:369-377

A. Serum amyloid A protein
B. Mutant transthyretin
C. β2-microglobulin
D. Light chains

1690. Amyloid A hereditary (AH) best relates to?

Clin Epidemiol. 2014;6:369-377

A. Serum amyloid A protein
B. Mutant transthyretin
C. β2-microglobulin
D. Light chains

1691. Which of the following diseases is related to serum amyloid A protein?

Harrison's 20th Ed. Chapter 308 Page 2146

A. Rheumatoid arthritis
B. Familial Mediterranean fever (FMF)
C. Muckle–Wells syndrome
D. All of the above

Autoimmune diseases such as rheumatoid arthritis, ankylosing spondylitis, chronic juvenile arthritis, and inflammatory bowel disease, or hereditary inflammatory diseases, such as FMF, TNF receptor-associated periodic syndrome, or Muckle–Wells syndrome, account for up to 90% of recent cases of AA amyloidosis.

1692. Which of the following is the most frequent clinical manifestation that should raise suspicion of AA amyloidosis?

Harrison's 20th Ed. Chapter 308 Page 2146

A. Hematuria
B. Proteinuria
C. Hepatosplenomegaly
D. Adrenal insufficiency

Proteinuria leading to nephrotic syndrome and renal insufficiency is the earliest and most frequent clinical manifestation that should raise suspicion of AA amyloidosis.

1693. Which of the following is the preferred site for biopsy for the diagnosis of amyloidosis?

Harrison's 20th Ed. Chapter 308 Page 2146

A. Rectal mucosa
B. Gingival mucosa
C. Abdominal fat pad aspirates
D. Minor salivary gland biopsy

In 1973, Westermark & Stenkvist described subcutaneous abdominal fat tissue aspiration as a new, noninvasive technique, and this has now become the preferred initial option in most centers throughout the world.

1694. Which of the following drugs is useful in the treatment for primary amyloidosis?

Harrison's 20th Ed. Chapter 308 Page 2146

A. Busulfan
B. Melphalan
C. Cyclophosphamide
D. Chlorambucil

The median survival of patients with primary amyloidosis is <2 years, with death usually from progressive congestive heart failure or renal failure. Chemotherapy with melphalan, prednisone, and colchicine, to reduce the concentration of monoclonal proteins, and autologous stem cell transplantation may prolong survival. Melphalan inhibits mitosis by cross-linking DNA strands. Colchicine decreases leukocyte motility and phagocytosis in inflammatory responses.

1695. Which of the following is false about fibrillary-immunotactoid glomerulopathy?

Harrison's 20th Ed. Chapter 308 Page 2146

A. Glomerular accumulation of nonbranching randomly arranged fibrils
B. Nonamyloid fibrillary disease not associated with a systemic illness
C. Congo red stains are negative
D. None of the above

The cause of this "nonamyloid" immunotactoid glomerulopathy is idiopathic, with an occasional association with chronic lymphocytic leukemia or B cell lymphoma.

1696. Which of the following best relates to Fabry's Disease?

Harrison's 20th Ed. Chapter 308 Page 2146

A. Glucosylceramide
B. Galactosylceramide
C. Globotriaosylceramide
D. Ceramide

Fabry disease is an X-linked inborn error of globotriaosylceramide metabolism secondary to deficient lysosomal α-galactosidase A activity (mutations in α-galactosidase gene), resulting in excessive intracellular storage of globotriaosylceramide.

1697. Organ affected in Fabry's disease is?

Harrison's 20th Ed. Chapter 308 Page 2146

A. Heart
B. Brain
C. Kidney
D. All of the above

Organs affected in Fabry's disease include the vascular endothelium, heart, brain, and kidneys.

1698. Classically, Fabry's disease presents with?

Harrison's 20th Ed. Chapter 308 Page 2146

A. Acroparesthesias
B. Angiokeratoma
C. Hypohidrosis
D. All of the above

Classically, Fabry's disease presents in childhood in males with acroparesthesias, angiokeratoma, and hypohidrosis.

1699. Clinical manifestations of Fabry's disease include all except?

Harrison's 20th Ed. Chapter 411 Page 3007, N Engl J Med. 2001;345:9-16

A. Angiokeratomas
B. Corneal and lenticular opacities
C. Small-vessel disease of the kidney
D. Macrocephaly

Fabry's disease is also known as angiokeratoma corpus diffusum or Anderson-Fabry disease. Clinically, Fabry's disease manifests as angiokeratomas (telangiectatic skin lesions), hypohidrosis, corneal and lenticular opacities (cornea verticillata), painful acroparesthesia, and small-vessel disease of kidney, heart, & brain.

1700. Which of the following is false about Fabry's disease?

Harrison's 20th Ed. Chapter 411 Page 3007

A. X-linked dominant disorder
B. Due to mutations in GALA that encodes α-galactosidase A
C. Accumulation of ceramide trihexoside in nerves, blood vessels
D. None of the above

1701. Angiokeratomas is a clinical feature of?
Br J Dermatol 1997;136594- 597

A. Fabry's disease
B. β-Mannosidosis
C. Fucosidosis
D. All of the above

Angiokeratomas are also seen in mannosidosis, fucosidosis, sialidosis, and β-galactosidase and β-hexosaminidase deficiency.

1702. In Fabry's disease, angiokeratomas are most dense?
Harrison's 20th Ed. Chapter 308 Page 2146

A. Over nape of the neck
B. Over fingertips
C. Between umbilicus and knees
D. Over forehead

In Fabry's disease, angiokeratomas (telangiectatic skin lesions) are most dense between umbilicus and knees "the bathing suit area" but may occur anywhere, including mucosal surfaces.

1703. In renal biopsy, "Zebra bodies" is a histopathological hallmark of?
Harrison's 20th Ed. Chapter 308 Page 2146

A. Fabry's disease
B. β-Mannosidosis
C. Fucosidosis
D. All of the above

In Fabry's disease, electron microscopy of renal biopsy shows enlarged glomerular visceral epithelial cells packed with vacuoles containing globotriaosylceramide in parallel arrays called zebra bodies.

1704. Nephropathy of Fabry's disease typically progresses to renal failure in which decade of life?
Harrison's 20th Ed. Chapter 308 Page 2146

A. First
B. Second
C. Third
D. Fourth

Nephropathy of Fabry's disease progresses to renal failure by the fourth or fifth decade. Nephropathy typically presents in the third decade of life as mild to moderate proteinuria, sometimes with microscopic hematuria or nephrotic syndrome.

1705. Which of the following is found in the urine of patients with Fabry's disease?
Harrison's 20th Ed. Chapter 308 Page 2146

A. Eosinophils
B. Maltese cross
C. Randall's plaque
D. Waxy casts

In Fabry's disease, urinalysis may reveal oval fat bodies and birefringent glycolipid globules under polarized light called maltese cross.

1706. In Fabry's disease, neutral glycosphingolipids accumulate in which orgenelle of glomerular cells?
Harrison's 20th Ed. Chapter 308 Page 2146

A. Mitochondria
B. Golgi apparatus
C. Lysosome
D. Nucleus

1707. The dose of recombinant α-galactosidase A in Fabry's disease is?
N Engl J Med. 2001;345:9-16

A. 1 mg/kg
B. 2 mg/kg
C. 3 mg/kg
D. 4 mg/kg

The dose of 1 mg of recombinant α-galactosidase A per kilogram every other week for about six months to one year safely and effectively reversed the accumulation of microvascular endothelial deposits of globotriaosylceramide in the kidneys, heart, and skin.

1708. Which of the following is included in pulmonary renal syndromes?
Harrison's 20th Ed. Chapter 308 Page 2146

A. Goodpasture's syndrome
B. Henoch-Schonlein purpura
C. Cryoglobulinemia
D. All of the above

Pulmonary renal syndromes present with catastrophic hemoptysis and glomerulonephritis associated with varying degrees of renal failure. The usual causes include Goodpasture's syndrome, granulomatosis with polyangiitis, microscopic polyangiitis, Churg-Strauss vasculitis and Henoch-Schonlein purpura or cryoglobulinemia.

1709. Which of the following is a component of glomerular basement membrane?
Harrison's 20th Ed. Chapter 308 Page 2146

A. Collagen IV
B. Laminins
C. Nidogen
D. All of the above

1710. Kidney basement membrane is made of?
Harrison's 20th Ed. Chapter 308 Page 2146

A. Collagen IV with laminins
B. Nidogen
C. Sulfated proteoglycans
D. All of the above

kidney epithelia, including podocytes, rest on basement membranes assembled into a planar surface through the interweaving of collagen IV with laminins, nidogen and sulfated proteoglycans.

1711. Which of the following triple-helical protomer is present in glomerular & tubular basement membrane?
Harrison's 20th Ed. Chapter 308 Page 2146

A. α1.α1.α2(IV) collagen
B. α3.α4.α5(IV) collagen
C. α5.α5.α6(IV) collagen
D. All of the above

1712. Which of the following triple-helical protomer is present along Bowman's capsule in the kidney?
Harrison's 20th Ed. Chapter 308 Page 2146

A. α1.α1.α2(IV) collagen
B. α3.α4.α5(IV) collagen
C. α5.α5.α6(IV) collagen
D. All of the above

All epithelial basement membranes early in human development are composed of interconnected triple-helical protomers rich in α1.α1.α2(IV) collagen. The α1 (IV) and α2 (IV) chains are ubiquitous in all basement membranes. Specialized tissues like kidney (glomerular and tubular basement membrane), lung, testis, cochlea, and eye undergo a developmental switch replacing α1.α1.α2(IV) protomers with an α3.α4.α5(IV) collagen network. In skin, smooth muscle, esophagus and along Bowman's capsule in the kidney, α5.α5.α6(IV) collagen network appears. This modification provides more resistance to proteases and ensures the structural longevity of critical tissues.

1713. Which of the following is false about Alport's syndrome?

Harrison's 20th Ed. Chapter 308 Page 2146

A. Hematuria
B. Thinning and splitting of GBMs
C. Mild proteinuria
D. None of the above

1714. The triad of clinical findings of Alport syndrome includes all except?

Harrison's 20th Ed. Chapter 308 Page 2147

A. Hemorrhagic nephritis
B. Proteinuria
C. Sensorineural hearing loss
D. Characteristic ocular findings

Alport syndrome is an oculo-renal syndrome characterized by a triad of clinical findings consisting of hemorrhagic nephritis, sensorineural hearing loss and characteristic ocular findings.

1715. Which of the following is false about Alport's syndrome?

Harrison's 20th Ed. Chapter 308 Page 2147

A. Inherited tubulointerstitial disease
B. Due to mutation in COL4A5 gene
C. Hematuria, glomerulosclerosis & renal failure
D. Usually X linked

Chronic glomerulosclerosis is a feature of Alport's syndrome. Mutations in COL4A5 (X-linked), COL4A3, or COL4A4 (both autosomal recessive) genes result in defective synthesis of collagen type IV with consequent dysfunction and inflammation of the glomerular basement membrane.

1716. Which of the following is related to Alport's syndrome?

Harrison's 20th Ed. Chapter 308 Page 2147

A. Ataxia
B. Sensorineural deafness
C. Alopecia
D. Jaundice

Alport's syndrome consists of hematuria, proteinuria (<1 to 2 gram/day), progressive renal failure and sensorineural deafness. In the early stages, hearing impairment is detectable only by audiometry, with bilateral hearing loss of high tones in frequencies ranging from 2000-8000 hertz (Hz).

1717. Ocular manifestations of Alport's syndrome include?

Harrison's 20th Ed. Chapter 308 Page 2147

A. Anterior lenticonus
B. Dot-and-fleck retinopathy
C. Temporal macular thinning
D. All of the above

In Alport's syndrome, central part of the lens projects anteriorly 3-4 mm in an axial projection as seen on biomicroscopic examination. The condition is usually bilateral & causes a slowly progressive axial myopia. Numerous bilateral, white and yellow perimacular dots and flecks occur in this condition. These spare the fovea but can spread to the periphery. No associated visual impairment or night blindness occurs. Typically, dot-and-fleck retinopathy does not fluoresce with angiography.

1718. Which of the following is considered pathognomonic of Alport's syndrome?

Harrison's 20th Ed. Chapter 308 Page 2147

A. Anterior lenticonus
B. Sensorineural hearing loss
C. Hematuria
D. Leiomyomatosis

Anterior lenticonus is the most specific & is pathognomonic extrarenal manifestation of Alport's syndrome (AS). It also is a valuable marker of the severity of AS, being consistently associated with both a rapid progression to renal failure and hearing loss. Lenticonus is never present at birth.

1719. Positive "oil droplet sign" in Alport's syndrome pertains to?

N Engl J Med. 2003;348:2543-56, Harrison's 20th Ed. Chapter 308 Page 2147

A. Ocular lens
B. Tongue
C. Nails
D. Nose

In Alport's syndrome, lenticonus of anterior lens capsule is termed as positive "oil droplet sign". Distinctive oil droplet appearance on the red reflex on slit lamp examination is characteristic of Alport's syndrome.

1720. Which of the following suggests a poorer prognosis in Alport's syndrome?

Harrison's 20th Ed. Chapter 308 Page 2147

A. Early severe deafness
B. Lenticonus
C. Proteinuria
D. All of the above

Early severe deafness, lenticonus, or proteinuria suggests a poorer prognosis.

1721. In Alport's syndrome, skin biopsy revealing the lack of which of the following collagen chain helps in diagnosis?

Harrison's 20th Ed. Chapter 308 Page 2147

A. $\alpha 2$(IV)
B. $\alpha 3$(IV)
C. $\alpha 4$(IV)
D. $\alpha 5$(IV)

Since α5(IV) collagen is expressed in the skin, some X-linked Alport's patients can be diagnosed with a skin biopsy revealing the lack of the α5(IV) collagen chain on immunofluorescent analysis.

1722. Hereditary disorder that may include renal involvement and hearing loss is?

Kidney International. 1999;56:760-775

A. Muckle-Wells syndrome
B. Cockayne's syndrome
C. Alström's syndrome
D. All of the above

1723. Hereditary disorder that may include renal involvement and hearing loss is?

Kidney International. 1999;56:760-775

A. Bardet-Biedl syndrome
B. Refsum's disease
C. Charcot-Marie-Tooth syndrome
D. All of the above

A specific mitochondrial DNA (mtDNA) mutation (a guanine for adenine substitution at position 3243) is responsible for a syndrome combining diabetes mellitus, sensorineural deafness, & progressive renal failure.

1724. Thin basement membrane disease (TBMD) is typically associated with?

Harrison's 20th Ed. Chapter 308 Page 2147

A. Proteinuria
B. Hypertension
C. Loss of renal function
D. None of the above

Thin basement membrane disease (TBMD) characterized by persistent or recurrent hematuria is not typically associated with proteinuria, hypertension, or loss of renal function or extrarenal disease.

1725. Which of the following is false about thin basement membrane disease (TBMD)?

Harrison's 20th Ed. Chapter 308 Page 2147

A. Also called benign familial hematuria
B. Genetic defects in type IV collagen
C. Diffuse thinning of GBM
D. None of the above

1726. Which of the following is a heritable form of CKD?

Harrison's 20th Ed. Chapter 308 Page 2147

A. Alport's syndrome
B. Fabry disease
C. Cystinosis
D. All of the above

Alport syndrome, Fabry disease and cystinosis are a heritable form of CKD.

1727. Which of the following statements about 'Nail-patella syndrome' is false?

N Engl J Med. 2006;354:1387-401, Harrison's 20th Ed. Chapter 308 Page 2147

A. It an autosomal dominant disease
B. More common in females
C. Primarily affect patella, elbows and nails
D. None of the above

Skeletal features include absent or hypoplastic patellae, patella dislocations, elbow abnormalities, talipes, and iliac horns on X-ray. NPS is caused by loss of function mutations in the transcription factor LMX1B at 9q34.

1728. Nail-patella syndrome (NPS) is also known as?

Journal of Medical Genetics 2003;40:153-162

A. Hereditary osteo-onychodysplasia (HOOD)
B. Fong disease
C. Turner-Kieser syndrome
D. All of the above

Nail-patella syndrome (NPS) (OMIM 161200), also known as hereditary osteo-onychodysplasia (HOOD), Fong disease, Turner-Kieser syndrome, and Österreicher-Turner syndrome, is a pleiotropic condition with a classical clinical tetrad involving the nails, knees, elbows, and the presence of iliac horns.

1729. Which of the following is a clinical feature of Nail-patella syndrome?

Journal of Medical Genetics. 2003;40:153-162

A. Abnormal muscle distribution in upper arms
B. Nails may be absent, hypoplastic, or dystrophic
C. Patellae may be small, irregularly shaped, or absent
D. All of the above

Lean body habitus, poorly developed biceps & triceps muscles with full development of deltoids & forearm muscles are seen in Nail-patella syndrome. The nail changes may be limited to triangular lunules. A sensitive sign of digital involvement in NPS is loss of the creases in the skin overlying the distal interphalangeal (DIP) joints of the fingers.

1730. Which of the following is a clinical feature of Nail-patella syndrome?

Journal of Medical Genetics. 2003;40:153-162

A. Iliac horns
B. High forehead and hairline
C. Irregular thickening of GBM ("moth eaten" appearance)
D. All of the above

Features of Nail-patella syndrome are iliac horns which are bilateral, conical, bony processes that project posteriorly & laterally from central part of iliac bones of the pelvis. Also, irregular thickening of GBM giving it a mottled "moth eaten" appearance is seen. Lester's sign consists of a zone of darker pigmentation around the central part of iris, which is roughly a cloverleaf or flower shaped.

1731. Which of the following is a clinical feature of Nail-patella syndrome?

Journal of Medical Genetics. 2003;40:153-162

A. Cleft lip and palate
B. Deafness
C. Mental retardation
D. None of the above

1732. Which of the following statements about Nail-patella syndrome is false?

N Engl J Med. 2006;354:1387-401, Harrison's 20th Ed. Chapter 308 Page 2147

A. Glomerular basement membrane is thickened with splitting and fibrillar collagen deposits
B. Caused by loss-of-function mutations in *LMX1B*
C. *LMX1B* is expressed in kidney primarily by podocytes
D. None of the above

1733. LMX1B regulates the expression of genes encoding?

Harrison's 20th Ed. Chapter 308 Page 2147

A. $\alpha3$ and $\alpha4$ chains of collagen IV
B. Interstitial type III collagen
C. Podocin
D. All of the above

LMX1B regulates the expression of genes encoding $\alpha3$ and $\alpha4$ chains of collagen IV, interstitial type III collagen, podocin and CD2AP that help form the slit-pore membranes connecting podocytes.

1734. Which of the following may be present in Nail-patella syndrome?

Harrison's 20th Ed. Chapter 308 Page 2148

A. Neural-sensory hearing impairment
B. Glaucoma
C. Iliac horns on the pelvis
D. All of the above

Iliac horns are bilateral, conical, bony processes that project posteriorly and laterally from the central part of the iliac bones of the pelvis and are considered "pathognomonic" of NPS.

1735. Which of the following is a finding in renal biopsy in Nail-patella syndrome?

Harrison's 20th Ed. Chapter 308 Page 2148

A. Focal sclerosing glomerulonephritis
B. Lucent damage to the lamina densa of GBM
C. Increase in collagen III fibrils along glomerular capillaries and in mesangium
D. All of the above

In Nail-patella syndrome, renal biopsy shows focal sclerosing glomerulonephritis with specific lucent damage to lamina densa of the GBM, an increase in collagen III fibrils along glomerular capillaries and in the mesangium, and damage to slit-pore membrane.

1736. What magnitude of glomeruli are normally sclerotic by the age of 60 years?

Harrison's 20th Ed. Chapter 308 Page 2148

A. 10%
B. 20%
C. 30%
D. 40%

~10% of glomeruli are normally sclerotic by age 40, rising to 20% by age 60 and 30% by age 80.

1737. Which of the following is false about apolipoprotein E (ApoE)?
Harrison's 20th Ed. Chapter 308 Page 2148

A. Plasma glycoprotein
B. Helps lipoprotein clearance from circulation
C. Structural protein of chylomicrons, VLDL, IDL, HDL
D. None of the above

Apolipoprotein E (ApoE) is a plasma glycoprotein and helps lipoprotein clearance from circulation. ApoE is a structural protein of chylomicrons, very-low-density lipoproteins, intermediate-density lipoproteins, and high-density lipoproteins, and serves as a ligand for the uptake of ApoE-containing lipoproteins by the hepatic ApoE receptor or low-density lipoprotein (LDL) receptor. ApoE gene polymorphisms are associated with atherosclerosis and play critical roles in lipid metabolism.

1738. Lipoprotein glomerulopathy best relates to?
Harrison's 20th Ed. Chapter 308 Page 2148

A. E2 allele
B. E3 allele
C. E4 allele
D. All of the above

E4 allele is accompanied by increases in serum cholesterol and is more closely associated with atherogenic profiles in patients with renal failure. Mutations in E2 alleles, particularly in Japanese patients, produces lipoprotein glomerulopathy associated with glomerular lipoprotein thrombi & capillary dilation.

1739. Systemic hypertension causes permanent damage to kidneys in what percentage of patients with elevated blood pressure?
Harrison's 20th Ed. Chapter 308 Page 2148

A. ~ 6%
B. ~ 14%
C. ~ 26%
D. ~ 46%

Systemic hypertension causes permanent damage to kidneys in ~6% of patients with elevated BP.

1740. What percentage of patients with end-stage kidney disease have hypertension as a primary cause?
Harrison's 20th Ed. Chapter 308 Page 2148

A. 27%
B. 38%
C. 52%
D. 70%

~27% of patients with end-stage kidney disease (ESRD) have hypertension as a primary cause.

1741. Risk alleles associated with APOL1, a functional gene for apolipoprotein L1, expressed in?
Harrison's 20th Ed. Chapter 308 Page 2148

A. Glomerular basement membrane
B. Tubular basement membrane
C. Podocytes
D. All of the above

Risk alleles associated with APOL1, a functional gene for apolipoprotein L1 expressed in podocytes.

1742. Systemic hypertension associated risk factor for progression to end-stage kidney disease is?
Harrison's 20th Ed. Chapter 308 Page 2148

A. Smoking
B. Low birth weight
C. Preexisting renal injury
D. All of the above

Systemic hypertension associated risk factors for progression to ESRD include increased age, male gender, race, smoking, hypercholesterolemia, duration of hypertension, low birth weight, and preexisting renal injury.

1743. Kidney biopsies in patients with hypertension, microhematuria, and moderate proteinuria show all except?
Harrison's 20th Ed. Chapter 308 Page 2148

A. Arteriolosclerosis
B. Chronic nephrosclerosis
C. Interstitial fibrosis
D. Immune deposits

Kidney biopsies in patients with hypertension, microhematuria, and moderate proteinuria demonstrate arteriolosclerosis, chronic nephrosclerosis, and interstitial fibrosis in the absence of immune deposits.

1744. Hemodynamic stress of malignant hypertension leads to?
Harrison's 20th Ed. Chapter 308 Page 2148

A. Fibrinoid necrosis of small blood vessels
B. Thrombotic microangiography
C. Acute renal failure
D. All of the above

The hemodynamic stress of malignant hypertension leads to fibrinoid necrosis of small blood vessels, thrombotic microangiography, a nephritic urinalysis, and acute renal failure.

1745. In atherosclerosis, cholesterol crystals are showered into the circulation due to?
Harrison's 20th Ed. Chapter 308 Page 2148

A. Spontaneously
B. Endovascular procedure with manipulation of aorta
C. With use of systemic anticoagulation
D. All of the above

1746. Release of cholesterol fragments from atherosclerotic plaques can lead to which of the following?
Harrison's 20th Ed. Chapter 308 Page 2148

A. Cerebral transient ischemic attacks
B. Livedo reticularis in lower extremities
C. Hollenhorst plaques in retina with visual field cuts
D. All of the above

Release of cholesterol fragments from atherosclerotic plaques can lead to cerebral transient ischemic attacks, livedo reticularis in lower extremities, Hollenhorst plaques in retina with visual field cuts, necrosis of toes, acute glomerular capillary injury leading to FSGS and fever, eosinophilia, or eosinophiluria.

1747. Which out of the following is false about sickle cell disease?
Harrison's 20th Ed. Chapter 308 Page 2148

A. Hyposthenuria
B. Infarction of the renal medulla
C. Predisposition to volume depletion
D. None of the above

Individuals with SA-hemoglobin are usually asymptomatic, but most will gradually develop hyposthenuria due to subclinical infarction of renal medulla, thus predisposing them to volume depletion.

1748. In sickle cell disease, vessel occlusion in kidney produces which of the following?
Harrison's 20th Ed. Chapter 308 Page 2148

A. Glomerular hypertension
B. FSGS
C. Interstitial nephritis
D. All of the above

In sickle cell disease, vessel occlusion in kidney produces glomerular hypertension, FSGS, interstitial nephritis, and renal infarction associated with hyposthenuria, microscopic hematuria, and even gross hematuria.

1749. TTP & HUS share features of?
Harrison's 20th Ed. Chapter 308 Page 2148

A. Idiopathic thrombocytopenic purpura
B. Preeclampsia/HELLP
C. Antiphospholipid syndrome
D. All of the above

1750. TTP/HUS is seen with the use of?
Harrison's 20th Ed. Chapter 308 Page 2149

A. Quinine
B. Calcineurin inhibitors
C. Ticlopidine and clopidogrel
D. All of the above

1751. TTP/HUS is seen in?
Harrison's 20th Ed. Chapter 308 Page 2149

A. Pregnancy
B. With the use of oral contraceptives
C. HIV infection
D. All of the above

1752. Shiga toxin best relates to which of the following?
Harrison's 20th Ed. Chapter 308 Page 2149

A. Tetrodotoxin
B. Verotoxin
C. Excitotoxin
D. Crinotoxin

Shiga toxin producing Escherichia coli (STEC) HUS is caused by the Shiga toxins (Stx1 and Stx2), which are also referred to as verotoxin.

1753. Shiga toxin binds to which of the following?
Harrison's 20th Ed. Chapter 308 Page 2149

A. Heparan sulfate–like surface receptors
B. Glycolipid surface receptor globotriaosylceramide (Gb3)
C. Low-density lipoprotein receptor–related proteins (LRPs)
D. vascular endothelial growth factor (VEGF)

Shiga toxin binds to glycolipid surface receptor globotriaosylceramide (Gb3), which is richly expressed on cells of the renal microvasculature.

1754. Shiga toxin inhibits the endothelial production of?
Harrison's 20th Ed. Chapter 308 Page 2149

A. Fibroblast growth factor (FGF)
B. ADAMTS13
C. Vascular endothelial growth factor (VEGF)
D. IL-1α, β

Shiga toxin inhibits the endothelial production of ADAMTS13.

1755. ADAMTS13 best relates to?
Harrison's 20th Ed. Chapter 308 Page 2149

A. Epidermal growth factor
B. Transcription factors STAT3 and STAT6
C. von Willebrand's factor
D. Factor H

ADAMTS13 metalloprotease cleaves large multimers of von Willebrand's factor. In the absence of ADAMTS13, large multimers cause platelet clumping and intravascular hemolysis.

1756. Atypical HUS (aHUS) best relates to?
Harrison's 20th Ed. Chapter 308 Page 2149

A. Shiga toxin (verotoxin)
B. Thrombospondin receptor
C. Complement protein deficiencies
D. Plasminogen-activator inhibitor 1 (PAI-1)

Atypical HUS or complement mediated HUS is the result of complement dysregulation which may be congenital or acquired. Affected patients have low C3 and normal C4 levels, characteristic of alternative pathway activation. Factor H deficiency is the most common defect.

1757. Adult TTP/HUS with ADAMTS13 antibodies is treated with?
Harrison's 20th Ed. Chapter 308 Page 2149

A. Rituximab
B. Steroids
C. Plasmapheresis
D. Splenectomy

Treatment of adult TTP/HUS with ADAMTS13 antibodies is daily plasmapheresis with fresh frozen plasma.

1758. The lesion in HIV-associated nephropathy (HIVAN) is resembles that of?
Harrison's 20th Ed. Chapter 308 Page 2149

A. Minimal change disease
B. Focal segmental glomerulosclerosis (FSGS)
C. Membranous glomerulonephritis
D. Renal amyloidosis

The lesion in HIVAN is FSGS, with characteristic collapsing glomerulopathy. There occurs visceral epithelial cell swelling, microcystic dilatation of renal tubules, and tubuloreticular inclusion. Tubular microcysts and interstitial inflammation distinguish it from idiopathic FSGS.

1759. HIVAN develops almost exclusively in patients of black race origin who have which of the following variant?
Harrison's 20th Ed. Chapter 308 Page 2149

A. PKHD1
B. APOL1
C. UMOD
D. IL28B

1760. Which of the following about HIV-associated nephropathy (HIVAN) is false?
Harrison's 20th Ed. Chapter 308 Page 2149

A. Significant proteinuria and rapidly progressive kidney disease
B. Normal blood pressure
C. Normal to enlarged kidneys
D. None of the above

HIVAN usually presents in patients with advanced HIV disease, with low CD4 count and detectable viral load. HIVAN occurs almost exclusively in patients who are of African descent.

1761. Which of the following is not present in nephrotic syndrome associated with HIV infection?
Harrison's 20th Ed. Chapter 308 Page 2149

A. Hypertension
B. Edema
C. Hyperlipidemia
D. All of the above

1762. Which of the following about HIV immune complex kidney disease (HIVICK) is false?

Harrison's 20th Ed. Chapter 308 Page 2149

A. Complication of active HIV viremia
B. Glomerular lesions
C. ART was not associated with improved renal outcomes
D. None of the above

HIVICK, HIV immune complex kidney disease is a group of immune complex-mediated glomerular lesions seen in HIV patients, and on biopsy can look like other glomerular lesions including postinfectious glomerulonephritis, MGN, MPGN, DPGN, MCD, and IgA nephropathy. The HIVICK effect is a complication of active HIV viremia.

1763. After what duration does HIV-associated nephropathy begin?

Harrison's 20th Ed. Chapter 308 Page 2149

A. ~ 3 months
B. ~ 6 months
C. ~ 1 year
D ~ 2.5 years

HIV-associated nephropathy begins ~ 2.5 years after HIV infection.

1764. HIV infection is most commonly associated with which of the following glomerulopathies?

Harrison's 20th Ed. Chapter 308 Page 2149

A. Aggressive focal segmental glomerulosclerosis
B. Acute diffuse proliferative glomerulonephritis
C. IgA nephropathy
D. Membranous glomerulopathy

1765. Term HIV-associated nephropathy (HIVAN) is used for?

Harrison's 20th Ed. Chapter 308 Page 2149

A. Aggressive focal segmental glomerulosclerosis
B. Acute diffuse proliferative glomerulonephritis
C. IgA nephropathy
D. Membranous glomerulopathy

1766. Which of the following is false for HIV-associated nephropathy (HIVAN)?

Harrison's 20th Ed. Chapter 308 Page 2149

A. May be the first manifestation of HIV infection
B. More common in blacks
C. More frequent in intravenous drug abusers
D. Slow clinical course

1767. HIV patients with FSGS present with nephrotic-range proteinuria & hypoalbuminemia but without?

Harrison's 20th Ed. Chapter 308 Page 2149

A. Hypertension
B. Edema
C. Hyperlipidemia
D. All of the above

HIV patients with FSGS typically present with nephrotic-range proteinuria and hypoalbuminemia, but without hypertension, edema, or hyperlipidemia.

1768. There is a close association between hepatitis B infection and?

Harrison's 20th Ed. Chapter 308 Page 2149

A. Renal amyloidosis
B. Lymphoma
C. Polyarteritis nodosa with vasculitis
D. Parvovirus infection

There is a close association between hepatitis B infection and polyarteritis nodosa with vasculitis appearing generally in the first 6 months following infection.

1769. Renal manifestations of hepatitis B infection include?

Harrison's 20th Ed. Chapter 308 Page 2149

A. Renal artery aneurysms
B. Renal infarction
C. Renal ischemic scars
D. All of the above

Renal manifestations of hepatitis B infection include renal artery aneurysms, renal infarction & renal ischemic scars.

1770. Glomerular lesion associated with HBV infection include?

Harrison's 20th Ed. Chapter 308 Page 2149

A. Membranous glomerulonephritis (MGN)
B. Membrane proliferative glomerulonephritis (MPGN)
C. Cryoglobulinemic glomerulonephritis
D. All of the above

1771. Which out of the following viral antigen is most commonly found in the renal deposits in HBV infection?

Harrison's 20th Ed. Chapter 308 Page 2149

A. HBsAG
B. HBeAG
C. HBcAG
D. All of the above

HBeAG viral antigen is most commonly found in the renal deposits in HBV infection.

1772. What proportion of children with HBV infection achieve spontaneous remission within 4 years?

Harrison's 20th Ed. Chapter 308 Page 2149

A. 40–45%
B. 50–55%
C. 60–65%
D. 70–75%

60 - 65% of children with HBV infection achieve spontaneous remission within 4 years.

1773. Renal lesion most commonly seen in chronic hepatitis C infection is?

Harrison's 20th Ed. Chapter 308 Page 2149

A. Cryoglobulinemic glomerulonephritis
B. Membranous glomerulonephritis (MGN)
C. Type I Membrane proliferative glomerulonephritis (MPGN)
D. IgA nephropathy

Renal lesions most commonly seen in chronic hepatitis C infection, in order of decreasing frequency, are cryoglobulinemic glomerulonephritis, MGN, and type I MPGN.

1774. HCV-induced immune-complex disease is associated with which of the following?

Harrison's 20th Ed. Chapter 308 Page 2149

A. Cryoglobulinemic glomerulonephritis
B. MPGN
C. Membranous glomerulopathy
D. All of the above

The renal lesions most commonly seen in chronic hepatitis C infection in order of decreasing frequency are cryoglobulinemic glomerulonephritis, MGN and type I MPGN.

1775. Dengue hemorrhagic fever causes?

Harrison's 20th Ed. Chapter 308 Page 2150

A. Anti-GBM disease
B. Mesangioproliferative glomerulonephritis
C. Endocapillary proliferative glomerulonephritis
D. Focal glomerulornephritis

Like measles, dengue hemorrhagic fever causes endocapillary proliferative glomerulonephritis.

1776. Leprosy is classified by which of the following criteria?

Harrison's 20th Ed. Chapter 308 Page 2150

A. Manning criteria
B. Bethesda criteria
C. Ridley Jopling criteria
D. Rome criteria

Leprosy is classified by Ridley Jopling criteria into tuberculoid, borderline tuberculoid, mid-borderline and borderline lepromatous and lepromatous.

1777. Renal involvement is more severe in infection with?

Harrison's 20th Ed. Chapter 308 Page 2150

A. Plasmodium falciparum
B. Plasmodium malariae
C. Plasmodium vivax
D. Plasmodium ovale

In quartan malaria from infection with Plasmodium malariae, children are more commonly affected and renal involvement is more severe.

1778. Which of the following cells of kidney do not proliferate?

Harrison's 16th Ed. 1678

A. Mesangial cells
B. Endothelial cells
C. Visceral epithelial cells
D. All of the above

1779. 'Crescents' are composed of?

A. Infiltrating monocytes
B. Proliferating parietal epithelial cells
C. Fibrin
D. All of the above

1780. Intrarenal vasoconstrictors include all except?

Am Fam Physician. 2012;86(7):631-639

A. Leukotrienes
B. Nitric oxide
C. Thromboxanes
D. Platelet-activating factor

1781. Intrarenal vasoconstrictors include all except?

Am Fam Physician. 2012;86(7):631-639

A. Endothelins
B. Prostacyclin
C. Adenosine
D. Angiotensin II

Intrarenal vasoconstrictors include Angiotensin II, Endothelin, Thromboxane, Adenosine, Leukotrienes, Platelet-activating factor. Intrarenal vasodilators are endothelium derived nitric oxide (EDNO), bradykinin and prostaglandin I2 (PGI2).

1782. Which of the following is true for Henoch Schonlein purpura?

A. Normal complement levels
B. Negative anti-GBM serology
C. Negative ANCA serology
D. All of the above

1783. Which of the following glomerulopathies is most commonly associated with Hodgkin's lymphoma?

A. FSGS
B. MCD
C. MPGN
D. Membranous glomerulopathy

Polycystic Kidney Disease and Other Inherited Disorders of Tubule Growth and Development

1784. Ciliary dysfunction in ciliopathies manifest as?
Pediatr Nephrol. 2011;26:1039-1056

A. Retinal degeneration
B. Renal disease
C. Cerebral anomalies
D. All of the above

Ciliopathies comprise a group of disorders associated with genetic mutations encoding defective proteins, which result in abnormal formation or function of cilia. As cilia are a component of almost all cells, ciliary dysfunction can manifest as a constellation of features that include primarily retinal degeneration, renal disease and cerebral anomalies.

1785. Which of the following is a renal ciliopathic syndrome?
Pediatr Nephrol. 2011;26:1039-1056

A. Polycystic kidney disease (PKD)
B. Renal medullary cystic disease
C. Cystic renal dysplasia
D. All of the above

1786. Characteristic clinical features of a "Ciliopathy" includes all except?
Pediatr Nephrol. 2011;26:1039-1056

A. Renal disease
B. Retinal disease
C. Cerebral malformations
D. Ectopic thyroid

1787. Ciliopathic syndromes include all except?
Pediatr Nephrol. 2011;26:1039-1056

A. Joubert syndrome
B. Bardet–Biedl syndrome
C. Orofaciodigital syndrome
D. Atypical hemolytic uremic syndrome

1788. Retinitis pigmentosa is a feature of which of the following inherited diseases associated with a cystic phenotype?
Harrison's 20th Ed. Chapter 309 Page 2151 Table 309-1

A. Bardet-Biedl syndrome
B. Sensenbrenner syndrome
C. Leber congenital amaurosis
D. All of the above

1789. Gout is a feature of which of the following inherited diseases associated with a cystic phenotype?
Harrison's 20th Ed. Chapter 309 Page 2151 Table 309-1

A. Autosomal dominant polycystic kidney disease
B. Medullary cystic kidney
C. Nephronophthisis
D. Tuberous sclerosis

1790. Polydactyly is a feature of which of the following inherited diseases associated with a cystic phenotype?
Harrison's 20th Ed. Chapter 309 Page 2151 Table 309-1

A. Sensenbrenner syndrome
B. Bardet-Biedl syndrome
C. Meckel-Gruber syndrome
D. All of the above

1791. Pheochromocytoma is a feature of which of the following inherited diseases associated with a cystic phenotype?
Harrison's 20th Ed. Chapter 309 Page 2151 Table 309-1

A. Tuberous sclerosis
B. Nephronophthisis
C. Von Hippel-Lindau disease
D. Medullary cystic kidney

1792. Liver fibrosis is a feature of which of the following inherited diseases associated with a cystic phenotype?
Harrison's 20th Ed. Chapter 309 Page 2151 Table 309-1

A. Autosomal recessive polycystic kidney disease
B. Medullary cystic kidney
C. Nephronophthisis
D. Tuberous sclerosis

1793. Renal cell carcinoma is a feature of which of the following inherited diseases associated with a cystic phenotype?
Harrison's 20th Ed. Chapter 309 Page 2151 Table 309-1

A. Autosomal recessive polycystic kidney disease
B. Medullary cystic kidney
C. Nephronophthisis
D. Tuberous sclerosis

1794. Obesity is a feature of which of the following inherited diseases associated with a cystic phenotype?
Harrison's 20th Ed. Chapter 309 Page 2151 Table 309-1

A. Bardet-Biedl syndrome
B. Sensenbrenner syndrome
C. Senior-Loken syndrome
D. Von Hippel-Lindau disease

1795. UMOD gene is associated with which of the following inherited diseases associated with a cystic phenotype?
Harrison's 20th Ed. Chapter 309 Page 2151 Table 309-1

A. Autosomal recessive polycystic kidney disease
B. Medullary cystic kidney
C. Nephronophthisis
D. Tuberous sclerosis

1796. Which of the following gene is associated with autosomal recessive polycystic kidney disease?
Harrison's 20th Ed. Chapter 309 Page 2151 Table 309-1

A. PKD1
B. PKD2
C. PKHD1
D. NPHP1-20

1797. Which of the following gene is associated with tuberous sclerosis?

Harrison's 20th Ed. Chapter 309 Page 2151 Table 309-1

A. TCTN2
B. TSC1
C. TMEM67
D. All of the above

1798. Which of the following is a monogenic disorder?

Harrison's 20th Ed. Chapter 309 Page 2150

A. Autosomal dominant polycystic kidney disease (ADPKD)
B. Glucocorticoid-remediable primary hyperaldosteronism
C. Cystic fibrosis (CF)
D. All of the above

Monogenic disorders include primary hyperoxaluria, cystinuria, monogenic forms of DM, mutations of the amyloid precursor protein in familial Alzheimer's disease, the microtubule-associated protein tau (MAPT) in frontotemporal dementia, α-synuclein in Parkinson's disease, cerebral autosomal recessive arteriopathy with subcortical infarcts and leukoencephalopathy (CARASIL), hereditary endotheliopathy, retinopathy, nephropathy and stroke (HERNS), Glucocorticoid-remediable primary hyperaldosteronism, cystic fibrosis (CF), autosomal dominant polycystic kidney disease (ADPKD).

1799. Which of the following statements is false about polycystic kidney disease?

Harrison's 20th Ed. Chapter 309 Page 2150

A. ADPKD is seen predominantly in childhood
B. ARPKD is mainly a disease of adults
C. They infrequently cause kidney failure
D. All of the above

Autosomal dominant polycystic kidney disease (ADPKD) is seen predominantly in adults, whereas autosomal recessive polycystic kidney disease (ARPKD) is mainly a disease of childhood. They frequently causes kidney failure.

1800. What percentage of total nephrons are involved in ADPKD?

Harrison's 20th Ed. Chapter 309 Page 2150

A. < 1%
B. < 2%
C. < 3%
D. < 5%

In ADPKD, <5% of total nephrons (tubules) are involved.

1801. The cellular defect in ADPKD is?

Harrison's 20th Ed. Chapter 309 Page 2150

A. Increased cell proliferation and fluid secretion
B. Decreased cell differentiation
C. Abnormal extracellular matrix
D. All of the above

The cellular defects in ADPKD are increased cell proliferation and fluid secretion, decreased cell differentiation, and abnormal extracellular matrix.

1802. Which of the following is a PKD-1 encoded protein?

Harrison's 20th Ed. Chapter 309 Page 2150

A. Fibrocystin
B. Polycystin-1
C. Caveolin 3
D. FMR-1 protein

ADPKD results from mutations in either PKD-1 (85% of cases) or PKD-2 gene. PKD-1 encodes polycystin-1 (PC1), whereas PKD-2 gene product is polycystin-2 (PC2).

1803. Which of the following statements about 'Autosomal dominant polycystic kidney disease is false?

Harrison's 20th Ed. Chapter 309 Page 2150

A. PC1 is a large 11-transmembrane protein that functions like a G-protein coupled receptor
B. PC2 is a Ca^{++}-permeable 6 transmembrane protein that belongs to transient receptor potential (TRP) cation channel family
C. PKD1 is called 1st disease gene & PKD2 2nd disease gene
D. PKD1 is on chromosome 16 and PKD2 is on chromosome 6

The first disease gene (PKD1) is localized to the region of the alpha-globin gene on chromosome 16p13, and a second disease gene (PKD2) locus is mapped to chromosome 4q21-q23.

1804. Which of the following statements about polycystin-1 (PC1) is false?

Harrison's 20th Ed. Chapter 309 Page 2150

A. Large 11-transmembrane protein that functions like a GPCR
B. Widely expressed in almost all tissues and organs
C. Expression is high in development and low in the adult
D. None of the above

1805. Which of the following statements about polycystin-2 (PC2) is false?

Harrison's 20th Ed. Chapter 309 Page 2150

A. Ca^{++}-permeable 6 transmembrane protein of transient receptor potential (TRP) cation channel family
B. Widely expressed in almost all tissues and organs
C. Expression is relatively constant
D. None of the above

1806. Which of the following statements about PC1/2 is false?

Harrison's 20th Ed. Chapter 309 Page 2151

A. Found on the primary cilium
B. PC1 & PC2 bind together to form receptor-channel complex
C. Defect causes ciliopathies
D. None of the above

1807. Which of the following statements about primary cilia is false?

Harrison's 20th Ed. Chapter 309 Page 2152 Figure 309-1

A. "9+0" organization of microtubule doublets
B. Proteins are transported into cilium by motor protein kinesin 2
C. Proteins are transported out of the cilium by dynein
D. None of the above

Primary cilia differ from motile cilia (9+2 cilia) in their lack of central microtubule doublet, so they are described as having a "9+0" arrangement. 9+0 cilia are immotile and do not beat. Ciliary axoneme (shaft) is only 0.25 μm in diameter but its length can be up to 2 mm. The basal body is a cylindrical structure measuring 0.4 by 0.2 μm positioned perpendicular to the cell membrane, anchoring cilium in the cytoplasm. It also acts as the nucleation point from which the cilium extends out from the cell. The basal body consists of nine triplets of microtubules arranged in a ring from which extend three microtubules: A, B, and C. All three fibres project from the basal body into the proximal region of the cilium known as the transition zone. This is the region from which a nascent cilium grows. Further along the cilium is the middle zone composed of nine doublets consisting of just A and B filaments. The axoneme terminates with the distal zone, comprised primarily of microtubule singlets.

1808. Which of the following statements about PC1/2 protein complex is false?

Harrison's 20th Ed. Chapter 309 Page 2151

A. Serves as a mechanosensor or chemical sensor
B. Regulates calcium and G protein signaling
C. Regulate cellular functions & signaling pathways
D. None of the above

PC1/2 protein complex serves as a mechanosensor or chemical sensor and regulates calcium and G protein signaling.

1809. Which of the following cellular functions is regulated by PC1/2 protein complex?

Harrison's 20th Ed. Chapter 309 Page 2151

A. Cell cycle
B. Actin cytoskeleton
C. Planar cell polarity (PCP)
D. All of the above

PC1/2 protein complex also directly regulates cellular functions including the cell cycle, the actin cytoskeleton, planar cell polarity (PCP), and cell migration.

1810. Which of the following signaling pathways is regulated by PC1/2 protein complex?

Harrison's 20th Ed. Chapter 309 Page 2151

A. Wnt
B. Mammalian target of rapamycin (mTOR)
C. STAT3
D. All of the above

1811. Which of the following signaling pathways is regulated by PC1/2 protein complex?

Harrison's 20th Ed. Chapter 309 Page 2151

A. cMET
B. Phosphoinositide 3-kinase (PI3K/Akt)
C. G protein–coupled receptor (GPCR)
D. All of the above

PC1/2 protein complex has also been implicated in regulating a number of signaling pathways, including Wnt, mammalian target of rapamycin (mTOR), STAT3, cMET, phosphoinositide 3-kinase (PI3K/Akt), G protein–coupled receptor (GPCR), and epidermal growth factor receptor (EGFR), as well as in the localization and activity of cystic fibrosis transmembrane conductance regulator (CFTR).

1812. Loss of ciliary function of PC1 and PC2 in ADPKD kidneys leads to?

Harrison's 20th Ed. Chapter 309 Page 2151

A. Aberrant calcium signaling
B. Cyst growth by promoting proliferation
C. Fluid secretion of cyst-lining cells through Cl^- & AQP channels
D. All of the above

Loss of ciliary function of PC1 and PC2 in ADPKD kidneys leads to aberrant Ca^{++} signaling and consequent increase of adenylyl cyclase activity & decrease of phosphodiesterase activity, which, in turn, causes increased cellular cAMP. Increased cAMP promotes protein kinase A activity, and, in turn, leads to cyst growth by promoting proliferation and fluid secretion of cyst-lining cells through chloride & aquaporin channels.

1813. Which of the following statements about autosomal dominant polycystic kidney disease (ADPKD) is false?

Harrison's 20th Ed. Chapter 309 Page 2151

A. Inherited as an autosomal dominant trait
B. Complete penetrance
C. Variable expressivity
D. None of the above

ADPKD is inherited as an autosomal dominant trait with complete penetrance, but variable expressivity.

1814. Which of the following gene causes autosomal dominant polycystic kidney disease (ADPKD)?

Harrison's 20th Ed. Chapter 309 Page 2151

A. IFT80
B. GANAB
C. REN
D. MKS1

A third gene GANAB, encoding glucosidase IIa subunit, can cause ADPKD through mutations. All have polycystic liver disease also, and their kidney disease is milder than that in classic ADPKD.

1815. Which of the following statements about 'autosomal dominant polycystic kidney disease (ADPKD)' is false?

Harrison's 20th Ed. Chapter 309 Page 2150

A. ADPKD-1 gene is on chromosome 16p13.3
B. ADPKD-2 gene is on chromosome 4q21-23
C. Cysts are distributed throughout cortex & medulla
D. Erythropoietin production is low

1816. In ADPKD, cyst formation begins?

Harrison's 20th Ed. Chapter 309 Page 2152

A. In utero
B. In early childhood
C. In adolescence
D. In adulthood

In ADPKD, cyst formation begins in utero. It is the most common, life-threatening single-gene disease in adults.

1817. Extrarenal manifestation of ADPKD is?

Harrison's 20th Ed. Chapter 309 Page 2152

A. Intracranial aneurysm
B. Cardiac valvular abnormalities
C. Colonic diverticulae
D. All of the above

Intracranial aneurysm, cardiac valvular abnormalities (MVPS, AR), hepatic cysts, colonic diverticulae, inguinal hernias occur with a higher frequency than in the general population in ADPKD.

1818. Which of the following is the most common extrarenal complication in ADPKD?

Harrison's 20th Ed. Chapter 309 Page 2152

A. Intracranial aneurysm
B. Colonic diverticulae
C. Liver cysts
D. Abdominal wall hernias

Liver cysts derived from the biliary epithelia are the most common extrarenal complication.

1819. Autosomal dominant polycystic liver disease (ADPLD) is caused by mutations in?

Harrison's 20th Ed. Chapter 309 Page 2152

A. CRTAP
B. FKBP10
C. PRKCSH
D. IFITM5

Polycystic liver disease associated with ADPKD is different from autosomal dominant polycystic liver disease (ADPLD) which is caused by mutations in PRKCSH & SEC63 genes, and does not progress to renal failure. Massive polycystic liver disease occurs almost exclusively in women with ADPKD, particularly those with multiple pregnancies.

1820. Which of the following statements about 'Autosomal dominant polycystic kidney disease (ADPKD)' is false?

Harrison's 20th Ed. Chapter 309 Page 2153

A. Standard diagnostic criteria is at least 3 to 5 cysts in each kidney
B. Cysts may be found in brain, thyroid
C. Mitral valve prolapse found in 30% of patients
D. Intracranial aneurysms are 4–5 times more frequent

1821. In ADPKD, cysts can also develop in?

Harrison's 20th Ed. Chapter 309 Page 2153

A. Liver
B. Pancreas
C. Arachnoid membranes
D. All of the above

Cysts can also develop in liver, pancreas, spleen, arachnoid membranes & seminal vesicles in men.

1822. Vascular abnormalities in ADPKD patients include?

Harrison's 20th Ed. Chapter 309 Page 2153

A. Diffuse arterial dolichoectasias of anterior & posterior cerebral circulation
B. Left ventricular hypertrophy (LVH)
C. Stroke
D. All of the above

Vascular abnormalities in ADPKD patients include diffuse arterial dolichoectasias of the anterior & posterior cerebral circulation, which can predispose to arterial dissection and stroke.

1823. Which of the following valvular abnormalities is seen in ADPKD patients?

Harrison's 20th Ed. Chapter 309 Page 2153

A. Mitral valve prolapse
B. Tricuspid valve prolapse
C. Aortic insufficiency
D. All of the above

Mitral valve prolapse occurs in ~30% of patients with ADPKD, tricuspid valve prolapse is less common. Other valvular abnormalities include insufficiency of mitral, aortic, and tricuspid valves.

1824. Which of the following abnormalities is seen in ADPKD?

Harrison's 20th Ed. Chapter 309 Page 2153

A. Colonic diverticulae
B. Abdominal wall hernias
C. Stroke
D. All of the above

The prevalence of colonic diverticulae & abdominal wall hernias are increased in ADPKD patients.

1825. Diagnostic criteria for ADPKD in young include?

Harrison's 20th Ed. Chapter 309 Page 2153

A. ≥ 2
B. ≥ 3
C. ≥ 4
D. ≥ 5

1826. Diagnostic criteria for ADPKD in > 60 year old include?

Harrison's 20th Ed. Chapter 309 Page 2153

A. ≥ 1
B. ≥ 2
C. ≥ 3
D. ≥ 4

Diagnostic criteria for ADPKD require two or more cysts in kidney (unilateral or bilateral) in young subjects (15 and 29 years), but four or more in subjects older than 60 years. Presence of at least two cysts in each kidney is required for the diagnosis among at-risk subjects aged 30–59 years.

1827. Which of the following clinical trials is related to control of hypertension in ADPKD?

Harrison's 20th Ed. Chapter 309 Page 2153

A. STOP-PKD
B. HALT-PKD
C. CONTROL-PKD
D. SLOW-PKD

The HALT-PKD trial was a prospective randomized study to test whether dual blockade of RAAS using ACEI and ARB combination therapy delay normal progression of kidney disease compared to ACEI monotherapy. Results showed that in the early stages of ADPKD, dual inhibition of RAAS did not significantly decrease the rate of total kidney volume growth.

1828. What level of BP is recommended by JNC VIII for reducing CV complications in ADPKD & renal disease progression?

Harrison's 20th Ed. Chapter 309 Page 2153

A. 110/70 mm Hg
B. 120/80 mm Hg
C. 140/80 mm Hg
D. 140/90 mm Hg

Blood pressure control to a target of 140/90 mm Hg is recommended according to the guidelines from the eighth report of the Joint National Committee on Prevention, Detection, Evaluation, and Treatment of High Blood Pressure (JNC VIII) for reducing cardiovascular complications in ADPKD and renal disease progression. More rigorous blood pressure control does not equal greater clinical benefits.

1829. Which of the following antibiotics is not preferred for cyst infection in ADPKD?

Harrison's 20th Ed. Chapter 309 Page 2153

A. Cephalosporins
B. Trimethoprim-sulfamethoxazole
C. Quinolones
D. Chloramphenicol

Lipid-soluble antibiotics against common gram-negative enteric organisms such as trimethoprim-sulfamethoxazole, quinolones and chloramphenicol are preferred for cyst infection because most renal cysts are not connected to glomerular filtration and antibiotics that are capable of penetrating the cyst walls are likely to be more effective. Treatment often requires 4–6 weeks.

1830. Which of the following drugs are useful in ADPKD?

Harrison's 20th Ed. Chapter 309 Page 2154

A. Sirolimus
B. Tolvaptan
C. Octreotide
D. All of the above

1831. Autosomal recessive polycystic kidney disease (ARPKD) gene is called?

Harrison's 20th Ed. Chapter 309 Page 2154

A. ARPKD-1
B. ARPKD-2
C. PKHD1
D. PKHD2

ARPKD gene, on chromosome 6p21.1-6p12.2, is called PKHD1 (polycystic kidney & hepatic disease 1) gene. Mutations in PKHD1 cause all the clinical presentations of ARPKD.

1832. Protein expressed by PKHD1 is termed?

Harrison's 20th Ed. Chapter 309 Page 2154

A. Nephrocystin
B. Inversin
C. Fibrocystin/polyductin (FPC)
D. Polycystin-3

Protein expressed by PKHD1 is termed fibrocystin/polyductin (FPC).

1833. Fibrocystin/polyductin (FPC) is localized on the primary cilia of epithelia cells of?

Harrison's 20th Ed. Chapter 309 Page 2154

A. Cortical collecting ducts
B. Medullary collecting ducts
C. Cholangiocytes of bile ducts
D. All of the above

Single transmembrane FPC is localized on the primary cilia of epithelia cells of cortical & medullary collecting ducts and cholangiocytes of bile ducts. FPC is also expressed on the basal body and plasma membrane.

1834. Which of the following relate to classic ARPKD?

Harrison's 20th Ed. Chapter 309 Page 2154

A. Oligohydraminos
B. Pulmonary hypoplasia
C. Biliary dysgenesis
D. All of the above

In classic ARPKD, reduced fetal urine production contributes to oligohydraminos and pulmonary hypoplasia. Biliary dysgenesis due to a primary ductal plate malformation with associated periportal fibrosis occurs (congenital hepatic fibrosis).

1835. Which of the following statements about 'autosomal recessive polycystic kidney disease (ARPKD)' is false?

Harrison's 20th Ed. Chapter 309 Page 2154

A. Distal tubules & collecting ducts are dilated
B. Portal hypertension & esophageal varices are frequent
C. Unilateral abdominal mass is common
D. Death in neonates is due to pulmonary hypoplasia

Enlarged kidneys are detected soon after birth as bilateral abdominal masses.

1836. Caroli's disease best relates to?

Harrison's 20th Ed. Chapter 309 Page 2154

A. Dilatation of intrahepatic bile ducts
B. Biliary dysgenesis
C. Liver cysts
D. All of the above

Caroli's disease refers to dilatation of intrahepatic bile ducts & may need porto-systemic shunting.

1837. The hallmark of ARPKD liver disease is?

Harrison's 20th Ed. Chapter 309 Page 2154

A. Liver cysts
B. Biliary dysgenesis
C. Cholangiocarcinoma
D. Hepatic steatosis

The hallmarks of ARPKD liver disease are biliary dysgenesis due to a primary ductal plate malformation with associated periportal fibrosis—congenital hepatic fibrosis (CHF) and dilatation of intrahepatic bile ducts (Caroli's disease).

1838. The slow progression of renal disease in ARPKD is due to?

Harrison's 20th Ed. Chapter 309 Page 2154

A. Increasing fibrosis
B. Development of cysts
C. Systemic hypertension
D. All of the above

The slow progression of renal disease in ARPKD is due to increasing fibrosis rather than development of cysts. Systemic hypertension is common in all ARPKD patients, even those with normal renal function.

1839. Which of the following about ultrasonography in ARPKD is false?

Harrison's 20th Ed. Chapter 309 Page 2154

A. Large, echogenic kidneys
B. Poor corticomedullary differentiation
C. Diagnosis can be made in utero >24 weeks of gestation
D. None of the above

USG in ARPKD reveals large, echogenic kidneys with poor corticomedullary differentiation. The diagnosis can be made in utero after 24 weeks of gestation in severe cases.

1840. Which of the following about Tuberous sclerosis (TS) is false?

Harrison's 20th Ed. Chapter 309 Page 2154

A. Autosomal recessive
B. Caused by mutations in TSC1 encoding hamartin
C. Caused by mutations in TSC2 encoding tuberin
D. Kidney cysts are frequent

Tuberous sclerosis (TS) is a rare autosomal dominant syndrome caused by mutations in one of two genes, TSC1 encoding hamartin or TSC2 encoding tuberin.

1841. Essentially all TS patients have associated?

Harrison's 20th Ed. Chapter 309 Page 2154

A. Skin lesions
B. Neurologic lesions
C. Cardiac lesions
D. Renal lesions

TS is a syndrome affecting multiple organ systems that includes benign growths in nervous system, eyes, heart, lung, liver, and skin. Essentially all TS patients have such skin lesions, and a large proportion of patients have neurologic and cognitive manifestations.

1842. Abnormalities of kidney in tuberous sclerosis (TS) include?

Harrison's 20th Ed. Chapter 309 Page 2154

A. Renal cysts
B. Renal angiomyolipomas
C. Renal cell carcinoma
D. All of the above

Renal TS occurs as renal cysts, renal angiomyolipomas & renal cell carcinoma.

1843. The TSC2 gene is adjacent to which of the following genes in the human genome?

Harrison's 20th Ed. Chapter 309 Page 2154

A. PKD1
B. PKD2
C. PKHD1
D. All of the above

The TSC2 gene is adjacent to PKD1 in the human genome. Inactivation of these two genes may have manifestations of both ADPKD and TS.

1844. The most common kidney finding in TS is the presence of?
Harrison's 20th Ed. Chapter 309 Page 2154

A. Angiomyolipomas
B. Renal cell carcinoma
C. Renal cyst
D. Nephrolithiasis

The most common kidney finding in TS is the presence of angiomyolipomas. Multiple, bilateral and benign, surgical removal is recommended for angiomyolipomas larger than 4 cm in diameter. In contrast to ADPKD, there is a clearly increased risk of renal cell carcinoma in TS patients.

1845. Which of the following about TS is false?
Harrison's 20th Ed. Chapter 309 Page 2155

A. May lead to significant CKD & progress to ESRD
B. Unremarkable urine sediment
C. Minimal to mild proteinuria
D. None of the above

1846. Which of the following about cysts in TS is false?
Harrison's 20th Ed. Chapter 309 Page 2155

A. Radiographically similar to those seen in ADPKD
B. Pose an increased risk of renal cell carcinoma
C. Rarely become large and hemorrhagic
D. None of the above

1847. Tuberin & hamartin protein complex is localized to?
Harrison's 20th Ed. Chapter 309 Page 2155

A. Base of the cilia
B. Transition zone of cilia
C. Ciliary membrane
D. Nucleus

1848. Tuberin & hamartin protein complex is best related to?
Harrison's 20th Ed. Chapter 309 Page 2155

A. Wnt
B. Mammalian target of rapamycin (mTOR)
C. STAT3
D. G protein–coupled receptor (GPCR)

TSC1 & TSC2 gene products tuberin & hamartin interact physically. This protein complex is localized to the base of the cilia and inhibits intracellular signaling processes mediated by mTOR (mammalian target of rapamycin), leading to abnormal growth in tissues.

1849. Which of the following is false about Von Hippel-Lindau disease (VHL)?
Harrison's 20th Ed. Chapter 309 Page 2155

A. Inherited cancer syndrome
B. Autosomal dominant
C. Caused by mutations in VHL tumor-suppressor gene
D. None of the above

Von Hippel-Lindau disease (VHL) is an inherited cancer syndrome with renal manifestations. VHL is an autosomal dominant condition caused by mutations in the VHL tumor-suppressor gene. VHL is localized to the primary cilia and is necessary for the formation of primary cilia.

1850. Which of the following is a manifestation of VHL?
Harrison's 20th Ed. Chapter 309 Page 2155

A. Multiple bilateral kidney cysts
B. Renal cell carcinoma
C. Pheochromocytoma
D. All of the above

1851. Which of the following is a manifestation of VHL?
Harrison's 20th Ed. Chapter 309 Page 2155

A. Cerebellar hemangioblastomas
B. Retinal hemangiomas
C. Pheochromocytoma
D. All of the above

Kidney manifestations of VHL include multiple bilateral kidney cysts & renal cell carcinomas. Kidney cysts & carcinoma affect the majority of VHL patients. Nonrenal features of VHL include pheochromocytoma, cerebellar hemangioblastomas and retinal hemangiomas.

1852. Large renal cysts are seen in?
Harrison's 20th Ed. Chapter 309 Page 2155

A. Von Hippel-Lindau disease (VHL)
B. Tuberous sclerosis (TS)
C. Autosomal dominant polycystic kidney disease (ADPKD)
D. All of the above

1853. Medullary Cystic Kidney Disease Type I is due to mutation in?
Harrison's 20th Ed. Chapter 309 Page 2155

A. MUC1
B. UMOD
C. REN
D. KIF3A

Patients with Medullary Cystic Kidney Disease Type I (MCKD I) have mutations in the mucin 1 gene (MUC1).

1854. UMOD mutations cause which of the following diseases?
Harrison's 20th Ed. Chapter 309 Page 2155

A. Medullary Cystic Kidney Disease Type II
B. Familial juvenile hyperuricemic nephropathy (HNFJ1)
C. Glomerulocystic kidney disease (GCKD)
D. All of the above

UMOD mutations cause Medullary Cystic Kidney Disease Type II, familial juvenile hyperuricemic nephropathy (HNFJ1) and glomerulocystic kidney disease (GCKD).

1855. Uromodulin is also known as?
Harrison's 20th Ed. Chapter 309 Page 2155

A. Hop protein
B. Bence-Jones protein
C. Tamm-Horsfall protein
D. R-binder protein

UMOD gene encodes protein uromodulin which is also known as Tamm-Horsfall protein.

1856. Uromodulin is found on?
Harrison's 20th Ed. Chapter 309 Page 2155

A. Centrosome
B. Mitotic spindle
C. Primary cilia
D. All of the above

Uromodulin is found on centrosome, mitotic spindle, and the primary cilia. It colocalizes with nephrocystin-1 & KIF3A on the cilia. The products of the NPHP genes are referred to as nephrocystins.

1857. Which of the following is false about Medullary Cystic Kidney Disease Type II?

Harrison's 20th Ed. Chapter 309 Page 2155

A. Benign urine sediments
B. Absence of significant proteinuria
C. Hyperuricemia
D. None of the above

MCKD II should be suspected clinically in patients with a family history of late onset kidney disease, benign urine sediments, absence of significant proteinuria and hyperuricemia.

1858. Presence of hyperuricemia and gout point towards the diagnosis of which of the following?

Harrison's 20th Ed. Chapter 309 Page 2155

A. Autosomal recessive polycystic kidney disease
B. Medullary cystic kidney disease 2
C. Bartter's syndrome
D. Nephronophthisis (NPHP)

Most patients with medullary cystic kidney disease 2 (MCKD2) have severe hyperuricemia and precocious onset of gout.

1859. Presence of hyperuricemia and gout point towards the diagnosis of which of the following?

Harrison's 20th Ed. Chapter 309 Page 2155

A. Autosomal recessive polycystic kidney disease
B. ADKTKD-REN
C. ADTKD-MUC1
D. Nephronophthisis (NPHP)

Patients with mutations in renin gene REN (leading to ADTKD-REN) demonstrate hyporeninemia with mild hyperkalemia, hyperuricemia and gout.

1860. Which of the following is the most common genetic cause of ESRD in childhood?

Harrison's 20th Ed. Chapter 309 Page 2155

A. Autosomal recessive polycystic kidney disease
B. Medullary sponge kidney (MSK)
C. Bartter's syndrome
D. Nephronophthisis (NPHP)

Nephronophthisis (NPHP) is the most common inherited childhood form of kidney failure requiring kidney replacement therapy.

1861. Which of the following relates to nephronophthisis (NPHP)?

Harrison's 20th Ed. Chapter 309 Page 2155

A. Autosomal recessive pattern of inheritance
B. Ciliopathy
C. Most common inherited childhood form of kidney failure
D. None of the above

1862. Which of the following is a feature of nephronophthisis?

Harrison's 20th Ed. Chapter 309 Page 2155

A. Tubulointerstitial fibrosis
B. Corticomedullary cysts
C. Progressive CKD leading to renal failure
D. All of the above

NPHP share common features, including tubulointerstitial fibrosis, corticomedullary cysts and progressive CKD leading to renal failure. Proteinuria is absent or mild and the urine sediment is not active.

1863. Products of the NPHP genes are referred to as?

Harrison's 20th Ed. Chapter 309 Page 2155

A. Nephronocystins
B. Nephrocystins
C. Nephricystins
D. Nephritic cystins

Products of the NPHP genes are referred to as nephrocystins.

1864. Which of the following form of NPHP is most frequent?

Harrison's 20th Ed. Chapter 309 Page 2156

A. Infantile
B. Juvenile
C. Adolescent
D. Adult

NPHP is divided into infantile, juvenile, and adolescent forms. The juvenile form is the most frequent.

1865. Infantile form NPHP is caused by mutations in?

Harrison's 20th Ed. Chapter 309 Page 2156

A. NPHP1 gene
B. NPHP2 gene
C. NPHP3 gene
D. NPHP4 gene

1866. Juvenile form NPHP is caused by mutations in?

Harrison's 20th Ed. Chapter 309 Page 2156

A. NPHP1 gene
B. NPHP2 gene
C. NPHP3 gene
D. NPHP4 gene

1867. Senior-Loken syndrome, besides juvenile nephronophthisis, best relates to?

Harrison's 20th Ed. Chapter 309 Page 2156

A. Intracranial aneurysm
B. Retinitis pigmentosa
C. Colonic diverticulae
D. All of the above

When juvenile NPHP has retinitis pigmentosa as an extrarenal manifestation, the syndrome is called Senior-Loken syndrome.

1868. Joubert's syndrome best relates to?

Harrison's 20th Ed. Chapter 309 Page 2156

A. Retinal dystrophy
B. Cystic dilatation of renal collecting ducts
C. Hypoplasia of the cerebellar vermis
D. All of the above

1869. Which of the following is not a feature of Bardet-Biedl syndrome (BBS)?

Harrison's 20th Ed. Chapter 309 Page 2156

A. Polydactyly
B. Retinal hemangioma
C. Kidney cysts
D. Truncal obesity

The multisystem disease Bardet-Biedl syndrome (BBS) features truncal obesity, cognitive impairment, retinal dystrophy, polydactyly, developmental urogenital abnormalities and kidney cysts.

1870. Which of the following is a disease of abnormal ciliary function?

Harrison's 20th Ed. Chapter 309 Page 2156

A. Autosomal dominant polycystic kidney disease (ADPKD)
B. Nephronophthisis (NPHP)
C. Bardet-Biedl syndrome (BBS)
D. All of the above

Tubulointerstitial Diseases of the Kidney

1871. Which of the following about tubulointerstitial nephritis (TIN) is false?
Harrison's 20th Ed. Chapter 310 Page 2157

A. Tubules & interstitium primarily affected
B. Relative sparing of glomeruli
C. Relative sparing of renal vessels
D. None of the above

Tubulointerstitial nephritis (TIN) is a group of disorders that primarily affect tubules & interstitium, with relative sparing of glomeruli & renal vessels. They can be acute and chronic.

1872. Tubulointerstitial diseases of the kidney can be due to?
Harrison's 20th Ed. Chapter 310 Page 2157 Table 310-1

A. Acute tubulointerstitial disorders
B. Chronic tubulointerstitial disorders
C. Cystic and hereditary disorders
D. All of the above

Tubulointerstitial diseases of the kidney can be due to acute tubulointerstitial disorders, chronic tubulointerstitial disorders, metabolic disturbances and cystic and hereditary disorders.

1873. Acute interstitial nephritis of the kidney can be due to?
Harrison's 20th Ed. Chapter 310 Page 2157 Table 310-1

A. Therapeutic agents
B. Infections
C. Autoimmune etiology
D. All of the above

Acute interstitial nephritis can be due to therapeutic agents, infections, autoimmune etiology, and acute obstructive causes.

1874. Which of the following about tubulointerstitial nephritis (TIN) is false?
Harrison's 20th Ed. Chapter 310 Page 2157

A. Acute TIN mostly presents as acute renal failure
B. Chronic TIN mostly presents as disorders of tubular function
C. Allergic reaction to a drug mostly cause acute interstitial nephritis (AIN)
D. None of the above

1875. Acute TIN caused by aggressive inflammatory infiltrates leads to?
Harrison's 20th Ed. Chapter 310 Page 2157

A. Tissue edema
B. Tubular cell injury
C. Compromised tubular flow
D. All of the above

1876. Frank obstruction of the tubules can be caused by?
Harrison's 20th Ed. Chapter 310 Page 2157

A. Casts
B. Cellular debris
C. Crystals
D. All of the above

Acute TIN that presents with acute renal failure is caused by aggressive inflammatory infiltrates that lead to tissue edema, tubular cell injury, and compromised tubular flow, or by Frank obstruction of the tubules with casts, cellular debris, or crystals.

1877. The clinical features of chronic TIN manifest with disorders of?
Harrison's 20th Ed. Chapter 310 Page 2157

A. Glomerular function
B. Tubular function
C. Interstitial function
D. All of the above

The clinical features of chronic TIN are more indolent and manifest with disorders of tubular function.

1878. Renal tubular dysfunction can manifest as?
Harrison's 20th Ed. Chapter 310 Page 2157

A. Polyuria
B. Non-anion-gap metabolic acidosis
C. Hyperkalemia
D. All of the above

1879. Which of the following is a feature of Fanconi's syndrome?
Harrison's 20th Ed. Chapter 310 Page 2157

A. Glycosuria
B. Phosphaturia
C. Aminoaciduria
D. All of the above

Disorders of tubular function can lead to polyuria from impaired concentrating ability (nephrogenic diabetes insipidus), defective proximal tubular reabsorption leading to features of Fanconi's syndrome (glycosuria, phosphaturia, aminoaciduria, hypokalemia and type II renal tubular acidosis [RTA] from bicarbonaturia) or non-anion-gap metabolic acidosis and hyperkalemia (type IV RTA) due to impaired ammonia genesis, as well as progressive azotemia (rising creatinine & blood urea nitrogen).

1880. On renal ultrasonography, which of the following is found in "medical renal disease"?
Harrison's 20th Ed. Chapter 310 Page 2157

A. Increased echogenicity of renal parenchyma
B. Loss of corticomedullary differentiation
C. Prominence of renal pyramids
D. All of the above

In Chronic TIN, renal ultrasonography may reveal "medical renal disease" which includes increased echogenicity of the renal parenchyma with loss of corticomedullary differentiation, prominence of the renal pyramids and cortical scarring.

1881. The predominant pathology in chronic TIN is?
Harrison's 20th Ed. Chapter 310 Page 2157

A. Interstitial fibrosis with patchy mononuclear cell infiltration
B. Widespread tubular atrophy & luminal dilation
C. Thickening of tubular basement membranes
D. All of the above

The predominant pathology in chronic TIN is interstitial fibrosis with patchy mononuclear cell infiltration & widespread tubular atrophy, luminal dilation, and thickening of tubular basement membranes.

1882. Which of the following is common in NSAID induced allergic interstitial nephritis?
Harrison's 20th Ed. Chapter 310 Page 2158

A. Fever
B. Rash
C. Eosinophilia
D. Proteinuria

In nonsteroidal anti-inflammatory drug (NSAID)-induced acute interstitial nephritis (AIN) fever, rash and eosinophilia are rare but acute renal failure with heavy proteinuria is common.

1883. Severe & rapid-onset allergic interstitial nephritis may occur on reintroduction after a drug-free period of which of the following drug?

Harrison's 20th Ed. Chapter 310 Page 2158

A. Proton pump inhibitors
B. Rifampin
C. Sulfasalazine
D. Indinavir

A particularly severe & rapid-onset AIN may occur upon reintroduction, after a drug-free period, of rifampin.

1884. Which of the following provide supporting evidence to the diagnosis of allergic interstitial nephritis?

Harrison's 20th Ed. Chapter 310 Page 2158

A. Peripheral blood eosinophilia
B. Pyuria with white blood cell casts
C. Hematuria
D. All of the above

1885. Which of the following may accelerate renal recovery in allergic interstitial nephritis?

Harrison's 20th Ed. Chapter 310 Page 2158

A. Diuretics
B. Glucocorticoids
C. N-acetyl cysteine
D. All of the above

Glucocorticoid therapy may accelerate renal recovery, but does not appear to impact long-term renal survival. It is best reserved for cases with severe renal failure in which dialysis is imminent or if renal function continues to deteriorate despite stopping the offending drug.

1886. Which of the following acute obstructive disorders cause acute interstitial nephritis?

Harrison's 20th Ed. Chapter 310 Page 2157 Table 310-1

A. Light chain cast nephropathy (myeloma kidney)
B. Acute phosphate nephropathy
C. Acute urate nephropathy
D. All of the above

1887. Which of the following autoimmune diseases can cause acute interstitial nephritis?

Harrison's 20th Ed. Chapter 310 Page 2157 Table 310-1

A. Sjogren's syndrome
B. Systemic lupus erythematosus
C. IgG4-related systemic disease
D. All of the above

1888. Which of the following drugs can cause chronic interstitial nephritis?

Harrison's 20th Ed. Chapter 310 Page 2157 Table 310-1

A. Rifampin
B. Acyclovir
C. Lithium
D. Valproate

1889. Which of the following can cause chronic interstitial nephritis?

Harrison's 20th Ed. Chapter 310 Page 2157 Table 310-1

A. Cyclosporine
B. Lead
C. Cadmium
D. All of the above

1890. Which of the following can cause chronic interstitial nephritis?

Harrison's 20th Ed. Chapter 310 Page 2157 Table 310-1

A. Radiation nephritis
B. Sickle cell disease
C. Nephronophthisis
D. All of the above

1891. Corticosteroids & immunosuppressives are absolutely indicated which of the following causes of interstitial nephritis?

Harrison's 20th Ed. Chapter 310 Page 2158 Table 310-2

A. Sjögren's syndrome
B. Sarcoidosis
C. SLE interstitial nephritis
D. All of the above

1892. Sjogren's syndrome is best related to?

Harrison's 20th Ed. Chapter 310 Page 2158

A. Dumping syndrome
B. Sinusoidal obstruction syndrome
C. Sicca syndrome
D. Tumor lysis syndrome

1893. Which of the following is false about Sjogren's syndrome?

Harrison's 20th Ed. Chapter 310 Page 2158

A. Autoimmune disorder that targets exocrine glands
B. Positive for anti-Ro (SS-A) & anti-La (SS- B) antibodies
C. Polyclonal hypergammaglobulinemia
D. None of the above

1894. Sjogren' s syndrome can be associated with?

Harrison's 20th Ed. Chapter 310 Page 2158

A. Aristolochic acid
B. Hyperuricemia
C. Nephrogenic diabetes insipidus
D. Nephrocalcinosis

1895. Sjogren' s syndrome can be associated with?

Harrison's 20th Ed. Chapter 310 Page 2158

A. Distal RTA
B. Nephrogenic diabetes insipidus
C. Renal failure
D. All of the above

Tubulointerstitial nephritis with a predominant lymphocytic infiltrate is the most common renal manifestation of Sjogren's syndrome and can be associated with distal RTA, nephrogenic diabetes insipidus and moderate renal failure.

1896. Which of the following drug is useful in Sjogren' s syndrome?
Harrison's 20th Ed. Chapter 310 Page 2158

A. Glucocorticoids
B. Azathioprine
C. Mycophenolate mofetil
D. All of the above

Treatment of Sjogren' s syndrome is initiated with glucocorticoids. Patients may require maintenance therapy with azathioprine or mycophenolate mofetil to prevent relapse.

1897. Which of the following about tubulointerstitial nephritis with uveitis (TINU) is false?
Harrison's 20th Ed. Chapter 310 Page 2158

A. Systemic autoimmune disease of unknown etiology
B. Affects females three times more often than males
C. Median age of onset is 15 years
D. None of the above

1898. Which of the following about tubulointerstitial nephritis with uveitis (TINU) is false?
Harrison's 20th Ed. Chapter 310 Page 2158

A. Posterior uveitis
B. Elevated creatinine, sterile pyuria, mild proteinuria
C. Features of Fanconi's syndrome
D. Clinical symptoms are self-limited in children

In addition to lymphocyte-predominant interstitial nephritis in TINU, the hallmark feature is a painful anterior uveitis, often bilateral and accompanied by blurred vision & photophobia. Ocular symptoms precede or accompany the renal disease.

1899. Cause of uveitis and renal disease is?
Harrison's 20th Ed. Chapter 310 Page 2158

A. Sjogren's syndrome
B. Sarcoidosis
C. Systemic lupus erythematosus
D. All of the above

Causes of uveitis and renal disease are tubulointerstitial nephritis with uveitis (TINU), Sjogren's syndrome, Behcet's disease, sarcoidosis and systemic lupus erythematosus.

1900. Chronic sclerosing sialadenitis is a feature of?
Harrison's 20th Ed. Chapter 310 Page 2158

A. Tubulointerstitial nephritis with uveitis (TINU)
B. Sarcoidosis
C. IgG4-related systemic disease
D. Systemic lupus erythematosus

1901. Urinalysis showing "sheaf of wheat" crystals best relates to?
Harrison's 20th Ed. Chapter 310 Page 2159

A. Intravenous acyclovir
B. Indinavir
C. Sulfonamide
D. Allopurinol

1902. Red-green birefringement needle-shaped crystals on urinalysis are of?
Harrison's 20th Ed. Chapter 310 Page 2159

A. Acyclovir
B. Indinavir
C. Sulfonamide
D. Allopurinol

1903. Oral phospho-soda best relates to?
Harrison's 20th Ed. Chapter 310 Page 2159

A. Diuretic
B. Antacid
C. Laxative
D. Sunscreen

Acute phosphate nephropathy is a serious complication of oral Phospho-soda used as a laxative or for bowel preparation for colonoscopy.

1904. Myeloma kidney best relates to?
Harrison's 20th Ed. Chapter 310 Page 2160

A. POEMS syndrome
B. Multiple myeloma
C. Waldenstrom's macroglobulinemia
D. All of the above

Myeloma kidney is also called light chain cast nephropathy (LCCN).

1905. Clinical clues to the diagnosis of myeloma cast nephropathy include?
Harrison's 20th Ed. Chapter 310 Page 2160

A. Hypercalcemia
B. Abnormally narrow anion gap
C. Hypoalbuminemia and hypergammaglobulinemia
D. All of the above

Clinical clues to the diagnosis of myeloma cast nephropathy include anemia, bone pain, hypercalcemia, and an abnormally narrow anion gap due to hypoalbuminemia and hypergammaglobulinemia.

1906. Chronic interstitial nephritis (CIN) occurs mostly due to?
Harrison's 20th Ed. Chapter 310 Page 2160

A. Secondary to a primary glomerular disease
B. Developmental anomalies
C. Inherited diseases
D. All of the above

Chronic interstitial nephritis (CIN) occurs mostly due to renal ischemia or secondary to a primary glomerular disease. Other important forms of CIN are the result of developmental anomalies or inherited diseases such as reflux nephropathy or sickle cell nephropathy.

1907. Tubulointerstitial disease affecting predominantly medullary & papillary structures is?
Harrison's 20th Ed. Chapter 310 Page 2160

A. Analgesic nephropathy
B. Lead nephropathy
C. Plasma cell dyscrasias
D. All of the above

Tubulointerstitial diseases that predominantly affect medullary & papillary structures are analgesic nephropathy & sickle cell disease.

1908. Renal papillary necrosis invariably produces?
Harrison's 20th Ed. Chapter 94 Page 693

A. Painless hematuria
B. Obstructive uropathy
C. Isosthenuria
D. Renal hematoma

Renal papillary necrosis invariably produces isosthenuria which refers to nonconcentrated urine that is isosmotic with plasma.

1909. Which of the following is a cause of papillary necrosis?
Harrison's 20th Ed. Chapter 310 Page 2162 Table 310-3

A. Analgesic nephropathy
B. Sickle cell nephropathy
C. Diabetes with urinary tract infection
D. All of the above

1910. "Ring sign" on the pyelogram is pathognomonic of?
J Clin Diagn Res. 2016;10(1):TD10-TD12

A. Polycystic kidney disease
B. Papillary necrosis
C. Transitional cell carcinoma
D. Medullary sponge kidney

"Ring sign" (radiolucent sloughed papilla surrounded by radiodense contrast material in calyx) on pyelogram is pathognomonic of papillary necrosis due to analgesic nephropathy. CT reveals papillary calcifications surrounding the central sinus complex in a "garland" pattern. Contrast-containing rice grain sized cavities in the papilla are the pathognomonic feature of the medullary form of renal papillary necrosis.

1911. Which of the following is false about aristolochic acid?
Harrison's 20th Ed. Chapter 310 Page 2162

A. Carcinogen, causes DNA damage
B. Cause of Balkan endemic nephropathy
C. Renal interstitial fibrosis with paucity of cellular infiltrates
D. None of the above

1912. Which of the following is false about aristolochic acid?
Harrison's 20th Ed. Chapter 310 Page 2162

A. Cause of Chinese herbal nephropathy
B. Causes severe anemia
C. Aristolactam-DNA adducts in kidney or urinary tract tissue
D. None of the above

1913. Which of the following gene is involved in karyomegalic tubulointerstitial nephritis?
Harrison's 20th Ed. Chapter 310 Page 2162

A. AGR2
B. cagA
C. FAN1
D. dupA

Karyomegalic tubulointerstitial nephritis is a recessive disorder caused by inheritance of two mutant copies of FAN1 gene. FAN1 encodes a component of a DNA repair machinery complex.

1914. Which of the following is the most common renal sequelae of lithium associated nephropathy?
Harrison's 20th Ed. Chapter 310 Page 2162

A. Secondary FSGS
B. Nephrogenic diabetes insipidus
C. Chronic tubulointerstitial nephritis
D. None of the above

Use of lithium salts has renal sequelae, the most common of which is nephrogenic diabetes insipidus.

1915. Lithium best relates to which of the following?
Harrison's 20th Ed. Chapter 310 Page 2162

A. Electroneutral thiazide-sensitive Na^+/Cl^- cotransporter
B. Epithelial sodium channel (ENaC)
C. Apical Ca^{++}-selective channels (TRPV5)
D. K^+/Cl^- cotransporter

Lithium accumulates in principal cells of collecting duct by entering through epithelial sodium channel (ENaC), where it inhibits glycogen synthase kinase 3β & downregulates vasopressin-regulated aquaporin water channels.

1916. Which of the following is highly characteristic of lithium associated nephropathy on renal biopsy?
Harrison's 20th Ed. Chapter 310 Page 2162

A. Glomerulosclerosis
B. Interstitial fibrosis
C. Tubular atrophy
C. Cysts or dilation of the distal tubule & collecting duct

1917. Which of the following is effective to prevent & treat lithium-induced nephrogenic diabetes insipidus?
Harrison's 20th Ed. Chapter 310 Page 2162

A. Amiloride
B. Thiazide diuretic
C. Dexamethasone
D. All of the above

The entry of lithium through amiloride-sensitive Na^+ channel ENaC is required for the effect of the drug on principal cells, such that combined therapy within lithium & amiloride can mitigate lithium-associated NDI.

1918. Which of the following cause blockade of epithelial sodium channel (ENaC)?
Harrison's 20th Ed. Chapter 49 Page 309 Table 49-5

A. Triamterene
B. Trimethoprim
C. Nafamostat
D. All of the above

Amiloride, triamterene, trimethoprim, pentamidine, & nafamostat cause blockade of epithelial sodium channel (ENaC).

1919. Acute renal injury with the use of calcineurin inhibitor (CNI) is due to?
Harrison's 20th Ed. Chapter 310 Page 2163

A. Vasoconstriction
B. Thrombotic microangiopathy
C. Toxic tubulopathy
D. All of the above

1920. Hyperkalemia as a complication of the use of calcineurin inhibitor (CNI) is caused by tubular resistance to?
Harrison's 20th Ed. Chapter 310 Page 2163

A. Renin
B. Aldosterone
C. Angiotensin II
D. All of the above

Hyperkalemia with use of calcineurin inhibitor (CNI) is caused by tubular resistance to aldosterone.

1921. Histologic change in renal tissue with the use of calcineurin inhibitor (CNI) is?
Harrison's 20th Ed. Chapter 310 Page 2163

A. Patchy interstitial fibrosis
B. Tubular atrophy in a "striped" pattern
C. Intrarenal vasculature hyalinosis
D. All of the above

The histologic changes in renal tissue include patchy interstitial fibrosis and tubular atrophy, in a "striped" pattern. In addition, the intrarenal vasculature demonstrates hyalinosis, and focal glomerulosclerosis.

1922. Lead exposure best relates to?
Harrison's 20th Ed. Chapter 310 Page 2163, Arch Intern Med. 1993;153(12):1501-4

A. Nip joint
B. Moonshine whiskey
C. Congener
D. Rum-running

Moonshine derives its name from production of illegal whiskey under cover of darkness with only the moon as a guide. It contained lead levels exceeding Environmental Protection Agency water guidelines of 15 parts per billion. Moonshine whiskey are distilled in lead-tainted containers & cause lead toxicity.

1923. Early signs of chronic lead intoxication are attributable to?
Harrison's 20th Ed. Chapter 310 Page 2163

A. Proximal tubule dysfunction
B. Loop of Henle dysfunction
C. Distal convoluted tubule dysfunction
D. Collecting duct dysfunction

Early signs of chronic lead intoxication are attributable to proximal tubule dysfunction.

1924. Which of the following is a characteristic finding in patients with chronic lead nephropathy?
Harrison's 20th Ed. Chapter 310 Page 2163

A. Hypokalemia
B. Hypercalcemia
C. Hyperuricemia
D. Hyponatremia

Patients with chronic lead nephropathy are characteristically hyperuricemic due to increased reabsorption of filtered urate leading to acute gouty arthritis called saturnine gout. Saturnine gout refers to development of hyperuricaemia & gout due to inhibiting effect of lead on the tubular urate transport.

1925. Which of the following is not a feature of lead intoxication?
Harrison's 20th Ed. Chapter 310 Page 2163

A. Chronic interstitial nephritis (CIN)
B. Gout
C. Hyperglycemia
D. Hypertension

1926. Lead exposure is likely if the diagnostic triad is present that consists of all except?
Harrison's 20th Ed. Chapter 310 Page 2163

A. Gout
B. Anemia
C. Hypertension
D. Renal insufficiency

1927. Chronic hypercalcemia occurs in?
Harrison's 20th Ed. Chapter 310 Page 2163

A. Sarcoidosis
B. Multiple myeloma
C. Metastatic bone disease
D. All of the above

Chronic hypercalcemia occurs in primary hyperparathyroidism, sarcoidosis, multiple myeloma, vitamin D intoxication, or metastatic bone disease. It causes tubulointerstitial disease & progressive renal failure.

1928. The earliest lesion in hypercalcemic nephropathy is?
Harrison's 20th Ed. Chapter 310 Page 2163

A. Calcium deposition in glomeruli
B. Calcium deposition in tubular cell
C. Calcium deposition in walls of renal arterioles
D. Focal degenerative change in renal epithelia

1929. In hypercalcemic nephropathy, initial focal degenerative change involves renal epithelia of?
Harrison's 20th Ed. Chapter 310 Page 2163

A. Collecting ducts
B. Distal tubules
C. Loops of Henle
D. All of the above

The earliest lesion in hypercalcemic nephropathy is a focal degenerative change in renal epithelia, primarily in collecting ducts, distal tubules & loops of Henle.

1930. Nephrocalcinosis refers to?
Harrison's 20th Ed. Chapter 310 Page 2163

A. Glomerular calcium deposition
B. Tubular calcium deposition
C. Interstitial calcium deposition
D. All of the above

Tubular epithelial cell necrosis leads to nephron obstruction and stasis of intrarenal urine, favoring precipitation of Ca^{++} salts and infection. Dilation & atrophy of tubules, interstitial fibrosis, mononuclear leukocyte infiltration, and interstitial calcium deposition eventually occur. Interstitial calcium deposition is called nephrocalcinosis.

1931. Which of the following occurs in hypercalcemic nephropathy?
Harrison's 20th Ed. Chapter 310 Page 2163

A. Reduced responsiveness to arginine vasopressin in CD
B. Defective transport of sodium & chloride in loop of Henle
C. Tubulointerstitial damage
D. All of the above

1932. Which of the following can cause prolonged and severe hypokalemia?
Harrison's 20th Ed. Chapter 310 Page 2163

A. Primary aldosteronism
B. Chronic laxative or diuretic abuse
C. Surreptitious vomiting
D. All of the above

Patients with prolonged and severe hypokalemia develop a reversible tubular lesion characterized by vacuolar degeneration of proximal and distal tubular cells.

Vascular Injury to the Kidney

1933. Thrombotic microangiopathy (TMA) is characterized by all except?

Harrison's 20th Ed. Chapter 311 Page 2164

A. Endothelial cell injury
B. Mainly of arterioles & capillaries
C. Occlusive platelet and hyaline thrombi
D. Thrombocytosis

TMA is usually accompanied by microangiopathic hemolytic anemia (MAHA) with its typical features of thrombocytopenia and schistocytes.

1934. Which of the following pattern is seen in the glomerulus in TMA?

Harrison's 20th Ed. Chapter 311 Page 2164

A. Minimal change
B. Membranous
C. Membranoproliferative
D. All of the above

1935. Which of the following is seen in the glomerulus in TMA?

Harrison's 20th Ed. Chapter 311 Page 2164

A. Endotheliosis
B. Fibrin thrombi & platelet plugs
C. Arterial intimal fibrosis
D. All of the above

In kidney, TMA is characterized by swollen endocapillary cells (endotheliosis), fibrin thrombi, platelet plugs, arterial intimal fibrosis and a membranoproliferative pattern in glomerulus. Fibrin thrombi may extend into arteriolar vascular pole, producing glomerular collapse and cortical necrosis. In kidneys that recover from acute TMA, secondary focal segmental glomerulosclerosis may develop.

1936. Diseases associated with TMA include?

Harrison's 20th Ed. Chapter 311 Page 2164

A. Antiphospholipid syndrome
B. HIV infection
C. Radiation nephropathy
D. All of the above

Diseases associated with TMA include thrombotic thrombocytopenic purpura (TTP), hemolytic-uremic syndrome (HUS), malignant hypertension, scleroderma renal crisis, antiphospholipid syndrome, preeclampsia/HELLP syndrome, HIV infection and radiation nephropathy.

1937. Thrombotic microangiopathy (TMA) can be seen in?

Harrison's 20th Ed. Chapter 311 Page 2164

A. Myeloproliferative neoplasm-related glomerulopathy
B. POEMS syndrome
C. Malignant hypertension
D. All of the above

TMA can be seen in myeloproliferative neoplasm (MPN)-related glomerulopathy and POEMS syndrome which are not associated with MAHA.

1938. Which of the following statements is false?

Harrison's 20th Ed. Chapter 311 Page 2164

A. HUS & TTP are the prototypes for MAHA
B. TTP develops more commonly in adults
C. HUS occurs more commonly in children
D. None of the above

TTP develops more commonly in adults and has more neurologic complications. HUS occurs more frequently in children, particularly when associated with hemorrhagic diarrhea.

1939. Shiga toxin is best related to which bacteria?

Harrison's 20th Ed. Chapter 311 Page 2164

A. Streptococcus viridans
B. Staphylococcus aureus
C. Escherichia coli
D. Enterococcus sp

Shiga toxins (Stx1 & Stx2) are also referred to as verotoxins. These toxins are produced by certain strains of E. coli and Shigella dysenteriae.

1940. Which is the most common variant of hemolytic-uremic syndrome (HUS)?

Harrison's 20th Ed. Chapter 311 Page 2164

A. Shiga toxin-producing Escherichia coli (STEC) HUS
B. D^+ HUS
C. Enterohemorrhagic E. coli (EHEC) HUS
D. All of the above

All of the above are the same entity.

1941. Hemolytic-uremic syndrome is associated with which pathotype of E. coli?

Harrison's 20th Ed. Chapter 311 Page 2164

A. STEC/EHEC/STEAEC
B. ETEC
C. EPEC
D. All of the above

ETEC (enterotoxigenic E. coli), STEAEC (Shiga toxin-producing enteroaggregative) E. coli, STEC (Shiga toxi n-producing E. coli), EPEC (enteropathogenic E. coli).

1942. Which of the following usually precedes MAHA?

Harrison's 20th Ed. Chapter 311 Page 2164

A. Diarrhea
B. Abdominal pain
C. Cramping
D. Vomiting

1943. Which of the following is typically absent in MAHA?

Harrison's 20th Ed. Chapter 311 Page 2164

A. Fever
B. Abdominal pain
C. Cramping
D. Vomiting

Diarrhea, often bloody, precedes MAHA within 1 week in >80% of cases. Abdominal pain, cramping, and vomiting are frequent whereas fever is typically absent.

1944. Verotoxin best relates to?
Harrison's 20th Ed. Chapter 311 Page 2164

A. Botulinum toxin
B. Hepatotoxin
C. Neurotoxin
D. Shiga toxin

1945. Which of the following is an action of Shiga toxin?
Harrison's 20th Ed. Chapter 311 Page 2164, Chapter 308 Page 2148

A. Binding to glycolipid surface receptor globotriaosylceramide (Gb3)
B. Inhibition of endothelial production of ADAMTS13
C. Inducing inflammatory cytokines & chemokine receptors
D. All of the above

1946. Which of the following is an inflammatory cytokine?
Harrison's 20th Ed. Chapter 311 Page 2164

A. Interleukin 8 (IL-8)
B. Monocyte chemotactic protein 1 (MCP-1)
C. Stromal cell–derived factor 1 (SDF-1)
D. All of the above

1947. Which of the following can also cause HUS?
Harrison's 20th Ed. Chapter 311 Page 2164

A. E. coli
B. Shigella dysenteriae
C. Streptococcus pneumoniae
D. All of the above

Streptococcus pneumoniae can also cause HUS.

1948. Which of the following about Thomsen-Friedenreich antigen is false?
Harrison's 20th Ed. Chapter 311 Page 2164

A. Present on platelets and endothelial cells
B. Normally covered by N-acetylneuraminic acid moieties
B. Exposure to preformed IgM results in severe MAHA
D. None of the above

1949. Thomsen–Friedenreich antigen best relates to?
Harrison's 20th Ed. Chapter 311 Page 2164, N Engl J Med. 2014; 371:1846-1848

A. S. pneumoniae-associated hemolytic-uremic syndrome
B. S. aureus-associated hemolytic-uremic syndrome
C. Enterococcus-associated hemolytic-uremic syndrome
D. Escherichia coli-associated hemolytic-uremic syndrome

1950. Thomsen-Friedenreich antigen (T-antigen) best relates to?
Harrison's 20th Ed. Chapter 311 Page 2164, Pediatr Infect Dis J 2011;30:1-4

A. Glucosaminidase
B. Neuraminidase
C. Hexosaminidase
D. Mannosidase

Streptococcus pneumoniae-associated hemolytic-uremic syndrome (SP-HUS) is a rare but severe complication that implicates binding of Thomsen–Friedenreich antigen (T-antigen) to preformed circulating IgM antibodies, owing to neuraminidase-mediated cleavage of sialic acid residues from the membrane of glomerular capillary endothelial cells, red cells, and platelets, leading to pneumococcal sepsis-mediated thrombotic microangiopathy and HUS. Neuraminidase-associated thrombotic microangiopathy is generally observed in pediatric patients with pneumonia and meningitis.

1951. Which STEC strain is mostly causes HUS?
Harrison's 20th Ed. Chapter 311 Page 2164

A. O157:H7
B. O145:H28
C. O157/H-
D. O111:H-

1952. Glomerular endotheliosis is a feature of?
Harrison's 20th Ed. Chapter 311 Page 2164

A. Preeclampsia
B. HELLP syndrome
C. HUS
D. All of the above

Glomerular endotheliosis is seen in HUS, preeclampsia/HELLP (hemolysis, elevated liver enzymes, and low platelet count syndrome), malignant hypertension and the antiphospholipid syndrome.

1953. Which of the following is related to "atypical HUS"?
Harrison's 20th Ed. Chapter 311 Page 2164

A. Complement dysregulation
B. Low C3 and normal C4 levels
C. Factor H deficiency
D. All of the above

The complement dysregulation can be congenital or acquired. Low C3 and a normal C4 levels are characteristic of alternative pathway activation.

1954. Which of the following about Factor H is false?
Harrison's 20th Ed. Chapter 311 Page 2164

A. Competes with factor B to prevent formation of C3bBb
B. Acts as a cofactor for factor I which degrades C3b
C. Deficiency linked to families with aHUS
D. None of the above

1955. DEAP HUS best relates to?
Harrison's 20th Ed. Chapter 311 Page 2165

A. Factor B
B. Factor H
C. Factor I
D. All of the above

DEAP refers to deficiency of CFHR plasma proteins and CFH autoantibody positive. HUS occurs when an autoantibody to factor H is formed, and blocks binding of factor H to C3b & surface-bound C3 convertase.

1956. Which of the following is not typical of TTP?
Harrison's 20th Ed. Chapter 311 Page 2165

A. Thrombocytopenia
B. Hemorrhagic tendency
C. Neurologic symptoms
D. Renal failure

Traditionally, TTP is characterized by the pentad: MAHA, thrombocytopenia, neurologic symptoms, fever and renal failure.

1957. Which of the following best relates to the pathophysiology of TTP?
Harrison's 20th Ed. Chapter 311 Page 2165

A. von Willebrand factor
B. Factor B
C. Factor H
D. All of the above

1958. Which of the following best relates to the pathophysiology of TTP?

Harrison's 20th Ed. Chapter 311 Page 2165

A. ADAMTS13
B. ADAMTS14
C. ADAMTS15
D. ADAMTS16

The pathophysiology of TTP involves accumulation of ultra-large multimers of von Willebrand factor due to the absence or markedly decreased activity of plasma protease ADAMTS13, a disintegrin and metalloproteinase with a thrombospondin type 1 motif, member 13. These ultra-large multimers form clots and damage erythrocytes, resulting in MAHA.

1959. TTP is defined as MAHA associated with ADAMTS13 activity of?

Harrison's 20th Ed. Chapter 311 Page 2165

A. < 5–10%
B. < 15–20%
C. < 35–40%
D. < 50–60%

TTP is defined as MAHA associated with ADAMTS13 activity of < 5–10%.

1960. Apart from low levels of ADAMTS13, which of the following is required to initiate clinical TTP?

Harrison's 20th Ed. Chapter 311 Page 2165

A. Infection
B. Surgery
C. Pregnancy
D. All of the above

Apart from low levels of ADAMTS13, an additional inflammatory trigger (infection, surgery, pancreatitis, or pregnancy) is required to initiate clinical TTP. This may be mediated by human neutrophil peptides that inhibit cleavage of von Willebrand factor by ADAMTS13.

1961. The median age of onset of TTP is?

Harrison's 20th Ed. Chapter 311 Page 2165

A. 20 years
B. 30 years
C. 40 years
D. 50 years

The median age of onset of TTP is 40 years.

1962. Which of the following about TTP is false?

Harrison's 20th Ed. Chapter 311 Page 2165

A. Incidence is higher among blacks than among non-blacks
B. Incidence is higher among women than among men
C. If untreated, TTP has a mortality rate exceeding 90%
D. None of the above

1963. Which of the following is a hereditary condition characterized by congenital deficiency of ADAMTS13?

Harrison's 20th Ed. Chapter 311 Page 2165

A. Boerhaave's syndrome
B. Upshaw-Schülman syndrome
C. Münchausen's syndrome
D. Chédiak-Higashi syndrome

Upshaw-Schülman syndrome is a hereditary condition characterized by congenital deficiency of ADAMTS13.

1964. TTP/HUS is seen in?

Harrison's 20th Ed. Chapter 311 Page 2165

A. Pregnancy
B. Use of oral contraceptives
C. HIV infection
D. All of the above

1965. TTP/HUS is seen with the use of?

Harrison's 20th Ed. Chapter 311 Page 2165

A. Quinine
B. Cyclosporine/tacrolimus
C. Ticlopidine/clopidogrel
D. All of the above

1966. Toxic or endothelial damage is the main cause of TMA produced by all of the following drugs except?

Harrison's 20th Ed. Chapter 311 Page 2165

A. Gemcitabine
B. Quinine
C. Interferon
D. Cyclosporine

1967. Quinine induces autoantibodies to all except?

Harrison's 20th Ed. Chapter 311 Page 2165

A. Granulocytes, lymphocytes
B. Endothelial cells
C. Platelet glycoprotein Ib/IX or IIb/IIIa complexes
D. ADAMTS13

Quinine induces autoantibodies to granulocytes, lymphocytes, endothelial cells, and platelet glycoprotein Ib/IX or IIb/IIIa complexes, but not to ADAMTS13.

1968. Autoantibody-mediated TTP and DEAP HUS respond to which of the following?

Harrison's 20th Ed. Chapter 311 Page 2165

A. Plasma exchange
B. Prednisone
C. Rituximab
D. All of the above

1969. Drug-induced TMA secondary to endothelial damage respond to?

Harrison's 20th Ed. Chapter 311 Page 2165

A. Plasma exchange
B. Prednisone
C. Rituximab
D. None of the above

Drug-induced TMA secondary to endothelial damage typically does not respond to plasma exchange and is treated primarily by discontinuing use of the offending agent and providing supportive care.

1970. STEC HUS respond to?

Harrison's 20th Ed. Chapter 311 Page 2165

A. Plasma exchange
B. Prednisone
C. Rituximab
D. None of the above

STEC HUS should be treated with supportive measures as plasma exchange is not effective.

1971. Which of the following is approved for use in aHUS?
Harrison's 20th Ed. Chapter 311 Page 2165

A. Golimumab
B. Bevacizumab
C. Eculizumab
D. Certolizumab pegol

Eculizumab is a monoclonal antibody to C5 that is approved for use in aHUS.

1972. Neuraminidase-associated HUS respond to?
Harrison's 20th Ed. Chapter 311 Page 2165

A. Antibiotics
B. Washed red cells
C. Plasmapheresis
D. All of the above

Antibiotics, washed red cells & plasmapheresis may be helpful in neuraminidase-associated HUS.

1973. Hematopoietic stem cell transplantation associated thrombotic microangiopathy (HSCT-TMA) usually occurs within how many days of HSCT?
Harrison's 20th Ed. Chapter 311 Page 2165

A. First 10 days
B. First 100 days
C. First 300 days
D. First 500 days

HSCT-TMA usually occurs within the first 100 days of HSCT.

1974. The incidence of HSCT-TMA developing after HSCT is?
Harrison's 20th Ed. Chapter 311 Page 2165

A. ~ 2%
B. ~ 4%
C. ~ 6%
D. ~ 8%

HSCT-TMA develops after HSCT, with an incidence of ~8%.

1975. Which of the following variables is not included in criteria for establishing microangiopathic kidney injury associated with HSCT by International Working Group?
Harrison's 20th Ed. Chapter 311 Page 2165 Table 311-1

A. Schistocytes in the blood
B. LDH concentration
C. Haptoglobin concentration
D. Coombs test

1976. Scleroderma renal crisis (SRC) includes?
Harrison's 20th Ed. Chapter 311 Page 2166

A. Accelerated hypertension
B. Rapid deterioration in renal function
C. Nephrotic proteinuria
D. All of the above

SRC is a rapid deterioration in renal function, usually accompanied by accelerated hypertension, oliguria, nephrotic range proteinuria, hematuria, fluid retention, microangiopathic hemolytic anemia, retinopathy and encephalopathy.

1977. Which of the following is rare in scleroderma renal crisis?
Harrison's 20th Ed. Chapter 311 Page 2166

A. Pericarditis
B. Retinopathy
C. Coagulopathy
D. Pulmonary edema

MAHA is present in > 50% patients of SRC, coagulopathy is rare.

1978. Renal lesion in scleroderma renal crisis is characterized by?
Harrison's 20th Ed. Chapter 311 Page 2166

A. Arcuate artery intimal proliferation
B. Arcuate artery medial proliferation
C. Luminal narrowing
D. All of the above

Renal lesion in scleroderma renal crisis is characterized by arcuate artery intimal and medial proliferation with luminal narrowing, described as "onion-skinning" and can be accompanied by glomerular collapse due to reduced blood flow.

1979. Onion-skin pattern best relates to?
Harrison's 20th Ed. Chapter 311 Page 2166

A. Intimal proliferation
B. Medial proliferation
C. Luminal narrowing
D. Hyalinosis

Patients with scleroderma renal crisis show acute fibrinoid necrosis of afferent arterioles, followed by intimal proliferation (onion-skin pattern), and ischemic collapse of glomeruli.

1980. Histologically, scleroderma renal crisis is indistinguishable from?
Harrison's 20th Ed. Chapter 311 Page 2166

A. Radiation nephropathy
B. HSCT-TMA
C. Malignant hypertension
D. HIV-related TMA

Histologically, scleroderma renal crisis is indistinguishable from malignant hypertension.

1981. Which of the following antibodies are strongly associated with scleroderma renal disease?
Harrison's 20th Ed. Chapter 311 Page 2166

A. P-ANCA
B. Smooth-muscle antibody (SMA)
C. anti-Jo-1 antibody
D. Anti-U3-RNP

Anti-U3-RNP antibodies are strongly associated with scleroderma renal disease. Anticentromere antibody is a negative predictor of this disorder.

1982. Which of the following is used for blood pressure management & improvement of renal perfusion in scleroderma renal crisis?
Harrison's 20th Ed. Chapter 311 Page 2166

A. Epoprostenol
B. Iloprost
C. Treprostinil
D. All of the above

Iloprost, epoprostenol & treprostinil are prostacyclin analogues.

1983. Which of the following is an antiphospholipid antibody?
Harrison's 20th Ed. Chapter 311 Page 2166

A. Anticardiolipin antibodies (IgG, IgM, IgA)
B. Lupus anticoagulant
C. Anti-β-2 glycoprotein I antibodies (antiβ2GPI)
D. All of the above

Patients with both anticardiolipin antibodies and antiβ2GPI have the highest risk of thrombosis.

1984. Anticardiolipin antibodies may belong to which of the following class of immunoglobulins?
Harrison's 20th Ed. Chapter 311 Page 2166

A. IgG
B. IgM
C. IgA
D. All of the above

1985. Which of the following is unusual in antiphospholipid syndrome?
Harrison's 20th Ed. Chapter 311 Page 2166

A. Systemic thrombosis (arterial and venous)
B. Fetal morbidity
C. Arteriosclerosis
D. Microangiopathic hemolytic anemia (MAHA)

In antiphospholipid syndrome, signs of MAHA and platelet consumption are usually absent.

1986. Which of the following is false about treatment in antiphospholipid syndrome?
Harrison's 20th Ed. Chapter 311 Page 2166

A. Lifelong anticoagulation
B. Glucocorticoids may be beneficial in accelerated hypertension
C. Immunosuppression and plasma exchange may be helpful
D. None of the above

1987. Which of the following about HELLP syndrome is false?
Harrison's 20th Ed. Chapter 311 Page 2166

A. Occurs in 0.2–0.9% of all pregnancies
B. Occurs in 10–20% of women with severe preeclampsia
C. Carries a mortality rate of 7.4–34%
D. None of the above

1988. Which of the following about HELLP syndrome is false?
Harrison's 20th Ed. Chapter 311 Page 2166

A. Most commonly develops in the third trimester
B. 10% of cases occur before week 27 of gestation
C. 30% cases occur post-partum
D. None of the above

1989. Risk factor HELLP syndrome is?
Harrison's 20th Ed. Chapter 311 Page 2166

A. Elevated levels of fetal mRNA for FLT1
B. Elevated levels of endoglin
C. Abnormal placentation
D. All of the above

1990. Patients with HELLP syndrome have higher levels of?
Harrison's 20th Ed. Chapter 311 Page 2166

A. C-reactive protein
B. IL-1 Ra
C. IL-6
D. All of the above

HELLP syndrome risk factors include abnormal placentation, family history, and elevated levels of fetal mRNA for FLT1 (vascular endothelial growth factor receptor 1) and endoglin. Patients with HELLP syndrome have higher levels of inflammatory markers (C-reactive protein, IL-1Ra, and IL-6) and soluble HLADR than do those with preeclampsia alone.

1991. Organ that defines HELLP syndrome is?
Harrison's 20th Ed. Chapter 311 Page 2166

A. Kidney
B. Lung
C. Liver
D. Brain

Although renal failure is common, the organ that defines HELLP syndrome is the liver.

1992. Potentially life-threatening complication of HELLP syndrome is?
Harrison's 20th Ed. Chapter 311 Page 2167

A. Spontaneous rupture of the liver
B. Cerebral infarction
C. Cerebral and brainstem hemorrhage
D. All of the above

In HELLP syndrome, subcapsular hepatic hematomas may produce spontaneous rupture of liver and can be life threatening.

1993. Which of the following is a complication of HELLP syndrome?
Harrison's 20th Ed. Chapter 311 Page 2167

A. Placental abruption
B. Permanent vision loss
C. Bleeding
D. All of the above

HELLP syndrome, nonfatal complications include placental abruption, permanent vision loss due to Purtscher-like retinopathy (hemorrhagic & vaso-occlusive vasculopathy), pulmonary edema, bleeding, and fetal demise.

1994. Which of the following can be triggered by pregnancy?
Harrison's 20th Ed. Chapter 311 Page 2167

A. HELLP syndrome
B. aHUS
C. TTP
D. All of the above

1995. Which of the following is false in HELLP syndrome?
Harrison's 20th Ed. Chapter 311 Page 2167

A. Serum levels of ADAMTS13 activity are reduced
B. Levels of antithrombin III are reduced
C. Levels of D-dimer are elevated
D. None of the above

Antithrombin III levels are decreased in HELLP syndrome (but not in TTP) and D-dimer levels are elevated in HELLP syndrome but not in TTP.

1996. Which of the following is a myeloproliferative neoplasm (MPN)?
Harrison's 20th Ed. Chapter 311 Page 2167

A. Chronic myelogenous leukemia (CML)
B. Polycythemia vera (PV)
C. Essential thrombocythemia (ET)
D. All of the above

1997. Which of the following is a myeloproliferative neoplasm (MPN)?
Harrison's 20th Ed. Chapter 311 Page 2167

A. Primary myelofibrosis (PMF)
B. Systemic mastocytosis
C. Chronic eosinophilic leukemia
D. All of the above

MPN represents a group of clonal disorders that includes chronic myelogenous leukemia (CML), polycythemia vera (PV), essential thrombocythemia (ET), primary myelofibrosis (PMF), systemic mastocytosis, chronic eosinophilic leukemia not otherwise specified, chronic neutrophilic leukemia, and unclassifiable MPN.

1998. Median time from diagnosis of MPN to MPN-related glomerulopathy is?
Harrison's 20th Ed. Chapter 311 Page 2167

A. ~ 1 year
B. ~ 3 years
C. ~ 5 years
D. ~ 7 years

MPN-related glomerulopathy usually occurs late in the course of the hematologic condition and median time from diagnosis of MPN to glomerulopathy is ~7.2 years.

1999. In POEMS syndrome, "O" stands for?
Harrison's 20th Ed. Chapter 311 Page 2167

A. Obesity
B. Organomegaly
C. Obstructive jaundice
D. Oliguria

POEMS syndrome is a systemic disease characterized by polyneuropathy, organomegaly, endocrinopathy, monoclonal gammopathy, and skin changes.

2000. Which of the following is the hallmark of POEMS syndrome?
Harrison's 20th Ed. Chapter 311 Page 2167

A. Peripheral neuropathy
B. Skin changes
C. Endocrinopathy
D. Monoclonal gammopathy

Peripheral neuropathy with severe motorsensory deficit is the hallmark of POEMS syndrome.

2001. In POEMS syndrome, majority of monoclonal light chain is of which isotype?
Harrison's 20th Ed. Chapter 311 Page 2167

A. Kappa
B. Lambda
C. Gamma
D. Theta

In POEMS syndrome, >95% of mono clonal light chain is of the lambda isotype. IgA also makes up about 50% of the monoclonal protein.

2002. Which of the following about POEMS syndrome is false?
Harrison's 20th Ed. Chapter 311 Page 2167

A. IgA constitutes ~50% of monoclonal protein
B. Lymphadenopathy is common
C. Unilateral hypertrophy of kidney frequent
D. None of the above

2003. Which of the following about POEMS syndrome is false?
Harrison's 20th Ed. Chapter 311 Page 2167

A. Glomerulomegaly
B. Low grade proteinuria
C. Progression to end stage renal disease is rare
D. None of the above

2004. Renal complications in sickle cell disease is due to occlusion of?
Harrison's 20th Ed. Chapter 311 Page 2167

A. Afferent arteriole
B. Efferent arteriole
C. Glomeruli
D. Vasa recta

Renal complications in sickle cell disease result from occlusion of the vasa recta in the renal medulla.

2005. Which of the following occur in sickle cell disease?
Harrison's 20th Ed. Chapter 311 Page 2167

A. Hyposthenuria
B. Hematuria
C. Papillary necrosis
D. All of the above

2006. Which of the following is true about sickle cell disease?
Harrison's 20th Ed. Chapter 311 Page 2167

A. Hypertension is uncommon
B. Glomeruli are typically enlarged
C. More prone to acute renal failure
D. All of the above

2007. Renal vein thrombosis can occur in?
Harrison's 20th Ed. Chapter 311 Page 2167

A. Antiphospholipid syndrome
B. Nephrotic syndrome
C. Proteins C, S and antithrombin deficiency
D. All of the above

2008. Renal vein thrombosis can occur in?
Harrison's 20th Ed. Chapter 311 Page 2167

A. Factor V Leiden
B. Disseminated malignancy
C. Oral contraceptives
D. All of the above

2009. Nephrotic syndrome due to which of the following predisposes to renal vein thrombosis?
Harrison's 20th Ed. Chapter 311 Page 2167

A. Minimal change disease
B. Membranous nephropathy
C. Membranoproliferative glomerulonephritis
D. Lupus nephropathy

Nephrotic syndrome due to membranous nephropathy predisposes to renal vein thrombosis.

2010. Which of the following threaten blood supply of the kidney?

N Engl J Med. 2009;361:1972-8

A. Fibromuscular diseases
B. Inflammatory disorders
C. Primary hematologic disorders
D. All of the above

Disorders that threaten blood supply of kidney include large vessel atherosclerosis, fibromuscular diseases, embolic, inflammatory, and primary hematologic disorders.

2011. Large-vessel renal artery occlusive disease result most commonly from?

N Engl J Med. 2009;361:1972-8

A. Extrinsic compression of the vessel
B. Fibromuscular dysplasias
C. Atherosclerotic disease
D. None of the above

Large vessel renal artery occlusive disease results most commonly from atherosclerotic disease and also from extrinsic compression of the vessel and fibromuscular dysplasias.

2012. What percentage of cases of hypertension are caused by renal artery stenosis (RAS)?

N Engl J Med. 2009;361:1972-8

A. ~ 1%
B. ~ 5%
C. ~ 7%
D. ~ 10%

~5% of cases of hypertension are caused by renal artery stenosis (RAS).

2013. Which of the following is not a characteristic of renal artery stenosis due to fibromuscular dysplasia?

N Engl J Med. 2009;361:1972-8

A. Usually young (<40 yr)
B. Usually male
C. Middle or distal lesion location
D. Good BP response to revascularization

Patients of RAS due to fibromuscular dysplasia are usually female (15–50 yrs).

2014. The clinical clues for the diagnosis of renal-artery stenosis include all except?

N Engl J Med. 2009;361:1972-8

A. Onset of stage 2 hypertension >30 years of age
B. Absence of family history of hypertension
C. Hypertension associated with renal insufficiency
D. Renal function worsens after ACE inhibitors

Classic clinical clues that suggest the diagnosis of RAS are onset of stage 2 hypertension (BP>160/100 mm Hg) after 50 years of age, absence of family history of HTN, HTN with renal insufficiency, renal function worsens after administration of renin–angiotensin–aldosterone system blocker, HTN with repeated hospital admissions for heart failure, and drug-resistant hypertension.

2015. Which of the following diagnostic imaging tests for renal-artery stenosis provide best image quality & anatomical information?

N Engl J Med. 2009;361:1972-8

A. Duplex ultrasonography
B. Magnetic resonance angiography
C. Computed tomographic angiography
D. Digital-subtraction angiography

2016. Which of the following is termed as renal enzyme?

N Engl J Med. 2009;361:1972-8

A. Serum aspartate aminotransferase (AST)
B. Serum lactate dehydrogenase (LDH)
C. Serum alkaline phosphatase
D. All of the above

Renal enzymes elevated in renal infarction are aspartate aminotransferase (AST), lactate dehydrogenase (LDH), and alkaline phosphatase.

2017. Most common cause of cholesterol crystal embolization in atheroembolic renal disease is?

N Engl J Med. 2009;361:1972-8

A. Vascular surgery
B. Arteriography
C. Anticoagulation with heparin
D. Thrombolytic therapy

Arteriographic procedures are the most common cause of cholesterol crystal embolization in atheroembolic renal disease.

2018. Which of the following is rare in cholesterol crystal embolization in atheroembolic renal disease?

N Engl J Med. 2009;361:1972-8

A. Livedo reticularis
B. "Purple" toes
C. Toe gangrene
D. Renal infarction

Renal infarction secondary to cholesterol embolization is rare.

2019. Lab. findings in cholesterol crystal embolization in atheroembolic renal disease include all except?

N Engl J Med. 2009;361:1972-8

A. Rising blood urea nitrogen & creatinine
B. Eosinopenia
C. Anemia
D. Hypocomplementemia

Lab. findings in cholesterol crystal embolization in atheroembolic renal disease include rising BUN & creatinine, eosinophilia, eosinophiluria, leukocytosis, elevated ESR, anemia & hypocomplementemia.

2020. Which of the following approaches in atheroembolic renal disease is not beneficial?

N Engl J Med. 2009;361:1972-8

A. Anticoagulation
B. Cholesterol-lowering agents
C. Steroid therapy
D. All of the above

Withdrawal of anticoagulation may be beneficial.

2021. In 'Benign arteriolar nephrosclerosis' the characteristic pathology 'Hyaline arteriolosclerosis' is in?

N Engl J Med. 2009;361:1972-8

A. Afferent arterioles
B. Capillaries
C. Efferent arterioles
D. All of the above

Characteristic pathology of arteriolar nephrosclerosis is in afferent arterioles that have thickened walls & narrowing of vascular lumen due to deposition of homogeneous eosinophilic material (hyaline arteriolosclerosis) resulting in ischemic injury to glomeruli & tubules.

2022. 'Flea-bitten appearance' of kidneys is seen in?

N Engl J Med. 2009;361:1972-8

A. Malignant arteriolar nephrosclerosis
B. Hemolytic uremic syndrome (HUS)
C. Thrombotic thrombocytopenic purpura (TTP)
D. All of the above

Flea-bitten appearance of kidneys is due to hemorrhages in surface capillaries.

2023. Which of the following is false regarding "onion-skin lesion"?

N Engl J Med. 2009;361:1972-8

A. Seen in malignant arteriolar nephrosclerosis
B. Involves interlobular arteries
C. Hyperplastic arteriolitis
D. None of the above

2024. In the natural course of malignant hypertension, death is almost always due to?

N Engl J Med. 2009;361:1972-8

A. CHF
B. Ischemic heart disease
C. Cerebrovascular accident
D. Uremia

Malignant hypertension is a medical emergency. Its natural course includes a death rate of 80–90% within 1 year of onset, almost always due to uremia.

2025. Acute bilateral cortical necrosis is associated with?

N Engl J Med. 2009;361:1972-8

A. Septic abortion
B. Abruptio placentae
C. Preeclampsia
D. All of the above

Acute bilateral cortical necrosis is associated with septic abortions, abruptio placentae & preeclampsia.

Nephrolithiasis

2026. Which of the following kidney stones are most common?
Harrison's 20th Ed. Chapter 312 Page 2168

A. Calcium oxalate
B. Calcium phosphate
C. Uric acid
D. Struvite

2027. Which of the following kidney stones is least common?
Harrison's 20th Ed. Chapter 312 Page 2168

A. Calcium oxalate
B. Calcium phosphate
C. Uric acid
D. Struvite

Calcium oxalate kidney stones are most common (~75%) followed by calcium phosphate (~15%), uric acid (~8%), struvite (~1%) and cystine (<1%).

2028. Kidney stones may be composed of which of the following medications?
Harrison's 20th Ed. Chapter 312 Page 2168

A. Acyclovir
B. Atazanavir
C. Triamterene
D. All of the above

Stones may be composed of medications like acyclovir, atazanavir and triamterene.

2029. Struvite best relates to?
Harrison's 20th Ed. Chapter 312 Page 2168

A. Calcium phosphate
B. Magnesium ammonium phosphate
C. Calcium oxalate dihydrate
D. Calcium oxalate monohydrate

2030. Apatite best relates to?
Harrison's 20th Ed. Chapter 312 Page 2168

A. Calcium phosphate
B. Magnesium ammonium phosphate
C. Calcium oxalate dihydrate
D. Calcium oxalate monohydrate

The main constituent of calcium stones is brushite (calcium hydrogen phosphate) or hydroxyapatite. Calcium oxalate crystals are of two types — the dihydrate (or Wedellite) and the monohydrate (or Whewellite).

2031. Which of the following duct is related to nephron?
Harrison's 20th Ed. Chapter 81 Page 616

A. Duct of Wirsung
B. Duct of Luschka
C. Duct of Rivinus
D. Duct of Bellini

2032. Which of the following about supersaturation (SS) is false?
Harrison's 20th Ed. Chapter 312 Page 2168

A. Driving force for crystallization in urine
B. Ratio of the concentration of dissolved salt to its solubility
C. Used to monitor response to medical & dietary interventions for stone prevention
D. None of the above

Supersaturation (SS) is the driving force for crystallization in urine and is defined as ratio of the concentration of dissolved salt to its solubility. The consequences of increased urinary SS are formation of crystalline particles that is the forerunner to stone formation. SSs are also used to monitor response to medical and dietary interventions for stone prevention.

2033. "Recurrent stone former" is defined as an increase in stone size during past?
Harrison's 20th Ed. Chapter 312 Page 2168

A. 1 year
B. 5 years
C. 10 years
D. 15 years

"Recurrent stone former" was defined as either a recurrent stone event or an increase in the stone size during the past five years confirmed by imaging modalities.

2034. Which of the following about nephrolithiasis is false?
Harrison's 20th Ed. Chapter 312 Page 2168

A. 19% men & 9% women will develop at least one stone in life
B. Prevalence is lower among black individuals than whites
C. Among white men, peak annual incidence at age 40
D. None of the above

2035. Which of the following about nephrolithiasis is false?
Harrison's 20th Ed. Chapter 312 Page 2168

A. Global disease
B. Systemic disorder
C. Incidence varies by age, sex, and race
D. None of the above

2036. Which of the following conditions predispose to stone formation?
Harrison's 20th Ed. Chapter 312 Page 2168

A. Crohn's disease
B. Gastric bypass surgery
C. Type 2 diabetes mellitus
D. All of the above

2037. Which of the following conditions predispose to stone formation?
Harrison's 20th Ed. Chapter 312 Page 2168

A. Gout
B. Cholelithiasis
C. Reduced bone mineral density
D. All of the above

Conditions that predispose to stone formation are Crohn's disease, gastric bypass surgery, primary hyperparathyroidism, obesity, type 2 diabetes mellitus and distal renal tubular acidosis. Medical conditions that are more likely to be present in individuals with a history of nephrolithiasis are hypertension, gout, cholelithiasis, reduced bone mineral density and chronic kidney disease.

2038. Term "pus under pressure" best relates to?
Harrison's 20th Ed. Chapter 312 Page 2168

A. Infected subcapsular renal infarct
B. Urinary tract infection in the setting of an obstructing stone
C. Urinary stone and renal papillary necrosis
D. All of the above

Nephrolithiasis does not directly cause upper urinary tract infections (UTIs). UTI in the setting of an obstructing stone is a urologic emergency and is referred to as "pus under pressure".

2039. Clinically, most important inhibitor of crystallization of calcium-containing stones is?
Harrison's 20th Ed. Chapter 312 Page 2168

A. Urine ammonia
B. Urine bicarbonate
C. Urine citrate
D. Urine phosphate

Clinically, most important inhibitor of calcium-containing stones is urine citrate.

2040. Renal biopsies of stone formers show which of the following?
Harrison's 20th Ed. Chapter 312 Page 2168

A. Calcium phosphate in the renal interstitium
B. Calcium phosphate in the renal glomerular mesangium
C. Calcium phosphate in the renal vessels
D. All of the above

Renal biopsies of stone formers reveal calcium phosphate in the renal interstitium.

2041. As an initial event, calcium phosphate deposits at?
Harrison's 20th Ed. Chapter 312 Page 2168

A. Thin limb of the loop of Henle
B. Thick limb of the loop of Henle
C. Distal convoluted tubuls
D. Collecting duct

It is hypothesized that as an initial event calcium phosphate deposits at the thin limb of loop of Henle, and then extends down to papilla and erodes through papillary epithelium, where it provides a site for deposition of calcium oxalate & calcium phosphate crystals.

2042. Randall's plaque best relates to?
Harrison's 20th Ed. Chapter 312 Page 2168

A. Renal interstitium
B. Renal papilla
C. Renal glomerulus
D. Renal vessels

Majority of calcium oxalate stones grow on calcium phosphate at the tip of renal papilla (Randall's plaque).

2043. Dietary factors that are associated with an increased risk of nephrolithiasis include all except?
Harrison's 20th Ed. Chapter 312 Page 2168

A. Dietary oxalate
B. Dietary sodium
C. Dietary calcium
D. Dietary sucrose

2044. Dietary factor associated with a lower risk of nephrolithiasis is?
Harrison's 20th Ed. Chapter 312 Page 2168

A. Calcium
B. Potassium
C. Phytate
D. All of the above

Dietary factors that are associated with an increased risk of nephrolithiasis include animal protein, oxalate, sodium, sucrose and fructose. Dietary factors associated with a lower risk include calcium, potassium and phytate. Higher dietary calcium intake is related to a lower risk of stone formation. Reduction in risk associated with higher calcium intake may be due to a reduction in intestinal absorption of dietary oxalate that results in lower urine oxalate.

2045. Which of the following increases the risk of stone formation?
Harrison's 20th Ed. Chapter 312 Page 2169

A. Vitamin C supplements
B. Sugar-sweetened carbonated beverage consumption
C. Higher intake of animal protein
D. All of the above

2046. Higher intake of animal protein leads to?
Harrison's 20th Ed. Chapter 312 Page 2169

A. Increased excretion of calcium
B. Increased excretion of uric acid
C. Decreased urinary excretion of citrate
D. All of the above

2047. Which of the following reduces risk of renal stones in type 1 primary hyperoxaluria?
Harrison's 20th Ed. Chapter 312 Page 2169

A. Supplemental vitamin B1
B. Supplemental vitamin B3
C. Supplemental vitamin B6
D. Supplemental vitamin B12

High doses of supplemental vitamin B6 may be beneficial in selected patients with type 1 primary hyperoxaluria, the risk is not reduced in other patients.

2048. Which of the following is false about renal stones?
Harrison's 20th Ed. Chapter 312 Page 2169

A. Risk increases as urine volume decreases
B. Higher dietary Ca^{++} intake lowers risk of stone formation
C. Urinary oxalate is a risk factor for Ca^{++} oxalate stone formation
D. Lower urine citrate excretion decreases the risk

When the urine output is <1 L/day, the risk of stone formation more than doubles. Lower urine volume results in higher concentrations of lithogenic factors and is a common & readily modifiable risk factor. Lower urine citrate excretion increases the risk.

2049. Which of the following is false about renal stones?
Harrison's 20th Ed. Chapter 312 Page 2169

A. Higher potassium intake decreases calcium excretion
B. Higher sodium & sucrose intake increases calcium excretion
C. Magnesium & phytate lower renal stone risk include
D. Higher urine uric acid increases risk of Ca^{++} oxalate stones

Higher urine levels of uric acid is a risk factor for uric acid stone formation but is not associated with the risk of calcium oxalate stone formation.

2050. Which of the following reduces risk of renal stones?
Harrison's 20th Ed. Chapter 312 Page 2169

A. Tea
B. Beer
C. Orange juice
D. All of the above

Coffee, tea, beer, wine, and orange juice are associated with a reduced risk of renal stone formation.

2051. Which of the following about urine pH and kidney stones is false?

Harrison's 20th Ed. Chapter 312 Page 2169

A. Uric acid stones form when urine pH is consistently ≤ 5.5
B. Ca^{++} phosphate stones form when urine pH is ≥ 6.5
C. Ca^{++} oxalate stones are not influenced by urine pH
D. None of the above

2052. Which of the following disorders cause nephrolithiasis?

Harrison's 20th Ed. Chapter 312 Page 2169

A. Hartnup disorder
B. Homocystinuria
C. Cystinuria
D. Dent disease

Two most common monogenic disorders that lead to kidney stone formation are primary hyperoxaluria and cystinuria.

2053. Which of the following about primary hyperoxaluria is false?

Harrison's 20th Ed. Chapter 312 Page 2169

A. Autosomal recessive disorder
B. Excessive endogenous oxalate generation by liver
C. Ca^{++} oxalate stone formation & crystal deposition in organs
D. None of the above

Primary hyperoxaluria is an autosomal recessive disorder that causes excessive endogenous oxalate generation by liver, with consequent calcium oxalate stone formation and crystal deposition in organs.

2054. Which of the following about cystinuria is false?

Harrison's 20th Ed. Chapter 312 Page 2169

A. Autosomal recessive disorder
B. Abnormal reabsorption of filtered basic amino acids
C. Excessive urinary excretion of cysteine
D. Cysteine stones are visible on plain radiographs and often manifest as staghorn calculi or multiple bilateral stones

Cystinuria is an autosomal recessive disorder that causes abnormal reabsorption of filtered basic amino acids. The excessive urinary excretion of cystine, which is poorly soluble, leads to cystine stone formation. Cystine stones are visible on plain radiographs and often manifest as staghorn calculi or multiple bilateral stones.

2055. Which of the following is a common presentation for individuals with an acute stone event?

Harrison's 20th Ed. Chapter 312 Page 2169

A. Syncope
B. Painless gross hematuria
C. Urinary urgency
D. Urinary burning

2056. Which of the following is false about renal colic?

Harrison's 20th Ed. Chapter 312 Page 2169

A. Sudden onset of unilateral flank pain
B. No alleviating factors
C. Accompanied by nausea and vomiting
D. None of the above

2057. Differential diagnosis of renal colic include?

Harrison's 20th Ed. Chapter 312 Page 2170

A. Acute cholecystitis
B. Acute appendicitis
C. Acute diverticulitis
D. All of the above

2058. Urinary urgency and frequency appear when the renal stone lodges at?

Harrison's 20th Ed. Chapter 312 Page 2170

A. Ureteral pelvic junction
B. Pelvic brim
C. Ureterovesical junction
D. All of the above

If the stone lodges in ureter at ureterovesical junction, patient experiences urinary urgency & frequency.

2059. Renal colic may be confused as acute diverticulitis when the stone lodges at?

Harrison's 20th Ed. Chapter 312 Page 2170

A. Ureteral pelvic junction
B. Pelvic brim
C. Ureterovesical junction
D. All of the above

2060. Renal colic may be confused as acute appendicitis when the stone lodges at?

Harrison's 20th Ed. Chapter 312 Page 2170

A. Ureteral pelvic junction
B. Pelvic brim
C. Ureterovesical junction
D. All of the above

2061. Which of the following stone is radiolucent?

Harrison's 20th Ed. Chapter 312 Page 2170

A. Calcium
B. Cystine
C. Struvite
D. Uric acid

Calcium, cystine & struvite stones are radiopaque on standard X-rays. Uric acid stones are radiolucent.

2062. The "gold standard" diagnostic test in nephrolithiasis is?

Harrison's 20th Ed. Chapter 312 Page 2170

A. Helical CT without contrast
B. Helical CT with contrast
C. Renal ultrasound
D. MRI

The "gold standard" diagnostic test in nephrolithiasis is helical CT without contrast. Helical CT detects stones as small as 1 mm.

2063. In helical CT, which of the following is the evidence of recent passage of a ureteral stone?

Harrison's 20th Ed. Chapter 312 Page 2170

A. Irregular ureteral lumen
B. Irregular urinary bladder neck
C. Perinephric stranding
D. All of the above

2064. In helical CT, which of the following is the evidence of recent passage of a ureteral stone?

Harrison's 20th Ed. Chapter 312 Page 2170

A. Irregular ureteral peristalsis
B. Hydronephrosis
C. Vesicoureteral reflux
D. All of the above

Helical CT reveals ureteral stone or evidence of recent passage (perinephric stranding or hydronephrosis).

2065. Use of which of the following may increase the rate of spontaneous renal stone passage?

Harrison's 20th Ed. Chapter 312 Page 2170

A. Alpha blocker
B. Beta blocker
C. NSAID
D. PDE-5 inhibitor

Use of alpha blockers (tamsulosin) may increase the rate of spontaneous renal stone passage.

2066. Renal stones of what size have a low probability of spontaneous passage?

Harrison's 20th Ed. Chapter 312 Page 2170

A. ≥ 3 mm
B. ≥ 6 mm
C. ≥ 8 mm
D. ≥ 10 mm

Renal stones measuring ≥ 6 mm have a low probability of spontaneous passage.

2067. Which of the following states suggest a low probability of spontaneous passage of renal stones?

Harrison's 20th Ed. Chapter 312 Page 2170

A. Renal stone measuring ≥ 6 mm
B. An urological anatomic abnormality
C. Intractable pain
D. All of the above

2068. More than half of first-time stone formers will have a recurrence within?

Harrison's 20th Ed. Chapter 312 Page 2171

A. 3 years
B. 5 years
C. 7 years
D. 10 years

More than half of first-time stone formers will have a recurrence within 10 years.

2069. Which of the following is a high-oxalate food?

Harrison's 20th Ed. Chapter 312 Page 2171

A. Spinach
B. Rhubarb
C. Potatoes
D. All of the above

High-oxalate foods are spinach, rhubarb, almonds, and potatoes.

2070. Levels of which of the following must be measured in concert with PTH?

Harrison's 20th Ed. Chapter 312 Page 2171

A. Calcium
B. Phosphorus
C. 25-hydroxy vitamin D
D. Uric acid

Elevated serum levels of parathyroid hormone (PTH) and a normal 25-hydroxy vitamin D level is rare. 25-hydroxy vitamin D is measured in concert with PTH to investigate the possible role of secondarily elevated PTH levels in the setting of vitamin D insufficiency. Similarly, primary renal Ca^{++} loss with lower serum Ca^{++} concentrations is rare.

2071. Which of the following renal stones can be identified by low Hounsfield units on CT?

Harrison's 20th Ed. Chapter 312 Page 2171

A. Calcium oxalate
B. Calcium phosphate
C. Uric acid
D. Struvite

Pure uric acid stones can be identified by low Hounsfield units on CT.

2072. Which of the following statements is false?

Harrison's 20th Ed. Chapter 312 Page 2171

A. ↑ed urine Ca^{++} excretion causes ↑ed absorption of ingested Ca^{++}
B. Crystalluria is a strong risk factor for new stone formation
C. Consistently diluted urine reduces likelihood of crystal formation
D. None of the above

Calcium oxalate dihydrate crystals are bipyramidally shaped, and cystine crystals are hexagonal

2073. For prevention of stone formation, urine volume should be?

Harrison's 20th Ed. Chapter 312 Page 2171

A. 1 liter per day
B. 2 liters per day
C. 3 liters per day
D. 4 liters per day

Urine volume goal is of 2 L/day for prevention of stone formation.

2074. Risk factor for calcium oxalate stones is?

Harrison's 20th Ed. Chapter 312 Page 2171

A. Higher urine calcium
B. Higher urine oxalate
C. Lower urine citrate
D. All of the above

Risk factors for calcium oxalate stones include higher urine calcium, higher urine oxalate, and lower urine citrate. This stone type is insensitive to pH in physiologic range.

2075. What quantity of calcium is recommended for a patient with or history of calcium oxalate stone?

Harrison's 20th Ed. Chapter 312 Page 2172

A. 400 mg/day
B. 800 mg/day
C. 1200 mg/day
D. 1600 mg/day

In men with high urine calcium & recurrent calcium oxalate stones, a diet of 1200 mg/day of calcium with low intake of sodium & animal protein significantly reduced subsequent stone formation from that with a low-calcium diet (400 mg/day). Excessive calcium intake (>1200 mg/day) should be avoided.

2076. Which of the following can substantially lower urine calcium excretion?

Harrison's 20th Ed. Chapter 312 Page 2172

A. Furosemide
B. Thiazide
C. Triamterene
D. Spironolactone

Thiazide diuretic (chlorthalidone), in doses higher than those used to treat hypertension (with sodium restriction), can substantially lower urine calcium excretion and consequently can reduce calcium oxalate stone recurrence.

2077. Which of the following is the only known strategy that reduces endogenous oxalate production?

Harrison's 20th Ed. Chapter 312 Page 2172

A. Overhydration
B. Avoiding nondairy animal protein
C. Avoiding high-dose vitamin C supplements
D. All of the above

Avoiding high-dose vitamin C supplements is the only known strategy that reduces endogenous oxalate production.

2078. Which of the following about calcium phosphate renal stones is false?

Harrison's 20th Ed. Chapter 312 Page 2172

A. ↑ed occurrence with higher urine pH (≥ 6.5)
B. More common in patients with distal renal tubular acidosis
C. More common in patients with primary hyperparathyroidism
D. None of the above

2079. Nephrocalcinosis best relates to?

Harrison's 20th Ed. Chapter 312 Page 2172

A. Primary hyperparathyroidism
B. Type 1 RTA
C. Primary oxalosis
D. All of the above

Multiple papillary calcifications are called nephrocalcinosis.

2080. Main risk factors for uric acid stones is?

Harrison's 20th Ed. Chapter 312 Page 2172

A. Persistently low urine pH
B. Persistently high urine pH
C. Persistently normal urine pH
D. All of the above

Two main risk factors for uric acid renal stones are persistently low urine pH & higher uric acid excretion.

2081. Mainstay of prevention of uric acid stone formation is?

Harrison's 20th Ed. Chapter 312 Page 2172

A. Avoiding nondairy animal protein
B. Increasing urine pH
C. Allopurinol therapy
D. All of the above

Mainstay of prevention of uric acid stone formation entails increasing urine pH. Recommended urine pH goal is of 6.5 throughout day and night.

2082. Which of the following drug increases cystine solubility and prevents cystine stone formation?

Harrison's 20th Ed. Chapter 312 Page 2172

A. Vitamin B6
B. Tiopronin
C. Terbinafine
D. Zinc

Tiopronin & penicillamine covalently bind to cystine.

2083. Which of the following are the most common cause of renal stones in children?

Harrison's 20th Ed. Chapter 414 Page 3022

A. Calcium oxalate
B. Calcium phosphate
C. Cystine
D. Struvite

Cystine stones account for 1–2% of all urinary tract calculi but are the most common cause of renal stones in children.

2084. Which of the following about struvite stones is false?

Harrison's 20th Ed. Chapter 312 Page 2172

A. Also known as infection stones or triple-phosphate stones
B. Grow quickly & fill the renal pelvis (staghorn calculi)
C. Form only when the upper urinary tract is infected with urease-producing bacteria
D. None of the above

2085. Which of the following renal stones form only when upper urinary tract is infected with urease-producing bacteria?

Harrison's 20th Ed. Chapter 312 Page 2172

A. Calcium oxalate
B. Calcium phosphate
C. Cystine
D. Struvite

Struvite stones, also known as infection stones or triple-phosphate stones, form only when the upper urinary tract is infected with urease-producing bacteria such as Proteus mirabilis, Klebsiella pneumoniae, or Providencia species. Urease produced by these bacteria hydrolyzes urea and may elevate the urine pH to a supraphysiologic level (>8.0).

2086. Infection due to bacteria that possess enzyme urease can cause stones composed of?

Harrison's 20th Ed. Chapter 312 Page 2172

A. Calcium
B. Cystine
C. Struvite
D. Uric acid

Infection due to bacteria that possess the enzyme urease can cause stones composed of struvite.

2087. Which of the following is false about 'Struvite stones'?

Harrison's 20th Ed. Chapter 312 Page 2172

A. Occur mainly in men
B. Occur in patients with chronic bladder catheterization
C. Due to UTI with urease-producing bacteria
D. May grow to produce a "staghorn" appearance

Struvite stones occur mainly in women.

2088. Which of the following is an urease inhibitor?
Harrison's 20th Ed. Chapter 312 Page 2172

A. Acetohydroxamic acid
B. Tranexamic acid
C. ε-aminocaproic acid
D. Pyroglutamic acid

2089. The element in 'Struvite' is?
Harrison's 20th Ed. Chapter 313 Page 2174

A. Calcium
B. Aluminium
C. Magnesium
D. Zinc

The chemical formula of struvite is Magnesium Ammonium Phosphate ($MgNH_4PO_4$).

2090. Causes of 'Hypercalciuria' include all except?
Harrison's 20th Ed. Chapter 403 Page 2932

A. Hypothyroidism
B. Cushing syndrome
C. Sarcoidosis
D. Immobilization

2091. Causes of 'Hypercalciuria' include?
Harrison's 20th Ed. Chapter 403 Page 2932

A. Vitamin D intoxication
B. Rapidly progressive bone disease
C. Paget's disease
D. All of the above

Hyperthyroidism, Cushing syndrome, sarcoidosis, malignant tumors, immobilization, vitamin D intoxication, rapidly progressive bone disease, and Paget's disease cause hypercalciuria.

2092. Basic constituents of most kidney stones include all except?
Nephrol Dial Transplant 1996;11:379-387

A. Alumina
B. Uric acid
C. Cystine
D. Struvite

2093. Urine crystals that are rectangular prisms and resemble 'coffin lids' are of?
Nephrol Dial Transplant 1996;11:379-387

A. Calcium
B. Uric acid
C. Cystine
D. Struvite

The typical shape of triple phosphate crystals is that of prisms ('coffin lid'), which are always strongly birefringent. Triple phosphate crystals are typical of infected urine, especially that caused by urea-splitting bacteria. For this reason they are frequently found also in patients with infected calculi.

2094. Urine crystals that are flat, rhomboidal shaped are of?
Nephrol Dial Transplant 1996;11:379-387

A. Calcium
B. Uric acid
C. Cystine
D. Struvite

Uric acid crystals are very pleiomorphic, but the amber coloured, constant polychromatic birefringence rhomboidal shape is the most frequent.

2095. Urine crystals that are rectangular prism shaped are of?
Nephrol Dial Transplant 1996;11:379-387

A. Calcium
B. Uric acid
C. Cystine
D. Struvite

2096. Urine crystals that are Hexagonal plate shaped are of?
Nephrol Dial Transplant 1996;11:379-387

A. Calcium
B. Uric acid
C. Cystine
D. Struvite

Cystine crystals precipitate as symmetrical hexagons, mostly aggregated, and are constantly birefringent.

2097. Urine crystals that are of dumbbell shape are of?
Nephrol Dial Transplant 1996;11:379-387

A. Calcium oxalate monohydrate
B. Calcium oxalate dihydrate
C. Cystine
D. Struvite

2098. Urine crystals that are of bipyramidal shape are of?
Nephrol Dial Transplant 1996;11:379-387

A. Calcium oxalate monohydrate
B. Calcium oxalate dihydrate
C. Calcium phosphate
D. Mixed calcium oxalate/uric acid

2099. Urine crystals that are of elongated, narrow shape are of?
Nephrol Dial Transplant 1996;11:379-387

A. Calcium oxalate monohydrate
B. Calcium oxalate dihydrate
C. Calcium phosphate
D. Mixed calcium oxalate/uric acid

Calcium phosphate crystals are pleiomorphic, appearing as birefringent stars or needles, in isolation or in clumps. Calcium phosphate crystals were the most frequent crystals in both normals and stone formers.

2100. 'Maltese crosses' urine crystals best relate to?
Nephrol Dial Transplant 1996;11:379-387

A. Acyclovir
B. Sulphadiazine
C. Triamterene
D. Primidone

Triamterene crystals are spherical & predominantly brown in colour, under polarized light they appear as 'Maltese crosses'. These crystals are associated with brown casts, which are also due to triamterene.

2101. Calcium oxalate monohydrate crystals in the urinary sediment are typical of?
N Engl J Med. 2006;354:1065-72

A. Antacid overdose
B. Ethylene glycol ingestion
C. Blunt abdominal trauma
D. Fat embolism

ANSWERS

1. C
2. D
3. B
4. D
5. B
6. D
7. C
8. B
9. C
10. D
11. D
12. B
13. C
14. A
15. D
16. C
17. B
18. B
19. A
20. A
21. A
22. A
23. D
24. D
25. D
26. D
27. B
28. A
29. D
30. C
31. D
32. B
33. B
34. D
35. D
36. D
37. A
38. B
39. B
40. D
41. D
42. D
43. D
44. D
45. A
46. D
47. B
48. D
49. C
50. B
51. D
52. D
53. D
54. D
55. C
56. D
57. D
58. D
59. B
60. D
61. B
62. D
63. D
64. D
65. C
66. C
67. C
68. D
69. D
70. C
71. A
72. A
73. A
74. D
75. D
76. B
77. C
78. D
79. D
80. C
81. D
82. D
83. D
84. A
85. A
86. D
87. C
88. D
89. D
90. D
91. A
92. C
93. B
94. D
95. B
96. D
97. B
98. D
99. D
100. D
101. D
102. D
103. C
104. D
105. D
106. B
107. A
108. B
109. C
110. B
111. C
112. C
113. B
114. A
115. A
116. D
117. D
118. A
119. C
120. D
121. D
122. B
123. C
124. D
125. B
126. C
127. D
128. B
129. A
130. C
131. D
132. D
133. D
134. B
135. D
136. D
137. A
138. D
139. B
140. C
141. D
142. C
143. A
144. A
145. B
146. B
147. C
148. D
149. D
150. C
151. D
152. D
153. A
154. D
155. B
156. B
157. B
158. A
159. D
160. A
161. B
162. C
163. D
164. D
165. B
166. A
167. D
168. C
169. D
170. D
171. A
172. B
173. D
174. C
175. A
176. D
177. A
178. C
179. D
180. D
181. B
182. D
183. C
184. A
185. D
186. C
187. A
188. D
189. D
190. D
191. D
192. B
193. C
194. B
195. D
196. C
197. D
198. B
199. D
200. D
201. A
202. B
203. D
204. C
205. A
206. D
207. B
208. D
209. A
210. B
211. C
212. B
213. B
214. D
215. D
216. D
217. D
218. C
219. D
220. D
221. D
222. D
223. D
224. D
225. A
226. B
227. B
228. D
229. D
230. A
231. D
232. D
233. D
234. D
235. C
236. A
237. D
238. A
239. D
240. D
241. D
242. D
243. D
244. D
245. D
246. D

ANSWERS

247. A
248. A
249. B
250. C
251. D
252. A
253. D
254. B
255. A
256. D
257. D
258. B
259. A
260. D
261. A
262. D
263. A
264. D
265. B
266. D
267. A
268. D
269. C
270. B
271. C
272. A
273. D
274. D
275. C
276. A
277. D
278. D
279. C
280. D
281. D
282. C
283. B
284. B
285. D
286. D
287. D
288. D
289. A
290. B
291. C
292. C
293. C
294. D
295. C
296. D
297. C
298. B
299. A
300. B
301. D
302. A
303. C
304. D
305. A
306. D
307. D
308. D
309. D
310. C
311. B
312. D
313. C
314. B
315. B
316. D
317. D
318. D
319. D
320. D
321. D
322. D
323. D
324. D
325. C
326. B
327. C
328. C
329. D
330. C
331. C
332. D
333. D
334. A
335. D
336. C
337. A
338. B
339. C
340. C
341. C
342. C
343. B
344. D
345. A
346. D
347. B
348. D
349. B
350. D
351. B
352. A
353. A
354. A
355. A
356. B
357. D
358. B
359. D
360. D
361. B
362. A
363. D
364. C
365. B
366. D
367. D
368. D
369. C
370. D
371. A
372. D
373. A
374. A
375. D
376. D
377. D
378. B
379. B
380. D
381. D
382. D
383. D
384. D
385. D
386. D
387. D
388. D
389. B
390. C
391. D
392. D
393. C
394. C
395. D
396. D
397. D
398. D
399. D
400. D
401. D
402. C
403. D
404. A
405. A
406. D
407. D
408. D
409. D
410. D
411. D
412. D
413. D
414. A
415. B
416. A
417. A
418. D
419. D
420. D
421. D
422. D
423. D
424. A
425. C
426. D
427. A
428. D
429. D
430. D
431. A
432. A
433. B
434. D
435. D
436. A
437. B
438. A
439. C
440. C
441. D
442. D
443. A
444. A
445. D
446. D
447. C
448. B
449. D
450. D
451. D
452. D
453. D
454. C
455. D
456. C
457. B
458. C
459. D
460. C
461. D
462. D
463. B
464. D
465. D
466. C
467. D
468. D
469. A
470. C
471. D
472. A
473. D
474. C
475. D
476. B
477. A
478. D
479. C
480. C
481. B
482. D
483. D
484. D
485. D
486. D
487. D
488. C
489. D
490. C
491. D
492. B

ANSWERS

493. B
494. D
495. D
496. C
497. C
498. D
499. D
500. D
501. A
502. D
503. B
504. B
505. D
506. B
507. B
508. B
509. B
510. B
511. B
512. D
513. D
514. D
515. D
516. D
517. B
518. C
519. D
520. D
521. D
522. C
523. D
524. D
525. A
526. D
527. B
528. D
529. D
530. D
531. D
532. D
533. B
534. C
535. D
536. C
537. D
538. D
539. D
540. D
541. D
542. A
543. D
544. C
545. C
546. D
547. B
548. C
549. D
550. D
551. A
552. D
553. D
554. A
555. D
556. D
557. B
558. B
559. B
560. B
561. C
562. D
563. B
564. D
565. B
566. B
567. C
568. A
569. D
570. D
571. B
572. B
573. D
574. D
575. A
576. D
577. D
578. D
579. D
580. D
581. A
582. B
583. C
584. C
585. D
586. C
587. B
588. C
589. C
590. A
591. D
592. C
593. C
594. A
595. C
596. B
597. D
598. A
599. D
600. A
601. D
602. B
603. A
604. C
605. D
606. B
607. C
608. A
609. B
610. C
611. D
612. C
613. D
614. C
615. B
616. D
617. D
618. A
619. D
620. C
621. D
622. A
623. A
624. D
625. D
626. D
627. A
628. C
629. D
630. D
631. D
632. D
633. C
634. B
635. A
636. A
637. D
638. D
639. D
640. A
641. C
642. C
643. D
644. D
645. D
646. D
647. C
648. A
649. A
650. D
651. A
652. C
653. C
654. A
655. D
656. B
657. D
658. C
659. C
660. A
661. D
662. A
663. C
664. D
665. B
666. A
667. A
668. D
669. D
670. C
671. D
672. D
673. C
674. B
675. C
676. B
677. B
678. D
679. B
680. A
681. D
682. D
683. C
684. C
685. D
686. D
687. D
688. A
689. C
690. D
691. D
692. D
693. B
694. C
695. D
696. D
697. D
698. C
699. B
700. A
701. A
702. B
703. C
704. D
705. C
706. A
707. D
708. D
709. D
710. D
711. B
712. D
713. D
714. A
715. D
716. D
717. D
718. C
719. D
720. D
721. D
722. D
723. C
724. D
725. D
726. D
727. A
728. C
729. A
730. D
731. B
732. B
733. D
734. B
735. D
736. D
737. C
738. D

ANSWERS

739. D
740. A
741. A
742. A
743. C
744. A
745. A
746. A
747. C
748. B
749. C
750. B
751. D
752. B
753. B
754. A
755. B
756. C
757. D
758. D
759. B
760. A
761. D
762. A
763. C
764. C
765. A
766. A
767. D
768. D
769. D
770. D
771. D
772. C
773. D
774. D
775. C
776. C
777. D
778. D
779. D
780. D
781. D
782. D
783. D
784. D
785. D
786. D
787. C
788. A
789. B
790. D
791. D
792. C
793. D
794. D
795. C
796. D
797. D
798. B
799. B
800. D
801. B
802. A
803. A
804. D
805. B
806. A
807. A
808. D
809. A
810. C
811. A
812. D
813. D
814. A
815. C
816. C
817. B
818. B
819. B
820. A
821. B
822. C
823. B
824. A
825. B
826. B
827. D
828. C
829. D
830. B
831. D
832. B
833. B
834. A
835. D
836. D
837. C
838. D
839. B
840. D
841. B
842. A
843. A
844. D
845. A
846. A
847. B
848. B
849. C
850. A
851. A
852. A
853. B
854. D
855. D
856. B
857. D
858. D
859. D
860. B
861. A
862. C
863. D
864. B
865. A
866. D
867. D
868. D
869. D
870. C
871. C
872. C
873. D
874. C
875. D
876. D
877. D
878. B
879. B
880. D
881. D
882. D
883. D
884. C
885. D
886. B
887. C
888. D
889. D
890. D
891. A
892. B
893. C
894. D
895. D
896. D
897. D
898. C
899. C
900. A
901. B
902. D
903. D
904. D
905. A
906. D
907. B
908. D
909. D
910. D
911. D
912. B
913. B
914. D
915. B
916. A
917. D
918. B
919. D
920. D
921. D
922. D
923. D
924. D
925. B
926. B
927. B
928. D
929. C
930. B
931. C
932. D
933. D
934. D
935. A
936. C
937. D
938. D
939. A
940. B
941. A
942. A
943. C
944. B
945. D
946. C
947. B
948. B
949. D
950. A
951. A
952. A
953. A
954. D
955. D
956. C
957. D
958. D
959. C
960. D
961. D
962. A
963. B
964. B
965. D
966. D
967. C
968. C
969. D
970. B
971. D
972. C
973. A
974. D
975. B
976. D
977. D
978. D
979. D
980. D
981. C
982. A
983. B
984. D

ANSWERS

985. A
986. A
987. D
988. A
989. B
990. D
991. D
992. D
993. C
994. D
995. D
996. C
997. D
998. D
999. B
1000. D
1001. D
1002. A
1003. D
1004. A
1005. D
1006. D
1007. B
1008. D
1009. D
1010. D
1011. C
1012. C
1013. A
1014. D
1015. D
1016. D
1017. B
1018. D
1019. D
1020. D
1021. D
1022. C
1023. C
1024. D
1025. D
1026. C
1027. A
1028. D
1029. D
1030. D
1031. D
1032. D
1033. D
1034. B
1035. D
1036. C
1037. D
1038. D
1039. D
1040. D
1041. D
1042. A
1043. D
1044. D
1045. B
1046. D
1047. B
1048. B
1049. A
1050. D
1051. D
1052. B
1053. D
1054. A
1055. C
1056. B
1057. A
1058. A
1059. A
1060. D
1061. D
1062. D
1063. D
1064. B
1065. D
1066. A
1067. B
1068. C
1069. C
1070. D
1071. D
1072. D
1073. D
1074. D
1075. D
1076. D
1077. D
1078. D
1079. D
1080. D
1081. D
1082. D
1083. D
1084. D
1085. D
1086. A
1087. C
1088. D
1089. D
1090. D
1091. D
1092. D
1093. D
1094. D
1095. A
1096. D
1097. C
1098. D
1099. D
1100. C
1101. D
1102. D
1103. D
1104. D
1105. D
1106. D
1107. D
1108. D
1109. D
1110. D
1111. D
1112. D
1113. B
1114. D
1115. D
1116. D
1117. C
1118. C
1119. B
1120. B
1121. C
1122. D
1123. A
1124. D
1125. D
1126. D
1127. C
1128. D
1129. D
1130. A
1131. A
1132. A
1133. A
1134. D
1135. C
1136. D
1137. C
1138. C
1139. D
1140. D
1141. D
1142. D
1143. B
1144. D
1145. D
1146. C
1147. A
1148. D
1149. D
1150. D
1151. D
1152. D
1153. D
1154. D
1155. D
1156. D
1157. A
1158. D
1159. D
1160. C
1161. D
1162. B
1163. D
1164. D
1165. D
1166. D
1167. D
1168. A
1169. A
1170. D
1171. D
1172. D
1173. C
1174. C
1175. D
1176. A
1177. A
1178. D
1179. C
1180. C
1181. B
1182. D
1183. D
1184. D
1185. D
1186. A
1187. D
1188. B
1189. D
1190. D
1191. D
1192. B
1193. D
1194. B
1195. D
1196. D
1197. D
1198. C
1199. C
1200. C
1201. B
1202. D
1203. D
1204. D
1205. B
1206. D
1207. D
1208. B
1209. C
1210. C
1211. D
1212. B
1213. C
1214. D
1215. D
1216. D
1217. B
1218. D
1219. D
1220. D
1221. A
1222. C
1223. D
1224. D
1225. D
1226. B
1227. D
1228. D
1229. B
1230. D

ANSWERS

1231. A
1232. D
1233. D
1234. D
1235. B
1236. D
1237. D
1238. D
1239. D
1240. D
1241. A
1242. B
1243. D
1244. C
1245. B
1246. D
1247. C
1248. C
1249. D
1250. B
1251. D
1252. C
1253. B
1254. D
1255. D
1256. D
1257. D
1258. B
1259. D
1260. D
1261. A
1262. B
1263. D
1264. D
1265. D
1266. D
1267. D
1268. D
1269. B
1270. A
1271. D
1272. D
1273. A
1274. B
1275. B
1276. A
1277. D
1278. D
1279. D
1280. B
1281. D
1282. D
1283. D
1284. B
1285. B
1286. D
1287. D
1288. B
1289. C
1290. A
1291. A
1292. B
1293. A
1294. C
1295. D
1296. D
1297. C
1298. B
1299. B
1300. B
1301. A
1302. D
1303. D
1304. D
1305. B
1306. D
1307. D
1308. A
1309. B
1310. D
1311. C
1312. D
1313. D
1314. D
1315. D
1316. D
1317. D
1318. A
1319. D
1320. D
1321. A
1322. B
1323. D
1324. D
1325. D
1326. D
1327. D
1328. D
1329. D
1330. D
1331. D
1332. B
1333. D
1334. D
1335. D
1336. D
1337. B
1338. D
1339. D
1340. D
1341. C
1342. D
1343. A
1344. B
1345. D
1346. D
1347. B
1348. A
1349. C
1350. D
1351. D
1352. D
1353. D
1354. D
1355. B
1356. C
1357. C
1358. D
1359. B
1360. C
1361. B
1362. A
1363. D
1364. C
1365. D
1366. D
1367. B
1368. A
1369. D
1370. B
1371. D
1372. C
1373. D
1374. B
1375. C
1376. A
1377. D
1378. D
1379. C
1380. D
1381. B
1382. D
1383. B
1384. B
1385. D
1386. C
1387. B
1388. C
1389. B
1390. D
1391. A
1392. B
1393. A
1394. B
1395. A
1396. D
1397. B
1398. D
1399. D
1400. A
1401. D
1402. B
1403. B
1404. D
1405. A
1406. D
1407. D
1408. D
1409. A
1410. D
1411. D
1412. B
1413. D
1414. D
1415. C
1416. B
1417. D
1418. A
1419. B
1420. B
1421. C
1422. C
1423. D
1424. D
1425. D
1426. C
1427. B
1428. D
1429. D
1430. D
1431. D
1432. D
1433. D
1434. D
1435. C
1436. B
1437. A
1438. D
1439. D
1440. B
1441. C
1442. C
1443. D
1444. B
1445. D
1446. A
1447. B
1448. D
1449. A
1450. D
1451. A
1452. A
1453. B
1454. C
1455. D
1456. D
1457. A
1458. C
1459. A
1460. B
1461. D
1462. B
1463. C
1464. B
1465. D
1466. B
1467. D
1468. D
1469. C
1470. B
1471. A
1472. D
1473. B
1474. D
1475. D
1476. D

ANSWERS

1477. D
1478. D
1479. C
1480. B
1481. D
1482. A
1483. C
1484. D
1485. D
1486. D
1487. B
1488. D
1489. D
1490. D
1491. B
1492. C
1493. A
1494. C
1495. B
1496. C
1497. C
1498. D
1499. C
1500. D
1501. D
1502. C
1503. A
1504. C
1505. D
1506. D
1507. D
1508. B
1509. D
1510. D
1511. D
1512. A
1513. B
1514. A
1515. C
1516. D
1517. D
1518. D
1519. D
1520. D
1521. B
1522. D
1523. B
1524. D
1525. D
1526. B
1527. D
1528. B
1529. D
1530. D
1531. D
1532. D
1533. A
1534. A
1535. D
1536. B
1537. D
1538. B
1539. C
1540. D
1541. D
1542. D
1543. D
1544. B
1545. D
1546. A
1547. D
1548. D
1549. B
1550. B
1551. B
1552. C
1553. B
1554. C
1555. D
1556. B
1557. D
1558. B
1559. D
1560. C
1561. D
1562. D
1563. C
1564. B
1565. C
1566. D
1567. D
1568. D
1569. A
1570. B
1571. B
1572. D
1573. D
1574. D
1575. D
1576. C
1577. D
1578. B
1579. A
1580. D
1581. D
1582. A
1583. D
1584. D
1585. D
1586. D
1587. D
1588. B
1589. D
1590. A
1591. D
1592. B
1593. D
1594. B
1595. D
1596. D
1597. D
1598. D
1599. D
1600. D
1601. D
1602. C
1603. B
1604. D
1605. D
1606. D
1607. D
1608. D
1609. A
1610. C
1611. B
1612. C
1613. A
1614. D
1615. D
1616. B
1617. B
1618. B
1619. B
1620. D
1621. D
1622. C
1623. D
1624. A
1625. D
1626. D
1627. D
1628. D
1629. A
1630. B
1631. D
1632. D
1633. D
1634. A
1635. A
1636. C
1637. B
1638. D
1639. D
1640. A
1641. D
1642. D
1643. D
1644. D
1645. D
1646. D
1647. C
1648. D
1649. D
1650. D
1651. D
1652. B
1653. D
1654. A
1655. C
1656. C
1657. D
1658. D
1659. D
1660. D
1661. D
1662. D
1663. C
1664. C
1665. A
1666. B
1667. D
1668. D
1669. B
1670. A
1671. C
1672. D
1673. D
1674. D
1675. C
1676. D
1677. C
1678. A
1679. D
1680. C
1681. D
1682. D
1683. B
1684. A
1685. D
1686. D
1687. D
1688. B
1689. B
1690. C
1691. D
1692. B
1693. C
1694. B
1695. D
1696. C
1697. D
1698. D
1699. D
1700. D
1701. D
1702. C
1703. A
1704. D
1705. B
1706. C
1707. A
1708. D
1709. D
1710. D
1711. B
1712. C
1713. D
1714. B
1715. A
1716. B
1717. D
1718. A
1719. A

ANSWERS

1720. D	1760. D	1800. D	1840. A	1880. D	1920. B
1721. D	1761. D	1801. D	1841. A	1881. D	1921. D
1722. D	1762. D	1802. B	1842. D	1882. D	1922. B
1723. D	1763. D	1803. D	1843. A	1883. B	1923. A
1724. D	1764. A	1804. D	1844. A	1884. D	1924. C
1725. D	1765. A	1805. D	1845. D	1885. B	1925. C
1726. D	1766. D	1806. D	1846. D	1886. D	1926. B
1727. D	1767. D	1807. D	1847. A	1887. D	1927. D
1728. D	1768. C	1808. D	1848. B	1888. C	1928. D
1729. D	1769. D	1809. D	1849. D	1889. D	1929. D
1730. D	1770. D	1810. D	1850. D	1890. B	1930. C
1731. D	1771. B	1811. D	1851. D	1891. D	1931. D
1732. D	1772. C	1812. D	1852. D	1892. C	1932. D
1733. D	1773. A	1813. D	1853. A	1893. D	1933. D
1734. D	1774. D	1814. B	1854. D	1894. C	1934. C
1735. D	1775. C	1815. D	1855. C	1895. D	1935. D
1736. B	1776. C	1816. A	1856. D	1896. D	1936. D
1737. D	1777. B	1817. D	1857. D	1897. D	1937. D
1738. A	1778. C	1818. C	1858. B	1898. A	1938. D
1739. A	1779. D	1819. C	1859. B	1899. D	1939. C
1740. A	1780. B	1820. B	1860. D	1900. C	1940. D
1741. C	1781. B	1821. D	1861. D	1901. C	1941. A
1742. D	1782. D	1822. D	1862. D	1902. A	1942. A
1743. D	1783. B	1823. D	1863. B	1903. C	1943. A
1744. D	1784. D	1824. D	1864. B	1904. B	1944. D
1745. D	1785. D	1825. A	1865. B	1905. D	1945. D
1746. D	1786. D	1826. D	1866. B	1906. A	1946. D
1747. D	1787. D	1827. B	1867. B	1907. A	1947. D
1748. D	1788. D	1828. D	1868. C	1908. C	1948. D
1749. D	1789. B	1829. A	1869. B	1909. D	1949. A
1750. D	1790. D	1830. D	1870. D	1910. B	1950. B
1751. D	1791. C	1831. C	1871. D	1911. D	1951. A
1752. B	1792. A	1832. C	1872. D	1912. D	1952. D
1753. B	1793. D	1833. D	1873. D	1913. C	1953. D
1754. B	1794. A	1834. D	1874. D	1914. B	1954. D
1755. C	1795. B	1835. C	1875. D	1915. B	1955. B
1756. C	1796. C	1836. A	1876. D	1916. C	1956. B
1757. C	1797. B	1837. B	1877. B	1917. A	1957. A
1758. B	1798. D	1838. A	1878. D	1918. D	1958. A
1759. B	1799. D	1839. D	1879. D	1919. D	1959. A

ANSWERS

1960. D	1984. D	2008. D	2032. D	2056. D	2080. A
1961. C	1985. D	2009. B	2033. B	2057. D	2081. B
1962. D	1986. D	2010. D	2034. D	2058. C	2082. B
1963. B	1987. D	2011. C	2035. D	2059. B	2083. C
1964. D	1988. D	2012. B	2036. D	2060. B	2084. D
1965. D	1989. D	2013. B	2037. D	2061. D	2085. D
1966. B	1990. D	2014. A	2038. B	2062. A	2086. C
1967. D	1991. C	2015. D	2039. C	2063. C	2087. A
1968. D	1992. D	2016. D	2040. A	2064. B	2088. A
1969. D	1993. D	2017. B	2041. A	2065. A	2089. C
1970. D	1994. D	2018. D	2042. B	2066. B	2090. A
1971. C	1995. D	2019. B	2043. C	2067. D	2091. D
1972. D	1996. D	2020. A	2044. D	2068. D	2092. A
1973. B	1997. D	2021. A	2045. D	2069. D	2093. D
1974. D	1998. D	2022. D	2046. D	2070. C	2094. B
1975. D	1999. B	2023. D	2047. C	2071. C	2095. D
1976. D	2000. A	2024. D	2048. D	2072. D	2096. C
1977. C	2001. B	2025. D	2049. D	2073. B	2097. A
1978. D	2002. D	2026. A	2050. D	2074. D	2098. B
1979. A	2003. D	2027. D	2051. D	2075. C	2099. C
1980. C	2004. D	2028. D	2052. C	2076. B	2100. C
1981. D	2005. D	2029. B	2053. D	2077. C	2101. B
1982. B	2006. D	2030. A	2054. A	2078. D	
1983. D	2007. D	2031. D	2055. B	2079. D	

Gastroenterology 5

Dysphagia

1. Dysphagia is defined as a sensation of "sticking" or obstruction of the passage of food through?
Harrison's 20th Ed. Chapter 40 Page 249

A. Mouth
B. Pharynx
C. Esophagus
D. All of the above

Dysphagia is defined as a sensation of "sticking" or obstruction of the passage of food through the mouth, pharynx or esophagus.

2. Foreign body sensation localized in the neck is termed as?
Harrison's 20th Ed. Chapter 40 Page 250

A. Odynophagia
B. Globus pharyngeus
C. Transfer dysphagia
D. Phagophobia

A foreign body sensation localized in the neck that does not interfere with swallowing and is sometimes relieved by swallowing is termed as "Globus pharyngeus" or a "lump in the throat" sensation.

3. Which of the following is characteristic of oropharyngeal dysphagia?
Harrison's 20th Ed. Chapter 40 Page 250

A. Odynophagia
B. Globus pharyngeus
C. Transfer dysphagia
D. Phagophobia

Transfer dysphagia frequently results in nasal regurgitation and pulmonary aspiration during swallowing and is characteristic of oropharyngeal dysphagia or "high" dysphagia.

4. Which of the following may have a psychogenic cause of dysphagia?
Harrison's 20th Ed. Chapter 40 Page 250

A. Globus pharyngeus
B. Transfer dysphagia
C. Phagophobia
D. All of the above

Phagophobia refers to fear of swallowing. Refusal to swallow thereby may be psychogenic.

5. Which of the following terms refers to an acute setting of esophageal foreign body impaction?
Harrison's 20th Ed. Chapter 40 Page 250

A. Globus pharyngeus
B. Odynophagia
C. Phagophobia
D. Aphagia

Aphagia refers to complete esophageal obstruction, most commonly encountered in acute setting of a food bolus or foreign body impaction.

6. "Deglutitive inhibition" best relates to which of the following?
Harrison's 20th Ed. Chapter 40 Page 250

A. Smell
B. Mastication
C. Peristaltic contraction of esophagus
D. Gastroesophageal reflux

Primary peristalsis refers to peristaltic contractions elicited in response to a swallow. It is an interplay of sequenced inhibition followed by contraction of the entire length of esophageal musculature. The inhibition that precedes peristaltic contraction is called deglutitive inhibition.

7. Deglutitive inhibition refers to?
Harrison's 20th Ed. Chapter 40 Page 250

A. Complete esophageal obstruction
B. Difficulty in initiating a swallow
C. Inhibition that precedes peristaltic contraction
D. Misdirection of food

Inhibition that precedes the peristaltic contraction is called deglutitive inhibition.

8. Which of the following esophageal contractions is nonperistaltic?
Harrison's 20th Ed. Chapter 40 Page 250

A. Primary peristalsis
B. Secondary peristalsis
C. Tertiary peristalsis
D. Any of the above

Tertiary esophageal contractions are nonperistaltic, disordered esophageal contractions that occur spontaneously during fluoroscopic observation.

9. Peristalsis that begins at the point of esophageal distention and proceeds distally is called?
Harrison's 20th Ed. Chapter 40 Page 250

A. Primary peristalsis
B. Secondary peristalsis
C. Tertiary peristalsis
D. Any of the above

Local distention of esophagus activates secondary peristalsis. It begins at the point of distention and proceeds distally as in gastroesophageal reflux.

10. Musculature of which of the following is striated?
Harrison's 20th Ed. Chapter 40 Page 250

A. Pharynx
B. Upper esophageal sphincter (UES)
C. Cervical esophagus
D. All of the above

The musculature of the oral cavity, pharynx, UES, and cervical esophagus is striated.

11. Lower esophageal sphincter (LES) relaxes when?
Harrison's 20th Ed. Chapter 40 Page 250

A. As the food enters esophagus
B. As the food travels through esophagus
C. As the food bolus is delivered into stomach
D. All of the above

Lower esophageal sphincter (LES) relaxes as the food enters esophagus and remains relaxed until the peristaltic contraction has delivered the food bolus into the stomach.

12. Which of the following is physiologically a part of upper esophageal sphincter (UES)?

Harrison's 20th Ed. Chapter 40 Page 250

A. Cricopharyngeus muscle
B. Inferior pharyngeal constrictor
C. Proximal portion of cervical esophagus
D. All of the above

Physiologically, UES consists of the cricopharyngeus muscle, the adjacent inferior pharyngeal constrictor, and the proximal portion of the cervical esophagus.

13. Innervation to the musculature acting on UES to facilitate its opening during swallowing comes from?

Harrison's 20th Ed. Chapter 40 Page 250

A. Fifth cranial nerve
B. Seventh cranial nerve
C. Twelfth cranial nerve
D. All of the above

14. UES innervation is derived from?

Harrison's 20th Ed. Chapter 40 Page 250

A. Fifth cranial nerve
B. Seventh cranial nerve
C. Twelfth cranial nerve
D. Tenth cranial nerve

UES innervation is derived from vagus nerve, whereas innervation to the musculature acting on UES to facilitate its opening during swallowing comes from fifth, seventh & twelfth cranial nerves.

15. Which of the following is involved in keeping UES closed at rest?

Harrison's 20th Ed. Chapter 40 Page 250

A. Cricopharyngeus muscle
B. Inferior pharyngeal constrictor
C. Proximal portion of cervical esophagus
D. All of the above

UES remains closed at rest due to its inherent elastic properties and neurogenically mediated contraction of cricopharyngeus muscle.

16. Which of the following muscle acts on the upper esophageal sphincter (UES)?

Harrison's 20th Ed. Chapter 40 Page 250

A. Cricopharyngeus muscle
B. Suprahyoid muscle
C. Geniohyoid muscle
D. All of the above

UES opening during swallowing involves cessation of vagal excitation to cricopharyngeus and simultaneous contraction of suprahyoid and geniohyoid muscles that pull open UES along with upward and forward displacement of larynx.

17. Which of the following muscle is involved in opening UES during swallowing?

Harrison's 20th Ed. Chapter 40 Page 250

A. Geniohyoid
B. Mylohyoid
C. Styloglossus
D. All of the above

UES opening during swallowing is due to relaxation of cricopharyngeus muscle (cessation of vagal excitation) and simultaneous contraction of suprahyoid & geniohyoid muscles.

18. Peristalsis in the proximal esophagus is governed by?

Harrison's 20th Ed. Chapter 40 Page 250

A. Lower motor neurons of the vagus nerve
B. Vagal motor neurons in the nucleus ambiguus
C. Neurons within the esophageal myenteric plexus
D. All of the above

Striated muscles of cervical esophagus are directly innervated by lower motor neurons of vagus nerve. Peristalsis in proximal esophagus is governed by sequential activation of vagal motor neurons in nucleus ambiguus. Distal esophagus & LES are composed of smooth muscle and are controlled by excitatory & inhibitory neurons within the esophageal myenteric plexus. Medullary preganglionic neurons from dorsal motor nucleus of vagus trigger peristalsis via these ganglionic neurons during primary peristalsis.

19. Neurotransmitter of the inhibitory ganglionic neurons during primary peristalsis is?

Harrison's 20th Ed. Chapter 40 Page 250

A. Vasoactive intestinal peptide
B. Acetylcholine
C. Substance P
D. All of the above

For during primary peristalsis, neurotransmitters of excitatory ganglionic neurons are acetylcholine & substance P. Those of inhibitory neurons are vasoactive intestinal peptide & nitric oxide.

20. Which of the following acts as an external sphincter in the functioning of LES?

Harrison's 20th Ed. Chapter 40 Page 250

A. Muscles of the right diaphragmatic crus
B. Muscle of the left diaphragmatic crus
C. Muscle of the central diaphragmatic crus
D. All of the above

Function of LES is supplemented by surrounding muscle of the right diaphragmatic crus, which acts as an external sphincter during inspiration, cough or abdominal straining.

21. Agents that increase LES pressure are all except?

Harrison's 20th Ed. Chapter 40 Page 250

A. Substance P
B. Prostaglandin $F_{2\alpha}$
C. Secretin
D. Gastrin

22. Agents that reduce LES pressure are all except?

Harrison's 20th Ed. Chapter 40 Page 250

A. Cholecystokinin
B. Secretin
C. Dopamine
D. Gastrin

23. Agents that reduce LES pressure are all except?

Harrison's 20th Ed. Chapter 40 Page 250

A. VIP
B. Calcitonin gene-related peptide (CGRP)
C. Prostaglandin E
D. Prostaglandin $F_{2\alpha}$

24. Agents that reduce LES pressure are all except?
Harrison's 20th Ed. Chapter 40 Page 250

A. Adenosine
B. Dopamine
C. Substance P
D. Nitrates

Reduction in LES sphincter pressure occurs with phosphodiesterase-5 inhibitors (sildenafil) use, fatty meals, smoking, and beverages with high xanthine content (tea, coffee, cola), nicotine, beta-adrenergic agonists, dopamine, cholecystokinin, secretin, vasoactive intestinal peptide (VIP), calcitonin gene–related peptide, adenosine, prostaglandin E, nitric oxide donors (nitrates). LES contraction occurs with GABA-B agonists (baclofen), muscarinic M_2 and M_3 receptor agonists, alpha-adrenergic agonists, gastrin, substance P & Pg $F_{2\alpha}$

25. Which of the following statements about upper esophageal sphincter (UES) is false?
Harrison's 20th Ed. Chapter 40 Page 250

A. Formed by cricopharyngeus & inferior pharyngeal constrictor muscles
B. These muscles exhibit myogenic tone
C. These muscles receive no inhibitory innervation
D. Opened by central inhibition of sphincter muscles

The UES remains closed at rest due to its inherent elastic properties and neurogenically mediated contraction of the cricopharyngeus muscle.

26. Which of the following statements about lower esophageal sphincter (LES) is false?
Harrison's 20th Ed. Chapter 40 Page 250

A. Innervated by parallel sets of parasympathetic excitatory & inhibitory pathways
B. Opens in response to activity of inhibitory nerves
C. Neurotransmitters of excitatory nerves are acetylcholine, substance P & nitric oxide
D. Neurotransmitters of inhibitory nerves is VIP

27. Motor dysphagia refers to?
Harrison's 20th Ed. Chapter 40 Page 251

A. Weakness of peristaltic contractions
B. Impaired deglutitive inhibition
C. Impaired sphincter relaxation
D. All of the above

Dysphagia caused by a large bolus or a narrow lumen is called structural dysphagia. Dysphagia due to weakness of peristaltic contractions or to impaired deglutitive inhibition causing nonperistaltic contractions & impaired sphincter relaxation is called propulsive or motor dysphagia.

28. Length of adult esophagus is?
Harrison's 20th Ed. Chapter 40 Page 251

A. 12 – 16 cm
B. 14 – 20 cm
C. 16 – 24 cm
D. 18 – 26 cm

Adult esophagus is 18 – 26 cm in length. Anatomically, it is divided into cervical esophagus (from pharyngoesophageal junction to suprasternal notch) and thoracic esophagus (up to the diaphragmatic hiatus).

29. In an adult, esophageal lumen can distend up to?
Harrison's 20th Ed. Chapter 40 Page 251

A. 2 cm in anteroposterior plane & 3 cm in lateral plane
B. 3 cm in anteroposterior plane & 4 cm in lateral plane
C. 4 cm in anteroposterior plane & 5 cm in lateral plane
D. 5 cm in anteroposterior plane & 6 cm in lateral plane

In adult, esophageal lumen can distend up to 4 cm in diameter or 2 cm in anteroposterior plane & 3 cm in lateral plane. When esophagus cannot dilate beyond 2.5 cm in diameter, dysphagia to normal solid food occurs. Dysphagia is always present when esophagus cannot distend beyond 1.3 cm.

30. Which of the following is a structural cause of dysphagia?
Harrison's 20th Ed. Chapter 40 Page 251

A. Schatzki's rings
B. Eosinophilic esophagitis
C. Peptic strictures
D. All of the above

The most common structural causes of dysphagia are Schatzki's rings, eosinophilic esophagitis and peptic strictures.

31. Hallmark of oropharyngeal dysphagia is?
Harrison's 20th Ed. Chapter 40 Page 251

A. Food impaction
B. Odynophagia
C. Nasal regurgitation
D. Hoarseness

Nasal regurgitation & tracheobronchial aspiration with swallowing are hallmarks of oropharyngeal dysphagia ("high" dysphagia) or a tracheoesophageal fistula.

32. Which of the following is important in medical history of a case of dysphagia?
Harrison's 20th Ed. Chapter 40 Page 252

A. Location
B. Types of foods and/or liquids
C. Progressive or intermittent, duration of symptoms
D. All of the above

In a case of dysphagia, key features to consider in medical history are : location, types of foods and/or liquids, progressive or intermittent and duration of symptoms.

33. Which of the following features suggest structural dysphagia?
Harrison's 20th Ed. Chapter 40 Page 252

A. Dysphagia caused by an oversized bolus or a narrow lumen
B. Intermittent dysphagia that occurs only with solid food
C. Food impaction with a prolonged inability to pass an ingested bolus even with ingestion of liquid
D. All of the above

34. Which of the following features suggest motor dysphagia?
Harrison's 20th Ed. Chapter 40 Page 252

A. Due to abnormalities of peristalsis
B. Due to impaired sphincter relaxation after swallowing
C. Constant dysphagia with both liquids & solids
D. All of the above

35. Malignancy is likely if there is?
Harrison's 20th Ed. Chapter 40 Page 252

A. Short duration (<4 months), disease progression
B. Dysphagia more for solids than for liquids
C. Weight loss
D. All of the above

Malignancy is likely if there is a short duration (<4 months), disease progression, dysphagia more for solids than for liquids and weight loss.

36. Bird's beak sign best relates to?
The American Journal of Medicine. 2015; 128(10):1138.e18

A. Achalasia
B. Zenker's diverticulum
C. Diffuse esophageal spasm (DES)
D. Schatzki's rings

Achalasia is characterized by dilation & sigmoidization of esophagus with classic bird's beak sign.

37. Achalasia is more likely if there is?
Harrison's 20th Ed. Chapter 40 Page 252

A. Dysphagia for both solids and liquids
B. Passive nocturnal regurgitation of mucus or food
C. Problem that has existed for several months or years
D. All of the above

Achalasia is more likely if there is dysphagia for both solids & liquids (dysphagia for liquids strongly suggests the diagnosis), there is passive nocturnal regurgitation of mucus or food, has existed for several months or years.

38. Chest pain frequently accompanies which of the following dysphagias?
Harrison's 20th Ed. Chapter 40 Page 252

A. Motor disorders
B. Structural disorders
C. Reflux disease
D. All of the above

Chest pain frequently accompanies dysphagia whether it is related to motor disorders, structural disorders or reflux disease.

39. Which of the following skin diseases may involve the esophagus?
Harrison's 20th Ed. Chapter 40 Page 252

A. Scleroderma
B. Pemphigoid
C. Epidermolysis bullosa
D. All of the above

Scleroderma, pemphigoid, lichen planus and epidermolysis bullosa can involve the esophagus.

40. Oropharyngeal dysphagia may be due to which of the following causes?
Harrison's 20th Ed. Chapter 40 Page 251

A. Neurologic cause
B. Muscular cause
C. Metabolic cause
D. All of the above

Oropharyngeal dysphagia may be due to neurologic (cerebrovascular accidents, Parkinson's disease, amyotrophic lateral sclerosis), muscular, structural (Zenker's diverticulum, cricopharyngeal bar, neoplasia), iatrogenic (surgery and radiation), infectious and metabolic causes.

41. Oropharyngeal dysphagia most commonly results from?
Harrison's 20th Ed. Chapter 40 Page 252

A. Neurologic cause
B. Muscular cause
C. Metabolic cause
D. All of the above

Oropharyngeal dysphagia most commonly results from functional deficits caused by neurologic disorders.

42. Zenker's diverticulum is best related to?
Harrison's 20th Ed. Chapter 40 Page 251

A. Glossopharyngeus
B. Hyoglossus
C. Cricopharyngeus
D. Mylohyoid

43. Zenker's diverticulum is best related to?
Harrison's 20th Ed. Chapter 40 Page 251

A. Diffuse esophageal spasm (DES)
B. Lower esophageal sphincter (LES)
C. Killian's dehiscence
D. Schatzki's rings

Zenker's diverticulum is typically seen in elderly patients. Its pathogenesis is related to stenosis of cricopharyngeus that causes diminished opening of UES leading to increased hypopharyngeal pressure during swallowing. This results in development of a pulsion diverticulum immediately above cricopharyngeus in a region of potential weakness known as Killian's dehiscence. Killian dehiscence is a posterior midline weakness of pharyngoesophageal segment just above cricopharyngeus.

44. Which of the following about Killian-Jamieson diverticulum is false?
Radiology 1983; 146: 117-22

A. Esophageal diverticulum
B. In anterolateral wall of cervical esophagus
C. Inferior to cricopharyngeus
D. None of the above

Killian-Jamieson diverticulum is a rare esophageal diverticulum protruding through a muscular gap, Killian-Jamieson space, in the anterolateral wall of cervical esophagus inferior to the cricopharyngeus and lateral to the longitudinal tendon of the esophagus.

45. Dysphagia lusoria is best related to?
N Engl J Med. 2016; 375:e4

A. Right carotid artery
B. Left carotid artery
C. Right subclavian artery
D. Left subclavian artery

Dysphagia lusoria (or Bayford-Autenrieth dysphagia) is an abnormal condition characterized by difficulty in swallowing caused by an aberrant right subclavian artery seen in cases of truncus bicaroticus (a vascular anomaly in which the carotid arteries have a common origin).

46. Dysphagia aortica is caused by?
N Engl J Med. 1941;225:490-94

A. Thoracic aortic aneurysm
B. Aortic dissection
C. Tortuous aorta
D. All of the above

Dysphagia aortica is caused by extrinsic compression of esophagus due to an ectatic, tortuous, aneurysmatic (true or pseudo) atherosclerotic thoracic aorta or dissection tracts of the aneurysm.

47. Cricopharyngeal myotomy is useful in?
Harrison's 20th Ed. Chapter 40 Page 253

A. Idiopathic cricopharyngeal bar
B. Zenker's diverticulum
C. Oculopharyngeal muscular dystrophy
D. All of the above

Usually, cricopharyngeal myotomy is not helpful except in the disorders mentioned above.

48. "Strawberry gums" is a pathognomonic sign of?
Harrison's 20th Ed. Chapter 32 Page 220

A. Granulomatosis with polyangiitis
B. Acute myelomonocytic leukemia
C. Down's syndrome
D. Diabetes mellitus

Pathognomonic sign of Granulomatosis with polyangiitis (Wegener's granulomatosis) is a red-purplish, granular gingivitis called strawberry gums.

Nausea, Vomiting, and Indigestion

49. Which of the following about vomiting is false?
Harrison's 20th Ed. Chapter 41 Page 253

A. No volitional control
B. Oral expulsion of gastrointestinal contents
C. Due to gut & thoracoabdominal wall contractions
D. None of the above

50. Dyspepsia encompasses a range of symptoms thought to originate in?
Harrison's 20th Ed. Chapter 41 Page 253

A. Gastroduodenum
B. Small intestines
C. Large intestines
D. Any of the above

Dyspepsia is a term encompassing symptoms thought to originate in the gastroduodenal region. It usually include nausea, vomiting, heartburn, regurgitation, and dyspepsia.

51. Which of the following coordinate initiation of emesis?
Harrison's 20th Ed. Chapter 41 Page 253

A. Nucleus tractus solitarius
B. Dorsal vagal nuclei
C. Phrenic nuclei
D. All of the above

52. Which of the following coordinate initiation of emesis?
Harrison's 20th Ed. Chapter 41 Page 253

A. Neurokinin NK_1 pathway
B. Serotonin 5-HT_3 pathway
C. Vasopressin pathway
D. All of the above

Brainstem nuclei, including nucleus tractus solitarius, dorsal vagal and phrenic nuclei, medullary nuclei regulating respiration and nuclei that control pharyngeal, facial & tongue movements coordinate initiation of emesis. Pathways involved include neurokinin NK_1, serotonin 5-HT_3, and vasopressin.

53. Chemoreceptor trigger zone best relates to?
Harrison's 20th Ed. Chapter 41 Page 253

A. Area postrema
B. Broca's area
C. Wernicke's area
D. All of the above

Area postrema, termed chemoreceptor trigger zone, is the vomiting center located in floor of IV ventricle.

54. Area postrema in medulla responds to which of the following stimuli?
Harrison's 20th Ed. Chapter 41 Page 253

A. Uremia
B. Hypoxia
C. Ketoacidosis
D. All of the above

Area postrema in medulla, responds to blood borne stimuli like emetogenic drugs, bacterial toxins, uremia, hypoxia, ketoacidosis.

55. Area postrema is served by nerves acting on?
Harrison's 20th Ed. Chapter 41 Page 253

A. 5-HT_3 receptors
B. Muscarinic M_1 receptors
C. Dopamine D_2 receptors
D. All of the above

56. Vagal afferent stimuli activate which of the following receptors?
Harrison's 20th Ed. Chapter 41 Page 253

A. Muscarinic M_1 receptors
B. Histaminergic H_1 receptors
C. Dopamine D_2 receptors
D. 5-HT_3 receptors

Vagal afferent stimuli activate 5-HT_3 receptors.

57. Labyrinthine disorders stimulate which of the following receptors?
Harrison's 20th Ed. Chapter 41 Page 253

A. Muscarinic M_1 receptors
B. Central NK_1 receptors
C. Dopamine D_2 receptors
D. 5-HT_3 receptors

Labyrinthine disorders stimulate vestibular muscarinic M_1 and histaminergic H_1 receptors.

58. Vomiting can be induced via activation of which of the following receptors?
Ther Adv Gastroenterol. 2016;9(1):98-112

A. μ opioid
B. Glucagon peptide 1
C. Vanilloid TRPV1
D. All of the above

Vomiting can be induced via the activation of several cell membrane bound receptors including: serotonergic 5-HT_3 and 5-HT_4, tachykininergic NK_1, dopaminergic D_2 and D_3; muscarinic M_1; histaminergic H_1; μ opioid; cysteinyl leukotriene 1; prostaglandin DP, FP, and EP; thromboxane TP; glucagon peptide 1, and vanilloid TRPV1.

59. In superior mesenteric artery syndrome, which of the following is compressed by the overlying superior mesenteric artery?
Harrison's 20th Ed. Chapter 41 Page 254

A. Stomach
B. Duodenum
C. Jejunum
D. Ileum

In superior mesenteric artery syndrome, duodenum is compressed by overlying superior mesenteric artery.

60. Which of the following causes gastroparesis?
Harrison's 20th Ed. Chapter 41 Page 254

A. Post vagotomy
B. Pancreatic carcinoma
C. Mesenteric vascular insufficiency
D. All of the above

Gastroparesis occurs after vagotomy, with pancreatic carcinoma, mesenteric vascular insufficiency. Also in diabetes, scleroderma, and amyloidosis. Idiopathic gastroparesis is the most common etiology.

61. Which of the following causes intestinal pseudoobstruction?
Harrison's 20th Ed. Chapter 41 Page 254

A. Scleroderma
B. Amyloidosis
C. Paraneoplastic consequence of malignancy
D. All of the above

62. Which of the following is a functional gastroduodenal disorder?
Harrison's 20th Ed. Chapter 41 Page 254

A. Chronic nausea vomiting syndrome
B. Cyclic vomiting syndrome
C. Cannabinoid hyperemesis syndrome
D. All of the above

63. Which of the following is often misdiagnosed as refractory vomiting?
Harrison's 20th Ed. Chapter 41 Page 254

A. Chronic nausea vomiting syndrome
B. Cyclic vomiting syndrome
C. Cannabinoid hyperemesis syndrome
D. Rumination syndrome

Vomiting occurring minutes after meal consumption prompts consideration of rumination syndrome.

64. Postoperative emesis occurs in what proportion of surgeries?
Harrison's 20th Ed. Chapter 41 Page 254

A. 10%
B. 25%
C. 40%
D. 60%

Postoperative emesis occurs in ~25% of surgeries, most commonly abdominal & orthopedic surgery.

65. Acute emesis from cisplatin is mediated by?
Harrison's 20th Ed. Chapter 41 Page 254

A. Muscarinic M_1 receptors
B. Central NK_1 receptors
C. Dopamine D_2 receptors
D. $5\text{-}HT_3$ receptors

66. Nausea during first trimester of pregnancy affects what proportion of women?
Harrison's 20th Ed. Chapter 41 Page 254

A. 25%
B. 50%
C. 70%
D. 90%

Pregnancy is the most common endocrinologic cause of nausea. It affects 70% of women in first trimester.

67. Brainstem dorsal vagal complex (DVC) comprises of?
Ther Adv Gastroenterol 2016;9(1):98-112

A. Area postrema (AP)
B. Nucleus of the solitary tract (NTS)
C. Dorsal motor nucleus of the vagus (DMNX)
D. All of the above

68. Nucleus tractus solitarius receives inputs from which of the following pathways?
Ther Adv Gastroenterol 2016;9(1):98-112

A. Vestibular and cerebellar
B. Cerebral cortex and limbic system
C. Area postrema
D. All of the above

Afferent information from various stimuli are relayed to nucleus tractus solitarius via four pathways: vestibular & cerebellar, cerebral cortex & limbic system, area postrema and gastrointestinal tract via vagus nerve.

69. Rise in which of the following hormones precede emesis?
Ther Adv Gastroenterol 2016;9(1):98-112

A. Vasopressin
B. Estrogen
C. Melanin
D. Cortisol

Rise in vasopressin level precedes emesis.

70. Which of the following evoke emesis via effects on the area postrema?
Harrison's 20th Ed. Chapter 41 Page 254

A. Fulminant liver failure
B. Exogenous enterotoxins
C. Ethanol intoxication
D. All of the above

71. Which of the following is used in gastric emptying breath test?
Harrison's 20th Ed. Chapter 41 Page 255

A. ^{11}C
B. ^{12}C
C. ^{13}C
D. ^{14}C

72. Which of the following has antiemetic effects?
Harrison's 20th Ed. Chapter 41 Page 255

A. Mirtazapine
B. Olanzapine
C. Gabapentin
D. All of the above

73. Which of the following is a NK1 antagonist?
Harrison's 20th Ed. Chapter 41 Page 256

A. Aprepitant
B. Granisetron
C. Gabapentin
D. Dimenhydrinate

74. Which of the following is a $5\text{-}HT_3$ antagonist?
Harrison's 20th Ed. Chapter 41 Page 256

A. Aprepitant
B. Granisetron
C. Gabapentin
D. Dimenhydrinate

75. Which of the following increases gastroduodenal motility by action on receptors for motilin?

Harrison's 20th Ed. Chapter 41 Page 256

A. Domperidone
B. Metoclopramide
C. Erythromycin
D. Prucalopride

Erythromycin increases gastroduodenal motility by action on receptors for motilin. Motilin is a GI peptide released from the duodenum and an endogenous fasting motor stimulant.

76. Which of the following is a combined 5-HT_4 agonist and D_2 antagonist?

Harrison's 20th Ed. Chapter 41 Page 256

A. Domperidone
B. Prucalopride
C. Metoclopramide
D. Octreotide

77. Which of the following is a 5-HT_4 agonist?

Harrison's 20th Ed. Chapter 41 Page 256

A. Domperidone
B. Prucalopride
C. Metoclopramide
D. Octreotide

78. Which of the following is a D_2 antagonist?

Harrison's 20th Ed. Chapter 41 Page 256

A. Domperidone
B. Prucalopride
C. Metoclopramide
D. Octreotide

79. Which of the following can induce dangerous cardiac arrhythmias?

Harrison's 20th Ed. Chapter 41 Page 256

A. Ondansetron
B. Domperidone
C. Erythromycin
D. All of the above

80. Which of the following is a prokinetic agent?

Harrison's 20th Ed. Chapter 41 Page 255 Table 41-2

A. Pyridostigmine
B. Octreotide
C. Erythromycin
D. All of the above

81. Which of the following is useful in anticipatory nausea and vomiting with chemotherapy?

Harrison's 20th Ed. Chapter 41 Page 255 Table 41-2

A. Lorazepam
B. Olanzapine
C. Pyridostigmine
D. Dexamethasone

82. Gastric fundus relaxation after eating is called?

Harrison's 20th Ed. Chapter 41 Page 256

A. Accommodation
B. Appetation
C. Rumination
D. Gastration

83. Which of the following promote gastroesophageal reflux?

Harrison's 20th Ed. Chapter 41 Page 256

A. Theophylline
B. Progesterone
C. Calcium channel blockers
D. All of the above

84. Which of the following promote LES relaxation?

Harrison's 20th Ed. Chapter 41 Page 256

A. Ethanol
B. Tobacco
C. Caffeine
D. All of the above

85. Alkaline reflux esophagitis produces GERD-like symptoms most often in?

Harrison's 20th Ed. Chapter 41 Page 257

A. Pregnancy
B. Patients who underwent surgery for peptic ulcer disease
C. Achalasia
D. All of the above

Alkaline reflux esophagitis produces GERD-like symptoms most often in patients who underwent surgery for peptic ulcer disease.

86. Epigastric pain syndrome is best related to?

Harrison's 20th Ed. Chapter 41 Page 257

A. Gastroesophageal reflux disease (GERD)
B. Functional dyspepsia
C. Peptic ulcer disease
D. Zollinger-Ellison syndrome

Functional dyspepsia is subdivided into postprandial distress syndrome and epigastric pain syndrome.

87. Barrett's metaplasia predisposes to?

Harrison's 20th Ed. Chapter 41 Page 257

A. Esophageal squamous cell carcinoma
B. Esophageal adenocarcinoma
C. Lymphoma
D. All of the above

8–20% of GERD patients exhibit esophageal intestinal metaplasia, termed Barrett's metaplasia, which predisposes to esophageal adenocarcinoma.

88. GERD classically produces which of the following?

Harrison's 20th Ed. Chapter 41 Page 257

A. Water brash
B. Heartburn
C. Hoarseness
D. Chest pain

GERD classically produces heartburn, a substernal warmth that moves up toward the neck.

89. Functional dyspepsia overlaps with which of the following disorders?

Harrison's 20th Ed. Chapter 41 Page 257

A. GERD
B. IBS
C. Idiopathic gastroparesis
D. All of the above

90. Odynophagia suggests which of the following?

Harrison's 20th Ed. Chapter 41 Page 257

A. Food bolus impaction
B. Esophageal infection
C. Zenker's diverticulum
D. Achalasia

Odynophagia suggests esophageal infection.

91. Alarm feature for malignant esophageal blockage is?

Harrison's 20th Ed. Chapter 41 Page 257

A. Recurrent vomiting
B. Occult or gross bleeding
C. Jaundice
D. All of the above

Malignant esophageal blockage leading to dysphagia is suggested by unexplained weight loss, recurrent vomiting, occult or gross bleeding, jaundice, palpable mass or adenopathy, and a family history of gastrointestinal neoplasm.

92. Which of the following about "Steakhouse syndrome" is true?

World J Gastrointest Endosc. 2011;3(5):101-104

A. Food impaction of the esophagus
B. Esophageal tear
C. Esophageal agenesis
D. Any of the above

Acute esophageal obstruction caused by the impaction of a large bolus of food is called the 'steakhouse syndrome'. It was first reported by Norton in 1963.

93. Complication of long-term PPI therapy is?

Harrison's 20th Ed. Chapter 41 Page 258

A. Hypomagnesemia
B. Interstitial nephritis
C. Impaired absorption of clopidogrel
D. All of the above

Complications of long-term PPI therapy include diarrhea (from Clostridium difficile infection or microscopic colitis), small-intestinal bacterial overgrowth, nutrient deficiency (vitamin B_{12}, iron, calcium), hypomagnesemia, bone demineralization, interstitial nephritis & impaired medication absorption (clopidogrel).

94. Which of the following is useful for functional dyspepsia?

Harrison's 20th Ed. Chapter 41 Page 258

A. Buspirone
B. Acotiamide
C. Tandospirone
D. All of the above

95. Which of the following reduces esophageal exposure to acid and nonacidic fluids by reducing TLESRs?

Harrison's 20th Ed. Chapter 41 Page 258

A. Buspirone
B. Acotiamide
C. Tandospirone
D. Baclofen

Baclofen is a γ-aminobutyric acid B (GABA-B) agonist.

96. Which of the following is a long-term complication of fundoplication?

Harrison's 20th Ed. Chapter 41 Page 258

A. Dysphagia
B. Gas-bloat syndrome
C. Gastroparesis
D. All of the above

Diarrhea and Constipation

97. Which of the following names is associated with neuro-gastroenterology?
Gut 1999;45(Suppl II):II6–II16

A. Rice
B. Bayliss and Starling
C. Edith Bülbring
D. Langley

English investigators William M. Bayliss & Ernest H. Starling demonstrated that application of pressure to intestinal lumen of anesthetized dogs resulted in oral contraction & anal relaxation, followed by a propulsive wave ("law of the intestine" and now called the peristaltic reflex).

98. Which of the following is false about myenteric (or Auerbach's plexus)?
Harrison's 20th Ed. Chapter 42 Page 259

A. Ganglionated plexus
B. Lies between longitudinal & circular muscle layers
C. Control activity of smooth muscle of the gut
D. None of the above

99. Which of the following is false about submucosal (or Meissner's plexus)?
Harrison's 20th Ed. Chapter 42 Page 259

A. Ganglionated plexus
B. Lies between circular muscle layer and the mucosa
C. Regulates mucosal secretion & blood flow
D. None of the above

The ENS is organized in two ganglionated plexuses, myenteric (or Auerbach's plexus) and submucosal (or Meissner's plexus), composed of neurons and enteric glial cells. myenteric (or Auerbach's plexus) lies between the external longitudinal & internal circular muscle layers.

100. Enteric nervous system comprises of which of the following?
Harrison's 20th Ed. Chapter 42 Page 259

A. Myenteric layer
B. Submucosal layer
C. Mucosal neuronal layer
D. All of the above

Small intestine & colon have intrinsic & extrinsic innervation. Intrinsic innervation or the enteric nervous system comprises myenteric, submucosal, and mucosal neuronal layers.

101. Which of the following is a neurotransmitter in the enteric nervous system?
Harrison's 20th Ed. Chapter 42 Page 259

A. Acetylcholine
B. Vasoactive intestinal peptide (VIP)
C. Norepinephrine
D. All of the above

102. Which of the following is a neurotransmitter in the enteric nervous system?
Harrison's 20th Ed. Chapter 42 Page 259

A. Serotonin
B. Adenosine triphosphate (ATP)
C. Nitric oxide (NO)
D. All of the above

The function of layers of enteric nervous system are modulated by "interneurons" through actions of neurotransmitter amines or peptides that include acetylcholine, vasoactive intestinal peptide (VIP), opioids, norepinephrine, serotonin, adenosine triphosphate (ATP), and nitric oxide (NO).

103. Interstitial cells of Cajal are best related to?
Harrison's 20th Ed. Chapter 42 Page 259

A. Myenteric layer
B. Submucosal layer
C. Mucosal neuronal layer
D. All of the above

104. Which of the following is called pacemakers in gastrointestinal muscles?
Harrison's 20th Ed. Chapter 42 Page 259

A. Auerbach's plexus
B. Meissner's plexus
C. Interstitial cells of Cajal
D. All of the above

Interstitial cells of Cajal (ICC) are distinctive populations of muscle-like cells. They make contact with each other & with muscle cells & nerve terminals & function as pacemakers in gastrointestinal muscles by initiating rhythmic electrical activity.

105. Which of the following affects secretion, absorption, and mucosal blood flow?
Harrison's 20th Ed. Chapter 42 Page 259

A. Myenteric layer
B. Submucosal layer
C. Mucosal neuronal layer
D. All of the above

Myenteric plexus regulates smooth-muscle function through intermediary pacemaker-like cells called "interstitial cells of Cajal". Submucosal plexus affects secretion, absorption, and mucosal blood flow.

106. Which of the following statements is false?
Harrison's 20th Ed. Chapter 42 Page 259

A. Parasympathetic nerves convey visceral sensations from small intestine & colon
B. Parasympathetic nerves convey excitatory motor impulses to small intestine & colon
C. Parasympathetic fibers reach small intestine & proximal colon along branches of superior mesenteric artery
D. None of the above

107. Which of the following statements is false?
Harrison's 20th Ed. Chapter 42 Page 259

A. Sympathetic nerve supply to gut modulates motor functions
B. Sympathetic input to gut is excitatory to sphincters
C. Sympathetic input to gut is inhibitory to non-sphincteric muscle
D. None of the above

108. On an average day, how much fluid enter the GI tract?
Harrison's 20th Ed. Chapter 42 Page 260

A. 6 liters
B. 9 liters
C. 12 liters
D. 15 liters

On an average day, 9 liters of fluid enter GI tract. About 1 liter of residual fluid reaches colon, and stool excretion of fluid constitutes about 0.2 liters/day.

109. Migrating motor complex (MMC) best relates to?
Harrison's 20th Ed. Chapter 42 Page 260

A. Motility of the stomach
B. Motility of the small intestine
C. Motility of the large intestine
D. All of the above

During fasting period, in order to clear nondigestible residue from small intestine, motility of small intestine is characterized by a cyclical event. This is referred to as migrating motor complex (MMC) or intestinal "housekeeper".

110. Which of the following about migrating motor complex (MMC) is false?
Harrison's 20th Ed. Chapter 42 Page 260

A. Organized, propagated series of contractions
B. Lasts for ~4 minutes & occurs every 60–90 minutes
C. Involves the entire small intestine
D. None of the above

111. Which of the following is true for distal ileum?
Harrison's 20th Ed. Chapter 42 Page 260

A. Acts as a reservoir
B. Empties intermittently by powerful contractions
C. MMC rarely continues into the colon
D. All of the above

112. Which of the following statements is false?
Harrison's 20th Ed. Chapter 42 Page 260

A. Ascending & transverse colons function as reservoirs
B. Descending colon acts as a conduit
C. Transit time in ascending & transverse colons is 15 hours
D. Transit time in descending colon is 8 hours

Ascending & transverse colons function as reservoirs and average transit time is 15 hours. The descending colon acts as a conduit and average transit time is 3 hours.

113. High-amplitude propagated contractions (HAPCs) with mass movements in colon occur how many times per day?
Harrison's 20th Ed. Chapter 42 Page 260

A. Four times
B. Five times
C. Six times
D. Eight times

High-amplitude (>75 mm Hg) propagated contractions (HAPCs) associated with mass movements of colon and normally occur ~five times per day, usually on awakening in morning & postprandially.

114. After meal ingestion, colonic phasic & tonic contractility increases for a period of?
Harrison's 20th Ed. Chapter 42 Page 260

A. ~ 30 minutes
B. ~ 1 hour
C. ~ 2 hours
D. ~ 3 hours

After meal ingestion, colonic phasic & tonic contractility increases for a period of ~2 hours. Initial phase (~10 minutes) is mediated by vagus nerve in response to mechanical distention of "stomach". Subsequent response of colon is by caloric stimulation (intake of at least 500 kcal) and is partly mediated by hormones like gastrin & serotonin.

115. Sling around the rectoanal junction is formed by?
Harrison's 20th Ed. Chapter 42 Page 260

A. Ischiocavernosus muscle
B. External anal sphincter muscle
C. Puborectalis muscle
D. All of the above

Puborectalis muscle forms a sling around the rectoanal junction to maintain continence by tonic contraction.

116. Continence is maintained by?
Harrison's 20th Ed. Chapter 42 Page 260 Figure 42-1

A. Normal rectal sensation
B. Tonic contraction of internal anal sphincter
C. Tonic contraction of puborectalis muscle
D. All of the above

117. Puborectalis muscle wraps around anorectum to maintain an anorectal angle between?
Harrison's 20th Ed. Chapter 42 Page 260 Figure 42-1

A. 35° and 60°
B. 60° and 90°
C. 80° and 110°
D. 100° and 140°

Puborectalis muscle wraps around anorectum to maintain an anorectal angle between 80° and 110°.

118. During defecation, the anorectal angle to straighten by at least?
Harrison's 20th Ed. Chapter 42 Page 260 Figure 42-1

A. 5°
B. 10°
C. 15°
D. 20°

During defecation, the anorectal angle straightens by at least 15°, perineum descends by 1–3.5 cm. and the external anal sphincter relaxes and reduces pressure on anal canal.

119. What weight of stool for adults on a typical Western diet is considered diarrheal?
Harrison's 20th Ed. Chapter 42 Page 261

A. >75 grams/day
B. >100 grams/day
C. >150 grams/day
D. >200 grams/day

>200 grams/day of stool for adults on a typical Western diet is considered diarrheal. Diarrhea is defined as acute if <2 weeks, persistent if 2–4 weeks, and chronic if >4 weeks in duration.

120. Which of the following may be confused with true diarrhea?
Harrison's 20th Ed. Chapter 42 Page 261

A. Pseudodiarrhea
B. Fecal incontinence
C. Overflow diarrhea
D. All of the above

Pseudodiarrhea is frequent passage of small volumes of stool. It is associated with rectal urgency, tenesmus, or a feeling of incomplete evacuation, and accompanies IBS or proctitis. Fecal incontinence is involuntary discharge of rectal contents and is caused by neuromuscular disorders or structural anorectal problems. Overflow diarrhea occurs due to fecal impaction.

121. Persons with hemochromatosis are especially prone to?
Harrison's 20th Ed. Chapter 42 Page 261

A. Yersinia infections
B. Chlamydia infections
C. Salmonella infections
D. Staphylococcus aureus infections

Persons with hemochromatosis are prone to enteric infections with Vibrio species and Yersinia infections and should avoid raw fish.

122. Profuse, watery diarrhea secondary to small-bowel hypersecretion occurs with?
Harrison's 20th Ed. Chapter 42 Page 261

A. Ingestion of preformed bacterial toxins
B. Ingestion of enterotoxin-producing bacteria
C. Ingestion of enteroadherent pathogens
D. All of the above

Profuse, watery diarrhea secondary to small-bowel hypersecretion occurs with ingestion of preformed bacterial toxins, enterotoxin-producing bacteria & enteroadherent pathogens.

123. Infection with which of the following can cause severe abdominal pain with tenderness mimicking acute appendicitis?
Harrison's 20th Ed. Chapter 42 Page 261

A. Yersinia infections
B. E. coli infections
C. Salmonella infections
D. Staphylococcus aureus infections

Yersinia invades terminal ileal & proximal colon mucosa. It may cause severe abdominal pain with tenderness mimicking acute appendicitis.

124. Reactive arthritis (Reiter's syndrome) may accompany or follow infections by?
Harrison's 20th Ed. Chapter 42 Page 261

A. Salmonella
B. Campylobacter
C. Shigella
D. All of the above

Reactive arthritis (Reiter's syndrome), may accompany or follow infections by Salmonella, Campylobacter, Shigella & Yersinia.

125. Yersiniosis may lead to?
Harrison's 20th Ed. Chapter 42 Page 261

A. Autoimmune-type thyroiditis
B. Pericarditis
C. Glomerulonephritis
D. All of the above

Yersiniosis may lead to autoimmune-type thyroiditis, pericarditis & glomerulonephritis.

126. Infection with which of the following can cause hemolytic-uremic syndrome?
Harrison's 20th Ed. Chapter 42 Page 261

A. E. coli (O113:H7)
B. E. coli (O121:H7)
C. E. coli (O145:H7)
D. E. coli (O157:H7)

127. Infection with which of the following can cause hemolytic-uremic syndrome?
Harrison's 20th Ed. Chapter 42 Page 261

A. Enterohemorrhagic E. coli (O157:H7)
B. Campylobacter
C. Salmonella
D. All of the above

Enterohemorrhagic E. coli (O157:H7) and Shigella can lead to the hemolytic-uremic syndrome with an attendant high mortality rate.

128. Which of the following pathotypes of intestinal pathogenic E. coli does not cause acute diarrheal disease?
Harrison's 20th Ed. Chapter 156 Page 1152

A. Shiga toxin–producing E. coli (STEC)
B. Enteroinvasive E. coli (EIEC)
C. Adherent invasive E. coli (AIEC)
D. Diffusely adherent E. coli (DAEC)

Pathotypes of intestinal pathogenic E. coli include Shiga toxin–producing E. coli (STEC), enterohemorrhagic E. coli (EHEC), Shiga toxin-producing enteroaggregative E. coli (ST-EAEC); enterotoxigenic E. coli (ETEC); enteropathogenic E. coli (EPEC); enteroinvasive E. coli (EIEC); enteroaggregative E. coli (EAEC); Diffusely adherent E. coli (DAEC); cytodetaching E. coli and adherent invasive E. coli (AIEC). AIEC is associated with Crohn's disease but does not cause acute diarrheal disease.

129. Acute diarrhea can be a major symptom of?
Harrison's 20th Ed. Chapter 42 Page 261

A. Viral hepatitis
B. Listeriosis
C. Legionellosis
D. All of the above

Acute diarrhea can be a major symptom of viral hepatitis, listeriosis, legionellosis & toxic shock syndrome.

130. Increased levels of which of the following signal intestinal inflammation?
Harrison's 20th Ed. Chapter 42 Page 261

A. Fecal hemoglobin
B. Lactoferrin
C. Neopterin
D. All of the above

131. Increased levels of which of the following signal intestinal inflammation?
Harrison's 20th Ed. Chapter 42 Page 261

A. Calprotectin
B. Protectin
C. Resolvin
D. All of the above

132. Which of the following is an abrupt onset diarrhea that persists for at least 4 weeks or longer?

Harrison's 20th Ed. Chapter 42 Page 263

A. Runner's diarrhea
B. Brainerd diarrhea
C. Traveler's diarrhea
D. Factitious diarrhea

Brainerd diarrhea was first described in Brainerd, Minnesota in 1983.

133. Nitazoxanide is active against?

Harrison's 20th Ed. Chapter 42 Page 263

A. Giardia
B. Cryptosporidium
C. E. histolytica
D. All of the above

Nitazoxanide is used for the treatment of cryptosporidiosis and giardiasis. It is active against other intestinal protozoa also.

134. Which of the following about Nitazoxanide is false?

Harrison's 20th Ed. Chapter 217 Page 1566

A. 1-nitrothiazole compound
B. 3-nitrothiazole compound
C. 5-nitrothiazole compound
D. 7-nitrothiazole compound

Nitazoxanide is a 5-nitrothiazole compound.

135. Which of the following is an active metabolite of Nitazoxanide?

Harrison's 20th Ed. Chapter 217 Page 1566

A. Dizoxanide
B. Tizoxanide
C. Nizoxanide
D. Rizoxanide

Nitazoxanide is hydrolyzed to an active metabolite, tizoxanide (desacetylnitazoxanide) which then undergoes conjugation, primarily by glucuronidation. It is is highly bound to plasma protein.

136. Mechanism of action of Nitazoxanide is related to which of the following?

Harrison's 20th Ed. Chapter 217 Page 1566

A. Pyruvate-ferredoxin oxidoreductase (PFOR)
B. P450 oxidoreductase (POR)
C. Ubiquinone oxidoreductase
D. All of the above

Antiprotozoal activity of nitazoxanide is due to interference with the pyruvate-ferredoxin oxidoreductase (PFOR) enzyme–dependent electron transfer reaction that is essential to anaerobic energy metabolism.

137. Which of the following is an active metabolite of Nitazoxanide?

Harrison's 20th Ed. Chapter 217 Page 1566

A. Approved for use in children between 1–11 years of age
B. Tizoxanide glucuronide is excreted in urine & bile
C. Tizoxanide is highly bound to plasma protein
D. None of the above

138. Which of the following is false about secretory diarrheas?

Harrison's 20th Ed. Chapter 42 Page 263

A. Due to derangements across enterocolonic mucosa
B. Watery, large-volume fecal outputs
C. Painless and respond to fasting
D. No fecal osmotic gap

Secretory diarrheas are due to derangements in fluid & electrolyte transport across enterocolonic mucosa, characterized by painless, watery, large-volume fecal outputs that persist with fasting. There is no fecal osmotic gap.

139. Which of the following is an endogenous laxative?

Harrison's 20th Ed. Chapter 42 Page 263 Table 42-3

A. Dihydroxy bile acids
B. Oxidized bile acids
C. Hydrolized bile acids
D. Dimethyl bile acids

140. Which of the following angiotensin-receptor blocker is associated with diarrhea?

Harrison's 20th Ed. Chapter 42 Page 264

A. Irbesartan
B. Losartan
C. Olmesartan
D. All of the above

Angiotensin-receptor blocker, olmesartan, is associated with diarrhea due to sprue-like enteropathy.

141. Which of the following is not a cause of secretory chronic diarrhea?

Harrison's 20th Ed. Chapter 42 Page 263 Table 42-3

A. Addison's disease
B. VIPoma
C. Lactase and other disaccharide deficiencies
D. Carcinoid syndrome

142. Mucosal malabsorption can be due to?

Harrison's 20th Ed. Chapter 42 Page 263 Table 42-3

A. Celiac sprue
B. Whipple's disease
C. Abetalipoproteinemia
D. All of the above

143. Which of the following does not cause diarrhea?

Harrison's 20th Ed. Chapter 42 Page 264

A. Ca^{2+} blockers
B. Chronic ethanol consumption
C. Olmesartan
D. Arsenic

Ca^{2+} blockers and antidepressants cause constipation in adults.

144. Which of the following is a negative regulator of bile acid synthesis?

Harrison's 20th Ed. Chapter 42 Page 264

A. FGF-7
B. FGF-11
C. FGF-13
D. FGF-19

Fibroblast growth factor 19 (FGF-19) is produced by ileal enterocytes and serves as a negative feedback of bile acid synthesis in hepatocytes.

145. Which of the following mediates the effect of FGF-19 on the hepatocyte?

Harrison's 20th Ed. Chapter 42 Page 264

A. α-klotho
B. β-klotho
C. γ-klotho
D. δ-klotho

146. Which of the following is the most common cause of unexplained chronic diarrhea?

Harrison's 20th Ed. Chapter 42 Page 264

A. Cystic fibrosis
B. Idiopathic bile acid malabsorption (BAM)
C. Metastatic gastrointestinal carcinoid tumors
D. Pancreatic cholera

147. Which of the following is an intestinal secretagogue?

Harrison's 20th Ed. Chapter 42 Page 264

A. Serotonin
B. Histamine
C. Prostaglandins
D. All of the above

148. Glucose-dependent insulinotropic peptide is also called?

Harrison's 20th Ed. Chapter 42 Page 264

A. Secretin
B. Gastrin-inhibitory polypeptide
C. Neurotensin
D. Calcitonin

149. Non-β cell pancreatic adenoma best relates to?

Harrison's 20th Ed. Chapter 42 Page 264

A. Watery diarrhea hypokalemia achlorhydria syndrome
B. Pancreatic cholera
C. VIPoma
D. All of the above

150. Mutation in NHE3 gene leads to?

Harrison's 20th Ed. Chapter 42 Page 264

A. Congenital chloridorrhea
B. Congenital sodium diarrhea
C. Addison's disease
D. All of the above

In congenital sodium diarrhea, mutation in NHE3 (sodium-hydrogen exchanger) gene causes defective Na^+/H^+ exchange resulting in diarrhea and acidosis.

151. One of the most common causes of chronic diarrhea in adults is?

Harrison's 20th Ed. Chapter 42 Page 264

A. Lactase deficiency
B. Ingestion of magnesium-containing antacids
C. Gastrinoma
D. Chronic ethanol consumption

152. In the acronym FODMAP, F stands for?

Harrison's 20th Ed. Chapter 42 Page 264

A. Fermentable
B. Food
C. Fecal
D. Free

153. In the acronym FODMAP, P stands for?

Harrison's 20th Ed. Chapter 42 Page 264

A. Polyol
B. Polysaccharide
C. Phenyl
D. Phenol

FODMAP stands for fermentable oligosaccharides, disaccharides, monosaccharides, and polyols.

154. Steatorrhea is defined as stool fat exceeding?

Harrison's 20th Ed. Chapter 42 Page 264

A. 3 grams/day
B. 4 grams/day
C. 6 grams/day
D. 7 grams/day

Steatorrhea is defined as stool fat exceeding the normal 7 grams/day.

155. Of the following, fecal fat excretion is most in?

Harrison's 20th Ed. Chapter 42 Page 264

A. Rapid-transit diarrhea
B. Small-intestinal diseases
C. Pancreatic exocrine insufficiency
D. Postmucosal lymphatic obstruction

156. Pancreatic exocrine insufficiency occurs when what percentage of pancreatic secretory function is lost?

Harrison's 20th Ed. Chapter 42 Page 264

A. > 30%
B. > 50%
C. > 75%
D. > 90%

Pancreatic exocrine insufficiency occurs when >90% of pancreatic secretory function is lost.

157. Most frequent cause of pancreatic insufficiency is?

Harrison's 20th Ed. Chapter 42 Page 264

A. Chronic pancreatitis
B. Cystic fibrosis
C. Pancreatic duct obstruction
D. Somatostatinoma

Ethanol abuse is the most common cause of chronic pancreatitis.

158. Mucosal malabsorption most commonly occurs from?

Harrison's 20th Ed. Chapter 42 Page 265

A. Giardiasis
B. Whipple's disease
C. Celiac disease
D. Tropical sprue

Mucosal malabsorption most commonly occurs from celiac disease.

159. Which of the following is associated with acanthocytic erythrocytes, ataxia & retinitis pigmentosa?

Harrison's 20th Ed. Chapter 42 Page 265

A. Abetalipoproteinemia
B. Whipple's disease
C. Celiac disease
D. Tropical sprue

Abetalipoproteinemia is a defect of chylomicron formation & fat malabsorption in children. It is associated with acanthocytic erythrocytes, ataxia & retinitis pigmentosa.

160. Which of the following medication may cause mucosal malabsorption?

Harrison's 20th Ed. Chapter 42 Page 265

A. Olmesartan
B. Mycophenolate mofetil
C. Cholestyramine
D. All of the above

161. Which of the following about postmucosal lymphatic obstruction is false?

Harrison's 20th Ed. Chapter 42 Page 265

A. Fat malabsorption with enteric losses of protein
B. Lymphocytopenia
C. Carbohydrate and amino acid absorption preserved
D. None of the above

162. Which of the following is a polyposis colonic syndrome?

Gastroenterol Hepatol (NY) 2012;8:197-201

A. Cowden syndrome
B. Peutz-Jeghers syndrome
C. Cronkhite-Canada syndrome
D. All of the above

163. Which of the following is a feature of Cronkhite-Canada syndrome (CCS)?

Gastroenterol Hepatol (NY) 2012;8:197-201

A. Gastrointestinal hamartomatous polyposis
B. Alopecia & onychodystrophy
C. Hyperpigmentation
D. All of the above

Cronkhite-Canada syndrome (CCS) is a noninherited condition characterized by gastrointestinal hamartomatous polyposis, alopecia, onychodystrophy, hyperpigmentation & diarrhea.

164. Which of the following is not a feature of irritable bowel syndrome (IBS)?

Harrison's 20th Ed. Chapter 42 Page 265

A. Stool frequency ceases at night
B. Abdominal pain relieved with defecation
C. Weight loss
D. Diarrhea alternating with periods of constipation

Irritable bowel syndrome (IBS) is characterized by stool frequency that ceases at night, alternates with periods of constipation, abdominal pain relieved with defecation, no weight loss.

165. Which of the following is recommended for the control of diabetic diarrhea?

Harrison's 20th Ed. Chapter 42 Page 267

A. Diphenoxylate
B. Codeine
C. Clonidine
D. Rifaximin

α^2-adrenergic agonist clonidine may be of use for the control of diabetic diarrhea.

166. Which of the following is useful for the treatment of diarrhea associated with IBS?

Harrison's 20th Ed. Chapter 42 Page 267

A. Alosetron
B. Rifaximin
C. Eluxadoline
D. All of the above

167. Which of the following may induce sphincter of Oddi spasm?

Harrison's 20th Ed. Chapter 42 Page 267

A. Alosetron
B. Rifaximin
C. Eluxadoline
D. All of the above

Eluxadoline may induce sphincter of Oddi spasm and lead to acute pancreatitis, mostly in patients with past h/o cholecystectomy.

168. Eluxadoline is an antagonist of which of the following opioid receptor?

Harrison's 20th Ed. Chapter 42 Page 267

A. μ
B. κ
C. δ
D. All of the above

Eluxadoline is an oral agent with mixed opioid effects i.e. μ- and κ-opioid receptor agonist and δ-opioid receptor (OR) antagonist.

169. In constipation, recommended quantity of dietary fiber as a supplement is?

Harrison's 20th Ed. Chapter 42 Page 268

A. 5 – 15 grams/day
B. 15 – 25 grams/day
C. 30 – 50 grams/day
D. 50 – 60 grams/day

170. Melanosis coli is best related to?

Harrison's 20th Ed. Chapter 42 Page 268

A. Anthraquinone
B. Benzoquinone
C. Naphthoquinone
D. Parietin

Plants with high levels of anthraquinones include aloe, cascara, sagrada, frangula (buckthorn), rhubarb, senna.

171. The dark pigment seen in melanosis coli is?

N Engl J Med. 2013; 368:2303

A. Melanin
B. Lipofuscin
C. Hemosiderin
D. Alizarin

Anthraquinone use causes injury to colonic epithelial cells resulting in the production of lipofuscin, the dark pigment seen in melanosis coli.

172. Which of the following about melanosis coli is false?

Harrison's 20th Ed. Chapter 42 Page 268

A. Due to use of anthraquinone laxatives
B. Pigmentation of colon mucosa
C. Benign and reversible
D. None of the above

173. Which of the following is not a osmotic laxative?

Harrison's 20th Ed. Chapter 42 Page 268

A. Lactulose
B. Sorbitol
C. Glycerin
D. Polyethylene glycol

174. Which of the following is a cause of constipation?

Harrison's 20th Ed. Chapter 42 Page 268

A. Descending perineum syndrome
B. Paradoxical contraction of puborectalis muscle
C. Rectocele
D. All of the above

175. Lubiprostone is best related to?

Harrison's 20th Ed. Chapter 42 Page 268

A. Guanylate cyclase C agonist
B. Chloride channel activator
C. μ-opioid receptor (OR) agonist
D. κ-opioid receptor (OR) agonist

Lubiprostone is a locally acting, bicyclic functional fatty acid derived from prostaglandin E1 that acts by specifically activating CIC-2 chloride channels on the apical aspect of enterocytes, thereby eliciting a chloride-rich fluid secretion. CIC refers to chronic idiopathic constipation.

176. Linaclotide is best related to?

Harrison's 20th Ed. Chapter 42 Page 268

A. Guanylate cyclase C agonist
B. Chloride channel activator
C. μ-opioid receptor (OR) agonist
D. κ-opioid receptor (OR) agonist

Linaclotide is a guanylate cyclase C agonist that activates chloride secretion. Plecanatide is also an oral, locally acting guanylate cyclase agonist.

177. Which of the following is a 5-HT4 agonist?

Harrison's 20th Ed. Chapter 42 Page 269

A. Lubiprostone
B. Linaclotide
C. Bisacodyl
D. Prucalopride

Gastrointestinal Bleeding

178. Risk-assessment score for upper gastrointestinal bleeding is done by?

N Engl J Med. 2016;374:2367-76

A. Glasgow - Barkun Score
B. Glasgow - Blatchford Score
C. Glasgow - Cooper Score
D. Glasgow - Hearnshaw Score

Risk assessment is performed to determine the severity of upper gastrointestinal bleeding by Glasgow - Blatchford Score.

179. Variables used in Glasgow - Blatchford Score include all except?

N Engl J Med. 2016;374:2367-76

A. Blood urea nitrogen
B. Serum creatinine
C. Melena
D. Syncope

Variables used in Glasgow - Blatchford Score include Blood urea nitrogen, Hemoglobin, Systolic blood pressure, Heart rate, Melena, Syncope, Hepatic disease and Cardiac failure. Glasgow–Blatchford scores range from 0 to 23, with higher scores indicating higher risk. High clinical risk is when Glasgow–Blatchford score is ≥12.

180. Risk-assessment score for upper gastrointestinal bleeding is done by?

Tropical Gastroenterology 2016;37(4):276-282

A. AIMS65 scoring system
B. Rockall score
C. Glasgow - Blatchford Score
D. All of the above

Rockall score (described in 1996) is more useful in non-variceal bleeding. It is used to predict mortality and consists of a pre-endoscopic clinical score and a complete endoscopic score after endoscopy. AIMS65 helps in predicting mortality using five factors including albumin levels, deranged INR, impaired mental status, SBP of 90 or less, age of 65 or more.

181. Risk-assessment score for upper gastrointestinal bleeding is done by?

World J Gastroenterol. 2013;19(22):3466-72

A. Rockall score
B. Baylor bleeding score
C. Cedars-Sinai Medical Centre Predictive Index
D. All of the above

182. Endoscopic findings in bleeding peptic ulcers are classified by?

Lancet. 1974;2:394.

A. Pateron classification
B. Forrest classification
C. Laursen classification
D. Barth classification

Endoscopic findings in patients with bleeding peptic ulcers are described using Forrest classification. Findings include spurting hemorrhage (class Ia), oozing hemorrhage (class Ib), a nonbleeding visible vessel (class IIa), an adherent clot (class IIb), a flat pigmented spot (class IIc), and a clean ulcer base (class III). The endoscopic appearance helps determine which lesions require endoscopic therapy.

183. Overt Gastrointestinal bleeding (GIB) is manifested by?

Harrison's 20th Ed. Chapter 44 Page 272

A. Hematemesis
B. Melena
C. Hematochezia
D. All of the above

184. Upper gastrointestinal bleeding (UGIB) is said to occur when the site of bleeding is from?

Harrison's 20th Ed. Chapter 44 Page 272, N Engl J Med. 2018;378:2506-16

A. Esophagus
B. Stomach
C. Duodenum
D. All of the above

Hemorrhage from upper gastrointestinal tract (esophagus, stomach, or duodenum) is defined as primary when it is the cause of hospital admission and is defined as secondary when it complicates the hospital course for patients who have been admitted for other reasons.

185. Lower gastrointestinal bleeding (LGIB) is said to occur when the site of bleeding is from?

Harrison's 20th Ed. Chapter 44 Page 272

A. Small intestine
B. Colon
C. Obscure
D. All of the above

186. Upper gastrointestinal tract is up to?

Harrison's 20 Ed. Chapter 322 Page 2293

A. Pylorus
B. Ampulla of Vater
C. Ligament of Treitz
D. End of jejunum

Upper GI is above the ligament of Treitz. Over 90% of patients with melena are bleeding proximal to the ligament of Treitz, and about 90% of patients with hematochezia are bleeding from the colon.

187. Most common cause of upper GI bleeding (UGIB) is?

Harrison's 20th Ed. Chapter 44 Page 272

A. Esophageal varices
B. Peptic ulcers
C. Gastroduodenal erosions
D. Erosive esophagitis

Peptic ulcers are the most common cause of UGIB, accounting for up to ~50% of cases of UGIB hospitalizations.

188. High-risk peptic ulcer refers to?

Harrison's 20th Ed. Chapter 44 Page 272

A. Active bleeding
B. Nonbleeding visible vessel
C. Adherent clot
D. All of the above

189. High-dose, constant-infusion IV proton pump inhibitor (PPI) applies to?

Harrison's 20th Ed. Chapter 44 Page 272

A. 40 mg bolus & 4 mg/hour infusion
B. 60 mg bolus & 6 mg/hour infusion
C. 80 mg bolus & 8 mg/hour infusion
D. 100 mg bolus & 10 mg/hour infusion

High-dose, constant-infusion IV proton pump inhibitor (PPI) means 80 mg bolus & 8 mg/hour infusion.

190. Objective of high-dose, constant IV infusion of proton pump inhibitor is to sustain intragastric pH at?

Harrison's 20th Ed. Chapter 44 Page 272

A. > 4
B. > 5
C. > 6
D. > 7

191. Prevention of recurrent bleeding focuses on?

Harrison's 20th Ed. Chapter 44 Page 272

A. Helicobacter pylori
B. Nonsteroidal anti-inflammatory drugs (NSAIDs)
C. Gastric acid
D. All of the above

192. Portal hypertension is responsible for bleeding from?

Harrison's 20th Ed. Chapter 44 Page 272

A. Varices in the small & large intestine
B. Portal hypertensive gastropathy
C. Enterocolopathy
D. All of the above

Portal hypertension is responsible for bleeding from gastric varices, varices in small & large intestine, portal hypertensive gastropathy and enterocolopathy. Endoscopic appearance of Gastric antral vascular ectasia (GAVE) syndrome resembles that in portal hypertensive gastropathy (PHG) or antral gastritis. PHG causes predominant changes in the fundus and corpus.

193. Watermelon stomach best relates to?

Harrison's 20th Ed. Chapter 44 Page 273

A. Gastric antral vascular ectasia (GAVE)
B. Hereditary hemorrhagic telangiectasias
C. Prolapse gastropathy
D. Hemosuccus pancreaticus

Gastric antral vascular ectasia (GAVE) was first described by Rider as "fiery red changes with marked hypertrophic mucosal changes, and scattered profuse bleeding" and later as columns of red tortuous ectatic vessels along longitudinal folds of the antrum resembling watermelon stripes.

194. Dieulafoy's lesion is also termed as?

Ann R Coll Surg Engl. 2010;92(7):548-554

A. Caliber persistent artery
B. Exulceratio simplex
C. Miliary aneurysms of the stomach
D. All of the above

Dieulafoy's lesion refers to an aberrant vessel in the mucosa that bleeds from a pinpoint mucosal defect.

195. The most common cause of LGIB in adults is?

Harrison's 20th Ed. Chapter 44 Page 273

A. NSAID-induced colitis
B. Diverticulosis
C. Ulcerative colitis
D. Crohn's disease

The most common cause of LGIB in adults is diverticulosis.

196. Which of the following is false about diverticular bleeding?

Harrison's 20th Ed. Chapter 44 Page 273

A. Abrupt in onset, usually painless
B. Commonly from right colon
C. Bleeding stops spontaneously
D. None of the above

197. In Heyde's syndrome, which of the following is a feature besides bleeding vascular ectasias?

Harrison's 20th Ed. Chapter 44 Page 273

A. Aortic stenosis
B. Mitral stenosis
C. Aortic regurgitation
D. Mitral regurgitation

Heyde's syndrome refers to bleeding vascular ectasias & aortic stenosis.

198. Blood transfusion is recommended in acute GIB when the hemoglobin drops below?

Harrison's 20th Ed. Chapter 44 Page 273

A. 5 grams/dL
B. 6 grams/dL
C. 7 grams/dL
D. 8 grams/dL

199. For melena, blood should be present in GI tract for what duration?

Harrison's 20th Ed. Chapter 44 Page 273

A. 3 hours
B. 7 hours
C. 14 hours
D. 22 hours

Melena indicates that blood has been present in the GI tract for at least 14 hours and as long as 3–5 days.

200. Clues to upper gastrointestinal bleed include?

Harrison's 20th Ed. Chapter 44 Page 273

A. Hyperactive bowel sounds
B. Melena
C. Elevated blood urea nitrogen
D. All of the above

Clues to UGIB include melena, hyperactive bowel sounds & elevated BUN level (due to volume depletion and blood proteins absorbed in the small intestine).

201. Rectal ulcer is found in what proportion of patients of solitary rectal ulcer syndrome?

World J Gastroenterol. 2014;20(3):738-744

A. 40%
B. 60%
C. 80%
D. 100%

Solitary rectal ulcer syndrome is a misnomer because ulcers are found in 40% of patients. Passage of blood during defecation is the hallmark.

202. Cirrhotic patients presenting with UGIB should be placed on?

Harrison's 20th Ed. Chapter 44 Page 274

A. Antibiotics
B. Tranquillizers
C. Lactulose
D. Domperidone

Cirrhotic patients presenting with UGIB should be placed on antibiotics (quinolone, ceftriaxone) and started on a vasoactive medication (octreotide, terlipressin, somatostatin, vapreotide) upon presentation, even before endoscopy. Antibiotics decrease bacterial infections, rebleeding, and mortality in this population, and vasoactive medications improve control of bleeding in the first 12 hours after presentation.

203. Which of the following is not a low-risk endoscopic lesion?

Harrison's 20th Ed. Chapter 44 Page 274, N Engl J Med. 2016;374:2367-76

A. Visible vessel
B. Clean-based ulcers
C. Erosions
D. Nonbleeding Mallory-Weiss tears

An adherent clot is also a high-risk endoscopic finding.

204. Which of the following statements is false?

N Engl J Med. 2016;374:2367-76

A. No advantage of nasogastric lavage in upper GI bleed
B. BUN / creatinine ratio helpful to identify upper GI bleed
C. Restrictive transfusion strategy is beneficial
D. None of the above

205. Tissue deposition of bilirubin occurs in?

Harrison's 20th Ed. Chapter 45 Page 276

A. Serum hyperbilirubinemia
B. Hemolytic disorder
C. Disorder of bilirubin metabolism
D. All of the above

Jaundice

206. Sclerae have affinity for bilirubin due to its?

Harrison's 20th Ed. Chapter 45 Page 276

A. High collagen content
B. High elastin content
C. High mucopolysaccharide content
D. All of the above

Sclerae have affinity for bilirubin due to its high elastin content.

207. Presence of scleral icterus indicates a serum bilirubin level of at least?

Harrison's 20th Ed. Chapter 45 Page 276

A. 1.5 mg/dL
B. 2 mg/dL
C. 2.5 mg/dL
D. 3 mg/dL

Presence of scleral icterus indicates a serum bilirubin level of at least 3 mg/dL (51 μmol/L). Jaundice is rarely detectable if the serum bilirubin level is <2.5 mg/dL but may remain detectable below this level during recovery from jaundice (because of protein and tissue binding of conjugated bilirubin).

208. A second site to detect icterus is?

Harrison's 20th Ed. Chapter 45 Page 276

A. Uvula
B. Hard palate
C. Nails
D. Underneath the tongue

A second site to detect icterus is underneath the tongue.

209. In long-standing deep jaundice, skin color may become?

Harrison's 20th Ed. Chapter 45 Page 276

A. Gray
B. Brown
C. Green
D. Orange

As serum bilirubin levels rises and the process is long-standing, skin becomes green due to oxidation of bilirubin to biliverdin.

210. Yellowing of the skin may occur in?

Harrison's 20th Ed. Chapter 45 Page 276

A. Carotenoderma
B. Quinacrine use
C. Excessive exposure to phenols
D. All of the above

211. Carotenoderma develops with ingestion of excessive amounts of?

Harrison's 20th Ed. Chapter 45 Page 276

A. Carrots
B. Leafy vegetables
C. Oranges
D. All of the above

Carotenoderma develops in healthy individuals who ingest excessive amounts of vegetables and fruits that contain carotene, such as carrots, leafy vegetables, squash, peaches, and oranges.

212. In carotenoderma, the pigment is concentrated on?

Harrison's 20th Ed. Chapter 45 Page 276

A. Palms & soles
B. Forehead
C. Nasolabial folds
D. All of the above

In carotenoderma, the pigment is concentrated on palms, soles, forehead & nasolabial folds but spares the sclerae ("pseudo-jaundice").

213. Pruritis may be seen when the bilirubin reaches?

Harrison's 20th Ed. Chapter 79 Page 593

A. 4 - 6 mg/dL
B. 6 - 8 mg/dL
C. 8 - 10 mg/dL
D. 10 - 12 mg/dL

Pruritis may be seen when the bilirubin reaches 6 - 8 mg/dL.

214. Which of the following is true for bilirubin?

Harrison's 20th Ed. Chapter 45 Page 276

A. Bipyrrole pigment
B. Tripyrrole pigment
C. Tetrapyrrole pigment
D. Pentapyrrole pigment

Bilirubin is a tetrapyrrole pigment. Heme is an iron-chelated tetrapyrrole or porphyrin.

215. What amount of bilirubin is produced each day?

Harrison's 20th Ed. Chapter 45 Page 276

A. 1 mg/kg body weight
B. 2 mg/kg body weight
C. 3 mg/kg body weight
D. 4 mg/kg body weight

216. Which of the following is a hemoprotein?

Harrison's 20th Ed. Chapter 45 Page 276

A. Heme
B. Myoglobin
C. Cytochrome
D. All of the above

217. Formation of bilirubin occurs in?

Harrison's 20th Ed. Chapter 45 Page 276

A. Bone marrow
B. Spleen
C. Kidneys
D. Intestine

Formation of bilirubin occurs in reticuloendothelial cells, primarily in spleen & liver.

218. Oxidative cleavage of α bridge of porphyrin group and opening of heme ring is catalyzed by?
Harrison's 20th Ed. Chapter 45 Page 276

A. Heme oxygenase
B. ALA-dehydratase
C. Hydroxymethylbilane synthase
D. PROTO-oxidase

Oxidative cleavage of α bridge of porphyrin group and opening of heme ring is catalyzed by heme oxygenase.

219. The end product of reaction catalyzed by heme oxygenase is?
Harrison's 20th Ed. Chapter 45 Page 276

A. Biliverdin
B. Carbon monoxide
C. Iron
D. All of the above

220. Which of the following about biliverdin reductase is false?
Harrison's 20th Ed. Chapter 45 Page 276

A. Cytosolic enzyme
B. Microsomal enzyme
C. Reduces central methylene bridge of biliverdin
D. Converts biliverdin to bilirubin

Biliverdin reductase is a cytosolic enzyme. Heme oxygenase is a microsomal enzyme.

221. Which of the following is a moiety of bilirubin?
Harrison's 20th Ed. Chapter 45 Page 276

A. Propionic acid carboxyl groups
B. Imino group
C. Lactam group
D. All of the above

222. Solubilization is accomplished by reversible, noncovalent binding of bilirubin to?
Harrison's 20th Ed. Chapter 45 Page 276

A. Albumin
B. Globulin
C. Biliverdin
D. All of the above

Solubilization is accomplished by the reversible, noncovalent binding of bilirubin to albumin.

223. Unconjugated bilirubin is bound in cytosol to proteins in?
Harrison's 20th Ed. Chapter 45 Page 276

A. Glutathione-S-transferase superfamily
B. Cystatin superfamily
C. Cytochrome P450 (CYP) monooxygenase superfamily
D. GPCR superfamily

Unconjugated bilirubin is bound in cytosol to proteins in the glutathione-S-transferase superfamily.

224. Bilirubin is made aqueous soluble by conjugation to glucuronic acid in?
Harrison's 20th Ed. Chapter 45 Page 276

A. Golgi apparatus
B. Endoplasmic reticulum
C. Mitochondria
D. Lysosome

In endoplasmic reticulum (ER), bilirubin is made aqueous soluble by conjugation to glucuronic acid by disrupting hydrophobic internal hydrogen bonds & formation of bilirubin monoglucuronide & diglucuronide.

225. Conjugation of glucuronic acid to bilirubin is catalyzed by?
Harrison's 20th Ed. Chapter 45 Page 276

A. Bilirubin uridine diphosphate-glucuronyl transferase
B. Bilirubin uridine diphosphate-glucuronosyl transferase
C. Bilirubin uridine diphosphate-glucuronidase transferase
D. Bilirubin uridine diphosphate-glucuronide transferase

Conjugation of glucuronic acid to bilirubin is catalyzed by bilirubin uridine diphosphate-glucuronosyl transferase (UDPGT).

226. Bilirubin monoglucuronide & diglucuronide are actively transported into canalicular bile by?
Harrison's 20th Ed. Chapter 45 Page 276

A. Macrophage associated protein type 2
B. Contactin-associated protein-like 2 (Caspr2)
C. Hemidesmosome-associated protein
D. Multidrug resistance-associated protein 2 (MRP2)

Bilirubin monoglucuronide & diglucuronide are actively transported into canalicular bile by multidrug resistance-associated protein 2 (MRP2).

227. Sinusoidal organic anion transport protein 1B1 and 1B3 best relate to?
Harrison's 20th Ed. Chapter 45 Page 276

A. Transportation of unconjugated bilirubin into hepatocytes
B. Transportation of bilirubin glucuronides into canalicular bile
C. Reuptake of bilirubin glucuronides into hepatocyte
D. Efflux of bilirubin back into serum

A portion of bilirubin glucuronides is transported into sinusoids & portal circulation by MRP3 from where reuptake into hepatocyte occurs by sinusoidal organic anion transport protein 1B1 (OATP1B1) & OATP1B3.

228. Which of the following statements is false?
Harrison's 20th Ed. Chapter 45 Page 276

A. Conjugated bilirubin is not reabsorbed by intestinal mucosa
B. Conjugated bilirubin is hydrolyzed to unconjugated bilirubin in distal ileum & colon
C. Conjugated bilirubin is hydrolyzed to unconjugated bilirubin by bacterial β-glucuronidases
D. None of the above

229. Which of the following about urobilinogen is false?
Harrison's 20th Ed. Chapter 45 Page 276

A. Colorless tetrapyrrole
B. Formed from conjugated bilirubin
C. Most of it is excreted in feces
D. Urobilins are oxidized urobilinogen

The "unconjugated" bilirubin is reduced by normal gut bacteria to colorless tetrapyrroles called urobilinogens, ~80 – 90% are excreted in feces, either unchanged or oxidized to orange derivatives called urobilins.

230. What percentage of urobilinogens undergo enterohepatic cycling?
Harrison's 20th Ed. Chapter 45 Page 276

A. 10 – 20%
B. 20 – 30%
C. 30 – 40%
D. 40 – 50%

10 - 20% of urobilinogens undergo enterohepatic cycling.

231. Increased urinary excretion of urobilinogen can be due to?
Harrison's 20th Ed. Chapter 45 Page 276

A. Increased bilirubin production
B. Increased hepatic reabsorption of urobilinogen from colon
C. Decreased hepatic clearance of urobilinogen
D. All of the above

232. Nationality of Abraham Albert Hijmans van den Bergh was?

A. Russian
B. Dutch
C. German
D. Spanish

Abraham Albert Hijmans van den Bergh (1869 - 1943) was a Dutch physician.

233. Serum bilirubin assay is best related to?
Harrison's 20th Ed. Chapter 45 Page 276

A. Azo pigment
B. Phthalocyanine pigment
C. Quinacridone pigment
D. Arylide yellow

In serum bilirubin assay, bilirubin is exposed to diazotized sulfanilic acid. It splits into two stable dipyrromethene azo pigments that allows photometric analysis at 540 nm.

234. Accelerator substance in van den Bergh reaction is?
Harrison's 20th Ed. Chapter 45 Page 276

A. Alcohol
B. HCl
C. H_2SO_4
D. HNO_3

In van den Bergh reaction, direct fraction is that which reacts with diazotized sulfanilic acid in absence of accelerator substance (alcohol). Direct fraction correlates with the conjugated bilirubin level in serum. Total serum bilirubin is the amount that reacts after addition of alcohol.

235. Unconjugated hyperbilirubinemia is present when direct fraction is what percentage of total serum bilirubin?
Harrison's 20th Ed. Chapter 45 Page 277

A. < 10%
B. < 15%
C. < 20%
D. < 25%

Unconjugated hyperbilirubinemia is said to be present when direct fraction is <15% of total serum bilirubin.

236. Which of the following statements about calculated indirect bilirubin is true?
Harrison's 20th Ed. Chapter 45 Page 277

A. Under estimates true amount of unconjugated bilirubin
B. Over estimates true amount of unconjugated bilirubin
C. Same as true amount of unconjugated bilirubin
D. Any of the above

Unconjugated bilirubin slowly reacts with diazo reagents, even without the accelerator. Thus, calculated indirect bilirubin is an underestimate of the true amount of unconjugated bilirubin in circulation.

237. In 95% of a normal population, total serum bilirubin concentrations are between?
Harrison's 20th Ed. Chapter 45 Page 277

A. 0.1 and 0.5 mg/dL
B. 0.2 and 0.9 mg/dL
C. 0.3 and 1.0 mg/dL
D. 0.4 and 1.1 mg/dL

With the van den Bergh method, the normal serum bilirubin concentration usually is between 1 and 1.5 mg/dL. Total serum bilirubin concentrations are between 0.2 and 0.9 mg/dL in 95% of a normal population.

238. Albumin-linked fraction of conjugated bilirubin is called?
Harrison's 20th Ed. Chapter 45 Page 277

A. Delta fraction
B. Delta bilirubin
C. Biliprotein
D. All of the above

239. Clearance rate of delta bilirubin is?
Harrison's 20th Ed. Chapter 45 Page 277

A. 1 – 4 days
B. 4 – 7 days
C. 7 – 10 days
D. 12 – 14 days

Because of the tight binding between bilirubin and albumin, the clearance rate of delta bilirubin from serum approximates half-life of albumin (12 - 14 days) rather than the short half-life of bilirubin (about 4 hours).

240. Biliprotein was undetectable in?
N Engl J Med. 1983; 309:1654-1655

A. Serum from horses
B. Icteric human fluids (cyst fluid, pleural exudate)
C. Serum from patients with hemolytic jaundice
D. All of the above

Biliprotein is undetectable in serum from horses (the animal model of Gilbert's syndrome) and in icteric human fluids (cyst fluid, pleural exudate, or serum from patients with hemolytic jaundice).

241. Which of the following about bilirubin is false?
Am J Physiol Endocrinol Metab. 2017;312(4):E244-E252

A. Antioxidant and anti-inflammatory molecule
B. Activates PPARα
C. Suppressor of PPARγ activity
D. None of the above

Bilirubin reduces lipid accumulation by PPARα activation and a reduction in PPARγ transcriptional activity. Patients with Gilbert's syndrome are protected from development of cardiovascular disease.

242. Which of the following statements is false?
Harrison's 20th Ed. Chapter 45 Page 277

A. Unconjugated bilirubin is always bound to albumin in serum
B. Unconjugated bilirubin is not found in urine
C. Most of conjugated bilirubin is reabsorbed by proximal tubules
D. None of the above

243. Hyperbilirubinemia may result from?
Harrison's 20th Ed. Chapter 45 Page 277

A. Overproduction of bilirubin
B. Impaired uptake, conjugation, or excretion of bilirubin
C. Regurgitation of unconjugated or conjugated bilirubin from damaged hepatocytes or bile ducts
D. All of the above

244. Increase in unconjugated bilirubin in serum results from?
Harrison's 20th Ed. Chapter 45 Page 277

A. Overproduction
B. Impaired uptake
C. Impaired conjugation of bilirubin
D. All of the above

245. An increase in conjugated bilirubin in serum is due to?
Harrison's 20th Ed. Chapter 45 Page 277

A. Overproduction
B. Impaired uptake
C. Impaired conjugation of bilirubin
D. Decreased excretion into bile ductules

An increase in conjugated bilirubin is due to decreased excretion into bile ductules or backward leakage of the pigment.

246. Ineffective erythropoiesis occurs in?
Harrison's 20th Ed. Chapter 45 Page 277

A. Cobalamin deficiency
B. Folate deficiency
C. Iron deficiency
D. All of the above

247. Impaired bilirubin conjugation occurs in?
Harrison's 20th Ed. Chapter 45 Page 277

A. Crigler-Najjar syndrome type I
B. Crigler-Najjar syndrome type II
C. Gilbert's syndrome
D. All of the above

248. In Crigler-Najjar type II, bilirubin UDPGT activity is reduced to?
Harrison's 20th Ed. Chapter 45 Page 278

A. < 10%
B. < 20%
C. < 30%
D. < 40%

Because of mutations in bilirubin UDPGT gene, there occurs reduction in enzyme's activity to ≤10% in patients of Crigler-Najjar type II.

249. In Gilbert's syndrome, bilirubin UDPGT activity is reduced to?
Harrison's 20th Ed. Chapter 45 Page 278

A. 2 – 10% of normal
B. 10 – 35% of normal
C. 35 – 50% of normal
D. 50 – 75% of normal

Gilbert's syndrome is marked by impaired conjugation of bilirubin due to reduced bilirubin UDPGT activity - typically 10 - 35% of normal.

250. Serum bilirubin level in patients with Gilbert's syndrome is almost always?
Harrison's 20th Ed. Chapter 45 Page 278

A. < 3 mg/dL
B. < 4 mg/dL
C. < 5 mg/dL
D. < 6 mg/dL

Patients with Gilbert's syndrome have mild unconjugated hyperbilirubinemia, with serum bilirubin levels almost always < 6 mg/dL (103 μmol/L).

251. In Gilbert's syndrome, serum bilirubin levels worsen with?
Harrison's 20th Ed. Chapter 45 Page 278

A. Stress, concurrent illness
B. Alcohol use
C. Fasting
D. All of the above

In Gilbert's syndrome, serum bilirubin levels worsen during periods of stress, concurrent illness, alcohol use, or fasting.

252. The reported incidence of Gilbert's syndrome is?
Harrison's 20th Ed. Chapter 45 Page 278

A. 0.3 – 0.7% of the population
B. 0.7 – 1.5% of the population
C. 1.5 – 3% of the population
D. 3 – 7% of the population

Reported incidence of Gilbert's syndrome is 3 - 7% of the population, with males predominating over females by a ratio of 1.5 - 7:1.

253. Which of the following is a more common condition?
Harrison's 20th Ed. Chapter 45 Page 278

A. Dubin-Johnson syndrome
B. Rotor syndrome
C. Gilbert's syndrome
D. Crigler-Najjar type II

254. Mutations in the gene for MRP2 best relates to?
Harrison's 20th Ed. Chapter 45 Page 278

A. Dubin-Johnson syndrome
B. Rotor syndrome
C. Gilbert's syndrome
D. All of the above

255. Deficiency of hepatic drug reuptake transporters OATP1B1 & OATP1B3 best relates to?
Harrison's 20th Ed. Chapter 45 Page 278

A. Dubin-Johnson syndrome
B. Rotor syndrome
C. Gilbert's syndrome
D. All of the above

256. Which of the following has a benign nature?
Harrison's 20th Ed. Chapter 45 Page 278

A. Dubin-Johnson syndrome
B. Rotor syndrome
C. Gilbert's syndrome
D. All of the above

257. Which of the following is true for Virchow's node?
Harrison's 20th Ed. Chapter 45 Page 279, 412

A. Enlarged right supraclavicular node
B. Enlarged left supraclavicular node
C. Enlarged right infraclavicular node
D. Enlarged left infraclavicular node

Virchow's node refers to an enlarged left supraclavicular node which is infiltrated with metastatic cancer from a gastrointestinal primary. Metastases to supraclavicular nodes also occur from lung, breast, testis, or ovarian cancers. Tuberculosis, sarcoidosis, and toxoplasmosis are nonneoplastic causes of supraclavicular adenopathy.

258. Location of Sister Mary Joseph's nodule is?
Harrison's 20th Ed. Chapter 45 Page 279

A. Neck
B. Chest
C. Abdomen
D. Lower limbs

Sister Mary Joseph's nodule refers to a periumbilical nodule & suggests an abdominal malignancy.

259. Murphy's sign best relates to?
Harrison's 20th Ed. Chapter 45 Page 279

A. Cholecystitis
B. Alcoholic hepatitis
C. Pancreatic cancer
D. Cirrhosis liver

Murphy's sign refers to severe right-upper-quadrant abdominal tenderness ("liver pain") with respiratory arrest on inspiration. It suggests cholecystitis.

260. Which of the following is a feature of cirrhosis liver?
Harrison's 20th Ed. Chapter 45 Page 279

A. Ascites in the presence of jaundice
B. Enlarged left lobe of the liver
C. Temporal and proximal muscle wasting
D. All of the above

261. Which of the following is not an enzyme test?
Harrison's 20th Ed. Chapter 45 Page 279

A. Serum bilirubin
B. Serum alanine aminotransferase (ALT)
C. Serum aspartate aminotransferase (AST)
D. Serum alkaline phosphatase (ALP)

262. Elevated prothrombin time indicates which of the following?
Harrison's 20th Ed. Chapter 45 Page 279

A. Vitamin K deficiency due to prolonged jaundice
B. Malabsorption of vitamin K
C. Significant hepatocellular dysfunction
D. All of the above

Failure of PT to correct with parenteral administration of vitamin K indicates severe hepatocellular injury.

263. In alcoholic hepatitis, AST-to-ALT ratio is at least?
Harrison's 20th Ed. Chapter 45 Page 279

A. 1:1.5
B. 1:2
C. 1.5:1
D. 2:1

In alcoholic hepatitis, AST-to-ALT ratio is at least 2:1. AST level rarely is > 300 U/L.

264. In acute hepatocellular disease, ALT & AST values are how many times higher than normal?
Harrison's 20th Ed. Chapter 45 Page 279

A. 5 times
B. 15 times
C. 25 times
D. 35 times

265. In cholestatic liver disease, ALT & AST values are how many times higher than normal?
Harrison's 20th Ed. Chapter 45 Page 279

A. < 8 times
B. < 12 times
C. < 16 times
D. < 20 times

266. Which of the following mushroom causes hepatotoxicity?
Harrison's 20th Ed. Chapter 45 Page 280

A. Amanita muscaria
B. Amanita pantherina
C. Amanita phalloides
D. All of the above

Mushrooms Amanita phalloides and A. verna contain highly hepatotoxic amatoxins and produces massive hepatic necrosis. The lethal dose of the toxin is ~10 mg,

267. Which of the following can cause cholestatic hepatitis?
Harrison's 20th Ed. Chapter 45 Page 280

A. Hepatitis A and E
B. Hepatitis B
C. Hepatitis C
D. All of the above

268. Which of the following can cause cholestatic hepatitis?
Harrison's 20th Ed. Chapter 45 Page 280

A. Alcoholic hepatitis
B. EBV infection
C. CMV infection
D. All of the above

269. Chronic cholestasis is associated with?
Harrison's 20th Ed. Chapter 45 Page 280

A. Chlorpromazine
B. Imipramine
C. Tolbutamide
D. Erythromycin estolate

Chronic cholestasis has been associated with chlorpromazine and prochlorperazine.

270. About 75% of patients with primary sclerosing cholangitis (PSC) have?
Harrison's 20th Ed. Chapter 45 Page 280

A. Diabetes mellitus
B. Retroperitoneal fibrosis
C. Budd-Chiari syndrome
D. Inflammatory bowel disease

Also, cholangiocarcinoma is most commonly associated with PSC.

271. Vanishing bile duct syndrome is seen in?
Harrison's 20th Ed. Chapter 45 Page 281

A. Graft-versus-host disease
B. Sarcoidosis
C. Chlorpromazine
D. All of the above

272. Which of the following is not a feature of benign recurrent intrahepatic cholestasis (BRIC)?
Harrison's 20th Ed. Chapter 45 Page 281

A. Episodic attacks of pruritus
B. Cholestasis
C. Jaundice beginning at any age
D. Chronic liver disease

Benign recurrent intrahepatic cholestasis (BRIC) types 1 and 2 are a familial form of intrahepatic cholestasis that does not lead to chronic liver disease. Serum bile acids are elevated during episodes, but serum γ-glutamyltransferase (γ-GT) activity is normal.

273. High levels of serum γ-glutamyltransferase are found in?
Harrison's 20th Ed. Chapter 45 Page 281

A. Benign recurrent intrahepatic cholestasis (BRIC)
B. Progressive familial intrahepatic cholestasis (PFIC) types 1
C. Progressive familial intrahepatic cholestasis (PFIC) types 2
D. Progressive familial intrahepatic cholestasis (PFIC) types 3

274. Which of the following is false about cholestasis of pregnancy?
Harrison's 20th Ed. Chapter 45 Page 281

A. Occurs in II & III trimesters, resolves after delivery
B. Probably inherited
C. Cholestasis can be triggered by estrogen administration
D. None of the above

275. Stauffer's syndrome best relates to?
Harrison's 20th Ed. Chapter 45 Page 281

A. Hodgkin's disease
B. Medullary thyroid cancer
C. Renal cell cancer
D. Prostate cancer

Stauffer's syndrome refers to intrahepatic cholestasis specifically associated with renal cell cancer.

276. "Shock liver" best relates to?
Harrison's 20th Ed. Chapter 45 Page 281

A. Ischemic hepatitis
B. Graft-versus-host disease
C. Heart failure
D. Sepsis

Ischemic hepatitis is a distinct entity of acute hypoperfusion characterized by acute (dramatic) elevation in serum aminotransferases followed by a gradual peak in serum bilirubin.

277. In severe cases of Plasmodium falciparum malaria, jaundice is due to?
Harrison's 20th Ed. Chapter 45 Page 281

A. Hemolysis
B. Cholestasis
C. Hepatocellular damage
D. All of the above

278. Weil's syndrome consists of?
Harrison's 20th Ed. Chapter 45 Page 281, 1290

A. Jaundice
B. Renal dysfunction
C. Hemorrhagic diathesis
D. All of the above

With or without jaundice, severe pulmonary hemorrhage is increasingly recognized as an important presentation of severe Weil's disease.

279. Which of the following malignancies has the highest surgical cure rate?
Harrison's 20th Ed. Chapter 45 Page 281

A. Ampullary carcinoma
B. Pancreatic tumor
C. Gallbladder tumor
D. Cholangiocarcinoma

Ampullary carcinoma has the highest surgical cure rate of all the tumors that present as painless jaundice.

280. Findings of which of the following is often identical to that of PSC?
Harrison's 20th Ed. Chapter 45 Page 281

A. Cholangiocarcinoma
B. AIDS cholangiopathy due to CMV
C. AIDS cholangiopathy due to cryptosporidia
D. All of the above

281. Which of the following is a cause of benign extrahepatic cholestatic conditions that may produce jaundice?
Harrison's 20th Ed. Chapter 45 Page 280 Table 45-3

A. Mirizzi's syndrome
B. AIDS cholangiopathy
C. Primary sclerosing cholangitis
D. All of the above

Mirizzi's syndrome is a rare complication in which a gallstone becomes impacted in cystic duct or neck of gallbladder compressing CBD, resulting in CBD obstruction & jaundice.

282. Jaundice is a feature of?
Harrison's 20th Ed. Chapter 45 Page 281

A. Babesiosis
B. Typhoid fever
C. Dengue hemorrhagic fever
D. All of the above

283. Charcot's triad in patients with ascending cholangitis & biliary sepsis consists of all except?
Harrison's 20th Ed. Chapter 315 Page 2200

A. Nausea, vomiting
B. Jaundice
C. Abdominal pain
D. Spiking fever

Charcot's triad of jaundice, abdominal pain, and fever is present in ~70% of patients with ascending cholangitis and biliary sepsis.

284. Which of the following statements about choledocholithiasis is false?
Harrison's 20th Ed. Chapter 339 Page 2431

A. Maximum bilirubin level is 15.0 mg/dL in choledocholithiasis
B. Rise in alkaline phosphatase often precedes clinical jaundice
C. Pancreatitis complicates choledocholithiasis in >30% cases
D. None of the above

285. Which of the following statements about choledocholithiasis is false?
Harrison's 20th Ed. Chapter 45 Page 281

A. Most common cause of extrahepatic cholestasis
B. ERCP is "gold standard" for identifying choledocholithiasis
C. Normal albumin level is suggestive of choledocholithiasis
D. None of the above

Abdominal Swelling and Ascites

286. Which of the following is not one of the six "F" that are the causes of abdominal swelling?
Harrison's 20th Ed. Chapter 46 Page 282

A. Flatus
B. Fat
C. Feces
D. Fertile

Causes of abdominal swelling can be remembered as the six Fs: flatus, fat, fluid, fetus, feces, or a "fatal growth" (often a neoplasm).

287. The normal small intestine contains how much gas?
Harrison's 20th Ed. Chapter 46 Page 282

A. ~ 100 mL
B. ~ 200 mL
C. ~ 300 mL
D. ~ 400 mL

288. Small intestinal gas is?
Harrison's 20th Ed. Chapter 46 Page 282

A. Oxygen
B. Hydrogen
C. Methane
D. All of the above

289. Which of the following gases is produced intraluminally by bacterial fermentation?
Harrison's 20th Ed. Chapter 46 Page 282

A. Carbon dioxide
B. Hydrogen
C. Methane
D. All of the above

Normal small intestine contains ~200 mL of gas made up of nitrogen, oxygen, carbon dioxide, hydrogen & methane. Nitrogen & oxygen are swallowed from outside) whereas carbon dioxide, hydrogen & methane are produced intraluminally by bacterial fermentation.

290. Which of the following is a cause of abdominal distention?
Harrison's 20th Ed. Chapter 46 Page 282

A. Impaired intestinal transit of gas
B. Lack of coordination between diaphragmatic contraction & anterior abdominal wall relaxation
C. Increased lumbar lordosis
D. All of the above

291. Increase in abdominal size is first noted at how many weeks of gestation?
Harrison's 20th Ed. Chapter 46 Page 282

A. 6 – 8
B. 8 – 10
C. 10 – 12
D. 12 – 14

292. A minimum of how much ascitic fluid is required for detection on physical examination?
Harrison's 20th Ed. Chapter 46 Page 282

A. 1000 mL
B. 1500 mL
C. 2000 mL
D. 2500 mL

A minimum of 1500 mL of ascitic fluid is required for detection on physical examination.

293. Abdominal ultrasonography can detect how much ascitic fluid?
Harrison's 20th Ed. Chapter 46 Page 282

A. 100 mL
B. 200 mL
C. 300 mL
D. 400 mL

Abdominal ultrasonography can detect as little as 100 mL of ascitic fluid.

294. Increased hepatic resistance occurs by which of the following mechanisms?
Harrison's 20th Ed. Chapter 46 Page 283

A. Development of hepatic fibrosis
B. Activation of hepatic stellate cells
C. Decrease in endothelial nitric oxide synthetase production
D. All of the above

295. Development of cirrhosis is associated with?
Harrison's 20th Ed. Chapter 46 Page 283

A. Increased systemic circulating levels of nitric oxide
B. Increased levels of vascular endothelial growth factor
C. Increased levels of tumor necrosis factor
D. All of the above

Development of cirrhosis is associated with increased systemic circulating levels of nitric oxide (contrary to decrease seen intrahepatically), increased levels of vascular endothelial growth factor and tumor necrosis factor that result in splanchnic arterial vasodilation.

296. Vasodilation of the splanchnic circulation results in?
Harrison's 20th Ed. Chapter 46 Page 283

A. Release of antidiuretic hormone
B. Activation of sympathetic nervous system
C. Activation of renin angiotensin aldosterone system
D. All of the above

297. Cirrhosis accounts for what percentage of cases of ascites?
Harrison's 20th Ed. Chapter 46 Page 283

A. 34%
B. 54%
C. 64%
D. 84%

Cirrhosis accounts for 84% of cases of ascites.

298. Out of the following which is a less common cause of ascites?
Harrison's 20th Ed. Chapter 46 Page 283

A. Cardiac ascites
B. Tuberculosis
C. Peritoneal carcinomatosis
D. Cirrhosis + a second disease

Cardiac ascites, peritoneal carcinomatosis, and "mixed" ascites (cirrhosis and a second disease) account for 10 – 15% of cases. Less common causes of ascites include massive hepatic metastasis, tuberculosis, Chlamydia infection, pancreatitis, and nephrotic syndrome. Rare causes of ascites include hypothyroidism & familial Mediterranean fever.

299. Dark brown ascitic fluid may indicate?
Harrison's 20th Ed. Chapter 46 Page 283

A. Familial Mediterranean fever
B. Chlamydia infection
C. Pancreatic necrosis
D. Biliary tract perforation

300. Black ascitic fluid may indicate?
Harrison's 20th Ed. Chapter 46 Page 283

A. Familial Mediterranean fever
B. Chlamydia infection
C. Pancreatic necrosis
D. Biliary tract perforation

301. The serum-ascites albumin gradient (SAAG) reflects the pressure within the?
Harrison's 20th Ed. Chapter 46 Page 283

A. Hepatic sinusoids
B. Hepatic artery
C. Hepatic vein
D. Portal vein

SAAG reflects pressure within hepatic sinusoids and correlates with hepatic venous pressure gradient. According to Starling's law, high SAAG reflects oncotic pressure that counterbalances portal pressure.

302. Which of the following is false about serum-ascites albumin gradient (SAAG)?
Harrison's 20th Ed. Chapter 46 Page 284

A. Calculated as ascitic albumin - serum albumin concentration
B. Does not change with diuresis
C. SAAG ≥1.1 g/dL reflects presence of portal hypertension
D. SAAG <1.1 g/dL suggests Budd-Chiari syndrome

303. Which of the following is a cause of a high SAAG?
Harrison's 20th Ed. Chapter 46 Page 284

A. Cardiac ascites
B. Hepatic vein thrombosis (Budd-Chiari syndrome)
C. Sinusoidal obstruction syndrome (veno-occlusive disease)
D. All of the above

304. Which of the following is a cause of SAAG <1.1 g/dL?
Harrison's 20th Ed. Chapter 46 Page 284

A. Tuberculous peritonitis
B. Peritoneal carcinomatosis
C. Pancreatic ascites
D. All of the above

305. Which of the following is a cause of ascitic protein level of ≥ 2.5 g/dL?
Harrison's 20th Ed. Chapter 46 Page 284

A. Cardiac ascites
B. Early Budd-Chiari syndrome
C. Sinusoidal obstruction syndrome
D. All of the above

306. Which of the following is a cause of ascitic protein level of <2.5 g/dL?
Harrison's 20th Ed. Chapter 46 Page 284

A. Cirrhosis
B. Late Budd-Chiari syndrome
C. Massive liver metastases
D. All of the above

307. Secondary peritonitis is suggested by?
Harrison's 20th Ed. Chapter 46 Page 284

A. Ascitic glucose level <50 mg/dL
B. Ascitic LDH level > serum LDH level
C. Detection of multiple pathogens on ascitic fluid culture
D. All of the above

308. In pancreatic ascites, ascitic amylase level is typically?
Harrison's 20th Ed. Chapter 46 Page 284

A. > 200 mg/dL
B. > 600 mg/dL
C. > 800 mg/dL
D. > 1000 mg/dL

309. Estimation of ascitic adenosine deaminase level is of value in?
Harrison's 20th Ed. Chapter 46 Page 284

A. Budd-Chiari syndrome
B. Tuberculous peritonitis
C. Veno-occlusive disease
D. Peritoneal carcinomatosis

310. Maximal daily dose of furosemide in cirrhotic ascites is?
Harrison's 20th Ed. Chapter 46 Page 284

A. 100 mg/day
B. 200 mg/day
C. 400 mg/day
D. 600 mg/day

Maximal daily dose of furosemide in cirrhotic ascites is 400 mg/day.

311. Maximal daily dose of spironolactone in cirrhotic ascites is?
Harrison's 20th Ed. Chapter 46 Page 284

A. 100 mg/day
B. 140 mg/day
C. 160 mg/day
D. 180 mg/day

Maximal daily dose of spironolactone in cirrhotic ascites is 160 mg/day.

312. In refractory ascites, which of the following is added to diuretic regimen?

Harrison's 20th Ed. Chapter 46 Page 284

A. Amiloride
B. Ethacrynic acid
C. Clonidine
D. Captopril

Refractory cirrhotic ascites is defined by the persistence of ascites despite sodium restriction and maximally tolerated diuretic use. Addition of midodrine (α1-adrenergic agonist) or clonidine (α2-adrenergic agonist) to diuretic therapy is beneficial. They act as vasoconstrictors, counteracting splanchnic vasodilation.

313. Post-paracentesis circulatory dysfunction is prevented by?

Harrison's 20th Ed. Chapter 46 Page 284

A. β-adrenergic blocking agents
B. Intravenous albumin
C. α1-adrenergic agonist - midodrine
D. All of the above

314. Spontaneous bacterial peritonitis is rare in?

Harrison's 20th Ed. Chapter 46 Page 284

A. Malignant ascites
B. Nephrotic syndrome
C. Heart failure
D. Acute liver failure

Spontaneous bacterial peritonitis is a common complication of cirrhotic ascites. SBP also complicates ascites caused by nephrotic syndrome, heart failure, acute hepatitis, and acute liver failure but is rare in malignant ascites.

315. Which of the following is false about spontaneous bacterial peritonitis (SBP)?

Harrison's 20th Ed. Chapter 46 Page 284

A. Abdominal tenderness is found in only 40% of patients, rebound tenderness is uncommon
B. New onset of or exacerbation of hepatic encephalopathy
C. Cultures of ascitic fluid typically reveal one bacterial pathogen
D. None of the above

SBP is the result of enteric bacteria that have translocated across an edematous bowel wall.

316. What polymorphonuclear neutrophil count in ascitic fluid denotes spontaneous bacterial peritonitis?

Harrison's 20th Ed. Chapter 46 Page 284

A. ≥ 50 / μL
B. ≥ 150 / μL
C. ≥ 250 / μL
D. ≥ 350 / μL

317. Which of the following antibiotic is recommended to prevent SBP?

Harrison's 20th Ed. Chapter 46 Page 284

A. Doxycycline
B. Norfloxacin
C. Azithromycin
D. Trimethoprim + sulfamethoxazole

318. Which of the following should be avoided in hepatic hydrothorax?

Harrison's 20th Ed. Chapter 46 Page 284

A. Diuretics
B. Thoracentesis
C. TIPS placement
D. Chest tube placement

Diseases of the Esophagus

319. The most common esophageal symptom is?
Harrison's 20th Ed. Chapter 316 Page 2209

A. Heartburn
B. Regurgitation
C. Water brash
D. Globus sensation

Heartburn is the most common esophageal symptom. It is characterized by a discomfort or burning sensation behind sternum arising from epigastrium and radiates toward neck.

320. In which of the following situations, heartburn is most commonly experienced?
Harrison's 20th Ed. Chapter 316 Page 2209

A. After eating
B. During exercise
C. While lying recumbent
D. All of the above

Heartburn is an intermittent symptom, most commonly experienced after eating, during exercise and while lying recumbent.

321. Pyrosis is best related to?
Harrison's 20th Ed. Chapter 316 Page 2209

A. Fever
B. Heartburn
C. Defervescence
D. Pain

Heartburn, or pyrosis, is characterized by burning retrosternal discomfort.

322. Which of the following is false about esophageal chest pain?
Harrison's 20th Ed. Chapter 316 Page 2210

A. Pressure type sensation in mid chest
B. Radiation to mid back or arms
C. Radiation to jaws
D. None of the above

Similarity of esophageal chest pain to cardiac pain is because the two organs share a nerve plexus and nerve endings in esophageal wall have poor discriminative ability among stimuli.

323. Most frequent esophageal cause of chest pain is?
Harrison's 20th Ed. Chapter 316 Page 2210

A. Gastroesophageal reflux
B. Diffuse esophageal spasm (DES)
C. Achalasia
D. Esophageal hypersensitivity syndrome

Gastroesophageal reflux is the most common cause of esophageal chest pain.

324. Dysphagia for liquids as well as solid food suggests?
Harrison's 20th Ed. Chapter 316 Page 2210

A. Esophageal stricture
B. Esophageal ring
C. Esophageal tumor
D. Esophageal motility disorder

325. Solid food dysphagia is suggestive of?
Harrison's 20th Ed. Chapter 316 Page 2210

A. Esophageal stricture
B. Esophageal ring
C. Esophageal tumor
D. Any of the above

326. Which of the following is not a concomitant symptom associated with oropharyngeal dysphagia?
Harrison's 20th Ed. Chapter 316 Page 2210

A. Odynophagia
B. Aspiration
C. Cough
D. Drooling

Concomitant symptoms associated with oropharyngeal dysphagia are aspiration, nasopharyngeal regurgitation, cough, drooling.

327. Odynophagia is unusual in?
Harrison's 20th Ed. Chapter 316 Page 2210

A. Pill-induced esophagitis
B. Nonreflux esophagitis
C. Esophageal perforation
D. Uncomplicated reflux esophagitis

Odynophagia (painful swallowing) is characteristic of nonreflux esophagitis, herpes & pill-induced esophagitis. Odynophagia may occur with peptic ulcer of esophagus (Barrett's ulcer), carcinoma with periesophageal involvement, caustic damage of esophagus, and esophageal perforation. Odynophagia is unusual in uncomplicated reflux esophagitis.

328. Globus sensation or "globus hystericus" is the perception of a lump or fullness in?
Harrison's 20th Ed. Chapter 316 Page 2210

A. Mouth
B. Throat
C. Chest
D. Abdomen

Globus sensation or "globus hystericus" is the perception of a lump or fullness in the throat that is felt irrespective of swallowing, often relieved by the act of swallowing.

329. Reflex salivary hypersecretion in response to acidification of the esophageal mucosa is called?
Harrison's 20th Ed. Chapter 316 Page 2210

A. Water brash
B. Salivary brash
C. Esophageal brash
D. Barret's brash

Water brash is excessive reflex salivation resulting from a vagal reflex triggered by acidification of the esophageal mucosa. It is not regurgitation which is effortless appearance of gastric or esophageal contents in the mouth.

330. Which of the following is an uncommon symptom of esophageal diseases?

Harrison's 20th Ed. Chapter 316 Page 2210

A. Water brash
B. Odynophagia
C. Globus sensation
D. Chest pain

331. Barium radiography is better than esophagogastro-duodenoscopy (EGD) in?

Harrison's 20th Ed. Chapter 316 Page 2210

A. Esophageal strictures
B. Esophageal function and morphology
C. Disorders of the cricopharyngeus muscle
D. All of the above

332. Endoscopic ultrasound (EUS) is useful in which of the following esophageal condition?

Harrison's 20th Ed. Chapter 316 Page 2210

A. To stage esophageal cancer
B. To evaluate dysplasia in Barrett's esophagus
C. To assess submucosal lesions
D. All of the above

Endoscopic ultrasound (EUS) is useful in which of the following esophageal conditions : to stage esophageal cancer, to evaluate dysplasia in Barrett's esophagus & to assess submucosal lesions.

333. Esophageal peristalsis is best studied in?

Harrison's 20th Ed. Chapter 316 Page 2210

A. Upright position
B. Recumbent position
C. Lateral position
D. Head down position

Esophageal peristalsis is best studied in the recumbent position, because in the upright position barium passage occurs largely by gravity alone.

334. Which of the following defines gastroesophageal reflux disease (GERD)?

Harrison's 20th Ed. Chapter 316 Page 2210

A. Heartburn
B. Esophageal chest pain
C. Esophageal dysphagia
D. Endoscopic esophagitis

335. Which is the most common type of hiatus hernia?

Harrison's 20th Ed. Chapter 316 Page 2211

A. Type I
B. Type II
C. Type III
D. Type IV

Type I or sliding hiatal hernia comprises ~95% of the overall total cases of hiatus hernia.

336. Sliding hiatal hernias enlarge with?

Harrison's 20th Ed. Chapter 316 Page 2211

A. Increased intraabdominal pressure
B. Swallowing
C. Respiration
D. All of the above

337. Sliding hiatal hernias are a result of weakening of?

Harrison's 20th Ed. Chapter 316 Page 2211

A. Phrenoesophageal ligament
B. Hepatophrenic ligament
C. Costotransverse ligament
D. All of the above

In sliding hiatal hernia, gastroesophageal junction & gastric cardia translocate cephalad due to weakening of phrenoesophageal ligament attaching gastroesophageal junction to diaphragm at the hiatus and dilatation of diaphragmatic hiatus.

338. The gastroesophageal junction remains fixed at the hiatus in which type of hiatal hernia?

Harrison's 20th Ed. Chapter 316 Page 2211

A. Type I
B. Type II
C. Type III
D. Type IV

In type II hiatal hernia, the gastroesophageal junction remains fixed at the hiatus.

339. When colon herniate into the mediastinum, the type of hiatus hernia is?

Harrison's 20th Ed. Chapter 316 Page 2211

A. Type I
B. Type II
C. Type III
D. Type IV

With type IV hiatal hernias, viscera other than stomach herniate into mediastinum, most commonly the colon.

340. Gastric cardia does not herniate into the mediastinum in which of the following hiatal hernias?

Harrison's 20th Ed. Chapter 316 Page 2211

A. Type II
B. Type III
C. Type IV
D. All of the above

Type II, III, and IV hiatal hernias are subtypes of paraesophageal hernia in which herniation into mediastinum includes a visceral structure other than the gastric cardia.

341. Intersection of squamous epithelium of tubular esophagus & columnar epithelium of stomach is termed?

Lancet 2009; 373:850 - 61

A. W line
B. X line
C. Y line
D. Z line

The intersection of squamous epithelium of the tubular esophagus & columnar epithelium of stomach is termed Z line, because of jagged appearance of the interface.

342. Lower esophageal mucosal ring is also called?

Harrison's 20th Ed. Chapter 316 Page 2211

A. A ring
B. B ring
C. C ring
D. D ring

A lower esophageal mucosal ring, also called B ring, is a thin membranous narrowing at the squamocolumnar mucosal junction.

343. Location of 'Schatzki ring' is?

Harrison's 20th Ed. Chapter 316 Page 2211

A. Hypopharyngeal
B. Mid esophageal
C. Lower esophageal
D. Any of the above

Schatzki ring is a lower esophageal mucosal ring. It is a thin, weblike constriction located at the squamo-columnar mucosal junction at or near the border of the LES. It may result from GERD or be congenital in origin.

344. Schatzki ring invariably produces dysphagia when the lumen diameter is?

Harrison's 20th Ed. Chapter 316 Page 2211

A. < 1.3 cm
B. < 2.3 cm
C. < 3.3 cm
D. < 4.3 cm

Schatzki ring invariably produces dysphagia when the lumen diameter is <1.3 cm.

345. "Steakhouse syndrome" best relates to?

Harrison's 20th Ed. Chapter 316 Page 2211

A. Mouth
B. Esophagus
C. Stomach
D. Colon

Schatzki ring is one of the most common causes of intermittent food impaction, also called "steakhouse syndrome" as meat is a typical instigator.

346. Which of the following is false about Plummer-Vinson syndrome?

Harrison's 20th Ed. Chapter 316 Page 2211

A. Young women
B. Symptomatic proximal esophageal web
C. Iron-deficiency anemia
D. All of the above

Symptomatic hypopharyngeal webs and iron-deficiency anemia in middle-aged women constitutes Plummer-Vinson syndrome.

347. Which of the following is false about Zenker's diverticula?

Harrison's 20th Ed. Chapter 316 Page 2211

A. Hypopharyngeal
B. False diverticula
C. Associated with distal obstruction
D. None of the above

348. Which of the following is false about Zenker's diverticulum?

Harrison's 20th Ed. Chapter 316 Page 2211

A. Occurs below the Killian's triangle
B. Causes halitosis & regurgitation of saliva & food
C. Nasogastric intubation may cause perforation
D. Symptomatic pt's treated by cricopharyngeal myotomy

Zenker's diverticulum appears in natural zone of weakness in posterior hypopharyngeal wall (Killian's triangle).

349. Epiphrenic diverticula are associated with?

Harrison's 20th Ed. Chapter 316 Page 2212

A. Achalasia
B. Esophageal hypercontractile disorders
C. Distal esophageal stricture
D. All of the above

350. Esophageal cancer has poor survival because of the?

Harrison's 20th Ed. Chapter 316 Page 2212

A. Constant proximity to acidic milieu
B. Nonconvoluted pipe like structure
C. Abundant esophageal lymphatics
D. All of the above

Esophageal cancer has poor survival because of the abundant esophageal lymphatics leading to regional lymph node metastases.

351. The most common congenital esophageal anomaly is?

Harrison's 20th Ed. Chapter 316 Page 2212

A. Esophageal atresia
B. Congenital esophageal stenosis
C. Esophageal webs
D. Esophageal duplications

The most common congenital esophageal anomaly is esophageal atresia, occurring in about 1 in 5000 live births.

352. Dysphagia lusoria best relates to which of the following?

Harrison's 20th Ed. Chapter 316 Page 2213

A. Artery of Adamkiewicz
B. Aberrant right subclavian artery
C. Aberrant mast cells
D. Dieulafoy's lesion

Dysphagia lusoria is a condition wherein the esophagus is compressed by an aberrant right subclavian artery arising from the descending aorta and passing behind the esophagus.

353. Esophageal inlet patch best relates to?

Harrison's 20th Ed. Chapter 316 Page 2213

A. Esophageal atresia
B. Benign esophageal tumor
C. Heterotopic gastric mucosa
D. Zenker's diverticula

Heterotopic gastric mucosa, also known as an esophageal inlet patch, is an area of gastric type epithelium in proximal cervical esophagus. The inlet patch is due to incomplete replacement of embryonic columnar epithelium with squamous epithelium. It produces acid as most contain fundic type gastric epithelium with parietal cells.

354. Which of the following is an esophageal motility disorder?

Harrison's 20th Ed. Chapter 316 Page 2213

A. Achalasia
B. Diffuse esophageal spasm (DES)
C. Gastroesophageal reflux disease (GERD)
D. All of the above

Esophageal motility disorders are diseases attributable to esophageal neuromuscular dysfunction. The major entities are achalasia, diffuse esophageal spasm (DES) and GERD.

355. Which of the following is a secondary esophageal motility disorder?
Harrison's 20th Ed. Chapter 316 Page 2213

A. Pseudoachalasia
B. Chagas' disease
C. Scleroderma
D. Diphtheria

Motility disorders can be secondary to pseudoachalasia, Chagas' disease and scleroderma.

356. Secondary achalasia may be caused by all except?
Harrison's 20th Ed. Chapter 316 Page 2213

A. Ulcerative colitis
B. Chagas' disease
C. Eosinophilic gastroenteritis
D. Neurodegenerative disorders

Secondary achalasia may be caused by gastric carcinoma that infiltrates the esophagus, lymphoma, Chagas' disease, certain viral infections, eosinophilic gastroenteritis & neurodegenerative disorders.

357. Which of the following statements about achalasia is false?
Harrison's 20th Ed. Chapter 316 Page 2213

A. Motor disorder of esophageal smooth muscle
B. UES & LES relax normally with swallowing
C. Nonperistaltic contractions in esophageal body
D. Underlying abnormality is loss of intramural neurons

With a swallow, pressure in sphincters falls and a contraction wave starts in pharynx and progresses down the esophagus. In achalasia, esophageal body loses peristaltic contractions & are replaced by simultaneous contractions with elevated resting pressure & LES does not relax normally in response to swallowing. Prominent loss of ganglion cells within the esophageal myenteric plexus is seen in achalasia.

358. Cause of ganglion cell degeneration in achalasia is infection with?
Harrison's 20th Ed. Chapter 316 Page 2213

A. Varicella zoster virus
B. Human herpes simplex virus 1
C. Cytomegalovirus
D. Epstein-Barr virus

Cause of ganglion cell degeneration in achalasia is an autoimmune process attributable to a latent infection with human herpes simplex virus 1 combined with genetic susceptibility.

359. Sigmoid deformity of esophagus with hypertrophy of LES is suggestive of?
Harrison's 20th Ed. Chapter 316 Page 2213

A. Achalasia
B. Diffuse esophageal spasm
C. Jackhammer esophagus
D. All of the above

Long-standing achalasia is characterized by progressive dilatation and sigmoid deformity of the esophagus with hypertrophy of LES.

360. Which of the following statements about achalasia is false?
Harrison's 20th Ed. Chapter 316 Page 2213

A. Impaired LES relaxation
B. Absent peristalsis
C. Presence of GE reflux goes against achalasia
D. None of the above

Inhibitory neurons containing VIP and nitric oxide synthase are predominantly involved.

361. Which of the following is not a feature of achalasia?
Harrison's 20th Ed. Chapter 316 Page 2213

A. Dysphagia
B. Gastroesophageal reflux
C. Chest pain
D. Regurgitation

Dysphagia, chest pain, regurgitation and weight loss are the main symptoms of achalasia. Presence of gastroesophageal reflux goes against achalasia.

362. Chest X-ray in achalasia may show all except?
Harrison's 20th Ed. Chapter 316 Page 2213

A. Absence of the gastric air bubble
B. Tubular mediastinal mass beside the aorta
C. Air-fluid level in mediastinum in upright position
D. Atelectasis

A chest X-ray shows absence of the gastric air bubble and sometimes a tubular mediastinal mass beside the aorta. An air-fluid level in the mediastinum in the upright position represents retained food in the esophagus. Barium swallow shows esophageal dilation, and in advanced cases the esophagus may become sigmoid. On fluoroscopy with barium swallow, normal peristalsis is lost in the lower two-thirds of the esophagus. The terminal part of the esophagus shows a persistent beaklike narrowing representing the nonrelaxing LES.

363. Which of the following is the most sensitive diagnostic test for achalasia?
Harrison's 20th Ed. Chapter 316 Page 2213

A. Esophageal manometry
B. Barium swallow X-ray
C. Esophagogastroduodenoscopy (EGD)
D. None of the above

364. Impaired lower esophageal sphincter (LES) relaxation & absent peristalsis are seen in?
Harrison's 20th Ed. Chapter 316 Page 2213

A. Classic achalasia
B. Achalasia with esophageal compression
C. Spastic achalasia
D. All of the above

365. In CCK test, paradoxical contraction of LES is found in?
Harrison's 17th Ed. 1850

A. Achalasia
B. Gastric carcinoma
C. Scleroderma
D. Diffuse esophageal spasm

In achalasia, Cholecystokinin (CCK) paradoxically causes contraction of LES (CCK test) because neurally transmitted inhibitory effect of CCK is absent & direct excitatory effect of CCK remains unopposed.

366. Which of the following is typical of esophageal chest pain?
Harrison's 20th Ed. Chapter 316 Page 2214

A. Nonexertional
B. Prolonged
C. Interrupts sleep, meal-related
D. All of the above

Features suggesting esophageal pain include nonexertional, prolonged, interrupts sleep, meal-related, relieved with antacids, and accompanied by heartburn, dysphagia, or regurgitation.

367. Which of the following drugs can be used in achalasia?
Harrison's 20th Ed. Chapter 316 Page 2213

A. Nitrates or calcium channel blockers
B. Botulinum toxin
C. Sildenafil
D. All of the above

368. In achalasia, which is the treatment of choice?
Harrison's 20th Ed. Chapter 316 Page 2213

A. Pneumatic dilatation
B. Esophageal resection with gastric pull-up
C. Laparoscopic Heller myotomy of LES
D. Open surgical myotomy of LES

Laparoscopic Heller myotomy is currently the procedure of choice.

369. "Corkscrew" esophagus is typical of?
Harrison's 20th Ed. Chapter 316 Page 2215

A. Diffuse esophageal spasm (DES)
B. Achalasia
C. Carcinoma esophagus
D. GERD

Barium swallow in DES shows curling or multiple ripples in the wall, sacculations, and pseudodiverticula - termed "corkscrew" esophagus and rosary bead esophagus. Diffuse esophageal spasm is primarily defined by a short latency (premature) contraction.

370. Which of the following about "corkscrew" esophagus is false?
Harrison's 20th Ed. Chapter 316 Page 2214 Figure 316-7

A. Radiographic term
B. Spastic tertiary contraction of circular muscle in esophageal wall
C. Normal deglutitive LES relaxation
D. None of the above

371. Which of the following about "Jackhammer" esophagus is false?
Harrison's 20th Ed. Chapter 316 Page 2215 Figure 316-8

A. Variant of esophageal spasm
B. Vigorous & repetitive contractions with normal peristaltic onset
C. Normal latency of the contraction
D. None of the above

Jackhammer esophagus is defined by the extraordinarily vigorous and repetitive contractions with normal peristaltic onset and normal latency of the contraction.

372. Which of the following is most efficacious in DES?
Harrison's 20th Ed. Chapter 316 Page 2215

A. Nitrates
B. Calcium channel blockers
C. Botulinum toxin
D. Anxiolytics

Nitrates, calcium channel blockers, hydralazine, botulinum toxin and anxiolytics have been tried in DES with anxiolytics most efficacious.

373. Which of the following is not a hypertensive motor disorder of esophagus?
Harrison's 20th Ed. Chapter 316 Page 2215

A. Diffuse esophageal spasm (DES)
B. Nutcracker esophagus
C. Hypercontracting LES
D. Hypertensive LES

The hypertensive disorders of esophagus include nutcracker esophagus, hypercontracting LES and hypertensive LES. DES is characterized by nonperistaltic contractions.

374. Motility pattern of esophagus showing reduced amplitude of contractions in lower esophagus, peristaltic or simultaneous in onset with hypotension of LES is suggestive of?
Harrison's 20th Ed. Chapter 316 Page 2215

A. Scleroderma
B. Achalasia
C. Diffuse esophageal spasm
D. None of the above

In scleroderma, thoracic esophagus shows reduced amplitude of contractions, which may be peristaltic or simultaneous in onset & hypotension of LES.

375. Motility pattern of esophagus showing reduced amplitude of contractions in lower esophagus, simultaneous in onset with hypertensive LES nonrelaxing on swallowing is suggestive of?
Harrison's 20th Ed. Chapter 316 Page 2215

A. Scleroderma
B. Achalasia
C. Diffuse esophageal spasm
D. None of the above

In achalasia, lower part of esophagus shows contractions that are reduced in amplitude & simultaneous in onset. In contrast to scleroderma, LES in achalasia is hypertensive and fails to relax in response to a swallow.

376. Motility pattern of esophagus showing large amplitude, prolonged and repetitive contractions in lower esophagus, simultaneous in onset is suggestive of?
Harrison's 20th Ed. Chapter 316 Page 2215

A. Scleroderma
B. Achalasia
C. Diffuse esophageal spasm
D. None of the above

In diffuse esophageal spasm, lower part of esophagus shows simultaneous-onset, large-amplitude, prolonged, repetitive contractions.

377. Esophageal motility studies are helpful in the diagnosis of all except?
Harrison's 20th Ed. Chapter 316 Page 2215

A. Achalasia
B. Diffuse esophageal spasm
C. Scleroderma
D. Mechanical dysphagia

Esophageal motility studies are helpful in the diagnosis of esophageal motor disorders (achalasia, spasm, and scleroderma) but are of little value in the differential diagnosis of mechanical dysphagia.

378. Esophageal contractions are normally peristaltic but hypertensive in?
Harrison's 19th Ed. 1905

A. Nutcracker esophagus
B. Hypercontracting LES
C. Hypertensive LES
D. All of the above

In nutcracker esophagus, esophageal contractions are normally peristaltic but hypertensive. In hypercontracting LES, normal sphincter relaxation is followed by hypertensive contraction. In hypertensive LES, basal LES pressure is elevated, but sphincter relaxation and contraction are normal.

379. Gastric distention-evoked transient lower esophageal sphincter relaxation (tLESR) is a?

Harrison's 20th Ed. Chapter 316 Page 2215

A. Stretch reflex
B. Chemical reflex
C. Vasovagal reflex
D. All of the above

Gastric distention - evoked transient lower esophageal sphincter relaxation (tLESR) is a vagovagal reflex.

380. Which of the following contributes to the development of gastroesophageal reflux disease (GERD)?

Harrison's 20th Ed. Chapter 316 Page 2215

A. Transient LES relaxations
B. LES hypotension
C. Anatomic distortion of esophagogastric junction
D. All of the above

381. Which of the following may have a protective effect in GERD patients?

Harrison's 20th Ed. Chapter 316 Page 2216

A. Zollinger-Ellison syndrome
B. Chronic H. pylori gastritis
C. Hiatus hernia
D. Scleroderma

Chronic H. pylori gastritis may have a protective effect in GERD by inducing atrophic gastritis with concomitant hypoacidity.

382. Which of the following acts as a cofactor in the pathogenesis of Barrett's metaplasia and esophageal adenocarcinoma?

Harrison's 20th Ed. Chapter 316 Page 2216

A. Pepsin
B. Bile
C. Pancreatic enzymes
D. All of the above

Bile persists in refluxate despite acid-suppressing medications. Bile can transverse the cell membrane, imparting severe cellular injury in a weakly acidic environment and acts as a cofactor in the pathogenesis of Barrett's metaplasia and adenocarcinoma.

383. Which out of the following conditions has associations with GERD?

Harrison's 20th Ed. Chapter 316 Page 2216

A. Pulmonary fibrosis
B. Chronic sinusitis
C. Cardiac arrhythmias
D. All of the above

Extraesophageal syndromes that have established association to GERD include chronic cough, laryngitis, asthma & dental erosions. Other conditions like pharyngitis, chronic bronchitis, pulmonary fibrosis, chronic sinusitis, cardiac arrhythmias, sleep apnea, and recurrent aspiration pneumonia have proposed associations with GERD.

384. Which of the following groups is at greatest risk of Barrett's metaplasia progressing to adenocarcinoma?

Harrison's 20th Ed. Chapter 316 Page 2216

A. Obese black males in fifth decade of life
B. Obese white males in fifth decade of life
C. Obese black males in sixth decade of life
D. Obese white males in sixth decade of life

Barrett's metaplasia can progress to adenocarcinoma and the group at greatest risk is obese white males in their sixth decade of life.

385. Which of the following foods is "refluxogenic"?

Harrison's 20th Ed. Chapter 316 Page 2217

A. Peppermint
B. Coffee and tea
C. Alcohol
D. All of the above

Foods that reduce lower esophageal sphincter pressure are called "refluxogenic". These include fatty foods, alcohol, spearmint, peppermint, tomato-based foods, coffee and tea.

386. Absorption of which of the following may be compromised on indefinite treatment with PPIs?

Harrison's 20th Ed. Chapter 316 Page 2217

A. Vitamin B12
B. Calcium
C. Iron
D. All of the above

With indefinite treatment with PPIs, Vitamin B12, calcium, and iron absorption may be compromised and susceptibility to enteric infections, particularly Clostridium difficile colitis increased.

387. Which of the following has been reported with indefinite treatment with PPIs?

Harrison's 20th Ed. Chapter 316 Page 2217

A. Interstitial nephritis
B. Severe, reversible hypomagnesemia
C. Clostridium difficile colitis
D. All of the above

388. Multiple esophageal mucosal rings are characteristic of?

Harrison's 20th Ed. Chapter 316 Page 2217

A. Eosinophilic esophagitis
B. Radiation esophagitis
C. Corrosive esophagitis
D. Candida esophagitis

Multiple mucosal rings (feline esophagus) are characteristic of eosinophilic esophagitis.

389. Characteristic endoscopic finding of Eosinophilic Esophagitis is?

Harrison's 20th Ed. Chapter 316 Page 2217

A. Multiple esophageal rings
B. Linear furrows
C. White punctate exudates
D. All of the above

The characteristic endoscopic findings of Eosinophilic Esophagitis (EoE) include multiple esophageal rings, linear furrows, and white punctate exudates.

390. For diagnosis of eosinophilic esophagitis, eosinophils in esophagal mucosa per high-power field should be?

Harrison's 20th Ed. Chapter 316 Page 2217

A. 5 or more
B. 10 or more
C. 15 or more
D. 20 or more

The diagnosis of eosinophilic esophagitis is made histologically, with 15 or more eosinophils per high-power field in the esophagal mucosa. Normal esophagus contains almost no eosinophils.

391. Preferred treatment of eosinophilic esophagitis is?

Harrison's 20th Ed. Chapter 316 Page 2218

A. H_2 receptor blocking agents
B. Nifedipine
C. Swallowed fluticasone propionate
D. Isosorbide dinitrate

Treatment of eosinophilic esophagitis consists of a 12-week course of swallowed fluticasone propionate using a metered dose inhaler. Anti human interleukin 5, systemic steroids, montelukast or cromolyn may be useful.

392. Risk of development of esophageal adenocarcinoma in Barrett's metaplasia is increased by?

N Engl J Med. 2006;354:1403-9

A. 5 fold
B. 10 fold
C. 15 fold
D. 20 fold

Risk of development of esophageal adenocarcinoma in Barrett's metaplasia is increased by 20 fold.

393. Esophageal mucosal biopsies should be taken at least?

N Engl J Med. 2006;354:1403-9

A. 2 cm above the LES
B. 5 cm above the LES
C. 7 cm above the LES
D. 9 cm above the LES

Mucosal biopsies should be performed at least 5 cm above LES, as esophageal mucosal changes of chronic esophagitis are frequent in the most distal esophagus in otherwise normal individuals.

394. Which of the following about Bernstein test is false?

N Engl J Med. 2006;354:1403-9

A. Infusion of 0.1 N HCl & saline in esophagus
B. Useful in diagnosing Barrett's esophagus that is not endoscopically obvious
C. In symptomatic esophagitis, infusion of acid, but not of saline, reproduces symptoms of heartburn
D. Infusion of acid in normal individuals produces no symptom

Bernstein test involves infusion of solutions of 0.1 N HCl or normal saline in esophagus. In symptomatic esophagitis, infusion of acid, but not of saline, reproduces the symptoms of heartburn. Infusion of acid in normal individuals usually produces no symptoms.

395. Which of the following statements about Barrett's esophagus is false?

N Engl J Med. 2006;354:1403-9

A. Barrett's esophagus is an acquired condition
B. Metaplasia occurs from esophageal columnar to squamous epithelium
C. Complication of severe reflux esophagitis
D. Risk factor for esophageal adenocarcinoma

Metaplasia of esophageal squamous epithelium to columnar epithelium (Barrett's esophagus) is a complication of severe reflux esophagitis. Finding intestinal metaplasia with goblet cells in esophagus is diagnostic of Barrett's esophagus.

396. Methods for mucosal ablation in Barrett's esophagus include all except?

N Engl J Med. 2006;354:1403-9

A. Electrocautery
B. Mucosal stripping
C. Argon-plasma-beam fulguration
D. Chemical fulguration

397. Methods for mucosal ablation in Barrett's esophagus include all except?

N Engl J Med. 2006;354:1403-9

A. Laser photothermal coagulation
B. Heater-probe ablation
C. Hyperbaric oxygen ablation
D. Cryotherapy

398. Photosensitizing agent used in photodynamic therapy for Barrett's esophagus is?

N Engl J Med. 2006;354:1403-9

A. Trigen sodium
B. Porfimer sodium
C. Sugran sodium
D. Mofetil sodium

399. Odynophagia is a characteristic symptom of?

Harrison's 20th Ed. Chapter 316 Page 2218

A. Pill-induced esophagitis
B. Reflux esophagitis
C. Esophageal perforation
D. Infectious esophagitis

Regardless of the infectious agent, odynophagia is a characteristic symptom of infectious esophagitis. Odynophagia is uncommon with reflux esophagitis.

400. Feline esophagus best relates to which of the following?

Harrison's 20th Ed. Chapter 315 Page 2203

A. Herpes simplex virus esophagitis
B. Candida esophagitis
C. Eosinophilic esophagitis
D. Radiation esophagitis

The presence of linear furrows and multiple corrugated rings throughout a narrowed esophagus (feline esophagus) should raise suspicion for eosinophilic esophagitis.

401. Which of the following is characteristic of Candida esophagitis?

Harrison's 20th Ed. Chapter 316 Page 2218

A. Bleeding
B. White plaques with friability
C. Perforation
D. Stricture

Candida esophagitis has a characteristic appearance of white plaques with friability. Rarely, Candida esophagitis is complicated by bleeding, perforation, stricture, or systemic invasion.

402. Candida esophagitis can be treated with?

Harrison's 20th Ed. Chapter 316 Page 2218

A. Fluconazole
B. Echinocandin
C. Voriconazole
D. Any of the above

Oral fluconazole, itraconazole, voriconazole or posaconazole are effective. Poorly responsive patients or those who cannot swallow medications can be treated with an intravenous echinocandin (caspofungin).

403. "Volcano-like" esophageal ulcerations are seen in?

N Engl J Med. 2006;354:1403-9

A. Candidiasis
B. HSV
C. CMV
D. Corrosive poisoning

In HSV (1 or 2) infection of esophagus, endoscopy shows vesicles & small, discrete, punched-out ("volcano-like") superficial ulcerations with or without a fibrinous exudate.

404. Eosinophilic Cowdry's type A inclusion bodies is related to?
Harrison's 20th Ed. Chapter 316 Page 2218

A. Herpes simplex esophagitis
B. Candida esophagitis
C. Radiation esophagitis
D. Cytomegalovirus esophagitis

Herpes simplex infections are limited to squamous epithelium. Biopsies shows characteristic ground-glass nuclei, eosinophilic Cowdry's type A inclusion bodies and giant cells.

405. Herpes simplex virus (HSV) esophagitis is treated with?
Harrison's 20th Ed. Chapter 316 Page 2218

A. Acyclovir
B. Valacyclovir
C. Famciclovir
D. All of the above

406. Which of the following infections occur primarily in immunocompromised patients?
Harrison's 20th Ed. Chapter 316 Page 2218

A. Herpes simplex virus (HSV) esophagitis
B. Varicella-zoster virus (VZV) esophagitis
C. Cytomegalovirus (CMV) esophagitis
D. Candida esophagitis

Cytomegalovirus (CMV) infections occur primarily in immunocompromised patients, particularly transplant recipients.

407. Serpiginous ulcers in an otherwise normal esophageal mucosa is a feature of?
Harrison's 20th Ed. Chapter 316 Page 2218

A. Herpes simplex virus (HSV) esophagitis
B. Varicella-zoster virus (VZV) esophagitis
C. Cytomegalovirus (CMV) esophagitis
D. Candida esophagitis

Endoscopically, CMV lesions appear as serpiginous ulcers in an otherwise normal mucosa, particularly in the distal esophagus.

408. Ganciclovir is the treatment of choice for?
Harrison's 20th Ed. Chapter 316 Page 2218

A. Herpes simplex virus (HSV) esophagitis
B. Varicella-zoster virus (VZV) esophagitis
C. Cytomegalovirus (CMV) esophagitis
D. Candida esophagitis

Ganciclovir, 5 mg/kg BD IV, is the treatment of choice for Cytomegalovirus (CMV) esophagitis.

409. Boerhaave's syndrome refers to?
Harrison's 20th Ed. Chapter 316 Page 2219

A. Esophagial damage due to instrumentation
B. Esophagial damage due to vomiting or retching
C. Esophagial damage due to external trauma
D. None of the above

Boerhaave's syndrome or spontaneous rupture refers to esophageal rupture at gastroesophageal junction caused by increased intraesophageal pressure associated with forceful vomiting or retching.

410. Instrumental perforation usually occurs in?
Harrison's 20th Ed. Chapter 316 Page 2219

A. Upper esophagus
B. Mid esophagus
C. Lower esophagus
D. Any of the above

Instrumental perforation occurs in pharynx or lower esophagus, just above diaphragm in posterolateral wall.

411. Esophageal perforation may cause?
Harrison's 20th Ed. Chapter 316 Page 2219

A. Pneumomediastinum
B. Subcutaneous emphysema
C. Mediastinitis
D. All of the above

412. Mallory-Weiss syndrome can be caused by?
Harrison's 20th Ed. Chapter 316 Page 2219

A. Vomiting
B. Retching
C. Vigorous coughing
D. All of the above

Vomiting, retching, or vigorous coughing can cause a nontransmural tear at the gastroesophageal junction that is Mallory-Weiss Syndrome.

413. Which of the following is false about Mallory-Weiss syndrome?
Harrison's 20th Ed. Chapter 316 Page 2219

A. Usually involves esophageal mucosa
B. Upper gastrointestinal bleeding
C. In most patients bleeding ceases spontaneously
D. Respond to vasopressin therapy

Mallory-Weiss Syndrome refers to nontransmural tear or mucosal tear involving gastric mucosa near the squamocolumnar mucosal junction caused by vomiting, retching or vigorous coughing. Upper gastrointestinal bleeding may be severe but in mostly bleeding ceases spontaneously. Respond to vasopressin therapy or angiographic embolization.

414. Which of the following increases the risk of radiation esophagitis?
Harrison's 20th Ed. Chapter 316 Page 2219

A. Doxorubicin
B. Bleomycin
C. Cyclophosphamide
D. All of the above

Radiosensitizing drugs such as doxorubicin, bleomycin, cyclophosphamide and cisplatin increase the risk of radiation esophagitis.

415. Treatment with which of the following can reduce esophagitis during radiation treatment?
Harrison's 20th Ed. Chapter 316 Page 2219

A. Cimetidine
B. Indomethacin
C. Allopurinol
D. Sucralfate

indomethacin treatment may reduce radiation damage of esophagus.

416. Patients with alkaline esophagitis are treated with?
Harrison's 20th Ed. Chapter 316 Page 2219

A. Cholestyramine
B. Aluminum hydroxide
C. Sucralfate
D. All of the above

Treatment of alkaline esophagitis includes neutralization of bile salts with cholestyramine, aluminum hydroxide, or sucralfate.

417. Pill-induced esophagitis can be caused by all except?
Harrison's 20th Ed. Chapter 316 Page 2219

A. Alendronate
B. Ferrous sulfate
C. Doxycycline
D. Medroxyprogesterone

Pill-induced esophagitis mostly occurs with ingestion of doxycycline, tetracycline, quinidine, phenytoin, potassium chloride, ferrous sulfate, nonsteroidal anti-inflammatory drugs (NSAIDs), and bisphosphonates.

418. Most common location for the pill to lodge is in?
Harrison's 20th Ed. Chapter 316 Page 2219

A. Upper esophagus
B. Mid esophagus
C. Lower esophagus
D. Any of the above.

The most common location for the pill to lodge is in the mid-esophagus near the crossing of the aorta or carina.

419. Which of the following is sometimes tried before endoscopic dislodgement of impacted food?
Harrison's 20th Ed. Chapter 316 Page 2219

A. Adrenaline
B. Isoprenaline
C. Glucagon
D. Atropine

420. Esophageal lesion in systemic sclerosis consist of?
Harrison's 20th Ed. Chapter 316 Page 2219

A. Atrophy of smooth muscle
B. Weakness in lower two-thirds of esophagus
C. Incompetence of LES
D. All of the above

Esophageal lesions in systemic sclerosis consist of atrophy of smooth muscle, manifested by weakness in lower two-thirds of esophagus & incompetence of LES.

421. Which of the following dermatologic disorders can cause esophagitis?
Harrison's 20th Ed. Chapter 316 Page 2219

A. Pemphigus vulgaris
B. Bullous pemphigoid
C. Cicatricial pemphigoid
D. All of the above

422. What is normal integrated relaxation pressure?
Cleveland Clinic Journal of Medicine 2017;84(6):446

A. < 5 mm Hg
B. < 15 mm Hg
C. < 25 mm Hg
D. < 35 mm Hg

Integrated relaxation pressure is a measurement of lower esophageal relaxation. Normal is <15 mm Hg.

423. What is normal distal latency?
Cleveland Clinic Journal of Medicine 2017;84(6):446

A. > 2.5 seconds
B. > 3.5 seconds
C. > 4.5 seconds
D. > 5.5 seconds

Distal latency is the time from onset to completion of the peristaltic wave during the swallow. Normal is greater than 4.5 seconds. Distal latency less than 4.5 seconds indicates a premature contraction. In distal esophageal spasm, there is normal lower esophageal sphincter relaxation (median integrated relaxation pressure < 15 mm Hg) and ≥ 20% of swallows are premature contraction in the distal esophagus (distal latency < 4.5 seconds).

424. What is normal distal contractile integral?
Cleveland Clinic Journal of Medicine 2017;84(6):446

A. 150 and 8,000 mm Hg· s· cm
B. 250 and 8,000 mm Hg· s· cm
C. 350 and 8,000 mm Hg· s· cm
D. 450 and 8,000 mm Hg· s· cm

Distal contractile integral is the measure of vigor of peristaltic contraction. Normal is between 450 and 8,000 mm Hg· s· cm. Hypercontractile ('jackhammer') esophagus is characterized by distal contractile integral > 8,000 mm Hg· s· cm in at least 2 swallows.

Peptic Ulcer Disease and Related Disorders

425. Rumination is best related to?

Harrison's 20th Ed. Chapter 41 Page 253

A. Nausea
B. Vomiting
C. Regurgitation
D. All of the above

Rumination refers to repeated voluntary regurgitation of stomach contents, which may be rechewed and reswallowed.

426. Under normal conditions, frequency of slow wave cycles in the stomach is?

Harrison's 20th Ed. Chapter 41 Page 253

A. 3 cycles / minute
B. 6 cycles / minute
C. 9 cycles / minute
D. 12 cycles / minute

427. Under normal conditions, frequency of slow wave cycles in the duodenum is?

Harrison's 20th Ed. Chapter 41 Page 253

A. 4 cycles / minute
B. 8 cycles / minute
C. 11 cycles / minute
D. 15 cycles / minute

Under normal conditions, distally migrating gut contractions, the slow wave, occur at 3 cycles/minute in the stomach and 11 cycles/minute in duodenum.

428. Which of the following is termed the chemoreceptor trigger zone?

Harrison's 20th Ed. Chapter 41 Page 253

A. Area postrema
B. Nucleus tractus solitarius
C. Dorsal vagal nuclei
D. Phrenic nuclei

Area postrema, a medullary nucleus, responds to bloodborne emetic stimuli and is termed the chemoreceptor trigger zone.

429. Which of the following act on the area postrema?

Harrison's 20th Ed. Chapter 41 Page 253

A. Uremia
B. Hypoxia
C. Ketoacidosis
D. All of the above

Uremia, hypoxia, and ketoacidosis act on the area postrema and are emetogenic.

430. Which of the following stimulate induction of vomiting in labyrinthine disorders is?

Harrison's 20th Ed. Chapter 41 Page 253

A. Muscarinic M_1 receptors
B. Histaminergic H_2 receptors
C. Serotonin 5-HT_3 receptors
D. Dopamine D_2 receptors

Neurotransmitters that mediate induction of vomiting in labyrinthine disorders is vestibular muscarinic M_1 and histaminergic H_1 receptors, whereas vagal afferent stimuli activate serotonin 5-HT_3 receptors. Area postrema is richly served by nerves acting on 5-HT_3, M_1, H_1, and dopamine D_2 subtypes.

431. Gastroparesis occurs after which of the following?

Harrison's 20th Ed. Chapter 41 Page 254

A. Pancreatic adenocarcinoma
B. Mesenteric vascular insufficiency
C. Scleroderma
D. All of the above

Gastroparesis or a delay in gastric emptying of food occurs after vagotomy, with pancreatic adenocarcinoma, with mesenteric vascular insufficiency, or in systemic diseases such as diabetes, scleroderma, and amyloidosis. Anorexia nervosa, bulimia nervosa, anxiety, and depression may cause significant nausea that may be associated with delayed gastric emptying.

432. Gastroparesis does not occur with which of the following?

Harrison's 20th Ed. Chapter 41 Page 254

A. Diabetes
B. Amyloidosis
C. Scleroderma
D. Cyclic vomiting syndrome

Cyclic vomiting syndrome produces periodic discrete episodes of relentless nausea & vomiting and has a strong association with migraine headaches. Cyclic vomiting is most common in children, although adult cases occur in association with rapid gastric emptying & with chronic cannabis use.

433. Which of the following drugs is a highly emetogenic agent?

Harrison's 20th Ed. Chapter 41 Page 254

A. Digoxin
B. Oral contraceptives
C. Cisplatin
D. Erythromycin

Acute emesis from intensely emetogenic cisplatin is mediated by 5-HT_3 pathways.

434. What proportion of pregnant women experience nausea in the first trimester?

Harrison's 20th Ed. Chapter 41 Page 254

A. 25%
B. 50%
C. 70%
D. 90%

Nausea affects 70% of pregnant women in first trimester.

435. Relief of abdominal pain by emesis is characteristic of?

Harrison's 20th Ed. Chapter 41 Page 255

A. Pancreatitis
B. Zenker's diverticulum
C. Gastric obstruction
D. Intestinal obstruction

Relief of abdominal pain by emesis characterizes intestinal obstruction, whereas vomiting has no effect on pancreatitis or cholecystitis pain.

436. Which of the following antiemetic agent is a Serotonin5-HT_3 antagonist?

Harrison's 20th Ed. Chapter 41 Page 256

A. Meclizine
B. Granisetron
C. Mirtazapine
D. Dimenhydrinate

Antiemetic agent ondansetron and granisetron are Serotonin5-HT_3 antagonists. Meclizine & dimenhydrinate are antihistamines. Scopolamine is an anticholinergic drug.

437. Which of the following is a combined 5-HT_4 agonist and D_2 antagonist?

Harrison's 20th Ed. Chapter 41 Page 256

A. Metoclopramide
B. Domperidone
C. Erythromycin
D. Octreotide

Metoclopramide is a combined 5-HT_4 agonist & D_2 antagonist. Domperidone is a D_2 antagonist. Erythromycin increases gastroduodenal motility by action on receptors for motilin. Somatostatin analogue octreotide induces propagative small intestinal motor complexes.

438. Which of the following is a Neurokinin NK_1 antagonist?

Harrison's 20th Ed. Chapter 41 Page 255 Table 41-2

A. Aprepitant
B. Kevetiracetam
C. Cyproheptadine
D. Sumatriptan

Aprepitant is a neurokinin NK_1 antagonist that has antiemetic & antinausea effects during acute and delayed periods after chemotherapy.

439. Gastric pits of stomach branch into?

Harrison's 20th Ed. Chapter 317 Page 2220

A. 1 or 2 gastric glands
B. 3 or 4 gastric glands
C. 4 or 5 gastric glands
D. 6 or 7 gastric glands

Microscopic gastric pits (foveolus) of gastric epithelial lining branch into four or five gastric glands made up of highly specialized epithelial cells.

440. Which of the following cells is found deepest in the oxyntic gastric gland?

Harrison's 20th Ed. Chapter 317 Page 2220 Figure 317-1

A. Mucous neck cells
B. Parietal cells
C. Endocrine cells
D. Chief cells

441. Parietal cell is also known as?

Harrison's 20th Ed. Chapter 317 Page 2220

A. Mucous cell
B. Oxyntic cell
C. Endocrine cell
D. Enterochromaffin-like (ECL) cell

Parietal cell is also known as oxyntic cell and is found in neck, or isthmus, or in oxyntic gland.

442. Peptic ulcer disease (PUD) occurs due to constant attack on gastroduodenal mucosa by all noxious agents except?

Harrison's 20th Ed. Chapter 317 Page 2220

A. Hydrochloric acid (HCl)
B. Pepsinogen/pepsin
C. Bile acids
D. Salivary amylase

443. PUD occurs due to constant attack on gastroduodenal mucosa by all noxious agents except?

Harrison's 20th Ed. Chapter 317 Page 2220

A. Pancreatic enzymes
B. Alcohol
C. Virus
D. Bacteria

PUD occurs due to constant attack on gastroduodenal mucosa by endogenous noxious agents like acid, pepsin, bile acids, pancreatic enzymes or exogenous substances like medications, alcohol & bacteria.

444. Which of the following is an element of gastric mucosal defense system?

Harrison's 20th Ed. Chapter 317 Page 2221

A. Preepithelial
B. Epithelial
C. Subepithelial
D. All of the above

Gastric mucosal defense is a 3-level barrier composed of preepithelial, epithelial & subepithelial elements.

445. First line of defense of gastric epithelium is?

Harrison's 20th Ed. Chapter 317 Page 2221

A. Mucus layer
B. Bicarbonate-phospholipid layer
C. Phospholipid layer
D. Mucus-bicarbonate-phospholipid layer

The first line of defense of gastric epithelium is a mucus-bicarbonate-phospholipid layer that serves as a physicochemical barrier. Surface epithelial cells provide the next line of defense.

446. Surface epithelial cells generate which of the following?

Harrison's 20th Ed. Chapter 317 Page 2221 Figure 317-3

A. Heat shock proteins
B. Trefoil peptides
C. Antimicrobial cathelicidins
D. All of the above

Surface epithelial cells generate heat shock proteins that prevent protein denaturation, trefoil factor family peptides and antimicrobial cathelicidins, which play a role in surface cell protection and regeneration.

447. Trefoil factor family (TFF) peptides were formerly known as?

Cellular and Molecular Life Sciences. 2009; 66(8):1350-1369

A. C-domain peptides
B. D-domain peptides
C. G-domain peptides
D. P-domain peptides

Trefoil factor family peptides (TFF1, TFF2, TFF3) were formerly called P-domain peptides promote wound healing in the gut through epithelial restitution. TFF peptides are found in mucous membranes of stomach, conjunctiva, Brunner's glands, intestine, salivary glands, uterus and respiratory tract.

448. Cathelicidin is best related to?

Mol Biol Rep. 2012; 39(12):10957-10970

A. P-domain peptides
B. Antimicrobial peptides (AMPs)
C. Angiogenesis
D. All of the above

Antimicrobial peptides (AMPs) have the capacity to rapidly inactivate infectious agents. The two major AMP families in mammals are the defensins and cathelicidin peptides.

449. Continuous cell renewal accomplished by proliferation of progenitor cells is regulated by?

Gastroenterology. 2008;135:41-60

A. Growth factors
B. PGE2
C. Survivin
D. All of the above

Survivin is a member of the inhibitor of apoptosis (IAP) protein family that inhibits caspases & blocks cell death. It is highly expressed in most cancers and is associated with a poor clinical outcome.

450. In seriously ill patients, which of the following cause reperfusion injury?

N Engl J Med. 2018;378:2506-16

A. Proinflammatory state
B. Splanchnic hypoperfusion
C. Impaired microcirculation
D. All of the above

In seriously ill patients, proinflammatory states, splanchnic hypoperfusion, and impaired microcirculation induce ischemia, reperfusion injury, and low gastric intramucosal pH.

451. Surface epithelial cells secrete which of the following?

N Engl J Med. 2018;378:2506-16

A. Mucus
B. Bicarbonate
C. Prostaglandins
D. All of the above

Beneath the layer of alkaline mucus gel lining are surface epithelial cells that secrete mucus, bicarbonate, prostaglandins. Surface epithelial cells are regenerated by mucosal progenitor cells.

452. Which of the following is a predictor of clinically important upper gastrointestinal bleeding in patients in ICU?

N Engl J Med. 2018;378:2506-16

A. Coagulopathy
B. Renal-replacement therapy
C. Use of acid suppressants
D. All of the above

Predictors of clinically important upper gastrointestinal bleeding in patients in the ICU include invasive mechanical ventilation for 48 hours or longer, coagulopathy, three or more coexisting diseases, liver disease, renal-replacement therapy, a high organ-failure score, & use of acid suppressants.

453. Which of the following define clinically important upper GI bleeding?

N Engl J Med. 2018;378:2506-16

A. Orthostatic increase in pulse of ≥20 beats/minute and decrease in systolic BP of 10 mm Hg
B. Decrease in hemoglobin of ≥2 g/dL over a 24-hour period
C. Transfusion of ≥2 units of PRBCs within 24 hour after start of bleeding
D. All of the above

454. With acid suppression, there is evidence of an increased risk of?

N Engl J Med. 2018;378:2506-16

A. Gastric perforation
B. Pancreatitis
C. Pneumonia
D. All of the above

Pharmacoepidemiologic studies provide support for an increased risk of pneumonia with acid suppression.

455. With acid suppression, there is evidence of an increased risk of?

N Engl J Med. 2018;378:2506-16

A. Achalasia
B. Duodenitis
C. C. difficile infection
D. Ileus

Hospital-acquired C. difficile infection showed an association with proton-pump inhibitors among patients in medical & surgical units.

456. Restitution of gastric mucosa means?

Harrison's 20th Ed. Chapter 317 Page 2221

A. Proliferation of damaged gastric mucosa
B. Regeneration of damaged gastric mucosa
C. Migration of normal gastric epithelium to damaged areas
D. All of the above

Restitution is migration of gastric epithelial cells bordering site of injury when preepithelial barrier is breached.

457. Which of the following statements about restitution is false?

Harrison's 20th Ed. Chapter 317 Page 2222

A. Occurs independent of cell division
B. Requires uninterrupted blood flow
C. Requires an alkaline pH in surroundings
D. None of the above

Restitution occurs independent of cell division and requires uninterrupted blood flow and an alkaline pH in the surrounding environment.

458. Restitution of gastric mucosa is modulated by?

Harrison's 20th Ed. Chapter 317 Page 2222

A. Epidermal growth factor (EGF)
B. Transforming growth factor alpha (TGF-α)
C. Fibroblast growth factor (FGF)
D. All of the above

Growth factors like epidermal growth factor (EGF), transforming growth factor (TGF) alpha and basic fibroblast growth factor (FGF) modulate restitution.

459. Gastric epithelial cell regeneration is regulated by?

Harrison's 20th Ed. Chapter 317 Page 2222

A. Prostaglandins
B. Epidermal growth factor (EGF)
C. Transforming growth factor-alpha (TGF-α)
D. All of the above

Larger defects not effectively repaired by restitution require cell proliferation. Epithelial cell regeneration is regulated by prostaglandins, EGF & TGF-alpha.

460. Angiogenesis in the gastric mucosa is regulated by?
Harrison's 20th Ed. Chapter 317 Page 2222

A. Fibroblast growth factor (FGF)
B. Vascular endothelial growth factor (VEGF)
C. Gastric peptide gastrin
D. All of the above

461. Bicarbonate secretion in stomach is stimulated by all except?
Harrison's 20th Ed. Chapter 317 Page 2222

A. Calcium
B. Prostaglandins
C. VIP
D. Luminal acidification

462. Which of the following plays a central role in gastric epithelial defense / repair?
Harrison's 20th Ed. Chapter 317 Page 2222

A. Mucosal bicarbonate
B. Mucus
C. Prostaglandins
D. Growth factor

463. Prostaglandins are important in gastric epithelial defense / repair due to all except?
Harrison's 20th Ed. Chapter 317 Page 2222

A. Release of mucosal bicarbonate and mucus
B. Inhibition of parietal cell secretion
C. Maintaining mucosal lymphatic flow
D. Epithelial cell restitution

Pg's in gastric mucosa play a central role in gastric epithelial defense/repair. Pg regulate release of mucosal bicarbonate & mucus, inhibit parietal cell secretion & maintain mucosal blood flow & epithelial cell restitution.

464. Key enzyme that controls the rate-limiting step in prostaglandin synthesis is?
Harrison's 20th Ed. Chapter 317 Page 2222

A. Thromboxane A_2 (TXA_2)
B. Phospholipase A_2
C. Cyclooxygenase (COX)
D. Prostacyclin (PGI_2)

Prostaglandins are derived from esterified arachidonic acid which is formed from phospholipids (cell membrane) by the action of phospholipase A2. Key enzyme that controls the rate-limiting step in prostaglandin synthesis is cyclooxygenase (COX) which is present in two isoforms - COX-1 & COX-2.

465. COX-1 is expressed in all except?
Harrison's 20th Ed. Chapter 317 Page 2222

A. Stomach
B. Platelets
C. Kidneys
D. Liver

COX-1 is expressed in stomach, platelets, kidneys, and endothelial cells. Gastro-intestinal mucosal ulceration & renal dysfunction is due to inhibition of COX-1.

466. COX-2 is expressed in all except?
Harrison's 20th Ed. Chapter 317 Page 2222

A. Macrophages
B. Leukocytes
C. Platelets
D. Synovial cells

COX-2, induced by inflammatory stimuli is expressed in macrophages, leukocytes, fibroblasts & synovial cells.

467. Selective COX-2 inhibitors increase the risk of?
Harrison's 20th Ed. Chapter 317 Page 2222

A. Myocardial infarction
B. Blindness
C. Acute renal failure
D. Fulminant hepatitis

Selective COX-2 inhibitors has adverse effects on the cardiovascular system, leading to increased risk of myocardial infarction. Valdecoxib and rofecoxib are banned by USFDA.

468. Which of the following is a function of Nitric oxide (NO)?
Harrison's 20th Ed. Chapter 317 Page 2222

A. Stimulates gastric mucus
B. Increases mucosal blood flow
C. Maintains epithelial cell barrier function
D. All of the above

Nitric oxide (NO) is important in the maintenance of gastric mucosal integrity. The key enzyme NO synthase is constitutively expressed in the mucosa and contributes to cytoprotection by stimulating gastric mucus, increasing mucosal blood flow and maintaining epithelial cell barrier function.

469. Gastric acid & pepsinogen play a physiologic role in?
Harrison's 20th Ed. Chapter 317 Page 2222

A. Protein digestion
B. Absorption of iron, calcium, magnesium & vitamin B_{12}
C. Killing ingested bacteria
D. All of the above

Gastric acid and pepsinogen play a physiologic role in protein digestion, absorption of iron, calcium, magnesium and vitamin B12 and killing ingested bacteria.

470. Which of the following is capable of inducing mucosal injury?
Harrison's 20th Ed. Chapter 317 Page 2222

A. Amylin
B. Phospholipase A_2
C. Pepsinogen
D. Ghrelin

Hydrochloric acid and pepsinogen are the two principal gastric secretory products capable of inducing mucosal injury.

471. Which of the following about acid production in stomach is false?
Harrison's 20th Ed. Chapter 317 Page 2222

A. Basal acid production occurs in a circadian pattern
B. Cholinergic & histaminergic input are the principal contributors to basal acid secretion
C. Stimulated gastric acid secretion occurs in cephalic, gastric & intestinal phases
D. Cephalic phase stimulates gastric secretion via hormones

Cephalic phase stimulates gastric secretion via vagus nerve.

472. Which of the following about acid production in stomach is false?

Harrison's 20th Ed. Chapter 317 Page 2222

A. Cephalic phase stimulates gastric secretion via vagus
B. Gastric phase is activated when food enters stomach
C. Amino acids stimulate vagus to release gastrin
D. Intestinal phase is mediated by luminal distention

Gastric phase is activated once food enters stomach. Amino acids and amines directly stimulate G cell to release gastrin, which in turn activate parietal cell.

473. Gastric acid production is inhibited by?

Harrison's 20th Ed. Chapter 317 Page 2222

A. Prostaglandins
B. Somatostatin
C. EGF
D. All of the above

Gastric acid production is inhibited by prostaglandins, somatostatin & epidermal growth factor (EGF).

474. Which of the following is a part of innate immune system?

Harrison's 20th Ed. Chapter 317 Page 2222

A. Dendritic cell
B. Epithelial cells
C. Macrophages
D. All of the above

475. Which of the following about basal acid secretion is false?

Harrison's 20th Ed. Chapter 317 Page 2222

A. Highest levels during night & lowest during morning hours
B. Cholinergic input via the vagus nerve play a role
C. Histaminergic input from local gastric sources play a role
D. None of the above

476. Histamine is released in stomach from?

Harrison's 20th Ed. Chapter 317 Page 2222

A. D cells
B. ECL cells
C. Gr cells
D. G cells

477. Somatostatin is released from D cells in response to?

Harrison's 20th Ed. Chapter 317 Page 2222

A. Pepsinogen
B. HCl
C. Secretin
D. All of the above

GI hormone somatostatin is released from endocrine cells in gastric mucosa (D cells) in response to HCl.

478. Somatostatin inhibits acid production by?

Harrison's 20th Ed. Chapter 317 Page 2222

A. Decreasing histamine release from ECL cells
B. Decreasing ghrelin release from Gr cells
C. Decreasing gastrin release from G cells
D. All of the above

479. Somatostatin acts by?

Harrison's 20th Ed. Chapter 317 Page 2222

A. Direct inhibition of parietal cells
B. Decreased histamine release from ECL cells
C. Decreased gastrin release from G cells
D. All of the above

Somatostatin is released from endocrine cells in gastric mucosa (D cells) in response to HCl. Somatostatin inhibits acid production by direct action on parietal cell, decreased histamine release from enterochromaffin-like (ECL) cells and gastrin release from G cells.

480. Which of the following hormone play a role in counterbalancing acid secretion?

Harrison's 20th Ed. Chapter 317 Page 2222

A. Atrial natriuretic peptide (ANP)
B. Cholecystokinin
C. Obestatin
D. All of the above

Amylin, atrial natriuretic peptide (ANP), cholecystokinin, ghrelin, interleukin 11 (IL-11, obestatin, secretin, and serotonin play a role in counterbalancing acid secretion.

481. Which of the following is the appetite-regulating hormone?

Harrison's 20th Ed. Chapter 317 Page 2222

A. Amylin
B. Obestatin
C. Secretin
D. Ghrelin

Ghrelin is the appetite-regulating hormone expressed in Gr cells in the stomach, may increase gastric acid secretion through stimulation of histamine release from ECL cells.

482. Which of the following about Ghrelin is false?

Journal of Clinical Endocrinology and Metabolism, 2005;90(4):2205-2211

A. Only peptide hormone modified by a fatty acid
B. Natural ligand for growth hormone secretagogue receptor (GHS-R)
C. Influences secretion of growth hormone
D. None of the above

Orexigenic Ghrelin is the only known peptide hormone modified by a fatty acid. Ghrelin is the natural ligand for the growth hormone secretagogue (GHS) receptor (GHS-R). Major biological functions of ghrelin include secretion of growth hormone, stimulation of appetite & food intake, modulation of gastric acid secretion & motility, and modulation of endocrine and exocrine pancreatic secretions.

483. Ghrelin is expressed in?

Journal of Clinical Endocrinology and Metabolism, 2005;90(4):2205-2211

A. Stomach
B. Lung
C. Testis
D. All of the above

Suffix "Ghre" means "to grow". It was discovered in 1999 as a peptide hormone. In addition to stomach, ghrelin is expressed in duodenum, jejunum, ileum, colon, lung, heart, pancreas, kidney, testis, pituitary, and hypothalamus.

484. Which of the following is called ghrelin's antagonistic hormone?

Journal of Clinical Endocrinology and Metabolism, 2005;90(4):2205-2211

A. Nucleobindin2 / Nesfatin-1
B. Leptin
C. Neuropeptide Y
D. All of the above

Orexigenic and anorexigenic peptides control appetite. Orexigenic peptides include neuropeptides Y (NPY), agoutirelated peptide (AGRP), orexins, melanin-concentrating hormone (MCH), galanin, & ghrelin. Ghrelin is the only one acting peripherally to stimulate appetite, while all other orexigenic peptides act centrally. Anorexigenic peptides includemelanocortin (a-MSH), cocaine- and amphetamine- regulated transcript (CART), corticotrophin-releasing hormone (CRH), cholecystokinin (CCK), gastrin-related peptide (GRP), glucagon like peptides 1 and 2 (GLP1, GLP2), pancreatic polypeptide (PP), peptide YY (PYY)), and leptin.

485. Which of the following is a cell type in gastric mucosa?
Journal of Clinical Endocrinology and Metabolism, 2005;90(4):2205-2211

A. Enterochromaffin-like cells (ECL)
B. D cells
C. P/D1 cell
D. All of the above

Gastric mucosa is composed of five endocrine cell types: enterochromaffin cells (EC), enterochromaffin-like cells (ECL), D cells, G cells, and X/A like cells or P/D1 cell which, respectively, secrete serotonin, histamine, somatostatin, gastrin, and ghrelin.

486. X/A-like cells or P/D1 cells release which of the following?
J Neurogastroenterol Motil. 2012;18(2):138-149

A. Desacyl ghrelin
B. Obestatin
C. Nesfatin-1
D. All of the above

X/A-like cells produce desacyl ghrelin, obestatin and nesfatin-1.

487. Which of the following about parietal cells is false?
Harrison's 20th Ed. Chapter 317 Page 2222

A. Located in oxyntic gland
B. Does not secrete intrinsic factor
C. Express receptors for histamine, gastrin & acetylcholine
D. Express receptors for ligands that inhibit acid production

Acid-secreting parietal cell secretes intrinsic factor (IF) and IL-11.

488. Activation of which of the following receptor on D-cells inhibits somatostatin release?
Harrison's 20th Ed. Chapter 317 Page 2223

A. H2 receptor
B. H3 receptor
C. M3 receptor
D. All of the above

489. Which of the following statements about enzyme H^+, K^+-ATPase is false?
Harrison's 20th Ed. Chapter 317 Page 2223

A. Responsible for generating large concentration of H^+
B. Membrane-bound protein consisting of α & β subunits
C. Active catalytic site is found within α subunit
D. Active catalytic site is found within β subunit

Active catalytic site is found within α subunit.

490. Which of the following statements about enzyme H^+, K^+-ATPase is false?
Harrison's 20th Ed. Chapter 317 Page 2223

A. Transfers H^+ ions from parietal cell cytoplasm to secretory canaliculi in exchange for K^+
B. Located within secretory canaliculus & in nonsecretory cytoplasmic tubulovesicles
C. Tubulovesicles are impermeable to K^+
D. At rest, 50% of pumps are within secretory canaliculus

Distribution of proton pumps between nonsecretory vesicles & secretory canaliculus varies according to parietal cell activity. They are recycled back to inactive state in cytoplasmic vesicles once parietal cell activation ceases.

491. Which of the following is an actin binding protein?
Harrison's 20th Ed. Chapter 317 Page 2223

A. Carin
B. Hamartin
C. Ezrin
D. Tuberin

492. Which of the following about chief cell is false?
Harrison's 20th Ed. Chapter 317 Page 2223

A. Found primarily in gastric fundus
B. Synthesize & secrete pepsinogen
C. Acid environment converts pepsinogen to pepsin
D. Pepsin activity is irreversibly inactivated & denatured at a pH of ≥4

Pepsin activity is significantly diminished at a pH of 4 and irreversibly inactivated and denatured at a pH of ≥7.

493. Which out of the following is the strongest risk factor for PUD?
Harrison's 20th Ed. Chapter 317 Page 2223

A. Chronic obstructive lung disease
B. Chronic renal insufficiency
C. Current tobacco use
D. Older age

Risk factors (odds ratio) for PUD are chronic obstructive lung disease (2.34), chronic renal insufficiency (2.29), current tobacco use (1.99), former tobacco use (1.55), older age (1.67), three or more doctor visits in a year (1.49), coronary heart disease (1.46), former alcohol use (1.29), African-American race (1.20), obesity (1.18) & diabetes (1.13).

494. All of the following about gastric ulcer are true except?
Harrison's 20th Ed. Chapter 317 Page 2223

A. A break in mucosal surface >5 mm in size
B. Depth to submucosa
C. More than half of gastric ulcers occur in males
D. Peak incidence is in the 4th decade of life

Gastric & duodenal ulcers are defined as breaks in mucosal surface >5 mm in size with depth to submucosa. Peak incidence of gastric ulcers is in the sixth decade & more than half of GUs occur in males.

495. ~90% of DU's occur within what distance from pylorus?
Harrison's 20th Ed. Chapter 317 Page 2223

A. 3 cm
B. 5 cm
C. 7 cm
D. 9 cm

~90% of DU's are located within 3 cm of the pylorus.

496. Which of the following statements about DU is false?
Harrison's 20th Ed. Chapter 317 Page 2223

A. Most often occur in first part of duodenum
B. Usually <=1 cm in diameter
C. Malignant DUs are extremely rare
D. Base of ulcer consists of neutrophilic necrosis with surrounding fibrosis

Base of DU consists of a zone of eosinophilic necrosis with surrounding fibrosis. Malignant DUs are rare.

497. Which of the following statements about GU is false?
Harrison's 20th Ed. Chapter 317 Page 2223

A. Can represent malignancy
B. Benign GUs are found distal to junction between antrum & acid secretory mucosa
C. Benign GUs are common in gastric fundus
D. Gastric acid output is normal or decreased in GU

Benign GUs are rare in the gastric fundus.

498. A chemical gastropathy is typified by?
Harrison's 20th Ed. Chapter 317 Page 2223

A. Foveolar hyperplasia
B. Edema of lamina propria
C. Epithelial regeneration in the absence of *H. pylori*
D. All of the above

499. Type IV Gastric Ulcers are found in?
Harrison's 20th Ed. Chapter 317 Page 2224

A. Cardia
B. Gastric body
C. Gastric antrum
D. Pylorus

Gastric ulcers are classified based on their location. Type I occur in gastric body, type II occur in antrum, type III occur within 3 cm of pylorus and type IV are found in the cardia.

500. Which of the following Gastric Ulcers has high gastric acid production?
Harrison's 20th Ed. Chapter 317 Page 2224

A. Type I
B. Type II
C. Type III
D. Type IV

Type III GU's occur within 3 cm of the pylorus and are commonly accompanied by duodenal ulcers and normal or high gastric acid production.

501. *Helicobacter pylori* was discovered by?
N Engl J Med. 2010;362:1597-604

A. Marshall B & Warren R
B. Julie Parsonnet & Jennings R
C. Banatvala N & Mayo K
D. Deeks JJ & Feldman RA

Helicobacter pylori is a gram-negative helical rod shaped bacterium found on the luminal surface of gastric epithelium. It was first isolated by Warren and Marshall in 1983.

502. Gastric infection with *H. pylori* can lead to?
Harrison's 20th Ed. Chapter 317 Page 2224

A. Peptic ulcer disease (PUD)
B. Gastric mucosal-associated lymphoid tissue lymphoma
C. Gastric adenocarcinoma
D. All of the above

H. pylori plays a role in the development of majority of PUD, gastric mucosal-associated lymphoid tissue (MALT) lymphoma and gastric adenocarcinoma.

503. Which of the following statements about *H. pylori* is false?
Harrison's 20th Ed. Chapter 317 Page 2224

A. It is a gram-positive microaerophilic rod
B. Found between mucous layer & gastric epithelium
C. Normally, it does not invade gastric epithelial cells
D. S-shaped & contains multiple sheathed flagella

H. pylori is a gram-negative microaerophilic rod found most commonly between the mucous layer and the gastric epithelium.

504. pH-gated urea channel in *H. pylori* bacterium is called?
N Engl J Med. 2002:347,1175

A. UreI
B. UreJ
C. UreK
D. UreL

505. Which of the following statements about *H. pylori* is false?
Harrison's 20th Ed. Chapter 317 Page 2224

A. Its genome contains 1.65 million base pairs
B. May transform into coccoid dormant form
C. Produces urease to convert urea to NH_3 and water
D. Single strain of *H. pylori* exist

Multiple strains of H. pylori exist. Different diseases related to H. pylori infection can be attributed to different strains with distinct pathogenic features.

506. Which of the following statements about *H. pylori* is false?
N Engl J Med. 2002:347,1175

A. 80% population by age 20 years is infected in developing countries
B. Transmission occurs through faeco-oral route
C. Infection is associated with chronic active gastritis
D. BabA is vital for entry into gastric epithelial cell

507. Which of the following statements about *H. pylori* is false?
Harrison's 20th Ed. Chapter 317 Page 2224

A. Express vacuolating cytotoxin VacA
B. Cag A and pic B are virulence factors
C. Its LPS has high immunologic activity
D. Neutrophil response is strong in acute & chronic *H. pylori* infection

508. Which out of the following factors has a central role in *H. pylori* infection?
N Engl J Med. 2002:347,1175

A. Interleukin-1β
B. Interleukin-2
C. Interleukin-6
D. Interleukin-8

509. Which of the following statements about *H. pylori* is false?
N Engl J Med. 2002:347, 1175

A. Most pathogenic strains contain VacA pathogenicity island
B. 5 of its genes are similar to Agrobacterium tumefaciens
C. Pathogenicity island proteins are involved in interleukin-8 production by gastric epithelial cells
D. Pathogenicity island proteins are involved in translocation of CagA from bacterium into host cell

510. Adhesins for *H. pylori* include all except?
N Engl J Med. 2002:347,1175

A. BabA
B. AlpA
C. AlpB
D. HopY

H. pylori expresses adhesins which facilitate attachment of the bacteria to gastric epithelial cells.

511. Which of the following statements about *H. pylori* is false?
N Engl J Med. 2002:347,1175

A. *H. pylori* is usually acquired in childhood
B. Acute infection causes transient hypochlorhydria
C. 80-90% with chronic gastritis will never have symptoms
D. After eradication, reinfection rates are high

Reinfection after successful eradication of H. pylori is rare in US. If recurrent infection occurs within first 6 months after completing therapy, most likely explanation is recrudescence and not reinfection.

512. Which of the following enzymes is not related to *H. pylori*–induced gastrointestinal disease?
Harrison's 20th Ed. Chapter 317 Page 2224 Table 317-6

A. Urease
B. Vac A
C. GAD
D. Cag A

Bacterial enzymes that cause H. pylori-induced gastrointestinal disease are Urease, Vac A & Cag A.

513. "cag" stands for?
Harrison's 20th Ed. Chapter 317 Page 2224

A. Cytotoxin-associated gene
B. Cytotoxin-assembly gene
C. Cytotoxin-augmented gene
D. Cytotoxin-apoptotic gene

514. Which of the following secretion system is associated with *H. pylori* infection?
N Engl J Med. 2002:347,1175

A. Type I
B. Type II
C. Type III
D. Type IV

515. Which of the following about Cag A is false?
Harrison's 20th Ed. Chapter 317 Page 2224

A. Virulence factor in pathogenicity island (cag-PAI)
B. Cytotoxin-associated gene A
C. Oncoprotein
D. None of the above

516. Chronic *H. pylori* infection may lead to?
Harrison's 20th Ed. Chapter 317 Page 2224 Figure 317-8

A. Antral predominant gastritis
B. Nonatrophic pangastritis
C. Corpus predominant atrophic gastritis
D. All of the above

517. Asymptomatic *H. pylori* infection may be a consequence of?
Harrison's 20th Ed. Chapter 317 Page 2224 Figure 317-8

A. Antral predominant gastritis
B. Nonatrophic pangastritis
C. Corpus predominant atrophic gastritis
D. All of the above

518. Which of the following consequences of chronic *H. pylori* infection leads to gastric cancer?
Harrison's 20th Ed. Chapter 317 Page 2224 Figure 317-8

A. Antral predominant gastritis
B. Nonatrophic pangastritis
C. Corpus predominant atrophic gastritis
D. All of the above

Chronic H. pylori infection leading to corpus predominant atrophic gastritis going on to intestinal metaplasia is an important predisposing factor for gastric cancer.

519. Which of the following consequences of chronic *H. pylori* infection leads to DU?
Harrison's 20th Ed. Chapter 317 Page 2224 Figure 317-8

A. Antral predominant gastritis
B. Nonatrophic pangastritis
C. Corpus predominant atrophic gastritis
D. All of the above

Presence of antral-predominant gastritis is associated with DU formation.

520. Which of the following consequences of chronic H. pylori infection leads to MALT lymphoma?
Harrison's 20th Ed. Chapter 317 Page 2224 Figure 317-8

A. Antral predominant gastritis
B. Nonatrophic pangastritis
C. Corpus predominant atrophic gastritis
D. All of the above

Chronic infection with H. pylori is associated with development of a low-grade B cell lymphoma, gastric MALT lymphoma. (MALT refers to mucosal-associated lymphoid tissue).

521. Which of the following in *H. pylori* may be associated with development of DUs?
Harrison's 20th Ed. Chapter 317 Page 2225

A. Cag A
B. dupA
C. pic B
D. Vac A

In H. pylori, bacterial factor DU-promoting gene A (dupA) may be associated with development of DUs.

522. Antral-predominant gastritis is associated with the development of?
Harrison's 20th Ed. Chapter 317 Page 2225

A. DU
B. GU
C. Gastric atrophy
D. Gastric carcinoma

523. Gastritis involving primarily corpus predisposes to development of?
Harrison's 20th Ed. Chapter 317 Page 2225

A. GU
B. Gastric atrophy
C. Gastric carcinoma
D. All of the above

524. Risk factors that increase morbidity and mortality related to NSAID usage are all except?
Harrison's 20th Ed. Chapter 317 Page 2226

A. Advanced age
B. History of PUD
C. Concomitant use of iron
D. Multisystem disease

525. Risk factors that increase morbidity and mortality related to NSAID usage are all except?
Harrison's 20th Ed. Chapter 317 Page 2226

A. High dose NSAIDs
B. Multiple NSAIDs
C. Concomitant use of anticoagulants
D. Spicy food

Established risk factors for serious gastrointestinal complications from NSAIDs include advanced age, history of ulcer, concomitant use of glucocorticoids, high-dose NSAIDs, multiple NSAIDs, concomitant use of anticoagulants, and serious or multisystem disease. Possible risk factors include concomitant infection with H. pylori, cigarette smoking, and alcohol consumption.

526. Disorders that are associated with PUD include all except?
Harrison's 20th Ed. Chapter 317 Page 2226

A. Systemic mastocytosis
B. Chronic pulmonary disease
C. Chronic renal failure
D. Acute pancreatitis

527. Disorders that are associated with PUD include all except?
Harrison's 20th Ed. Chapter 317 Page 2226

A. Cirrhosis
B. Nephrolithiasis
C. Hyperthyroidism
D. α1 antitrypsin deficiency

Chronic disorders that have a strong association with PUD are systemic mastocytosis, chronic pulmonary disease, chronic renal failure, cirrhosis, nephrolithiasis, and alpha$_1$-antitrypsin deficiency. Those with a possible association are hyperparathyroidism, coronary artery disease, polycythemia vera, and chronic pancreatitis.

528. Which of the following blood group has been implicated in the pathogenesis of PUD?
Harrison's 20th Ed. Chapter 317 Page 2226

A. Blood group A
B. Blood group B
C. Blood group AB
D. Blood group O

Increased frequency of blood group O has been implicated as genetic risk factors for peptic diathesis.

529. The typical pain pattern in DU occurs?
Harrison's 20th Ed. Chapter 317 Page 2227

A. 15 minutes to 1 hour after a meal
B. 30 minutes to 2 hour after a meal
C. 60 minutes to 3 hour after a meal
D. 90 minutes to 3 hour after a meal

Typical pain pattern in DU occurs 90 minutes to 3 hours after a meal and is frequently relieved by antacids or food.

530. Which of the following is a feature of pain pattern in GU?
Harrison's 20th Ed. Chapter 317 Page 2227

A. Awakes patient from sleep between midnight and 3 AM
B. Discomfort may be precipitated by food
C. Nausea & weight loss occur more commonly
D. All of the above

Pain that awakes the patient from sleep (between midnight and 3 AM) is the most discriminating symptom. In GU, nausea & weight loss occur more commonly & discomfort may be precipitated by food.

531. Which of the following infectious agents can cause PUD?
Harrison's 20th Ed. Chapter 317 Page 2227 Table 317-1

A. Cytomegalovirus
B. Herpes simplex virus
C. Helicobacter heilmannii
D. All of the above

532. Which of the following is the most frequent finding in patients with GU or DU?
Harrison's 20th Ed. Chapter 317 Page 2227

A. Succussion splash
B. Epigastric tenderness
C. Dehydration secondary to vomiting
D. Abdominal distension

533. Most common complication observed in PUD is?
Harrison's 20th Ed. Chapter 317 Page 2227

A. Gastrointestinal bleeding
B. Perforation
C. Gastric Outlet Obstruction
D. Malignancy

Gastrointestinal bleeding is the most common complication observed in PUD followed by perforation and gastric outlet obstruction. >50% of patients with ulcer-related hemorrhage bleed without any preceding warning signs or symptoms.

534. Which of the following is the least common cause of mortality in PUD-related bleeding?
Harrison's 20th Ed. Chapter 317 Page 2227

A. Exsanguination
B. Multiorgan failure
C. Pulmonary complications
D. Malignancy

Most of the mortality in PUD-related bleeding is due to nonbleeding causes like multiorgan failure (24%), pulmonary complications (24%), and malignancy (34%).

535. Out of the following, which is the least common ulcer-related complication?
Harrison's 20th Ed. Chapter 317 Page 2227

A. Gastric outlet obstruction
B. Gastrointestinal bleeding
C. Perforation
D. Malignancy

Gastric outlet obstruction is the least common ulcer-related complication.

536. GUs tend to perforate into?
Harrison's 20th Ed. Chapter 317 Page 2227

A. Spleen
B. Pancreas
C. Left hepatic lobe
D. Left kidney

537. DUs tend to perforate into?
Harrison's 20th Ed. Chapter 317 Page 2227

A. Spleen
B. Pancreas
C. Right hepatic lobe
D. Left kidney

GUs tend to penetrate into the left hepatic lobe while DUs tend to penetrate posteriorly into pancreas.

538. Functional dyspepsia or essential dyspepsia is typified by?
Harrison's 20th Ed. Chapter 317 Page 2227

A. Heartburn
B. Upper abdominal pain
C. Water brash
D. Loss of appetite

NUD (functional dyspepsia / essential dyspepsia) is typified by upper abdominal pain without presence of ulcer.

539. Postprandial distress syndrome & epigastric pain syndrome are a type of?
Harrison's 20th Ed. Chapter 317 Page 2227

A. Functional dyspepsia
B. Gastric outlet obstruction
C. Coronary artery disease
D. Neuroticism

Postprandial distress syndrome (PDS) and epigastric pain syndrome (EPS) are subcategories of functional dyspepsia (FD).

540. Ulcers are more often malignant when their size is?
Harrison's 20th Ed. Chapter 317 Page 2228

A. > 1 cm
B. > 2 cm
C. > 3 cm
D. > 4 cm

Ulcers are more often malignant when their size is > 3 cm or those associated with a mass.

541. Tests for diagnosing *H. pylori* include?
Harrison's 20th Ed. Chapter 317 Page 2229 Table 317-2

A. Biopsy urease test
B. Fecal *H. pylori* antigen test
C. ^{13}C- or ^{14}C-urea breath test
D. All of the above

Tests for diagnosing H. pylori include serologic testing, ^{13}C- or ^{14}C-urea breath test& fecal H. pylori (Hp) antigen test (monoclonal antibody test). Urinary Hp antigen test appear promising.

542. Rapid urease invasive test for detection of *H. pylori* is false negative with recent use of?
Harrison's 20th Ed. Chapter 317 Page 2229 Table 317-2

A. PPIs
B. Antibiotics
C. Bismuth compounds
D. All of the above

543. Milk-alkali syndrome includes all except?
Harrison's 20th Ed. Chapter 317 Page 2229

A. Hypercalcemia
B. Hypophosphatemia
C. Renal calcinosis
D. Progression to renal insufficiency

Milk-alkali syndrome comprises of hypercalcemia, hyperphosphatemia, renal calcinosis & progression to renal insufficiency.

544. Initial mild hypercalcemia in Milk-alkali syndrome first leads to?
Harrison's 20th Ed. Chapter 403 Page 2933

A. Alkalosis
B. Bicarbonate retention
C. Renal calcium retention
D. Severe hypercalcemia

545. Burnett's syndrome is best related to?
Harrison's 20th Ed. Chapter 403 Page 2933

A. Aluminum intoxication
B. Vitamin A intoxication
C. Milk-alkali syndrome
D. Hypethyroidism

The chronic form of Milk-alkali syndrome is termed as Burnett's syndrome. It is associated with irreversible renal damage.

546. Phrase "no acid, no ulcer" is best related to?
N Engl J Med. 1971; 285:620

A. Palmer
B. Piper
C. Schwarz
D. Bralow

"No acid - no ulcer" statement has been referred to as Schwarz's dictum. Dragutin (Carl) Schwarz (1868-1917) is primarily remembered for his dictum 'No acid, no ulcer' (1910).

547. Structure of H_2 receptor antagonists share structural homology with?
Harrison's 20th Ed. Chapter 317 Page 2229

A. Pepsin
B. Secretin
C. Gastrin
D. Histamine

H_2 receptor antagonists (cimetidine, ranitidine, famotidine & nizatidine) have structural homology with histamine.

548. Which of the following about cimetidine is false?
Harrison's 20th Ed. Chapter 317 Page 2229

A. First H_2 receptor antagonist used in acid peptic disorders
B. Antiandrogenic side effects
C. Inhibit cytochrome P450
D. None of the above

549. Monitoring of which of the following drugs is needed when used with cimetidine?
Harrison's 20th Ed. Chapter 317 Page 2229

A. Warfarin
B. Phenytoin
C. Theophylline
D. All of the above

Caution is needed when using theophylline, warfarin, diazepam, atazanavir & phenytoin with PPIs.

550. Which of the following H_2 receptor antagonist does not bind to hepatic cytochrome P450?
Harrison's 20th Ed. Chapter 317 Page 2229

A. Cimetidine
B. Ranitidine
C. Famotidine
D. All of the above

Famotidine and nizatidine do not bind to hepatic cytochrome P450.

551. Which of the following is the most recent PPI approved for clinical use?
Harrison's 20th Ed. Chapter 317 Page 2229

A. Esomeprazole
B. Dexlansoprazole
C. Tenatoprazole
D. Rabeprazole

Dexlansoprazole is an R-isomer of lansoprazole, and is the most recent PPI approved for clinical use.

552. The half-life of PPIs is?
Harrison's 20th Ed. Chapter 317 Page 2229

A. ~ 8 hours
B. ~ 12 hours
C. ~ 14 hours
D. ~ 18 hours

The half-life of PPIs is ~18 hours.

553. Which of the following occurs with the use of PPIs?
Harrison's 20th Ed. Chapter 317 Page 2229

A. Hypergastrinemia
B. IF production is inhibited
C. Hypomagnesemia
D. All of the above

Long-term use of PPIs may lead to development of iron, vitamin B12, and magnesium deficiency.

554. Proton pump inhibitors may interfere with absorption of?
Harrison's 20th Ed. Chapter 317 Page 2230

A. Ketoconazole
B. Iron
C. Digoxin
D. All of the above

PPIs may interfere with absorption of ketoconazole, ampicillin, iron & digoxin.

555. Hepatic cytochrome P450 can be inhibited by?
Harrison's 20th Ed. Chapter 317 Page 2230

A. Lansoprazole
B. Rabeprazole
C. Pantoprazole
D. Esomeprazole

Hepatic cytochrome P450 can be inhibited by omeprazole & lansoprazole and not by rabeprazole, pantoprazole and esomeprazole.

556. Long-term acid suppression with PPIs has been associated with a higher incidence of?
Harrison's 20th Ed. Chapter 317 Page 2230

A. Bacterial meningitis
B. Community-acquired pneumonia
C. Urinary tract infection
D. Gall stones

557. Long-term acid suppression with PPIs has been associated with a higher incidence of?
Harrison's 20th Ed. Chapter 317 Page 2230

A. Nail dystrophy
B. Clostridium difficile - associated disease
C. Gingivitis
D. Cataract

Long-term acid suppression with PPIs is associated with higher incidence of community-acquired pneumonia and community and hospital acquired Clostridium difficile-associated disease.

558. Which of the following cytochrome P450 is involved in the competition of PPI & clopidogrel?
Harrison's 20th Ed. Chapter 317 Page 2230

A. CYP2B6
B. CYP2D6
C. CYP2C19
D. CYP3A

PPIs may exert a negative effect on the antiplatelet effect of clopidogrel. If PPIs are to be given, there should be a 12 hour separation between administration of PPI & clopidogrel.

559. PPI containing an imidazopyridine ring instead of a benzimidazole ring is?
Harrison's 20th Ed. Chapter 317 Page 2230

A. Rabeprazole
B. Pantoprazole
C. Tenatoprazole
D. Esomeprazole

Tenatoprazole is a PPI containing an imidazopyridine ring instead of a benzimidazole ring.

560. Which of the following is a potassium-competitive acid pump antagonists (P-CABs)?
Harrison's 20th Ed. Chapter 317 Page 2230

A. Vilazodone
B. Revaprazan
C. Gadoteridol
D. All of the above

Revaprazan & venoprazan are potassium-competitive acid pump antagonists (P-CABs).

561. Sucralfate is a complex sucrose salt in which hydroxyl groups are substituted by?

Harrison's 20th Ed. Chapter 317 Page 2231

A. Aluminum acetate
B. Aluminum chloride
C. Aluminum hydroxide
D. Aluminum phosphate

Sucralfate is a complex sucrose salt in which the hydroxyl groups are substituted by aluminum hydroxide & sulfate.

562. Which of the following is false about Sucralfate?

Harrison's 20th Ed. Chapter 317 Page 2231

A. Complex sucrose salt
B. Insoluble in water
C. To be avoided in chronic renal insufficiency
D. None of the above

563. Sir William Osler considered which of the following the drug of choice for treating PUD?

Harrison's 20th Ed. Chapter 317 Page 2231

A. Antacids
B. Bismuth-containing compounds
C. Sucralfate
D. H_2 receptor antagonists

Sir William Osler considered bismuth-containing compounds the drug of choice for treating PUD.

564. Black stools & darkening of tongue are adverse effects of?

Harrison's 20th Ed. Chapter 317 Page 2231

A. Misoprostol
B. Sucralfate
C. Colloidal bismuth subcitrate (CBS)
D. Proton Pump Inhibitors (PPI)

Adverse effects with short-term usage of Colloidal bismuth subcitrate (CBS) and bismuth subsalicylate (BSS) include black stools, constipation and darkening of tongue.

565. Maastricht IV/Florence Consensus Report recommends a test-and-treat approach for patients with uninvestigated dyspepsia if the local incidence of *H. pylori* is?

Harrison's 20th Ed. Chapter 317 Page 2231

A. > 10%
B. > 20%
C. > 30%
D. > 40%

566. ACG clinical guidelines recommend testing & offering H. pylori eradication to patients with?

Harrison's 20th Ed. Chapter 317 Page 2231

A. Enteric fever
B. Idiopathic thrombocytopenic purpura
C. Nephrolithiasis
D. Asthma

ACG clinical guidelines recommend testing & offering H. pylori eradication to patients with unexplained iron deficiency anemia & idiopathic thrombocytopenic purpura.

567. Which of the following about therapy of *H. pylori* is false?

Harrison's 20th Ed. Chapter 317 Page 2231

A. No single agent is effective in eradicating the organism
B. Combination therapy for 14 days provides greatest efficacy
C. Aim for initial eradication rates should be 85 – 90%
D. None of the above

568. Combination therapy for *H. pylori* infection should be given for a period of?

Harrison's 20th Ed. Chapter 317 Page 2231

A. 7 days
B. 14 days
C. 21 days
D. 28 days

Combination therapy for H. pylori infection for 14 days provides the greatest efficacy.

569. First triple regimen therapy against *H. pylori* was?

Harrison's 20th Ed. Chapter 317 Page 2231

A. Amoxicillin + omeprazole + metronidazole
B. Bismuth + metronidazole + tetracycline
C. Clarithromycin + omeprazole + metronidazole
D. Lansoprazole + clarithromycin + amoxicillin

First triple regimen therapy against H. pylori was bismuth, metronidazole & tetracycline.

570. Most feared complication with amoxicillin is?

Harrison's 20th Ed. Chapter 317 Page 2232

A. Antibiotic-associated diarrhea
B. Pseudomembranous colitis
C. Hepatotoxicity
D. Anaphylaxis

571. Which of the following statements about *H. pylori* is false?

Harrison's 20th Ed. Chapter 317 Page 2232

A. *H. pylori* should be eradicated in documented PUD
B. No single agent is effective in eradicating *H. pylori*
C. Rifabutin used to treat resistant strains of *H. pylori*
D. *H. pylori* is implicated in pathogenesis of acute pancreatitis

572. Which of the following is a treatment regimen for eradication of *H. pylori* infection?

Harrison's 20th Ed. Chapter 317 Page 2232

A. Triple therapy
B. Quadruple therapy
C. Sequential therapy
D. All of the above

573. Which of the following drugs can be used for eradication of *H. pylori*?

Harrison's 20th Ed. Chapter 317 Page 2232

A. Tinidazole
B. Levofloxacin
C. Furazolidone
D. All of the above

574. Which of the following drugs can be used for eradication of *H. pylori*?

Harrison's 20th Ed. Chapter 317 Page 2234

A. N-acetylcysteine
B. Lactobacillus spp.
C. Saccharomyces spp.
D. All of the above

575. Which of the following can heal GUs or DUs, independent of whether NSAIDs are discontinued?

Harrison's 20th Ed. Chapter 317 Page 2234

A. H_2 receptor antagonist
B. PPIs
C. Misoprostol
D. Sucralfate

Only PPIs can heal GUs or DUs, independent of whether NSAIDs are discontinued.

576. H. pylori eradication should be documented how many weeks after completing antibiotics?

Harrison's 20th Ed. Chapter 317 Page 2235

A. 1
B. 2
C. 3
D. 4

H. pylori eradication should be documented 4 weeks after completing antibiotics.

577. Test of choice for documenting eradication of *H. pylori* is?

Harrison's 20th Ed. Chapter 317 Page 2235

A. Biopsy urease test
B. Fecal *H. pylori* antigen test
C. ^{13}C- or ^{14}C-urea breath test
D. Urinary Hp antigen test

The test of choice for documenting eradication is the urea breath test (UBT).

578. A GU is considered refractory if it fails to heal after how many weeks of therapy?

Harrison's 20th Ed. Chapter 317 Page 2235

A. 4 weeks
B. 8 weeks
C. 12 weeks
D. 16 weeks

579. A DU is considered refractory if it fails to heal after how many weeks of therapy?

Harrison's 20th Ed. Chapter 317 Page 2235

A. 4 weeks
B. 8 weeks
C. 12 weeks
D. 16 weeks

GU that fails to heal >12 weeks & a DU that does not heal >8 weeks of therapy is considered refractory.

580. Etiologies of refractory ulcers (GU / DU) include all except?

Harrison's 20th Ed. Chapter 317 Page 2235

A. Ischemia
B. Crohn's disease
C. Ulcerative colitis
D. Amyloidosis

581. Etiologies of refractory ulcers (GU / DU) include all except?

Harrison's 20th Ed. Chapter 317 Page 2235

A. Sarcoidosis
B. Lymphoma
C. Eosinophilic gastroenteritis
D. HIV

582. Etiologies of refractory ulcers (GU / DU) include all except?

Harrison's 20th Ed. Chapter 317 Page 2235

A. Leprosy
B. Cytomegalovirus (CMV)
C. Tuberculosis
D. Syphilis

Rare etiologies of refractory GU/DU's include ischemia, Crohn's disease, amyloidosis, sarcoidosis, lymphoma, eosinophilic gastroenteritis, cytomegalovirus (CMV), tuberculosis or syphilis.

583. Posterior DU can penetrate into?

Harrison's 20th Ed. Chapter 317 Page 2236

A. Pancreas
B. Colon
C. Liver
D. All of the above

Posterior DU can penetrate into pancreas, colon, liver or biliary tree.

584. Which of the following is a component of Zollinger–Ellison Syndrome (ZES)?

Harrison's 20th Ed. Chapter 317 Page 2238

A. Severe peptic ulcer diathesis
B. Gastric acid hypersecretion
C. Unregulated gastrin from a non-β cell neuroendocrine tumor
D. None of the above

ZES is typified by severe peptic ulcer diathesis secondary to gastric acid hypersecretion due to unregulated gastrin release from gastrinoma - a non-β cell well-differentiated neuroendocrine tumor.

585. Which of the following is not a typical feature of Zollinger–Ellison Syndrome (ZES)?

Harrison's 20th Ed. Chapter 317 Page 2238

A. Gastrin release from beta cell endocrine tumor
B. Hypergastrinemia
C. Erosive esophagitis
D. Diarrhea

The increased gastric acid output leads to peptic ulcer diathesis, erosive esophagitis, and diarrhea.

586. In ZES, majority of patients are diagnosed between ages of?

Harrison's 20th Ed. Chapter 317 Page 2238

A. 01 and 10 years
B. 10 and 30 years
C. 30 and 50 years
D. 50 and 70 years

In ZES, males are more commonly affected than females, and majority of patients are diagnosed between the ages of 30 and 50 years.

587. Average time from symptom onset to diagnosis of Zollinger–Ellison syndrome is?

N Engl J Med. 2018;378:73-9

A. > 3 years
B. > 5 years
C. > 7 years
D. > 10 years

Average time from symptom onset to diagnosis of Zollinger–Ellison syndrome is more than 5 years.

588. Multiple endocrine neoplasia (MEN) type 1 is characterized by all except?

Harrison's 20th Ed. Chapter 369 Page 2649

A. Parathyroid tumor
B. Pancreatic islet tumor
C. Pheochromocytoma
D. Pituitary tumor

Gastrinomas are classified into sporadic tumors (80%) and those associated with multiple endocrine neoplasia (MEN) type 1.

589. Which of the following is the action of gastrin?

Harrison's 20th Ed. Chapter 317 Page 2238

A. Stimulates acid secretion through gastrin receptors on parietal cells
B. Stimulates acid secretion by inducing histamine release from ECL cells
C. Has a trophic action on gastric epithelial cells
D. All of the above

Gastrin stimulates acid secretion through gastrin receptors on parietal cells and by inducing histamine release from ECL cells. Gastrin also has a trophic action on gastric epithelial cells.

590. 'Gastrinoma triangle' is formed by all except?

Harrison's 20th Ed. Chapter 317 Page 2238

A. Cystic and common bile ducts
B. Junction of II and III portions of duodenum
C. Inferior surface of liver
D. Junction of neck & body of pancreas

Hypothetical gastrinoma triangle is formed by confluence of cystic & common bile ducts superiorly, junction of second & third portions of duodenum inferiorly, and junction of neck & body of pancreas medially.

591. What proportion of gastrinoma are found within the hypothetical gastrinoma triangle?

Harrison's 20th Ed. Chapter 317 Page 2238

A. 20%
B. 40%
C. 60%
D. 80%

Gastrinomas occur within pancreas or may be extrapancreatic. Over 80% of gastrinoma are found within the hypothetical gastrinoma triangle.

592. Which of the following is the most common extrapancreatic site of gastrinoma?

Harrison's 20th Ed. Chapter 317 Page 2238

A. Stomach
B. Duodenum
C. Liver
D. Lymph nodes

Duodenal gastrinoma tumors constitute the most common nonpancreatic lesion (50 to75%). Less-common extrapancreatic sites include stomach, bones, ovaries, heart, liver, and lymph nodes.

593. What proportion of gastrinoma are malignant?

Harrison's 20th Ed. Chapter 317 Page 2238

A. 20%
B. 40%
C. 60%
D. 80%

More than 60% of gastrinoma tumors are considered malignant, with up to 30–50% of patients having multiple lesions or metastatic disease at presentation.

594. Marker typically found in endocrine neoplasms is?

Harrison's 20th Ed. Chapter 74 Page 538

A. Chromogranin
B. Neuron-specific enolase
C. Synaptophysin
D. All of the above

Markers for neuroendocrine differentiation within a tumor are neuron-specific enolase (NSE), CD56 or NCAM, synaptophysin, chromogranin, and Leu7.

595. Which of the following suggest the diagnosis of ZES?

Harrison's 20th Ed. Chapter 317 Page 2238

A. Ulcer in second part of duodenum & beyond
B. Ulcers refractory to standard medical therapy
C. Ulcer presenting with frank complication
D. All of the above

Gastrinoma should be suspected when ulcers occur unusual locations like II part of duodenum & beyond, ulcers refractory to standard medical therapy, ulcer recurrence after acid-reducing surgery, ulcers presenting with frank complications (bleeding, obstruction, and perforation), or ulcers in the absence of H. pylori or NSAID ingestion.

596. What proportion of ZES patients have diarrhea?

Harrison's 20th Ed. Chapter 317 Page 2238

A. 25%
B. 50%
C. 75%
D. 100%

After peptic ulcer (90%), diarrhea is the next most common clinical manifestation after peptic ulcer and is found in up to 50% of patients of ZES.

597. Etiology of the diarrhea in ZES is?

Harrison's 20th Ed. Chapter 317 Page 2238

A. Volume overload to the small bowel
B. Pancreatic enzyme inactivation by acid
C. Damage of the intestinal epithelial surface by acid
D. All of the above

In ZES, etiology of diarrhea is multifactorial, resulting from marked volume overload to small bowel, pancreatic enzyme inactivation by acid & damage of intestinal epithelial surface by acid.

598. Gastrinomas develop in the presence of MEN 1 syndrome in what percentage of patients?

Harrison's 20th Ed. Chapter 317 Page 2238

A. ~ 10%
B. ~ 25%
C. ~ 50%
D. ~ 75%

Gastrinomas can develop in the presence of MEN 1 syndrome in ~25% of patients.

599. Organs involved in MEN 1 syndrome are all except?
Harrison's 20th Ed. Chapter 317 Page 2238

A. Parathyroid
B. Thyroid
C. Pancreas
D. Pituitary

MEN I syndrome (autosomal dominant) involves parathyroid glands (80–90%), pancreas (40–80%), pituitary gland (30–60%) and gastrinomas (~25%).

600. Genetic defect in MEN 1 is in?
Harrison's 20th Ed. Chapter 317 Page 2238

A. Short arm of chromosome 11
B. Long arm of chromosome 11
C. Short arm of chromosome 12
D. Long arm of chromosome 12

The genetic defect in MEN I is in the long arm of chromosome 11 (11q11-q13).

601. MEN1 tumor suppressor gene encodes for?
Harrison's 20th Ed. Chapter 317 Page 2238

A. β-catenin
B. Parafibromin
C. Menin
D. Neurokinin B

MEN1 tumor suppressor gene encodes for Menin, 610-amino-acid protein. Pathophysiology of MEN 1 follows the Knudson two-hit hypothesis.

602. Distinguishing feature between MEN I associated ZES & sprodic ZES is?
Harrison's 20th Ed. Chapter 317 Page 2239

A. Incidence of gastric carcinoid tumor
B. Size, number & location of gastrinoma
C. Disease free period after surgery
D. All of the above

Gastrinomas tend to be smaller, multiple, and located in the duodenal wall more often than is seen in patients with sporadic ZES. An additional distinguishing feature in ZES patients with MEN I is the higher incidence of gastric carcinoid tumor development (as compared to patients with sporadic gastrinomas). Gastrinomas tend to be smaller, multiple, and located in the duodenal wall more often than is seen in patients with sporadic ZES.

603. First step in the evaluation of a patient suspected of ZES is?
Harrison's 20th Ed. Chapter 317 Page 2239

A. Assess acid secretion
B. Obtain a fasting gastrin level
C. Secretin stimulation test
D. Calcium infusion study

The first step in evaluation of a patient suspected of ZES is to obtain a fasting gastrin level.

604. Patients with gastrinoma have gastrin level more than?
Harrison's 20th Ed. Chapter 317 Page 2239

A. 25 pg/mL
B. 50 pg/mL
C. 100 pg/mL
D. 150 pg/mL

Fasting gastrin levels are <150 pg/mL. All gastrinoma patients have a gastrin level >150 – 200 pg/mL.

605. The most frequent condition that leads to an elevated fasting gastrin level is?
Harrison's 20th Ed. Chapter 317 Page 2239

A. Nonsteroidal antiinflammatory drug ingestion
B. *H. pylori* infection
C. Gastric hypochlorhydria and achlorhydria
D. Hypercalcemia

Most frequent condition that leads to an elevated fasting gastrin level is gastric hypochlorhydria / achlorhydria, with or without pernicious anemia.

606. PPI should be stopped for a minimum of how many days before estimation of fasting gastrin level?
Harrison's 20th Ed. Chapter 317 Page 2239

A. 3
B. 7
C. 10
D. 14

PPI should be stopped for a minimum of 7 days before fasting gastrin level testing.

607. Elevated fasting gastrin level are due to all except?
Harrison's 20th Ed. Chapter 317 Page 2239

A. Hypochlorhydria
B. Renal insufficiency
C. Diabetes mellitus
D. Hypertension

608. Elevated fasting gastrin level are due to all except?
Harrison's 20th Ed. Chapter 317 Page 2239

A. Rheumatoid arthritis
B. Ankylosing arthritis
C. Pheochromocytoma
D. Vitiligo

Elevated fasting gastrin level are due to gastric hypochlorhydria or achlorhydria, renal insufficiency, massive small-bowel obstruction, rheumatoid arthritis, vitiligo, diabetes mellitus & pheochromocytoma.

609. Patients with gastrinoma have a BAO level more than?
Harrison's 20th Ed. Chapter 317 Page 2239

A. 4 meq/hour
B. 8 meq/hour
C. 12 meq/hour
D. 15 meq/hour

Normal BAO in nongastric surgery patients is typically <5 meq/hour.

610. What value of BAO / MAO is highly suggestive of ZES?
Harrison's 20th Ed. Chapter 317 Page 2239

A. < 0.3
B. < 0.6
C. > 0.3
D. > 0.6

BAO/MAO ratio using pentagastrin infusion of >0.6 is highly suggestive of ZES.

611. What level of basal gastric pH excludes gastrinoma?
Harrison's 20th Ed. Chapter 317 Page 2239

A. ≥ 1
B. ≥ 1.5
C. ≥ 2
D. ≥ 3

A basal gastric pH ≥ 3 virtually excludes a gastrinoma.

612. Which of the following is the most sensitive & specific gastrin provocative test?

Harrison's 20th Ed. Chapter 317 Page 2239

A. Secretin stimulation test
B. Calcium infusion study
C. Standard meal test
D. None of the above

Most sensitive & specific gastrin provocative test for diagnosis of gastrinoma is secretin study. Increase in gastrin of ≥120 pg within 15 minutes of secretin injection has a sensitivity & specificity of >90% for ZES. Calcium infusion study is less sensitive & specific with greater potential for adverse effects.

613. Which of the following tests has maximum sensitivity in detecting primary gastrinoma?

Harrison's 20th Ed. Chapter 317 Page 2240 Table 317-10

A. Selective arterial secretin injection (SASI)
B. Octreoscan imaging with ^{111}In-pentreotide
C. Endoscopic ultrasonography (EUS)
D. Magnetic resonance imaging

Sensitivity of EUS in Zollinger-Ellison Syndrome is 80 – 100%.

614. In surgery-naive ZES patients, PPI dosing should be adjusted to achieve a BAO of?

Harrison's 20th Ed. Chapter 317 Page 2240

A. <1 meq/hour
B. <3 meq/hour
C. <7 meq/hour
D. <10 meq/hour

615. Which of the following is a favorable prognostic indicator in ZES?

Harrison's 20th Ed. Chapter 317 Page 2240

A. Primary duodenal wall tumor
B. Isolated lymph node tumor
C. Undetectable tumor upon surgical exploration
D. All of the above

In ZES, favorable prognostic indicators include primary duodenal wall tumors, isolated lymph node tumor, and undetectable tumor upon surgical exploration. Poor outcome indicators are shorter disease duration; higher gastrin levels (>10,000 pg/mL); large pancreatic primary tumors (>3 cm); metastatic disease to lymph nodes, liver, and bone and Cushing's syndrome. Rapid growth of hepatic metastases is also predictive of poor outcome.

616. Procedure that provides the lowest rates of peptic ulcer recurrence but has highest complication rate is?

Harrison's 20th Ed. Chapter 317 Page 2236

A. Vagotomy
B. Billroth I
C. Vagotomy in combination with antrectomy
D. Billroth II

617. Cushing's ulcer refers to?

Harrison's 20th Ed. Chapter 317 Page 2241

A. Stress ulceration after head trauma
B. Stress ulceration after severe burns
C. Stress ulceration after mechanical ventilation
D. Stress ulceration after sepsis

Elevated gastric acid secretion may be noted in patients with stress ulceration after head trauma (Cushing's ulcer).

618. Curling's ulcer refers to?

Harrison's 20th Ed. Chapter 317 Page 2241

A. Stress ulceration after head trauma
B. Stress ulceration after severe burns
C. Stress ulceration after mechanical ventilation
D. Stress ulceration after sepsis

Elevated gastric acid secretion may be noted in patients with stress ulceration after severe burns (Curling's ulcer).

619. To avoid stress ulceration, gastric pH should be maintained at?

Harrison's 20th Ed. Chapter 317 Page 2241

A. > 1.5
B. > 2.0
C. > 2.5
D. > 3.5

Maintenance of gastric pH >3.5 with continuous infusion of H_2 blockers or liquid antacids administered every 2–3 hours are viable options to avoid stress ulceration.

620. Treatment of choice for stress ulcer prophylaxis is?

Harrison's 20th Ed. Chapter 317 Page 2241

A. H_2 blocker
B. PPI
C. Sucralfate
D. All of the above

PPIs are the treatment of choice for stress ulcer prophylaxis.

621. 'Phlegmonous gastritis' refers to?

Harrison's 20th Ed. Chapter 317 Page 2241

A. Viral infection of stomach
B. Bacterial infection of stomach
C. Vascular congestion of stomach
D. All of the above

Bacterial infection of the stomach or phlegmonous gastritis although rare is a potentially life-threatening disorder characterized by marked & diffuse acute inflammatory infiltrates of entire gastric wall, at times accompanied by necrosis.

622. Which of the following are affected by phlegmonous gastritis?

Harrison's 20th Ed. Chapter 317 Page 2241

A. Elderly individuals
B. Alcoholics
C. AIDS patients
D. All of the above

Elderly individuals, alcoholics, and AIDS patients may be affected by Phlegmonous gastritis.

623. Organism associated with phlegmonous gastritis is?

Harrison's 20th Ed. Chapter 317 Page 2241

A. Staphylococci
B. Escherichia coli
C. Haemophilus
D. All of the above

Organisms associated with Phlegmonous gastritis include streptococci, staphylococci, Escherichia coli, Proteus, and Haemophilus species.

624. Bouveret's Syndrome best relates to?

N Engl J Med. 2018:378,1335

A. Pneumoperitoneum
B. Retroperitoneal fibrosis
C. Situs inversus
D. Gallstone ileus

625. Rigler's triad includes all except?

N Engl J Med. 2018:378,1335

A. Pneumobilia
B. Small-bowel obstruction
C. Large-bowel obstruction
D. Ectopic gallstone

Bouveret's syndrome is a form of gallstone ileus that is characterized by gastric outlet obstruction caused by impaction of a gallstone in pylorus or proximal duodenum after its passage through a cholecystoduodenal fistula. Patients with gallstone ileus may present with radiographic findings of Rigler's triad i.e., pneumobilia, small-bowel obstruction, and ectopic gallstone.

626. The final stage of chronic gastritis is?

Harrison's 20th Ed. Chapter 317 Page 2241

A. Superficial gastritis
B. Atrophic gastritis
C. Gastric atrophy
D. Intestinal metaplasia

Early phase of chronic gastritis is superficial gastritis in which inflammatory changes are limited to lamina propria and intact gastric glands. Next stage is atrophic gastritis in which inflammatory infiltrate extends deeper into mucosa, with destruction of gastric glands. Final stage of chronic gastritis is gastric atrophy in which glandular structures are lost, and there is a paucity of inflammatory infiltrates. Endoscopically, mucosa is thin and underlying blood vessels can be visualized. Intestinal metaplasia refers to the conversion of gastric glands to small-bowel mucosal glands containing goblet cells. Intestinal metaplasia is an important predisposing factor for gastric cancer.

627. Antral-predominant form of chronic gastritis is called?

Harrison's 20th Ed. Chapter 317 Page 2241

A. Type A gastritis
B. Type B gastritis
C. Type AB gastritis
D. Type O gastritis

Chronic gastritis is also classified according to the predominant site of involvement. Type A refers to fundus and body predominant form , with antral sparing (autoimmune) and type B is the antral-predominant form (H. pylori–related). AB gastritis refers to a mixed antral/body picture.

628. Which of the following types of chronic gastritis is associated with pernicious anemia?

Harrison's 20th Ed. Chapter 317 Page 2241

A. Type A gastritis
B. Type B gastritis
C. Type AB gastritis
D. Type O gastritis

Type A gastritis, also called autoimmune gastritis is associated with pernicious anemia with circulating antibodies against parietal cells and IF.

629. Parietal cell antibodies are directed against which of the following?

Harrison's 20th Ed. Chapter 317 Page 2242

A. Gastrin receptors
B. Acetylcholine receptors
C. Histamine receptors
D. H^+,K^+-ATPase

Antibodies to parietal cells are detected in >90% of patients with pernicious anemia and in up to 50% of patients with type A gastritis. The parietal cell antibody is directed against H^+,K^+-ATPase.

630. Varioliform gastritis best relates to?

Harrison's 20th Ed. Chapter 317 Page 2242

A. Lymphocytic gastritis
B. Eosinophilic gastritis
C. Granulomatous gastritis
D. Sarcoidosis

A subgroup of patients with lymphocytic gastritis have thickened folds noted on endoscopy. These folds are often capped by small nodules that contain a central depression or erosion; this form of the disease is called varioliform gastritis.

631. Which of the following is false about Ménétrier's disease?

Harrison's 20th Ed. Chapter 317 Page 2243

A. Protein-losing gastropathy
B. Large gastric mucosal folds in body and fundus
C. Hyperplasia of surface & glandular mucous cells
D. None of the above

Ménétrier's disease is not considered a form of gastritis. It is characterized by large, tortuous gastric mucosal folds.

632. Large gastric folds can be seen in?

Harrison's 20th Ed. Chapter 317 Page 2243

A. ZES
B. Gastric malignancy
C. Sarcoidosis
D. All of the above

Large gastric folds are due to ZES, malignancy (lymphoma, infiltrating carcinoma), infectious etiologies (CMV, histoplasmosis, syphilis, tuberculosis), gastritis polyposa profunda & infiltrative disorders like sarcoidosis.

633. Which of the following is most useful in the treatment of Ménétrier's disease?

Harrison's 20th Ed. Chapter 317 Page 2243

A. Octreotide
B. Prednisone
C. Cetuximab
D. PPIs

Medical therapy with EGF inhibitory antibody cetuximab, anticholinergic agents, prostaglandins, octreotide, PPIs, prednisone, and H_2 receptor antagonists yields varying results. Anticholinergics decrease protein loss.

Disorders of Absorption

634. In malabsorption syndrome, intestinal absorption is increased in?

Harrison's 20th Ed. Chapter 318 Page 2244

A. Cirrhosis
B. Jejunal diverticulosis
C. Hemochromatosis
D. Crohn's disease

635. In malabsorption syndrome, intestinal absorption is increased in?

Harrison's 20th Ed. Chapter 318 Page 2244

A. Cirrhosis
B. Jejunal diverticulosis
C. Wilson's disease
D. Crohn's disease

Only clinical malabsorption situations in which absorption is increased are hemochromatosis & Wilson's disease, where absorption of iron and copper is increased respectively.

636. Steatorrhea is defined as an increase in stool fat excretion of how much of dietary fat intake?

Harrison's 20th Ed. Chapter 318 Page 2244

A. > 2%
B. > 4%
C. > 5%
D. > 7%

Most malabsorption syndrome disorders are associated with an increase in stool fat excretion of >7% of dietary fat intake (steatorrhea).

637. Malabsorption disorder that is not associated with steatorrhea is?

Harrison's 20th Ed. Chapter 318 Page 2244

A. Primary lactase deficiency
B. Celiac sprue
C. Abetalipoproteinemia
D. Intestinal lymphangiectasia

638. Malabsorption disorder that is not associated with steatorrhea is?

Harrison's 20th Ed. Chapter 318 Page 2244

A. Tropical sprue
B. Celiac sprue
C. Pernicious anemia
D. Bacterial overgrowth syndrome

Most, but not all, malabsorption syndromes are associated with steatorrhea. Primary lactase deficiency and pernicious anemia are not associated with steatorrhea.

639. In a western-type diet, diarrhea as a sign is a quantitative increase in stool water or weight of?

Harrison's 20th Ed. Chapter 318 Page 2244

A. > 100 – 200 gram/day
B. > 200 – 225 gram/day
C. > 300 – 425 gram/day
D. > 400 – 500 gram/day

Diarrhea as a sign quantitative increase in stool weight of >200–225 mL or gram per day, when a western-type diet is consumed.

640. Which of the following diarrhea would undoubtedly cease during a prolonged fast?

Harrison's 20th Ed. Chapter 318 Page 2244

A. Enterotoxin-induced traveler's diarrhea
B. Primary lactase deficiency
C. VIPoma
D. All of the above

Diarrhea secondary to lactose malabsorption in primary lactase deficiency ceases during a prolonged fast.

641. Stool osmolality is?

Harrison's 20th Ed. Chapter 318 Page 2244

A. 250 mosmol/kg H_2O
B. 275 mosmol/kg H_2O
C. 300 mosmol/kg H_2O
D. 325 mosmol/kg H_2O

Stool osmotic gap = 2 x (stool Na + stool K). Stool osmolality is assumed to be 300 mosmol/kg H_2O.

642. Fecal osmotic gap is calculated as?

Gastroenterology. 1999;116:1461-1463

A. 90 - 2([Na^+] + [K^+])
B. 190 - 2([Na^+] + [K^+])
C. 290 - 2([Na^+] + [K^+])
D. 390 - 2([Na^+] + [K^+])

Osmotic diarrheas are characterized by osmotic gaps >125 mOsm/kg (nonelectrolytes account for most of the osmolality of stool water), whereas secretory diarrheas typically have osmotic gaps <50 mOsm/kg (electrolytes account for most of stool osmolality).

643. The lengths of the small intestine and colon are?

Harrison's 20th Ed. Chapter 318 Page 2244

A. ~200 cm and ~50 cm, respectively
B. ~250 cm and ~70 cm, respectively
C. ~300 cm and ~80 cm, respectively
D. ~400 cm and ~100 cm, respectively

Lengths of small intestine and colon are ~300 cm and ~80 cm respectively.

644. Effective functional surface area of intestines is about how many times greater than that of a hollow tube?

Harrison's 20th Ed. Chapter 318 Page 2244

A. 200 times
B. 400 times
C. 600 times
D. 800 times

Effective functional surface area is about 600-fold greater than that of a hollow tube due to the presence of folds, villi (in small intestine), and microvilli.

645. Intestinal mucosa synthesizes & secretes which of the following immunoglobulin?

Harrison's 20th Ed. Chapter 318 Page 2244

A. Secretory IgA
B. Secretory IgG
C. Secretory IgM
D. Secretory IgE

Intestinal mucosa synthesizes and secretes secretory IgA.

646. Daily salivary, gastric, pancreatic, biliary, and intestinal fluid amounts to?

Harrison's 20th Ed. Chapter 318 Page 2244

A. 3 to 4 L/day
B. 5 to 6 L/day
C. 6 to 7 L/day
D. 7 to 8 L/day

The intestine absorbs ~7 to 8 liters of fluid daily, comprising dietary fluid intake (1 to 2 L/day) and salivary, gastric, pancreatic, biliary, and intestinal fluid (6 to 7 L/day).

647. The intestine produces which of the following?

Harrison's 20th Ed. Chapter 318 Page 2245

A. IgA
B. Apolipoproteins
C. 5-hydroxytryptophan
D. All of the above

648. Which of the following statements is false?

Harrison's 20th Ed. Chapter 318 Page 2245

A. Villi are present in small intestine & colon
B. Nutrient digestion & absorption occurs in small intestine but not in colon
C. Digestive hydrolytic enzymes are present in brush border of villus epithelial cells
D. Secretory function is present in crypts of both small & large intestine

Villi are present in small intestine but are absent in colon.

649. Na^+, K^+ - ATPase in the Na^+ pump is located on?

Harrison's 20th Ed. Chapter 318 Page 2245

A. Apical membrane
B. Basolateral membrane
C. Basomedial membrane
D. All of the above

Na^+ pump is located on the basolateral membrane, which expels Na^+ and maintains a low intracellular Na^+ through Na^+,K^+ - ATPase.

650. Transport protein SGLT is located on?

Harrison's 20th Ed. Chapter 318 Page 2245

A. Apical membrane
B. Basolateral membrane
C. Basomedial membrane
D. All of the above

Active glucose (monosaccharide) absorption & glucose-stimulated Na^+ absorption require both apical membrane transport protein SGLT (sodium/glucose cotransporter) & basolateral Na^+,K^+ - ATPase. A competitive inhibitor of SGLT, phlorizin exerts a hypoglycemic effect in diabetics. Gene for SGLT is SLC5A.

651. Which of the following about bile acids is false?

Harrison's 20th Ed. Chapter 318 Page 2245

A. Primary bile acids are synthesized in liver from cholesterol
B. Secondary bile acids are synthesized from primary in intestine
C. Cholic & deoxycholic acids are primary bile acids
D. Lithocholic acid is a secondary bile acid

Bile acids are not present in the diet but are synthesized in liver. Primary bile acids are synthesized in liver from cholesterol and secondary bile acids are synthesized from primary bile acids in intestine by colonic bacterial enzymes. Primary bile acids are cholic acid & chenodeoxycholic acid. Secondary bile acids are deoxycholic acid and lithocholic acid.

652. What quantity of bile acids are synthesized in liver every day?

Harrison's 20th Ed. Chapter 318 Page 2245

A. 200 mg
B. 300 mg
C. 400 mg
D. 500 mg

About 500 mg bile acids are synthesized in liver daily, conjugated to either taurine or glycine to form tauro-conjugated or glyco-conjugated bile acids, respectively, and then secreted into duodenum as bile.

653. Primary functions of bile acids is?

Harrison's 20th Ed. Chapter 318 Page 2245

A. To promote bile flow
B. To solubilize cholesterol & phospholipid in gallbladder
C. To enhance dietary lipid digestion & absorption
D. All of the above

Primary functions of bile acids are to promote bile flow, to solubilize cholesterol and phospholipid in gallbladder and to enhance dietary lipid digestion and absorption by forming mixed micelles in proximal small intestine.

654. Bile acids are primarily absorbed "actively" in?

Harrison's 20th Ed. Chapter 318 Page 2245

A. Duodenum
B. Jejunum
C. Ileum
D. Colon

Bile acids are primarily absorbed by an active, Na^+-dependent process exclusively in ileum. To a lesser extent, they are absorbed by non-carrier-mediated transport processes in the jejunum, ileum and colon.

655. The bile acid pool size is approximately?

Harrison's 20th Ed. Chapter 318 Page 2245

A. 4 grams
B. 8 grams
C. 12 grams
D. 16 grams

656. How many times bile acid pool is circulated via enterohepatic circulation?

Harrison's 20th Ed. Chapter 318 Page 2245

A. 2 to 4 times / day
B. 4 to 6 times / day
C. 6 to 8 times / day
D. 8 to 12 times / day

Bile acid pool size is ~4 grams and is circulated via the enterohepatic circulation about twice during each meal, or six to eight times daily.

657. Daily bile acids excretion in stool (fecal loss) equals?

Harrison's 20th Ed. Chapter 318 Page 2245

A. Half of total fat intake
B. Half of enterohepatic circulation
C. Hepatic bile acid synthesis
D. None of the above

A relatively small quantity of bile acids (~500 mg) is not absorbed and is excreted in stool daily; this fecal loss is matched by hepatic bile acid synthesis.

658. Secondary bile acids are formed in?

Harrison's 20th Ed. Chapter 318 Page 2245

A. Duodenum
B. Jejunum
C. Ileum
D. Colon

Colonic bacterial enzymes dehydroxylate bile acids to secondary bile acids.

659. Bile acid synthesis is autoregulated by?

Harrison's 20th Ed. Chapter 318 Page 2245

A. 7 α-hydroxylase
B. 7 β-hydroxylase
C. 7 δ-hydroxylase
D. 7 γ-hydroxylase

Bile acid synthesis is autoregulated by 7 alpha-hydroxylase, an initial enzyme in cholesterol degradation.

660. Steatorrhea can be caused by abnormalities in?

Harrison's 20th Ed. Chapter 318 Page 2245

A. Bile-acid synthesis & excretion
B. Physical state of bile-acids in the intestinal lumen
C. Bile-acid reabsorption
D. All of the above

661. Small ileal dysfunction leads to?

Harrison's 20th Ed. Chapter 318 Page 2246

A. Bile acid diarrhea
B. Fatty acid diarrhea
C. Chloride diarrhea
D. Protein diarrhea

Due to limited ileal disease or resection increased amount of bile acids are delivered into colon that stimulate active Cl^- secretion producing diarrhea but not steatorrhea because hepatic synthesis of bile acids increases to compensate for the rate of fecal bile acid losses up to a limit. It is called bile acid diarrhea, or cholorrheic enteropathy. It responds promptly to cholestyramine until ileal size is severely reduced.

662. Large ileal dysfunction leads to?

Harrison's 20th Ed. Chapter 318 Page 2246

A. Bile acid diarrhea
B. Fatty acid diarrhea
C. Carbohydrate diarrhea
D. Protein diarrhea

Patients with greater degrees of ileal disease and/or resection have diarrhea & steatorrhea that do not respond to cholestyramine. Increased quantities of bile acids enter colon. Hepatic synthesis proves insufficient resulting in impaired micelle formation and steatorrhea. This is called fatty acid diarrhea. Low-fat diet can be effective.

663. Reabsorption defect in enterohepatic circulation of bile acids is due to?

Harrison's 20th Ed. Chapter 318 Page 2246

A. Cirrhosis
B. Primary biliary cirrhosis
C. Jejunal diverticulosis
D. Crohn's disease

Ileal dysfunction caused by Crohn's disease results in a decrease in bile acid reabsorption in ileum and an increase in the delivery of bile acids to large intestine leading to diarrhea with or without steatorrhea.

664. Which of the following is not a feature of bile acid diarrhea?

Harrison's 20th Ed. Chapter 318 Page 2246 Table 318-2

A. Normal bile acid pool size
B. None or mild steatorrhea
C. Responds to cholestyramine
D. Responds to low-fat diet

Features of bile acid diarrhea are—extent of ileal disease is limited, Ileal bile acid absorption is reduced, fecal bile acid excretion is increased, fecal bile acid loss is compensated by hepatic synthesis, bile acid pool size is normal, steatorrhea is absent or mild, response obtained with cholestyramine & no response to low-fat diet.

665. Which of the following is not a feature of fatty acid diarrhea?

Harrison's 20th Ed. Chapter 318 Page 2246 Table 318-2

A. Reduced bile acid pool size
B. Steatorrhea
C. Responds to cholestyramine
D. Responds to low-fat diet

Features of fatty acid diarrhea are extensive ileal disease, ileal bile acid absorption reduced, fecal bile acid excretion increased, fecal bile acid loss is not compensated by hepatic synthesis, bile acid pool size is reduced, steatorrhea (>20 grams) that does not respond to cholestyramine but responds to a low-fat diet.

666. Which of the following is a negative regulator of bile acid synthesis?

Harrison's 20th Ed. Chapter 318 Page 2246

A. FGF17
B. FGF18
C. FGF19
D. FGF20

FGF19 is a negative regulator of bile acid synthesis. Bile acids in intestine release fibroblast growth factor 19 (FGF19) into circulation, which is transported to liver where it suppresses synthesis of bile acids from cholesterol by inhibiting the rate-limiting enzyme cytochrome P450 7A1 (CYP7A1) and also promotes gallbladder relaxation.

667. Which of the following type of fatty acids compose fats?

Harrison's 20th Ed. Chapter 318 Page 2246

A. Long-chain fatty acids (LCFAs)
B. Medium-chain fatty acids (MCFAs)
C. Short-chain fatty acids (SCFAs)
D. All of the above

Three types of fatty acids compose fats: long-chain fatty acids (LCFAs), medium-chain fatty acids (MCFAs), and short-chain fatty acids (SCFAs).

668. Dietary fat is in the form of?

Harrison's 20th Ed. Chapter 318 Page 2246

A. Long-chain triglycerides (LCTs)
B. Medium-chain fatty acids (MCFAs)
C. Short-chain fatty acids (SCFAs)
D. All of the above

Dietary fat is exclusively composed of long-chain triglycerides (LCTs), i.e., glycerol that is bound via ester-linkages to three LCFAs.

669. Majority of dietary long chain fatty acids (LCFAs) have carbon chain lengths of?

Harrison's 20th Ed. Chapter 318 Page 2246 Table 318-3

A. 6 - 8
B. 8 - 10
C. 10 - 12
D. > 12

3 types of fatty acids compose fats—long chain fatty acids (LCFAs), medium-chain fatty acids (MCFAs) & short-chain fatty acids (SCFAs). Majority of dietary LCFAs have carbon chain lengths of 16 or 18.

670. Dietary MCFAs have carbon chain lengths of?

Harrison's 20th Ed. Chapter 318 Page 2246 Table 318-3

A. 6 - 8
B. 8 - 12
C. 12 - 16
D. 16 - 20

Medium-chain triglycerides (MCTs) or medium-chain fatty acids, composed of fatty acids with carbon chain lengths of 8 to 10, are present in large amounts in coconut oil.

671. Which of the following fatty acids requires pancreatic lipolysis?

Harrison's 20th Ed. Chapter 318 Page 2246 Table 318-3

A. Long-chain fatty acids (LCFAs)
B. Medium-chain fatty acids (MCFAs)
C. Short-chain fatty acids (SCFAs)
D. All of the above

672. Which of the following fatty acids requires micelle formation?

Harrison's 20th Ed. Chapter 318 Page 2246 Table 318-3

A. Long-chain fatty acids (LCFAs)
B. Medium-chain fatty acids (MCFAs)
C. Short-chain fatty acids (SCFAs)
D. All of the above

673. Which of the following fatty acids is not present in diet?

Harrison's 20th Ed. Chapter 318 Page 2246 Table 318-3

A. Long-chain fatty acids (LCFAs)
B. Medium-chain fatty acids (MCFAs)
C. Short-chain fatty acids (SCFAs)
D. All of the above

674. Colon is the primary site of absorption of which of the following fatty acids?

Harrison's 20th Ed. Chapter 318 Page 2246 Table 318-3

A. Long-chain fatty acids (LCFAs)
B. Medium-chain fatty acids (MCFAs)
C. Short-chain fatty acids (SCFAs)
D. All of the above

675. Substantial amounts of which of the fatty acids is present in stool?

Harrison's 20th Ed. Chapter 318 Page 2246 Table 318-3

A. Long-chain fatty acids (LCFAs)
B. Medium-chain fatty acids (MCFAs)
C. Short-chain fatty acids (SCFAs)
D. All of the above

676. Steatorrhea results due to defect in which phase of dietary lipid assimilation?

Harrison's 20th Ed. Chapter 318 Page 2246

A. Intraluminal or digestive phase
B. Mucosal or absorptive phase
C. Delivery or postabsorptive phase
D. Any of the above

Assimilation of dietary lipid occurs in intraluminal or digestive phase, mucosal or absorptive phase and delivery or postabsorptive phase. An abnormality at any site of this process can cause steatorrhea.

677. "Micellar formation" belongs to which phase of dietary lipid assimilation?

Harrison's 20th Ed. Chapter 318 Page 2246

A. Intraluminal or digestive phase
B. Mucosal or absorptive phase
C. Delivery or postabsorptive phase
D. Any of the above

The digestive phase has two components, lipolysis and micellar formation.

678. Which of the following statements is false?

Harrison's 20th Ed. Chapter 318 Page 2247

A. Dietary lipid is in the form of long-chain triglycerides (LCTs)
B. Intestinal mucosa does not absorb triglycerides
C. All fatty acids of carbon chain length >12 are metabolized in the same manner
D. None of the above

679. Lipolysis is initiated in?

Harrison's 20th Ed. Chapter 318 Page 2247

A. Stomach
B. Duodenum
C. Jejunum
D. Iliem

680. In lipolysis, hydrolysis of triglycerides by lipase leads to the formation of?

Harrison's 20th Ed. Chapter 318 Page 2247

A. Free fatty acids
B. Monoglycerides
C. Glycerol
D. All of the above

Lipolysis i.e. hydrolysis of Tg to free fatty acids, β-monoglycerides & glycerol by lipase is "initiated" in stomach by gastric lipase. ~20 – 30% of total lipolysis occurs in stomach.

681. Pancreatic lipolysis is greatly enhanced by?

Harrison's 20th Ed. Chapter 318 Page 2247

A. Gastric lipase
B. Pancreatic lipase
C. Colipase
D. All of the above

Pancreatic lipolysis is greatly enhanced by the presence of pancreatic enzyme, colipase, which facilitates the movement of lipase to triglyceride.

682. Normal lipolysis can be maintained by what percentage of maximal pancreatic lipase secretion?

Harrison's 20th Ed. Chapter 318 Page 2247

A. 5%
B. 15%
C. 25%
D. 35%

Normal lipolysis can be maintained by ~5% of maximal pancreatic lipase secretion.

683. Pancreatic lipase is inactivated at?

Harrison's 20th Ed. Chapter 318 Page 2247

A. pH < 7
B. pH < 7.5
C. pH < 8
D. pH < 8.5

Lipolysis is completed in the duodenum and jejunum by pancreatic lipase, which is inactivated by pH <7.0 leading to altered lipolysis.

684. Mixed micelles are molecular aggregates composed of all except?

Harrison's 20th Ed. Chapter 318 Page 2247

A. Fatty acids
B. Triglycerides
C. Cholesterol
D. Conjugated bile acids

Mixed micelles are molecular aggregates composed of fatty acids, monoglycerides, phospholipids, cholesterol, and conjugated bile acids. Mixed micelles are formed when concentration of conjugated bile acids is greater than its CMC.

685. Which of the following relates best with absorptive phase of lipid digestion-absorption?

Harrison's 20th Ed. Chapter 318 Page 2247

A. Micellar formation
B. Uptake and reesterification
C. Formation of chylomicrons
D. Colonic bacterial enzymes

Uptake and reesterification constitute the absorptive phase of lipid digestion-absorption.

686. In which form lipids exit from intestinal epithelial cell?

Harrison's 20th Ed. Chapter 318 Page 2247

A. Free fatty acids
B. Reesterified triglyceride
C. Cholesterol
D. Monoglyceride

Fatty acids and monoglycerides are reesterified by a series of enzymatic steps in the endoplasmic reticulum to form triglycerides, the form in which lipid exits from the intestinal epithelial cell. Reesterified triglycerides require formation of chylomicrons for their exit from small-intestinal epithelial cell & their delivery to liver via lymphatics.

687. Chylomicrons are composed of?

Harrison's 20th Ed. Chapter 318 Page 2247

A. α-lipoprotein
B. β-lipoprotein
C. δ-lipoprotein
D. γ-lipoprotein

688. Chylomicrons contain?

Harrison's 20th Ed. Chapter 318 Page 2247

A. Triglyceride
B. Cholesterol and Cholesterol ester
C. Phospholipid
D. All of the above

689. Reesterified triglyceride exit from intestinal epithelial cell into?

Harrison's 20th Ed. Chapter 318 Page 2247

A. Lymphatics
B. Portal vein
C. Systemic vein
D. All of the above

Chylomicrons are composed of beta-lipoprotein and contain triglycerides, cholesterol, cholesterol esters, and phospholipids and enter the lymphatics, not the portal vein.

690. In abetalipoproteinemia, the defect is in?

Harrison's 20th Ed. Chapter 318 Page 2247

A. Lipolysis
B. Micelle formation
C. Lipid uptake
D. Reesterified triglyceride exit from epithelial cell

691. Which of the following is normal in patients with abetalipoproteinemia?

Harrison's 20th Ed. Chapter 318 Page 2247

A. Lipolysis
B. Micelle formation
C. Lipid uptake
D. All of the above

Abetalipoproteinemia, or acanthocytosis is a disorder of impaired synthesis of beta-lipoprotein. In abetalipoproteinemia, lipolysis, micelle formation & lipid uptake are all normal, but reesterified triglyceride cannot exit from intestinal epithelial cell because of the failure to produce chylomicrons.

692. Coconut oil contains mainly?

Harrison's 20th Ed. Chapter 318 Page 2247

A. Long-chain triglycerides (LCTs)
B. Medium-chain triglycerides (MCT)
C. Short-chain fatty acids (SCFA)
D. All of the above

Medium-chain triglycerides (MCTs), composed of fatty acids with carbon chain lengths of 8 to 10, are present in large amounts in coconut oil and are used as a nutritional supplement.

693. Which of the following statements about Medium-chain triglycerides (MCTs) is false?

Harrison's 20th Ed. Chapter 318 Page 2248

A. Do not require pancreatic lipolysis
B. Micelle formation is not necessary for absorption
C. Following absorption, not reesterified
D. Route of exit is via lymphatics

Unlike LCTs, MCTs do not require pancreatic lipolysis as Tg can be absorbed intact by intestinal epithelial cell & micelle formation is not necessary for absorption of MCTs, following absorption are not reesterified, do not require chylomicron formation for their exit from intestinal epithelial cells, & their route of exit is via portal vein & not via lymphatics.

694. The SCFA present in stool is?
Harrison's 20th Ed. Chapter 318 Page 2248

A. Acetate
B. Propionate
C. Butyrate
D. All of the above

The SCFAs present in stool are primarily acetate, propionate, and butyrate, whose carbon chain lengths are 2, 3, and 4, respectively.

695. The primary nutrient for colonic epithelial cells is?
Harrison's 20th Ed. Chapter 318 Page 2248

A. Acetate
B. Propionate
C. Butyrate
D. All of the above

Butyrate is the primary nutrient for colonic epithelial cells & its deficiency may be associated with colitis.

696. Which of the following statements about SCFAs is false?
Harrison's 20th Ed. Chapter 318 Page 2248

A. SCFAs are dietary lipids
B. Synthesized by colonic bacterial enzymes from nonabsorbed carbohydrate
C. SCFAs in stool are acetate, propionate, & butyrate
D. SCFAs are rapidly absorbed & stimulate colonic Na-Cl & fluid absorption

SCFAs are not dietary lipids but are synthesized by colonic bacterial enzymes from nonabsorbed carbohydrate. SCFAs present in stool are primarily acetate, propionate, and butyrate. SCFAs are rapidly absorbed and stimulate colonic Na-Cl and fluid absorption.

697. C. difficile accounts for what percentage of all antibiotic-associated diarrhea?
Harrison's 20th Ed. Chapter 318 Page 2248

A. ~ 10 - 15%
B. ~ 25 - 40%
C. ~ 40 - 75%
D. ~ 75 - 95%

C. difficile accounts for ~10 - 15% of all antibiotic-associated diarrhea.

698. Carbohydrates in the diet are present in the form of?
Harrison's 20th Ed. Chapter 318 Page 2248

A. Starch
B. Disaccharides (sucrose & lactose)
C. Glucose
D. All of the above

Carbohydrates in the diet are present in the form of starch, disaccharides (sucrose and lactose), and glucose.

699. Which of the following statements about carbohydrates is false?
Harrison's 20th Ed. Chapter 318 Page 2248

A. Absorbed only in the small intestine
B. Absorbed only in the form of monosaccharides
C. Absorption occurs by a Na-dependent process
D. None of the above

700. Brush border transport protein that mediates monosaccharide absorption is?
Harrison's 20th Ed. Chapter 318 Page 2248

A. AGLT1
B. MGLT1
C. SGLT1
D. TGLT1

Carbohydrates are absorbed only in the small intestine and only in the form of monosaccharides whose absorption occurs by a Na-dependent process mediated by the brush border transport protein SGLT1.

701. Which of the following about lactose malabsorption is false?
Harrison's 20th Ed. Chapter 318 Page 2248

A. Glucose and galactose are constituents of lactose
B. Primary lactase deficiency patients have severe symptoms
C. Secondary lactase deficiency is seen in celiac sprue
D. Symptoms may be similar to IBS

Most individuals with primary lactase deficiency do not have symptoms.

702. Congenital absence of SGLT leads to?
Harrison's 20th Ed. Chapter 318 Page 2248

A. Glucose, galactose malabsorption
B. Lactose malabsorption
C. Maltose malabsorption
D. Sucrose malabsorption

Congenital absence of SGLT leads to glucose-galactose or monosaccharide malabsorption diarrhea.

703. Which of the following carbohydrate is absorbed by brush border transport protein - GLUT 5?
Harrison's 20th Ed. Chapter 318 Page 2248

A. Glucose
B. Galactose
C. Fructose
D. Sorbitol

Fructose is absorbed by the brush border transport protein GLUT 5, a facilitated diffusion process that is not Na-dependent and is distinct from SGLT.

704. Actively transported monosaccharides are all except?
Harrison's 20th Ed. Chapter 318 Page 2248

A. Glucose
B. Galactose
C. Fructose
D. All of the above

Actively transported monosaccharides are glucose and galactose.

705. Sugar used in diabetic candy is?
Harrison's 20th Ed. Chapter 318 Page 2248

A. Sorbitol
B. Galactose
C. Fructose
D. None of the above

Sugar used in diabetic candy is sorbitol which is only minimally absorbed due to absence of an intestinal absorptive transport mechanism for sorbitol.

706. What value of stool pH is consistent with carbohydrate malabsorption?

Gastroenterology 1999;116:1461-1463

A. < 5.6
B. < 6.6
C. < 7.6
D. < 8.6

Stool pH <5.6 is consistent with carbohydrate malabsorption.

707. Protein is present in food almost exclusively as?

Harrison's 20th Ed. Chapter 318 Page 2248

A. Polypeptides
B. Dipeptides
C. Tripeptides
D. Amino acids

Protein is present in food almost exclusively as polypeptides and requires extensive hydrolysis to di- and tripeptides and amino acids before absorption.

708. Brush border enzyme that converts the proenzyme trypsinogen to trypsin is?

Harrison's 20th Ed. Chapter 318 Page 2249

A. Enterokinase
B. Colipase
C. Pepsinogen
D. Amylase

Proenzyme trypsinogen is activated to trypsin by the intestinal brush border enzyme enterokinase, and subsequently by trypsin.

709. Alterations in protein or amino acid digestion and absorption is seen in which of the following?

Harrison's 20th Ed. Chapter 318 Page 2249

A. Enterokinase deficiency
B. Hartnup syndrome
C. Cystinuria
D. All of the above

Enterokinase deficiency leads to failure to convert proenzyme trypsinogen to trypsin and is manifested as diarrhea, growth retardation and hypoproteinemia. Hartnup syndrome, a defect in neutral amino acid transport, is characterized by a pellagra-like rash and neuropsychiatric symptoms. Cystinuria, a defect in dibasic amino acid transport, is associated with renal calculi and chronic pancreatitis.

710. The proximal small intestine is the site for the absorption of all of the following except?

Harrison's 20th Ed. Chapter 318 Page 2249

A. Calcium
B. Iron
C. Folic acid
D. Bile acids

Calcium, iron and folic acid are exclusively absorbed by active transport processes in proximal small intestine especially the duodenum.

711. Ileum is the absorption site of all of the following except?

Harrison's 20th Ed. Chapter 318 Page 2249

A. Cobalamin
B. Bile acids
C. Calcium
D. None of the above

Active transport mechanisms for cobalamin & bile acids are present only in ileum.

712. Glucose, amino acids and lipids are absorbed in?

Harrison's 20th Ed. Chapter 318 Page 2249

A. Duodenum
B. Jejunum
C. Ileum
D. Throughout the small intestine

Glucose, amino acids & lipids are absorbed throughout the small intestine, although their rate of absorption is greater in the proximal than in the distal segments.

713. Which of the following is critical for survival of individuals with massive resection of small intestine and/or colon?

Harrison's 20th Ed. Chapter 318 Page 2249

A. Adaptation
B. Acclimation
C. Adaption
D. Accommodation

After segmental resection of small intestine/colon, remaining segments undergo morphologic & functional "adaptation" to enhance absorption.

714. Estimation of which of the following in stool helps distinguish pancreatic from nonpancreatic etiologies of steatorrhea?

Harrison's 20th Ed. Chapter 318 Page 2249

A. Stool trypsin
B. Stool chymotrypsin
C. Stool lipase
D. All of the above

Assays for stool chymotrypsin & elastase can distinguish pancreatic from nonpancreatic etiologies of steatorrhea. Indirect tests like assay of fecal elastase or chymotrypsin activity or a bentiromide test have fallen out of favor because of low sensitivity & specificity.

715. Which of the following is false about urinary D-xylose test?

Harrison's 20th Ed. Chapter 318 Page 2249

A. Assesses proximal small-intestinal mucosal function
B. D-Xylose is a pentose carbohydrate
C. 25 g of D-xylose & collecting urine for 5 hours
D. < 12 g excretion means an abnormal test

D-Xylose is a pentose absorbed almost exclusively in proximal small intestine. Urinary D-xylose test (<4.5 gram excretion) reflects presence of duodenal / jejunal mucosal disease.

716. Samples of which of the following are collected in the D-xylose test?

Harrison's 20th Ed. Chapter 318 Page 2249

A. Urine
B. Stool
C. Blood
D. All of the above

D-xylose test is performed by administering 25 grams of D-xylose and collecting urine for 5 hours.

717. Urinary D-xylose test can be false-positive in?

Harrison's 20th Ed. Chapter 318 Page 2249

A. Head injury
B. Myocardial infarction
C. Ascitis
D. Pneumonia

Urinary D-xylose test is false-positive in large fluid collections in third space (ascites, pleural fluid).

718. D-Xylose Test is normal in which of the following?
Harrison's 20th Ed. Chapter 318 Page 2252 Table 318-7

A. Chronic pancreatitis
B. Ileal disease
C. Intestinal lymphangiectasia
D. All of the above

719. Which of the following is suspected when macrophages in lamina propria contain material positive on PAS staining?
Harrison's 20th Ed. Chapter 318 Page 2251 Table 318-6

A. Amyloidosis
B. Celiac disease
C. Whipple's disease
D. Crohn's disease

720. Short villi, decreased mitosis in crypts and megalocytosis is a feature of all except?
Harrison's 20th Ed. Chapter 318 Page 2251 Table 318-6

A. Folate deficiency
B. Vitamin B12 deficiency
C. Radiation enteritis
D. Drug-induced enteritis

721. Noncaseating granulomas in small-intestinal mucosal biopsies is a feature of?
Harrison's 20th Ed. Chapter 318 Page 2251 Table 318-6

A. Tropical sprue
B. Crohn's disease
C. Intestinal lymphangiectasia
D. Amyloidosis

722. Normal villi with epithelial cells vacuolated with fat postprandially in small-intestinal mucosal biopsies is a feature of?
Harrison's 20th Ed. Chapter 318 Page 2251 Table 318-6

A. Whipple's disease
B. Agammaglobulinemia
C. Abetalipoproteinemia
D. Protein-calorie malnutrition

723. Clubbed villi in small-intestinal mucosal biopsies is a feature of?
Harrison's 20th Ed. Chapter 318 Page 2251 Table 318-6

A. Tropical sprue
B. Crohn's disease
C. Intestinal lymphangiectasia
D. Amyloidosis

724. Schilling test is performed to determine the cause for?
Harrison's 20th Ed. Chapter 327 Page 2323 Table 327-2

A. Cobalamin malabsorption
B. Folic acid malabsorption
C. Iron malabsorption
D. All of the above

Schilling test is performed to determine the cause for cobalamin malabsorption.

725. Cobalamin is present primarily in?
Harrison's 20th Ed. Chapter 95 Page 699

A. Fruits
B. Green vegetables
C. Meat
D. Egg

Cobalamin is present primarily in meat.

726. Cyanide toxicity is a possibility with which of the following forms of vitamin B12?
N Engl J Med. 2013;368:2041

A. Cyanocobalamin
B. Hydroxocobalamin
C. Methylcobalamin
D. All of the above

A 1000-μg dose of cyanocobalamin contains 20 μg (0.78 μmol) of cyanide. Oral vitamin B12 at a daily dose of 2000 μg (20 μg absorbed on average) is equivalent to weekly injections of cyanocobalamin at a dose of 1000 μg (150 μg retained).

727. Haptocorrin was previously named as?
BMC Res Notes. 2011; 4: 208

A. Transcobalamin I
B. Transcobalamin III
C. R-binder
D. All of the above

Haptocorrin (previously named transcobalamin I and III, and R-binder) is a glycoprotein, which is present in human milk in relatively large amounts. It is characterized by its ability to bind vitamin B12 and other corrinoids, and exists in two forms in human milk - apo-haptocorrin, which is unsaturated with vitamin B12, and holo-haptocorrin, which is saturated with vitamin B12.

728. Intrinsic factor is synthesized and released by?
Harrison's 20th Ed. Chapter 317 Page 2222

A. Gastric parietal cells
B. Gastric oxyntic cells
C. Gastric chief cells
D. Gastric G cells

Intrinsic factor (IF) is absolutely required for the absorption of cobalamin. IF is a glycoprotein synthesized & released by gastric parietal cells, to promote its uptake by specific cobalamin receptors on the brush border of ileal enterocytes. Pancreatic protease enzymes split the cobalamin–R binder complex to release cobalamin in proximal small intestine, where cobalamin is then bound by intrinsic factor (IF).

729. Cobalamin absorption may be abnormal in which of the following?
Harrison's 20th Ed. Chapter 95 Page 707

A. Pernicious anemia
B. Chronic pancreatitis
C. Bacterial overgrowth syndromes
D. All of the above

Cobalamin absorption may be abnormal in pernicious anemia, chronic pancreatitis, achlorhydria, bacterial overgrowth syndromes, and Ileal dysfunction.

730. Which isotope is used in Schilling test?
Harrison's 20th Ed. Chapter 95 Page 703

A. ^{58}Co-labeled cobalamin
B. ^{68}Co-labeled cobalamin
C. ^{78}Co-labeled cobalamin
D. ^{88}Co-labeled cobalamin

Schilling test is performed by administering ^{58}Co-labeled cobalamin orally and collecting urine for 24 hours. It is dependent on normal renal and bladder function. Radioactive B_{12} is no longer available, and Schilling tests are no longer performed.

731. Synonym of Celiac sprue is?

Harrison's 20th Ed. Chapter 318 Page 2251

A. Nontropical sprue
B. Celiac disease
C. Gluten sensitive enteropathy
D. All of the above

Celiac sprue has also been known as nontropical sprue, celiac disease (in children), adult celiac disease, and gluten sensitive enteropathy.

732. Which of the following about Celiac disease is false?

N Engl J Med. 2012;367:2419-26

A. Systemic disorder
B. Immune-mediated disorder
C. Triggered by dietary gluten
D. None of the above

Celiac disease is a systemic immune-mediated disorder triggered by dietary gluten in genetically susceptible persons.

733. The word "sprue" comes from which language?

N Engl J Med. 2007;357:1731-43

A. Dutch
B. Latin
C. Greek
D. English

734. Which of the following respond to elimination of gluten from the diet in celiac sprue?

Harrison's 20th Ed. Chapter 318 Page 2251

A. Symptoms
B. Evidence of malabsorption
C. Histopathologic changes in small-intestinal biopsy
D. All of the above

In celiac sprue, symptoms, evidence of malabsorption and histopathologic changes on small-intestinal biopsy respond to elimination of gluten from diet.

735. Gliadin (a component of gluten) is present in all except?

Harrison's 20th Ed. Chapter 318 Page 2252

A. Wheat
B. Barley
C. Rice
D. Rye

Gluten is a protein complex. Gliadin is a component of gluten present in wheat, barley, rye & in smaller amounts in oats. Antiendomysial antibody tTG deaminates gliadin.

736. Which of the following is considered as "safe grains" (gluten-free)?

N Engl J Med. 2007;357:1731-43

A. Rice
B. Corn
C. Millet
D. All of the above

Safe grains (gluten-free) include rice, amaranth, buckwheat, corn, millet, quinoa, sorghum, teff (an Ethiopian cereal grain), & oats.

737. Gliadin is which component of gluten?

N Engl J Med. 2007;357:1731-43

A. Heat resistant fraction
B. Alcohol-soluble fraction
C. Water soluble fraction
D. Contaminated fraction

"Gluten" refers to the entire protein component of wheat. Gliadin is the alcohol-soluble fraction of gluten that contains bulk of toxic components.

738. Which of the following enzyme in intestine deamidates gliadin peptides?

N Engl J Med. 2007;357:1731-43

A. Tissue transaminase
B. Tissue transmurase
C. Tissue transglutaminase
D. Tissue transpeptidase

Enzyme tissue transglutaminase in intestine deamidates gliadin peptides increasing their immunogenicity.

739. The most sensitive antibody tests for the diagnosis of celiac disease are of which class?

N Engl J Med. 2007;357:1731-43

A. IgA
B. IgG
C. IgM
D. IgE

Most sensitive antibody tests for diagnosis of celiac disease are of IgA class.

740. Serum antibodies found in celiac sprue include all except?

Harrison's 20th Ed. Chapter 318 Page 2252

A. IgA antigliadin
B. IgA antiendomysial antibodies
C. IgA anti-tissue transglutaminase
D. IgA anti-tissue transpeptidase

"Celiac serologies" in celiac sprue include serum antibodies like IgA antigliadin, IgA antiendomysial and IgA anti-tTG antibodies are present suggesting an immunologic component to etiology.

741. Antiendomysial antibodies are directed against?

N Engl J Med. 2007;357:1731-43

A. Epithelial tissue
B. Enzyme
C. Connective-tissue
D. All of the above

Serological tests in celiac disease include antigliadin antibodies, connective-tissue antibodies (antireticulin & antiendomysial antibodies), & antibodies against tissue transglutaminase, enzyme responsible for deamidation of gliadin in lamina propria.

742. Antigen recognized by the antiendomysial antibody test is?

Harrison's 20th Ed. Chapter 318 Page 2252

A. Tissue transaminase
B. Tissue transmurase
C. Tissue transglutaminase
D. Tissue transpeptidase

In celiac sprue, antigen recognized by antiendomysial antibody test is tissue transglutaminase (tTG).

743. Negative predictive value of which of the following HLA allele is almost 100% in celiac sprue?

N Engl J Med. 2007;357:1731-43

A. HLA-DQ2
B. HLA-DQ3
C. HLA-DQ4
D. HLA-DQ5

In patients with doubtful celiac sprue, HLA-DQ2 or HLA-DQ8 typing is useful, since negative predictive value of this test is almost 100%. Almost all patients with celiac sprue express HLA-DQ2 allele. Absence of DQ2 excludes the diagnosis of celiac sprue. All patients with celiac disease express the HLA-DQ2 or HLA-DQ8 allele.

744. The *HLA-DQ2* haplotype (*DQA1*0501/DQB1*0201*) is expressed in what proportion of the general population?

N Engl J Med. 2012;367:2419-26

A. One third
B. One half
C. Three fourth
D. None

*The HLA-DQ2 haplotype (DQA1*0501/DQB1*0201) is expressed in the majority of patients with celiac disease (90%), whereas it is expressed in one third of the general population. In another 5% of patients with celiac disease, the HLA-DQ8 haplotype (DQA1*0301/DQB1*0302) is expressed, whereas almost all the remaining 5% of patients have at least one of the two genes encoding DQ2 (DQB1*0201 or DQA1*0501). DQ2 & DQ8 haplotypes are necessary but not sufficient for the development of celiac disease. At least 39 non-HLA genes that predispose to celiac disease have been identified, mostly involved in inflammatory and immune responses.*

745. Which of the following tests have a high negative predictive value in the diagnosis of celiac disease?

N Engl J Med. 2012;367:2419-26

A. IgA anti-tTG antibodies
B. IgG anti-tTG antibodies
C. IgA antiendomysial antibodies
D. HLA-DQ2 or HLA-DQ8

Testing for HLA-DQ2 and HLA-DQ8 may be useful in at-risk persons (e.g., family members of patients with celiac disease). Such testing has a high negative predictive value, which means that the disease is very unlikely to develop in persons who are negative for both HLA-DQ2 and HLA-DQ8. Absence of HLA DQ2/DQ8 excludes the diagnosis of celiac disease.

746. Which of the following tests have usefulness in patients with IgA deficiency?

N Engl J Med. 2012;367:2419-26

A. IgA anti-tTG antibodies
B. IgG anti-tTG antibodies
C. IgA antiendomysial antibodies
D. HLA-DQ2 or HLA-DQ8

747. Which of the following tests have usefulness in patients with an uncertain diagnosis?

N Engl J Med. 2012;367:2419-26

A. IgA anti-tTG antibodies
B. IgG anti-tTG antibodies
C. IgA antiendomysial antibodies
D. HLA-DQ2 or HLA-DQ8

748. Absence of DQ2/DQ8 which of the following excludes the diagnosis of celiac disease?

Harrison's 20th Ed. Chapter 318 Page 2253

A. DQ1 / DQ8
B. DQ2 / DQ8
C. DQ3 / DQ8
D. DQ4 / DQ8

All patients with celiac disease express HLA-DQ2 or HLA-DQ8 allele. Absence of DQ2/DQ8 excludes the diagnosis of celiac disease.

749. Which of the following is false about duodenal/jejunal biopsy histopathology in celiac sprue?

Harrison's 20th Ed. Chapter 318 Page 2253

A. Reduced height of villi
B. Crypt hyperplasia
C. Increased lymphocytes & plasma cells in lamina propria
D. None of the above

A small-intestinal biopsy is required to establish a diagnosis of celiac disease. In celiac sprue, changes seen on duodenal/jejunal biopsy are restricted to mucosa and include absence or reduced height of villi (flat appearance), crypt hyperplasia and villus atrophy and increased lymphocytes and plasma cells in the lamina propria.

750. Histopathologic features characteristic of celiac sprue can also be seen in all except?

Harrison's 20th Ed. Chapter 318 Page 2253

A. Tropical sprue
B. Ulcerative colitis
C. Milk-protein intolerance in children
D. Eosinophilic enteritis

751. Histopathologic features characteristic of celiac sprue can also be seen in all except?

Harrison's 20th Ed. Chapter 318 Page 2253

A. Lymphoma
B. Intestinal lymphangiectasis
C. Crohn's disease
D. Gastrinoma with acid hypersecretion

Histopathologic features of celiac sprue is seen in tropical sprue, eosinophilic enteritis & milk-protein intolerance in children, lymphoma, bacterial overgrowth, Crohn's disease & gastrinoma with acid hypersecretion.

752. Which of the following about "Celiac crisis" is false?

N Engl J Med. 2012;367:2419-26

A. Mostly observed in adults
B. Severe diarrhea
C. Hypoproteinemia
D. Metabolic and electrolyte imbalances

Celiac crisis is a rare life-threatening syndrome, mostly observed in children, characterized by severe diarrhea, hypoproteinemia, and metabolic and electrolyte imbalances.

753. After how many months of a strict gluten free diet, celiac disease is termed refractory?

N Engl J Med. 2012;367:2419-26

A. 3 months
B. 6 months
C. 9 months
D. 12 months

Refractory celiac disease is diagnosed when there are persistent or recurrent malabsorptive symptoms and signs with villous atrophy detected on biopsy despite maintenance of a strict gluten free diet for more than 12 months.

754. Which of the following is true for refractory celiac disease type 2?

N Engl J Med. 2012;367:2419-26

A. Abnormal intraepithelial lymphocytes
B. Clonal intraepithelial lymphocytes without CD3
C. Clonal intraepithelial lymphocytes without CD8
D. All of the above

Refractory celiac disease can be classified as type 1 (normal intraepithelial lymphocytes) or type 2 (abnormal intraepithelial lymphocytes; clonal intraepithelial lymphocytes lacking surface markers CD3, CD8, and T-cell receptors; or both). Type 2 is associated with a higher risk of ulcerative jejunoileitis and lymphoma than type 1.

755. In celiac disease, the lowest amount of daily gluten that causes damage to celiac intestinal mucosa over time (gluten threshold) is?

N Engl J Med. 2012;367:2419-26

A. 1 to 5 mg per day
B. 10 to 50 mg per day
C. 100 to 500 mg per day
D. 1000 to 2500 mg per day

In celiac disease, the lowest amount of daily gluten that causes damage to celiac intestinal mucosa over time (gluten threshold) is 10 to 50 mg per day (a 25 gram slice of bread contains ~1.6 grams of gluten). New Codex Alimentarius regulation permits a maximum gluten contamination of 20 ppm in gluten-free products.

756. Interval between exposure to gluten and onset of symptoms in Celiac disease is?

N Engl J Med. 2012;367:2419-26

A. Minutes to hours
B. Hours to days
C. Weeks to years
D. Any of the above

757. Interval between exposure to gluten and onset of symptoms in wheat allergy is?

N Engl J Med. 2012;367:2419-26

A. Minutes to hours
B. Hours to days
C. Weeks to years
D. Any of the above

758. Interval between exposure to gluten and onset of symptoms in gluten sensitivity is?

N Engl J Med. 2012;367:2419-26

A. Minutes to hours
B. Hours to days
C. Weeks to years
D. Any of the above

759. Mechanism of diarrhea in celiac disease is?

Harrison's 20th Ed. Chapter 318 Page 2253

A. Steatorrhea
B. Secondary lactase deficiency
C. Bile acid malabsorption
D. All of the above

The diarrhea in celiac disease may be secondary to steatorrhea (due to changes in jejunal mucosal function), secondary lactase deficiency (due to changes in jejunal brush border enzymatic function), bile acid malabsorption (due to bile acid–induced fluid secretion in the colon) and endogenous fluid secretion resulting from crypt hyperplasia.

760. The diarrhea in celiac sprue is due to all except?

Harrison's 20th Ed. Chapter 318 Page 2253

A. Steatorrhea
B. Lipase deficiency
C. Bile acid malabsorption
D. Endogenous fluid secretion

Diarrhea in celiac sprue may be secondary to steatorrhea, secondary lactase deficiency, bile acid malabsorption and endogenous fluid secretion.

761. Celiac disease patients may improve temporarily with restriction of?

Harrison's 20th Ed. Chapter 318 Page 2253

A. Soy
B. Dietary lactose
C. Fat
D. All of the above

762. Celiac sprue may be associated with following diseases except?

Harrison's 20th Ed. Chapter 318 Page 2253, N Engl J Med. 2002;346:181

A. Dermatitis herpetiformis (DH)
B. Type 1 diabetes mellitus
C. IgA deficiency
D. Chronic pancreatitis

Celiac disease is associated with dermatitis herpetiformis (DH), diabetes mellitus type 1, IgA deficiency, Down syndrome, Turner's syndrome, Autoimmune thyroid disease, Sjögren's syndrome, Microscopic colitis, Rheumatoid arthritis.

763. Patients with DH have characteristic papulovesicular lesions that respond to?

Harrison's 20th Ed. Chapter 318 Page 2253

A. Azathioprine
B. Dapsone
C. Thalidomide
D. All of the above

764. Prevalence of celiac disease is increased in which of the following conditions?

N Engl J Med. 2012;367:2419-26

A. Hashimoto's thyroiditis
B. Turner's syndrome
C. IgA deficiency
D. All of the above

Prevalence of celiac disease is 1.5 to 2 times as high among women as among men and is increased among persons who have an affected first-degree relative (10 to 15%), type 1 diabetes (3 to 16%), Hashimoto's thyroiditis (5%) or other autoimmune diseases (including autoimmune liver diseases, Sjögren's syndrome, and IgA nephropathy), Down's syndrome (5%), Turner's syndrome (3%), and IgA deficiency (9%).

765. Complications of Celiac sprue include all except?

Harrison's 20th Ed. Chapter 318 Page 2253

A. Malignancy
B. Intestinal ulceration
C. Collagenous sprue
D. Fistulas

Complications of celiac sprue include gastrointestinal and nongastrointestinal neoplasms, intestinal ulceration and collagenous sprue.

766. Complications associated with untreated celiac disease include?

Harrison's 20th Ed. Chapter 318 Page 2253, N Engl J Med. 2012;367:2419-26

A. Infertility or recurrent abortion
B. Impaired splenic function
C. Neurologic disorders
D. All of the above

Complications associated with untreated celiac disease include osteoporosis, impaired splenic function, neurologic disorders, infertility or recurrent abortion, ulcerative jejunoileitis, and cancer. Enteropathy-associated T-cell lymphoma and adenocarcinoma of the jejunum are rare complications of celiac disease.

767. Endocrine and metabolic disorders that can cause malabsorption syndrome include?

Harrison's 20th Ed. Chapter 318 Page 2257, Table 318-8

A. Hypoparathyroidism
B. Hyperthyroidism
C. Carcinoid syndrome
D. All of the above

Endocrine & metabolic disorders that can cause malabsorption syndrome include diabetes, hypoparathyroidism, adrenal insufficiency, hyperthyroidism & carcinoid syndrome.

768. Circulatory disorders that can cause malabsorption syndrome include?

Harrison's 20th Ed. Chapter 318 Page 2257, Table 318-8

A. Congestive heart failure
B. Constrictive pericarditis
C. Mesenteric artery atherosclerosis
D. All of the above

769. Dermatitis in malabsorption syndrome is due to deficiency of?

Harrison's 20th Ed. Chapter 318 Page 2257, Table 318-9

A. Vitamin A
B. Zinc
C. Essential fatty acid
D. All of the above

770. Glossitis, cheilosis, stomatitis in malabsorption syndrome is due to deficiency of?

Harrison's 20th Ed. Chapter 318 Page 2257, Table 318-9

A. Iron
B. Vitamin B12, folate
C. Vitamin A
D. All of the above

771. Tropical sprue is manifested by all except?

Harrison's 20th Ed. Chapter 318 Page 2253

A. Acute diarrhea
B. Steatorrhea
C. Weight loss
D. Nutritional deficiencies

Tropical sprue is manifested by chronic diarrhea, steatorrhea, weight loss, and nutritional deficiencies.

772. Chronic diarrhea in a tropical environment is most often caused by all except?

Harrison's 20th Ed. Chapter 318 Page 2253

A. Yersinia enterocolitica
B. Cryptosporidium parvum
C. Giardia lamblia
D. Entamoeba histolytica

Chronic diarrhea in a tropical environment is most often caused by G. lamblia, Yersinia enterocolitica, C. difficile, Cryptosporidium parvum and Cyclospora cayetanensis.

773. Which of the following is similar to Tropical sprue?

Harrison's 20th Ed. Chapter 318 Page 2254

A. Sprue-like enteropathy
B. Environmental enteropathy
C. Protein-wasting enteropathy
D. Autoimmune enteropathy

Environmental enteropathy ("impoverished gut"; blunted small-intestinal villi with lamina propria inflammation) is observed in tropical developing areas with endemic enteric infections like amebiasis.

774. Patients of Tropical sprue are rarely found in?

Harrison's 20th Ed. Chapter 318 Page 2254

A. South India
B. Philippines
C. Caribbean islands
D. Africa

Tropical sprue is found in South India, Philippines and Caribbean islands, but is rarely observed in Africa, Jamaica, or Southeast Asia.

775. Which of the following in tropical sprue differentiate it from celiac disease?

Harrison's 20th Ed. Chapter 318 Page 2254

A. More mononuclear cell infiltrate in the lamina propria
B. Less villous architectural alteration
C. Similar degree of severity throughout small intestine
D. All of the above

Further, gluten-free diet does not result in either clinical or histologic improvement in tropical sprue.

776. Treatment of tropical sprue includes?

Harrison's 20th Ed. Chapter 318 Page 2254

A. Vitamin B12
B. Folic acid
C. Iron
D. Calcium

777. Treatment of tropical sprue includes?

Harrison's 20th Ed. Chapter 318 Page 2254

A. Gluten-free diet
B. Broad-spectrum antibiotics
C. Glucocorticoids
D. All of the above

Broad-spectrum antibiotics and folic acid are curative in tropical sprue.

778. In tropical sprue, tetracycline should be used for up to?

Harrison's 20th Ed. Chapter 318 Page 2254

A. 4 weeks
B. 12 weeks
C. 24 weeks
D. 48 weeks

In tropical sprue, tetracycline should be used for up to 6 months.

779. Diseases that may arise following small-intestinal resection include all except?

Harrison's 20th Ed. Chapter 318 Page 2254

A. Colonic diverticulosis
B. Cholesterol gallstones
C. Gastric hypersecretion of acid
D. Hyperoxaluria

Following large resections of small intestine, enteric hyperoxaluria, cholesterol gallstones and gastric hypersecretion of acid occurs.

780. "Intestinal failure" best relates to?

Harrison's 20th Ed. Chapter 318 Page 2255

A. Inability to maintain nutrition with parenteral support
B. Inability to maintain nutrition without parenteral support
C. Inability to maintain nutrition by all means
D. All of the above

Intestinal failure refers to an inability to maintain nutrition without parenteral support.

781. Enteric hyperoxaluria is best treated with?

Harrison's 20th Ed. Chapter 318 Page 2255

A. Allopurinol
B. Aspirin
C. Codeine
D. Cholestyramine

Cholestyramine, an anion-binding resin & calcium are useful in reducing hyperoxaluria.

782. Which of the following hormones has a role in the treatment of short bowel syndrome?

Harrison's 20th Ed. Chapter 318 Page 2255

A. Glucagon-like peptide 2 (GLP-2)
B. VIP
C. Cholecystokinin
D. TSH

A recombinant analogue of glucagon - like peptide 2 (teduglutide) is approved for short bowel syndrome.

783. Which of the following is not a presentation of bacterial overgrowth syndrome?

Harrison's 20th Ed. Chapter 318 Page 2255

A. Diarrhea
B. Steatorrhea
C. Macrocytic anemia
D. Microcytic anemia

Bacterial overgrowth syndromes comprise a group of disorders with diarrhea, steatorrhea & macrocytic anemia. The common feature is proliferation of colonic-type bacteria within small intestine like E. coli or Bacteroides.

784. Stagnant bowel or blind loop syndrome refers to?

Harrison's 20th Ed. Chapter 318 Page 2255

A. Stasis due to impaired peristalsis
B. Changes in intestinal anatomy
C. Direct communication between small & large intestine
D. All of the above

Bacterial proliferation in bacterial overgrowth syndrome or stagnant bowel syndrome or blind loop syndrome is due to stasis caused by impaired peristalsis (functional stasis), changes in intestinal anatomy (anatomic stasis) or direct communication between small and large intestine.

785. In bacterial overgrowth syndromes, macrocytic anemia is due to deficiency of?

Harrison's 20th Ed. Chapter 318 Page 2255

A. Cobalamin
B. Folate
C. Cobalamin + Folate
D. Any of the above

In bacterial overgrowth syndromes, macrocytic anemia is due to cobalamin, not folate deficiency.

786. Diagnosis of the bacterial overgrowth syndrome is done by all except?

Harrison's 20th Ed. Chapter 318 Page 2255

A. Low serum cobalamin level
B. Low serum folate level
C. Increased aerobic &/or anaerobic colonic-type bacteria in jejunal aspirate
D. Schilling test

Diagnosis of the bacterial overgrowth syndrome is done by a low serum cobalamin level, elevated serum folate level, increased levels of aerobic and/or anaerobic colonic-type bacteria in a jejunal aspirate, Schilling test. Following tetracycline for 5 days, Schilling test will become normal.

787. For frequent recurrences of bacterial overgrowth syndrome, which of the following treatment strategies is most effective?

Harrison's 20th Ed. Chapter 318 Page 2255

A. Antibiotics for 1 week per month
B. Antibiotics for ~3 weeks
C. Antibiotics until symptoms remit
D. Antibiotics continuously

In the presence of frequent recurrences, use of antibiotics for 1 week per month whether or not symptoms are present is most effective.

788. Bacterial overgrowth may occur in?

Harrison's 20th Ed. Chapter 318 Page 2256

A. Scleroderma
B. Crohn's disease
C. Radiation enteritis
D. All of the above

789. Whipple's disease is caused by the bacteria named?

Harrison's 20th Ed. Chapter 318 Page 2256

A. Tropheryma whippeli
B. Treponema whippeli
C. Toxoplasma whippeli
D. Trenoderma whippeli

Whipple's disease is a chronic multisystem disease that presents as diarrhea, steatorrhea, weight loss, arthralgia & CNS and cardiac problems. It is caused by bacteria Tropheryma whipplei.

790. Which of the following statements about Tropheryma whippeli is false?

Harrison's 20th Ed. Chapter 318 Page 2256

A. Gram-positive
B. Actinobacterium
C. Low virulence, low infectivity
D. PAS+ macrophages in small intestine

Hallmark of Whipple's disease is the presence of PAS-positive macrophages in small intestine. T. whipplei is a small gram-positive, actinobacterium bacillus, with low virulence but high infectivity.

791. Which of the following about Whipple's disease is false?
Harrison's 20th Ed. Chapter 318 Page 2256

A. Multisystem disease
B. T. whippelii outside macrophages indicates active disease
C. T. whipplei cannot be grown on culture
D. Drug of first choice is TMP/SMX for 1 year

Presence of T. whipplei bacillus outside of macrophages is a more important indicator of active disease than within macrophages. T. whipplei has been grown in culture. The current drug of choice is double-strength trimethoprim/sulfamethoxazole for ~1 year.

792. Which of the following about Whipple's disease is false?
Harrison's 20th Ed. Chapter 318 Page 2256

A. Drug of second choice is Chloramphenicol
B. Antibiotic therapy has to be prolonged
C. Disease recurrence with dementia is a poor prognostic sign
D. None of the above

If TMP/SMX is not tolerated, chloramphenicol is an appropriate second choice. Recurrence of disease activity, especially with dementia, is an extremely poor prognostic sign.

793. Which of the following is the most common neurologic manifestations of classic Whipple's disease?
N Engl J Med. 2007;356:55-66

A. Cognitive change
B. Supranuclear ophthalmoplegia
C. Oculomasticatory or oculofacioskeletal myorhythmia
D. Ataxia

Cognitive changes and later dementia are commonest neurologic signs. Movement disorders of eye muscles (oculomasticatory or oculofacioskeletal myorhythmia) are considered pathognomonic for Whipple's disease.

794. Which of the following about protein-losing enteropathy is false?
Harrison's 20th Ed. Chapter 318 Page 2256

A. Hypoproteinemia
B. Edema
C. Proteinuria
D. No defects in protein synthesis

Protein-losing enteropathy is not a specific disease but rather a group of gastrointestinal & nongastrointestinal disorders with hypoproteinemia & edema in absence of either proteinuria or defects in protein synthesis.

795. Normally, what percentage of total protein catabolism occurs via gastrointestinal tract?
Harrison's 20th Ed. Chapter 318 Page 2256

A. ~ 5%
B. ~ 10%
C. ~ 15%
D. ~ 20%

Normally, ~10% of total protein catabolism occurs via the gastrointestinal tract.

796. Which of the following about protein-losing enteropathy is false?
Harrison's 20th Ed. Chapter 318 Page 2256

A. Excess protein loss into gastrointestinal tract
B. Low serum albumin & globulin both in absence of renal & hepatic disease
C. α_1-antitrypsin clearance can be useful in diagnosis
D. Lymphocytosis supports diagnosis

Protein-losing enteropathy is characterized by excess protein loss into gastrointestinal tract. With loss of protein, peripheral lymphocytes are also lost via lymphatics, resulting in a relative lymphopenia. Thus, presence of lymphopenia in a patient with hypoproteinemia supports the presence of increased loss of protein into gastrointestinal tract.

797. Which of the following can cause protein-losing enteropathy?
Harrison's 20th Ed. Chapter 318 Page 2256

A. Peripheral vascular disease
B. Chronic pericarditis
C. Hemolytic uremic syndrome
D. Hypothyroidism

798. Hypoproteinemia in intestinal lymphangiectasia should be treated with?
Harrison's 20th Ed. Chapter 318 Page 2256

A. SCFA
B. MCT
C. LCFA
D. All of the above

Treatment of hypoproteinemia in intestinal lymphangiectasia is done by low-fat diet and administration of MCTs, which do not exit from intestinal epithelial cells via lymphatics but are delivered to the body via portal vein.

799. Which of the following disorders is associated with lymphedema?
Harrison's 20th Ed. Chapter 276 Page 1934

A. Meige's disease
B. Milroy's disease
C. Yellow nail syndrome
D. All of the above

800. Mutations in which of the following genes causes Milroy's disease?
Harrison's 20th Ed. Chapter 276 Page 1933

A. LSC1
B. FOXC2
C. VEGFR3
D. CCBE1

Mutations in genes expressing vascular endothelial growth factor receptor 3 (VEGFR3), which is a determinant of lymphangiogenesis, cause Milroy's disease.

801. Adherence to colonic mucin by E. histolytica trophozoites is mediated by?
N Engl J Med. 2003;348:16

A. Gal/GalNAc–specific lectin
B. Gal/GalNAc–specific pepsin
C. Gal/GalNAc–specific trypsin
D. Gal/GalNAc–specific capsin

Inflammatory Bowel Disease

802. Which of the following about IBD is false?
Harrison's 20th Ed. Chapter 319 Page 2258

A. Immune-mediated
B. Chronic intestinal condition
C. Dysregulated tridirectional relationship between commensal (microbiota), intestinal epithelial cells (IEC) and mucosal immune system
D. None of the above

803. Which out of the following countries has the highest incidence of IBD?
Harrison's 20th Ed. Chapter 319 Page 2258

A. Canada
B. Israel
C. Greece
D. China

The highest reported incidence rates are in Canada (19.2 per 100,000 for UC and 20.2 per 1 00,000 for CD. ~0.6% of the Canadian population has IBD.

804. Out of the following, which ethnic group has the highest prevalence of IBD?
Harrison's 20th Ed. Chapter 319 Page 2258 Table 319-1

A. Jewish
B. African American
C. Hispanic
D. Asian

Prevalence of IBD in Ashkenazi Jews is ~twice that of Israeli-born, Sephardic, or Oriental Jews. Prevalence decreases progressively in non-Jewish Caucasian, African-American, Hispanic, and Asian populations.

805. All of the following are predisposing factors for UC except?
Harrison's 20th Ed. Chapter 319 Page 2258

A. Jewish ethnicity
B. High socio-economic status
C. Smoking
D. Hermansky-Pudlak syndrome

806. Which of the following statements about ulcerative colitis (UC) and Crohn's disease (CD) is false?
Harrison's 20th Ed. Chapter 319 Page 2258

A. Peak age of onset of UC & CD is second to fourth decades
B. Second peak occurs in seventh and ninth decades
C. Appendectomy aggravates UC
D. IBD is not gender specific

Appendectomy is protective against UC but increases the risk of CD.

807. Very early onset IBD (VEOIBD) is defined as IBD that occurs in children below the age of?
Harrison's 20th Ed. Chapter 319 Page 2258

A. 4 years
B. 6 years
C. 8 years
D. 10 years

Very early onset IBD (VEOIBD) is defined as IBD that occurs in children below the age of <6 years.

808. Infantile IBD is defined as IBD that occurs in children below the age of?
Harrison's 20th Ed. Chapter 319 Page 2258

A. 3 months
B. 12 months
C. 18 months
D. 24 months

Infantile IBD is defined as IBD that occurs in children below the age of <2 years.

809. Which of the following is false about VEOIBD and infantile IBD?
Harrison's 20th Ed. Chapter 319 Page 2258

A. Mainly affect the colon
B. Resistant to standard medications
C. Patients have a strong family history of IBD
D. None of the above

810. What percentage of patients with VEOIBD and infantile IBD have underlying immunodeficiency?
Harrison's 20th Ed. Chapter 319 Page 2258

A. 10%
B. 15%
C. 25%
D. 40%

Twenty-five percent of patients with VEOIBD and infantile IBD have an underlying immunodeficiency. In some cases, infantile IBD or VEOIBD can be caused by rare, single genetic mutations.

811. Which of the following is not associated with increased risk of UC?
Harrison's 20th Ed. Chapter 319 Page 2258

A. Urban domicile
B. High socio-economic status
C. Former smoker
D. Appendectomy

Urban areas, high socioeconomic classes have a higher prevalence of IBD. Former smokers have a 1.7-fold increased risk for UC than people who have never smoked. Appendectomy is protective against UC.

812. If a patient has IBD, the lifetime risk that a first degree relative will be similarly affected is?
Harrison's 20th Ed. Chapter 319 Page 2258

A. 10%
B. 20%
C. 30%
D. 40%

Lifetime risk of a first-degree relative of IBD patient is ~10%. If two parents have IBD, each child has a 36% chance of being affected. In twin studies, 58% of monozygotic twins are concordant for CD and 6% are concordant for UC, whereas 4% of dizygotic twins are concordant for CD and none are concordant for UC.

813. If two parents have IBD, what chance does each child has of being affected?
Harrison's 20th Ed. Chapter 319 Page 2258

A. 36%
B. 45%
C. 66%
D. 72%

If two parents have IBD, each child has a 36% chance of being affected.

814. Term "supraorganism" in IBD is best related to?
Harrison's 20th Ed. Chapter 319 Page 2259

A. Microbiota
B. IECs
C. Immune cells
D. All of the above

Under normal physiologic conditions, homeostasis exists between commensal microbiota, intestinal epithelial cells and immune cells within tissues. They function together as an integrated "supraorganism". They are affected by specific environmental (smoking, antibiotics, enteropathogens) and genetic factors in a susceptible host, cumulatively & interactively disrupting homeostasis. This leads to a chronic state of dysregulated inflammation, i.e. IBD.

815. Nonmalignant mortality in IBD cases is maximum during?
Harrison's 18th Ed. 2477

A. First year of disease
B. After five years of disease
C. After ten years of disease
D. After fifteen years of disease

Highest mortality is during first year of IBD & in long-duration disease due to risk of colon cancer.

816. Which genetic disorder is a predisposing factor for IBD?
Harrison's 20th Ed. Chapter 319 Page 2260 Table 319-2

A. Turner's syndrome
B. Down syndrome
C. Patau syndrome
D. Edward syndrome

817. IBD is associated with all of the following except?
Harrison's 20th Ed. Chapter 319 Page 2260 Table 319-2

A. Turner's syndrome
B. Down syndrome
C. Hermansky-Pudlak syndrome
D. Wiskott-Aldrich syndrome

UC and CD are associated with Turner's syndrome and Hermansky-Pudlak syndrome, Wiskott-Aldrich syndrome and chronic granulomatous disease. Immunodeficiency disorders like hypogammaglobulinemia, selective IgA deficiency and hereditary angioedema also have increased association with IBD.

818. Disease that are shares genetic risk factors with IBD is?
Harrison's 20th Ed. Chapter 319 Page 2261

A. Rheumatoid arthritis
B. Psoriasis
C. Systemic lupus erythematosus
D. All of the above

Diseases and genetic risk factors that are shared with IBD include rheumatoid arthritis (TNFAIP3), psoriasis (IL23R,IL12B), ankylosing spondylitis (IL23R), type 1 diabetes mellitus (IL10,PTPN2), asthma (ORMDL3), and systemic lupus erythematosus (TNFAIP3, IL10).

819. Which of the following single gene defects can cause IBD?
Harrison's 20th Ed. Chapter 319 Page 2260

A. IL10
B. CTLA4
C. NCF2
D. All of the above

IBD occurs with genetic syndromes and development of severe, refractory IBD in early life in single gene defects that affect the immune system. These include mutations in genes encoding interleukin-10 (IL-10), IL-10 receptor (IL-10R), cytotoxic T-lymphocyte associated protein-4 (CTLA4), neutrophil cytosolic factor 2 protein (NCF2), X linked inhibitor of apoptosis protein (XIAP), lipopolysaccharide responsive and beige-like anchor protein (LRBA), or tetratricopeptide repeat domain 7A protein (TTC7).

820. Which of the following genes is associated with innate immunity and autophagy?
Harrison's 20th Ed. Chapter 319 Page 2260 Table 319-3

A. NOD2
B. ATG16L1
C. IRGM
D. All of the above

Genes that are associated with innate immunity and autophagy are NOD2, ATG16L1, IRGM, JAK2, STAT3 that function in innate immune cells (both parenchymal and hematopoietic) to respond to and clear bacteria, mycobacteria and viruses.

821. Which of the following genes is associated with endoplasmic reticulum (ER) and metabolic stress?
Harrison's 20th Ed. Chapter 319 Page 2261

A. XBP1
B. ORMDL3
C. OCTN
D. All of the above

Genes that are associated with endoplasmic reticulum (ER) and metabolic stress are XBP1, ORMDL3, OCTN, which serve to regulate the secretory activity of cells involved in responses to the commensal microbiota such as Paneth and goblet cells and the manner in which intestinal cells respond to the metabolic products of bacteria.

822. Which of the following genes is associated with regulation of adaptive immunity?
Harrison's 20th Ed. Chapter 319 Page 2260 Table 319-3

A. IL23R
B. IL12B
C. IL10
D. All of the above

Genes that are associated with regulation of adaptive immunity are IL23R, IL12B, IL10, PTPN2, which regulate the balance between inflammatory and regulatory cytokines.

823. Which of the following genes is involved in the development and resolution of inflammation?
Harrison's 20th Ed. Chapter 319 Page 2260 Table 319-3

A. MST1
B. CCR6
C. TNFAIP3
D. All of the above

Genes that are involved in the development and resolution of inflammation are MST1, CCR6, TNFAIP3, PTGER4 and ultimately leukocyte recruitment and inflammatory mediator production.

824. NOD1 gene is now known as?

A. CARD1
B. CARD2
C. CARD3
D. CARD4

825. NOD2 gene is now known as?
Harrison's 20th Ed. Chapter 355 Page 2573

A. CARD1
B. CARD5
C. CARD15
D. CARD18

Gene CARD4 was formerly called NOD1, and CARD15 was formerly called NOD2. CARD15 means caspase-associated recruitment domain containing protein 15, while NOD2 refers to nucleotide oligomerisation domain 2 or NOTCH protein domain.

826. The disease-related gene of IBD1 on chromosome 16 is?
N Engl J Med. 2002;347:417

A. NOD-1
B. NOD-2
C. NOD-3
D. NOD-4

The IBD1 locus encodes NOD2 (nucleotide-binding oligomerization domain also designated CARD 15 or caspase recruitment domain protein 15) found in approximately one-half of patients with CD.

827. Which of the following syndromes is associated with NOD2 mutation?
Harrison's 20th Ed. Chapter 362 Page 2613

A. Muckle-Wells syndrome (MWS)
B. Blau's syndrome
C. Syndrome of pyogenic arthritis with pyoderma gangrenosum and acne (PAPA)
D. Schnitzler's syndrome

Blau's syndrome is caused by mutations in CARD15 (also known as NOD2), which regulates nuclear factor-κB activation. Blau's syndrome is characterized by granulomatous dermatitis, uveitis and arthritis. Distinct CARD15 variants predispose to Crohn's disease.

828. Intracellular NOD1 and NOD2 proteins are best related to?
N Engl J Med. 2002;347:417

A. FoxP3 transcription factor
B. Antitumor necrosis factor
C. Pattern-recognition proteins
D. All of the above

Pattern-recognition proteins that are important for sensing microbes include the intracellular NOD1 and NOD2 proteins which recognize discrete fragments of bacterial peptidoglycan.

829. Which of the following IBD subtype has its loci on chromosome 16?
N Engl J Med. 2002;347:417, Indian J Gastroenterol. 2008;27:8-11

A. IBD 6
B. IBD 7
C. IBD 8
D. IBD 9

IBD loci are on chromosomes 16q12 (IBD1), 12q13 (IBD2), 6p13 (IBD3), 14q11 (IBD4), 5q31-33 (IBD5), 19p13 (IBD6), 1p36 (IBD7), 16p (IBD8), 3p (IBD9). Three alleles of the NOD2/CARD15 gene on chromosome 16 have been found in ~one-half of patients with CD.

830. CARD15 is constitutively expressed in?
N Engl J Med. 2002;347:417

A. Paneth cells
B. Parietal or oxyntic cells
C. G cells
D. D cells

Paneth cells are specialized epithelial cells selectively expressed in ileum, located mainly in crypts in close proximity to epithelial stem cells. Paneth cells secrete antibacterial substances. Main antimicrobial factors secreted by Paneth cell include lysozyme, phospholipase A2, trypsin, alpha-defensins & angiogenins.

831. CARD15 protein is expressed in the cytoplasm of?
N Engl J Med. 2002;347:417

A. Peripheral blood monocytes
B. Paneth cells
C. Dendritic cells
D. All of the above

CARD15 (caspase activation and recruitment domain) is expressed by intestinal epithelial cells (Paneth cells, monocytes, macrophages & dendritic cells).

832. Which of the following is false about CARD15 protein?
N Engl J Med. 2002;347:417

A. CARD15 was formerly called NOD1
B. Intracellular recognition protein for bacterial components
C. Activates nuclear factor kappa B pathway
D. Gain-of-function mutations are associated with CD

CARD15 protein acts as an intracellular recognition protein for bacterial components such as peptidoglycans and activates nuclear factor kappa B pathway which regulates apoptosis and inflammation. Loss-of-function mutations in CARD15 are highly associated with CD.

833. Signaling adaptor protein MyD88 is related to which of the following?
N Engl J Med. 2002;347:417

A. Goblet cells
B. Paneth cells
C. Enteroendocrine cell
D. All of the above

Paneth cells directly sense the presence of a microbiota through expression of the signaling adaptor protein MyD88, which helps transduce signals to host cells upon recognition of microbial products through Toll-like receptors (TLRs). This recognition drives expression of antibacterial products (the lectin RegIIIγ) that act to prevent microbial translocation across the gut mucosal barrier.

834. Which of the following stimulates Paneth cells to produce RegIII-γ?
N Engl J Med. 2002;347:417

A. Porphyromonas asaccharolytica
B. B. fragilis
C. Prevotella bivia
D. B. thetaiotaomicron

B. thetaiotaomicron stimulates Paneth cells to produce RegIII-γ, a bactericidal lectin that can result in killing of gram-positive bacteria.

835. Which of the following is an anti-inflammatory bacterial species?
Harrison's 20th Ed. Chapter 319 Page 2261

A. Faecalibacterium prausnitzii
B. Eggerthella lenta
C. Ruminococcus gnavus
D. All of the above

Faecalibacterium prausnitzii belongs to anti-inflammatory bacterial species. Ruminococcus gnavus belongs to pro-inflammatory bacterial species. Digoxin is inactivated by the human gut bacterium Eggerthella lenta.

836. Which of the following bacterial species prevents growth impairment?

Harrison's 20th Ed. Chapter 459 Page 3385

A. Faecalibacterium prausnitzii
B. Ruminococcus gnavus
C. Clostridium nexile
D. All of the above

Investigators have identified five bacterial species (Faecalibacterium prausnitzii, Ruminococcus gnavus, Clostridium nexile, Clostridium symbiosum, and Dorea formicigenerans) that when administered together as a "cocktail" were able to prevent growth impairments.

837. Lack of immune responsiveness of gut mucosal immune system to dietary antigens is best related to?

Harrison's 20th Ed. Chapter 319 Page 2261

A. Intestinal tolerance
B. Gastric tolerance
C. Oral tolerance
D. All of the above

The gut mucosal immune system is normally unreactive to luminal contents due to oral (mucosal) tolerance. In IBD this suppression of inflammation is altered, leading to uncontrolled inflammation.

838. Which of the following is an anti-inflammatory cytokine?

Harrison's 20th Ed. Chapter 319 Page 2261

A. IL-10
B. IL-35
C. Transforming growth factor β (TGF-β)
D. All of the above

In IBD, suppression of inflammation is altered, leading to uncontrolled inflammation.

839. Which of the following is related to regulation of responses to commensal bacteria?

Harrison's 20th Ed. Chapter 319 Page 2261

A. XBP1
B. Mucus glycoproteins
C. Nuclear factor-κB (NF-κB)
D. All of the above

840. In unstimulated cells, NF-κB is found in?

N Engl J Med. 1997;336:1067

A. Nucleus
B. Cytoplasm
C. Cell membrane
D. All of the above

NF-κB (nuclear factor kappa-light-chain-enhancer of activated B cells) is located in the cytosol complexed with the inhibitory protein IκB.

841. In unstimulated cells, NF-κ B remains bound to?

N Engl J Med. 1997;336:1067

A. G-κ B
B. H-κ B
C. I-κ B
D. J-κ B

In unstimulated cells, the NF-κB dimers are sequestered in cytoplasm by a family of inhibitors, called IκB (Inhibitor of κB). Activation of NF-κB is initiated by signal-induced degradation of IκB which occurs via activation of a kinase called the IκB kinase (IKK). With degradation of IκB inhibitor, NF-κB complex is freed to enter the nucleus where it activates expression of genes that have DNA-binding sites for NF-κB leading to physiological responses like inflammatory or immune response, cell survival response, cellular proliferation and activating expression of its own repressor, IκB. IκB then re-inhibits NF-κB (auto feedback loop).

842. Which of the following can activate NF-κ B?

N Engl J Med. 1997;336:1067

A. Cytokines
B. Activators of protein kinase C
C. Viruses
D. All of the above

NF-κB is a rapidly acting primary transcription factor found in all cell types. It is activated through TLR-4 by cytokines, activators of protein kinase C, bacteria / viruses, stress, UV.

843. CD4⁺ T helper (T_H) cell that promotes inflammation is?

Harrison's 20th Ed. Chapter 319 Page 2261

A. T_H1 cells
B. T_H2 cells
C. T_H17 cells
D. All of the above

CD4⁺ T helper (T_H) cells that promote inflammation are of three major types namely T_H1 cells, T_H2 cells and T_H17 cells.

844. Which of the following is a type of CD4+ T cell?

Harrison's 20th Ed. Chapter 319 Page 2261

A. T_H1 cells
B. T_H2 cells
C. T_H17 cells
D. All of the above

CD4+ T cells are of three major types : T_H1 cells, T_H2 cells and T_H17 cells.

845. T_H2 of CD4 + T cells produce all except?

Harrison's 20th Ed. Chapter 319 Page 2261

A. Interferon-γ (IFN-γ)
B. Interleukin -4 (IL-4)
C. Interleukin -5 (IL-5)
D. Interleukin -13 (IL-13)

CD4+ T cells are composed of Th1 cells, that produce interferon-gamma (IFN-γ), and Th2 cells that produce interleukin-4, IL-5 and IL-13.

846. Interferon (IFN) gamma is secreted by which of the following?

Harrison's 20th Ed. Chapter 319 Page 2261

A. T_H1 cells
B. T_H2 cells
C. T_H17 cells
D. All of the above

T_H1 cells secrete interferon (IFN) gamma, T_H2 cells secrete IL-4, IL-5, IL-13, and T_H17 cells secrete IL-17, IL-21.

847. Which of the following cells induce transmural granulomatous inflammation that resembles CD?

Harrison's 20th Ed. Chapter 319 Page 2261

A. T_H1 cells
B. T_H2 cells
C. T_H17 cells
D. All of the above

T_H1 cells induce transmural granulomatous inflammation that resembles CD.

848. Which of the following cells induce superficial mucosal inflammation resembling UC?

Harrison's 20th Ed. Chapter 319 Page 2261

A. T_H1 cells
B. T_H2 cells
C. T_H17 cells
D. All of the above

T_H2 cells, & related natural killer T cells that secrete IL-13 induce superficial mucosal inflammation resembling UC. T_H17 cells may be responsible for neutrophilic recruitment.

849. The T_H1 cytokine pathway is initiated by?

Harrison's 20th Ed. Chapter 319 Page 2262

A. IL-4
B. IL-6
C. IL-12
D. IL-23

The T_H1 cytokine pathway is initiated by IL-12. IL-4 and IL-23, together with IL-6 and TGF-beta, induce T_H2 and T_H17 cells, respectively.

850. Which of the following is also called "lymphotoxin"?

Harrison's 20th Ed. Chapter 343 Page 2482

A. TNF-α
B. TNF-β
C. IFN-α
D. IFN-γ

Tumor-necrosis factor-beta (TNF-β) is also known as lymphotoxin.

851. Levels of which of the following is elevated in IBD?

N Engl J Med. 2009;361:2066-78

A. Tumor necrosis factor α (TNF-α)
B. Interleukin-1β
C. Interferon-γ
D. All of the above

Levels of tumor necrosis factor α (TNF-α), interleukin-1β, interferon-γ, and cytokines of the interleukin-23–Th17 pathway are elevated in IBD.

852. Which of the following is not a probiotic?

Harrison's 20th Ed. Chapter 317 Page 2234

A. Lactobacillus spp.
B. Bifidobacterium spp.
C. Campylobacter spp.
D. Saccharomyces spp.

Salmonella sp., Shigella sp., Campylobacter sp., Clostridium difficile are pathogens that may initiate IBD by triggering an inflammatory response. While Faecalibacterium prausnitzii, Lactobacillus, Bifidobacterium and Saccharomyces boulardii are probiotics that may inhibit inflammation.

853. What proportion of UC patients have involvement of whole colon?

Harrison's 20th Ed. Chapter 319 Page 2262

A. 10%
B. 20%
C. 30%
D. 40%

~40-50% of UC patients have disease limited to rectum & rectosigmoid, 30-40% have disease extending beyond sigmoid but not involving whole colon. 20% have a total colitis.

854. Backwash ileitis occurs when which part of colon is involved in UC?

Harrison's 20th Ed. Chapter 319 Page 2262

A. Ascending colon
B. Transverse colon
C. Descending colon
D. Whole colon

UC is a mucosal disease that almost always involves rectum and extends proximally to involve colon in continuity without areas of uninvolved mucosa. When "whole colon" is involved, inflammation extends 1-2 cm into terminal ileum in 10–20% of patients. This is called backwash ileitis.

855. Psychosocial factors can contribute to worsening of symptoms in following illnesses except?

Harrison's 20th Ed. Chapter 319 Page 2262

A. Malabsorption syndrome
B. Fibromyalgia
C. Amyotrophic lateral sclerosis
D. Bipolar mood disorder

856. Which of the following statements about pathology of Ulcerative colitis (UC) is false?

Harrison's 20th Ed. Chapter 319 Page 2262

A. Mucosal disease involving rectum and colon
B. Proximal spread occurs in continuity
C. Sandpaper like appearance of mucosa reflects severe inflammation
D. Inflammatory polyps (pseudopolyps) are due to epithelial regeneration

In UC, with "mild inflammation" mucosa is erythematous & has a fine granular surface that looks like sandpaper.

857. Which of the following statements about pathology of Ulcerative colitis (UC) is false?

Harrison's 20th Ed. Chapter 319 Page 2262

A. Limited to mucosa & superficial submucosa
B. Crypt architecture of colon is preserved
C. Basal lymphoplasmacytosis suggests chronicity
D. Cryptitis and crypt atrophy

UC process is limited to mucosa and superficial submucosa, with deeper layers unaffected except in fulminant disease. Histologic features that suggest chronicity are that crypt architecture of colon is distorted and presence of basal plasma cells and multiple basal lymphoid aggregates.

858. Which of the following statements about pathology of Crohn's disease (CD) is false?

Harrison's 20th Ed. Chapter 319 Page 2262

A. Can affect any part of gastrointestinal tract
B. Terminal ileum involved in 90% of patients
C. Rectum is always involved in CD
D. Segmental with skip areas

Unlike UC, which almost always involves the rectum, the rectum is often spared in CD.

859. Which of the following statements about pathology of Crohn's disease (CD) is false?

Harrison's 20th Ed. Chapter 319 Page 2262

A. Perirectal fistulas, abscesses & anal stenosis common
B. Never involves liver & pancreas
C. Transmural process
D. "Cobblestone" appearance on endoscopy

In CD, granulomas are seen in lymph nodes, mesentery, peritoneum, liver & pancreas.

860. Which of the following statements is false?
Harrison's 20th Ed. Chapter 319 Page 2262

A. CD is a transmural process
B. Between lesions, mucosa is histologically normal
C. Thickening of the colon wall
D. None of the above

861. "Cobblestone mucosa" in CD is mainly seen in?
Harrison's 20th Ed. Chapter 319 Page 2262

A. Sigmoid colon
B. Transverse colon
C. Ileum
D. Rectum

Unlike UC, CD is a transmural process. CD is segmental with skip areas in the midst of diseased intestine. In CD, stellate ulcerations fuse longitudinally & transversely to demarcate islands of mucosa that are histologically normal. This "cobblestone" appearance is characteristic of CD, endoscopically and by barium radiography. Oral mucosal lesions in CD include aphthous stomatitis & "cobblestone" lesions of the buccal mucosa.

862. Which of the following statements about pathology of Crohn's disease (CD) is false?
Harrison's 20th Ed. Chapter 319 Page 2263

A. Earliest lesions are aphthoid ulcerations & focal crypt abscesses
B. Caseating granulomas in all bowel wall layers common
C. Granulomas can be seen in liver & pancreas
D. Granulomas can be seen in lymph nodes, mesentery, peritoneum

In CD, earliest lesions are aphthoid ulcerations & focal crypt abscesses with loose aggregations of macrophages, forming "noncaseating" granulomas in all layers of bowel wall.

863. In CD, "creeping fat" is the term given to?
Harrison's 20th Ed. Chapter 319 Page 2263

A. Excessive enlargement of omentum
B. Necrosis of omentum
C. Projections of thickened mesentery encasing bowel
D. Fatty adhesions

Projections of thickened mesentery encase the bowel is termed as "creeping fat".

864. Which of the following is a feature of UC?
Harrison's 20th Ed. Chapter 319 Page 2263

A. Bowel wall thickening
B. Cobblestoning
C. Pseudopolyps
D. Skip areas in the midst of diseased intestine

865. Which of the following is not a major symptom of UC?
Harrison's 20th Ed. Chapter 319 Page 2263

A. Rectal bleeding
B. Constipation
C. Crampy abdominal pain
D. Tenesmus

The major symptoms of UC are diarrhea, rectal bleeding, tenesmus, passage of mucus, and crampy abdominal pain. Other symptoms in moderate to severe disease include anorexia, nausea, vomiting, fever, and weight loss. With proctitis or proctosigmoiditis, proximal transit slows, which may account for the constipation commonly seen in patients with distal disease.

866. Which of the following statements about clinical features of Ulcerative colitis (UC) is false?
Harrison's 20th Ed. Chapter 319 Page 2263

A. Tenesmus is a major symptom
B. Severity of symptoms do not correlate with extent of disease
C. Constipation seen in patients with distal disease
D. Diarrhea is often nocturnal and/or postprandial

Severity of symptoms correlates with the extent of disease.

867. Which of the following is not a manifestion severe UC?
Harrison's 20th Ed. Chapter 319 Page 2263 Table 319-4

A. Bowel movements 4-6/day
B. Mean body temperature >37.5ºC
C. Mean pulse rate > 90 / minute
D. ESR > 30 mm in first hour

In severe UC, bowel movements are >6 per day.

868. In severe ulcerative colitis, number of bowel movements per day is?
Harrison's 20th Ed. Chapter 319 Page 2263 Table 319-4

A. 2 – 3
B. 3 – 4
C. 4 – 5
D. > 6

869. Which of the following about investigative features of Ulcerative colitis (UC) is false?
Harrison's 20th Ed. Chapter 319 Page 2263

A. CRP levels may rise in active disease
B. Orosomucoid levels may rise in active disease
C. Leukocytosis is a specific indicator of disease activity
D. Proctitis or proctosigmoiditis rarely cause rise in CRP

In UC, leukocytosis occurs but is not a specific indicator of disease activity. Proctitis or proctosigmoiditis rarely causes a rise in CRP.

870. Which of the following is a highly sensitive & specific marker for detecting intestinal inflammation?
Harrison's 20th Ed. Chapter 319 Page 2263

A. Fecal lactoferrin
B. Fecal transferrin
C. Fecal hemolysin
D. Fecal reactin

Fecal lactoferrin is a highly sensitive and specific marker of fecal leukocytes and for detecting intestinal inflammation, tested by latex agglutination & enzyme-linked immunosorbent assays.

871. Which of the following about fecal calprotectin is false?
Harrison's 20th Ed. Chapter 319 Page 2263

A. Levels correlate well with histologic inflammation
B. Predict relapses
C. Detects pouchitis
D. None of the above

Fecal calprotectin levels correlate well with histologic inflammation, predict relapses, and detect pouchitis.

872. Which of the following is fecal marker of GI tract inflammation?
Clinical and Experimental Gastroenterology 2016:9 21–29

A. Lactoferrin
B. S100A12
C. M2-PK
D. All of the above

Fecal marker of GI tract inflammation include calprotectin, lactoferrin, S100A12, polymorphonuclear elastase, and M2-PK, which is an isoform of pyruvate kinase expressed by rapidly dividing cells.

873. Which of the following is false about "fecal calprotectin"?
Harrison's 20th Ed. Chapter 319 Page 2263

A. Neutrophilic cytosolic protein
B. Resistant to colonic bacterial degradation
C. Formerly called L1 protein
D. None of the above

874. Which of the following is false about "fecal calprotectin"?
Clinical and Experimental Gastroenterology 2016:9 21–29

A. Calcium binding
B. Has antimicrobial properties
C. Predict relapses in IBD
D. None of the above

Fecal Calprotectin is a neutrophilic cytosolic protein, first isolated from granulocytes by Fagerhol and named L1 protein. It was renamed calprotectin upon identification of its calcium binding, antimicrobial properties and resistance to colonic bacterial degradation. Calprotectin, although present in blood, enters bowel lumen as part of an inflammatory process. It is positive in stools of IBD and colorectal cancer patients. Fecal calprotectin & lactoferrin is useful in predicting impending clinical relapse in CD & UC patients.

875. Which of the following statements about complications of Ulcerative colitis (UC) is false?
Harrison's 20th Ed. Chapter 319 Page 2264

A. Toxic megacolon means a transverse colon with diameter > 6 cm, with loss of haustration
B. Toxic megacolon can be triggered by electrolyte abnormalities and narcotics
C. In toxic colitis and severe ulcerations, bowel may perforate without first dilating
D. UC patients never develop anal fissures, perianal abscesses

UC patients occasionally develop anal fissures, perianal abscesses, or hemorrhoids, but occurrence of extensive perianal lesions should suggest CD.

876. Which of the following statements about clinical features of Crohn's disease (CD) is false?
Harrison's 20th Ed. Chapter 319 Page 2264

A. Can be of fibrostenotic-obstructing or penetrating-fistulous pattern
B. Most common site of inflammation is caecum
C. Presentation may mimic acute appendicitis
D. Radiographic "string sign" refers to narrowed intestinal lumen

In CD, the most common site of inflammation is terminal ileum.

877. Which of the following is not a feature of pain in CD?
Harrison's 20th Ed. Chapter 319 Page 2264

A. Colicky
B. Precedes defecation
C. Relieved by defecation
D. Continues after defecation

Pain is colicky, precedes and is relieved by defecation.

878. Right lower quadrant abdominal inflammatory mass in CD is composed of?
Harrison's 20th Ed. Chapter 319 Page 2264

A. Inflamed bowel
B. Adherent and indurated mesentery
C. Enlarged abdominal lymph nodes
D. All of the above

Abdominal mass in CD is composed of inflamed bowel, adherent and indurated mesentery, and enlarged abdominal lymph nodes.

879. Radiographic "string sign" of a narrowed intestinal lumen in CD is due to?
Harrison's 20th Ed. Chapter 319 Page 2264

A. Edema of bowel wall
B. Bowel wall thickening
C. Fibrosis of bowel wall
D. All of the above

Transmural inflammation of CD causes decreased luminal diameter & limited distensibility. Radiographic "string sign" represents long areas of circumferential inflammation & fibrosis causing long segments of luminal narrowing. Edema, bowel wall thickening & fibrosis of bowel wall account for the radiographic "string sign" of a narrowed intestinal lumen.

880. Factors recognized to exacerbate CD include?
Am J Gastroenterol 2009; 104:465-483

A. Intercurrent infections
B. Cigarette smoking
C. Non-steroidal anti-infl ammatory drugs
D. All of the above

Factors recognized to exacerbate CD include intercurrent infections (both upper respiratory tract & enteric infections, including C. difficile), cigarette smoking & non-steroidal anti-inflammatory drugs.

881. Which of the following statements about clinical features of Crohn's disease (CD) is false?
Harrison's 20th Ed. Chapter 319 Page 2264

A. Pneumaturia may be present
B. Fecaluria may be present
C. Enterocutaneous fistulas may be present
D. Enterocholedocal fistulas may be present

Severe inflammation of ileocecal region may lead to microperforation and fistula formation to adjacent bowel, skin, urinary bladder, to abscess cavity in mesentery, or vagina.

882. In Crohn's disease (CD), intestinal malabsorption can cause all except?
Harrison's 20th Ed. Chapter 319 Page 2264

A. Hyperoxaluria
B. Hypocalcemia
C. Hypomagnesemia
D. Hypokalemia

In CD, intestinal malabsorption can cause anemia, hypoalbuminemia, hypocalcemia, hypomagnesemia, coagulopathy, hyperoxaluria, vitamin D deficiency and vitamin B_{12} deficiency.

883. Diarrhea in active CD is caused by?
Harrison's 20th Ed. Chapter 319 Page 2264

A. Bacterial overgrowth
B. Bile-acid malabsorption
C. Intestinal inflammation
D. All of the above

Causes of diarrhea in active CD include bacterial overgrowth in obstructive stasis or fistulization, bile-acid malabsorption due to diseased or resected terminal ileum & intestinal inflammation with decreased water absorption, increased secretion of electrolytes and decreased rectal compliance.

884. Which of the following about CD is false?
Harrison's 20th Ed. Chapter 319 Page 2265

A. Epigastric pain
B. *H. pylori* negative gastritis
C. Second part of duodenum more commonly involved than bulb
D. None of the above

885. Which of the following statements about investigations of Crohn's disease (CD) is false?
Harrison's 20th Ed. Chapter 319 Page 2265

A. Elevated ESR
B. Elevated CRP
C. Leucopenia
D. Hypoalbuminemia

Laboratory abnormalities in CD include elevated ESR & CRP, hypoalbuminemia, anemia & leukocytosis.

886. Which of the following about endoscopic features of Crohn's disease (CD) is false?
Harrison's 20th Ed. Chapter 319 Page 2265

A. Rectal sparing
B. Aphthous ulcerations & skip lesions
C. Fistulas
D. None of the above

Endoscopic features of CD include rectal sparing, aphthous ulcerations, fistulas, and skip lesions.

887. Earliest macroscopic findings of colonic CD is?
Harrison's 20th Ed. Chapter 319 Page 2265

A. Aphthous ulcers
B. Longitudinal stellate, serpiginous, & linear ulcers
C. Fistulas
D. Polyps

Earliest macroscopic findings of colonic CD are aphthous ulcers which are small, multiple ulcers separated by normal intervening mucosa.

888. Which out of the following is the first-line test for evaluation of suspected CD and its complications?
Harrison's 20th Ed. Chapter 319 Page 2265

A. USG
B. MRI
C. CT enterography
D. Endoscopy

CT enterography permits visualization of entire small bowel for inflammation associated with CD by displaying mural hyperenhancement, interloop sinus tracts, mesenteric fat stranding, engorged vasa recta and perienteric inflammatory changes. MRI may superior for demonstrating pelvic lesions like ischiorectal abscesses.

889. Which of the following statements about complications of Crohn's disease (CD) is false?
Harrison's 20th Ed. Chapter 319 Page 2265

A. Serosal adhesions common
B. Free perforation common in duodenum
C. Systemic glucocorticoid therapy increase risk of intraabdominal & pelvic abscesses
D. Perianal disease common

Perforation occur usually in ileum but occasionally in jejunum.

890. Which of the following antibody reactivity to antigens is associated with CD?
Harrison's 20th Ed. Chapter 319 Page 2266

A. Bacterial flagellin (CBir1)
B. Outer membrane porin C (OmpC)
C. Bacterial sequence I2 (anti-I2)
D. All of the above

Presence of antibody reactivity to antigens like oligomannan (ASCA, anti-Saccharomyces cerevisiae antibody) is seen in CD. Antibodies associated with CD include antibodies to bacterial proteins (Omp-C and I2), flagellin (CBir1) and bacterial carbohydrates, including laminaribioside (ALCA), chitobioside (ACCA) and mannobioside (SMCA).

891. Autoantibody found in cases of UC is?
Harrison's 20th Ed. Chapter 319 Page 2266

A. Anti dsDNA
B. cANCA
C. pANCA
D. Antimitochondrial

pANCA positivity is found in about 60 – 70% of UC patients and 5 – 10% of CD patients.

892. Which of the following statements about serological diagnosis of IBD is false?
Harrison's 20th Ed. Chapter 319 Page 2266

A. pANCA (+) in 5-10% of UC & 60-70% of CD patients
B. 5-15% of I° relatives of UC patients are pANCA (+)
C. pANCA positivity is associated with pancolitis, early surgery, and primary sclerosing cholangitis
D. pANCA in CD is associated with colonic disease

pANCA positivity is found in about 60–70% of UC patients and 5–10% of CD patients.

893. Which of the following about ASCA in IBD is false?
Harrison's 20th Ed. Chapter 319 Page 2266

A. ASCA is associated with large bowel CD
B. 60–70% of CD, 10–15% of UC patients are ASCA (+)
C. ASCA positivity is associated with increased & early CD complications
D. Saccharomyces cerevisiae is Brewer's or Baker's yeast

The presence of both Anti-Saccharomyces cerevisiae antibodies (ASCA) IgG and IgA is highly specific for the presence of Crohn's disease. ASCA is the most sensitive serologic marker of Crohn's disease. Saccharomyces cerevisiae is Brewer's or Baker's yeast.

894. Which of the following about serology of CD is false?
Harrison's 20th Ed. Chapter 319 Page 2266

A. Omp C (+) patients more likely to have internal perforating disease
B. I_2 (+) patients more likely to have fibrostenosing disease

C. Anti-CBir1 expression is associated with small-bowel disease, fibrostenosing, and internal penetrating disease
D. None of the above

Omp C–positive patients are more likely to have internal perforating disease; and I_2 positive patients are more likely to have fibrostenosing disease. Anti-Cbir1 expression is associated with small-bowel disease, fibrostenosing, and internal penetrating disease.

895. Cases of IBD that cannot be categorized as UC or CD are termed?
Harrison's 20th Ed. Chapter 319 Page 2266

A. Indeterminate colitis
B. Lymphocytic colitis
C. Diversion colitis
D. Collagenous colitis

Cases of IBD that cannot be categorized as UC or CD are called indeterminate colitis. IBD cases cannot be distinguished between UC & CD in ~15% of cases.

896. Which of the following is independently associated with disabling CD after 5 years?
Harrison's 20th Ed. Chapter 319 Page 2266

A. Age at diagnosis below 40 years
B. ASCA positivity
C. pANCA positivity
D. Rectal involvement

Features of CD that have been shown to be independently associated with subsequent disabling CD after 5 years are initial requirement for glucocorticoid use, age at diagnosis below 40 years and presence of perianal disease at diagnosis.

897. All of the following are true for CD except?
Harrison's 20th Ed. Chapter 319 Page 2267 Table 319-5

A. Abdominal mass
B. pANCA positivity
C. Response to antibiotics
D. Recurrence after surgery

898. Which of the following can mimic the endoscopic appearance of severe UC?
Harrison's 20th Ed. Chapter 319 Page 2266

A. Herpes simplex infection
B. Yersinia enterocolitica infection
C. Campylobacter colitis
D. Mycobacterium avium-intracellulare complex infection

Campylobacter colitis can mimic the endoscopic appearance of severe UC and can cause a relapse of established UC.

899. Which of the following can cause watery diarrhea?
Harrison's 20th Ed. Chapter 319 Page 2266

A. Salmonella
B. Shigella
C. C. difficile
D. All of the above

Apart from above three, the main symptom in Collagenous colitis is chronic watery diarrhea.

900. Which of the following can cause proctitis?
Harrison's 20th Ed. Chapter 319 Page 2266

A. Gonorrhea
B. Chlamydia
C. Syphilis
D. All of the above

Gonorrhea, Chlamydia, and syphilis can cause proctitis.

901. CMV infection occurs least commonly in?
Harrison's 20th Ed. Chapter 319 Page 2267

A. Esophagus
B. Small intestine
C. Colon
D. Rectum

902. Herpes simplex infection occurs most commonly in?
Harrison's 20th Ed. Chapter 319 Page 2267

A. Oropharynx
B. Anorectum
C. Perianal areas
D. All of the above

903. Parasitic infections that mimic IBD include all except?
Harrison's 20th Ed. Chapter 319 Page 2267

A. Necator americanus
B. Trichuris trichiura
C. Strongyloides stercoralis
D. Enterobius vermicularis

Parasitic infections that may mimic IBD include hookworm (Necator americanus), whipworm (Trichuris trichiura), Strongyloides stercoralis, Isospora belli and Entamoeba histolytica.

904. Mucosal abnormalities in diverticular-associated colitis are limited to?
Harrison's 20th Ed. Chapter 319 Page 2268

A. Caecum
B. Ascending colon
C. Transverse colon
D. Sigmoid and descending colon

Diverticular-associated colitis is similar to CD, but mucosal abnormalities are limited to the sigmoid and descending colon.

905. Patients of ischemic colitis usually present with sudden onset of pain in?
Harrison's 20th Ed. Chapter 319 Page 2268

A. Epigastrium
B. Periumbilical region
C. Right lower quadrant
D. Left lower quadrant

Patients of ischemic colitis usually present with sudden onset of left lower quadrant pain, urgency to defecate and the passage of bright red blood per rectum. Endoscopic examination often demonstrates a normal-appearing rectum and a sharp transition to an area of inflammation in the descending colon and splenic flexure.

906. Which of the following is typical of effects of radiotherapy on the GI tract?
Harrison's 20th Ed. Chapter 319 Page 2268

A. Abscesses
B. Mucus fistula
C. Telangiectasia
D. Ulceration

Flexible sigmoidoscopy reveals mucosal granularity, friability, numerous telangiectasias and occasionally discrete ulcerations.

907. Use of which of the following drugs can mimic IBD?
Harrison's 20th Ed. Chapter 319 Page 2268

A. Azathioprine
B. Mycophenolate mofetil
C. Cyclosporine
D. Rituximab

Use of ipilimumab, mycophenolate mofetil (MMF) & entanercept can mimic IBD.

908. Ipilimumab-induced colitis is typically treated with?
Harrison's 20th Ed. Chapter 319 Page 2268

A. Rituximab
B. Infliximab
C. Tacrolimus
D. Belatacept

Ipilimumab-induced colitis is typically treated with glucocorticoids or infliximab.

909. Patients with inflammatory bowel disease are at risk for?
N Engl J Med. 2009;361:2066-78

A. Primary sclerosing cholangitis
B. Ankylosing spondylitis
C. Psoriasis
D. All of the above

Patients with IBD are at risk for primary sclerosing cholangitis, ankylosing spondylitis, and psoriasis.

910. Which of the following is false about collagenous colitis?
Harrison's 20th Ed. Chapter 319 Page 2268

A. Increased subepithelial collagen deposition
B. Male to female ratio is 9:1
C. Most patients present in 6th or 7th decades
D. Main symptom is chronic watery diarrhea

Female to male ratio is 9:1.

911. Sertraline is a risk factor for which of the following?
Harrison's 20th Ed. Chapter 319 Page 2268

A. Diversion colitis
B. Collagenous colitis
C. Lymphocytic colitis
D. All of the above

912. The frequency of celiac disease is increased in which of the following?
Harrison's 20th Ed. Chapter 319 Page 2268

A. Diversion colitis
B. Collagenous colitis
C. Lymphocytic colitis
D. All of the above

The frequency of celiac disease is increased in lymphocytic colitis and ranges from 9 to 27%.

913. Which of the following is false about Erythema nodosum (EN) in IBD?
Harrison's 20th Ed. Chapter 319 Page 2268

A. Correlate with bowel activity
B. Develop after onset of bowel symptoms
C. Concomitant active peripheral arthritis
D. None of the above

EN occurs in ~15% of CD and 10% of UC patients. Attacks correlate with bowel activity, develop after onset of bowel symptoms, and frequently have concomitant active peripheral arthritis.

914. Which of the following is false about Erythema nodosum?
Harrison's 20th Ed. Chapter 319 Page 2268

A. Erythematous tender nodules
B. 1-5 cm in diameter
C. Found on anterior surface of lower legs and arms
D. None of the above

Lesions of EN are hot, red, tender nodules measuring 1 to 5 cm in diameter and found on anterior surface of lower legs, ankles, calves, thighs and arms.

915. Which of the following is false about Pyoderma gangrenosum (PG) in IBD?
Harrison's 20th Ed. Chapter 319 Page 2268

A. May occur years before onset of bowel symptoms
B. Independent of the bowel disease
C. Respond poorly to colectomy
D. None of the above

PG occurs years before the onset of bowel symptoms, is independent of bowel disease & respond poorly to colectomy, usually associated with severe disease.

916. Which of the following is false about Pyoderma gangrenosum (PG)?
Harrison's 20th Ed. Chapter 319 Page 2268

A. Found on dorsal surface of feet and legs
B. Usually begins as a macule
C. May be single or multiple
D. Difficult to treat

PG usually begins as a pustule and then spreads concentrically to rapidly undermine healthy skin.

917. Dermatologic manifestations of IBD include all except?
Harrison's 20th Ed. Chapter 319 Page 2268

A. Erythema nodosum (EN)
B. Pyoderma gangrenosum (PG)
C. Pyoderma vegetans
D. Erythema marginatum

918. Dermatologic manifestations of IBD include all except?
Harrison's 20th Ed. Chapter 319 Page 2268

A. Pyostomatitis vegetans
B. Alopecia
C. Perianal skin tags
D. Psoriasis

919. Which of the following skin lesions is most frequent in CD?
Harrison's 20th Ed. Chapter 319 Page 2268

A. Erythema nodosum (EN)
B. Pyoderma gangrenosum (PG)
C. Psoriasis
D. Perianal skin tags

Perianal skin tags are found in 75 – 80% of patients with CD, especially those with colon involvement.

920. Which of the following is sometimes associated with Crohn's disease?

Harrison's 20th Ed. Chapter 55 Page 359

A. Epidermolysis bullosa acquisita (EBA)
B. Dermatitis herpetiformis (DH)
C. Pemphigoid gestationis (PG)
D. Mucous membrane pemphigoid (MMP)

921. Peripheral arthritis that develops in IBD patients involves which of the following joints?

Harrison's 20th Ed. Chapter 319 Page 2268

A. Small joints of upper & lower extremities
B. Large joints of upper & lower extremities
C. Small joints of upper extremity
D. Small joints of lower extremity

Peripheral arthritis of IBD patients is asymmetric, polyarticular and migratory and affects large joints of upper and lower extremities.

922. Rheumatologic manifestations of IBD include all except?

Harrison's 20th Ed. Chapter 319 Page 2269

A. Peripheral arthritis
B. Ankylosing spondylitis (AS)
C. Osteopetrosis
D. Sacroiliitis

923. Rheumatologic manifestations of IBD include all except?

Harrison's 20th Ed. Chapter 319 Page 2269

A. Hypertrophic osteoarthropathy
B. Pelvic/femoral osteomyelitis
C. Relapsing polychondritis
D. Osteitis

924. Which of the following skeletal disease occurs equally in UC and CD?

Harrison's 20th Ed. Chapter 319 Page 2269

A. Peripheral arthritis
B. Ankylosing spondylitis (AS)
C. Sacroiliitis
D. All of the above

Symmetric sacroiliitis occurs equally in UC & CD. Peripheral arthritis and ankylosing spondylitis are more common in CD than UC.

925. Ocular manifestations of IBD include all except?

Harrison's 20th Ed. Chapter 319 Page 2269

A. Conjunctivitis
B. Anterior uveitis / iritis
C. Episcleritis
D. Retinitis

Ocular manifestations of IBD include conjunctivitis, anterior uveitis/iritis, and episcleritis.

926. Which of the following is false about ocular complications in IBD?

Harrison's 20th Ed. Chapter 319 Page 2269

A. Uveitis may be found during periods of remission
B. May develop in IBD patients following bowel resection
C. Episcleritis is a benign disorder more common in Crohn's colitis
D. None of the above

927. Common hepatobiliary manifestations of IBD include all except?

Harrison's 20th Ed. Chapter 319 Page 2269

A. Hepatic steatosis
B. Pancreatitis
C. Cholelithiasis
D. Primary sclerosing cholangitis (PSC)

Pancreatitis is a rare extraintestinal manifestation of IBD and results from duodenal fistulas, ampullary CD, gallstones, PSC, autoimmune pancreatitis and primary CD of the pancreas.

928. All are complications of UC except?

Harrison's 20th Ed. Chapter 319 Page 2269

A. Hemorrhage
B. Malignant change
C. Intusucception
D. Polyposis

929. Urologic manifestations of IBD include all except?

Harrison's 20th Ed. Chapter 319 Page 2269

A. Calculi
B. Ureteral obstruction
C. Ileal bladder fistulas
D. Glomerulonephritis

930. Hypercoagulable state in IBD is due to all except?

Harrison's 20th Ed. Chapter 319 Page 2269

A. Reactive thrombocytosis
B. Increased fibrinopeptide A, factor V, VIII & fibrinogen
C. Decreased thromboplastin generation
D. Antithrombin III deficiency

In IBD, risk of venous & arterial thrombosis increases even when disease is not active due to abnormalities of platelet-endothelial interaction, hyperhomocysteinemia, alterations in coagulation cascade, impaired fibrinolysis, involvement of tissue factor-bearing microvesicles, disruption of normal coagulation system by autoantibodies, vasculitides and genetic predisposition.

931. Cardiopulmonary manifestations of IBD include all except?

Harrison's 20th Ed. Chapter 319 Page 2269

A. Endocarditis / Myocarditis
B. Pleuropericarditis
C. Interstitial lung disease (ILD)
D. Obstructive lung disease

In IBD, cardiopulmonary manifestations include endocarditis, myocarditis, pleuropericarditis, & ILD.

932. Most common extraintestinal pulmonary complication of IBD is?

Harrison's 20th Ed. Chapter 319 Page 2269

A. ILD
B. Pneumonitis
C. Malignancy
D. Obstructive lung disease

933. Which of the following studies is related to patients of IBD?
Harrison's 20th Ed. Chapter 319 Page 2276

A. CESAME study
B. IDEAL trial
C. TONIC study
D. BLOOM study

In the prospective observational CESAME study in a cohort of IBD patients in France, the standardized incidence ratios of colorectal cancer were 2.2 for all IBD patients and 7.0 for patients with long-standing extensive colitis (both Crohn's and UC).

934. Risk of colorectal cancer in patients with IBD is relatively small during the initial?
Harrison's 20th Ed. Chapter 319 Page 2276

A. 2 years
B. 5 years
C. 10 years
D. 20 years

Risk of colorectal cancer in patients with IBD is relatively small during initial 10 years of the disease, but increases at a rate of ~0.5-1% per year. Cancer may develop in 8-30% of patients after 25 years of disease. The risk is higher in younger patients with pancolitis.

935. Role of sulfasalazine is not clear in which of the following?
Harrison's 20th Ed. Chapter 319 Page 2270

A. Inducing remission in UC
B. Maintaining remission in UC
C. Inducing remission in CD
D. Maintaining remission in CD

Sulfasalazine and other 5-ASA agents are effective at inducing and maintaining remission in UC with limited role in inducing remission in CD but no clear role in maintenance of CD. The most convincing evidence for use of sulfasalazine is treatment of active CD involving colon.

936. Which of the following is commonly referred to as sulphasalazine (SASP)?
Mediators of Inflammation. 1992;1:151-165

A. Salicylazosulphanilamide
B. Salicylazosulphapyridine
C. Salicylazosulphaguanidine
D. Salicylazosulphasuxidine

Salicylazosulphapyridine is also referred to as sulphasalazine (SASP) and consisting of 5-aminosalicylic acid (5-ASA) and sulphapyridine (SP) joined together by a diazo bond.

937. Enzymatic oxidation of arachidonic acid gives rise to?
Mediators of Inflammation. 1992;1:151-165

A. Prostaglandins & thromboxanes by cyclooxygenase pathway
B. Leukotrienes & intermediate hydroxyeicosatetraenoic acids (HETEs) from lipoxygenase pathway
C. Lipoxins
D. All of the above

938. Which of the following is a functional receptor mediating aminosalicylate activities in IBD?
World Journal of Gastroenterology. 2011;17(2):197-206

A. Steroidogenic factor 1 (SF1)
B. Peroxisome proliferator activated receptor-γ (PPAR-γ)
C. Retinoic acid receptor (RAR)
D. All of the above

PPAR-γ is the key receptor for 5-ASA that mediates its main effects in the colon Activation of PPAR-γ can antagonize nuclear factor κB (NFκB) action in macrophages resulting in downregulation of proinflammatory cytokines.

939. Very high expression levels of PPAR-γ are found in?
World Journal of Gastroenterology. 2011;17(2):197-206

A. Colonic epithelium
B. Macrophages, lymphocytes
C. Hepatocytes
D. Skeletal muscle

940. Nuclear receptor PPAR-γ controls expression of regulatory genes in?
World Journal of Gastroenterology. 2011;17(2):197-206

A. Lipid metabolisms
B. Insulin sensitization
C. Inflammation
D. All of the above

PPAR-γ is an essential nuclear receptor that controls expression of regulatory genes in lipid metabolisms, insulin sensitization, inflammation, and cell proliferation.

941. PPAR-γ interferes with inflammatory pathways by interactions with which of the following transcription factors?
World Journal of Gastroenterology. 2011;17(2):197-206

A. Nuclear factor kappa B (NF-κB)
B. Activating protein-1 (AP-1)
C. Signal transducer and activator of transcription (STAT)
D. All of the above

PPAR-γ interferes with inflammatory pathways by interactions with transcription factors like nuclear factor kappa B (NF-κB), activating protein-1 (AP-1), signal transducer and activator of transcription (STAT), and nuclear factor-activated T cell (NFAT).

942. Which of the following is critical in colonic steady state PPAR-γ expression through Toll-like receptor (TLR)?
Journal of Advances in Internal Medicine. 2012;01(1):33-38

A. Polyunsaturated fatty acids intake
B. Eicosanoids
C. Lipopolysaccharide (LPS) of Gram negative bacteria
D. Lipopolysaccharide (LPS) of Gram positive bacteria

Lipopolysaccharide (LPS) of Gram negative bacteria is critical in colonic steady state PPAR-γ expression through Toll-like receptor (TLR).

943. Which of the following is a dual acting PPAR-α/γ agonist?
Journal of Advances in Internal Medicine. 2012;01(1):33-38

A. Trogliazone
B. Rosiglitazone
C. Pioglitazone
D. Glitazar

Glitazar is a dual acting PPAR-α/γ agonist used for oral treatment for insulin resistance related glucose & lipid abnormalities associated with T2DM & metabolic syndrome.

944. Name of the bond linking the sulfa and 5-ASA moieties in Sulfasalazine is?

Harrison's 20th Ed. Chapter 319 Page 2270

A. Azo bond
B. Thio bond
C. Tau bond
D. Conn bond

Sulphasalazine (SASP) consists of 5-aminosalicylic acid (5-ASA) and sulphapyridine (SP) joined together by a diazo bond. Sulfasalazine is broken down in colon by bacterial azo reductases. They cleave the azo bond linking the sulfa and 5-ASA moieties.

945. Which of the following about sulphasalazine (SASP) is false?

Mediators of Inflammation. 1992;1:151-165

A. SASP acts as a pro-drug
B. Sulphapyridine (SP) acts as a carrier
C. 5-ASA is the active moiety
D. None of the above

Sulfasalazine, the azo-bonded 5-ASA prodrug, undergoes metabolism by bacterial azoreductase enzymes in colonic lumen to release the active 5-ASA moiety and the therapeutically inactive sulfapyridine. 5-ASA acts on and is metabolised by intestinal epithelial cells.

946. Sulfasalazine intolerable side effects are attributable to?

Harrison's 20th Ed. Chapter 319 Page 2270

A. Sulfapyridine moiety
B. Sulfasialic moiety
C. Sulfaphenol moiety
D. All of the above

Allergic reactions or intolerable side effects of sulfasalazine are attributable to sulfapyridine moiety.

947. With sulfasalazine therapy, which of the following should be supplemented?

Harrison's 20th Ed. Chapter 319 Page 2270

A. Iron
B. Folic acid
C. Vitamin B_{12}
D. Pyridoxine

Sulfasalazine can also impair folate absorption, and patients should be given folic acid supplements.

948. Which of the following is a folic acid antagonist?

N Engl J Med. 2000;343:1608-14

A. Trimethoprim
B. Triamterene
C. Carbamazepine
D. All of the above

949. Which of the following is a folic acid antagonist?

N Engl J Med. 2000;343:1608-14

A. Phenytoin
B. Phenobarbital
C. Primidone
D. All of the above

Folic acid antagonists include trimethoprim, triamterene, carbamazepine, phenytoin, phenobarbital, and primidone. These folic acid antagonists affect various enzymes in folate metabolism, impair absorption of folate, or increase degradation of folate.

950. Which of the following is a dihydrofolate reductase inhibitor?

N Engl J Med. 2000;343:1608-14

A. Methotrexate
B. Sulfasalazine
C. Pyrimethamine
D. All of the above

Dihydrofolate reductase inhibitors include aminopterin, methotrexate, sulfasalazine, pyrimethamine, triamterene, and trimethoprim, which displace folate from the enzyme and thereby block conversion of folate to its more active metabolites.

951. Use of folic acid antagonists in early pregnancy may increase the risk of?

N Engl J Med. 2000;343:1608-14

A. Cardiovascular defects
B. Oral clefts
C. Urinary tract defects
D. All of the above

Use of folic acid antagonists in early pregnancy may increase the risk of cardiovascular defects, oral clefts, and urinary tract defects.

952. Hypersensitivity reactions to sulfasalazine include all except?

Harrison's 20th Ed. Chapter 319 Page 2270

A. Hepatitis
B. Thrombocytosis
C. Worsening of colitis
D. Reversible sperm abnormalities

Hypersensitivity reactions of sulfasalazine include rash, fever, hepatitis, agranulocytosis, hypersensitivity pneumonitis, pancreatitis, worsening of colitis and reversible sperm abnormalities.

953. Most common adverse effect reported with 5-ASA agents is?

Gastroenterology & Hepatology. 2008; 4(11), Supplement 24:5

A. Headache
B. Skin rash
C. Constipation
D. Teeth discoloration

The most common adverse effects reported with 5-ASA agents include headaches and GI symptoms such as diarrhea, gas, and nausea.

954. Which out of the following mesalamine formulation has ethylcellulose coating?

Harrison's 20th Ed. Chapter 319 Page 2270

A. Asacol
B. Balsalazide
C. Claversal
D. Pentasa

Pentasa is a mesalamine formulation that has an ethylcellulose coating to allow water absorption into small beads containing mesalamine.

955. Which of the following is a pH-independent formulation mesalamine formulation to deliver 5-ASA?

Gastroenterology & Hepatology. 2008; 4(11), Supplement 24:5

A. Asacol
B. Lialda
C. Pentasa
D. All of the above

Lialda consists of a core of lipophilic & hydrophilic matrices (multimatrix core, MMX) enclosed within a pH-dependent coating. Like Asacol, pH-dependent coating delays release of mesalamine until the tablet is exposed to a pH of 7 or greater. Pentasa is a controlled-released, pH-independent formulation containing microspheres of 5-ASA enclosed within a moisture-sensitive, methylcellulose, semipermeable membrane.

956. Which of the following is a azo-bonded prodrugs of 5-ASA?
Gastroenterology & Hepatology. 2008; 4(11), Supplement 24:5

A. Sulfasalazine
B. Olsalazine
C. Balsalazide
D. All of the above

Olsalazine & balsalazide are prodrugs that deliver 5-ASA to colon without using a sulfapyridine carrier.

957. Which of the following is composed of two 5-ASA radicals linked by an azo bond?
Harrison's 20th Ed. Chapter 319 Page 2270

A. Asacol
B. Balsalazide
C. Claversal
D. Olsalazine

Olsalazine is composed of two 5-ASA radicals linked by an azo bond, which is split in colon by bacterial reduction and two 5-ASA molecules are released. Balsalazide links 5-ASA via a diazo bond to an inactive carrier molecule, 4-aminobenzoyl-β-alanine.

958. 5-ASA agents act within what period of time?
Harrison's 20th Ed. Chapter 319 Page 2270

A. 6-12 hours
B. 1-7 days
C. 2-4 weeks
D. 4-6 weeks

As a general rule, 5-ASA agents act within 2-4 weeks.

959. Which of the following about budesonide is false?
Harrison's 20th Ed. Chapter 319 Page 2271

A. Released entirely in colon
B. Has minimal to no glucocorticoid side effects
C. No taper is required
D. None of the above

Budesonide is useful in UC. It is released entirely in colon and has minimal to no glucocorticoid side effects. Dose is 9 mg/day for 8 weeks, and no taper is required.

960. Which of the following is false regarding treatment of IBD?
Harrison's 20th Ed. Chapter 319 Page 2271

A. Antibiotics have no role in treatment of active or quiescent UC
B. Glucocorticoids useful in maintenance therapy in UC & CD
C. 5-ASA effective in inducing remission in UC & CD
D. 5-ASA useful in maintaining remission in UC

Glucocorticoids play no role in maintenance therapy in UC or CD. 5-ASA is effective in inducing remission in UC & CD & maintaining remission in UC. Its role in remission maintenance in CD is not established. Topica 5-ASA therapy is more effective than topical steroid therapy in the treatment of distal UC.

961. Which of the following side effects of glucocorticoid therapy in IBD is not related to dose & duration of therapy?
Harrison's 20th Ed. Chapter 319 Page 2271

A. Abdominal striae
B. Subcapsular cataract
C. Osteonecrosis
D. Emotional disturbances

Most of these side effects of glucocorticoids, other than osteonecrosis, are related to dose and duration of therapy.

962. First line treatment in active inflammatory, fistulizing and perianal CD is?
Harrison's 20th Ed. Chapter 319 Page 2271

A. 5-ASA
B. Azathioprine
C. Metronidazole
D. Glucocorticoids

Metronidazole is effective in active inflammatory, fistulous, and perianal CD and may prevent recurrence after ileal resection.

963. First line treatment in active inflammatory, fistulizing and perianal CD is?
Harrison's 20th Ed. Chapter 319 Page 2271

A. 5-ASA
B. Azathioprine
C. Ciprofloxacin
D. Glucocorticoids

Both ciprofloxacin and metronidazole antibiotics can be used as first-line drugs for short periods of time in active inflammatory, fistulizing and perianal CD.

964. Achilles tendinitis and rupture is associated with which of the following medicines?
Harrison's 20th Ed. Chapter 319 Page 2271

A. Azathioprine
B. Glucocorticoids
C. Ciprofloxacin
D. Metronidazole

Ciprofloxacin has recently been associated with Achilles tendinitis and rupture.

965. Active end product of Azathioprine is?
Harrison's 20th Ed. Chapter 319 Page 2271

A. 6-MP
B. Thioinosinic acid
C. Inosinic acid
D. Thioguanic acid

Azathioprine is converted to 6-MP, which is metabolized to active end product, thioinosinic acid, an inhibitor of purine ribonucleotide synthesis and cell proliferation.

966. Which of the following is the end product of 6-MP metabolism?
Harrison's 20th Ed. Chapter 319 Page 2271

A. 6-thymidine-mercaptopurine
B. 6-methyl-mercaptopurine
C. 6-propyl-mercaptopurine
D. 6-ethyl-mercaptopurine

Azathioprine therapy adherence can be monitored by levels of 6-thioguanine & 6-methyl-mercaptopurine, end products of 6-MP metabolism. 1 in 300 individuals lacks thiopurine methyltransferase, the enzyme responsible for drug metabolism to inactive end-products (6-methylmercaptopurine).

967. Which of the following drugs is used for postoperative prophylaxis of CD?
Harrison's 20th Ed. Chapter 319 Page 2271

A. 5-ASA
B. Azathioprine
C. Metronidazole
D. Salicylates

6-MP or azathioprine is effective for postoperative prophylaxis of CD.

968. Which of the following statements about azathioprine use in IBD is false?

Harrison's 20th Ed. Chapter 319 Page 2271

A. Pancreatitis as a side effect is completely reversible on stopping drug
B. Thiopurine methyltransferase is the enzyme responsible for its metabolism
C. No increased risk of cancer in IBD patients chronically taking azathioprine
D. Leukopenia is dose-related and delayed

IBD patients treated with azathioprine/6-MP are at a fourfold increased risk of developing a lymphoma due to medications, underlying disease, or both.

969. Methotrexate (MTX) inhibits which of the following?

Harrison's 20th Ed. Chapter 319 Page 2271

A. Dihydrofolate reductase
B. HMG-CoA reductase
C. Trypanothione reductase
D. Fumarate reductase

Methotrexate (MTX) inhibits dihydrofolate reductase, resulting in impaired DNA synthesis. Additional anti-inflammatory properties may be related to decreased IL-1 production.

970. Potential toxicities of Methotrexate include all except?

Harrison's 20th Ed. Chapter 319 Page 2271

A. Leukopenia
B. Hepatic fibrosis
C. Hypersensitivity pneumonitis
D. Cholelithiasis

Potential toxicities of MTX include leukopenia, hepatic fibrosis and hypersensitivity pneumonitis (rarely).

971. Which of the following drugs is a lipophilic peptide?

Harrison's 20th Ed. Chapter 319 Page 2271

A. Azathioprine
B. Methotrexate
C. Cyclosporine
D. Tacrolimus

Cyclosporine (CSA) is a lipophilic peptide with inhibitory effects on both the cellular and humoral immune systems.

972. Cyclosporine (CSA) acts by inhibition of?

Harrison's 20th Ed. Chapter 319 Page 2271

A. IL-1
B. IL-2
C. IFN-α
D. All of the above

973. Cyclosporine (CSA) binds to?

Harrison's 20th Ed. Chapter 319 Page 2271

A. Cyclocysteine
B. Cyclopurine
C. Cyclophilin
D. Cycloserine

974. CSA inhibits which of the following?

Harrison's 20th Ed. Chapter 319 Page 2271

A. Calcitriol
B. Calcineurin
C. Osteocalcin
D. Calcitonin

CSA blocks production of IL-2 by T-helper lymphocytes. CSA binds to cyclophilin, and this complex inhibits calcineurin, a cytoplasmic phosphatase enzyme involved in activation of T cells. CSA also indirectly inhibits B cell function by blocking helper T cells.

975. Which of the following about cyclosporine is false?

Harrison's 20th Ed. Chapter 307 Page 2128 Table 307-3

A. Forms trimolecular complex with cyclophilin & calcineurin
B. Blocks cytokine IL-2 production
C. Stimulates TGF-β production
D. None of the above

976. Blood levels of cyclosporine should be maintained between?

Harrison's 20th Ed. Chapter 319 Page 2271

A. 50 and 50 ng/mL
B. 50 and 150 ng/mL
C. 150 and 350 ng/mL
D. 350 and 550 ng/mL

Blood levels of cyclosporine should be maintained between 150 and 350 ng/mL.

977. Severe UC patients that are refractory to IV glucocortcoids, should be treated with?

Harrison's 20th Ed. Chapter 319 Page 2271

A. IV Cyclosporine
B. Oral cyclosporine
C. Azathioprine
D. 6 Mercaptopurine

CSA is given intravenously in severe UC that is refractory to intravenous glucocorticoids.

978. Which of the following is not a side effect of cyclosporine therapy?

Harrison's 20th Ed. Chapter 319 Page 2271

A. Hypertension
B. Gingival hyperplasia
C. Alopecia
D. Paresthesias

Creatinine elevation, hypertension, gingival hyperplasia, hypertrichosis, paresthesias, tremors, headaches, electrolyte abnormalities and seizures are common side effects of cyclosporine therapy.

979. Seizures may complicate cyclosporine therapy if there is?

Harrison's 20th Ed. Chapter 319 Page 2271

A. Hypocholesterolemia
B. Hypercholesterolemia
C. Hypertriglyceridemia
D. All of the above

Seizures may complicate CSA therapy if the patient is hypomagnesemic or if serum cholesterol levels are <120 mg/dL.

980. Opportunistic infection that commonly occurs with cyclosporine therapy is?

Harrison's 20th Ed. Chapter 319 Page 2271

A. Pneumocystis carnii infection
B. M. tuberculosis infection
C. Klebsiella infection
D. Pseudomonas infection

Opportunistic infections, most often Pneumocystis carinii pneumonia, may occur with CSA combination immunosuppressive treatment.

981. Tacrolimus has immunomodulatory properties similar to?

Harrison's 20th Ed. Chapter 319 Page 2271

A. Methotrexate
B. Cyclosporine
C. Mycophenolate mofetil
D. Thalidomide

Tacrolimus is a macrolide antibiotic with immunomodulatory properties similar to CSA.

982. Which of the following drugs is a macrolide antibiotic?

Harrison's 20th Ed. Chapter 319 Page 2271

A. Azathioprine
B. Methotrexate
C. Cyclosporine
D. Tacrolimus

Tacrolimus is a macrolide antibiotic, 100 times as potent as CSA. It is not dependent on bile or mucosal integrity for absorption.

983. First biologic therapy approved for CD & UC is?

Harrison's 20th Ed. Chapter 319 Page 2272

A. Adalimumab
B. Infliximab
C. Natalizumab
D. Etanercept

The first biologic therapy approved for Crohn's disease & UC was infliximab.

984. Infliximab is?

Harrison's 20th Ed. Chapter 319 Page 2272

A. IgG_1 chimeric monoclonal antibody against TNF-α
B. IgG_1 fully human monoclonal antibody against TNF-α
C. IgG_4 chimeric monoclonal antibody against TNF-α
D. P75 TNF receptor fusion protein

Infliximab is a chimeric mouse-human monoclonal antibody against TNF-α. It blocks TNF in serum and at cell surface and lyses TNF-producing macrophages & T cells.

985. Which of the following trials evaluated infliximab in CD?

Harrison's 20th Ed. Chapter 319 Page 2272

A. PRECISE II
B. ACCENT I
C. CHARM
D. GEMINI I

The ACCENT I (A Crohn's Disease Clinical Trial Evaluating Infliximab in a New Long-Term Treatment Regimen) study showed that of the patients who experience an initial response, 40% will maintain remission for at least 1 year with repeated infusions of infliximab every 8 weeks.

986. Which of the following trials evaluated infliximab in CD?

Harrison's 20th Ed. Chapter 319 Page 2272

A. ACCENT I
B. ACCENT II
C. SONIC
D. All of the above

987. Adalimumab is a?

Harrison's 20th Ed. Chapter 319 Page 2272

A. IgG_1 chimeric monoclonal antibody against TNF
B. IgG_1 recombinant human monoclonal antibody against TNF
C. IgG_4 chimeric monoclonal antibody against TNF
D. P75 TNF receptor fusion protein

Less immunogenic than Infliximab, Adalimumab is a recombinant human monoclonal IgG1 antibody containing only human peptide sequences. Adalimumab binds TNF and neutralizes its function by blocking the interaction between TNF and its cell-surface receptor.

988. Anti-TNF monoclonal antibody useful in treatment of moderate to severely active CD in patients is?

Harrison's 20th Ed. Chapter 319 Page 2272

A. Infliximab
B. Adalimumab
C. Certolizumab pegol
D. All of the above

Anti-TNF monoclonal antibodies, infliximab, adalimumab, certolizumab pegol and golimumab are effective in the treatment of moderate to severely active CD in patients who have not responded despite complete & adequate therapy with a corticosteroid or an immunosuppressive agent.

989. Infusion reaction that occur with Infliximab therapy is due to?

Harrison's 20th Ed. Chapter 319 Page 2272

A. Antibody to Infliximab
B. Concurrent Methotrexate therapy
C. Anti ds-DNA antibody
D. Antinuclear factor

The development of antibodies to infliximab (ATI) is associated with an increased risk of infusion reactions and a decreased response to treatment.

990. Which one of the following is considered to be useful additional therapy with treatment of CD with Infliximab?

Harrison's 20th Ed. Chapter 319 Page 2272

A. Oral steroids
B. 5-ASA
C. Azathioprine
D. Elemental diet

If infliximab is used episodically for flares, concomitant immunosuppression with AZA, 6-MP or methotrexate in therapeutic doses is recommended to reduce clinical consequences of immunogenicity of chimeric antibodies. SONIC (Study of Biologic and Immunomodulator-Naïve Patients with Crohn's Disease) Trial compared infliximab plus azathioprine, infliximab alone and azathioprine alone in moderate-to-severe Crohn's disease with infliximab plus azathioprine group showing best results and no greater adverse events.

991. Risk of which of the following is increased with anti-TNF therapy?

Harrison's 20th Ed. Chapter 319 Page 2272

A. Non-Hodgkin's Lymphoma (NHL)
B. Hepatosplenic T Cell Lymphoma (HSTCL)
C. Melanoma
D. All of the above

992. Infliximab is not useful in?

Harrison's 20th Ed. Chapter 319 Page 2272

A. Crohn's disease
B. Rheumatoid arthritis
C. Ankylosing spondilitis
D. Primary sclerosing cholangitis

993. Which one of the following specifically blocks Integrin-α_4 and prevents lymphocyte trafficking to the intestine in IBD?

Harrison's 20th Ed. Chapter 319 Page 2273

A. Anti IL-12 P40 antibody
B. Anti-gamma interferon
C. Natalizumab
D. Basiliximab

Humanized monoclonal antibody to alpha-4 integrin - Natalizumab inhibits lymphocyte trafficking and is effective in treatment of moderate to severely active CD who have had an inadequate response or are unable tolerate conventional CD therapies and anti-TNF monoclonal antibody therapy.

994. Natalizumab is a?

Harrison's 20th Ed. Chapter 319 Page 2273

A. IgG_1 chimeric monoclonal antibody against TNF
B. IgG_1 recombinant human monoclonal antibody against TNF
C. Recombinant humanized IgG_4 antibody against α4 integrin
D. P75 TNF receptor fusion protein

Natalizumab is a recombinant humanized immunoglobulin G4 antibody against α4 integrin that is effective in the induction and maintenance of remission in CD patients.

995. Natalizumab causes progressive multifocal leukoencephalopathy (PML) by reactivation of which virus?

Harrison's 20th Ed. Chapter 319 Page 2273, Am J Gastroenterol 2009; 104:465.483

A. Hepatitis B
B. Human JC polyoma virus
C. Hepatitis C
D. Cytomegalovirus (CMV)

Natalizumab reactivates the human John Cunningham (JC) polyoma virus, which can lead to progressive multifocal leukoencephalopathy (PML). It is not used in combination with any immunosuppressant medications.

996. Which of the following provides gut-selective immuno-suppresslon?

Harrison's 20th Ed. Chapter 319 Page 2273

A. Natalizumab
B. Vedolizumab
C. Ustekinumab
D. Tofacitinib

Vedolizumab is a leukocyte trafficking inhibitor. It does not cross the blood-brain barrier. It is a monoclonal antibody directed against α4β7 integrin specifically and has the ability to convey gut-selective immunosuppression.

997. Which of the following biologic therapy agents blocks the biologic activity of IL-12 & IL-23?

Harrison's 20th Ed. Chapter 319 Page 2273

A. Natalizumab
B. Vedolizumab
C. Ustekinumab
D. All of the above

Ustekinumab is a fully human IgG1 monoclonal antibody that blocks the biologic activity of IL-12 & IL-23.

998. Which of the following is a infliximab biosimilar?

Harrison's 20th Ed. Chapter 319 Page 2273

A. CT-P12
B. CT-P13
C. CT-P14
D. CT-P15

Biosimilars are biological products that are replicas of their innovator biopharmaceuticals, developed after patent expiration and are submitted for separate marketing approval. Biosimilars should not be considered as "biological generics". Infliximab biosimilar CT-P13 is approved & available for use.

999. Which of the following is an oral inhibitor of Janus kinases 1?

Harrison's 20th Ed. Chapter 319 Page 2273

A. Ozanimod
B. Tofacitinib
C. Tocilizumab
D. Omalizumab

1000. Which of the following causes peripheral lymphocyte sequestration?

Harrison's 20th Ed. Chapter 319 Page 2273

A. Ozanimod
B. Tofacitinib
C. Tocilizumab
D. Omalizumab

Ozanimod is an oral agonist of the sphingosine-1-phosphate receptor subtypes 1 and 5 that causes peripheral lymphocyte sequestration.

1001. Which of the following is false about ileoanal J pouch anastomosis (IPAA)?

Harrison's 20th Ed. Chapter 319 Page 2273

A. Most frequent complication is pouchitis
B. Ileum serves as a neorectum
C. Contraindicated in CD
D. None of the above

1002. Which of the following is false in females with IBD?

Harrison's 20th Ed. Chapter 319 Page 2275

A. Normal fertility rates in quiescent IBD
B. Fallopian tubes scarred by inflammatory process of CD, especially on right side
C. Fallopian tubes scarred by inflammatory process of CD, especially on left side
D. Dyspareunia common

Fallopian tubes can be scarred by inflammatory process of CD, especially on right side because of the proximity of terminal ileum.

1003. In IBD, which of following drugs is safe for use in pregnancy?

Harrison's 20th Ed. Chapter 319 Page 2275

A. Sulfasalazine
B. Mesalamine
C. Balsalazide
D. All of the above

Sulfasalazine, mesalamine, and balsalazide are safe for use in pregnancy and nursing, but additional folate supplementation must be given with sulfasalazine. Topical 5-ASA agents are also safe during pregnancy and nursing. Glucocorticoids are generally safe for use during pregnancy.

1004. The safe antibiotics to use for short periods in pregnant CD patients are all except?

Harrison's 20th Ed. Chapter 319 Page 2275

A. Ampicillin
B. Cephalosporin
C. Ciprofloxacin
D. Metronidazole

Safest antibiotics in CD in pregnancy for weeks, not months are ampicillin and cephalosporin. Metronidazole can be used in the second or third trimester. Ciprofloxacin causes cartilage lesions and should be avoided.

1005. In treatment of IBD with pregnancy, which of the following drugs is contraindicated?

Harrison's 20th Ed. Chapter 319 Page 2275

A. 6-Mercaptopurine
B. Azathioprine
C. Methotrexate
D. Cyclosporine

Methotrexate is contraindicated in pregnancy and nursing. 6-MP and azathioprine pose minimal or no risk during pregnancy. In severe IBD treated with IV CSA during pregnancy, 80% of pregnancies were successfully completed without development of renal toxicity, congenital malformations, or developmental defects.

1006. In pregnancy, exacerbation in Crohn's disease is seen in?

Harrison's 20th Ed. Chapter 466 Page 3444

A. First trimester
B. Second and third trimesters
C. Postpartum period
D. All of the above

1007. In pregnancy, exacerbation in Ulcerative colitis is seen in?

Harrison's 20th Ed. Chapter 466 Page 3444

A. First trimester
B. Second trimester
C. Third trimester
D. All of the above

Crohn's disease may be associated with exacerbations in the second and third trimesters. Ulcerative colitis is associated with disease exacerbations in first trimester & during early postpartum period.

1008. Patients with CD have an increased risk of developing which of the following cancers?

Harrison's 20th Ed. Chapter 319 Page 2275

A. Non-Hodgkin's lymphoma
B. Hodgkin's lymphoma
C. Bronchogenic carcinoma
D. Carcinoma cervix

1009. Patients with CD have an increased risk of developing which of the following cancers?

Harrison's 20th Ed. Chapter 319 Page 2275

A. Hodgkin's lymphoma
B. Endometrial carcinoma
C. Bronchogenic carcinoma
D. Squamous cell cancers

Patients with CD may have an increased risk of non-Hodgkin's lymphoma, leukemia, and myelodysplastic syndromes. Severe chronic, complicated perianal disease in CD patients may be associated with an increased risk of cancer in lower rectum and anal canal (squamous cell cancers).

1010. Mucosal ulcerations of the gut resembling Crohn's disease can be seen in?

Harrison's 20th Ed. Chapter 357 Page 2590

A. Sjogren's syndrome
B. Behcet's syndrome
C. Hypereosinophilic syndrome
D. All of the above

In Behcet's syndrome, gastrointestinal involvement is seen more frequently in patients from Japan and consists of mucosal ulcerations of the gut, resembling Crohn's disease.

1011. Rectal biopsy findings of which of the following resemble those in Crohn's disease?

Harrison's 20th Ed. Chapter 131 Page 989

A. Herpes
B. Lymphogranuloma venereum (LGV)
C. Chancroid
D. Donovanosis

In LGV, rectal biopsy typically shows crypt abscesses, granulomas and giant cells - findings resembling those in Crohn's disease.

1012. Presentation of which of the following may mimic that of ulcerative colitis or Crohn's disease?

Harrison's 20th Ed. Chapter 162 Page 1186

A. Shigella-induced dysentery
B. Cholera
C. Campylobacter enteritis
D. Salmonella gastroenteritis

Presentation of Campylobacter enteritis may mimic that of ulcerative colitis or Crohn's disease.

1013. Before making a diagnosis of IBD, which of the following infections should be ruled out?

Harrison's 20th Ed. Chapter 162 Page 1186

A. Campylobacter
B. Arcobacter
C. Helicobacter
D. All of the above

Presentation of Campylobacter enteritis may mimic UC or CD. As Campylobacter enteritis is much more common than UC and CD among young adults, a diagnosis of IBD should not be made until Campylobacter infection has been ruled out.

1014. Ulcerative colitis and Crohn's disease may be complicated by?

Harrison's 20th Ed. Chapter 438 Page 3214

A. SLE
B. Sjogren's syndrome
C. GBS
D. All of the above

Ulcerative colitis and Crohn's disease may be complicated by GBS, CIDP, generalized axonal sensory or sensorimotor polyneuropathy, small-fiber neuropathy or mononeuropathy.

1015. Which of the following seronegative arthropathies is strongly associated with HLA-B27 histocompatibility antigen?

Harrison's 20th Ed. Chapter 355 Page 2573

A. Ankylosing spondylitis
B. Psoriatic arthritis
C. Arthritides associated with ulcerative colitis
D. All of the above

Seronegative arthropathies like ankylosing spondylitis, reactive arthritis, psoriatic arthritis and arthritides associated with ulcerative colitis and regional enteritis are all strongly associated with the HLA-B27 histocompatibility antigen.

Irritable Bowel Syndrome

1016. Which of the following is a criteria for the diagnosis of Irritable Bowel Syndrome (IBS)?

Harrison's 20th Ed. Chapter 320 Page 2276

A. Paris
B. Rome
C. Helsinki
D. Warsaw

Rome IV criteria is useful for the diagnosis of IBS.

1017. In which year, Rome III criteria for diagnosis of IBS was updated to Rome IV?

Harrison's 20th Ed. Chapter 320 Page 2276

A. 2012
B. 2014
C. 2016
D. 2018

In 2016, the Rome III criteria for the diagnosis of IBS were updated to Rome IV. Rome II criteria for diagnosis of IBS was revised in 2006.

1018. Which of the following is not included in the Rome IV criteria for the diagnosis of IBS?

Harrison's 20th Ed. Chapter 320 Page 2276 Table 320-1

A. Recurrent abdominal pain related to defecation
B. Recurrent abdominal pain related to nausea & vomiting
C. Recurrent abdominal pain with change in frequency of stool
D. Recurrent abdominal pain with change in form of stool

Rome IV diagnostic criteria for IBS includes recurrent abdominal pain at least 1 day per week in the last 3 months associated with two or more of the following-related to defecation, associated with change in frequency of stool and associated with a change in form or appearance of stool. Painless diarrhea or constipation are not included in the criteria.

1019. Which of the following is a key symptom for the diagnosis of IBS?

Harrison's 20th Ed. Chapter 320 Page 2276

A. Abdominal pain
B. Frequency of stool
C. Form (appearance) of stool
D. Feeling of incomplete bowel movement and bloating

1020. Which of the following is not included in the criteria for the diagnosis of IBS?

Harrison's 20th Ed. Chapter 320 Page 2276

A. Painless diarrhea or constipation
B. Feeling of incomplete bowel movement
C. Passing mucus in stool
D. All of the above

Abdominal pain is a key symptom for the diagnosis of IBS. Supportive symptoms that are not part of the diagnostic criteria include defecation straining, urgency or a feeling of incomplete bowel movement, passing mucus and bloating.

1021. IBS symptoms often overlap with which of the following functional disorders?

Harrison's 20th Ed. Chapter 320 Page 2276

A. Fibromyalgia
B. Headache
C. Genitourinary symptoms
D. All of the above

IBS symptoms have a tendency to come & go over time and often overlap with other functional disorders such as fibromyalgia, headache, backache and genitourinary symptoms.

1022. Which of the following about IBS is false?

Harrison's 20th Ed. Chapter 320 Page 2276

A. Most patients have their first symptoms before 45 years
B. Women make up to 80% of severe IBS patients
C. Rome II criteria for diagnosis of IBS was revised in 2006
D. None of the above

1023. Which of the following about abdominal pain in IBS is false?

Harrison's 20th Ed. Chapter 320 Page 2276

A. Sleep deprivation is usual
B. Exacerbated by eating
C. Improved by passage of flatus or stools
D. Worsens during the premenstrual & menstrual phases

Sleep deprivation is unusual and abdominal pain is almost uniformly present only during waking hours.

1024. Which of the following is a prerequisite clinical feature of IBS?

Harrison's 20th Ed. Chapter 320 Page 2276

A. Abdominal pain
B. Alteration in bowel habits
C. Gas and Flatulence
D. Dyspepsia

1025. Abdominal pain in IBS is exacerbated by?

Harrison's 20th Ed. Chapter 320 Page 2276

A. Eating
B. Emotional stress
C. During premenstrual & menstrual phases in female patients
D. All of the above

1026. Which of the following is the most consistent clinical feature in IBS?

Harrison's 20th Ed. Chapter 320 Page 2277

A. Abdominal pain or discomfort
B. Alteration in bowel habits
C. Gas and Flatulence
D. Dyspepsia

Abdominal pain or discomfort is a prerequisite clinical feature of IBS. While, alteration in bowel habits is the most consistent clinical feature in IBS.

1027. Which of the following is rare in IBS?

Harrison's 20th Ed. Chapter 320 Page 2276

A. Malnutrition
B. Weight loss
C. Sleep deprivation
D. All of the above

1028. Which of the following about diarrhea in IBS is false?
Harrison's 20th Ed. Chapter 320 Page 2277

A. Small volume
B. Nocturnal
C. Aggravated by emotional stress
D. Aggravated by eating

Nocturnal diarrhea or steatorrheal stools do not occur in IBS and malabsorption or weight loss does not occur. Stool volume >200–300 mL/day argues against IBS.

1029. Which of the following IBS subgroup is most prevalent?
Harrison's 20th Ed. Chapter 320 Page 2277

A. IBS-diarrhea predominant (IBS-D)
B. IBS-constipation predominant (IBS-C)
C. IBS-mixed (IBS-M)
D. None of the above

On the basis of the predominant bowel habit, IBS has been categorized into one of the following subgroups: IBS with diarrhea (more common in men), IBS with constipation (more common in women), and IBS with mixed bowel habits. Each group accounts for about one third of all patients.

1030. What percentage of IBS patients change subtypes over 1 year?
Harrison's 20th Ed. Chapter 320 Page 2277

A. 25%
B. 50%
C. 75%
D. 100%

75% of IBS patients change subtypes and 29% switch between IBS-C and IBS-D over 1 year.

1031. Which of the following is false in IBS patients?
Harrison's 20th Ed. Chapter 320 Page 2277

A. Impaired transit of intestinal gas loads
B. Impaired tolerance of intestinal gas loads
C. Gas reflux from distal to more proximal intestine
D. None of the above

1032. Motor abnormalities under stimulated conditions in IBS are seen in?
Harrison's 20th Ed. Chapter 320 Page 2277

A. Transverse colon
B. Descending colon
C. Sigmoid colon
D. All of the above

Colonic myoelectrical & motor activity under "unstimulated" conditions do not show consistent abnormalities in IBS. IBS patients exhibit increased rectosigmoid motor activity for up to 3 hours after eating.

1033. Which of the following myoelectrical and motor abnormality is seen in IBS under stimulated conditions?
Harrison's 20th Ed. Chapter 320 Page 2277

A. Increased rectosigmoid motor activity
B. Prolonged distention-evoked contractile activity
C. Increased peak amplitude of high-amplitude propagating contractions (HAPCs)
D. All of the above

1034. In IBS, postprandial pain is temporally related to entry of food bolus into which of the following?
Harrison's 20th Ed. Chapter 320 Page 2277

A. Stomach
B. Duodenum
C. Jejunum
D. Cecum

Postprandial pain is temporally related to entry of the food bolus into cecum in IBS.

1035. Which of the following lower the thresholds for the first sensation of gas, discomfort & pain in IBS patients?
Harrison's 20th Ed. Chapter 320 Page 2277

A. Carbohydrates
B. Proteins
C. Lipids
D. Water

Lipids lower the thresholds for the first sensation of gas, discomfort and pain in IBS patients. Thus, postprandial symptoms in IBS patients are explained by a nutrient-dependent exaggerated sensory component of the gastrocolonic response. Afferent pathway disturbances in IBS are selective for visceral innervation with sparing of somatic pathways.

1036. In IBS, mechanisms responsible for visceral hypersensitivity may be?
Harrison's 20th Ed. Chapter 320 Page 2277

A. Recruitment of "silent" nociceptors
B. Spinal hyperexcitability
C. Neuroplasticity
D. All of the above

1037. Brain region concerned with attention processes & response selection is?
Harrison's 20th Ed. Chapter 320 Page 2278

A. Amygdala
B. Mid-cingulate cortex
C. Perigenual anterior cingulated cortex
D. Hippocampus

Mid-cingulate cortex is a region in brain that is concerned with attention processes & response selection. This region shows greater activation in IBS patients. Modulation of this region produces changes in subjective unpleasantness of pain. Also, in IBS patients there occurs preferential activation of the prefrontal lobe that increases alertness.

1038. Which of the following is the most important risk factor for developing post-infectious IBS?
Harrison's 20th Ed. Chapter 320 Page 2278

A. Toxicity of infecting bacterial strain
B. Smoking
C. Prolonged duration of initial illness
D. Depression

Risk factors for developing postinfectious IBS include, in order of importance, prolonged duration of initial illness, toxicity of infecting bacterial strain, smoking, mucosal markers of inflammation, female gender, depression, hypochondriasis and adverse life events in the preceding 3 months.

1039. Which of the following protects against post-infectious IBS?
Harrison's 20th Ed. Chapter 320 Page 2278

A. Age > 60 years
B. Treatment with antibiotics
C. Presence of mucosal markers of inflammation
D. Female sex

Age older than 60 years might protect against post-infectious IBS.

1040. Microbe involved in the initial infection of post-infectious IBS is?

Harrison's 20th Ed. Chapter 320 Page 2278

A. Campylobacter
B. Salmonella
C. Shigella
D. All of the above

Microbes involved in the initial infection of post-infectious IBS are Campylobacter, Salmonella & Shigella.

1041. Functional Bowel Disorder Severity Index (FBDSI) was developed and published by?

Gastroenterology 2016;150:1262

A. Talley
B. Eswaran
C. Drossman
D. Mayer

1042. Which of the following is a nonselective cation channel expressed in nociceptive neurons?

Harrison's 20th Ed. Chapter 320 Page 2278

A. TRPV 1
B. TRPV 2
C. TRPV 3
D. TRPV 4

TRPV 1 is a nonselective cation channel expressed in nociceptive neurons and are central to the initiation & persistence of visceral hypersensitivity.

1043. TRPV stands for?

Harrison's 20th Ed. Chapter 320 Page 2278

A. Transient receptor potential cation channel
B. Terminal receptor potential cation channel
C. Total receptor potential cation channel
D. Timed receptor potential cation channel

TRPV4 stands for transient receptor potential cation channel subfamily V, member 4. TRPV5 and TRPV6 are calcium transporters expressed by intestinal epithelia whose expression is controlled principally by 1,25(OH)$_2$D.

1044. TRP channels are cellular sensors involved in?

Br J Pharmacol. 2014;171(10):2474-2507

A. Nociception
B. Taste perception
C. Thermosensation
D. All of the above

TRP channels are cellular sensors involved in nociception, taste perception, thermosensation, mechano- and osmolarity sensing.

1045. Which of the following is a member of the TRP channels?

Br J Pharmacol. 2014;171(10):2474-2507

A. TRPC (Canonical)
B. TRPV (Vanilloid)
C. TRPM (Melastatin)
D. All of the above

TRP channels comprise 28 members and are divided into six subfamilies: TRPC (Canonical), TRPV (Vanilloid), TRPM (Melastatin), TRPP (Polycystin), TRPML (Mucolipin) and TRPA (Ankyrin).

1046. Which of the following is a TRP channelopathy?

Br J Pharmacol. 2014;171(10):2474-2507

A. Focal segmental glomerular sclerosis (FSGS)
B. ADPKD
C. Scapuloperoneal spinal muscular atrophy
D. All of the above

'TRP channelopathies' include focal segmental glomerular sclerosis (FSGS), ADPKD and scapuloperoneal spinal muscular atrophy.

1047. In healthy adults, 80% of the identified fecal microbiota belong to phyla?

BMC Microbiology 2009;9:123

A. Bacteroidetes
B. Firmicutes
C. Actinobacteria
D. All of the above

In healthy adults, 80% of the identified fecal microbiota can be classified into three dominant phyla: Bacteroidetes, Firmicutes and Actinobacteria. They predominantly influence human nutrition & metabolism.

1048. Firmicutes best relate to?

BMC Microbiology 2009;9:123

A. Prevotella
B. Bifidobacterium
C. Clostridium
D. All of the above

The Firmicutes include a large number of genera that belong to Clostridium clusters IV and XIV. Some prominent members being Eubacterium, Faecalibacterium, Roseburia & Ruminococcus.

1049. Which of the following is false in IBS patients?

Harrison's 20th Ed. Chapter 320 Page 2278

A. Decreased Bifidobacterium proportion
B. Decreased Lactobacillus proportion
C. Increased ratio of Firmicutes : Bacteroidetes
D. None of the above

1050. Which of the following pathways is abnormal in IBS?

Harrison's 20th Ed. Chapter 320 Page 2278

A. Serotonin
B. Dopamine
C. Norepinephrine
D. All of the above

1051. Which of the following is the rate-limiting enzyme in enterochromaffin cell 5-HT biosynthesis?

Harrison's 20th Ed. Chapter 320 Page 2278

A. Tryptophan hydroxylase 1
B. Tryptophan hydroxylase 2
C. Tryptophan hydroxylase 3
D. Tryptophan hydroxylase 4

Tryptophan hydroxylase 1 (TPH1) is the rate-limiting enzyme in enterochromaffin cell 5-HT biosynthesis.

1052. Which of the following is a diagnostic criteria for IBS?

Harrison's 20th Ed. Chapter 320 Page 2278

A. Manning's criteria
B. Barbara's criteria
C. Mayer's criteria
D. Talley's criteria

1053. Which of the following argue against the diagnosis of IBS?
Harrison's 20th Ed. Chapter 320 Page 2279

A. Appearance for the first time in old age
B. Persistent diarrhea after a 48 hour fast
C. Nocturnal diarrhea or steatorrheal stools
D. All of the above

Appearance of the disorder for the first time in old age, progressive course from time of onset, persistent diarrhea after a 48-hour fast, and presence of nocturnal diarrhea or steatorrheal stools argue against the diagnosis of IBS.

1054. Which of the following argue against the diagnosis of IBS?
Harrison's 20th Ed. Chapter 320 Page 2279

A. Anemia
B. Presence of leukocytes or blood in stool
C. Stool volume > 200 - 300 mL/day
D. All of the above

Laboratory features that argue against IBS include evidence of anemia, elevated sedimentation rate, presence of leukocytes or blood in stool and stool volume >200-300 mL/day.

1055. Which of the following abnormality is pathognomonic of IBS?
Harrison's 20th Ed. Chapter 320 Page 2279

A. Abdominal pain
B. Abdominal bloating
C. Alteration in bowel habits
D. None of the above

IBS is a disorder for which no pathognomonic abnormality has been identified.

1056. Painful constipation is a major complaint in which of the following?
Harrison's 20th Ed. Chapter 320 Page 2279

A. Acute intermittent porphyria
B. Hypothyroidism
C. Hypoparathyroidism
D. All of the above

Painful constipation is a major complaint in acute intermittent porphyria and lead poisoning.

1057. Which of the following is a FODMAP?
Harrison's 20th Ed. Chapter 320 Page 2279

A. Lactose
B. Fructose
C. Sorbitol
D. All of the above

FODMAP stands for fermentable oligosaccharides, disaccharides, monosaccharides and polyols such as lactose, fructose or sorbitol. FODMAPs are poorly absorbed by the small intestine and fermented by bacteria in colon to produce gas and osmotically active carbohydrates. A diet low in FODMAPs has been shown to be helpful in IBS patients.

1058. Fiber can exacerbate which of the following?
Harrison's 20th Ed. Chapter 320 Page 2280

A. Bloating
B. Flatulence
C. Diarrhea
D. All of the above

Fiber can exacerbate bloating, flatulence, constipation and diarrhea.

1059. In IBS, the best time to give antispasmodics for postprandial pain is?
Harrison's 20th Ed. Chapter 320 Page 2280

A. 30 minutes before meals
B. Along with meals
C. Immediately following meals
D. 1 hour after meals

Antispasmodics are most effective when prescribed in anticipation of predictable pain. To inhibit gastrocolic reflex and postprandial pain, antispasmodics are given 30 minutes before meals.

1060. Which of the following is an antidiarrheal agent?
Harrison's 20th Ed. Chapter 320 Page 2280

A. Loperamide
B. Paregoric
C. Cholestyramine
D. All of the above

1061. Which of the following antibiotic is useful for the treatment of IBS?
Harrison's 20th Ed. Chapter 320 Page 2281

A. Neomycin
B. Amoxycillin
C. Azithromycin
D. Levofloxacin

Neomycin and nonabsorbed oral antibiotic Rifaximin are useful in IBS.

1062. Which of the following about rifaximin is false?
Harrison's 20th Ed. Chapter 320 Page 2281

A. Oral drug
B. Nonsystemic, broad-spectrum antibiotic
C. Not absorbed
D. None of the above

Rifaximin is a minimally absorbed oral antimicrobial agent that is concentrated in gastrointestinal tract. It has broad-spectrum in vitro activity against gram-positive, gram-negative aerobic and anaerobic enteric bacteria, and has a low risk of inducing bacterial resistance.

1063. Which of the following probiotics has shown significant benefit in IBS patients?
Harrison's 20th Ed. Chapter 320 Page 2281

A. Faecalibacterium prausnitzii
B. Bifidobacterium breve
C. Taenia suis
D. All of the above

Probiotics naturally alter the gut flora. Bifidobacterium breve, B. longum and Lactobacillus acidophilus species showed significant improvement in the composite score for IBS.

1064. Alosetron was withdrawn from the market due to the increased incidence of?
Harrison's 20th Ed. Chapter 320 Page 2282

A. Depression & suicidal tendency
B. Dyslipidemia
C. Ischemic colitis
D. Myocardial infarction

Alosetron is a 5-HT3 receptor antagonist that reduces perception of painful visceral stimulation in IBS. Alosetron was withdrawn from the market due to the increased incidence of ischemic colitis.

1065. Which of the following is a 5-HT4 receptor antagonist?

Harrison's 20th Ed. Chapter 320 Page 2282

A. Alosetron
B. Rifaximin
C. Tegaserod
D. Lubiprostone

Tegaserod is a 5-HT4 receptor agonist that exhibits prokinetic activity by stimulating peristalsis.

1066. Tegaserod was withdrawn from the market due to increased incidence of?

Harrison's 20th Ed. Chapter 320 Page 2282

A. Seizure events
B. Cardiovascular events
C. Hematologic diathesis
D. Depression & suicidal tendency

1067. Which of the following is a chloride channel activator?

Harrison's 20th Ed. Chapter 320 Page 2282

A. Alosetron
B. Rifaximin
C. Tegaserod
D. Lubiprostone

1068. Which of the following about Lubiprostone is false?

Harrison's 20th Ed. Chapter 320 Page 2282

A. Bicyclic fatty acid
B. Stimulates Cl^- channels in intestinal epithelial cells
C. Oral administration
D. None of the above

Lubiprostone is a bicyclic fatty acid that stimulates chloride channels in the apical membrane of intestinal epithelial cells. Chloride secretion induces passive movement of sodium & water into bowel lumen & improves bowel function in constipation-predominant IBS patients. Alosetron is a 5-HT3 receptor antagonist. Rifaximin is a non-absorbed oral antibiotic. Tegaserod is a 5-HT4 receptor agonists.

1069. Which of the following about Linaclotide is false?

Harrison's 20th Ed. Chapter 320 Page 2282

A. Guanylate cyclase-C (GC-C) agonist
B. Action mediated by cGMP
C. Minimally absorbed
D. None of the above

Novel agents that induce secretion or intestinal secretagogues are lubiprostone (chloride channel activator) and linaclotide (a guanylate cyclase C agonist).

1070. Which of the following is an osmotic laxative?

Harrison's 20th Ed. Chapter 42 Page 268

A. Magnesium salts
B, Lactulose
C. Polyethylene glycol
D. All of the above

Osmotic laxatives are magnesium salts, lactulose, sorbitol and polyethylene glycol.

Mesenteric Vascular Insufficiency

1071. Mesenteric circulation consists of?
N Engl J Med. 2016;374:959-68

A. Celiac artery
B. Superior mesenteric artery
C. Inferior mesenteric artery
D. All of the above

Three primary vessels contributing to mesenteric circulation are the celiac artery (foregut), superior mesenteric artery (midgut), and inferior mesenteric artery (hindgut). They are interconnect through collateral networks between visceral & nonvisceral circulations. These interconnections ensure that the loss of a single vessel does not lead to catastrophic malperfusion of the viscera.

1072. Which of the following is a category of intestinal ischemia?
Harrison's 20th Ed. Chapter 322 Page 2291

A. Arterioocclusive mesenteric ischemia (AOMI)
B. Nonocclusive mesenteric ischemia (NOMI)
C. Mesenteric venous thrombosis (MVT)
D. All of the above

Arterial obstruction, the most common cause of mesenteric ischemia, has both acute and chronic forms.

1073. Risk factors for acute intestinal arterial ischemia include?
Harrison's 20th Ed. Chapter 322 Page 2291

A. Atrial fibrillation
B. Recent myocardial infarction
C. Valvular heart disease
D. All of the above

Risk factors for acute intestinal arterial ischemia include atrial fibrillation, recent myocardial infarction, valvular heart disease, and recent cardiac or vascular catheterization.

1074. "Intestinal angina" best applies to?
Harrison's 20th Ed. Chapter 322 Page 2291

A. Arterioocclusive mesenteric ischemia (AOMI)
B. Nonocclusive mesenteric ischemia (NOMI)
C. Mesenteric venous thrombosis (MVT)
D. All of the above

1075. Nonocclusive mesenteric ischemia is seen in?
Harrison's 20th Ed. Chapter 322 Page 2292

A. Patients receiving high-dose vasopressor infusions
B. Patients presenting with cardiogenic or septic shock
C. Cocaine overdose
D. All of the above

The mesenteric circulation is a high-resistance vascular bed in which impaired regional perfusion owing to vasospasm can develop. The resulting ischemia is referred to as nonocclusive mesenteric ischemia.

1076. Mesenteric venous thrombosis is associated with?
Harrison's 20th Ed. Chapter 322 Page 2292

A. Antithrombin III deficiency
B. Polycythemia vera
C. Carcinoma
D. All of the above

Mesenteric venous thrombosis is associated with the presence of a hypercoagulable state like protein C or S deficiency, antithrombin III deficiency, polycythemia vera, and carcinoma.

1077. Which of the following is a watershed area within the colonic blood supply and common location for intestinal ischemia?
Harrison's 20th Ed. Chapter 322 Page 2292

A. Matsumoto point
B. Griffiths' point
C. Wyers point
D. Mitchell point

1078. Which of the following is a watershed area within the colonic blood supply and common location for intestinal ischemia?
Harrison's 20th Ed. Chapter 322 Page 2292

A. Shih point
B. Sudeck's point
C. Hsu point
D. Sise point

Collateral vessels within small bowel meet within duodenum & bed of pancreas. Collateral vessels within colon meet at splenic flexure & descending/sigmoid colon. These watershed areas are inherently at risk for decreased blood flow and are known as Griffiths' point and Sudeck's point respectively and are the most common locations for colonic ischemia.

1079. Nationality of Jean Riolan was?

A. French
B. German
C. Spanish
D. Portugese

Arch of Riolan is named after Jean Riolan, French anatomist (1580–1657). It connects the proximal superior mesenteric artery (SMA) or one of its primary branches (middle colic artery) to the proximal inferior mesenteric artery (IMA) or one of its primary branches and runs close to the root of the mesentery.

1080. Emboli originating from heart preferentially lodge in?
Harrison's 20th Ed. Chapter 322 Page 2292

A. Superior mesenteric artery
B. Inferior mesenteric artery
C. Celiac trunk
D. Arc of Riolan

In >75% of cases, emboli originate from heart & preferentially lodge in superior mesenteric artery (SMA) just distal to the origin of middle colic artery.

1081. "Pain out of proportion to examination," with an epigastric bruit is indicative of?
N Engl J Med. 2016;374:959-68

A. Acute mesenteric ischemia
B. Chronic mesenteric ischemia
C. Mesenteric venous thrombosis
D. Nonocclusive mesenteric ischemia

1082. Patients with chronic mesenteric ischemia can present as?
N Engl J Med. 2016;374:959-68

A. Postprandial pain
B. Early satiety
C. Weight loss
D. Any of the above

Patients with chronic mesenteric ischemia can present with abdominal pain, postprandial pain, nausea or vomiting, early satiety, diarrhea or constipation & weight loss. Abdominal pain 30 to 60 minutes after eating is common and is often self-treated with food restriction ("food fear" or sitophobia), resulting in weight loss.

1083. Postprandial pain is a feature of?
N Engl J Med. 2016;374:959-68

A. Peptic ulcer disease
B. Pancreatitis
C. Irritable bowel syndrome
D. All of the above

Postprandial pain may be associated with biliary disease, peptic ulcer disease, pancreatitis, diverticular disease, gastric reflux, irritable bowel syndrome, and gastroparesis.

1084. Which of the following is an ominous pathological findings in patients with mesenteric ischemia?
N Engl J Med. 2016;374:959-68

A. Pneumatosis
B. Free intraabdominal air
C. Portal venous gas
D. All of the above

1085. Progressive thrombosis of at least how many major vessels supplying intestine is required for chronic intestinal angina?
Harrison's 20th Ed. Chapter 322 Page 2292

A. One
B. Two
C. Three
D. Four

Progressive thrombosis of at least two of the major vessels supplying the intestine is required for the development of chronic intestinal angina.

1086. Mortality rate in intestinal ischemia is?
Harrison's 20th Ed. Chapter 322 Page 2292

A. > 10%
B. > 20%
C. > 30%
D. > 50%

The most critical factor influencing outcomes in patients with mesenteric ischemia is the speed of diagnosis and intervention.

1087. Which of the following is a feature of intestinal ischemia?
Harrison's 20th Ed. Chapter 322 Page 2292

A. Thumbprinting
B. Pneumatosis intestinalis
C. Air within the portal venous system
D. All of the above

Features of intestinal ischemia include bowel-wall edema ("thumbprinting"), air within the bowel wall (pneumatosis intestinalis) and within the portal venous system.

1088. The gold standard for confirmation of acute mesenteric arterial occlusion is?
Harrison's 20th Ed. Chapter 322 Page 2292

A. Mesenteric angiography
B. Duplex ultrasound
C. Magnetic resonance angiography
D. Abdominal spiral CT

Gold standard for confirmation of mesenteric arterial occlusion is mesenteric angiography. Duplex ultrasound evaluation of the mesenteric vessels is used as a screening test for patients with symptoms suggestive of chronic mesenteric ischemia.

1089. Which of the following is spared in superior mesenteric artery (SMA) occlusion?
Harrison's 20th Ed. Chapter 322 Page 2293

A. Jejunum
B. Terminal ileum
C. Caecum
D. Ascending colon

In SMA occlusion, where embolus usually lies just proximal to the origin of middle colic artery, proximal jejunum is often spared while remainder of the small bowel up to transverse colon becomes ischemic.

1090. Markers for intestinal ischemia include all except?
Harrison's 20th Ed. Chapter 322 Page 2293

A. D-dimer
B. Glutathione S-transferase
C. UDP-glucuronosyltransferase
D. Platelet-activating factor (PAF)

Markers for intestinal ischemia include D-dimer, glutathione S-transferase, platelet-activating factor (PAF), and mucosal pH monitoring.

1091. Which of the following is associated with the best prognosis?
Harrison's 20th Ed. Chapter 322 Page 2294

A. Arterioocclusive mesenteric ischemia (AOMI)
B. Nonocclusive mesenteric ischemia (NOMI)
C. Mesenteric venous thrombosis (MVT)
D. All of the above

1092. Which of the following is not a feature of chronic mesenteric angina?
Harrison's 20th Ed. Chapter 322 Page 2294

A. Abdominal cramping & pain following ingestion of meal
B. Weight loss
C. Constipation
D. Chronic diarrhea

Patients of chronic intestinal ischemia (intestinal angina) presents with abdominal cramping and pain following ingestion of a meal, weight loss and chronic diarrhea. Abdominal pain without weight loss is not chronic mesenteric angina.

Approach to the Patient with Liver Disease

1093. The liver weighs about?
Harrison's 20th Ed. Chapter 329 Page 2332

A. 0.5 - 1.0 kg
B. 1.0 - 1.5 kg
C. 1.5 - 2.0 kg
D. 2.0 - 2.5 kg

1094. The liver represents what percentage of lean body mass?
Harrison's 20th Ed. Chapter 329 Page 2332

A. 0.5 - 1.0%
B. 1.0 - 1.5%
C. 1.5 - 2.5%
D. 2.5 - 3.5%

The liver is the largest organ of body, weighing 1–1.5 kg & representing 1.5-2.5% of the lean body mass.

1095. The contribution of blood supply to liver from hepatic artery and portal vein is?
Harrison's 20th Ed. Chapter 329 Page 2332

A. 50% and 50% respectively
B. 40% and 60% respectively
C. 60% and 40% respectively
D. 20% and 80% respectively

Liver receives a dual blood supply, ~20% of blood flow is oxygen-rich blood from hepatic artery and 80% is nutrient-rich blood from the portal vein arising from stomach, intestines, pancreas & spleen.

1096. From a metabolic perspective, the functional unit of liver is?
Diseases of liver & biliary system, Sheila Sherlock 9th Ed. 1

A. Hepatic lobule
B. Hepatic acinus
C. Portal lobule
D. All of the above

1097. Which of the following statements is false?
Diseases of liver & biliary system, Sheila Sherlock 9th Ed. 1

A. Shape of hepatic lobule is polygonal
B. Shape of portal lobule is triangular
C. Shape of hepatic acinus is elliptical
D. None of the above

1098. Which of the following statements is true?
Diseases of liver & biliary system, Sheila Sherlock 9th Ed. 1

A. Central vein is at the center of hepatic acinus
B. Central vein is at the center of hepatic lobule
C. Central vein is at the center of portal lobule
D. All of the above

1099. Which of the following hepatic zones is most oxygenated?
Diseases of liver & biliary system, Sheila Sherlock 9th Ed. 1

A. Zone 1
B. Zone 2
C. Zone 3
D. All of the above

Hepatic zone 3 is least oxygenated.

1100. Right lobe of liver is about how many times bigger than the left lobe?
Diseases of liver & biliary system, Sheila Sherlock 9th Ed. 1

A. 2 times
B. 4 times
C. 6 times
D. 8 times

1101. Pressure in the free hepatic vein is about?
Diseases of liver & biliary system, Sheila Sherlock 9th Ed. 1

A. 3 mm Hg
B. 6 mm Hg
C. 9 mm Hg
D. 12 mm Hg

1102. All are true regarding hepatic venous system except?
Diseases of liver & biliary system, Sheila Sherlock 9th Ed. 1

A. Hepatic venous blood in ~67% saturated with oxygen
B. Hepatic venous blood is usually sterile
C. Hepatic veins are seven in number
D. Hepatic veins begin as zone 3 veins

1103. Blood of caudate lobe of liver drains into?
Diseases of liver & biliary system, Sheila Sherlock 9th Ed. 1

A. Right hepatic vein
B. Left hepatic vein
C. Middle hepatic vein
D. Inferior vena cava

1104. Right & left lobes of liver are separated inferiorly by?
Diseases of liver & biliary system, Sheila Sherlock 9th Ed. 1

A. Falciform ligament
B. Fissure for ligamentum venosum
C. Fissure for ligamentum teres
D. All of the above

The right and left lobes of liver are separated anteriorly by falciform ligament, posteriorly by fissure for ligamentum venosum and inferiorly by fissure for ligamentum teres.

1105. Capacity of gallbladder is about?
Diseases of liver & biliary system, Sheila Sherlock 9th Ed. 3

A. 20 ml
B. 30 ml
C. 40 ml
D. 50 ml

Gallbladder is a pear shaped bag, ~9 cm long with a capacity of about 50 ml.

1106. Rokitansky-Aschoff sinuses are related to which of the following organs?

Diseases of liver & biliary system, Sheila Sherlock 9th Ed. 4

A. Liver
B. Pancreas
C. Gallbladder
D. Intestine

Rokitansky-Aschoff sinuses are branching evaginations from the lumen into the mucosa and muscularis of the gallbladder.

1107. Which of the following is not a cell type in liver?

Harrison's 20th Ed. Chapter 329 Page 2332

A. Hepatocyte
B. Rho cells
C. Kupffer cells
D. Ito cells

Hepatocytes constitute two-thirds of mass of liver. The remaining cell types are Kupffer cells (RE system), stellate (Ito or fat-storing) cells, endothelial cells and blood vessels, bile ductular cells and supporting structures.

1108. Portal areas from which zone of the hepatic acinus?

Harrison's 20th Ed. Chapter 329 Page 2332

A. Zone 1
B. Zone 2
C. Zone 3
D. Zone 4

Functionally, liver is organized into acini. Hepatic arterial and portal venous blood enter acinus from portal areas (zone 1) and flow through the sinusoids to terminal hepatic veins (zone 3). Intervening hepatocytes constitute zone 2.

1109. "Central veins" in liver are also called?

Harrison's 20th Ed. Chapter 329 Page 2332

A. Terminal hepatic veins
B. Terminal portal veins
C. Terminal sinusoidal veins
D. All of the above

Blood from portal areas is distributed through sinusoids, passing from zone 1 to zone 3 of acinus and draining into terminal hepatic veins ("central veins").

1110. In hepatic acinus, secreted bile flows in which of the following direction?

Harrison's 20th Ed. Chapter 329 Page 2332

A. Zone 1 to zone 3
B. Zone 3 to zone 1
C. Zone 1 to zone 2
D. Zone 2 to zone 1

In hepatic acinus, secreted bile flows in a counter current pattern from zone 3 to zone 1.

1111. Which of the following is false about subendothelial space of Disse?

Harrison's 20th Ed. Chapter 329 Page 2332

A. Plasma is in direct contact with hepatocytes
B. Lined by basolateral side of the hepatocyte
C. Stellate cells are located in it
D. None of the above

The plasma is in direct contact with hepatocytes in the subendothelial space of Disse.

1112. Kupffer cells are best described as?

Harrison's 20th Ed. Chapter 329 Page 2332

A. Peripheral T lymphocytes
B. Circulating B lymphocytes
C. Fixed macrophages
D. None of the above

Kupffer cells lie within sinusoidal vascular space & represent largest group of fixed macrophages in body.

1113. Hepatocytes produce which of the following?

Harrison's 20th Ed. Chapter 329 Page 2332

A. Cholesterol
B. Lecithin
C. Phospholipids
D. All of the above

Hepatocytes produce bile and its carriers i.e. bile acids, cholesterol, lecithin, phospholipids.

1114. Liver regulates which of the following nutrients?

Harrison's 20th Ed. Chapter 329 Page 2332

A. Glycogen
B. Cholesterol
C. Amino acids
D. All of the above

1115. Which out of the following is the more liver-specific symptom?

Harrison's 20th Ed. Chapter 329 Page 2333

A. Nausea
B. Bloating
C. Poor appetite
D. Malaise

Constitutional symptoms of liver disease include fatigue, weakness, nausea, poor appetite, and malaise. More liver-specific symptoms include jaundice, dark urine, light stools, itching, abdominal pain, and bloating.

1116. Most common & most characteristic symptom of liver disease is?

Harrison's 20th Ed. Chapter 329 Page 2333

A. Fatigue
B. Nausea
C. Poor appetite
D. Itching

Fatigue is the most common & most characteristic symptom of liver disease. It typically arises after activity or exercise & is rarely present or severe in the morning after adequate rest. Fatigue in liver disease is often intermittent and variable in severity from hour to hour and day to day.

1117. Severe right upper quadrant pain ("liver pain") is most typical of all except?

Harrison's 20th Ed. Chapter 329 Page 2333

A. Gallbladder disease
B. Liver abscess
C. Severe veno-occlusive disease
D. Acute hepatitis

Right upper quadrant severe pain is most typical of gallbladder disease, liver abscess, and severe veno-occlusive disease but is an occasional accompaniment of acute hepatitis.

1118. Which of the following is the most reliable marker of severity of liver disease?
Harrison's 20th Ed. Chapter 329 Page 2333

A. Jaundice
B. Serum albumin
C. Prothrombin time
D. Hepatic enzymes

Jaundice is the hallmark symptom of liver disease & perhaps the most reliable marker of severity.

1119. Jaundice without dark urine indicates which of the following?
Harrison's 20th Ed. Chapter 329 Page 2333

A. Hemolytic anemia
B. Gilbert's syndrome
C. Crigler-Najjar syndrome
D. All of the above

Jaundice without dark urine indicates indirect (unconjugated) hyperbilirubinemia and is typical of hemolytic anemia, Gilbert's syndrome and Crigler-Najjar syndrome.

1120. In Gilbert's syndrome, jaundice is more noticeable after which of the following?
Harrison's 20th Ed. Chapter 329 Page 2333

A. Fasting
B. Overnight sleep
C. Exposure to sun
D. All of the above

In Gilbert's syndrome, jaundice is more noticeable after fasting and with stress.

1121. Which of the following statements about hepatitis C is false?
Harrison's 20th Ed. Chapter 329 Page 2333

A. Sexual exposure is a rare mode of spread
B. Maternal-infant transmission occurs
C. No means of prevention of vertical spread
D. None of the above

Vertical spread of hepatitis C occurs uncommonly. Sexual exposure is a common mode of spread of hepatitis B and hepatitis C.

1122. Single most common risk factor for hepatitis C is?
Harrison's 20th Ed. Chapter 329 Page 2333

A. Blood transfusion
B. Injection drug use
C. Maternal-infant transmission
D. Sexual exposure

Injection drug use is now the single most common risk factor for hepatitis C.

1123. Screening for antibody to hepatitis B & C was introduced in?
Harrison's 20th Ed. Chapter 329 Page 2333

A. 1982 & 1990 respectively
B. 1984 & 1991 respectively
C. 1986 & 1992 respectively
D. 1988 & 1993 respectively

Screening for antibody to hepatitis B core antigen was introduced 1986 and for hepatitis C in 1992.

1124. An average drink representing how many grams of alcohol?
Harrison's 20th Ed. Chapter 329 Page 2334

A. 5 - 10 grams
B. 8 - 12 grams
C. 11 - 15 grams
D. 15 - 19 grams

An average drink representing 11–15 grams of alcohol.

1125. What quantity of alcohol consumption per day is associated with an increased rate of alcoholic liver disease in men?
Harrison's 20th Ed. Chapter 329 Page 2334

A. 10 to 25 grams
B, 25 to 33 grams
C. 33 to 45 grams
D. 45 to 62 grams

1126. What quantity of alcohol consumption per day is associated with an increased rate of alcoholic liver disease in women?
Harrison's 20th Ed. Chapter 329 Page 2334

A. 10 to 22 grams
B, 22 to 30 grams
C. 33 to 45 grams
D. 45 to 62 grams

Alcohol consumption associated with an increased rate of alcoholic liver disease is probably more than 22–30 gram per day in women and 33–45 gram in men.

1127. Alcoholism is usually defined by the?
Harrison's 20th Ed. Chapter 329 Page 2334

A. Amount of alcohol
B. Type of alcohol
C. Consequences of alcohol intake
D. All of the above

Alcoholism is usually defined by behavioral patterns & consequences of alcohol intake, not by the amount.

1128. Of the following, which is considered the more serious & advanced form of alcoholism?
Harrison's 20th Ed. Chapter 329 Page 2334

A. Abuse
B. Binge
C. Dependence
D. All of the above

Abuse is defined by a repetitive pattern of drinking alcohol that has adverse effects on social, family, occupational or health status. Dependence is defined by alcohol-seeking behavior, despite its adverse effects. Dependence is considered the more serious & advanced form of alcoholism.

1129. CAGE questionnaire is used for?
Harrison's 20th Ed. Chapter 329 Page 2334 Table 329-2

A. Sexual behaviour
B. Cigarette smoking
C. Alcohol dependence & abuse
D. None of the above

One "yes" response of the four questions in CAGE questionnaire should raise suspicion of an alcohol use problem, and more than one is a strong indication that alcohol abuse or dependence exists.

1130. In CAGE questionnaire, "C" refers to?
Harrison's 20th Ed. Chapter 329 Page 2334 Table 329-2

A. Continuous
B. Cut
C. Craving
D. Constant

C = Cut, A = Annoyed, G = Guilty, E = Eyeopener. One "yes" response should raise suspicion of an alcohol use problem, and more than one is a strong indication that abuse or dependence exists.

1131. Which of the following is an inherited liver disease?
Harrison's 20th Ed. Chapter 329 Page 2334

A. Wilson's disease
B. Hemochromatosis
C. a_1 antitrypsin (a1AT) deficiency
D. All of the above

1132. Which of the following is an inherited pediatric liver disease?
Harrison's 20th Ed. Chapter 329 Page 2334

A. Familial intrahepatic cholestasis
B. Benign recurrent intrahepatic cholestasis
C. Alagille syndrome
D. All of the above

1133. Which of the following mutations is typical of genetic hemochromatosis?
Harrison's 20th Ed. Chapter 329 Page 2334

A. 167delT
B. G1896A
C. H63D
D. FIC1

C282Y & H63D mutations in HFE gene are typical of genetic hemochromatosis.

1134. Which of the following statements is false?
Harrison's 20th Ed. Chapter 329 Page 2334

A. Muscle wasting is a sign of advanced liver disease
B. Palmar erythema occurs in acute liver disease
C. Jaundice may be detectable with S. bilirubin <2.5 mg/dL
D. None of the above

Signs of advanced liver disease include muscle wasting, ascites, edema, bruising, dilated abdominal veins, hepatic fetor, asterixis, mental confusion, stupor, and coma. During recovery phase, jaundice may be detectable with S. bilirubin <2.5 mg/dL. Spider angiomata & palmar erythema occur in both acute & chronic liver disease.

1135. Which of the following best relates to asterixis?
Harrison's 20th Ed. Chapter 428 Page 3138

A. Action myoclonus
B. Negative myoclonus
C. Dystonia
D. Paroxysmal dyskinesia

Negative myoclonus consists of a brief loss of muscle activity, exemplified by asterixis in hepatic failure.

1136. Asterixis is seen in which of the following?
Harrison's 20th Ed. Chapter 300 Page 2071

A. Hepatic encephalopathy
B. Hypercapnia
C. Uremia
D. All of the above

Asterixis is not specific to liver disease but also appears in encephalopathy from other causes like hypercapnia, uremia or drug intoxication. Unilateral asterixis indicates structural disease in the contralateral brain.

1137. Which of the following about spider angiomata is false?
Harrison's 20th Ed. Chapter 329 Page 2334

A. Occur in acute & chronic liver disease
B. Occur during pregnancy
C. Occur only on arms, face & upper torso
D. None of the above

Spider angiomata occur only on the arms, face, and upper torso. Spider angiomata and palmar erythema occur in both acute and chronic liver disease and are prominent in cirrhosis, but they can occur in normal individuals and are frequently present during pregnancy.

1138. The nature of vessel involved in spider angiomata is?
Harrison's 20th Ed. Chapter 329 Page 2334

A. Artery
B. Arteriole
C. Vein
D. Capillary

Spider angiomata are superficial, tortuous arterioles & fill from center outwards & can be pulsatile. Spider telangiectasia has three components: (1) central arteriole ("body" of the spider) that can be seen to pulsate when compressed slightly with a glass slide; (2) multiple radiating "legs"; and (3) surrounding erythema, which may encompass the entire lesion or only its central portion. After blanching, returning blood fills central arteriole first before traveling to the peripheral tips of each leg.

1139. Spiders are most numerous on?
Harrison's 20th Ed. Chapter 329 Page 2334

A. Face
B. Palms
C. Soles
D. Scalp

Spiders are most numerous on face & neck, followed by shoulders, thorax, arms, and hands. They are rare on palms, scalp, and below the umbilicus. This peculiar distribution may reflect the neurohormonal properties of the microcirculation, because it is similar to the distribution of where blushing is most intense.

1140. Acquired vascular spiders are associated with?
Harrison's 20th Ed. Chapter 329 Page 2334

A. Liver disease
B. Pregnancy
C. Malnutrition
D. All of the above

Acquired vascular spiders are associated with liver disease, pregnancy and malnutrition. Vascular spiders were first described by the English physician Erasmus Wilson in 1867.

1141. Marked hepatomegaly is typical of?
Harrison's 20th Ed. Chapter 329 Page 2334

A. Cirrhosis
B. Sinusoidal obstruction syndrome
C. Alcoholic hepatitis
D. All of the above

Marked hepatomegaly is typical of cirrhosis, sinusoidal obstruction syndrome, infiltrative disorders (amyloidosis, metastatic, or primary cancers of the liver) and alcoholic hepatitis.

1142. Most reliable physical finding in examining the liver is?

Harrison's 20th Ed. Chapter 329 Page 2334

A. Size
B. Shape
C. Tenderness
D. Liver edge

Most reliable physical finding in examining the liver is hepatic tenderness.

1143. Foetor hepaticus best relates to?

Harrison's 20th Ed. Chapter 337 Page 2413

A. Vaptan
B. Mercaptan
C. Mercaptoethane
D. Mercaptoethanesulfonate

1144. Foetor hepaticus best relates to?

Br J Gen Pract. 2012;62(605):652-653

A. Dimethylformamide
B. Dimethylarginine
C. Dimethyl disulphide
D. Dimethyltryptamine

Foetor hepaticus is a feature of severe liver disease; a sweet & musty smell both on breath and in urine. It is caused by excretion of dimethyl disulphide & methyl mercaptan (CH_3SH), arising from an excess of methionine.

1145. In chronic liver disease, encephalopathy is triggered by?

Harrison's 20th Ed. Chapter 329 Page 2335

A. Infection
B. Constipation
C. Use of narcotic analgesics
D. All of the above

In chronic liver disease, encephalopathy is triggered by gastrointestinal bleeding, over-diuresis, uremia, dehydration, electrolyte imbalance, infection, constipation, or use of narcotic analgesics.

1146. Which of the following is a test of mental status in hepatic encephalopathy?

Harrison's 20th Ed. Chapter 329 Page 2335

A. Trail-making test
B. Comparison of signatures
C. Drawing abstract objects
D. All of the above

Mental status examination for hepatic encephalopathy include trail-making test, drawing abstract objects or comparison of a signature to previous ones.

1147. Which of the following is false about trail-making test?

Harrison's 20th Ed. Chapter 329 Page 2335

A. Series of 10 numbered circles
B. Normal time for connect-the-dot test is 15-30 seconds
C. Considerable delay means early hepatic encephalopathy
D. None of the above

Mental status examination by trail-making test consists of a series of 25 numbered circles that the patient is asked to connect as rapidly as possible using a pencil. Normal range for connect-the-dot test is 15-30 seconds. Delay means early hepatic encephalopathy.

1148. Which of the following is not a feature of hepatopulmonary syndrome?

Harrison's 20th Ed. Chapter 329 Page 2335

A. Hypoxemia
B. Pulmonary arteriovenous shunting
C. Orthodeoxia
D. Hypercarbia

Hepatopulmonary syndrome is defined by the triad of liver disease, hypoxemia and pulmonary arteriovenous shunting. It is characterized by platypnea and orthodeoxia, representing shortness of breath and oxygen desaturation that occur upon assuming an upright position.

1149. Slate-gray pigmentation to the skin also occurs with?

Harrison's 20th Ed. Chapter 329 Page 2335

A. Primary biliary cirrhosis
B. Sclerosing cholangitis
C. Xanthelasma
D. Hemochromatosis

A slate-gray pigmentation of the skin occurs in hemochromatosis, if iron levels are high for a prolonged period.

1150. Mucocutaneous vasculitis with palpable purpura is typical of?

Harrison's 20th Ed. Chapter 329 Page 2335

A. Primary biliary cirrhosis
B. Primary hepatocellular carcinoma
C. Cryoglobulinemia of chronic hepatitis C
D. Wilsons disease

Mucocutaneous vasculitis with palpable purpura on lower extremities is typical of cryoglobulinemia of chronic hepatitis C.

1151. Kayser-Fleischer rings are a finding in?

Harrison's 20th Ed. Chapter 329 Page 2335

A. Primary biliary cirrhosis
B. Primary hepatocellular carcinoma
C. Wilson's disease
D. Hemochromatosis

Kayser-Fleischer rings occur in Wilson's disease also called hepatolenticular degeneration/ Westphal-Strumpell disease/Westphal pseudosclerosis. Bernhard Kayser and Bruno Fleischer were German ophthalmologists.

1152. Which of the following statements about Kayser-Fleischer ring is false?

Br J Ophthalmol 2002;86:114

A. Found in 95% of patients of Wilson's disease
B. All patients with KF rings have neurological manifestations
C. Density of a KF ring correlates with severity of WD
D. None of the above

K-F-like ring has been reported in many other conditions like cryptogenic cirrhosis, chronic active hepatitis, neonatal hepatitis, primary biliary cirrhosis, cholestatic cirrhosis, hepatocellular disorders (when bilirubin rises acutely above 20mg/dl), alcoholic liver disease, galactosialidosis, schistosoma infection, multiple myeloma and intraocular foreign body containing copper.

1153. The color of Kayser-Fleischer ring is?

Harrison's 20th Ed. Chapter 329 Page 2335

A. Yellow-red
B. Yellow-green
C. Golden-brown
D. Green-brown

Kayser-Fleischer rings consist of a golden-brown copper pigment deposited in Descemet's membrane at the periphery of the cornea—sclero-corneal junction. It may regress or disappear when systemic condition is well treated. It is usually bilateral & appears initially superiorly at 10 to 2 o'clock position, then inferiorly and later becomes circumferential.

1154. Wilson's disease is due to defect in?
Harrison's 20th Ed. Chapter 408 Page 2982

A. ATP6B gene
B. ATP7B gene
C. ATP8B gene
D. ATP9B gene

Wilson disease is an autosomal recessive disorder caused by mutations in the ATP7B gene, a membrane-bound copper-transporting ATPase. ATP7B facilitates the transfer of copper into Golgi apparatus where it combines with ceruloplasmin. Failure of this process leads to instability and decreased half life of ceruloplasmin and paradoxical ceruloplasmin deficiency. Free circulating copper accumulates in liver cytosol resulting in hepatocyte degeneration and cirrhosis. Other hepatic conditions as listed above that prevent elimination of copper, or intraocular foreign bodies containing copper, lead to elevated free copper concentrations and K-F ring.

1155. Wilson's disease can produce a cataract described as?
Harrison's 20th Ed. Chapter 408 Page 2983

A. Christmas tree
B. Palm tree
C. Sunflower
D. Rose flower

Sunflower cataracts & Kayser-Fleischer rings (copper deposits in the outer rim of cornea) are seen in Wilson's disease.

1156. Testing for P-ANCA is for the diagnosis of which of the following?
Harrison's 20th Ed. Chapter 329 Page 2335 Table 329-3

A. Primary biliary cirrhosis
B. Primary sclerosing cholangitis
C. Autoimmune hepatitis
D. Nonalcoholic steatohepatitis

1157. Most common causes of chronic liver disease is?
Harrison's 20th Ed. Chapter 329 Page 2335

A. Chronic hepatitis C
B. Alcoholic liver disease
C. Chronic hepatitis B
D. Autoimmune hepatitis

Most common causes of chronic liver disease in general order of frequency are chronic hepatitis C, alcoholic liver disease, nonalcoholic steatohepatitis, chronic hepatitis B, autoimmune hepatitis, sclerosing cholangitis, primary biliary cirrhosis, hemochromatosis, and Wilson disease.

1158. Liver biopsy plays an important role in the diagnosis of?
Harrison's 20th Ed. Chapter 329 Page 2335

A. Autoimmune hepatitis
B. Primary biliary cholangitis
C. Nonalcoholic and alcoholic steatohepatitis
D. All of the above

Liver biopsy plays an important role in the diagnosis of autoimmune hepatitis, primary biliary cholangitis, nonalcoholic & alcoholic steatohepatitis and Wilson disease.

1159. γ-glutamyl transpeptidase (γGT) best relates to?
Harrison's 20th Ed. Chapter 329 Page 2335

A. Serum alanine aminotransferase (ALT)
B. Serum aspartate aminotransferase (AST)
C. Serum alkaline phosphatase (AlkP)
D. Serum bilirubin

γ-glutamyl transpeptidase (γGT) estimation helps to define whether alkaline phosphatase (AlkP) elevations are due to liver disease.

1160. ERCP is more valuable in evaluating which of the following?
Harrison's 20th Ed. Chapter 329 Page 2336

A. Pancreatitis
B. Primary sclerosing cholangitis
C. Choledocholithiasis
D. Fatty liver

ERCP is more valuable in evaluating ampullary lesions and primary sclerosing cholangitis.

1161. Which of the following liver cells is the primary source of extracellular matrix?
N Engl J Med. 2015;372:1138-49

A. Kupffer cell
B. Hepatic stellate cell
C. Endothelial cell
D. All of the above

Hepatic stellate cells appear to be the primary source of extracellular matrix. Stellate cell is pericyte-like, undergoing transformation into myofibroblast in response to injury.

1162. Hepatic stellate cells or HSCs are also called?
Biomarker Insights. 2012;7:105-117

A. Vitamin A-storing cells
B. Lipocytes
C. Ito cells
D. All of the above

1163. Vitamin A is stored in the cytoplasm of Hepatic stellate cells (HSCs) as?
Biomarker Insights. 2012;7:105-117

A. Retinyl sialate
B. Retinyl palmitate
C. Retinyl stearate
D. Retinyl fumarate

Hepatic stellate cells (HSCs) are the key fibrogenic cells and their 'activation' is the dominant event in fibrogenesis. Activation of HSCs refers to conversion of quiescent, vitamin A-storing cells into proliferative, fibrogenic & contractile myofibroblasts which can synthesize & secrete large amounts of fibril-forming collagens, particularly collagen type I and III. HSCs, also called vitamin A-storing cells, lipocytes, interstitial cells, fat-storing cells, Ito cells, exist in the space between parenchymal cells & sinusoidal endothelial cells of hepatic lobule, and store 80% of vitamin A in the whole body as retinyl palmitate in lipid droplets in the cytoplasm.

1164. Which of the following is the major stimulus for HSCs to synthesize extracellular matrix (ECM)?
Biomarker Insights. 2012;7:105-117

A. TNF-α
B. TGF-β
C. IL-6
D. INF-γ

TGF-β is the major stimulus for HSCs to synthesize ECM. Platelet-derived growth factor (PDGF), mainly produced by Kupffer cells, is a potent fibrogenic growth factor known to synergize with TGF-β.

1165. Normal AST/ALT ratio in healthy subjects is?
Biomarker Insights. 2012;7:105-117

A. 0.4
B. 0.6
C. 0.8
D. 1.0

Ratio of AST to ALT tends to increase with advancing stages of fibrosis from ~0.8 in healthy subjects. A ratio of more than 1 suggests the presence of cirrhosis.

1166. Which of the following variable is used in calculating AST-to-platelet ratio index (APRI)?

Harrison's 20th Ed. Chapter 329 Page 2337, Biomarker Insights. 2012;7:105-117

A. AST value
B. Upper limit of normal range of AST
C. Platelet count
D. All of the above

The AST-to-platelet ratio index (APRI) is calculated as (AST/upper limit of normal range)/platelet count (10^9/L) × 100.

1167. Which of the following is a serum biochemical marker associated with hepatic fibrosis?

Harrison's 20th Ed. Chapter 329 Page 2337 Table 329-4

A. Alpha-2-macroglobulin
B. Apolipoprotein A1
C. Haptoglobin
D. All of the above

The fibrotest is a composite of five serum biochemical markers i.e. alpha-2-macroglobulin, apolipoprotein A1, haptoglobin, γ-glutamyl transpeptidase, and bilirubin associated with hepatic fibrosis.

1168. Which of the following is a numerical scales for grading activity in chronic liver disease?

Harrison's 20th Ed. Chapter 329 Page 2337

A. METAVIR
B. Knodell histology activity index
C. Ishak fibrosis scale
D. All of the above

Numerical scales for grading activity in chronic liver disease, the most commonly used are the METAVIR, Knodell histology activity index, Ishak fibrosis scale (modified Knodell score) and International Association for Study of the Liver system.

1169. Stage F4 on the METAVIR fibrosis score means?

N Engl J Med. 2014;371:2375-82

A. No fibrosis
B. Portal fibrosis without septa
C. Fibrosis consistent with compensated cirrhosis
D. Fibrosis consistent with decompensated cirrhosis

METAVIR fibrosis score for chronic hepatitis ranges from F0 to F4, with F0 indicating no fibrosis and F4 fibrosis consistent with compensated cirrhosis. F0 (no fibrosis), F1 (portal fibrosis without septa), F2 (portal fibrosis with few septa), F3 (numerous septa without cirrhosis) and F4 (cirrhosis). Also, A0 (No activity), A1 (Mild activity), A2 (Moderate activity) and A3 (Severe activity).

1170. METAVIR stands for?

N Engl J Med. 2014;371:2375-82

A. Meta-analysis of Histological Data in Viral Hepatitis
B. Meta-analysis of Histological Data in Virology
C. Meta-analysis of Histological Data in Viral diseases
D. Meta-analysis of Histological Data in Viral infections

1171. Which of the following is activated on the surface of stellate cells triggering fibrogenesis?

N Engl J Med. 2015;372:1138-49

A. Toll-like receptor 1 (TLR1)
B. Toll-like receptor 2 (TLR2)
C. Toll-like receptor 3 (TLR3)
D. Toll-like receptor 4 (TLR4)

A pathway that is unique to liver involves toll-like receptor 4 (TLR4) that is activated on surface of stellate cells by intestinal bacterial LPS derived from gut, triggering cell activation & fibrogenesis. TLR4 expression is associated with portal inflammation & fibrosis in patients with fatty liver disease.

1172. Which of the following is often the first indication of worsening fibrosis in liver cirrhosis?

Harrison's 20th Ed. Chapter 329 Page 2337

A. Mild elevations of bilirubin
B. Prolongation of prothrombin time
C. Slight decreases in serum albumin
D. Mild thrombocytopenia

Noninvasive tests that suggest advanced liver fibrosis include mild elevations of bilirubin, prolongation of prothrombin time, slight decreases in serum albumin, and mild thrombocytopenia (which is often the first indication of worsening fibrosis).

1173. Which of the following is not a factor in Child-Pugh classification of cirrhosis liver?

Harrison's 20th Ed. Chapter 329 Page 2337

A. Serum bilirubin
B. SGPT
C. Ascites
D. Hepatic encephalopathy

Factors included in Child-Pugh classification of cirrhosis liver are serum bilirubin, serum albumin, prothrombin time, ascites & hepatic encephalopathy.

1174. Child-Pugh score can predict which of the following?

Harrison's 20th Ed. Chapter 329 Page 2337

A. Bleeding from varices
B. Spontaneous bacterial peritonitis
C. Need for liver transplantation
D. All of the above

Child-Pugh score is a reliable predictor of bleeding from varices, spontaneous bacterial peritonitis and need for liver transplantation.

1175. Decompensation indicates cirrhosis with a Child-Pugh score of?

Harrison's 20th Ed. Chapter 329 Page 2337 Table 329-4

A. 4
B. 5
C. 6
D. 7

The Child-Pugh score is calculated by adding the scores of the five factors and can range from 5 to 15. Child-Pugh class is either A (a score of 5 to 6), B (7 to 9), or C (10 or above). Decompensation indicates cirrhosis with a Child-Pugh score of 7 or more (Class B).

1176. MELD score is used for?

Harrison's 20th Ed. Chapter 329 Page 2337

A. Assessing bleeding from varices
B. Assessing hepatocellular carcinoma
C. Assessing spontaneous bacterial peritonitis
D. Assessing need for liver transplantation

Model for end-stage liver disease (MELD) score is used for assessing the need for liver transplantation.

1177. Variables for calculation of MELD score include all except?

Harrison's 20th Ed. Chapter 329 Page 2337

A. Prothrombin time

B. Serum bilirubin

C. Blood urea

D. Serum creatinine

MELD score is a prospectively derived scoring system calculated using three noninvasive variables—prothrombin time (INR), serum bilirubin and serum creatinine.

1178. System similar to MELD used for children below the age of 12 is termed?

Harrison's 20th Ed. Chapter 329 Page 2337

A. CELD

B. SELD

C. PELD

D. KELD

System similar to MELD using bilirubin, INR, serum albumin, age, and nutritional status is used for children below the age of 12 is PELD.

Evaluation of Liver Function

1179. Which of the following liver function tests do not measure liver function at all?
Harrison's 20th Ed. Chapter 330 Page 2338

A. S. Bilirubin
B. S. Aminotransferases
C. S. Albumin
D. Prothrombin time

Aminotransferases or alkaline phosphatase do not measure liver function at all.

1180. Upper limit of normal for conjugated bilirubin is?
Harrison's 20th Ed. Chapter 330 Page 2338

A. 0.2 mg/dL
B. 0.3 mg/dL
C. 0.4 mg/dL
D. 0.5 mg/dL

The most frequently reported upper limit of normal for conjugated bilirubin is 0.3 mg/dL. If the direct-acting fraction is <15% of the total, all bilirubin can be considered to be indirect.

1181. Which of the following statements is false?
Harrison's 20th Ed. Chapter 330 Page 2338

A. Elevation of unconjugated bilirubin is rarely due to liver disease
B. Conjugated hyperbilirubinemia almost always implies liver or biliary tract disease
C. Rate-limiting step in bilirubin metabolism is bilirubin conjugation
D. In most liver diseases, both conjugated & unconjugated bilirubin are elevated

The rate-limiting step in bilirubin metabolism is not conjugation of bilirubin, but transport of conjugated bilirubin into bile canaliculi.

1182. Which of the following about liver functions is false?
Harrison's 20th Ed. Chapter 330 Page 2338

A. Increased unconjugated bilirubin is rarely due to liver disease
B. Conjugated hyperbilirubinemia almost always implies liver or biliary tract disease
C. In most liver diseases, both conjugated & unconjugated bilirubin are elevated
D. None of the above

1183. Isolated elevation of unconjugated bilirubin is seen in?
Harrison's 20th Ed. Chapter 330 Page 2338

A. Hemolytic disorders
B. Crigler-Najjar syndrome
C. Gilbert's syndrome
D. All of the above

Isolated elevation of unconjugated bilirubin is seen in hemolytic disorders, Crigler-Najjar & Gilbert's syndromes.

1184. Total serum bilirubin correlates with poor outcomes in?
Harrison's 20th Ed. Chapter 330 Page 2338

A. Alcoholic hepatitis
B. Autoimmune hepatitis
C. Hepatocellular carcinome
D. All of the above

Total serum bilirubin correlates with poor outcomes in alcoholic hepatitis.

1185. In isolated unconjugated hyperbilirubinemia, of the total bilirubin, the direct bilirubin is?
Harrison's 20th Ed. Chapter 330 Page 2338

A. < 15%
B. < 20%
C. < 25%
D. < 30%

In isolated unconjugated hyperbilirubinemia, serum bilirubin is elevated but direct bilirubin is <15%.

1186. In liver disease, rate-limiting step in bilirubin metabolism is?
Harrison's 20th Ed. Chapter 330 Page 2338

A. Entry of bilirubin in hepatocyte
B. Conjugation of bilirubin in hepatocyte
C. Transport of conjugated bilirubin into bile canaliculi
D. All of the above

Rate-limiting step in bilirubin metabolism is not conjugation of bilirubin, but transport of conjugated bilirubin into the bile canaliculi.

1187. Total serum bilirubin correlates with poor outcomes in?
Harrison's 20th Ed. Chapter 330 Page 2338

A. Viral hepatitis
B. Alcoholic hepatitis
C. Drug-induced liver disease
D. All of the above

Serum bilirubin serves as a prognostic marker in viral hepatitis, alcoholic hepatitisin MELD score, drug-induced liver disease indicates more severe injury.

1188. Bilirubin found in urine is?
Harrison's 20th Ed. Chapter 330 Page 2338

A. Unconjugated
B. Conjugated
C. Unconjugated + conjugated
D. All of the above

Unconjugated bilirubin always binds to albumin in serum and is not filtered by kidney. Therefore, any bilirubin found in urine is conjugated bilirubin and bilirubinuria implies the presence of liver disease.

1189. Which of the following may give a false-positive reading with Ictotest tablet?
Harrison's 20th Ed. Chapter 330 Page 2338

A. Barbiturates
B. Phenothiazines
C. Antacids
D. NSAIDs

Phenothiazines may give a false-positive reading with Ictotest tablet.

1190. Which of the following is true in patients recovering from jaundice?

Harrison's 20th Ed. Chapter 330 Page 2338

A. Urine bilirubin clears prior to serum bilirubin
B. Serum bilirubin clears prior to urine bilirubin
C. Urine and serum bilirubin clear simultaneously
D. Any of the above

In patients recovering from jaundice, the urine bilirubin clears prior to the serum bilirubin.

1191. Aspartate aminotransferase (AST) found in all except?

Harrison's 20th Ed. Chapter 330 Page 2339

A. Skeletal muscle
B. Kidneys
C. Spleen
D. Lungs

1192. Aspartate aminotransferase (AST) not found in?

Harrison's 20th Ed. Chapter 330 Page 2339

A. Leukocytes
B. Erythrocytes
C. Platelets
D. All of the above

1193. Least concentration of AST is in?

Harrison's 20th Ed. Chapter 330 Page 2339

A. Brain
B. Erythrocytes
C. Lungs
D. Pancreas

AST is found in liver, cardiac muscle, skeletal muscle, kidneys, brain, pancreas, lungs, leukocytes, & erythrocytes in decreasing order of concentration.

1194. Aminotransferase level elevation up to what level are considered nonspecific?

Harrison's 20th Ed. Chapter 330 Page 2339

A. 100 U/L
B. 200 U/L
C. 300 U/L
D. 400 U/L

1195. Elevation of aminotransferases to >1000 U/L occurs in which of the following disorders?

Harrison's 20th Ed. Chapter 330 Page 2339

A. Viral hepatitis
B. Ischemic liver injury
C. Toxin or drug-induced liver injury
D. All of the above

Aminotransferase levels of up to 300 U/L are nonspecific and may be found in any type of liver disorder. Aminotransferases levels of >1000 U/L occur in disorders associated with extensive hepatocellular injury like viral hepatitis, ischemic liver injury, and toxin or drug induced liver injury.

1196. What AST : ALT ratio is highly suggestive of alcoholic liver disease?

Harrison's 20th Ed. Chapter 330 Page 2339

A. > 1.5:1
B. > 2:1
C. > 2.5:1
D. > 3:1

An AST:ALT ratio >2:1 is suggestive while a ratio >3:1 is highly suggestive of alcoholic liver disease.

1197. Which of the following about alcoholic liver disease is false?

Harrison's 20th Ed. Chapter 330 Page 2339

A. AST rarely > 300 U/L
B. ALT often normal
C. Increase in IgA levels
D. None of the above

AST in alcoholic liver disease is rarely >300 U/L and ALT is often normal. Increases in IgA levels occur in alcoholic liver disease.

1198. Which of the following about aminotransferases is false?

Harrison's 20th Ed. Chapter 330 Page 2339

A. Aminotransferases are present in serum in low concentrations
B. Liver cell necrosis not required for release of aminotransferases
C. Absolute elevation of aminotransferases is of no prognostic significance in acute hepatocellular disorders
D. None of the above

1199. Low serum ALT in alcoholic liver disease is due to alcohol-induced deficiency of?

Harrison's 20th Ed. Chapter 330 Page 2339

A. Pyridoxal sulphate
B. Pyridoxal phosphate
C. Pyridoxal gluconate
D. Pyridoxal chloride

A low level of ALT in the serum is due to an alcohol-induced deficiency of pyridoxal phosphate.

1200. Which of the following enzymes is elevated in cholestasis?

Harrison's 20th Ed. Chapter 330 Page 2340

A. Alkaline phosphatase
B. 5'-nucleotidase
C. Gamma glutamyl transpeptidase (GGT)
D. All of the above

Alkaline phosphatase, 5'-nucleotidase & GGT are usually elevated in cholestasis.

1201. Which of the following is located in endoplasmic reticulum of hepatocytes?

Harrison's 20th Ed. Chapter 330 Page 2340

A. Alkaline phosphatase
B. 5'-nucleotidase
C. Gamma glutamyl transpeptidase (GGT)
D. All of the above

Alkaline phosphatase and 5'-nucleotidase are found in or near the bile canalicular membrane of hepatocytes, while GGT is located in the endoplasmic reticulum and in bile duct epithelial cells. Serum 5'-nucleotidase or GGT are rarely elevated in conditions other than liver disease.

1202. Elevated heat-stable fraction of serum alkaline phosphatase suggests its origin from?

Harrison's 20th Ed. Chapter 330 Page 2340

A. Liver
B. Bone
C. Placenta
D. Intestine

Elevated heat-stable fraction of serum alkaline phosphatase strongly suggests its placental or tumor source. Bone alkaline phosphatase is most susceptible to inactivation by heat.

1203. Individuals of which of the following blood group can have an elevation of serum alkaline phosphatase after eating a fatty meal?

Harrison's 20th Ed. Chapter 330 Page 2340

A. A
B. B
C. AB
D. All of the above

Individuals with blood types O & B can have an elevation of serum alkaline phosphatase after eating a fatty meal due to influx of intestinal alkaline phosphatase into the blood.

1204. In cholestatic liver disorders, alkaline phosphatase elevations are how many times greater than normal?

Harrison's 20th Ed. Chapter 330 Page 2340

A. 2 times
B. 3 times
C. 4 times
D. None of the above

Alkaline phosphatase elevations greater than four times normal occur primarily in cholestatic liver disorders, infiltrative liver diseases and Paget's disease.

1205. Conditions causing isolated elevations of serum alkaline phosphatase include all except?

Harrison's 20th Ed. Chapter 330 Page 2340

A. Hodgkin's disease
B. Inflammatory bowel disease
C. Hypothyroidism
D. Congestive heart failure

Isolated elevations of serum alkaline phosphatase is seen in Hodgkin's disease, diabetes, hyperthyroidism, CHF, amyloidosis and inflammatory bowel disease. Simultaneous measurement of serum 5'-nucleotidase or GGT enzymes helps to differentiate liver disease from others.

1206. Which of the following is not a cause of intrahepatic cholestasis?

Harrison's 20th Ed. Chapter 330 Page 2340

A. Drug-induced hepatitis
B. Sclerosing cholangitis
C. Primary biliary cirrhosis
D. Alcohol-induced steatohepatitis

Intrahepatic cholestasis is due to drug-induced hepatitis, primary biliary cirrhosis, rejection of transplanted livers and alcohol-induced steatohepatitis.

1207. Serum albumin is synthesized by?

Harrison's 20th Ed. Chapter 330 Page 2340

A. Hepatocyte
B. Kidney
C. Intestinal epithelial cells
D. All of the above

Serum albumin is synthesized exclusively by hepatocytes.

1208. Serum albumin has a half-life of?

Harrison's 20th Ed. Chapter 330 Page 2340

A. 18 to 20 days
B. 28 to 35 days
C. 35 to 45 days
D. > 60 days

1209. What proportion of albumin is degraded per day?

Harrison's 20th Ed. Chapter 330 Page 2340

A. 2%
B. 4%
C. 6%
D. 8%

Serum albumin has a half-life of 18 to 20 days with approximately 4% degraded per day.

1210. Minimal changes in the serum albumin are seen in?

Harrison's 20th Ed. Chapter 330 Page 2340

A. Viral hepatitis
B. Drug-related hepatotoxicity
C. Obstructive jaundice
D. All of the above

Minimal changes in the serum albumin are seen in acute liver conditions such as viral hepatitis, drug-related hepatotoxicity and obstructive jaundice.

1211. Albumin synthesis is inhibited by?

Harrison's 20th Ed. Chapter 330 Page 2340

A. Serum interleukin 1
B. Cholecystokinin
C. Lipase
D. All of the above

Prolonged increases in levels of serum cytokines IL-1 &/or tumor necrosis factor inhibit albumin synthesis.

1212. Which of the following serum globulins is not produced by hepatocytes?

Harrison's 20th Ed. Chapter 330 Page 2340

A. Alpha globulin
B. Beta globulin
C. Gamma globulin
D. All of the above

Gamma globulins (immunoglobulins) are produced by B lymphocytes and alpha and beta globulins are produced in hepatocytes.

1213. Which of the following statements is false?

Harrison's 20th Ed. Chapter 330 Page 2340

A. Gamma globulins are increased in chronic liver disease
B. IgG levels increase in autoimmune hepatitis
C. IgM levels increase in primary biliary cirrhosis
D. None of the above

In cirrhosis, increased serum gamma globulin concentration is due to increased synthesis of antibodies, some directed against intestinal bacteria because cirrhotic liver fails to clear bacterial antigens. Diffuse polyclonal increases in IgG levels are common in autoimmune hepatitis. Increases in IgM levels are common in primary biliary cirrhosis, while increases in IgA levels occur in alcoholic liver disease.

1214. Which of the following blood clotting factors is not made by hepatocytes?
Harrison's 20th Ed. Chapter 330 Page 2340

A. II
B. V
C. VIII
D. X

With the exception of factor VIII (produced by vascular endothelial cells), blood clotting factors are made exclusively in hepatocytes.

1215. Serum half-life of factor VII is?
Harrison's 20th Ed. Chapter 330 Page 2340

A. 6 hours
B. 24 hours
C. 48 hours
D. 72 hours

Serum half life of factor VII is 6 hours.

1216. Serum half-life of fibrinogen is?
Harrison's 20th Ed. Chapter 330 Page 2340

A. 2 days
B. 3 days
C. 5 days
D. 7 days

Serum half life of fibrinogen is 5 days.

1217. Serum prothrombin time does not measure which of the following factor?
Harrison's 20th Ed. Chapter 330 Page 2340

A. II
B. V
C. IX
D. X

Serum prothrombin time collectively measures factors II, V, VII and X.

1218. Single best acute measure of hepatic synthetic function is?
Harrison's 20th Ed. Chapter 330 Page 2340

A. Serum albumin
B. Serum globulins
C. Clotting factors
D. Serum bilirubin

Because of their rapid turnover, measurement of the clotting factors is the single best acute measure of hepatic synthetic function.

1219. Biosynthesis of factors which of the following factors depends on vitamin K?
Harrison's 20th Ed. Chapter 330 Page 2340

A. II
B. IX
C. X
D. All of the above

Biosynthesis of factors II, VII, IX, and X depends on vitamin K.

1220. Which of the following play a role in detoxification of ammonia?
Harrison's 20th Ed. Chapter 330 Page 2341

A. Spleen
B. Pancreas
C. Striated muscle
D. Cartilage

Liver converts ammonia to urea which is excreted by kidneys. Striated muscles detoxify ammonia by combining it with glutamic acid to form glutamine.

1221. Which of the following tests is useful in diagnosing advanced liver fibrosis?
Harrison's 20th Ed. Chapter 330 Page 2341

A. Haptoglobin
B. Apolipoprotein A-I
C. α2-macroglobulin
D. All of the above

Haptoglobin, bilirubin, GGT, apolipoprotein A-I and α2-macroglobulin are used for diagnosing advanced fibrosis in patients with chronic hepatitis C, chronic hepatitis B, alcoholic liver disease and patients taking methotrexate for psoriasis.

1222. First test ordered in patients suspected of having Budd-Chiari syndrome is?
Harrison's 20th Ed. Chapter 330 Page 2341

A. Percutaneous biopsy of the liver
B. Ultrasonography with Doppler imaging
C. Magnetic resonance cholangiopancreatography (MRCP)
D. Computerized tomography (CT)

Ultrasound with Doppler imaging is the first test ordered in patients suspected of having Budd-Chiari syndrome.

1223. Which of the following about Gilbert's syndrome is false?
Harrison's 20th Ed. Chapter 330 Page 2341 Table 330-1

A. Healthy patient
B. Isolated, unconjugated hyperbilirubinemia
C. Absence of hemolysis
D. None of the above

1224. Which of the following is elevated in Gilbert's syndrome?
Harrison's 20th Ed. Chapter 330 Page 2341 Table 330-1

A. S. Aminotransferases
B. S. Alkaline phosphatase
C. Prothrombin time
D. None of the above

In Hemolysis/Gilbert's syndrome, aminotransferases, alkaline phosphatase, albumin and prothrombin time are normal. There is no bilirubinuria.

Hyperbilirubinemias

1225. Which of the following chemical structure represents bilirubin?

A. $C_{30}H_{36}N_4O_6$
B. $C_{31}H_{36}N_4O_6$
C. $C_{32}H_{36}N_4O_6$
D. $C_{33}H_{36}N_4O_6$

Word bilirubin comes from Latin bilis + ruber meaning red. Bilirubin a a reddish-yellow pigment $C_{33}H_{36}N_4O_6$ that is formed by the breakdown of heme (ferroprotoporphyrin IX). Chemical structure of biliverdin is $C_{33}H_{34}N_4O_6$.

1226. Which of the following contain four pyrrolic rings?

A. Bilirubin
B. Phycobilin
C. Phytochrome
D. All of the above

1227. Which of the following about biliverdin is true?

A. Green tetrapyrrolic bile pigment
B. Red tetrapyrrolic bile pigment
C. Yellow tetrapyrrolic bile pigment
D. Blue tetrapyrrolic bile pigment

1228. Which of the following about urobilinogen is true?
Harrison's 20th Ed. Chapter 45 Page 276

A. Yellow tetrapyrrole
B. Orange tetrapyrrole
C. Green tetrapyrrole
D. Colorless tetrapyrrole

Urobilinogens are colorless because each of the bridges connecting the pyrrole rings is saturated, and the conjugation of double bonds is limited to individual rings.

1229. Which of the following about Heme is true?
Harrison's 20th Ed. Chapter 57 Page 377

A. Iron-chelated tetrapyrrole
B. Zinc-chelated tetrapyrrole
C. Iron-Zinc chelated tetrapyrrole
D. All of the above

Heme is an iron-chelated tetrapyrrole or porphyrin. The most complex known tetrapyrrole is cobalt-containing cobalamin (vitamin B12).

1230. Term linear tetrapyrrole best relates to?
Harrison's 20th Ed. Chapter 409 Page 2987

A. Uroporphyrinogen III
B. Hydroxymethylbilane
C. Coproporphyrinogen III
D. 5-aminolevulinic acid

In contrast to cyclic tetrapyrroles, linear tetrapyrroles do not contain a tightly bound metal. Light-responsive regulatory systems utilize linear tetrapyrroles as cofactors.

1231. What proportion of bilirubin is derived from degradation of the hemoglobin of senescent red blood cells?
Harrison's 20th Ed. Chapter 331 Page 2342

A. ~ 30 - 50%
B. ~ 50 - 70%
C. ~ 70 - 90%
D. ~ 100%

About 70–90% of bilirubin is derived from degradation of the hemoglobin of senescent red blood cells. Rest comes from degradation of cytochromes and others.

1232. In a normal adult, what quantity of bilirubin is produced daily?
Front. Pharmacol. 2017;8:887

A. 50 – 150 mg
B. 200 – 300 mg
C. 300 – 500 mg
D. 500 – 7500 mg

Bilirubin (BR) is a tetrapyrrolic pigment found in plasma as an albumin-bound reversible complex. It is derived from catabolism of heme, released by hemoglobin (75%) and cytochromes (25%), with a daily production of about 200–300 mg. in a normal healthy adult.

1233. Glutathione-S-transferase (GST) is related to which of the following steps in bilirubin metabolism?
Harrison's 20th Ed. Chapter 331 Page 2342

A. Hepatocellular uptake
B. Intracellular binding
C. Conjugation
D. Biliary excretion

After hepatocellular uptake, bilirubin is kept in solution by binding to glutathione-S-transferases formerly called ligandins.

1234. Bilirubin-UDP-glucuronosyltransferase (UGT1A1) is related to which of the following steps in bilirubin metabolism?
Harrison's 20th Ed. Chapter 331 Page 2342

A. Hepatocellular uptake
B. Intracellular binding
C. Conjugation
D. Biliary excretion

Bilirubin is conjugated with one or two glucuronic acid moieties by a specific UDP-glucuronosyltransferase to form bilirubin mono- and diglucuronide, respectively.

1235. Aqueous insolubility of bilirubin is due to which of the following?
Harrison's 20th Ed. Chapter 331 Page 2342

A. Internal phosphate bonding
B. Internal hydrogen bonding
C. Internal sulphate bonding
D. Internal glucoronate bonding

Conjugation of bilirubin with glucuronic acid moieties disrupts internal hydrogen bonding that limits aqueous solubility of bilirubin & the resulting glucuronide conjugates are highly soluble in water.

1236. Which of the following are the four common exons that encode the shared carboxyl-terminal half of all UGT1 isoforms?

Harrison's 20th Ed. Chapter 331 Page 2342

A. Exons 1 - 4
B. Exons 2 - 5
C. Exons 3 - 6
D. Exons 4 - 7

Exons 2–5 are four common exons that encode the shared carboxyl-terminal half of all UGT1 isoforms. A mutation in exons 2–5 will alter all isoforms encoded by the UGT1 gene complex. Mutations in a first exon affect only a single isoform.

1237. UDP-glucuronosyltransferases (UGT) that conjugate bilirubin belong to which UGT family?

Harrison's 20th Ed. Chapter 331 Page 2342

A. UGT1
B. UGT2
C. UGT3
D. UGT4

UDP-glucuronosyltransferases (UGT) that conjugate bilirubin belong to the UGT1 family. Exon A1 and the four common exons, collectively designated the UGT1A1 gene, encode the physiologically critical enzyme bilirubin-UDP-glucuronosyltransferase (UGT1A1).

1238. Human UGT1 gene complex is on which of the following chromosomes?

Harrison's 20th Ed. Chapter 331 Page 2343 Figure 331-2

A. 2
B. 4
C. 6
D. 8

Human UGT1 gene complex is on chromosome 2. It contains at least 13 substrate-specific first exons (A1, A2, etc.). Since four of these are pseudogenes, nine UGT1 isoforms with differing substrate specificities are expressed. Mutations in a first exon affect only a single isoform. Those in exons 2–5 affect all enzymes encoded by the UGT1 complex.

1239. Multidrug resistance-associated protein 2 (MRP2) is related to which of the following steps in bilirubin metabolism?

Harrison's 20th Ed. Chapter 331 Page 2342

A. Hepatocellular uptake
B. Intracellular binding
C. Conjugation
D. Biliary excretion

Bilirubin mono- and diglucuronides are excreted across canalicular plasma membrane into bile canaliculus by ATP-dependent transport process mediated by a canalicular membrane protein called multidrug resistance-associated protein 2 (MRP2). Mutations of MRP2 result in Dubin-Johnson syndrome.

1240. Which of the following is false about urobilinogen?

Harrison's 20th Ed. Chapter 331 Page 2342

A. Made from unconjugated bilirubin in gut
B. Water-soluble
C. Colorless
D. Undergoes enterohepatic cycling

"Conjugated bilirubin" is converted by bacterial metabolism in gut to water-soluble colorless urobilinogen. Urobilinogen undergoes enterohepatic cycling. Urobilinogen not taken up by liver reaches systemic circulation, from which some is cleared by kidneys.

1241. Which of the following interrupts bilirubin enterohepatic cycling?

Harrison's 20th Ed. Chapter 331 Page 2343

A. Aluminum hydroxide
B. Magnesium sulphate
C. Calcium phosphate
D. Calcium carbonate

Oral administration of calcium phosphate with or without the lipase inhibitor orlistat may be an efficient means to interrupt bilirubin enterohepatic cycling.

1242. In response to hemolytic stress, bone marrow is capable of increasing erythrocyte production by?

Harrison's 20th Ed. Chapter 331 Page 2343

A. Two fold
B. Four fold
C. Six fold
D. Eight fold

In response to hemolytic stress, bone marrow is capable of a sustained eight fold increase in erythrocyte production.

1243. Hemolysis alone cannot result in a sustained hyperbilirubinemia of more than?

Harrison's 20th Ed. Chapter 331 Page 2343

A. ~ 2 mg/dL
B. ~ 4 mg/dL
C. ~ 6 mg/dL
D. ~ 8 mg/dL

Hemolysis alone cannot result in a sustained hyperbilirubinemia of more than ~ 4 mg/dL.

1244. Direct-reacting fraction is how much of total serum bilirubin in isolated hemolysis?

Harrison's 20th Ed. Chapter 331 Page 2343

A. ≤ 10%
B. ≤ 12%
C. ≤ 15%
D. ≤ 18%

Hemolysis results in pure unconjugated hyperbilirubinemia, with direct-reacting fraction being ≤15% of total serum bilirubin.

1245. Ineffective erythropoiesis is seen in all except?

Harrison's 20th Ed. Chapter 331 Page 2343

A. Thalassemia major
B. Congenital erythropoietic porphyria
C. Crigler-Najjar syndrome
D. Lead poisoning

In thalassemia major, megaloblastic anemias due to folate or vitamin B12 deficiency, congenital erythropoietic porphyria, lead poisoning, and congenital & acquired dyserythropoietic anemias, the fraction of total bilirubin production derived from ineffective erythropoiesis is increased, reaching as much as 70% of the total producing modest degrees of unconjugated hyperbilirubinemia.

1246. Which of the following produces hyperbilirubinemia due to decreased hepatic bilirubin uptake?

Harrison's 20th Ed. Chapter 331 Page 2343

A. Pregnanediol
B. Chloramphenicol
C. Gentamicin
D. Cholecystographic contrast agents

Apart from Gilbert's syndrome, flavaspidic acid, novobiocin, rifampin and cholecystographic contrast agents produce defects in bilirubin uptake. Pregnanediol, novobiocin, chloramphenicol, and gentamicin produce unconjugated hyperbilirubinemia by inhibiting UGT1A1 activity.

1247. Fetal bilirubin is cleared by?

Harrison's 20th Ed. Chapter 331 Page 2343

A. Fetal liver
B. Fetal kidney
C. Placenta
D. All of the above

Bilirubin produced by the fetus is cleared by the placenta and eliminated by the maternal liver.

1248. Most neonates develop mild unconjugated hyperbilirubinemia between days?

Harrison's 20th Ed. Chapter 331 Page 2343

A. 1 and 3 after birth
B. 2 and 5 after birth
C. 5 and 7 after birth
D. 7 and 10 after birth

Immediately after birth, due to incompletely developed hepatic physiologic processes like low levels of UGT1A1, undeveloped intestinal flora that convert bilirubin to urobilinogen, most neonates develop mild unconjugated hyperbilirubinemia between days 2 and 5 after birth.

1249. What are the peak levels of physiologic neonatal jaundice?

Harrison's 20th Ed. Chapter 331 Page 2343

A. 3 - 5 mg/dL
B. 5 - 10 mg/dL
C. 10 - 15 mg/dL
D. 15 - 20 mg/dL

Peak levels of physiologic neonatal jaundice are typically 5–10 mg/dL.

1250. Bilibubin levels of physiologic neonatal jaundice return to normal adult concentrations within?

Harrison's 20th Ed. Chapter 331 Page 2343

A. 1 week
B. 2 weeks
C. 3 weeks
D. 4 weeks

Bilibubin levels of physiologic neonatal jaundice return to normal adult concentrations within 2 weeks as mechanisms required for bilirubin disposition mature.

1251. Which of the following is false for bilirubin encephalopathy, or kernicterus?

Harrison's 20th Ed. Chapter 331 Page 2343

A. Rapidly rising unconjugated bilirubin concentration
B. Immature blood-brain barrier
C. Deposition in the basal ganglia
D. None of the above

A rapidly rising unconjugated bilirubin concentration, or absolute levels >20 mg/dL, exposed the infant to the at risk of bilirubin encephalopathy, or kernicterus.

1252. Which of the following drugs may produce unconjugated hyperbilirubinemia by inhibiting UGT1A1 activity?

Harrison's 20th Ed. Chapter 331 Page 2343

A. Pregnanediol
B. Chloramphenicol
C. Gentamicin
D. All of the above

Pregnanediol, novobiocin, chloramphenicol, atazanavir and gentamicin may produce unconjugated hyperbilirubinemia by inhibiting UGT1A1 activity.

1253. 'Breast milk jaundice' in neonates is due to presence of what in breast milk?

Harrison's 20th Ed. Chapter 331 Page 2343

A. Immunoglobulins
B. Proteins
C. Fatty acids
D. Carbohydrates

Bilirubin conjugation may be inhibited by certain fatty acids that are present in breast milk but not serum of mothers whose infants have excessive neonatal hyperbilirubinemia (breast milk jaundice).

1254. Lucey-Driscoll syndrome is related to?

Harrison's 20th Ed. Chapter 331 Page 2343

A. UGT1A1 inhibitor in breast milk
B. UGT1A1 inhibitor in maternal serum
C. Low UGT1A1 levels at birth
D. All of the above

In transient familial neonatal hyperbilirubinemia (Lucey-Driscoll syndrome) there is a UGT1A1 inhibitor in maternal serum.

1255. Which of the following about Crigler-Najjar Syndrome, Type I is false?

Harrison's 20th Ed. Chapter 331 Page 2344

A. Unconjugated hyperbilirubinemia of ~ 20-45 mg/dL
B. Appears in the neonatal period
C. Persists for life
D. Bilirubin is found in the urine

No bilirubin is found in the urine.

1256. Which of the following about Crigler-Najjar Syndrome, Type I is false?

Harrison's 20th Ed. Chapter 331 Page 2344

A. Normal serum aminotransferases
B. Normal alkaline phosphatase
C. No evidence of hemolysis
D. None of the above

1257. Which of the following is false about Crigler-Najjar Syndrome Type I?

Harrison's 20th Ed. Chapter 331 Page 2344

A. Unconjugated hyperbilirubinemia
B. Absent UGT1A1 activity in liver
C. Kernicterus common
D. Responds to phenobarbital

Crigler-Najjar Syndrome, Type I (CN-I) is characterized by unconjugated hyperbilirubinemia of ~20 to 45 mg/dL that appears in neonatal period and persists for life. Bilirubin glucuronides are absent from bile and there is no UGT1A1 activity in hepatic tissue. There is no response to phenobarbital or any enzyme inducer.

1258. Causative mutation is in the bilirubin-specific exon A1 of which variety of Crigler-Najjar Syndrome Type I?

Harrison's 20th Ed. Chapter 331 Page 2344

A. Crigler-Najjar syndrome Type IA
B. Crigler-Najjar syndrome Type IB
C. Crigler-Najjar syndrome Type IC
D. Crigler-Najjar syndrome Type ID

In Crigler-Najjar Syndrome Type IB, the defect is limited to bilirubin conjugation, and the causative mutation is in the bilirubin-specific exon A1.

1259. Which of the following is false about Crigler-Najjar Syndrome Type I?

Harrison's 20th Ed. Chapter 331 Page 2344

A. Rare (estimated prevalence = 0.6 - 1.0 per million)
B. Autosomal recessive pattern of inheritance
C. Estrogen glucuronidation is defective
D. Liver transplantation not helpful

In Crigler-Najjar Syndrome Type I, early liver transplantation remains the best hope to prevent brain injury and death.

1260. Crigler-Najjar Syndrome Type I (CN-I) differs from Crigler-Najjar Syndrome, Type II (CN-II) is which of the following?

Harrison's 20th Ed. Chapter 331 Page 2344

A. Average bilirubin concentrations are lower in CN-II
B. CN-II is infrequently associated with kernicterus
C. CN-II responds to phenobarbital
D. All of the above

Crigler-Najjar Syndrome Type II (CN-II) is characterized by marked unconjugated hyperbilirubinemia with normal conventional hepatic biochemical tests, hepatic histology and no hemolysis. Average bilirubin concentrations are lower in CN-II. CN-II is infrequently associated with kernicterus. Bile in CN-II contains bilirubin glucuronides mostly monoglucuronides. UGT1A1 in liver is present at reduced levels in CN-II and bilirubin concentrations fall with phenobarbital therapy.

1261. Which of the following is false about Gilbert's Syndrome?

Harrison's 20th Ed. Chapter 331 Page 2344

A. Conjugated hyperbilirubinemia
B. UGT1A1 activity - 10-35% of normal
C. Phenobarbital normalizes serum bilirubin
D. Aggravated by alcohol use

In Gilbert's Syndrome, UGT1A1 activity is typically reduced to 10 - 35% of normal, and bile pigments exhibit a characteristic increase in bilirubin monoglucuronides.

1262. Gilbert's Syndrome is a close clinical entity to which of the following?

Harrison's 20th Ed. Chapter 331 Page 2344

A. Crigler-Najjar syndrome Type I
B. Crigler-Najjar syndrome Type II
C. Lucey-Driscoll syndrome
D. Benign recurrent intrahepatic cholestasis (BRIC)

The clinical spectrum of Gilbert's Syndrome hyperbilirubinemia fades into that of CN-II at serum bilirubin concentrations of 5 - 8 mg/dL.

1263. Which of the following pigment is increased in hepatic histology of patients of Gilbert's Syndrome?

Harrison's 20th Ed. Chapter 331 Page 2345

A. Melanopsin
B. Lipofuscin
C. Hemosiderin
D. Oxidized homogentisic acid

1264. In GS, elevated bilirubin concentrations are associated with?

Harrison's 20th Ed. Chapter 331 Page 2345

A. Stress
B. Alcohol use
C. Reduced caloric intake
D. All of the above

In GS, elevated bilirubin concentrations particularly bilirubin monoglucuronides are associated with stress, fatigue, alcohol use, reduced caloric intake and intercurrent illness while increased caloric intake or administration of enzyme-inducing agents produces lower bilirubin levels.

1265. Which of the following drugs is glucuronidated specifically by bilirubin-UDP-glucuronosyltransferase?

Harrison's 20th Ed. Chapter 331 Page 2345

A. Estradiol benzoate
B. Acetaminophen
C. Tolbutamide
D. Irinotecan

In Gilbert's Syndrome, toxicity occurs upon administration of antitumor agent irinotecan (CPT-11) because its active metabolite (SN-38) is glucuronidated specifically by bilirubin-UDP-glucuronosyltransferase.

1266. Which of the following drugs used in HIV patients inhibits UGT1A1?

Harrison's 20th Ed. Chapter 331 Page 2345

A. Zidovudine
B. Indinavir
C. Enfuvirtide
D. All of the above

HIV protease inhibitors indinavir and atazanavir inhibit UGT1A1, resulting in hyperbilirubinemia that is most pronounced in patients with preexisting Gilbert's Syndrome.

1267. Which of the following are examples of familial defects in hepatic excretory function?

Harrison's 20th Ed. Chapter 331 Page 2345

A. Dubin-Johnson syndrome
B. Rotor syndrome
C. Benign recurrent intrahepatic cholestasis
D. All of the above

1268. Which of the following does not manifest as predominantly conjugated hyperbilirubinemia?

Harrison's 20th Ed. Chapter 331 Page 2345

A. Dubin-Johnson syndrome
B. Crigler-Najjar syndrome
C. Rotor syndrome
D. Benign recurrent intrahepatic cholestasis

1269. In Dubin-Johnson Syndrome, degree of hyperbilirubinemia may be increased by?

Harrison's 20th Ed. Chapter 331 Page 2345

A. Intercurrent illness
B. Oral contraceptive use
C. Pregnancy
D. All of the above

In Dubin-Johnson Syndrome, degree of hyperbilirubinemia may be increased by intercurrent illness, oral contraceptive use, and pregnancy.

1270. Liver is grossly black in appearance in which of the following?

Harrison's 20th Ed. Chapter 331 Page 2346

A. Dubin-Johnson syndrome
B. Rotor syndrome
C. Progressive familial intrahepatic cholestasis
D. Benign recurrent intrahepatic cholestasis (BRIC)

In DJS, due to accumulation in lysosomes of centrilobular hepatocytes of dark, coarsely granular pigment, liver is grossly black in appearance. This pigment is thought to be derived from epinephrine metabolites that are not excreted normally.

1271. Which of the following is false about Dubin-Johnson Syndrome?
Harrison's 20th Ed. Chapter 331 Page 2346

A. Conjugated hyperbilirubinemia
B. Bilirubinuria present
C. Liver grossly black
D. Pruritus common

DJS patients have normal serum & biliary bile acid concentrations & do not have pruritus.

1272. Dark, coarsely granular pigment in hepatocytes in Dubin-Johnson Syndrome disappears during?
Harrison's 20th Ed. Chapter 331 Page 2346

A. Enteric fever
B. Viral hepatitis
C. Malaria
D. All of the above

Dark, coarsely granular pigment in hepatocytes in Dubin-Johnson Syndrome disappears during bouts of viral hepatitis, only to reaccumulate slowly after recovery.

1273. Pigment producing grossly black liver in DJS is best related to?
Harrison's 20th Ed. Chapter 331 Page 2346

A. Tryptophan
B. Melanin
C. Epinephrine
D. Glutathione

A cardinal feature of DJS is the accumulation in the lysosomes of centrilobular hepatocytes of dark, coarsely granular pigment. As a result, liver is grossly black in appearance. This pigment is thought to be derived from epinephrine metabolites that are not excreted normally.

1274. Mutation in which of the following genes produce the Dubin-Johnson phenotype?
Harrison's 20th Ed. Chapter 331 Page 2346

A. ABCC2
B. NTCP
C. MRP2
D. FIC1

MRP2 is an ATP-dependent canalicular membrane transporter and mutations in the MRP2 gene produce the Dubin-Johnson phenotype, which has an autosomal recessive pattern of inheritance.

1275. In urine from Dubin-Johnson Syndrome patients, which is the predominant coproporphyrin isomer?
Harrison's 20th Ed. Chapter 331 Page 2346

A. Coproporphyrin isomer I
B. Coproporphyrin isomer II
C. Coproporphyrin isomer III
D. Coproporphyrin isomer IV

Naturally occurring coproporphyrin isomers are I and III. Normally, 75% of the coproporphyrin in urine is isomer III. In urine from DJS patients, total coproporphyrin content is normal, but >80% of the total is isomer I.

1276. Which of the following is typical of Dubin-Johnson Syndrome?
Harrison's 20th Ed. Chapter 331 Page 2346

A. Liver is grossly black in appearance
B. Gallbladder not visualized on oral cholecystography
C. Total urinary coproporphyrin excretion normal
D. All of the above

1277. Which of the following is an autosomal recessive disorder?
Harrison's 20th Ed. Chapter 331 Page 2346

A. Crigler-Najjar syndrome
B. Gilbert's syndrome
C. Rotor syndrome
D. All of the above

1278. Rotor Syndrome is clinically similar to?
Harrison's 20th Ed. Chapter 331 Page 2346

A. Dubin-Johnson syndrome
B. Crigler-Najjar syndrome
C. Gilbert's syndrome
D. Lucey-Driscoll syndrome

Rotor Syndrome is a benign, autosomal recessive disorder clinically similar to DJS.

1279. Which of the following is false about Rotor Syndrome?
Harrison's 20th Ed. Chapter 331 Page 2346

A. Conjugated hyperbilirubinemia
B. Gallbladder visualized on oral cholecystography
C. Liver normal in appearance
D. Total urinary coproporphyrin excretion normal

In Rotor syndrome, the gallbladder is visualized on oral cholecystography, in contrast to nonvisualization that is typical of DJS. Total urinary coproporphyrin excretion is substantially increased in Rotor syndrome, in contrast to the normal levels seen in DJS.

1280. Which of the following is related to transportation of bilirubin glucuronides into the portal circulation?
Harrison's 20th Ed. Chapter 331 Page 2346

A. MRP2
B. MRP3
C. Bilirubin-UDP-glucuronosyltransferase (UGT1A1)
D. All of the above

In addition to direct excretion of bilirubin glucuronides, a portion is transported into the portal circulation by MRP3 and subjected to reuptake into the hepatocyte by OATP1B1 and OATP1B3. Recent studies indicate that the molecular basis of Rotor syndrome results from simultaneous deficiency of the plasma membrane transporters OATP1B1 and OATP1B3. This results in reduced reuptake of conjugated bilirubin that has been pumped out of the cell into the portal circulation by MRP3.

1281. Which of the following is false about Benign Recurrent Intrahepatic Cholestasis (BRIC)?
Harrison's 20th Ed. Chapter 331 Page 2346

A. Recurrent attacks of pruritus and jaundice
B. Normal serum aminotransferase levels
C. Elevations in alkaline phosphatase
D. Does not lead to cirrhosis

BRIC is characterized by recurrent attacks of pruritus and jaundice. Laboratory findings include elevations in serum conjugated bilirubin, aminotransferase and alkaline phosphatase levels. BRIC is an autosomal recessive benign disorder in that it does not lead to cirrhosis or end-stage liver disease.

1282. Mutation in which of the following genes produce the Benign Recurrent Intrahepatic Cholestasis (BRIC)?
Harrison's 20th Ed. Chapter 331 Page 2346

A. ABCC2
B. NTCP
C. MRP2
D. FIC1

Gene FIC1 is mutated in patients with BRIC.

1283. Gene FIC1 is mainly expressed in?

Harrison's 20th Ed. Chapter 331 Page 2346

A. Liver

B. Small intestine

C. Kidney

D. Heart

Gene FIC1 is mainly expressed strongly in the small intestine but only weakly in the liver.

1284. Byler disease is also known as?

Harrison's 20th Ed. Chapter 331 Page 2347

A. Progressive familial intrahepatic cholestasis type 1

B. Progressive familial intrahepatic cholestasis type 2

C. Progressive familial intrahepatic cholestasis type 3

D. Progressive familial intrahepatic cholestasis type 4

Byler disease is also termed as Progressive Familial Intrahepatic Cholestasis (FIC) type 1. This is also a consequence of an FIC1 mutation and may progresses to malnutrition, growth retardation, and end-stage liver disease during childhood.

1285. Mutation of MDR3 gene results in?

Harrison's 20th Ed. Chapter 331 Page 2347

A. Progressive familial intrahepatic cholestasis type 1

B. Progressive familial intrahepatic cholestasis type 2

C. Progressive familial intrahepatic cholestasis type 3

D. Progressive familial intrahepatic cholestasis type 4

Progressive FIC type 3 has been associated with a mutation of MDR3, a protein that is essential for normal hepatocellular excretion of phospholipids across the bile canaliculus.

Acute Viral Hepatitis

1286. World Hepatitis Day is observed on?

A. October 01
B. December 01
C. February 04
D. July 28

World Hepatitis Day is recognized annually on July 28th, the birthday of Dr. Baruch Blumberg (1925-2011). Dr. Blumberg discovered hepatitis B virus in 1967 and two years later developed the first hepatitis B vaccine and for these achievements won the Nobel Prize. World Hepatitis Awareness Day - October 01, World AIDS Day - December 1, World Cancer Day - February 04.

1287. DANE particle is the name given to?
N Engl J Med. 1973; 288:1409

A. Hepatitis A virion
B. Hepatitis B virion
C. Hepatitis C virion
D. Hepatitis D virion

D.S. Dane and others discovered the HBV virus particle in 1970 by electron microscopy.

1288. Which of the following is not a RNA virus?
Harrison's 20th Ed. Chapter 332 Page 2347

A. Hepatitis A virus
B. Hepatitis B virus
C. Hepatitis C virus
D. Hepatitis D virus

A, C, D, E human hepatitis viruses are RNA viruses.

1289. Which of the following viruses is a DNA virus?
Harrison's 20th Ed. Chapter 332 Page 2347

A. Hepatitis A
B. Hepatitis B
C. Hepatitis C
D. Hepatitis D

Hepatitis B is a DNA virus but replicates like a retrovirus.

1290. Which of the following is not a bloodborne type virus?
Harrison's 20th Ed. Chapter 332 Page 2347

A. Hepatitis A
B. Hepatitis B
C. Hepatitis C
D. Hepatitis D

HBV, HCV, and HDV are bloodborne type viruses.

1291. Which of the following about Hepatitis A virus is false?
Harrison's 20th Ed. Chapter 332 Page 2347

A. Enveloped
B. Heat resistant
C. Acid resistant
D. Ether resistant

Hepatitis A virus is a nonenveloped 27-nm, heat, acid, and ether-resistant RNA virus in the hepatovirus genus of the picornavirus family.

1292. Four capsid polypeptides of Hepatitis A virion are designated as?
Harrison's 20th Ed. Chapter 332 Page 2347

A. SP1 to SP4
B. HP1 to HP4
C. VP1 to VP4
D. WP1 to WP4

Hepatitis A virion contains four capsid polypeptides, designated VP1 to VP4. These are cleaved posttranslationally from the polyprotein product of a 7500-nucleotide genome.

1293. Inactivation of Hepatitis A virus can be achieved by?
Harrison's 20th Ed. Chapter 332 Page 2347

A. Formaldehyde
B. Chlorine
C. Ultraviolet irradiation
D. All of the above

Inactivation of viral activity can be achieved by boiling for 1 minute, by formaldehyde and chlorine, or by ultraviolet irradiation.

1294. Hepatitis A has an incubation period of?
Harrison's 20th Ed. Chapter 332 Page 2347

A. ~ 2 weeks
B. ~ 4 weeks
C. ~ 6 weeks
D. ~ 8 weeks

Hepatitis A has an incubation period of ~4 weeks.

1295. Replication of Hepatitis A virus occurs in?
Harrison's 20th Ed. Chapter 332 Page 2347

A. Liver
B. Bile
C. Blood
D. All of the above

Hepatitis A virus replication is limited to liver. But, the virus is present in liver, bile, stools, and blood during the late incubation period and acute preicteric phase of illness.

1296. Which of the following statements about Hepatitis A virus is false?
Harrison's 20th Ed. Chapter 332 Page 2347

A. HAV can be cultivated reproducibly in vitro
B. Virus is present in liver, bile, stools and blood during late incubation period & acute preicteric phase of illness
C. Viral shedding in feces, viremia and infectivity diminish rapidly once jaundice becomes apparent
D. None of the above

Despite persistence of virus in liver, viral shedding in feces, viremia, and infectivity diminish rapidly once jaundice becomes apparent.

1297. After acute illness, anti-HAV of IgM class remains detectable for?

Harrison's 20th Ed. Chapter 332 Page 2347

A. Up to 3 months
B. Up to 6 months
C. Up to 12 months
D. Up to 18 months

Early antibody response to HAV infection is predominantly of the IgM class and persists for ~3 months, rarely for 6-12 months.

1298. After acute illness, anti-HAV of IgG class remains detectable for?

Harrison's 20th Ed. Chapter 332 Page 2347

A. 3 months
B. 6 months
C. 12 months
D. Indefinitely

After acute illness, anti-HAV of the IgG class remains detectable indefinitely.

1299. Which of the following has the largest virus particle size?

Harrison's 20th Ed. Chapter 332 Page 2348 Figure 332-1

A. Hepatitis A
B. Hepatitis D
C. Hepatitis C
D. Hepatitis E

1300. Which of the following has the smallest virus particle size?

Harrison's 20th Ed. Chapter 332 Page 2348 Figure 332-1

A. Hepatitis A
B. Hepatitis D
C. Hepatitis C
D. Hepatitis E

Hepatitis A virus (27-nm), Hepatitis B virus (42-nm), Hepatitis C virus (55-nm), Hepatitis D virus (35–37 nm) and Hepatitis E virus (32–34 nm)

1301. Which of the following has the largest viral genome size?

Harrison's 20th Ed. Chapter 332 Page 2348 Figure 332-1

A. Hepatitis A
B. Hepatitis B
C. Hepatitis C
D. Hepatitis E

1302. Which of the following has the smallest viral genome size?

Harrison's 20th Ed. Chapter 332 Page 2348 Table 332-1

A. Hepatitis A
B. Hepatitis B
C. Hepatitis C
D. Hepatitis D

1303. Which of the following has the smallest viral genome size?

Harrison's 20th Ed. Chapter 332 Page 2348 Table 332-1

A. Hepatitis A
B. Hepatitis B
C. Hepatitis C
D. Hepatitis E

HAV - 7.5 kb, HBV 3.2 kb, HCV - 9.4 kb, HDV - 1.7 kb, HEV - 7.6 kb.

1304. HBV belongs to which family of viruses?

Harrison's 20th Ed. Chapter 332 Page 2347

A. Hepadnaviruses
B. Hepatovirus
C. Hepacivirus
D. Hepevirus

HBV belongs to hepadnaviruses family of viruses, type 1 ("hepa" from hepatotrophic and "dna" because it is a DNA virus), HAV is a Hepatovirus, HCV is Hepacivirus and HEV is a Hepevirus. HDV resembles viroids and plant satellite viruses.

1305. The four overlapping genes of encoding proteins in Hepatitis B virus are?

Harrison's 20th Ed. Chapter 332 Page 2347

A. S, C, P and X
B. S, T, U and V
C. S, O, M and Z
D. S, Q, C, and Y

In Hepatitis B virus, the four overlapping genes encoded by the genome are S, C, P and X.

1306. Hepadnaviruses also infect which of the following?

Harrison's 20th Ed. Chapter 332 Page 2347

A. Woodchucks
B. Ground and tree squirrels
C. Pekin ducks
D. All of the above

Hepadnavirus type 1 viruses infect species of woodchucks, ground & tree squirrels, and Pekin ducks.

1307. Out of the following, who is related to the discovery of Australia antigen?

N Engl J Med. 1970; 283:349-354

A. Alter MJ
B. Baruch Blumberg
C. Bouchard MJ
D. Zuckerman AJ

In 1965, American physician & geneticist Baruch Blumberg (1925-2011), working at National Institutes of Health (NIH), discovered the Australia antigen (later known to be Hepatitis B surface antigen, or HBsAg) in the blood of Australian aboriginal people. He was the co-recipient of the 1976 Nobel Prize in Physiology or Medicine.

1308. Additional name for Australia antigen is?

N Engl J Med. 1970; 283:349-354

A. Hepatitis antigen
B. SH antigen
C. Hepatitis-associated antigen
D. All of the above

1309. Which of the following is false about HBV genome?

Harrison's 20th Ed. Chapter 332 Page 2348

A. Circular genome
B. Partially double-strand and partially single-strand
C. Replicates through an RNA intermediate form by reverse transcription
D. None of the above

Hepatitis B is a non-retroviral virus which uses reverse transcription for its replication.

1310. Which of the following about Hepatitis B virus is false?

N Engl J Med. 2004;351:2832-8

A. Enveloped, double-stranded DNA virus
B. Smallest dsDNA virus known to infect humans
C. Primary reservoir is chronically infected people
D. Insects can transmit HBV

1311. Which of the following about Hepatitis B virus is false?

N Engl J Med. 2004;351:2832-8

A. Blood contains highest concentrations of virus
B. Not transmitted by fecal-oral route
C. Vertical transmission from mother to child possible
D. Breast milk can cause viral transmission

1312. Which of the following about Hepatitis B virus is false?

N Engl J Med. 2004;350:1118-29

A. Replication of DNA genome by reverse transcription of RNA intermediate
B. Covalently closed circular DNA (cccDNA) is formed in hepatocyte nucleus
C. Most abundant protein in HBV genome is S protein
D. Risk of development of chronicity is directly related to age at time of infection

1313. Entry of HBV into hepatocytes is mediated by binding to?

Harrison's 20th Ed. Chapter 332 Page 2348

A. Sodium taurocholate cotransporting polypeptide receptor
B. Sodium deoxycholate cotransporting polypeptide receptor
C. Sodium lithocholate cotransporting polypeptide receptor
D. All of the above

Entry of HBV into hepatocytes is mediated by binding to the sodium taurocholate cotransporting polypeptide receptor. Hepatitis B virus entry into hepatocytes requires the binding of myristolated N-terminal pre-S1 peptide of large HBsAg to sodium taurocholate co-transporting peptide, the functional receptor for HBV into hepatocytes.

1314. Which is the largest overlapping gene in Hepatitis B virus?

Harrison's 20th Ed. Chapter 332 Page 2348 Figure 332-3

A. S
B. C
C. P
D. X

The P gene of HBV is the largest gene and codes for DNA polymerase.

1315. Which of the following statements about overlapping genes in Hepatitis B virus is false?

Harrison's 20th Ed. Chapter 332 Page 2348 Figure 332-3

A. S gene codes for HBsAg
B. P gene codes for DNA polymerase
C. C gene codes for HBeAg
D. X gene codes for HBcAg

1316. Which of the following may bind to p53?

Harrison's 20th Ed. Chapter 332 Page 2348 Figure 332-3

A. HBsAg
B. HBcAg
C. HBeAg
D. HBxAg

The S gene codes for the "major" envelope protein, HBsAg. The largest gene, P, codes for DNA polymerase. C gene codes for nucleocapsid proteins—HBeAg and HBcAg. X gene codes for HBxAg which can transactivate the transcription of cellular and viral genes and may contribute to carcinogenesis by binding to p53.

1317. Which particulate form of HBV is most numerous in blood?

Harrison's 20th Ed. Chapter 332 Page 2348

A. 22-nm
B. 27-nm
C. 42-nm
D. All of the above

Of the three particulate forms of HBV, the most numerous are the 22-nm particles, which appear as spherical or long filamentous forms. These are antigenically indistinguishable from outer surface or envelope protein of HBV and are thought to represent excess viral envelope protein.

1318. Which of the following represents the intact hepatitis B virion?

Harrison's 20th Ed. Chapter 332 Page 2348

A. 22-nm
B. 27-nm
C. 42-nm
D. All of the above

Large, 42-nm, double-shelled spherical particles represent the intact hepatitis B virion.

1319. Which of the following about hepatitis B surface antigen (HBsAg) is false?

Harrison's 20th Ed. Chapter 332 Page 2348

A. It is the product of the S gene of HBV
B. Envelope protein
C. Expressed on outer surface of virion and on smaller spherical & tubular structures
D. None of the above

1320. Which is the common group-reactive antigen in different HBsAg subdeterminants?

Harrison's 20th Ed. Chapter 332 Page 2348

A. a
B. b
C. c
D. d

In different HBsAg subdeterminants, common group-reactive antigen, "a" is shared by all HBsAg isolates.

1321. Number of genotypes in Hepatitis B isolates is?

Harrison's 20th Ed. Chapter 332 Page 2348

A. 4
B. 10
C. 12
D. 16

In 1988, hepatitis B virus (HBV) was classified into four genotypes by a sequence divergence in the entire genome exceeding 8%, and designated by capital letters of the alphabet from A to D. Later, six more were added from E to J. Genotype H is phylogenetically closely related to genotype F.

1322. Genotypes of HBV were defined by a sequence divergence greater than what percentage in the entire genome?

Harrison's 20th Ed. Chapter 332 Page 2348

A. 2
B. 4
C. 6
D. 8

Genotypes of HBV were defined by a sequence divergence greater than 8% in the entire genome.

1323. Which of the following is not a major serotype of HBV?

Harrison's 20th Ed. Chapter 332 Page 2348

A. add
B. adw
C. ayr
D. ayw

HBV virus is divided into 4 major serotypes (adr, adw, ayr, ayw) based on antigenic epitopes present on its envelope proteins, and into ten genotypes (A-J) according to overall nucleotide sequence variation of the genome. Genotypes of HBV were defined by a sequence divergence > 8% in the entire genome. HBsAg serotypes adw, adr, ayw and ayr are readily determined by immunological methods, and they were regarded the phenotypic expression of HBV genotypes. All HBV isolates of genotype A or B isolates were adw and all genotype D isolates were ayw. Isolates of genotype C were heterogeneous and covered adw, adr and ayr.

1324. The protein product of S region in Hepatitis B virus is?

Harrison's 20th Ed. Chapter 332 Page 2348

A. Major protein
B. Middle protein
C. Large protein
D. All of the above

1325. The protein product of S gene in Hepatitis B virus is?

Harrison's 20th Ed. Chapter 332 Page 2348

A. Major protein
B. Middle protein
C. Large protein
D. All of the above

1326. The protein product of S region plus pre-S2 region in Hepatitis B virus is?

Harrison's 20th Ed. Chapter 332 Page 2348

A. Major protein
B. Middle protein
C. Large protein
D. All of the above

1327. The protein product of pre-S1 plus pre-S2 plus S regions in Hepatitis B virus is?

Harrison's 20th Ed. Chapter 332 Page 2348

A. Major protein
B. Middle protein
C. Large protein
D. All of the above

The envelope protein, HBsAg, is the product of the S gene of HBV. HBsAg gene is one long open reading frame but contains 3 in frame "start" (ATG) codons that divide the gene into 3 sections, pre-S1, pre-S2, and S. S gene codes for the "major" envelope protein - HBsAg. "Large" protein is the product of pre-S1 + pre-S2 + S. "Middle" protein is the product of pre-S2 + S.

1328. HBsAg is also called?

Harrison's 20th Ed. Chapter 332 Page 2348

A. Major protein
B. Middle protein
C. Large protein
D. All of the above

The S gene codes for the "major" envelope protein, HBsAg.

1329. Nucleocapsid proteins are coded for by?

Harrison's 20th Ed. Chapter 332 Page 2348

A. Pre-S1 gene
B. Pre-S2 gene
C. S gene
D. C gene

Nucleocapsid proteins are coded for by the C gene. The C gene codes for two nucleocapsid proteins, HBeAg, a soluble, secreted protein (initiation from the pre-C region of the gene), and HBcAg, the intracellular core protein (initiation after pre-C).

1330. Which of the following is not a nucleocapsid protein?

Harrison's 20th Ed. Chapter 332 Page 2348

A. HBsAg
B. HBeAg
C. HBcAg
D. All of the above

The C gene codes for two nucleocapsid proteins, HBeAg and HBcAg. If translation is initiated at the precore region of C gene, the protein product is HBeAg, while if translation begins with the core region of C gene, HBcAg is the protein product.

1331. Which of the following represents excess virus coat material?

Harrison's 20th Ed. Chapter 332 Page 2348

A. HBsAg
B. HBeAg
C. HBcAg
D. HBxAg

1332. In Hepatitis B virus, which of the following is a 'secreted' nucleocapsid protein?

Harrison's 20th Ed. Chapter 332 Page 2348

A. HBsAg
B. HBeAg
C. HBcAg
D. HBxAg

HBeAg is a soluble, secreted nucleocapsid protein. HBeAg provides a convenient, readily detectable, qualitative marker of HBV replication and relative infectivity. HBeAg has a signal peptide that binds it to the smooth endoplasmic reticulum and leads to its secretion into the circulation.

1333. Which of the following is qualitative marker of HBV replication & relative infectivity?

Harrison's 20th Ed. Chapter 332 Page 2349

A. HBsAg
B. HBeAg
C. HBcAg
D. HBxAg

HBsAg-positive serum containing HBeAg is highly infectious and associated with presence of hepatitis B virions than HBeAg-negative or anti-HBe-positive serum. Anti-HBeAg positivity usually indicates low infectivity and no replication, unless patient is precore mutant.

1334. Persistence of HBeAg in serum beyond how many months of acute infection is predictive of chronic infection?
Harrison's 20th Ed. Chapter 332 Page 2349

A. 1 month
B. 2 month
C. 3 month
D. Any of the above

HBeAg appears transiently and early during acute hepatitis B infection. Persistence of HBeAg in serum beyond the first three months of acute infection may be predictive of the development of chronic infection.

1335. HBsAg-positive mothers rarely infect their offspring, if their serum contains?
Harrison's 20th Ed. Chapter 332 Page 2349

A. HBsAg
B. HBeAg
C. Anti-HBs
D. Anti-HBe

HBsAg-positive mothers who are HBeAg-positive almost invariably (>90%) transmit hepatitis B infection to their offspring, whereas HBsAg-positive mothers with anti-HBe rarely infect their offspring.

1336. Presence of HBeAg during chronic hepatitis B tends to be associated with?
Harrison's 20th Ed. Chapter 332 Page 2349

A. Ongoing viral replication
B. Infectivity
C. Inflammatory liver injury
D. All of the above

1337. Which of the following particles of HBV do not circulate in the serum?
Harrison's 20th Ed. Chapter 332 Page 2349

A. HBsAg
B. HBcAg
C. HBeAg
D. All of the above

HBcAg is intracellular. When in serum, it is within an HBsAg coat. Therefore, naked HBcAg particles do not circulate in serum and are not detectable routinely in serum of patients with HBV infection.

1338. Hepatitis B patients contain which of the following circulating antibodies?
Harrison's 20th Ed. Chapter 332 Page 2349

A. Anti-HBe Ag
B. Anti-HBs Ag
C. Anti HBcAg
D. All of the above

Hepatitis B patients contain circulating antibodies against HBcAg (hepatitis B core antigen), & develop antibodies against HBeAg & HBsAg (anti-HBe & anti-HBs) at later stages.

1339. Which of the following HBV genes codes for DNA polymerase?
Harrison's 20th Ed. Chapter 332 Page 2349

A. S
B. C
C. P
D. X

Gene P of the HBV genes is the largest and codes for DNA polymerase which has both DNA-dependent DNA polymerase and RNA-dependent reverse transcriptase activities.

1340. Which of the following about HBV DNA polymerase is false?
Harrison's 20th Ed. Chapter 332 Page 2349

A. Encoded by P gene
B. Has DNA-dependent DNA polymerase activity
C. Has RNA-dependent reverse transcriptase activity
D. None of the above

1341. Which of the following is a nonparticulate protein of HBV?
Harrison's 20th Ed. Chapter 332 Page 2349

A. HBeAg
B. HBcAg
C. HBxAg
D. All of the above

1342. Which of the following HBV antigens stimulates HBV reverse transcription and HBV DNA replication?
Harrison's 20th Ed. Chapter 332 Page 2349

A. HBsAg
B. HBeAg
C. HBcAg
D. HBxAg

Hepatitis B x antigen (HBxAg) activates signal-transduction pathways that lead to stimulation of HBV reverse transcription and HBV DNA replication.

1343. Clinical association is observed between expression of which of the following & severe chronic hepatitis & hepatocellular carcinoma?
Harrison's 20th Ed. Chapter 332 Page 2349

A. HBsAg
B. HBeAg
C. HBcAg
D. HBxAg

Because HBxAg transactivation enhances replication of HBV, clinical association is observed between its expression with severe chronic hepatitis and hepatocellular carcinoma.

1344. Expression of which of the following HBV antigens induces programmed cell death (apoptosis)?
Harrison's 20th Ed. Chapter 332 Page 2349

A. HBsAg
B. HBeAg
C. HBcAg
D. HBxAg

Expression of HBxAg induces programmed cell death (apoptosis).

1345. Which of the following is transactivated by expression of HBxAg?
Harrison's 20th Ed. Chapter 332 Page 2350

A. Transcription & replication of HIV
B. Transactivation of human interferon gene
C. Transactivation of class I major histocompatibility genes
D. All of the above

1346. After infection with HBV, the first virologic marker detectable in serum is?

Harrison's 20th Ed. Chapter 332 Page 2350

A. HBsAg
B. HBeAg
C. HBcAg
D. HBxAg

Upon HBV infection, the first virologic marker detectable in serum within 1-12 weeks, usually between 8–12 weeks is HBsAg.

1347. Which of the following statements is true?

Harrison's 20th Ed. Chapter 332 Page 2350

A. Circulating HBsAg precedes elevations of SGOT/SGPT
B. Circulating HBsAg follow elevations of SGOT/SGPT
C. Circulating HBsAg coincide with elevations of SGOT/SGPT
D. None of the above

Circulating HBsAg precedes elevations of serum aminotransferase activity and clinical symptoms by 2–6 weeks and remains detectable during the entire icteric or symptomatic phase of acute hepatitis B and beyond.

1348. After the onset of jaundice, HBsAg rarely persists beyond how many months?

Harrison's 20th Ed. Chapter 332 Page 2350

A. 1 month
B. 3 months
C. 6 months
D. 9 months

In typical cases, HBsAg becomes undetectable 1–2 months after the onset of jaundice and rarely persists beyond 6 months.

1349. Of the following antibodies against HBV, which one is first to appear?

Harrison's 20th Ed. Chapter 332 Page 2350

A. Anti-HBc
B. Anti-HBs
C. Anti-HBe
D. None of the above

1350. Of the following antibodies against HBV, which one is detected last?

Harrison's 20th Ed. Chapter 332 Page 2350

A. Anti-HBc
B. Anti-HBs
C. Anti-HBe
D. None of the above

Of the 3 antibodies against HBV, anti-HBc develops first, whereas anti-HBs antibody is detected last. Anti-HBc appears in serum within the first 1–2 weeks after appearance of HBsAg & preceding anti-HBs by weeks to months. Anti-HBs becomes detectable after HBsAg disappears in serum and remains detectable indefinitely thereafter.

1351. Which of the following about HBsAg in acute HBV infection is false?

Harrison's 20th Ed. Chapter 332 Page 2350

A. Precedes rise in ALT
B. Precedes clinical symptoms
C. Detectable during entire icteric or symptomatic phase
D. Rarely persists beyond 3 months

Circulating HBsAg precedes rise in serum aminotransferase levels & clinical symptoms by 2–6 weeks and remains detectable during the entire icteric or symptomatic phase of acute hepatitis B & beyond. HBsAg becomes undetectable 1–2 months after onset of jaundice & rarely persists beyond 6 months.

1352. Which of the following about serology in acute HBV infection is false?

Harrison's 20th Ed. Chapter 332 Page 2350

A. Anti-HBs appears after HBsAg disappears
B. Anti-HBs remains detectable indefinitely
C. Anti-HBs precedes appearance of anti-HBc
D. HBeAg appears almost concurrently with HBsAg

After HBsAg disappears, antibody to HBsAg (anti-HBs) becomes detectable in serum & remains detectable indefinitely. HBcAg naked core particles do not circulate in serum & therefore, HBcAg is not detectable routinely in serum of patients with HBV infection. Anti-HBc is readily demonstrable in serum, beginning within first 1–2 weeks after appearance of HBsAg & preceding detectable levels of anti-HBs by weeks to months. HBeAg appears concurrently with or shortly after HBsAg.

1353. Which of the following is true during "gap" or "window" period in acute HBV infection?

Harrison's 20th Ed. Chapter 332 Page 2350

A. Absence of HBsAg
B. Absence of anti-HBs
C. Presence of IgM anti-HBc
D. All of the above

At times a gap of several weeks or longer may separate disappearance of HBsAg & appearance of anti-HBs. During this "gap" or "window" period, anti-HBc may be the only serologic evidence of current or recent HBV infection & blood containing IgM anti-HBc in the absence of HBsAg & anti-HBs has been implicated in development of transfusion-associated hepatitis B. HBV DNA may be low or undetected.

1354. Presence of which of the following represents hepatitis B infection in remote past?

Harrison's 20th Ed. Chapter 332 Page 2350

A. Anti-HBc
B. Anti-HBs
C. Anti-HBe
D. Any of the above

Isolated anti-HBc represent hepatitis B infection in the remote past. IgM anti-HBc predominates during the first six months after acute infection, whereas IgG anti-HBc persists beyond six months. Generally, in persons who have recovered from hepatitis B, anti-HBs and anti-HBc persist indefinitely.

1355. Isolated presence of which of the following suggests hepatitis B infection in remote past?

Harrison's 20th Ed. Chapter 332 Page 2350

A. HBsAg
B. Anti-HBs
C. IgM anti-HBc
D. IgG anti-HBc

After HBV infection, anti-HBc may persist in circulation longer than anti-HBs. Isolated anti-HBc does not indicate active virus replication but indicates HBV infection in remote past.

1356. Recent and remote HBV infections can be distinguished by determination of?

Harrison's 20th Ed. Chapter 332 Page 2350

A. Anti-HBs
B. IgM anti-HBc

C. IgG anti-HBc

D. All of the above

IgM anti-HBc predominates in first 6 months after acute infection, whereas IgG anti-HBc predominates beyond 6 months. In persons who have recovered from hepatitis B, anti-HBs & anti-HBc persist indefinitely.

1357. Presence of isolated anti-HBc suggests?
Harrison's 20th Ed. Chapter 332 Page 2350

A. Hepatitis B infection in the remote past

B. Low-level hepatitis B viremia (HBsAg below threshold)

C. Cross-reacting or false-positive immunologic specificity

D. Any of the above

Isolated anti-HBc does not necessarily indicate active virus replication.

1358. Which of the following genotype of HBV is frequent in India?
Hepatol Res. 2009;39(2):157-63

A. A

B. B

C. C

D. Any of the above

1359. Which of the following is false about the serology in first stage of HBV patient?
Harrison's 20th Ed. Chapter 332 Page 2350

A. Presence of HBsAg

B. Presence of HBeAg

C. Presence of anti-HBs antibody

D. Presence of IgM anti-HBc antibody

First stage of HBV infection is characterized by presence of HBsAg, HBeAg, and IgM class of anti-HBc antibodies. In intermediate stage, patients lose HBeAg, develop anti-HBe antibodies & enter into clinical remission. Finally, loss of HBsAg & rise of the anti-HBs antibody indicate recovery from infection.

1360. Which of the following about HBV viremia titer is false?
Int. J. Med. Sci. 2005;2(1)

A. Highest during HBeAg phase of infection

B. Declines during the anti-HBe phase

C. Disappears at the anti-HBs phase

D. None of the above

1361. Which of the following is false about expression of core protein and HBeAg?
Int. J. Med. Sci. 2005;2(1)

A. Core protein is translated from pregenomic mRNA, using the ATG codon at 1901 as initiation site

B. HBeAg is translated from precore mRNA, using ATG at 1814

C. G1896A nonsense mutation in precore region specifically prevents translation of HBeAg

D. None of the above

Core protein is translated from pregenomic mRNA, using the ATG codon at 1901 as initiation site. HBeAg is translated from the precore mRNA, using ATG at 1814. G1896A nonsense mutation in the precore region specifically prevents translation of HBeAg.

1362. HBeAg differs from HBcAg by a?
Journal of General Virology. 1995;76(4):1041-5

A. Longer N-terminus and longer C-terminal tail

B. Shorter N-terminus and shorter C-terminal tail

C. Shorter N-terminus and longer C-terminal tail

D. Longer N-terminus and shorter C-terminal tail

HBeAg differs from core protein (HBcAg) by a longer N-terminus and shorter C-terminal tail. HBeAg is a 15 kDa soluble antigen derived from a precursor protein (precore protein) by two processing events, cleavage of the N-terminal signal peptide and cleavage of the C-terminal 34 amino acids.

1363. Which of the following statements about HBV is false?
Harrison's 20th Ed. Chapter 332 Page 2350

A. HBeAg is not part of the virus particle

B. Anti-HBc antibody rises soon after infection

C. HBeAg expression is not essential for virus replication

D. None of the above

1364. HBeAg-negative chronic hepatitis B or e-CHB is characterised by all except?
Harrison's 20th Ed. Chapter 332 Page 2350

A. HBsAg-positive for at least 6 months

B. HBeAg-positive

C. Anti-HBe-positive

D. HBV DNA detectable in serum unamplified assays

e-CHB or HBeAg-negative chronic hepatitis B patients are HBsAg-positive for at least 6 months, HBeAg-negative, anti-HBe-positive, with HBV DNA detectable in serum unamplified assays, and active liver disease (elevated AST or ALT, liver histology showing chronic hepatitis with or without cirrhosis).

1365. Which of the following is expressed during periods of peak replication?
Harrison's 20th Ed. Chapter 332 Page 2350

A. HBeAg

B. Pre-S1 proteins

C. Pre-S2 proteins

D. All of the above

HBeAg, appears concurrently with or shortly after HBsAg and its appearance coincides expression of pre-S1 and pre-S2 proteins marking high levels of virus replication and presence of circulating intact virions and detectable HBV DNA.

1366. Which of the following is the qualitative marker of the replicative stage of HBV infection?
Harrison's 20th Ed. Chapter 332 Page 2351

A. HBsAg

B. HBcAg

C. HBeAg

D. HBxAg

Replicative stage of HBV infection is the time of maximal infectivity & liver injury. HBeAg is a qualitative marker & HBV DNA a quantitative marker of replicative phase, during which all three forms of HBV circulate, including intact virions.

1367. Replicative phase of chronic HBV infection converts to relatively nonreplicative phase at a rate of?
Harrison's 20th Ed. Chapter 332 Page 2351

A. 10% per year

B. 20% per year

C. 30% per year

D. 40% per year

Replicative phase of chronic HBV infection converts to a relatively nonreplicative phase at a rate of 10% per year accompanied by seroconversion from HBeAg-positive to anti-HBe-positive.

1368. Seroconversion from HBeAg-positive to anti-HBe-positive is accompanied by which of the following?

Harrison's 20th Ed. Chapter 332 Page 2351

A. Acute elevation in alanine aminotransferase (ALT) activity
B. Hemoglobinuria
C. Anemia
D. All of the above

Seroconversion from HBeAg-positive to anti-HBe-positive is accompanied by a transient, acute hepatitis-like elevation in aminotransferase activity, believed to reflect cell-mediated immune clearance of virus-infected hepatocytes.

1369. Spontaneous reactivation of replicative HBV infection from nonreplicative phase is marked by which of the following?

Harrison's 20th Ed. Chapter 332 Page 2351

A. Re-expression of HBeAg
B. Re-expression of HBV DNA
C. Reappearance of IgM anti-HBc
D. All of the above

Spontaneous reactivations i.e. nonreplicative HBV infection converting back to replicative infection is accompanied by re-expression of HBeAg and HBV DNA, IgM anti-HBc and exacerbations of liver injury.

1370. HBV infections is self-limited if?

Harrison's 20th Ed. Chapter 332 Page 2351

A. HBeAg becomes undetectable after peak rise in ALT
B. HBeAg becomes undetectable before disappearance of HBsAg
C. Anti-HBe becomes detectable before disappearance of HBsAg
D. All of the above

1371. Which of the following about HBeAg in acute HBV infection is false?

Harrison's 20th Ed. Chapter 332 Page 2351

A. Appears with HBsAg
B. Appearance coincides with high viral replication
C. Undetectable after peak rise in ALT
D. Undetectable after disappearance of HBsAg

HBeAg presence coincides with high levels of virus replication and reflects the presence of circulating intact virions and detectable HBV DNA. In self-limited HBV infections, HBeAg becomes undetectable shortly after peak elevations in aminotransferase activity, before the disappearance of HBsAg, and anti-HBe then becomes detectable, coinciding with a period of relatively lower infectivity.

1372. Which of the following about chronic HBV infection is false?

Harrison's 20th Ed. Chapter 332 Page 2351

A. HBsAg detectable > 6 months
B. IgG anti-HBc present
C. Anti-HBs low to absent
D. None of the above

In chronic HBV infection, HBsAg remains detectable beyond 6 months, anti-HBc is primarily of the IgG class, and anti-HBs is either undetectable or detectable at low levels.

1373. Replicative chronic hepatitis B in the absence of HBeAg occurs in which of the following situations?

Harrison's 20th Ed. Chapter 332 Page 2351

A. Patients with core mutations
B. Patients with precore mutations
C. Patients with pre S1 mutations
D. Patients with pre S2 mutations

Replicative chronic hepatitis B in the absence of HBeAg occurs in patients with precore mutations who cannot synthesize HBeAg.

1374. HBeAg-negative chronic hepatitis with mutations in the precore region is now the most frequently encountered form of hepatitis B in which region of the world?

Harrison's 20th Ed. Chapter 332 Page 2351

A. North America
B. South America
C. Mediterranean countries
D. Southeast Asia

HBeAg-negative chronic hepatitis with mutations in the precore region is now the most frequently encountered form of hepatitis B in Mediterranean countries and in Europe.

1375. Which of the following is false about severe chronic HBV infection due to precore region HBV mutant?

Harrison's 20th Ed. Chapter 332 Page 2351

A. Detectable HBV DNA
B. HBeAg negative
C. Anti-HBe positive
D. None of the above

Molecular variants of HBV may not express typical viral proteins i.e. nucleocapsid proteins, envelope proteins, or both. Severe chronic HBV infection due to precore region HBV mutantion have detectable HBV DNA (> 105 copies/ml), and anti-HBe but no HBeAg as the mutant virus is incapable of encoding HBeAg. This is an example of single base substitution, from G to A, which occurs in the second to last codon of pre-C gene at nucleotide 1896 results in the replacement of the TGG tryptophan codon by a stop codon (TAG), which prevents the translation of HBeAg.

1376. HBV escape mutants best relate to which of the following?

Harrison's 20th Ed. Chapter 332 Page 2351

A. Single base substitution
B. Single base addition
C. Single amino acid substitution
D. Single amino acid addition

In escape mutants of HBV there occurs a single amino acid substitution, from glycine to arginine at position 145 of the immunodominant "a" determinant common to all subtypes of HBsAg. This change in HBsAg leads to a loss of neutralizing activity by anti-HBs. This HBV/a mutant is seen in active and passive immunization, and in liver transplant recipients who underwent the procedure for hepatitis B and who were treated with a high-potency human monoclonal anti-HBs preparation.

1377. Extrahepatic site where Hepatitis B antigen and HBV DNA has been identified is?

Harrison's 20th Ed. Chapter 332 Page 2351

A. Bone marrow
B. Spleen
C. Pancreas
D. All of the above

Although not associated with tissue injury, extrahepatic site where Hepatitis B antigens and HBV DNA have been identified include lymph nodes, bone marrow, circulating lymphocytes, spleen, and pancreas.

1378. Which of the following is a member of the genus Deltavirus?

Harrison's 20th Ed. Chapter 332 Page 2351

A. Hepatitis D virus
B. Marburg virus
C. California encephalitis virus
D. All of the above

Delta hepatitis agent (HDV) is the only member of the genus Deltavirus.

1379. Which of the following is false about delta hepatitis virus?
Harrison's 20th Ed. Chapter 332 Page 2351

A. Defective RNA virus
B. 35- to 37-nm in size
C. 1700-nucleotide genome
D. Has antigenic homology with HBV antigens

HDV is a defective RNA virus that coinfects with and requires the helper function of HBV for its replication & expression. It is formalin-sensitive, 35- to 37-nm virus with a hybrid structure. Its genome is a 1700-nucleotide, circular, single-strand RNA. Delta antigen bears no antigenic homology with any of the HBV antigens.

1380. Delta core of HDV is "encapsidated" by an outer envelope of?
Harrison's 20th Ed. Chapter 332 Page 2351

A. HBcAg
B. HBsAg
C. HBeAg
D. None of the above

The delta core of HDV is "encapsidated" by an outer envelope of HBsAg quite like that of HBV.

1381. The single-stranded RNA genome of HDV is homologous to an extent with which gene of HBV?
Harrison's 20th Ed. Chapter 332 Page 2351

A. S
B. C
C. P
D. X

HDV genome is a small, 1700-nucleotide, circular, single-strand RNA of negative polarity that is nonhomologous with HBV DNA, except for a small area of the polymerase gene.

1382. HDV RNA requires which of the following for its replication?
Harrison's 20th Ed. Chapter 332 Page 2351

A. Host RNA polymerase I
B. Viral RNA polymerase I
C. Host RNA polymerase II
D. Viral RNA polymerase II

HDV RNA requires host RNA polymerase II for its replication via RNA-directed RNA synthesis by transcription of genomic RNA to a complementary antigenomic (plus strand) RNA. The antigenomic RNA, in turn, serves as a template for subsequent genomic RNA synthesis.

1383. When HDV infects a person simultaneously with HBV, it is called?
Harrison's 20th Ed. Chapter 332 Page 2352

A. Super-infection
B. Co-infection
C. Multiple infection
D. Sub-infection

Co-infection means HDV infecting a person simultaneously with HBV. Superinfection means HDV infecting a person already infected with HBV.

1384. Which of the following is false about delta hepatitis virus?
Harrison's 20th Ed. Chapter 332 Page 2352

A. HDV relies absolutely on HBV
B. HDV replication tends to suppress HBV replication
C. In chronic HDV infection, anti-HDV circulates in high titer
D. None of the above

1385. Which of the following is false about delta hepatitis virus?
Harrison's 20th Ed. Chapter 332 Page 2352

A. HDV antigen is expressed in hepatocyte nuclei
B. Intracellular replication of HDV RNA can occur without HBV
C. Duration of HDV infection determined by duration of HBV infection
D. In acute HDV infection, anti-HDV detected before symptoms appear

In acute HDV infection, anti-HDV is detected 30–40 days after symptoms appear.

1386. Which of the following is an HDV protein?
Harrison's 20th Ed. Chapter 332 Page 2352

A. HDAg
B. HDsAg
C. HDeAg
D. All of the above

HDV RNA has only one open reading frame, and delta antigen (HDAg), a product of the antigenomic strand is the only known HDV protein. When HDV infection is transmitted from a donor with a particular HBsAg subtype to an HBsAg-positive recipient with a different subtype, HDV assumes the HBsAg subtype of the recipient, rather than the donor.

1387. Which of the following hepatitis was earlier called "non-A, non-B hepatitis"?
Harrison's 20th Ed. Chapter 332 Page 2352

A. Hepatitis A
B. Hepatitis B
C. Hepatitis C
D. Hepatitis E

Before its identification, Hepatitis C virus was labeled as "non-A, non-B hepatitis".

1388. Hepatitis C virus was first identified in which year?
Liver Int. 2009;29(1):82-8

A. 1986
B. 1989
C. 1992
D. 1995

The non-A, non-B hepatitis virus, later known as Hepatitis C virus was first identified in 1989 by scientists at a California biotechnology company called Chiron Corporation who were collaborating with investigators at the Centers for Disease Control and Prevention (CDC).

1389. Which of the following genera belong to the family Flaviviridae?
Harrison's 20th Ed. Chapter 332 Page 2352

A. Pestivirus
B. Hepacivirus
C. Flavivirus
D. All of the above

The genera Pestivirus, Hepacivirus and Flavivirus are grouped together in the family Flaviviridae.

1390. Which of the following is a hepacivirus?
Harrison's 20th Ed. Chapter 332 Page 2352

A. Hepatitis C virus
B. Hepatitis D virus
C. Hepatitis E virus
D. All of the above

HCV is the only member of the genus Hepacivirus in the family Flaviviridae.

1391. Which of the following is a member of family Flaviviridae?
Harrison's 20th Ed. Chapter 332 Page 2352

A. Yellow fever virus
B. Dengue virus
C. Hepatitis C virus
D. All of the above

Members of family Flaviviridae are Yellow fever virus, Dengue virus, St. Louis encephalitis virus, West Nile virus, Hepatitis C virus (HCV) and Hepatitis G virus.

1392. Which of the following is a structural protein in HCV?
Harrison's 20th Ed. Chapter 332 Page 2352

A. C
B. E1
C. E2
D. All of the above

The three structural genes at the 5' end of hepatitis C virus genome are C - which codes for nucleocapsid, and E1 and E2 - which code for envelope glycoproteins.

1393. In hepatitis C virus genome, which of the following functions as an ion channel?
Harrison's 20th Ed. Chapter 332 Page 2352

A. C
B. E1
C. E2
D. p7

Placed adjacent to the structural proteins, p7 is a membrane protein that appears to function as an ion channel.

1394. Which of the following is present between structural & nonstructural regions of hepatitis C virus genome?
Harrison's 20th Ed. Chapter 332 Page 2352 Figure 332-6

A. NS3
B. NS4
C. NS5A
D. p7

1395. NS2 codes for which of the following enzymes?
Harrison's 20th Ed. Chapter 332 Page 2352 Figure 332-6

A. Cysteine protease
B. Serine protease
C. RNA helicase
D. All of the above

NS2 codes for a cysteine protease. NS3 codes for a serine protease and an RNA helicase.

1396. Which of the following nonstructural regions of hepatitis C virus genome codes for RNA-dependent RNA polymerase?
Harrison's 20th Ed. Chapter 332 Page 2352 Figure 332-6

A. NS3
B. NS4
C. NS5A
D. NS5B

At 3' end are seven nonstructural (NS) proteins: p7, NS2, NS3, NS4A, NS4B, NS5A, and NS5B. NS5B codes for an RNA-dependent RNA polymerase.

1397. Which of the following is false about HCV?
Harrison's 20th Ed. Chapter 332 Page 2352

A. 40–60 nm in diameter
B. 9600-nucleotide RNA virus
C. Its half-life is 2.7 hours
D. None of the above

1398. Which of the following is false about HCV?
Harrison's 20th Ed. Chapter 332 Page 2352

A. HCV enters hepatocyte via CD81 receptor
B. Does not induce lasting immunity against reinfection
C. Most sensitive indicator is the presence of HCV RNA
D. None of the above

HCV gains entry into the hepatocyte via the nonliver-specific CD81 receptor and the liver-specific tight junction protein claudin-1. Most sensitive indicator of HCV infection is presence of HCV RNA, that requires molecular amplification by PCR or transcription-mediated amplification (TMA).

1399. Host receptor to which HCV binds on cell entry is?
Harrison's 20th Ed. Chapter 332 Page 2352

A. Occludin
B. Scavenger receptor B1
C. Epidermal growth factor receptor
D. All of the above

Other host receptors to which HCV binds on cell entry includes occludin, low-density lipoprotein receptors, glycosaminoglycans, scavenger receptor B1 and epidermal growth factor receptor.

1400. HCV masquerades as which of the following?
Harrison's 20th Ed. Chapter 332 Page 2352

A. Viroid
B. Nucleocapsid protein
C. Lipoprotein
D. CD81 receptor

HCV is a lipoviroparticle and masquerades as a lipoprotein.

1401. Internal ribosomal entry site (IRES) is situated at which end of the HCV genome?
Harrison's 20th Ed. Chapter 332 Page 2352

A. 3' end
B. 5' end
C. Both 3' end and 5' end
D. Any of the above

The 5' end of HCV genome consists of an untranslated region containing an internal ribosomal entry site (IRES) adjacent to the genes for three structural proteins, C, E1 and E2.

1402. Host cofactor involved in HCV replication is?
Harrison's 20th Ed. Chapter 332 Page 2352

A. Cyclophilin A
B. Cyclophilin B
C. Cyclophilin C
D. Cyclophilin D

1403. Which of the following is a liver-specific host microRNA?
Harrison's 20th Ed. Chapter 332 Page 2352

A. miR-122
B. miR-146a

C. miR-155
D. miR-21

Host cofactors involved in HCV replication include cyclophilin A (which binds to NS5A), and liver-specific host microRNA miR-122.

1404. Number of HCV genotypes identified is?
Harrison's 20th Ed. Chapter 332 Page 2352

A. 2
B. 3
C. 4
D. 6

Till date HCV genotypes identified are 6 as well as >50 subtypes within genotypes.

1405. HCV genotypes differ one from another in sequence homology by?
Harrison's 20th Ed. Chapter 332 Page 2352

A. 10%
B. 20%
C. 30%
D. 40%

1406. HCV subtypes differ one from another in sequence homology by?
Harrison's 20th Ed. Chapter 332 Page 2352

A. 10%
B. 20%
C. 30%
D. 40%

Genotypes differ one from another in sequence homology by 30%, subtypes differ by ~ 20%. Those with less differences in sequence homology are referred to as quasispecies.

1407. Which of the following interferes with effective humoral immunity in HCV infection?
Harrison's 20th Ed. Chapter 332 Page 2352

A. High replication rate
B. Large hypervariable region
C. High mutation rate
D. Intragenotypic differences

High mutation rate of HCV virus interferes with effective humoral immunity. Neither heterologous nor homologous immunity develops commonly after acute HCV infection.

1408. In which HCV genotype, hepatic steatosis & clinical progression are more likely?
Harrison's 20th Ed. Chapter 332 Page 2352

A. 1
B. 2
C. 3
D. 4

In HCV genotype 3, hepatic steatosis & clinical progression are more likely.

1409. Differences exist among HCV genotypes in as regards?
Harrison's 20th Ed. Chapter 332 Page 2352

A. Responsiveness to antiviral therapy
B. Pathogenicity
C. Clinical progression
D. All of the above

There are no differences among HCV genotypes in pathogenicity or clinical progression. However, differences exist among HCV genotypes in responsiveness to antiviral therapy.

1410. In acute HCV infection, immunoassays detect anti-HCV antibodies against which of the following proteins?
Harrison's 20th Ed. Chapter 332 Page 2352

A. Core
B. NS3 region
C. NS5 region
D. All of the above

1411. HCV RNA is reported as?
Harrison's 20th Ed. Chapter 332 Page 2353

A. International units (IUs) per milliliter
B. Microgram per milliliter
C. Copies per milliliter
D. Virions per milliliter

HCV RNA is reported as international units (IUs) per milliliter.

1412. Which of the following is useful to detect the presence of HCV RNA?
Harrison's 20th Ed. Chapter 332 Page 2353

A. Transcription-mediated amplification (TMA)
B. Ligase chain reaction (LCR)
C. Enzyme immunoassays (EIAs)
D. Gas liquid chromatography assays

The most sensitive indicator of HCV infection is the presence of HCV RNA, which requires molecular amplification by PCR or transcription-mediated amplification (TMA).

1413. Which of the following is the first detectable event during acute hepatitis C progressing to chronicity?
Harrison's 20th Ed. Chapter 332 Page 2353 Figure 332-7

A. HCV RNA
B. HCV DNA
C. Elevated alanine aminotransferase (ALT)
D. Elevation and appearance of anti-HCV

During acute hepatitis C progressing to chronicity, HCV RNA is the first detectable event, preceding alanine aminotransferase (ALT) elevation and the appearance of anti-HCV.

1414. "Epidemic, non-A, non-B hepatitis" relates to which of the following?
N Engl J Med. 2012;367:1237-44, Harrison's 20th Ed. Chapter 332 Page 2353

A. Hepatitis A
B. Hepatitis B
C. Hepatitis C
D. Hepatitis E

Hepatitis E was initially identified in 1980 as "epidemic or enterically transmitted, non-A, non-B hepatitis", an infectious, waterborne illness similar to hepatitis A.

1415. In India, most common cause of acute hepatitis is?
Harrison's 20th Ed. Chapter 332 Page 2353

A. Hepatitis A
B. Hepatitis B

C. Hepatitis C
D. Hepatitis E

In India, enterically transmitted HEV is the most common cause of acute hepatitis.

1416. Which of the following about HEV is false?
N Engl J Med. 2012;367:1237-44, Harrison's 20th Ed. Chapter 332 Page 2353

A. Enveloped virus
B. Single-stranded, positive-sense RNA genome
C. Genome is 7.2 kb in length
D. Genome contains three open reading frames (ORFs)

HEV is a small (32- to 34-nm), nonenveloped virus with a single-strand, positive-sense RNA genome (7.2 kb in length) which contains three partially overlapping open reading frames (ORFs) bracketed by short 5' and 3' nontranslated regions.

1417. ORF1 encodes which of the following nonstructural proteins?
N Engl J Med. 2012;367:1237-44

A. Methyl transferase (MT)
B. Cysteine protease (Pro)
C. Helicase (Hel)
D. All of the above

ORF1 encodes nonstructural proteins namely methyl transferase (MT), cysteine protease (Pro), helicase (Hel), and RNA polymerase (Pol). ORF1 also encodes three regions of unknown function (Y, H, and X).

1418. Which of the following ORF in Hepatitis E virus genome encodes the nonstructural, enzymatic activities required for viral replication?
N Engl J Med. 2012;367:1237-44, Harrison's 20th Ed. Chapter 332 Page 2353

A. ORF1
B. ORF2
C. ORF3
D. All of the above

Largest of three ORFs, ORF1 encodes the nonstructural, enzymatic activities required for viral replication.

1419. In HEV, which of the following genes encode the nucleocapsid protein?
Harrison's 20th Ed. Chapter 332 Page 2353

A. ORF1
B. ORF2
C. ORF3
D. All of the above

The middle-sized open reading frame 2 (ORF2) gene in HEV encodes the nucleocapsid protein. Largest ORF1 encodes nonstructural proteins involved in virus replication. The smallest ORF3, encodes a structural protein whose function remains undetermined.

1420. ORF gene relates to?
Harrison's 20th Ed. Chapter 332 Page 2353

A. Hepatitis A
B. Hepatitis B
C. Hepatitis C
D. Hepatitis E

HEV has three open reading frames (ORF) genes.

1421. Which of the following acts as an animal reservoir contributing to the perpetuation of HEV?
Harrison's 20th Ed. Chapter 332 Page 2353

A. Swine
B. Bird
C. Fish
D. Dog

Contributing to the perpetuation of HEV are animal reservoirs, most notably in swine. Others include camels, deer, rats, and rabbits.

1422. Which of the following best relates to HEV?
N Engl J Med. 2012;367:1237-44, Harrison's 20th Ed. Chapter 332 Page 2353

A. Flaviviridae
B. Hepeviridae
C. Rhabdoviridae
D. Arenaviridae

HEV was the first member to be identified in the Hepeviridae family.

1423. Which of the following about HEV is false?
N Engl J Med. 2012;367:1237-44

A. HEV replicates in cytoplasm
B. Genotypes 1 and 2 are human viruses
C. Genotypes 3 and 4 are swine viruses
D. None of the above

HEV replicates in cytoplasm. Four genotypes of HEV have been categorized into two major groups. Genotypes 1 and 2 are human viruses that cause epidemic hepatitis with waterborne and fecal-oral transmission. Genotypes 3 and 4 are swine viruses.

1424. Which of the following about HEV infection is false?
N Engl J Med. 2012;367:1237-44

A. HEV RNA is detectable in stool during incubation period
B. HEV RNA is detectable in serum during incubation period
C. IgM antibody is undetectable during recovery
D. None of the above

Both IgM anti-HEV and IgG anti-HEV appear early during acute infection, but both fall rapidly after acute infection, reaching low levels within 9–12 months.

1425. Incubation period of acute hepatitis E infection is?
N Engl J Med. 2012;367:1237-44

A. 1 to 2 weeks
B. 2 to 4 weeks
C. 3 to 8 weeks
D. 6 to 12 weeks

Acute hepatitis E has an incubation period of 3 to 8 weeks.

1426. Average case fatality rate in acute HEV infections is?
N Engl J Med. 2012;367:1237-44

A. 0%
B. 2%
C. 3%
D. 5%

Acute hepatitis E is mostly self-limited without progression to chronic hepatitis. Average case fatality rate is ~ 5%.

1427. Clinical features of autochthonous hepatitis E include all except?
N Engl J Med. 2012;367:1237-44

A. Disease rates highest among older adults
B. Hepatitis E is preventable by vaccination

C. No neurologic complications

D. Ribavirin, peginterferon indicated

In endemic, or autochthonous hepatitis E, the average age was more than 60 years, and men outnumbered women by at least 3 to 1. Hepatitis E is preventable by vaccination. Autochthonous HEV infection is usually subclinical and mild. Autochthonous hepatitis E has frequent serious complications, including "acute-on-chronic" liver failure, neurologic disorders (polyradiculopathy, the GBS, Bell's palsy, peripheral neuropathy, ataxia, and mental confusion), and chronic hepatitis. Chronic hepatitis E is also susceptible to antiviral therapy (peginterferon, ribavirin, or a combination of two).

1428. Chronic infection in Hepatitis E has been identified almost exclusively among?

N Engl J Med. 2012;367:1237-44

A. Pre-existing liver disease

B. Blood transfusion recipients

C. Pork eaters

D. Immunocompromised persons

Chronic HEV infection has been identified almost exclusively among immunocompromised persons (organ transplant recipients, patients receiving cancer chemotherapy, and HIV-infected persons). Blood transfusion is a potential but rare route of HEV transmission. Chronic hepatitis E is characterized by the persistence of HEV RNA in serum & stool, accompanied by fluctuating, mild-to-moderate elevations in serum ALT levels and low or moderate titers of IgG and IgM anti-HEV antibodies.

1429. Which of the following hepatitis viruses is directly cytopathic to hepatocytes?

Harrison's 20th Ed. Chapter 332 Page 2353

A. Hepatitis A

B. Hepatitis B

C. Hepatitis C

D. None of the above

None of the hepatitis viruses is directly cytopathic to hepatocytes.

1430. Which of the following statements is false?

Harrison's 20th Ed. Chapter 332 Page 2353

A. Hepatitis B virus is not directly cytopathic

B. HBcAg invites cytolytic T cells to destroy hepatocytes

C. Inactive hepatitis B carriers can have normal liver histology

D. None of the above

1431. Which of the following nucleocapsid protein of HBV invites cytolytic T cells to destroy HBV-infected hepatocytes?

Harrison's 20th Ed. Chapter 332 Page 2353

A. HBsAg

B. HBcAg

C. HBxAg

D. All of the above

Nucleocapsid proteins (HBcAg and HBeAg) on the cell membrane are the viral target antigens that, with host antigens, invite cytolytic T cells to destroy HBV-infected hepatocytes.

1432. Acute hepatitis B patients who would recover or progress to chronic hepatitis is determined by?

Harrison's 20th Ed. Chapter 332 Page 2353

A. HBV-specific helper CD4+ T cells levels

B. Polyclonality of CD8+ cytolytic T cell responsiveness

C. Antiviral cytokine elaboration by T cells

D. All of the above

Whether or not, acute hepatitis B patient would recover or progress to chronic hepatitis is determined by differences in robustness & broad polyclonality of CD8+ cytolytic T cell responsiveness; in HBV-specific helper CD4+ T cells level; in virus-specific T cells level; in viral T cell epitope escape mutations; and in elaboration of antiviral cytokines by T cells.

1433. Which of the following participate in the early immune response to HBV infection?

Harrison's 20th Ed. Chapter 332 Page 2353

A. Cytopathic antiviral mechanisms

B. Innate immune system

C. Inflammatory cytokines

D. All of the above

Early immune response to HBV infection leads to elimination of HBV replicative intermediates from cytoplasm & covalently closed circular viral DNA from the nucleus of infected hepatocytes.

1434. Which of the following participates in innate immune response to HBV infection?

Harrison's 20th Ed. Chapter 332 Page 2353

A. Natural killer (NK) cell cytotoxicity

B. Interleukin 10 (IL10) & transforming growth factor β (TGFβ)

C. Major histocompatibility complex

D. All of the above

Ultimately, HBV-HLA–specific cytolytic T cell responses of the adaptive immune system are responsible for recovery from HBV infection.

1435. Fibrosing cholestatic hepatitis best relates to?

Harrison's 20th Ed. Chapter 332 Page 2353

A. Gallstones

B. Liver transplantation

C. HIV infection

D. Cholangiocarcinoma

In patients who undergo liver transplantation for end-stage chronic hepatitis B, occasionally, rapidly progressive liver injury appears in the new liver with an unusual histologic pattern - fibrosing cholestatic hepatitis. Ultrastructurally, it represents a choking of the cell with overwhelming quantities of HBsAg.

1436. Which of the following statements is false?

Harrison's 20th Ed. Chapter 332 Page 2353

A. Patients with defects in cellular immune competence are more likely to remain chronically infected with HBV

B. Chronic HBV infection can occur in the absence of serum hepatitis Be antigen (HBeAg)

C. Most characteristic histologic feature of chronic HBV infection is "ground-glass hepatocyte" due to intracellular accumulation of HBsAg

D. None of the above

1437. Which of the following is associated with a more severe outcome of HBV infection?

Harrison's 20th Ed. Chapter 332 Page 2353

A. Infection with precore genetic mutants of HBV

B. Concomitant HDV and HBV infections

C. In liver transplantation for end-stage chronic hepatitis B

D. All of the above

1438. HBV infection in neonatal period is associated with all except?
Harrison's 20th Ed. Chapter 332 Page 2354

A. Acquisition of immunologic tolerance to HBV
B. Absence of acute-hepatitis illness
C. Almost invariable establishment of chronic infection
D. Never go into cirrhosis & hepatocellular carcinoma

Neonatally acquired HBV infection can may culminate into cirrhosis & hepatocellular carcinoma.

1439. HBV infection acquired during adolescence or early adulthood is associated with all except?
Harrison's 20th Ed. Chapter 332 Page 2354

A. Robust host-immune response
B. Acute hepatitis-like illness
C. Failure to recover is the exception
D. Chronicity is common

Chronicity is uncommon and risk of hepatocellular carcinoma is very low.

1440. Which of the following is a HBV infection phase?
Harrison's 20th Ed. Chapter 332 Page 2354

A. "Immunotolerant" phase
B. "Immunoreactive" phase
C. "Inactive" phase
D. All of the above

1441. In which of the following, there is no period of immunologic tolerance?
Harrison's 20th Ed. Chapter 332 Page 2354

A. Babies born to mothers with replicative chronic HBV infection
B. Adulthood-acquired HBV infection
C. Elderly-acquired HBV infection
D. All of the above

A typical adult living in West has self-limited acute hepatitis B. There is no period of immunologic tolerance.

1442. Which of the following HLA allele has been linked with self-limited hepatitis C?
Harrison's 20th Ed. Chapter 332 Page 2354

A. HLA-B*1501
B. HLA-B*5701
C. Single nucleotide polymorphism T allele at IL28B locus
D. C/C haplotype of the IL28B gene

*C/C haplotype of the IL28B gene has been linked with self-limited hepatitis C. It codes for interferon l3, a component of innate immune antiviral defense. The IL28B association is even stronger when combined with HLA class II DQB1*03:01.*

1443. Which of the following is type II interferon (IFN)?
Clin Microbiol Infect. 2014;20:1237-1245

A. IFN-α
B. IFN-β
C. IFN-γ
D. IFN-λ

IFNs are categorized into three different families: type I IFNs (IFN-α and IFN-β, with least 13 subtypes), type II IFN (IFN-γ), and type III IFN (IFN-λ1–4).

1444. Interleukin (IL)-28B is also known as?
Clin Microbiol Infect. 2014;20:1237-1245

A. IFN-λ1
B. IFN-λ2
C. IFN-λ3
D. IFN-λ4

1445. IL-28B gene resides on the short arm of chromosome?
Clin Microbiol Infect. 2014;20:1237-1245

A. 11
B. 15
C. 19
D. 21

IL-28B gene resides on the short arm of chromosome 19 (19q13.13) and encodes IFN-λ3, which, together with IFN-λ1 (IL-29), IFN-λ2 (IL-28A), and IFN-λ4, constitutes the IFN-λ family.

1446. Which of the following is related to the association between hepatitis C and autoimmune hepatitis?
Harrison's 20th Ed. Chapter 332 Page 2354

A. HCV NS3
B. HCV NS5A
C. Cytochrome P450 2D6
D. All of the above

Cross-reactivity between viral antigens (HCV NS3 & NS5A) and host autoantigens (cytochrome P450 2D6) explain the association between hepatitis C & patients with autoimmune hepatitis and antibodies to liver-kidney microsomal (LKM) antigen (anti-LKM).

1447. Which of the following plays a pathogenetic role in the extrahepatic manifestations of acute hepatitis B?
Harrison's 20th Ed. Chapter 332 Page 2354

A. Cytopathic role of virus
B. Immune complex - mediated tissue damage
C. Cryoprecipitable immune complexes
D. All of the above

Immune complex - mediated tissue damage (HBsAg-anti-HBs with activation of complement system) plays a pathogenetic role in the extrahepatic manifestations of acute hepatitis B.

1448. Which of the following is an extrahepatic manifestation of chronic hepatitis B?
Harrison's 20th Ed. Chapter 332 Page 2354

A. Glomerulonephritis with nephrotic syndrome
B. Polyarteritis nodosa
C. Essential mixed cryoglobulinemia (EMC)
D. All of the above

1449. Deposition of which of the following occurs in glomerular basement membrane in patients of chronic hepatitis B?
Harrison's 20th Ed. Chapter 332 Page 2354

A. HBsAg
B. Immunoglobulin
C. C3
D. All of the above

Glomerulonephritis with nephrotic syndrome seen in chronic hepatitis B is due to deposition of HBsAg, immunoglobulin, and C3 in the glomerular basement membrane.

1450. What percentage of patients with polyarteritis nodosa have HBsAg in their serum?

Harrison's 20th Ed. Chapter 332 Page 2354

A. 5–10%
B. 10–20%
C. 20–30%
D. 30–40%

20–30% of patients with polyarteritis nodosa have HBsAg in their serum.

1451. Which of the following is strongly associated with HCV infection?

N Engl J Med. 2011; 364:1479-80

A. Necrolytic acral erythema
B. Porphyria cutanea tarda
C. Leucocytoclastic vasculitis
D. Lichen planus (LP)

1452. Necrolytic acral erythema closely resembles?

N Engl J Med. 2011; 364:1479-80

A. Atopic dermatitis
B. Pemphigus vulgaris
C. Psoriasis
D. Scleroderma

1453. Necrolytic acral erythema is best related to?

N Engl J Med. 2011; 364:1479-80

A. Calcific chronic pancreatitis
B. Penicillamine therapy
C. Myeloproliferative disorders
D. Zinc deficiency

Necrolytic acral erythema, first described in 1996, is strongly associated with hepatitis C, often an early cutaneous marker of HCV infection. It is described as a well-defined, pruritic or burning, hyperkeratotic erythematous eruption that most often affects the acral surfaces. The pathogenesis of necrolytic acral erythema is related to zinc dysregulation due to hepatitis C induced metabolic alteration. Necrolytic acral erythema closely resembles psoriasis.

1454. Mixed cryoglobulinemia (MC) is associated with which of the following?

Harrison's 20th Ed. Chapter 308 Page 2149

A. HAV
B. HCV
C. HDV
D. HEV

Mixed cryoglobulinemia (MC) is unequivocally associated with HCV. Cryoglobulinemia can be seen with multiple myeloma, lymphoproliferative disorders, connective tissue diseases, infection & liver disease, in many instances it is idiopathic. When there is apparent absence of an underlying disease and presence of cryoprecipitate containing oligoclonal / polyclonal immunoglobulins, this entity is called essential mixed cryoglobulinemia (EMC). Vast majority of patients who were considered to have EMC have cryoglobulinemic vasculitis related to hepatitis C infection.

1455. Monoclonal cryoglobulinemia is associated with which of the following?

Harrison's 20th Ed. Chapter 54 Page 354

A. Plasma cell dyscrasias
B. Chronic lymphocytic leukemia
C. Lymphoma
D. All of the above

Monoclonal cryoglobulinemia is associated with plasma cell dyscrasias, chronic lymphocytic leukemia and lymphoma.

1456. Classic triad of cryoglobulinemic syndrome includes all except?

Harrison's 20th Ed. Chapter 356 Page 2586

A. Purpura
B. Arthralgias
C. Weakness
D. Acrocyanosis

Classic triad of cryoglobulinemic syndrome consists of palpable purpura, arthralgias & weakness. Others are glomerulonephritis, peripheral neuropathy, generalized vasculitis, livedo reticularis, ischemic ulcers, acrocyanosis and hemorrhagic bullae.

1457. What percentage of patients with chronic hepatitis C will develop cryoglobulinemic vasculitis?

Harrison's 20th Ed. Chapter 356 Page 2586

A. 5%
B. 10%
C. 20%
D. 40%

5% of patients with chronic hepatitis C will develop cryoglobulinemic vasculitis.

1458. Which of the following glomerulonephritis is responsible for most renal lesions in cryoglobulinemic vasculitis?

Harrison's 20th Ed. Chapter 356 Page 2586

A. Minimal change glomerulonephritis
B. Membranoproliferative glomerulonephritis
C. Membranous glomerulonephritis (MGN)
D. Mesangioproliferative glomerulonephritis

Membranoproliferative glomerulonephritis is responsible for 80% of all renal lesions in cryoglobulinemic vasculitis.

1459. In cryoglobulinemic vasculitis, immune complexes consisting of?

Harrison's 20th Ed. Chapter 356 Page 2586

A. Hepatitis C antigens
B. Polyclonal hepatitis C-specific IgG
C. Monoclonal IgM rheumatoid factor
D. All of the above

Cryoglobulinemic vasculitis occurs when an aberrant immune response to hepatitis C infection leads to the formation of immune complexes consisting of hepatitis C antigens, polyclonal hepatitis C-specific IgG, and monoclonal IgM rheumatoid factor. The deposition of these immune complexes in blood vessel walls triggers an inflammatory cascade that results in cryoglobulinemic vasculitis.

1460. Which of the following is almost always found in cryoglobulinemic vasculitis?

Harrison's 20th Ed. Chapter 356 Page 2586

A. Antinuclear antibodies
B. Anti-smooth muscle antibodies
C. Antiplatelet antibodies
D. Rheumatoid factor

Rheumatoid factor is almost always found in cryoglobulinemic vasculitis and may be a useful clue to the disease when cryoglobulins are not detected. Hypocomplementemia occurs in 90% of patients An elevated ESR and anemia occur frequently. Evidence for hepatitis C infection must be sought in all patients by testing for hepatitis C antibodies and hepatitis C RNA.

1461. Which of the following about cryoglobulins is false?
Harrison's 20th Ed. Chapter 107 Page 802

A. Mixed cryoglobulins are not associated with malignancy
B. 10% of macroglobulins are cryoglobulins
C. For cryoglobulins, blood is drawn into a warm syringe
D. None of the above

Mixed cryoglobulins are composed of IgM or IgA complexed with IgG, for which they are specific.

1462. Morphologic lesions of viral hepatitis are all except?
Harrison's 20th Ed. Chapter 332 Page 2355

A. Panlobular mononuclear cells infiltration
B. Hepatic cell necrosis
C. Cholestasis
D. Atrophy of Kupffer cells

Typical morphologic lesions of all types of viral hepatitis are panlobular infiltration with mononuclear cells, hepatic cell necrosis, Kupffer cells hyperplasia & variable cholestasis. Hepatic cell regeneration is present.

1463. Hepatic cell regeneration is evidenced by?
Harrison's 20th Ed. Chapter 332 Page 2355

A. Numerous mitotic figures
B. Multinucleated cells
C. "Rosette" or "pseudoacinar" formation
D. All of the above

Hepatic cell regeneration is evidenced by numerous mitotic figures, multinucleated cells and "rosette" or "pseudoacinar" formation.

1464. Panlobular mononuclear infiltration in viral hepatitis consists "primarily" of?
Harrison's 20th Ed. Chapter 332 Page 2355

A. Plasma cells
B. Small lymphocytes
C. Large lymphocytes
D. Eosinophils

Panlobular mononuclear infiltration in viral hepatitis consists "primarily" of small lymphocytes. Plasma cells & eosinophils are present occasionally.

1465. William Thomas Councilman (1854-1933) was of which nationality?
Science. 1933;77(2009):613-18

A. British
B. American
C. Ireland
D. Canadian

Councilman bodies are named after American pathologist William Thomas Councilman (1854-1933) who discovered them. His work included study of amebiasis, diphtheria, smallpox, and yellow fever.

1466. Councilman bodies are best related to?
Harrison's 20th Ed. Chapter 332 Page 2355

A. Fibrosis
B. Liver cell regeneration
C. Apoptosis
D. Growth arrest

Liver cell damage leads to acidophilic degeneration of hepatocytes called Councilman or apoptotic bodies.

1467. Liver cell damage in viral hepatitis consists of?
Harrison's 20th Ed. Chapter 332 Page 2355

A. Hepatic cell degeneration and necrosis
B. Cell dropout, ballooning of cells
C. Acidophilic degeneration of hepatocytes
D. All of the above

Liver cell damage in viral hepatitis consists of hepatic cell degeneration and necrosis, cell dropout, ballooning of cells, and acidophilic degeneration of hepatocytes (Councilman or apoptotic bodies).

1468. Which of the following is seen in chronic but not in acute HBV infection?
Harrison's 20th Ed. Chapter 332 Page 2355

A. Acidophilic degeneration of hepatocytes
B. Ballooning of hepatocytes
C. Hepatocyte dropout
D. Large hepatocytes with ground-glass appearance of cytoplasm

Large hepatocytes with a ground-glass appearance of the cytoplasm may be seen in chronic but not in acute HBV infection.

1469. Ground-glass appearance of the cytoplasm in chronic HBV infection is due to?
Harrison's 20th Ed. Chapter 332 Page 2355

A. HBsAg
B. HBeAg
C. HBcAg
D. HBxAg

1470. Hepatocytes containing HBsAg can be identified histochemically with?
Harrison's 20th Ed. Chapter 332 Page 2355

A. Orcein or aldehyde fuchsin
B. Congo red
C. Nitroblue tetrazolium (NBT)
D. Crystal violet

Ground-glass appearance of the cytoplasm in chronic HBV infection is due to HBsAg and can be identified histochemically with orcein or aldehyde fuchsin.

1471. In hepatitis C, the most remarkable histologic feature is?
Harrison's 20th Ed. Chapter 332 Page 2355

A. Marked increase in activation of sinusoidal lining cells
B. Relative paucity of inflammation
C. Lymphoid aggregates
D. Bile duct lesions

In hepatitis C, the histologic lesion is remarkable for a relative paucity of inflammation.

1472. In Hepatitis C, which of the following histologic lesion is linked to increased fibrosis?
Harrison's 20th Ed. Chapter 332 Page 2355

A. Increase in activation of sinusoidal lining cells
B. Lymphoid aggregates
C. Presence of fat
D. Bile duct lesions

In hepatitis C, apart from the most notable histologic lesion i.e. relative paucity of inflammation, there is marked increase in activation of sinusoidal lining cells, lymphoid aggregates, presence of fat (more frequent in genotype 3 & linked to increased fibrosis), and, occasionally, bile duct lesions.

1473. Marked cholestasis is a feature of?

Harrison's 20th Ed. Chapter 332 Page 2355

A. HAV
B. HCV
C. HDV
D. HEV

Marked cholestasis is a common histologic feature of hepatitis E.

1474. Bridging hepatic necrosis is also called?

Harrison's 20th Ed. Chapter 332 Page 2355

A. Subacute necrosis
B. Confluent necrosis
C. Interface hepatitis
D. All of the above

In acute hepatitis, bridging hepatic necrosis, also termed subacute or confluent necrosis or interface hepatitis is observed occasionally.

1475. What was earlier called piecemeal necrosis is now called?

Harrison's 20th Ed. Chapter 334 Page 2375

A. Gradual hepatitis
B. Interface hepatitis
C. Coupled hepatitis
D. Destruction hepatitis

Piecemeal necrosis or limiting plate necrosis is now called "interface hepatitis".

1476. In bridging hepatic necrosis, the bridge consists of?

Harrison's 20th Ed. Chapter 332 Page 2355

A. Condensed reticulum
B. Inflammatory debris
C. Degenerating liver cells
D. All of the above

1477. The bridge in bridging hepatic necrosis spans?

Harrison's 20th Ed. Chapter 332 Page 2355

A. Adjacent portal areas
B. Portal to central veins
C. Central vein to central vein
D. Any of the above

In bridging hepatic necrosis, the bridge consists of condensed reticulum, inflammatory debris, and degenerating liver cells that span adjacent portal areas, portal to central veins, or central vein to central vein. There is collapse of the reticulin framework.

1478. Postmortem examination finding of a small, shrunken, soft liver is seen in?

Harrison's 20th Ed. Chapter 332 Page 2355

A. Massive hepatic necrosis
B. Fulminant hepatitis
C. Acute yellow atrophy
D. All of the above

Massive hepatic necrosis, fulminant hepatitis and acute yellow atrophy are synonymous.

1479. Which of the following histologic changes occur in liver injury?

World J Gastroenterol. 2011;17(17):2172-77

A. Ballooned hepatocytes
B. Mallory–Denk bodies
C. Apoptotic hepatocytes
D. All of the above

In liver disease, histologic examination of biopsied liver tissue may demonstrate steatosis, inflammation, ballooned hepatocytes, Mallory–Denk bodies, apoptotic hepatocytes, and fibrosis or cirrhosis.

1480. Mallory-Denk Bodies (MDB) are seen in?

World J Gastroenterol. 2011;17(17):2172-77

A. Hepatitis C
B. Primary biliary cirrhosis (PBC)
C. Nonalcoholic fatty liver disease (NAFLD)
D. All of the above

1481. Which of the following is localized to hepatocyte nucleus?

Harrison's 20th Ed. Chapter 332 Page 2355

A. HAV antigen
B. HCV antigen
C. HDV antigen
D. HEV antigen

1482. Which of the following antigens are localized to the cytoplasm?

Harrison's 20th Ed. Chapter 332 Page 2355

A. HAV
B. HCV
C. HEV
D. All of the above

HDV antigen is localized to hepatocyte nucleus, while HAV, HCV & HEV antigens are localized to the cytoplasm. HBsAg is localized to the cytoplasm & plasma membrane of infected liver cells.

1483. Which of the following hepatitis can be transmitted by fecal-oral route?

Harrison's 20th Ed. Chapter 332 Page 2356 Table 332-2

A. Hepatitis B
B. Hepatitis C
C. Hepatitis D
D. None of the above

Hepatitis A is transmitted almost exclusively by the fecal-oral route.

1484. Hepatitis virus with longest incubation period is?

Harrison's 20th Ed. Chapter 332 Page 2356 Table 332-2

A. Hepatitis A
B. Hepatitis B
C. Hepatitis C
D. Hepatitis E

1485. Hepatitis virus with an incubation period of ~2 weeks is?

Harrison's 20th Ed. Chapter 332 Page 2356 Table 332-2

A. Hepatitis A
B. Hepatitis C
C. Hepatitis E
D. All of the above

Incubation period in days: HAV - 15–45, mean 30, HBV - 30–180, mean 60–90, HCV - 15–160, mean 50, HDV - 30–180, mean 60–90, HEV - 14–60, mean 40.

1486. Viral hepatitis with an insidious onset only is?
Harrison's 20th Ed. Chapter 332 Page 2356 Table 332-2

A. Hepatitis A
B. Hepatitis B
C. Hepatitis C
D. Hepatitis E

Onset : HAV - acute, HBV - insidious or acute, HCV - insidious, HDV - insidious or acute, HEV - acute

1487. Chronicity is invariable in which of the following infections?
Harrison's 20th Ed. Chapter 332 Page 2356 Table 332-2

A. HBV / HDV coinfection
B. HBV / HDV superinfection
C. HBV / HIV co-infection
D. All of the above

1488. Which of the following hepatitis is not transmitted by sexual route?
Harrison's 20th Ed. Chapter 332 Page 2356 Table 332-2

A. Hepatitis A
B. Hepatitis B
C. Hepatitis D
D. Hepatitis E

1489. Which of the following hepatitis, perinatal transmission is least likely?
Harrison's 20th Ed. Chapter 332 Page 2356 Table 332-2

A. Hepatitis A
B. Hepatitis B
C. Hepatitis C
D. Hepatitis D

1490. Which of the following hepatitis, fulminant progression is most common in?
Harrison's 20th Ed. Chapter 332 Page 2356 Table 332-2

A. Hepatitis A
B. Hepatitis B
C. Hepatitis C
D. Hepatitis D

1491. Which of the following hepatitis, prognosis is excellent?
Harrison's 20th Ed. Chapter 332 Page 2356 Table 332-2

A. Hepatitis A
B. Hepatitis B
C. Hepatitis C
D. Hepatitis E

1492. Food material incriminated in transmission of HAV is?
Harrison's 20th Ed. Chapter 332 Page 2355

A. Frozen raspberries & strawberries
B. Green onions imported from Mexico
C. Shellfish
D. All of the above

HAV large outbreaks as well as sporadic cases have been traced to contaminated food, water, milk, frozen raspberries and strawberries, green onions imported from Mexico and shellfish.

1493. Hepatitis A infections tend to occur in?
Harrison's 20th Ed. Chapter 332 Page 2355

A. Early summer
B. Spring
C. Mid - monsoon
D. Late fall and early winter

Epidemiologic observations point towards the fact that hepatitis A infections tend to occur in late fall and early winter.

1494. Which of the following about HAV infections is false?
Harrison's 20th Ed. Chapter 332 Page 2355

A. Intrafamily & intrainstitutional spread common
B. No HAV carrier state identified after acute hepatitis A
C. Hepatitis A tends to be more symptomatic in adults
D. Hepatis A is never bloodborne

Hepatitis A is rarely bloodborne, several outbreaks have been recognized in recipients of clotting-factor concentrates.

1495. Which of the following body fluid from infected persons is most infectious?
Harrison's 20th Ed. Chapter 332 Page 2355

A. Semen
B. Saliva
C. Serum
D. All are equally infectious

HBsAg is identified in almost every body fluid from infected persons. Semen & saliva are infectious though less than serum.

1496. Which of the following is the mode of HBV transmission?
Harrison's 20th Ed. Chapter 332 Page 2356

A. Percutaneous inoculation
B. Sexual contact
C. Perinatal transmission
D. All of the above

HBV transmission by oral ingestion has been documented as a potential but inefficient route of exposure.

1497. What is not true for Hepatitis B virus infections?
Harrison's 20th Ed. Chapter 332 Page 2356, N Engl J Med. 2004;351:2832-8

A. Can be transmitted through breast milk
B. Incubation period for acute infection is 45 to 160 days
C. Risk of chronicity in infected neonates is 90%
D. No known animal reservoirs

~10% of HBV infections are acquired in utero. Most infections occur at the time of delivery and early postpartum period & are not related to breastfeeding.

1498. Perinatal transmission occurs in infants born to HBsAg carrier mothers during?
Harrison's 20th Ed. Chapter 332 Page 2356

A. First trimester of pregnancy
B. Second trimester of pregnancy
C. Third trimester of pregnancy
D. Any of the above

Perinatal transmission occurs primarily in infants born to HBsAg carrier mothers or mothers with acute hepatitis B during third trimester of pregnancy or during the early postpartum period.

1499. Which of the following mothers almost invariably transmit hepatitis B infection to their offspring?
Harrison's 20th Ed. Chapter 332 Page 2356

A. HBsAg-positive + HBeAg-positive
B. HBsAg-negative + HBeAg-negative
C. HBsAg-positive + HBeAg-negative
D. HBsAg-negative + HBeAg-positive

HBsAg positive mothers who are HBeAg-positive almost invariably (>90%) transmit hepatitis B infection to their offspring, whereas HBsAg carrier mothers with anti-HBe rarely (10-15%) infect their offspring.

1500. Likelihood of perinatal transmission of HBV correlates with the presence of?
Harrison's 20th Ed. Chapter 332 Page 2356

A. HBsAg
B. HBcAg
C. HBeAg
D. HBxAg

Likelihood of perinatal transmission of HBV correlates with presence of HBeAg. 90% of HBeAg-positive mothers but only 10–15% of anti-HBe-positive mothers transmit HBV infection to their offspring.

1501. Hepatitis B virus (HBV) chronically infects how many people worldwide?
Harrison's 20th Ed. Chapter 332 Page 2356

A. ~50 million
B. ~100 million
C. ~250 million
D. ~350 million

Hepatitis B virus (HBV) chronically infects over 350 million people worldwide.

1502. Prevalence of HBV sero-positivity is more in?
Harrison's 20th Ed. Chapter 332 Page 2356

A. Down's syndrome
B. Lepromatous leprosy
C. Hodgkin's disease
D. All of the above

Increased prevalence of serum HBsAg is found in Down's syndrome, lepromatous leprosy, leukemia, Hodgkin's disease, polyarteritis nodosa, CKD patients on dialysis and IDUs.

1503. Risk of acquiring HBV infection from a blood transfusion is?
Harrison's 20th Ed. Chapter 332 Page 2356

A. 1 in 50,000
B. 1 in 140,000
C. 1 in 230,000
D. 1 in 320,000

Because of highly sensitive virologic screening of donor blood, risk of acquiring HBV infection from a blood transfusion is 1 in 230,000 while it is 1 in 2.3 million for transfusion-associated HCV infection.

1504. HDV infection is endemic among those with hepatitis B in?
Harrison's 20th Ed. Chapter 332 Page 2357

A. Northern African countries
B. Southern European countries
C. Middle East countries
D. All of the above

1505. Which of the following is related to hepatitis D?
Harrison's 20th Ed. Chapter 332 Page 2357

A. Haverhill fever
B. Lábrea fever
C. Hibernian fever
D. Lassa fever

1506. Hepatitis C virus (HCV) infects how many people worldwide?
Harrison's 20th Ed. Chapter 332 Page 2357

A. ~80 million
B. ~120 million
C. ~170 million
D. ~250 million

1507. Extraordinarily high prevalences of HCV infection occur in?
Harrison's 20th Ed. Chapter 332 Page 2357

A. Thailand
B. Venezuala
C. Egypt
D. Haiti

Extraordinarily high prevalences of HCV infection occur in Egypt.

1508. Baby boomer generation refers to persons born between?
Harrison's 20th Ed. Chapter 332 Page 2358, N Engl J Med. 2006; 355:758-60

A. 1943 and 1961
B. 1944 and 1962
C. 1945 and 1963
D. 1946 and 1964

The term "baby boomer" refers to individuals born in the United States between mid-1946 and mid-1964.

1509. By 2012, HCV mortality had surpassed deaths from?
Harrison's 20th Ed. Chapter 332 Page 2358

A. HIV
B. Tuberculosis
C. Hepatitis B
D. All of the above

By 2012, HCV mortality had surpassed deaths from HIV, tuberculosis, hepatitis B, and 57 other notifiable infectious diseases (i.e. all infectious diseases)

1510. Which of the following about HCV infection is false?
Harrison's 20th Ed. Chapter 332 Page 2358

A. Accounts for 40% of chronic liver disease
B. Most frequent indication for liver transplantation
C. Worldwide, genotype 1 is the most common
D. Breastfeeding increases risk of HCV vertical infection

Worldwide, genotype 1 is the most common. Genotype 4 predominates in Egypt; genotype 5 is localized to South Africa, and genotype 6 to Hong Kong. Breastfeeding does not increase the risk of HCV infection between an infected mother and her infant.

1511. Which of the following about HEV infection is false?
Harrison's 20th Ed. Chapter 332 Page 2358

A. Enteric mode of spread
B. Secondary person-to-person spread rare

C. Swine is the zoonotic reservoir for HEV
D. None of the above

An epidemiologic feature that distinguishes HEV from other enteric agents is the rarity of secondary person-to-person spread from infected persons to their close contacts.

1512. Which of the following about presentation of acute viral hepatitis is false?
Harrison's 20th Ed. Chapter 332 Page 2359

A. Constitutional symptoms may precede onset of jaundice by 1 - 2 weeks
B. Dark urine & clay-colored stools occur 1 - 5 days before onset of clinical jaundice
C. Alterations in olfaction and taste
D. None of the above

1513. Which of the following is a presentation of acute viral hepatitis?
Harrison's 20th Ed. Chapter 332 Page 2359

A. Splenomegaly
B. Cervical adenopathy
C. Spider angiomas
D. All of the above

1514. Acute hepatitis B is self-limited in what proportion of cases?
Harrison's 20th Ed. Chapter 332 Page 2359

A. 50–69%
B. 69–79%
C. 79–89%
D. 95–99%

Acute hepatitis B is self-limited in 95 - 99% of infections.

1515. Acute hepatitis C is self-limited in what proportion of cases?
Harrison's 20th Ed. Chapter 332 Page 2359

A. 5–9%
B. 15–20%
C. 35–45%
D. 55–75%

Acute hepatitis C is self-limited in 15–20%.

1516. Which of the following is false about infection with HDV?
Harrison's 20th Ed. Chapter 332 Page 2359

A. Can occur in the presence of acute HBV infection
B. Can occur in the presence of chronic HBV infection
C. Duration of HBV infection determines duration of HDV infection
D. None of the above

1517. Acute hepatitis-like clinical events in chronic hepatitis B may be due to?
Harrison's 20th Ed. Chapter 332 Page 2359

A. HDV superinfection
B. Spontaneous HBeAg to anti-HBe seroconversion
C. Reversion from relatively nonreplicative to replicative infection
D. All of the above

Apart from the above conditions, acute clinical exacerbations of chronic hepatitis B may be due to emergence of a precore mutant.

1518. Therapy with which of the following can lead to reactivation of both hepatitis B and C?
Harrison's 20th Ed. Chapter 332 Page 2359

A. Anti-TNF-α therapy
B. Glucocorticoid therapy
C. Extracorporeal liver-assist devices
D. Plasmapheresis

Anti-TNF-α therapy can lead to reactivation of both hepatitis B and C.

1519. The diagnosis of anicteric hepatitis is based on?
Harrison's 20th Ed. Chapter 332 Page 2359

A. S. Aminotransferase levels
B. S. Bilirubin levels
C. S. Alkaline phosphatase levels
D. S. GGT levels

The diagnosis of anicteric hepatitis is based on clinical features & on aminotransferase elevations.

1520. In acute hepatitis, very high serum bilirubin level (20–30 mg/dL) occur in?
Harrison's 20th Ed. Chapter 332 Page 2359

A. Severe disease
B. Glucose-6-phosphate dehydrogenase deficiency
C. Sickle cell anemia
D. All of the above

Bilirubin levels >20 mg/dL persisting late into the course of viral hepatitis is associated with severe disease. Patients with underlying hemolytic anemia, like glucose-6-phosphate dehydrogenase deficiency and sickle cell anemia, also have high serum bilirubin levels (>30 mg/dL) due to superimposed hemolysis.

1521. Which of the following occur transiently in acute viral hepatitis?
Harrison's 20th Ed. Chapter 332 Page 2359

A. Neutropenia
B. Lymphopenia
C. Steatorrhea
D. All of the above

Neutropenia and lymphopenia are transient and are followed by a relative lymphocytosis. Also, mild and transient steatorrhea, microscopic hematuria and minimal proteinuria have been noted.

1522. Prognostically, which of the following is relevant in acute hepatitis?
Harrison's 20th Ed. Chapter 332 Page 2359

A. Levels of serum bilirubin
B. Levels of aminotransferases
C. Prothrombin time (PT) prolongation
D. All of the above

Prothrombin time (PT) prolongation in acute viral hepatitis reflects a severe hepatic synthetic defect, signify extensive hepatocellular necrosis, and indicates a worse prognosis.

1523. Which of the following is characteristically elevated during acute hepatitis A?
Harrison's 20th Ed. Chapter 332 Page 2359

A. Serum IgG
B. Serum IgM
C. Serum IgA
D. Serum IgE

A diffuse but mild elevation of the gamma globulin fraction is common during acute viral hepatitis. Serum IgM level is elevated more characteristically during acute hepatitis A.

1524. Which of the following antibodies may be present during the acute phase of viral hepatitis?

Harrison's 20th Ed. Chapter 332 Page 2359

A. Rheumatoid factor

B. Nuclear antibody

C. Heterophil antibody

D. All of the above

During the acute phase of viral hepatitis, antibodies to smooth muscle and other cell constituents may be present, and low titers of rheumatoid factor, nuclear antibody, and heterophil antibody can also be found. In hepatitis C and D, antibodies to LKM may be found.

1525. Which of the following can give rise to false-positive results for IgM anti-HAV during acute illness?

Harrison's 20th Ed. Chapter 332 Page 2359

A. Antibodies to LKM

B. Rheumatoid factor

C. Antiphospholipid antibodies

D. Cytoplasmic antineutrophil cytoplasmic antibody (c-ANCA)

1526. If levels of HBsAg are too low to be detected during acute HBV infection, which of the following establishes its diagnosis?

Harrison's 20th Ed. Chapter 332 Page 2359

A. IgM anti-HBc

B. IgG anti-HBc

C. IgM & IgG anti-HBc

D. HBeAg

If levels of HBsAg are too low to be detected during acute HBV infection, presence of IgM anti-HBc establishes its diagnosis. HBeAg is invariably present during early acute hepatitis B, HBeAg testing is indicated primarily during follow-up of chronic infection.

1527. Which of the following about HBsAg is false?

Harrison's 20th Ed. Chapter 332 Page 2359

A. HBsAg titer is not related to severity of clinical disease

B. HBsAg titers are highest in immunosuppressed patients

C. HBsAg titers are very low in acute fulminant hepatitis

D. None of the above

1528. Which of the following about HBeAg is false?

Harrison's 20th Ed. Chapter 332 Page 2360

A. It is an indicator of relative infectivity

B. HBeAg is invariably present during early acute hepatitis B

C. HBeAg testing is indicated primarily in chronic infection

D. None of the above

1529. Which of the following is true in chronic HBV infection?

Harrison's 20th Ed. Chapter 332 Page 2360

A. IgM anti-HBc-positive, IgG anti-HBc-positive

B. IgM anti-HBc-negative, IgG anti-HBc-negative

C. IgM anti-HBc-negative, IgG anti-HBc-positive

D. IgM anti-HBc-positive, IgG anti-HBc-negative

IgM anti-HBc may be useful to distinguish between acute or recent infection (IgM anti-HBc-positive) and chronic HBV infection (IgM anti-HBc-negative, IgG anti-HBc-positive).

1530. A false-positive test for IgM anti-HBc may be found in patients with?

Harrison's 20th Ed. Chapter 332 Page 2360

A. Glucose-6-phosphate dehydrogenase deficiency

B. High-titer rheumatoid factor

C. Sickle cell anemia

D. All of the above

A false-positive test for IgM anti-HBc may be encountered in patients with high-titer rheumatoid factor.

1531. Presence of anti-HBs in the presence of HBsAg in patients with acute hepatitis B indicates which of the following?

Harrison's 20th Ed. Chapter 332 Page 2360

A. Fulminant hepatitis

B. Chronicity

C. Imminent HBsAg clearance

D. None of the above

Anti-HBs is rarely detectable in the presence of HBsAg in patients with acute hepatitis B. When this happens, its of no recognized clinical significance.

1532. After hepatitis B vaccination, which is the only serologic marker to appear?

Harrison's 20th Ed. Chapter 332 Page 2360

A. Anti-HBs

B. Anti-HBe

C. Anti-HBc

D. All of the above

After immunization with hepatitis B vaccine, which consists of HBsAg alone, anti-HBs is the only serologic marker to appear.

1533. In hepatitis B, threshold for infectivity and liver injury is?

Harrison's 20th Ed. Chapter 332 Page 2360

A. 10^1 - 10^2 IU/mL

B. 10^2 - 10^3 IU/mL

C. 10^3 - 10^4 IU/mL

D. 10^5 - 10^6 IU/mL

1534. Which of the following is related to HBV replication?

Harrison's 20th Ed. Chapter 332 Page 2360

A. Hepatitis D virus

B. HBeAg

C. Serum HBV DNA

D. All of the above

Patients with hepatitis D tend to have lower levels of HBV replication. In hepatitis B is HBeAg. Its principal clinical usefulness is as an indicator of relative infectivity. Serum HBV DNA is an indicator of HBV replication.

1535. In chronic hepatitis B, high levels of HBV DNA indicate increased risk of?

Harrison's 20th Ed. Chapter 332 Page 2360

A. Cirrhosis

B. Hepatic decompensation

C. Hepatocellular carcinoma

D. All of the above

In chronic hepatitis B, high levels of HBV DNA increase the risk of cirrhosis, hepatic decompensation, and hepatocellular carcinoma.

1536. Presence of which of the following confirms that HBV infection is acute?

Harrison's 20th Ed. Chapter 332 Page 2360

A. IgM anti-HBcAg
B. IgM anti-HBsAg
C. IgM anti-HBeAg
D. IgM anti-HBxAg

Presence of HBsAg, with or without IgM anti-HBc, represents HBV infection. If IgM anti-HBc is present, the HBV infection is considered acute even in the absence of HBsAg. If IgM anti-HBc is absent, the HBV infection is considered chronic.

1537. HBsAg (+), Anti-HBs (–), IgM Anti-HBc (+), HBeAg (+), Anti-HBe (–) is indicative of?

Harrison's 20th Ed. Chapter 332 Page 2360 Table 332-5

A. Acute hepatitis B, high infectivity
B. Chronic hepatitis B, high infectivity
C. Low-level hepatitis B carrier
D. Hepatitis B in remote past

1538. HBsAg (+), Anti-HBs (–), IgG Anti-HBc (+), HBeAg (+), Anti-HBe (–) is indicative of?

Harrison's 20th Ed. Chapter 332 Page 2360 Table 332-5

A. Acute hepatitis B, high infectivity
B. Chronic hepatitis B, high infectivity
C. Low-level hepatitis B carrier
D. Hepatitis B in remote past

1539. HBsAg (+), Anti-HBs (–), IgG Anti-HBc (+), HBeAg (–), Anti-HBe (+) is indicative of?

Harrison's 20th Ed. Chapter 332 Page 2360 Table 332-5

A. Acute hepatitis B, high infectivity
B. Late acute or chronic hepatitis B, low infectivity
C. Anti-HBc "window"
D. Hepatitis B in remote past

1540. HBsAg (–), Anti-HBs (–), IgM Anti-HBc (+), HBeAg (±), Anti-HBe (±) is indicative of?

Harrison's 20th Ed. Chapter 332 Page 2360 Table 332-5

A. Acute hepatitis B, high infectivity
B. Late acute or chronic hepatitis B, low infectivity
C. Anti-HBc "window"
D. Recovery from hepatitis B

1541. HBsAg (–), Anti-HBs (–), IgG Anti-HBc (+), HBeAg (–), Anti-HBe (±) is indicative of?

Harrison's 20th Ed. Chapter 332 Page 2360 Table 332-5

A. Recovery from hepatitis B
B. Immunization with HBsAg
C. Low-level hepatitis B carrier
D. Anti-HBc "window"

1542. HBsAg (–), Anti-HBs (+), IgG Anti-HBc (+), HBeAg (–), Anti-HBe (±) is indicative of?

Harrison's 20th Ed. Chapter 332 Page 2360 Table 332-5

A. Recovery from hepatitis B
B. Immunization with HBsAg
C. Low-level hepatitis B carrier
D. Anti-HBc "window"

1543. HBsAg (–), Anti-HBs (+), IgG Anti-HBc (–), HBeAg (–), Anti-HBe (–) is indicative of?

Harrison's 20th Ed. Chapter 332 Page 2360 Table 332-5

A. Recovery from hepatitis B
B. Immunization with HBsAg
C. Low-level hepatitis B carrier
D. Anti-HBc "window"

1544. HBsAg (–), Anti-HBs (+), IgG Anti-HBc (–), HBeAg (–), Anti-HBe (–) is indicative of?

Harrison's 20th Ed. Chapter 332 Page 2360 Table 332-5

A. Hepatitis B in the remote past
B. Immunization with HBsAg
C. False-positive
D. Any of the above

1545. Which of the following may reappear during acute reactivation of chronic hepatitis B?

Harrison's 20th Ed. Chapter 332 Page 2360 Table 332-5

A. HBsAg
B. HBeAg
C. IgM anti-HBc
D. IgG anti-HBc

IgM anti-HBc may reappear during acute reactivation of chronic hepatitis B.

1546. Which of the following about anti-HCV is false?

Harrison's 20th Ed. Chapter 332 Page 2360

A. Detected in acute hepatitis C
B. Remains detectable during chronic infection
C. False positive in persons with circulating rheumatoid factor
D. None of the above

1547. Which of the following about HCV RNA in HCV infections is false?

Harrison's 20th Ed. Chapter 332 Page 2360

A. Most sensitive test for HCV infection - "gold standard"
B. Can be detected before acute elevation of aminotransferases
C. Can be detected before appearance of anti-HCV
D. None of the above

1548. Which of the following about HCV RNA in HCV infections is false?

Harrison's 20th Ed. Chapter 332 Page 2360

A. Remains detectable indefinitely in chronic hepatitis C
B. Values expressed in IU/mL
C. Reliable marker of disease severity or prognosis
D. Helps in predicting relative responsiveness to antiviral therapy

Determination of HCV RNA level is not a reliable marker of disease severity or prognosis.

1549. Which of the following is true for "cured" hepatitis C?
Harrison's 20th Ed. Chapter 332 Page 2361

A. Anti-HCV (–), HCV RNA (–)
B. Anti-HCV (+), HCV RNA (–)
C. Anti-HCV (–), HCV RNA (+)
D. Anti-HCV (+), HCV RNA (+)

Detectable anti-HCV in the absence of HCV RNA signifies spontaneous or therapeutically induced recovery from hepatitis C i.e. "cured".

1550. Which of the following is false about HDV infection?
Harrison's 20th Ed. Chapter 332 Page 2361

A. Intrahepatic HDV antigen demonstrable
B. Circulating HDV antigen is detectable only briefly
C. Anti-HDV is undetectable once HBsAg disappears
D. None of the above

Anti-HDV appears after a delay of up to 30–40 days in acute HDV infection.

1551. Which of the following helps to differentiate whether HBV and HDV infections are simultaneous or superimposed?
Harrison's 20th Ed. Chapter 332 Page 2361

A. HBeAg
B. Anti-HDV
C. Anti-HBc
D. Anti-HBe

In simultaneous acute HBV and HDV infections, IgM anti-HBc will be detectable. In acute HDV infection superimposed on chronic HBV infection, anti-HBc will be of IgG class.

1552. HBsAg (+), IgM Anti-HAV (–), IgM Anti-HBc (+), Anti-HCV (–) indicates?
Harrison's 20th Ed. Chapter 332 Page 2361 Table 332-6

A. Acute hepatitis B
B. Chronic hepatitis B
C. Acute hepatitis A superimposed on chronic hepatitis B
D. Acute hepatitis A and B

1553. HBsAg (+), IgM Anti-HAV (–), IgM Anti-HBc (–), Anti-HCV (–) indicates?
Harrison's 20th Ed. Chapter 332 Page 2361 Table 332-6

A. Acute hepatitis B
B. Chronic hepatitis B
C. Acute hepatitis A superimposed on chronic hepatitis B
D. Acute hepatitis A and B

1554. HBsAg (+), IgM Anti-HAV (+), IgM Anti-HBc (–), Anti-HCV (–) indicates?
Harrison's 20th Ed. Chapter 332 Page 2361 Table 332-6

A. Acute hepatitis B
B. Chronic hepatitis B
C. Acute hepatitis A superimposed on chronic hepatitis B
D. Acute hepatitis A and B

1555. HBsAg (+), IgM Anti-HAV (+), IgM Anti-HBc (+), Anti-HCV (-) indicates?
Harrison's 20th Ed. Chapter 332 Page 2361 Table 332-6

A. Acute hepatitis B
B. Chronic hepatitis B
C. Acute hepatitis A superimposed on chronic hepatitis B
D. Acute hepatitis A and B

1556. HBsAg (–), IgM Anti-HAV (+), IgM Anti-HBc (–), Anti-HCV (–) indicates?
Harrison's 20th Ed. Chapter 332 Page 2361 Table 332-6

A. Acute hepatitis A
B. Acute hepatitis A and B (HBsAg below detection threshold)
C. Acute hepatitis B (HBsAg below detection threshold)
D. Acute hepatitis C

1557. HBsAg (–), IgM Anti-HAV (+), IgM Anti-HBc (+), Anti-HCV (–) indicates?
Harrison's 20th Ed. Chapter 332 Page 2361 Table 332-6

A. Acute hepatitis A
B. Acute hepatitis A and B (HBsAg below detection threshold)
C. Acute hepatitis B (HBsAg below detection threshold)
D. Acute hepatitis C

1558. HBsAg (–), IgM Anti-HAV (–), IgM Anti-HBc (+), Anti-HCV (–) indicates?
Harrison's 20th Ed. Chapter 332 Page 2361 Table 332-6

A. Acute hepatitis A
B. Acute hepatitis A and B (HBsAg below detection threshold)
C. Acute hepatitis B (HBsAg below detection threshold)
D. Acute hepatitis C

1559. HBsAg (–), IgM Anti-HAV (–), IgM Anti-HBc (–), Anti-HCV (+) indicates?
Harrison's 20th Ed. Chapter 332 Page 2361 Table 332-6

A. Acute hepatitis A
B. Acute hepatitis A and B (HBsAg below detection threshold)
C. Acute hepatitis B (HBsAg below detection threshold)
D. Acute hepatitis C

1560. Which of the following hepatitis is more likely to be anicteric?
Harrison's 20th Ed. Chapter 332 Page 2361

A. Hepatitis A
B. Hepatitis B
C. Hepatitis C
D. All of the above

1561. Pregnant women with hepatitis E have a case fatality rate of?
Harrison's 20th Ed. Chapter 332 Page 2361

A. 1–2%
B. 5–10%
C. 10–20%
D. 20–30%

In outbreaks of hepatitis E in India, case fatality rate is 1–2% and up to 10–20% in pregnant women.

1562. Relapsing hepatitis is a feature of?
Harrison's 20th Ed. Chapter 332 Page 2361

A. Acute hepatitis A
B. Acute hepatitis B

C. Acute hepatitis C
D. Hepatitis D superinfection

Complications of hepatitis A include relapsing hepatitis appearing weeks to months after apparent recovery from acute hepatitis, cholestatic hepatitis and rarely fulminant hepatitis.

1563. Relapses in relapsing hepatitis are characterized by?
Harrison's 20th Ed. Chapter 332 Page 2362

A. Recurrence of symptoms
B. Aminotransferase elevations
C. Fecal excretion of HAV
D. All of the above

Relapses are characterized by recurrence of symptoms, aminotransferase elevations, occasionally jaundice and fecal excretion of HAV.

1564. Cholestatic hepatitis is unusual variant of?
Harrison's 20th Ed. Chapter 332 Page 2362

A. Acute hepatitis A
B. Acute hepatitis B
C. Acute hepatitis C
D. Hepatitis D superinfection

Cholestatic hepatitis is an unusual variant of acute hepatitis A characterized by protracted cholestatic jaundice and pruritus.

1565. Prodromal phase of acute hepatitis B is often diagnosed erroneously as?
Harrison's 20th Ed. Chapter 332 Page 2362

A. Hematological diseases
B. Sexually transmitted diseases
C. Rheumatologic diseases
D. Malignancy

During prodromal phase of acute hepatitis B, a serum sickness-like syndrome characterized by arthralgia or arthritis, rash, angioedema and rarely hematuria and proteinuria may develop in 5–10% of patients. It occurs before the onset of clinical jaundice and is often diagnosed erroneously as rheumatologic diseases.

1566. Extrahepatic manifestations of HCV include?
Harrison's 20th Ed. Chapter 332 Page 2362

A. Mixed cryoglobulinemia
B. Porphyria cutanea tarda
C. Lichen planus (LP)
D. All of the above

Well-accepted extrahepatic manifestations of HCV include pruritus, mixed cryoglobulinemia & necrolytic acral erythema. Frequently associated conditions include porphyria cutanea tarda, leucocytoclastic vasculitis, lichen planus, sicca syndrome & polyarteritis nodosa.

1567. Which of the following is a complication of HCV infection?
Harrison's 20th Ed. Chapter 332 Page 2362

A. Hepatic steatosis
B. Hypercholesterolemia
C. Insulin resistance
D. All of the above

HCV infection may be complicated by hepatic steatosis, hypercholesterolemia, insulin resistance (and other manifestations of the metabolic syndrome) and type 2 diabetes mellitus.

1568. Which of the following complications of HCV infection blunts responsiveness to antiviral therapy?
Harrison's 20th Ed. Chapter 332 Page 2362

A. Hepatic steatosis
B. Hypercholesterolemia
C. Hepatitis B co-infection
D. All of the above

Hepatic steatosis & insulin resistance accelerate hepatic fibrosis & blunt antiviral therapy response.

1569. Which of the following is false in the original definition of "fulminant hepatic failure"?
N Engl J Med. 2013;369:2525-34

A. Severe liver injury
B. Potentially reversible in nature
C. Hepatic encephalopathy within 2 weeks of first symptoms
D. Absence of pre-existing liver disease

The original term "fulminant hepatic failure" was defined as "a severe liver injury, potentially reversible in nature and with onset of hepatic encephalopathy within 8 weeks of the first symptoms in the absence of pre-existing liver disease."

1570. Which of the following is the most common cause of acute liver failure in United States?
N Engl J Med. 2013;369:2525-34

A. Drug-induced liver injury
B. Hepatitis A, B, and E
C. Autoimmune hepatitis
D. Cocaine use

Drug-induced liver injury is the most common cause of acute liver failure in United States and much of Western Europe.

1571. Which of the following viral infection can cause acute liver failure?
N Engl J Med. 2013;369:2525-34

A. Cytomegalovirus
B. Epstein - Barr virus
C. Parvoviruses
D. All of the above

Rare viral causes of acute liver failure include herpes simplex virus, cytomegalovirus, Epstein–Barr virus, and parvoviruses.

1572. Which of the following is a classification system for acute liver failure?
N Engl J Med. 2013;369:2525-34

A. O'Grady System
B. Bernuau System
C. Japanese System
D. All of the above

1573. Which of the following criteria is used for selection of patients with acute liver failure for transplantation?
N Engl J Med. 2013;369:2525-34

A. King's College criteria
B. Clichy criteria
C. Japanese criteria
D. All of the above

The King's College criteria are from O'Grady et al., the Clichy criteria from Bernuau et al., and Japanese criteria from Mochida et al.

1574. Which of the following is a cause of acute liver failure?
N Engl J Med. 2013;369:2525-34

A. Heatstroke
B. Mushroom ingestion
C. Wilson's disease
D. All of the above

Causes of acute liver failure also include neoplastic infiltration, acute Budd–Chiari syndrome, heatstroke, mushroom ingestion, Wilson's disease and pregnancy.

1575. Which of the following is decreased in acute liver failure?
N Engl J Med. 2013;369:2525-34

A. Gluconeogenesis
B. Lactate clearance
C. Ammonia clearance
D. All of the above

1576. In acute liver failure, which of the following is more common particularly in acetaminophen-related disease?
N Engl J Med. 2013;369:2525-34

A. Acute lung injury
B. Pancreatitis
C. Bone marrow suppression
D. Coagulopathy

Substantial renal dysfunction and pancreatitis more common in patients with acetaminophen-induced acute liver failure.

1577. In acute liver failure and hypotension despite volume repletion, which vasopressor is preferred?
N Engl J Med. 2013;369:2525-34

A. Norepinephrine
B. Vasopressin
C. Vasopressin analogue
D. Any of the above

In acute liver failure patients who continue to have hypotension despite volume repletion, norepinephrine is the preferred vasopressor, with or without adjunctive use of vasopressin or vasopressin analogues.

1578. Fulminant hepatitis is rare in?
Harrison's 20th Ed. Chapter 332 Page 2362

A. Hepatitis A
B. Hepatitis B & D
C. Hepatitis E
D. All of the above

Fulminant hepatitis is primarily seen in hepatitis B and D, and hepatitis E. It is rare in hepatitis A.

1579. Which of the following predispose to fulminant cases of hepatitis A?
Harrison's 20th Ed. Chapter 332 Page 2362

A. Older adults
B. Chronic hepatitis B
C. Chronic hepatitis C
D. All of the above

1580. Out of the following, fulminant hepatitis is most common in?
Harrison's 20th Ed. Chapter 332 Page 2362

A. Hepatitis A
B. Hepatitis B
C. Hepatitis C
D. Hepatitis E

Hepatitis B accounts for >50% of fulminant cases of viral hepatitis.

1581. Fulminant hepatitis is hardly ever seen in?
Harrison's 20th Ed. Chapter 332 Page 2362

A. Hepatitis A
B. Hepatitis B
C. Hepatitis C
D. Hepatitis E

Fulminant hepatitis is hardly ever seen in hepatitis C.

1582. Which of the following variables does not indicate impending hepatic failure with encephalopathy?
Harrison's 20th Ed. Chapter 332 Page 2362

A. Shrunken liver
B. Excessively prolonged PT
C. Rapidly rising bilirubin level
D. Rapidly rising aminotransferase levels

Aminotransferase levels may register a fall due to reduced hepatocyte mass in massive hepatic necrosis.

1583. Likelihood of remaining chronically infected after acute HBV infection is high in all except?
Harrison's 20th Ed. Chapter 332 Page 2362

A. Old
B. Down's syndrome
C. Chronically hemodialyzed patients
D. HIV infection

Likelihood of remaining chronically infected after acute HBV infection is high among neonates, Down's syndrome, chronically hemodialyzed patients & immunosuppressed patients, including those with HIV infection.

1584. Progression of acute to chronic hepatitis B is likely if?
Harrison's 20th Ed. Chapter 332 Page 2362

A. HBeAg persists for >3 months
B. HBsAg persists for >6 months
C. AST/ALT do not normalise within 6–12 months
D. All of the above

Progression of acute hepatitis to chronic hepatitis is likely if clinical symptoms do not resolve, AST/ALT, bilirubin and globulin levels fail to normalise within 6–12 months, HBeAg persists for >3 months and HBsAg persists for >6 months.

1585. Which of the following is false about hepatitis D superinfection?
Harrison's 20th Ed. Chapter 332 Page 2362

A. Can transform inactive chronic hepatitis B into severe, progressive chronic hepatitis and cirrhosis
B. Can accelerate course of chronic hepatitis B
C. Can potentiate chronic hepatitis B to fulminant hepatitis
D. Can increase likelihood of chronicity of acute hepatitis B

Acute hepatitis D infection does not increase likelihood of chronicity of simultaneous acute hepatitis B.

1586. The annual rate of cirrhosis in patients with chronic hepatitis D is?

Harrison's 20th Ed. Chapter 332 Page 2362

A. 1%
B. 2%
C. 3%
D. 4%

The annual rate of cirrhosis in patients with chronic hepatitis D is 4%.

1587. Likelihood of remaining chronically infected after acute HCV infection is?

Harrison's 20th Ed. Chapter 332 Page 2362

A. 25–40%
B. 40–60%
C. 65–75%
D. 85–90%

After acute HCV infection, the likelihood of remaining chronically infected approaches 85–90%.

1588. Progression of chronic hepatitis C is be influenced by?

Harrison's 20th Ed. Chapter 332 Page 2362

A. Advanced age of acquisition
B. Coexisting excessive alcohol use
C. HIV coinfection
D. All of the above

Progression of chronic hepatitis C may be influenced by advanced age of acquisition, long duration of infection, immunosuppression, coexisting excessive alcohol use, concomitant hepatic steatosis, other hepatitis virus infection or HIV coinfection.

1589. Condition leading to chronicity in hepatitis E is?

Harrison's 20th Ed. Chapter 332 Page 2362

A. Immunosuppressed organ-transplant recipients
B. Persons receiving cytotoxic chemotherapy
C. Persons with HIV infection
D. All of the above

1590. Enhanced risk of hepatocellular carcinoma in chronic hepatitis B is more in?

Harrison's 20th Ed. Chapter 332 Page 2362

A. Those infected in infancy or early childhood
B. Those with HBeAg
C. Those with high-level HBV DNA
D. All of the above

1591. The annual rate of hepatocellular carcinoma in patients with chronic hepatitis D and cirrhosis is?

Harrison's 20th Ed. Chapter 332 Page 2362

A. ~ 1%
B. ~ 2%
C. ~ 3%
D. ~ 4%

1592. Annual risk of hepatocellular carcinoma in cirrhotic patients with chronic hepatitis C is?

Harrison's 20th Ed. Chapter 332 Page 2362

A. ~ 1–4%
B. ~ 4–8%
C. ~ 8–12%
D. ~ 12–14%

1593. Gianotti-Crosti syndrome is best related to?

Harrison's 20th Ed. Chapter 332 Page 2363

A. Hepatitis A
B. Hepatitis B
C. Hepatitis C
D. Hepatitis E

Gianotti-Crosti syndrome or papular acrodermatitis of childhood refers to hepatitis B that presents with anicteric hepatitis, nonpruritic papular rash of face, buttocks & limbs & lymphadenopathy.

1594. Autoimmune hepatitis can be triggered by?

Harrison's 20th Ed. Chapter 332 Page 2363

A. Hepatitis A
B. Hepatitis B
C. Hepatitis C
D. All of the above

1595. Which of the following is a heterophile test?

Harrison's 20th Ed. Chapter 332 Page 2363

A. Weil Felix test
B. Paul Bunnel test or mononuclear spot test
C. Cold agglutination test
D. All of the above

Similar antigens present on dissimilar organisms are heterophile antigens. Antibodies thus produced are called hererophile antibodies or an antibody that reacts with antigens other than the antigen that stimulated it, i.e. an antibody that cross reacts.

1596. Clinical condition that may mimic acute hepatitis is?

Harrison's 20th Ed. Chapter 332 Page 2363

A. Right ventricular failure
B. Hypoperfusion syndromes
C. Budd-Chiari syndrome
D. All of the above

1597. Clinical condition that may mimic acute hepatitis is?

Harrison's 20th Ed. Chapter 332 Page 2363

A. Constrictive pericarditis
B. Right atrial myxoma
C. Venoocclusive disease
D. All of the above

Clinical constellation that may mimic acute hepatitis is right ventricular failure with passive hepatic congestion or hypoperfusion syndromes (shock, severe hypotension and severe left ventricular failure), right atrial myxoma, constrictive pericarditis, hepatic vein occlusion (Budd-Chiari syndrome) or venoocclusive disease. Others include acute fatty liver of pregnancy, cholestasis of pregnancy, eclampsia, and HELLP syndrome. Very rarely, malignancies metastatic to liver can mimic acute or even fulminant viral hepatitis. Genetic or metabolic liver disorders (Wilson's disease, α1 antitrypsin deficiency) and nonalcoholic fatty liver disease are confused with acute viral hepatitis.

1598. For severe acute hepatitis B, which of the following drugs is useful?

Harrison's 20th Ed. Chapter 332 Page 2363

A. Tenofovir
B. Ribavirin
C. Telaprevir
D. Boceprevir

1599. Which of the following is false about antiviral therapy for severe acute hepatitis B?

Harrison's 20th Ed. Chapter 332 Page 2363

A. Nucleoside analogue tenofovir is potent & least resistance prone agent
B. To be continued till 3 months after HBsAg seroconversion
C. To be continued till 6 months after HBeAg seroconversion
D. None of the above

Recovery occurs in ~99% of patients with acute hepatitis B. Rarely, for severe, not mild-moderate, acute hepatitis B, treatment has been attempted successfully with nucleoside analogue (entecavir or tenofovir). Treatment should continue until 3 months after HBsAg seroconversion or 6 months after HBeAg seroconversion. Other drugs used are Interferon, Lamivudine, Adefovir, Pegylated interferon, Telbivudine.

1600. Which of the following drugs provides high efficacy in treatment of acute hepatitis C?

Harrison's 20th Ed. Chapter 332 Page 2363

A. Ribavirin
B. Pegylated interferon
C. Telaprevir
D. Boceprevir

In typical cases of acute hepatitis C, recovery is rare and progression to chronic hepatitis is the rule. Pegylated interferon-based therapy for acute hepatitis C is efficacious.

1601. Sofosbuvir is best related to which of the following?

Cleveland Clinic Journal of Medicine. 2014;81(3):159

A. NS3 protease inhibitor
B. NS5A inhibitor
C. NS5B nucleoside inhibitor
D. NS5B non-nucleoside inhibitor

Sofosbuvir is a uridine nucleotide analogue that selectively inhibits HCV NS5B RNA-dependent RNA polymerase. It targets the highly conserved nucleotide binding pocket of this enzyme and functions as a chain terminator.

1602. Simeprevir is best related to which of the following?

Cleveland Clinic Journal of Medicine. 2014;81(3):159

A. NS3 protease inhibitor
B. NS5A inhibitor
C. NS5B nucleoside inhibitor
D. NS5B non-nucleoside inhibitor

Simeprevir belongs to the macrocyclic class with FDA approval only for HCV genotype 1 and in combination with interferon alfa and ribavirin. It is a weak inhibitor of the CYP3A4 enzyme and hence has less drug-drug interactions. Patients infected with HCV genotype 1a should be screened for the NS3 Q80K polymorphism at baseline, as it has been associated with substantially reduced response to simeprevir.

1603. Complications of Ribavirin treatment include which of the following?

Cleveland Clinic Journal of Medicine. 2014;81(3):159

A. Hemolysis
B. Skin complications
C. Teratogenicity
D. All of the above

Ribavirin causes hemolysis and skin complications and is teratogenic.

1604. Complications of Interferon treatment include which of the following?

Cleveland Clinic Journal of Medicine. 2014;81(3):159

A. Seizures
B. Peripheral neuropathy
C. Bone marrow suppression
D. All of the above

Interferon causes fatigue, flu-like symptoms, psychiatric symptoms (including depression or psychosis), weight loss, seizures, peripheral neuropathy, and bone marrow suppression.

1605. Patients with which of the following *IL28B* HCV genotype have a better chance of sustained virologic response with interferon?

Cleveland Clinic Journal of Medicine. 2014;81(3):159

A. IL28B CC
B. IL28B CT
C. IL28B TT
D. All of the above

When using interferon for HCV infected patient, information of IL28B genotype is essential i.e. single-nucleotide polymorphism (C or T) on chromosome 19q13 (rs12979860) upstream of the IL28B gene encoding for interferon lambda-3. Patients with the IL28B CC genotype have a much better chance of a sustained virologic response with interferon than do patients with CT or TT.

1606. Boceprevir and telaprevir are best related to which of the following?

Cleveland Clinic Journal of Medicine. 2014;81(3):159

A. NS3/4 protease inhibitor
B. NS5A inhibitor
C. NS5B nucleoside inhibitor
D. NS5B non-nucleoside inhibitor

Telaprevir & boceprevir are NS3/A4 protease inhibitors that belong to the alfa-ketoamid derivative class. In May 2011, the FDA approved NS3/4A protease inhibitors boceprevir & telaprevir for treating HCV genotype 1 being highly specific for the amino acid target sequence of the NS3 region. These direct-acting antiviral agents had to be used in combination with interferon alfa and ribavirin.

1607. Dysgeusia is a adverse effect of which of the following drugs used to treat HCV infection?

Cleveland Clinic Journal of Medicine. 2014;81(3):159

A. Boceprevir
B. Telaprevir
C. Sofosbuvir
D. Simeprevir

Dysgeusia is seen with boceprevir, rash with telaprevir, and anemia with both.

1608. Principal enzyme responsible for boceprevir & telaprevir metabolism is?

Cleveland Clinic Journal of Medicine. 2014;81(3):159

A. CYP2C9
B. CYP2D6
C. CYP3A4
D. CYP2C19

Serious drug-drug interactions occur with the use of boceprevir & telaprevir with other medications that interact with CYP3A4, the principal enzyme responsible for their metabolism.

1609. Which of the following improves survival in patients of fulminant hepatitis?

Harrison's 20th Ed. Chapter 332 Page 2364

A. Protein intake restriction
B. Glucocorticoid therapy
C. Prophylactic antibiotic coverage
D. Plasmapheresis

Orthotopic liver transplantation provides excellent results in patients with fulminant hepatitis.

1610. Active immunization with vaccines is the preferable approach for prevention of?

Harrison's 20th Ed. Chapter 332 Page 2364

A. Hepatitis A
B. Hepatitis B
C. Hepatitis E
D. All of the above

1611. Hepatitis A vaccination is recommended for?

Harrison's 20th Ed. Chapter 332 Page 2364

A. Patients with chronic hepatitis B
B. Patients with chronic hepatitis C
C. Patients receiving clotting-factor concentrates
D. All of the above

1612. Hepatitis A vaccines provide adequate protection how many weeks after a primary inoculation?

Harrison's 20th Ed. Chapter 332 Page 2364

A. 1 week
B. 2 weeks
C. 3 weeks
D. 4 weeks

Formalin-inactivated vaccines made from strains of HAV attenuated in tissue culture are safe, immunogenic, and effectively prevent hepatitis A. Hepatitis A vaccines provide adequate protection beginning 4 weeks after a primary inoculation.

1613. Hepatitis A vaccine is administered by which route?

Harrison's 20th Ed. Chapter 332 Page 2364

A. Intradermal
B. Subcutenuous
C. Intramuscular
D. Intravenous

Hepatitis A vaccine is administered intramuscularly.

1614. The first vaccine for hepatitis B active immunization was prepared from?

Harrison's 20th Ed. Chapter 332 Page 2365

A. 22-nm spherical forms of HBsAg
B. 27-nm spherical forms of HBsAg
C. 42-nm spherical forms of HBsAg
D. All of the above

First vaccine for active immunization (1982) was prepared from purified, noninfectious 22-nm spherical forms of HBsAg derived from plasma of healthy HBsAg carriers.

1615. Which of the following is the difference between plasma-derived vaccine and genetically engineered Hepatitis B vaccine?

Harrison's 20th Ed. Chapter 332 Page 2365

A. Nonglycosylated
B. Hydrolyzed
C. Oxidized
D. Heat attenuated

Plasma-derived Hepatitis B vaccine is prepared from purified, noninfectious 22-nm spherical forms of HBsAg derived from plasma of healthy HBsAg carriers, while genetically engineered Hepatitis B vaccine is derived from recombinant yeast and consists of HBsAg particles that are nonglycosylated but are otherwise indistinguishable from natural HBsAg;

1616. Hepatitis B vaccine is administered?

Harrison's 20th Ed. Chapter 332 Page 2365

A. Intradermally
B. Subcuteneously
C. Intramuscularly
D. Intravenously

1617. In adults, recommended site of Hepatitis B vaccine is?

Harrison's 20th Ed. Chapter 332 Page 2365

A. Thigh muscle
B. Triceps muscle
C. Deltoid muscle
D. Gluteal muscle

1618. After the first dose of Hepatitis B vaccine, the third dose is given after?

Harrison's 20th Ed. Chapter 332 Page 2365

A. One month
B. Three months
C. Six months
D. Twelve months

For preexposure prophylaxis against hepatitis B, three IM injections of hepatitis B vaccine in deltoid, not gluteal muscle are recommended at 0, 1, and 6 months.

1619. Engerix-B for adults contains what amount of HBsAg in 1 mL?

Harrison's 20th Ed. Chapter 332 Page 2365

A. 5 μg
B. 10 μg
C. 15 μg
D. 20 μg

1620. For postexposure HBV prophylaxis, dose of HbIg is?

Harrison's 20th Ed. Chapter 332 Page 2365

A. 0.02 mL/kg
B. 0.04 mL/kg
C. 0.06 mL/kg
D. 0.08 mL/kg

For postexposure HBV prophylaxis, dose of HbIg is a single intramuscular dose of HbIg, 0.06 mL/kg, administered as soon after exposure as possible and followed by a complete course of hepatitis B vaccine to begin within the first week.

1621. Which of the following statements about Hepatitis B vaccination is false?

Harrison's 20th Ed. Chapter 332 Page 2365

A. Pregnancy is not a contraindication to vaccination
B. Booster immunizations are not recommended routinely
C. Booster recommended if anti-HBs levels are <10 mIU/mL
D. None of the above

1622. True nonresponse after proper HBV vaccination means antibody level of less than?

Harrison's 20th Ed. Chapter 332 Page 2365, N Engl J Med. 2004;351:2832-8

A. 10 mIU/mL
B. 15 mIU/mL

C. 20 mIU/mL

D. 50 mIU/mL

Booster immunizations are not recommended routinely in immunocompetent persons. Booster doses are recommended when anti-HBs levels fall to <10 mIU/mL.

1623. HBV inactive carriers have serum HBV DNA level below?

N Engl J Med. 2008;359:1486-500

A. 1000 IU per milliliter

B. 10000 IU per milliliter

C. 100000 IU per milliliter

D. 1000000 IU per milliliter

Persons with a serum HBV DNA level below 1000 IU per milliliter and a normal ALT level consistently are considered to be inactive carriers.

1624. Hepatitis B immune globulin (Hblg) is used in?

N Engl J Med. 2004;351:2832-8

A. Infants born to HBsAg + mothers

B. Contact with HBsAg + blood / bodily fluid

C. Sexual contact with person who is HBsAg +

D. All of the above

1625. Groups for whom Hepatitis B vaccine is recommended include all except?

N Engl J Med. 2004;351:2832-8

A. All infants

B. Patients on peritoneal dialysis

C. Persons at occupational risk

D. Clients & staff of institutions for developmentally disabled

1626. Groups for whom Hepatitis B vaccine is recommended include all except?

N Engl J Med. 2004;351:2832-8

A. Recipients of clotting-factor concentrates

B. Household members & sexual partners of HBV carriers

C. Adoptees from countries where HBV infection is endemic

D. Travelers spending > 6 weeks in HBV endemic areas

1627. Which of the following is false about hepatitis C vaccination?

Harrison's 20th Ed. Chapter 332 Page 2366

A. IG is ineffective in preventing hepatitis C

B. Hepatitis C vaccination is not feasible practically

C. No special precautions are recommended for babies born to mothers with hepatitis C

D. Breastfeeding to be restricted

Breastfeeding does not have to be restricted.

1628. Leser-Trelat sign mostly points towards which pathology?

Harrison's 20th Ed. Chapter 54 Page 346

A. Infection

B. Neoplasm

C. Nutritional deficiency

D. Environmental toxin

Leser-Trelat sign refers to multiple pruritic seborrheic keratoses of sudden onset. Mostly associated with gastrointestinal adenocarcinomas, breast, lung, urinary tract cancers & lymphoid malignancies.

1629. Which drug should be included in ART regimen when Hepatitis B and HIV occur together?

Harrison's 20th Ed. Chapter 334 Page 2379

A. Interferon alpha

B. Entecavir

C. Tenofovir

D. None of the above

1630. Wickman's striae are best related to?

N Engl J Med. 2018;379:567

A. Necrolytic acral erythema

B. Porphyria cutanea tarda

C. Leucocytoclastic vasculitis

D. Lichen planus (LP)

LP is an inflammatory disease of skin & mucous membranes, characterized by pruritic, purple, polygonal, papules with an overlying fine reticulate pattern of dots and lines called Wickman's striae. Lichen planus has a known association with HCV infection.

Toxic and Drug-induced Hepatitis

1631. Drugs affect a normal hepatocyte by?
Harrison's 20th Ed. Chapter 333 Page 2368 Figure 333-1

A. Disruption of intracellular calcium homeostasis
B. Disruption of actin filaments next to the canaliculus
C. Covalent binding of cytochrome P450 enzyme
D. All of the above

1632. Drugs affect a normal hepatocyte by?
Harrison's 20th Ed. Chapter 333 Page 2368 Figure 333-1

A. Stimulating immune response by cytolytic T cells & cytokines
B. Activation of apoptotic pathways by TNF-α receptor or Fas
C. Inhibition of mitochondrial function
D. All of the above

1633. Phase I reaction in drug metabolism include which of the following chemical process?
N Engl J Med. 2005;352:2211-21

A. Oxidation
B. Reduction
C. Hydrolysis
D. All of the above

1634. Phase II reaction in drug metabolism include which of the following chemical process?
N Engl J Med. 2005;352:2211-21

A. Glucuronidation
B. Sulfation
C. Acetylation
D. All of the above

1635. Phase II reactions in drug metabolism include all except?
N Engl J Med. 2005;352:2211-21

A. Sulfation
B. Glucuronidation
C. Acetylation
D. Hydrolysis

Drugs may be metabolized by sequential or competitive chemical processes involving oxidation, reduction & hydrolysis (phase I reactions) or glucuronidation, sulfation, acetylation & methylation (phase II reactions). CYP is important for phase I metabolism and are located primarily in endoplasmic reticulum, while phase 2 conjugation enzymes are cytosolic.

1636. Which of the following is not a feature of direct toxic hepatitis?
Harrison's 20th Ed. Chapter 333 Page 2367

A. Predictable regularity
B. Dose-dependent
C. Latent period usually long
D. Morphologic abnormalities reproducible for each toxin

In direct toxic hepatitis, latent period between exposure and liver injury is usually short (often several hours), although clinical manifestations may be delayed for 24–48 hours.

1637. Which of the following is not a feature of idiosyncratic drug hepatotoxicity?
Harrison's 20th Ed. Chapter 333 Page 2367

A. Unpredictability
B. Not dose-dependent
C. Extrahepatic manifestations of hypersensitivity
D. None of the above

1638. Which of the following is involved in the pathogenesis of drug-induced cholestasis?
Harrison's 20th Ed. Chapter 333 Page 2367, J Clin Exp Hepatol. 2012;2(3):247-259

A. Farnesoid X receptor (FXR)
B. Pregnane X receptor (PXR)
C. Constitutive androstane receptor (CXR)
D. All of the above

1639. Hepatocellular injury produced by idiosyncratic reactions resembles that observed in?
Harrison's 20th Ed. Chapter 333 Page 2367

A. Acute viral hepatitis A
B. Acute viral hepatitis B
C. Acute viral hepatitis C
D. All of the above

1640. Antibody to liver-kidney microsomes associated with drug induced hepatitis is?
Harrison's 20th Ed. Chapter 333 Page 2367

A. Anti LKM 1
B. Anti LKM 2
C. Anti LKM 3
D. All of the above

Drug hepatotoxicity may be associated with the appearance of autoantibodies, including a class of antibodies to liver-kidney microsomes, anti-LKM2, directed against a cytochrome P450 enzyme.

1641. Amoxicillin-clavulanic acid produces which type of drug-induced cholestasis?
Harrison's 20th Ed. Chapter 333 Page 2367

A. Bland cholestasis
B. Inflammatory cholestasis
C. Sclerosing cholangitis
D. Ductopenic cholestasis

1642. Distinction between hepatocellular and cholestatic reaction is indicated by?
Harrison's 20th Ed. Chapter 333 Page 2367

A. Q value
B. R value
C. S value
D. T value

Distinction between hepatocellular and cholestatic reaction is indicated by R value which is the ratio of alanine aminotransferase (ALT) to alkaline phosphatase values, both expressed as multiples of the upper limit of normal. An R value of >5.0 is indicative of hepatocellular injury, R <2.0 of cholestatic injury, and R between 2.0 and 5.0 of mixed hepatocellular-cholestatic injury. R value was established by the Council for International Organizations of Medical Sciences. R = (ALT value ÷ ALT ULN) ÷ (Alk P value ÷ Alk P ULN).

1643. Which of the following is a causality assessment method for assessing causality in drug-induced liver injury (DILI)?

Harrison's 20th Ed. Chapter 333 Page 2367

A. Benichou Causality Assessment Method
B. Roussel Uclaf Causality Assessment Method
C. Lachin Danan Causality Assessment Method
D. Watkins Navarro Causality Assessment Method

The Roussel Uclaf Causality Assessment Method (RUCAM) was developed to quantify the strength of association between a liver injury and the medication implicated as causing the injury. RUCAM is composed of seven different criteria including time to onset, clinical course, risk factors, concomitant drugs, non-drug-causes, published information on hepatotoxicity, and the response to any re-administration. RUCAM score ranges from −8 to + 14, with higher values signifying a greater degree of association.

1644. Which of the following is a causality assessment method for assessing causality in drug-induced liver injury (DILI)?

J Clin Exp Hepatol. 2012;2(3):247-59

A. Roussel Uclaf Causality Assessment Method (RUCAM)
B. Maria and Victorino (M and V) method
C. DILIN (Drug-Induced Liver Injury Network) expert opinion
D. All of the above

1645. Name of the prognostic law stating that a pure drug-induced liver injury (DILI) leading to jaundice, without a hepatic transplant, has a case fatality rate of 10% to 50% is?

Harrison's 20th Ed. Chapter 333 Page 2367

A. Zy's law
B. Ky's law
C. Hy's law
D. Wy's law

Hy's Law criteria: >3x ULN AST or ALT + >2x ULN TBL, no initial cholestasis (normal AP), no other prior or concomitant reason for liver function abnormality. Rezulin Rule is also a prognostic rule of DILI. Rezulin is the trade name of banned drug troglitazone.

1646. Portal hypertension in the absence of cirrhosis may result from the use of?

Harrison's 20th Ed. Chapter 333 Page 2369

A. Vitamin A
B. Arsenic intoxication
C. Exposure to vinyl chloride
D. All of the above

1647. Which of the following are associated with angiosarcoma of the liver?

Harrison's 20th Ed. Chapter 333 Page 2369

A. Arsenic intoxication
B. Vinyl chloride
C. Thorium dioxide
D. All of the above

Arsenic intoxication, industrial exposure to vinyl chloride, or administration of thorium dioxide have been associated with angiosarcoma of the liver.

1648. Peliosis hepatis refers to?

Harrison's 20th Ed. Chapter 333 Page 2369

A. Trauma of liver
B. Blood cysts of liver
C. Ectopic liver
D. Unilobular liver

Peliosis hepatis refers to blood cysts of the liver.

1649. Peliosis hepatis is seen in patients treated with?

Harrison's 20th Ed. Chapter 333 Page 2369

A. Halothane
B. Anabolic steroids
C. Chlorpromazine
D. Methotrexate

Peliosis hepatis has been observed in some patients treated with anabolic steroids.

1650. Which of the following about acetaminophen metabolism is false?

N Engl J Med. 2008;359:285-92

A. >90% is metabolized by glucuronidation or sulfation
B. ~5% is metabolized by cytochrome P450 2E1 to NAPQI
C. NAPQI is detoxified by glutathione to cysteine & mercapturic acid
D. None of the above

As long as sufficient glutathione is present, the liver is protected from injury. N-acetylcysteine prevents hepatic injury primarily by restoring hepatic glutathione, improving hemodynamics and oxygen use, increasing clearance of indocyanine green and decreasing cerebral edema.

1651. Which of the following histopathologic changes occur after toxic quantity of acetaminophen ingestion?

Harrison's 20th Ed. Chapter 333 Page 2371

A. Periportal hepatic necrosis
B. Centrilobular hepatic necrosis
C. Massive hepatic necrosis
D. Bridging hepatic necrosis

Acetaminophen causes dose-related centrilobular hepatic necrosis after single time-point ingestions.

1652. Fatal fulminant liver disease is usually associated with ingestion of what amount of acetaminophen?

Harrison's 20th Ed. Chapter 333 Page 2371

A. 5 grams
B. 10 grams
C. 20 grams
D. 25 grams

A single dose of 10–15 grams may produce clinical evidence of liver injury. Fatal fulminant liver disease is usually associated with ingestion of over 25 grams of acetaminophen.

1653. What level of acetaminophen in blood is predictive of severe liver damage?

Harrison's 20th Ed. Chapter 333 Page 2371

A. > 100 μg/mL
B. > 150 μg/mL
C. > 200 μg/mL
D. > 300 μg/mL

Blood levels of acetaminophen of >300 μg/mL, 4 hours after ingestion are predictive severe liver damage. Levels <150 μg/mL suggest that hepatic injury is highly unlikely.

1654. Maximal hepatic injury and hepatic failure occurs after how many days of acetaminophen ingestion?

Harrison's 20th Ed. Chapter 333 Page 2371

A. 1–2 days
B. 2–3 days
C. 3–5 days
D. 7–9 days

Maximal hepatic injury & hepatic failure appear 3–5 days after acetaminophen ingestion. Extremely high aminotransferase levels in association with low bilirubin levels are characteristic.

1655. Which of the following is "hepatoprotective"?

Harrison's 20th Ed. Chapter 333 Page 2371

A. Activated charcoal
B. Cholestyramine
C. Glutathione
D. All of the above

Alcohol suppresses hepatic glutathione production.

1656. Glutathione is synthesized from which of the following amino acids?

N Engl J Med. 2008;359:285-92

A. Cysteine
B. Glutamate
C. Glycine
D. All of the above

Glutamate & glycine are present in abundance in hepatocytes. Availability of cysteine is the rate-limiting factor in glutathione synthesis. Cysteine itself is not well absorbed after oral administration. Acetylcysteine, in contrast, is readily absorbed & rapidly enters cells, where it is hydrolyzed to cysteine, thus providing the limiting substrate for glutathione synthesis.

1657. Nomogram to define risk of acetaminophen hepatotoxicity is called?

N Engl J Med. 2008;359:285-92

A. Makin-Mitchell nomogram
B. Rumack-Matthew nomogram
C. Jollow-Devlin nomogram
D. Trey-Daly nomogram

The Rumack–Matthew nomogram was first published in 1975. It estimates the likelihood of hepatic injury due to acetaminophen toxicity for patients with a single ingestion at a known time.

1658. Which of the following is the hepatotoxic metabolite formed from acetaminophen?

Harrison's 20th Ed. Chapter 333 Page 2371

A. 4-pentenoic acid
B. Electrophilic arene oxides
C. NAPQI
D. Betaine

N-acetyl-p-benzoquinone imine (NAPQI) is the hepatotoxic metabolite formed from acetaminophen by cytochrome P450 CYP2E1 by a phase 1 reaction. When excessive amounts of NAPQI are formed or when glutathione levels are low, glutathione levels are depleted and overwhelmed, permitting covalent binding to nucleophilic hepatocyte macromolecules forming acetaminophen-protein "adducts" which can be measured in serum by high performance liquid chromatography.

1659. N-acetyl-benzoquinone-imine (NAPQI) is best related to which of the following?

Harrison's 20th Ed. Chapter 333 Page 2371

A. Acetaminophen
B. Quinidine
C. Azathioprine
D. Carbamazine

1660. Which of the following is the end product of acetaminophen metabolism?

Harrison's 20th Ed. Chapter 333 Page 2371

A. Gamma-aminobutyric acid
B. Mercapturic acid
C. Boric acid
D. Butyric acid

Most of acetaminophen is metabolized by phase II reaction to sulfate & glucuronide metabolites. Phase I reaction by CYP2E1 metabolizes a small amount of acetaminophen to N-acetyl-benzoquinone-imine (NAPQI) which is hepatotoxic. However, "hepatoprotective" glutathione binds NAPQI to form harmless mercapturic acid that is excreted through kidneys. Alcohol induces cytochrome P450 CYP2E1.

1661. With acetaminophen, hepatic injury may be potentiated by?

Harrison's 20th Ed. Chapter 333 Page 2371

A. Alcohol
B. Phenobarbital
C. INH
D. All of the above

Hepatic injury may be potentiated by prior administration of alcohol, phenobarbital, INH, & starvation.

1662. Which of the following about alcohol is false?

Harrison's 20th Ed. Chapter 333 Page 2371

A. Direct hepatotoxin
B. Induces cytochrome P450 CYP2E1
C. Suppresses hepatic glutathione production
D. None of the above

1663. Oral activated charcoal or cholestyramine is useless how much time after acetaminophen ingestion?

Harrison's 20th Ed. Chapter 333 Page 2371

A. > 30 minutes
B. > 60 minutes
C. > 90 minutes
D. > 120 minutes

Oral activated charcoal or cholestyramine to prevent absorption of residual drug is useless if given >30 minutes after acetaminophen ingestion.

1664. Which of the following has a role in the management of acetaminophen hepatotoxicity?

Harrison's 20th Ed. Chapter 333 Page 2371

A. Cysteamine
B. Cysteine
C. N-acetylcysteine
D. All of the above

If given within 8 hours of ingestion of acetaminophen, administration of sulfhydryl compounds (cysteamine, cysteine, or N-acetylcysteine) reduces the severity of hepatic necrosis. These agents act by providing a reservoir of sulfhydryl groups to bind toxic metabolites or by stimulating synthesis and repletion of hepatic glutathione. If these fail, liver transplantation may be the only option.

1665. Patients of acetaminophen hepatotoxicity who present with hepatic failure have a mortality rate of?
N Engl J Med. 2008;359:285-92

A. 5 to 20%
B. 20 to 40%
C. 40 to 60%
D. 60 to 80%

Acetaminophen hepatotoxicity patients presenting with hepatic failure have a mortality rate of 20 to 40%.

1666. In acute acetaminophen ingestion, oral acetylcysteine is given as a loading dose of?
N Engl J Med. 2008;359:285-92

A. 40 mg per kilogram of body weight
B. 140 mg per kilogram of body weight
C. 240 mg per kilogram of body weight
D. 340 mg per kilogram of body weight

1667. In acute acetaminophen ingestion, maintenance dose of oral acetylcysteine is?
N Engl J Med. 2008;359:285-92

A. 40 mg per kilogram of body weight
B. 50 mg per kilogram of body weight
C. 60 mg per kilogram of body weight
D. 70 mg per kilogram of body weight

Oral acetylcysteine is given as a loading dose of 140 mg per kilogram of body weight, with maintenance doses of 70 mg per kilogram that are repeated every 4 hours for a total of 17 doses. Rechecking the alanine aminotransferase & serum acetaminophen concentrations is particularly important to increase the duration of treatment.

1668. In acute acetaminophen ingestion, intravenous loading dose of acetylcysteine is?
N Engl J Med. 2008;359:285-92

A. 120 mg per kilogram of body weight
B. 150 mg per kilogram of body weight
C. 200 mg per kilogram of body weight
D. 220 mg per kilogram of body weight

The intravenous loading dose of acetylcysteine in acute acetaminophen ingestion is 150 mg per kilogram, followed by an infusion of 12.5 mg per kilogram per hour over a 4-hour period, and finally an infusion of 6.25 mg per kilogram per hour over a 16-hour period.

1669. Which of the following is an adverse effect of intravenous acetylcysteine?
N Engl J Med. 2008;359:285-92

A. Pruritus
B. Angioedema, bronchospasm
C. Tachycardia, hypotension
D. All of the above

The most commonly reported adverse effects of intravenous acetylcysteine are anaphylactoid reactions, including rash, pruritus, angioedema, bronchospasm, tachycardia, and hypotension.

1670. In acetaminophen hepatotoxicity, which of the following may identify patients highly likely to require liver transplantation?
Harrison's 20th Ed. Chapter 333 Page 2372

A. Arterial blood ammonia levels
B. Arterial blood mercaptan levels
C. Arterial blood lactate levels
D. All of the above

Early arterial blood lactate levels of >3.5 mmol/L in patients with acute liver failure due to acetaminophen hepatotoxicity may distinguish patients highly likely to require liver transplantation from those likely to survive without liver replacement.

1671. Which of the following about isoniazid is false?
Clin Infect Dis. 2016;63:e147

A. Also called isonicotinylhydrazide or isonicotinic acid hydrazine
B. Synthetic antibiotic
C. Bactericidal against replicating Mycobacterium tuberculosis
D. None of the above

1672. In USA, which of the following is the commonest cause of drug-induced acute liver failure (ALF)?
J Clin Exp Hepatol. 2012;2(3):247-259

A. Paracetamol
B. Antituberculosis drugs
C. Antiepileptic drugs
D. Herbal drugs

1673. In India, which of the following is the commonest cause of drug-induced acute liver failure (ALF) in adults and children?
J Clin Exp Hepatol. 2012;2(3):247-259

A. Paracetamol
B. Antituberculosis drugs
C. Antiepileptic drugs
D. Herbal drugs

In India antituberculosis drugs are the commonest cause of drug-induced ALF in adults and children.

1674. Isoniazid hepatotoxicity is enhanced by?
Harrison's 20th Ed. Chapter 333 Page 2372

A. Alcohol
B. Rifampin
C. Pyrazinamide
D. All of the above

Isoniazid hepatotoxicity is enhanced by alcohol, barbiturates, rifampin & pyrazinamide.

1675. Highest frequency of substantial liver injury due to INH use is in patients over the age of?
Harrison's 20th Ed. Chapter 333 Page 2372

A. 20 years
B. 30 years
C. 40 years
D. 50 years

Substantial liver injury appears to be age-related, increasing substantially after age 35. Highest frequency is in patients over age 50 years and the lowest is in patients under the age of 20.

1676. Which of the following drugs produce toxic and idiosyncratic reactions?
Harrison's 20th Ed. Chapter 333 Page 2372

A. Isoniazid
B. Sodium valproate

C. Amiodarone
D. All of the above

1677. Which of the following drugs act as a direct toxin in liver?
Harrison's 20th Ed. Chapter 333 Page 2372

A. Acetaminophen
B. Nitrofurantoin
C. Amoxicillin-clavulanate
D. Simvastatin

Acetaminophen causes dose-related centrilobular hepatic necrosis after single-time-point ingestions.

1678. IV administration of carnitine may be ameliorate hepatotoxicity due to?
Harrison's 20th Ed. Chapter 333 Page 2372

A. Valproate
B. Isoniazid
C. Halothane
D. Acetaminophen

Valproate hepatotoxicity may be ameliorated by IV administration of carnitine. Valproate inhibits biosynthesis of carnitine, by affecting the beta-oxidation of fatty acids. Carnitine supplementation circumvents the defect by increasing the beta-oxidation of valproate.

1679. Which metabolite of sodium valproate may be responsible for hepatic injury?
Harrison's 20th Ed. Chapter 333 Page 2372

A. 1-pentenoic acid
B. 2-pentenoic acid
C. 3-pentenoic acid
D. 4-pentenoic acid

Sodium valproate is not directly hepatotoxic, but its metabolite 4-pentenoic acid may be responsible for hepatic injury.

1680. Which of the following drugs is associated with moderate to severe chronic hepatitis with autoimmune features?
Harrison's 20th Ed. Chapter 333 Page 2372

A. Nitrofurantoin
B. Hydralazine
C. Methyldopa
D. All of the above

Nitrofurantoin, minocycline, hydralazine and methyldopa have been associated with moderate to severe chronic hepatitis with autoimmune features.

1681. "Vanishing bile duct syndrome" best relates to?
Harrison's 20th Ed. Chapter 333 Page 2372

A. Amoxicillin-clavulanate hepatotoxicity
B. Oral contraceptive hepatotoxicity
C. Anabolic steroid hepatotoxicity
D. All of the above

1682. "Vanishing bile duct syndrome" best relates to?
Harrison's 20th Ed. Chapter 45 Page 280, Chapter 338 Page 2420

A. Chronic liver transplant rejection
B. Graft-versus-host disease after bone marrow transplantation
C. Sarcoidosis
D. All of the above

1683. Pure cholestasis is due to which of the following drug toxicity?
Harrison's 20th Ed. Chapter 45 Page 280 Table 45-3

A. Chlorpromazine
B. Erythromycin estolate
C. Anabolic and contraceptive steroids
D. Prochlorperazine

1684. Cholestatic hepatitis is due to which of the following drug toxicity?
Harrison's 20th Ed. Chapter 45 Page 280 Table 45-3

A. Anabolic steroids
B. Erythromycin estolate
C. Contraceptive steroids
D. Prochlorperazine

1685. Chronic cholestasis is due to which of the following drug toxicity?
Harrison's 20th Ed. Chapter 45 Page 280 Table 45-3

A. Anabolic steroids
B. Erythromycin estolate
C. Contraceptive steroids
D. Chlorpromazine

1686. Which of the following about halothane hepatotoxicity is false?
Hepat Mon. 2011;11(1):3-6

A. Idiosyncratic reaction
B. Halothane is not a direct hepatotoxin
C. Cause severe centrilobular hepatic necrosis
D. Cross-reactions between halothane & methoxyflurane

The pathologic changes produced by halothane hepatotoxicity are indistinguishable from massive hepatic necrosis resulting from viral hepatitis. Severe centrilobular hepatic necrosis is typical of acetaminophen toxicity.

1687. Which of the following is false about methyldopa hepatotoxicity?
The American Journal of Medicine. 1976;60(7):941-948

A. Toxic reaction
B. Idiosyncratic reaction
C. Resolves with discontinuation of drug
D. None of the above

1688. A defect in epoxide hydrolase activity could cause hepatotoxicity due to which drug?
Harrison's 20th Ed. Chapter 333 Page 2372

A. Valproate
B. Phenytoin
C. Halothane
D. Acetaminophen

A defect in epoxide hydrolase activity could cause hepatotoxicity due to Phenytoin.

1689. Stevens-Johnson syndrome may be a presentation of toxicity due to?
Harrison's 20th Ed. Chapter 333 Page 2372

A. Valproate
B. Phenytoin

C. Halothane
D. Acetaminophen

Apart from drug induced hepatitis, fever, lymphadenopathy, rash (Stevens-Johnson syndrome or exfoliative dermatitis), leukocytosis & eosinophilia may manifest in hepatotoxicity due to Phenytoin.

1690. Histopathologically, abundance of eosinophils in liver points towards the toxicity with which of the following drug?
Harrison's 20th Ed. Chapter 333 Page 2372

A. Valproate
B. Phenytoin
C. Halothane
D. Acetaminophen

1691. Hepatic injury manifests within what period after beginning phenytoin therapy?
Harrison's 20th Ed. Chapter 333 Page 2372

A. First day
B. First week
C. First month
D. Two months

Hepatic injury manifests within the first 2 months after beginning phenytoin therapy.

1692. Which of the following is a major metabolite of Amiodarone?
Harrison's 20th Ed. Chapter 333 Page 2373

A. Desmethylamiodarone
B. Desethylamiodarone
C. Levomethylamiodarone
D. Levoethylamiodarone

1693. Amiodarone metabolite desethylamiodarone accumulate in which of the following?
Harrison's 20th Ed. Chapter 333 Page 2373

A. Hepatocyte lysosomes
B. Hepatocyte mitochondria
C. Bile duct epithelium
D. All of the above

1694. Pseudoalcoholic liver injury best relates to toxicity with?
Harrison's 20th Ed. Chapter 333 Page 2373

A. Valproate
B. Phenytoin
C. Halothane
D. Amiodarone

In amiodarone toxicity, pseudoalcoholic liver injury can range from steatosis, to alcoholic hepatitis like neutrophilic infiltration and Mallory's hyaline, to cirrhosis.

1695. Phospholipidosis is best related to which of the following drug toxicity?
Harrison's 20th Ed. Chapter 333 Page 2373

A. Valproate
B. Phenytoin
C. Halothane
D. Amiodarone

Electron-microscopic demonstration of phospholipid-laden lysosomal lamellar bodies (ultrastructural phospholipidosis) can help to distinguish amiodarone hepatotoxicity from typical alcoholic hepatitis.

1696. Toxicity with which of the following produces cholestatic idiosyncratic reaction?
Harrison's 20th Ed. Chapter 333 Page 2373

A. Acetaminophen
B. Erythromycin
C. Azathioprine
D. Carbamazine

1697. Drugs producing cholestatic reaction and portal inflammation is?
Harrison's 20th Ed. Chapter 333 Page 2373

A. Erythromycin
B. Oral contraceptive
C. Amiodarone
D. 17, α-Alkyl-Substituted Anabolic Steroids

1698. Which of the following rises most in liver injury due to anabolic steroids?
Harrison's 20th Ed. Chapter 333 Page 2373

A. Serum aminotransferases
B. Serum alkaline phosphatase
C. Serum bilirubin
D. Serum globulin

In liver injury due to anabolic steroids, serum aminotransferase levels are usually <100 IU/L, serum alkaline phosphatase levels are generally moderately elevated with bilirubin levels frequently exceeding 20 mg/dL.

1699. In Trimethoprim-Sulfamethoxazole toxicity, hepatotoxicity is attributable to which component of the drug?
Harrison's 20th Ed. Chapter 333 Page 2373

A. Sulfamethoxazole
B. Trimethoprim
C. Sulfamethoxazole + Trimethoprim
D. None of the above

The hepatotoxicity with the use of Trimethoprim-Sulfamethoxazole is attributable to the sulfamethoxazole component of the drug.

1700. The risk of trimethoprim-sulfamethoxazole hepatotoxicity is increased in persons with?
Harrison's 20th Ed. Chapter 333 Page 2373

A. HIV infection
B. Severe anemia
C. Chronic renal failure
D. Congestive heart failure

Risk of trimethoprim-sulfamethoxazole hepatotoxicity is increased in persons with HIV infection.

1701. Statin hepatotoxicity is increased in which of the following patients?
Harrison's 20th Ed. Chapter 333 Page 2374

A. Chronic hepatitis C
B. Hepatic steatosis
C. Other underlying liver diseases
D. None of the above

Statin hepatotoxicity is "not" increased in patients with chronic hepatitis C, hepatic steatosis, or other underlying liver diseases, and statins can be used safely in these patients.

1702. In Total Parenteral Nutrition (TPN), steatosis or steatohepatitis may result due to an excess of?

Harrison's 20th Ed. Chapter 333 Page 2374

A. Carbohydrate calories
B. Protein calories
C. Fat calories
D. Deficiency of minerals

In Total Parenteral Nutrition (TPN), steatosis or steatohepatitis may result due to an excess of carbohydrate calories. This complication has reduced substantially by introduction of balanced TPN formulas that rely on lipid as an alternative caloric source.

1703. Herbal remedies associated with toxic hepatitis is?

Harrison's 20th Ed. Chapter 333 Page 2374

A. Jin Bu Huan
B. Xiao-chai-hutang
C. Ma huang
D. All of the above

Jin Bu Huan, xiao-chai-hutang, germander, chaparral, senna, mistletoe, skullcap, gentian, comfrey (containing pyrrolizidine alkaloids), ma huang, bee pollen, valerian root, pennyroyal oil, kava, celandine, Impila (Callilepis laureola), LipoKinetix, Hydroxycut, herbal nutritional supplements and herbal teas containing Camellia sinensis (green tea extract).

1704. Which of the following drugs is implicated in the development of cirrhosis?

Harrison's 20th Ed. Chapter 333 Page 2369

A. Oxyphenisatin
B. Methyldopa
C. Isoniazid
D. Methotrexate

Methotrexate, tamoxifen and amiodarone have been implicated in the development of cirrhosis.

1705. Most common cause of liver enzyme elevation is?

Cleveland Clinic Journal of Medicine. 2018;85(8):612

A. Alcohol toxicity
B. Medication overdose
C. Fatty liver disease
D. All of the above

Most common causes of liver enzyme elevation are alcohol toxicity, medication overdose, & fatty liver disease.

1706. Cytochrome P450 (CYP) was first discovered in 1954 by?

J Adv Pract Oncol. 2013;4(4):263-268

A. Wilhelm Kuhnz & Hille Gieschen
B. Bernhardt
C. Martin Klingenberg & David Garfinkel
D. Akio Suzuki

1707. Cytochrome P-450 enzymes (CYPs) are important in the biosynthesis and degradation of?

N Engl J Med. 2005;352:2211-21

A. Steroids
B. Lipids
C. Vitamins
D. All of the above

Cytochrome P-450 enzymes (CYPs) are important in biosynthesis & degradation of endogenous compounds like steroids, lipids, and vitamins.

1708. Cytochrome P-450 enzymes (CYPs) are important in the biosynthesis & degradation of endogenous compounds like?

N Engl J Med. 2005;352:2211-21

A. Steroids
B. Lipids
C. Vitamins
D. All of the above

1709. The P in P450 stands for?

Am Fam Phys 1998;57:107-16

A. Particle
B. Pigment
C. Pattern
D. Protein

The P in P450 stands for "pigment".

1710. "450" in Cytochrome P450 isoenzymes is related to?

J Adv Pract Oncol. 2013;4(4):263-268

A. Number of isoenzymes in liver
B. Number of chemical reactions
C. Number of electron needed for its activity
D. Spectrophotometric absorption peak

Name cytochrome P450 is derived from the fact that these are colored ('chrome') cellular ('cyto') proteins, with a "pigment at 450 nm", so named for the characteristic spectrophotometric absorption peak formed by absorbance of light at wavelengths near 450 nm when the heme iron is reduced and complexed to carbon monoxide.

1711. In CYP2E1, letter '2' indicates?

J Adv Pract Oncol. 2013;4(4):263-268

A. Gene family
B. Gene subfamily
C. Individual gene
D. None of the above

"CYP" stands for cytochrome P450, followed by a numeral indicating gene family, a capital letter indicating subfamily and another numeral for the individual gene.

1712. Which of the following about cytochrome P450 is false?

J Adv Pract Oncol. 2013;4(4):263-268

A. Hemoprotein
B. Monooxygenases
C. Pigment at 450 nm
D. None of the above

Cytochrome P450 belongs to a superfamily of hemoproteins. Most common reaction catalysed by cytochrome P450 is a monooxygenase reaction, i.e. insertion of one atom of oxygen into an organic substrate (RH) while the other oxygen atom is reduced to water: $RH + O_2 + 2H^+ + 2e^- = ROH + H_2O$

1713. The catalytic activity of CYP2D6 in humans is best assessed by using which of the following drug?

Pharmacogenomics. 2009;10(1):17-28

A. Debrisoquine
B. Fluoxetine
C. Perphenazine
D. Dextromethorphan

CYP2D6 or Debrisoquine hydroxylase is second to CYP3A4 in the number of commonly used drugs that it metabolizes. Debrisoquine is a derivative of guanidine. It is an antihypertensive drug similar to guanethidine. Debrisoquine is frequently used for phenotyping the CYP2D6 enzyme.

1714. Which of the following cytochrome P-450 is present in enterocytes?

N Engl J Med. 2005;352:2211-21

A. CYP1A2
B. CYP2D6
C. CYP2C9
D. CYP3A

CYP3A is present in the enterocytes.

1715. Which of the following CYP is found mainly in the glomerulosa zone of adrenal gland?

Harrison's 20th Ed. Chapter 379 Page 2723

A. CYP11B2
B. CYP3A5
C. CYP2D6
D. CYP2C19

CYP11B2 is found mainly if not exclusively in the glomerulosa zone of the adrenal gland.

1716. Which of the following is the primary isoenzyme expressed during the prenatal period?

J Pediatr Pharmacol Ther. 2014;19(4):262-276

A. CYP1A2
B. CYP3A7
C. CYP2D6
D. CYP2C19

CYP3A7 is the primary isoenzyme expressed during the prenatal period. It declines rapidly after birth and is barely measurable in adults.

1717. Which of the following CYP is not expressed in neonates?

J Pediatr Pharmacol Ther. 2014;19(4):262-276

A. CYP1A2
B. CYP3A5
C. CYP2D6
D. CYP2C19

CYP1A2 is not expressed in neonates, making them susceptible to toxicity from drugs such as caffeine.

1718. Drugs having a narrow range between the plasma levels yielding therapeutic and adverse effects include all except?

A. Digoxin
B. Theophylline
C. Lidocaine
D. Amiodarone

1719. Which of the following anti-HIV agent is not a CYP3A inhibitor?

N Engl J Med. 2005;352:2211-21

A. Indinavir
B. Ritonavir
C. Saquinavir
D. Nevirapine

1720. Which of the following macrolide antibiotics is not a CYP3A inhibitor?

N Engl J Med. 2005;352:2211-21

A. Clarithromycin
B. Erythromycin
C. Troleandomycin
D. Azithromycin

1721. Which of the following anticonvulsant agent is not a CYP3A inducer?

N Engl J Med. 2005;352:2211-21

A. Carbamazepine
B. Phenobarbital
C. Phenytoin
D. Lamotrigine

1722. Which of the following enzyme is responsible for metabolism of most of the drugs used?

Harrison's 20th Ed. Chapter 64 Page 430

A. CYP3A4
B. CYP3A5
C. CYP2D6
D. CYP2C19

CYP3A4 is the most abundant hepatic and intestinal CYP and is also the enzyme responsible for metabolism of the greatest number of drugs in therapeutic use. CYP2D6 is second to CYP3A4 in the number of commonly used drugs that it metabolizes. Families or enzymes that are of greatest importance in metabolism of drugs are CYP3A4, 2D6, 2C9, 2C19, 1A2, 2E1, and 2B6.

1723. In liver, the family of cytochrome P450 (CYP) isoforms is present in?

J Adv Pract Oncol. 2013;4(4):263-268

A. Endoplasmic reticulum
B. Cell membrane
C. Golgi bodies
D. Nucleus

1724. Which of the following does not inhibit CYP3A4?

Harrison's 20th Ed. Chapter 139 Page 1053

A. Azithromycin
B. Erythromycin
C. Clarithromycin
D. Telithromycin

Erythromycin, clarithromycin and telithromycin inhibit CYP3A4 hepatic drug metabolizing enzyme and can result in increased levels of coadministered drugs, including benzodiazepines, statins, warfarin, cyclosporine and tacrolimus. Azithromycin does not inhibit CYP3A4 and lacks these drug-drug interactions.

1725. Major hepatic isoenzyme involved in warfarin metabolism is?

Harrison's 20th Ed. Chapter 63 Page 421 Table 63-1

A. CYP 2C9
B. CYP 2C19
C. CYP 2D6
D. CYP 3A

1726. Major hepatic isoenzyme involved in phenytoin metabolism is?

Harrison's 20th Ed. Chapter 63 Page 421 Table 63-1

A. CYP 2C9
B. CYP 2C19

C. CYP 2D6
D. CYP 3A

1727. Major hepatic isoenzyme in omeprazole metabolism is?
Harrison's 20th Ed. Chapter 63 Page 421 Table 63-1

A. CYP 2C9
B. CYP 2C19
C. CYP 2D6
D. CYP 3A

1728. Major hepatic isoenzyme in metoprolol metabolism is?
Harrison's 20th Ed. Chapter 63 Page 421 Table 63-1

A. CYP 2C9
B. CYP 2C19
C. CYP 2D6
D. CYP 3A

1729. Major hepatic isoenzyme in tricyclic antidepressants metabolism is?
Harrison's 20th Ed. Chapter 63 Page 421 Table 63-1

A. CYP 2C9
B. CYP 2C19
C. CYP 2D6
D. CYP 3A

1730. Major hepatic isoenzyme involved in selective serotonin reuptake inhibitors metabolism is?
Harrison's 20th Ed. Chapter 63 Page 421 Table 63-1

A. CYP 2C9
B. CYP 2C19
C. CYP 2D6
D. CYP 3A

1731. Major hepatic isoenzyme involved in codeine metabolism is?
Harrison's 20th Ed. Chapter 63 Page 421 Table 63-1

A. CYP 2C9
B. CYP 2C19
C. CYP 2D6
D. CYP 3A

1732. Major hepatic isoenzyme in cyclosporine metabolism is?
Harrison's 20th Ed. Chapter 63 Page 421 Table 63-1

A. CYP 2C9
B. CYP 2C19
C. CYP 2D6
D. CYP 3A

1733. Major hepatic isoenzyme in statin metabolism is?
Harrison's 20th Ed. Chapter 63 Page 421 Table 63-1

A. CYP 2C9
B. CYP 2C19
C. CYP 2D6
D. CYP 3A

1734. Major hepatic isoenzyme in lidocaine metabolism is?
Harrison's 20th Ed. Chapter 63 Page 421 Table 63-1

A. CYP 2C9
B. CYP 2C19
C. CYP 2D6
D. CYP 3A

1735. Major hepatic isoenzyme in quinidine metabolism is?
Harrison's 20th Ed. Chapter 63 Page 421 Table 63-1

A. CYP 2C9
B. CYP 2C19
C. CYP 2D6
D. CYP 3A

1736. Which of the following has been used in mushroom (Amanita phalloides) toxicity?
J Clin Exp Hepatol. 2012;2(3):247-259

A. N-acetylcysteine (NAC)
B. Silymarin
C. S-adenosine methionine
D. Ursodeoxycholic acid

Silymarin alone or silymarin combination with benzylpenicillin has been used in mushroom (Amanita phalloides) toxicity

Chronic Hepatitis

1737. In chronic hepatitis, hepatic inflammation and necrosis continue for at least?
Harrison's 20th Ed. Chapter 334 Page 2375

A. 3 months
B. 6 months
C. 9 months
D. 12 months

In chronic hepatitis, hepatic inflammation & necrosis continue for at least 6 months.

1738. Chronic hepatitis is due to?
Harrison's 20th Ed. Chapter 334 Page 2375

A. Virus
B. Drug-induced
C. Autoimmune
D. All of the above

Chronic viral hepatitis, drug-induced chronic hepatitis & autoimmune chronic hepatitis can cause chronicity.

1739. Chronic hepatitis is due to?
Harrison's 20th Ed. Chapter 334 Page 2375

A. Wilson's disease
B. α1 antitrypsin deficiency
C. Nonalcoholic fatty liver disease
D. All of the above

1740. Which of the following is the more severe form of chronic hepatitis?
Harrison's 20th Ed. Chapter 334 Page 2375

A. Chronic persistent hepatitis
B. Chronic lobular hepatitis
C. Chronic active hepatitis
D. All of the above

Earlier, chronic hepatitis was defined histopathologically as Chronic persistent hepatitis, chronic lobular hepatitis and chronic active hepatitis. Out of these chronic active hepatitis was considered as the more sever form.

1741. Classification of chronic hepatitis is based on?
Harrison's 20th Ed. Chapter 334 Page 2375

A. Cause
B. Histologic activity, or grade
C. Degree of progression, or stage
D. All of the above

Classification of chronic hepatitis is based on its cause, its histologic assessment of necroinflammatory activity, or grade and its degree of progression, or stage.

1742. Which of the following histologic features is accounted for in grading chronic hepatitis?
Harrison's 20th Ed. Chapter 334 Page 2375

A. Periportal necrosis
B. Bridging necrosis
C. Portal inflammation
D. All of the above

1743. Staging of chronic hepatitis is based on?
Harrison's 20th Ed. Chapter 334 Page 2375

A. Hepatic necrosis
B. Hepatic fibrosis
C. Hepatic inflammation
D. All of the above

The stage of chronic hepatitis is based on the degree of hepatic fibrosis.

1744. Histologic activity index (HAI) scoring for necroinflammatory activity (grade) is done out of?
Harrison's 20th Ed. Chapter 334 Page 2376 Table 334-2

A. 10
B. 14
C. 18
D. 20

Out of a maximum of 18, individual scoring is degree of periportal necrosis (max. 4), degree of intralobular confluent necrosis (max. 6), degree of intralobular focal necrosis (max. 4) & degree of portal inflammation (max. 4).

1745. Histologic activity index (HAI) scoring for fibrosis (stage) is done out of?
Harrison's 20th Ed. Chapter 334 Page 2376 Table 334-2

A. 3
B. 4
C. 6
D. 8

Staging is based on the degree of fibrosis as categorized on a numerical scale from 0-6 (HAI) or 0-4 (METAVIR).

1746. Histologic activity index (HAI) scoring for necroinflammatory activity (grade) includes all except?
Harrison's 20th Ed. Chapter 334 Page 2376 Table 334-2

A. Degree of periportal necrosis
B. Portal fibrosis
C. Intralobular necrosis
D. Degree of portal inflammation

Grade, a histologic assessment of necroinflammatory activity, is done by examination of liver biopsy. It includes assessment of degree of periportal necrosis, degree of hepatocyte degeneration and focal necrosis within lobule and degree of portal inflammation.

1747. In Europe, scoring system for assessment of necroinflammatory activity in liver is?
Harrison's 20th Ed. Chapter 334 Page 2375

A. Child-Pugh
B. Ishak
C. METAVIR
D. All of the above

1748. The likelihood of chronicity after acute hepatitis B depends on?
Harrison's 20th Ed. Chapter 334 Page 2375

A. Mode of transmission
B. Quantum of viral infection
C. Associated medical conditions
D. Age at the time of infection

The likelihood of chronicity after acute hepatitis B varies as a function of age at the time of acquisition. Perinatal transmission can be dramatically reduced by the administration of hepatitis B immunoglobulin at childbirth and the hepatitis B vaccine.

1749. What percentage of HBV infection acquired at birth will become chronic?
Harrison's 20th Ed. Chapter 334 Page 2376

A. 10%
B. 40%
C. 75%
D. 90%

HBV infection at birth is associated with clinically silent acute infection but a 90% chance of chronic infection.

1750. What percentage of HBV infection acquired in immunocompetent young adulthood will become chronic?
Harrison's 20th Ed. Chapter 334 Page 2376

A. ~ 1%
B. ~ 4%
C. ~ 7%
D. ~ 9%

HBV infection in immunocompetent young adulthood carry a risk of chronicity of ~ 1%.

1751. Which of the following has prognostic importance among adults with chronic hepatitis B?
Harrison's 20th Ed. Chapter 334 Page 2376

A. HBV serology
B. HLA DR3 or DR4 markers
C. AST and ALT
D. Liver histology

Among adults with chronic hepatitis B, histologic features are of prognostic importance. Distinctions in HBV replication and in histologic category do not always coincide.

1752. Replicative phase of chronic HBV infection is characterized by?
Harrison's 20th Ed. Chapter 334 Page 2376

A. Presence of HBeAg in serum
B. HBV DNA levels > 10^5–10^6 virions/mL
C. Presence of intrahepatocyte HBcAg in liver
D. All of the above

Replicative phase is characterized by presence of HBeAg & HBV DNA levels over 10^5–10^6 virions/mL in serum, by presence of HBcAg in liver, by high infectivity & by accompanying liver injury.

1753. Nonreplicative phase of chronic HBV infection is characterized by all except?
Harrison's 20th Ed. Chapter 334 Page 2376

A. Absence of HBeAg in serum
B. HBV DNA levels < 10^3 virions/mL
C. Presence of anti-HBe
D. Presence of intrahepatocyte HBcAg in liver

Nonreplicative phase is characterized by the absence of the conventional serum marker of HBV replication (HBeAg), the appearance of anti-HBe, levels of HBV DNA below a threshold of ~10^3 virions/mL, the absence of intrahepatocytic HBcAg, limited infectivity, and minimal liver injury.

1754. What percentage of HBeAg-reactive chronic hepatitis B convert spontaneously from replicative to nonreplicative infection per year?
Harrison's 20th Ed. Chapter 334 Page 2376

A. ~ 5%
B. ~ 10%
C. ~ 15%
D. ~ 20%

~10% patients of HBeAg-reactive chronic hepatitis B convert spontaneously from relatively replicative to nonreplicative infection per year.

1755. Most important risk factor for development of cirrhosis & HCC in chronic HBV infection is?
Harrison's 20th Ed. Chapter 334 Page 2376

A. Levels of HBV DNA
B. Level of HBV replication
C. Levels of aminotransferase activity
D. All of the above

Level of HBV replication is the most important risk factor for the ultimate development of cirrhosis & HCC in both HBeAg-reactive and HBeAg-negative patients.

1756. HBV inactive carriers is characterized by all except?
Harrison's 20th Ed. Chapter 334 Page 2377

A. Circulating HBsAg
B. Raised serum aminotransferase levels
C. Undetectable HBeAg
D. Almost undetectable levels of HBV DNA

Inactive HBV carriers have circulating HBsAg, normal serum aminotransferase levels, undetectable HBeAg, and almost undetectable levels of HBV DNA. This serologic profile occurs also in patients with HBeAg-negative chronic hepatitis B during periods of relative inactivity.

1757. Which of the following is not a complication of chronic hepatitis B?
Harrison's 20th Ed. Chapter 334 Page 2377

A. Hyperglobulinemia
B. Immune-complex glomerulonephritis
C. Generalized vasculitis
D. Leukocytoclastic vasculitis

Hyperglobulinemia & detectable circulating autoantibodies are distinctly absent in chronic hepatitis B in contrast to autoimmune hepatitis.

1758. HBV DNA can be detected in serum at levels as low as?
N Engl J Med. 2008;359:1486-500

A. 20 IU/mL
B. 40 IU/mL
C. 60 IU/mL
D. 80 IU/mL

HBV DNA can be detected in the serum at levels as low as 60 IU/mL.

1759. Histologic improvement is defined as a reduction of 2 or more points in the histologic activity index at?
N Engl J Med. 2008;359:1486-500

A. Month 3
B. Month 6
C. Year 1
D. Year 2

1760. Serum HBV DNA undetectable by PCR is defined as?
N Engl J Med. 2008;359:1486-500

A. < 100 to 200 copies per milliliter
B. < 300 to 400 copies per milliliter
C. < 500 to 1000 copies per milliliter
D. < 1000 to 2000 copies per milliliter

Serum HBV DNA undetectable by PCR is defined as <300 to 400 copies per milliliter (<1000 copies / mL for adefovir) at the end of year 1.

1761. Immunity to HBV infection is characterized by all except?
N Engl J Med. 2008;359:1486-500

A. Loss of HBV surface antigen
B. Loss of HBV e antigen
C. Loss of anti-core antigen IgM
D. Loss of anti-core antigen IgG

Immunity to HBV infection is characterized by loss of HBV surface antigen, DNA, e antigen, & anti-core antigen IgM with development of anti-surface antigen antibody & anti-core antigen IgG (total anti-core antigen antibody).

1762. Which of the following differentiates natural immunity by resolved HBV infection from that which is acquired through vaccination?
N Engl J Med. 2008;359:1486-500

A. Presence of Anti HBs + IgM anti HBc
B. Presence of Anti HBs + IgG anti HBc
C. Presence of Anti HBs + anti HBe
D. All of the above

Presence of anti HBs & IgG anti Hbc together differentiates natural immunity through resolved infection from that which is acquired through vaccination, which is denoted by isolated anti-surface antigen antibody.

1763. Which of the following phase is seen almost exclusively in those who acquired HBV infection vertically or during early childhood?
N Engl J Med. 2008;359:1486-500

A. Immune tolerance phase
B. Immune clearance phase
C. Inactive carrier phase
D. Reactivation phase

Immune tolerance phase, the initial phase of chronic HBV infection, is seen almost exclusively in those who acquired HBV infection vertically or during early childhood.

1764. Predictor of spontaneous e antigen seroconversion is?
N Engl J Med. 2008;359:1486-500

A. Old age
B. Elevated ALT level
C. Acute exacerbation
D. All of the above

The strongest predictors of spontaneous e antigen seroconversion are old age, an elevated ALT level, and an acute exacerbation.

1765. Which of the following phase is also called HBV e antigen negative chronic hepatitis?
N Engl J Med. 2008;359:1486-500

A. Immune tolerance phase
B. Immune clearance phase
C. Inactive carrier phase
D. Reactivation phase

Reactivation phase is also termed as HBV e antigen negative chronic hepatitis.

1766. Liver biopsy findings are normal or nonspecific in which of the following phase of HBV infection?
N Engl J Med. 2008;359:1486-500

A. Immune tolerance phase
B. Immune clearance phase
C. Inactive carrier phase
D. Reactivation phase

Liver biopsy shows findings of chronic hepatitis in immune clearance and reactivation phase. Nonsignificant hepatitis is observed in inactive carrier phase.

1767. e antibody is positive in which of the following phase of HBV infection?
N Engl J Med. 2008;359:1486-500

A. Immune tolerance phase
B. Immune clearance phase
C. Inactive carrier phase
D. All of the above

e antibody is negative in immune tolerance and immune clearance phase.

1768. HBV DNA is high in which of the following phase of HBV infection?
N Engl J Med. 2008;359:1486-500

A. Immune tolerance phase
B. Immune clearance phase
C. Inactive carrier phase
D. Reactivation phase

1769. Inactive HBV carriers with a low risk of clinical progression are those with a serum HBV DNA level below?
N Engl J Med. 2008;359:1486-500

A. 1000 IU per milliliter
B. 5000 IU per milliliter
C. 10000 IU per milliliter
D. 10000 IU per milliliter

Persons with a serum HBV DNA level below 1000 IU per milliliter and a normal ALT level consistently are considered to be inactive carriers with a low risk of clinical progression.

1770. Which of the following drug is beneficial in severe acute hepatitis B?
Harrison's 20th Ed. Chapter 334 Page 2377

A. Lamivudine
B. Interferon monotherapy
C. Ribavirin
D. Glucocorticoid

Oral drugs that have been approved for treatment of chronic hepatitis B include lamivudine, adefovir dipivoxil, entecavir, telbivudine and tenofovir.

1771. Which of the following is approved for treatment of chronic HBV infection?
Harrison's 20th Ed. Chapter 334 Page 2377, Lancet Infect Dis 2005;5:374–82

A. PEG IFN
B. Adefovir dipivoxil
C. Entecavir
D. All of the above

Drugs approved for treatment of chronic hepatitis B are injectable interferon (IFN) α and pegylated interferon (PEG IFN), lamivudine, adefovir dipivoxil, entecavir, telbivudine and tenofovir disoproxil fumarate (TDF).

1772. Which of the following drugs was the first to be approved for treatment of chronic HBV infection?
Harrison's 20th Ed. Chapter 334 Page 2377, Lancet Infect Dis 2005;5:374–82

A. Interferon α
B. Lamivudine
C. Adefovir
D. Entecavir

IFN-α was the first approved therapy for chronic hepatitis B in 1992, Lamivudine in 1998, Adefovir dipivoxil in 2002.

1773. Which of the following is the standard therapy for Interferon α?
Harrison's 20th Ed. Chapter 334 Page 2377

A. 5 million units subcutaneously per day for 12 weeks
B. 5 million units subcutaneously per day for 14 weeks
C. 5 million units subcutaneously per day for 16 weeks
D. 5 million units subcutaneously per day for 18 weeks

Standard therapy by immunomodulator Interferon α in chronic hepatitis B is 16-week course of IFN, subcutaneously at a daily dose of 5 million units, or three times a week at a dose of 10 million units.

1774. IFN-α therapy is not effective in which of the following groups of CHB patients?
Harrison's 20th Ed. Chapter 334 Page 2378

A. Very young children infected at birth
B. Immunosuppressed persons
C. Decompensated chronic hepatitis B
D. All of the above

IFN therapy has not been effective in very young children infected at birth, in immunosuppressed persons, Asian patients with minimal-to-mild ALT elevations, or patients with decompensated chronic hepatitis B.

1775. Which of the following side effects of IFN-α therapy is not reversible upon dose lowering or cessation of therapy?
Harrison's 20th Ed. Chapter 334 Page 2378

A. Autoimmune thyroiditis
B. Bone marrow suppression
C. Alopecia
D. Numbness & tingling of extremities

Except autoimmune thyroiditis, all side effects are reversible upon dose lowering / cessation of IFN-α.

1776. Which of the following is a 'Nucleoside analogue'?
Harrison's 20th Ed. Chapter 334 Page 2378, Lancet Infect Dis 2005;5:374–82

A. Lamivudine
B. Adefovir
C. Entecavir
D. Emtricitabine

Adefovir dipivoxil and Tenofovir are nucleotide analogues. Lamivudine - nucleoside analogue, Entecavir - guanosine analogue polymerase inhibitor, Telbivudine - cytosine analogue, Emtricitabine - fluorinated cytosine analogue, Clevudine - pyrimidine nucleoside analogue.

1777. Lamivudine was approved for hepatitis B treatment in?
Harrison's 20th Ed. Chapter 334 Page 2378

A. 1994
B. 1996
C. 1998
D. 2000

1778. Which of the following about Lamivudine is false?
Harrison's 20th Ed. Chapter 334 Page 2378

A. Dideoxynucleoside
B. Inhibits reverse transcriptase activity of HBV
C. Inhibits reverse transcriptase activity of HIV
D. None of the above

1779. HBV DNA level of ~10^3 IU/mL is equivalent to?
Harrison's 20th Ed. Chapter 334 Page 2378

A. <10^2 copies/mL
B. <10^3 copies/mL
C. <10^4 copies/mL
D. <10^5 copies/mL

HBV DNA level of ~10^3 IU/mL is equivalent to <10^4 copies/mL.

1780. Which of the following statements about lamivudine is false?
Harrison's 20th Ed. Chapter 334 Page 2378, Lancet Infect Dis. 2005;5:374–82

A. Anti-HIV & anti-HBV activity
B. Dose lower for blocking HIV replication than HBV replication
C. Not be used as monotherapy in HBV/HIV co-infected patients
D. Anti-HBe seroconversion occurs in minority of patients

1781. The inhibitory dose of Lamivudine for treating HBV/HIV co-infected patients is?
Harrison's 20th Ed. Chapter 334 Page 2379, Lancet Infect Dis 2005;5:374–82

A. 100 mg/day
B. 200 mg/day
C. 300 mg/day
D. 400 mg/day

The inhibitory dose of Lamivudine for blocking HBV replication is 100 mg/day. 300 mg/day should be given when treating HBV/HIV co-infected patients, and should always be combined with at least two other anti-HIV agents.

1782. YMDD mutation best relates to?
Harrison's 20th Ed. Chapter 334 Page 2378

A. Lamivudine-resistant virus
B. IFN nonresponders
C. Lamivudine and IFN nonresponders
D. Any of the above

The term YMDD mutant is applied to patients taking lamivudine who initially become hepatitis B DNA negative and subsequently manifest hepatitis DNA in their serum while on therapy. YMDD mutation can be thought of as lamivudine-resistant virus.

1783. Long-term monotherapy with lamivudine is associated with mutation in which motif of HBV DNA polymerase?
Harrison's 20th Ed. Chapter 334 Page 2378

A. Chemokine (C-C motif) receptor 6
B. RNA-binding motif (RBM)

C. YMDD
D. All of the above

Long-term monotherapy with lamivudine is associated with methionine-to-valine (M204V) or methionine-to-isoleucine (M204I) mutations, primarily at amino acid 204 in the tyrosine-methionine-aspartate-aspartate (YMDD) motif (codons 203~206 of the reverse transcriptase) of HBV DNA polymerase.

1784. YMDD mutation after lamivudine therapy best relates to?
Harrison's 20th Ed. Chapter 334 Page 2379

A. Tyrosine-methionine-aspartate-aspartate
B. Tyrosine-aspartate-methionine-aspartate
C. Tyrosine-aspartate-aspartate-methionine
D. All of the above

The greatest drawback with lamivudine treatment is the emergence of drug-resistant HBV mutants with concomitant rise in ALT, DNA and worsening histology in some patients. This mutation of tyrosine-methionine-aspartate-aspartate (YMDD) motif in the C domain of the HBV DNA polymerase gene is also associated with flares of liver disease.

1785. Which of the following about Lamivudine is false?
Harrison's 20th Ed. Chapter 334 Page 2379

A. Effective in patients with decompensated hepatitis B
B. Not teratogenic
C. Reduces the likelihood of perinatal transmission of hepatitis B
D. None of the above

1786. Which of the following about adefovir dipivoxil is false?
Harrison's 20th Ed. Chapter 334 Page 2379

A. Acyclic nucleotide analogue
B. Prodrug of adefovir
C. Oral formulation, daily dose of 10 mg. for 48-week course
D. None of the above

1787. Adefovir dipivoxil is effective in?
Harrison's 20th Ed. Chapter 334 Page 2379

A. IFN nonresponders
B. Lamivudine-resistant, YMDD mutant HBV
C. Among patients co-infected with HBV and HIV
D. All of the above

1788. Which of the following drugs is least likely to result in HBeAg seroconversion?
Harrison's 20th Ed. Chapter 334 Page 2379

A. Lamivudine
B. Adefovir
C. Tenofovir
D. Entecavir

1789. Which of the following is false for HBV treatment in HIV positive patient?
Lancet Infect Dis 2005;5:374–82

A. Response to Interferon α is lower
B. Indefinite treatment with nucleoside/nucleotide analogues
C. Co-infection with hepatitis C rare
D. Frequent "Flares" while on HAART

1790. Which of the following has the highest rates of co-infection with HBV & HIV?
Lancet Infect Dis 2005;5:374–82

A. Men who have sex with men
B. Intravenous drug users
C. Infection through heterosexual contacts
D. Blood transfusion

1791. Markers of successful anti HBV therapy include?
N Engl J Med. 2004;350:1118-29

A. Loss of HBeAg
B. Seroconversion to anti-HBe antibodies
C. Reduction of circulating viral load
D. All of the above

1792. In CHB, factor that is not predictive of a response to antiviral therapy is?
N Engl J Med. 2008;359:1492

A. Low ALT level
B. Low HBV DNA level
C. Mild-to-moderate histologic activity and stage
D. HBV genotype A>B>C>D

Factors that are most predictive of a response include a high ALT level, a low HBV DNA level, and mild-to-moderate histologic activity & stage. Likelihood of HBeAg loss in PEG IFN alfa-2b treated HBeAg-reactive patients is associated with HBV genotype A > B > C > D.

1793. Which hepatitis virus infection leads to the most severe form of chronic viral hepatitis?
J Viral Hepat. 2010;17(11):749-56

A. Hepatitis A virus (HAV)
B. Hepatitis B virus (HBV)
C. Hepatitis C virus (HCV)
D. Hepatitis D virus (HDV)

Hepatitis D virus (HDV) infection leads to the most severe form of chronic viral hepatitis

1794. For HBeAg-reactive chronic HBV infection, antiviral therapy is indicated for patients with?
N Engl J Med. 2008;359:1492

A. ALT level more than two times upper limit of normal
B. HBV DNA > 20,000 IU per milliliter
C. Risk factors for progression
D. All of the above

For HBeAg-reactive chronic HBV, antiviral therapy is indicated if ALT levels are more than twice the upper limit of normal and HBV DNA >20,000 IU/mL. Risk factors for progression (older than 40 years, family history of HCC, or ALT level in high normal range (up to twice the upper limit of normal).

1795. For HBeAg-negative chronic HBV infection, antiviral therapy is indicated for patients with?
N Engl J Med. 2008;359:1492

A. ALT level more than two times upper limit of normal
B. HBV DNA > 20,000 IU per milliliter
C. Moderate-to-severe necroinflammatory activity or fibrosis
D. All of the above

For HBeAg-negative chronic HBV, antiviral therapy is indicated if ALT levels are more than twice the upper limit of normal and HBV DNA >20,000 IU/mL. If ALT is <2X with HBV DNA >20,000 IU/mL, liver biopsy is indicated. Moderate-to-severe necroinflammatory activity or fibrosis favours antiviral therapy.

1796. Conversion factor for HBV DNA between international units (IU) per milliliter and copies per milliliter is about?
N Engl J Med. 2008;359:1492

A. 2.6
B. 3.6
C. 4.6
D. 5.6

Conversion factor HBV DNA between international units /mL & copies/mL is ~ 5.6 (1 IU/mL is ~ 5.6 copies/mL). Treatment thresholds in copies/mL are 5 times higher than international units/mL.

1797. Nephrotoxicity of adefovir is best related to?
Therapeutic Advances in Gastroenterology 2008; 1; 61-75

A. Acute glomerulonephritis
B. Goodpasteur's syndrome
C. Fanconi-like syndrome
D. All of the above

Adefovir at 30 mg has higher antiviral potency. It's potential nephrotoxicity manifests as a Fanconi-like syndrome with phosphaturia and proteinuria.

1798. PEG stands for?
Harrison's 20th Ed. Chapter 334 Page 2379

A. Polyethylene glycerol
B. Perethylene glycerol
C. Polyethylene glycol
D. Perethylene glycol

Pegylated interferon (PEG IFN) is a long-acting IFN bound to polyethylene glycol (PEG).

1799. Pegylated IFN-α was approved by FDA for chronic hepatitis B in which year?
Harrison's 20th Ed. Chapter 334 Page 2380

A. 2000
B. 2002
C. 2003
D. 2005

1992 - Interferon alfa (IFN-α), 1998 - Lamivudine (LAM), 2002 - Adefovir (ADV), 2005 - Entecavir (ETV), Pegylated IFN-α, 2006 - Telbivudine (LDT), 2008 - Tenofovir (TDF).

1800. The recommended regimen of peg IFNa-2a for CHB is?
Harrison's 20th Ed. Chapter 334 Page 2380

A. 180 μg subcutaneously weekly for 24 weeks
B. 180 μg subcutaneously weekly for 36 weeks
C. 180 μg subcutaneously weekly for 48 weeks
D. 180 μg subcutaneously weekly for 51 weeks

Recommended regimen for peg IFNa-2a in CHB is 180 μg subcutaneously weekly for one year.

1801. Which of the following HBV genotype has the highest rate of IFN-induced HBeAg loss?
Harrison's 20th Ed. Chapter 334 Page 2380

A. Genotype A
B. Genotype B
C. Genotype C
D. Genotype D

Patients with HBV genotype A have the highest rate of IFN-induced HBeAg loss. Genotype A is most common in North America & Europe. HBeAg clearance associated with nucleos(t)ide analogues is independent of HBV genotype (HBV genotype A > B > C > D).

1802. PEG IFN therapy should be discontinued if HBsAg levels fail to reach <20,000 IU/mL by?
Harrison's 20th Ed. Chapter 334 Page 2380

A. Week 12
B. Week 24
C. Week 36
D. Week 48

If HBsAg levels fail to fall within first 12–24 weeks or to reach levels <20,000 IU/mL by week 24, PEG IFN therapy is unlikely to be effective and should be discontinued.

1803. The most potent of the HBV antiviral is?
Harrison's 20th Ed. Chapter 334 Page 2380

A. Entecavir
B. Telbivudine
C. Tenofovir
D. Adefovir Dipivoxil

1804. Which of the following is false about Entecavir?
Harrison's 20th Ed. Chapter 334 Page 2380

A. Oral cyclopentyl guanosine analogue polymerase inhibitor
B. Oral dose 0.5 mg daily
C. Effective against lamivudine-resistant HBV infection
D. Entecavir does not have antiviral activity against HIV

Entecavir is an oral cyclopentyl guanosine analogue polymerase inhibitor and is the most potent of the HBV antivirals. Its high barrier to resistance coupled with its high potency and an excellent safety profile renders entecavir a first-line drug for patients with chronic hepatitis B. Entecavir has low-level antiviral activity against HIV and cannot be used as monotherapy to treat HBV infection in HIV/HBV co-infected persons.

1805. Which of the following is false about Tenofovir?
Harrison's 20th Ed. Chapter 334 Page 2381

A. Acyclic nucleotide analogue
B. Antiretroviral agent
C. Oral once-daily dose of 300 mg
D. None of the above

1806. Tenofovir (TDF) is similar to which of the following?
Harrison's 20th Ed. Chapter 334 Page 2381

A. Entecavir
B. Telbivudine
C. Tenofovir
D. Adefovir Dipivoxil

Tenofovir disoproxil fumarate, an acyclic nucleotide analogue similar to adefovir.

1807. Very high HBV DNA levels refers to?
Harrison's 20th Ed. Chapter 334 Page 2381

A. $\geq 10^4$ IU/mL
B. $\geq 10^6$ IU/mL
C. $\geq 10^8$ IU/mL
D. $\geq 10^{10}$ IU/mL

1808. Which of the following is very similar to lamivudine in structure, efficacy, and resistance profile?
Harrison's 20th Ed. Chapter 334 Page 2381

A. Tenofovir
B. Emtricitabine

C. Clevudine

D. Telbivudine

1809. Which of the following is a prodrug of tenofovir?
Harrison's 20th Ed. Chapter 334 Page 2381

A. Tenofovir rufinamide

B. Tenofovir thionamide

C. Tenofovir alafenamide

D. Tenofovir prolinamide

Tenofovir alafenamide (TAF) is a prodrug of tenofovir that is metabolized to the active agent in its target organ (liver for HBV infection), thus permitting higher dose delivery to liver with reduced systemic exposure.

1810. Inactive "nonreplicative" hepatitis B carriers have?
Harrison's 20th Ed. Chapter 334 Page 2382

A. Undetectable HBeAg

B. Normal ALT

C. HBV DNA $\leq 10^3$ IU/mL

D. All of the above

Inactive "nonreplicative" hepatitis B carriers have undetectable HBeAg with normal ALT and HBV DNA $\leq 10^3$ IU/mL documented serially over time.

1811. Treatment for chronic hepatitis B is recommended by the AASLD for those with?
Harrison's 20th Ed. Chapter 334 Page 2383

A. Detectable HBeAg

B. HBV DNA levels $>2 \times 10^4$ IU/mL

C. ALT levels above 2 × the upper limit of normal

D. All of the above

Antiviral therapy is not recommended currently by American association for the study of the liver diseases (AASLD) for HBeAg-positive patients with ALT ≤2 × the upper limit of normal, in whom sustained responses are not likely.

1812. Which of the following is recommended as first-line therapy in Chronic Hepatitis B?
Harrison's 20th Ed. Chapter 334 Page 2384

A. PEG IFN

B. Entecavir

C. Tenofovir

D. All of the above

Among the drugs for hepatitis B, PEG IFN has supplanted standard IFN, entecavir has supplanted lamivudine, and tenofovir has supplanted adefovir. PEG IFN, entecavir, or tenofovir are recommended as first-line therapy.

1813. Therapy with which of the following is least likely to foster emergence of viral mutations?
Harrison's 20th Ed. Chapter 334 Page 2384

A. Lamivudine

B. Tenofovir

C. Telbivudine

D. Adefovir

Lamivudine and telbivudine foster the emergence of viral mutations, adefovir somewhat less so, and entecavir (except in lamivudine-experienced patients) and tenofovir rarely at all.

1814. For treatment of chronic hepatitis B, which of the following can be used safely during pregnancy?
Harrison's 20th Ed. Chapter 334 Page 2384

A. Tenofovir

B. Entecavir

C. Emtricitabine

D. All of the above

Telbivudine and tenofovir are both pregnancy category B drugs and can be used safely during pregnancy. Despite its Class C designation, lamivudine has an extensive pregnancy safety record in women with HIV/AIDS.

1815. Which of the following should be avoided or used with extreme caution during pregnancy?
Harrison's 20th Ed. Chapter 334 Page 2384

A. PEG IFN

B. Adefovir

C. Entecavir

D. All of the above

Except for lamivudine, other antivirals for hepatitis B should be avoided or used with extreme caution during pregnancy.

1816. Which of the following should not be used in patients with compensated or decompensated cirrhosis?
Harrison's 20th Ed. Chapter 334 Page 2384

A. PEG IFN

B. Entecavir

C. Tenofovir

D. All of the above

PEG IFN should not be used in patients with compensated or decompensated cirrhosis due to unfavorable resistance profile.

1817. In patients with HBV-HIV infection, which of the should never be used as monotherapy?
Harrison's 20th Ed. Chapter 334 Page 2385

A. Lamivudine

B. Adefovir

C. Entecavir

D. Tenofovir

Lamivudine should never be used as monotherapy in HBV-HIV infection, because HIV resistance emerges rapidly to both viruses. Adefovir, entecavir, Tenofovir and tenofovir + emtricitabine can be used for treating HBV infection in HBV-HIV co-infected patients.

1818. Which of the following antiviral drugs has dual antiviral activity against HBV & HIV?
Harrison's 20th Ed. Chapter 334 Page 2385, Lancet Infect Dis 2005;5:374–82

A. Emtricitabine

B. Adefovir

C. Entecavir

D. All of the above

1819. Which of the following antiviral drugs has dual antiviral activity against HBV & HIV?
Harrison's 20th Ed. Chapter 334 Page 2385, Lancet Infect Dis 2005;5:374–82

A. Tenofovir

B. Emtricitabine

C. Lamivudine

D. All of the above

Besides lamivudine, tenofovir and emtricitabine have antiviral activity against HBV & HIV.

1820. Which combination of antiviral drugs is recommended for HBV-HIV co-infected patients?

Harrison's 20th Ed. Chapter 334 Page 2385

A. Lamivudine and Adefovir
B. Tenofovir and Emtricitabine
C. Entecavir and Emtricitabine
D. Lamivudine and Entecavir

Combination of tenofovir and emtricitabine is an excellent choice for treating HBV infection in HBV-HIV co-infected patients.

1821. Which of the following drugs is used for chemotherapy-associated reactivation of hepatitis B?

Harrison's 20th Ed. Chapter 334 Page 2385

A. Lamivudine
B. Entecavir
C. Tenofovir
D. All of the above

1822. Variables that favour the treatment of HBV/HIV co-infected patients with pegylated interferon are all except?

Lancet Infect Dis 2005;5:374–82

A. HBeAg-positive
B. Elevated aminotransferases
C. High CD4 counts
D. Psychiatric disorders

1823. Which of the following about chronic hepatitis D virus (HDV) is false?

Harrison's 20th Ed. Chapter 334 Page 2385

A. HDV co-infection can increase severity of acute hepatitis B
B. Does not increase progression of acute to chronic hepatitis B
C. Long-term HDV infection is the rule if HDV infects chronically infected with HBV patients
D. None of the above

1824. Chronic hepatitis B plus D is similar to chronic hepatitis B alone in all respects except?

Harrison's 20th Ed. Chapter 334 Page 2385

A. Severity
B. Clinical features
C. Laboratory features
D. Route of infection

1825. Anti-LKM antibodies are seen in patients with?

Harrison's 20th Ed. Chapter 334 Page 2385

A. Hepatitis D
B. Autoimmune hepatitis
C. Chronic hepatitis C
D. All of the above

1826. Which of the following antibody is seen in chronic hepatitis D?

Harrison's 20th Ed. Chapter 334 Page 2385

A. Anti-LKM1
B. Anti-LKM2
C. Anti-LKM3
D. Anti-LKM4

A distinguishing serologic feature of chronic hepatitis D is the presence in the circulation of anti-LKM3 directed against uridine diphosphate glucuronosyltransferase.

1827. Which of the following drugs has a role in the treatment of chronic hepatitis D?

Harrison's 20th Ed. Chapter 334 Page 2385

A. IFN-α & PEG IFN
B. Lonafarnib
C. Myrcludex B
D. All of the above

1828. Which of the following is a nucleoside analogue antiviral agent for hepatitis B?

Harrison's 20th Ed. Chapter 334 Page 2385

A. Lamivudine
B. Entecavir
C. Telbivudine
D. All of the above

1829. Which of the following drugs has a role in the treatment of chronic hepatitis D?

Harrison's 20th Ed. Chapter 334 Page 2385

A. Glucocorticoids
B. Lamivudine
C. Entecavir
D. None of the above

None of the nucleoside analogue antiviral agents for hepatitis B is effective in hepatitis D.

1830. Dose of IFN-α in the treatment of chronic hepatitis D is?

Harrison's 20th Ed. Chapter 334 Page 2385

A. 3 million units three times a week for 12 months
B. 6 million units three times a week for 12 months
C. 9 million units three times a week for 12 months
D. 12 million units three times a week for 12 months

High-dose IFN-α i.e. 9 million units three times a week for 12 months is associated with a sustained loss of HDV replication and clinical improvement.

1831. Which of the following is an oral prenylation inhibitor?

Harrison's 20th Ed. Chapter 334 Page 2385

A. Tipifarnib
B. Lonafarnib
C. Sorafenib
D. Sunitinib

Lonafarnib (LNF) is an oral prenylation inhibitor.

1832. Which of the following about prenylation is false?

Harrison's 20th Ed. Chapter 334 Page 2385

A. Posttranslational
B. Irreversible covalent addition of prenyl lipid farnesyl to HDV antigen
C. Required for HDV protein to interact & form secreted viral particles with HBsAg
D. None of the above

Prenylation is the posttranslational covalent addition of prenyl lipid farnesyl to large HDV antigen. It is required for HDV protein to interact & form secreted viral particles with HBsAg.

1833. Which of the following prenyltransferase enzymes catalyze prenylation?

ACS Chem. Biol. 2015;10(1):51-62

A. Farnesyltransferase (FTase)
B. Geranylgeranyltransferase type 1 (GGTase-I)
C. Geranylgeranyltransferase type 2 (GGTase-II or Rab geranylgeranyltransferase
D. All of the above

Protein prenylation modification is necessary to maintain malignant activity of oncogenic Ras proteins. Inhibition of prenylation has provided an attractive strategy to inhibit oncogenic activity of Ras and achieve antitumor effects.

1834. Which of the following is the structure of myristic acid?

Immunology. 2016;149(2):139-145

A. 12-carbon saturated fatty acid
B. 13-carbon saturated fatty acid
C. 14-carbon saturated fatty acid
D. 15-carbon saturated fatty acid

1835. Which of the following plays a central role in the interaction between viruses and the receptors?

Immunology. 2016;149(2):139-145

A. Pre-S1 domain
B. Pre-S2 domain
C. Post-S1 domain
D. Post-S2 domain

Unlike bacteria, viruses do not produce their own lipids. However, some viral proteins are lipid modified by using the host cellular machinery through a protein lipidation modification process, referred to as N-myristoylation. Hepatitis B virus entry into hepatocytes requires the binding of myristolated N-terminal pre-S1 peptide of large HBsAg to sodium taurocholate co-transporting peptide, the functional receptor for HBV into hepatocytes.

1836. Sodium taurocholate cotransporting polypeptide is also named as?

Immunology. 2016;149(2):139-145

A. STCP
B. NTCP
C. MTCP
D. PTCP

Sodium taurocholate co-transporting peptide is the functional receptor for HBV into hepatocytes. This HBV receptor has been identified to be sodium taurocholate cotransporting polypeptide, also known as NTCP. When the gene that codes for NTCP is silenced, HBV infection is greatly reduced.

1837. Which of the following about sodium taurocholate cotransporting polypeptide (NTCP) is false?

Harrison's 20th Ed. Chapter 334 Page 2385

A. Multiple transmembrane transporter mainly expressed in liver
B. Interacts specifically with the L proteins of HBV & HDV
C. Functions as a common receptor for both viruses
D. None of the above

1838. Which of the following about NTCP (Slc10a1) is false?

Immunology. 2016;149(2):139-145

A. Solute carrier protein
B. Hepatic Na^+ bile acid symporter
C. Localizes to sinusoidal (basolateral) plasma membrane of hepatocytes
D. None of the above

Interaction between NTCP and L protein of HBV is highly specific, and NTCP is crucial for productive viral entry of hepatocytes.

1839. Which of the following has the capacity to mediate lipopeptide antigen presentation?

Immunology. 2016;149(2):139-145

A. MHC class I
B. MHC class II
C. MHC class III
D. MHC class IV

'Classical' MHC class I molecules have the capacity to mediate lipopeptide antigen presentation.

1840. Which of the following is known to be susceptible to infection by human HBV & HDV?

Immunology. 2016;149(2):139-145

A. Chimpanzees
B. Treeshrew
C. Humans
D. All of the above

In addition to humans, only two species are known to be susceptible to infection by human HBV and HDV - chimpanzees and a small mammal known as the treeshrew.

1841. Which of the following processes is related to post-translational modification (PTM) of proteins?

Immunology. 2016;149(2):139-145

A. Phosphorylation
B. O-linked glycosylation
C. Acetylation
D. All of the above

Phosphorylation, O-linked glycosylation, Acetylation, Formylation, N-myristoylation, Citrullination, Methylation, Deamidation and Cysteinylation are involved in post-translational modification (PTM) of proteins.

1842. Which of the following is a synthetic homologous myristolated lipopeptide?

Harrison's 20th Ed. Chapter 334 Page 2385

A. Myrcludex A
B. Myrcludex B
C. Myrcludex C
D. Myrcludex D

Myrcludex B is a synthetic homologous myristolated lipopeptide that competes for binding with HBsAg. Myrcludex B acts as a hepatitis B and D virus entry inhibitor blocking sodium taurocholate cotransporting polypeptide (SLC10A1).

1843. What is the likelihood of patients having chronic HCV infection after acute hepatitis C?

Harrison's 20th Ed. Chapter 334 Page 2386

A. ~ 15%
B. ~ 35%
C. ~ 55%
D. ~ 85%

From 70% to 80% of acute hepatitis C virus infections persist and become chronic, while 20% to 30% spontaneously resolve.

1844. Which of the following distinguishes between responders & nonresponders to IFN-based antiviral therapy for HCV?

Harrison's 20th Ed. Chapter 334 Page 2386

A. IL25B
B. IL27B
C. IL28B
D. IL29B

Located on chromosome 19, IL28B, which codes for IFN-λ3, distinguishes between responders and nonresponders to IFN-based antiviral therapy for HCV.

1845. The human genome contains how many base pairs?

Cleveland Clinic Journal of Medicine. 2015;82(2):97

A. > 1 billion
B. > 2 billion
C, > 3 billion
D. > 4 billion

The human genome contains more than 3 billion base pairs of nucleotides. Of theses, fewer than 1% differ between individuals, but this 1% is responsible for the diversity of human beings. Differences in genetic sequences among individuals are called genetic polymorphisms. A single-nucleotide polymorphism is a DNA sequence variation that occurs in a single nucleotide in the genome.

1846. Which genotype of hepatitis C virus is more likely to clear the virus spontaneously?

Cleveland Clinic Journal of Medicine. 2015;82(2):97

A. IL28B CC
B. IL28B CT
C. IL28B TT
D. All of the above

In hepatitis C virus infection, people born with nucleotide cytosine (C) at location rs12979860 in both alleles of the gene that codes for interleukin 28B (IL28B CC genotype) are luckier than those born with thymine (T) in this location in one of their alleles (CT genotype) or both of their alleles (TT genotype). Those with CC genotype are more likely to clear the virus spontaneously, and even if infection persists, it is less likely to progress to liver cancer and more likely to respond to treatment with interferon. People who have the IL28B CC genotype are three times more likely to spontaneously clear the virus than those with the CT or TT genotype.

1847. Interferon lambda family consists of which of the following cytokines?

Cleveland Clinic Journal of Medicine 2015;82(2):97

A. Interleukin 29 (interferon lambda 1)
B. Interleukin 28A (interferon lambda 2)
C. Interleukin 28B (interferon lambda 3)
D. All of the above

1848. Which of the following statements about HCV is false?

Harrison's 20th Ed. Chapter 334 Page 2386

A. Most frequent indication for liver transplantation
B. HCV infection always recurs after liver transplantation
C. Tends to be very slowly and insidiously progressive
D. None of the above

1849. Which of the following antibody is prevalent in patients with chronic hepatitis C virus (HCV) infection?

Harrison's 20th Ed. Chapter 334 Page 2386

A. Smooth muscle antibodies (SMA)
B. Antinuclear (ANA) antibodies
C. Anti-liver kidney microsomal type 1 (LKM1) antibody
D. All of the above

Non-organ specific autoantibodies (NOSA), particularly smooth muscle antibodies (SMA) and antinuclear (ANA) antibodies are highly prevalent in patients with chronic hepatitis C virus (HCV) infection. Occasionally, Anti-liver kidney microsomal type 1 (LKM1) antibody, Anti-liver cytosol type 1 (LC1) are found.

1850. Out of the following, which one is the most important as regards progression of liver disease in chronic hepatitis C?

Harrison's 20th Ed. Chapter 334 Page 2386

A. Older age
B. Longer duration of infection
C. HIV infection
D. Obesity

Progression of liver disease in chronic hepatitis C is more likely in older age, longer duration of infection, advanced histologic stage and grade, genotype 1, more complex quasispecies diversity, increased hepatic iron, concomitant other liver disorders (alcoholic liver disease, chronic hepatitis B, hemochromatosis, α_1-antitrypsin deficiency, and steatohepatitis), HIV infection, and obesity. Out of these, duration of infection is the most important.

1851. Which of the following features of chronic hepatitis C is predictive of eventual outcome?

Harrison's 20th Ed. Chapter 334 Page 2386

A. Level of aminotransferase activity
B. Level of HCV RNA
C. Presence or absence of jaundice during acute hepatitis
D. None of the above

No other epidemiologic or clinical features of chronic hepatitis C like severity of acute hepatitis, level of aminotransferase activity, level of HCV RNA, presence or absence of jaundice during acute hepatitis, is predictive of eventual outcome.

1852. Annual rate of HCC in cirrhotic patients with hepatitis C is?

Harrison's 20th Ed. Chapter 334 Page 2386

A. 0.2–0.4%
B. 0.4–1%
C. 1–4%
D. 2.3–5.8%

Annual rate of HCC in cirrhotic patients with hepatitis C is 1–4% in those patients who have had HCV infection for 30 years or more.

1853. Best prognostic indicator in chronic hepatitis C is?

Harrison's 20th Ed. Chapter 334 Page 2386

A. Liver histology
B. Severity of jaundice
C. Levels of aminotransferases
D. HIV status

Best prognostic indicator in chronic hepatitis C is liver histology.

1854. The pace of fibrosis progression in chronic HCV may be accelerated by?

Harrison's 20th Ed. Chapter 334 Page 2386

A. Concomitant HIV infection
B. Excessive alcohol use
C. Hepatic steatosis
D. All of the above

Pace of fibrosis progression may be accelerated by such factors as concomitant HIV infection, excessive alcohol use and hepatic steatosis.

1855. Among HCV patients with compensated cirrhosis associated, which of the following is false?
Harrison's 20th Ed. Chapter 334 Page 2386

A. 10-year survival rate is ~80%
B. Mortality occurs at a rate of 2–6% per year
C. Decompensation occurs at a rate of 4–5% per year
D. None of the above

Among hepatitis C patients with compensated cirrhosis, 10-year survival rate is close to 80%, mortality occurs at a rate of 2–6% per year, decompensation occurs at a rate of 4–5% per year and HCC at a rate of 1–4% per year.

1856. The peak prevalence of chronic HCV was estimated to have occurred in?
Harrison's 20th Ed. Chapter 334 Page 2386

A. 2013
B. 2014
C. 2015
D. 2016

1857. Estimated peak mortality due to chronic HCV has been predicted to occur in?
Harrison's 20th Ed. Chapter 334 Page 2386

A. 2026
B. 2028
C. 2032
D. 2035

1858. Which of the following is the most common symptom in chronic hepatitis C?
Harrison's 20th Ed. Chapter 334 Page 2386

A. Fatigue
B. Jaundice
C. Fever
D. Weight loss

Fatigue is the most common symptom of chronic hepatitis C. Jaundice is rare.

1859. Extrahepatic complications unrelated to immune-complex injury in chronic hepatitis C are all except?
Harrison's 20th Ed. Chapter 334 Page 2387

A. Sjögren's syndrome
B. Porphyria cutanea tarda
C. Essential mixed cryoglobulinemia
D. Lichen planus

Essential mixed cryoglobulinemia is an immune complex–mediated extrahepatic complications of chronic hepatitis C. While those unrelated to immune-complex injury are Sjögren's syndrome, lichen planus, porphyria cutanea tarda, type-2 diabetes mellitus and metabolic syndrome (including insulin resistance & steatohepatitis).

1860. Which of the following in a laboratory feature of chronic hepatitis C?
Harrison's 20th Ed. Chapter 334 Page 2387

A. Fluctuating aminotransferase levels
B. Jaundice is rare
C. Circulating anti-LKM1 antibodies
D. All of the above

1861. Anti-LKM1 are directed against which of the following?
Harrison's 20th Ed. Chapter 334 Page 2387

A. Cytochrome P450 2D6
B. Cytochrome P450 3A4
C. Cytochrome P450 2C9
D. Cytochrome P450 2B6

1862. Which of the following enhances the efficacy of IFN?
Harrison's 20th Ed. Chapter 334 Page 2387

A. Ribavirin
B. Adefovir
C. Entecavir
D. Tenofovir

Oral guanosine nucleoside ribavirin is ineffective when used alone. But, ribavirin enhances the efficacy of IFN by reducing the likelihood of sustained virologic response (SVR) after the achievement of an end-treatment response (ETR) i.e. response measured during, and maintained to the end of treatment.

1863. Which of the following statements is false?
Harrison's 20th Ed. Chapter 334 Page 2387

A. Hepatitis C proteins inhibit JAK-STAT signaling
B. JAK-STAT regulates interferon-stimulated genes
C. Interferon lambda signal through IL10R-IL28R receptor
D. None of the above

1864. Which of the following sustained virologic response (SVR) is now the new standard?
Harrison's 20th Ed. Chapter 334 Page 2387

A. SVR_{12}
B. SVR_{24}
C. SVR_{36}
D. SVR_{48}

SVR_{12} has now become the new standard for therapy responses.

1865. Interferon therapy results in activation of?
Harrison's 20th Ed. Chapter 334 Page 2387

A. Cytokines
B. Chemokines
C. JAK-STAT signal transduction pathway
D. All of the above

Interferon therapy results in activation of the JAK-STAT signal transduction pathway, which results in the intracellular elaboration of genes & their protein products with antiviral properties. Hepatitis C proteins inhibit JAK-STAT signaling pathway, and exogenous interferon restores expression of interferon-stimulated genes and their antiviral effects.

1866. Which of the following is a nucleoside analogue?
Harrison's 20th Ed. Chapter 334 Page 2387

A. Telaprevir
B. Boceprevir
C. Sofosbuvir
D. Ribavirin

Sofosbuvir was the first nucleoside analogue approved in 2013 for the treatment of chronic hepatitis C.

1867. Which of the following variable does not correlate favourably in the IFN-based treatment of chronic hepatitis C?

Harrison's 20th Ed. Chapter 334 Page 2387

A. Genotypes 2 and 3
B. Genotypes 1 and 4
C. Low baseline HCV RNA level
D. Histologically mild hepatitis

Patient variables that tend to correlate with sustained virologic responsiveness to IFN-based therapy include favorable genotype (genotypes 2 and 3 as opposed to genotypes 1 and 4), low baseline HCV RNA level (<2 million copies/mL, which is equivalent to 800,000 IU/ml), histologically mild hepatitis and minimal fibrosis, age <40, absence of obesity as well as insulin resistance and type-II diabetes mellitus, and female gender. Patients with cirrhosis respond less favourably.

1868. Duration of IFN-ribavirin therapy have in patients with genotype 1 should last for?

Harrison's 20th Ed. Chapter 334 Page 2388

A. 12 weeks
B. 24 weeks
C. 48 weeks
D. 72 weeks

1869. Duration of IFN-ribavirin therapy have in patients with genotype 2 and 3 should last for?

Harrison's 20th Ed. Chapter 334 Page 2388

A. 12 weeks
B. 24 weeks
C. 48 weeks
D. 72 weeks

Combination IFN-ribavirin therapy in chronic hepatitis C with genotype 1 should for 48 weeks, while in those with genotypes 2 and 3, a 24-week course of therapy suffices.

1870. Which of the following is relevant for patients treated with PEG IFN and ribavirin?

Harrison's 20th Ed. Chapter 334 Page 2388

A. SLCO1B1
B. HLA-B*1501
C. IL15
D. IL28B

In studies of patients treated with PEG IFN and ribavirin, variants of the IL28B SNP that code for IFN-λ3 correlate significantly with responsiveness. Patients homozygous for the C allele at this locus have the highest frequency of achieving an SVR (80%), those homozygous for the T allele at this locus are least likely to achieve an SVR (25%), and those heterozygous at this locus (C/T) have an intermediate level of responsiveness (SVRs in 35%).

1871. The most pronounced side effect of ribavirin therapy is?

Harrison's 20th Ed. Chapter 334 Page 2388

A. Seizure
B. Agranulocytosis
C. Hemolysis
D. All of the above

The most pronounced side effect of ribavirin therapy is hemolysis.

1872. Which of the following is a side effect of ribavirin therapy?

Harrison's 20th Ed. Chapter 334 Page 2388

A. Pruritus
B. Gout
C. Anemia
D. All of the above

1873. Half-life in serum of Hepatitis C virion is?

Harrison's 20th Ed. Chapter 334 Page 2388

A. 2–3 hours
B. 2–3 days
C. 2–3 monhs
D. 2–3 years

Despite a Hepatitis C virion half life in serum of only 2–3 hours, the level of HCV is maintained by a high replication rate of 10^{12} hepatitis C virions per day.

1874. Null responders are the ones who after therapy have HCV RNA reduction of?

Harrison's 20th Ed. Chapter 334 Page 2387, Figure 334-2

A. < 1 $\log_{10}$ IU/mL
B. < 2 $\log_{10}$ IU/mL
C. < 3 $\log_{10}$ IU/mL
D. < 4 $\log_{10}$ IU/mL

Null responders are the ones who after therapy have HCV RNA reduction of < 2 $\log_{10}$ IU/mL by week 24 of therapy.

1875. Rapid virologic response (RVR) is estimated at what time after institution of therapy in Hepatitis C?

Harrison's 20th Ed. Chapter 334 Page 2387, Figure 334-2

A. 2 weeks
B. 4 weeks
C. 8 weeks
D. 12 weeks

RVR (Rapid virologic response) refers to undetectable HCV RNA at week 4 in responders as shown with sensitive amplification assays.

1876. Early virologic response (EVR) is estimated at what time after institution of therapy in Hepatitis C?

Harrison's 20th Ed. Chapter 334 Page 2387, Figure 334-2

A. 2 weeks
B. 4 weeks
C. 8 weeks
D. 12 weeks

EVR refers to ≥2 $\log_{10}$ IU/mL HCV RNA reduction by week 12. If HCV RNA is undetectable at 12 weeks, the designation is "complete" EVR; or at the end of therapy, 48 weeks (ETR, end-treatment response).

1877. Responder status is estimated at what time after institution of therapy in Hepatitis C?

Harrison's 20th Ed. Chapter 334 Page 2387, Figure 334-2

A. 12 weeks
B. 24 weeks
C. 48 weeks
D. 72 weeks

1878. Sustained virologic response (SVR) is estimated at what time after institution of therapy in Hepatitis C?

Harrison's 20th Ed. Chapter 334 Page 2387, Figure 334-2

A. 12 weeks
B. 24 weeks
C. 48 weeks
D. 72 weeks

In responders, if HCV RNA remains undetectable for 24 weeks after ETR, week 72, the patient has a sustained virologic response (SVR).

1879. Elimination time of PEG IFN is how many times longer than standard IFN?

Harrison's 20th Ed. Chapter 334 Page 2388

A. Three times
B. Five times
C. Seven times
D. Nine times

For the treatment of chronic hepatitis C, standard IFNs have now been supplanted by PEG IFNs and these have elimination times up to seven fold longer than standard IFNs, permitting once a week dosage.

1880. The standard treatment of chronic hepatitis C before 2011 was?

Harrison's 20th Ed. Chapter 334 Page 2388

A. PEG IFN
B. Ribavirin
C. PEG IFN + Ribavirin
D. All of the above

The standard treatment of chronic hepatitis C before 2011 was the combination of long acting pegylated IFN (PEG IFN) and ribavirin for all HCV genotypes.

1881. Dose of PEG IFN α-2a is?

Harrison's 20th Ed. Chapter 334 Page 2388

A. 180 μg daily subcutaneously
B. 180 μg weekly subcutaneously
C. 180 μg daily intramuscularly
D. 180 μg weekly intramuscularly

Two PEG IFNs are available: PEG IFN α-2b and α-2a. PEG IFN α-2a is given 180 μg weekly subcutaneously.

1882. Dose of PEG IFN α-2b is?

Harrison's 20th Ed. Chapter 334 Page 2388

A. 0.5 μg / kg weekly subcutaneously
B. 1.5 μg / kg weekly subcutaneously
C. 2.5 μg / kg weekly subcutaneously
D. 3.5 μg / kg weekly subcutaneously

PEG IFN α-2b is given 1.5 μg / kg weekly subcutaneously.

1883. Duration of PEG IFN / ribavirin therapy in chronic hepatitis C of genotypes 1 and 4 is?

Harrison's 20th Ed. Chapter 334 Page 2388

A. 12 weeks
B. 24 weeks
C. 48 weeks
D. 72 weeks

1884. Duration of PEG IFN / ribavirin therapy in chronic hepatitis C of genotypes 2 and 3 is?

Harrison's 20th Ed. Chapter 334 Page 2388

A. 12 weeks
B. 24 weeks
C. 48 weeks
D. 72 weeks

1885. Telaprevir and boceprevir best relate to?

Harrison's 20th Ed. Chapter 334 Page 2389

A. NS3/4A
B. NS4B
C. NS5A
D. NS5B

Telaprevir and boceprevir are serine protease inhibitors that target NS3/4A.

1886. Triple therapy for chronic HCV includes all except?

Harrison's 20th Ed. Chapter 334 Page 2389

A. PEG IFN
B. Ribavirin
C. Telaprevir
D. Tenofovir

Because resistance developed rapidly during monotherapy with telaprevir & boceprevir, these drugs had to be used in combination with PEG IFN and ribavirin.

1887. Dual therapy for chronic HCV refers to?

Harrison's 20th Ed. Chapter 334 Page 2389

A. PEG IFN plus ribavirin
B. PEG IFN plus telaprevir
C. PEG IFN plus boceprevir
D. Any of the above

Telaprevir and boceprevir regimens consisted of periods of triple therapy and periods of dual therapy based on HCV RNA status at weeks 4 and 12 ("response-guided therapy").

1888. Which of the following is a NS5A inhibitor?

Harrison's 20th Ed. Chapter 334 Page 2390

A. Ledipasvir
B. Velpatasvir
C. Daclatasvir
D. All of the above

NS5A inhibitors include Ledipasvir, velpatasvir, daclatasvir, elbasvir, & ombitasvir. NS5A is a membrane-associated phosphoprotein that is part of the HCV RNA replication complex and is essential for viral replication & assembly.

1889. Which of the following is a NS3/4 protease inhibitor?

Harrison's 20th Ed. Chapter 334 Page 2393

A. Ombitasvir
B. Grazoprevir
C. Dasabuvir
D. Ribavirin

Grazoprevir and Paritaprevir are NS3/4 protease inhibitors.

1890. Sofosbuvir-containing combinations are contraindicated with which of the following drugs?

Harrison's 20th Ed. Chapter 334 Page 2390

A. Cyclosporine
B. Ramipril
C. Amiodarone
D. All of the above

sofosbuvir containing regimens can be associated with severe bradycardia in patients taking the antiarrhythmic agent amiodarone and therefore contraindicated.

1891. Sofosbuvir / ledipasvir fixed-dose regimen for chronic HCV is not effective for which genotype?

Harrison's 20th Ed. Chapter 334 Page 2396

A. 3
B. 4
C. 5
D. 6

The most popular of the regimens for chronic HCV is sofosbuvir / ledipasvir, which is effective for all genotypes except 2 and 3.

1892. For HCV genotypes 2 and 3, which of the following is the combination of choice?

Harrison's 20th Ed. Chapter 334 Page 2396

A. Paritaprevir / ritonavir
B. Elbasvir / grazoprevir
C. Sofosbuvir / velpatasvir
D. All of the above

For HCV genotypes 2 and 3, fixed dose, single-pill sofosbuvir / velpatasvir is the combination of choice.

1893. Standard indication for antiviral therapy of chronic hepatitis C is?

Harrison's 20th Ed. Chapter 334 Page 2391 Table 334-6

A. Detectable HCV RNA (with or without elevated ALT)
B. Portal/bridging fibrosis on liver biopsy
C. Moderate to severe hepatitis on liver biopsy
D. All of the above

1894. Antiviral therapy is not recommended in which of the following patients of chronic hepatitis C?

Harrison's 20th Ed. Chapter 334 Page 2391 Table 334-6

A. Age > 70 years
B. Mild hepatitis on liver biopsy
C. Persons with severe renal insufficiency
D. All of the above

1895. Which of the following patients of chronic hepatitis C are not candidates for IFN-based antiviral therapy?

Harrison's 20th Ed. Chapter 334 Page 2391 Table 334-6

A. Decompensated cirrhosis
B. Pregnancy
C. Contraindications to use of interferon or ribavirin
D. All of the above

Patients with decompensated cirrhosis are not candidates for IFN-based antiviral therapy but should be referred for liver transplantation. Interferons are antiproliferative and ribavirin is teratogenic.

1896. Which of the following is recommended for the success of therapy with PEG IFN / ribavirin in chronic hepatitis C?

Harrison's 20th Ed. Chapter 334 Page 2395

A. HCV genotype should be determined prior to therapy
B. Measure HCV RNA at 12 weeks
C. Pretreatment liver biopsy
D. All of the above

1897. Which of the following is advocated in those who have not responded to treatment with PEG IFN/ribavirin in chronic hepatitis C?

Harrison's 20th Ed. Chapter 334 Page 2395

A. Longer duration of treatment
B. Higher doses of either PEG IFN, ribavirin, or both
C. Switching to a different IFN preparation
D. All of the above

For those who have not responded to treatment with PEG IFN / ribavirin in chronicn hepatitis C, following may be tried : longer duration of treatment; higher doses of either PEG IFN, ribavirin, or both and switching to a different IFN preparation. However, none of these approaches achieves more than a marginal benefit.

1898. Which of the following associated with hepatitis C may respond to antiviral therapy?

Harrison's 20th Ed. Chapter 334 Page 2395

A. Essential mixed cryoglobulinemia
B. Porphyria cutanea tarda
C. Lichen planus
D. All of the above

1899. Which of the following drug is beneficial in acute hepatitis C?

Harrison's 20th Ed. Chapter 334 Page 2395

A. Lamivudine
B. Interferon monotherapy
C. Ribavirin
D. Glucocorticoid

In acute hepatitis C, interferon monotherapy (3 million units SC three times a week) is beneficial. Long-acting pegylated interferon plus ribavirin is superior to interferon monotherapy.

1900. Drugs that have been recommended in acute liver failure are all except?

Harrison's 20th Ed. Chapter 334 Page 2395

A. Lamivudine
B. Telbivudine
C. Adefovir
D. Entecavir

Nucleoside/nucleotide analogues recommended in acute liver failure are lamivudine, telbivudine and entecavir. Adefovir has a slow action & potential nephrotoxicity. Interferon drugs are contraindicated because they can worsen hepatitis.

Autoimmune Hepatitis

1901. Autoimmune hepatitis is a kind of?

Harrison's 20th Ed. Chapter 334 Page 2396

A. Acute hepatitis
B. Subacute hepatitis
C. Chronic hepatitis
D. Any of the above

Autoimmune hepatitis is a chronic disorder characterized by continuing hepatocellular necrosis & inflammation, usually with fibrosis, which can progress to cirrhosis & liver failure.

1902. Which of the following is prominent in cases of autoimmune hepatitis?

Harrison's 20th Ed. Chapter 334 Page 2396

A. Extrahepatic features of autoimmunity
B. Serologic abnormalities
C. Immunologic abnormalities
D. All of the above

In autoimmune hepatitis, extrahepatic features of autoimmunity & seroimmunologic abnormalities are prominent & supports an autoimmune process in its pathogenesis, though autoantibodies do not occur in all cases.

1903. Which class of serum globulins is elevated in autoimmune hepatitis?

Harrison's 20th Ed. Chapter 334 Page 2396, N Engl J Med. 2006;354:54-66

A. Alpha globulin
B. Beta globulin
C. Gamma globulin
D. Delta globulin

One characteristic laboratory feature of autoimmune hepatitis is a generalized elevation of serum globulins, particularly gamma globulin and IgG, which are generally 1.2 to 3.0 times normal.

1904. Which of the following virus has been implicated in pathogenesis of autoimmune hepatitis?

N Engl J Med. 2006;354:54-66, Harrison's 20th Ed. Chapter 334 Page 2396

A. Hepatitis viruses
B. Measles virus
C. Epstein–Barr virus
D. All of the above

Measles virus, hepatitis viruses, cytomegalovirus, and Epstein–Barr virus have been implicated as initiators of autoimmune hepatitis in genetically predisposed. Most evidence is related to hepatitis viruses - A, B, or C.

1905. Which of the following drug has been implicated in pathogenesis of autoimmune hepatitis?

N Engl J Med. 2006;354:54-66, Harrison's 20th Ed. Chapter 334 Page 2396

A. Minocycline
B. Atorvastatin
C. Interferon
D. All of the above

Oxyphenisatin, methyldopa, nitrofurantoin, diclofenac, interferon, pemoline, minocycline & atorvastatin can induce hepatocellular injury that mimics autoimmune hepatitis.

1906. Autoimmune disorder that occur with increased frequency in autoimmune hepatitis patients is?

Harrison's 20th Ed. Chapter 334 Page 2396

A. Thyroiditis
B. Rheumatoid arthritis
C. Autoimmune hemolytic anemia
D. All of the above

Autoimmune disorders that occur with increased frequency in autoimmune hepatitis patients are thyroiditis, rheumatoid arthritis, autoimmune hemolytic anemia, ulcerative colitis, membranoproliferative glomerulonephritis, type 1 diabetes mellitus, celiac disease & Sjögren's syndrome.

1907. Which of the following autoantibody is present in patients of autoimmune hepatitis?

Harrison's 20th Ed. Chapter 334 Page 2396

A. Antinuclear antibodies (ANAs)
B. Anti-LKM
C. Antibodies to soluble liver antigen
D. All of the above

Autoantibodies found in autoimmune hepatitis patients are antinuclear antibodies (ANAs), anti-smooth-muscle antibodies (directed at actin, vimentin and skeletin), antibodies to F-actin, anti-LKM, antibodies to "soluble liver antigen/liver pancreas antigen" (SLA/LP autoantibodies), antibodies to α-actinin, antibodies to liver-specific asialoglycoprotein receptor ("hepatic lectin").

1908. Which of the following statements about anti-soluble liver antigen is false?

Harrison's 20th Ed. Chapter 334 Page 2396

A. Associated with a more severe disease course
B. Present in nonhepatic autoimmune disorders
C. Target of anti-SLA is $tRNP^{(Ser)Sec}$
D. Specific serologic marker for autoimmune liver diseases

Anti-SLA is serologic marker for autoimmune liver diseases, is associated with a more severe disease course, it is virtually absent in nonhepatic autoimmune disorders. Target of anti-SLA is a UGA serine tRNA-associated protein complex [$tRNP^{(Ser)Sec}$].

1909. In autoimmune hepatitis, immunoregulatory dysfunction of which of the following occurs?

Harrison's 20th Ed. Chapter 334 Page 2396

A. CD8+CD24+ regulatory T cells
B. CD8+CD25+ regulatory T cells
C. CD4+CD24+ regulatory T cells
D. CD4+CD25+ regulatory T cells

Immunoregulatory dysfunction characterized by decreased numbers of CD4+CD25+ regulatory T cells and decreased levels of scurfin, the protein product of FOXP3 gene occurs in autoimmune hepatitis.

1910. Scurfin is the protein product of which gene?

Nature Immunology. 2003;4:337-342

A. FOXP1 gene
B. FOXP2 gene
C. FOXP3 gene
D. FOXP4 gene

In autoimmune hepatitis, levels of scurfin are decreased. Scurfin is the protein product of FOXP3 gene that is a member of forkhead family of transcription factors.

1911. Extrahepatic manifestation of autoimmune hepatitis is?
Harrison's 20th Ed. Chapter 334 Page 2396

A. Arthritis
B. Cutaneous vasculitis
C. Glomerulonephritis
D. All of the above

Extrahepatic manifestations of autoimmune hepatitis include arthralgias, arthritis, cutaneous vasculitis and glomerulonephritis.

1912. In the clinical presentation suggestive of acute viral hepatitis, which of the following point towards autoimmune hepatitis?
Harrison's 20th Ed. Chapter 334 Page 2396

A. Young to middle-aged women
B. Marked hyperglobulinemia (>2.5 g/dL)
C. High-titer circulating ANAs
D. All of the above

1913. Poor prognostic sign in autoimmune hepatitis is?
Harrison's 20th Ed. Chapter 334 Page 2397

A. Multilobular collapse histopathologically at initial presentation
B. Failure of serum bilirubin to improve after 2 weeks of therapy
C. Bridging necrosis or multilobular necrosis on liver biopsy
D. All of the above

Poor prognostic signs in autoimmune hepatitis are the presence of multilobular collapse at the time of initial presentation on histopathologically and failure of serum bilirubin to improve after 2 weeks of therapy.

1914. Type 1 autoimmune hepatitis is associated with which HLA-DR serotype?
Harrison's 20th Ed. Chapter 334 Page 2397

A. HLA-DR1
B. HLA-DR2
C. HLA-DR3
D. None of the above

Type I autoimmune hepatitis is associated with HLA-DR3 or HLA-DR4.

1915. Type 2 autoimmune hepatitis is associated with which HLA haplotype?
Harrison's 20th Ed. Chapter 334 Page 2397

A. HLA-DRB1
B. HLA-DRB2
C. HLA-DRB3
D. HLA-DRB4

Type II autoimmune hepatitis is linked to HLA-DRB1 & HLA-DQB1 haplotypes.

1916. Feature of HLA-DR3 associated autoimmune hepatitis include?
N Engl J Med. 2006;354:54-66

A. Early-onset
B. Severe form
C. In girls and young women
D. All of the above

HLA-DR3–associated disease is more common in the early-onset, severe form of autoimmune hepatitis, which often occurs in girls and young women.

1917. Feature of HLA-DR4 associated autoimmune hepatitis include?
N Engl J Med. 2006;354:54-66

A. Common in adults
B. Extrahepatic manifestations
C. Better response to corticosteroid therapy
D. All of the above

HLA-DR4 associated autoimmune hepatitis is more common in adults and associated with increased incidence of extrahepatic manifestations, milder disease & a better response to corticosteroid therapy.

1918. Type I autoimmune hepatitis is associated with which of the following antibodies?
Harrison's 20th Ed. Chapter 334 Page 2397

A. Antinuclear antibodies (ANA)
B. Atypical perinuclear antineutrophilic cytoplasmic antibodies
C. Antiactin antibodies
D. All of the above

Type I autoimmune hepatitis is associated with circulating ANAs, autoantibodies against actin, atypical perinuclear antineutrophilic cytoplasmic antibodies (pANCA) & SLA/LP autoantibodies. Antiactin antibodies are more specific for type 1 autoimmune hepatitis. Anti–LKM-1 & anti–LC-1 characterize type 2 disease.

1919. Which of the following is the most specific autoantibody identified in type 1 autoimmune hepatitis?
N Engl J Med. 2006;354:54-66

A. Antiactin antibodies
B. SLA/LP autoantibodies
C. Antinuclear antibodies (ANA)
D. Anti-LKM1

SLA/LP autoantibodies are the most specific autoantibody identified in type 1 autoimmune hepatitis but is found in only 10 to 30 percent of cases.

1920. Type II autoimmune hepatitis is associated with which of the following antibodies?
Harrison's 20th Ed. Chapter 334 Page 2397

A. Antinuclear antibodies (ANA)
B. Antiactin antibodies
C. Anti-LKM1
D. Atypical perinuclear antineutrophilic cytoplasmic antibodies

1921. Type II autoimmune hepatitis is associated with which of the following antibodies?
Harrison's 20th Ed. Chapter 334 Page 2397

A. Antinuclear antibodies (ANA)
B. Antiactin antibodies
C. Anti-liver cytosol 1 (anti–LC-1)
D. Atypical perinuclear antineutrophilic cytoplasmic antibodies

Type II autoimmune hepatitis is associated not with ANA but with anti-LKM1. Also seen is autoantibody directed against liver cytosol formiminotransferase cyclodeaminase, a liver-specific 58-kD metabolic enzyme (anti-liver cytosol 1).

1922. In type II autoimmune hepatitis, the anti-LKM1 antibody is directed against which cytochrome?
Harrison's 20th Ed. Chapter 334 Page 2397

A. P450 2D6
B. P450 2C9

C. P450 2C19
D. P450 3A

In type II autoimmune hepatitis, the anti-LKM1 antibody is directed against cytochrome P450 2D6 (CYP2D6).

1923. Anti-LKM antibody seen in Type II autoimmune hepatitis is also seen in which of the following?
Harrison's 20th Ed. Chapter 334 Page 2397

A. Drug-induced hepatitis
B. Chronic hepatitis C
C. Chronic hepatitis D
D. All of the above

Anti-LKM1 antibody seen in type II autoimmune hepatitis is seen in some patients with chronic hepatitis C. Anti-LKM2 is seen in drug-induced hepatitis & anti-LKM3 is seen in patients with chronic hepatitis D.

1924. Which of the following statements is false?
Harrison's 20th Ed. Chapter 334 Page 2397

A. Anti-LKM1 is seen in type II autoimmune hepatitis
B. Anti-LKM2 is seen in drug-induced hepatitis
C. Anti-LKM3 is seen in chronic hepatitis D
D. None of the above

1925. Type III autoimmune hepatitis is associated with which of the following antibodies?
Harrison's 20th Ed. Chapter 334 Page 2397

A. Antinuclear antibodies (ANA)
B. Antibodies to soluble liver antigen/liver pancreas antigen
C. Anti-LKM1
D. All of the above

Type III autoimmune hepatitis patients lack ANA and anti-LKM1 but have circulating antibodies to soluble liver antigen/liver pancreas antigen.

1926. Which of the following is false about histopathological features of liver in autoimmune hepatitis?
Harrison's 20th Ed. Chapter 334 Page 2397

A. Mononuclear-cell infiltrate
B. Interface hepatitis or piecemeal necrosis
C. Sparing of the biliary tree
D. None of the above

Autoimmune hepatitis is characterized by a mononuclear-cell infiltrate (plasma cells + eosinophils) invading the limiting plate (piecemeal necrosis or interface hepatitis). Biliary tree is generally spared and fibrosis is present.

1927. Which of the following feature goes against the diagnosis of autoimmune hepatitis?
Harrison's 20th Ed. Chapter 334 Page 2397

A. Female gender
B. Predominant aminotransferase elevation
C. Mitochondrial antibodies
D. Globulin level elevation

Features that favor diagnosis of autoimmune hepatitis include female gender, predominant aminotransferase elevation, globulin level elevation, presence of nuclear, smooth muscle, LKM1, and other autoantibodies, concurrent other autoimmune diseases, characteristic histologic features (interface hepatitis, plasma cells, rosettes), HLA DR3 or DR4 markers, & response to treatment. Features against the diagnosis are predominant alkaline phosphatase elevation, mitochondrial antibodies, markers of viral hepatitis, history of hepatotoxic drugs or excessive alcohol, histologic evidence of bile duct injury, or such atypical histologic features as fatty infiltration, iron overload, and viral inclusions. Antimitochondrial antibody (AMA) is the sine qua non of primary biliary cirrhosis (PBC) but may be observed in the so-called overlap syndrome with autoimmune hepatitis.

1928. Mainstay of management in autoimmune hepatitis is?
Harrison's 20th Ed. Chapter 334 Page 2398

A. Azathioprine
B. Glucocorticoid
C. Cyclosporine
D. Mycophenolate mofetil

Mainstay of management in autoimmune hepatitis is daily glucocorticoid therapy. Azathioprine alone is not effective in achieving remission. Patients refractory to this regimen may be treated with cyclosporine, tacrolimus, or mycophenolate mofetil.

1929. Severe autoimmune hepatitis is defined as?
Harrison's 20th Ed. Chapter 334 Page 2398

A. Serum AST ≥ 10 times upper limit of normal
B. Serum AST ≥ 5 times upper limit of normal and gamma-globulin level ≥ twice normal
C. Bridging necrosis or multiacinar necrosis on liver biopsy
D. All of the above

1930. Therapy for autoimmune hepatitis should continue for at least?
Harrison's 20th Ed. Chapter 334 Page 2398

A. 3 - 6 months
B. 6 - 12 months
C. 12 - 18 months
D. 18 - 24 months

Therapy for autoimmune hepatitis should continue for at least 12–18 months. After tapering and cessation of therapy, the likelihood of relapse is at least 50%. Majority of patients require therapy at maintenance doses indefinitely.

1931. Which of the following is useful in refractory autoimmune hepatitis?
Harrison's 20th Ed. Chapter 334 Page 2398

A. Infliximab
B. Rituximab
C. Cyclosporine, tacrolimus, or mycophenolate mofetil
D. All of the above

Alcoholic Liver Disease

1932. Alcoholic Liver Disease (ALD) includes?
Clin Liver Dis. 2016 ;20(3):445-456

A. Hepatic steatosis
B. Acute alcoholic hepatitis with or without cirrhosis
C. Hepatocellular carcinoma as a complication of cirrhosis
D. All of the above

1933. Which of the following is the major lesion in the pathology of alcoholic liver disease?
Harrison's 20th Ed. Chapter 335 Page 2399

A. Fatty liver
B. Alcoholic hepatitis
C. Cirrhosis
D. All of the above

Major lesions in the pathology of alcoholic liver disease are fatty liver, alcoholic hepatitis & cirrhosis.

1934. Which of the following is considered to be a precursor to cirrhosis?
Harrison's 20th Ed. Chapter 335 Page 2399

A. Fatty liver
B. NASH
C. Alcoholic hepatitis
D. All of the above

Alcoholic hepatitis is thought to be a precursor to cirrhosis.

1935. Fatty liver is present in what proportion of daily as well as binge drinkers?
Harrison's 20th Ed. Chapter 335 Page 2399

A. > 30%
B. > 50%
C. > 70%
D. > 90%

Fatty liver is present in >90% of daily as well as binge drinkers.

1936. Which of the following can predict individual susceptibility to alcoholic liver disease?
Harrison's 20th Ed. Chapter 335 Page 2399

A. Quantity of alcohol consumed per day
B. Total duration of alcohol consumed
C. Obesity
D. None of the above

There are no diagnostic tools that can predict individual susceptibility to alcoholic liver disease.

1937. One beer (12 oz), four ounces of wine or one ounce of 80% spirits contain how many grams of alcohol?
Harrison's 20th Ed. Chapter 335 Page 2399

A. ~ 8 grams
B. ~ 10 grams
C. ~ 12 grams
D. ~ 14 grams

One beer, four ounces of wine, or one ounce of 80% spirits all contain ~12 grams of alcohol.

1938. In men, what quantity of ethanol produces fatty liver?
Harrison's 20th Ed. Chapter 335 Page 2399 Table 335-1

A. 10 - 20 gm/day
B. 20 - 40 gm/day
C. 40 - 80 gm/day
D. 80 - 120 gm/day

In men, 40–80 gram/day of ethanol produces fatty liver.

1939. In men, what quantity & duration of ethanol consumption causes hepatitis or cirrhosis?
Harrison's 20th Ed. Chapter 335 Page 2399 Table 335-1

A. 80 gm/day for 5 - 10 years
B. 160 gm/day for 5 - 10 years
C. 80 gm/day for 10 - 20 years
D. 160 gm/day for 10 - 20 years

In men, 160 gm/day for 10-20 years of ethanol consumption causes hepatitis or cirrhosis.

1940. What proportion of alcoholics develop alcoholic liver disease?
Harrison's 20th Ed. Chapter 335 Page 2399 Table 335-1

A. 15%
B. 30%
C. 45%
D. 75%

Only 15% of alcoholics develop alcoholic liver disease.

1941. Which of the following statements about alcohol consumption is false?
Harrison's 20th Ed. Chapter 335 Page 2399 Table 335-1

A. Alcohol is a direct hepatotoxin
B. Men more susceptible to alcoholic liver injury than women
C. Alcohol injury does not require malnutrition
D. 15% of alcoholics develop alcoholic liver disease

Women are more susceptible to alcoholic liver disease than men.

1942. Alcohol stimulates lipogenesis by the upregulation of?
Clin Liver Dis. 2016 ;20(3):445-456

A. Sterol regulatory element-binding transcription factor 1a
B. Sterol regulatory element-binding transcription factor 1b
C. Sterol regulatory element-binding transcription factor 1c
D. All of the above

Alcohol stimulates lipogenesis by upregulation of sterol regulatory element-binding transcription factor 1c (SREBP-1c). Alcohol also downregulates the negative regulators of SREBP-1c, including 5' adenosine monophosphate-activated protein kinase (AMPK), Sirtuin 1, adiponectin, and signal transducer and activator of transcription 3 (STAT3).

1943. Which of the following about alcohol is false?
Clin Liver Dis. 2016 ;20(3):445-456

A. Alcohol downregulates PPAR-α
B. Alcohol activates the complement system (C3, C4)
C. Alcohol disrupts intestinal tight junction integrity, "leaky gut"
D. None of the above

1944. Which of the following about alcohol is false?
Clin Liver Dis. 2016 ;20(3):445-456

A. KRT7 is a marker of ductular reaction in liver disease
B. Prominin-1 (PROM1) is a marker of progenitor cells from liver
C. Plasma miRNA-155 correlates with alcohol induced liver inflammation
D. None of the above

1945. Which of the following is related to the genetic risk factors for alcoholic liver disease?
Harrison's 20th Ed. Chapter 335 Page 2399 Table 335-1, N Engl J Med. 2018;379:1251-61

A. ATP8B1
B. IL28B
C. PNPLA3
D. ORMDL3

Patatin-like phospholipase domain-containing protein 3 (PNPLA3, rs738409C>G) has been associated with alcoholic cirrhosis.

1946. Which of the following is considered as a strong genetic risk locus for both alcoholic cirrhosis and AH?
Gut Liver. 2017;11:173-188

A. Patatin-like phospholipase encoding 3 (PNPLA3)
B. Membrane bound O-acyltransferase domain containing 7 (MBOAT7)
C. Transmembrane 6 superfamily member 2 (TM6SF2)
D. All of the above

Both PNPLA3 & TM6SF2 are implicated in hepatic lipid trapping, while MBOAT7 mediates the transfer of fatty acid between phospholipids and lysophospholipids, a potent driver of hepatic inflammation.

1947. Cytochrome P-450 2E1 (CYP2E1) converts alcohol to?
Gut Liver. 2017;11:173-188

A. Acetate
B. Carbon dioxide
C. Free fatty acids
D. Acetaldehyde

In liver, there are two main pathways of alcohol metabolism, alcohol dehydrogenase and cytochrome P-450 2E1. They converts alcohol to acetaldehyde. Acetaldehyde subsequently is metabolized to acetate via acetaldehyde dehydrogenase.

1948. Which of the following accelerates progression of alcoholic liver disease to cirrhosis in chronic and excessive drinkers?
Harrison's 20th Ed. Chapter 335 Page 2399

A. Acute hepatitis B
B. Acute hepatitis C
C. Chronic hepatitis B
D. Chronic hepatitis C

Chronic infection with hepatitis C (HCV) is an important comorbidity in the progression of alcoholic liver disease to cirrhosis in chronic and excessive drinkers. Alcohol intake also decreases efficacy of interferon-based antiviral therapy in them.

1949. Which of the following initiates the pathogenic process in alcoholic liver injury?
Harrison's 20th Ed. Chapter 335 Page 2399

A. Fatty acid oxidation
B. Intestinal-derived endotoxin
C. Microbiome dysbiosis
D. Proinflammatory cytokines

In the pathogenesis of alcoholic liver injury, intestinal-derived endotoxin initiates a pathogenic process through toll-like receptor 4 and tumor necrosis factor α (TNF-α) that facilitates hepatocyte apoptosis & necrosis.

1950. Initial and most common histologic response to hepatotoxic stimuli is?
Harrison's 20th Ed. Chapter 335 Page 2399

A. Fatty liver
B. NASH
C. Steatohepatitis
D. All of the above

1951. Chronic alcohol ingestion lead to which of the following?
Harrison's 20th Ed. Chapter 335 Page 2399

A. Autoimmune response
B. Fibrotic response
C. Inflammatory response
D. All of the above

Hepatocyte injury and impaired regeneration following chronic alcohol ingestion are ultimately associated with stellate cell activation and collagen production, which are key events in fibrogenesis.

1952. Major enzyme responsible for alcohol metabolism is?
Harrison's 20th Ed. Chapter 335 Page 2399

A. Alcohol dehydrogenase
B. Alcohol reductase
C. Alcohol oxidase
D. All of the above

In fatty liver secondary to alcohol induced liver injury, accumulation of fat within the perivenular hepatocytes coincides with the location of alcohol dehydrogenase which is the major enzyme responsible for alcohol metabolism.

1953. Which of the following about Damage-Associated Molecular Patterns (DAMPs) is false?
Clin Liver Dis. 2016 ;20(3):445-456

A. Endogenous, hidden from extracellular environment
B. Activate cellular pattern recognition receptors
C. Result in sterile inflammation (inflammasome)
D. None of the above

1954. Steatosis is characterized by the accumulation of which of the following in hepatocytes?
Clin Liver Dis. 2016 ;20(3):445-456

A. Triglycerides
B. Phospholipids

C. Cholesterol esters
D. All of the above

Steatosis refers to accumulation of triglycerides, phospholipids, and cholesterol esters in hepatocytes.

1955. Which of the following hepatic pathologic features may be associated with progressive liver injury?
Harrison's 20th Ed. Chapter 335 Page 2399

A. Giant mitochondria
B. Perivenular fibrosis
C. Macrovesicular fat
D. All of the above

1956. Histologically, the earliest changes in alcoholic hepatitis are located predominantly in?
Harrison's 20th Ed. Chapter 335 Page 2399

A. Zone 1
B. Zone 2
C. Zone 3
D. All of the above

Histologically, the earliest changes in alcoholic hepatitis are located predominantly around the central vein i.e. centrilobular (perivenular) areas (zone 3 of Rappaport).

1957. The hallmark features of hepatocyte injury in alcoholic hepatitis are all except?
Harrison's 20th Ed. Chapter 335 Page 2400

A. Polymorphonuclear infiltrate
B. Ballooning degeneration
C. Mallory-Denk bodies
D. Fibrosis in perisinusoidal space of Disse

Hallmark of alcoholic hepatitis is hepatocyte injury characterized by ballooning degeneration, spotty necrosis, polymorphonuclear infiltrate, and fibrosis in the perivenular and perisinusoidal space of Disse. Mallory-Denk bodies are often present in florid cases but are neither specific nor necessary for substantiating diagnosis.

1958. Which of the following is false about Terry's nails?
Indian J Dermatol. 2017;62(3):309-311

A. Ground glass appearance of fingernails
B. No lunula
C. Frequent in severe liver disease
D. None of the above

Terry's nails (a type of leukonychia) refers to finger/toe nails that have a "ground glass" appearance, with no lunula (white crescent-shaped area of finger). It frequently occurs in hepatic failure, cirrhosis, DM, CHF, hyperthyroidism, malnutrition.

1959. Skin texture of cheeks & nasolabial folds in patient with alcohol-related liver disease is called?
Cleveland Clinic Journal of Medicine. 2009;76(10):601

A. Gooseberry skin
B. Cheese wind skin
C. Weather heat skin
D. Paper-money skin

Paper-money skin (or "Dollar-paper" markings) seen in alcoholic cirrhosis describes the condition in which the upper trunk is covered with many randomly scattered, needle-thin superficial capillaries.

1960. Which of the following are found in patients with liver disease?
Cleveland Clinic Journal of Medicine. 2009;76(10):601

A. Xanthelasma
B. Bier spots
C. "Paper-money" skin
D. All of the above

Bier spots are small, irregularly shaped, hypopigmented patches on the arms and legs. Bier spots are a sign of liver disease.

1961. In alcoholic hepatitis, which of the following can occur in the absence of cirrhosis?
Harrison's 20th Ed. Chapter 335 Page 2400

A. Portal hypertension
B. Ascites
C. Variceal bleeding
D. All of the above

In alcoholic hepatitis, portal hypertension, ascites, or variceal bleeding can occur in the absence of cirrhosis. Patients with alcoholic cirrhosis often exhibit clinical features identical to other causes of cirrhosis.

1962. In alcoholic hepatitis, AST: ALT ratio is?
Harrison's 20th Ed. Chapter 335 Page 2400

A. > 0.25
B. > 0.50
C. > 0.75
D. > 1

In alcoholic hepatitis, the AST : ALT ratio is >1. AST:ALT ratio is higher in pericentral hepatocytes than other regions in liver lobule & pericentral zone is more selectively affected in acute alcoholic hepatitis.

1963. In alcoholic hepatitis, AST and ALT are rarely more than?
Harrison's 20th Ed. Chapter 335 Page 2400

A. 100 IU/L
B. 200 IU/L
C. 300 IU/L
D. 400 IU/L

In alcoholic hepatitis, AST & ALT are usually elevated 2-7 fold. They are rarely >400 IU/L.

1964. Which of the following is a laboratory feature alcoholic fatty liver?
Harrison's 20th Ed. Chapter 335 Page 2400

A. Increased gamma-glutamyl transpeptidase (GGTP)
B. Hypertriglyceridemia,
C. Hypercholesterolemia
D. All of the above

1965. Which of the following in ultrasonography indicates serious liver injury with less potential for complete reversal?
Harrison's 20th Ed. Chapter 335 Page 2400

A. Portal vein flow reversal
B. Ascites
C. Intra-abdominal collaterals
D. All of the above

1966. Discriminant function (DF) formula predicting the outcome of severe alcoholic hepatitis is named after?
Harrison's 20th Ed. Chapter 335 Page 2400

A. Nathan
B. Cushin
C. Maddrey
D. George

The discriminant function (DF) formula of Maddrey is based on PT and bilirubin.

1967. Which of the following is the correct formula of Discriminant function (DF)?

Harrison's 20th Ed. Chapter 335 Page 2400

A. 2.6 x PT prolongation + total S. bilirubin in mg/dL
B. 3.6 x PT prolongation + total S. bilirubin in mg/dL
C. 4.6 x PT prolongation + total S. bilirubin in mg/dL
D. 5.6 x PT prolongation + total S. bilirubin in mg/dL

Modified Maddrey's discriminant function predicts prognosis in alcoholic hepatitis. It is calculated as 4.6 x [prothombin time - control value (seconds)] + serum bilirubin (mg/dL). A value >32 implies poor outcome with one month mortality > 50% if only supportive treatment is given. Cut off value of 32 &/or hepatic encephalopathy has been used as a threshold to consider corticosteroid treatment.

1968. Formula for assessment of prognosis of alcoholic hepatitis is?

Gut Liver. 2017;11:173-188

A. Age, Bilirubin, INR, Creatinine (ABIC) score
B. Model for end-stage liver disease (MELD) score
C. Glasgow alcoholic hepatitis score (GAHS)
D. All of the above

Besides the above ones and also the classical Child-Turcotte-Pugh (CTP) score, Asymmetric dimethylarginine (ADMA) score is the most recently proposed predictor of adverse clinical outcome in patients with severe alcoholic hepatitis.

1969. Variables included in Glasgow alcoholic hepatitis score (GAHS) are all except?

Gut Liver. 2017;11:173-188

A. Age
B. Hemoglobin
C. Bilirubin
D. BUN

Five variables included in GAHS are age, bilirubin, BUN, PT, and TLC. Glasgow Alcoholic Hepatitis score ≥ 9 requires treatment.

1970. MELD score is calculated based on all except?

N Engl J Med. 2009;361:1279-90

A. Prothrombin time
B. Serum albumin
C. Serum creatinine
D. Serum bilirubin

MELD score is based on a patient's prothrombin time, serum creatinine & bilirubin.

1971. Model for End-Stage Liver Disease (MELD) score was introduced in USA in year?

N Engl J Med. 2009;361:1279-90

A. 1995
B. 1998
C. 2002
D. 2005

In 2002, MELD score derived from measurements of serum bilirubin, international normalized ratio of prothrombin time and serum creatinine to evaluate pretransplantation renal function was introduced as an aid to organ allocation among candidates for liver transplantation.

1972. The presence of which of the following in alcoholic hepatitis predicts a dismal prognosis?

Harrison's 20th Ed. Chapter 335 Page 2400

A. Ascites
B. Variceal hemorrhage
C. Hepatorenal syndrome
D. All of the above

The presence of ascites, variceal hemorrhage, deep encephalopathy, or hepatorenal syndrome predicts a dismal prognosis in patients with alcoholic hepatitis.

1973. Severe alcoholic hepatitis is defined as a discriminant function of?

Harrison's 20th Ed. Chapter 335 Page 2400

A. > 24
B. > 28
C. > 30
D. > 32

1974. Severe alcoholic hepatitis is defined as an MELD of?

Harrison's 20th Ed. Chapter 335 Page 2400

A. > 20
B. > 30
C. > 40
D. > 50

Patients with severe alcoholic hepatitis are defined as a discriminant function >32 or MELD >20.

1975. Which of the following score is used to identify alcoholic hepatitis patients unresponsive to therapy?

Harrison's 20th Ed. Chapter 335 Page 2400

A. Sanyal score
B. Lille score
C. Thurz score
D. Mathurin score

A Lille score >0.45 uses pretreatment variables plus change in total bilirubin at day 7 of glucocorticoids to identify those patients unresponsive to therapy.

1976. Which of the following drugs has been approved by Food and Drug Administration for treatment of alcohol-use disorder?

N Engl J Med. 2018;379:1251-61

A. Naltrexone
B. Disulfiram
C. Acamprosate
D. All of the above

Three medications (naltrexone, disulfiram, and acamprosate) have been approved by the Food and Drug Administration for the treatment of alcohol-use disorder. Nalmefene has been approved in many European countries for the reduction of alcohol consumption.

1977. Which of the following about Naltrexone is false?

N Engl J Med. 2018;379:1251-61

A. Mu-opioid and kappa-opioid receptor antagonist
B. Reduces alcohol-related dopamine release in nucleus accumbens
C. Reduces the reward sensation
D. None of the above

Naltrexone is a mu-opioid & kappa-opioid receptor antagonist. It reduces alcohol-related dopamine release in nucleus accumbens thereby reducing the reward sensation, thus making patients less motivated to drink.

1978. Which of the following about Acamprosate is false?

N Engl J Med. 2018;379:1251-61

A. Acts as N-methyl-D-aspartate receptor antagonist
B. Acts as a modulator of GABA type A receptor

C. Reduces symptoms of protracted abstinence
D. None of the above

Acamprosate acts as N-methyl-D-aspartate receptor antagonist and a modulator of γ-aminobutyric acid (GABA) type A receptor and reduces symptoms of protracted abstinence. Acamprosate has no hepatic metabolism.

1979. Which of the following about Acamprosate is false?
N Engl J Med. 2018;379:1251-61

A. Mu-opioid and delta-opioid receptor antagonist
B. Kappa-opioid receptor partial agonist
C. No evidence of hepatotoxicity
D. None of the above

1980. Which of the following about Baclofen is false?
N Engl J Med. 2018;379:1251-61

A. Selective GABA type B receptor antagonist
B. Also used to control spasticity
C. No liver toxicity
D. None of the above

1981. Which of the following drugs has been tested in patients with alcohol-use disorder?
N Engl J Med. 2018;379:1251-61

A. Gabapentin
B. Ondansetron
C. Varenicline
D. All of the above

Four other treatments that have been tested in patients with alcohol-use disorder include gabapentin, ondansetron, topiramate, and varenicline.

1982. Acetaldehyde syndrome consists of?
N Engl J Med. 2018;379:1251-61

A. Facial flushing
B. Nausea, vomiting
C. Tachycardia, hypotension
D. All of the above

Disulfiram inhibits acetaldehyde dehydrogenase, thus provoking acetaldehyde syndrome (facial flushing, nausea, vomiting, tachycardia, and hypotension) when disulfiram is consumed with alcohol. Use of disulfiram is contraindicated in patients with liver cirrhosis, especially in those with synthetic dysfunction.

1983. Which of the following is used as a pharmaceutical approaches to treat alcohol use disorders (AUD)?
N Engl J Med. 2018;379:1251-61

A. Baclofen
B. Disulfiram
C. Nalmefene
D. All of the above

Pharmaceutical approaches to treat AUD include baclofen, disulfiram, naltrexone and nalmefene. FDA-approved disulfiram & naltrexone are contraindicated in ALD patients due to possible hepatotoxicity. Nalmefene, a μ- and δ-opioid receptor antagonist and κ-opioid receptor partial-agonist was approved for AUD by FDA, but safety data in patients with ALD is limited.

1984. Which of the following is advocated for severe alcoholic hepatitis?
Harrison's 20th Ed. Chapter 335 Page 2400

A. Glucocorticoids
B. Thiamine
C. Proton pump inhibitors
D. All of the above

Patients with severe alcoholic hepatitis, Women with encephalopathy in particular, should be given prednisone, 40 mg/day, or prednisolone, 32 mg/day, for 4 weeks, followed by a steroid taper.

1985. Use of which of the following improves survival in severe alcoholic hepatitis?
Harrison's 20th Ed. Chapter 335 Page 2400

A. Pentoxifylline
B. Propylthiouracil
C. Infliximab
D. Colchicine

1986. Pentoxifylline improves survival in severe alcoholic hepatitis primarily due to a decrease in development of?
Harrison's 20th Ed. Chapter 335 Page 2400

A. Pancreatitis
B. Encephalopathy
C. Hepatorenal syndrome
D. All of the above

The nonspecific TNF inhibitor, pentoxifylline (orally absorbed nonselective phosphodiesterase inhibitor) improves survival in severe alcoholic hepatitis was primarily due to a decrease in the development of hepatorenal syndrome.

1987. Use of Infliximab in severe alcoholic hepatitis was stopped due to the increased risk of?
N Engl J Med. 2018;379:1251-61

A. Bone marrow suppression
B. Seizure
C. Infection
D. Jaundice

Use of Infliximab in severe alcoholic hepatitis was stopped due to the increased risk of increased deaths secondary to infection and renal failure.

1988. Most liver transplantation centers require alcoholics to have documented abstinence of at least?
N Engl J Med. 2018;379:1251-61

A. 3 months
B. 6 months
C. 9 months
D. 12 months

Most transplantation centers currently require patients with a history of alcohol abuse to have documented abstinence of at least 6 months before undergoing transplantation ("6-month abstinence rule").

Nonalcoholic Fatty Liver Disease and Nonalcoholic Steatohepatitis

1989. Accumulation of which of the following occurs within hepatocytes in hepatic steatosis?

Harrison's 20th Ed. Chapter 336 Page 2401

A. Cholesterol

B. Chylomicrons

C. Triglyceride

D. All of the above

Accumulation of triglyceride occurs within hepatocytes in hepatic steatosis.

1990. Which of the following statements about chronic hepatic steatosis is false?

Harrison's 20th Ed. Chapter 336 Page 2401

A. Risk of developing cirrhosis is extremely low

B. May become complicated by NASH

C. NAFLD-related cirrhosis may produce primary liver cancer

D. None of the above

Isolated hepatic steatosis is entirely benign. The risk of death from liver disease increases by a factor of 50 to 80 for patients with nonalcoholic steatohepatitis who have F3 or F4 fibrosis.

1991. "Cryptogenic" ALT elevations increase with which of the following?

Harrison's 20th Ed. Chapter 336 Page 2401

A. Alcohol consumption

B. Malnutrition

C. Body mass index

D. All of the above

"Cryptogenic" ALT elevations increase with body mass index. Serum ALT elevations that cannot be explained by excessive alcohol consumption, other known causes of fatty liver disease, viral hepatitis, drug-induced or congenital liver diseases are termed "cryptogenic".

1992. Nonalcoholic Steatohepatitis (NASH) is defined by a constellation of features that include?

Cleveland Clinic Journal of Medicine. 2017;84(4):273

A. Steatosis

B. Lobular & portal inflammation

C. Liver cell injury (hepatocyte ballooning)

D. All of the above

NAFLD remains a diagnosis of exclusion of other liver diseases.

1993. Which of the following can be a consequence of Nonalcoholic steatohepatitis?

N Engl J Med. 2017;377:2063-72

A. Can regress to isolated steatosis

B. Can smolder at a relatively constant level of activity

C. Can cause progressive fibrosis leading to cirrhosis (F4 fibrosis)

D. Any of the above

NASH is a potentially progressive type of nonalcoholic fatty liver disease (NAFLD). Nonalcoholic steatohepatitis is a dynamic condition that can regress to isolated steatosis, smolder at a relatively constant level of activity, or cause progressive fibrosis that leads to cirrhosis (F4 fibrosis). Nonalcoholic steatohepatitis is the sum of injury and repair responses triggered by lipotoxicity.

1994. Which of the following promote the development of nonalcoholic steatohepatitis?

N Engl J Med. 2017;377:2063-72

A. PDZ domain–containing protein

B. SCR homology 2 domain-containing leukocyte protein

C. Toll-interleukin 1 receptor domain-containing adapter protein

D. Patatin-like phospholipase domain–containing 3 (PNPLA3)

Polymorphisms in patatin-like phospholipase domain - containing 3 (PNPLA3) and transmembrane 6 superfamily, member 2 (TM6SF2) promote development of nonalcoholic steatohepatitis and related liver damage (cirrhosis, primary liver cancer).

1995. PNPLA3 encodes which of the following?

N Engl J Med. 2017;377:2063-72

A. Adipocytokine leptin (LEPR)

B. Adiponutrin

C. Adiponectin

D. Kisspeptin

PNPLA3 encodes adiponutrin, a lipase that regulates both triglyceride and retinoid metabolism. PNPLA3 polymorphisms (I148M) are strongly associated with hepatic steatosis, steatohepatitis, fibrosis & cancer.

1996. Hepatic cirrhosis develops in what percentage of individuals with NAFLD?

Harrison's 20th Ed. Chapter 336 Page 2401

A. ~ 1%

B. ~ 3%

C. ~ 6%

D. ~ 9%

Hepatic cirrhosis develops in about 6% of individuals with NAFLD. The risk for advanced liver fibrosis is highest in individuals with NASH who are older than 45–50 years of age and overweight/obese or afflicted with type 2 diabetes.

1997. Prevalence of hepatitis C-related cirrhosis in the United States is?

Harrison's 20th Ed. Chapter 336 Page 2401

A. ~ 0.1%

B. ~ 0.5%

C. ~ 1%

D. ~ 1.8%

Prevalence of hepatitis C-related cirrhosis in the United States is about 0.5%.

1998. Which of the following have been well documented in children?

Harrison's 20th Ed. Chapter 336 Page 2401

A. NAFLD

B. NASH

C. NAFLD-related cirrhosis

D. All of the above

NAFLD, NASH and NAFLD-related cirrhosis are well documented in children. As in adults, obesity and insulin resistance are the main risk factors for pediatric NAFLD.

1999. Hyperinsulinemia promotes which of the following?

Harrison's 20th Ed. Chapter 336 Page 2401

A. Lipid uptake
B. Fat synthesis
C. Fat storage
D. All of the above

Hyperglycemia in insulin resistance promotes pancreas to produce more insulin. Hyperinsulinemia promotes lipid uptake, fat synthesis and fat storage. This results in hepatic triglyceride accumulation (steatosis).

2000. Which of the following damage hepatocytes?

Harrison's 20th Ed. Chapter 336 Page 2402

A. Fatty acids
B. Diacylglycerols
C. Reactive oxygen species
D. All of the above

Triglyceride per se is not hepatotoxic. Its precursors (fatty acids and diacylglycerols) and metabolic by-products (reactive oxygen species) may damage hepatocytes leading to hepatocyte lipotoxicity, cell death and consequent cell healing and repair efforts. NASH is the morphologic manifestation of lipotoxicity and resultant wound healing responses or futile repair.

2001. One drink is defined as having how much ethanol?

Harrison's 20th Ed. Chapter 336 Page 2402

A. 5 grams
B. 10 grams
C. 14 grams
D. 18 grams

One drink is defined as having 10 grams of ethanol equivalent to one can of beer, 4 ounces of wine or 1.5 ounces (one shot) of distilled spirits.

2002. NAFLD risk factors include?

Harrison's 20th Ed. Chapter 336 Page 2402

A. Body mass index
B. Hyperuricemia/gout
C. Systemic hypertension
D. All of the above

NAFLD risk factors include increased body mass index, insulin resistance/type 2 diabetes mellitus, systemic hypertension, dyslipidemia, hyperuricemia/gout, cardiovascular disease in the patient or family members.

2003. NAFLD is associated with which of the following?

Harrison's 20th Ed. Chapter 336 Page 2403

A. Obstructive sleep apnea
B. Thyroid dysfunction
C. Chronic pain syndrome
D. All of the above

2004. Which of the following is an acceptable first-line test for diagnosis of NASH?

Harrison's 20th Ed. Chapter 336 Page 2403

A. Ultrasound scan
B. Computed tomography (CT)
C. Magnetic resonance imaging (MRI)
D. Liver biopsy

Ultrasound is an acceptable first-line test. Liver biopsy is the gold standard for establishing the severity of liver injury and fibrosis.

2005. Which of the following differentiates individuals with NASH from those with simple steatosis or normal livers?

Hepatology. 2004;40(2):459-66

A. D8/18
B. F8/18
C. J8/18
D. K8/18

Serum levels of keratins 8 and 18 (K8/18) are epithelial cytoskeletal proteins that undergo cleavage during programmed cell death (apoptosis). Both cleaved and full-length K8/18 are released into blood as hepatocytes die. Serum levels of K8/18 differentiate individuals with NASH from those with simple steatosis or normal livers more reliably than do serum aminotransferase levels.

2006. Which of the following tests must be done in every patient of NAFLD?

Cleveland Clinic Journal of Medicine. 2017;84(4):273

A. Viral hepatitis panel
B. Antinuclear antibody (ANA)
C. Antismooth muscle antibody (ASMA)
D. All of the above

2007. Which of the following tests must be done in every patient of NAFLD?

Cleveland Clinic Journal of Medicine. 2017;84(4):273

A. Iron studies
B. Alpha-1 antitrypsin level
C. Ceruloplasmin level
D. All of the above

Initial evaluation of a patient with suspected NAFLD should include a thorough serologic evaluation to exclude coexisting causes of chronic liver disease. Tests include: viral hepatitis panel, antinuclear antibody (ANA), antismooth muscle antibody (ASMA), antimitochondrial antibody (AMA), iron studies, alpha-1 antitrypsin level, and ceruloplasmin level. Liver biopsy is the gold standard for diagnosing steatohepatitis and fibrosis.

2008. Which of the following improve necroinflammation associated with NASH?

Cleveland Clinic Journal of Medicine 2017;84(4):273

A. Vitamin E
B. Thiazolidinediones
C. Obeticholic acid
D. All of the above

Pentoxifylline and obeticholic acid improve fibrosis, while vitamin E, thiazolidinediones, and obeticholic acid improve necroinflammation associated with NASH.

2009. Which is the best dietary regimen for patients with NAFLD?

World J Gastroenterol. 2014;20(26):8341-8350

A. Chinese diet
B. Lebanese diet
C. Mediterranean diet
D. Japanese diet

Mediterranean diet seems to be the best dietary regimen for patients with NAFLD.

2010. Which of the following stimulate hepatic lipid accumulation and progression in NASH?

World J Gastroenterol. 2014;20(26):8341-8350

A. Choline
B. High-protein diets rich in isoflavones
C. Antioxidants
D. Fructose

Saturated fat & fructose stimulate hepatic lipid accumulation & progression in NASH. Unsaturated fat, choline, antioxidants and high-protein diets rich in isoflavones have a preventive effect. Among polyunsaturated fatty acids, n-3 fatty acids reduce the accumulation of triglycerides & ameliorate hepatic steatosis.

Cirrhosis and its Complications

2011. Reversal of fibrosis in cirrhosis liver can be achieved with treatment in which of the following diseases?
Harrison's 20th Ed. Chapter 337 Page 2405

A. Chronic hepatitis C
B. Hemochromatosis
C. Alcoholic liver disease
D. All of the above

Upon successful treatment of chronic hepatitis C, hemochromatosis and alcoholic liver disease liver fibrosis can be reversed.

2012. The cardinal pathologic features of cirrhosis liver are?
Harrison's 20th Ed. Chapter 337 Page 2405

A. Irreversible chronic injury of hepatic parenchyma
B. Extensive fibrosis
C. Formation of regenerative nodules
D. All of the above

The cardinal pathologic features reflect irreversible chronic injury of the hepatic parenchyma and include extensive fibrosis in association with the formation of regenerative nodules.

2013. The pathologic features of cirrhosis liver result from?
Harrison's 20th Ed. Chapter 337 Page 2405

A. Hepatocyte necrosis
B. Destruction of the supporting reticulin network
C. Distortion of the vascular bed
D. All of the above

The pathologic features result from hepatocyte necrosis, collapse of the supporting reticulin network with subsequent connective tissue deposition, distortion of the vascular bed, and nodular regeneration of remaining liver parenchyma.

2014. Central event leading to hepatic fibrosis in cirrhosis liver is?
Harrison's 20th Ed. Chapter 337 Page 2405

A. Activation of the hepatic stellate cell
B. Activation of the CD 8+ cells
C. Activation of Kupffer cells
D. All of the above

The central event leading to hepatic fibrosis is activation of the hepatic stellate cell resulting in the formation of increased amounts of collagen and other components of the extracellular matrix.

2015. Alcohol induced liver injury refers to?
Harrison's 20th Ed. Chapter 337 Page 2405

A. Alcoholic cirrhosis
B. Alcoholic fatty liver
C. Alcoholic hepatitis
D. All of the above

Alcohol-induced liver injury includes consequences resulting from chronic alcohol ingestion like alcoholic fatty liver, alcoholic hepatitis and alcoholic cirrhosis.

2016. Alcoholic cirrhosis is also called?
Harrison's 20th Ed. Chapter 337 Page 2405

A. Gaucher's cirrhosis
B. Johnson's cirrhosis
C. Gilbert's cirrhosis
D. Laennec's cirrhosis

Alcoholic cirrhosis, historically referred to as Laennec's cirrhosis is the most common type of cirrhosis encountered in North America, western Europe and South America.

2017. Use of excessive alcohol can contribute to liver damage in patients with?
Harrison's 20th Ed. Chapter 337 Page 2405

A. Hepatitis C
B. Hemochromatosis
C. Fatty liver disease related to obesity
D. All of the above

Use of excessive alcohol can contribute to liver damage in patients with other liver diseases like hepatitis C, hemochromatosis and fatty liver disease related to obesity.

2018. Hepatic fibrosis secondary to chronic alcohol use is?
Harrison's 20th Ed. Chapter 337 Page 2405

A. Centrilobular
B. Pericellular
C. Periportal
D. Any of the above

Chronic alcohol use can produce fibrosis in the absence of accompanying inflammation and/or necrosis. Fibrosis can be centrilobular, pericellular, or periportal.

2019. The diameter of nodules in alcoholic cirrhosis is?
Harrison's 20th Ed. Chapter 337 Page 2405

A. < 0.5 mm
B. < 1 mm
C. < 2 mm
D. < 3 mm

In alcoholic cirrhosis, nodules are usually <3 mm in diameter (micronodular). With cessation of alcohol use, larger nodules may form, resulting in a mixed micronodular and macronodular cirrhosis.

2020. Ethanol is mainly absorbed in?
Harrison's 20th Ed. Chapter 337 Page 2405

A. Stomach
B. Small intestine
C. Large intestine
D. All of the above

Ethanol is mainly absorbed by small intestine and to a lesser degree through stomach.

2021. Which of the following initiates alcohol metabolism?
Harrison's 20th Ed. Chapter 337 Page 2405

A. Cytosolic alcohol dehydrogenase (ADH)
B. Microsomal ethanol-oxidizing system (MEOS)
C. Peroxisomal catalase
D. Gastric alcohol dehydrogenase (ADH)

Gastric alcohol dehydrogenase (ADH) initiates alcohol metabolism.

2022. Enzyme system for metabolism of alcohol in the liver is?
Harrison's 20th Ed. Chapter 337 Page 2405

A. Cytosolic alcohol dehydrogenase (ADH)
B. Microsomal ethanol oxidizing system (MEOS)
C. Peroxisomal catalase
D. All of the above

Three enzyme systems metabolize alcohol in liver. These are cytosolic ADH, the microsomal-oxidizing system (MEOS), and peroxisomal catalase.

2023. Which of the following is a hepatic consequence of intake of ethanol?
Harrison's 20th Ed. Chapter 440 Page 3238

A. Increases intracellular accumulation of triglycerides
B. Impairment of protein synthesis, glycosylation, and secretion
C. Production of excess collagen and extracellular matrix
D. All of the above

2024. Ethanol is oxidized to acetaldehyde by?
Harrison's 20th Ed. Chapter 337 Page 2405

A. Cytosolic alcohol dehydrogenase (ADH)
B. Microsomal-oxidizing system (MEOS)
C. Peroxisomal catalase
D. Gastric alcohol dehydrogenase (ADH)

Majority of ethanol oxidation occurs via ADH to form acetaldehyde.

2025. Which out of the following is a highly reactive molecule?
Harrison's 20th Ed. Chapter 337 Page 2405

A. Alcohol
B. Acetaldehyde
C. Acetate
D. All of the above

2026. Acetaldehyde is metabolized to acetate by?
Harrison's 20th Ed. Chapter 337 Page 2405

A. Succinic semialdehyde dehydrogenase
B. α-Aminoadipic semialdehyde synthase
C. Aldehyde dehydrogenase
D. All of the above

Ethanol oxidation occurs via ADH to form acetaldehyde which is metabolized to acetate by aldehyde dehydrogenase (ALDH). Acetaldehyde combines with proteins to form protein-acetaldehyde adducts that lead to hepatocyte damage like interference with specific enzyme activities (microtubular formation & hepatic protein trafficking), Kupffer cell activation. As a result, profibrogenic cytokines are produced that initiate and perpetuate stellate cell activation, with the resultant production of excess collagen and extracellular matrix.

2027. Aldehyde dehydrogenase is also expressed by?
Harrison's 20th Ed. Chapter 440 Page 3238

A. Cardiomyocytes
B. Hematopoietic precursors (stem cells)
C. Renal mesangial cells
D. Synovial fibroblasts

At high doses, cyclophosphamide eliminates mature lymphocytes but spares hematopoietic precursors (stem cells), because they express the enzyme aldehyde dehydrogenase, which hydrolyzes cyclophosphamide.

2028. In alcoholic cirrhosis, clinical findings include?
Harrison's 20th Ed. Chapter 337 Page 2406

A. Palmar erythema
B. Spider angiomas
C. Lacrimal gland enlargement
D. All of the above

2029. In alcoholic cirrhosis, clinical findings include all except?
Harrison's 20th Ed. Chapter 337 Page 2406

A. Clubbing of fingers
B. Muscle wasting
C. Signs of virilization in women
D. Xanthoma

2030. Which of the following findings are associated with alcoholism but are not specifically related to cirrhosis?
Harrison's 20th Ed. Chapter 337 Page 2406

A. Palmar erythema
B. Spider angiomas
C. Gynecomastia
D. Dupuytren's contractures

Frequent findings in alcoholic cirrhosis include jaundice, palmar erythema, spider angiomas, parotid and lacrimal gland enlargement, clubbing of fingers, splenomegaly, muscle wasting, and ascites with or without peripheral edema. Increased peripheral formation of estrogen due to diminished hepatic clearance of the precursor androstenedione leads to gynecomastia, testicular atrophy and decreased body hair in men. In women, signs of virilization or menstrual irregularities may occur. Dupuytren's contractures resulting from fibrosis of the palmar fascia with resulting flexion contracture of digits are associated with alcoholism but are not specifically related to cirrhosis.

2031. Which of the following is false about palmar erythema?
Harrison's 20th Ed. Chapter 337 Page 2406

A. Occurs in patients of alcoholic cirrhosis
B. Erythema is peripheral over the palm with central pallor
C. Frequently found during pregnancy
D. None of the above

Spider angiomata and palmar erythema occur in both acute and chronic liver disease. These manifestations may be especially prominent in persons with cirrhosis but can develop in normal individuals and are frequently found during pregnancy.

2032. Anemia in alcoholic cirrhosis may be due to?
Harrison's 20th Ed. Chapter 337 Page 2406

A. Acute/chronic GI blood loss
B. Coexistent folic acid & vitamin B_{12} deficiency
C. Hypersplenism
D. All of the above

2033. Anemia in alcoholic cirrhosis may be due to?
Harrison's 20th Ed. Chapter 337 Page 2406

A. Psychogenic factors
B. Direct suppressive effect of alcohol on bone marrow
C. Deficiency of iron
D. All of the above

Anemia results from acute & chronic gastrointestinal blood loss, coexistent folic acid & vitamin B12 deficiency, hypersplenism, & suppressive effect of alcohol on bone marrow.

2034. Zieve's syndrome in alcoholics is best related to?
Harrison's 20th Ed. Chapter 337 Page 2406

A. Diarrhea
B. Myocardial infarction
C. Hemolytic anemia
D. Pneumonia

ZS is an acute metabolic condition that can occur in severe alcoholic hepatitis and during withdrawal from prolonged alcohol abuse. It consists of hemolytic anemia (spur cells and acanthocytes), hyperlipoproteinemia, jaundice, and abdominal pain. The underlying cause is liver delipidization.

2035. Zieve's syndrome in alcoholics is best related to?
Harrison's 20th Ed. Chapter 337 Page 2406

A. Acanthocytes
B. Dacrocytes
C. Schistocytes
D. Echinocytes

A unique form of hemolytic anemia (with spur cells and acanthocytes) called Zieve 's syndrome can occur in patients with severe alcoholic hepatitis.

2036. Acanthocyte is best related to?
Harrison's 20th Ed. Chapter 428 Page 3137

A. Chorea
B. Seizure
C. Blindness
D. Mania

Chorea-acanthocytosis (neuroacanthocytosis) is a progressive and typically fatal autosomal recessive disorder that is characterized by chorea coupled with red cell abnormalities on peripheral blood smear (acanthocytes).

2037. Acanthocytosis is best related to?
Harrison's 20th Ed. Chapter 109 Page 810

A. Pelger-Huet anomaly
B. Chediak-Higashi syndrome
C. McLeod phenotype
D. Severe uremia

The Kell protein is very large (720 amino acids) and its secondary structure contains many different antigenic epitopes. The immunogenicity of Kell is third behind the ABO and Rh systems. The absence of the Kell precursor protein (controlled by a gene on X) is associated with acanthocytosis, shortened RBC survival and a progressive form of muscular dystrophy that includes cardiac defects. This rare condition is called the McLeod phenotype.

2038. Acanthocytes reflect which of the following?
Harrison's 20th Ed. Chapter 58 Page 379, N Engl J Med. 2018;379:774

A. Renal disease
B. Abetalipoproteinemia
C. Splenectomy
D. All of the above

Acanthocytes are spiculated red cells with the spikes irregularly distributed. This process tends to be irreversible and reflects underlying renal disease, abetalipoproteinemia or splenectomy. Spur-cell anemia is associated with a poor prognosis and is definitively treated by liver transplantation.

2039. Apart from acanthocytosis, which of the following is a feature of abetalipoproteinemia?
Harrison's 20th Ed. Chapter 438 Page 3221

A. Steatorrhea
B. Pigmentary retinopathy
C. Progressive ataxia
D. All of the above

Abetalipoproteinemia is a rare autosomal dominant hereditary disorder characterized by steatorrhea, pigmentary retinopathy, acanthocytosis and progressive ataxia.

2040. Laboratory finding unusual in alcoholic cirrhosis is?
Harrison's 20th Ed. Chapter 335 Page 2400

A. Hemolytic anemia
B. Hyperbilirubinemia
C. Elevated serum alkaline phosphatase
D. Serum AST levels > 400 units

Hemolytic anemia due to effects of hypercholesterolemia or erythrocyte membranes resulting in unusual spurlike projections (acanthocytosis) may occur. Hyperbilirubinemia is found in association with elevated serum alkaline phosphatase levels. Levels of serum AST are frequently elevated, but levels > 400 units are unusual.

2041. The ratio of serum activities of AST and ALT is called as?
Clin Biochem Rev. 2013;34:117

A. Rathbone ratio
B. Josephine ratio
C. Langworthy ratio
D. De Ritis ratio

De Ritis ratio of AST to ALT has much clinical utility in detecting the cause of injury to the liver.

2042. Which of the following about AST and ALT is false?
Clin Biochem Rev. 2013;34:117

A. ALT is only present in hepatocyte cytoplasm
B. AST is present in both hepatocyte cytoplasm & mitochondria
C. 80% of total AST activity in human liver is contributed by Mitochondrial AST
D. None of the above

2043. Which of the following is false about alcoholic cirrhosis?
Harrison's 20th Ed. Chapter 337 Page 2406

A. Serum alanine aminotransferase (ALT) elevated
B. Serum aspartate aminotransferase (AST) elevated
C. AST levels > ALT levels, usually by a 2:1 ratio
D. None of the above

2044. In alcoholic liver disease, AST levels > ALT are due to?
Harrison's 20th Ed. Chapter 337 Page 2406

A. Greater inhibition of ALT synthesis by ethanol
B. Greater production of AST by ethanol
C. Greater clearance of ALT by ethanol
D. Lesser clearance of AST by ethanol

In alcoholic liver disease & in contrast to viral hepatitis, serum AST is usually disproportionately elevated relative to ALT (AST/ALT ratio >2) due to proportionally greater inhibition of ALT synthesis by ethanol which may be partially reversed by pyridoxal phosphate.

2045. Which of the following about alcoholic cirrhosis is true?
Harrison's 20th Ed. Chapter 337 Page 2406

A. Glucocorticoids are helpful in severe alcoholic hepatitis & encephalopathy
B. Survival benefit has been reported for S-adenosyl methionine in alcoholic cirrhosis

C. Diuretics, sedatives, aspirin, acetaminophen should be used with caution
D. All of the above

Glucocorticoids in moderately large doses for 4 weeks are helpful in patients with severe alcoholic hepatitis and encephalopathy but have no role in the treatment of established alcoholic cirrhosis. S-adenosyl methionine decreases proinflammatory cytokines and has survival benefit in alcoholic cirrhosis. Diuretics, sedatives, aspirin, acetaminophen should be used with caution.

2046. In patients with severe alcoholic hepatitis, treatment with glucocorticoids is restricted to patients with a discriminant function (DF) value of?
Harrison's 20th Ed. Chapter 337 Page 2406

A. > 24
B. > 28
C. > 30
D. > 32

In patients with severe alcoholic hepatitis, treatment with glucocorticoids is restricted to patients with a discriminant function (DF) value of >32.

2047. Which of the following medications is approved for treating alcoholism by reducing craving?
Harrison's 20th Ed. Chapter 337 Page 2407

A. Pentoxifylline
B. Acamprosate calcium
C. Colchicine
D. Penicillamine

Tiapride is a dopamine antagonist. Acamprosate reduces craving for alcohol, helps restore balance of excitatory & inhibitory neurotransmission in nucleus accumbens by blocking GABA receptors and Glutamate receptors and activating GABA-A receptors. Naltrexone is an opioid antagonist.

2048. In alcoholics, which concomitant hepatitis infection accelerates development of alcoholic cirrhosis?
Harrison's 20th Ed. Chapter 337 Page 2407

A. Acute hepatitis A
B. Acute hepatitis B
C. Chronic hepatitis B
D. Chronic hepatitis C

Concomitant chronic hepatitis C virus (HCV) infection significantly accelerates development of alcoholic cirrhosis. Of patients exposed to the hepatitis C virus (HCV), about 80% develop chronic hepatitis C and of those about 20–30% will develop cirrhosis over 20–30 years. Of adult patients exposed to hepatitis B, about 5% develop chronic hepatitis B and about 20% of those patients will go on to develop cirrhosis.

2049. Steatosis is present in patients with which HCV genotype?
Harrison's 20th Ed. Chapter 337 Page 2407

A. 1
B. 2
C. 3
D. 4

In patients with HCV genotype 3, steatosis is often present.

2050. Nonalcoholic steatohepatitis (NASH) is nowadays diagnosed as what was earlier diagnosed as?
Harrison's 20th Ed. Chapter 337 Page 2407

A. Autoimmune cholangiopathy
B. Cardiac cirrhosis
C. Cryptogenic cirrhosis
D. Autoimmune hepatitis

Many patients who were thought to have cryptogenic cirrhosis in fact have nonalcoholic steatohepatitis.

2051. Which of the following presentation result from both hepatocellular insufficiency and portal hypertension?
Harrison's 20th Ed. Chapter 337 Page 2407

A. Ascites
B. Jaundice
C. Coagulopathy
D. Splenomegaly

2052. Which of the following presentation result from both hepatocellular insufficiency and portal hypertension?
Harrison's 20th Ed. Chapter 337 Page 2407

A. Splenomegaly
B. Jaundice
C. Coagulopathy
D. Hepatic encephalopathy

Jaundice, edema, coagulopathy, and certain metabolic abnormalities are due to loss of functioning hepatocellular mass. Gastroesophageal varices and splenomegaly are due to portal hypertension. Ascites & hepatic encephalopathy result from both hepatocellular insufficiency & portal hypertension.

2053. Which of the following is a cause of chronic cholestatic syndrome?
Harrison's 20th Ed. Chapter 337 Page 2407

A. Primary biliary cirrhosis (PBC)
B. Autoimmune cholangitis (AIC)
C. Primary sclerosing cholangitis (PSC)
D. All of the above

Causes of chronic cholestatic syndromes are primary biliary cirrhosis (PBC), autoimmune cholangitis, primary sclerosing cholangitis (PSC) and idiopathic adulthood ductopenia.

2054. Histopathologic features of chronic cholestasis are all except?
Harrison's 20th Ed. Chapter 337 Page 2407

A. Copper deposition
B. Xanthomatous transformation of hepatocytes
C. Iron deposition
D. Biliary fibrosis

Histopathologic features of chronic cholestasis are cholate stasis, copper deposition, xanthomatous transformation of hepatocytes, and biliary fibrosis. There may also be chronic portal inflammation, interface activity and chronic lobular inflammation. Ductopenia is a result of this progressive disease as patients develop cirrhosis.

2055. Stauffer's syndrome refers to intrahepatic cholestasis specifically associated with?
J Gen Intern Med. 2006;21(7): 11-C13

A. Sarcoidosis
B. Carcinoma pancreas
C. Renal cell cancer
D. Halothane

Non-metastatic (paraneoplastic) hepatic dysfunction in patients suffering from renal cell carcinoma is known as Stauffer's syndrome. It is characterized by elevated AlkP, ESR, α-2-globulin, and γ-glutamyl transferase, thrombocytosis, prolongation of prothrombin time, and hepatosplenomegaly, in the absence of hepatic metastasis and jaundice.

2056. Primary biliary cholangitis (PBC) is characterized by?

Harrison's 20th Ed. Chapter 337 Page 2408

A. Fibrous obliteration of intrahepatic bile ductules
B. Fibrous obliteration of larger extrahepatic ducts
C. Fibrous obliteration of intrahepatic bile ductules and larger extrahepatic ducts both
D. None of the above

PBC is characterized by portal inflammation & necrosis of cholangiocytes in small and medium-sized bile ducts.

2057. Which of the following about primary biliary cholangitis (PBC) is false?

N Engl J Med. 2005;353:1261-73

A. Most prevalent in northern Europe
B. Slowly progressive autoimmune disease of liver
C. Primarily affects men
D. Peak incidence is in fifth decade of life

Among patients with symptomatic disease, 90% are women between age 35 to 60 years.

2058. Which of the following represent the pathological Stage I of PBC?

Harrison's 20th Ed. Chapter 337 Page 2408

A. Chronic nonsuppurative destructive cholangitis
B. Reduction in number of bile ducts and proliferation of smaller bile ductules
C. Decrease in interlobular ducts, loss of liver cells, and expansion of periportal fibrosis into a network of connective tissue scars
D. Micronodular or macronodular cirrhosis

PBC is divided morphologically into 4 stages. Stage I is termed chronic nonsuppurative destructive cholangitis. It is a necrotizing inflammatory process of portal triads characterized by destruction of medium & small bile ducts, a dense infiltrate of acute & chronic inflammatory cells, mild fibrosis & occasionally, bile stasis. In stage II, inflammatory infiltrate becomes less prominent, number of bile ducts are reduced & smaller bile ductules proliferate. Over months to years there is a decrease in interlobular ducts, loss of liver cells & expansion of periportal fibrosis into a network of connective tissue scars marking stage III. Stage IV represents cirrhosis - micronodular or macronodular.

2059. Antimitochondrial antibody (AMA) found in primary biliary cirrhosis is of which type of immunoglobulin?

Harrison's 20th Ed. Chapter 337 Page 2408

A. IgG
B. IgM
C. IgA
D. IgE

A circulating IgG antimitochondrial antibody (AMA) is detected in ~90% of patients with PBC and only rarely in other forms of liver disease.

2060. Which of the following is an autoreactive mitochondrial antigen in primary biliary cholangitis?

Harrison's 20th Ed. Chapter 337 Page 2408

A. Pyruvate dehydrogenase complex (PDC)
B. 2-oxoglutarate dehydrogenase complex (OGDC)
C. Branched-chain 2-oxoacid dehydrogenase complex
D. All of the above

In PBC, circulating IgG antimitochondrial autoantibodies (AMA) recognize inner mitochondrial membrane proteins identified as enzymes of the pyruvate dehydrogenase complex (PDC), branched chain 2-oxoacid dehydrogenase complex (BCOADC), and 2-oxoglutarate dehydrogenase complex (OGDC).

2061. T cells infiltrating the liver in primary biliary cholangitis are specific for?

N Engl J Med. 2005;353:1261-73

A. Pyruvate dehydrogenase E2 complex (PDC-E2)
B. E3-binding protein (E3-BP)
C. Ketoglutaric acid dehydrogenase E2 complex (OGDC-E2)
D. Branched-chain 2-oxo-acid dehydrogenase E2 complex (BCKD-E2)

The major autoantigen in PBC (90%) is 74-kDa E2 component of PDC, dihydrolipoamide acetyltransferase. Antibodies are directed to a region essential for binding of a lipoic acid cofactor and inhibit the overall enzymatic activity of the PDC. Other AMA autoantibodies in PBC patients are directed to similar constituents of BCOADC and OGDC and also inhibit their enzymatic function.

2062. In PBC, pruritus is most bothersome in?

Harrison's 20th Ed. Chapter 337 Page 2408

A. Morning
B. Afternoon
C. Evening
D. Night

Pruritus is seen in approximately 50% of PBC patients. Pruritus is most bothersome in evening.

2063. Features unique to PBC include all except?

Harrison's 20th Ed. Chapter 337 Page 2408

A. Hypopigmentation
B. Xanthelasma
C. Xanthomata
D. Bone pain

Features unique to PBC include hyperpigmentation, xanthelasma, xanthomata & bone pain. The first three are related to the altered cholesterol metabolism seen in PBC.

2064. In PBC, hyperpigmentation is evident on?

Harrison's 20th Ed. Chapter 337 Page 2408

A. Trunk
B. Face
C. Areas of exfoliation and lichenification
D. All of the above

In PBC, hyperpigmentation is evident on trunk and arms and in areas of exfoliation and lichenification.

2065. Which of the following about primary biliary cholangitis (PBC) is true?

N Engl J Med. 2005;353:1261-73

A. Antimitochondrial antibodies are present in ~90%
B. Antimitochondrial antibodies are detectable years before clinical signs appear
C. Autoantibodies recognize three to five inner mitochondrial membrane proteins
D. All of the above

2066. Which of the following about primary biliary cholangitis (PBC) is true?

N Engl J Med. 2005;353:1261-73

A. Fatigue & pruritus are the commonest presenting symptoms
B. Pruritus precedes onset of jaundice by months to years

C. Pruritus is usually worse at night and is exacerbated by contact with wool, other fabrics, or heat
D. All of the above

In PBC, the earliest symptom is pruritus, which may be either generalized or limited initially to palms and soles. Fatigue is a prominent early symptom.

2067. Which of the following is true for "autoimmune cholangitis"?
Harrison's 19th Ed. 2061

A. Histological features similar to PBC
B. Negative AMA
C. Antinuclear or smooth-muscle antibodies present
D. All of the above

In autoimmune cholangitis, histological features are similar to PBC. The AMA titre is negative. Antinuclear or smooth-muscle antibodies are present.

2068. Asymptomatic patients of PBC are initially detected by?
Harrison's 20th Ed. Chapter 337 Page 2408

A. Elevated serum alkaline phosphatase levels
B. Elevated AST levels
C. Elevated ALT levels
D. All of the above

Most patients with PBC are asymptomatic, and the disease is initially detected by elevated serum alkaline phosphatase levels during routine screening.

2069. Which of the following is increased in patients of PBC?
Harrison's 20th Ed. Chapter 337 Page 2408

A. γ-glutamyl transpeptidase
B. Alkaline phosphatase (ALP)
C. IgM Immunoglobulins
D. All of the above

Laboratory findings in PBC show cholestatic liver enzyme abnormalities with an elevation in γ-glutamyl transpeptidase and alkaline phosphatase (ALP) along with mild elevations in aminotransferases (ALT and AST). Immunoglobulins, particularly IgM, are typically increased.

2070. Which of the following is false about ursodiol therapy in PBC?
Harrison's 20th Ed. Chapter 337 Page 2408

A. Dose is 13 to 15 mg/kg per day
B. Should be given with food
C. As a single dose daily
D. None of the above

Ursodiol is given in doses of 13 to 15 mg/kg per day, with food and as a single dose daily.

2071. Which of the following drugs is useful in treatment of PBC patients with an inadequate response to UDCA?
Harrison's 20th Ed. Chapter 337 Page 2408

A. Aniticholic acid
B. Afoticholic acid
C. Obeticholic acid
D. Neoticholic acid

In 2016, obeticholic acid was approved for use in PBC patients with an inadequate response to UDCA.

2072. Drugs used to treat pruritus in PBC include all except?
Harrison's 20th Ed. Chapter 337 Page 2408

A. Cholestyramine
B. Naltrexone
C. Rifampin
D. Tetracycline

Rifampin, opiate antagonists (naloxone or naltrexone), ondansetron, plasmapheresis, and ultraviolet light have been tried for control of pruritus with varying results. Cholestyramine, an oral bile salt sequestering resin, may be helpful in doses of 12 to 16 gm/day to decrease both pruritus and hypercholesterolemia.

2073. The only established "cure" in the treatment of primary biliary cholangitis is?
Harrison's 20th Ed. Chapter 337 Page 2408

A. Liver transplantation
B. Long term Cyclosporine therapy
C. Long term Tacrolimus therapy
D. All of the above

Ursodiol therapy may not prevent ultimate progression of PBC and the only established 'cure' is liver transplantation.

2074. Secondary biliary cirrhosis (SBC) is characterized by?
Harrison's 20th Ed. Chapter 339 Page 2431

A. Fibrous obliteration of intrahepatic bile ductules
B. Fibrous obliteration of larger extrahepatic ducts
C. Fibrous obliteration of intrahepatic bile ductules and larger extrahepatic ducts both
D. None of the above

Biliary cirrhosis results from injury to or prolonged obstruction of either the intrahepatic or extrahepatic biliary system. It is associated with impaired biliary excretion, destruction of hepatic parenchyma, and progressive fibrosis. Primary biliary cirrhosis (PBC) is characterized by chronic inflammation and fibrous obliteration of intrahepatic bile ductules. Secondary biliary cirrhosis (SBC) is the result of longstanding obstruction of the larger extrahepatic ducts.

2075. Which of the following about Primary Sclerosing Cholangitis (PSC) is false?
Harrison's 20th Ed. Chapter 337 Page 2408

A. Chronic cholestatic syndrome
B. Obliteration of intrahepatic biliary tree
C. Obliteration of extrahepatic biliary tree
D. None of the above

PSC is a chronic cholestatic syndrome that is characterized by diffuse inflammation and fibrosis involving the entire biliary tree (intra- and extrahepatic), resulting in chronic cholestasis.

2076. Pathologic change occurs in PSC is?
Harrison's 20th Ed. Chapter 337 Page 2408

A. Bile duct proliferation
B. Ductopenia
C. Fibrous cholangitis (pericholangitis)
D. All of the above

Pathologic changes that can occur in PSC show bile duct proliferation as well as ductopenia and fibrous cholangitis (pericholangitis).

2077. Which of the following antibody is seen frequently in Primary Sclerosing Cholangitis (PSC)?
Harrison's 20th Ed. Chapter 337 Page 2409

A. Anti-DNA antibody
B. Cryoglobulins
C. Perinuclear antineutrophil cytoplasmic antibody (p-ANCA)
D. Antiphospholipid antibody

Perinuclear antineutrophil cytoplasmic antibody (p-ANCA), is positive in ~65% of patients of PSC.

2078. Which of the following is seen frequently in Primary Sclerosing Cholangitis (PSC)?

Harrison's 20th Ed. Chapter 337 Page 2409

A. Hodgkin's lymphoma
B. Ulcerative colitis (UC)
C. Azoospermia
D. Amenorrhea

Over 50% of patients with PSC also have ulcerative colitis (UC). PSC occurs less often in patients with CD. ~5% of patients with UC have PSC, but 50–75% of patients with PSC have IBD. IBD and PSC are commonly pANCA positive.

2079. Typical cholangiographic findings in PSC is?

Harrison's 20th Ed. Chapter 337 Page 2409

A. Multiple calculi in biliary tree
B. Multifocal stricturing & beading of biliary tree
C. Diffuse fibrotic narrowing of biliary tree
D. All of the above

Typical cholangiographic findings in PSC are multifocal stricturing and beading with intervening segments of normal or dilated ducts involving both the intrahepatic and extrahepatic biliary tree. Scarring prevents the intrahepatic ducts from dilating.

2080. Primary or idiopathic sclerosing cholangitis may be associated with?

Harrison's 20th Ed. Chapter 339 Page 2431

A. Autoimmune pancreatitis
B. Multifocal fibrosclerosis syndromes
C. Riedel's struma
D. All of the above

Primary or idiopathic sclerosing cholangitis may be associated with autoimmune pancreatitis; multifocal fibrosclerosis syndromes (retroperitoneal, mediastinal, and/or periureteral fibrosis), Riedel's struma or pseudotumor of the orbit.

2081. Which of the following has biochemical & cholangiographic features indistinguishable from PSC?

Harrison's 20th Ed. Chapter 339 Page 2431

A. Immunoglobulin G1 - associated cholangitis
B. Immunoglobulin G2 - associated cholangitis
C. Immunoglobulin G3 - associated cholangitis
D. Immunoglobulin G4 - associated cholangitis

Immunoglobulin G4–associated cholangitis is a recently described biliary disease of unknown etiology that presents with biochemical and cholangiographic features indistinguishable from PSC. Often associated with autoimmune pancreatitis & other fibrosing conditions but not inflammatory bowel disease, it is characterized by elevated serum IgG4 and infiltration of IgG4-positive plasma cells in bile ducts and liver tissue. Glucocorticoids and/or azathioprine are helpful.

2082. Independent predictor of a bad prognosis in PSC is?

Harrison's 20th Ed. Chapter 339 Page 2432

A. Age
B. Serum bilirubin concentration
C. Liver histologic changes
D. All of the above

Independent predictors of a bad prognosis in PSC are age, serum bilirubin concentration, liver histologic changes and splenomegaly. Cholangiocarcinoma is a dreaded consequence.

2083. Patients of PSC are more vulnerable to which of the following malignancies?

Harrison's 20th Ed. Chapter 319 Page 2269

A. Gallbladder polyp
B. Cervical cancer
C. Endometrial cancer
D. All of the above

Gallbladder polyps in patients with PSC have a high incidence of malignancy and cholecystectomy is recommended, even if a mass lesion is <1 cm in diameter.

2084. Which of the following malignancy is most commonly associated with PSC?

Harrison's 20th Ed. Chapter 337 Page 2409

A. Cholangiocarcinoma
B. Carcinoma pancreas
C. Carcinoma gallbladder
D. Ampullary cancer

Cholangiocarcinoma is most commonly associated with PSC and is exceptionally difficult to diagnose because its appearance is often identical to that of PSC. PSC patients have a 10–15% lifetime risk of developing cholangiocarcinoma.

2085. Cholangiography is normal in which variant of PSC?

Harrison's 20th Ed. Chapter 319 Page 2269

A. Pauci primary sclerosing cholangitis
B. Small duct primary sclerosing cholangitis
C. Hereditary sclerosing cholangitis
D. Drug induced sclerosing cholangitis

Cholangiography is normal in small duct primary sclerosing cholangitis - a variant of PSC. This variant is sometimes referred to as "pericholangitis" and involves small-caliber bile ducts. It has similar biochemical and histologic features to classic PSC and has significantly better prognosis than classic PSC, although it may evolve into classic PSC.

2086. Histopathologically, which of the following is helpful in making the diagnosis of PSC?

Harrison's 20th Ed. Chapter 337 Page 2409

A. Bile duct proliferation
B. Ductopenia
C. Periductal fibrosis
D. Xanthomatous transformation of hepatocytes

2087. Which of the following has cholangiographic appearance similar to that of PSC?

Harrison's 20th Ed. Chapter 339 Page 2432

A. AIDS cholangiopathy
B. Traumatic biliary injury
C. Chronic pancreatitis
D. All of the above

AIDS cholangiopathy is a condition, usually due to infection of the bile duct epithelium with CMV or cryptosporidia, which has a cholangiographic appearance similar to that of PSC. These patients usually present with greatly elevated serum alkaline phosphatase levels (mean, 800 IU/L), but the bilirubin is often near normal. These patients do not typically present with jaundice.

2088. Diagnosis of PSC is best made with?

Harrison's 20th Ed. Chapter 337 Page 2409

A. Ultrasound
B. MRCP
C. CT Scan
D. Liver biopsy

Primary sclerosing cholangitis is characterized by the destruction and fibrosis of larger bile ducts. Diagnosis of PSC is made with cholangiography (MRCP or ERCP), which demonstrates the pathognomonic segmental strictures.

2089. Which of the following is efficacious in PSC?
Harrison's 20th Ed. Chapter 337 Page 2409, Harrison's 20th Ed. Chapter 339 Page 2433

A. Glucocorticoids
B. Methotrexate
C. Cyclosporine
D. UDCA

Glucocorticoids, methotrexate, and cyclosporine have not been shown to be efficacious in PSC. UDCA in high dosage (20 mg/kg) improves serum liver tests, but an effect on survival has not been documented. Ultimate treatment is liver transplantation except when complicated by cholangiocarcinoma.

2090. "Nutmeg liver" is the term used to describe liver in?
Clin Liver Dis. 2002;6(4):947-67

A. Cardiac cirrhosis
B. Primary Biliary Cirrhosis
C. Secondary Biliary Cirrhosis
D. None of the above

In right heart failure, hepatic sinusoids become dilated & engorged with blood, along with hepatic ischemia from poor perfusion leading to necrosis of centrilobular hepatocytes with fibrosis in central areas. Centrilobular fibrosis extends outward in a characteristic stellate pattern from central vein.

2091. In "nutmeg liver", gross examination of liver shows which of the following?
Clin Liver Dis. 2002;6(4):947-67

A. Nodules on the surface of liver
B. Alternating red and pale areas
C. Pyramid like elevations on surface of liver
D. Brownish black discoloration of liver

In nutmeg liver, gross examination shows alternating red (congested) & pale (fibrotic) areas.

2092. Levels of which of the following is characteristically elevated in cardiac cirrhosis?
Harrison's 20th Ed. Chapter 337 Page 2409

A. S. Bilirubin
B. SGOT
C. SGPT
D. S. Alkaline phosphatase

ALP levels are characteristically elevated in cardiac cirrhosis, Aminotransferases may be normal or slightly increased with AST usually higher than ALT.

2093. Which of the following is false in cardiac cirrhosis?
Harrison's 20th Ed. Chapter 337 Page 2409

A. Pericentral fibrosis
B. Unlikely that patients will develop variceal hemorrhage
C. Unlikely that patients will develop encephalopathy
D. None of the above

2094. Inherited metabolic liver disease that can progress to cirrhosis is?
Harrison's 20th Ed. Chapter 337 Page 2409

A. Hemochromatosis
B. Wilson's disease
C. Cystic fibrosis
D. All of the above

Inherited metabolic liver diseases that can progress to cirrhosis include hemochromatosis, Wilson's disease, α_1 antitrypsin deficiency, and cystic fibrosis.

2095. Which of the following points is against the diagnosis of Budd-Chiari syndrome?
Harrison's 20th Ed. Chapter 337 Page 2409

A. Tender hepatomegaly
B. Intractable ascites
C. Right-sided heart failure
D. Centrilobular congestion & sinusoidal dilatation on liver biopsy

In Budd-Chiari syndrome, liver is grossly enlarged, tender & severe intractable ascites is present. Signs & symptoms of heart failure are notably absent. Hepatic venography or liver biopsy showing centrilobular congestion & sinusoidal dilatation in absence of right heart failure characterize Budd-Chiari syndrome.

2096. Toxicity of which of the following vitamins can cause veno-occlusive disease of liver?
Sherlock

A. A
B. D
C. E
D. K

2097. Acute Budd-Chiari syndrome has all the features except?
Sherlock

A. Abdominal pain
B. Jaundice
C. Ascites
D. Caudate lobe hypertrophy

2098. Initial investigation of choice in suspected Budd-Chiari syndrome is?
Sherlock

A. USG abdomen
B. Doppler studies
C. CT abdomen
D. MR angiography

2099. Portal hypertension is defined as elevation of hepatic venous pressure gradient (HVPG) to?
Harrison's 20th Ed. Chapter 337 Page 2410

A. > 2 mm Hg
B. > 3 mm Hg
C. > 4 mm Hg
D. > 5 mm Hg

Portal hypertension is defined as elevation of hepatic venous pressure gradient (HVPG) to >5 mm Hg. Varices may develop but do not bleed if HVPG is <12 mm Hg. HVPG is equal to wedged hepatic venous pressure (portal venous pressure) minus free hepatic venous pressure (intra-abdominal pressure).

2100. In variceal hemorrhage, mortality associated with each episode of bleeding is?
Harrison's 20th Ed. Chapter 337 Page 2410

A. 10 - 20%
B. 20 - 30%
C. 30 - 40%
D. 40 - 50%

Mortality associated with each episode of variceal bleeding is 20–30%. Even if the patient survives an initial episode of variceal bleeding, probability of another episode is high. Rebleeding rate without treatment is 70% within 1 year. The mortality rate with rebleeding is 33%.

2101. Portal vein is formed by the confluence of splenic vein with?
Harrison's 20th Ed. Chapter 337 Page 2410

A. Superior mesenteric vein
B. Inferior mesenteric vein
C. Gastric vein
D. All of the above

Portal vein is formed by the confluence of superior mesenteric and splenic veins.

2102. Which of the following is a posthepatic cause of portal hypertension?
Harrison's 20th Ed. Chapter 337 Page 2410

A. Portal vein thrombosis
B. Veno-occlusive disease
C. Splenic vein thrombosis
D. All of the above

2103. Which of the following is a posthepatic cause of portal hypertension?
Harrison's 20th Ed. Chapter 337 Page 2410

A. Budd-Chiari syndrome (BCS)
B. Veno-occlusive disease
C. Chronic right-sided cardiac congestion
D. All of the above

2104. Which of the following accounts for most cases of portal hypertension?
Harrison's 20th Ed. Chapter 337 Page 2410

A. Prehepatic
B. Intrahepatic
C. Posthepatic
D. Any of the above

Intrahepatic causes of portal hypertension account for over 95% of cases of portal hypertension and are represented by the major forms of cirrhosis.

2105. Esophageal varices are present in what percentage of compensated and decompensated cirrhosis?
Gastroenterol Hepatol (N Y). 2006;2(2):124-133

A. 10 & 40%
B. 20 & 50%
C. 30 & 60%
D. 40 & 70%

Esophageal varices are present in 30% of patients with compensated cirrhosis and in up to 60% of those with decompensated cirrhosis (with evidence of ascites or encephalopathy).

2106. Budd-Chiari syndrome is an example of?
Harrison's 20th Ed. Chapter 337 Page 2410

A. Presinusoidal obstruction
B. Sinusoidal obstruction
C. Post-sinusoidal obstruction
D. Any of the above

Postsinusoidal obstruction may also occur outside the liver at the level of the hepatic veins (Budd-Chiari syndrome), the inferior vena cava so that the liver parenchyma is exposed to elevated venous pressures.

2107. Which of the following is a presinusoidal cause of portal hypertension?
Harrison's 20th Ed. Chapter 337 Page 2410

A. Schistosomiasis
B. Chronic right-sided cardiac congestion
C. Cirrhosis liver
D. All of the above

Presinusoidal causes of portal hypertension include congenital hepatic fibrosis and schistosomiasis. Sinusoidal causes are related to cirrhosis from various causes.

2108. When cirrhosis is complicated by portal hypertension, the increased resistance is?
Harrison's 20th Ed. Chapter 337 Page 2410

A. Presinusoidal
B. Sinusoidal
C. Post-sinusoidal
D. All of the above

Portal hypertension (>10 mm Hg) mostly results from increased resistance to portal blood flow. When hepatic cirrhosis is complicated by portal hypertension, increased resistance is usually sinusoidal.

2109. 'Symmers' clay-pipe stem fibrosis in liver is due to?
Harrison's 20th Ed. Chapter 229 Page 1638

A. Brucellosis
B. Toxoplasmosis
C. Echinococcosis
D. Schistosomiasis

Intrahepatic presinusoidal causes of portal hypertension include congenital hepatic fibrosis and schistosomiasis. Schistosomiasis alone results in pure fibrotic lesions in liver. Cirrhosis occurs when other nutritional or infectious agents (hepatitis B or C virus) are involved. It is characteristically periportal (Symmers' clay pipe-stem fibrosis).

2110. Portal vein obstruction may occur in association with?
Harrison's 20th Ed. Chapter 337 Page 2410

A. Cirrhosis
B. Abdominal trauma
C. Pancreatitis
D. All of the above

Portal vein obstruction may be idiopathic or occur in association with cirrhosis, infection, pancreatitis, or abdominal trauma.

2111. Portal vein thrombosis may develop in?
Harrison's 20th Ed. Chapter 337 Page 2410

A. Polycythemia vera
B. Deficiencies of protein C, protein S, or antithrombin III
C. Factor V Leiden
D. All of the above

Idiopathic portal vein thrombosis may develop in hypercoagulable states like polycythemia vera, essential thrombocythemia, deficiencies of protein C / protein S / antithrombin III, resistance to activated protein C (factor V Leiden) & mutation of prothrombin gene (G20210A).

2112. Primary complication of portal hypertension is?
Harrison's 20th Ed. Chapter 337 Page 2410

A. Gastroesophageal varices with hemorrhage
B. Ascites
C. Hypersplenism
D. All of the above

Three primary complications of portal hypertension are gastroesophageal varices with hemorrhage, ascites, and hypersplenism.

2113. On screening of histologically confirmed cirrhosis cases, what proportion of patients have esophageal varices?

Harrison's 20th Ed. Chapter 337 Page 2410

A. One - fourth
B. One - third
C. One - half
D. Three - fourth

On screening of histologically confirmed cirrhosis cases, one - third of patients have esophageal varices.

2114. In cirrhosis, factor that predicts the risk of esophageal variceal bleeding is?

Harrison's 20th Ed. Chapter 337 Page 2410

A. Severity of cirrhosis
B. Wedged-hepatic vein pressure
C. Tense ascites
D. All of the above

In cirrhosis, factors that predict risk of esophageal variceal bleeding include severity of cirrhosis (Child's class, MELD score), height of wedged-hepatic vein pressure, size of varix, location of varix, endoscopic stigmatas (red wale signs, hematocystic spots, diffuse erythema, bluish color, cherry red spots, or white-nipple spots and tense ascites.

2115. Marker of the presence of cirrhosis in a patient being followed for chronic liver disease is?

Harrison's 20th Ed. Chapter 337 Page 2410

A. Progressive decrease in platelet count
B. Progressive increase in platelet count
C. Progressive decrease in lymphocyte count
D. Progressive increase in lymphocyte count

Progressive decrease in platelet count serves as a marker of the presence of cirrhosis in a patient being followed for chronic liver disease. A low-normal platelet count can be the first clue to progression to cirrhosis.

2116. Marker of the presence of cirrhosis in a patient being followed for chronic liver disease is?

Harrison's 20th Ed. Chapter 337 Page 2410

A. Appearance of an enlarged spleen
B. Development of ascites
C. Hepatic encephalopathy
D. All of the above

Progressive decrease in platelet count, appearance of enlarged spleen, development of ascites, encephalopathy, and/or esophageal varices with or without bleeding serve as markers of the presence of cirrhosis in a patient being followed for chronic liver disease.

2117. The risk of variceal hemorrhage is related to?

Harrison's 20th Ed. Chapter 337 Page 2410

A. Size of varices
B. Appearance of varices
C. Severity of liver dysfunction
D. All of the above

Risk of variceal hemorrhage is related to size of varices (varices ≤ 5 mm in diameter have a 7% risk of bleeding in 2 years, while those >5 mm have a 30% risk of bleeding within 2 years), appearance of the varices (red wale sign i.e. red streaks of mucosa overlying varix) have an increased risk of hemorrhage & severity of liver dysfunction (high Child-Pugh score - B or C represents decompensated cirrhosis & is associated with an increased risk of bleeding).

2118. In liver disease, development of portal hypertension is revealed by the appearance of which of the following?

Harrison's 20th Ed. Chapter 337 Page 2410

A. Splenomegaly
B. Ascites
C. Encephalopathy
D. All of the above

In patients with liver disease, development of portal hypertension is revealed by the appearance of splenomegaly, ascites, encephalopathy, and/or esophageal varices.

2119. Which of the following statements about free and wedged hepatic vein pressure is false?

Harrison's 20th Ed. Chapter 337 Page 2410

A. Wedged hepatic vein pressure is usually normal in presinusoidal portal hypertension
B. Wedged hepatic vein pressure is elevated in sinusoidal portal hypertension
C. Wedged hepatic vein pressure is elevated in postsinusoidal portal hypertension
D. None of the above

Wedged hepatic vein pressure is elevated in sinusoidal and postsinusoidal portal hypertension, it is normal in presinusoidal portal hypertension.

2120. What level of portal hypertension threatens bleeding from gastroesophageal varices?

Harrison's 20th Ed. Chapter 337 Page 2410

A. > 6 mm Hg
B. > 8 mm Hg
C. > 10 mm Hg
D. > 12 mm Hg

Wedged and free hepatic vein pressures allow calculation of a wedged-to-free gradient, which is equivalent to the portal pressure. Average normal wedged-to-free gradient is 5 mm Hg, and patients with a gradient >12 mm Hg are at risk for variceal hemorrhage.

2121. Apart from propranolol, which other β-adrenergic blocker is used to reduce portal pressure?

Harrison's 20th Ed. Chapter 337 Page 2411

A. Atenolol
B. Nadolol
C. Sotalol
D. Carvedilol

β-adrenergic blockade with nonselective agents (propranolol or nadolol) reduces portal pressure through vasoconstrictive effects on both splanchnic arterial bed & portal venous system in combination with reduced cardiac output. Such therapy is effective in preventing both a first variceal bleed & subsequent episodes.

2122. Doses of propranolol to treat portal hypertension should aim to reduce the resting pulse rate by?

Gut Liver. 2007;1(2):159-164

A. 5%
B. 10%
C. 25%
D. 33%

In treatment of portal hypertension, especially variceal bleeding, reduction of resting pulse through β-adrenergic blockade with nonselective agents such as propranolol by 25% is reasonable.

2123. The goal of treatment in patients of portal hypertension is to reduce hepatic venous pressure gradient (HVPG) to?

Gut Liver. 2007;1(2):159-164

A. <20 mm Hg or by 50% from baseline
B. <15 mm Hg or by 40% from baseline

C. <12 mm Hg or by 20% from baseline

D. <6 mm Hg or by 10% from baseline

Treatment of patients with clinically significant sequelae of portal hypertension, especially variceal bleeding, is titrated to reduce the hepatic venous pressure gradient (HVPG = wedged hepatic venous pressure – free hepatic venous pressure) to <12 mm Hg or by 20% from baseline.

2124. "Caput medusae" is best related to?
N Engl J Med. 2005; 353:e19

A. Cardioesophageal junction
B. Rectum
C. Retroperitoneal space
D. Falciform ligament of liver

Major sites of portalsystemic collateral flow are veins around cardioesophageal junction (esophagogastric varices), rectum (hemorrhoids), retroperitoneal space & falciform ligament of liver (periumbilical or abdominal wall collaterals). Abdominal wall collaterals appear as tortuous epigastric vessels that radiate from umbilicus toward xiphoid & rib margins (caput medusae).

2125. Which of the following is false about Dieulafoy's lesion?
Harrison's 20th Ed. Chapter 315 Page 2197

A. Large-caliber arteriole beneath gastrointestinal mucosa
B. Bleeds through a pinpoint mucosal erosion
C. Most common on greater curvature of proximal stomach
D. Also called persistent caliber artery

Dieulafoy's lesion is seen most commonly on the lesser curvature of the proximal stomach.

2126. Gastric antral vascular ectasia is the cause of?
Harrison's 20th Ed. Chapter 315 Page 2198

A. Washermen stomach
B. Watermelon stomach
C. Windmill stomach
D. Windshield stomach

Watermelon stomach is seen in gastric antral vascular ectasia (GAVE).

2127. Which of the following should be the first-line treatment to control bleeding acutely?
Harrison's 20th Ed. Chapter 337 Page 2411

A. Somatostatin/octreotide
B. Balloon tamponade
C. Emergency portal-systemic nonselective shunts
D. Endoscopic intervention

Endoscopic intervention should be the first-line treatment to control bleeding acutely. Treatment of acute bleeding requires both fluid and blood-product replacement as well as prevention of subsequent bleeding with Endoscopic variceal ligation (EVL).

2128. Sengstaken-Blakemore tube has how many lumens?
Harrison's 20th Ed. Chapter 337 Page 2411

A. 1
B. 2
C. 3
D. 4

2129. Minnesota tube has how many lumens?
Harrison's 20th Ed. Chapter 337 Page 2411

A. 1
B. 2
C. 3
D. 4

Balloon tamponade of bleeding gastroesophageal varices may be accomplished with a triple-lumen (Sengstaken-Blakemore) or four-lumen (Minnesota) tube with esophageal and gastric balloons.

2130. "TIPS" stands for?
Harrison's 20th Ed. Chapter 337 Page 2411

A. Transcuteneous intrahepatic portosystemic shunt
B. Transvenous intrahepatic portosystemic shunt
C. Transjugular intrahepatic portosystemic shunt
D. Transarterial intrahepatic portosystemic shunt

Decompression procedure to lower portal pressure is accomplished without surgery through percutaneous placement of a portal-systemic shunt, termed transjugular intrahepatic portosystemic shunt (TIPS).

2131. Hepatic encephalopathy occurs in what proportion of patients after TIPS?
Harrison's 20th Ed. Chapter 337 Page 2411

A. 10%
B. 20%
C. 30%
D. 40%

Hepatic encephalopathy occur in 20% of patients after TIPS.

2132. Somatostatin and octreotide are?
Harrison's 20th Ed. Chapter 337 Page 2411

A. Generalized vasoconstrictors
B. Direct splanchnic vasoconstrictors
C. Direct systemic vasoconstrictors
D. None of the above

Somatostatin and its analogue, octreotide, are direct splanchnic vasoconstrictors.

2133. Which of the following agents is useful in the treatment of portal hypertensive gastropathy?
Harrison's 20th Ed. Chapter 337 Page 2411

A. Proton pump inhibitors
B. H2 receptor blockers
C. Sucralfate
D. None of the above

Congestive gastropathy due to the venous hypertension is a complication of portal hypertension. Nonselective beta-adrenergic blockade is sometimes effective. Proton pump inhibitors or other agents useful in the treatment of peptic disease are usually not helpful.

2134. Theories proposed for ascites include?
Gastroenterol Hepatol (NY). 2009;5(9):647-656

A. "Underfilling" theory
B. "Overflow" theory
C. "Peripheral arterial vasodilation" theory
D. All of the above

2135. Hepatic hydrothorax is more common on which side?
Harrison's 20th Ed. Chapter 337 Page 2412

A. Right side
B. Left side
C. Bilateral
D. Any of the above

Hepatic hydrothorax is more common on right side due to a rent in the diaphragm with free flow of ascitic fluid into the thoracic cavity.

2136. What does SAAG stand for?

Harrison's 20th Ed. Chapter 337 Page 2412

A. Serum ascites-to-albumin gradient
B. Serum albumin-to-ascites gradient
C. Serum albumin-to-anion gradient
D. Serum anion-to-albumin gradient

In cirrhosis, protein concentration of ascitic fluid is low (<1 g/dL). With the use of serum ascites-to-albumin gradient (SAAG), terms like exudative or transudative fluid have been replaced. Cirrhosis leading to portal hypertension leading to ascitis, gradient between serum albumin level and ascitic fluid albumin level is >1.1 g/dL. When the gradient is <1.1 g/dL, infectious or malignant causes of ascites should be considered.

2137. There is an increased risk for developing which of the following when levels of ascitic fluid proteins are very low?

Harrison's 20th Ed. Chapter 337 Page 2412

A. Refractory ascites
B. Hepatic Encephalopathy
C. Spontaneous Bacterial Peritonitis (SBP)
D. Hepatocellular cancer

When levels of ascitic fluid proteins are very low, patients are at increased risk for developing SBP.

2138. What absolute level of polymorphonuclear leukocytes count suggests ascitic fluid infection?

Harrison's 20th Ed. Chapter 337 Page 2412

A. > 100/μL
B. > 150/μL
C. > 200/μL
D. > 250/μL

A high level of red blood cells in the ascitic fluid signifies a traumatic tap or perhaps a hepatocellular cancer or a ruptured omental varix. When the absolute level of polymorphonuclear leukocytes is >250/μL, ascitic fluid infection should be strongly considered.

2139. The recommended amount of sodium per day in the management of ascites is?

Harrison's 20th Ed. Chapter 337 Page 2412

A. < 2 gram
B. < 4 gram
C. < 6 gram
D. < 8 gram

< 2 gram of sodium per day is the recommended amount in the management of ascites.

2140. Which of the following about refractory ascites is false?

Gastroenterol Hepatol (NY). 2009;5(9):647-656

A. Ascites that does not recede despite sodium restriction and diuretic treatment
B. Ascites that recurs shortly after therapeutic paracentesis
C. Prognosis for patients with cirrhosis with ascites is poor
D. None of the above

Refractory ascites is defined as ascites that does not recede or that recurs shortly after therapeutic paracentesis, despite sodium restriction and diuretic treatment. To date, there is no approved medical therapy specifically for refractory ascites. Management is based on large-volume paracentesis (LVP) and transjugular intrahepatic portosystemic shunts (TIPS), which temporarily alleviate symptoms, but are not curative. The only curative treatment is liver transplantation.

2141. Maximal doses of spironolactone and furosemide are?

Gastroenterol Hepatol (NY). 2009;5(9):647-656

A. Spironolactone 100 mg/day & furosemide 160 mg/day
B. Spironolactone 200 mg/day & furosemide 160 mg/day
C. Spironolactone 300 mg/day & furosemide 160 mg/day
D. Spironolactone 400 mg/day & furosemide 160 mg/day

Maximal doses of spironolactone and furosemide are 400 mg/day and 160 mg/day respectively.

2142. Which of the following is used to determine the likelihood that a patient with ascites will respond to therapy?

Gastroenterol Hepatol (NY). 2009;5(9):647-656

A. U_{Cr}/P_{Cr} ratio
B. Fractional excretion of sodium (Fe_{Na})
C. Serum vasopressin (AVP) level
D. All of the above

Initial fractional excretion of sodium (FeNa) >0.2% may predict the development of refractory ascites in patients receiving diuretic therapy.

2143. Which of the following statements about spontaneous bacterial peritonitis (SBP) is false?

Harrison's 20th Ed. Chapter 337 Page 2413

A. Develops without obvious primary source of infection
B. Ascitic fluid has high concentrations of albumin
C. In ascitic fluid, >250 PMN/μL is diagnostic
D. Monomicrobial nonneutrocytic bacterascites is a variant of SBP

SBP is characterized by spontaneous infection of ascitic fluid in absence of intra-abdominal source of infection. Bacterial translocation is the presumed mechanism for development of SBP, with gut flora traversing the intestine into mesenteric lymph nodes, leading to bacteremia and seeding of the ascitic fluid.

2144. Which of the following statements about spontaneous bacterial peritonitis (SBP) is false?

Harrison's 20th Ed. Chapter 337 Page 2413, N Engl J Med. 2004;350:1646-54

A. Escherichia coli are most commonly isolated
B. A single organism is typically isolated
C. Anaerobes are found less frequently
D. Recurrent episodes are relatively uncommon

SBP involves translocation of bacteria from intestinal lumen to lymph nodes, with subsequent bacteremia & infection of ascitic fluid. After resolution, SBP frequently recurs, with an estimated 70% probability of recurrence at one year.

2145. Which of the following statements about spontaneous bacterial peritonitis (SBP) is false?

Harrison's 20th Ed. Chapter 337 Page 2413

A. Therapy is for 10 to 14 days
B. Prophylactic norfloxacin reduces recurrences
C. Primary prevention recommended in high-risk cirrhotics
D. Empirical coverage for anaerobes is necessary

In patients with variceal hemorrhage, frequency of SBP is significantly increased, and prophylaxis against SBP is recommended when a patient presents with upper GI bleeding. Patients who have had an episode(s) of SBP and recovered, once-weekly administration of antibiotics is used as prophylaxis for recurrent SBP.

2146. Hepatorenal syndrome (HRS) occurs in what percentage of patients with advanced cirrhosis or acute liver failure?

Harrison's 20th Ed. Chapter 337 Page 2413

A. ~ 5%
B. ~ 10%
C. ~ 20%
D. ~ 30%

HRS is a type of functional renal failure "without renal pathology" that occurs in ~10% of patients with advanced cirrhosis or acute liver failure.

2147. Which of the following about hepatorenal syndrome is false?
Harrison's 20th Ed. Chapter 337 Page 2413

A. Splanchnic vasodilation
B. Arteriovenous shunting
C. Profound renal vasoconstriction
D. None of the above

In HRS, kidneys are structurally normal but fail due to splanchnic vasodilation & arteriovenous shunting, resulting in profound renal vasoconstriction resulting from extreme underfilling of arterial circulation.

2148. Renal failure in cirrhosis is defined as serum creatinine above?
N Engl J Med. 2009;361:1279-90

A. 1.2 mg/dL
B. 1.3 mg/dL
C. 1.4 mg/dL
D. 1.5 mg/dL

Most studies & consensus conferences have defined renal failure in cirrhosis as a serum creatinine concentration above 1.5 mg /dL.

2149. Which of the following about hepatorenal syndrome is false?
Harrison's 20th Ed. Chapter 337 Page 2413

A. Type I HRS is the more aggressive form
B. Type I HRS carries a mortality rate of >90%
C. HRS is seen in patients with refractory ascites
D. None of the above

HRS is a unique form of prerenal ARF that complicates advanced cirrhosis and acute liver failure and is seen in in patients with refractory ascites. Type I HRS is the more aggressive form of the disease & carries a mortality rate of >90%.

2150. Type 1 HRS is characterized by doubling of serum creatinine level to > 2.5 mg/dL in?
N Engl J Med. 2009;361:1279-90

A. < 2 weeks
B. < 4 weeks
C. < 6 weeks
D. < 8 weeks

Type 1 HRS is characterized by a doubling of serum creatinine level to > 2.5 mg/dL in < 2 weeks. Type 2 is characterized by a stable or less rapidly progressive course than in type 1.

2151. Which of the following is true for type 1 hepatorenal syndrome?
N Engl J Med. 2004;350:1646-54

A. Progressive oliguria
B. Rapid rise of serum creatinine
C. Common precipitating event is SBP
D. All of the above

Type 1 hepatorenal syndrome is characterized by progressive oliguria and a rapid rise of the serum creatinine. A common precipitating event is spontaneous bacterial peritonitis (SBP).

2152. Which of the following is true for type 2 hepatorenal syndrome?
N Engl J Med. 2004;350:1646-54

A. Most have refractory ascites
B. Increase in serum creatinine is moderate
C. No tendency of serum creatinine to progress over time
D. All of the above

In type 2 hepatorenal syndrome, most patients have refractory ascites, increase in serum creatinine is moderate and has no tendency to progress over time.

2153. Type 2 HRS is mainly characterized by?
N Engl J Med. 2009;361:1279-90

A. Hepatic encephalopathy
B. Refractory ascites
C. Hypotension
D. All of the above

Type 1 hepatorenal syndrome has severe multiorgan dysfunction, which affects not only the kidneys but also the heart, systemic circulation, brain, adrenal glands, and liver, whereas the clinical course of patients with type 2 hepatorenal syndrome is mainly characterized by refractory ascites.

2154. Which of the following treatments have a role in hepatorenal syndrome?
Harrison's 20th Ed. Chapter 337 Page 2413

A. Midodrine
B. Octreotide
C. Intravenous albumin
D. All of the above

Currently, patients of HRS are treated with midodrine, an α-agonist, along with octreotide & IV albumin. The best therapy for HRS is liver transplantation.

2155. Which of the following is a vasoconstrictor drug?
N Engl J Med. 2009;361:1279-90

A. Terlipressin
B. Norepinephrine
C. Midodrine
D. All of the above

Best approach in management of HRS is administration of vasoconstrictor drugs. Treatment with renal vasodilators like dopamine or prostaglandins is ineffective.

2156. Long-term administration of which of the following reduces the risk of hepatorenal syndrome & improves survival?
N Engl J Med. 2009;361:1279-90

A. Norfloxacin
B. Eplerenone
C. Torsemide
D. Vitamin E

Long-term oral norfloxacin reduces risk of hepatorenal syndrome & improves survival.

2157. Which of the following statements about hepatorenal syndrome (HRS) is false?
Harrison's 20th Ed. Chapter 337 Page 2413

A. Worsening azotemia
B. Avid sodium retention
C. Oliguria without identifiable causes of renal dysfunction
D. Kidneys are structurally smaller

2158. Which of the following statements about hepatorenal syndrome (HRS) is false?
Harrison's 20th Ed. Chapter 337 Page 2413

A. Urinalysis normal
B. Renal biopsy is normal
C. Kidneys can be used for renal transplantation
D. Hypernatremia

2159. Which of the following statements about hepatorenal syndrome (HRS) is false?

Harrison's 20th Ed. Chapter 337 Page 2413

A. Treatment is usually unsuccessful
B. Vasodilator therapy with intravenous infusions of low dose dopamine is effective
C. TIPS can improve renal function
D. Treatment of choice is liver transplantation

2160. Which of the following is false about hepatic encephalopathy?

Harrison's 20th Ed. Chapter 337 Page 2413

A. More common in chronic liver disease
B. Essential for diagnosis of fulminant hepatic failure
C. Diagnosis of hepatic encephalopathy is clinical
D. None of the above

2161. Which of the following characteristics about hepatic encephalopathy is false?

Harrison's 20th Ed. Chapter 337 Page 2413

A. Disturbances in consciousness
B. Behavior & personality changes
C. Fluctuating neurologic signs
D. No electroencephalographic changes

2162. Which of the following statements about hepatic encephalopathy is false?

Harrison's 20th Ed. Chapter 337 Page 2413

A. Blood-brain barrier is intact
B. Ammonia is incriminated in its pathogenesis
C. Many patients have elevated blood ammonia levels
D. Mercaptans, short-chain fatty acids, & phenol are incriminated in its pathogenesis

2163. Which of the following is the most common predisposing factor for hepatic encephalopathy?

Harrison's 20th Ed. Chapter 337 Page 2413

A. Gastrointestinal bleeding
B. Increased dietary protein
C. Electrolyte disturbances
D. Injudicious use of CNS-depressing drugs

2164. Which of the following is the most common predisposing factor for hepatic encephalopathy?

Harrison's 20th Ed. Chapter 337 Page 2413

A. Gastrointestinal bleeding
B. Surgery
C. Superimposed acute viral hepatitis
D. Alcoholic hepatitis

2165. Which of the following is the most common predisposing factor for hepatic encephalopathy?

Harrison's 20th Ed. Chapter 337 Page 2413

A. Gastrointestinal bleeding
B. Extrahepatic bile duct obstruction
C. Constipation
D. Surgery

In chronic liver disease, encephalopathy is usually triggered by a medical complication such as gastrointestinal bleeding, over-diuresis, uremia, dehydration, electrolyte imbalance, infection, constipation or use of narcotic analgesics.

2166. Astrocytic glutamine synthetase converts ammonia & glutamate into?

N Engl J Med. 2016;375:1660-70

A. Inositol
B. Taurine
C. Arginine
D. Glutamine

At high levels, ammonia can cross blood–brain barrier, where astrocytic glutamine synthetase converts ammonia & glutamate into glutamine, which acts as an osmolyte & increases cerebral volume.

2167. Which of the following elements is a possible contributor to hepatic encephalopathy?

N Engl J Med. 2016;375:1660-70

A. Molybdenum
B. Manganese
C. Nickel
D. Silicon

A possible contributor to hepatic encephalopathy, particularly in patients with long-standing cirrhosis, is manganese toxicity. Mercaptans, short fatty acids, decreased glutaminergic synaptic function, lactate & dopamine metabolites have also been implicated.

2168. The MELD score determination does not include?

Harrison's 20th Ed. Chapter 338 Page 2416

A. Bilirubin
B. Urea
C. Creatinine
D. Prothrombin time

The MELD score is based on a mathematical model that includes bilirubin, creatinine and prothrombin time expressed as international normalized ratio (INR). The formula is 3.78 x $\log_e$ bilirubin (mg/100 mL) ± 11.2 x $\log_e$ international normalized ratio (INR) ± 9.57 x $\log_e$ creatinine (mg/100 mL) ± 6.43.

2169. Neurologic signs in hepatic encephalopathy includes all except?

Harrison's 20th Ed. Chapter 337 Page 2413

A. Rigidity
B. Decreased DTR
C. Extensor plantar signs
D. Seizures

2170. Earliest sign of hepatic encephalopathy is?

Harrison's 20th Ed. Chapter 337 Page 2413

A. EEG changes
B. Asterixis
C. Reversal of sleep/wake cycle
D. Deterioration in handwriting

The first signs of hepatic encephalopathy are subtle & nonspecific like change in sleep patterns, change in personality, irritability and mental dullness. Thereafter, confusion, disorientation, stupor and eventually coma supervene.

2171. Typical smell in fetor hepaticus is due to?

Br J Gen Pract. 2012;62(605):652-653, Harrison's 16th Ed. 1867

A. Mercaptans
B. Ammonia

C. Bilirubin

D. All of the above

Fetor hepaticus refers to the slightly sweet, ammoniacal odor that can develop in patients with liver failure, particularly if there is portal-venous shunting of blood around the liver.

2172. Mercaptans are derived from intestinal metabolism of?

Br J Gen Pract. 2012;62(605):652-653, Harrison's 16th Ed. 1867

A. Threonine

B. Methionine

C. Leucine

D. Isoleucine

Fetor hepaticus is a feature of severe liver disease; a sweet and musty smell both on the breath and in urine. It is caused by the excretion of dimethyl disulphide and methyl mercaptan (CH_3SH), arising from an excess of methionine.

2173. For diagnosis of hepatic encephalopathy, which of the following tests has most relevance?

Harrison's 20th Ed. Chapter 337 Page 2413

A. Elevated arterial ammonia level

B. Examination of the cerebrospinal fluid

C. Computed tomography of brain

D. MRI of brain

Elevated arterial ammonia levels have been shown to correlate with outcome in fulminant hepatic failure.

2174. In hepatic encephalopathy, risk of cerebral edema increases with arterial ammonia levels that exceed?

N Engl J Med. 2016;375:1660-70

A. 140 µg per deciliter

B. 240 µg per deciliter

C. 340 µg per deciliter

D. 440 µg per deciliter

The correlation between serum ammonia levels and severity of hepatic encephalopathy appears to be stronger in patients with fulminant hepatic failure, and the risk of cerebral edema increases with arterial ammonia levels that exceed 200 µmol per liter (340 µg per deciliter).

2175. In Greek, sterixis means?

N Engl J Med. 2016;375:1660-70

A. Movement

B. Regular

C. Fixed position

D. Happy

In Greek language sterixis, means "fixed position," The term "asterixis" with the prefix a, meaning "without" denoted an inability to keep outstretched arms and hands in place.

2176. Which of the following is characteristic of the earlier stages of hepatic encephalopathy?

N Engl J Med. 2016;375:1660-70

A. Reduced awareness of surroundings and stimuli

B. Yawning

C. Dozing off

D. All of the above

Reduced awareness of surroundings & stimuli, yawning and dozing off are characteristic of the earlier stages. New irritability & maniacal excitement have also been reported.

2177. Hepatologists have graded severity of hepatic encephalopathy by?

N Engl J Med. 2016;375:1660-70

A. Milan criteria

B. West Haven criteria

C. University of California, San Francisco (UCSF) criteria

D. CURB-65 criteria

2178. Which of the following is a scoring method to grade severity of hepatic encephalopathy?

N Engl J Med. 2016;375:1660-70

A. Full Outline of Unresponsiveness (FOUR) score

B. Glasgow coma score

C. Karnofsky performance scores

D. Agatston score

Full Outline of Unresponsiveness (FOUR) score is more discriminating than the West Haven grading system because it includes brainstem and respiration assessment, which are not further differentiated in the West Haven system.

2179. Restless tossing & muscle or limb twitching seen in progressive hepatic encephalopathy is termed?

N Engl J Med. 2016;375:1660-70

A. Flotation

B. Fragmentation

C. Hypermutation

D. Jactitations

Jactitations refers to restless tossing & muscle or limb twitching common with progressive hepatic encephalopathy and may merge with multifocal myoclonus. Abnormal movements such as dystonia, orofacial dyskinesias, and parkinsonian features favour the diagnosis of Wilson's disease, which in rare cases may be characterized by acute hepatic failure.

2180. Main practical use of EEG in assessing patients for hepatic encephalopathy is to rule out?

N Engl J Med. 2016;375:1660-70

A. Nonconvulsive status epilepticus

B. Multifocal myoclonus

C. Hysterical conversion reaction

D. All of the above

The main practical use of EEG in assessing patients for hepatic encephalopathy is to rule out nonconvulsive status epilepticus.

2181. Outcome in hepatic encephalopathy worsens when which of the following happens in EEG?

N Engl J Med. 2016;375:1660-70

A. Dyssynchronization of fast activity

B. Appearance of triphasic waves

C. Increased dysrhythmicity

D. Slower delta activity

The outcome worsens in the setting of hepatic encephalopathy, once triphasic waves appear. Triphasic-wave patterns appear as generalized, bilaterally synchronous, bifrontal periodic waves, with background slowing. They appear in grade 2 or 3 of hepatic encephalopathy but disappear in comatose state.

2182. Disorders that can mimic the clinical features of hepatic encephalopathy are all except?

N Engl J Med. 2016;375:1660-70

A. Acute alcohol intoxication

B. Sedative overdose

C. Delirium tremens
D. Encephalitis

2183. Disorders that can mimic the clinical features of hepatic encephalopathy are all except?
N Engl J Med. 2016;375:1660-70

A. Wernicke's encephalopathy
B. Korsakoff's psychosis
C. Subdural hematoma
D. Schizophrenia

2184. Disorders that can mimic the clinical features of hepatic encephalopathy are all except?
N Engl J Med. 2016;375:1660-70

A. Meningitis
B. Hypoglycemia
C. Hypocalcemia
D. Wilson's disease

2185. Which of the following disease has hyperammonemia with neuropsychiatric symptoms resembling hepatic encephalopathy?
Harrison's 20th Ed. Chapter 414 Page 3022

A. "Punch-drunk" syndrome
B. Hashimoto's encephalopathy
C. Citrullinemia type 2
D. Posterior reversible encephalopathy syndrome (PRES)

Citrullinemia type 2 usually presents with sudden onset between 20 & 50 years of age with recurring episodes of hyperammonemia with associated neuropsychiatric symptoms such as altered mental status, irritability, seizures or coma resembling hepatic encephalopathy.

2186. Citrullinemia type 2 is caused by molecular defect in?
Harrison's 20th Ed. Chapter 414 Page 3022

A. Dibasic transporter SLC7A7
B. Carnitine transporter OCTN2
C. Mitochondrial apartate/glutamate carrier 2 SLC25A13
D. Lysosomal cystine transporter

Citrullinemia type 2 (Citrin deficiency) is a recessive condition caused by deficiency of mitochondrial aspartate-glutamate carrier AGC2 (citrin). A defect in this transporter reduces availability of cytoplasmic aspartate to combine with citrullin impairing urea cycle & decreasing transfer of reducing equivalents from cytosol to mitochondria through malate-aspartate NADH shuttle. Mutation is in SLC25A13 gene. Presentation is recurring episodes of hyperammonemia with associated neuropsychiatric symptoms like altered mental status, irritability, seizures or coma resembling hepatic encephalopathy. Without therapy, most patients die due to cerebral edema within a few years of onset.

2187. Which of the following is an ammonia scavenger?
N Engl J Med. 2017; 376:186

A. Sodium butyrate
B. Glycerol phenylbutyrate
C. Sodium phenylacetate
D. All of the above

Various ammonia scavengers are sodium butyrate, glycerol phenylbutyrate, sodium phenylacetate and sodium benzoate.

2188. Which of the following about lactulose is false?
Harrison's 20th Ed. Chapter 337 Page 2413

A. Nonabsorbable
B. Disaccharide
C. Leads to colonic acidification
D. None of the above

The mainstay of treatment for encephalopathy is lactulose (25 mL twice daily). It is a nonabsorbable disaccharide, which results in colonic acidification. Consequent catharsis eliminates nitrogenous products in gut that are responsible for the development of encephalopathy.

2189. Goal of lactulose therapy is to promote how many soft stools per day?
Harrison's 20th Ed. Chapter 337 Page 2414

A. 2 - 3
B. 4 - 6
C. 6 - 8
D. 8 - 10

The goal of lactulose therapy is to promote 2 - 3 soft stools per day.

2190. Which of the following has a role in the treatment of hepatic encephalopathy?
Harrison's 20th Ed. Chapter 337 Page 2414

A. Azithromycin
B. Ritonavir
C. Rifaximin
D. Lumefantrine

Rifaximin (550 mg twice daily) is very effective in treating encephalopathy without the known side effects of neomycin (renal insufficiency and ototoxicity) or metronidazole (peripheral neuropathy). Rifaximin is a poorly absorbed rifampin derivative & is highly effective against noninvasive bacterial pathogens (toxigenic & enteroaggregative E. coli).

2191. Supplementation of which of the following is recommended in patients with hepatic encephalopathy?
Harrison's 20th Ed. Chapter 337 Page 2414

A. Copper
B. Zinc
C. Calcium
D. Magnesium

Zinc supplementation is at times helpful in patients with hepatic encephalopathy.

2192. First clotting factor to be depleted in cirrhosis liver is?
Harrison's 20th Ed. Chapter 337 Page 2414

A. Factor V
B. Factor VII
C. Factor VIII
D. Factor IX

2193. In hepatic cirrhosis, which clotting factor is not reduced?
Harrison's 20th Ed. Chapter 337 Page 2414

A. Factor II
B. Factor V
C. Factor VII
D. Factor XI

2194. Reduction in levels of which clotting factor is not worsened by the coincident malabsorption of vitamin K?
Harrison's 20th Ed. Chapter 337 Page 2414

A. Factor II
B. Factor V

C. Factor VII

D. Factor XI

Vitamin K–dependent clotting factors are Factors II, VII, IX, and X. Because of a decrease in hepatic mass, administration of parenteral vitamin K does not improve clotting factors or prothrombin time.

2195. Coagulopathy in liver disease results due to?

Harrison's 20th Ed. Chapter 337 Page 2414

A. Decreased synthesis of clotting factors

B. Impaired clearance of anticoagulants

C. Thrombocytopenia due to hypersplenism

D. All of the above

Coagulopathy is almost universal in patients with cirrhosis. There is decreased synthesis of clotting factors and impaired clearance of anticoagulants. Patients may have thrombocytopenia from hypersplenism due to portal hypertension.

2196. The triad of hepatopulmonary syndrome includes all except?

Harrison's 20th Ed. Chapter 329 Page 2335

A. Liver disease

B. Hypoxemia

C. Hypercarbia

D. Pulmonary arteriovenous shunting

Patients with long-standing cirrhosis and portal hypertension are prone to develop the hepatopulmonary syndrome, defined by the triad of liver disease, hypoxemia, and pulmonary arteriovenous shunting. The defect in oxygenation is due to a ventilation perfusion mismatch.

2197. Hepatopulmonary syndrome is manifested by?

Harrison's 20th Ed. Chapter 329 Page 2335

A. Hypoxemia

B. Platypnea

C. Orthodeoxia

D. All of the above

Hepatopulmonary syndrome is characterized by platypnea and orthodeoxia, representing shortness of breath and oxygen desaturation that occur paradoxically upon assuming an upright position. If the partial pressure of oxygen in arterial blood decreases by 5% or more or by 4 mm Hg (0.5 kPa) or more when the patient moves from a supine to an upright position (called orthodeoxia), he or she may describe worsening dyspnea (platypnea) related to further ventilation perfusion mismatch.

2198. Platypnea is a clinical presentation of?

Harrison's 20th Ed. Chapter 33 Page 227

A. Constrictive pericarditis

B. Budd-Chiari Syndrome

C. Left atrial myxoma

D. HOCM

Platypnea (dyspnea in upright position with relief in supine position) is also a feature of left atrial myxoma. Left atrial myxoma or hepatopulmonary syndrome should be considered when the patient complains of platypnea or dyspnea in upright position with relief in the supine position.

2199. Which of the following is not a part of hepatopulmonary syndrome?

N Engl J Med. 2008;358:2378-87

A. Liver disease

B. Pulmonary vascular dilatation

C. Pulmonary vascular constriction

D. Defect in oxygenation

Hepatopulmonary syndrome has three components - liver disease, pulmonary vascular dilatation, and a defect in oxygenation.

2200. The unique striking pathological feature of hepatopulmonary syndrome is?

N Engl J Med. 2008;358:2378-87

A. Gross dilatation of pulmonary pre- & capillary vessels

B. Absolute increase in number of dilated vessels

C. Pleural & pulmonary arteriovenous shunts

D. All of the above

The unique striking pathological feature of hepatopulmonary syndrome is gross dilatation of pulmonary precapillary & capillary vessels (15 to 100 μm diameter), coupled with an absolute increase in number of dilated vessels. Also, pleural and pulmonary arteriovenous shunts and portopulmonary venous anastomoses can be seen. in a healthy person, diameter of capillary ranges between 8 and 15 μm.

2201. Which of the following has clinical similarities to hepatopulmonary syndrome?

N Engl J Med. 2008;358:2378-87

A. Blue rubber bleb syndrome

B. Chiari malformation

C. Dandy-Walker malformations

D. Type 1 Abernethy malformation

Rare congenital cardiac disorders without liver injury in which either hepatic venous blood flow does not reach the lung or portal venous blood reaches the inferior vena cava without passing through the liver (Type 1 Abernethy malformation) have clinical similarities to hepatopulmonary syndrome. This provides support for the hypothesis that blood from the gut must cross liver to prevent pulmonary vascular dilatation.

Hepatocellular Carcinoma

2202. Which of the following statements is false?
N Engl J Med. 2011;365:1118-27

A. Liver cancer is the fifth most common cancer in men and the seventh in women
B. Highest incidence rates of liver cancer is in regions where infection with hepatitis B virus (HBV) is endemic
C. Hepatocellular carcinoma rarely occurs before 40 years of age
D. Hepatocellular carcinoma incidence reaches a peak at approximately 50 years of age

Hepatocellular carcinoma incidence reaches a peak at approximately 70 years of age. Rates of liver cancer among men are two to four times as high as the rates among women.

2203. Which of the following is associated with a reduced risk of hepatocellular carcinoma?
N Engl J Med. 2011;365:1118-27

A. Coffee drinking
B. Tea drinking
C. Alcohol drinking
D. Tobacco chewing

Studies conducted in Japan and southern Europe found that coffee drinking is associated with a reduced risk of hepatocellular carcinoma. Coffee drinking has also been associated with reduced insulin levels and a reduced risk of type 2 diabetes.

2204. Major risk factors for hepatocellular carcinoma (HCC) include infection with all except?
N Engl J Med. 2011;365:1118-27

A. HBV
B. HCV
C. HIV
D. Alcoholic liver disease

Major risk factors for HCC include infection with HBV or HCV, alcoholic liver disease & nonalcoholic fatty liver disease. Less common causes include hereditary hemochromatosis, alpha 1-antitrypsin deficiency, autoimmune hepatitis, some porphyrias, and Wilson's disease.

2205. Liver cancer comprises of?
Harrison's 20th Ed. Chapter 78 Page 578

A. Hepatocellular carcinoma
B. Intrahepatic cholangiocarcinoma
C. Epithelioid hemangiothelioma
D. All of the above

Liver cancer comprises of hepatocellular carcinoma, intrahepatic cholangiocarcinoma, fibrolamellar HCC, mixed HCCiCCA, epithelioid hemangiothelioma, and pediatric cancer hepatoblastoma.

2206. HCC is less common in cirrhosis associated with?
Harrison's 20th Ed. Chapter 78 Page 578

A. Alcohol abuse
B. Metabolic syndrome
C. Alpha-1 antitrypsin deficiency
D. Hemochromatosis

2207. HCC is less common in cirrhosis associated with?
Harrison's 20th Ed. Chapter 78 Page 578

A. Autoimmune hepatitis
B. Wilson's disease
C. Cholestatic liver disorders
D. All of the above

HCC is less common in cirrhosis associated with alpha-1 antitrypsin deficiency, autoimmune hepatitis, Wilson's disease, and cholestatic liver disorders.

2208. Factor associated with an increased risk of developing HCC is?
Harrison's 20th Ed. Chapter 78 Page 578

A. Hepatitis B or C chronic infection
B. Cirrhosis from any cause
C. Nonalcoholic steatohepatitis (NASH)
D. All of the above

Factor associated with an increased risk of developing HCC include hepatitis, alcohol, autoimmune chronic active hepatitis, cryptogenic cirrhosis and NASH/NAFL. Less common association is with primary biliary cirrhosis and several metabolic diseases including hemochromatosis, Wilson disease, alpha$_1$-antitrypsin deficiency, tyrosinemia, porphyria cutanea tarda, glycogenesis types 1 and 3, citrullinemia. and orotic aciduria.

2209. Predictors of liver cancer development among cirrhotic patients include?
Harrison's 20th Ed. Chapter 78 Page 579

A. Platelet count of <100,000/mm^3
B. Presence of portal hypertension
C. Higher degree of liver stiffness on transient elastography (TE)
D. All of the above

Predictors of liver cancer development among cirrhotic patients is associated with liver disease severity i.e. platelet count of <100,000/mm^3, presence of portal hypertension, degree of liver stiffness as measured by transient elastography (TE), and liver gene signatures capturing the cancer field effect.

2210. Which country has the highest incidence of HCC globally?
Harrison's 20th Ed. Chapter 78 Page 579 Figure 78-2

A. Sudan
B. Egypt
C. Mongolia
D. China

Mongolia has the highest incidence of HCC globally, with 78 cases per 100,000 inhabitants.

2211. Which country has the highest prevalence of HCV infection?
Harrison's 20th Ed. Chapter 78 Page 579 Figure 78-2

A. Sudan
B. Egypt
C. Mongolia
D. China

2212. Aflatoxin B$_1$ is the cause of development of HCC in which country?
Harrison's 20th Ed. Chapter 78 Page 579 Figure 78-2

A. Sudan
B. Egypt

C. Mongolia
D. China

2213. HCC occurrence with HCV infection is greater if?
Harrison's 20th Ed. Chapter 78 Page 579

A. Advanced hepatic fibrosis is present
B. HCV genotype is 1b
C. Polymorphism that activates EGF receptor is present
D. All of the above

2214. Which polymorphism is strongly associated with fatty and alcoholic chronic liver diseases & HCC occurrence?
Harrison's 20th Ed. Chapter 78 Page 580

A. GPIV T13254C
B. PI A2
C. PNPLA3
D. MTHFR C677T

Patatin-like phospholipase domain-containing protein 3 (PNPLA3) polymorphism is strongly associated with fatty and alcoholic chronic liver diseases and HCC occurrence.

2215. Aflatoxin B_1 is related to which of the following pathogen?
Harrison's 20th Ed. Chapter 78 Page 580

A. Aspergillus
B. Nocardia
C. Candida
D. Cryptococcus

Aflatoxin B_1 is a product of the Aspergillus fungus. It is a most potent ubiquitous natural chemical carcinogen producing signature mutations in p53 (mutation of arginine to serine at codon 249) and leads to hepatocellular carcinoma.

2216. Which of the following predispose to HCC development?
Harrison's 20th Ed. Chapter 78 Page 580

A. Infection with adeno-associated virus 2
B. Tobacco
C. Aflatoxin B_1
D. All of the above

2217. Which of the following about HCC is false?
Harrison's 20th Ed. Chapter 78 Page 580

A. Inflammation-associated cancer
B. Mutations in telomere reverse transcriptase (TERT) gene
C. Wnt/β-catenin pathway activation
D. All of the above

In HCC, the most common mutations are in the telomerase reverse transcriptase (TERT) promoter, TP53, CTNNB1, ARID2, ARID1A and AXIN1 genes.

2218. Which of the following genes is mutated in HCC?
Harrison's 20th Ed. Chapter 78 Page 580

A. HER2
B. PIK3CA
C. BRAF
D. None of the above

Solid tumors such as EGFR, HER2, PIK3CA, BRAF, or KRAS are rarely mutated in HCC.

2219. HCV infection & alcohol abuse are significantly associated with which mutation?
Harrison's 20th Ed. Chapter 78 Page 581

A. MLL4
B. CTNNB1
C. CCNE1
D. TP53

HBV integrates into the genome of driver genes, like TERT promoter, MLL4 & cyclin E1 (CCNE1). HCV infection & alcohol abuse are significantly associated with CTNNB1 mutations. TP53 mutations are the most frequent alterations with a specific hotspot of mutation (R249S) in patients with aflatoxin B1 exposure.

2220. Serum "quad" test consists of all except?
Harrison's 20th Ed. Chapter 456 Page 3367

A. α-fetoprotein
B. β human chorionic gonadotropin
C. Inhibin-A
D. Conjugated estriol

Serum "quad" test consists of α-fetoprotein, β human chorionic gonadotropin, inhibin-A & unconjugated estriol.

2221. α-fetoprotein is found in patients of?
Harrison's 20th Ed. Chapter 74 Page 553

A. Germ cell tumor
B. Medullary cancer of the thyroid
C. Hodgkin's disease
D. All of the above

2222. Use of which of the following is associated with a reduced risk of HCC?
Harrison's 20th Ed. Chapter 78 Page 581

A. Coffee consumption
B. Statins
C. Metformin
D. All of the above

2223. Which of the following is recommended as a method of surveillance for HCC?
Harrison's 20th Ed. Chapter 78 Page 581

A. Ultrasonography
B. Computed tomography (CT)
C. Magnetic resonance imaging (MRI)
D. All of the above

2224. Which of the following imaging modality is most recommended for hepatocellular carcinoma surveillance?
Harrison's 20th Ed. Chapter 78 Page 581, N Engl J Med. 2011;365:1118-27

A. Ultrasonographic imaging
B. Computed tomography (CT)
C. Magnetic resonance imaging (MRI)
D. All of the above

CT and MRI are not generally recommended for hepatocellular carcinoma surveillance. Their sensitivity, specificity, and positive and negative predictive values for this purpose are unknown, and their use is associated with high cost as well as possible harm.

2225. Which of the following is of no use in the diagnosis of HCC?

Harrison's 20th Ed. Chapter 78 Page 581

A. Triphasic CT
B. Gadolinium-enhanced MRI
C. Ultrasound
D. PET imaging

Positron emission tomography (PET)-scan performs poorly for early diagnosis.

2226. Serum biomarker that identifies patients with HCC is?

Harrison's 20th Ed. Chapter 78 Page 581

A. Alpha-fetoprotein (AFP)
B. L3 fraction of AFP (AFP-L3)
C. Des-γ carboxyprothrombin (DCP)
D. All of the above

AFP levels ≥ 400 ng/dL are highly suspicious, but not diagnostic of HCC according to guidelines.

2227. Which of the following is a protein induced by vitamin K absence?

J Adv Res. 2013;4(6):539-546

A. PIVKA-I
B. PIVKA-II
C. PIVKA-III
D. PIVKA-IV

Prothrombin induced by vitamin K absence-II (PIVKA-II) is also known as Des-gamma carboxyprothrombin (DCP) is an abnormal prothrombin protein that is increased in the sera of patients with HCC. This protein is increased in as many as 80% of HCC patients but may also be elevated in patients with vitamin K deficiency. It is always elevated after Coumadin use. It may predict for portal vein invasion.

2228. Radiological diagnosis of HCC with a high degree of confidence is established if on contrast-enhanced imaging techniques?

Harrison's 20th Ed. Chapter 78 Page 581

A. Lesion is ≥2 cm in diameter
B. Vascular uptake of the nodule in the arterial phase
C. Washout in the portal venous or delayed phases
D. All of the above

The above radiological pattern captures the hypervascular nature characteristic of HCC and the diagnostic specificity is ~95–100% and a biopsy is not necessary.

2229. For HCC, the most accepted staging system is?

Harrison's 20th Ed. Chapter 78 Page 582

A. Anderson-Clinic-Liver Cancer (ACLC) Classification
B. Barcelona-Clinic-Liver Cancer (BCLC) Classification
C. Cleveland-Clinic-Liver Cancer (CCLC) Classification
D. Detroit-Clinic-Liver Cancer (DCLC) Classification

For HCC, the most accepted staging system is the Barcelona-Clinic-Liver Cancer (BCLC) Classification, which is endorsed by U.S. and European clinical practice guidelines.

2230. Which of the following treatments have improved survival in HCC?

Harrison's 20th Ed. Chapter 78 Page 582

A. Surgical resection, liver transplantation
B. Radiofrequency (RF) ablation, chemoembolization
C. Systemic therapies
D. All of the above

2231. Which of the following drugs is used for systemic therapy of HCC?

Harrison's 20th Ed. Chapter 78 Page 582

A. Sorafenib
B. Regorafenib
C. Lenvatinib
D. All of the above

Agents used for systemic therapy in HCC include sorafenib, regorafenib, lenvatinib, cabozantinib, & ramucirumab. Sorafenib is the standard of care systemic therapy for HCC.

2232. TACE stands for?

N Engl J Med. 2011;365:1118-27

A. Transarterial catheter embolization
B. Transarterial cryoembolization
C. Transarterial chemoembolization
D. Transarterial cavity embolization

Transarterial chemoembolization (TACE) is useful in intermediate-stage hepatocellular carcinoma. TACE improves survival among patients with preserved liver function, particularly those with Child-Pugh class A cirrhosis who do not have extrahepatic metastases, vascular invasion, or prominent cancer-related symptoms.

2233. A typical interval between HCV-associated transfusion and subsequent HCC is approximately?

Harrison's 20th Ed. Chapter 332 Page 2362

A. 10 years
B. 20 years
C. 30 years
D. 40 years

A typical interval between HCV-associated transfusion and subsequent HCC is approximately 30 years. HCV-associated HCC patients tend to have more frequent and advanced cirrhosis, but in HBV-associated HCC, only half the patients have cirrhosis; the remainder having chronic active hepatitis.

2234. Worldwide, chronic HBV infection accounts for what percentage of all cases of hepatocellular carcinoma?

N Engl J Med. 2011;365:1118-27

A. ~ 25%
B. ~ 50%
C. ~ 75%
D. ~ 100%

Worldwide, chronic HBV infection accounts for ~50% of all cases of hepatocellular carcinoma and virtually all childhood cases.

2235. What percentage of patients with HBV-related hepatocellular carcinoma have cirrhosis?

N Engl J Med. 2011;365:1118-27

A. ~ 25%
B. ~ 50%
C. ~ 75%
D. ~ 100%

HBV can cause hepatocellular carcinoma in the absence of cirrhosis. However, majority (70 to 80%) of patients with HBV-related hepatocellular carcinoma have cirrhosis.

2236. Which of the following is a paraneoplastic syndrome in HCC?

N Engl J Med. 2011;365:1118-27

A. Erythrocytosis
B. Hypercalcemia
C. Hypercholesterolemia
D. All of the above

Most paraneoplastic syndromes in HCC are biochemical abnormalities without associated clinical consequences. They include hypoglycemia, erythrocytosis, hypercalcemia, hypercholesterolemia, dysfibrinogenemia, carcinoid syndrome, increased thyroxin-binding globulin, changes in secondary sex characteristics (gynecomastia, testicular atrophy & precocious puberty) & porphyria cutanea tarda.

2237. Which of the following estimations are useful in the surveillance for hepatocellular carcinoma?

N Engl J Med. 2011;365:1118-27

A. Serum alpha-fetoprotein (AFP)

B. Des-gamma-carboxyprothrombin (DCP)

C. Lens culinaris agglutinin-reactive fraction of AFP (AFP-L3)

D. All of the above

Combined measurement of alpha-fetoprotein, with des-gamma-carboxyprothrombin or lectin-bound alpha-fetoprotein, provide limited additional benefit as compared with the measurement of alpha-fetoprotein alone.

2238. Which of the following imaging feature is diagnostic of hepatocellular carcinoma?

N Engl J Med. 2011;365:1118-27

A. Focal hepatic mass >2 cm in diameter in cirrhotics

B. Areas of early arterial enhancement

C. Areas of delayed washout

D. All of the above

In patients with cirrhosis and a focal hepatic mass larger than 2 cm in diameter, areas of early arterial enhancement and delayed washout in venous or delayed phase of four-phase multidetector CT or in dynamic contrast-enhanced MRI have high predictive value for HCC.

2239. Child-Pugh scoring system uses how many clinical measures of liver disease?

N Engl J Med. 2011;365:1118-27

A. 3

B. 4

C. 5

D. 6

The Child-Pugh scoring system uses five clinical measures of liver disease.

2240. How many points in Child-Pugh scoring system denote class A disease?

N Engl J Med. 2011;365:1118-27

A. 5 or 6 points

B. 7 to 9 points

C. 10 to 15 points

D. 16 to 20 points

A sum of 5 or 6 points Child-Pugh scoring system indicate class A disease, 7 to 9 points class B, and 10 to 15 points class C, or the most severe disease.

Liver Transplantation

2241. Who pioneered liver transplantation?

Harrison's 20th Ed. Chapter 338 Page 2414

A. PW Angus
B. Thomas Starzl
C. JA Fishman
D. KF Murray

Pioneered in 1960s by Thomas Starzl at the University of Colorado and, later, at the University of Pittsburgh and by Roy Calne in Cambridge, England, liver transplantation is now performed routinely worldwide. Success measured as 1-year survival has improved from 30% in the 1970s to 90% today.

2242. Routine candidates for liver transplantation are patients with?

Harrison's 20th Ed. Chapter 338 Page 2415

A. Alcoholic cirrhosis
B. Chronic viral hepatitis
C. Primary hepatocellular malignancies
D. All of the above

Routine candidates for liver transplantation are patients with alcoholic cirrhosis, chronic viral hepatitis, and primary hepatocellular malignancies.

2243. Currently, which of the following is the most common indications for liver transplantation in adults?

Harrison's 20th Ed. Chapter 338 Page 2415

A. Fulminant hepatitis
B. Primary sclerosing cholangitis
C. Chronic hepatitis C
D. Primary biliary cirrhosis

Currently, chronic hepatitis C & alcoholic liver disease are the most common indications for liver transplantation, accounting for over 40% of all adult candidates who undergo the procedure.

2244. Which of the following is false about chronic HCV patients after transplantation?

Harrison's 20th Ed. Chapter 338 Page 2415

A. Reinfection in the donor organ is universal
B. Allograft cirrhosis develops in 20–30% at 5 years
C. Cirrhosis occur at a higher frequency beyond 5 years
D. None of the above

2245. Patients with which of the following nonmetastatic primary hepatobiliary tumors have undergone liver transplantation?

Harrison's 20th Ed. Chapter 338 Page 2415

A. Cholangiocarcinoma
B. Hepatoblastoma
C. Angiosarcoma
D. All of the above

Patients with nonmetastatic primary hepatobiliary tumors like primary hepatocellular carcinoma (HCC), cholangiocarcinoma, hepatoblastoma, angiosarcoma, epithelioid hemangioendothelioma, and multiple or massive hepatic adenomata have undergone liver transplantation.

2246. Which of the following hepatic malignancies have a likelihood of recurrence after liver transplantation?

Harrison's 20th Ed. Chapter 338 Page 2415

A. Hepatoblastoma
B. Angiosarcoma
C. Epithelioid hemangioendothelioma
D. Cholangiocarcinoma

2247. Arteriohepatic dysplasia, with paucity of bile ducts, and congenital malformations, including pulmonary stenosis is called?

Harrison's 20th Ed. Chapter 338 Page 2415, Table 338-1

A. Alagille's syndrome
B. Byler's disease
C. Caroli's disease
D. Budd-Chiari syndrome

2248. Intrahepatic cholestasis, progressive liver failure, mental and growth retardation is called?

Harrison's 20th Ed. Chapter 338 Page 2415, Table 338-1

A. Alagille's syndrome
B. Byler's disease
C. Caroli's disease
D. Budd-Chiari syndrome

2249. Multiple cystic dilatations of the intrahepatic biliary tree is called?

Harrison's 20th Ed. Chapter 338 Page 2415, Table 338-1

A. Alagille's syndrome
B. Byler's disease
C. Caroli's disease
D. Budd-Chiari syndrome

2250. The most common indication for transplantation in children is?

Harrison's 20th Ed. Chapter 338 Page 2415

A. Congenital hepatic fibrosis
B. Biliary atresia
C. Crigler-Najjar disease type I
D. Neonatal hepatitis

The most common indication for transplantation in children is biliary atresia.

2251. Postoperative anticoagulation after liver transplantation is essential for which disease?

Harrison's 20th Ed. Chapter 338 Page 2415

A. Autoimmune hepatitis
B. Budd-Chiari syndrome
C. Caroli's disease
D. Nonalcoholic steatohepatitis

Postoperative anticoagulation is essential in patients who undergo transplantation for hepatic vein thrombosis (Budd-Chiari syndrome, underlying myeloproliferative disorders.

2252. Which of the following is not an absolute contraindication for liver transplantation?

Harrison's 20th Ed. Chapter 338 Page 2415

A. Advanced age (>70 years)
B. Metastatic malignancy

C. Active drug abuse

D. Active alcohol abuse

Absolute contraindications for transplantation include life-threatening systemic diseases, uncontrolled extrahepatic bacterial or fungal infections, preexisting advanced cardiovascular or pulmonary disease, multiple uncorrectable life-threatening congenital anomalies, metastatic malignancy, and active drug or alcohol abuse. Advanced age (>70 years) should be considered a relative contraindication.

2253. Cadaver donor livers for liver transplantation are procured primarily from victims of?

Harrison's 20th Ed. Chapter 338 Page 2416

A. Head trauma

B. Jail deaths

C. Suicide deaths

D. Voluntary donors

Cadaver donor livers for transplantation are procured primarily from victims of head trauma.

2254. Which of the following about cadaver donor livers for liver transplantation is false?

Harrison's 20th Ed. Chapter 338 Page 2416

A. Compatibility in ABO blood group is essential

B. Human leukocyte antigen (HLA) matching is not required

C. University of Wisconsin (UW) solution used for preservation

D. None of the above

2255. University of Wisconsin (UW) solution is rich in?

Harrison's 20th Ed. Chapter 338 Page 2416

A. Lactobiotin

B. Parobionate

C. Raffinose

D. Sobrinose

The use of University of Wisconsin (UW) solution is rich in lactobionate & raffinose. It permits extension of cold ischemic time up to 20 hours, preferably 12 hours.

2256. UNOS stands for?

Harrison's 20th Ed. Chapter 338 Page 2416

A. United Network for Organ Selection

B. United Network for Organ Sharing

C. United Network for Organ Surgery

D. United Network for Organ Substitution

UNOS stands for United Network for Organ Sharing. It was adopted in 2002. It is designed to allocate available organs based on regional considerations and recipient acuity.

2257. Liver recipients with what MELD scores experienced higher post-transplantation mortality rates?

Harrison's 20th Ed. Chapter 338 Page 2416

A. < 15

B. < 20

C. < 25

D. < 30

Liver recipients with MELD scores <15 experienced higher post-transplantation mortality rates. The MELD scale is continuous, with 34 levels ranging between 6 and 40. Donor organs usually do not become available unless the MELD score exceeds 20.

2258. Model for End-Stage Liver Disease (MELD) scale uses which of the following variables?

Harrison's 20th Ed. Chapter 338 Page 2416 Table 338-3

A. Bilirubin (mg/100 mL)

B. International normalized ratio (INR)

C. Creatinine (mg/100 mL)

D. All of the above

MELD = 3.78 × $\log_e$ bilirubin (mg/100 mL) ± 11.2 × $\log_e$ international normalized ratio (INR) ± 9.57 × $\log_e$ creatinine (mg/100 mL) + 6.43

2259. Which of the following is an important predictor of survival in liver transplantation candidates?

Harrison's 20th Ed. Chapter 338 Page 2416

A. Serum sodium

B. Serum potassium

C. Serum uric acid

D. Serum creatinine

In 2016, MELD score was modified to include serum sodium which is another important predictor of survival in liver transplantation candidates (MELD-Na score). MELD-Na = MELD + 1.59 x (135 – Na [mEq/L]). There is an increase in mortality by 5% for each millimole decrease in serum sodium between 125 and 140 mmol/L

2260. Pediatric End-Stage Liver Disease (PELD) scale uses which of the following variables?

Harrison's 20th Ed. Chapter 338 Page 2416 Table 338-3

A. Albumin

B. Bilirubin

C. INR

D. All of the above

For children <18 years of age, the Pediatric End-Stage Liver Disease (PELD) scale is used. This scale is based on albumin, bilirubin, INR, growth failure, and age.

2261. The highest priority (status 1) for liver transplantation is?

Harrison's 20th Ed. Chapter 338 Page 2416 Table 338-3

A. Severe acute alcoholic hepatitis

B. Hepatic vein thrombosis

C. Fulminant hepatic failure

D. Primary hepatocellular carcinoma (HCC)

Highest priority (status 1) is reserved for patients with fulminant hepatic failure or primary graft nonfunction.

2262. Disease-specific MELD exceptions include?

Harrison's 20th Ed. Chapter 338 Page 2417

A. Hepatocellular carcinoma (HCC)

B. Portopulmonary hypertension

C. Hepatopulmonary syndrome

D. All of the above

2263. What is the risk of death to the healthy donor in living donor transplantation?

Harrison's 20th Ed. Chapter 338 Page 2417

A. 0.02 - 0.04%

B. 0.06 - 0.1%

C. 0.2 - 0.4%

D. 0.6 - 1.3%

2264. For living donor transplantation, characteristics of the donor includes?

Harrison's 20th Ed. Chapter 338 Page 2417

A. 18 - 60 years old

B. Compatible blood type with the recipient

C. Related genetically or emotionally to the recipient
D. All of the above

Donors for living donor transplantation should be 18 - 60 years old; have a compatible blood type with recipient; have no chronic medical problems or history of major abdominal surgery; should be related genetically or emotionally to recipient; and normal clinical, biochemical, and serologic evaluations.

2265. Which of the following anastomosis is performed last in liver transplantation?
Harrison's 20th Ed. Chapter 338 Page 2417

A. Caval
B. Portal vein
C. Hepatic artery
D. Common bile duct

Caval, portal vein, hepatic artery, and bile duct anastomoses are performed in succession, the last by end-to-end suturing of the donor and recipient common bile ducts.

2266. Which immunosuppressive agent can be given after liver transplantation?
Harrison's 20th Ed. Chapter 338 Page 2417

A. Cyclosporine
B. Tacrolimus
C. Mycophenolic acid
D. All of the above

2267. Which of the following is true about Cyclosporine?
Harrison's 20th Ed. Chapter 338 Page 2417

A. Isolated from Streptomyces tsukubaensis
B. Calcineurin inhibitor (CNI)
C. Nonnucleoside purine metabolism inhibitor
D. Monoclonal antibodies to T cells

Cyclosporine is a calcineurin inhibitor (CNI). It blocks early activation of T cells & is specific for T cell functions that result from the interaction of T cell with its receptor and that involve the calcium-dependent signal transduction pathway. Activity of cyclosporine leads to inhibition of lymphokine gene activation, blocking interleukins 2, 3, and 4, tumor necrosis factor α, and other lymphokines. Cyclosporine also inhibits B cell functions. This process occurs without affecting rapidly dividing cells in the bone marrow, thus reducing frequency of posttransplantation systemic infections.

2268. Which of the following is a macrolide lactone antibiotic?
Harrison's 20th Ed. Chapter 338 Page 2417

A. Cyclosporine
B. Tacrolimus
C. Mycophenolic acid
D. Rapamycin

Tacrolimus is a macrolide lactone antibiotic isolated from a Japanese soil fungus, Streptomyces tsukubaensis.

2269. Which of the following side effects are not present with use of Tacrolimus, but present with use of Cyclosporine?
Harrison's 20th Ed. Chapter 338 Page 2417

A. Nephrotoxicity
B. Hypertension
C. Hirsutism
D. Diabetes mellitus

Tacrolimus does not cause hirsutism or gingival hyperplasia.

2270. Which of the following is used occasionally to help boost tacrolimus levels?
Harrison's 20th Ed. Chapter 338 Page 2418

A. Carbamazepine
B. Rifampin
C. Itraconazole
D. Phenobarbital

Drugs that inhibit cytochrome P450 increase cyclosporine and tacrolimus blood levels. Itraconazole is used occasionally to help boost tacrolimus levels.

2271. Which of the following is a nonnucleoside purine metabolism inhibitor?
Harrison's 20th Ed. Chapter 338 Page 2418

A. Cyclosporine
B. Tacrolimus
C. Mycophenolic acid
D. Rapamycin

Mycophenolic acid, a nonnucleoside purine metabolism inhibitor derived as a fermentation product from several Penicillium species.

2272. Induction or maintenance of immunosuppression in renal dysfunction, which of the following is preferred?
Harrison's 20th Ed. Chapter 338 Page 2418

A. Cyclosporine
B. Tacrolimus
C. Mycophenolic acid
D. Antithymocyte globulin (ATG, thymoglobulin)

2273. Hemolytic uremic syndrome can be associated with?
Harrison's 20th Ed. Chapter 338 Page 2419

A. Cyclosporine
B. Tacrolimus
C. OKT3
D. All of the above

Hemolytic uremic syndrome can be associated with cyclosporine, tacrolimus, or OKT3.

2274. Hepatic artery thrombosis in post-transplantation period is an adverse effect of?
Harrison's 20th Ed. Chapter 338 Page 2419

A. OKT3
B. Sirolimus
C. Antithymocyte globulin
D. Cyclosporine

2275. Which of the following neoplasms appear at increased frequency after liver transplantation?
Harrison's 20th Ed. Chapter 338 Page 2420

A. Carcinoma pancreas
B. Squamous cell carcinoma
C. Carcinoma of lung
D. Carcinoma esophagus

De novo neoplasms appear at increased frequency after liver transplantation, particularly squamous cell carcinomas of the skin.

2276. Which of the following accounts for most of the mortality after liver transplantation?

Harrison's 20th Ed. Chapter 338 Page 2420

A. Hepatic complications
B. Renal failure
C. Cardiovascular disease
D. Cerebrovascular disease

Hepatic complications account for most of the mortality after liver transplantation.

2277. Rejection of the transplanted liver begins how many weeks after surgery?

Harrison's 20th Ed. Chapter 338 Page 2420

A. 1 - 2 weeks
B. 2 - 3 weeks
C. 3 - 4 weeks
D. 4 - 5 weeks

Rejection of the transplanted liver occurs in a proportion of patients, beginning 1–2 weeks after surgery, despite the use of immunosuppressive drugs.

2278. Morphologic features of acute rejection after liver transplantation include?

Harrison's 20th Ed. Chapter 338 Page 2420

A. Mixed portal cellular infiltrate
B. Bile duct injury
C. Endothelial inflammation ("endothelialitis")
D. All of the above

2279. Morphologic features of acute rejection after liver transplantation include?

Harrison's 20th Ed. Chapter 338 Page 2420

A. Progressive cholestasis
B. Vanishing bile duct syndrome
C. Hepatic fibrosis
D. All of the above

Morphologically, chronic rejection after liver transplantation is characterized by progressive cholestasis, focal parenchymal necrosis, mononuclear infiltration, vascular lesions and fibrosis. Also, vanishing bile duct syndrome more common in patients undergoing liver transplantation for autoimmune liver disease.

2280. Survival rate for patients undergoing liver transplantation is?

Harrison's 20th Ed. Chapter 338 Page 2420

A. 55 - 70%
B. 75 - 80%
C. 85 - 90%
D. 95 - 99%

2281. The 5-year survival rate for patients undergoing liver transplantation is?

Harrison's 20th Ed. Chapter 338 Page 2420

A. ~ 40%
B. ~ 50%
C. ~ 60%
D. ~ 70%

Failures within the first 3 months are due to technical complications, postoperative infections, and hemorrhage. Transplant failures after the first 3 months are due to infection, rejection, or recurrent disease (malignancy or viral hepatitis).

2282. Feature of which of the following overlap with those of rejection or posttransplantation bile duct injury?

Harrison's 20th Ed. Chapter 338 Page 2420

A. Autoimmune hepatitis
B. Primary sclerosing cholangitis
C. Primary biliary cirrhosis
D. All of the above

2283. Which of the following do not recur after liver transplantation?

Harrison's 20th Ed. Chapter 338 Page 2420

A. Wilson's disease
B. α1-antitrypsin deficiency
C. Hemophiliacs
D. All of the above

2284. Which of the following recur after liver transplantation?

Harrison's 20th Ed. Chapter 338 Page 2420

A. Hemochromatosis
B. Budd-Chiari syndrome
C. Cholangiocarcinoma
D. All of the above

Diseases of the Gallbladder and Bile Ducts

2285. Electrolyte composition of hepatic bile resembles that of?
Harrison's 20th Ed. Chapter 339 Page 2422

A. Cerebrospinal fluid
B. Blood plasma
C. Lymph
D. Ascitic fluid

Hepatic bile is an isotonic fluid with an electrolyte composition resembling blood plasma.

2286. Total solute concentration of hepatic bile is?
Harrison's 20th Ed. Chapter 339 Page 2422

A. 1 - 2 gram/dL
B. 2 - 3 gram/dL
C. 3 - 4 gram/dL
D. 4 - 5 gram/dL

2287. Total solute concentration of gallbladder bile is?
Harrison's 20th Ed. Chapter 339 Page 2422

A. 5 - 10 gram/dL
B. 10 - 15 gram/dL
C. 15 - 20 gram/dL
D. 20 - 25 gram/dL

The electrolyte composition of gallbladder bile differs from that of hepatic bile because most of the inorganic anions, chloride, and bicarbonate are removed by reabsorption across gallbladder epithelium. As a result of water reabsorption, total solute concentration of bile increases from 3–4 gram/dL in hepatic bile to 10–15 gram/dL in gallbladder bile.

2288. Which of the following is the most abundant solute component of bile?
Harrison's 20th Ed. Chapter 339 Page 2422

A. Bile acids
B. Lecithin and other phospholipids
C. Unesterified cholesterol
D. Albumin

Major solute components of bile are bile acids (80%), lecithin and phospholipids (16%), and unesterified cholesterol (4%).

2289. Human cystic bile does not contain?
World J Gastroenterol 2013;19(42):7341-7360

A. Vitamins
B. Mineral salts
C. Trace elements
D. Triglycerides

Human cystic bile is virtually free of triglycerides.

2290. In the lithogenic state, the cholesterol level in bile can be?
Harrison's 20th Ed. Chapter 339 Page 2422

A. 8 - 10%
B. 12 - 18%
C. 18 - 30%
D. 30 - 40%

In the lithogenic state, the cholesterol value can be 8–10%.

2291. The total daily basal secretion of hepatic bile is?
Harrison's 20th Ed. Chapter 339 Page 2422

A. ~ 50 - 100 mL
B. ~ 100 - 250 mL
C. ~ 250 - 400 mL
D. ~ 500 - 600 mL

The total daily basal secretion of hepatic bile is ~500–600 mL.

2292. Which of the following is synthesized de novo in hepatocyte?
Harrison's 20th Ed. Chapter 339 Page 2422

A. Phospholipids
B. Primary bile acids
C. Cholesterol
D. All of the above

Phospholipids, portion of primary bile acids & some cholesterol are synthesized de novo in hepatocyte.

2293. Which of the following is a secretin-mediated and cyclic AMP–dependent mechanism?
Harrison's 20th Ed. Chapter 339 Page 2422

A. Active transport of bile acids from hepatocytes into bile canaliculi
B. Active transport of other organic anions
C. Cholangiocellular secretion
D. All of the above

Cholangiocellular secretion is a secretin-mediated and cyclic AMP dependent mechanism that results in the secretion of a sodium- and bicarbonate-rich fluid into the bile ducts.

2294. Which of the following is located on the apical plasma membrane of the hepatocyte?
Harrison's 20th Ed. Chapter 339 Page 2422

A. Na^+/taurocholate cotransporter (NTCP, SLC10A1)
B. Organic anion–transporting proteins (OATPs)
C. Anionic conjugate export pump (MRP2, ABCC2)
D. All of the above

2295. Which of the following is a solute carrier (SLC) transporter on basolateral (sinusoidal) end of hepatocyte?
Harrison's 20th Ed. Chapter 339 Page 2422

A. OAT (Organic anion transporter)
B. OCT (Organic cation transporter)
C. NTCP (Na^+/taurocholate co-transporting polypeptide)
D. All of the above

2296. Which of the following is an ATP-binding cassette transporter?
Harrison's 20th Ed. Chapter 339 Page 2422

A. MRP2 (Multidrug resistance protein 2)
B. BSEP (Bile salt export pump)
C. BRCP (Breast cancer resistance protein)
D. All of the above

On the basolateral (sinusoidal) end of hepatocyte, Na^+/taurocholate cotransporter (NTCP, SLC10A1) and the organic anion–transporting proteins (OATPs) are present. On the canalicular apical plasma membrane of hepatocyte, "export pumps" (ATP-binding cassette transport proteins) are present. Bile *salt export pump (BSEP, ABCB11); the anionic conjugate export pump (MRP2, ABCC2), which mediates the canalicular excretion of various amphiphilic conjugates formed by phase II conjugation (e.g., bilirubin mono- and diglucuronides and drugs); the multidrug export pump (MDR1, ABCB1) for hydrophobic cationic compounds; and the phospholipid export pump (MDR3, ABCB4).*

2297. The solute carrier (SLC) families encode membrane proteins that have been identified as?
Current Pharmaceutical Design. 2010;16(2):224

A. Passive transporters
B. Ion coupled transporters
C. Exchangers
D. All of the above

The two most commonly studied membrane transporters include members of the ATP-binding cassette transporters and solute carriers (SLCs). Their prototype representative is organic anion transporting polypeptides (OATP) which mediate the sodium-independent transport.

2298. Which of the following is not a primary bile acid?
Harrison's 20th Ed. Chapter 339 Page 2423

A. Cholic acid
B. Chenodeoxycholic acid
C. Deoxycholate
D. All of the above

2299. The primary bile acids are synthesized from?
Harrison's 20th Ed. Chapter 339 Page 2423

A. Lipopolysaccharide
B. Cholesterol
C. Secondary bile acids
D. Heme

The primary bile acids are cholic acid and chenodeoxycholic acid (CDCA), are synthesized from cholesterol in the liver, conjugated with glycine or taurine, and secreted into the bile. Bile acid synthesis is a major pathway for hepatic cholesterol catabolism. Bile acids are biological detergents that facilitate intestinal absorption of lipids and fat-soluble vitamins.

2300. Which of the following is not a secondary bile acid?
Harrison's 20th Ed. Chapter 339 Page 2423

A. Deoxycholate
B. Ursodeoxycholic acid
C. Lithocholate
D. All of the above

Secondary bile acids are deoxycholate and lithocholate. They are formed in colon as bacterial metabolites of the primary bile acids. Ursodeoxycholic acid (UDCA), a stereoisomer of CDCA, is also a secondary bile acid found in low concentration.

2301. Which of the following is a secondary bile acid?
World J Gastroenterol. 2013;19(42):7341-7360

A. Lithocholic acid
B. Ursodeoxycholic acid
C. Sulfolithocholic acid
D. All of the above

Biliary secondary bile acids are deoxycholic, lithocholic, ursodeoxycholic and sulfolithocholic acids.

2302. Whose name is associated with the discovery of bile acids?
World J Gastroenterol. 2013;19(42):7341-7360

A. Shaffer
B. Strecker
C. Trauner
D. Crawford

In 1848 Strecker discovered bile acids.

2303. In healthy subjects, the ratio of glycine to taurine conjugates in bile is?
Harrison's 20th Ed. Chapter 339 Page 2423

A. ~1 : 1
B. ~2 : 1
C. ~3 : 1
D. ~4 : 1

In healthy subjects, the ratio of glycine to taurine conjugates in bile is ~3:1.

2304. Molecular aggregates (micelles) are formed above what level of critical concentration of bile acids?
Harrison's 20th Ed. Chapter 339 Page 2423

A. ~ 1 mM
B. ~ 2 mM
C. ~ 3 mM
D. ~ 4 mM

2305. Which of the following is false about bile acids?
Harrison's 20th Ed. Chapter 339 Page 2423

A. Detergent-like molecules
B. Above a concentration of ~2 mM form micelles
C. Facilitate normal intestinal absorption of dietary fats
D. None of the above

2306. Passive diffusion for unconjugated bile acids occurs in?
Harrison's 20th Ed. Chapter 339 Page 2423

A. Jejunum
B. Ileum
C. Colon
D. All of the above

2307. Active transport mechanism for conjugated bile acids occurs in?
Harrison's 20th Ed. Chapter 339 Page 2423

A. Jejunum
B. Proximal ileum
C. Distal ileum
D. Colon

Unconjugated, and to a lesser degree conjugated, bile acids are absorbed by passive diffusion along the entire gut. Active transport mechanism for conjugated bile acids (95%) occurs in distal ileum by apical sodium-dependent bile acid transporter (ASBT) located in the brush border membrane.

2308. Enterohepatic circulation includes which of the following?
Harrison's 20th Ed. Chapter 339 Page 2423

A. Reabsorption of bile acids
B. Reconjugation in hepatocytes
C. Resecreted into bile
D. All of the above

Enterohepatic circulation refers to the sequesnce of events i.e. reabsorption of bile acids, rapid reconjugation by hepatocytes, and resecretion into bile.

2309. The normal bile acid pool size is?

Harrison's 20th Ed. Chapter 339 Page 2423

A. ~ 2 - 4 gram
B. ~ 10 - 14 gram
C. ~ 20 - 40 gram
D. ~ 40 - 60 gram

The normal bile acid pool size is ~2 - 4 gram.

2310. Normally, the bile acid pool circulates how many times daily?

Harrison's 20th Ed. Chapter 339 Page 2423

A. ~ 2 - 3 times
B. ~ 3 - 5 times
C. ~ 5 - 10 times
D. ~ 10 - 12 times

Normally, the bile acid pool circulates ~5 - 10 times daily.

2311. Fecal loss of bile acids is about?

Harrison's 20th Ed. Chapter 339 Page 2423

A. 0.2 - 0.4 gram/day
B. 0.8 - 2.4 gram/day
C. 2.4 - 4.4 gram/day
D. 5.2 - 7.4 gram/day

Fecal loss of bile acids is ~ 0.2–0.4 gram/day. Normally, this fecal loss is compensated by an equal daily synthesis of bile acids by liver.

2312. The maximum rate of synthesis by bile acids by liver is?

Harrison's 20th Ed. Chapter 339 Page 2423

A. ~ 2 gram/day
B. ~ 3 gram/day
C. ~ 4 gram/day
D. ~ 5 gram/day

The maximum rate of synthesis by bile acids by liver is ~ 5 gram/day. Synthesis of BAs from cholesterol occurs either via the classical pathway (7α-hydroxylation of cholesterol; CYP7A1) or via the alternate pathway (CYP39A1 or CYP7B1). BAs induce FXR, which inhibits CYP7A1 transcription by activation of SHP (small heterodimer partner) and inhibition of HNF4α transactivation.

2313. Bile acids release fibroblast growth factor 19 (FGF19) in?

Harrison's 20th Ed. Chapter 339 Page 2423

A. Liver
B. Bile ducts
C. Intestine
D. All of the above

Bile acids in intestine release fibroblast growth factor 19 (FGF19) into circulation, which is transported to the liver.

2314. Rate-limiting enzyme that suppresses synthesis of bile acids is?

Harrison's 20th Ed. Chapter 339 Page 2423

A. CYP3A4
B. CYP24A1
C. CYP2C19
D. CYP7A1

Fibroblast growth factor 19 (FGF19) in liver suppresses synthesis of bile acids from cholesterol by inhibiting the rate-limiting enzyme cytochrome P450 7A1 (CYP7A1, cholesterol 7α-hydroxylase) and also promotes gallbladder relaxation.

2315. Which of the following is a acid sensor?

Harrison's 20th Ed. Chapter 339 Page 2423

A. Farnesoid X receptor (FXR)
B. Constitutive androstane receptor (CAR)
C. Pregnane X receptor (PXR)
D. All of the above

The nuclear receptor farnesoid X receptor (FXR) is the master regulator of bile acids (BAs) homeostasis since it transcriptionally drives modulation of BA synthesis, influx, efflux, and detoxification along the enterohepatic axis. FXR is encoded by NR1H4 gene. It is activated by bile acids. The hepatic BSEP (ABCB11) is upregulated by farnesoid X receptor (FXR), a bile acid sensor that also represses bile acid synthesis. FXR regulates the BSEP and MDR3 phospholipid flippase.

2316. Which of the following is a cholesterol transporter?

Harrison's 20th Ed. Chapter 339 Page 2423

A. ABCC2
B. ATP8B1
C. ABCG5/G8
D. ABCB4

ABCG5/G8 are two hemitransporters that function as a couple and constitute the canalicular cholesterol and phytosterol transporter.

2317. Liver X receptor (LXR) best relates to?

Harrison's 20th Ed. Chapter 339 Page 2423

A. Bile acid sensor
B. Oxysterol sensor
C. Intracellular microbial sensor
D. Calcium sensor

The expression of the cholesterol transporter, ABCG5/G8, is upregulated by the liver X receptor (LXR), which is an oxysterol sensor. LXR regulates ABCG5/G8 cholesterol transport protein. Oxysterols are potent regulators of cholesterol synthesis and lipid metabolism. Oxysterols are derived from cholesterol, and the intermediates of the cholesterol and bile acid synthesis pathways by either enzymatic or nonenzymatic oxidations. The most abundant oxysterol in circulation is 27-hydroxycholesterol.

2318. Which of the following nuclear receptors is involved in the regulation of lipogenesis?

Harrison's 20th Ed. Chapter 339 Page 2423

A. Peroxisome proliferator-activated receptors (PPARs)
B. Liver X receptors (LXRs)
C. Farnesoid X receptor (FXR)
D. All of the above

Peroxisome proliferator-activated receptors (PPARs), liver X receptors (LXRs), farnesoid X receptor (FXR) and hepatocyte nuclear factor 4α (HNF4α) are the nuclear receptors involved in the regulation of lipogenesis.

2319. Which of the following is a bile acid-activated nuclear receptor?

Harrison's 20th Ed. Chapter 339 Page 2423

A. Farnesoid X receptor (FXR)
B. Pregnane X receptor (PXR)
C. Vitamin D receptor (VDR)
D. All of the above

Bile acid-activated nuclear receptors, farnesoid X receptor (FXR), pregnane X receptor (PXR), & vitamin D receptor (VDR), play critical roles in regulation of key regulatory genes involved in bile acid metabolism in the liver and intestine.

2320. Cholecystokinin (CCK) is released from?

Harrison's 20th Ed. Chapter 339 Page 2423

A. Stomach mucosa
B. Duodenal mucosa

C. Jejunal mucosa
D. All of the above

2321. Which of the following is a function of cholecystokinin (CCK)?
Harrison's 20th Ed. Chapter 339 Page 2423

A. Powerful contraction of the gallbladder
B. Decreased resistance of the sphincter of Oddi (SOD)
C. Enhanced flow of biliary contents into duodenum
D. All of the above

Major factor controlling evacuation of gallbladder is the peptide hormone cholecystokinin (CCK), which is released from the duodenal mucosa in response to the ingestion of fats & amino acids.

2322. How much is the normal capacity of the gallbladder of bile?
Harrison's 20th Ed. Chapter 339 Page 2423

A. ~ 15 mL
B. ~ 30 mL
C. ~ 45 mL
D. ~ 60 mL

The normal capacity of the gallbladder is ~30 mL of bile.

2323. Phrygian cap best relates to?
Harrison's 20th Ed. Chapter 339 Page 2423

A. Agenesis of the gallbladder
B. Rudimentary or oversized "giant" gallbladders
C. Diverticula of the gallbladder
D. None of the above

In Phrygian cap, a partial or complete septum separates the fundus from the body.

2324. Which of the following about gallstones is false?
Harrison's 20th Ed. Chapter 339 Page 2423

A. Gallstone formation increases after age 50
B. Gallstones are formed because of abnormal bile composition
C. Cholesterol stones account for >90% of all gallstones in West
D. None of the above

2325. >50% content of cholesterol gallstones is?
Harrison's 20th Ed. Chapter 339 Page 2423

A. Cholesterol monohydrate
B. Cholesterol dinohydrate
C. Cholesterol trihydrate
D. Cholesterol tetrahydrate

Cholesterol gallstones usually contain >50% cholesterol monohydrate plus an admixture of calcium salts, bile pigments, proteins and fatty acids.

2326. Pigment stones contain how much cholesterol?
Harrison's 20th Ed. Chapter 339 Page 2423

A. < 20%
B. < 30%
C. < 40%
D. < 50%

Pigment stones are composed primarily of calcium bilirubinate. They contain <20% cholesterol.

2327. Gallstones forming secondary to chronic biliary infection are?
Harrison's 20th Ed. Chapter 339 Page 2423

A. Black colored
B. Brown colored
C. Yellow colored
D. White colored

Gallstones forming secondary to chronic biliary infection are brown colored.

2328. Black gallstones are associated with?
Surgical Clinics of North America. 2008;88(6):1175-1194

A. Chronic hemolytic states
B. Cirrhosis
C. Gilbert syndrome
D. All of the above

Pigment stones are formed by the precipitation of bilirubin in bile, with black stones associated with chronic hemolytic states, cirrhosis, Gilbert syndrome, or cystic fibrosis, and brown stones associated with chronic bacterial or parasitic infections.

2329. Which of the following about gallstones is false?
Harrison's 20th Ed. Chapter 339 Page 2423

A. More frequent in females
B. Major types include cholesterol and pigment stones
C. Hemolytic anemia causes gallstones
D. None of the above

2330. Mixed micelles consist of?
Harrison's 20th Ed. Chapter 339 Page 2423

A. Bile acids
B. Phospholipids (lecithin)
C. Cholesterol
D. All of the above

2331. Mixed micelles are formed due to the action of?
Harrison's 20th Ed. Chapter 339 Page 2423

A. Lipase
B. Bile acids
C. Cholecystokinin (CCK)
D. All of the above

Cholesterol & phospholipids are secreted into bile and are converted into mixed micelles consisting of bile acids, phospholipids, and cholesterol by the action of bile acids.

2332. Higher incidence of gallstones is reported in?
Harrison's 20th Ed. Chapter 339 Page 2423

A. Subtotal gastrectomy
B. Chronic hemolytic disease
C. Octreotide treatment
D. All of the above

2333. Which of the following favor cholesterol gallstone formation?
Harrison's 20th Ed. Chapter 339 Page 2424 Figure 339-1

A. ↑ Cholesterol
B. ↓ Bile acids
C. ↓ Lecithin
D. All of the above

2334. Which of the following favor cholesterol gallstone formation?
Harrison's 20th Ed. Chapter 339 Page 2424 Figure 339-1

A. ↑ ABCG5/G8
B. ↓ CYP7A1
C. ↓ MDR3 (ABCB4)
D. All of the above

2335. Which of the following is called phospholipid export pump?
Harrison's 20th Ed. Chapter 339 Page 2424 Figure 339-1

A. Multidrug resistance protein 1 (MDR1)
B. Multidrug resistance protein 2 (MDR2)
C. Multidrug resistance protein 3 (MDR3)
D. Multidrug resistance protein 4 (MDR4)

2336. Most important mechanism in the formation of lithogenic bile is?
Harrison's 20th Ed. Chapter 339 Page 2423

A. High-caloric and cholesterol-rich diets
B. Genetic factors
C. Increased biliary secretion of cholesterol
D. Gallbladder hypomotility

The most important mechanism in the formation of lithogenic (stone-forming) bile is increased biliary secretion of cholesterol.

2337. Increased biliary secretion of cholesterol may be due to?
Harrison's 20th Ed. Chapter 339 Page 2423

A. Increased activity of HMG-CoA reductase
B. High-caloric and cholesterol-rich diets
C. Clofibrate
D. All of the above

2338. Cholesterol crystal formation requires the presence of?
Surgical Clinics of North America. 2008;88(6):1175-1194

A. Cholesterol supersaturation
B. Accelerated nucleation
C. Gallbladder hypomotility/bile stasis
D. Any of the above

Cholesterol crystal formation requires the presence of one or more of the following: (a) cholesterol supersaturation, (b) accelerated nucleation, or (c) gallbladder hypomotility/bile stasis.

2339. Mutation in which of the following causes defective phospholipid secretion into bile?
Harrison's 20th Ed. Chapter 339 Page 2424

A. CYP7A1
B. MDR3 (ABCB4)
C. ABCG5/G8
D. All of the above

Mutations in the MDR3 (ABCB4) gene (encodes the phospholipid export pump in the canalicular membrane of the hepatocyte) may cause defective phospholipid secretion into bile, resulting in cholesterol supersaturation of bile and formation of cholesterol gallstones in the gallbladder and in the bile ducts.

2340. Which of the following state is associated with gallstones?
Harrison's 20th Ed. Chapter 339 Page 2424

A. Hypersecretion of cholesterol
B. Hyposecretion of bile acids
C. Hyposecretion of phospholipids
D. All of the above

2341. Which of the following state is associated with hypersecretion of cholesterol into bile?
Harrison's 20th Ed. Chapter 339 Page 2424

A. Enhanced conversion of cholic acid to deoxycholic acid
B. Gain of function of the cholesterol transporter ABCG5/G8
C. Increased activity of HMG-CoA reductase
D. All of the above

2342. Nucleating factor of cholesterol monohydrate crystals is?
Harrison's 20th Ed. Chapter 339 Page 2424

A. Mucin
B. Apolipoprotein A-I
C. Apolipoprotein A-II
D. All of the above

Cholesterol monohydrate crystal nucleation & crystal growth occur within the mucin gel layer.

2343. Condition associated with infrequent or impaired gallbladder emptying is?
Harrison's 20th Ed. Chapter 339 Page 2424

A. Fasting
B. Parenteral nutrition
C. Pregnancy
D. All of the above

The incidence of gallstones is increased in conditions associated with infrequent or impaired gallbladder emptying like fasting, parenteral nutrition, pregnancy and drugs that inhibit gallbladder motility.

2344. Biliary sludge contains which of the following?
Harrison's 20th Ed. Chapter 339 Page 2424

A. Lecithin-cholesterol liquid crystals
B. Cholesterol monohydrate crystals
C. Calcium bilirubinate
D. All of the above

Biliary sludge is a thick, mucous material that contains lecithin-cholesterol liquid crystals, cholesterol monohydrate crystals, calcium bilirubinate and mucin gels. Presence of biliary sludge implies supersaturation of bile with either cholesterol or calcium bilirubinate.

2345. Which of the following can occur to biliary sludge?
Harrison's 20th Ed. Chapter 339 Page 2424

A. May disappear and not recur
B. May disappear and reappear
C. May form gallstones
D. All of the above

2346. Gallbladder hypomotility is caused by?
Harrison's 20th Ed. Chapter 339 Page 2424

A. Total parenteral nutrition
B. Pregnancy
C. Oral contraceptives, octreotide
D. All of the above

2347. During pregnancy, gallbladder sludge develops in what proportion of women?
Harrison's 20th Ed. Chapter 339 Page 2425

A. 2 - 3%
B. 5 - 10%
C. 10 - 20%
D. 20 - 30%

During pregnancy, gallbladder sludge develops in 20 - 30% of women and gallstones in 5 - 12%. it is usually asymptomatic and resolves spontaneously after delivery.

2348. In persons with rapid weight reduction through dieting, gallstones develop in what proportion of persons?
Harrison's 20th Ed. Chapter 339 Page 2425

A. 2 - 3%
B. 5 - 10%
C. 10 - 20%
D. 20 - 30%

~10–20% of persons with rapid weight reduction through very-low-calorie dieting develop gallstones. 600 mg/day of UDCA is highly effective in preventing gallstone formation.

2349. Pigment stones develop in which of the following conditions?
Harrison's 20th Ed. Chapter 339 Page 2425 Table 339-1

A. Primary biliary cirrhosis
B. Alcoholic liver cirrhosis
C. Genetic defect of the CYP7A1 gene
D. Clofibrate therapy

2350. Pigment stones develop in which of the following conditions?
Harrison's 20th Ed. Chapter 339 Page 2425 Table 339-1

A. Pernicious anemia
B. Cystic fibrosis
C. Ileal disease, ileal resection or bypass
D. All of the above

2351. Which of the following is false about biliary sludge?
Harrison's 20th Ed. Chapter 339 Page 2425

A. Material of low echogenic activity
B. In the most dependent position of the gallbladder
C. Shifts with postural changes
D. Produces acoustic shadowing

On USG, biliary sludge has low echogenic activity. It forms a layer in the most dependent position of gallbladder. This layer shifts with postural changes but does not produce acoustic shadowing.

2352. Which of the following about biliary colic is false?
Harrison's 20th Ed. Chapter 339 Page 2426

A. Intermittent
B. May persist with severe intensity for 30 minutes to 5 hours
C. Nocturnal
D. Precipitated by eating a fatty meal

Biliary colic begins quite suddenly and may persist with severe intensity for 30 minutes to 5 hours, subsiding gradually or rapidly. It is steady rather than intermittent. Pain persisting beyond 5 hours should raise the suspicion of acute cholecystitis.

2353. Biliary colic pain may radiate to?
Harrison's 20th Ed. Chapter 339 Page 2426

A. Interscapular area
B. Right scapula
C. Shoulder
D. All of the above

2354. Patients with gallstones remaining asymptomatic for how many years are unlikely to develop symptoms during follow up?
Harrison's 20th Ed. Chapter 339 Page 2426

A. 5 years
B. 10 years
C. 15 years
D. 20 years

Patients with gallstones remaining asymptomatic for 15 years are unlikely to develop symptoms during further follow-up.

2355. Prophylactic cholecystectomy is recommended in?
Harrison's 20th Ed. Chapter 339 Page 2427

A. Gallstones >3 cm in diameter
B. Gallstones in a congenitally anomalous gallbladder
C. Young patients with silent gallstones
D. All of the above

2356. Which of the following about gallstone treatment is false?
Harrison's 20th Ed. Chapter 339 Page 2427

A. Radiolucent stones <10 mm dissolve with UDCA therapy
B. Pigment stones are not responsive to UDCA therapy
C. Dose of UDCA is 10–15 mg/kg per day
D. None of the above

2357. Ursodeoxycholic acid (UDCA) is recommended in which of the following conditions?
Harrison's 20th Ed. Chapter 339 Page 2427

A. Primary biliary cholangitis (PBC)
B. Primary Sclerosing Cholangitis
C. Cholangiocarcinoma
D. All of the above

2358. Chemical inflammation in acute cholecystitis best relates to?
Harrison's 20th Ed. Chapter 339 Page 2427

A. Isolecithin
B. Lysolecithin
C. Phylolecithin
D. All of the above

In acute cholecystitis, chemical inflammation is caused by the release of lysolecithin due to the action of phospholipase on lecithin in bile.

2359. Cholecystectomy is recommended in porcelain gallbladder because of the increased risk of?
Harrison's 20th Ed. Chapter 339 Page 2429

A. Perforation
B. Carcinoma
C. Chronic infection
D. All of the above

2360. Biliary obstruction due to extrinsic compression of the ducts is mostly because of?
Harrison's 20th Ed. Chapter 339 Page 2431

A. Carcinoma of the head of the pancreas
B. Lymphoma
C. Metastatic carcinoma
D. Hepatocellular carcinoma

2361. Low phospholipid-associated cholelithiasis (LPAC) is best related to?
Orphanet J Rare Dis. 2007; 2:29

A. ABCB1
B. ABCB2
C. ABCB3
D. ABCB4

Low phospholipid-associated cholelithiasis (LPAC) is characterized by the association of ABCB4 mutations and low biliary phospholipid concentration with symptomatic and recurring cholelithiasis.

Approach to the Patient with Pancreatic Disease

2362. The mortality rate of acute pancreatitis is?
Harrison's 20th Ed. Chapter 340 Page 2433

A. ~ 1%
B. ~ 2%
C. ~ 3%
D. ~ 4%

The incidence of acute pancreatitis is ~5 - 35 per 100,000 new cases per year worldwide, with a mortality rate of about 3%.

2363. In US, which of the following is the most common gastrointestinal diagnosis requiring hospitalization?
Harrison's 20th Ed. Chapter 340 Page 2433

A. Peptic ulcer disease
B. Ulcerative colitis
C. Acute pancreatitis
D. Acute cholecystitis

In USA, acute pancreatitis is the most common gastrointestinal diagnosis requiring hospitalization.

2364. How much of pancreas must be damaged before maldigestion of fat and protein is manifested?
Harrison's 20th Ed. Chapter 340 Page 2433

A. ~ 25%
B. ~ 50%
C. ~ 75%
D. ~ 90%

Pancreas has a large secretory reserve capacity. > 90% of pancreas must be damaged before maldigestion of fat & protein is manifested.

2365. Which of the following is the enzyme measurement of choice for diagnosis of acute pancreatitis?
Harrison's 20th Ed. Chapter 340 Page 2434 Table 340-1

A. Serum lipase
B. Serum lipase amylase
C. Urine amylase
D. Fecal elastase

Lipase is the single best enzyme to measure for the diagnosis of acute pancreatitis.

2366. In acute pancreatitis, serum amylase rises within?
Harrison's 20th Ed. Chapter 340 Page 2433

A. 24 hours
B. 36 hours
C. 48 hours
D. 72 hours

2367. In acute pancreatitis, serum amylase remains elevated for?
Harrison's 20th Ed. Chapter 340 Page 2433

A. 1 - 3 days
B. 3 - 7 days
C. 7 - 9 days
D. 9 - 14 days

In acute pancreatitis, the serum amylase is usually elevated within 24 hours of onset and remains so for 3 - 7 days. Levels usually return to normal within 7 days unless there is pancreatic ductal disruption, ductal obstruction, or pseudocyst formation.

2368. Patients with proven pancreatitis have spuriously low levels of amylase in?
Harrison's 20th Ed. Chapter 340 Page 2433

A. Incomplete ductal obstruction
B. Pseudocyst formation
C. Hypertriglyceridemia
D. All of the above

Serum amylase level may be normal if hypertriglyceridemia is present.

2369. Amylase is not found in which of the followng?
Harrison's 20th Ed. Chapter 340 Page 2433

A. Fallopian tubes
B. Thyroid
C. Tonsils
D. Cornea

In addition to pancreas & salivary glands, small quantities of amylase are found in the tissues of fallopian tubes, lung, thyroid, and tonsils.

2370. Hyperamylasemia is found in?
Harrison's 20th Ed. Chapter 340 Page 2436, Table 340-2

A. Acute Pancreatitis
B. Diabetic ketoacidosis
C. Perforated peptic ulcer
D. All of the above

2371. Hyperamylasemia is found in which of the following?
Harrison's 20th Ed. Chapter 340 Page 2436, Table 340-2

A. Carcinoma of lung
B. Carcinoma of esophagus
C. Breast carcinoma
D. All of the above

"Tumor" hyperamylasemia is seen in Carcinoma of lung, Carcinoma of esophagus, Breast carcinoma and ovarian carcinoma.

2372. Hyperamylasemia is found in which of the following?
Harrison's 20th Ed. Chapter 340 Page 2436, Table 340-2

A. Pregnancy
B. Aortic aneurysm
C. Morphine
D. All of the above

2373. Abdominal disorder that can simulate pancreatitis is?
Harrison's 20th Ed. Chapter 340 Page 2434

A. Intestinal obstruction
B. Intestinal infarction

C. Perforated peptic ulcer
D. All of the above

2374. Which of the following blood test is reliable for diagnosis of acute pancreatitis in patients with renal failure?
Harrison's 20th Ed. Chapter 340 Page 2434

A. Serum amylase
B. Serum lipase
C. Serum trypsinogen
D. None of the above

No single blood test is reliable for the diagnosis of acute pancreatitis in patients with renal failure. Trypsinogen, amylase & lipase are excreted by kidney therefore are elevated in renal failure.

2375. The recommended screening test for acute pancreatitis in renal disease is?
Harrison's 20th Ed. Chapter 340 Page 2434

A. Serum lipase
B. Serum amylase
C. Serum trypsinogen
D. None of the above

The recommended screening test for acute pancreatitis in renal disease is serum lipase. Also, serum lipase is the single best enzyme to measure for the diagnosis of acute pancreatitis.

2376. Serum amylase levels are elevated when creatinine clearance is less than?
Harrison's 20th Ed. Chapter 340 Page 2434

A. < 100 mL/minute
B. < 85 mL/minute
C. < 75 mL/minute
D. < 50 mL/minute

Serum amylase levels are elevated in patients with renal dysfunction when creatinine clearance is < 50 mL/minute. They are invariably <500 IU/L in the absence of acute pancreatitis.

2377. In acute pancreatitis, serum amylase values are highly specific if they are more than?
Harrison's 20th Ed. Chapter 340 Page 2434

A. Two times normal
B. Three times normal
C. Four times normal
D. Five times normal

In acute pancreatitis, serum amylase values > 3 times normal are highly specific.

2378. Which of the following is a finding of acute pancreatitis by Computed tomography (CT)?
Harrison's 20th Ed. Chapter 340 Page 2435

A. Enlargement of the pancreatic outline
B. Distortion of the pancreatic contour
C. Pancreatic fluid with different attenuation coefficient than normal pancreas
D. All of the above

The major benefit of CT in acute pancreatitis is the diagnosis of pancreatic necrosis in patients not responding to conservative management within 72 hours

2379. What is the incidence of post-ERCP pancreatitis?
Harrison's 20th Ed. Chapter 340 Page 2435

A. 1 - 5%
B. 5 - 10%
C. 10 - 15%
D. 15 - 20%

2380. Which of the following can be performed by endoscopic ultrasonography?
Harrison's 20th Ed. Chapter 340 Page 2435

A. HR imaging of pancreatic parenchyma and pancreatic duct
B. Pancreatic biopsy
C. Nerve-block anesthesia
D. All of the above

2381. Which of the following is not included in the endoscopic ultrasonographic criteria for chronic pancreatitis?
Harrison's 20th Ed. Chapter 340 Page 2436 Table 340-3

A. Main duct irregularity
B. Visible side branches
C. Main duct dilatation
D. Main duct not visible

2382. Which of the following is included in the endoscopic ultrasonographic criteria for chronic pancreatitis?
Harrison's 20th Ed. Chapter 340 Page 2436 Table 340-3

A. Echogenic strands
B. Echogenic foci
C. Lobular contour
D. All of the above

Criteria for ductal imaging includes: Stones, Hyperechoic main duct margins, Main duct irregularity, Main duct dilatation and Visible side branches. Criteria for parenchymal imaging includes: Echogenic strands, Echogenic foci, Lobular contour and Cyst. Presence of five or more of the nine criteria is highly predictive of chronic pancreatitis.

2383. Which of the following statements is false?
Harrison's 20th Ed. Chapter 340 Page 2436

A. Secondary ducts are not visualized in normal pancreas by MRI
B. Secretin-enhanced MRCP is better to evaluate ductal changes
C. T2 imaging can differentiate necrotic debris from fluid
D. T2 imaging can diagnose hemorrhage

2384. ERCP in today's time is meant for?
Harrison's 20th Ed. Chapter 340 Page 2436

A. Clarification of equivocal findings of imaging techniques
B. Primarily of therapeutic value
C. Should not be done for diagnostic purposes
D. All of the above

2385. Double-duct sign best relates to?
Harrison's 20th Ed. Chapter 340 Page 2436

A. Acute pancreatitis
B. Chronic pancreatitis
C. Pancreatic carcinoma
D. All of the above

Pancreatic carcinoma is characterized by stenosis or obstruction of either pancreatic duct or common bile duct. Double-duct sign is present when both ductal systems are abnormal.

2386. In the Cambridge classification, mild chronic pancreatitis is defined as?

World J Gastroenterol. 2008;14(8):1218-1221

A. Normal main pancreatic duct
B. > 3 abnormal side branches
C. No cysts
D. All of the above

2387. In the Cambridge classification, severe chronic pancreatitis is defined as?

World J Gastroenterol. 2008;14(8):1218-1221

A. Gross irregularity of main pancreatic duct
B. Intraductal calculus
C. Large cysts > 10 mm
D. All of the above

2388. Which of the following can decrease the incidence of ERCP-induced pancreatitis?

Harrison's 20th Ed. Chapter 340 Page 2436

A. Glucose-Insulin therapy
B. Methylprednisolone
C. Octreotide
D. Rectal indomethacin

Elevated serum amylase after ERCP occur in majority of patients and clinical pancreatitis in 5 to 10% of patients. Pancreatic duct stenting & rectal indomethacin can decrease incidence of ERCP-induced pancreatitis.

2389. Which of the following is false about secretin test?

Harrison's 20th Ed. Chapter 340 Page 2436

A. Pancreatic ductal secretory function test
B. Synthetic human secretin is given IV, 0.2 μg/kg as a bolus
C. Maximal bicarbonate concentration is most useful variable
D. None of the above

2390. Normal value for the standard secretin test is?

Harrison's 20th Ed. Chapter 340 Page 2436

A. Volume output > 2 mL / kg per hour
B. Bicarbonate concentration > 80 mmol / L
C. Bicarbonate output > 10 mmol / L in 1 hour
D. All of the above

In the standard assay, secretin is given IV in a dose of 0.2 μg/kg of synthetic human secretin as a bolus.

2391. What solid fecal level of elastase-1 activity (FE-1) is definitive for pancreatic exocrine insufficiency (PEI)?

Harrison's 20th Ed. Chapter 340 Page 2436

A. < 50 μg/gram
B. < 100 μg/gram
C. < 150 μg/gram
D. < 200 μg/gram

FE-1 levels >200 μg/gram are normal. Fecal levels <50 μg/gram are definitive for pancreatic exocrine insufficiency (PEI).

2392. The newer lipase assays relate best to which of the following?

Harrison's 20th Ed. Chapter 341 Page 2437

A. Trypsin
B. Chymotrypsin
C. Colipase
D. Phospholipase A_2

Lipase is the single best enzyme to measure for diagnosis of acute pancreatitis. The newer lipase assays have colipase as a cofactor and are fully automated.

2393. Enzyme trypsinogen is present in which of the following?

Harrison's 20th Ed. Chapter 341 Page 2437

A. Gallbladder
B. Pancreas
C. Intestine
D. All of the above

Pancreas is the only organ that contains trypsinogen.

2394. "Sentinel loop" refers to a localized ileus of which part of intestine in acute pancreatitis?

N Engl J Med. 1954; 251(13):497

A. Duodenum
B. Jejunum
C. Ileum
D. Colon

"Sentinel loop" refers to a localized ileus of jejunum in acute pancreatitis. A sentinel loop is a short segment of adynamic ileus close to an intra-abdominal inflammatory process. The sentinel loop sign may aid in localising the source of inflammation. For example, a sentinel loop in the upper abdomen may indicate pancreatitis, while one in the right lower quadrant may be due to appendicitis.

2395. "Colon cutoff sign" refers to isolated distention of which part of intestine in acute pancreatitis?

N Engl J Med. 2018; 378:1621

A. Ascending colon
B. Transverse colon
C. Descending colon
D. Sigmoid colon

Abrupt termination of gas within the descending colon is referred to as a colon cutoff sign. The colon cutoff sign is classically described in association with acute pancreatitis, when inflammation causes spasm or narrowing at the splenic flexure and isolated distention of transverse colon.

2396. In chronic pancreatitis, pancreatic calcification on radiological examination is superimposed on which lumbar vertebra?

World J Gastrointest Pathophysiol. 2014;5(3):252-270

A. I
B. II
C. III
D. IV

In chronic pancreatitis, radiographic pancreatic calcification is superimposed on 2nd lumbar vertebra.

Acute and Chronic Pancreatitis

2397. The quantity of pancreatic secretion per day is?
Harrison's 20th Ed. Chapter 341 Page 2437

A. 1000 - 1500 ml
B. 1500 - 3000 ml
C. 3000 - 4500 ml
D. About 5000 ml

2398. The pancreatic secretion contain about?
Harrison's 20th Ed. Chapter 341 Page 2437

A. 10 enzymes and zymogens
B. 20 enzymes and zymogens
C. 30 enzymes and zymogens
D. 40 enzymes and zymogens

2399. The pancreatic secretion is?
Harrison's 20th Ed. Chapter 341 Page 2437

A. Isosmotic alkaline
B. Isosmotic acidic
C. Hyposmotic alkaline
D. Hyposmotic acidic

Pancreas secretes 1500 - 3000 mL of isosmotic alkaline (pH > 8.0) fluid / day containing ~20 enzymes & zymogens.

2400. Which of the following about secretin is false?
Harrison's 20th Ed. Chapter 341 Page 2437

A. Gastric acid is a stimulus for release of secretin
B. Secretin is a peptide with 27 amino acids
C. pH threshold for release of secretin from duodenum & jejunum is 6.5
D. Secretin stimulates secretion of pancreatic juice rich in water & electrolytes

2401. Which of the following cells of the duodenal mucosa secrete secretin?
Harrison's 20th Ed. Chapter 341 Page 2437

A. S cells
B. T cells
C. U cells
D. V cells

Gastric acid is the stimulus for the release secretin from the duodenal mucosa (S cells) which in turn stimulates the secretion of water and electrolytes from pancreatic ductal cells.

2402. Ito cells are located in?
Harrison's 20th Ed. Chapter 341 Page 2437

A. Gastric antral mucosa
B. Proximal jejunal mucosa
C. Distal jejunal mucosa
D. Proximal ileal mucosa

Cholecystokinin (CCK) is released from the duodenal and proximal jejunal mucosa (Ito cells).

2403. Which of the following essential amino acids trigger release of Cholecystokinin (CCK)?
Harrison's 20th Ed. Chapter 341 Page 2437

A. Tryptophan
B. Phenylalanine
C. Methionine
D. All of the above

Essential amino acids - tryptophan, phenylalanine, valine and methionine trigger release of Cholecystokinin (CCK).

2404. Which of the following about cholecystokinin (CCK) is false?
Harrison's 20th Ed. Chapter 341 Page 2437

A. CCK evokes an enzyme-rich secretion from pancreas
B. Release of CCK is triggered by short-chain fatty acids
C. Release of CCK is triggered by essential amino acids
D. Release of CCK is triggered by gastric acid

Release of CCK from duodenum & jejunum is triggered by long-chain fatty acids, essential amino acids (tryptophan, phenylalanine, valine, methionine), and gastric acid itself.

2405. Which of the following statements is false?
Harrison's 20th Ed. Chapter 341 Page 2437

A. Bile salts stimulate pancreatic secretion
B. Parasympathetic nervous system exerts significant control over pancreatic secretion
C. Vasoactive intestinal peptide (VIP) is a CCK agonist
D. H_2O and HCO_3^- secretion by pancreas is dependent secretin and CCK

Vagal stimulation leads to release of VIP which is a secretin agonist.

2406. The quantity of bicarbonate from pancreas needed to neutralize gastric acid is?
Harrison's 20th Ed. Chapter 341 Page 2437

A. 20 to 30 mmol/day
B. 50 to 100 mmol/day
C. 120 to 300 mmol/day
D. About 500 mmol/day

2407. In acini and in ducts, which hormone causes the cells to add water and bicarbonate to pancreatic fluid?
Harrison's 20th Ed. Chapter 341 Page 2437

A. Insulin
B. Secretin
C. Somatostatin
D. Gastrin

Gastric acid is the stimulus for release of secretin which stimulates secretion of pancreatic juice rich in water and electrolytes. CCK evokes an enzyme-rich secretion from the pancreas.

2408. How much exocrine function of pancreas must be lost before secretin stimulation test is abnormal?
Harrison's 20th Ed. Chapter 341 Page 2437

A. ~ 15%
B. ~ 20%

C. ~ 40%
D. ~ 60%

Secretin stimulation test for assessing pancreatic exocrine function is abnormal when >60% of exocrine function has been lost.

2409. Which of the following is an inhibitory neuropeptide?
Harrison's 20th Ed. Chapter 341 Page 2437

A. Somatostatin
B. Neuropeptide Y
C. Calcitonin gene - related peptides
D. All of the above

2410. Pancreatic exocrine secretion is influenced by?
Harrison's 20th Ed. Chapter 341 Page 2437

A. Somatostatin
B. Neuropeptide Y
C. Calcitonin gene - related peptides
D. All of the above

Pancreatic exocrine secretion is influenced by inhibitory neuropeptides like somatostatin, pancreatic polypeptide, peptide YY, neuropeptide Y, enkephalin, pancreastatin, calcitonin gene–related peptides, glucagon, and galanin.

2411. Which of the following correlates best between stimulation with secretin and the pancreatic mass?
Harrison's 20th Ed. Chapter 341 Page 2437

A. Maximal sodium output
B. Maximal chloride output
C. Maximal acid output
D. Maximal bicarbonate output

2412. Bicarbonate in pancreatic secretion is related to?
Harrison's 20th Ed. Chapter 341 Page 2437

A. Insulin
B. Glucagon
C. Cystic fibrosis transmembrane conductance regulator
D. All of the above

2413. Which of the following plays an important role in ductal cell secretion?
Harrison's 20th Ed. Chapter 341 Page 2437

A. CCK
B. Secretin and VIP
C. Acetylcholine
D. All of the above

Bicarbonate enters the duct lumen through the sodium bicarbonate cotransporter with depolarization caused by chloride efflux through the cystic fibrosis transmembrane conductance regulator (CFTR). Secretin and VIP bind at the basolateral surface and cause an increase in secondary messenger intracellular cyclic AMP, and act on the apical surface of the ductal cells opening the CFTR in promoting secretion. CCK, acting as a neuromodulator, markedly potentiates the stimulatory effects of secretin. Acetylcholine also plays an important role in ductal cell secretion.

2414. Pancreas secretes which of the following enzymes?
Harrison's 20th Ed. Chapter 341 Page 2437

A. Amylolytic
B. Lipolytic
C. Proteolytic
D. All of the above

The pancreas secretes amylolytic, lipolytic, and proteolytic enzymes.

2415. The lipolytic enzymes secreted by pancreas are?
Harrison's 20th Ed. Chapter 341 Page 2437

A. Lipase
B. Phospholipase A
C. Cholesterol esterase
D. All of the above

Lipolytic enzymes secreted by pancreas include lipase, phospholipase A & cholesterol esterase.

2416. Which of the following about bile salts is false?
Harrison's 20th Ed. Chapter 341 Page 2437

A. Inhibit lipase in isolation
B. Colipase binds to lipase & prevents inhibition by bile salts
C. Activate phospholipase A and cholesterol esterase
D. None of the above

Bile salts inhibit lipase in isolation, but colipase of pancreatic secretion, binds to lipase and prevents this inhibition. Bile salts activate phospholipase A and cholesterol esterase.

2417. Which of the following statements is false?
Harrison's 20th Ed. Chapter 341 Page 2437

A. Bile salts inhibit lipase
B. Colipase binds to lipase
C. Bile salts activate phospholipase A & cholesterol esterase
D. None of the above

Bile salts inhibit lipase. Colipase in pancreatic secretion binds to lipase and prevents this inhibition. Bile salts activate phospholipase A and cholesterol esterase.

2418. Proteolytic enzymes secreted as inactive precursors are called?
Harrison's 20th Ed. Chapter 341 Page 2437

A. Zymogens
B. Proteogens
C. Amylogens
D. Chymogens

Proteolytic enzymes are secreted as inactive precursors called zymogens.

2419. Which of the following is an endopeptidase?
Harrison's 20th Ed. Chapter 341 Page 2437

A. Carboxypeptidases
B. Aminopeptidases
C. Chymotrypsin
D. Elastase

Proteolytic enzymes include endopeptidases, exopeptidases and elastase. Endopeptidases like trypsin & chymotrypsin act on internal peptide bonds of proteins and polypeptides. Exopeptidases are carboxypeptidases & aminopeptidases, which act on the free carboxyl- and amino-terminal ends of peptides, respectively.

2420. Enzyme that cleaves lysine-isoleucine bond of trypsinogen to form trypsin is?
Harrison's 20th Ed. Chapter 341 Page 2437

A. Duodenokinase
B. Enterokinase

C. Gastrokinase
D. Trypsokinase

2421. Bond that is cleaved to form trypsin from trypsinogen is?
Harrison's 20th Ed. Chapter 341 Page 2437

A. Lysine-isoleucine bond
B. Arginine-Threonine bond
C. Arginine-Lysine bond
D. Threonine-Lysine bond

2422. Enzyme enterokinase is found in?
Harrison's 20th Ed. Chapter 341 Page 2437

A. Gastric mucosa
B. Duodenal mucosa
C. Jejunal mucosa
D. Ileal mucosa

Enterokinase is an enzyme found in duodenal mucosa. It cleaves lysine-isoleucine bond of trypsinogen to form trypsin.

2423. Which of the following is the pH optima range of pancreatic enzymes?
Harrison's 20th Ed. Chapter 341 Page 2437

A. 7.1 to 7.2
B. 7.2 to 7.3
C. 7.3 to 7.4
D. 7.4 to 7.5

All pancreatic enzymes have pH optima in the alkaline range.

2424. Which of the following initiates pancreatic enzyme secretion?
Harrison's 20th Ed. Chapter 341 Page 2437

A. Acetylcholine
B. VIP
C. CCK
D. Secretin

The nervous system initiates pancreatic enzyme secretion. Neurologic stimulation is cholinergic, involving extrinsic innervation by vagus nerve & subsequent innervation by intrapancreatic cholinergic nerves. Stimulatory neurotransmitters are acetylcholine & gastrin-releasing peptides. These neurotransmitters activate calcium-dependent secondary messenger systems, resulting in the release of zymogens into pancreas duct.

2425. VIP in intrapancreatic nerves potentiates the effect of?
Harrison's 20th Ed. Chapter 341 Page 2437

A. Acetylcholine
B. Enterokinase
C. CCK
D. Secretin

VIP is present in intrapancreatic nerves and potentiates the effect of acetylcholine.

2426. In humans, receptors of which of the following are absent on acinar cells?
Harrison's 20th Ed. Chapter 341 Page 2437

A. Acetylcholine
B. Gastrin-releasing peptides
C. CCK
D. VIP

In contrast to other species, there are no CCK receptors on acinar cells in humans. CCK in physiologic concentrations stimulates pancreatic secretion by stimulating afferent vagal and intrapancreatic nerves.

2427. Which of the following can lyse and inactivate trypsin?
Harrison's 20th Ed. Chapter 341 Page 2437

A. Mesotrypsin
B. Chymotrypsin C
C. Enzyme Y
D. All of the above

Mesotrypsin, chymotrypsin C, and enzyme Y can also lyse and inactivate trypsin.

2428. Protease inhibitors are found in?
Harrison's 20th Ed. Chapter 341 Page 2438

A. Pancreatic acinar cells
B. Pancreatic secretions
C. a_1- and a_2-globulin fractions of plasma
D. All of the above

Protease inhibitors, that prevent autodigestion of pancreas, are found in the acinar cells, the pancreatic secretions, and the a_1- and a_2-globulin fractions of plasma.

2429. Autodigestion of the pancreas is prevented by which of the following?
Harrison's 20th Ed. Chapter 341 Page 2438

A. Low intracellular sodium in cytosol of acinar cell
B. Low intracellular potassium in cytosol of acinar cell
C. Low intracellular calcium in cytosol of acinar cell
D. Low intracellular chloride in cytosol of acinar cell

Low intracellular calcium in the cytosol of the acinar cell promotes the destruction of spontaneously activated trypsin.

2430. Kazal type 1 (SPINK1) is best related to?
Lancet 2008;371:143-52

A. Pancreatic hyperstimulation
B. Alcohol abuse
C. Anti-inflammatory cytokine
D. Serine protease inhibitor

Autodigestion of the pancreas is prevented by the packaging of proteases in precursor form and by the synthesis of protease inhibitors, i.e., pancreatic secretory trypsin inhibitor (PSTI) and serine protease inhibitor, kazal type 1 (SPINK1) that prevents conversion of trypsinogen to trypsin.

2431. SPINK1 is synthesised in?
Lancet 2008;371:143-52

A. Gallbladder
B. Duodenum
C. Stomach
D. Pancreas

Pancreas synthesises SPINK1, a specific trypsin inhibitor, the function of which can be lost by mutation. In pancreatic ductal cells, CFTR controls chloride and bicarbonate fluxes. SPINK1 and CFTR mutations together may cause pancreatitis.

2432. Which of the following is not a type of trypsinogen in human pancreatic juice?
Gastroenterology 2007;132:1557-1573

A. Telotrypsinogen
B. Cationic trypsinogen
C. Anionic trypsinogen
D. Mesotrypsinogen

Three different trypsinogens in human pancreatic juice have been designated according to their electrophoretic mobility, as cationic trypsinogen (PRSS1), anionic trypsinogen (PRSS2) & mesotrypsinogen (PRSS3). Compared with the anionic isoenzyme, cationic trypsinogen autoactivates more easily and is more resistant to autolysis.

2433. Which of the following is the most common PRSS1 mutation?

Gastroenterology 2007;132:1557-1573

A. R122A
B. R122C
C. R122H
D. R122K

R122H is the most common PRSS1 mutation observed worldwide. Mutations in PRSS1 gene are seen in most patients with hereditary pancreatitis.

2434. CFTR and SPINK1 genetic mutations causing acute pancreatitis are frequent in?

Lancet 2008;371:143-52

A. Thalassemia patients
B. HIV-positive patients
C. COPD patients
D. Leukemia patients

Genetic mutations such as those in CFTR and SPINK1 genes are frequent in HIV-positive patients with acute pancreatitis.

2435. CCK-releasing factor (CCK-RF) is present in?

Harrison's 20th Ed. Chapter 341 Page 2438

A. Stomach
B. Duodenum
C. Jejunum
D. All of the above

Duodenum contains a peptide CCK-releasing factor that is involved in stimulating CCK release.

2436. Which of the following statements is false?

Harrison's 20th Ed. Chapter 341 Page 2438

A. Serine proteases inhibit pancreatic secretion
B. Secretin activates bicarbonate secretion
C. CCK acts to increase pancreatic enzyme secretion
D. None of the above

Acidification of the duodenum releases secretin, which stimulates vagal and other neural pathways to activate pancreatic duct cells, which secrete bicarbonate. CCK in blood in physiologic concentrations acts primarily through neural pathways (vagal-vagal) leading to acetylcholine mediated pancreatic enzyme secretion. Serine proteases inhibit pancreatic secretion by inactivating CCK-releasing peptide in the lumen of the small intestine.

2437. Which of the following is the most common cause of acute pancreatitis?

Harrison's 20th Ed. Chapter 341 Page 2438

A. Gallstones
B. Alcohol
C. Drugs
D. ERCP

Cause of acute pancreatitis include gallstones (30-60%), alcohol (15-30%), ERCP (5-10%), hypertriglyceridemia (1.3-3.8%) and drug-related (0.1-2%).

2438. Risk factors for post-ERCP pancreatitis include?

Harrison's 20th Ed. Chapter 341 Page 2438

A. Sphincter of Oddi dysfunction
B. Age < 60 years
C. > 2 contrast injections into pancreatic duct
D. All of the above

Risk factors for post-ERCP pancreatitis include minor papilla sphincterotomy, sphincter of Oddi dysfunction, prior history of post-ERCP pancreatitis, age <60 years, >2 contrast injections into the pancreatic duct, and endoscopic trainee involvement.

2439. What level of hypertriglyceridemia causes acute pancreatitis?

Harrison's 20th Ed. Chapter 341 Page 2438

A. > 250 mg / dL
B. > 500 mg / dL
C. > 750 mg / dL
D. > 1000 mg / dL

Hypertriglyceridemia can cause acute pancreatitis in 1.3 - 3.8% of cases when serum triglyceride levels are usually > 1000 mg/dL. The goal is to reduce fasting plasma triglycerides to below 500 mg/dL to prevent the risk of acute pancreatitis.

2440. Deficiency of which of the following have an increased incidence of pancreatitis?

Harrison's 20th Ed. Chapter 341 Page 2438

A. ApoA-I
B. ApoB-100
C. ApoC-I
D. ApoC-II

Both LPL & apoC-II deficiency usually present in childhood with recurrent episodes of severe abdominal pain due to acute pancreatitis. Apolipoprotein CII activates lipoprotein lipase. Triglycerides of chylomicrons are hydrolyzed by LPL, and free fatty acids are released. ApoC-II, which is transferred to circulating chylomicrons from HDL, acts as a required cofactor for LPL in this reaction.

2441. Deficiency of which of the following poses an increased incidence of pancreatitis?

Harrison's 20th Ed. Chapter 341 Page 2438

A. Apolipoprotein CII
B. Apolipoprotein A-I
C. Apolipoprotein A-II
D. All of the above

Patients with deficiency of apolipoprotein CII have an increased incidence of pancreatitis. Apolipoprotein CII activates lipoprotein lipase, which is important in clearing chylomicrons from bloodstream.

2442. Which of the following statements is false?

Harrison's 20th Ed. Chapter 341 Page 2438

A. Hypertriglyceridemia can precede & cause pancreatitis
B. >80% patients of acute pancreatitis do not have hypertriglyceridemia
C. Patients with pancreatitis & hypertriglyceridemia have preexisting abnormalities in lipoprotein metabolism
D. Fasting Tg levels of < 500 mg/dL pose no risk of pancreatitis

Fasting Tg levels of < 300 mg/dL pose no risk of pancreatitis.

2443. Drugs that can elevate serum triglycerides include all except?

Harrison's 20th Ed. Chapter 341 Page 2438

A. Progesterone
B. Vitamin A
C. Thiazide diuretics
D. Beta-blockers

Drugs that can elevate serum Tg are estrogens, vitamin A, thiazides and propanolol.

2444. What percentage of acute pancreatitis are drug-related?
Harrison's 20th Ed. Chapter 341 Page 2439

A. 0.1 to 2%
B. 2 to 5%
C. 5 to 10%
D. About 15%

~ 0.1 - 2% of acute pancreatitis are drug-related.

2445. Which of the following statements about interstitial pancreatitis is false?
Harrison's 20th Ed. Chapter 341 Page 2439

A. Acute pancreatitis
B. Self-limited
C. Blood supply to pancreas maintained
D. None of the above

Pathologically, acute pancreatitis varies from interstitial pancreatitis (pancreas blood supply maintained), which is generally self-limited to necrotizing pancreatitis in which pancreas blood supply is interrupted and the extent of necrosis may correlate with severity of attack & its systemic complications.

2446. Which of the following is a proteolytic enzyme?
Harrison's 20th Ed. Chapter 341 Page 2439

A. Trypsinogen
B. Chymotrypsinogen
C. Proelastase
D. All of the above

Autodigestion is a currently accepted pathogenic theory of acute pancreatitis in which pancreatitis results when proteolytic enzymes (trypsinogen, chymotrypsinogen, proelastase) and lipolytic enzymes such as phospholipase A2 are activated in the pancreas acinar cell rather than in the intestinal lumen.

2447. Which of the following factors facilitate premature activation of trypsin?
Harrison's 20th Ed. Chapter 341 Page 2439

A. Oxidative stress
B. Direct trauma
C. Lysosomal calcium
D. All of the above

A number of factors (endotoxins, exotoxins, viral infections, ischemia, oxidative stress, lysosomal calcium and direct trauma) are believed to facilitate premature activation of trypsin.

2448. Activation, chemoattraction & sequestration of neutrophils in pancreas occur in which phase of pancreatitis?
Harrison's 20th Ed. Chapter 341 Page 2439

A. Phase 1
B. Phase 2
C. Phase 3
D. Phase 4

Pancreatitis evolves in three phases. Initial phase is characterized by intrapancreatic digestive enzyme activation & acinar cell injury. Second phase involves activation, chemoattraction & sequestration of neutrophils in pancreas resulting in intrapancreatic inflammatory reaction. Third phase is due to effects of activated proteolytic enzymes & cytokines released by inflamed pancreas on distant organs.

2449. Cathepsin B is best related to?
Harrison's 20th Ed. Chapter 341 Page 2439

A. Fat necrosis
B. Activation of elastase & phospholipase
C. Lysosomal hydrolases
D. Chemoattraction of neutrophils

Zymogen activation is mediated by lysosomal hydrolases (cathepsin B) which become co-localized with digestive enzymes in intracellular organelles leading to pancreatic acinar cell injury.

2450. In pancreatitis, cellular injury results in liberation of?
Harrison's 20th Ed. Chapter 341 Page 2439

A. Bradykinin peptides
B. Vasoactive substances
C. Histamine
D. All of the above

Cellular injury and death result in the liberation of bradykinin peptides, vasoactive substances, and histamine that can produce vasodilation, increased vascular permeability and edema with profound effects on many organs.

2451. Which of the following is an accurate predictor of severity & death when measured early in the course of acute pancreatitis?
Harrison's 20th Ed. Chapter 341 Page 2439

A. Bradykinin peptides
B. Vasoactive substances
C. Histamine
D. MCP-1 levels

Monocyte chemotactic protein (MCP-1) levels measured early in the course of acute pancreatitis are an accurate predictor of severity and death.

2452. Which of the following susceptibility gene is a determinant of occurrence of pancreatitis?
Harrison's 20th Ed. Chapter 341 Page 2439

A. PRSS1
B. CFTR
C. SPINK1
D. All of the above

Five genetic variants have been identified as being associated with susceptibility to pancreatitis. The genes that have been identified include (1) cationic trypsinogen gene (PRSSI), (2) pancreatic secretory trypsin inhibitor (SPINK1), (3) the cystic fibrosis transmembrane conductance regulator gene (CFTR), (4) the chymotrypsin C gene (CTRC) and (5) the calcium-sensing receptor (CASR).

2453. Which of the following is false about abdominal pain of acute pancreatitis?
Harrison's 20th Ed. Chapter 341 Page 2439

A. Colicky
B. Radiates to back
C. Radiate to chest, flanks, and lower abdomen
D. Located in epigastrium & periumbilical region

Abdominal pain of acute pancreatitis is steady & boring in character.

2454. Abdominal pain due to pancreatitis may have which of the following location?
Harrison's 20th Ed. Chapter 341 Page 2439

A. Right upper quadrant
B. Epigastric
C. Left upper quadrant
D. Any of the above

2455. Exudation of blood & plasma proteins into retroperitoneal space due to activated proteolytic enzymes in acute pancreatitis is termed as?

Harrison's 20th Ed. Chapter 341 Page 2439

A. Retroperitoneal abscess
B. Retroperitoneal tan
C. Retroperitoneal quinsy
D. Retroperitoneal burn

Exudation of blood & plasma proteins into retroperitoneal space due to activated proteolytic enzymes in acute pancreatitis is termed as retroperitoneal burn.

2456. Pleural effusion in acute pancreatitis is most frequently?

Harrison's 20th Ed. Chapter 341 Page 2439

A. Left-sided
B. Right-sided
C. Bilateral
D. Any of the above

Pleural effusion in acute pancreatitis is most frequently left-sided.

2457. Erythematous skin nodules in acute pancreatitis is due to?

Harrison's 20th Ed. Chapter 341 Page 2439

A. Vasculitis
B. Subcutaneous fat necrosis
C. Thromboembolism
D. All of the above

Erythematous skin nodules in acute pancreatitis is due to subcutaneous fat necrosis.

2458. Fat necrosis associated with pancreatic disease is seen in?

Harrison's 20th Ed. Chapter 341 Page 2439

A. Pancreatic carcinoma
B. Acute pancreatitis
C. Chronic pancreatitis
D. All of the above

Fat necrosis associated with pancreatic disease is secondary to circulating lipases and is seen in pancreatic carcinoma and acute & chronic pancreatitis.

2459. Cullen's sign of severe necrotizing pancreatitis is due to?

Harrison's 20th Ed. Chapter 341 Page 2439

A. Pancreatic pseudocyst
B. DIC
C. Intestinal ischemia
D. Hemoperitoneum

Cullen's sign in severe necrotizing pancreatitis refers to a faint blue discoloration around umbilicus as the result of hemoperitoneum.

2460. Turner's sign of severe necrotizing pancreatitis is due to?

Harrison's 20th Ed. Chapter 341 Page 2439

A. Tissue catabolism of hemoglobin
B. Pyoperitoneum
C. Intestinal ischemia
D. DIC

Turner's sign of severe necrotizing pancreatitis refers to a blue-red-purple or green-brown discoloration of flanks and reflects tissue catabolism of hemoglobin.

2461. Pearson syndrome is characterized by?

Harrison's 20th Ed. Chapter 472 Page 3483

A. Diabetes mellitus from pancreatic insufficiency
B. Pancytopenia
C. Lactic acidosis
D. All of the above

Pearson syndrome is characterized by diabetes mellitus from pancreatic insufficiency with pancytopenia & lactic acidosis, caused by large-scale sporadic deletion of several mtDNA genes. Kearns-Sayre syndrome (KSS), sporadic progressive external ophthalmoplegia (PEO) and Pearson syndrome are three disease phenotypes caused by large-scale mtDNA rearrangements including partial deletions or partial duplication.

2462. Which of the following about pancreatitis is false?

Harrison's 20th Ed. Chapter 341 Page 2439

A. Risk of acute pancreatitis is greater with gallstone <5 mm than larger stones
B. ~ 25% of acute pancreatitis will have recurrence
C. Cystic fibrosis is a cause of recurrent pancreatitis
D. None of the above

Gallstones with a diameter of ~ 5 mm can migrate in bile duct & trigger acute pancreatitis. Gallstones with diameter of >8 mm remain in gallbladder.

2463. Which of the following about acute pancreatitis is false?

Harrison's 20th Ed. Chapter 341 Page 2439

A. Pancreatic isoamylase & lipase remain elevated for 7-14 days
B. Serum amylase is higher in gallstone pancreatitis
C. Serum lipase higher in alcohol-associated pancreatitis
D. None of the above

2464. Patients with which of the following may have spurious elevations in serum amylase?

Harrison's 20th Ed. Chapter 341 Page 2439

A. Acidemia
B. Hyponatremia
C. Hyperkalemia
D. All of the above

Patients with acidemia (arterial pH <=7.32) may have spurious elevations in serum amylase.

2465. Which of the following is a significant risk factor for mortality in acute pancreatitis?

Harrison's 20th Ed. Chapter 341 Page 2439

A. Azotemia
B. Hemoconcentration
C. Hyperglycemia
D. All of the above

In acute pancreatitis, hemoconcentration may be the harbinger of more severe disease (pancreatic necrosis) whereas azotemia is a significant risk factor for mortality.

2466. Hyperglycemia in acute pancreatitis is due to?

Harrison's 20th Ed. Chapter 341 Page 2439

A. Decreased insulin release
B. Increased glucagon release
C. Increased output of adrenal glucocorticoids & catecholamines
D. All of the above

Hyperglycemia in acute pancreatitis is due to decreased insulin release, increased glucagon release and increased output of adrenal glucocorticoids and catecholamines.

2467. Hypocalcemia may occur in which of the following conditions?
Harrison's 20th Ed. Chapter 403 Page 2937

A. Burns
B. Tumor lysis
C. Pancreatitis
D. All of the above

Hypocalcemia may occur with severe tissue injury like burns, rhabdomyolysis, tumor lysis, or pancreatitis. Cause of hypocalcemia includes a combination of low albumin, hyperphosphatemia, tissue deposition of calcium, and impaired PTH secretion.

2468. Markers of poor prognosis in severe pancreatitis is?
Harrison's 20th Ed. Chapter 341 Page 2439

A. Elevated serum LDH levels (> 500 U/dL)
B. Azotemia
C. Hypoxemia (arterial PO_2 <=60 mm Hg)
D. All of the above

Azotemia is a significant risk factor for mortality.

2469. Serum amylase levels are elevated in all except?
Harrison's 20th Ed. Chapter 341 Page 2439

A. Pregnancy
B. Hypertriglyceridemia
C. Aortic aneurysm
D. Ruptured ectopic pregnancy

Serum amylase levels in patients with hypertriglyceridemia are often spuriously normal.

2470. Revised Atlanta criteria best relates to which of the following?
Harrison's 20th Ed. Chapter 341 Page 2440

A. Clinical features of acute pancreatitis
B. Morphologic features of acute pancreatitis on CT scan
C. Histopathologic features of acute pancreatitis
D. All of the above

Revised Atlanta criteria clearly outlines the morphologic features of acute pancreatitis on computed tomography (CT) scan.

2471. The Revised Atlanta Classification defines which of the following?
Harrison's 20th Ed. Chapter 341 Page 2440

A. Phases of acute pancreatitis
B. Severity of acute pancreatitis
C. Clarifies imaging definitions
D. All of the above

The Revised Atlanta Classification defines phases of acute pancreatitis, defines severity of acute pancreatitis and clarifies imaging definitions.

2472. Laboratory studies in acute pancreatitis may show?
Harrison's 20th Ed. Chapter 341 Page 2440

A. Leukocytosis
B. Hypocalcemia
C. Hyperglycemia
D. All of the above

2473. Risk factor for severity in acute pancreatitis is?
Harrison's 20th Ed. Chapter 341 Page 2441 Table 341-3

A. Age > 60 years
B. Obesity (BMI > 30)
C. Comorbid disease
D. All of the above

2474. Which of the following is a Comorbidity Index?
J Chronic Dis 1987;40(5):373-383

A. Andresen
B. Romano
C. Charlson
D. Grasso

The Charlson Comorbidity Index is a method of categorizing comorbidities of patients based on the International Classification of Diseases (ICD) diagnosis codes. It has 17 categories.

2475. Which of the following is not included in the bedside index of severity (BISAP) in acute pancreatitis?
Harrison's 20th Ed. Chapter 341 Page 2441 Table 341-3

A. PaO_2 < 60 mmHg
B. Blood urea nitrogen (BUN) > 25 mg%
C. Age > 60 years
D. Impaired mental status

BISAP or bedside index of severity in acute pancreatitis includes (B) Blood urea nitrogen (BUN) >25 mg%, (I) Impaired mental status, (S) SIRS: 2/4 present, (A) Age >60 years, (P) Pleural effusion

2476. Bedside Index of Severity in Acute Pancreatitis (BISAP) incorporates how many clinical and laboratory parameters?
Harrison's 20th Ed. Chapter 341 Page 2441 Table 341-3

A. 3
B. 5
C. 7
D. 9

Bedside Index of Severity in Acute Pancreatitis (BISAP), incorporates five clinical and laboratory parameters obtained within the first 24 hours of hospitalization. Presence of three or more of these factors is associated with substantially increased risk for in-hospital mortality in acute pancreatitis.

2477. Indicators of a severe attack of pancreatitis are all except?
Harrison's 20th Ed. Chapter 341 Page 2443

A. Age > 60 years
B. Body mass index (BMI) < 25
C. Hematocrit > 44%
D. Admission BUN (>22 mg/dL)

Indicators of a severe attack of pancreatitis are age > 60 years, BMI > 30, Hct > 44% & admission BUN (>22 mg/dL).

2478. Differential diagnosis of acute pancreatitis include?
Harrison's 20th Ed. Chapter 341 Page 2440

A. Perforated viscus
B. Dissecting aortic aneurysm
C. Connective tissue disorders with vasculitis
D. All of the above

Differential diagnosis of acute pancreatitis includes perforated viscus, acute cholecystitis, acute intestinal obstruction, mesenteric vascular occlusion, renal colic, myocardial infarction, dissecting aortic aneurysm, connective tissue disorders with vasculitis, pneumonia & diabetic ketoacidosis.

2479. Which of the following is true in diabetic ketoacidosis?
Harrison's 20th Ed. Chapter 341 Page 2440

A. Elevated total serum amylase levels
B. Pancreatic isoamylase levels not elevated

C. Serum lipase not elevated
D. All of the above

Diabetic ketoacidosis is accompanied by abdominal pain & elevated total serum amylase levels. Serum lipase level is not elevated in DKA.

2480. Which investigation is most helpful in differentiating acute cholecystitis from acute pancreatitis?
Harrison's 20th Ed. Chapter 341 Page 2440

A. Serum Lipase
B. Upper GI Endoscopy
C. Radionuclide scanning
D. FP abdomen

Pain of biliary tract origin is more right-sided or epigastric than periumbilical, ileus is usually absent. Sonography & radionuclide scanning are helpful in diagnosis of cholelithiasis & cholecystitis.

2481. Multiple factor scoring system for acute pancreatitis is?
Harrison's 20th Ed. Chapter 315 Page 2201

A. Ranson
B. Glasgow
C. APACHE II
D. All of the above

Ranson, Glasgow, Imrie & Apache II are multiple factor scoring systems for predicting outcome of acute pancreatitis.

2482. SOFA score stands for?
Lancet 2008; 371: 143-52

A. Septic organ failure assessment
B. Surgical organ failure assessment
C. Symptomatic organ failure assessment
D. Sequential organ failure assessment

2483. Test that is more specific for acute pancreatitis than serum amylase and lipase is?
N Engl J Med. 2006;354:2142-50

A. Urine Trypsinogen activation peptide (TAP)
B. Trypsinogen-2
C. Abdominal CT & MRI
D. All of the above

2484. Which of the following tests is more specific for the diagnosis of acute pancreatitis?
N Engl J Med. 2006;354:2142-50

A. Serum amylase
B. Serum lipase
C. Trypsinogen activation peptide
D. Trypsinogen-4

2485. At 24 hours after admission, the most sensitive & specific predictor of severe acute pancreatitis is?
N Engl J Med. 2006;354:2142-50

A. APACHE II score >=8
B. C-reactive protein level >150 mg/dl
C. PMN elastase >300 μg/liter
D. Urinary TAP >35 nmol/liter

2486. Pancreatic-duct disruption is suspected when?
N Engl J Med. 2006;354:2142-50

A. Fluid collections with very high levels of pancreatic enzymes
B. Pseudocysts
C. Ascites or pleural effusions
D. All of the above

2487. Recurrent pancreatitis in the absence of biliary disease, alcoholism, and toxic or metabolic causes suggests?
N Engl J Med. 2006;354:2142-50

A. Pancreas divisum
B. Duct-obstructing masses
C. Genetic susceptibility
D. Any of the above

2488. Test that identifies early pancreatic duct disruption is?
N Engl J Med. 2006;354:2142-50

A. CT abdomen
B. MRI abdomen
C. Transabdominal ultrasound
D. All of the above

2489. Biliary sludge is made up of?
Lancet 2008; 371: 143-52

A. Cholesterol crystals
B. Calcium bilirubinate granules
C. Gallbladder mucus
D. All of the above

Biliary sludge refers to a viscous bile suspension that contains cholesterol crystals and calcium bilirubinate granules embedded in strands of gallbladder mucus.

2490. Which test is more sensitive for identifying gallstones and sludge and for detecting bile-duct dilatation?
N Engl J Med. 2006;354:2142-50

A. Transabdominal ultrasonography
B. CT abdomen
C. MRI abdomen
D. ERCP

2491. Transabdominal ultrasonography is insensitive for detecting?
N Engl J Med. 2006;354:2142-50

A. Gallstones and sludge
B. Bile-duct dilatation
C. Stones in the distal bile duct
D. Stones in the proximal bile duct

2492. Which of the following genes may predict severity of acute pancreatitis?
N Engl J Med. 2006;354:2142-50

A. RET
B. MCP-1
C. MEN-1
D. VHL

2493. Recognized markers of risk of severe acute pancreatitis include all except?

N Engl J Med. 2006;354:2142-50

A. Elevated C-reactive protein
B. Ranson's & APACHE II scores
C. Obesity
D. High reticulocyte index

2494. Biliary sludge is associated with which of the following?

Lancet 2008; 371: 143-52

A. Total parenteral feeding
B. Long-lasting fast
C. Distal bile duct obstruction
D. All of the above

2495. Risk factors for post-ERCP pancreatitis include all except?

Lancet 2008; 371: 143-52

A. Old age
B. Female sex
C. Number of cannulation attempts of papilla
D. Poor emptying of pancreatic duct after opacification

Risk of acute pancreatitis is higher when ERCP is done to treat Oddi sphincter dysfunction than to remove bile duct stones. Other risk factors for post-ERCP pancreatitis include young age, female sex, number of cannulation attempts of papilla before success & poor emptying of pancreatic duct after opacification.

2496. The median prevalence of organ failure in necrotizing pancreatitis is?

Harrison's 20th Ed. Chapter 341 Page 2442

A. ~ 25%
B. ~ 50%
C. ~ 75%
D. ~ 95%

The median prevalence of organ failure is 54% in necrotizing pancreatitis.

2497. The mortality in acute pancreatitis with single organ system failure is?

Harrison's 20th Ed. Chapter 341 Page 2442

A. ~ 5%
B. ~ 10%
C. ~ 25%
D. ~ 50%

2498. The mortality in acute pancreatitis with multisystem organ system failure is?

Harrison's 20th Ed. Chapter 341 Page 2442

A. ~ 5%
B. ~ 10%
C. ~ 25%
D. ~ 50%

With single organ system failure, the mortality is 3–10% but increases to 47% with multisystem organ failure.

2499. What proportion of patients with acute pancreatitis have necrotizing pancreatitis?

Harrison's 20th Ed. Chapter 341 Page 2442

A. ~ 5%
B. ~ 10%
C. ~ 25%
D. ~ 50%

Necrotizing pancreatitis occurs in ~10% of all patients with acute pancreatitis.

2500. Necrosis is present in what percentage of patients with acute pancreatitis?

Harrison's 20th Ed. Chapter 341 Page 2442

A. 5 - 10%
B. 12 - 20%
C. 25 - 45%
D. 50 - 70%

Necrosis is present in 12 - 20% of patients with acute pancreatitis.

2501. In what proportion of acute pancreatitis, the disease is self-limited and subsides spontaneously?

Harrison's 20th Ed. Chapter 341 Page 2441

A. ~ 25%
B. ~ 50%
C. ~ 75%
D. ~ 90%

In most patients (85–90%) with acute pancreatitis, the disease is self-limited and subsides spontaneously, usually within three to seven days after treatment is instituted.

2502. In pancreatitis, oral intake is started by considering all of the following factors except?

Harrison's 20th Ed. Chapter 341 Page 2442

A. Resolution of abdominal pain
B. Patient is hungry
C. Organ dysfunction
D. Elevated levels of serum amylase / lipase

Inflammatory changes on CT scan or persistent elevations in serum amylase/lipase may not resolve for weeks to months & should not discourage feeding a hungry asymptomatic patient of pancreatitis.

2503. Which of the following is used in the management of pancreatitis?

Harrison's 20th Ed. Chapter 49 Page 309 Table 49-5

A. Nafamostat
B. Pentamidine
C. Tacrolimus
D. Aliskiren

Nafamostat, a protease inhibitor is utilized in the management of pancreatitis, disseminated intravascular coagulation, and extracorporeal circulation (ECC), such as during hemodialysis therapy (HD), plasmapheresis, and cardiopulmonary bypass. It inhibits aldosterone-induced proteases that activate ENaC by proteolytic cleavage. It may cause hyperkalemia.

2504. Preferred method of nutritional support in patients of necrotizing pancreatitis is?

Harrison's 20th Ed. Chapter 341 Page 2443

A. Total parenteral nutrition (TPN)
B. Feeding with a nasogastric tube
C. Enteral-feeding with a nasojejunal tube
D. PEG

Enteral-feeding with a nasojejunal tube has fewer infectious complications than with total parenteral nutrition (TPN) and is the preferred method of nutritional support. Also, enteral feeding helps to maintain integrity of the intestinal tract during severe acute pancreatitis.

2505. What proportion of patients of acute pancreatitis have a recurrence?

Harrison's 20th Ed. Chapter 341 Page 2444

A. ~ 25%
B. ~ 50%
C. ~ 75%
D. ~ 90%

~25% of patients who have had an attack of acute pancreatitis have a recurrence.

2506. Which of the following occult biliary tract diseases can lead to acute pancreatitis?

Harrison's 20th Ed. Chapter 341 Page 2444

A. Microlithiasis
B. Pancreatic cancer
C. Pancreas divisum
D. All of the above

If a cause could not be found in patients with recurrent pancreatitis, occult biliary tract disease should be looked at. These include microlithiasis, hypertriglyceridemia, drugs, pancreatic cancer, sphincter of Oddi dysfunction, pancreas divisum, cystic fibrosis, hereditary pancreatitis, choledochocele; ampullary tumors, pancreatic duct stones, stricture, and tumor.

2507. "Walled-off Necrosis" occurs how many weeks after necrotizing pancreatitis?

Harrison's 20th Ed. Chapter 341 Page 2440 Table 341-2

A. > 2 weeks
B. > 4 weeks
C. > 6 weeks
D. > 8 weeks

"Walled-off necrosis" or WON is a mature encapsulated collection of pancreatic and/or peripancreatic necrosis that has developed a well-defined inflammatory wall. WON usually occurs >4 weeks after onset of necrotizing pancreatitis.

2508. Which of the following is false about pancreatic pseudocysts?

Harrison's 20th Ed. Chapter 341 Page 2440 Table 341-2

A. Extrapancreatic
B. Minimal or no necrosis
C. Occurs >4 weeks after interstitial edematous pancreatitis
D. None of the above

An encapsulated collection of fluid with a well-defined inflammatory wall usually outside pancreas with minimal or no necrosis. It usually occurs >4 weeks after onset of interstitial edematous pancreatitis.

2509. After acute pancreatitis, pseudocysts of pancreas develop over a period of?

Harrison's 20th Ed. Chapter 341 Page 2440 Table 341-2

A. 1 - 2 weeks
B. 2 - 3 weeks
C. 3 - 4 weeks
D. 4 - 6 weeks

Pseudocysts of pancreas are collections of tissue, fluid, debris, pancreatic enzymes & blood that develop over 4-6 weeks after acute pancreatitis.

2510. Which of the following about pseudocysts of pancreas is false?

Harrison's 20th Ed. Chapter 341 Page 2440

A. Preceded by pancreatitis in 90% of cases
B. Mostly located in body or tail of pancreas
C. Abdominal pain is the usual presenting complaint
D. Serum amylase level is mostly normal

Serum amylase level is elevated in 75% of pseudocysts of pancreas at some point during their illness and may fluctuate markedly.

2511. Significant number of pancreatic pseudocysts resolve spontaneously how many weeks after their formation?

Harrison's 20th Ed. Chapter 341 Page 2443

A. > 1 week
B. > 2 weeks
C. > 4 weeks
D. > 6 weeks

Significant number of pancreatic pseudocysts resolve spontaneously >6 weeks after their formation.

2512. Which of the following statements is false for Purtscher's retinopathy?

Optom Vis Sci. 2014;91(2):e43-51

A. Due to occlusion of anterior retinal artery
B. Sudden and severe loss of vision
C. Cotton wool spots & hemorrhages in optical fundus
D. It is a complication of acute pancreatitis

Purtscher's retinopathy in acute pancreatitis is due to occlusion of posterior retinal artery with aggregated granulocytes. Optical fundus shows cotton-wool spots & hemorrhages confined to an area limited by optic disk & macula.

2513. Which of the following is a classification system for Chronic Pancreatitis and Pancreatic Exocrine Insufficiency?

Harrison's 20th Ed. Chapter 341 Page 2445 Table 341-5

A. RICOR
B. TEMNA
C. TIGAR-O
D. PROZE

TIGAR-O stands for toxic-metabolic, idiopathic, genetic, autoimmune, recurrent and obstructive.

2514. Complication of chronic pancreatitis is?

Harrison's 20th Ed. Chapter 341 Page 2445

A. Abdominal pain
B. Steatorrhea
C. Diabetes mellitus
D. All of the above

Complications of chronic pancreatitis are abdominal pain, steatorrhea, weight loss & diabetes mellitus.

2515. Which of the following is best related to chronic pancreatitis?

Harrison's 20th Ed. Chapter 341 Page 2445

A. Fluctuating symptomatology
B. Risk of malignancy
C. Irreversible damage to pancreas
D. All of the above

Chronic pancreatitis is characterized by irreversible damage to pancreas.

2516. There is a strong association of which of the following and chronic pancreatitis?

Harrison's 18th Ed. 2643

A. Smoking
B. Intravenous drug use

C. Prolonged fasting

D. Obesity

There is a strong independent, dose-dependent association of smoking and chronic and recurrent acute pancreatitis. Cigarette smoke leads to an increased susceptibility to pancreatic self-digestion and predisposes to dysregulation of duct cell CFTR function. It increases severity in alcohol-induced chronic pancreatitis.

2517. Which of the following plays a key role in the development of chronic pancreatitis?

Harrison's 20th Ed. Chapter 341 Page 2445

A. Islet cells of Langerhans

B. Pancreatic stellate cells (PSC)

C. Acinar epithelial cells

D. All of the above

Pancreatic stellate cells (PSC) play a role in maintaining normal pancreatic architecture that can shift toward fibrogenesis in the case of chronic pancreatitis.

2518. Which of the following hypothesis describes events in the pathogenesis of chronic pancreatitis?

Harrison's 20th Ed. Chapter 341 Page 2445

A. Sentinel acute pancreatitis event

B. Sentinel chronic pancreatitis event

C. Sequential acute pancreatitis event

D. Sequential chronic pancreatitis event

The sentinel acute pancreatitis event (SAPE) hypothesis uniformly describes the events in the pathogenesis of chronic pancreatitis.

2519. Which of the following induces pancreatic stellate cells (PSC) activity with subsequent new collagen synthesis?

Harrison's 20th Ed. Chapter 341 Page 2445

A. Proinflammatory cytokines

B. Oxidants

C. Growth factors

D. All of the above

Proinflammatory cytokines, tumor necrosis factor (TNF-α), interleukin 1 (IL-1), and interleukin 6 (IL-6) as well as oxidant complexes & growth factors are able to induce PSC activity with subsequent new collagen synthesis.

2520. Which of the following plays a role in self-activating autocrine pathways that lead to progression in chronic pancreatitis?

Harrison's 20th Ed. Chapter 341 Page 2445

A. Tumor necrosis factor (TNF-α)

B. Interleukin 1 (IL-1)

C. Interleukin 6 (IL-6)

D. Transforming growth factor (TGF-β)

PSCs also possess transforming growth factor (TGF-β)–mediated self-activating autocrine pathways that may explain disease progression in chronic pancreatitis even after removal of noxious stimuli.

2521. Which of the following is the most frequent cause of clinically apparent chronic pancreatitis in children?

Harrison's 20th Ed. Chapter 341 Page 2445

A. Cystic fibrosis

B. Hereditary pancreatitis

C. Isolated autoimmune chronic pancreatitis

D. Pancreas divisum

In United States, alcoholism is the most common cause of clinically apparent chronic pancreatitis in adults, while cystic fibrosis is the most frequent cause in children.

2522. In hereditary chronic pancreatitis, defect in gene encoding for which of the following is found?

Harrison's 20th Ed. Chapter 341 Page 2445

A. Pepsin

B. Chymotrypsin

C. Trypsinogen

D. All of the above

In hereditary chronic pancreatitis, a genetic defect that affects the gene encoding for trypsinogen was identified. The defect prevents the destruction of trypsinogen and allows it to be resistant to the effect of trypsin inhibitor, become spontaneously activated, and to remain activated leading to continual activation of digestive enzymes within the gland causing acute injury and eventually chronic pancreatitis.

2523. Which of the following mutation increases the risk of chronic pancreatitis?

Harrison's 20th Ed. Chapter 341 Page 2445

A. N32S SPINK1

B. N33S SPINK1

C. N34S SPINK1

D. N35S SPINK1

Presence of an N34S SPINK1 mutation increased the risk of chronic pancreatitis by twentyfold. A combination of two CFTR mutations and an N34S SPINK1 mutation increased the risk of chronic pancreatitis 900-fold.

2524. Autoimmune Pancreatitis (AIP) is which form of pancreatitis?

N Engl J Med. 2006;355:2670-6

A. Acute

B. Chronic

C. Recurrent

D. All of the above

2525. Autoimmune Pancreatitis (AIP) is also called?

N Engl J Med. 2006;355:2670-6

A. Sclerosing pancreatitis

B. Tumefactive pancreatitis

C. Nonalcoholic destructive pancreatitis

D. All of the above

AIP is also referred to as sclerosing pancreatitis, tumefactive pancreatitis and nonalcoholic destructive pancreatitis.

2526. Autoimmune pancreatitis is frequently associated with?

Harrison's 20th Ed. Chapter 341 Page 2446

A. Rheumatoid arthritis

B. Sjögren's syndrome

C. Ulcerative colitis

D. All of the above

AIP is associated with primary sclerosing cholangitis, primary biliary sclerosis, rheumatoid arthritis, Sjögren's syndrome, ulcerative colitis, mediastinal adenopathy, autoimmune thyroiditis, tubulointerstitial nephritis, and retroperitoneal fibrosis.

2527. Majority of patients with AIP present with?

Harrison's 20th Ed. Chapter 341 Page 2446

A. Obstructive jaundice

B. Acute pancreatitis

C. Recurrent pancreatitis
D. Malabsorption syndrome

In the United States, 50–75% of patients with AIP present with obstructive jaundice.

2528. Immunologic abnormalities in autoimmune pancreatitis include?
N Engl J Med. 2006;355:2670-6

A. Hypergammaglobulinemia
B. Autoantibodies against carbonic anhydrase
C. Autoantibodies against lactoferrin
D. All of the above

Autoimmune pancreatitis is characterized by the presence of increased serum gammaglobulin levels (IgG4), presence of autoantibodies (antinuclear antibodies, antilactoferrin antibodies, anticarbonic anhydrase antibodies & rheumatoid factor), pancreatic fibrosis with lymphocytic infiltration & an absence of pancreatic calcification, an association with other autoimmune diseases and response to steroid therapy.

2529. Serum levels of which of the following immunoglobulin is elevated in AIP?
Harrison's 20th Ed. Chapter 341 Page 2446

A. Immunoglobulin G1
B. Immunoglobulin G2
C. Immunoglobulin G3
D. Immunoglobulin G4

IgG constitutes ~75–85% of total serum immunoglobulin. The four IgG subclasses are numbered in order of their level in serum, IgG1 being found in greatest amounts and IgG4 the least. Serum IgG4 normally accounts for only 5–6% of the total IgG in healthy patients but is elevated at least twofold higher than 135 mg/dL in those with AIP.

2530. Which of the following syndrome is related to IgG4?
Harrison's 20th Ed. Chapter 341 Page 2446

A. IgG4-related immunologic disease
B. IgG4-related systemic disease
C. IgG4-related pulmonary disease
D. IgG4-related neuronal disease

IgG4-related systemic disease is a variety of acute tubulointerstitial disorder and a form of Acute Interstitial Nephritis (AIN). It is characterized by a dense inflammatory infiltrate containing IgG4-expressing plasma cells. Glucocorticoids lead to response.

2531. Which of the following syndrome is related to IgG4?
Harrison's 20th Ed. Chapter 341 Page 2446

A. Immunoglobulin G4–associated carditis
B. Immunoglobulin G4–associated neuritis
C. Immunoglobulin G4–associated pneumonitis
D. Immunoglobulin G4–associated cholangitis

Immunoglobulin G4–associated cholangitis is a biliary disease of unknown etiology with biochemical & cholangiographic features indistinguishable from PSC. It is associated with autoimmune pancreatitis and is characterized by elevated serum IgG4 and infiltration of IgG4-positive plasma cells in bile ducts and liver tissue. In contrast to PSC, it is not associated with inflammatory bowel disease.

2532. Which of the following is characteristic imaging finding in AIP?
Harrison's 20th Ed. Chapter 341 Page 2446

A. Enlargement at the head of pancreas
B. Strictures in bile duct
C. Narrowing of pancreatic bile duct
D. All of the above

2533. Which of the following drug is useful in AIP?
Harrison's 20th Ed. Chapter 341 Page 2446

A. Glucocorticoids
B. Azathioprine
C. 6-mercaptopurine
D. All of the above

Glucocorticoids, azathioprine, 6-mercaptapurine, rituximab, cyclosporine and cyclophosphamide are useful in AIP.

2534. Which of the following is false about chronic pancreatitis?
Harrison's 20th Ed. Chapter 341 Page 2446

A. Deficiencies of fat-soluble vitamins are uncommon
B. Serum amylase & lipase levels are raised
C. Best diagnostic test is secretin stimulation test
D. Vitamin B_{12} malabsorption is corrected by oral pancreatic enzymes

Serum amylase & lipase levels are normal.

2535. Which of the following tests is useful in identifying severe pancreatic exocrine insufficiency?
Harrison's 20th Ed. Chapter 341 Page 2446

A. D-xylose excretion test
B. Fecal elastase
C. Serum amylase
D. Serum lipase

Fecal elastase levels of < 100 µg per gram of stool strongly suggests severe pancreatic exocrine insufficiency.

2536. Severe pancreatic exocrine insufficiency is obvious when serum trypsinogen levels are?
Harrison's 19th Ed. 2099

A. < 20 mg/mL
B. < 40 mg/mL
C. < 60 mg/mL
D. < 80 mg/mL

Decrease of serum trypsinogen level to < 20 mg/mL strongly suggests severe pancreatic exocrine insufficiency.

2537. Absence of pancreatic calcification is a feature of?
Harrison's 20th Ed. Chapter 341 Page 2446, Gastroenterology 2007;132:1557-1573

A. Idiopathic chronic pancreatitis
B. Islet cell tumors
C. Autoimmune pancreatitis
D. Severe protein-calorie malnutrition

2538. In chronic pancreatitis, secretin stimulation test is abnormal when how much of pancreatic exocrine function is lost?
Harrison's 20th Ed. Chapter 341 Page 2446

A. 20%
B. 40%
C. 60%
D. 80%

In chronic pancreatitis, secretin stimulation test becomes abnormal when 60% of the pancreatic exocrine function has been lost. This correlates well with the onset of chronic abdominal pain.

2539. Most common cause of pancreatic calcification is?
Harrison's 20th Ed. Chapter 341 Page 2446

A. Idiopathic chronic pancreatitis
B. Hypercalcemic pancreatitis
C. Alcohol
D. Severe protein-calorie malnutrition

Alcohol is the most common cause of pancreatic calcification. Diffuse pancreatic calcifications on FP abdomen indicates ~80% damage to pancreas. Pancreatic calcification is also seen in severe protein-calorie malnutrition, hereditary pancreatitis, posttraumatic pancreatitis, hypercalcemic pancreatitis, islet cell tumors, idiopathic chronic pancreatitis and tropical pancreatitis.

2540. Tropical pancreatitis is characterized by all except?
Gastroenterology 2007;132:1557-1573

A. Early onset
B. Slow progression
C. Severe pancreatic damage
D. No history of alcohol abuse or biliary disease

Tropical pancreatitis is characterized by early onset, rapid progression & severe pancreatic damage in the absence of a history of alcohol abuse or biliary disease. Both exocrine & endocrine insufficiency is evident at very early stages, often at the time of presentation in majority (70%) of patients.

2541. Which of the following is an uncommon complication of chronic pancreatitis?
Harrison's 20th Ed. Chapter 341 Page 2447

A. Diabetic ketoacidosis
B. Pancreatic cancer
C. Gastrointestinal bleeding
D. Biliary cirrhosis

In chronic pancreatitis, most patients have impaired glucose tolerance, diabetic ketoacidosis and coma are uncommon.

2542. According to the American Diabetes Association, which of the following diabetes in found in chronic pancreatitis?
Gastroenterology 2007;132:1557-1573

A. Type I
B. Type II
C. Type IIIc
D. Any of the above

Diabetes of chronic pancreatitis is classified as type IIIc according to ADA & is characterized by destruction of both insulin & glucagon-producing cells.

2543. Hemosuccus pancreaticus best relates to?
Harrison's 20th Ed. Chapter 341 Page 2447

A. Pseudocyst eroding into the duodenum
B. Arterial bleeding into pancreatic duct
C. Ruptured varices secondary to splenic vein thrombosis
D. Pseudocyst eroding into the stomach

2544. Increased incidence of pancreatic carcinoma is seen in which of the following?
Harrison's 20th Ed. Chapter 341 Page 2447

A. Idiopathic chronic pancreatitis
B. Hypercalcemic pancreatitis
C. Hereditary pancreatitis
D. Severe protein-calorie malnutrition

Patients with hereditary pancreatitis develop pancreatic calcification, diabetes mellitus & steatorrhea. They have a tenfold higher risk of pancreatic carcinoma (40% by 70 years).

2545. Which of the following significantly relieves pain in severe refractory large-duct chronic pancreatitis?
Harrison's 20th Ed. Chapter 341 Page 2448

A. UDCA
B. Cholestyramine
C. Domperidone
D. Pregabalin

2546. The ideal pancreatic enzyme preparation is?
Harrison's 20th Ed. Chapter 341 Page 2448

A. Enteric-coated lipase & free proteases
B. Enteric-coated lipase & enteric-coated proteases
C. Free lipase & enteric-coated proteases
D. Free lipase & free proteases

Ideal pancreatic enzyme preparation is enteric-coated lipase & free proteases. Free proteases enter duodenum & evoke a positive feedback control mechanism & enteric-coated lipase open beyond duodenum & enhance fat absorption. Recent data suggests that dosages up to 80,000–100,000 units of lipase per meal may be necessary to normalize nutritional parameters in malnourished chronic pancreatitis patients.

2547. The major cause of death in alcoholic CP is?
Gastroenterology 2007;132:1557-1573

A. Cardiovascular disease
B. Severe infection
C. Malignancy
D. All of the above

Major causes of death in alcoholic CP are cardiovascular disease, infection & malignancy.

2548. The most common congenital anatomic variant of human pancreas is?
Harrison's 20th Ed. Chapter 341 Page 2449

A. Annular pancreas
B. Pancreas divisum
C. Sphincter of Oddi disorders
D. Pancreatic duct scars

Pancreas divisum is the most common congenital anatomic variant of the human pancreas.

2549. Which of the following does not predispose to the development of pancreatitis?
Harrison's 20th Ed. Chapter 341 Page 2449

A. Hereditary pancreatitis
B. Annular pancreas
C. Pancreas divisum
D. All of the above

Pancreas divisum does not predispose to the development of pancreatitis in the great majority of patients who harbor it.

2550. Macroamylasaemia is characterised by formation of large molecular complexes between amylase and?
Harrison's 20th Ed. Chapter 341 Page 2449

A. Urea
B. Haem
C. Clotting factors
D. Abnormal immunoglobulins

Macroamylasaemia is a syndrome characterised by formation of large molecular complexes between amylase & abnormal immunoglobulins.

2551. Paraduodenal pancreatitis is also called?

World J Gastrointest Pathophysiol. 2014;5(3):252-270

A. Ectopic pancreatitis

B. Groove pancreatitis

C. Minimal pancreatitis

D. Sentinel pancreatitis

Groove pancreatitis is a rare form of focal chronic pancreatitis involving the anatomic groove between the pancreatic head, duodenum and common bile duct.

2552. Which of the following about Tropical chronic pancreatitis (TCP) is false?

Indian J Pediatr 2006;73 (10):907-912

A. Juvenile form of chronic pancreatitis

B. Higher risk of pancreatic calculi, diabetes & pancreatic malignancy

C. Highly associated with SPINK1 N34S mutation

D. None of the above

Tropical chronic pancreatitis (TCP) is a juvenile form of chronic pancreatitis prevalent in tropical developing countries. TCP differs from temperate zone pancreatitis in its younger age of onset, more accelerated course, higher prevalence of pancreatic calculi and diabetes, and greater propensity to pancreatic malignancy. TCP involves the main pancreatic duct resulting in large ductal calculi & is highly associated with SPINK1 N34S mutation.

ANSWERS

1. D
2. B
3. C
4. C
5. D
6. C
7. C
8. C
9. B
10. D
11. D
12. D
13. D
14. D
15. A
16. D
17. A
18. B
19. A
20. A
21. C
22. D
23. D
24. C
25. B
26. C
27. D
28. D
29. A
30. D
31. C
32. D
33. D
34. D
35. D
36. A
37. D
38. D
39. D
40. D
41. A
42. C
43. C
44. D
45. C
46. D
47. D
48. A
49. D
50. A
51. D
52. D
53. A
54. D
55. D
56. D
57. A
58. D
59. B
60. D
61. D
62. D
63. D
64. B
65. D
66. C
67. D
68. D
69. A
70. D
71. C
72. D
73. A
74. B
75. C
76. C
77. B
78. A
79. D
80. D
81. A
82. A
83. D
84. D
85. B
86. B
87. B
88. B
89. D
90. B
91. D
92. A
93. D
94. D
95. D
96. D
97. B
98. D
99. D
100. D
101. D
102. D
103. A
104. C
105. B
106. D
107. D
108. B
109. B
110. D
111. D
112. D
113. B
114. C
115. C
116. D
117. C
118. C
119. D
120. D
121. A
122. D
123. A
124. D
125. D
126. D
127. A
128. C
129. D
130. D
131. A
132. B
133. D
134. C
135. B
136. A
137. D
138. C
139. A
140. C
141. C
142. D
143. A
144. D
145. B
146. B
147. D
148. B
149. D
150. B
151. A
152. A
153. A
154. D
155. C
156. D
157. A
158. C
159. A
160. D
161. D
162. D
163. D
164. C
165. C
166. D
167. C
168. C
169. B
170. A
171. B
172. D
173. C
174. D
175. B
176. A
177. D
178. B
179. B
180. D
181. D
182. B
183. D
184. D
185. D
186. C
187. B
188. D
189. C
190. C
191. D
192. D
193. A
194. D
195. B
196. D
197. A
198. C
199. C
200. D
201. A
202. A
203. A
204. D
205. D
206. B
207. D
208. D
209. C
210. D
211. D
212. D
213. B
214. C
215. D
216. D
217. B
218. A
219. D
220. B
221. D
222. A
223. A
224. B
225. B
226. D
227. C
228. D
229. B
230. A
231. D
232. B
233. A
234. A
235. B
236. A
237. B
238. D
239. D
240. D
241. D
242. D
243. D
244. D
245. D
246. D
247. D
248. A
249. B
250. D
251. D
252. D
253. C
254. A
255. B
256. D
257. B
258. C
259. A
260. D
261. A
262. D
263. D
264. C
265. A
266. C
267. D
268. D
269. A
270. D

ANSWERS

271. D
272. D
273. D
274. D
275. C
276. A
277. D
278. D
279. A
280. D
281. D
282. D
283. A
284. D
285. D
286. D
287. B
288. D
289. D
290. D
291. D
292. B
293. A
294. D
295. D
296. D
297. D
298. B
299. D
300. C
301. A
302. D
303. D
304. D
305. D
306. D
307. D
308. D
309. B
310. C
311. C
312. C
313. B
314. A
315. D
316. C
317. B
318. D
319. A
320. D
321. B
322. D
323. A
324. D
325. D
326. A
327. D
328. B
329. A
330. A
331. D
332. D
333. B
334. D
335. A
336. D
337. A
338. B
339. D
340. D
341. D
342. B
343. C
344. A
345. B
346. A
347. D
348. A
349. D
350. C
351. A
352. B
353. C
354. D
355. D
356. A
357. B
358. B
359. A
360. D
361. B
362. D
363. A
364. D
365. A
366. D
367. D
368. C
369. A
370. D
371. D
372. D
373. A
374. A
375. B
376. C
377. D
378. A
379. C
380. D
381. B
382. B
383. D
384. D
385. D
386. D
387. D
388. A
389. D
390. C
391. C
392. D
393. B
394. B
395. B
396. D
397. C
398. B
399. D
400. C
401. B
402. D
403. B
404. A
405. D
406. C
407. C
408. C
409. B
410. C
411. D
412. D
413. A
414. D
415. B
416. D
417. D
418. B
419. C
420. D
421. D
422. B
423. C
424. D
425. C
426. A
427. C
428. A
429. D
430. A
431. D
432. D
433. C
434. C
435. D
436. B
437. A
438. A
439. C
440. D
441. B
442. D
443. C
444. D
445. D
446. D
447. D
448. B
449. D
450. D
451. D
452. D
453. D
454. C
455. C
456. C
457. D
458. D
459. D
460. D
461. C
462. C
463. C
464. C
465. D
466. C
467. A
468. D
469. D
470. C
471. D
472. C
473. D
474. D
475. D
476. B
477. B
478. D
479. D
480. D
481. D
482. D
483. D
484. B
485. D
486. D
487. B
488. B
489. D
490. D
491. C
492. D
493. A
494. D
495. A
496. D
497. C
498. D
499. A
500. C
501. A
502. D
503. A
504. A
505. D
506. D
507. C
508. D
509. A
510. D
511. D
512. C
513. A
514. D
515. D
516. D
517. D
518. C
519. A
520. B
521. B
522. A
523. D
524. C
525. D
526. D
527. C
528. D
529. D
530. D
531. D
532. B
533. A
534. A
535. A
536. C
537. B
538. B
539. A
540. C

ANSWERS

541. D
542. D
543. B
544. B
545. C
546. C
547. D
548. D
549. D
550. C
551. B
552. D
553. D
554. D
555. A
556. B
557. B
558. C
559. C
560. B
561. C
562. D
563. B
564. C
565. B
566. B
567. D
568. B
569. B
570. B
571. D
572. D
573. D
574. D
575. B
576. D
577. C
578. C
579. B
580. C
581. D
582. A
583. D
584. D
585. A
586. C
587. B
588. C
589. D
590. C
591. D
592. B
593. C
594. D
595. D
596. B
597. D
598. B
599. B
600. B
601. C
602. D
603. B
604. D
605. C
606. B
607. D
608. B
609. D
610. D
611. D
612. A
613. C
614. D
615. D
616. C
617. A
618. B
619. D
620. B
621. B
622. D
623. D
624. D
625. C
626. C
627. B
628. A
629. D
630. A
631. D
632. D
633. C
634. C
635. C
636. D
637. A
638. C
639. B
640. B
641. C
642. C
643. C
644. C
645. A
646. C
647. D
648. A
649. B
650. A
651. C
652. D
653. D
654. C
655. A
656. C
657. C
658. D
659. A
660. D
661. A
662. B
663. D
664. D
665. C
666. C
667. D
668. A
669. D
670. B
671. A
672. A
673. C
674. C
675. C
676. D
677. A
678. D
679. A
680. D
681. C
682. A
683. A
684. B
685. B
686. B
687. B
688. D
689. A
690. D
691. D
692. B
693. D
694. D
695. C
696. A
697. A
698. D
699. D
700. C
701. B
702. A
703. C
704. C
705. A
706. A
707. A
708. A
709. D
710. D
711. C
712. D
713. A
714. B
715. D
716. A
717. C
718. D
719. C
720. D
721. B
722. C
723. C
724. A
725. C
726. A
727. D
728. A
729. D
730. A
731. D
732. D
733. A
734. D
735. C
736. D
737. B
738. C
739. A
740. D
741. C
742. C
743. A
744. A
745. D
746. B
747. C
748. B
749. D
750. B
751. B
752. A
753. D
754. D
755. B
756. C
757. A
758. B
759. D
760. B
761. D
762. D
763. B
764. D
765. D
766. D
767. D
768. D
769. D
770. D
771. A
772. D
773. B
774. D
775. D
776. B
777. B
778. C
779. A
780. B
781. D
782. A
783. D
784. D
785. A
786. B
787. A
788. D
789. A
790. C
791. C
792. D
793. A
794. C
795. B
796. D
797. B
798. B
799. D
800. C
801. A
802. D
803. A
804. A
805. C
806. C
807. B
808. D
809. D
810. C

ANSWERS

811. D
812. A
813. A
814. D
815. A
816. A
817. B
818. D
819. D
820. D
821. D
822. D
823. D
824. D
825. C
826. B
827. B
828. C
829. C
830. A
831. D
832. D
833. B
834. D
835. A
836. D
837. C
838. D
839. D
840. B
841. C
842. D
843. D
844. D
845. A
846. A
847. A
848. B
849. C
850. B
851. D
852. C
853. B
854. D
855. A
856. C
857. B
858. C
859. B
860. D
861. C
862. B
863. C
864. C
865. B
866. B
867. A
868. D
869. C
870. A
871. D
872. D
873. D
874. D
875. D
876. B
877. D
878. D
879. D
880. D
881. D
882. D
883. D
884. D
885. C
886. D
887. A
888. C
889. B
890. D
891. C
892. A
893. A
894. D
895. A
896. A
897. B
898. C
899. D
900. D
901. B
902. D
903. D
904. D
905. D
906. C
907. B
908. B
909. D
910. B
911. C
912. C
913. D
914. D
915. D
916. B
917. D
918. B
919. D
920. A
921. B
922. C
923. D
924. C
925. D
926. D
927. B
928. C
929. D
930. C
931. D
932. A
933. A
934. C
935. D
936. B
937. D
938. B
939. A
940. D
941. D
942. C
943. D
944. A
945. D
946. A
947. B
948. D
949. D
950. D
951. D
952. B
953. A
954. D
955. C
956. D
957. D
958. C
959. D
960. B
961. C
962. C
963. C
964. C
965. B
966. B
967. B
968. C
969. A
970. D
971. C
972. B
973. C
974. B
975. D
976. C
977. A
978. C
979. A
980. A
981. B
982. D
983. B
984. A
985. B
986. D
987. B
988. D
989. A
990. C
991. D
992. D
993. C
994. C
995. B
996. B
997. C
998. B
999. B
1000. A
1001. D
1002. C
1003. D
1004. C
1005. C
1006. B
1007. A
1008. A
1009. D
1010. B
1011. B
1012. C
1013. A
1014. C
1015. D
1016. B
1017. C
1018. B
1019. A
1020. D
1021. D
1022. D
1023. A
1024. A
1025. D
1026. B
1027. D
1028. B
1029. D
1030. C
1031. D
1032. C
1033. D
1034. D
1035. C
1036. D
1037. B
1038. C
1039. A
1040. D
1041. C
1042. A
1043. A
1044. D
1045. D
1046. D
1047. D
1048. C
1049. D
1050. A
1051. A
1052. A
1053. D
1054. D
1055. D
1056. A
1057. D
1058. D
1059. A
1060. D
1061. A
1062. D
1063. B
1064. C
1065. C
1066. B
1067. D
1068. D
1069. D
1070. D
1071. D
1072. D
1073. D
1074. B
1075. D
1076. D
1077. B
1078. B
1079. A
1080. A

ANSWERS

1081. A
1082. D
1083. D
1084. D
1085. B
1086. D
1087. D
1088. A
1089. A
1090. C
1091. C
1092. C
1093. B
1094. C
1095. D
1096. B
1097. D
1098. B
1099. A
1100. C
1101. B
1102. C
1103. D
1104. C
1105. D
1106. C
1107. B
1108. A
1109. A
1110. B
1111. D
1112. C
1113. D
1114. D
1115. B
1116. A
1117. D
1118. A
1119. D
1120. A
1121. D
1122. B
1123. C
1124. C
1125. C
1126. B,
1127. C
1128. C
1129. C
1130. B
1131. D
1132. D
1133. C
1134. D
1135. B
1136. D
1137. D
1138. B
1139. A
1140. D
1141. D
1142. C
1143. B
1144. C
1145. D
1146. D
1147. A
1148. D
1149. D
1150. C
1151. C
1152. D
1153. C
1154. B
1155. C
1156. B
1157. A
1158. D
1159. C
1160. B
1161. B
1162. D
1163. B
1164. B
1165. C
1166. D
1167. D
1168. D
1169. C
1170. A
1171. D
1172. D
1173. B
1174. D
1175. D
1176. D
1177. C
1178. C
1179. B
1180. B
1181. C
1182. D
1183. D
1184. A
1185. A
1186. C
1187. D
1188. B
1189. B
1190. A
1191. C
1192. C
1193. B
1194. C
1195. D
1196. D
1197. D
1198. D
1199. B
1200. D
1201. C
1202. C
1203. B
1204. C
1205. C
1206. B
1207. A
1208. A
1209. B
1210. D
1211. A
1212. C
1213. D
1214. C
1215. A
1216. C
1217. C
1218. C
1219. D
1220. C
1221. D
1222. B
1223. D
1224. D
1225. D
1226. D
1227. A
1228. D
1229. A
1230. B
1231. C
1232. B
1233. B
1234. C
1235. B
1236. B
1237. A
1238. A
1239. D
1240. A
1241. C
1242. D
1243. B
1244. C
1245. C
1246. D
1247. C
1248. B
1249. B
1250. B
1251. D
1252. D
1253. C
1254. B
1255. D
1256. D
1257. D
1258. B
1259. D
1260. D
1261. A
1262. B
1263. B
1264. D
1265. D
1266. B
1267. D
1268. B
1269. D
1270. A
1271. D
1272. B
1273. C
1274. C
1275. A
1276. D
1277. D
1278. A
1279. D
1280. B
1281. B
1282. D
1283. B
1284. A
1285. C
1286. D
1287. B
1288. B
1289. B
1290. A
1291. A
1292. C
1293. D
1294. B
1295. A
1296. D
1297. C
1298. D
1299. C
1300. A
1301. C
1302. D
1303. B
1304. A
1305. A
1306. D
1307. B
1308. D
1309. D
1310. D
1311. D
1312. D
1313. A
1314. C
1315. D
1316. D
1317. A
1318. C
1319. D
1320. A
1321. B
1322. D
1323. A
1324. D
1325. A
1326. B
1327. C
1328. A
1329. D
1330. A
1331. A
1332. B
1333. B
1334. C
1335. D
1336. D
1337. B
1338. D
1339. C
1340. D
1341. D
1342. D
1343. D
1344. D
1345. D
1346. A
1347. A
1348. C
1349. A
1350. B

ANSWERS

1351. D
1352. C
1353. D
1354. A
1355. D
1356. D
1357. D
1358. A
1359. C
1360. D
1361. D
1362. D
1363. D
1364. B
1365. D
1366. C
1367. A
1368. A
1369. D
1370. D
1371. D
1372. D
1373. B
1374. C
1375. D
1376. C
1377. D
1378. A
1379. D
1380. B
1381. C
1382. C
1383. B
1384. D
1385. D
1386. A
1387. C
1388. B
1389. D
1390. A
1391. D
1392. D
1393. D
1394. D
1395. A
1396. D
1397. D
1398. D
1399. D
1400. C
1401. B
1402. A
1403. A
1404. D
1405. C
1406. B
1407. C
1408. C
1409. A
1410. D
1411. A
1412. A
1413. A
1414. D
1415. D
1416. A
1417. D
1418. A
1419. B
1420. D
1421. A
1422. B
1423. D
1424. D
1425. C
1426. D
1427. C
1428. D
1429. D
1430. D
1431. B
1432. D
1433. D
1434. D
1435. B
1436. D
1437. D
1438. D
1439. D
1440. D
1441. B
1442. D
1443. C
1444. C
1445. C
1446. D
1447. B
1448. D
1449. D
1450. C
1451. A
1452. C
1453. D
1454. B
1455. D
1456. D
1457. A
1458. B
1459. D
1460. D
1461. D
1462. D
1463. D
1464. B
1465. B
1466. C
1467. D
1468. D
1469. A
1470. A
1471. B
1472. C
1473. D
1474. D
1475. B
1476. D
1477. D
1478. D
1479. D
1480. D
1481. C
1482. D
1483. D
1484. B
1485. D
1486. C
1487. B
1488. D
1489. A
1490. D
1491. A
1492. D
1493. D
1494. D
1495. C
1496. D
1497. A
1498. C
1499. A
1500. C
1501. D
1502. D
1503. C
1504. D
1505. B
1506. C
1507. C
1508. D
1509. D
1510. D
1511. D
1512. D
1513. D
1514. D
1515. B
1516. D
1517. D
1518. A
1519. A
1520. D
1521. D
1522. C
1523. B
1524. D
1525. B
1526. A
1527. D
1528. D
1529. C
1530. B
1531. D
1532. A
1533. C
1534. D
1535. D
1536. A
1537. A
1538. B
1539. B
1540. C
1541. C
1542. A
1543. B
1544. D
1545. C
1546. D
1547. D
1548. C
1549. B
1550. D
1551. C
1552. A
1553. B
1554. C
1555. D
1556. A
1557. B
1558. C
1559. D
1560. C
1561. C
1562. A
1563. D
1564. A
1565. C
1566. D
1567. D
1568. A
1569. C
1570. A
1571. D
1572. D
1573. D
1574. D
1575. D
1576. B
1577. A
1578. A
1579. D
1580. B
1581. C
1582. D
1583. A
1584. D
1585. D
1586. D
1587. D
1588. D
1589. D
1590. D
1591. C
1592. A
1593. B
1594. D
1595. D
1596. D
1597. D
1598. A
1599. D
1600. B
1601. C
1602. A
1603. D
1604. D
1605. A
1606. A
1607. A
1608. C
1609. C
1610. D
1611. D
1612. D
1613. C
1614. A
1615. A
1616. C
1617. C
1618. C
1619. D
1620. C

ANSWERS

1621. D
1622. A
1623. A
1624. D
1625. B
1626. D
1627. D
1628. B
1629. C
1630. D
1631. D
1632. D
1633. D
1634. D
1635. D
1636. C
1637. D
1638. D
1639. D
1640. B
1641. B
1642. B
1643. B
1644. D
1645. C
1646. D
1647. D
1648. B
1649. B
1650. D
1651. B
1652. D
1653. D
1654. C
1655. C
1656. D
1657. B
1658. C
1659. A
1660. B
1661. D
1662. D
1663. A
1664. D
1665. B
1666. B
1667. D
1668. B
1669. D
1670. C
1671. D
1672. A
1673. B
1674. D
1675. D
1676. D
1677. A
1678. A
1679. D
1680. D
1681. A
1682. D
1683. C
1684. B
1685. D
1686. C
1687. D
1688. B
1689. B
1690. B
1691. D
1692. B
1693. D
1694. D
1695. D
1696. B
1697. A
1698. C
1699. A
1700. A
1701. D
1702. A
1703. D
1704. D
1705. D
1706. C
1707. D
1708. D
1709. B
1710. D
1711. A
1712. D
1713. A
1714. D
1715. A
1716. B
1717. A
1718. D
1719. D
1720. D
1721. D
1722. A
1723. A
1724. A
1725. A
1726. A
1727. B
1728. C
1729. C
1730. C
1731. C
1732. D
1733. D
1734. D
1735. D
1736. B
1737. B
1738. D
1739. D
1740. C
1741. D
1742. D
1743. B
1744. C
1745. C
1746. B
1747. C
1748. D
1749. D
1750. A
1751. D
1752. D
1753. D
1754. B
1755. B
1756. B
1757. A
1758. C
1759. C
1760. B
1761. D
1762. B
1763. A
1764. D
1765. D
1766. A
1767. C
1768. A
1769. A
1770. A
1771. D
1772. A
1773. C
1774. D
1775. A
1776. A
1777. C
1778. D
1779. C
1780. B
1781. C
1782. A
1783. C
1784. A
1785. D
1786. D
1787. D
1788. B
1789. C
1790. A
1791. D
1792. A
1793. D
1794. D
1795. D
1796. D
1797. C
1798. C
1799. D
1800. C
1801. A
1802. B
1803. A
1804. D
1805. D
1806. D
1807. C
1808. B
1809. C
1810. D
1811. D
1812. D
1813. B
1814. A
1815. D
1816. A
1817. A
1818. D
1819. D
1820. B
1821. D
1822. D
1823. D
1824. A
1825. D
1826. C
1827. D
1828. D
1829. D
1830. C
1831. B
1832. D
1833. D
1834. C
1835. A
1836. B
1837. D
1838. D
1839. A
1840. D
1841. D
1842. B
1843. D
1844. C
1845. C,
1846. A
1847. D
1848. D
1849. D
1850. B
1851. D
1852. C
1853. A
1854. D
1855. D
1856. C
1857. C
1858. A
1859. C
1860. D
1861. A
1862. A
1863. D
1864. A
1865. C
1866. C
1867. B
1868. C
1869. B
1870. D
1871. C
1872. D
1873. A
1874. B
1875. B
1876. D
1877. B
1878. D
1879. C
1880. C
1881. B
1882. B
1883. C
1884. B
1885. A
1886. D
1887. A
1888. D
1889. B
1890. C

ANSWERS

1891. A
1892. C
1893. D
1894. D
1895. D
1896. D
1897. D
1898. D
1899. B
1900. C
1901. C
1902. D
1903. C
1904. D
1905. D
1906. D
1907. D
1908. B
1909. D
1910. C
1911. D
1912. D
1913. D
1914. C
1915. A
1916. D
1917. D
1918. D
1919. B
1920. C
1921. C
1922. A
1923. B
1924. D
1925. B
1926. D
1927. C
1928. B
1929. D
1930. C
1931. D
1932. D
1933. D
1934. C
1935. D
1936. D
1937. C
1938. C
1939. D
1940. A
1941. B
1942. C
1943. D
1944. D
1945. C
1946. D
1947. D
1948. D
1949. B
1950. A
1951. D
1952. A
1953. D
1954. D
1955. D
1956. C
1957. C
1958. D
1959. D
1960. D
1961. D
1962. D
1963. D
1964. D
1965. D
1966. C
1967. C
1968. D
1969. B
1970. B
1971. C
1972. D
1973. D
1974. A
1975. B
1976. D
1977. D
1978. D
1979. D
1980. D
1981. D
1982. D
1983. D
1984. A
1985. A
1986. C
1987. C
1988. B
1989. C
1990. D
1991. D
1992. D
1993. D
1994. D
1995. B
1996. C
1997. B
1998. D
1999. D
2000. D
2001. B
2002. D
2003. D
2004. A
2005. D
2006. D
2007. D
2008. D
2009. C
2010. D
2011. D
2012. D
2013. D
2014. A
2015. D
2016. D
2017. D
2018. D
2019. D
2020. B
2021. D
2022. D
2023. D
2024. A
2025. B
2026. C
2027. B
2028. D
2029. D
2030. D
2031. D
2032. D
2033. B
2034. C
2035. A
2036. A
2037. C
2038. D
2039. D
2040. D
2041. D
2042. D
2043. D
2044. A
2045. D
2046. D
2047. B
2048. D
2049. C
2050. C
2051. A
2052. D
2053. D
2054. C
2055. C
2056. A
2057. C
2058. A
2059. A
2060. D
2061. A
2062. C
2063. A
2064. D
2065. D
2066. D
2067. D
2068. A
2069. D
2070. D
2071. C
2072. D
2073. A
2074. B
2075. D
2076. D
2077. C
2078. B
2079. B
2080. D
2081. D
2082. D
2083. A
2084. A
2085. B
2086. C
2087. A
2088. B
2089. D
2090. A
2091. B
2092. D
2093. D
2094. D
2095. C
2096. A
2097. D
2098. B
2099. D
2100. B
2101. A
2102. B
2103. D
2104. B
2105. C
2106. C
2107. A
2108. B
2109. D
2110. D
2111. D
2112. D
2113. B
2114. D
2115. A
2116. D
2117. D
2118. D
2119. D
2120. D
2121. B
2122. C
2123. C
2124. D
2125. C
2126. B
2127. D
2128. C
2129. D
2130. C
2131. B
2132. B
2133. D
2134. D
2135. A
2136. A
2137. C
2138. D
2139. A
2140. D
2141. D
2142. B
2143. B
2144. D
2145. D
2146. B
2147. D
2148. D
2149. D
2150. A
2151. D
2152. D
2153. B
2154. D
2155. D
2156. C
2157. D
2158. D
2159. B
2160. D

ANSWERS

2161. D
2162. A
2163. A
2164. A
2165. A
2166. D
2167. B
2168. B
2169. B
2170. C
2171. A
2172. B
2173. A
2174. C
2175. C
2176. D
2177. B
2178. A
2179. D
2180. A
2181. B
2182. D
2183. D
2184. C
2185. C
2186. C
2187. D
2188. D
2189. A
2190. C
2191. B
2192. B
2193. D
2194. B
2195. D
2196. C
2197. D
2198. C
2199. C
2200. D
2201. D
2202. D
2203. A
2204. C
2205. D
2206. C
2207. D
2208. D
2209. D
2210. C
2211. B
2212. A
2213. D
2214. C
2215. A
2216. D
2217. D
2218. D
2219. B
2220. D
2221. A
2222. D
2223. A
2224. A
2225. D
2226. D
2227. B
2228. D
2229. B
2230. D
2231. D
2232. C
2233. C
2234. B
2235. C
2236. D
2237. D
2238. D
2239. C
2240. A
2241. B
2242. D
2243. C
2244. D
2245. D
2246. D
2247. A
2248. B
2249. C
2250. B
2251. B
2252. A
2253. A
2254. D
2255. C
2256. B
2257. A
2258. D
2259. A
2260. D
2261. C
2262. D
2263. C
2264. D
2265. D
2266. D
2267. B
2268. B
2269. C
2270. C
2271. C
2272. D
2273. D
2274. B
2275. B
2276. A
2277. A
2278. D
2279. D
2280. C
2281. C
2282. D
2283. D
2284. D
2285. B
2286. C
2287. B
2288. A
2289. D
2290. A
2291. D
2292. D
2293. C
2294. C
2295. D
2296. D
2297. D
2298. D
2299. B
2300. D
2301. D
2302. B
2303. C
2304. B
2305. D
2306. D
2307. C
2308. D
2309. A
2310. B
2311. A
2312. D
2313. C
2314. D
2315. A
2316. C
2317. B
2318. D
2319. D
2320. B
2321. D
2322. B
2323. D
2324. D
2325. A
2326. A
2327. B
2328. D
2329. D
2330. D
2331. B
2332. D
2333. D
2334. D
2335. C
2336. C
2337. D
2338. D
2339. B
2340. D
2341. D
2342. A
2343. D
2344. D
2345. D
2346. D
2347. D
2348. C
2349. B
2350. D
2351. D
2352. A
2353. D
2354. C
2355. D
2356. D
2357. A
2358. B
2359. B
2360. A
2361. D
2362. C
2363. C
2364. D
2365. A
2366. A
2367. B
2368. C
2369. D
2370. D
2371. D
2372. D
2373. D
2374. D
2375. A
2376. D
2377. B
2378. D
2379. B
2380. D
2381. D
2382. D
2383. D
2384. D
2385. C
2386. D
2387. D
2388. D
2389. D
2390. D
2391. A
2392. C
2393. B
2394. B
2395. B
2396. B
2397. B
2398. B
2399. A
2400. C
2401. A
2402. B
2403. D
2404. B
2405. C
2406. C
2407. B
2408. D
2409. D
2410. D
2411. D
2412. C
2413. D
2414. D
2415. D
2416. D
2417. D
2418. A
2419. C
2420. B
2421. A
2422. B
2423. D
2424. A
2425. A
2426. C
2427. D
2428. D
2429. C
2430. D

ANSWERS

2431. D	2451. D	2471. D	2491. C	2511. D	2531. D
2432. A	2452. D	2472. D	2492. B	2512. A	2532. D
2433. C	2453. A	2473. D	2493. D	2513. C	2533. D
2434. B	2454. D	2474. C	2494. D	2514. D	2534. B
2435. B	2455. D	2475. A	2495. A	2515. C	2535. B
2436. D	2456. A	2476. B	2496. B	2516. A	2536. A
2437. A	2457. B	2477. B	2497. A	2517. B	2537. C
2438. D	2458. D	2478. D	2498. D	2518. A	2538. C
2439. D	2459. D	2479. D	2499. B	2519. D	2539. C
2440. D	2460. A	2480. C	2500. B	2520. D	2540. B
2441. A	2461. D	2481. D	2501. D	2521. A	2541. A
2442. D	2462. D	2482. D	2502. D	2522. C	2542. C
2443. A	2463. D	2483. D	2503. A	2523. C	2543. B
2444. A	2464. A	2484. C	2504. C	2524. B	2544. C
2445. D	2465. A	2485. C	2505. A	2525. D	2545. D
2446. D	2466. D	2486. A	2506. D	2526. D	2546. A
2447. D	2467. D	2487. D	2507. B	2527. A	2547. D
2448. B	2468. D	2488. B	2508. D	2528. D	2548. B
2449. C	2469. B	2489. D	2509. D	2529. D	2549. C
2450. D	2470. B	2490. A	2510. D	2530. B	2550. D
					2551. B
					2552. D

Endocrinology 6

Approach to the Patient with Endocrine Disorders

1. Term 'endocrine' was coined by?
Harrison's 20th Ed. Chapter 369 Page 2649

A. Jameson
B. Smith
C. Starling
D. Keith

2. The term hormone, derived from a Greek phrase meaning?
Harrison's 20th Ed. Chapter 369 Page 2649

A. "To synchronize"
B. "To set in motion"
C. "To rewind"
D. "To speak"

Starling differentiated between endocrine & exocrine secretions. Word "Hormone" is derived from a Greek phrase meaning "to set in motion".

3. Classic endocrine glands communicate with other organs through?
Harrison's 20th Ed. Chapter 369 Page 2649

A. Hormones
B. Cytokines
C. Growth factors
D. All of the above

The classic endocrine glands (pituitary, thyroid, parathyroid, pancreatic islets, adrenals & gonads) communicate broadly with other organs through the nervous system, hormones, cytokines & growth factors.

4. Which of the following is caused by dysregulation of immune surveillance and tolerance?
Harrison's 20th Ed. Chapter 369 Page 2649

A. Autoimmune thyroid disease
B. Addison's disease
C. Lymphocytic hypophysitis
D. Polyglandular failure

5. Which of the following is a vasoactive substance?
Harrison's 20th Ed. Chapter 369 Page 2649

A. Angiotensin II
B. Endothelin
C. Nitric oxide
D. All of the above

Vasoactive substances include catecholamines, angiotensin II, endothelin, and nitric oxide.

6. Which of the following is produced by adipose tissue?
Harrison's 20th Ed. Chapter 369 Page 2649

A. Leptin
B. Adiponectin
C. Resistin
D. All of the above

7. Endocrine diseases include those due to?
Harrison's 20th Ed. Chapter 369 Page 2649

A. Hormone excess
B. Hormone deficiency
C. Hormone resistance
D. All of the above

8. Syndromes of hormone excess can be caused by?
Harrison's 20th Ed. Chapter 369 Page 2649

A. Neoplastic growth of endocrine cells
B. Autoimmune disorders
C. Excess hormone administration
D. All of the above

9. Which of the following is a "set point defect" endocrine tumor?
Harrison's 20th Ed. Chapter 369 Page 2649

A. Cushing's disease
B. Parathyroid adenoma
C. Autonomously functioning thyroid nodule
D. All of the above

10. MEN1 is characterized by all except?
Harrison's 20th Ed. Chapter 369 Page 2649

A. Parathyroid tumor
B. Pancreatic islet tumor
C. Pituitary tumor
D. Pheochromocytoma

11. MEN2 is characterized by all except?
Harrison's 20th Ed. Chapter 369 Page 2649

A. Medullary thyroid carcinoma
B. Pituitary tumor
C. Pheochromocytoma
D. Hyperparathyroidism

12. Which of the following is false about MEN1 gene?
Harrison's 20th Ed. Chapter 369 Page 2649

A. Located on chromosome 11q13
B. Encodes menin
C. Menin is a putative tumor-suppressor gene
D. None of the above

13. MEN2 best relates to?
Harrison's 20th Ed. Chapter 369 Page 2649

A. Homozygous inactivating mutation
B. Heterozygous inactivating mutation
C. Activating mutations in a single allele
D. Recessive inactivating mutation

MEN2 is caused by activating mutations in a single allele.

14. Medullary thyroid carcinoma best relates to?
Harrison's 20th Ed. Chapter 369 Page 2649

A. PRAD 1 proto-oncogene
B. RET proto-oncogene
C. KIT proto-oncogene
D. Proto-oncogene c-fos

RET protooncogene, which encodes a receptor tyrosine kinase, leads to thyroid C cell hyperplasia in childhood before the development of medullary thyroid carcinoma.

15. Which of the following is a disease of activating mutation?
Harrison's 20th Ed. Chapter 369 Page 2650

A. Male limited precocious puberty
B. McCune-Albright syndrome
C. Acromegaly
D. All of the above

16. Most severe hormone resistance syndromes are due to?
Harrison's 20th Ed. Chapter 369 Page 2650

A. Inherited defects in membrane receptors
B. Inherited defects in nuclear receptors
C. Inherited defects in pathways that transduce receptor signals
D. All of the above

17. Which of the following is an acquired form of functional hormone resistance?
Harrison's 20th Ed. Chapter 369 Page 2650

A. Insulin resistance in type 2 diabetes mellitus
B. Leptin resistance in obesity
C. GH resistance in catabolic states
D. All of the above

The pathogenesis of functional resistance involves receptor down regulation & postreceptor desensitization of signaling pathways. Functional forms of resistance are generally reversible.

18. Which of the following methods for estimating hormone concentration is now used rarely?
Harrison's 20th Ed. Chapter 369 Page 2650

A. Immunoassay
B. Mass spectroscopy
C. Chromatography
D. Bioassay

19. Urine determination of which of the following is useful?
Harrison's 20th Ed. Chapter 369 Page 2650

A. 17-hydroxycorticosteroid
B. 17-ketosteroid
C. Vanillylmandelic acid
D. All of the above

Urine determination of free cortisol, 17-hydroxycorticosteroids, 17-ketosteroids, vanillylmandelic acid, metanephrine, catecholamines, 5-hydroxyindoleacetic acid, and calcium is useful.

20. What is the approximate prevalence of Type 2 diabetes mellitus in adults?
Harrison's 20th Ed. Chapter 369 Page 2651 Table 369-2

A. > 4%
B. > 6%
C. > 8%
D. > 10%

21. What is the approximate prevalence of metabolic syndrome in adults?
Harrison's 20th Ed. Chapter 369 Page 2651 Table 369-2

A. > 15%
B. > 22%
C. > 35%
D. > 46%

22. What is the approximate prevalence of hyperlipidemia in adults?
Harrison's 20th Ed. Chapter 369 Page 2651 Table 369-2

A. ~ 15%
B. ~ 22%
C. ~ 35%
D. ~ 46%

Mechanisms of Hormone Action

23. Which of the following is not an amino acid derivative?
Harrison's 20th Ed. Chapter 370 Page 2653

A. Dopamine
B. Catecholamines
C. Somatostatin
D. Thyroid hormone

24. Which of the following is not a 'small neuropeptide' class of hormone?
Harrison's 20th Ed. Chapter 370 Page 2653

A. Gonadotropin-releasing hormone (GnRH)
B. Thyrotropin-releasing hormone (TRH)
C. Somatostatin
D. Luteinizing hormone (LH)

25. Which of the following is not a 'large protein' class of hormone?
Harrison's 20th Ed. Chapter 370 Page 2653

A. Vasopressin
B. Insulin
C. Luteinizing hormone (LH)
D. PTH

26. Which of the following hormone is "lipid-soluble"?
Harrison's 20th Ed. Chapter 370 Page 2653

A. Steroids
B. Thyroid hormones
C. Vitamin D
D. All of the above

27. The glycoprotein hormone family consists of?
Harrison's 20th Ed. Chapter 370 Page 2653

A. Thyroid-stimulating hormone (TSH)
B. Follicle-stimulating hormone (FSH) & Luteinizing hormone (LH)
C. Human chorionic gonadotropin (hCG)
D. All of the above

Hormones are divided into 5 major classes—amino acid derivatives (dopamine, catecholamines & thyroid hormone), small neuropeptides (GnRH, TRH, somatostatin & vasopressin), large proteins (insulin, LH & PTH), steroid hormones (cortisol & estrogen) & vitamin derivatives (vitamin A & D). Amino acid derived & peptide hormones interact with cell-surface membrane receptors. Steroids, thyroid hormones, vitamin D & retinoids are lipid-soluble & interact with intracellular nuclear receptors. Glycoprotein hormones are thyroid-stimulating hormone (TSH), FSH, LH & human chorionic gonadotropin (hCG).

28. Which of the following is about glycoprotein hormones?
Harrison's 20th Ed. Chapter 370 Page 2653

A. Heterodimers
B. Share the α subunit in common
C. β subunits are distinct and confer specific biologic actions
D. None of the above

29. Very high levels of hCG during pregnancy stimulate which of the following receptor?
Harrison's 20th Ed. Chapter 370 Page 2653

A. TSH
B. LH
C. FSH
D. All of the above

Very high levels of hCG during pregnancy stimulate the TSH receptor & increase thyroid hormone levels.

30. High degree of specificity is seen with?
Harrison's 20th Ed. Chapter 370 Page 2653

A. Glycoprotein hormones
B. Insulin and insulin-like growth factor I (IGF-I) and IGF-II
C. PTH and parathyroid hormone-related peptide (PTHrP)
D. All of the above

31. Which of the following is not type 1 of nuclear receptor family?
Harrison's 20th Ed. Chapter 370 Page 2653

A. Glucocorticoid receptor
B. Mineralocorticoid receptor
C. Androgen receptor
D. Thyroid hormone receptor

32. Which of the following is not type 2 of nuclear receptor family?
Harrison's 20th Ed. Chapter 370 Page 2653

A. Progesterone receptor
B. Peroxisome proliferator activated receptor
C. Retinoic acid receptor
D. Vitamin D receptor

According to their specificities for DNA binding sites, nuclear receptor family is classified into type 1 receptors (glucocorticoid receptor, mineralocorticoid receptor, androgen receptor, estrogen receptor, progesterone receptor) that bind steroids & type 2 receptors (thyroid hormone receptor, vitamin D receptor, retinoic acid receptor, peroxisome proliferator activated receptor) that bind thyroid hormone, vitamin D, retinoic acid.

33. Which of the following is highly conserved in nuclear receptors?
Harrison's 20th Ed. Chapter 370 Page 2653

A. Hormone-binding domains
B. Zinc finger DNA-binding domains
C. Ligand-binding domain
D. Ubiquitin-binding domain

34. Which of the following has relaxed nuclear receptor specificity?
Harrison's 20th Ed. Chapter 370 Page 2654

A. Androgen receptor
B. Retinoic acid receptor
C. Estrogen receptor
D. Peroxisome proliferator activated receptor

Estrogen receptor can bind an array of compounds, some of which have little apparent structural similarity to the high-affinity ligand estradiol. ER is susceptible to activation by "environmental estrogens".

35. Which of the following hormones is produced from precursor polypeptides?

Harrison's 20th Ed. Chapter 370 Page 2654

A. ACTH
B. Glucagon
C. PTH
D. All of the above

36. Which out of the following is the last step in synthesis of peptide hormones?

Harrison's 20th Ed. Chapter 370 Page 2654

A. Transcription
B. Protein
C. Intracellular sorting
D. Post-translational protein processing

The synthesis of peptide hormones occurs through a classic pathway of gene expression: transcription → mRNA → protein → posttranslational protein processing → intracellular sorting, followed by membrane integration or secretion.

37. Which of the following hormone precursors generate multiple biologically active peptides?

Harrison's 20th Ed. Chapter 370 Page 2654

A. Proopiomelanocortin (POMC)
B. Proinsulin
C. Pro-PTH
D. All of the above

POMC and proglucagon are hormone precursors that generate multiple biologically active peptides.

38. Hormones that are stored in secretory granules before release are all except?

Harrison's 20th Ed. Chapter 370 Page 2654

A. GnRH
B. Insulin
C. Steroid hormones
D. GH

Peptide hormones (GnRH, insulin, GH) are stored in secretory granules before a releasing factor or a neural signal stimulates their release. Steroid hormones diffuse into circulation as they are synthesized.

39. "StAR" refers to?

Harrison's 20th Ed. Chapter 370 Page 2654

A. Steroidogenic active regulatory protein
B. Steroidogenic acute regulatory protein
C. Steroidogenic action regulatory protein
D. Steroidogenic augmenting regulatory protein

StAR (steroidogenic acute regulatory protein) transports cholesterol into mitochondrion upon stimulation by ACTH and LH in the steroidogenic pathway.

40. Which of the following hormones has a short half-life?

Harrison's 20th Ed. Chapter 370 Page 2654

A. TSH
B. Somatostatin
C. Prolactin
D. PTH

41. Which of the following hormones has the longest half-life?

Harrison's 20th Ed. Chapter 370 Page 2654

A. LH
B. ACTH
C. T3
D. T4

Most protein hormones (ACTH, GH, prolactin, PTH, LH) have relatively short half-lives (<20 minutes). Somatostatin hormone signals are evanescent. T4 has a circulating half-life of 7 days.

42. T4 & T3 bind to which of the following serum-binding proteins?

Harrison's 20th Ed. Chapter 370 Page 2654

A. Thyroxine-binding globulin (TBG)
B. Albumin
C. Thyroxine-binding prealbumin (TBPA)
D. All of the above

T4 & T3 bind to thyroxine-binding globulin (TBG), albumin, and thyroxine-binding prealbumin (TBPA).

43. Follistatin bind which of the following?

Harrison's 20th Ed. Chapter 370 Page 2654

A. Activin
B. IGF-I and II
C. Cortisol
D. Estrogen

Activin binds to follistatin.

44. Hormone association with serum-binding proteins leads to?

Harrison's 20th Ed. Chapter 370 Page 2654

A. Provide a hormonal reservoir, prevent rapid degradation
B. Restrict hormone access to certain sites
C. Modulate the unbound or "free" hormone concentrations
D. All of the above

45. Which of the following displaces T4 from TBG?

Harrison's 20th Ed. Chapter 370 Page 2655

A. Insulin
B. Salicylates and salsalate
C. Testosterone
D. Ciprofloxacin

46. Which of the following is an endocytotic receptor for thyroglobulin?

Harrison's 20th Ed. Chapter 370 Page 2655

A. Megalin
B. Cubilin
C. Inulin
D. All of the above

47. Megalin is an endocytotic receptor for?

Harrison's 20th Ed. Chapter 370 Page 2655

A. Thyroglobulin
B. Carrier-bound vitamins A and D
C. SHBG-bound androgens & estrogens
D. All of the above

48. Which of the following inactivates glucocorticoids in renal tubular cells?
Harrison's 20th Ed. Chapter 370 Page 2655

A. 3β-hydroxysteroid dehydrogenase
B. 11β-hydroxysteroid dehydrogenase
C. 17β-hydroxysteroid dehydrogenase
D. All of the above

49. Which of the following about hormone receptors is false?
Harrison's 20th Ed. Chapter 370 Page 2655

A. Membrane receptors bind peptide hormones & catecholamine
B. Nuclear receptors bind small molecules
C. Low concentrations of free hormone rapidly associate and dissociate from receptors
D. None of the above

50. Which of the following about hormone receptors is false?
Harrison's 20th Ed. Chapter 370 Page 2655

A. ACTH receptors are located exclusively in adrenal cortex
B. FSH receptors are found only in gonads
C. Insulin receptors are widely distributed
D. Thyroid hormone receptors are found only in thyroid gland

Hormone receptors are either membrane or nuclear. Membrane receptors bind peptide hormones & catecholamines. Nuclear receptors bind small molecules that can diffuse across cell membrane like thyroid hormone, steroids & vitamin D. ACTH receptors are located almost exclusively in adrenal cortex, & FSH receptors are found only in gonads. Insulin & thyroid hormone receptors are widely distributed.

51. T4 & T3 bind to all except?
Harrison's 20th Ed. Chapter 370 Page 2655

A. Thyroxine-binding globulin (TBG)
B. Albumin
C. Thyroxine-binding prealbumin (TBPA)
D. Globulin

T4 & T3 bind to thyroxine-binding globulin (TBG), albumin & thyroxine-binding prealbumin (TBPA).

52. Which of the following is a membrane receptor for hormones?
Harrison's 20th Ed. Chapter 370 Page 2655

A. GPCR
B. Tyrosine kinase receptors
C. Serine kinase receptors
D. All of the above

Membrane receptors for hormones are 7 transmembrane GPCRs, tyrosine kinase receptors, cytokine receptors & serine kinase receptors. Membrane receptors bind peptide hormones & catecholamines.

53. G proteins are so named because?
Harrison's 20th Ed. Chapter 370 Page 2655

A. By alphabetical order
B. Growth phase of cell division
C. They bind guanine nucleotides (GTP, GDP)
D. None of the above

G proteins are a large family that form a heterotrimeric complex composed of various α and βγ subunits. The α subunit contains the guanine nucleotide—binding site & hydrolyzes GTP to GDP. The βγ subunits modulate the activity of the α subunit besides mediating their own effector signaling pathways.

54. Which of the following about G proteins (guanine nucleotide-binding proteins) is false?
N Engl J Med 2013; 368:2515-2516

A. Heterotrimers
B. Composed of guanosine triphosphate binding alpha subunits and tightly linked beta and gamma subunits
C. Couple G-protein–coupled receptors
D. None of the above

55. Which of the following about GNAS is false?
N Engl J Med 2013; 368:2515-2516

A. Human alpha-subunit gene
B. Expressed ubiquitously
C. Gs is the G protein encoded by GNAS
D. None of the above

56. Which of the following mediates signal transduction through adenylate cyclase or phospholipase C?
Harrison's 20th Ed. Chapter 370 Page 2655

A. GTP
B. GDP
C. Gα
D. Gbg

Hormone binding to the receptor induces GDP dissociation, allowing Gα to bind GTP & dissociate from the complex. Then, the Gα subunit is activated and mediates signal transduction through adenylate cyclase or phospholipase C. GTP hydrolysis to GDP allows reassociation with the βγ subunits and restores the inactive state.

57. Which of the following is an isoform of Gα subunit?
Harrison's 20th Ed. Chapter 370 Page 2655

A. Gsα
B. Giα
C. Gqα
D. All of the above

There are more than a dozen isoforms of Gα subunit. Gsα stimulates, whereas Giα inhibits adenylate cyclase that generates second messenger cyclic AMP leading to activation of protein kinase A. Gq subunits couple to phospholipase C generating diacylglycerol & inositol triphosphate leading to activation of protein kinase C & release of intracellular calcium.

58. Which of the following receptors transduce signals for insulin?
Harrison's 20th Ed. Chapter 370 Page 2655

A. GPCR
B. Tyrosine kinase receptors
C. Serine kinase receptors
D. Cytokine receptors

Tyrosine kinase receptors transduce signals for insulin & growth factors like IGF-I, epidermal growth factor (EGF), nerve growth factor, platelet-derived growth factor & fibroblast growth factor. Tyrosine kinase receptors play a prominent role in cell growth, differentiation & in intermediary metabolism.

59. Growth hormone (GH) acts via which of the following membrane receptor for hormones?
Harrison's 20th Ed. Chapter 370 Page 2655

A. GPCR
B. Tyrosine kinase receptors
C. Serine kinase receptors
D. Cytokine receptor-linked kinase

GH & PRL receptors belong to the cytokine receptor family.

60. The seven transmembrane GPCR family binds all of the following except?

Harrison's 20th Ed. Chapter 370 Page 2655

A. LH
B. TRH
C. Calcium
D. Activin

The seven transmembrane GPCR family binds large proteins (LH, PTH), small peptides (TRH, somatostatin), catecholamines (epinephrine, dopamine), and minerals (calcium).

61. Intracellular Janus kinases (JAKs) is related to which of the following receptors?

Harrison's 20th Ed. Chapter 370 Page 2656

A. GPCR
B. Tyrosine kinase receptors
C. Serine kinase receptors
D. Cytokine receptors

Janus kinases (JAKs) phosphorylate members of signal transduction & activators of transcription (STAT) family and other signaling pathways (Ras, PI3-K, MAPK). Activated STAT proteins translocate to the nucleus & stimulate expression of target genes.

62. Serine kinase receptors mediate the action of?

Harrison's 20th Ed. Chapter 370 Page 2657

A. Activins
B. Transforming growth factor
C. Müllerian-inhibiting substance
D. All of the above

Serine kinase receptors mediate the actions of activins, transforming growth factor, Müllerian-inhibiting substance (MIS or anti-Müllerian hormone-AMH), and bone morphogenic proteins (BMPs).

63. Smads is related to which of the following membrane receptor for hormones?

Harrison's 20th Ed. Chapter 370 Page 2657

A. GPCR
B. Tyrosine kinase receptors
C. Serine kinase receptors
D. Cytokine receptors

Serine kinase receptors (type I & II subunits) signal through proteins called smads (fusion of Caenorhabditis elegans *sma + mammalian mad).*

64. Short stature may be due to?

Harrison's 20th Ed. Chapter 370 Page 2658

A. GH deficiency
B. Hypothyroidism
C. Cushing's syndrome
D. All of the above

GH deficiency, hypothyroidism, Cushing's syndrome, precocious puberty, malnutrition, chronic illness or genetic abnormalities affecting epiphyseal growth plates (FGFR3 or SHOX mutations) cause short stature.

65. Which of the following does not stimulate growth?

Harrison's 20th Ed. Chapter 370 Page 2658

A. GH
B. IGF-I
C. Thyroid hormone
D. Sex steroids

GH, IGF-I & TH stimulate growth, whereas sex steroids lead to epiphyseal closure.

66. Feedback regulation for which of the following does not involve pituitary gland?

Harrison's 20th Ed. Chapter 370 Page 2659

A. Leptin
B. IGF-I
C. Thyroid hormones
D. Cortisol

Feedback regulation for endocrine systems that do not involve pituitary gland are calcium feedback on PTH, glucose inhibition of insulin secretion, and leptin feedback on the hypothalamus.

67. Which of the following is not a negative hormonal feedback regulatory system?

Harrison's 20th Ed. Chapter 370 Page 2659

A. Thyroid hormones on TRH-TSH axis
B. Estrogen-mediated stimulation of mid-cycle LH surge
C. Cortisol on CRH-ACTH axis
D. Gonadal steroids on GnRH-LH/FSH axis

Following are the negative feedback regulatory systems—thyroid hormones on TRH-TSH axis, cortisol on CRH-ACTH axis, gonadal steroids on GnRH-LH/FSH axis and IGF-I on GHRH-GH axis, calcium feedback on PTH, glucose inhibition of insulin secretion, and leptin feedback on hypothalamus. Positive feedback control is estrogen-mediated stimulation of mid-cycle LH surge.

68. Which of the following is false?

Harrison's 20th Ed. Chapter 370 Page 2659

A. Paracrine regulation means factors released by one cell that act on an adjacent cell in the same tissue
B. Autocrine regulation means action of a factor on the same cell from which it is produced
C. Levels of paracrine & autocrine control factors cannot be readily measured
D. None of the above

69. IGF-I acts on?

Harrison's 20th Ed. Chapter 370 Page 2659

A. Chondrocytes
B. Breast epithelium
C. Gonadal cells
D. All of the above

IGF-I acts on many cells that produce it like chondrocytes, breast epithelium & gonadal cells (autocrine regulation).

Physiology of Anterior Pituitary Hormones

70. The number of major hormones produced by anterior pituitary gland is?

Harrison's 20th Ed. Chapter 371 Page 2659

A. 4
B. 5
C. 6
D. 7

Six major hormones produced by anterior pituitary gland are Prolactin (PRL), Growth hormone (GH), Adrenocorticotropin hormone (ACTH), Luteinizing hormone (LH), Follicle-stimulating hormone (FSH) & Thyroid-stimulating hormone (TSH).

71. Which of the following about pituitary gland is false?

Harrison's 20th Ed. Chapter 371 Page 2659

A. Pituitary hormones are secreted in pulsatile manner
B. Posterior pituitary is supplied by superior hypophyseal arteries
C. Posterior lobe is innervated by hypothalamic neurons
D. Posterior pituitary hormones come from direct neural extensions

Major blood supply for anterior pituitary is hypothalamic-pituitary portal plexus which allows effective transmission of hypothalamic peptide pulses to it without significant systemic dilution. Posterior pituitary is supplied by inferior hypophyseal arteries.

72. The pituitary gland weighs about?

Harrison's 20th Ed. Chapter 371 Page 2660

A. 100 mg
B. 300 mg
C. 600 mg
D. 800 mg

Pituitary gland weighs ~600 mg. Located within sella turcica ventral to the diaphragma sella, it comprises anatomically & functionally distinct anterior & posterior lobes.

73. Which of the following is false?

Harrison's 20th Ed. Chapter 371 Page 2660

A. Hypothalamic neural cells synthesize releasing hormones
B. Hypothalamic neural cells synthesize inhibiting hormones
C. Hypothalamic hormones are secreted into portal vessels of pituitary stalk
D. None of the above

74. Which of the following is present in the pituitary stalk?

Harrison's 20th Ed. Chapter 371 Page 2660

A. Mediohypophyseal nerve tract
B. Opticohypophyseal nerve tract
C. Tuberohypophyseal nerve tract
D. Hypothalamohypophyseal nerve tract

The posterior lobe is directly innervated by hypothalamic neurons (supraopticohypophyseal and tuberohypophyseal nerve tracts) via the pituitary stalk.

75. "Median eminence" is best described as?

Guyton's Textbook of Medical Physiology 11th Ed. 921

A. Lowermost portion of hypothalamus
B. Uppermost portion of pituitary
C. Lowermost portion of pituitary
D. Anteriormost portion of pituitary

76. "Tuber cinereum" is best described as?

Guyton's Textbook of Medical Physiology 11th Ed. 921

A. Extension of pituitary tissue into pituitary stalk
B. Extension of hypothalamic tissue into pituitary stalk
C. Extension of anterior pituitary tissue into pars intermedia
D. Extension of posterior pituitary tissue into pars intermedia

Pituitary gland is also called hypophysis (anterior pituitary - adenohypophysis, posterior pituitary - neurohypophysis). It is connected to hypothalamus by pituitary (or hypophysial) stalk. Between these two portions of pituitary is a small, relatively avascular zone called pars intermedia. Lowermost portion of hypothalamus is called median eminence, which connects inferiorly with pituitary stalk. Tuber cinereum is an extension of hypothalamic tissue into pituitary stalk. Embryologically, anterior pituitary originates from Rathke's pouch, which is an embryonic invagination of the pharyngeal epithelium, while posterior pituitary originates from a neural tissue outgrowth from hypothalamus.

77. Fetal appearance of which of the following is earliest?

Harrison's 20th Ed. Chapter 371 Page 2660 Table 371-1

A. Gonadotrope
B. Lactotrope
C. Corticotrope
D. Thyrotrope

Corticotrope appear at 6 weeks, somatotrophs at 8 weeks & rest at 12 weeks in fetus.

78. Which of the following is an inhibitor of thyrotrope?

Harrison's 20th Ed. Chapter 371 Page 2660 Table 371-1

A. Dopamine
B. Somatostatin
C. Glucocorticoids
D. All of the above

79. Which of the following is a trophic effect on thyrotrope?

Harrison's 20th Ed. Chapter 371 Page 2660 Table 371-1

A. T3 synthesis and secretion
B. T4 synthesis and secretion
C. TSH synthesis and secretion
D. All of the above

80. Which of the following is a stimulator of gonadotrope?

Harrison's 20th Ed. Chapter 371 Page 2660 Table 371-1

A. GnRH
B. Activins
C. Estrogen
D. All of the above

81. Which of the following is a stimulator of lactotrope?

Harrison's 20th Ed. Chapter 371 Page 2660 Table 371-1

A. Estrogen
B. TRH
C. VIP
D. All of the above

82. Which of the following secrete a polypeptide?
Harrison's 20th Ed. Chapter 371 Page 2660 Table 371-1

A. Lactotrope
B. Somatotrope
C. Corticotrope
D. All of the above

83. SF-1 is the tissue-specific transcription factor for?
Harrison's 20th Ed. Chapter 371 Page 2660 Table 371-1

A. Thyrotrope
B. Lactotrope
C. Gonadotrope
D. Corticotrope

84. T-Pit is the tissue-specific transcription factor for?
Harrison's 20th Ed. Chapter 371 Page 2660 Table 371-1

A. Thyrotrope
B. Lactotrope
C. Gonadotrope
D. Corticotrope

85. Prop-1 is the tissue-specific transcription factor for?
Harrison's 20th Ed. Chapter 371 Page 2660 Table 371-1

A. Thyrotrope
B. Lactotrope
C. Somatotrope
D. All of the above

86. AVP is the stimulator for?
Harrison's 20th Ed. Chapter 371 Page 2660 Table 371-1

A. Thyrotrope
B. Lactotrope
C. Gonadotrope
D. Corticotrope

87. Ghrelin is the stimulator for?
Harrison's 20th Ed. Chapter 371 Page 2660 Table 371-1

A. Thyrotrope
B. Lactotrope
C. Gonadotrope
D. Somatotrope

88. Pituitary development best relates to?
Harrison's 20th Ed. Chapter 371 Page 2660

A. Hartmann's pouch
B. Indiana pouch
C. Rathke's pouch
D. Morrison's pouch

89. Pituitary gland secrete highly specific trophic hormones in response to?
N Engl J Med 2006;355:2558-73

A. Hypothalamic
B. Intrapituitary
C. Peripheral hormonal and growth factor signals
D. All of the above

Distinct cellular compartments within the pituitary gland secrete highly specific trophic hormones in response to hypothalamic, intrapituitary, and peripheral hormonal and growth factor signals.

90. Pit-1, Prop-1, SF-1, and DAX-1 are related to?
Harrison's 20th Ed. Chapter 371 Page 2660

A. Hypothalamus development
B. Pituitary development
C. Pancreatic development
D. All of the above

Anterior pituitary gland develops from nasopharyngeal Rathke's pouch. Pit-1, Prop-1, SF-1, and DAX-1 are lineage-specific transcription factors in pluripotential stem cells during embryonic differentiation. Pit-1 determines cell-specific expression of GH (somatotropes), PRL (lactotropes) & TSH (thyrotropes). Prop-1 induces the pituitary development of Pit-1-specific lineages, as well as gonadotropes. Gonadotrope cell development is further defined by the cell-specific expression of nuclear receptors, steroidogenic factor (SF-1) & DAX-1. Corticotropin upstream transcription element (CUTE) & PTX-1 transcription factor play a role in development of corticotrope cells.

91. Which of the following is the correct sequential expression pattern of pituitary-specific transcription factors?
Int. J. Mol. Sci. 2019;20(8):1875

A. PIT-1→PROP1→HESX-1→SOX2→SOX3→LHX-3→LHX-4
B. PROP1→PIT-1→HESX-1→SOX2→SOX3→LHX-3→LHX-4
C. PROP1→PIT-1→SOX2→HESX-1→SOX3→LHX-3→LHX-4
D. PROP1→PIT-1→SOX2→SOX3→HESX-1→LHX-3→LHX-4

Embryonic development of pituitary follows a well-defined pattern of sequential expression of pituitary-specific transcription factors such as Prophet of PIT-1 (PROP1), PIT-1 (POU1FI), HESX-1, SOX2, SOX3, LHX-3, and LHX-4.

92. Which of the following statements about PROP1 is false?
Harrison's 20th Ed. Chapter 371 Page 2660

A. PROP1 is a transcription factor for developing anterior pituitary
B. PROP1 expression precedes & is required for PIT-1 expression
C. PROP1 is located on chromosome 5q35.3
D. None of the above

The transcription factor PROP1 is a key regulator of the differentiation of pluripotent anterior pituitary cells into distinct cell lines with characteristic secretory profiles. Generally, hormone deficiencies present a typical temporal pattern: first GH and TSH and then FSH, LH, and ACTH. The human Pit1 gene has been mapped to chromosome 3.

93. Which of the following statements about PROP1 is false?
The Journal of Clinical Endocrinology & Metabolism. 2004; 89(10):5256-65

A. PROP1 is an acronym for "Prophet of PIT1"
B. Appears early in embryonic development
C. PROP-1 gene is expressed only in the anterior pituitary lobe
D. None of the above

94. Nuclear transcription factor PIT-1 is now called?
N Engl J Med 2006;355:2558-73

A. POU1F1
B. POU1F2
C. POU1F3
D. POU1F4

POU1F1 stands for POU domain, class 1 homeobox 1. PIT-1 is a pituitary lineage determining factor.

95. Which of the following statements about PIT-1 is false?
N Engl J Med 2006;355:2558-73

A. Pit-1 expression is restricted to the anterior pituitary lobe
B. Essential for the development of somatotrophs, lactotrophs, and thyrotrophs
C. R271W in one allele of Pit-1 gene is most common mutation
D. None of the above

96. Pit-1 mutations can cause deficiency of?
Harrison's 20th Ed. Chapter 371 Page 2660

A. GH
B. Prolactin
C. TSH
D. All of the above

Autosomal dominant or recessive Pit-1 mutations cause combined GH, PRL & TSH deficiencies resulting in growth failure & hypothyroidism.

97. Hypopituitarism in patients with PROP1 mutations typically includes deficiencies of?
The Journal of Clinical Endocrinology & Metabolism. 2004; 89(10):5256-65

A. LH/FSH
B. TSH
C. PRL
D. All of the above

Hypopituitarism in patients with PROP1 mutations includes deficiencies of GH, TSH, PRL, and LH/FSH.

98. PROP-1 mutations result in deficiency of all except?
Harrison's 20th Ed. Chapter 371 Page 2660

A. GH
B. Prolactin
C. ACTH
D. Gonadotropin

During development, Prop-1 is essential for Pit-1 function. Prop-1 mutations result in combined GH, PRL, TSH & gonadotropin deficiency with preservation of ACTH.

99. Which of the following about combined pituitary hormone deficiency (CPHD) is false?
Int. J. Mol. Sci. 2019;20(8):1875

A. Defined as impaired production of ≥ 2 anterior and/or posterior pituitary hormones
B. May result from acquired or from genetically defined conditions
C. PROP1 mutations are most common genetic cause of CPHD
D. None of the above

CPHD due to PROP1 mutations present with growth failure in late infancy or childhood with no neonatal sign of GH deficiency, such as hypoglycemia, seizures, and prolonged jaundice. c.301-302delAG and c.150delA are the most common PROP1 mutations and represent more than 90% of the mutated alleles in the Eastern European cohorts.

100. Lactotropes constitute what percentage of anterior pituitary cells?
Harrison's 20th Ed. Chapter 371 Page 2660

A. 5%
B. 10%
C. 15%
D. 20%

Lactotropes constitute ~20% of anterior pituitary cells. Lactotropes & somatotropes are derived from a common precursor cell.

101. Which of the following is false about prolactin (PRL)?
Harrison's 20th Ed. Chapter 371 Page 2660

A. Weakly homologous to GH
B. Weakly homologous to human placental lactogen (hPL)
C. Transient functional changes in lactotrope population during pregnancy are induced by estrogen
D. Transient functional changes in lactotrope population during first few months of lactation are induced by progesterone

Marked lactotrope cell hyperplasia develops during pregnancy and the first few months of lactation. These transient functional changes in the lactotrope population are induced by estrogen.

102. Which of the following is false about prolactin (PRL)?
Harrison's 20th Ed. Chapter 371 Page 2660

A. Normal adult serum PRL levels is 10–25 µg/L in women
B. Normal adult serum PRL levels is 10–20 µg/L in men
C. PRL secretion is pulsatile
D. PRL secretory peaks occur during NREM sleep

103. Which of the following is false about prolactin (PRL)?
Harrison's 20th Ed. Chapter 371 Page 2660

A. Peak serum PRL levels occur between 4–6 AM
B. Circulating half-life of PRL is 50 minutes
C. Predominant central control mechanism is inhibitory
D. None of the above

Normal adult serum PRL levels are ~10 to 25 µg/L in women & 10 to 20 µg/L in men. PRL secretion is pulsatile, with the highest secretory peaks occurring during rapid eye movement sleep. Peak serum PRL levels occur between 4 & 6 AM. Circulating half-life of PRL is ~50 minutes. Central control mechanism of PRL is inhibitory.

104. Which of the following is false about prolactin secretion?
Harrison's 20th Ed. Chapter 371 Page 2660

A. PRL hypersecretion occurs with pituitary stalk section
B. Pituitary dopamine type 2 (D2) receptors inhibit PRL synthesis
C. Pituitary dopamine type 2 (D2) receptors inhibit PRL secretion
D. None of the above

105. Which of the following is false about prolactin secretion?
Harrison's 20th Ed. Chapter 371 Page 2660

A. Thyrotropin-releasing hormone (TRH) elicits PRL release
B. Vasoactive intestinal peptide (VIP) induces PRL release
C. Glucocorticoids & thyroid hormone suppress PRL secretion
D. None of the above

106. Which of the following cause an increase in prolactin level?
Harrison's 20th Ed. Chapter 371 Page 2661

A. Exercise
B. Sexual intercourse
C. General anesthesia
D. All of the above

107. Which of the following cause an increase in prolactin level?
Harrison's 20th Ed. Chapter 371 Page 2661

A. Acute myocardial infarction
B. Acute stress
C. Chest wall injury
D. All of the above

Serum PRL levels rise transiently after exercise, meals, sexual intercourse, minor surgical procedures, general anesthesia, chest wall injury, acute myocardial infarction and other forms of acute stress. PRL levels increase markedly (about tenfold) during pregnancy & decline rapidly within two weeks of parturition.

108. Breast suckling increases PRL levels that last for about?
Harrison's 20th Ed. Chapter 371 Page 2661

A. 5–10 minutes
B. 10–30 minutes
C. 30–45 minutes
D. 45–60 minutes

Breast suckling stimulates transient reflex increases in PRL levels that last for about 30–45 minutes.

109. Which of the following belong to type 1 cytokine receptor family?
Harrison's 20th Ed. Chapter 371 Page 2661

A. PRL receptor
B. GH receptors
C. Interleukin (IL) 6 receptors
D. All of the above

PRL receptor, GH receptor & interleukin (IL) 6 receptor are members of type 1 cytokine receptor family.

110. In the breast, lobuloalveolar epithelium proliferates in response to?
Harrison's 20th Ed. Chapter 371 Page 2661

A. Estrogen
B. Progesterone
C. Insulin-like growth factor I (IGF-I)
D. All of the above

In the breast, the lobuloalveolar epithelium proliferates in response to PRL, placental lactogens, estrogen, progesterone, and insulin-like growth factor I (IGF-I).

111. Which of the following is the function of prolactin?
Harrison's 20th Ed. Chapter 371 Page 2661

A. Induce & maintain lactation
B. Decrease reproductive function
C. Suppress sexual drive
D. All of the above

PRL acts to induce & maintain lactation, decrease reproductive function and suppress sexual drive.

112. Which of the following is the function of prolactin?
Harrison's 20th Ed. Chapter 371 Page 2661

A. PRL blocks folliculogenesis in ovary
B. PRL inhibits granulosa cell aromatase activity in ovary
C. PRL suppresses hypothalamic gonadotropin-releasing hormone (GnRH)
D. All of the above

PRL inhibits reproductive function by suppressing hypothalamic gonadotropin-releasing hormone (GnRH) & pituitary gonadotropin secretion and by impairing gonadal steroidogenesis in both women and men. In ovary, PRL blocks folliculogenesis and inhibits granulosa cell aromatase activity, leading to hypoestrogenism and anovulation. PRL also has a luteolytic effect, generating a shortened, or inadequate, luteal phase of the menstrual cycle.

113. The most abundant anterior pituitary hormone is?
Harrison's 20th Ed. Chapter 371 Page 2662

A. Prolactin
B. TSH
C. GH
D. ACTH

Of the six anterior pituitary hormones, GH is the most secreted hormone from the GH-secreting somatotrope cells and mammosomatotrope cells, which coexpress PRL with GH.

114. GH-secreting somatotrope cells constitute what percentage of the total anterior pituitary cell population?
Harrison's 20th Ed. Chapter 371 Page 2662

A. 10%
B. 25%
C. 50%
D. 75%

GH-secreting somatotrope cells constitute up to 50% of the total anterior pituitary cell population.

115. Development & proliferation of somatotrophs is determined by which gene?
Harrison's 20th Ed. Chapter 371 Page 2662

A. Prophet of Pit-1 (PROP1)
B. Prophet of Pit-2 (PROP2)
C. Prophet of Pit-3 (PROP3)
D. Prophet of Pit-4 (PROP4)

Cell-specific Pit-1 nuclear transcription factor is responsible for development of somatotropes & subsequent transcription of GH. Mutations in transcription factors Pit-1 & Prop-1, which control somatotrope development, cause GH deficiency in combination with other pituitary hormone deficiencies.

116. Gene that encode GH is located on which chromosome?
Harrison's 20th Ed. Chapter 371 Page 2662

A. 9
B. 12
C. 17
D. 21

117. The name for pituitary GH gene is?
Harrison's 20th Ed. Chapter 371 Page 2662

A. hGH-G
B. hGH-N
C. hGH-P
D. hGH-Z

GH & related proteins are produced by five genes on chromosome 17. The pituitary GH gene (hGH-N) produces two kinds of GH (22-kDa & 20-kDa), both with similar biologic activity. GH variant gene (hGH-V) is expressed by placental syncytiotrophoblast.

118. Which of the following is GH related hormone?
Harrison's 20th Ed. Chapter 371 Page 2662

A. Human chorionic gonadotropin (hCG)
B. Human chorionic somatotropin (hCS)
C. Somatomedin
D. All of the above

119. Which of the following directly stimulate GH release?

Harrison's 20th Ed. Chapter 371 Page 2662

A. Leptin
B. Neuropeptide Y
C. Ghrelin
D. Kisspeptin

The stimulatory effects of ghrelin on growth hormone (GH) secretion and feeding are exclusively mediated through ghrelin receptor named growth hormone secretagogue 1a receptor (GHS-R1a).

120. Which of the following stimulate GH release?

Harrison's 20th Ed. Chapter 371 Page 2662

A. GH-releasing hormone (GHRH)
B. Ghrelin
C. Synthetic agonists of the GHS-R
D. All of the above

Ghrelin and synthetic agonists of GHS-R induce GHRH and also directly stimulate GH release.

121. Growth hormone secretagogue receptor (GHS-R) is a component of?

Curr Pharm Des. 2012;18(31):4749-54

A. Ghrelin signaling pathway
B. TSH-R signaling pathway
C. WNT signaling pathway
D. RET-RAS-BRAF signaling pathway

The growth hormone secretagogue receptor (GHS-R) is a component of the ghrelin signaling pathway and is involved in mediating the pleiotropic effects of ghrelin. Potent induction of GH secretion and stimulation of appetite are the functions of its isomer GHS-R1a.

122. Ghrelin is synthesized mainly in?

N Engl J Med 2006;355:2558-73

A. Gastrointestinal tract
B. Peripheral nervous system
C. Lungs
D. All of the above

Ghrelin, or octylated gastric-derived peptide, as well as synthetic agonists of the GHRP receptor stimulate GHRH & also directly stimulate GH release.

123. Somatotropin-release inhibiting factor (SRIF) is synthesized in which area of hypothalamus?

Harrison's 20th Ed. Chapter 371 Page 2662

A. Medial preoptic
B. Ventromedial nuclei
C. Central
D. All of the above

Somatostatin [somatotropin-release inhibiting factor (SRIF)] is synthesized in the medial preoptic area of the hypothalamus & inhibits GH secretion.

124. Which of the following sets basal GH secretory tone?

Harrison's 20th Ed. Chapter 371 Page 2662

A. Somatotropin-release inhibiting factor (SRIF)
B. GH-releasing hormone (GHRH)
C. Human chorionic somatotropin (hCS)
D. Ghrelin

GHRH is secreted as discrete spikes that elicit GH pulses, whereas SRIF sets basal GH tone.

125. Somatotropin-release inhibiting factor (SRIF) or somatostatin is expressed by which of the following?

Harrison's 20th Ed. Chapter 371 Page 2662

A. CNS
B. Gastrointestinal tract
C. Pancreas
D. All of the above

SRIF is also expressed in CNS, gastrointestinal tract & pancreas, where it also acts to inhibit islet hormone secretion. IGFI, the peripheral target hormone for GH, feeds back to inhibit GH. Estrogen induces GH whereas glucocorticoid excess suppresses GH release.

126. Which somatostatin receptor subtype preferentially suppresses GH secretion?

Harrison's 20th Ed. Chapter 371 Page 2662

A. SSTR1
B. SSTR2
C. SSTR3
D. SSTR4

127. Which somatostatin receptor subtype preferentially suppresses TSH secretion?

Harrison's 20th Ed. Chapter 371 Page 2662

A. SSTR1
B. SSTR2
C. SSTR3
D. SSTR4

Somatostatin binds to five distinct receptor subtypes (SSTR1 to SSTR5). SSTR2 & SSTR5 subtypes preferentially suppress GH & TSH secretion. Somatostatin analogues exert their therapeutic effects through SSTR2 & SSTR5 receptors, both of which are expressed by GH-secreting tumors.

128. Which somatostatin receptor subtype preferentially suppresses ACTH secretion?

Harrison's 20th Ed. Chapter 371 Page 2662

A. SSTR2
B. SSTR3
C. SSTR4
D. SSTR5

129. Elevated GH levels occur in all of the following except?

Harrison's 20th Ed. Chapter 371 Page 2662

A. Obesity
B. Exercise
C. Deep sleep
D. Sepsis

GH secretion is pulsatile, with greatest levels at night correlating with onset of sleep. By middle age, GH secretory rates is ~15% than that during puberty. GH secretion is reduced in obese individuals. Elevated GH levels occur within an hour of deep sleep onset as well as after exercise, physical stress, trauma & during sepsis.

130. Random GH measurements are undetectable in?

Harrison's 20th Ed. Chapter 371 Page 2662

A. Daytime samples from healthy subjects
B. Most obese subjects
C. Most elderly subjects
D. All of the above

131. GH secretion is stimulated by?

Harrison's 20th Ed. Chapter 371 Page 2662

A. Intravenous L-arginine
B. Dopamine
C. Apomorphine
D. All of the above

132. GH secretion is induced by all except?

Harrison's 20th Ed. Chapter 371 Page 2662

A. α-adrenergic pathways
B. Apomorphine
C. β-adrenergic blockade
D. Glucose load

GH secretion is induced by dopamine & apomorphine, as well as by α-adrenergic pathways. β-adrenergic blockade induces basal GH and enhances GHRH- and insulin-evoked GH release.

133. Somatostatin is best described as?

Guyton's Textbook of Medical Physiology 11th Ed. 921

A. Corticotropin-releasing hormone (CRH)
B. Growth hormone releasing hormone (GHRH)
C. Growth hormone inhibitory hormone (GHIH)
D. Prolactin inhibitory hormone (PIH)

Growth hormone inhibitory hormone (somatostatin) is a single chain of 14 amino acids Inhibits secretion of growth hormone by somatotropes.

134. Somatomedin C is best described as?

Guyton's Textbook of Medical Physiology 11th Ed. 924

A. Growth hormone releasing hormone (GHRH)
B. Growth hormone inhibitory hormone (GHIH)
C. Insulin-like growth factor (IGF-1)
D. None of the above

Growth hormone exerts its effect through intermediate substances called Somatomedins - also called "Insulin-Like Growth Factors" formed in liver under the influence of GH.

135. Which of the following organs has the greatest number of GH receptors?

Harrison's 20th Ed. Chapter 371 Page 2662

A. Pancreas
B. Liver
C. Heart
D. Muscle

Liver & cartilage contain the greatest number of GH receptors. GH binding induces receptor dimerization, followed by signaling through JAK/STAT pathway. Activated STAT proteins translocate to the nucleus, where they modulate expression of GH-regulated target genes.

136. Pegvisomant is best described as?

Harrison's 20th Ed. Chapter 371 Page 2662

A. GH receptor protein
B. GH receptor antagonist
C. GHRH receptor
D. GHRH antagonist

Pegvisomant is a GH receptor antagonist approved for treatment of acromegaly.

137. Which of the following is an action of GH?

Harrison's 20th Ed. Chapter 371 Page 2662

A. Induces protein synthesis
B. Promotes nitrogen retention
C. Impairs glucose tolerance by antagonizing insulin action
D. All of the above

138. Which of the following is an action of GH?

Harrison's 20th Ed. Chapter 371 Page 2662

A. Stimulates lipolysis
B. Promotes sodium, potassium, and water retention
C. Stimulates epiphyseal prechondrocyte differentiation
D. All of the above

139. Which of the following is an action of IGF-I?

Harrison's 20th Ed. Chapter 371 Page 2662

A. Induces hypoglycemia
B. Enhances nitrogen retention
C. Lowers cholesterol level
D. All of the above

GH impairs glucose tolerance by antagonizing insulin action. While, injected IGF-I induces hypoglycemia, and lower doses improve insulin sensitivity in patients with severe insulin resistance and diabetes.

140. The major source of circulating IGF-I is?

Harrison's 20th Ed. Chapter 371 Page 2662

A. Pancreas
B. Liver
C. Heart
D. Muscle

Major source of circulating IGF-I is liver. IGF-I is a potent growth & differentiation factor. Peripheral tissue IGF-I exerts local paracrine actions that appear to be both dependent & independent of GH.

141. Which fraction of circulating IGF-binding proteins (IGFBP) is a major carrier for circulating IGF-I?

Harrison's 20th Ed. Chapter 371 Page 2662

A. IGFBP1
B. IGFBP2
C. IGFBP3
D. All of the above

Both IGF-I and -II are bound to high-affinity circulating IGF-binding proteins (IGFBPs) that regulate IGF bioactivity. Levels of IGFBP3 are GH-dependent, and it serves as the major carrier protein for circulating IGF-I. IGFBP1 & 2 regulate local tissue IGF action but do not bind circulating IGF-I.

142. Which of the following about serum IGF-1 concentration is false?

Harrison's 20th Ed. Chapter 371 Page 2662

A. Levels peak at 16 years of age
B. Higher in males than in females
C. Levels low in sepsis
D. Levels high in acromegaly

Serum IGF-I levels increase during puberty, peak at 16 years & then decline. IGF-I concentrations are higher in females than in males. GH is the major determinant of hepatic IGF-I synthesis. IGF-I levels are low with cachexia, malnutrition & sepsis (hypocaloric states are associated with GH resistance). Though GH levels are increased in sepsis, IGF-I levels decrease due to GH resistance. In acromegaly, IGF-I levels are invariably high.

143. Which of the following is a side effect of IGF-I?
Harrison's 20th Ed. Chapter 371 Page 2662

A. Temporomandibular jaw pain
B. Increased intracranial pressure
C. Avascular femoral head necrosis
D. All of the above

144. Which of the following statements is false?
Harrison's 20th Ed. Chapter 371 Page 2662

A. GH mediate its physiologic effects through IGF-I
B. GH is the major determinant of hepatic IGF-I synthesis
C. Levels of IGFBP3 are GH-dependent
D. None of the above

145. Hormones promoting growth include all except?
Harrison's 20th Ed. Chapter 371 Page 2662

A. GH
B. IGF-I
C. IGF-II
D. Cytokines

Skeletal maturation & somatic growth is promoted by hormonal stimuli like GH, IGF-I, sex steroids, thyroid hormones, paracrine growth factors & cytokines.

146. What proportion of pituitary cell population are ACTH-secreting corticotrope cells?
Harrison's 20th Ed. Chapter 371 Page 2662

A. ~ 10%
B. ~ 20%
C. ~ 30%
D. ~ 40%

ACTH-secreting corticotrope cells constitute ~20% of pituitary cell population.

147. Besides ACTH, POMC precursor protein also produces which of the following peptides?
Harrison's 20th Ed. Chapter 371 Page 2663

A. β-lipotropin
B. β-endorphin
C. Met-enkephalin
D. All of the above

148. Besides ACTH, POMC precursor protein also produces which of the following peptides?
Harrison's 20th Ed. Chapter 371 Page 2663

A. α melanocyte-stimulating hormone (α-MSH)
B. β-endorphin
C. Corticotropin-like intermediate lobe protein (CLIP)
D. All of the above

ACTH (39 amino acids) is derived from POMC precursor protein (266 amino acids) that also produces β-lipotropin, β-endorphin, met-enkephalin, α-melanocyte-stimulating hormone (α-MSH) & corticotropin-like intermediate lobe protein (CLIP).

149. POMC gene is induced by?
Harrison's 20th Ed. Chapter 371 Page 2663

A. CRH
B. Arginine vasopressin (AVP)
C. IL-6
D. All of the above

POMC gene is powerfully suppressed by glucocorticoids & induced by CRH, arginine vasopressin (AVP) & proinflammatory cytokines, including IL-6 & leukemia inhibitory factor.

150. Peak ACTH secretion occurs at?
Harrison's 20th Ed. Chapter 371 Page 2663

A. 4 AM
B. 6 AM
C. 8 AM
D. 10 AM

ACTH secretion is pulsatile with circadian rhythm, peaking at 6 AM & reaching a nadir around midnight.

151. ACTH levels are increased by?
Harrison's 20th Ed. Chapter 371 Page 2663

A. Exercise
B. Physical stress
C. Insulin-induced hypoglycemia
D. All of the above

ACTH circadian rhythmicity is determined by variations in secretory pulse amplitude rather than changes in pulse frequency. ACTH levels are increased by AVP, physical stress, exercise, acute illness & insulin-induced hypoglycemia.

152. ACTH-inducing cytokine is?
Harrison's 20th Ed. Chapter 371 Page 2663

A. Tumor necrosis factor (TNF)
B. IL-1
C. IL-2
D. All of the above

ACTH-inducing cytokines include tumor necrosis factor (TNF), IL-1, IL-2, IL-6 & leukemia inhibitory factor.

153. ACTH-inducing cytokine activate?
Harrison's 20th Ed. Chapter 371 Page 2663

A. Hypothalamic CRH secretion
B. Hypothalamic AVP secretion
C. Pituitary POMC gene expression
D. All of the above

154. The receptor for ACTH is?
Harrison's 20th Ed. Chapter 371 Page 2663

A. Melanocortin-1 receptor
B. Melanocortin-2 receptor
C. Melanocortin-3 receptor
D. Melanocortin-4 receptor

Receptor for ACTH is melanocortin-2 receptor, a member of GPCR group, that induces steroidogenesis by stimulating a cascade of steroidogenic enzymes in adrenal cells.

155. What percentage of anterior pituitary cells are gonadotrope cells?

Harrison's 20th Ed. Chapter 371 Page 2663

A. 5%
B. 10%
C. 15%
D. 20%

Gonadotrope cells comprise ~10% of anterior pituitary cells and produce two gonadotropins LH & FSH.

156. Specificity of gonadotropins, LH and FSH, is conferred by which subunit?

Harrison's 20th Ed. Chapter 371 Page 2663

A. α
B. β
C. γ
D. δ

LH & FSH are glycoprotein hormones (like TSH & hCG) & consist of α & β subunits. The α subunit is common to these glycoprotein hormones, specificity is conferred by the β subunits, which are expressed by separate genes.

157. Which of the following is the smallest amino-acid peptide?

Harrison's 20th Ed. Chapter 371 Page 2663

A. Hypothalamic GnRH
B. ACTH
C. Corticotropin releasing hormone (CRH)
D. POMC precursor protein

Hypothalamic GnRH is a 10-amino-acid peptide. ACTH has 39 amino acids derived from POMC precursor protein which has 266 amino acids. CRH is a 41-amino-acid hypothalamic peptide synthesized in paraventricular nucleus.

158. Which of the following regulates hypothalamic GnRH release?

Harrison's 20th Ed. Chapter 371 Page 2663

A. Brain copeptin
B. Brain cryopeptin
C. Brain kisspeptin
D. Brain synpeptin

Brain kisspeptin, a product of the KISSI gene regulates hypothalamic GnRH release.

159. GnRH is secreted in discrete pulses every?

Harrison's 20th Ed. Chapter 371 Page 2663

A. 5 to 10 minutes
B. 10 to 30 minutes
C. 30 to 60 minutes
D. 60 to 120 minutes

Hypothalamic GnRH regulates synthesis & secretion of both LH & FSH. GnRH is secreted in discrete pulses every 60 to 120 minutes, which in turn elicit LH & FSH pulses. Pulsatile mode of GnRH release prime gonadotrope responsiveness, whereas continuous GnRH exposure induces desensitization.

160. FSH synthesis is under control of which of the following?

Harrison's 20th Ed. Chapter 371 Page 2663

A. Inhibin
B. Activin
C. GnRH
D. All of the above

Inhibin selectively suppresses FSH synthesis, whereas activin stimulates FSH synthesis. GnRH induces FSH secretion. Inhibin & activin are gonadal peptides & are members of transforming growth factor β (TGF-β) family.

161. Which of the following statements is false?

Harrison's 20th Ed. Chapter 371 Page 2663

A. Inhibin selectively suppresses FSH
B. Activin stimulates FSH synthesis
C. FSH stimulates ovarian estrogen production
D. None of the above

162. Which of the following statements is false?

Harrison's 20th Ed. Chapter 371 Page 2663

A. In women, FSH stimulates ovarian estrogen production
B. In women, LH helps maintain corpus luteum
C. In men, LH induces testosterone synthesis & secretion by Leydig cells
D. None of the above

163. TSH-secreting thyrotrope cells comprise what percentage of anterior pituitary cell population?

Harrison's 20th Ed. Chapter 371 Page 2663

A. 2%
B. 5%
C. 8%
D. 12%

TSH-secreting thyrotrope cells comprise 5% of the anterior pituitary cell population. Gonadotrope cells comprise about 10% of anterior pituitary cells. GH-secreting somatotrope cells constitute up to 50% of the total anterior pituitary cells. Lactotropes comprise about 20% of anterior pituitary cells.

164. TSH is structurally related to?

Harrison's 20th Ed. Chapter 371 Page 2663

A. GH
B. PRL
C. FSH
D. ACTH

TSH is structurally related to LH & FSH. It shares a common α subunit with these hormones but contains a specific TSH β subunit.

165. Hypothalamic tripeptide-TRH is also called?

Harrison's 20th Ed. Chapter 371 Page 2663

A. Pyroglutamyl histidylprolinamide
B. Proglutamyl histidylprolinamide
C. Pentaglutamyl histidylprolinamide
D. Preglutamyl histidylprolinamide

TRH is a hypothalamic tripeptide (pyroglutamyl histidylprolinamide) that acts through a GPCR to stimulate TSH synthesis & secretion.

166. Besides TSH, TRH also stimulates secretion of?

Harrison's 20th Ed. Chapter 371 Page 2663

A. PRL
B. GH
C. ACTH
D. Vasopressin

TRH also stimulates the lactotrope cell to secrete PRL.

167. TSH secretion is suppressed by?

Harrison's 20th Ed. Chapter 371 Page 2663

A. Dopamine
B. SRIF
C. Glucocorticoids
D. All of the above

TSH secretion is stimulated by TRH, whereas thyroid hormones, dopamine, somatostatin & glucocorticoids suppress TSH by overriding TRH induction.

168. Which of the following is secreted in pulses?

Harrison's 20th Ed. Chapter 371 Page 2663

A. GnRH
B. ACTH
C. GH
D. All of the above

Like TSH, GnRH, ACTH, GH, LH & FSH are secreted in pulses.

169. Which of the following has the longest half life?

Harrison's 20th Ed. Chapter 371 Page 2663

A. TSH
B. ACTH
C. GH
D. Prolactin (PRL)

TSH has a prolonged half-life with relatively constant serum levels, even though it is secreted in discrete pulses. ACTH, GH, prolactin, PTH, LH have relatively short half-lives (<20 min) with sharp peaks of secretion & decay.

Hypopituitarism

170. Which out of the following is the first hormone to reduce in pituitary compression or destruction?
Harrison's 20th Ed. Chapter 372 Page 2664 Table 371-1

A. Thyroid-stimulating hormone
B. Adrenocorticotropic hormone
C. Follicle-stimulating hormone
D. Luteinizing hormone

171. Which out of the following is the last hormone to reduce in pituitary compression or destruction?
Harrison's 20th Ed. Chapter 372 Page 2664 Table 371-1

A. Thyroid-stimulating hormone
B. Adrenocorticotropic hormone
C. Follicle-stimulating hormone
D. Luteinizing hormone

Trophic hormone failure associated with pituitary compression or destruction occurs sequentially: GH → FSH → LH → TSH → ACTH.

172. Which the following statements about hypopituitarism is false?
Harrison's 20th Ed. Chapter 372 Page 2664 Table 371-1

A. More commonly, adult hypopituitarism is acquired
B. During childhood, growth retardation is the presenting feature
C. In adults, hypogonadism is the earliest feature
D. None of the above

During childhood, growth retardation is the presenting feature, & in adults, hypogonadism is the earliest symptom.

173. Pituitary dysplasia may result in?
Harrison's 20th Ed. Chapter 372 Page 2664

A. Aplastic pituitary gland development
B. Hypoplastic pituitary gland development
C. Ectopic pituitary gland development
D. Any of the above

Pituitary dysplasia may result in aplastic, hypoplastic, or ectopic pituitary gland development. This is because pituitary development follows midline cell migration from nasopharyngeal Rathke's pouch and midline craniofacial disorders may be associated with pituitary dysplasia.

174. Acquired pituitary failure in the newborn can be caused by?
Harrison's 20th Ed. Chapter 372 Page 2664

A. Birth trauma
B. Birth asphyxia
C. Breech delivery
D. All of the above

175. Patients of septo-optic dysplasia have mutations in which of the following gene?
Harrison's 20th Ed. Chapter 372 Page 2664

A. Pit-1
B. Prop-1
C. HESX1
D. All of the above

Hypothalamic dysfunction and consequent hypopituitarism may result from dysgenesis of septum pellucidum or corpus callosum. Affected children have mutations in HESX1 gene, which is involved in early development of the ventral prosencephalon.

176. Children with septo-optic dysplasia have all of the following features except?
Harrison's 20th Ed. Chapter 372 Page 2664

A. Syndactyly
B. Atrial septal defect
C. Micropenis
D. Ear deformities

177. Children with septo-optic dysplasia present with?
Harrison's 20th Ed. Chapter 372 Page 2664

A. Diabetes insipidus
B. Short stature
C. Hypothyroidism
D. All of the above

Children septo-optic dysplasia present with a variable combination of cleft palate, syndactyly, ear deformities, hypertelorism, optic nerve hypoplasia, micropenis, and anosmia. Pituitary dysfunction leads to diabetes insipidus, growth hormone deficiency & short stature, and thyroid-stimulating hormone (TSH) deficiency.

178. Pit-1 mutations cause combined deficiency of?
Harrison's 20th Ed. Chapter 372 Page 2664

A. GH + prolactin + ACTH
B. GH + prolactin + TSH
C. GH + prolactin
D. GH + FSH + LH

Pit-1 mutations cause combined GH, prolactin (PRL), and TSH deficiencies.

179. Pit-1 mutations cause combined deficiency of?
Harrison's 20th Ed. Chapter 372 Page 2664

A. GH + PRL
B. GH + PRL + TSH
C. GH + PRL + TSH + gonadotropin
D. Any of the above

Familial & sporadic PROP1 mutations lead to combined GH, PRL, TSH, and gonadotropin deficiency.

180. ACTH deficiency associated with hypocortisolism is due to mutations in?
Harrison's 20th Ed. Chapter 372 Page 2664

A. Pit-1
B. Prop-1
C. TPIT
D. All of the above

TPIT mutations lead to ACTH deficiency associated with hypocortisolism.

181. Kallmann syndrome is due congenital synthesis defect of?
Harrison's 20th Ed. Chapter 372 Page 2664

A. LH
B. FSH
C. Testosterone
D. GnRH

182. Which of the following gene is associated with Kallmann syndrome?

Harrison's 20th Ed. Chapter 372 Page 2664

A. KLL
B. KAL
C. KLM
D. KLN

Kallmann syndrome is due to defective hypothalamic gonadotropin-releasing hormone (GnRH) synthesis. KAL gene defect on chromosome Xp22.3 is the culprit. Embryonic migration of GnRH neurons from hypothalamic olfactory placode to hypothalamus is prevented due to this genetic defect. GnRH deficiency prevents progression through puberty.

183. KAL1 gene encodes which of the following protein?

Harrison's 20th Ed. Chapter 372 Page 2664

A. Makorin ring-finger protein 3
B. Megalin
C. Anosmin
D. Neurokinin B

KAL1 gene encodes anosmin, a protein that mediates migration of neural progenitors of olfactory bulb and GnRH-producing neurons.

184. Which of the following genes is associated with GnRH deficiency?

Harrison's 20th Ed. Chapter 372 Page 2664

A. GNRH1
B. PROK2
C. CHD7
D. All of the above

Autosomal recessive (GPR54, KISS1) and dominant (FGFR1) modes of transmission have been described. In addition to KAL mutations, genes associated with GnRH deficiency include GNRH1, PROK2, PROKR2, CHD7, PCSK1, FGF8, NELF, WDR11, TAC3, TACR3, and SEMA3E.

185. GnRH neurons are located in?

Harrison's 20th Ed. Chapter 372 Page 2664

A. Preoptic region of hypothalamus
B. Suprachiasmatic nucleus of hypothalamus
C. Medial basal hypothalamus
D. Anteromedial hypothalamus

GnRH neurons, which are about 7000 in number, are scattered throughout the medial basal hypothalamus. They establish contacts with capillaries of pituitary portal system in the median eminence.

186. Which of the following is known as the GnRH receptor?

Harrison's 20th Ed. Chapter 372 Page 2664

A. Adrenopeptin
B. Gonopeptin
C. Kisspeptin
D. Copeptin

Brain Kisspeptin is a product of the KISSI gene and is known as the GnRH receptor. Kisspeptin regulates hypothalamic GnRH release.

187. Kallmann syndrome best relates to?

Harrison's 20th Ed. Chapter 372 Page 2664

A. Metastatic tumors
B. Diabetes insipidus
C. Olfactory bulb agenesis
D. Empty sella

Kallmann's syndrome is the anosmic form of GnRH deficiency. It results from mutations in genes associated with olfactory bulb morphogenesis and migration of GnRH neurons from their origin in the olfactory placode, along the scaffold established by the olfactory nerves, through cribriform plate into their final location into the preoptic region of hypothalamus.

188. Which of the following is not a feature of Kallmann syndrome?

Harrison's 20th Ed. Chapter 372 Page 2664

A. Hyposmia
B. Color blindness
C. Nerve deafness
D. Precocious puberty

Features of Kallmann syndrome include anosmia or hyposmia (due to olfactory bulb agenesis or hypoplasia), color blindness, optic atrophy, nerve deafness, cleft palate, renal abnormalities, cryptorchidism & neurologic abnormalities (mirror movements).

189. Hormone profile of Kallmann syndrome includes?

Harrison's 20th Ed. Chapter 372 Page 2664

A. Low LH
B. Low FSH
C. Low levels of sex steroids (testosterone or estradiol)
D. All of the above

GnRH deficiency prevents progression through puberty. Males present with delayed puberty & hypogonadism. Females present with primary amenorrhea & failure of secondary sexual development. Repetitive GnRH administration restores normal pituitary gonadotropin responses. Fertility may be restored in men with long-term treatment with human chorionic gonadotropin (hCG) or testosterone. Women are treated with cyclic estrogen & progestin.

190. Which of the following neurologic abnormalities is best related to Kallmann syndrome?

Harrison's 20th Ed. Chapter 372 Page 2664

A. Choreoathetotic movements
B. Dystonia
C. Mirror movements
D. Myoclonus

GnRH deficiency and variable combinations of anosmia or hyposmia, renal defects and neurologic abnormalities including mirror movements.

191. Bardet-Biedl syndrome is characterized by?

Harrison's 20th Ed. Chapter 372 Page 2665

A. Hexadactyly
B. Brachydactyly
C. Syndactyly
D. Any of the above

192. Bardet-Biedl syndrome is characterized by?

Harrison's 20th Ed. Chapter 372 Page 2665

A. Mental retardation
B. Renal abnormalities
C. Obesity
D. All of the above

Bardet-Biedl syndrome is characterized by mental retardation, renal abnormalities, obesity, and hexadactyly, brachydactyly, or syndactyly.

193. Which of the following is a feature of?

Harrison's 20th Ed. Chapter 372 Page 2665

A. Central diabetes insipidus
B. GnRH deficiency
C. Retinal degeneration
D. All of the above

194. Deficiencies of leptin or its receptor cause which of the following?

Harrison's 20th Ed. Chapter 372 Page 2665

A. Hyperphagia
B. Obesity
C. Central hypogonadism
D. All of the above

195. Which of the following gene is associated with Prader Willi syndrome?

Harrison's 20th Ed. Chapter 372 Page 2665

A. GNRH1
B. PROK2
C. CH7
D. SNRPN

196. Which of the following is not a feature of Prader Willi syndrome?

Harrison's 20th Ed. Chapter 372 Page 2665

A. Hypogonadotropic hypogonadism
B. Hyperphagia-obesity
C. Mental retardation
D. Type 1 diabetes mellitus

Prader Willi syndrome is a contiguous gene syndrome that results from deletion of the paternal copies of the imprinted SNRPN gene, the NECDIN gene and possibly other genes on chromosome 15q. Prader Willi syndrome is associated with hypogonadotropic hypogonadism, hyperphagia-obesity, chronic muscle hypotonia, mental retardation and adult-onset diabetes mellitus.

197. Which of the following conditions frequently involve both hypothalamic & pituitary neuronal and neurochemical tracts?

Harrison's 20th Ed. Chapter 372 Page 2665

A. Sarcoidosis
B. Histiocytosis X
C. Hemochromatosis
D. All of the above

Sarcoidosis, histiocytosis X, amyloidosis, and hemochromatosis frequently involve both hypothalamic & pituitary neuronal and neurochemical tracts.

198. Which of the following may occur when hypothalamic & pituitary neuronal and neurochemical tracts are involved?

Harrison's 20th Ed. Chapter 372 Page 2665

A. Diabetes insipidus
B. Hypogonadotropic hypogonadism
C. Hyperprolactinemia
D. All of the above

199. Acquired hypogonadotropic disorders can be due to?

Harrison's 20th Ed. Chapter 372 Page 2665

A. Severe illness
B. Malnutrition
C. Exercise
D. All of the above

Acquired hypogonadotropic disorders can be due to severe illness, stress, anorexia nervosa, malnutrition and exercise.

200. Main regulator of LH and FSH secretion is?

Harrison's 20th Ed. Chapter 372 Page 2665

A. GnRH
B. Inhibin
C. Activin
D. Progesterone

201. GnRH deficiency is found in which of the following?

Harrison's 20th Ed. Chapter 372 Page 2665

A. Prader-Willi Syndrome
B. Bardet-Biedl Syndrome
C. Frohlich Syndrome
D. All of the above

Bardet-Biedl Syndrome, Frohlich Syndrome & Prader-Willi Syndrome have GnRH deficiency with obesity. Patients of Bardet-Biedl Syndrome have mental retardation, defects of fingers, retinal degeneration & central diabetes insipidus. Patients of Frohlich Syndrome have hyperphagia, obesity & central hypogonadism. Patients of Prader-Willi Syndrome have mental retardation, adult-onset diabetes mellitus, hyperphagia, obesity & hypogonadotropic hypogonadism.

202. Retinal degeneration is a clinical feature of?

Harrison's 20th Ed. Chapter 372 Page 2665

A. Prader-Willi Syndrome
B. Bardet-Biedl Syndrome
C. Frohlich Syndrome
D. All of the above

203. What median dose of cranial irradiation can lead to development of hypopituitarism?

Harrison's 20th Ed. Chapter 372 Page 2665

A. 2000 rad
B. 3000 rad
C. 4000 rad
D. 5000 rad

Up to two-thirds of patients ultimately develop hormone insufficiency after a cranial irradiation median dose of 50 Gy (5000 rad) directed at skull base.

204. After cranial irradiation, hypopituitarism occurs over what period of time?

Harrison's 20th Ed. Chapter 372 Page 2665

A. 3 months to 2 years
B. 2–5 years
C. 5–15 years
D. > 20 years

After cranial irradiation, hypopituitarism occurs over 5 - 15 years and usually reflects hypothalamic damage rather than primary destruction of pituitary cells.

205. Which hormone deficiency is most common after cranial irradiation?

Harrison's 20th Ed. Chapter 372 Page 2665

A. GH
B. Gonadotropin
C. ACTH
D. ADH

After cranial irradiation, GH deficiency is most common, followed by gonadotropin & ACTH deficiency.

206. Lymphocytic hypophysitis occurs mainly in?

Harrison's 20th Ed. Chapter 372 Page 2665

A. Unmarried female
B. Postpartum female
C. Short statured female
D. Infertile female

Lymphocytic hypophysitis occurs mainly in post-partum women & presents with hyperprolactinemia & a pituitary mass on MRI. Resolves after prolonged glucocorticoid treatment.

207. Which of the following is a CTLA-4 blocker?
Harrison's 20th Ed. Chapter 372 Page 2665

A. Ipilumumab
B. Ramucirumab
C. Bevacizumab
D. Denosumab

Cytotoxic T-lymphocyte antigen-4 (CTLA-4), a T cell immunoregulatory gene like CD25, PTPN22, FCRL3, and CD226. Ipilumumab (a fully human IgG1 anti-CTLA-4 antibody) blocks CTLA-4 preventing interaction with CD80/86 and T cell inhibition. It can cause hypophysitis with associated thyroid adrenal & gonadal failure.

208. Pituitary apoplexy is associated with?
Harrison's 20th Ed. Chapter 372 Page 2665

A. Diabetes
B. Hypertension
C. Sickle cell anemia
D. All of the above

209. Sheehan's syndrome refers to pituitary apoplexy during?
Harrison's 20th Ed. Chapter 372 Page 2665

A. Antenatal period
B. Intra-partum period
C. Postpartum period
D. All of the above

Pituitary Apoplexy (acute intrapituitary hemorrhage) may occur spontaneously in a preexisting adenoma, postpartum (Sheehan's syndrome), diabetes, hypertension, sickle cell anemia or acute shock. It presents as severe headache with signs of meningeal irritation, bilateral visual changes, ophthalmoplegia, hypoglycemia, hypotension, CNS hemorrhage & death. Hypopituitarism is very common after apoplexy. Pituitary CT / MRI is diagnostic.

210. Indication for urgent surgical decompression after pituitary apoplexy is?
Harrison's 20th Ed. Chapter 372 Page 2665

A. Hypotension
B. Visual loss
C. Seizure
D. All of the above

Patients of pituitary apoplexy with significant or progressive visual loss, severe ophthalmoplegia or loss of consciousness require urgent surgical decompression. Rest can be managed with high-dose glucocorticoids.

211. Pituitary apoplexy occurs as a consequence of?
Harrison's 20th Ed. Chapter 379 Page 2735

A. Infarcted pituitary adenoma
B. Transient reduction in blood supply of pituitary during surgery
C. After rapid blood loss associated with parturition
D. All of the above

Pituitary apoplexy, either as a consequence of an infarcted pituitary adenoma or transient reduction in the blood supply of the pituitary during surgery or after rapid blood loss associated with parturition, also termed Sheehan's syndrome.

212. Pituitary apoplexy presents as?
Harrison's 20th Ed. Chapter 28 Page 189

A. Acute retrobulbar visual loss
B. Headache, nausea
C. Ocular motor nerve palsies
D. All of the above

Sudden expansion of a pituitary adenoma from infarction and bleeding (pituitary apoplexy) causes acute retrobulbar visual loss, with headache, nausea, and ocular motor nerve palsies.

213. In pituitary apoplexy, pituitary CT or MRI may show?
Harrison's 20th Ed. Chapter 372 Page 2665

A. Signs of intratumoral or sellar hemorrhage
B. Pituitary stalk deviation
C. Compression of pituitary tissue
D. All of the above

In pituitary apoplexy, pituitary computed tomography (CT) or MRI may show signs of intratumoral or sellar hemorrhage, with pituitary stalk deviation and compression of pituitary tissue.

214. In 'Empty Sella Syndrome', pituitary functions are usually?
Harrison's 20th Ed. Chapter 372 Page 2665

A. Normal
B. Decreased
C. Increased
D. Any of the above

Empty Sella patients usually have normal pituitary function. Peripheral rim of pituitary tissue is enough for hormone production, though with time hypopituitarism may develop.

215. Empty sella may be associated with?
Harrison's 20th Ed. Chapter 372 Page 2665

A. Meningitis
B. Intracranial hypertension
C. Ocular motor nerve palsies
D. Pituitary stalk deviation

Empty sella is often an incidental MRI finding, and may be associated with intracranial hypertension.

216. Which of the following best relates to empty sella?
Harrison's 20th Ed. Chapter 372 Page 2665

A. Dural perforation
B. Dural herniation
C. Dural hypoplasia
D. Dural hyperplasia

217. In patients with long-standing pituitary damage, epidemiologic studies show an increased mortality rate, primarily from?
Harrison's 20th Ed. Chapter 372 Page 2666

A. Road traffic accidents
B. Malignancies
C. Cardiovascular disease
D. Suicide

In patients with long-standing pituitary damage, epidemiologic studies document an increased mortality rate, primarily from increased cardiovascular and cerebrovascular disease.

218. Which of the following can be used to assess GH reserve?
Harrison's 20th Ed. Chapter 372 Page 2666

A. Insulin-induced hypoglycemia
B. Arginine
C. L-dopa
D. All of the above

GH responses to insulin-induced hypoglycemia, arginine, L-dopa, growth hormone releasing hormone (GHRH) or growth hormone releasing peptides (GHRPs) can be used to assess GH reserve.

219. In insulin tolerance test, what level of GH suggests a normal response?

Harrison's 20th Ed. Chapter 372 Page 2666 Table 372-2

A. > 1 μg/L
B. > 2 μg/L
C. > 3 μg/L
D. > 4 μg/L

In insulin tolerance test, regular insulin is given IV in doses of 0.05–0.15 U/kg to reduce blood glucose levels to <40 mg/dL. Blood glucose and GH are estimated 30 minutes before the test and again for next two hours at 30 minutes interval after insulin (total 5 samples). GH level of > 3 μg/L is considered as a normal response.

220. ACTH reserve is most reliably assessed by?

Harrison's 20th Ed. Chapter 379 Page 2736

A. CRH test
B. Metyrapone test
C. Insulin-induced hypoglycemia
D. Standard ACTH stimulation test

ACTH reserve is most reliably assessed during insulin-induced hypoglycemia.

221. Which of the following is used to assess prolactin reserve?

Harrison's 20th Ed. Chapter 372 Page 2666 Table 372-2

A. Insulin tolerance test
B. TRH test
C. GnRH test
D. Metyrapone test

222. In TRH test, what level of prolactin suggests a normal response?

Harrison's 20th Ed. Chapter 372 Page 2666 Table 372-2

A. > 1 μg/L
B. > 2 μg/L
C. > 3 μg/L
D. > 4 μg/L

In TRH test, TRH is given IV in doses of 200–500 μg. Blood for TSH and PRL is analyzed at 0, 20, and 60 minutes. PRL level of > 2 μg/L and increase >200% of baseline is considered as a normal response.

223. Which of the following is estimated in Metyrapone test?

Harrison's 20th Ed. Chapter 372 Page 2666 Table 372-2

A. 11-deoxycortisol
B. 21-deoxycortisol
C. 11-deoxycorticosterone
D. 17-Hydroxyprogesterone

224. Which of the following is estimated in Metyrapone test?

Harrison's 20th Ed. Chapter 372 Page 2666 Table 372-2

A. 11-deoxycortisol
B. Cortisol
C. ACTH
D. All of the above

225. Which of the following indicate a normal response in Metyrapone test?

Harrison's 20th Ed. Chapter 372 Page 2666 Table 372-2

A. 11-deoxycortisol >7.5 μg/dL
B. ACTH >75 pg/mL
C. Plasma cortisol <4 g/dL
D. All of the above

226. What level of cortisol indicates a normal response in standard ACTH stimulation test?

Harrison's 20th Ed. Chapter 372 Page 2666 Table 372-2

A. > 21 ng/dL
B. > 21 μg/dL
C. > 21 mg/dL
D. > 21 g/dL

227. In combined anterior pituitary test, which of the following is not included?

Harrison's 20th Ed. Chapter 372 Page 2666 Table 372-2

A. GHRH
B. CRH
C. GnRH
D. TSH

228. The growth plate is dependent on?

Harrison's 20th Ed. Chapter 372 Page 2667

A. GH
B. Insulin-like growth factor (IGF)-I
C. Thyroid hormones
D. All of the above

229. The growth plate is dependent on?

Harrison's 20th Ed. Chapter 372 Page 2667

A. Sex steroids
B. Paracrine growth factors
C. Cytokines
D. All of the above

The growth plate is dependent on hormonal stimuli like GH, insulin-like growth factor (IGF)-I, sex steroids, thyroid hormones, paracrine growth factors, and cytokines.

230. Growth-promoting process requires which of the following?

Harrison's 20th Ed. Chapter 372 Page 2667

A. Amino acids
B. Fatty acids
C. Glucose
D. All of the above

231. The growth-promoting process consumes what proportion of normal energy production?

Harrison's 20th Ed. Chapter 372 Page 2667

A. ~ 10%
B. ~ 20%
C. ~ 30%
D. ~ 40%

Growth-promoting process requires caloric energy, amino acids, vitamins, and trace metals and consumes about 10% of normal energy production.

232. Malnutrition impairs growth-promoting process by all except?
Harrison's 20th Ed. Chapter 372 Page 2667

A. Reducing osteophyte activity
B. Increasing GH resistance
C. Reducing circulating IGF-I
D. Reducing IGF binding protein (IGBP)-3 levels

233. In later childhood, mean growth velocity is about?
Harrison's 20th Ed. Chapter 372 Page 2667

A. 2 cm/year
B. 4 cm/year
C. 6 cm/year
D. 8 cm/year

Linear bone growth rates are very high in infancy & are pituitary dependent. Mean growth velocity is ~6 cm/year in later childhood. Peak growth rates occur during mid-puberty when bone age is 12 (girls) or 13 (boys). Secondary sexual development is associated with elevated sex steroids that cause progressive epiphyseal growth plate closure.

234. Normal bone age in a child with short stature is suggestive of?
Harrison's 20th Ed. Chapter 372 Page 2667

A. Hormonal disorder
B. Systemic disorder
C. Genetic cartilage dysplasia or growth plate disorder
D. All of the above

235. Delayed bone age in a child with short stature is suggestive of?
Harrison's 20th Ed. Chapter 372 Page 2667

A. Hormonal disorder or systemic disorder
B. Genetic cartilage dysplasia
C. Growth plate disorder
D. All of the above

Bone age is delayed in patients with all forms of true GH deficiency or GH receptor defects that result in attenuated GH action. Bone age is delayed by thyroid hormone deficiency. Elevated pubertal sex steroid levels (estrogen) induce GHRH-GH-IGF-I axis & directly stimulate epiphyseal growth. High doses of estrogen lead to epiphyseal closure. Glucocorticoid excess inhibits growth.

236. Characteristic voice in isolated GH deficiency is?
Harrison's 20th Ed. Chapter 372 Page 2667

A. High-pitched
B. Low-pitched
C. Hoarse
D. Any of the above

Isolated GH deficiency is characterized by short stature, micropenis, increased fat, high-pitched voice & a tendency for hypoglycemia.

237. Mode of inheritance of isolated GH deficiency is?
Harrison's 20th Ed. Chapter 372 Page 2667

A. Autosomal dominant
B. Autosomal recessive
C. X-linked
D. Any of the above

238. GH levels can be stimulated by exogenous?
Harrison's 20th Ed. Chapter 372 Page 2667

A. Growth hormone releasing hormone (GHRH)
B. Growth hormone releasing peptide (GHRP)
C. Insulin-induced hypoglycemia
D. All of the above

GH levels can be stimulated by exogenous GHRH, GHRP, or insulin-induced hypoglycemia.

239. Which of the following is false about Laron syndrome?
Harrison's 20th Ed. Chapter 372 Page 2667

A. GH insensitivity
B. Normal or high GH levels
C. Decreased circulating GHBP
D. High IGF-I levels

240. Which of the following is the laboratory finding in Laron's syndrome?
Harrison's 20th Ed. Chapter 372 Page 2667

A. Normal or high GH levels
B. Decreased circulating GH-binding protein (GHBP)
C. Low IGF-I levels
D. All of the above

Laron syndrome is caused by mutation defects of GH receptor structure or signaling leading to partial or complete GH insensitivity & growth failure. The diagnosis is based on normal or high GH levels, with decreased circulating GH-binding protein (GHBP), and low IGF-I levels.

241. STAT5B mutations best relate to?
Harrison's 20th Ed. Chapter 372 Page 2667

A. Allergy
B. Color blindness
C. Immunodeficiency
D. Anosmia

STAT5B mutations result in immunodeficiency and abrogated GH signaling.

242. Emotional and social deprivation can lead to?
Harrison's 20th Ed. Chapter 372 Page 2667

A. Growth retardation
B. Delayed speech
C. Discordant hyperphagia
D. All of the above

243. Short stature should be evaluated comprehensively if a patient's height is?
Harrison's 20th Ed. Chapter 372 Page 2667

A. > 1 standard deviations (SD) below the mean for age
B. > 2 standard deviations (SD) below the mean for age
C. > 3 standard deviations (SD) below the mean for age
D. > 4 standard deviations (SD) below the mean for age

Short stature should be evaluated comprehensively if a patient's height is >3 standard deviations (SD) below the mean for age or if the growth rate has decelerated.

244. Final height of children can be predicted by?
Harrison's 20th Ed. Chapter 372 Page 2667

A. Bayley-Pinneau scale
B. Tanner-Whitehouse scale
C. Midparental height
D. All of the above

Final height can be predicted using standardized scales (Bayley-Pinneau or Tanner-Whitehouse) or estimated by adding 6.5 cm (boys) or subtracting 6.5 cm (girls) from the midparental height.

245. Following provocative stimuli, GH levels normally increase to how much in children?
Harrison's 20th Ed. Chapter 372 Page 2667

A. > 3 μg/L
B. > 5 μg/L
C. > 7 μg/L
D. > 9 μg/L

As GH secretion is released in pulses, GH deficiency is best assessed by examining the response to exercise, insulin-induced hypoglycemia wherein GH levels normally increase to >7 μg/L in children.

246. Treatment with IGF-I is recommended for which of the following?
Harrison's 20th Ed. Chapter 372 Page 2667

A. Turner syndrome
B. Chronic renal failure
C. Growth retardation due to mutations of GH receptor
D. All of the above

In patients with GH insensitivity & growth retardation due to mutations of GH receptor, treatment with IGF-I bypasses the dysfunctional GH receptor. GH treatment is moderately effective for accelerating growth rates in children with Turner syndrome & chronic renal failure.

247. Which is the "last" hormone to be lost in acquired pituitary hormone deficiency?
Harrison's 20th Ed. Chapter 372 Page 2668

A. TSH
B. GH
C. ACTH
D. FSH/LH

Sequential order of hormone loss in acquired pituitary hormone deficiency is GH > FSH / LH > TSH > ACTH.

248. Adult GH deficiency (AGHD) is defined by a peak GH response to insulin-induced hypoglycemia of?
Harrison's 20th Ed. Chapter 372 Page 2668

A. <3 μg/L
B. <5 μg/L
C. <7 μg/L
D. <9 μg/L

Most validated test to distinguish pituitary-sufficient patients from those with AGHD is insulin induced (0.05–0.1 U/kg) hypoglycemia. After glucose reduction to ~40 mg/dL, most individuals experience neuroglycopenic symptoms, and peak GH release occurs at 60 minutes & remains elevated for up to 2 hours. ~90% of healthy adults exhibit GH responses >5 μg/L. AGHD is defined by a peak GH response to hypoglycemia of <3 μg/L.

249. Which of the following evokes GH secretion and used as a stimulatory test?
Harrison's 20th Ed. Chapter 372 Page 2668

A. Intravenous arginine
B. GHRP-6
C. Glucagon
D. All of the above

Alternative GH stimulatory tests are IV arginine (30 gram), GHRH (1 μg/kg), GHRP-6 (90 μg) & glucagon (1 mg). Combinations of these tests may evoke GH secretion in subjects who are not responsive to a single test.

250. Contraindications to GH therapy include?
Harrison's 20th Ed. Chapter 372 Page 2668

A. Presence of active neoplasm
B. Intracranial hypertension
C. Uncontrolled diabetes
D. All of the above

Contraindications to GH replacement therapy include presence of an active neoplasm, intracranial hypertension or uncontrolled diabetes & retinopathy.

251. Which of the following is a feature of secondary adrenal insufficiency?
Harrison's 20th Ed. Chapter 372 Page 2669

A. Hypocortisolism
B. Hyperpigmentation
C. Mineralocorticoid deficiency
D. All of the above

In contrast to primary adrenal failure, hypocortisolism associated with pituitary failure usually is not accompanied by hyperpigmentation or mineralocorticoid deficiency.

252. Which of the following is the most common presenting feature of adult hypopituitarism?
Harrison's 20th Ed. Chapter 372 Page 2669

A. Hypogonadism
B. Adrenal insufficiency
C. Adult Growth Hormone Deficiency
D. Diabetes insipidus

Hypogonadism is the most common presenting feature of adult hypopituitarism even when other pituitary hormones are also deficient.

253. Which of the following is associated with Kallmann's syndrome?
Harrison's 20th Ed. Chapter 372 Page 2669

A. Functional hypothalamic amenorrhea (HA)
B. Isolated hypogonadotropic hypogonadism (IHH)
C. Primary ovarian insufficiency (POI)
D. Polycystic ovarian syndrome (PCOS)

IHH presents with primary amenorrhea. IHH is associated with anosmia in about 50% of women (Kallmann's syndrome).

254. Acquired form of GnRH deficiency leading to hypogonadotropism is seen in association with?
Harrison's 20th Ed. Chapter 372 Page 2669

A. Anorexia nervosa
B. Stress and extreme exercise
C. Starvation
D. All of the above

255. In hypogonadal adult men, which of the following is the characteristic feature of secondary testicular failure?
Harrison's 20th Ed. Chapter 372 Page 2669

A. Reduced beard
B. Reduced body hair growth
C. Fine facial wrinkles
D. Soft testes

Pituitary Tumor Syndromes

256. Which of the following is "rare" in the process of expansion of an intrasellar mass?
Harrison's 20th Ed. Chapter 373 Page 2670 Table 373-1

A. Compression of intrasellar pituitary tissue
B. Invasion of dura to lift the optic chiasm
C. Lateral invasion to impinge on cavernous sinus
D. Bony erosion

When an intrasellar mass expands, bony erosion & direct brain compression is rare. Compression of intrasellar pituitary tissue is the first event.

257. Visual loss due to suprasellar extension of an intrasellar mass is due to?
Harrison's 20th Ed. Chapter 373 Page 2670

A. Compression of optic chiasm
B. Direct invasion of optic nerves
C. Obstruction of CSF flow
D. All of the above

Visual loss due to suprasellar extension of an intrasellar mass is due to compression of optic chiasm (most common), direct invasion of the optic nerves or obstruction of cerebrospinal fluid (CSF) flow leading to secondary visual disturbances.

258. "Stalk section" phenomenon may be caused by?
Harrison's 20th Ed. Chapter 373 Page 2670

A. Compression by hormonally active or inactive intrasellar mass
B. Whiplash injury with posterior clinoid stalk compression
C. Skull base fractures
D. All of the above

Pituitary stalk compression or "stalk section" phenomenon may be caused by a hormonally active or inactive intrasellar mass, trauma, whiplash injury with posterior clinoid stalk compression, or skull base fractures. It leads to compression of portal vessels, disrupting pituitary access to hypothalamic hormones and dopamine. This results in early hyperprolactinemia and later concurrent loss of other pituitary hormones.

259. Lateral mass invasion of an intrasellar mass damage all of the following except?
Harrison's 20th Ed. Chapter 373 Page 2670

A. Ophthalmic branches of the fifth cranial nerve
B. Maxillary branches of the fifth cranial nerve
C. Mandibular branches of the fifth cranial nerve
D. Fourth cranial nerve

260. Lateral mass invasion of an intrasellar mass damage which of the following?
Harrison's 20th Ed. Chapter 373 Page 2670

A. III cranial nerve
B. IV cranial nerve
C. VI cranial nerve
D. All of the above

Lateral mass invasion of an intrasellar mass may impinge on the cavernous sinus & compress its neural contents, leading to cranial nerve III, IV & VI palsies as well as ophthalmic & maxillary branches of fifth cranial nerve.

261. Feature of sellar mass lesion involving optic chiasm include?
Harrison's 20th Ed. Chapter 373 Page 2670 Table 373-1

A. Loss of red perception
B. Bitemporal hemianopia
C. Scotoma
D. All of the above

262. Patients with lateral mass invasion of an intrasellar mass may present with?
Harrison's 20th Ed. Chapter 373 Page 2670

A. Diplopia
B. Ptosis
C. Ophthalmoplegia
D. All of the above

Patients with lateral mass invasion of an intrasellar mass may present with diplopia, ptosis, ophthalmoplegia, and decreased facial sensation.

263. Invasive pituitary mass may encroach upon all except?
Harrison's 20th Ed. Chapter 373 Page 2670

A. Sphenoid sinus
B. Palate roof
C. Hypothalamus
D. Parietal lobe

Invasive pituitary mass may encroach upon sphenoid sinus, palate roof, temporal and frontal lobes and hypothalamus.

264. Hypothalamic encroachment by an invasive pituitary mass may lead to?
Harrison's 20th Ed. Chapter 373 Page 2670

A. Precocious puberty or hypogonadism
B. Diabetes insipidus
C. Appetite disorders
D. All of the above

Direct hypothalamic encroachment by an invasive pituitary mass may cause precocious puberty or hypogonadism, diabetes insipidus, sleep disturbances, dysthermia, appetite and thirst disorders, obesity, and autonomic dysfunction.

265. Which of the following is an abnormal feature of pituitary MRI?
Harrison's 20th Ed. Chapter 373 Page 2670

A. Pituitary gland height is <8 mm in adults
B. Convex upper aspect of adult pituitary
C. Vertical pituitary stalk
D. Slightly heterogeneous soft tissue consistency

Pituitary gland height is ~6 mm in children to 8 mm in adults. It increases during pregnancy & puberty to ~10 - 12 mm. Upper aspect of adult pituitary is flat or slightly concave, becomes convex in adolescent & pregnant.

266. On MRI, "pituitary bright spot" is due to?
Harrison's 20th Ed. Chapter 373 Page 2670

A. Anterior pituitary
B. Posterior pituitary
C. Pituitary stalk
D. None of the above

267. On MRI, "pituitary bright spot" is due to high content in the posterior pituitary of?

Harrison's 20th Ed. Chapter 373 Page 2670

A. Tryptophan
B. Glucose
C. Phospholipid
D. Ascorbic acid

High phospholipid content of posterior pituitary results in a "pituitary bright spot" on MRI.

268. Which of the following is false regarding "nonadenomatous pituitary lesions"?

Harrison's 20th Ed. Chapter 373 Page 2671

A. Meningiomas are associated with bony hyperostosis
B. Craniopharyngiomas may be calcified & are hypodense
C. Gliomas are hyperdense on T2-weighted images
D. None of the above

When larger pituitary masses (>1 cm) are encountered, they must be distinguished from nonadenomatous lesions like meningioma, craniopharyngiomas & gliomas.

269. Which of the following visual field defect occurs due to prechiasmal compression by an expanding intrasellar mass?

Harrison's 20th Ed. Chapter 373 Page 2671

A. Bitemporal hemianopia
B. Homonymous hemianopia
C. Monocular temporal field loss
D. All of the above

270. Which of the following visual field defect occurs due to postchiasmal compression by an expanding intrasellar mass?

Harrison's 20th Ed. Chapter 373 Page 2671

A. Bitemporal hemianopia
B. Homonymous hemianopia
C. Monocular temporal field loss
D. All of the above

Bitemporal hemianopia is observed classically when a sellar mass lesions impinges the optic chiasm. Homonymous hemianopia occurs from postchiasmal compression & monocular temporal field loss occurs from prechiasmal compression.

271. Presenting clinical features of functional pituitary adenomas can be?

Harrison's 20th Ed. Chapter 373 Page 2671

A. Acromegaly
B. Prolactinomas
C. Cushing syndrome
D. All of the above

272. When a pituitary adenoma is suspected on MRI, initial hormonal evaluation includes?

Harrison's 20th Ed. Chapter 373 Page 2671

A. Basal prolactin (PRL)
B. Insulin-like growth factor (IGF)-I
C. α subunit, FSH and LH
D. All of the above

When a pituitary adenoma is suspected based on MRI, initial hormonal evaluation usually includes basal prolactin (PRL), insulin-like growth factor (IGF)-I, 24 hour urinary free cortisol (UFC) and/or overnight oral dexamethasone (1 mg) suppression test, α subunit, FSH and LH and thyroid function tests.

273. Which of the following is false about pituitary tumors?

Harrison's 20th Ed. Chapter 373 Page 2671

A. Most pituitary tumors are benign
B. Most pituitary tumors are slow-growing
C. Life-long management & follow-up is necessary
D. None of the above

274. Somatostatin analogues are useful in treating patients with?

Harrison's 20th Ed. Chapter 373 Page 2672

A. Acromegaly
B. TSH-secreting tumors
C. ACTH-secreting tumors
D. All of the above

For prolactinomas, dopamine agonists are the treatment of choice.

275. Sellar masses may arise from?

Harrison's 20th Ed. Chapter 373 Page 2672

A. Brain
B. Hypothalamus
C. Pituitary
D. All of the above

Sellar masses other than pituitary adenomas may arise from brain, hypothalamic, or pituitary tissues.

276. Hyperthermia results due to lesion in which part of hypothalamus?

Harrison's 20th Ed. Chapter 373 Page 2673

A. Anterior and preoptic hypothalamus
B. Posterior hypothalamus
C. Ventromedial nuclei
D. Central hypothalamus

Hemorrhage in anterior & preoptic hypothalamus may cause acute hyperthermia accompanied by paradoxical vasoconstriction & tachycardia.

277. Periodic hypothermia syndrome results due to lesion in which part of hypothalamus?

Harrison's 20th Ed. Chapter 373 Page 2673

A. Anterior and preoptic hypothalamus
B. Posterior hypothalamus
C. Ventromedial nuclei
D. Central hypothalamus

Periodic hypothermia syndrome refers to episodic attacks of hypothermia, along with sweating, vasodilation, vomiting & bradycardia. It is due to lesion in posterior hypothalamus.

278. Hyperphagia and obesity results due to lesion in which part of hypothalamus?

Harrison's 20th Ed. Chapter 373 Page 2673

A. Anterior and preoptic hypothalamus
B. Posterior hypothalamus
C. Ventromedial nuclei
D. Central hypothalamus

Ventromedial nuclei of hypothalamus contain the energy-satiety responsive melanocortin receptors which are influenced by leptin, insulin, POMC & its products & gastrointestinal peptides. Craniopharyngiomas, trauma or inflammation can cause damage to ventromedial nuclei of hypothalamus leading to hyperphagia & obesity.

279. Central osmo-receptors are located in which part of hypothalamus?

Harrison's 20th Ed. Chapter 373 Page 2673

A. Preoptic nulcei of hypothalamus
B. Posterior hypothalamus
C. Ventromedial nuclei
D. Central hypothalamus

Central osmo-receptors are located in preoptic nuclei of hypothalamus. Damage to them is associated with polydipsia & hypodipsia.

280. Elevated serum catecholamine and cortisol levels result due to lesion in which part of hypothalamus?

Harrison's 20th Ed. Chapter 373 Page 2673

A. Anterior and preoptic hypothalamus
B. Posterior hypothalamus
C. Ventromedial nuclei
D. Central hypothalamus

Stimulation of sympathetic neurons with consequent elevation of serum catecholamine & cortisol levels occurs due to lesions of central hypothalamus and are predisposed to cardiac arrhythmias, hypertension & gastric erosions.

281. Which of the following about craniopharyngiomas is false?

Harrison's 20th Ed. Chapter 373 Page 2673

A. Benign
B. Suprasellar
C. Cystic
D. None of the above

Craniopharyngiomas are benign, suprasellar cystic masses.

282. Craniopharyngiomas arise near which of the following?

Harrison's 20th Ed. Chapter 373 Page 2673

A. Pituitary stalk
B. Anterior pituitary
C. Posterior pituitary
D. Hypothalamus

Craniopharyngiomas, derived from Rathke's pouch, arise near the pituitary stalk & extend into suprasellar cistern. They are often large, cystic, locally invasive & partially calcified. They present frequently before age 20, with signs of increased intracranial pressure. Other presentations include visual field abnormalities, personality changes & cognitive deterioration, growth retardation, cranial nerve damage, sleep difficulties, weight gain, anterior pituitary dysfunction & diabetes insipidus.

283. Hypopituitarism can be documented in what percentage of patients with craniopharyngioma?

Harrison's 20th Ed. Chapter 373 Page 2673

A. 20%
B. 40%
C. 60%
D. 90%

Hypopituitarism can be documented in about 90%, and diabetes insipidus occurs in about 10% of patients with craniopharyngioma.

284. Which of the following is not a feature of Hand-Schuller-Christian disease?

Harrison's 20th Ed. Chapter 373 Page 2673

A. Diabetes mellitus
B. Exophthalmos
C. Punched-out lytic bone lesions
D. Axillary skin rash

Foci of eosinophilic granulomas are a typical feature of Histiocytosis X. Hand-Schuller-Christian disease refers to a constellation of diabetes insipidus, exophthalmos, punched-out lytic bone lesions & typical axillary skin rash.

285. Blood-borne metastatic deposits in pituitary gland are found almost exclusively in?

Harrison's 20th Ed. Chapter 373 Page 2673

A. Anterior pituitary
B. Posterior pituitary
C. Pituitary stalk
D. Any of the above

Pituitary metastases occur in ~3% of cancer patients and blood-borne metastatic deposits are found almost exclusively in posterior pituitary. Diabetes insipidus is the presenting feature.

286. Hypothalamic hamartomas and gangliocytomas may overexpress which of the following hypothalamic neuropeptides?

Harrison's 20th Ed. Chapter 373 Page 2673

A. Gonadotropin releasing hormone (GnRH)
B. Growth hormone releasing hormone (GHRH)
C. Corticotropin releasing hormone (CRH)
D. All of the above

Hypothalamic hamartomas and gangliocytomas may arise from astrocytes, oligodendrocytes, and neurons. These tumors may overexpress hypothalamic neuropeptides, including gonadotropin-releasing hormone (GnRH), growth hormone–releasing hormone (GHRH), and corticotropin-releasing hormone (CRH).

287. Laughing seizure is also called?

Neuropsychiatr Dis Treat. 2008;4(6):1021–1031, Harrison's 20th Ed. Chapter 373 Page 2673

A. Psychogenic non-epileptic seizures (PNES)
B. Infantile spasms
C. Gelastic seizure
D. Dacrystic seizure

Hypothalamic hamartomas are rare congenital lesions presenting with the classic triad of gelastic epilepsy, precocious puberty and developmental delay.

288. Pallister-Hall syndrome is associated with?

Harrison's 20th Ed. Chapter 373 Page 2673

A. Hypothalamic gliomas
B. Hypothalamic hamartomas
C. Pituitary metastases
D. Rathke's cysts

Pituitary failure secondary to lesions around pituitary due to hamartoma along with craniofacial abnormalities, imperforate anus, cardiac, renal & lung disorders is called Pallister-Hall syndrome which is caused by mutations in the carboxy terminus of the GLI3 gene.

289. Pituitary adenomas account for what percentage of all intracranial neoplasms?

Harrison's 20th Ed. Chapter 373 Page 2673

A. ~ 2%
B. ~ 5%
C. ~ 15%
D. ~ 20%

Pituitary adenomas account for ~15% of all intracranial neoplasms. At autopsy, 25% of all pituitary glands have microadenoma (<10 mm diameter). Pituitary imaging detects small pituitary lesions in at least 10% of normal individuals.

290. Which of the following is false about pituitary adenomas?

Harrison's 20th Ed. Chapter 373 Page 2673

A. Monoclonal in origin
B. Benign neoplasms
C. Hormone production does not correlate with tumor size
D. None of the above

Almost all pituitary adenomas are monoclonal in origin due to somatic mutation leading to increased growth. Pituitary adenomas are benign uni- or plurihormonal neoplasms. Pituitary carcinomas with documented extracranial metastases are very rare. Hormone production does not always correlate with tumor size. ~One-third of all adenomas are clinically nonfunctioning & produce no distinct clinical hypersecretory syndrome.

291. Which out of the following is the most common cell type producing pituitary adenoma?

Harrison's 20th Ed. Chapter 373 Page 2674 Table 373-3

A. Thyrotrope
B. Gonadotrope
C. Somatotrope
D. Corticotrope

Hyperprolactinemia is the most common pituitary hormone hypersecretion syndrome in men and women.

292. Which out of the following is the least common cell type producing pituitary adenoma?

Harrison's 20th Ed. Chapter 373 Page 2674 Table 373-3

A. Thyrotrope
B. Gonadotrope
C. Somatotrope
D. Corticotrope

293. Loss of red perception is due to pressure on?

Harrison's 20th Ed. Chapter 373 Page 2670

A. Optic nerve
B. Optic chiasm
C. Optic tract
D. All of the above

Loss of red perception is an early sign of optic tract pressure. Bitemporal hemianopia or superior bitemporal defects are seen due to pressure of the expanding pituitary tumour because these tracts are located within inferior & posterior part of chiasm. Homonymous field defects are postchiasmal & monocular field cuts are prechiasmal.

294. Acidophil stem cell pituitary adenoma can lead to?

Harrison's 20th Ed. Chapter 373 Page 2674 Table 373-3

A. Hypogonadism
B. Galactorrhea
C. Acromegaly
D. All of the above

In patients with acidophilic stem-cell adenomas, features of hyperprolactinemia (hypogonadism & galactorrhea) predominate over the less clinically evident signs of acromegaly.

295. Mammosomatotrope pituitary adenoma can lead to?

Harrison's 20th Ed. Chapter 373 Page 2674 Table 373-3

A. Hypogonadism
B. Galactorrhea
C. Acromegaly
D. All of the above

Mammosomatotrope produce GH, PRL & can present with a clinical syndrome of acromegaly, hypogonadism & galactorrhea of varying degrees.

296. "CREB" stands for?

Harrison's 20th Ed. Chapter 373 Page 2674

A. Cholesterol response element binding protein
B. Cyclic AMP response element binding protein
C. Calcium response element binding protein
D. Cancer response element binding protein

CREB (cyclic adenosine monophosphate responsive element-binding) protein, is a critical transcription factor for neuronal survival which plays an important role in memory in the hippocampus.

297. Factors involved in initiation and promotion of pituitary tumors include?

Harrison's 20th Ed. Chapter 373 Page 2674

A. Basic fibroblast growth factor (bFGF)
B. Loss of negative-feedback inhibition
C. Estrogen-mediated or paracrine angiogenesis
D. All of the above

Basic fibroblast growth factor (bFGF) stimulate pituitary cell mitogenesis. Other factors involved in initiation & promotion of pituitary tumors include loss of negative-feedback inhibition & estrogen-mediated or paracrine angiogenesis.

298. Which of the following is a genetic syndrome associated with pituitary tumors?

Harrison's 20th Ed. Chapter 373 Page 2674

A. Multiple endocrine neoplasia (MEN) 1
B. Carney syndrome
C. McCune-Albright syndrome
D. All of the above

Genetic predisposition to parathyroid, pancreatic islet & pituitary adenomas occurs in autosomal dominant Multiple endocrine neoplasia (MEN) 1 because "MENIN", the tumor-suppressor gene on chromosome 11q13, is inactivated by mutation. Loss of heterozygosity (LOH)of the remaining normal MENIN allele, leads to tumorigenesis. Carney syndrome is due to mutations in R1a regulatory subunit of protein kinase A (PRKAR1A). Testicular, adrenal & pituitary adenomas along with spotty skin pigmentation & myxomas are the characteristic features. McCune-Albright syndrome refers to polyostotic fibrous dysplasia, pigmented skin patches, and GH-secreting pituitary tumors, adrenal and ovarian tumours. Hormonal hypersecretion is secondary to to cyclic AMP overproduction caused by postzygotic inactivation of GTPase activity of Gsα.

299. Which of the following gene is implicated in the causation of familial acromegaly?

Harrison's 20th Ed. Chapter 373 Page 2674

A. AIP
B. PRKAR1A
C. CDKNIB
D. MEN1

300. Systemic disorder associated with hyperprolactinemia is?

Harrison's 20th Ed. Chapter 373 Page 2675 Table 373-5

A. Chronic renal failure
B. Hypothyroidism
C. Cirrhosis
D. All of the above

Chronic renal failure, hypothyroidism, cirrhosis, pseudocyesis and epileptic seizures are the systemic disorders leading to hyperprolactinemia. Chronic renal failure elevates prolactin by decreasing peripheral prolactin clearance. Primary hypothyroidism causes hyperprolactinemia because of enhanced TRH secretion.

301. The most common pituitary hormone hypersecretion syndrome in both males and females is?

Harrison's 20th Ed. Chapter 373 Page 2675

A. Acromegaly
B. Hyperprolactinemia
C. Secondary hyperthyroidism
D. Cushing's syndrome

302. When PRL level is >200 μg/L, the most common cause is?

Harrison's 20th Ed. Chapter 373 Page 2675

A. Pituitary stalk compression
B. Prolactinoma
C. Antipsychotic and antidepressant drugs
D. Pregnancy and lactation

Prolactinomas are the most common cause of PRL levels >200 μg/L. Hypothalamus stimulates production of all anterior pituitary hormones except prolactin, where it has an inhibitory effect. Prolactin inhibitory hormone resembles catecholamine dopamine, secreted by arcuate nuclei of hypothalamus and decreases prolactin secretion. Thus, damage to hypothalamus or blockage of hypothalamic-hypophyseal portal system increases prolactin secretion.

303. Sleep-associated hyperprolactinemia reverts to normal within how much time after awakening?

Harrison's 20th Ed. Chapter 373 Page 2675

A. 1 hour
B. 2 hours
C. 3 hours
D. 6 hours

Sleep-associated hyperprolactinemia reverts to normal within an hour of awakening.

304. "Colostrum" does not contain which of the following?

Guyton's Textbook of Medical Physiology 11th Ed. 1040

A. Protein
B. Lactose
C. Fats
D. Calcium

305. Hormonal agents that induce prolactin include?

Harrison's 20th Ed. Chapter 373 Page 2675 Table 373-5

A. Estrogens
B. Antiandrogens
C. TRH
D. All of the above

306. Which of the following produce "drug-induced hyperprolactinemia" by blocking dopamine receptors?

Harrison's 20th Ed. Chapter 373 Page 2675 Table 373-5

A. Chlorpromazine
B. Haloperidol
C. Metoclopramide
D. All of the above

307. Which of the following produce "drug-induced hyperprolactinemia" by inhibiting dopamine synthesis?

Harrison's 20th Ed. Chapter 373 Page 2675 Table 373-5

A. Alpha-Methyldopa
B. Metoclopramide
C. Chlorpromazine
D. Haloperidol

308. Which of the following produce "drug-induced hyperprolactinemia" by depleting catecholamine?

Harrison's 20th Ed. Chapter 373 Page 2675 Table 373-5

A. Alpha-Methyldopa
B. Metoclopramide
C. Chlorpromazine
D. Reserpine

309. Which of the following produce "drug-induced hyperprolactinemia" by blocking dopamine release?

Harrison's 20th Ed. Chapter 373 Page 2675 Table 373-5

A. Alpha-Methyldopa
B. Metoclopramide
C. Verapamil
D. Reserpine

Dopamine receptors are blocked by phenothiazines like chlorpromazine, perphenazine, butyrophenones like haloperidol, thioxanthenes & metoclopramide. α-methyldopa inhibits dopamine synthesis. Reserpine is a catecholamine depletor. Verapamil blocks dopamine release. Estrogens, antiandrogens & TRH induce prolactin.

310. Which of the following is a hallmark of hyperprolactinemia in women?

Harrison's 20th Ed. Chapter 373 Page 2675

A. Amenorrhea
B. Galactorrhea
C. Infertility
D. All of the above

311. Sustained hyperprolactinemia is demonstrated by?

Harrison's 20th Ed. Chapter 373 Page 2675

A. Decreased libido
B. Reduced vertebral bone mineral density
C. Weight gain
D. Hirsutism

312. Which out of the following is the usual presenting symptom of hyperprolactinemia in men?

Harrison's 20th Ed. Chapter 373 Page 2675

A. Decreased beard growth
B. Visual loss
C. Osteopenia
D. Reduced muscle mass

313. Galactorrhea is present in what percentage of hyperprolactinemic women?

Harrison's 20th Ed. Chapter 373 Page 2675

A. Up to 80%
B. Up to 85%
C. Up to 90%
D. Up to 95%

314. Which of the following in not a presenting feature of hyperprolactinemia in women?

Harrison's 20th Ed. Chapter 373 Page 2675

A. Reduced vertebral bone density
B. Decreased libido
C. Weight loss
D. Hirsutism

Chief presentations of hyperprolactinemia in women are oligomenorrhea / amenorrhea, galactorrhea, infertility, reduced vertebral bone mineral density due to hypoestrogenemia, decreased libido, weight gain & hirsutism.

315. Breast milk secretion is considered abnormal if it persists for?

Harrison's 20th Ed. Chapter 373 Page 2675

A. > 3 months after childbirth or discontinuation of breastfeeding
B. > 6 months after childbirth or discontinuation of breastfeeding
C. > 9 months after childbirth or discontinuation of breastfeeding
D. > 12 months after childbirth or discontinuation of breastfeeding

Galactorrhea, the inappropriate discharge of milk-containing fluid from the breast, is considered abnormal if it persists for > 6 months after childbirth or discontinuation of breastfeeding.

316. What is the normal basal, fasting morning prolactin level?

Harrison's 20th Ed. Chapter 373 Page 2676

A. < 5 μg/L
B. < 10 μg/L
C. < 15 μg/L
D. < 20 μg/L

317. Which of the following is false about macroprolactinemia?

Harrison's 20th Ed. Chapter 373 Page 2676

A. Causes falsely elevated prolactin values
B. Usually biologically inactive
C. Aggregated forms of circulating PRL
D. None of the above

Basal, fasting morning PRL levels are normally <20 g/L. Prolactin secretion occurs in a pulsatile manner & levels vary widely. Assays on multiple occasions may be needed to document hyperprolactinemia. "Macroprolactinemia" refers to biologically inactive aggregated forms of circulating prolactin. It is a cause of false elevation of prolactin levels.

318. Which of the following is the least common hormone secreted by mixed tumors that secrete prolactin?

Harrison's 20th Ed. Chapter 373 Page 2676

A. GH
B. ACTH
C. TSH
D. None of the above

Tumors arising from lactotrope cells account for ~ half of all functioning pituitary tumors. Mixed tumors secreting combinations of GH & PRL, ACTH & PRL & rarely TSH & PRL are also seen.

319. The female : male ratio for microprolactinomas is?

Harrison's 20th Ed. Chapter 373 Page 2676

A. 1:1
B. 5:1
C. 10:1
D. 20:1

320. The female:male ratio for macroadenomas is?

Harrison's 20th Ed. Chapter 373 Page 2676

A. 1:1
B. 5:1
C. 10:1
D. 20:1

Female:male ratio for microprolactinomas is 20:1, whereas it is 1:1 for macroadenomas. Males tend to present with larger macroadenomas than females because of delay in appreciating signs & symptoms.

321. For defining "microadenoma" of pituitary gland, what is its cutoff diameter?

Harrison's 20th Ed. Chapter 373 Page 2676

A. < 0.2 cm
B. < 0.5 cm
C. < 0.8 cm
D. < 1.0 cm

Pituitary tumours <1 cm in diameter are termed microadenomas. They do not invade parasellar structures. Macroadenomas are >1 cm in diameter and are locally invasive & encroach on surrounding structures.

322. Which of the following statements about prolactinoma is false?

Harrison's 20th Ed. Chapter 373 Page 2676

A. Tumor size correlates directly with PRL concentrations
B. PRL >250 μg/L are associated with macroadenomas
C. PRL levels remain stable
D. None of the above

323. "High-dose hook effect" in prolactin macroadenomas best relates to?

J Hum Reprod Sci. 2010;3(3):160-161, Neurol India 2001;49:78-80

A. Raynaud's phenomenon
B. Koebner phenomenon
C. Prozone phenomenon
D. Tullio phenomenon

Very high prolactin (PRL) concentrations can interfere with immunoassay systems resulting in falsely low PRL determination. This is called the 'high dose hook effect' or the 'prozone phenomenon'.

324. If fertility is not desired, what should be the line of management of microadenomas?

Harrison's 20th Ed. Chapter 373 Page 2676

A. Dopamine agonists
B. Surgery
C. Radiation
D. No treatment

Pituitary microadenomas are slow growing tumours and only ~5% go on to be macroadenomas. In ~30% of microadenomas, hyperprolactinemia resolves spontaneously. Such asymptomatic patients should be monitored by regular serial prolactin and MRI. No treatment is advocated, if fertility is not desired. However, estrogen replacement may be given to prevent bone loss.

325. Dopamine agonists act by?
Harrison's 20th Ed. Chapter 373 Page 2676

A. Suppressing prolactin secretion
B. Suppressing prolactin synthesis
C. Suppressing lactotrope cell proliferation
D. All of the above

326. Which of the following is a nonergot oral dopamine agonist?
Hum Reprod. 2010;25(4):995-1004

A. Pergolide mesylate
B. Lisuride
C. Quinagolide
D. Bromocriptine

327. Fungus that produces "Ergot alkaloids" is?
Toxins. 2015;7(3):659-678

A. Hortaea werneckii
B. Trichosporon asahii
C. Sporothrix schenckii
D. Claviceps purpurea

Claviceps purpurea is known for epidemics of ergot poisoning (ergotism or St. Anthony's fire). Besides ergot alkaloids, this fungus synthesizes histamine, acetylcholine & tyramine. Bromocriptine, cabergoline & pergolide are ergot alkaloids that have the highest suppressive selectivity for pituitary dopamine D2 receptors. Quinagolide is a nonergot drug with similar D2 receptor affinity. Lysergic acid diethylamide (LSD) is a synthetic ergot compound & its behavioral effects are mediated by agonist effects at prejunctional or postjunctional 5-HT2 receptors in CNS. Cabergoline has a half-life of 63–69 hours.

328. Treatment may be withdrawn after what length of time in microadenoma responders to dopamine agonists?
Harrison's 20th Ed. Chapter 373 Page 2676

A. 3 months
B. 6 months
C. 1 year
D. 2 years

In patients with microadenomas who have achieved normoprolactinemia and significant reduction of tumor mass, the dopamine agonist may be withdrawn after 2 years.

329. Which of the following about cabergoline is false?
Harrison's 20th Ed. Chapter 373 Page 2676

A. Ergoline derivative
B. Long-acting dopamine agonist
C. High D2 receptor affinity
D. None of the above

330. Which of the following about cabergoline is false?
Harrison's 20th Ed. Chapter 373 Page 2676

A. May be effective in patients resistant to bromocriptine
B. Adverse effects less than with bromocriptine
C. Drug intolerance less than with bromocriptine
D. None of the above

331. Which of the following investigation should be done before initiating standard-dose cabergoline therapy?
Harrison's 20th Ed. Chapter 373 Page 2677

A. Electrocardiogram
B. Echocardiogram
C. X-ray chest
D. Ultrasonography abdomen

Patients who receive at least 3 mg of cabergoline daily have been reported to be at risk for development of cardiac valve regurgitation.

332. Which of the following about bromocriptine is false?
Harrison's 20th Ed. Chapter 373 Page 2676

A. Ergot alkaloid
B. Short-acting
C. Preferred when pregnancy is desired, no teratogenic effect
D. None of the above

Because cabergoline is long-acting with a high D2-receptor affinity, it is not recommended for use in women when fertility is desired.

333. Salt of bromocriptine used as dopamine receptor agonist for treatment of hyperprolactinemia is?
Harrison's 20th Ed. Chapter 373 Page 2676

A. Acetate
B. Mesylate
C. Cryptate
D. Sulphate

Ergot alkaloid bromocriptine mesylate is a dopamine receptor agonist that suppresses prolactin secretion. Because it is short-acting, the drug is preferred when pregnancy is desired. It is administered at bedtime with a snack.

334. Which of the following pituitary adenomas secrete GH?
Harrison's 20th Ed. Chapter 373 Page 2678

A. Somatotrope adenomas
B. Mammosomatotrope cell adenoma
C. Acidophilic stem-cell adenoma
D. All of the above

335. In which of the following pituitary adenomas, features of hyperprolactinemia predominate over those of acromegaly?
Harrison's 20th Ed. Chapter 373 Page 2678

A. Somatotrope adenomas
B. Mammosomatotrope cell adenoma
C. Acidophilic stem-cell adenoma
D. All of the above

336. Ectopic pituitary tissue remnants are reported in?
Harrison's 20th Ed. Chapter 373 Page 2678

A. Cavernous sinus
B. Nasopharynx
C. Dura mater
D. Trigeminal ganglion

Ectopic pituitary tissue remnants are reported in the nasopharynx or midline sinuses.

337. Ectopic GH secretion has been reported by tumors of?
Harrison's 20th Ed. Chapter 373 Page 2678

A. Pancreas
B. Ovary
C. Lung
D. All of the above

Ectopic GH secretion has been reported by tumors of pancreatic, ovarian, lung or hematopoietic origin.

338. Which of the following can lead to excess GHRH secretion?
Harrison's 20th Ed. Chapter 373 Page 2678 Table 373-6

A. Hypothalamic hamartoma
B. Choristoma
C. Ganglioneuroma
D. All of the above

339. Which of the following can lead to excess GHRH secretion?
Harrison's 20th Ed. Chapter 373 Page 2678 Table 373-6

A. Pancreatic islet cell tumor
B. Medullary thyroid carcinoma
C. Pheochromocytoma
D. All of the above

340. The most common cause of GHRH-mediated acromegaly is?
Harrison's 20th Ed. Chapter 373 Page 2678

A. Abdominal carcinoid tumor
B. Pancreatic cancer
C. Ovarian cancer
D. Lung cancer

The most common cause of GHRH-mediated acromegaly is a chest or abdominal carcinoid tumor.

341. The most common cause of GHRH-mediated acromegaly is?
Harrison's 20th Ed. Chapter 373 Page 2678

A. Pancreatic islet cell tumor
B. Pheochromocytoma
C. Chest carcinoid tumor
D. Medullary thyroid carcinoma

Most common cause of GHRH-mediated acromegaly is a chest or abdominal carcinoid tumor. Excessive GHRH may be secreted by hypothalamic tumors, usually choristomas or neuromas.

342. Normal daytime circulating levels of Growth Hormone is?
N Engl J Med 2006;355:2558-73

A. < 0.2 μg/liter
B. < 0.3 μg/liter
C. < 0.4 μg/liter
D. < 0.5 μg/liter

343. The production of IGF-I is suppressed in?
N Engl J Med 2006;355:2558-73

A. Liver disease
B. Hypothyroidism
C. Poorly controlled diabetes mellitus
D. All of the above

344. Familial syndromes associated with acromegaly include?
N Engl J Med 2006;355:2558-73

A. MEN type 1
B. McCune-Albright syndrome
C. Carney's syndrome
D. All of the above

345. Which of the following organs is not enlarged in acromegaly?
N Engl J Med 2006;355:2558-73

A. Tongue
B. Thyroid gland
C. Parotid gland
D. Heart

346. Which of the following organs is not enlarged in acromegaly?
N Engl J Med 2006;355:2558-73

A. Liver
B. Pancreas
C. Kidney
D. Prostate

Generalized visceromegaly occurs in acromegaly, including cardiomegaly, macroglossia, and thyroid gland enlargement.

347. Prognathism is due to enlargement of?
Harrison's 20th Ed. Chapter 373 Page 2678

A. Maxilla
B. Mandible
C. Nasal bones
D. All of the above

348. Acromegaly is associated with an increased risk of which of the following malignancies?
Harrison's 20th Ed. Chapter 373 Page 2678

A. Pancreatic
B. Colonic
C. Breast
D. Thyroid

Acromegaly is associated with an increased risk of colon polyps and colonic malignancy. Polyps are diagnosed in up to one-third of acromegalic patients.

349. Which of the following regarding acromegaly is false?
Harrison's 20th Ed. Chapter 373 Page 2678

A. Often clinically not diagnosed for 10 years or more
B. Without treatment, survival is reduced by ~10 years
C. Hypertension occur in about 75% of patients
D. Diabetes mellitus develops in 25% of patients

In acromegaly, cardiovascular system is most severely affected. Coronary heart disease, cardiomyopathy with arrhythmias, left ventricular hypertrophy, decreased diastolic function & hypertension occur in about 30% of patients. Diabetes mellitus develops in 25% of patients with acromegaly. Overall mortality is increased ~threefold and is due primarily to cardiovascular & cerebrovascular disorders, malignancy & respiratory disease. Without proper treatment, survival is reduced by an average of 10 years compared with an age-matched control population.

350. For the diagnosis of acromegaly, measurement of which of the following is most useful?
Harrison's 20th Ed. Chapter 373 Page 2679

A. GH
B. GHRH
C. IGF-I
D. IGF-II

Due to the pulsatility of GH secretion, measurement of a single random GH level is not useful for the diagnosis or exclusion of acromegaly and does not correlate with disease severity. IGF-I level provides a useful laboratory screening measure when clinical features raise the possibility of acromegaly.

351. In acromegaly, following oral glucose load, GH levels remain?
Harrison's 20th Ed. Chapter 373 Page 2679

A. > 0.1 μg/liter
B. > 0.2 μg/liter
C. > 0.3 μg/liter
D. > 0.4 μg/liter

Diagnosis of acromegaly is confirmed by demonstrating failure of GH suppression to <0.4 μg/L within 1 to 2 hours of 75 gram oral glucose load.

352. Which of the following about acromegaly is false?

Harrison's 20th Ed. Chapter 373 Page 2679

A. ~20% exhibit a paradoxical GH rise after glucose
B. PRL is elevated in ~25% of patients with acromegaly
C. Overall mortality is increased about threefold
D. None of the above

353. In GH-secreting microadenomas, which of the following is the preferred primary treatment for most patients?

Harrison's 20th Ed. Chapter 373 Page 2679

A. Surgical resection
B. Somatostatin analogues
C. Dopamine agonists
D. Irradiation

Surgery is the preferred primary treatment for GH secreting microadenomas. The high frequency of GH hypersecretion after macroadenoma resection usually necessitates adjuvant or primary medical therapy for these larger tumors. Patients unable to receive or respond to medical treatment can be offered radiation.

354. Which of the following is a somatostatin analogue?

Harrison's 20th Ed. Chapter 373 Page 2679

A. Octreotide
B. Lanreotide
C. Pasireotide
D. All of the above

355. Which of the following somatostatin analogue exhibits preferential SST5 binding?

Harrison's 20th Ed. Chapter 373 Page 2680

A. Octreotide
B. Lanreotide
C. Pasireotide
D. All of the above

356. Which of the following is false about Octreotide?

Harrison's 20th Ed. Chapter 373 Page 2679

A. Synthetic somatostatin analogue
B. 40 times more potent than native somatostatin
C. Administered subcutaneously
D. None of the above

357. Which of the following is a side effect of Octreotide?

Harrison's 20th Ed. Chapter 373 Page 2680

A. Tachycardia
B. Cholesterol gallstones
C. Hypoglycemia
D. All of the above

Octreotide suppresses postprandial gallbladder contractility & delays GB emptying. ~30% of patients treated with long-term Octreotide develop echogenic sludge or asymptomatic cholesterol gallstones. Octreotide suppresses gastrointestinal motility & secretion. It may also produce mild glucose intolerance due to transient insulin suppression, asymptomatic bradycardia, hypothyroxinemia & local pain at the injection site.

358. Which of the following somatostatin analogues has higher prevalence of glucose intolerance or new-onset diabetes?

Harrison's 20th Ed. Chapter 373 Page 2680

A. Octreotide
B. Lanreotide
C. Pasireotide
D. All of the above

359. Which of the following act by antagonizing endogenous GH binding to its receptor?

Harrison's 20th Ed. Chapter 373 Page 2680

A. Cabergoline
B. Lanreotide
C. Octreotide acetate
D. Pegvisomant

Pegvisomant is a GH analogue that antagonizes endogenous GH action by blocking peripheral GH binding to its receptor. Consequently, serum IGF-I levels are suppressed, potentially reducing the deleterious effects of excess endogenous GH. Cabergoline suppresses GH. Bromocriptine suppresses GH secretion particularly those with cosecretion of PRL. Lanreotide is a cyclic somatostatin octapeptide analogue that suppresses GH & IGF-I hypersecretion. Sandostatin-LAR is a long-acting formulation of octreotide causing GH suppression.`

360. In ACTH deficiency, total daily dose of hydrocortisone replacement therapy should not exceed?

Harrison's 20th Ed. Chapter 373 Page 2680

A. 10 mg daily
B. 20 mg daily
C. 25 mg daily
D. 40 mg daily

In ACTH deficiency, total daily dose of hydrocortisone replacement should not exceed 25 mg daily.

361. Most common cause of cushingoid features is?

Harrison's 20th Ed. Chapter 373 Page 2680

A. Pituitary corticotrope adenoma
B. Iatrogenic hypercortisolism
C. Ectopic tumor ACTH production
D. Cortisol-producing adrenal adenoma

Pituitary corticotrope adenomas (Cushing's disease) account for 70% of patients with endogenous causes of Cushing's syndrome. Iatrogenic hypercortisolism is the most common cause of cushingoid features.

362. Which of the following is the least common cause of Cushing's syndrome?

Harrison's 20th Ed. Chapter 373 Page 2680

A. Ectopic tumor ACTH production
B. Ectopic tumor CRH production
C. Cortisol-producing adrenal adenomas
D. Adrenal carcinoma

363. What percentage of all pituitary tumors are ACTH-producing adenomas?

Harrison's 20th Ed. Chapter 373 Page 2680

A. 2 to 5%
B. 5 to 10%
C. 10 to 15%
D. 15 to 20%

ACTH-producing adenomas account for ~10 to 15% of all pituitary tumors.

364. Hematopoietic features of hypercortisolism include?

Harrison's 20th Ed. Chapter 373 Page 2680

A. Leukocytosis
B. Lymphopenia
C. Eosinopenia
D. All of the above

Hematopoietic features of hypercortisolism include leukocytosis, lymphopenia, and eosinopenia.

365. Which of the following features make pathologic cause of hypercortisolism more likely?

Harrison's 20th Ed. Chapter 373 Page 2680

A. Central redistribution of fat
B. Thin skin with striae and bruising
C. Proximal muscle weakness
D. All of the above

366. Primary cause of death in patients of Cushing's syndrome is?

Harrison's 20th Ed. Chapter 373 Page 2680

A. Cardiovascular disease
B. Infections
C. Suicide
D. Renal failure

Primary cause of death in Cushing's syndrome is cardiovascular disease, but infections and risk of suicide are also increased.

367. Rapid development of skin hyperpigmentation and severe myopathy suggests the possibility of?

Harrison's 20th Ed. Chapter 373 Page 2681

A. Pituitary corticotrope adenoma
B. Iatrogenic hypercortisolism
C. Ectopic tumor ACTH production
D. Cortisol-producing adrenal adenoma

Rapid development of features of hypercortisolism associated with skin hyperpigmentation & severe myopathy suggests ectopic production of ACTH. Hypertension, hypokalemic alkalosis, glucose intolerance & edema are also more pronounced. Serum potassium levels <3.3 mmol/L are evident in ~70% of patients with ectopic ACTH secretion but are seen in <10% of patients with pituitary-dependent Cushing's disease.

368. Most reliable test for confirmation of pituitary ACTH-secreting adenomas is?

Harrison's 20th Ed. Chapter 373 Page 2681

A. 24-h urine free cortisol (UFC)
B. Bilateral inferior petrosal sinus ACTH sampling
C. Overnight 1-mg dexamethasone suppression test
D. Basal plasma ACTH levels

Small pituitary ACTH-secreting adenomas (<2 mm) may go undetected by gadolinium enhancement pituitary MRI. Bilateral inferior petrosal sinus ACTH sampling distinguishes pituitary ACTH-secreting adenomas from ectopic ACTH-secreting tumors. An increased ratio (>2) of inferior petrosal : peripheral vein ACTH confirms pituitary Cushing's disease.

369. Mean basal ACTH levels are about how many times higher in patients with ectopic ACTH secretion as compared to pituitary ACTH-secreting adenomas?

Harrison's 20th Ed. Chapter 373 Page 2681

A. 3
B. 5
C. 8
D. 12

Mean basal ACTH levels are about eightfold higher in patients with ectopic ACTH secretion compared to those with pituitary ACTH-secreting adenomas.

370. Diameter of most ACTH-secreting pituitary tumors is?

Harrison's 20th Ed. Chapter 373 Page 2681

A. < 2 mm
B. < 5 mm
C. < 8 mm
D. < 10 mm

Most ACTH-secreting pituitary tumors are <5 mm in diameter & about half are undetectable by sensitive MRI.

371. Endocrinopathies that frequently have associated hyperpigmentation include?

Harrison's 20th Ed. Chapter 54 Page

A. Addison's disease
B. Nelson syndrome
C. Ectopic ACTH syndrome
D. All of the above

Endocrinopathies that frequently have associated hyperpigmentation include Addison's disease, Nelson syndrome & ectopic ACTH syndrome.

372. Which of the following is false about Nelson's syndrome?

Harrison's 20th Ed. Chapter 373 Page 2682

A. Pituitary enlargement
B. Increased skin pigmentation
C. High ACTH levels
D. None of the above

Nelson's syndrome is a disorder characterized by rapid pituitary tumor enlargement and increased pigmentation secondary to high ACTH levels. Adrenalectomy in the setting of residual corticotrope adenoma tissue predisposes to its development. Radiation therapy may be indicated to prevent the development of Nelson's syndrome after adrenalectomy.

373. Which of the following is useful in the treatment of ACTH-secreting pituitary tumors?

Harrison's 20th Ed. Chapter 373 Page 2682

A. Pasireotide
B. Trilostane
C. Mifepristone
D. All of the above

Pasireotide (600 or 900 μg/day subcutaneously) is a somatostatin analog with high affinity for SST5 > SST2 receptors. It is approved for treating patients with ACTH-secreting pituitary tumors when surgery is not an option or has been unsuccessful. Mifepristone (300- 1 200 mg/d)¡A a glucocorticoid receptor antagonist¡A blocks peripheral cortisol action and is approved to treat hyperglycemia in Cushing's disease.

374. In treatment of Cushing's disease, which of the following drugs is useful?

Harrison's 20th Ed. Chapter 373 Page 2682

A. Ketoconazole
B. Metyrapone
C. Mitotane
D. All of the above

In Cushing's disease, steroidogenic inhibitors are used in combination with pituitary irradiation to block the adrenal effects of persistently high ACTH levels. Ketoconazole is an antimycotic drug that inhibits several P450 enzymes, Metyrapone inhibits 11b-hydroxylase activity & Mitotane suppresses cortisol hypersecretion by inhibiting 11b-hydroxylase and cholesterol side-chain cleavage enzymes & by destroying adrenocortical cells.

375. In treatment of Cushing's disease, which of the following drugs is useful?

Harrison's 20th Ed. Chapter 373 Page 2682

A. Aminoglutethimide
B. Cyproheptadine
C. Etomidate
D. All of the above

Aminoglutethimide, trilostane, cyproheptadine & etomidate block steroidogenesis and are useful in treatment of Cushing's disease.

376. Which out of the following clinical features of Cushing's syndrome is most common?

Harrison's 20th Ed. Chapter 373 Page 2680 Table 373-7

A. Hypertension
B. Purple skin striae
C. Thin skin
D. Truncal obesity

377. Which out of the following clinical features of Cushing's Syndrome is most common?

Harrison's 20th Ed. Chapter 373 Page 2680 Table 373-7

A. Acne
B. Hirsutism
C. Hyperpigmentation
D. Bruising

Clinical features of Cushing's Syndrome in order of frequency are : Obesity, Thin skin, Moon facies, Hypertension, Purple skin striae, Hirsutism, Menstrual disorders, Plethora, Abnormal glucose tolerance, Impotence, Proximal muscle weakness, Truncal obesity, Acne, Bruising, Mental changes, Osteoporosis, Edema of lower extremities, Hyperpigmentation, Hypokalemic alkalosis, Diabetes mellitus.

378. Most common presenting feature of adult hypopituitarism is?

Harrison's 20th Ed. Chapter 372 Page 2669

A. Hypothyroidism
B. Hypogonadism
C. Addison's disease
D. Hyperprolactinemia

Hypogonadism is the most common presenting feature of adult hypopituitarism, even when other pituitary hormones are also deficient.

379. Acquired GnRH deficiency causing hypogonadotropism can be due to?

Harrison's 20th Ed. Chapter 372 Page 2669

A. Anorexia nervosa
B. Stress
C. Starvation
D. All of the above

Acquired forms of GnRH deficiency leading to hypogonadotropism are seen in association with anorexia nervosa, stress, starvation & extreme exercise, but may also be idiopathic. Hypogonadotropic hypogonadism in these disorders is reversed by removal of the stressful stimulus.

380. Which of the following is the characteristic skin change in hypogonadal adult males?

Harrison's 20th Ed. Chapter 372 Page 2669

A. Petechiae
B. Fine facial wrinkles
C. Coarse thickened skin
D. Skin tags

In hypogonadal adult males, secondary testicular failure is associated with decreased libido & potency, infertility, decreased muscle mass with weakness, reduced beard and body hair growth, soft testes, and characteristic fine facial wrinkles.

381. Most clinically nonfunctioning adenomas originate from?

Harrison's 20th Ed. Chapter 373 Page 2682

A. Somatotroph cells
B. Corticotrope cells
C. Gonadotrope cells
D. Lactotroph cells

Most clinically nonfunctioning adenomas originate from gonadotrope cells. These tumors typically produce small amounts of intact gonadotropins (usually FSH) as well as uncombined α and LH β and FSH β subunits. Tumor secretion may lead to elevated α & FSH β subunits and, rarely, to increased LH β subunit levels. Some adenomas express a subunits without FSH or LH.

382. In patients with gonadotrope adenomas, administration of which of the following stimulates LH β subunit secretion?

Harrison's 20th Ed. Chapter 373 Page 2682

A. TRH
B. TSH
C. ACTH
D. CRH

In majority of patients with gonadotrope adenomas, TRH administration stimulates LH β subunit secretion. This response is not seen in normal individuals.

383. Which of the following is false in men with gonadotropin-secreting tumors?

Harrison's 20th Ed. Chapter 373 Page 2682

A. Increased gonadotropins (LH > FSH)
B. Pituitary mass
C. Low testosterone levels
D. None of the above

In men, gonadotropin-secreting tumors may be diagnosed because of slightly increased gonadotropins (FSH > LH) in the setting of a pituitary mass. Testosterone levels are usually low, despite the normal or increased LH level, perhaps reflecting reduced LH bioactivity or the loss of normal LH pulsatility.

384. Clinically inapparent somatotrope adenoma is best excluded by?

Harrison's 20th Ed. Chapter 373 Page 2682

A. Normal IGF-I value
B. Normal IGF-II value
C. Normal GH value
D. All of the above

Clinically inapparent somatotrope or corticotrope adenomas can be excluded by a normal IGF-I value and normal 24-hour urinary free cortisol levels. If PRL levels are <100 g/L in a patient with pituitary mass, a nonfunctioning adenoma causing pituitary stalk compression should be considered.

385. In the treatment of nonfunctioning pituitary tumors, which of the following reduces adenoma size?

Harrison's 20th Ed. Chapter 373 Page 2683

A. Dopamine agonists
B. Octreotide
C. Nal-Glu GnRH
D. None of the above

Nonfunctioning pituitary tumors respond poorly to dopamine agonists, octreotide and selective GnRH antagonist, Nal-Glu GnRH.

386. Which of the following is not useful in suppressing TSH secretion in TSH-producing macroadenomas?

Harrison's 20th Ed. Chapter 373 Page 2683

A. Dopamine agonists
B. Octreotide
C. Lanreotide
D. All of the above

Dopamine agonists are rarely effective for suppressing TSH secretion from TSH-secreting adenomas. Octreotide markedly suppresses TSH, causing biochemical hypothyroidism that requires concomitant thyroid hormone replacement. Lanreotide, a long acting somatostatin analogue, effectively suppresses TSH.

Disorders of the Neurohypophysis

387. Which of the following statements is false?
Harrison's 20th Ed. Chapter 374 Page 2684

A. Neurohypophysis is formed by axons that originate in supraoptic & paraventricular nuclei of hypothalamus
B. Neurohypophysis produces arginine vasopressin & oxytocin
C. Oxytocin reduces postpartum milk letdown
D. AVP concentrates urine

388. Which of the following is false about arginine vasopressin?
Harrison's 20th Ed. Chapter 374 Page 2684

A. Pentapeptide
B. Hexapeptide
C. Nonapeptide
D. Decapeptide

AVP is a nine-amino-acid peptide that is synthesized in the magnocellular nerve cell bodies of the supraoptic and paraventricular nuclei. AVP is enzymatically cleaved from its carrier protein, neurophysin II, as it is axonally transported to the synaptic terminal in the posterior pituitary.

389. Structure of arginine vasopressin (AVP) is?
Harrison's 20th Ed. Chapter 374 Page 2684

A. Five-membered disulfide ring with tripeptide tail
B. Six-membered disulfide ring with tripeptide tail
C. Seven-membered disulfide ring with tripeptide tail
D. Eight-membered disulfide ring with tripeptide tail

AVP is a nona-peptide composed of a six-membered disulfide ring and a tripeptide tail.

390. Which of the following is not synthesized via a polypeptide precursor?
Harrison's 20th Ed. Chapter 374 Page 2684

A. AVP
B. Neurophysin
C. Neuroptin
D. Copeptin

AVP secretion is synthesized via a polypeptide precursor that includes AVP, neurophysin & copeptin—all encoded by a single gene on chromosome 20..

391. Neuropeptide arginine vasopressin gene codes for?
N Engl J Med 2015;372:1349-58

A. 9-amino acid peptide arginine vasopressin
B. Carrier protein neurophysin-2
C. Small glycoprotein copeptin
D. All of the above

Neuropeptide arginine vasopressin gene codes for three peptides. They are the 9-amino acid peptide arginine vasopressin, a carrier protein called neurophysin-2, and a small glycoprotein called copeptin.

392. ADH is synthesized in which of the following?
Harrison's 20th Ed. Chapter 374 Page 2684

A. Hypothalamus
B. Anterior pituitary gland
C. Posterior pituitary gland
D. All of the above

393. ADH is released in peripheral blood by which of the following?
Harrison's 20th Ed. Chapter 374 Page 2684

A. Hypothalamus
B. Anterior pituitary gland
C. Posterior pituitary gland
D. All of the above

Antidiuretic hormone (ADH) is synthesized in supraoptic nuclei of hypothalamus and released by the posterior pituitary gland.

394. Absence of AVP produces which of the following?
Harrison's 20th Ed. Chapter 374 Page 2684

A. Osmotic diuresis
B. Water diuresis
C. Electrolyte diuresis
D. Ionic diuresis

Without AVP, cells that line distal tubule & medullary collecting ducts of kidney reabsorb little of the large volume of dilute filtrate that enters from proximal nephron resulting in excretion of very large volumes (0.2 mL/kg per min) of maximally dilute urine (specific gravity ~1.000 & osmolarity 50 mosmol/L). This is called "Water diuresis".

395. Osmoreceptors are present in?
Harrison's 20th Ed. Chapter 374 Page 2684, N Engl J Med 2015;372:1349-58

A. Hypothalamus
B. Posterior pituitary
C. Kidney
D. All of the above

Osmoreceptors are specialized hypothalamic cells that control AVP secretion through 'effective' osmotic pressure of body fluids.

396. Osmoreceptors are extremely sensitive to small changes in the plasma concentration of which of the following?
Harrison's 20th Ed. Chapter 374 Page 2684, N Engl J Med 2015;372:1349-58

A. Sodium
B. Urea
C. Glucose
D. All of the above

Osmoreceptors are extremely sensitive to small changes in plasma concentration of sodium but are insensitive to solutes like urea or glucose. "Osmosensing" is, in part, dependent on activation of nonselective calcium-permeable cation channels in osmosensing neurons that can serve as stretch receptors.

397. Below set point threshold, plasma AVP is?
Harrison's 20th Ed. Chapter 374 Page 2684

A. Suppressed
B. Stimulated
C. No response
D. Any of the above

Below set point threshold, plasma AVP is suppressed to levels that permit development of a maximum water diuresis. Above it, plasma AVP rises steeply in direct proportion to plasma osmolarity, quickly reaching levels sufficient to effect a maximum antidiuresis.

398. Which of the following is called a "second antidiuretic hormone"?
N Engl J Med 2015;372:1349-58

A. Desmopressin
B. Oxytocin
C. Vasopressinase
D. All of the above

399. The average threshold, or set point, for AVP release corresponds to a plasma osmolarity of about?

Harrison's 20th Ed. Chapter 374 Page 2684

A. 280 mosmol/L
B. 285 mosmol/L
C. 290 mosmol/L
D. 295 mosmol/L

Average threshold or set point for AVP release corresponds to a plasma osmolarity of ~ 280 mosmol/L.

400. The average threshold or set point for AVP release corresponds to a plasma sodium of about?

Harrison's 20th Ed. Chapter 374 Page 2684

A. 125 meq/L
B. 130 meq/L
C. 135 meq/L
D. 140 meq/L

Average threshold or set point for AVP release corresponds to a plasma sodium of about 135 meq/L.

401. Which of the following is related to the action of AVP?

Harrison's 20th Ed. Chapter 374 Page 2684

A. Aquaporin 1
B. Aquaporin 2
C. Aquaporin 3
D. Aquaporin 4

AVP action is mediated via binding to G protein coupled V2 receptors on the serosal surface of the cells that line distal tubule & medullary collecting ducts of kidney, activation of adenyl cyclase & insertion into luminal surface of water channels composed of a protein called aquaporin 2.

402. AV3V region that controls osmolarity is located in?

Harrison's 20th Ed. Chapter 374 Page 2684

A. Hypothalamus
B. Anterior pituitary gland
C. Posterior pituitary gland
D. Third ventricle

AV3V region is located along the anteroventral region of third ventricle and plays a role in controlling osmolarity and ADH secretion.

403. Which of the following stimuli increase ADH secretion?

Harrison's 20th Ed. Chapter 374 Page 2684

A. Increased blood osmolarity
B. Decreased arterial pressure
C. Decreased blood volume
D. All of the above

In addition to increased blood osmolarity, decreased arterial pressure and decreased blood volume increase ADH secretion.

404. In healthy adults, the set point of osmoregulatory system can be lowered by?

Harrison's 20th Ed. Chapter 374 Page 2684

A. Pregnancy
B. Menstrual cycle
C. Acute reductions in blood pressure or volume
D. All of the above

Set point of osmoregulatory system can be lowered by pregnancy, menstrual cycle, relatively large acute reductions in blood pressure or volume.

405. Which of the following stimulate AVP secretion?

Harrison's 20th Ed. Chapter 374 Page 2684

A. Nausea
B. Acute hypoglycemia
C. Glucocorticoid deficiency
D. All of the above

AVP secretion is stimulated by nausea, acute hypoglycemia, glucocorticoid deficiency, smoking and hyperangiotensinemia.

406. Emetic center is located in?

Harrison's 20th Ed. Chapter 374 Page 2684

A. Medulla
B. Midbrain
C. Pons
D. Cerebellum

Nausea is an extremely potent stimuli & causes immediate, 50- to 100-fold increases in plasma AVP. Emetic stimuli act via emetic center in medulla & can be completely blocked by antiemetics.

407. Of the fluid filtered by the kidneys, what percentage is reabsorbed isosmotically in proximal tubules?

Harrison's 20th Ed. Chapter 374 Page 2685 Figure 374-2

A. 30%
B. 50%
C. 80%
D. 95%

In a 70-kg healthy adult, kidney filters about 180 L/day of plasma. Of this, ~144 L (80%) is reabsorbed osmotically in proximal tubule & 8 L (4–5%) is reabsorbed without solute in descending limb of Henle's loop. Remainder is diluted to an osmolarity of ~60 mmol/kg by selective reabsorption of sodium & chloride in the ascending limb.

408. Under AVP influence, solute-free water is reabsorbed osmotically through which of the following cells?

Harrison's 20th Ed. Chapter 374 Page 2685 Figure 374-2

A. Principal cells
B. Intercalated cells
C. Mesangial cells
D. All of the above

Under AVP influence, solute-free water is reabsorbed osmotically through principal cells of collecting ducts.

409. Which of the following aquaporin water channels is located on apical membrane of principal cells of the collecting duct?

Harrison's 20th Ed. Chapter 374 Page 2685 Figure 374-2

A. Aquaporin 1
B. Aquaporin 2
C. Aquaporin 3
D. Aquaporin 4

Aquaporin 2 (AQP 2) water channels are located on the apical membrane. AQP 3 and AQP 4 water channels are located on the basal-lateral surface and water diffuses out of the cell through them.

410. The V2 receptors are encoded by genes on chromosome?

Harrison's 20th Ed. Chapter 374 Page 2685 Figure 374-2

A. 11
B. 17
C. 21
D. X

The V2 receptors and aquaporin 2 are encoded by genes on chromosome Xq28 and 12q13, respectively.

411. Antidiuretic effect of AVP is mediated via which of the following receptors?

Harrison's 20th Ed. Chapter 374 Page 2685 Figure 374-2

A. Receptor tyrosine kinase
B. Cytokine receptor–linked kinase
C. G protein–coupled seven-transmembrane (GPCR)
D. Serine Kinase

Antidiuretic effect of AVP is mediated via a G protein–coupled V2 receptor that increases intracellular cyclic AMP, thereby inducing translocation of aquaporin 2 (AQP 2) water channels into the apical membrane resulting in an increase in permeability that permits influx of water that diffuses out of the cell through AQP 3 and AQP 4 water channels on the basal-lateral surface.

412. At high concentrations, AVP action includes?

Harrison's 20th Ed. Chapter 374 Page 2684

A. Smooth muscle contraction of blood vessels & GI tract
B. Glycogenolysis in liver
C. Potentiates ACTH release by corticotropin-releasing factor
D. All of the above

All the above effects are mediated by V1a or V1b receptors that are coupled to phospholipase C.

413. AVP clearance is due to degradation in?

Harrison's 20th Ed. Chapter 374 Page 2684

A. Liver
B. Kidneys
C. Placenta
D. All of the above

AVP has a half life of 10 to 30 minutes. Most AVP clearance is due to degradation in liver and kidneys. During pregnancy, metabolic clearance of AVP is increased three- to four fold due to placental production of an N-terminal peptidase.

414. Thirst osmostat is 'set' about how much higher than the AVP osmostat?

Harrison's 20th Ed. Chapter 374 Page 2684

A. 2%
B. 3%
C. 4%
D. 5%

Thirst is regulated primarily by an osmostat that is located in anteromedial hypothalamus. Thirst osmostat is 'set' ~3% higher than AVP osmostat.

Diabetes Insipidus

415. Which of the following is included in 'polyuria-polydipsia syndrome'?

Hormone research in paediatrics. 2012;77(2):69–84

A. Central DI
B. Nephrogenic DI
C. Primary polydipsia
D. All of the above

Polyuria-polydipsia disorders include central DI, nephrogenic DI and primary polydipsia. They are characterized by hypotonic polyuria. Primary polydipsia is not a true DI state, but long-standing primary polydipsia can give rise to a DI-like picture on laboratory evaluation. One or more forms of polyuria-polydipsia syndrome can co-exist in a single individual.

416. Which of the following is the hallmark of DI?

Hormone research in paediatrics. 2012;77(2):69–84

A. Normotonic polyuria
B. Hypertonic polyuria
C. Hypotonic polyuria
D. Any of the above

Hypotonic polyuria (typically over 4 liters per day) is the hallmark of DI.

417. Polyuria is defined as excretion of a urinary volume more than?

Hormone research in paediatrics. 2012;77(2):69–84

A. 150 mL/kg/24 hours at birth
B. 100-110 mL/kg/24 hours up to the age of 2 years
C. 50 mL/Kg/24 hours in older children and adults
D. All of the above

Polyuria is defined as excretion of a urinary volume >150 mL/Kg/24 hours at birth, >100–110 mL/Kg/24 hours up to the age of 2 years, and >50 mL/Kg/24 hours in older children and adults.

418. What value of urine osmolality indicates optimal plasma AVP levels and appropriate renal response to AVP?

The Journal of Clinical Endocrinology & Metabolism. 2012;97(10):3426–3437

A. > 300 mOsm/Kg
B. > 500 mOsm/Kg
C. > 800 mOsm/Kg
D. > 1000 mOsm/Kg

A urine osmolality of >800 mOsm/Kg indicates optimal plasma AVP levels and appropriate renal response to AVP, therefore ruling out any form of DI.

419. Which of the following is a type of diabetes insipidus (DI)?

Harrison's 20th Ed. Chapter 374 Page 2685

A. Central DI
B. Nephrogenic DI
C. Gestational DI
D. All of the above

DI is typically classified into 3 forms : Central DI, Nephrogenic DI and Gestational DI.

420. How much decrease in the secretion or action of AVP results in diabetes insipidus (DI)?

Harrison's 20th Ed. Chapter 374 Page 2685

A. 10%
B. 25%
C. 50%
D. 75%

A decrease of ≥75% in the secretion or action of AVP usually results in diabetes insipidus (DI).

421. In diabetes insipidus (DI), 24 hour urine volume exceeds?

Harrison's 20th Ed. Chapter 374 Page 2685

A. 20 mL/kg body weight
B. 30 mL/kg body weight
C. 40 mL/kg body weight
D. 50 mL/kg body weight

422. In diabetes insipidus (DI), urine osmolarity is?

Harrison's 20th Ed. Chapter 374 Page 2685

A. < 300 mosmol/L
B. < 310 mosmol/L
C. < 320 mosmol/L
D. < 330 mosmol/L

In diabetes insipidus (DI), 24 hour urine volume exceeds 40 mL/kg body weight, and urine osmolarity is <300 mosmol/L.

423. Which of the following clinical features of diabetes insipidus is false?

Harrison's 20th Ed. Chapter 374 Page 2685

A. Daily urine volume is >40 mL/kg body weight
B. Urine osmolarity is <300 mosmol/L
C. Dehydration is common
D. Enuresis is common

In diabetes insipidus, due to decreased secretion or action of AVP urine volume is >50 mL/kg body weight/day & urine osmolarity is <300 mosmol/L. Polyuria produces urinary frequency, enuresis, and/or nocturia, thirst & polydipsia. Clinical signs of dehydration are uncommon unless fluid intake is impaired. Patients with an attenuated thirst response have reduced urge to drink water despite rising plasma osmolality and loss of large volumes of water in the urine, resulting in 'adipsic DI', classically associated with craniopharyngioma.

424. Primary deficiency of AVP is called?

Harrison's 20th Ed. Chapter 374 Page 2685

A. Neurohypophyseal DI
B. Pituitary DI
C. Central DI
D. Any of the above

Primary deficiency of AVP secretion results from agenesis or irreversible destruction of neuro-hypophysis and is also called neurohypophyseal DI, neurogenic DI, pituitary DI, cranial DI, or central DI.

425. Which of the following is the most common cause of pituitary DI?

Harrison's 20th Ed. Chapter 374 Page 2685

A. Congenital disorders
B. Acquired disorders
C. Genetic disorders
D. Idiopathic

Pituitary DI can be caused by congenital, acquired, or genetic disorders, but it is idiopathic in ~ ½ of all adult patients.

426. Wolfram's syndrome includes?

Harrison's 20th Ed. Chapter 374 Page 2685

A. Diabetes insipidus
B. Diabetes mellitus
C. Optic atrophy
D. All of the above

Wolfram's syndrome includes diabetes insipidus, diabetes mellitus, optic atrophy, and neural deafness (DIDMOAD)]. It is an autosomal recessive disorder due to mutations of WFS 1 gene.

427. Drug that stimulate release of AVP or enhance its action is?

N Engl J Med 2007;356:2064-72

A. Carbamazepine
B. Nicotine
C. Nonsteroidal antiinflammatory drugs
D. All of the above

Drugs that stimulate release of AVP or enhance its action include Chlorpropramide, SSRIs, Tricyclic antidepressants, Clofibrate, Carbamazepine, Vincristine, Nicotine, Narcotics, Antipsychotic drugs, Ifosfamide, Cyclophosphamide, Nonsteroidal anti-inflammatory drugs, Ecstasy.

428. Pituitary diabetes insipidus can be caused by?

Harrison's 20th Ed. Chapter 374 Page 2686 Table 374-1

A. Craniopharyngioma
B. Pituitary adenoma (suprasellar)
C. Meningioma
D. All of the above

429. Pituitary diabetes insipidus can be caused by?

Harrison's 20th Ed. Chapter 374 Page 2686 Table 374-1

A. Sarcoidosis
B. Histiocytosis X
C. Xanthoma disseminatum
D. All of the above

430. Pituitary diabetes insipidus can be caused by?

Harrison's 20th Ed. Chapter 374 Page 2686 Table 374-1

A. Tetrodotoxin
B. Snake venom
C. Hypoxic encephalopathy
D. All of the above

431. Pituitary diabetes insipidus can be caused by?

Harrison's 20th Ed. Chapter 374 Page 2686 Table 374-1

A. Pituitary metastases
B. Lymphoma
C. Leukemia
D. All of the above

432. In gestational DI, offending substance that produces deficiency of AVP comes from?

Harrison's 20th Ed. Chapter 374 Page 2685

A. Placenta
B. Fetus
C. Uterus
D. All of the above

A primary deficiency of plasma AVP can also result from increased metabolism by an N-terminal aminopeptidase produced by the placenta. It is referred to as gestational DI. Gestational DI results from the enzymatic breakdown of the endogenous AVP by a placental cysteine aminopeptidase. This enzymatic degradation of plasma AVP during pregnancy can unmask sub-clinical DI in those women with borderline-low plasma AVP levels.

433. Which of the following is false about gestational diabetes insipidus?

Harrison's 20th Ed. Chapter 374 Page 2686 Table 374-1

A. Due to increased metabolism by an N-terminal aminopeptidase
B. Occurs during first trimester of pregnancy
C. Signs & symptoms remit several weeks after delivery
D. Primary deficiency of plasma AVP

434. Drugs that can produce nephrogenic diabetes insipidus include?

Harrison's 20th Ed. Chapter 374 Page 2686 Table 374-1

A. Lithium
B. Aminoglycosides
C. Rifampin
D. All of the above

Drugs that can produce nephrogenic diabetes insipidus include Lithium, Demeclocycline, Methoxyflurane, Amphotericin B, Aminoglycosides, Cisplatin, Rifampin, Foscarnet.

435. Metabolic states that can produce nephrogenic diabetes insipidus include?

Harrison's 20th Ed. Chapter 374 Page 2686 Table 374-1

A. Hypercalcemia
B. Hypercalciuria
C. Hypokalemia
D. All of the above

436. Conditions that can produce primary polydipsia include?
Harrison's 20th Ed. Chapter 374 Page 2686 Table 374-1

A. Schizophrenia
B. Obsessive compulsive disorder
C. Tuberculous meningitis
D. All of the above

437. Urine concentration ceases when secretion or action of AVP is reduced to what level of normal?
Harrison's 20th Ed. Chapter 374 Page 2685

A. 30%
B. 50%
C. 75%
D. 100%

When secretion or action of AVP is reduced to ~75% of normal, urine concentration ceases & the rate of output increases to symptomatic levels.

438. Which of the following leads to secondary deficiencies of AVP secretion?
Harrison's 20th Ed. Chapter 374 Page 2685

A. Dipsogenic DI
B. Psychogenic polydipsia
C. Iatrogenic polydipsia
D. All of the above

439. Deficiencies of AVP secretion resulting from inhibition by excessive intake of fluids is called?
Harrison's 20th Ed. Chapter 374 Page 2685

A. Primary polydipsia
B. Central DI
C. Nephrogenic DI
D. All of the above

In chronic primary polydipsia, long-standing water diuresis blunts the renal medullary concentration gradient and also causes down-regulation of the aquaporin-2 channels in the proximal tubule and the collecting duct due to suppressed endogenous AVP, thus creating a state mimicking nephrogenic DI.

440. Which of the following is a primary polydipsia?
Harrison's 20th Ed. Chapter 374 Page 2685

A. Dipsogenic DI
B. Psychogenic polydipsia
C. Iatrogenic polydipsia
D. All of the above

Secondary deficiency of AVP due to inhibition of AVP secretion by excessive intake of fluids is called primary polydipsia. Dipsogenic DI is characterized by an inappropriate increase in thirst caused by a reduction in the 'set' of osmoregulatory mechanism. Psychogenic polydipsia is not associated with thirst & polydipsia is a feature of psychosis. In iatrogenic polydipsia there is increase fluid intake on recommendations of health professionals or media.

441. Primary deficiencies in the antidiuretic action of AVP result in?
Harrison's 20th Ed. Chapter 374 Page 2685

A. Central DI
B. Nephrogenic DI
C. Primary polydipsia
D. All of the above

Primary deficiencies in the antidiuretic action of AVP result in nephrogenic DI.

442. Hypernatremia and overt physical or laboratory signs of dehydration develop in patients with?
Harrison's 20th Ed. Chapter 374 Page 2686

A. Pituitary DI
B. Gestational DI
C. Nephrogenic DI
D. None of the above

Hypernatremia and other overt physical or laboratory signs of dehydration do not develop in pituitary, gestational, or nephrogenic DI, unless the patient also has a defect in thirst or fails to increase fluid intake for some other reason.

443. Which of the following increases plasma AVP levels?
Harrison's 20th Ed. Chapter 374 Page 2686

A. Nausea
B. Smoking
C. Vasovagal reaction
D. All of the above

Nausea, smoking & vasovagal reaction increases plasma AVP to produce profound antidiuresis.

444. In primary polydipsia, the pathogenesis of polydipsia and polyuria is the reverse of that in?
Harrison's 20th Ed. Chapter 374 Page 2686

A. Pituitary DI
B. Nephrogenic DI
C. Gestational DI
D. All of the above

In primary polydipsia, the pathogenesis of the polydipsia and polyuria is the reverse of that in pituitary, nephrogenic, and gestational DI.

445. Possibility of inaccurate collection of 24 hour urine is determined by measurement of?
Harrison's 20th Ed. Chapter 374 Page 2686

A. Total urinary sodium
B. Total urinary potassium
C. Total urinary creatinine
D. Total urinary ammonium

Total urinary creatinine is 20–30 mg/kg/day for the size of the patient. A 24 hours urine creatinine ensures an appropriate sample collection.

446. Basal plasma arginine vasopressin (AVP) is normal or elevated (>1 pg/mL) in patients with?
Harrison's 20th Ed. Chapter 374 Page 2686

A. Nephrogenic DI
B. Pituitary DI
C. Primary polydipsia
D. All of the above

Basal plasma arginine vasopressin (AVP) is normal or elevated (>1 pg/mL) in nephrogenic DI.

447. Which of the following investigation is useful in differentiating between pituitary DI and primary polydipsia?
Harrison's 20th Ed. Chapter 374 Page 2687

A. Plasma AVP
B. 24-hour urine volume
C. Urine osmolarity
D. Magnetic resonance imaging (MRI) of the brain

Magnetic resonance imaging (MRI) of the brain differentiates between pituitary DI or primary polydipsia. Normal posterior pituitary bright spot is visible on T1-weighted midsagittal images. This "bright spot" is almost always present in patients with primary polydipsia but is always absent or abnormally small in patients with pituitary DI. Patients with nephrogenic DI also lack a posterior pituitary bright spot, probably because they have an abnormally high rate of AVP secretion and turnover.

448. Pituitary bright spot is almost always present in patients with?
Harrison's 20th Ed. Chapter 374 Page 2687

A. Pituitary diabetes insipidus
B. Nephrogenic diabetes insipidus
C. Primary polydipsia
D. All of the above

In MRI of pituitary & hypothalamus of healthy beings, posterior pituitary emits a hyperintense signal in T1-weighted mid-sagittal images. This "pituitary bright spot" is almost always present in patients with primary polydipsia but is invariably absent or abnormally small in patients with pituitary DI, it is small or absent in nephrogenic DI because of high secretion & turnover of vasopressin. 'Bright spot' in the posterior pituitary is a result of phospholipid-rich granules that store arginine vasopressin (AVP) and oxytocin.

449. Pituitary bright spot is absent in patients with?
Harrison's 20th Ed. Chapter 374 Page 2687

A. Pituitary diabetes insipidus
B. Nephrogenic diabetes insipidus
C. Empty sella who do not have diabetes insipidus
D. All of the above

A normal pituitary bright spot on MRI excludes pituitary DI, is against nephrogenic DI and strongly suggests primary polydipsia. It is absent not only in pituitary and nephrogenic DI but also in some normal persons and in patients with empty sella who do not have DI.

450. Which of the following is false about nephrogenic diabetes insipidus?
Harrison's 20th Ed. Chapter 374 Page 2687 Figure 374-4

A. Urinary frequency, enuresis, nocturia
B. Urine osmolarity < 300 mosmol/L
C. Urine volume > 40 mL/kg per day
D. Basal plasma arginine vasopressin (AVP) <1 pg/mL

451. Which of the following is false about pituitary diabetes insipidus?
Harrison's 20th Ed. Chapter 374 Page 2687 Figure 374-4

A. Urinary frequency, enuresis, nocturia
B. Urine osmolarity < 300 mosmol/L
C. Urine volume > 40 mL/kg per day
D. Basal plasma arginine vasopressin (AVP) > 1 pg/mL

452. Which of the following is false about primary polydipsia?
Harrison's 20th Ed. Chapter 374 Page 2687 Figure 374-4

A. Urine volume > 40 mL/kg per day
B. Basal plasma arginine vasopressin (AVP) < 1 pg/mL
C. Pituitary bright spot present
D. None of the above

453. Which of the following is false about primary polydipsia?
Harrison's 20th Ed. Chapter 374 Page 2687 Figure 374-4

A. Low normal or low serum sodium (<135 mmol/L)
B. Normal or low plasma osmolality (≤280 mOsm/Kg)
C. Low serum sodium / plasma osmolality
D. None of the above

454. Which of the following electrolyte abnormality gives rise to a clinical picture of nephrogenic DI?
The American journal of the medical sciences. 1998;316(5):291–99

A. Hyperkalemia
B. Hypokalemia
C. Hypernatremia
D. Hyponatremia

Electrolyte abnormalities including hypokalemia and hypercalcemia can give rise to polyuria due to down-regulation of aquaporin-2 channels giving rise to a clinical picture of nephrogenic DI.

455. In water deprivation test, patients of which of the following can concentrate their urine?
Harrison's 20th Ed. Chapter 374 Page 2687

A. Primary polydipsia
B. Central DI
C. Nephrogenic DI
D. All of the above

Deprivation of water intake should allow patients with primary polydipsia to concentrate their urine while those with central or nephrogenic DI continue to excrete dilute urine.

456. Desmopressin administration can distinguish between?
Harrison's 20th Ed. Chapter 374 Page 2687

A. Central DI and nephrogenic DI
B. Central DI and primary polydipsia
C. Nephrogenic DI and primary polydipsia
D. All of the above

Desmopressin administration can distinguish between central DI and nephrogenic DI. In central DI, once the deficient action of AVP is substituted with desmopressin administration, urine osmolality increases while in nephrogenic DI, desmopressin is ineffective due to lack of renal response to its actions, the low urine osmolality persists.

457. Diuresis can be induced by?
Harrison's 20th Ed. Chapter 374 Page 2687

A. Sodium
B. Urea
C. Mannitol
D. All of the above

458. The duration of overnight water deprivation (in hours) can be determined by which of the following formula?
Endocrine Practice. 2018;24(11):963–72

A. Patient's weight (Kg) × 0.02 × 1000 (mL)/urine output (mL/hour)
B. Patient's weight (Kg) × 0.03 × 1000 (mL)/urine output (mL/hour)
C. Patient's weight (Kg) × 0.04 × 1000 (mL)/urine output (mL/hour)
D. Patient's weight (Kg) × 0.05 × 1000 (mL)/urine output (mL/hour)

The goal of water deprivation test is to achieve ~3% loss of body weight. The duration of overnight water deprivation (in hours) can be determined by using the following formula: patient's weight (Kg) x 0.03 x 1000 (mL)/urine output (mL/hour).

459. The dehydration phase should be discontinued if?
Endocrine Practice. 2018;24(11):963–972

A. Loss of > 3% of body weight
B. Elevation of serum sodium to ≥ 146 – 150 mmol/L
C. Orthostatic hypotension / symptoms
D. All of the above

The dehydration phase should be discontinued if one of the following occur: loss of >3% of body weight, elevation of serum Na^+ to ≥146 – 150 mmol/L), orthostatic hypotension or orthostatic symptoms (dizziness), or intractable thirst.

460. Dose of desmopressin used to identify the type of DI is?
Endocrine Practice. 2018;24(11):963–972

A. 1 µg
B. 2 µg
C. 3 µg
D. 4 µg

An injection of 2 µg desmopressin (synthetic analogue of AVP) is administered either through intravenous or intramuscular route.

461. In normal individuals, with dehydration, the urine osmolality usually increases up to?

Williams Textbook of Endocrinology, 13th Ed 13;2015:300-332

A. 300 – 400 mOsm/Kg
B. 400 – 600 mOsm/Kg
C. 600 – 800 mOsm/Kg
D. 800 – 1200 mOsm/Kg

In normal individuals, with dehydration, the urine osmolality usually increases up to 800 – 1200 mOsm/Kg.

462. What level of increase in urine osmolality after desmopressin administration suggests complete central DI?

Williams Textbook of Endocrinology, 13th Ed 13;2015:300-332

A. At least > 20%
B. At least > 30%
C. At least > 40%
D. At least > 50%

An increase of at least >50% in urine osmolality after desmopressin administration suggests complete central DI, while a <50% increase points towards complete nephrogenic DI.

463. Plasma concentration of AVP is expressed in?

Harrison's 20th Ed. Chapter 374 Page 2687 Figure 374-3

A. mg/mL
B. μg/mL
C. pg/mL
D. ng/mL

Plasma concentration of AVP (measured in pg/mL) is one of the lowest among all hormones. Plasma copeptin measurement is a better test when compared with plasma AVP measurement.

464. Desmopressin (DDAVP) can be administered by?

Harrison's 20th Ed. Chapter 374 Page 2687

A. SC injection
B. Nasal inhalation
C. Oral tablet
D. All of the above

DDAVP is a synthetic analogue of AVP that can be given IV or SC, nasal inhalation or orally.

465. DDAVP acts selectively at?

Harrison's 20th Ed. Chapter 374 Page 2687

A. V1 receptors
B. V2 receptors
C. V3 receptors
D. V4 receptors

DDAVP acts selectively at V2 receptors to increase urine concentration and decrease urine flow in a dose-dependent manner.

466. Treating primary polydipsia with DDAVP is associated with a risk of?

Harrison's 20th Ed. Chapter 374 Page 2687

A. Hyponatremia
B. Hypernatremia
C. Hypokalemia
D. Hyperkalemia

Primary polydipsia cannot be treated safely with DDAVP because it invariably produces hyponatremia and/or other signs of water intoxication.

467. Nephrogenic DI is treated by?

Harrison's 20th Ed. Chapter 374 Page 2688

A. Thiazide diuretic
B. Indomethacin
C. Amiloride
D. All of the above

Nephrogenic DI does not respond to desmopressin but may be reduced with thiazide diuretic and/or amiloride with low-sodium diet. Inhibitors of prostaglandin synthesis (indomethacin) are effective.

468. The most common cause of an increase in total body sodium is?

Harrison's 20th Ed. Chapter 374 Page 2688

A. Severe congestive heart failure
B. SIADH
C. Primary hyperaldosteronism
D. Cirrhosis

The most common cause of an increase in total body sodium is primary hyperaldosteronism.

469. Which of the following is false about hypodipsic hypernatremia?

Harrison's 20th Ed. Chapter 374 Page 2688

A. Hypovolemia
B. Hypokalemia
C. Hyperuricemia
D. None of the above

470. Hypodipsic hypernatremia is associated with?

Harrison's 20th Ed. Chapter 374 Page 2688

A. Primary hyperaldosteronism
B. Secondary hyperaldosteronism
C. Glucocorticoid remediable hyperaldosteronism
D. Syndrome of apparent mineralocorticoid excess

Adipsic hypernatremia is a state of chronic or recurrent hypertonic dehydration due to deficiency in osmoregulation of thirst. Hypernatremia is associated with hypovolemia presenting as tachycardia, postural hypotension, azotemia, hyperuricemia & hypokalemia (secondary hyperaldosteronism). Muscle weakness, pain, rhabdomyolysis, hyperglycemia, hyperlipidemia & acute renal failure may also occur. DI is usually not present, at least at presentation.

471. Hypodipsia is usually due to hypogenesis or destruction of osmoreceptors in?

Harrison's 20th Ed. Chapter 374 Page 2688

A. Anterior hypothalamus
B. Posterior hypothalamus
C. Anterior pituitary
D. Posterior pituitary

Hypodipsia is usually due to hypogenesis or destruction of the osmoreceptors in the anterior hypothalamus that regulate thirst.

472. Hypodipsia can arise due to occlusion of?

Harrison's 20th Ed. Chapter 374 Page 2688

A. Anterior communicating artery
B. Posterior communicating artery
C. Anterior inferior cerebellar artery
D. Posterior inferior cerebellar artery

473. In hypodipsic hypernatremia, AVP secretion responds poorly or not at all to?

Harrison's 20th Ed. Chapter 374 Page 2688

A. Hyperosmotic stimulation
B. Nausea
C. Large reductions in blood volume or blood pressure
D. All of the above

In hypodipsic hypernatremia, AVP secretion responds poorly or not at all to hyperosmotic stimulation but, in most cases, increases normally to nonosmotic stimuli like nausea or large reductions in blood volume or blood pressure, indicating that the neurohypophysis is intact.

474. Which of the following is false about hypodipsic hypernatremia?

Harrison's 20th Ed. Chapter 374 Page 2688

A. Due to destruction of neurohypophysis
B. Hypernatremic
C. Hypertonic dehydration
D. Develop hyponatremia if overhydrated

Hypodipsic hypernatremia is caused by agenesis or destruction of the hypothalamic osmoreceptors that normally regulate thirst & AVP secretion.

475. The free water deficit (ΔFW) can be estimated by which of the following formula?

Harrison's 20th Ed. Chapter 374 Page 2689

A. 0.3 body weight in Kg. × ([SNa – 140] / 140)
B. 0.4 body weight in Kg. × ([SNa – 140] / 140)
C. 0.5 body weight in Kg. × ([SNa – 140] / 140)
D. 0.6 body weight in Kg. × ([SNa – 140] / 140)

476. Serum sodium concentration decreases by how much for every 100 mg/dL increase in glucose concentration?

Diabetes Care 2010 Jul; 33(7): e91-e91

A. 1.2 mEq/L
B. 1.4 mEq/L
C. 1.6 mEq/L
D. 1.8 mEq/L

The serum sodium concentration decreases by 1.6 mEq/l for every 100 mg/dL increase in glucose concentration due to water shifts from the intracellular to the extracellular compartment. Serum sodium decreases ~1 meq/L for each 36 mg/dL rise in glucose.

477. By which of the following formula, measured SNa should be corrected, if serum glucose (SGlu) is elevated?

Harrison's 20th Ed. Chapter 374 Page 2689

A. SNa + ([SGlu–90]/30)
B. SNa + ([SGlu–90]/32)
C. SNa + ([SGlu–90]/34)
D. SNa + ([SGlu–90]/36)

If serum glucose is elevated, the measured serum sodium should be corrected by the formula S_{Na} + ($[S_{Glu}$–90]/36).

478. Decrease in serum sodium of 1 meq/L reduces plasma osmolarity by about?

N Engl J Med 1973; 289: 843–844

A. 1 mosmol/L
B. 2 mosmol/L
C. 3 mosmol/L
D. 4 mosmol/L

Each decrease in serum sodium of 1 meq/L reduces plasma osmolarity by about 2 mosmol/L. When serum triglycerides are above 100 mg/dL, for every 500 mg/dL rise in serum triglycerides, fall in serum sodium will be about 1.0 mEq/L. When serum protein is above 8 gm/dL, for every 1 gm/dL rise in serum protein, fall in serum sodium will be about 4.0 mEq/L.

479. The Schwartz and Bartter clinical criterion for SIADH includes all except?

Nephron Clin Pract 2011;119:c62–c73

A. Serum sodium < 135 mEq/L
B. Serum osmolality < 275 mOsm/kg
C. Urine sodium > 40 mEq/L
D. Urine osmolality < 100 mOsm/kg

The Schwartz and Bartter Clinical Criterion for SIADH includes Serum sodium <135mEq/L, Serum osmolality <275 mOsm/kg, Urine sodium >40 mEq/L and Urine osmolality >100 mOsm/kg.

480. SIADH was first described in patients with?

N Engl J Med 2007;356:2064-72

A. Sepsis
B. Head trauma
C. Bronchogenic carcinoma
D. Schizophrenia

SIADH was first detected in bronchogenic carcinoma patients by William Schwartz and Frederic Bartter in 1967. A physiologic stimulus for release of antidiuretic hormone was lacking and the level of secretion of ADH was deemed "inappropriate". After the syndrome was described, ADH in humans was found to be arginine vasopressin.

481. Which of the following is false about patients of SIADH with "reset osmostat"?

Harrison's 20th Ed. Chapter 374 Page 2689

A. AVP secretion fully responsive to changes in plasma osmolarity
B. AVP secretion fully responsive to changes in plasma sodium
C. Threshold of osmoregulatory system is abnormally low
D. None of the above

482. Syndrome of inappropriate antidiuretic hormone (SIADH) is due to all except?

Harrison's 20th Ed. Chapter 374 Page 2689

A. Malignancy
B. Cortisol deficiency
C. Stroke
D. Pneumonia

Nonhemodynamic stimulus (nausea or cortisol deficiency) impaires urine dilution by a defect in the osmotic suppression of AVP. Term SIADH is for a primary defect in osmoregulation caused by another disorder such as malignancy, stroke, or pneumonia.

483. Which of the following about SIADH is false?

Harrison's 20th Ed. Chapter 374 Page 2689

A. Euvolemic hypotonic hyponatremia
B. Urine osmolality ≥ 100 mOsm/kg
C. Urine sodium ≥ 30 mmol/L
D. None of the above

U_{Na} < 30 mmol/L can be used to identify both hypovolemic and hypervolemic hyponatremia. U_{Na} > 30 mmol/L, FE_{Urea} > 55% and $FE_{Uric\ Acid}$ >12% had the highest sensitivity and specificity to diagnose SIAD.

484. Which of the following is low in cases of SIADH?

Harrison's 20th Ed. Chapter 374 Page 2691 Table 374-3

A. Serum potassium
B. Serum albumin
C. Serum cortisol
D. Plasma renin activity

485. Which of the following is false about nephrogenic inappropriate antidiuresis or NSIAD?

Harrison's 20th Ed. Chapter 374 Page 2689

A. Euvolemic hyponatremia
B. Hypotonic hyponatremia
C. AVP-independent activation of renal V2 receptors
D. Inappropriate antidiuresis is transient

Hereditary SIADH, also known as nephrogenic SIADH, has been ascribed to the gain of function mutation in vasopressin 2 (V2) receptors in kidneys resulting in a spontaneously active receptor and unregulated water reabsorption. NSIAD is a rare X-linked recessive genetic disease. Inappropriate antidiuresis in NSIAD patients appears to be permanent. It should be suspected if the hyponatremia occurs in a child or several members of the family or is refractory to treatment with a vaptan.

486. Water intoxication can lead to?

Harrison's 20th Ed. Chapter 374 Page 2689

A. Headache
B. Anorexia, nausea, vomiting
C. Confusion, coma, convulsions
D. All of the above

Severe hyponatremia (serum sodium <125 mmol per liter), especially when the condition develops rapidly (within 48 hours), has serious sequelae, including confusion, hallucinations, seizures, coma, decerebrate posture & respiratory arrest, leading to death. Vomiting is an ominous sign for patients with acute hyponatremia.

487. Overt signs of volume expansion or contraction are absent in?

Harrison's 20th Ed. Chapter 374 Page 2689

A. SIADH
B. SIAD
C. NSIAD
D. All of the above

Overt signs of volume expansion or contraction are absent in SIADH, SIAD, NSIAD, and other forms of euvolemic hyponatremia.

488. In primary or metastatic malignancies, ectopic AVP production results from abnormal expression of which gene?

Harrison's 20th Ed. Chapter 374 Page 2689

A. AVP-NPI
B. AVP-NPII
C. AVP-NPIII
D. AVP-NPIV

Ectopic production of AVP result from abnormal expression of AVP-NPII gene by primary or metastatic malignancies.

489. In acute symptomatic SIADH, the aim should be to raise plasma osmolarity at a rate of?

Harrison's 20th Ed. Chapter 374 Page 2690

A. ~ 1% an hour
B. ~ 2% an hour
C. ~ 3% an hour
D. ~ 4% an hour

In acute symptomatic SIADH, the aim is to raise plasma osmolarity and/or plasma sodium at a rate ~1% an hour until they reach levels of ~270 mosmol/L or 130 meq/L, respectively. Regulating fluid intake so that it under replaces urine output by 5mL/kg body weight/hour will raise serum sodium at a rate of about 1% an hour.

490. Central pontine myelinolysis or osmotic demyelination syndrome is characterized by all except?

Harrison's 20th Ed. Chapter 49 Page

A. Quadriparesis
B. Diplopia
C. Paresthesias
D. Locked-in syndrome

Central pontine myelinolysis presents 1 or more days after overcorrection of hyponatremia with paraparesis or quadriparesis, dysphagia, dysarthria, diplopia, "locked-in syndrome" and/or loss of consciousness.

491. Central pontine myelinolysis is characterized by all except?

Harrison's 20th Ed. Chapter 374 Page 2691

A. Quadriparesis
B. Sensoneural hearing loss
C. Ataxia
D. Abnormal extraocular movements

Central pontine myelinolysis is an acute, potentially fatal neurologic syndrome characterized by quadriparesis, ataxia and abnormal extraocular movements.

492. Which of the following drugs induces a reversible form of nephrogenic DI?

Harrison's 20th Ed. Chapter 374 Page 2691

A. Fludrocortisone
B. Tolvaptan
C. Demeclocycline
D. Urea

Demeclocycline induces a reversible form of nephrogenic DI in 1–2 weeks by inhibiting vasopressin action on the renal distal tubule.

493. In treatment of hyponatremia in SIADH with hypertonic saline, maximum rise in serum sodium level should not be more than?

Harrison's 20th Ed. Chapter 49 Page

A. 6 mmol/L
B. 8 mmol/L
C. 10 mmol/L
D. 12 mmol/L

494. Most common electrolyte disorder in hospitalized patients is?

N Engl J Med 2007;356:2064-72

A. Hypokalemia
B. Hyponatremia
C. Hypocalcemia
D. Hypomagnesemia

Hyponatremia, defined as an excess of water in relation to sodium in extra-cellular fluid, is the most common electrolyte disorder in hospitalized patients.

495. Which of the following is an AVP analogue?

N Engl J Med 2007;356:2064-72

A. Desmopressin
B. Oxytocin
C. Vasopressin
D. All of the above

Thyroid Gland Physiology and Testing

496. Which of the following statements is false?
Harrison's 20th Ed. Chapter 375 Page 2692

A. α and β are thyroid hormone receptors
B. Thyroxine (T4) contains four iodine atoms
C. Deiodination of T4 produces reverse T3
D. None of the above

Deiodination of T4 produces a potent hormone triiodothyronine (T3) or the inactive hormone reverse T3.

497. Word thyroid is derived from Greek word "thyreos" meaning?
Harrison's 20th Ed. Chapter 375 Page 2692

A. Cone shaped
B. Shield
C. Superficial
D. Essential

Word thyroid is derived from a Greek word thyreos meaning "shield" plus eidos meaning "form".

498. What is the normal weight of human thyroid gland?
Harrison's 20th Ed. Chapter 375 Page 2692

A. 6 to 12 grams
B. 12 to 20 grams
C. 20 to 30 grams
D. 30 to 50 grams

Normal thyroid is 12–20 grams in weight.

499. Which of the following statements about thyroid gland is false?
Harrison's 20th Ed. Chapter 375 Page 2692

A. Placed between cricoid cartilage and suprasternal notch
B. Parathyroid glands are located posterior to each pole of thyroid
C. Recurrent laryngeal nerves traverse lateral borders of thyroid
D. None of the above

500. Thyroid hormone synthesis normally begins at what time of gestation?
Harrison's 20th Ed. Chapter 375 Page 2692

A. About 6 weeks'
B. About 11 weeks'
C. About 16 weeks'
D. About 21 weeks'

The thyroid gland develops from the floor of the primitive pharynx during the third week of gestation. Thyroid hormone synthesis normally begins at about 11 weeks' gestation.

501. Which of the following statements about thyroid medullary C cells is false?
Harrison's 20th Ed. Chapter 375 Page 2692

A. Neural crest derivative
B. Produce calcitonin
C. Interspersed throughout the thyroid gland
D. None of the above

502. Density of C cells in thyroid gland is greatest at?
Harrison's 20th Ed. Chapter 375 Page 2692

A. Junction of upper two-third & lower one-thirds
B. Junction of upper one-third & lower two-thirds
C. Junction of upper & lower halves
D. At the poles

Density of C cells in thyroid gland is greatest at the junction of upper one-third & lower two-thirds. Thyroid medullary C cells are neural crest derivatives & produce a calcium-lowering hormone - calcitonin.

503. Which of the following is thyroid gland developmental transcription factor?
Harrison's 20th Ed. Chapter 375 Page 2692

A. TTF-1 (NKX2A)
B. TTF-2 (FKHL15)
C. Paired homeobox-8 (PAX-8)
D. All of the above

Thyroid gland development is orchestrated by coordinated expression of developmental transcription factors like Thyroid transcription factor (TTF) 1, TTF-2, NKX2-1 & paired homeobox-8 (PAX-8).

504. Thyroid gland developmental transcription factors dictate induction of which of the following thyroid-specific genes?
Harrison's 20th Ed. Chapter 375 Page 2692

A. Thyroglobulin (Tg)
B. Thyroid peroxidase (TPO)
C. Thyroid-stimulating hormone receptor (TSH-R)
D. All of the above

Thyroid gland developmental transcription factors dictate thyroid cell development and induction of thyroid-specific genes such as thyroglobulin (Tg), thyroid peroxidase (TPO), the sodium iodide symporter (Na^+/I^-, NIS), and the thyroid-stimulating hormone receptor (TSH-R).

505. What is the prevalence of congenital hypothyroidism in newborns?
Harrison's 20th Ed. Chapter 375 Page 2692

A. 1 in 4000
B. 1 in 8000
C. 1 in 16000
D. 1 in 20000

Congenital hypothyroidism occurs in ~1 in 4000 newborns. It may be transient if mother has TSH-R blocking antibodies or has received antithyroid drugs. But, permanent hypothyroidism occurs in the majority. Transplacental passage of maternal thyroid hormone occurs before the fetal thyroid gland begins to function.

506. Which of the following surface of thyroid follicular cells is in contact with bloodstream?
Harrison's 20th Ed. Chapter 375 Page 2692

A. Apical
B. Basolateral
C. Basal
D. Lateral

Basolateral surface of thyroid follicular cells is apposed to bloodstream and apical surface faces the follicular lumen.

507. Which of the following is the protein precursor of thyroid hormones?

Harrison's 20th Ed. Chapter 375 Page 2692

A. TRH
B. TSH
C. Thyroglobulin
D. All of the above

508. Which of the following is false about "secreted" colloid?

Harrison's 20th Ed. Chapter 375 Page 2692

A. Surrounded by thyroid follicular cells
B. Proteinaceous fluid
C. Contains large amounts of thyroglobulin
D. None of the above

509. Which of the following occurs when TSH binds to its receptor on basolateral surface of follicular cells?

Harrison's 20th Ed. Chapter 375 Page 2692

A. Thyroglobulin reabsorbed into thyroid follicular cells
B. Proteolysis within cytoplasm of thyroid follicular cells
C. Secretion of thyroid hormones into bloodstream
D. All of the above

510. Which of the following statements is false?

Harrison's 20th Ed. Chapter 375 Page 2692

A. T4 & T3 inhibit hypothalamic production of TRH
B. T4 & T3 inhibit pituitary production of TSH
C. TRH stimulates thyroid gland production of T4 & T3
D. TSH stimulates thyroid gland production of T4 & T3

511. TSH is secreted by the thyrotrope cells of?

Harrison's 20th Ed. Chapter 375 Page 2692

A. Anterior pituitary
B. Posterior pituitary
C. Stalk of pituitary
D. All of the above

TSH is secreted by the thyrotrope cells of the anterior pituitary gland.

512. TSH secreting thyrotrope cells constitute what percentage of anterior pituitary cell population?

Harrison's 20th Ed. Chapter 371 Page 2663

A. 1%
B. 3%
C. 5%
D. 7%

TSH secreting thyrotrope cells constitute 5% of the anterior pituitary cell population.

513. Most useful physiologic marker of thyroid hormone action is?

Harrison's 20th Ed. Chapter 375 Page 2692

A. T3
B. T4
C. TSH
D. All of the above

TSH is the most useful physiologic marker of thyroid hormone action.

514. The size of thyroid-stimulating hormone (TSH) is?

Harrison's 20th Ed. Chapter 375 Page 2692

A. 11-kDa
B. 21-kDa
C. 31-kDa
D. 41-kDa

515. The α subunit of thyroid-stimulating hormone (TSH) is common to which of the following hormones?

Harrison's 20th Ed. Chapter 375 Page 2692

A. Luteinizing hormone
B. Follicle-stimulating hormone
C. Human chorionic gonadotropin (hCG)
D. All of the above

516. The β subunit of thyroid-stimulating hormone is common to which of the following hormones?

Harrison's 20th Ed. Chapter 375 Page 2692

A. Luteinizing hormone
B. Follicle-stimulating hormone
C. Human chorionic gonadotropin (hCG)
D. None of the above

TSH is a 31-kDa hormone composed of α & β subunits. α subunit is common to other glycoprotein hormones like luteinizing hormone, follicle-stimulating hormone, human chorionic gonadotropin (hCG), whereas TSH β subunit is unique to TSH.

517. Thyroid hormones act via which of the following to inhibit TRH & TSH production?

Harrison's 20th Ed. Chapter 375 Page 2692

A. TRβ1
B. TRβ2
C. TRβ3
D. TRβ4

Thyroid hormones act via negative feedback through thyroid hormone receptor β2 (TRβ2) to inhibit TRH and TSH production.

518. The "set-point" in thyroid axis (endocrine feedback loop) is established by?

Harrison's 20th Ed. Chapter 375 Page 2692

A. TRH
B. TSH
C. T3
D. T4

The "set-point" in thyroid axis is established by TSH.

519. Which of the following is the major positive regulator of TSH synthesis & secretion?

Harrison's 20th Ed. Chapter 375 Page 2693

A. T3
B. T4
C. TRH
D. All of the above

TRH is the major positive regulator of TSH synthesis and secretion.

520. On administration of exogenous TRH, after what time does peak TSH secretion occur?

Harrison's 20th Ed. Chapter 375 Page 2693

A. About 5 minutes
B. About 10 minutes
C. About 15 minutes
D. About 20 minutes

Peak TSH secretion occurs ~15 minutes after administration of exogenous TRH.

521. Which of the following suppress TSH?

Harrison's 20th Ed. Chapter 375 Page 2693

A. Dopamine
B. Glucocorticoids
C. Somatostatin
D. All of the above

Dopamine, glucocorticoids, and somatostatin, when administered in pharmacologic doses, suppress TSH.

522. Which of the following about TSH secretion is false?

Harrison's 20th Ed. Chapter 375 Page 2693

A. Released in pulsatile manner
B. Exhibits diurnal rhythm
C. Highest levels occur at night
D. None of the above

TSH is released in a pulsatile manner & exhibits diurnal rhythm with highest levels occurring at night.

523. Plasma half-life of TSH is?

Harrison's 20th Ed. Chapter 375 Page 2693

A. 10 minutes
B. 30 minutes
C. 50 minutes
D. 80 minutes

TSH has a relatively long plasma half-life of 50 minutes.

524. Single measurement of TSH is adequate for assessing its circulating level because of?

Harrison's 20th Ed. Chapter 375 Page 2693

A. No diurnal variation
B. Relatively long plasma half-life
C. Non pulsatile release
D. Low protein binding

Single measurements of TSH are adequate for assessing its circulating level due to its relatively long plasma half-life.

525. Which of the following is related to thyroid hormone synthesis?

Harrison's 20th Ed. Chapter 375 Page 2693

A. Iodination
B. Tyrosine residues
C. Ether linkage
D. All of the above

Thyroglobulin is a glycoprotein synthesized within endoplasmic reticulum (ER) of thyroid follicular cells. It forms exocytotic vesicles that migrate into colloid via the apical membrane. The tyrosine residues on thyroglobulin are used as substrates for the synthesis of thyroid hormone. The generation of iodothyronine residue involves the formation of an ether bond between the iodophenol part of a donor tyrosyl and the hydroxyl group of the acceptor tyrosyl.

526. Which of the following is the first step in thyroid hormone synthesis?

Ann Pediatr Endocrinol Metab 2018;23:169-75

A. Thyroid iodide transport
B. Thyroglobulin synthesis
C. Oxidation and organification
D. H_2O_2 generation

527. Which of the following statements is false?

Harrison's 20th Ed. Chapter 375 Page 2693

A. Iodide in colloid undergoes oxidation to iodine
B. Oxidation of iodide is catalyzed by thyroid peroxidase (TPO) and hydrogen peroxide (H_2O_2)
C. Iodine is covalently bound (organified) to tyrosine residues in Tg to form MIT and DIT
D. None of the above

Iodide that has been transported to colloid undergoes oxidation to iodine, which is then covalently bound (organified) to the tyrosine residues in thyroglobulin to form monoiodotyrosine (MIT) and diiodotyrosine (DIT). The oxidation of iodide is catalyzed by thyroid peroxidase (TPO), and hydrogen peroxide (H_2O_2).

528. Which of the following statements about coupling of iodotyrosyl residues of thyroglobulin is false?

Harrison's 20th Ed. Chapter 375 Page 2693

A. In thyroglobulin molecules, T4 forms when two DITs combine
B. T3 forms when one MIT combines with one DIT
C. These reactions are catalyzed by TPO
D. None of the above

529. Which of the following statements about recycling of iodide is false?

Ann Pediatr Endocrinol Metab 2018;23:169-75

A. DIT & MIT are converted to free iodide & tyrosine by iodotyrosine deiodinase (IYD)
B. Iodotyrosine deiodinase (IYD) is also known as iodotyrosine dehalogenase 1 (DEHAL1)
C. Free iodide & tyrosine are utilized inside of follicular cells
D. None of the above

DIT & MIT released following the hydrolysis of thyroglobulin are converted into free iodide and tyrosine by iodotyrosine deiodinase (IYD) (also known as iodotyrosine dehalogenase 1 (DEHAL1)), and the free iodide and tyrosine are then utilized inside of follicular cells.

530. Which of the following statements about iodotyrosine deiodinase (IYD) is false?

Ann Pediatr Endocrinol Metab 2018;23:169-175

A. Transmembrane protein
B. Located in the apical membrane of thyroid follicular cells
C. Releases free iodide from MIT and DIT
D. None of the above

IYD is a transmembrane protein located in the apical membrane of thyroid follicular cells, and releases free iodide from MIT and DIT, allowing it to be used again in thyroid hormone synthesis.

531. T4 & T3 are formed from thyroglobulin by what mechanism?

Harrison's 20th Ed. Chapter 375 Page 2693

A. Coupling
B. Proteolysis
C. Iodination
D. All of the above

Thyroid hormones are derived from a large iodinated glycoprotein thyroglobulin (Tg). After secretion into thyroid follicle, Tg is iodinated on tyrosine residues that are subsequently coupled via an ether linkage. Reuptake of Tg into thyroid follicular cell allows "proteolysis" & release of newly synthesized T4 & T3.

532. Which of the following about ingested iodine is false?
Harrison's 20th Ed. Chapter 375 Page 2693

A. Bound to albumin
B. Unbound iodine excreted in urine
C. Iodide uptake is mediated by Na+/I- symporter (NIS)
D. None of the above

Ingested iodine is bound to serum albumin. Unbound iodine is excreted in urine. Thyroid gland extracts iodine from circulation mediated by the Na^+/I^- symporter (NIS) which is expressed at the basolateral membrane of thyroid follicular cells.

533. Sodium iodide symporter (NIS; SLC5A5) in basolateral membrane actively transports which of the following?
Ann Pediatr Endocrinol Metab 2018;23:169-75

A. Iodide
B. Perchlorate
C. Pertechnetate
D. All of the above

Iodide accumulates in thyroid follicular cells via sodium iodide symporter (NIS; SLC5A5), an intrinsic transmembrane protein, in the basolateral membrane of thyroid follicular cells, together with sodium. Perchlorate & pertechnetate are also transported to thyroid gland by NIS act as competitive inhibitors of iodide transport. Inside thyroid follicular cells, iodide rapidly diffuses to the apical membrane, where it is transported into colloid by pendrin (PDS; SLC26A4) channels.

534. What proportion of radioactive iodine (^{123}I) is taken up by normal thyroid gland over 24 hours in an iodine-replete state?
Harrison's 20th Ed. Chapter 375 Page 2693

A. 10–25%
B. 25–40%
C. 40–60%
D. 60–75%

10–25% of radioactive iodine (^{123}I) is taken up by normal thyroid gland over 24 hours in an iodine-replete state. This value rises to 70–90% in Graves' disease.

535. Na^+/I^- symporter (NIS) is expressed in all of the following tissues except?
Harrison's 20th Ed. Chapter 375 Page 2693

A. Thyroid gland
B. Salivary glands
C. Placenta
D. Testicles

NIS is highly expressed in thyroid gland, but low levels are present in the salivary glands, lactating breast & placenta.

536. Iodine transporter-pendrin is located on which surface of thyroid cells?
Harrison's 20th Ed. Chapter 375 Page 2693

A. Apical
B. Basolateral
C. Basal
D. Lateral

537. Pendrin, a multifunctional anion exchanger expressed in?
Ann Pediatr Endocrinol Metab 2018;23:169-75

A. Thyroid
B. Inner ear
C. Kidney
D. All of the above

538. Pendrin is encoded by which of the following gene?
Ann Pediatr Endocrinol Metab 2018;23:169-75

A. SLC26A1
B. SLC26A2
C. SLC26A3
D. SLC26A4

Pendrin is a multifunctional anion exchanger expressed in the thyroid, inner ear, and kidney. In thyroid, pendrin is located in the apical membrane of follicular cells and is thought to mediate apical iodide transport. Pendrin is encoded by the SLC26A4 gene.

539. Which of the following is false about 'Pendred syndrome'?
Harrison's 20th Ed. Chapter 375 Page 2693

A. Due to deficiency of iodine transporter - pendrin
B. Due to mutation of PENDRIN gene
C. Characterized by goiter & sensorineural deafness
D. None of the above

Iodine transporter - pendrin mediates iodine efflux into the lumen. Mutation of PENDRIN gene causes Pendred syndrome characterized by defective organification of iodine, goiter & sensorineural deafness. It is the most common cause of syndromic deafness.

540. Which of the following is false about thyroid peroxidase (TPO)?
Ann Pediatr Endocrinol Metab 2018;23:169-75

A. A membrane-bound heme protein
B. Located in the apical membrane of thyroid follicular cells
C. Involved in coupling & tyrosyl iodination of thyroglobulin
D. None of the above

541. Mutations in TPO produce hypothyroidism characterized by?
Ann Pediatr Endocrinol Metab 2018;23:169-75

A. High radioiodine uptake in scintigraphy
B. Elevated serum thyroglobulin
C. Positive perchlorate discharge test
D. All of the above

542. Iodine-deficiency data of WHO is based on?
Harrison's 20th Ed. Chapter 375 Page 2693

A. Urinary excretion of iodine
B. Anthropometry
C. Serum levels of thyroid hormones
D. Symptoms & signs

Based on urinary excretion data, WHO estimates that ~ 2 billion people are iodine-deficient.

543. Concomitant deficiency of which element contributes to neurologic manifestations of cretinism?
Harrison's 20th Ed. Chapter 375 Page 2693

A. Manganese
B. Cobalt
C. Selenium
D. Copper

Concomitant selenium deficiency contributes to the neurologic manifestations of cretinism.

544. For adults, recommended average daily intake of iodine is?
Harrison's 20th Ed. Chapter 375 Page 2693

A. 100 μg/day
B. 150 μg/day
C. 200 μg/day
D. 250 μg/day

545. For pregnant women, recommended average daily intake of iodine is?

Harrison's 20th Ed. Chapter 375 Page 2693

A. 100 μg/day
B. 150 μg/day
C. 220 μg/day
D. 300 μg/day

546. For breast feeding women, recommended average daily intake of iodine is?

Harrison's 20th Ed. Chapter 375 Page 2693

A. 100 μg/day
B. 150 μg/day
C. 220 μg/day
D. 290 μg/day

RDA is 220 μg iodine per day for pregnant women and 290 μg iodine per day for breast feeding women.

547. In iodine-sufficient populations, urinary iodine level is?

Harrison's 20th Ed. Chapter 375 Page 2693

A. > 2 μg/dL
B. > 5 μg/dL
C. > 8 μg/dL
D. > 10 μg/dL

Urinary iodine is >10 μg/dL in iodine-sufficient populations.

548. Oversupply of iodine is associated with an increased incidence of?

Harrison's 20th Ed. Chapter 375 Page 2693

A. Autoimmune thyroid disease
B. Thyroid malignancy
C. Hypothyroidism
D. Any of the above

Oversupply of iodine is associated with an increased incidence of autoimmune thyroid disease.

549. Which of the following is false about thyroglobulin (Tg)?

Harrison's 20th Ed. Chapter 375 Page 2694

A. 660 kDa size
B. Dimeric protein
C. Consists of 2769 amino acids
D. None of the above

Thyroglobulin (Tg) is a large (660 kDa) dimeric protein that consists of 2769 amino acids.

550. Organification defect is due to defect in which gene protein?

Harrison's 20th Ed. Chapter 375 Page 2694

A. PROP-1
B. PIT- 1
C. PAX-8
D. DUOX

After iodide enters the thyroid, it is trapped and transported to the apical membrane of thyroid follicular cells, where it is oxidized in an organification reaction that involves TPO and hydrogen peroxide produced by dual oxidase (DUOX) and DUOX maturation factor (DUOXA).

551. Dual oxidases (DUOX1 and DUOX2) play a crucial role in the generation of?

J Clin Endocrinol Metab. 2011;96(5):E841-5

A. Hydrogen peroxide
B. Iodine
C. Iodide
D. All of the above

Dual oxidases (DUOX1 & DUOX2) are NADPH oxidases. They play a crucial role in the generation of hydrogen peroxide required in the oxidation of iodide and the synthesis of thyroid hormone or thyroid hormonogenesis. Heterodimerization with specific maturation factors (DUOXA1 & DUOXA2) is essential for the maturation and function of the DUOX enzyme complexes.

552. Thyroid dysgenesis is due to defect in which gene protein?

Harrison's 20th Ed. Chapter 376 Page 2699 Table 376-2

A. PROP-1
B. PIT- 1
C. PAX-8
D. DUOX2

553. Thyroid dysgenesis is due to defect in which gene protein?

Harrison's 20th Ed. Chapter 376 Page 2699 Table 376-2

A. PAX-8
B. NKX2-1
C. NKX2-5
D. All of the above

554. Loss of iodide reutilization is due to defect in which gene protein?

Harrison's 20th Ed. Chapter 376 Page 2699 Table 376-2

A. PROP-1
B. PIT- 1
C. Pendrin
D. Dehalogenase 1

555. Thyroglobulin is processed to T4 & T3 in which structure of thyroid cell?

Harrison's 20th Ed. Chapter 375 Page 2694

A. Mitochondria
B. Golgi apparatus
C. Lysosome
D. All of the above

After coupling, Tg is taken back into thyroid cell, where it is processed in "lysosomes" to release T4 & T3.

556. Congenital hypothyroidism is mostly due to mutations in?

Harrison's 20th Ed. Chapter 375 Page 2694

A. TPO
B. NIS
C. Dehalogenase
D. Pendrin

Majority of congenital hypothyroidism are due to recessive mutations in TPO or Tg. Defects have also been identified in TSH-R, NIS, pendrin, hydrogen peroxide generation, and dehalogenase.

557. Factors that influence thyroid hormone synthesis & release include all except?

Harrison's 20th Ed. Chapter 375 Page 2694

A. Insulin-like growth factor I (IGF-I)
B. Prolactin
C. Epidermal growth factor
D. Transforming growth factor β (TGF-β)

TSH is the dominant hormonal regulator of thyroid gland growth & function, but growth factors produced locally in thyroid gland also influence thyroid hormone synthesis which include insulin-like growth factor I (IGF-I), epidermal growth factor, transforming growth factor (TGF-β) & endothelins.

558. Wolff-Chaikoff effect is related to?

Harrison's 20th Ed. Chapter 375 Page 2694

A. Iodine deficiency
B. Excess iodide
C. Developmental abnormality of thyroid
D. All of the above

Excess iodide transiently inhibits thyroid iodide organification (apparently by inhibiting H_2O_2 generation), a phenomenon known as the Wolff-Chaikoff effect. Normal thyroid gland escapes from this inhibitory effect & iodide organification resumes. In patients with underlying autoimmune thyroid disease, suppressive action of high iodide may persist.

559. Which of the following factors alter thyroid function in pregnancy?

Harrison's 20th Ed. Chapter 375 Page 2694

A. Increase in hCG with reciprocal fall in TSH
B. Estrogen-induced rise in TBG
C. Increased thyroid hormone metabolism by the placenta
D. All of the above

Five factors alter thyroid function in pregnancy. They are transient increase in hCG during the first trimester, which weakly stimulates TSH-R, estrogen-induced rise in TBG during first trimester, which is sustained during pregnancy, alterations in immune system, leading to the onset, exacerbation, or amelioration of an underlying autoimmune thyroid disease, increased thyroid hormone metabolism by placenta and increased urinary iodide excretion.

560. Which of the following statements is false?

Harrison's 20th Ed. Chapter 375 Page 2694

A. TSH ↓ during 1st trimester & then ↑ as gestation progresses
B. Total T4 & T3 levels are ~1.5 times higher in pregnancy
C. Free T4 progressively decreases in pregnancy
D. None of the above

The rise in circulating hCG levels during the first trimester is accompanied by a reciprocal fall in TSH that persists into the middle of pregnancy. This reflects the weak binding of hCG, which is present at very high levels, to the TSH-R. Rare individuals have variant TSH-R sequences that enhance hCG binding and TSH-R activation. hCG-induced changes in thyroid function can result in transient gestational hyperthyroidism that may be associated with hyperemesis gravidarum, a condition characterized by severe nausea and vomiting and risk of volume depletion. However, since the hyperthyroidism is not causal, antithyroid drugs are not indicated unless concomitant Graves' disease is suspected. Parenteral fluid replacement usually suffices until the condition resolves. Normative values for most thyroid function tests differ during pregnancy and, if available, trimester specific reference ranges should be used when diagnosing thyroid dysfunction during pregnancy.

561. Targeted TSH testing for hypothyroidism is recommended for women planning a pregnancy if they have?

Harrison's 20th Ed. Chapter 375 Page 2695

A. A strong family history of autoimmune thyroid disease
B. Are older than 30 years
C. Infertility, prior preterm delivery or recurrent miscarriage
D. All of the above

562. Thyroid hormone requirements are increased by how much in pregnancy in levothyroxine-treated hypothyroid women?

Harrison's 20th Ed. Chapter 375 Page 2695

A. Up to 25%
B. Up to 45%
C. Up to 65%
D. Up to 75%

Thyroid hormone requirements are increased by up to 45% during pregnancy in levothyroxine-treated hypothyroid women.

563. T3 & T4 hormones circulate bound to which plasma protein?

Harrison's 20th Ed. Chapter 375 Page 2695

A. Thyroxine-binding globulin (TBG)
B. Transthyretin (TTR)
C. Albumin
D. All of the above

T4 & T3 are bound to plasma proteins which include thyroxine-binding globulin (TBG), transthyretin (TTR, formerly known as thyroxine-binding prealbumin, or TBPA) and albumin.

564. Function of serum-binding proteins is?

Harrison's 20th Ed. Chapter 375 Page 2695

A. To increase pool of circulating hormone
B. To delay hormone clearance
C. To modulate hormone delivery
D. All of the above

Plasma-binding proteins increase the pool of circulating hormone, delay hormone clearance, and may modulate hormone delivery to selected tissue sites.

565. Which of the following serum-binding proteins carries most of the thyroid bound hormones?

Harrison's 20th Ed. Chapter 375 Page 2695

A. Thyroxine-binding globulin (TBG)
B. Transthyretin (TTR)
C. Albumin
D. All of the above

TBG carries ~80% of the bound hormones because of its high affinity for thyroid hormones, despite of the fact that its concentration is relatively low (1-2 mg/dL). Albumin has relatively low affinity for thyroid hormones but has a high plasma concentration (~3.5 g/dL), and it binds up to 10% of T4 and 30% of T3. TTR carries about 10% of T4 but little T3. A minor proportion of the THs is bound on serum lipoproteins. Immunoglobulins also may bind thyroid hormones. Only 0.3% or less of T3 & T4 circulates unbound, it is this free hormone fraction that is metabolically active at the tissue and cellular level.

566. Which of the following about thyroxine-binding globulin (TBG) is false?

AACE Clinical Case Rep. 2017;3:e134-e139

A. Synthesized in the liver
B. Member of serine protease inhibitor (SERPIN) superfamily
C. Has a serum half-life of 5 days
D. None of the above

567. Which of the following belong to the serine protease inhibitor (SERPIN) superfamily?

AACE Clinical Case Rep. 2017;3:e134-e139, Genome Biol. 2006; 7(5): 216

A. Cortisol-binding globulin (CBG)
B. Antithrombin
C. Angiotensinogen
D. All of the above

The serine protease inhibitor (SERPIN) superfamily includes thyroxine-binding globulin (SERPINA7), cortisol-binding globulin (SERPINA6), antithrombin (SERPINC1), angiotensinogen (SERPINA8), antitrypsin (SERPINA1), plasminogen activator inhibitor I (SERPINE1).

568. Serum T4 has a plasma half-life of?

Harrison's 20th Ed. Chapter 375 Page 2695 Table 375-1

A. 1 day
B. 3 days
C. 7 days
D. 10 days

569. Serum T3 has a plasma half-life of about?

Harrison's 20th Ed. Chapter 375 Page 2695 Table 375-1

A. 2 days
B. 5 days
C. 7 days
D. 10 days

570. What fraction of circulating T3 comes directly from thyroid gland?

Harrison's 20th Ed. Chapter 375 Page 2695 Table 375-1

A. 10%
B. 20%
C. 30%
D. 40%

571. What fraction of circulating T4 comes directly from thyroid gland?

Harrison's 20th Ed. Chapter 375 Page 2695 Table 375-1

A. 25%
B. 50%
C. 75%
D. 100%

572. Normally, secretion ratio from thyroid gland of T3 & T4 is?

Harrison's 20th Ed. Chapter 375 Page 2695

A. 1 : 10
B. 1 : 20
C. 1 : 30
D. 1 : 40

573. In normal serum, what percentage of TBG is usually saturated with T4?

AACE Clinical Case Rep. 2017;3:e134-e139

A. 25%
B. 50%
C. 75%
D. 100%

In normal serum, TBG usually is only 25% saturated with T4.

574. Which of the following receptors mediate thyroglobulin (Tg) endocytosis by thyroid cells?

Harrison's 20th Ed. Chapter 370 Page 2655

A. Cubilin
B. Clathrin
C. Megalin
D. Adaptin

Megalin is a transmembrane glycoprotein that mediates endocytosis of Tg by thyroid cells resulting in its transcytosis, thereby avoiding the lysosomal pathway, where proteolytic cleavage of Tg results in hormone release. Transcytosis of Tg endocytosed from the colloid is thought to be one of the mechanisms that account for the presence of intact Tg in the circulation, where the levels have been shown to be increased under conditions with heightened TSH stimulation.

575. Megalin is also known as?

Endocrinology. 1998;139(3):1462-5

A. gp280
B. gp310
C. gp330
D. gp360

Megalin (gp330) is a large glycoprotein receptor found mainly on a group of absorptive epithelial cells, including renal proximal tubule, epididymal and thyroid cells.

576. Megalin belongs to which of the following?

Harrison's 20th Ed. Chapter 370 Page 2655

A. LDL-receptor family
B. Toll-like receptor family
C. EGF receptor family
D. Secretin receptor family

Megalin belongs to the LDL-receptor family, sharing common features with LDL receptor, LDL-receptor-related protein (LRP), very-low-density lipoprotein (VLDL) receptor, and the apolipoprotein E (apo E) receptor-2. Megalin serves as an endocytotic receptor for carrier bound vitamins A and D and SHBG-bound androgens and estrogens. After internalization, the carrier proteins are degraded in lysosomes and release their bound ligands within the cells. Membrane transporters have also been identified for thyroid hormones.

577. Homeostatic mechanisms regulating thyroid axis are directed toward maintenance of normal concentrations of?

Harrison's 20th Ed. Chapter 375 Page 2695

A. Unbound T3 and T4
B. Protein bound T3 and T4
C. TSH
D. TRH

Homeostatic mechanisms that regulate the thyroid axis are directed toward maintenance of normal concentrations of unbound hormones.

578. In X-linked Thyroxine-binding globulin (TBG) deficiency, patients are?

Harrison's 20th Ed. Chapter 375 Page 2695

A. Hypothyroid
B. Hyperthyroid
C. Euthyroid
D. Any of the above

X-linked TBG deficiency is associated with very low levels of total T4 and T3. However, because unbound hormone levels are normal, patients are euthyroid and TSH levels are normal. Efforts to normalize total T4 levels should be avoided, as it may lead to thyrotoxicosis.

579. A deficiency in thyroid hormone (TH) binding proteins is suspected when?

Harrison's 20th Ed. Chapter 375 Page 2695

A. Abnormally low serum total TH concentrations
B. Clinically euthyroid subject
C. Normal serum thyroid-stimulating hormone (TSH)
D. All of the above

A deficiency in TH-binding proteins is suspected when abnormally low serum total TH concentrations are encountered in clinically euthyroid subjects in the presence of normal serum thyroid-stimulating hormone (TSH). More specifically, low TBG is suggested because this protein carries the majority of the serum TH.

580. Thyroid function tests (TFTs) in patients with TBG deficiency show?

Harrison's 20th Ed. Chapter 375 Page 2695

A. Normal TSH
B. Normal free T4
C. Low total T4
D. All of the above

Thyroid function tests (TFTs) in patients with TBG deficiency show normal TSH and free T4, but low total T4 and, occasionally, low total T3 serum concentrations. The most important clinical aspect of TBG deficiency states is recognition of these disorders and avoidance of unnecessary and potentially harmful TH replacement therapy.

581. Acquired causes of TBG deficiency include?

N Engl J Med 2014; 370:533-42

A. Hyperthyroidism
B. Nephrotic syndrome
C. Chronic renal failure
D. All of the above

Acquired causes of TBG deficiency include hyperthyroidism, nephrotic syndrome, chronic renal failure, chronic liver disease, severe systemic illness (but not in HIV/AIDS or acute intermittent porphyria), malnutrition, acromegaly, Cushing syndrome and drugs (androgens, glucocorticoids, L-asparaginase).

582. Acquired TBG excess occurs due to all except?

Harrison's 20th Ed. Chapter 375 Page 2695 Table 375-2

A. Pregnancy
B. CHF
C. Cirrhosis
D. Estrogen treatment

Acquired TBG excess is seen with estrogen, pregnancy, cirrhosis & hepatitis.

583. Which of the following causes inherited TBG deficiency?

N Engl J Med 2014; 370:533-42

A. Ortiga syndrome
B. Jaeken syndrome
C. Stoupa syndrome
D. Zimmermann syndrome

Inherited TBG deficiency also has been described in congenital disorder of glycosylation type 1 (CDG1), or Jaeken syndrome. CDG1 is caused by mutations in phosphomannomutase 2. CDG1 gene locus is located on chromosomal band 16p13 in humans.

584. Which of the following statements about familial dysalbuminemic hyperthyroxinemia (FDH) is false?

Harrison's 20th Ed. Chapter 375 Page 2695

A. Due to mutations in albumin
B. Autosomal dominant transmission
C. Increased total T4 &/or T3, but free hormone levels are normal
D. TSH levels are decreased

Mutations in TBG, TTR, and albumin may increase the binding affinity for T4 and/or T3 and cause disorders known as euthyroid hyperthyroxinemia or familial dysalbuminemic hyperthyroxinemia (FDH). Total T4 and/or T3 are increased but unbound hormone levels are normal. Familial nature with normal TSH levels suggest this diagnosis. Unbound hormone levels (ideally measured by dialysis) are normal in FDH.

585. Which of the following is associated with euthyroid hyperthyroxinemia?

Harrison's 20th Ed. Chapter 375 Page 2695 Table 375-2

A. Propranolol
B. Iopanoic acid
C. Amiodarone
D. All of the above

586. Which of the following is associated with euthyroid hyperthyroxinemia?

Harrison's 20th Ed. Chapter 375 Page 2695 Table 375-2

A. TBG excess
B. Transthyretin excess
C. Resistance to thyroid hormone (RTH)
D. All of the above

587. Which of the following about deiodinases is false?

Harrison's 20th Ed. Chapter 375 Page 2695

A. T4 is converted to T3 by deiodinase enzymes
B. Type I deiodinase is located in thyroid, liver & kidney
C. Type I deiodinase has a relatively low affinity for T4
D. None of the above

T4 is converted to T3 by deiodinase enzymes. Type I deiodinase, which is located primarily in thyroid, liver, and kidney, has a relatively low affinity for T4.

588. Which of the following about deiodinases is false?

Harrison's 20th Ed. Chapter 375 Page 2695

A. Type II deiodinase found in pituitary, brown fat, brain & thyroid
B. Type II deiodinase has higher affinity for T4
C. Type III deiodinase inactivates T4 & T3
D. None of the above

Type II deiodinase has a higher affinity for T4 and is found primarily in the pituitary gland, brain, brown fat, and thyroid gland. Expression of type II deiodinase allows it to regulate T3 concentrations locally. Type III deiodinase inactivates T4 and T3.

589. Type I deiodinase is located in all except?

Harrison's 20th Ed. Chapter 375 Page 2695

A. Thyroid
B. Liver
C. Prostate
D. Kidney

Type I deiodinase is located primarily in thyroid, liver, and kidney.

590. Which of the following deiodinases is the most important source of reverse T3 (rT3)?

Harrison's 20th Ed. Chapter 375 Page 2696

A. Type I deiodinase
B. Type II deiodinase
C. Type III deiodinase
D. All of the above

Type III deiodinase inactivates T4 and T3 and is the most important source of reverse T3 (rT3). Massive hemangiomas that express type III deiodinase are a rare cause of hypothyroidism in infants.

591. T4 to T3 conversion may be impaired by?
Harrison's 20th Ed. Chapter 375 Page 2696

A. Fasting
B. Systemic illness
C. Acute trauma
D. All of the above

592. T4 to T3 conversion may be impaired by?
Harrison's 20th Ed. Chapter 375 Page 2696

A. Oral contrast agents
B. Amiodarone
C. Glucocorticoids
D. All of the above

T4 to T3 conversion is impaired by fasting, systemic illness or acute trauma, oral contrast agents, and medications like propylthiouracil, propranolol, amiodarone, glucocorticoids.

593. Which of the following is a thyroid hormone (TH) transporter?
Harrison's 20th Ed. Chapter 375 Page 2696

A. MCT2
B. MCT4
C. MCT6
D. MCT8

Circulating thyroid hormones enter cells by passive diffusion and via the monocarboxylate 8 (MCT8) transporter. Mutations in MCT8 cause neurologic deficits & thyroid function abnormalities (low T4, high T3, and high TSH).

594. Which of the following is a thyroid hormone (TH) transporter?
Harrison's 20th Ed. Chapter 375 Page 2696

A. Monocarboxylate 8 transporter (MCT8)
B. Monocarboxylate 10 transporter (MCT10)
C. Organic anion-transporting polypeptide 1C1
D. All of the above

595. Thyroid hormones act through?
Harrison's 20th Ed. Chapter 375 Page 2696

A. Nuclear receptors
B. Mitochondrial enzymes
C. Integrin receptors
D. All of the above

After entering cells, thyroid hormones act primarily through nuclear receptors. They also have nongenomic actions through stimulating mitochondrial enzymatic responses and may act directly on blood vessels & heart through integrin receptors.

596. Which of the following X-linked syndromes is related to mutation in MCT8 gene?
Clin Thyroidol. 2012;24:2-3

A. Gustavsson syndrome
B. Brooks-Wisniewski-Brown syndrome
C. Allan-Herndon-Dudley syndrome
D. Schimke syndrome

Allan-Herndon-Dudley syndrome is an X-linked mental retardation condition caused by mutations in the monocarboxylate transporter 8 (MCT8) gene. Its features include moderate-severe mental retardation, impaired speech, hypotonia, muscle weakness, and contractures. Mutations in this gene, located at Xq13.2, impair transport of T3 into neurons (elevated free T3 & decreased free T4 in blood).

597. Thyroid hormones act through?
Harrison's 20th Ed. Chapter 375 Page 2696

A. Cell membrane hormone receptors
B. Nuclear hormone receptors
C. Mitochondrial hormone receptors
D. All of the above

Thyroxine (T4) and triiodothyronine (T3) act through nuclear receptors.

598. Thyroid hormone receptor β (TRβ) is more abundant than TRα in which of the following organs?
Harrison's 20th Ed. Chapter 375 Page 2696

A. Brain
B. Kidney
C. Gonads
D. Pituitary

599. Thyroid hormone receptor β (TRβ) is more abundant than TRα in which of the following organs?
Harrison's 20th Ed. Chapter 375 Page 2696

A. Muscle
B. Kidney
C. Liver
D. Heart

Thyroid hormones bind with high affinity to nuclear thyroid hormone receptors (TR) alpha & beta—expressed in most tissues. TR-alpha is particularly abundant in brain, kidney, gonads, muscle, and heart, whereas TR - beta expression is relatively high in the pituitary and liver.

600. Which of the following plays a role in feedback control of the thyroid axis in hypothalamus and pituitary?
Harrison's 20th Ed. Chapter 375 Page 2696

A. TRα1
B. TRβ1
C. TRα2
D. TRβ2

The TRβ2 isoform, which has a unique amino terminus, is selectively expressed in the hypothalamus and pituitary, where it plays a role in feedback control of the thyroid axis.

601. Which of the following prevents thyroid hormone binding?
Harrison's 20th Ed. Chapter 375 Page 2696

A. TRα1
B. TRβ1
C. TRα2
D. TRβ2

TR - α2 isoform contains a unique carboxy terminus that precludes thyroid hormone binding.

602. Thyroid receptor (TR) binds to which of the following in the promoter region of target genes?
Harrison's 20th Ed. Chapter 375 Page 2696

A. Thyroid recruiting elements
B. Thyroid receptor elements
C. Thyroid response elements
D. Thyroid reacting elements

603. Thyroid receptor (TR) binds to which of the following receptor?
Harrison's 20th Ed. Chapter 375 Page 2696 Figure 375-4

A. Retinoic acid X receptors
B. TSH receptors
C. Orphan nuclear receptor SF1
D. Interleukin 1 receptors

In nucleus, thyroid hormone receptor (TR) & retinoid X receptor (RXR) form heterodimers that bind specifically to thyroid hormone response elements (TRE) in promoter regions of target genes.

604. In the absence of hormone, TR binds to which of the following?
Harrison's 20th Ed. Chapter 375 Page 2696 Figure 375-4

A. Co-repressor
B. Co-activator
C. Co-modulator
D. Any of the above

In the absence of hormone, TR binds co-repressor (CoR) proteins that silence gene expression.

605. Which of the following statements about resistance to thyroid hormone (RTH) is false?
Harrison's 20th Ed. Chapter 375 Page 2696

A. Autosomal dominant disorder
B. Due to mutation in TRβ receptor gene
C. Elevated free thyroid hormone levels
D. Presents as hypothyroidism

Resistance to thyroid hormone (RTH) is an autosomal dominant disorder characterized by elevated thyroid hormone levels & inappropriately normal or elevated TSH. Individuals with RTH do not exhibit signs & symptoms of hypothyroidism because hormone resistance is partial and is compensated by increased levels of thyroid hormone. RTH is caused by mutations in the TRβ gene.

606. Which of the following statements about resistance to thyroid hormone (RTH) is false?
Harrison's 20th Ed. Chapter 375 Page 2696

A. Goiter
B. Tachycardia
C. Impaired metabolic responses to thyroid hormone
D. Treated with thyroid replacement drugs

Clinical features of RTH include goiter, attention deficit disorder, mild reduction in IQ, delayed skeletal maturation, tachycardia & impaired metabolic responses to thyroid hormone. Mostly no treatment is indicated, rather inappropriate treatment of mistaken hyperthyroidism should be avoided.

607. Which of the following best relates to resistance to thyroid hormone (RTH)?
Harrison's 20th Ed. Chapter 375 Page 2696

A. Dominant negative activity
B. Dominant positive activity
C. Dominant neutral activity
D. All of the above

Classical forms of RTH are caused by mutations in the TRβ gene causing loss of receptor function and consequently working as antagonists of the remaining normal TRβ and TRα receptors. This property is referred to as "dominant negative" activity.

608. Which of the following best defines resistance to thyroid hormone (RTH)?
Harrison's 20th Ed. Chapter 375 Page 2696

A. ↑ unbound thyroid hormone levels without suppression of TSH
B. ↓ unbound thyroid hormone levels without suppression of TSH
C. ↑ unbound thyroid hormone levels with excess of TSH
D. ↓ unbound thyroid hormone levels with excess of TSH

609. ↑ unbound thyroid hormone levels without suppression of TSH is seen in?
Harrison's 20th Ed. Chapter 375 Page 2696

A. Resistance to thyroid hormone (RTH)
B. Familial dysalbuminemic hyperthyroxinemia (FDH)
C. TSH-secreting pituitary adenomas
D. All of the above

610. Which of the following is false about RTH caused by mutations in TRα gene?
Harrison's 20th Ed. Chapter 375 Page 2696

A. Normal TSH
B. Low or normal T4
C. Normal or elevated T3 levels
D. None of the above

611. Pemberton's sign is elicited by?
Harrison's 20th Ed. Chapter 375 Page 2697

A. Act of swallowing
B. Raising of arms
C. Extrusion of tongue
D. All of the above

Large retrosternal goiters can cause venous distention over the neck and difficulty breathing, especially when the arms are raised (Pemberton's sign). With any central mass above the thyroid, the tongue should be extended, as thyroglossal cysts then move upward.

612. Free T3 index is calculated by?
Harrison's 20th Ed. Chapter 375 Page 2697

A. Thyroid hormone binding ratio (THBR) × Total T3
B. Thyroid hormone binding ratio (THBR) / Total T3
C. Thyroid hormone binding ratio (THBR) × Free T3
D. Thyroid hormone binding ratio (THBR) / Free T3

The product of THBR and total T3 or T4 provides the free T3 or T4 index. In effect, the index corrects for anomalous total hormone values caused by abnormalities in hormone-protein binding.

613. TBG is increased due to all except?
Harrison's 20th Ed. Chapter 375 Page 2697

A. Pregnancy
B. Hormone replacement therapy
C. Nephrotic syndrome
D. Tamoxifen

Total thyroid hormone levels are elevated when TBG is increased due to estrogens (pregnancy, oral contraceptives, hormone therapy, tamoxifen, selective estrogen receptor modulators, inflammatory liver disease). TBG is reduced by androgens & in nephrotic syndrome.

614. In pregnancy, circulating free T4, free T3 and TSH are?
Harrison's 20th Ed. Chapter 375 Page 2697

A. Normal
B. Increased
C. Decreased
D. Any of the above

615. TSH levels are elevated in all except?
Harrison's 20th Ed. Chapter 375 Page 2697

A. Hypothyroidism
B. Thyroid hormone resistance
C. First trimester of pregnancy
D. TSH-secreting pituitary tumor

616. TSH levels are suppressed in all except?
Harrison's 20th Ed. Chapter 375 Page 2697

A. Thyrotoxicosis
B. First trimester of pregnancy
C. Insulin
D. Dopamine

Elevated TSH levels occur in hypothyroidism most commonly, and also in TSH-secreting pituitary tumor, thyroid hormone resistance & assay artifact. Suppressed TSH level (<0.1 mU/L) indicates thyrotoxicosis but are also seen during first trimester of pregnancy (due to hCG secretion), after treatment of hyperthyroidism & in response to high doses of glucocorticoids or dopamine.

617. What percentage of patients with autoimmune hypothyroidism have TPO antibodies?
Harrison's 20th Ed. Chapter 375 Page 2697

A. 40%
B. 60%
C. 80%
D. 100%

618. What percentage of patients with Graves' disease have TPO antibodies?
Harrison's 20th Ed. Chapter 375 Page 2697

A. 40%
B. 60%
C. 80%
D. 100%

Almost all patients with autoimmune hypothyroidism, and up to 80% of those with Graves' disease, have high levels of TPO antibodies.

619. Main use of thyroid-stimulating immunoglobulins (TSI) assays is to predict?
Harrison's 20th Ed. Chapter 375 Page 2697

A. Thyroiditis
B. Thyrotoxicosis factitia
C. Neonatal thyrotoxicosis
D. Thyroid cancer

Thyroid-stimulating immunoglobulins (TSI) are antibodies that stimulate the TSH-R in Graves' disease. They are most commonly measured by commercially available tracer displacement assays called TRAb (TSH receptor antibody) with the assumption that elevated levels in the setting of clinical hyperthyroidism reflect stimulatory effects on the TSH receptor. The main use of these assays is to predict neonatal thyrotoxicosis caused by high maternal levels of TRAb or TSI (>3x upper limit of normal) in the last trimester of pregnancy.

620. The main role for serum Tg measurement is in?
Harrison's 20th Ed. Chapter 375 Page 2697

A. Thyroiditis
B. Thyrotoxicosis factitia
C. Follow-up of thyroid cancer
D. All of the above

The main role for Tg measurement is in the follow-up of thyroid cancer patients. After total thyroidectomy and radioablation, serum Tg levels should be undetectable. In the absence of anti-Tg antibodies, measurable levels indicate incomplete ablation or recurrent cancer.

621. Which of the following radioisotopes of iodine is used for thyroid imaging?
Harrison's 20th Ed. Chapter 375 Page 2698

A. ^{123}I
B. ^{125}I
C. ^{131}I
D. All of the above

Thyroid gland selectively transports radioisotopes of iodine (^{123}I, ^{125}I, ^{131}I) and ^{99m}Tc pertechnetate, allowing thyroid imaging & quantitation of radioactive tracer fractional uptake.

622. Which of the following statements is false?
Harrison's 20th Ed. Chapter 375 Page 2698

A. Euthyroid individuals with thyroid antibodies are at increased risk of developing thyroid dysfunction
B. Serum Tg levels are increased in thyrotoxicosis factitia
C. Functioning or "hot" nodules are almost never malignant
D. Thyroid nodules do not produce thyroid hormone

Serum Tg levels are increased in all types of thyrotoxicosis except thyrotoxicosis factitia caused by self-administration of thyroid hormone.

623. What frequency of transducer is best for thyroid ultrasonography?
Harrison's 20th Ed. Chapter 375 Page 2698

A. 2.5 MHz
B. 5 MHz
C. 7.5 MHz
D. 10 MHz

A 10–12 MHz ultrasound probe can detect thyroid nodules and cysts >3 mm.

624. Which of the following sonographic patterns of thyroid is highly suggestive of malignancy?
Harrison's 20th Ed. Chapter 375 Page 2698

A. Hypoechoic solid nodules with infiltrative borders & microcalcifications
B. Hyperechoic solid nodules with infiltrative borders & microcalcifications
C. Spongiform nodules (multiple small internal cystic areas)
D. All of the above

On sonography of thyroid, hypoechoic solid nodules with infiltrative borders & microcalcifications are highly suggestive of malignancy. Spongiform nodules defined as multiple small internal cystic areas correlates with benignity. Heterogeneous thyroid enlargement is typical of Hashimoto's thyroiditis.

Hypothyroidism

625. Which of the following is a cause of autoimmune hypothyroidism?

Harrison's 20th Ed. Chapter 376 Page 2698 Table 376-1

A. Atrophic thyroiditis
B. Riedel's thyroiditis
C. Silent thyroiditis
D. Subacute thyroiditis

Autoimmune hypothyroidism may be associated with a goiter (Hashimoto's, or goitrous thyroiditis) or, at the later stages of the disease, minimal residual thyroid tissue (atrophic thyroiditis).

626. Which of the following is a cause of primary hypothyroidism?

Harrison's 20th Ed. Chapter 376 Page 2698 Table 376-1

A. Iodine excess
B. Iodine deficiency
C. ^{131}I treatment
D. All of the above

627. Which of the following drugs can cause primary hypothyroidism?

Harrison's 20th Ed. Chapter 376 Page 2698 Table 376-1

A. Lithium
B. p-aminosalicylic acid
C. Interferon α
D. All of the above

628. Which of the following drugs can cause congenital hypothyroidism?

Harrison's 20th Ed. Chapter 376 Page 2698 Table 376-1

A. Absent or ectopic thyroid gland
B. Dyshormonogenesis
C. TSH-R mutation
D. All of the above

629. Which of the following about Bexarotene is false?

Acta Derm Venereol. 2012;92(3):258-63

A. Oral retinoid
B. Used in cutaneous T-cell lymphoma (CTCL)
C. Can cause secondary hypothyroidism
D. None of the above

630. What is the prevalence of hypothyroidism in newborns?

Harrison's 20th Ed. Chapter 376 Page 2698

A. 1 in 4000
B. 1 in 8000
C. 1 in 16000
D. 1 in 20000

Hypothyroidism occurs in about 1 in 4000 newborns. It may be transient if the mother has TSH-R blocking antibodies or has received anti-thyroid drugs. But, permanent hypothyroidism occurs in the majority.

631. Neonatal hypothyroidism is most frequently due to?

Harrison's 20th Ed. Chapter 376 Page 2698

A. Thyroid gland dysgenesis
B. Inborn errors of thyroid hormone synthesis
C. TSH-R antibody-mediated
D. Idiopathic

Neonatal hypothyroidism is due to thyroid gland dysgenesis in 80–85%, to inborn errors of thyroid hormone synthesis in 10–15% & TSH-R antibody-mediated in 5% of affected newborns. They are twice more common in girls.

632. Clinical feature for diagnosis of congenital hypothyroidism is?

Harrison's 20th Ed. Chapter 376 Page 2699

A. Prolonged jaundice
B. Enlarged tongue
C. Umbilical hernia
D. All of the above

The majority of infants with congenital hypothyroidism appear normal at birth. Clinical features include prolonged jaundice, feeding problems, hypotonia, enlarged tongue, delayed bone maturation and umbilical hernia. Other congenital malformations, especially cardiac, are four times more common in congenital hypothyroidism.

633. Which of the following gene protein is defective in combined deficiencies of GH, prolactin and TSH?

Harrison's 20th Ed. Chapter 376 Page 2699 Table 376-2

A. PROP-1
B. PIT-1
C. PAX-8
D. NKX2-1

634. Which of the following gene protein is defective in combined pituitary hormone deficiencies with preservation of ACTH?

Harrison's 20th Ed. Chapter 376 Page 2699 Table 376-2

A. PROP-1
B. PIT-1
C. PAX-8
D. NKX2-1

635. Which of the following gene protein is defective in thyroid hypoplasia, choreoathetosis, pulmonary problems?

Harrison's 20th Ed. Chapter 376 Page 2699 Table 376-2

A. TTF-1
B. TTF-2
C. PAX-8
D. NKX2-1

636. Which of the following gene protein is defective in thyroid agenesis, choanal atresia, spiky hair?

Harrison's 20th Ed. Chapter 376 Page 2699 Table 376-2

A. TTF-1
B. TTF-2
C. PAX-8
D. NKX2-1

637. Which of the following gene protein is defective in thyroid dysgenesis, kidney abnormalities?

Harrison's 20th Ed. Chapter 376 Page 2699 Table 376-2

A. TTF-1
B. TTF-2
C. PAX-8
D. NKX2-1

638. Which of the following gene protein is defective in thyroid dysgenesis, brain, lung abnormalities?

Harrison's 20th Ed. Chapter 376 Page 2699 Table 376-2

A. TTF-1
B. TTF-2
C. PAX-8
D. NKX2-1

639. Which of the following gene protein is defective in thyroid dysgenesis, heart abnormalities?

Harrison's 20th Ed. Chapter 376 Page 2699 Table 376-2

A. TTF-1
B. TTF-2
C. PAX-8
D. NKX2-5

640. Pendred's syndrome best relates to?

Harrison's 20th Ed. Chapter 376 Page 2699 Table 376-2

A. SLC2A2
B. SLC22A12
C. SLC26A4
D. SLC22A13

Pendred's syndrome is related to Pendrin - SLC26A4 anion exchanger (Chloride/iodide transporter), FOXI1 (Transcriptional activator of SLC26A4) and KCNJ10 (Inwardly rectifying K^+ channel).

641. Thyroid peroxidase best relates to?

Harrison's 20th Ed. Chapter 376 Page 2699 Table 376-2

A. Inability to transport iodide
B. Defective synthesis of thyroid hormone
C. Loss of iodide reutilization
D. Defective organification of iodide

642. Thyroglobulin best relates to?

Harrison's 20th Ed. Chapter 376 Page 2699 Table 376-2

A. Inability to transport iodide
B. Defective synthesis of thyroid hormone
C. Loss of iodide reutilization
D. Defective organification of iodide

643. Na^+/I^- symporter (SLC5A5) best relates to?

Harrison's 20th Ed. Chapter 376 Page 2699 Table 376-2

A. Inability to transport iodide
B. Defective synthesis of thyroid hormone
C. Loss of iodide reutilization
D. Defective organification of iodide

644. For congenital hypothyroidism, dose of T4 is?

Harrison's 20th Ed. Chapter 376 Page 2699

A. 1–2 μg / kg per day
B. 2–5 μg / kg per day
C. 5–10 μg / kg per day
D. 10–15 μg / kg per day

For congenital hypothyroidism, dose of T4 is instituted at a dose of 10–15 μg/kg per day.

645. Symptoms of hypothyroidism become more readily apparent at TSH levels of?

Harrison's 20th Ed. Chapter 376 Page 2699

A. > 7 mIU/L
B. > 8 mIU/L
C. > 9 mIU/L
D. > 10 mIU/L

Symptoms of hypothyroidism become more readily apparent at when TSH is >10 mIU/L. This stage is referred to as clinical hypothyroidism or overt hypothyroidism.

646. Which of the following is false about autoimmune hypothyroidism?

Harrison's 20th Ed. Chapter 376 Page 2699

A. More common in women
B. More common in Japanese
C. More common in chronic exposure to a high-iodine diet
D. None of the above

647. Mean age at diagnosis of autoimmune hypothyroidism is?

Harrison's 20th Ed. Chapter 376 Page 2699

A. 30 years
B. 40 years
C. 50 years
D. 60 years

Mean age at diagnosis of autoimmune hypothyroidism is 60 years and the prevalence of overt hypothyroidism increases with age.

648. Which of the following is false about Hashimoto's or goitrous thyroiditis?

Harrison's 20th Ed. Chapter 376 Page 2699

A. Lymphocytic infiltration
B. Atrophy of thyroid follicles
C. No fibrosis
D. May progress to atrophic thyroiditis

In Hashimoto's thyroiditis, there is a marked lymphocytic infiltration of thyroid with germinal center formation, atrophy of thyroid follicles accompanied by oxyphil metaplasia, absence of colloid & mild to moderate fibrosis. Atrophic thyroiditis represents the end stage of Hashimoto's thyroiditis rather than a distinct disorder.

649. Which of the following gene polymorphism contributes to autoimmune thyroiditis?

Harrison's 20th Ed. Chapter 376 Page 2699

A. STAT4
B. TREX-1
C. CTLA4
D. ITGAM

A weak association exists between polymorphisms in CTLA-4, a T cell - regulatory gene and autoimmune hypothyroidism.

650. Which of the following blocks cytotoxic T-lymphocyte antigen-4 (CTLA-4)?

Harrison's 20th Ed. Chapter 376 Page 2699

A. Ofatumumab
B. Ipilimumab
C. Adalimumab
D. Golimumab

CTLA-4 is a member of the B7-CD28 family. Ipilimumab is a fully human monoclonal IgG1 antibody that blocks the immune checkpoint cytotoxic T-lymphocyte antigen-4 (CTLA-4).

651. Autoimmune hypothyroidism is associated with which of the following autoimmune diseases?

Harrison's 20th Ed. Chapter 376 Page 2699

A. Type 1 diabetes mellitus
B. Addison's disease
C. Pernicious anemia
D. All of the above

Autoimmune hypothyroidism is associated with other autoimmune diseases like type 1 diabetes mellitus, Addison's disease, pernicious anemia and vitiligo.

652. Autoimmune hypothyroidism is associated with which of the following conditions?

Harrison's 20th Ed. Chapter 376 Page 2699

A. Down's syndrome
B. Turner's syndrome
C. Low selenium intake
D. All of the above

653. Lymphocytic infiltrate in autoimmune hypothyroidism is composed of?

Harrison's 20th Ed. Chapter 376 Page 2700

A. Activated CD4+ T cells
B. Activated CD8+ T cells
C. B cells
D. All of the above

T cell-mediated injury is required to initiate autoimmune damage to the thyroid. Thyroid lymphocytic infiltrate in autoimmune hypothyroidism is composed of activated CD4+, CD8+ T cells and B cells. Thyroid cell destruction is primarily mediated by CD8+ cytotoxic T cells.

654. Patients with autoimmune hypothyroidism have antibodies against?

Harrison's 20th Ed. Chapter 376 Page 2700

A. TPO
B. TSH-R
C. Thyroglobulin (Tg)
D. All of the above

655. Out of the following, which is the most common symptom of hypothyroidism?

Harrison's 20th Ed. Chapter 376 Page 2699 Table 376-3

A. Dry skin
B. Hair loss
C. Constipation
D. Weight gain with poor appetite

656. Out of the following, which is the most common symptom of hypothyroidism?

Harrison's 20th Ed. Chapter 376 Page 2699 Table 376-3

A. Bradycardia
B. Diffuse alopecia
C. Dry coarse skin
D. Peripheral oedema

657. Which of the following about clinical features of hypothyroidism is false?

Harrison's 20th Ed. Chapter 376 Page 2700

A. Goiter is usually irregular & firm in consistency
B. Pyramidal lobe usually palpable
C. Painless
D. None of the above

658. Skin thickening in hypothyroidism best relates to which of the following?

Harrison's 20th Ed. Chapter 376 Page 2700

A. Glycolipid
B. Glycosaminoglycan
C. Amyloid P
D. Vitronectin

Increased dermal glycosaminoglycan content traps water, giving rise to skin thickening without pitting (myxedema).

659. Yellow tinge to the skin in patients of hypothyroidism is due to accumulation of?

Harrison's 20th Ed. Chapter 376 Page 2700

A. Bilirubin
B. Heme
C. Carotene
D. All of the above

In patients of hypothyroidism, there is pallor with a yellow tinge to the skin due to carotene accumulation.

660. Which of the following is a clinical feature of hypothyroidism?

Harrison's 20th Ed. Chapter 376 Page 2700

A. Nail growth is retarded
B. Thinning of outer third of eyebrows
C. Weight gain is due to fluid retention in myxedematous tissues
D. All of the above

Nail growth is retarded and there is thinning of the outer third of the eyebrows.

661. Hung up reflex (Woltman's sign) seen in hypothyroidism is best observed at?

N Engl J Med 2018; 379:e23

A. Ankle reflex
B. Knee reflex
C. Triceps reflex
D. All of the above

In hypothyroidism, the relaxation phase of muscle stretch reflexes is characteristically prolonged and best observed at the ankle or biceps brachii reflexes. Woltman's sign, which refers to the delayed relaxation phase of a deep-tendon reflex, is a neurologic manifestation of hypothyroidism. This delayed relaxation can also be associated with pregnancy, anorexia nervosa, diabetes mellitus, and advanced age.

662. Pericardial effusions occur in what percentage of patients of hypothyroidism?

Harrison's 20th Ed. Chapter 376 Page 2700

A. 10%
B. 30%
C. 50%
D. 75%

Pericardial effusions occur in ~30% of patients of hypothyroidism but rarely compromises cardiac function.

663. Which of the following is a clinical feature of hypothyroidism?

Harrison's 20th Ed. Chapter 376 Page 2700

A. Pseudomyotonia
B. Memory and concentration impairment
C. Carpal tunnel syndrome
D. All of the above

664. PET scans examining glucose metabolism in hypothyroid subjects show lower regional activity in?

Harrison's 20th Ed. Chapter 376 Page 2700

A. Amygdala
B. Hippocampus
C. Perigenual anterior cingulated cortex
D. All of the above

665. Which of the following is false about Hashimoto's encephalopathy?

Harrison's 20th Ed. Chapter 376 Page 2700

A. Grand Mal seizure
B. Slow-wave activity on EEG
C. Steroid-responsive
D. May occur in autoimmune thyroiditis without hypothyroidism

Hashimoto's encephalopathy is a steroid-responsive syndrome associated with TPO antibodies, myoclonus & slow-wave activity on EEG.

666. Fluid accumulation in hypothyroidism produces which of the following?

Harrison's 20th Ed. Chapter 376 Page 2700

A. Hoarse voice
B. Skin thickening
C. Conductive deafness
D. All of the above

Fluid accumulation in middle ear gives rise to conductive deafness. Hoarse voice and clumsy speech of hypothyroidism reflect fluid accumulation in the vocal cords and tongue.

667. Autoimmune hypothyroidism is less commonly associated with which of the following autoimmune diseases?

Harrison's 20th Ed. Chapter 376 Page 2701

A. Rheumatoid arthritis
B. Addison's disease
C. Pernicious anemia
D. Vitiligo

Autoimmune hypothyroidism may be associated with other autoimmune diseases, particularly vitiligo, pernicious anemia, Addison's disease, alopecia areata, and type 1 diabetes mellitus. Less common associations include celiac disease, dermatitis herpetiformis, chronic active hepatitis, rheumatoid arthritis, systemic lupus erythematosus (SLE), myasthenia gravis and Sjogren's syndrome.

668. Abnormal laboratory findings in hypothyroidism may include?

Harrison's 20th Ed. Chapter 376 Page 2701

A. Increased creatine phosphokinase
B. Elevated triglycerides
C. Macrocytic anemia
D. All of the above

Abnormal laboratory findings in hypothyroidism may include increased creatine phosphokinase, elevated cholesterol and triglycerides and anemia (normocytic or macrocytic). EMG is typically normal.

669. Which of the following can cause hypothyroidism?

Harrison's 20th Ed. Chapter 376 Page 2701

A. Iodine deficiency
B. Selenium deficiency
C. Chronic iodine excess
D. All of the above

670. Consumption of which of the following can cause hypothyroidism?

Harrison's 20th Ed. Chapter 376 Page 2701

A. Thiocyanates in cassava
B. Amiodarone
C. Lithium
D. All of the above

671. Which of the following systemic disorders can affect taste?

Harrison's 20th Ed. Chapter 376 Page 2701

A. Chronic renal failure
B. Diabetes mellitus
C. Hypothyroidism
D. All of the above

Systemic disorders can affect taste include chronic renal failure, end-stage liver disease, vitamin and mineral deficiencies, diabetes mellitus and hypothyroidism.

672. Which of the following systemic disorders can affect smell?

Harrison's 20th Ed. Chapter 376 Page 2701

A. Chronic renal failure
B. Diabetes mellitus
C. Hypothyroidism
D. All of the above

Medical conditions associated with smell impairment are renal failure, liver disease, hypothyroidism, diabetes and dementia.

673. Women treated with radioactive iodine should not become pregnant for how many months after treatment?

Harrison's 20th Ed. Chapter 376 Page 2701

A. 3–6 months
B. 6–12 months
C. 12–24 months
D. 24–36 months

Women treated with radioactive iodine should not become pregnant for 6–12 months after treatment.

674. Hypothyroidism can occur in?

Harrison's 20th Ed. Chapter 376 Page 2701

A. AL amyloidosis
B. Ethionamide therapy
C. Asthma
D. All of the above

675. Which of the following is found in hypothyroidism?

Harrison's 20th Ed. Chapter 376 Page 2702

A. "Water bottle" configuration of heart on CxR
B. Prolongation of QT interval in ECG
C. Pericardial effusion
D. All of the above

676. Which of the following can cause constipation?

Harrison's 20th Ed. Chapter 376 Page 2702

A. Hypothyroidism
B. Hypoparathyroidism
C. Lead poisoning
D. All of the above

677. Short stature may be caused by?

Harrison's 20th Ed. Chapter 376 Page 2702

A. GH deficiency
B. Hypothyroidism
C. Cushing's syndrome
D. All of the above

Short stature may be caused by GH deficiency, hypothyroidism, Cushing's syndrome, precocious puberty, malnutrition, chronic illness or genetic abnormalities that affect the epiphyseal growth plates (FGFR3 and SHOX mutations).

678. Subclinical hypothyroidism is defined by an elevated serum thyroid-stimulating hormone level along with normal levels of?

Cleveland clinic J of Med 2019;86(2):101

A. T3
B. T4
C. Free T3
D. Free T4

Subclinical hypothyroidism is defined by an elevated serum thyroid-stimulating hormone (TSH) level along with a normal free thyroxine (T4) level.

679. Subclinical hypothyroidism is defined as a thyrotropin level of ≥3 mU per liter and a free T4 level of?

N Engl J Med 2017;376:815-25

A. 0.86 to 1.90 pg per deciliter
B. 0.86 to 1.90 ng per deciliter
C. 0.86 to 1.90 μg per deciliter
D. 0.86 to 1.90 mg per deciliter

Subclinical hypothyroidism is defined as a thyrotropin level of ≥ 3 mU per liter (which correspond to the 97.5th percentile) and a free T4 level in the normal range (0.86 to 1.90 ng per deciliter).

680. Subclinical hypothyroidism is associated with?

N Engl J Med 2017;376:815-25

A. Impaired fetal neuropsychological development
B. Increased risks of preterm birth
C. Placental abruption
D. All of the above

Subclinical hypothyroidism is associated with impaired fetal neuropsychological development, increased risks of preterm birth, placental abruption, admission to the intensive care nursery (or neonatal intensive care unit).

681. Hypothyroxinemia is defined as a thyrotropin level in normal range and a free T4 level of less than?

N Engl J Med 2017;376:815-25

A. 0.66 ng per deciliter
B. 0.76 ng per deciliter
C. 0.86 ng per deciliter
D. 0.96 ng per deciliter

Hypothyroxinemia is defined as a thyrotropin level in the normal range (0.08 to 3.99 mU per liter) and a free T4 level of less than 0.86 ng per deciliter.

682. Evidence in favor of treating subclinical hypothyroidism is in patients with TSH levels higher than?

Cleveland clinic J of Med 2019;86(2):101

A. 4 mIU/L
B. 6 mIU/L
C. 8 mIU/L
D. 10 mIU/L

The strongest evidence in favor of treating subclinical hypothyroidism is in patients with TSH levels higher than 10 mIU/L.

683. Levothyroxine therapy is advised in pregnancy who have TSH levels higher than?

Cleveland clinic J of Med 2019;86(2):101

A. 2.5 mIU/L
B. 3.5 mIU/L
C. 4.5 mIU/L
D. 5.5 mIU/L

Due to the concern for possible adverse maternal & fetal outcomes and low IQ in children of pregnant patients with subclinical hypothyroidism, levothyroxine therapy is advised in pregnancy or planning pregnancy who have TSH levels ≥2.5 mIU/L, especially if they have thyroid peroxidase antibody.

684. Substances that interfere with TSH assays include?

Cleveland clinic J of Med 2019;86(2):101

A. Heterophile antibodies
B. Rheumatoid factor
C. Macro-TSH
D. All of the above

Substances that interfere with TSH assays include heterophile antibodies, rheumatoid factor, biotin & macro-TSH.

685. The most common cause of subclinical hypothyroidism is?

Cleveland clinic J of Med 2019;86(2):101

A. Autoimmune (Hashimoto) thyroiditis
B. Drugs
C. Recovery phase of euthyroid sick syndrome
D. Obesity

The most common cause of subclinical hypothyroidism, accounting for 60% to 80% of cases, is Hashimoto (autoimmune) thyroiditis, in which thyroid peroxidase antibodies are usually present. Other causes include suboptimal treatment of hypothyroidism due to other reasons such as thyroidectomy, radioactive iodine treatment, external radiation, infiltrative diseases (e.g., amyloidosis, sarcoidosis, hemochromatosis), and drugs (e.g., iodinated contrast, amiodarone, lithium, tyrosine kinase inhibitors).

686. Which of the following is used to monitor therapy in secondary hypothyroidism?

Harrison's 20th Ed. Chapter 376 Page 2702

A. T3
B. T4
C. TSH
D. All of the above

The goal of treatment in secondary hypothyroidism is to maintain T4 levels in the upper half of the reference range because TSH levels cannot be used to monitor therapy.

687. Daily replacement dose of levothyroxine is usually?

Harrison's 20th Ed. Chapter 376 Page 2702

A. 1.6 µg / kg body weight
B. 1.8 µg / kg body weight
C. 2.0 µg / kg body weight
D. 2.2 µg / kg body weight

If there is no residual thyroid function, daily replacement dose of levothyroxine is usually 1.6 µg/kg body weight (typically 100 - 150 µg) ideally taken at least 30 minutes before breakfast.

688. TSH responses should be measured after what time upon levothyroxine treatment?

Harrison's 20th Ed. Chapter 376 Page 2702

A. 7 days
B. 15 days
C. 1 month
D. 2 months

TSH responses to levothyroxine therapy are gradual & should be measured ~ 2 months after instituting treatment.

689. If TSH is high, levothyroxine dosage should be increased by?

Harrison's 20th Ed. Chapter 376 Page 2702

A. 6.25–12.5 µg increments
B. 12.5–25 µg increments
C. 25–75 µg increments
D. 75–100 µg increments

Adjustment of levothyroxine dosage is made in 12.5 or 25 µg increments if the TSH is high.

690. Upon normalization of TSH levels, patients experience full relief from symptoms after?

Harrison's 20th Ed. Chapter 376 Page 2702

A. 15 days to 2 months
B. 2 to 3 months
C. 3 to 6 months
D. 6 months to 1 year

Patients experience full relief from symptoms 3–6 months after normal TSH levels are restored.

691. Which of the following treatments is least recommended in hypothyroidism?

Harrison's 20th Ed. Chapter 376 Page 2702

A. T4 alone
B. T3 alone
C. T3 & T4 combined
D. T3 & T4 alternately

There is no place for liothyronine alone as long-term replacement due to its short half-life which necessitates multiple dosage per day and is associated with fluctuating T3 levels.

692. In patients taking Levothyroxine (> 200 µg/day) with elevated TSH level suggests the possibility of?

Harrison's 20th Ed. Chapter 376 Page 2702

A. Poor compliance
B. Inappropriate TSH secretion
C. Malabsorption
D. Any of the above

693. Drugs that interfere with T4 absorption / clearance are all except?

Harrison's 20th Ed. Chapter 376 Page 2702

A. Cholestyramine
B. Ferrous sulfate
C. Calcium supplements
D. Isoniazid

694. Drugs that interfere with T4 absorption / clearance are all except?

Harrison's 20th Ed. Chapter 376 Page 2702

A. Lovastatin
B. Aluminum hydroxide
C. Cimetidine
D. Rifampicin

695. Drugs that interfere with T4 absorption/clearance are all except?

Harrison's 20th Ed. Chapter 376 Page 2702

A. Lidocaine
B. Amiodarone
C. Carbamazepine
D. Phenytoin

Causes of increased levothyroxine requirements are malabsorption (celiac disease, small-bowel surgery), estrogen therapy, or selective estrogen receptor modulator therapy, ingestion with a meal, & drugs that interfere with T4 absorption or clearance like cholestyramine, ferrous sulfate, calcium supplements, proton pump inhibitors, lovastatin, aluminum hydroxide, rifampicin, amiodarone, carbamazepine, phenytoin and tyrosine kinase inhibitors.

696. During pregnancy, dose of levothyroxine may need to be?

Harrison's 20th Ed. Chapter 376 Page 2702

A. Increased
B. Decreased
C. Stopped
D. All of the above

The dose of levothyroxine may need to be increased by ~45% during pregnancy and returned to previous levels after delivery.

697. Thyroxine doses in elderly patients should be less than younger patients by?

Harrison's 20th Ed. Chapter 376 Page 2702

A. 10%
B. 20%
C. 30%
D. 50%

698. In elderly patients with CAD, the starting dose of levothyroxine is?

Harrison's 20th Ed. Chapter 376 Page 2702

A. 12.5 to 25 µg/day
B. 25 to 37.5 µg/day
C. 37.5 to 50 µg/day
D. 50 to 62.5 µg/day

Elderly patients may require up to 20% less thyroxine than younger patients. In elderly with coronary artery disease, starting dose of levothyroxine is 12.5 - 25 µg/day with similar increments every 2–3 months until TSH is normalized.

699. Myxedema coma almost always occurs in?

Harrison's 20th Ed. Chapter 376 Page 2702

A. Neonates
B. Adolescents
C. Adults
D. Elderly

Myxedema coma, rather myxedema crisis, is state of decompensated long standing severe untreated hypothyroidism. The three key features of myxedema coma are—altered mental status, defective thermoregulation (hypothermia) and a precipitating event. Myxedema coma is a medical emergency and is associated with a high mortality rate.

700. Myxedema coma is precipitated by?

Harrison's 20th Ed. Chapter 376 Page 2702

A. Sedatives
B. Anesthetics
C. Antidepressants
D. All of the above

Myxedema coma almost always occurs in the elderly & is usually precipitated by factors that impair respiration, such as drugs (sedatives, anesthetics, antidepressants), pneumonia, CHF, MI, GI bleeding, Sepsis or CVAs. Exposure to cold, hypoventilation, hypoglycemia & dilutional hyponatremia also contribute to the development of myxedema coma.

701. Initial dose of levothyroxine in myxedema coma given by nasogastric tube is?

Harrison's 20th Ed. Chapter 376 Page 2702

A. 200 µg
B. 300 µg
C. 400 µg
D. 500 µg

In myxedema coma, 500 µg of Levothyroxine can be given either as intravenous bolus or by nasogastric tube.

702. Which of the following is not indicated while treating myxedema coma?

Harrison's 20th Ed. Chapter 376 Page 2702

A. External warming
B. Parenteral hydrocortisone
C. Broad-spectrum antibiotics
D. Hypotonic intravenous fluids

In myxedema coma, hypotonic intravenous fluids should be avoided as they may exacerbate water retention secondary to reduced renal perfusion & inappropriate vasopressin secretion. Metabolism of most medications is impaired so reduced doses are recommended.

Hyperthyroidism

703. Which of the following about thyrotoxicosis is false?
Harrison's 20th Ed. Chapter 377 Page 2703

A. Result of excessive thyroid function
B. State of thyroid hormone excess
C. Not synonymous with hyperthyroidism
D. None of the above

Thyrotoxicosis is defined as a state of thyroid hormone excess as a result of excessive thyroid function. It is not synonymous with hyperthyroidism.

704. Major etiology of thyrotoxicosis is hyperthyroidism caused by?
Harrison's 20th Ed. Chapter 377 Page 2703

A. Graves' disease
B. Toxic multinodular goiter (MNG)
C. Toxic adenomas
D. All of the above

Major etiologies of thyrotoxicosis are hyperthyroidism caused by Graves' disease, toxic multinodular goiter (MNG), and toxic adenomas.

705. Which of the following is not a cause of primary hyperthyroidism?
Harrison's 20th Ed. Chapter 377 Page 2703 Table 377-1

A. Functioning thyroid carcinoma metastases
B. Struma ovarii
C. Gestational thyrotoxicosis
D. Iodine excess

706. Which of the following is not a cause of primary hyperthyroidism?
Harrison's 20th Ed. Chapter 377 Page 2703 Table 377-1

A. Activating mutation of the TSH receptor
B. Thyroid hormone resistance syndrome
C. McCune-Albright syndrome
D. Jod-Basedow phenomenon

707. Which of the following is a cause of thyrotoxicosis without hyperthyroidism?
Harrison's 20th Ed. Chapter 377 Page 2703 Table 377-1

A. Subacute thyroiditis
B. Silent thyroiditis
C. Thyrotoxicosis factitia
D. All of the above

708. Which of the following is a cause of thyrotoxicosis without hyperthyroidism?
Harrison's 20th Ed. Chapter 377 Page 2703 Table 377-1

A. Amiodarone
B. Radiation
C. Infarction of adenoma
D. All of the above

709. Which of the following is not a cause of thyrotoxicosis without hyperthyroidism?
Harrison's 20th Ed. Chapter 377 Page 2703 Table 377-1

A. Subacute thyroiditis
B. Silent thyroiditis
C. Toxic adenoma
D. Thyrotoxicosis factitia

Hyperthyroidism means that thyroid gland is functioning more than normal. Therefore, a hyperthyroid patient is thyrotoxic, but a thyrotoxic patient may not have an overactive thyroid and is not actually hyperthyroid.

710. Which of the following is not a cause of primary hyperthyroidism?
Harrison's 20th Ed. Chapter 377 Page 2703 Table 377-1

A. Toxic multinodular goiter
B. Toxic adenoma
C. Subacute thyroiditis
D. Functioning thyroid carcinoma metastases

711. Which of the following is not a cause of secondary hyperthyroidism?
Harrison's 20th Ed. Chapter 377 Page 2703 Table 377-1

A. TSH-secreting pituitary adenoma
B. Thyroid hormone resistance syndrome
C. Chorionic gonadotropin-secreting tumors
D. All of the above

712. Circulating TSH levels are low in which of the following causes of secondary hyperthyroidism?
Harrison's 20th Ed. Chapter 377 Page 2703 Table 377-1

A. Gestational thyrotoxicosis
B. Thyrotoxicosis factitia
C. Struma ovarii
D. Jod-Basedow phenomenon

Circulating TSH levels are low in chorionic gonadotropin-secreting tumors and gestational thyrotoxicosis.

713. Graves' disease accounts for what percentage of thyrotoxicosis?
Harrison's 20th Ed. Chapter 377 Page 2703

A. 20–30%
B. 30–50%
C. 50–60%
D. 60–80%

Graves' disease accounts for 60-80% of thyrotoxicosis.

714. Which of the following about Graves' disease is false?
Harrison's 20th Ed. Chapter 377 Page 2703

A. Graves' disease more with high iodine intake
B. More frequent in women
C. Rarely begins before adolescence
D. None of the above

715. Graves' disease typically occurs between the age of?

Harrison's 20th Ed. Chapter 377 Page 2703

A. 5 and 20 years
B. 10 and 30 years
C. 20 and 30 years
D. 20 and 50 years

Graves' disease typically occurs between 20 and 50 years of age. It can also occur in the elderly.

716. Which of the following contribute to Graves' disease susceptibility?

Harrison's 20th Ed. Chapter 377 Page 2703

A. Polymorphisms in HLA-DR
B. Polymorphisms in immunoregulatory genes
C. Polymorphisms in gene encoding TSH-R
D. All of the above

Polymorphisms in HLA-DR, immunoregulatory genes (CTLA-4, CD25, PTPN22, FCRL3, and CD226), and gene encoding thyroid-stimulating hormone receptor (TSH-R), contributes to Graves' disease susceptibility.

717. Which of the following contribute in the occurrence of Graves' disease?

Harrison's 20th Ed. Chapter 377 Page 2703

A. Stress
B. Smoking
C. Sudden increases in iodine intake
D. All of the above

718. Which of the following is a major risk factor for the development of ophthalmopathy in Graves' disease?

Harrison's 20th Ed. Chapter 377 Page 2703

A. Alcohol
B. Smoking
C. Coffee
D. Tea

Smoking is a minor risk factor for Graves' disease and a major risk factor for the development of ophthalmopathy.

719. Which of the following contribute in the occurrence of Graves' disease?

Harrison's 20th Ed. Chapter 377 Page 2703

A. Postpartum period
B. During immune reconstitution phase after HAART
C. Alemtuzumab treatment
D. All of the above

720. Toxicity of Alemtuzumab includes?

Harrison's 20th Ed. Chapter 436 Page

A. Thyroiditis
B. Graves' disease
C. Thyroid cancer
D. All of the above

721. Alemtuzumab is a humanized monoclonal antibody directed against?

Harrison's 20th Ed. Chapter 436 Page

A. CD20 antigen
B. CD34 antigen
C. CD40 antigen
D. CD52 antigen

Alemtuzumab is a humanized monoclonal antibody directed against the CD52 antigen that is expressed on both monocytes and lymphocytes causing depletion of both B and T cells.

722. Alemtuzumab is of use in?

Harrison's 20th Ed. Chapter 436 Page

A. Chronic lymphoid leukemia
B. T-cell malignancies
C. Myelodysplastic syndromes (MDS)
D. All of the above

723. Thyroid-stimulating immunoglobulin (TSI) are synthesized in all except?

Harrison's 20th Ed. Chapter 377 Page 2703

A. Thyroid gland
B. Spleen
C. Bone marrow
D. Lymph nodes

Hyperthyroidism of Graves' disease is caused by thyroid-stimulating immunoglobulins (TSI) that are synthesized in the thyroid gland as well as in bone marrow & lymph nodes.

724. In thyrotoxicosis, presence of thyroid-stimulating immunoglobulin (TSI) is detected by?

Harrison's 20th Ed. Chapter 377 Page 2703

A. Thyroid peroxidase (TPO) antibody
B. Thyroglobulin (Tg) antibody
C. Thyrotropin-binding inhibitory immunoglobulin (TBII)
D. All of the above

The presence of thyrotropin-binding inhibitory immunoglobulin (TBII) in a patient with thyrotoxicosis implies the existence of thyroid-stimulating immunoglobulin (TSI).

725. Increased synthesis of which of the following leads to characteristic extraocular muscle swelling in Graves' disease?

Harrison's 20th Ed. Chapter 377 Page 2703

A. Proteoglycan
B. Glycosaminoglycan
C. Sarcoglycan
D. Dystroglycan

In Graves' disease, increased synthesis of glycosaminoglycans that trap water, thereby leading to characteristic extraocular muscle swelling.

726. Which of the following plays a major role in thyroid-associated ophthalmopathy.?

Harrison's 20th Ed. Chapter 377 Page 2703

A. Cytokines
B. Adipokines
C. Myokines
D. Chemokines

Cytokines appear to play a major role in thyroid-associated ophthalmopathy.

727. Which of the following occurs in thyroid-associated ophthalmopathy?
Harrison's 20th Ed. Chapter 377 Page 2703

A. Infiltration of extraocular muscles by activated T cells
B. Release of cytokines IFN-γ, TNF, and IL-1
C. Fibroblast activation & increased synthesis of glycosaminoglycans
D. All of the above

728. Clinical presentation of thyrotoxicosis depends on?
Harrison's 20th Ed. Chapter 377 Page 2703

A. Severity of thyrotoxicosis
B. Duration of disease
C. Patient's age
D. All of the above

Clinical presentation of thyrotoxicosis depends on the severity of thyrotoxicosis, the duration of disease, individual susceptibility to excess thyroid hormone, and the patient's age.

729. Which of the following about apathetic thyrotoxicosis is false?
Harrison's 20th Ed. Chapter 377 Page 2703

A. Elderly
B. Fatigue and weight loss
C. Features of thyrotoxicosis may be subtle or masked
D. None of the above

Absence of hyperkinetic motor activity, hand tremor & ocular signs, typical of Graves' disease is noteworthy. Apathetic thyrotoxicosis may be mistaken for depression in the elderly.

730. Thyrotoxicosis may be associated with?
Harrison's 20th Ed. Chapter 377 Page 2704

A. Hyperkalemic periodic paralysis
B. Hypokalemic periodic paralysis
C. Myotonia congenita
D. Potassium aggravated myotonia

Thyrotoxicosis is sometimes associated with a form of hypokalemic periodic paralysis that is particularly common in Asian males with thyrotoxicosis.

731. Thyrotoxicosis may be associated with?
Harrison's 20th Ed. Chapter 377 Page 2704

A. Proximal myopathy without fasciculation
B. Chorea
C. Hypokalemic periodic paralysis
D. All of the above

732. Out of the following, which is the most common symptom of hyperthyroidism?
Harrison's 20th Ed. Chapter 377 Page 2703 Table 377-2

A. Palpitation
B. Heat intolerance and sweating
C. Weight loss and increased appetite
D. Diarrhea

733. Out of the following, which is the most common symptom of hyperthyroidism?
Harrison's 20th Ed. Chapter 377 Page 2703 Table 377-2

A. Tremor
B. Warm, moist skin
C. Tachycardia
D. Lid retraction or lag

734. In hyperthyroidism, von Graefe's sign refers to?
Del J Ophthalmol 2012;22(4):249-55

A. Lagging of upper eye lid on looking downward
B. Retracted lids causing wide palpebral opening
C. Diminished frequency of blinking
D. Inability to maintain convergence for close vision

735. In hyperthyroidism, Stellwag's sign refers to?
Del J Ophthalmol 2012;22(4):249-255

A. Lagging of upper eye lid on looking downward
B. Retracted lids causing wide palpebral opening
C. Diminished frequency of blinking
D. Inability to maintain convergence for close vision

736. In hyperthyroidism, Dalrymple's sign refers to?
Del J Ophthalmol 2012;22(4):249-55

A. Lagging of upper eye lid on looking downward
B. Retracted lids causing wide palpebral opening
C. Diminished frequency of blinking
D. Inability to maintain convergence for close vision

737. In hyperthyroidism, Moebius' sign refers to?
Del J Ophthalmol 2012;22(4):249-55

A. Lagging of upper eye lid on looking downward
B. Retracted lids causing wide palpebral opening
C. Diminished frequency of blinking
D. Inability to maintain convergence for close vision

738. In hyperthyroidism, Abadie's sign refers to?
Del J Ophthalmol 2012;22(4):249-55

A. Involuntary twitching or spasm of LPS muscle
B. Retracted lids causing wide palpebral opening
C. Diminished frequency of blinking
D. Inability to maintain convergence for close vision

Signs associated with Grave's orbitopathy include von Graefe's sign - lid lag in down gaze, Joffroy sign - absent creases in the forehead on superior gaze, Grove sign - resistance to pulling down the retracted upper lid, Stellwag sign - incomplete and infrequent blinking, Boston sign - Jerky irregular movement on downgaze, Vigouroux sign - eyelid fullness, Dalrymple's sign - a widened palpebral fissure during fixation, Kocher's sign - eye globe lag in up gaze, Möbius sign - poor convergence, Ballet sign - restriction of one or more extraocular muscles, Gifford sign - Difficulty in everting upper lid, Griffith sign - Lower lid lag on downgaze, Jellink's sign - Increased pigmentation on the lids.

739. Swellings that move with deglutition include?
Malaysian Family Physician 2014;9(2):61-63

A. Thyroglossal cyst
B. Subhyoid bursitis
C. Pretracheal lymph nodes
D. All of the above

740. Which of the following method is used in clinical examination of the thyroid gland?

A. Pizzillo's method
B. Lahey's method
C. Crile's method
D. All of the above

741. Which of the following is relevant to clinical examination of the thyroid gland?

A. Berry's Sign
B. Naffziger method
C. Scabbard trachea
D. All of the above

742. Which of the following about thyroid examination in Graves' disease is false?

Harrison's 20th Ed. Chapter 377 Page 2704

A. Diffusely enlarged-two to three times
B. No nodules
C. Thrill / bruit, best at inferolateral margins of thyroid lobes
D. None of the above

743. The earliest manifestation of ophthalmopathy in Graves' disease is?

Harrison's 20th Ed. Chapter 377 Page 2704

A. Sensation of grittiness
B. Eye discomfort
C. Excess tearing
D. All of the above

In Graves' disease, the earliest manifestations of ophthalmopathy are usually a sensation of grittiness, eye discomfort, and excess tearing.

744. Proptosis refers to visualization of sclera between border of iris and?

Harrison's 20th Ed. Chapter 377 Page 2704

A. Lower eyelid
B. Upper eyelid
C. Both the eyelids
D. Any of the above

With eyes in primary position, proptosis is best detected by visualization of sclera between the lower border of iris and the lower eyelid.

745. In Graves' disease, diplopia results when the patient looks?

Harrison's 20th Ed. Chapter 377 Page 2704

A. Up and medially
B. Up and laterally
C. Down and medially
D. Down and laterally

In Graves' disease, diplopia results, typically, but not exclusively, when the patient looks up & laterally.

746. In Graves' disease, compression of optic nerve at the apex of orbit leads to?

Harrison's 20th Ed. Chapter 377 Page 2704

A. Papilledema
B. Peripheral field defects
C. Permanent loss of vision
D. All of the above

747. In "NO SPECS" scoring system to evaluate ophthalmopathy, "P" stands for?

Harrison's 20th Ed. Chapter 377 Page 2704

A. Periorbital edema
B. Papilledema
C. Proptosis
D. Peripheral field defects

748. Which of the following is a scoring system to evaluate ophthalmopathy in Graves' disease?

Harrison's 20th Ed. Chapter 377 Page 2704

A. EOSS system
B. Bethesda system
C. EUGOGO system
D. TNM system

EUGOGO system was developed by European Group On Graves' Orbitopathy. It assesses disease activity and is preferable for monitoring and treatment purposes.

749. Hess chart best relates to?

Harrison's 20th Ed. Chapter 377 Page 2704

A. Evaluation of extraocular muscle function
B. Lid-fissure width
C. Corneal staining with fluorescein
D. Color vision

750. Which of the following about thyroid dermopathy is false?

Harrison's 20th Ed. Chapter 377 Page 2704

A. Almost always occurs in presence of ophthalmopathy
B. Over anterior & lateral aspects of lower leg
C. "Orange skin" appearance
D. None of the above

Thyroid dermopathy in Graves' disease occurs almost always in the presence of moderate or severe ophthalmopathy. It is most frequent over anterior & lateral aspects of lower leg, called pretibial myxedema.

751. Which of the following about the typical lesion in thyroid dermopathy is false?

Harrison's 20th Ed. Chapter 377 Page 2704

A. Noninflamed plaque
B. Indurated plaque
C. Deep pink or purple color plaque
D. None of the above

The typical lesion in thyroid dermopathy is a noninflamed, indurated plaque with a deep pink or purple color and an "orange skin" appearance.

752. Thyroid acropachy best relates to?

Harrison's 20th Ed. Chapter 377 Page 2704

A. Pretibial myxedema
B. Nails
C. Clubbing
D. All of the above

Thyroid acropachy refers to a form of clubbing found in <1% of patients with Graves' disease. It is so strongly associated with thyroid dermopathy.

753. Which of the following is true in Graves' disease?

Harrison's 20th Ed. Chapter 377 Page 2704

A. TSH level is suppressed
B. Total thyroid hormone levels are increased
C. Unbound thyroid hormone levels are increased
D. All of the above

In Graves' disease, TSH level is suppressed, and total and unbound thyroid hormone levels are increased.

754. Which of the following is true about T3 toxicosis?

Harrison's 20th Ed. Chapter 377 Page 2704

A. Occurs in 2–5% of thyrotoxicosis patients
B. More in areas of borderline iodine intake
C. Only T3 levels are increased
D. All of the above

755. Which of the following is true about T4 toxicosis?

Harrison's 20th Ed. Chapter 377 Page 2704

A. Normal T3 levels
B. Total and unbound T4 levels increased
C. Seen when hyperthyroidism is induced by excess iodine
D. All of the above

In T4 toxicosis, total & unbound T4 are elevated and T3 levels are normal. It is occasionally seen when hyperthyroidism is induced by excess iodine, providing surplus substrate for thyroid hormone synthesis.

756. Which of the following is increased in thyrotoxicosis?

Harrison's 20th Ed. Chapter 377 Page 2705

A. Bilirubin
B. Liver enzymes
C. Ferritin
D. All of the above

757. Which of the following is increased in thyrotoxicosis?

Harrison's 20th Ed. Chapter 377 Page 2705

A. Increased ferritin
B. Microcytic anemia
C. Thrombocytopenia
D. All of the above

758. Which of the following is a feature of subclinical hyperthyroidism?

Harrison's 20th Ed. Chapter 377 Page 2705 Table 377-2

A. Low TSH
B. Normal unbound T4
C. Normal unbound T3
D. All of the above

759. Low radionuclide uptake by thyroid is a feature of?

Harrison's 20th Ed. Chapter 377 Page 2705 Table 377-2

A. Destructive thyroiditis
B. Ectopic thyroid tissue
C. Factitious thyrotoxicosis
D. All of the above

760. Which of the following excludes Graves' disease as a cause of diffuse goiter?

Harrison's 20th Ed. Chapter 377 Page 2705 Table 377-2

A. T3
B. T4
C. TSH
D. TPO

A normal TSH also excludes Graves' disease as a cause of diffuse goiter.

761. Which of the following is an environmental goitrogen?

Harrison's 20th Ed. Chapter 377 Page 2705

A. Cassava root
B. Cabbage
C. Cauliflower
D. All of the above

762. In Graves' disease, ophthalmopathy typically worsens during?

Harrison's 20th Ed. Chapter 377 Page 2705

A. Initial 1–3 months
B. Initial 3–6 months
C. Initial 6–9 months
D. Initial 9–12 months

In Graves' disease, ophthalmopathy typically worsens over the initial 3–6 months, followed by a plateau phase over the next 12 –18 months, and then spontaneous improvement, particularly in soft tissue changes.

763. In Graves' disease, thyroid dermopathy appears how many months after development of Graves' hyperthyroidism?

Harrison's 20th Ed. Chapter 377 Page 2705

A. 1–3 months
B. 3–6 months
C. 6–12 months
D. 12–24 months

Thyroid dermopathy appears 1–2 years after the development of Graves' hyperthyroidism. It may improve spontaneously.

764. Hyperthyroidism of Graves' disease is treated by?

Harrison's 20th Ed. Chapter 377 Page 2705

A. Reducing thyroid hormone synthesis by antithyroid drug
B. Reducing amount of thyroid tissue with radioiodine (^{131}I)
C. Reducing amount of thyroid tissue by thyroidectomy
D. Any of the above

No single approach for treating hyperthyroidism of Graves' disease is optimal and that patients may require multiple treatments to achieve remission.

765. Which of the following antithyroid drugs is a thionamide?
Harrison's 20th Ed. Chapter 377 Page 2706

A. Propylthiouracil
B. Carbimazole
C. Methimazole
D. All of the above

766. All thionamide antithyroid drugs inhibit?
Harrison's 20th Ed. Chapter 377 Page 2706

A. TSH
B. TSHR
C. TPO
D. NIS

All thionamide antithyroid drugs inhibit the function of TPO, reducing oxidation & organification of iodide.

767. Indication for the use of propylthiouracil is?
Harrison's 20th Ed. Chapter 377 Page 2706

A. In first trimester of pregnancy
B. Treatment of thyroid storm
C. In patients with minor adverse reactions to methimazole
D. All of the above

768. Which of the following is the main toxicity of propylthiouracil?
Harrison's 20th Ed. Chapter 377 Page 2706

A. Nephrotoxicity
B. Hepatotoxicity
C. Hematotoxicity
D. Neurotoxicity

Propylthiouracil use has limited indications because of hepatotoxicity and shorter duration of action - 90 minutes. First trimester of pregnancy, treatment of thyroid storm, and patients with minor adverse reactions to methimazole are the main indications.

769. Titration of doses of anti-thyroid drugs is best based on?
Harrison's 20th Ed. Chapter 377 Page 2706

A. Unbound T3 levels
B. Unbound T4 levels
C. TSH
D. Any of the above

In hyperthyroidism, thyroid function tests & clinical manifestations are reviewed 4–6 weeks after starting treatment & the dose is titrated based on unbound T4 levels.

770. Which of the following regimen is used in prescribing antithyroid drugs?
Harrison's 20th Ed. Chapter 377 Page 2706

A. Combination regimen
B. Block-replace regimen
C. Basal/bolus regimen
D. Progressive regimen

In titration regimen, starting dose of an antithyroid drug is gradually reduced as thyrotoxicosis improves. Less commonly, in block-replace regimen, high doses of an antithyroid drug may be given combined with levothyroxine supplementation to avoid drug-induced hypothyroidism. The titration regimen is preferred to minimize the dose of antithyroid drug and provide an index of treatment response.

771. Maximum remission rates are achieved by how many months for the titration regimen?
Harrison's 20th Ed. Chapter 377 Page 2706

A. 3–12 months
B. 12–18 months
C. 18–24 months
D. 24–36 months

Maximum remission rates are achieved by 12–18 months for the titration regimen.

772. In Graves' disease, which of the following patients is most likely to relapse when treatment stops?
Harrison's 20th Ed. Chapter 377 Page 2706

A. Young
B. Males
C. Smokers
D. All of the above

Younger patients, males, smokers, and patients with a history of allergy, severe hyperthyroidism or large goiters are most likely to relapse when anti-thyroid drug treatment stops.

773. Agranulocytosis due to anti-thyroid drugs is?
Harrison's 20th Ed. Chapter 377 Page 2706

A. Idiosyncratic
B. Dose related
C. Duration related
D. All of the above

When using antithyroid drugs, it is not useful to monitor blood counts prospectively, as the onset of agranulocytosis is idiosyncratic and abrupt.

774. In atrial fibrillation due to thyrotoxicosis, dose of digoxin is?
Harrison's 20th Ed. Chapter 377 Page 2706

A. More
B. Less
C. Same
D. Any of the above

In atrial fibrillation due to thyrotoxicosis, increased doses of digoxin are needed.

775. Which of the following is useful in patients with thyrotoxic periodic paralysis?
Harrison's 20th Ed. Chapter 377 Page 2706

A. Warfarin
B. Beta blockers
C. Clonazepam
D. Digoxin

Beta blockers are useful in patients with thyrotoxic periodic paralysis, pending correction of thyrotoxicosis with antithyroid drugs or radioiodine.

776. Which of the following statements about atrial fibrillation in patients with thyrotoxicosis?
Harrison's 20th Ed. Chapter 377 Page 2706

A. Anticoagulation with warfarin
B. Decreased warfarin doses required in thyrotoxicosis
C. Increased digoxin doses required in thyrotoxicosis
D. None of the above

777. To avoid thyrotoxic crisis after radioiodine therapy, pretreatment with antithyroid drugs should be done for at least?

Harrison's 20th Ed. Chapter 377 Page 2706

A. 7 days
B. 14 days
C. 21 days
D. 1 month

Risk of thyrotoxic crisis after radioiodine therapy can be minimized by pretreatment with antithyroid drugs for at least a month before treatment.

778. Antithyroid drugs must be stopped how many days before administration of radioiodine?

Harrison's 20th Ed. Chapter 377 Page 2706

A. At least 1 day
B. At least 2 days
C. At least 3 days
D. At least 7 days

779. Antithyroid drugs can be restarted how many days after administration of radioiodine?

Harrison's 20th Ed. Chapter 377 Page 2706

A. 1–2 days
B. 3–7 days
C. 7–14 days
D. 14–21 days

Carbimazole or methimazole must be stopped at least 2 days before radioiodine administration to achieve optimum iodine uptake. They can be restarted 3–7 days after radioiodine, if needed. Propylthiouracil has a prolonged radioprotective effect & is stopped several weeks before radioiodine is given, or a larger dose of radioiodine will be necessary.

780. Calculated dose of radioiodine depends on?

Harrison's 20th Ed. Chapter 377 Page 2706

A. Severity of thyrotoxicosis
B. Size of the goiter
C. Level of radioiodine uptake
D. All of the above

781. Radioactive ^{131}I dose used for thyrotoxicosis is?

Harrison's 20th Ed. Chapter 377 Page 2706

A. 10 mCi–15 mCi
B. 15 mCi–25 mCi
C. 25 mCi–35 mCi
D. 35 mCi–45 mCi

^{131}I dosage generally ranges between 370 MBq (5 mCi) to 555 MBq (15 mCi).

782. Most authorities favor which of the following approach regarding radioiodine treatment for thyrotoxicosis?

Harrison's 20th Ed. Chapter 377 Page 2706

A. Hypothyroid state
B. Lesser hyperthyroid state
C. Euthyroid state
D. Any of the above

783. After radioiodine treatment for thyrotoxicosis, most patients ultimately progress to hypothyroidism over?

Harrison's 20th Ed. Chapter 377 Page 2706

A. 1–3 years
B. 3–5 years
C. 5–10 years
D. 10–15 years

After radioiodine treatment for thyrotoxicosis, most patients ultimately progress to hypothyroidism over 5–10 years. The risk of hypothyroidism after radioiodine depends on the dosage but is at least 10 –20% in the first year and 5% per year thereafter.

784. Hyperthyroidism can persist for how long before radioiodine takes full effect?

Harrison's 20th Ed. Chapter 377 Page 2706

A. 1 to 2 months
B. 2 to 3 months
C. 3 to 4 months
D. 4 to 5 months

Hyperthyroidism can persist for 2–3 months before radioiodine takes full effect.

785. Usually, second dose of radioiodine can be given after what duration in persistent hyperthyroidism?

Harrison's 20th Ed. Chapter 377 Page 2706

A. 1 month
B. 3 months
C. 6 months
D. 9 months

Persistent hyperthyroidism is treated with a 2nd dose of radioiodine, ~6 months after first dose.

786. Women can conceive safely how many months after radioiodine treatment?

Harrison's 20th Ed. Chapter 377 Page 2706

A. 1 month
B. 3 months
C. 6 months
D. 9 months

While pregnancy & breast feeding are absolute contraindications to radioiodine treatment, patients can conceive safely 6 months after treatment.

787. Which of the following drug prevents exacerbation of ophthalmopathy after radioiodine treatment for thyrotoxicosis?

Harrison's 20th Ed. Chapter 377 Page 2706

A. Prednisone
B. Colchicine
C. Thalidomide
D. All of the above

Prednisone given at the time of radioiodine treatment for Graves' disease, may prevent exacerbation of ophthalmopathy.

788. Which of the following is false about radioiodine treatment for Graves' disease?

Harrison's 20th Ed. Chapter 377 Page 2706

A. Breastfeeding is an absolute contraindication
B. Risk of cancer is not increased in adults
C. Can be used safely in older children
D. None of the above

789. Which anti-thyroid drug is preferred in pregnancy with Graves' disease?

Harrison's 20th Ed. Chapter 377 Page 2707

A. Propylthiouracil
B. Carbimazole
C. Methimazole
D. Any of the above

Propylthiouracil is titrated to lowest effective dose to manage Graves' disease in pregnancy because of relatively low transplacental transfer and its ability to block T4 to T3 conversion. Carbimazole & methimazole rarely cause fetal aplasia cutis and choanal atresia.

790. Hyperthyroidism is most difficult to control in which trimester of pregnancy?

Harrison's 20th Ed. Chapter 377 Page 2707

A. First
B. Second
C. Third
D. All of the above

791. Thyroid storm can develop in patients with?

Harrison's 20th Ed. Chapter 377 Page 2707

A. Graves' disease
B. Toxic multinodular goiter
C. Solitary toxic adenoma
D. All of the above

Thyroid storm represents the extreme manifestation of thyrotoxicosis as a true endocrine emergency.

792. Thyrotoxic crisis is precipitated by?

Harrison's 20th Ed. Chapter 377 Page 2707

A. Acute illness
B. Surgery (Thyroid / Non-thyroid surgery)
C. Radioiodine treatment
D. All of the above

793. Which of the following contribute to the development of thyroid storm?

Thyroid emergencies. Rev Endocr Metab Disord 2003;4:129

A. Rapid rate of increase in serum thyroid hormone levels
B. Increased responsiveness to catecholamines
C. Enhanced cellular responses to thyroid hormone
D. All of the above

794. Mortality in thyrotoxic crisis, or thyroid storm is due to?

Harrison's 20th Ed. Chapter 377 Page 2707

A. Cardiac failure
B. Arrhythmia
C. Hyperthermia
D. All of the above

In thyrotoxic crisis, or thyroid storm, mortality rate due to cardiac failure, arrhythmia, or hyperthermia is as high as 30%, even with treatment. CNS involvement is a poor prognostic factor for increased mortality.

795. Which of the following is used in the management of thyrotoxic crisis?

Harrison's 20th Ed. Chapter 377 Page 2707

A. Propylthiouracil
B. Stable iodide
C. β-adrenergic blockers
D. All of the above

The approach to the management of thyrotoxic crisis includes therapy to control increased adrenergic tone: Beta-blocker, therapy to reduce thyroid hormone synthesis: Thionamide, therapy to reduce release of thyroid hormone: Iodine solution, therapy to block peripheral conversion of T4 to T3: Iodinated radiocontrast agent, glucocorticoid, PTU, propranolol and therapy to reduce enterohepatic recycling of thyroid hormone: Bile acid sequestrant. An hour after the administration of propylthiouracil or methimazole, five drops of SSKI (super saturated potassium iodide) is given by mouth every 6 hours.

796. Which of the following is used in the management of thyrotoxic crisis?

Harrison's 20th Ed. Chapter 377 Page 2707

A. Colchicine
B. Simvastatin
C. Cholestyramine
D. Ezetimibe

Oral Cholestyramine (4 grams four times daily) is used to sequester thyroid hormones. Plasmapheresis is the last resort if all other measures fail.

797. Which of the following is a scoring system for the diagnosis of thyroid storm?

Endocrinol. Metab. Clin. North Am. 1993;22(2):263-77

A. Lake Louise Scoring System
B. Burch-Wartofsky Point Scale (BWPS)
C. 4T scoring system
D. SOI scoring system

798. Which of the following may be beneficial in thyroid dermopathy?

Harrison's 20th Ed. Chapter 377 Page 2707

A. Aprepitant
B. Octreotide
C. Cabergoline
D. Vitamin D

799. Which of the following is a cause of thyrotoxicosis with low or absent thyroid radionuclide uptake?

Harrison's 20th Ed. Chapter 377 Page 2707

A. Thyrotoxicosis factitia
B. Struma ovarii
C. Functional metastatic follicular carcinoma
D. All of the above

Causes of thyrotoxicosis with low or absent thyroid radionuclide uptake include thyrotoxicosis factitia, iodine excess, and, rarely, ectopic thyroid tissue, particularly teratomas of the ovary (struma ovarii) and functional metastatic follicular carcinoma.

800. Which of the following is false about destructive thyroiditis?

Harrison's 20th Ed. Chapter 377 Page 2707

A. Increased thyroid hormones
B. Low radionuclide uptake
C. Increased circulating thyroglobulin levels
D. None of the above

801. Estimation of which of the following supports the diagnosis of TSH-secreting pituitary adenoma?

Harrison's 20th Ed. Chapter 377 Page 2708

A. α-subunit of TSH
B. β-subunit of TSH
C. γ-subunit of TSH
D. δ-subunit of TSH

Diagnosis of TSH-secreting adenoma is supported by demonstrating elevated levels of α-subunit of TSH. α-subunit is nearly identical to that of human chorionic gonadotropin (hCG), luteinizing hormone (LH), and follicle-stimulating hormone (FSH). β-subunit is unique and specific to TSH.

802. Which of the following best relates to acute thyroiditis?

Harrison's 20th Ed. Chapter 377 Page 2708

A. Petrosal sinus
B. Piriform sinus
C. Urogenital sinus
D. Cavernous sinus

Piriform sinus, a remnant of the fourth branchial pouch that connects the oropharynx with the thyroid. It can cause acute thyroiditis in children and young adults.

803. Which of the following is not a cause of chronic thyroiditis?

Harrison's 20th Ed. Chapter 377 Page 2708 Table 377-3

A. Riedel's thyroiditis
B. Hashimoto's thyroiditis
C. Radiation thyroiditis after ^{131}I treatment
D. Parasitic thyroiditis (Echinococcosis)

804. Which of the following can cause acute, subacute or chronic thyroiditis?

Harrison's 20th Ed. Chapter 377 Page 2708 Table 377-3

A. ^{131}I treatment
B. Amiodarone
C. Mycobacterial infection
D. Riedel's thyroiditis

805. de Quervain's thyroiditis is a type of?

Harrison's 20th Ed. Chapter 377 Page 2708

A. Acute thyroiditis
B. Subacute thyroiditis
C. Chronic thyroiditis
D. Any of the above

806. Subacute thyroiditis is also termed as?

Harrison's 20th Ed. Chapter 377 Page 2708

A. de Quervain's thyroiditis
B. Granulomatous thyroiditis
C. Viral thyroiditis
D. All of the above

Subacute Thyroiditis is also termed de Quervain's thyroiditis, granulomatous thyroiditis, or viral thyroiditis.

807. Which of the following viruses has been implicated in the causation of subacute thyroiditis?

Harrison's 20th Ed. Chapter 377 Page 2708

A. Mumps
B. Coxsackie
C. Influenza
D. All of the above

Many viruses have been implicated in the causation of subacute thyroiditis, including mumps, coxsackie, influenza, adenoviruses, and echoviruses.

808. Symptoms of subacute thyroiditis mimic?

Harrison's 20th Ed. Chapter 377 Page 2708

A. Otitis media
B. Pharyngitis
C. GERD
D. Glossitis

The diagnosis of subacute thyroiditis is often overlooked because the symptoms can mimic pharyngitis.

809. Which of the following about Hashitoxicosis is false?

Thyroid Res Pract 2013;10:5-6

A. Transient hyperthyroid phase of chronic autoimmune thyroiditis
B. Normal / slightly increased vascularity of thyroid
C. May be caused by pegylated interferon-α2b and ribavirin
D. None of the above

Crucial USG difference between Graves' disease & Hashitoxicosis rests on assessment of vascularity.

810. In subacute thyroiditis, pain is referred to?

Harrison's 20th Ed. Chapter 377 Page 2708

A. Jaw
B. Retrosternum
C. Axilla
D. Occiput

In subacute thyroiditis, pain is referred to the jaw or ear.

811. Which of the following is the initial phase in the course of subacute thyroiditis?

Harrison's 20th Ed. Chapter 377 Page 2708

A. Thyrotoxic phase
B. Hypothyroid phase
C. Recovery phase
D. Any of the above

In the course of subacute thyroiditis, thyroid function tests characteristically evolve through three distinct phases over about 6 months—thyrotoxic phase, hypothyroid phase and recovery phase.

812. Which of the following is false about subacute thyroiditis?

Harrison's 20th Ed. Chapter 377 Page 2708

A. High ESR
B. Low radioiodine uptake
C. Aspirin is effective
D. Thyroid antibodies present

In subacute thyroiditis, diagnosis is confirmed by a high ESR, low radioiodine uptake and thyroid antibodies are negative.

813. In subacute thyroiditis, which of the following thyroid function should be monitored?

Harrison's 20th Ed. Chapter 377 Page 2708

A. Total T4 levels
B. Unbound T4 levels
C. Total T3 levels
D. Unbound T3 levels

Thyroid function should be monitored every 2–4 weeks using TSH and unbound T4 levels.

814. Painless thyroiditis, or "silent" thyroiditis, occurs in patients with underlying?

Harrison's 20th Ed. Chapter 377 Page 2708

A. Malignancy
B. Autoimmune thyroid disease
C. Granulomatous disease
D. Iodine deficiency

Painless thyroiditis, or "silent" thyroiditis, occurs in patients with underlying autoimmune thyroid disease.

815. Postpartum thyroiditis occurs how many months after pregnancy?

Harrison's 20th Ed. Chapter 377 Page 2708

A. 1 to 3 months
B. 3 to 6 months
C. 6 to 9 months
D. Any of the above

Postpartum thyroiditis occurs 3–6 months after pregnancy.

816. Which of the following is false about silent thyroiditis?

Harrison's 20th Ed. Chapter 377 Page 2708

A. High ESR
B. Low radioiodine uptake
C. No thyroid tenderness
D. Presence of TPO antibodies

Silent thyroiditis features a painless goiter, normal ESR and presence of TPO antibodies.

817. Which of the following is not indicated for silent thyroiditis?

Harrison's 20th Ed. Chapter 377 Page 2708

A. Glucocorticoid
B. Propranolol
C. Thyroxine
D. All of the above

Glucocorticoid treatment is not indicated for silent thyroiditis.

818. Which of the following can cause thyroiditis?

Harrison's 20th Ed. Chapter 377 Page 2708

A. IFN-a
B. IL-2
C. Amiodarone
D. All of the above

Patients receiving IFN-a, IL-2 or amiodarone may develop painless thyroiditis.

819. Which of the following is false about Riedel's thyroiditis?

Harrison's 20th Ed. Chapter 377 Page 2708

A. Painless goiter
B. Dense fibrosis of thyroid
C. Thyroid dysfunction common
D. Tamoxifen therapy beneficial

Riedel's thyroiditis is seen in middle-aged women. Presents insidiously as painless goiter with local symptoms due to compression of esophagus, trachea, neck veins or recurrent laryngeal nerves. Dense fibrosis disrupts normal gland architecture that can extend outside thyroid capsule. Despite extensive histologic changes, thyroid dysfunction is uncommon. Tamoxifen may be beneficial.

820. Riedel's thyroiditis is associated with which of the following?

Harrison's 20th Ed. Chapter 377 Page 2708

A. Multiple myeloma
B. IgG4-related disease
C. Primary biliary cirrhosis
D. Sarcoidosis

821. Riedel's thyroiditis is associated with fibrosis of?

Harrison's 20th Ed. Chapter 377 Page 2708

A. Retroperitoneum
B. Mediastinum
C. Lung
D. All of the above

Riedel's thyroiditis is associated with idiopathic fibrosis in retroperitoneum, mediastinum, biliary tree, lung, and orbit.

822. Which of the following is false about sick euthyroid syndrome?

Harrison's 20th Ed. Chapter 377 Page 2708

A. Decreased total & unbound T3 levels
B. Normal T4 levels
C. Normal TSH levels
D. None of the above

In sick euthyroid syndrome (SES), there is a decrease in total & unbound T3 levels (low T3 syndrome) with normal levels of T4 and TSH.

823. Which of the following is increased in sick euthyroid syndrome?

Harrison's 20th Ed. Chapter 377 Page 2708

A. Total T3 levels
B. Unbound T3 levels
C. Reverse T3 levels
D. TSH levels

T4 conversion to T3 via peripheral deiodination is impaired, leading to increased reverse T3 (rT3).

824. Increased rT3 is found in?

Harrison's 20th Ed. Chapter 377 Page 2708

A. Sick euthyroid syndrome (SES)
B. Nonthyroidal illness (NTI)
C. Low T3 syndrome
D. All of the above

825. Increased rT3 in sick euthyroid syndrome is due to?

Harrison's 20th Ed. Chapter 377 Page 2708

A. Decreased clearance of rT3
B. Increased production of rT3
C. T4 metabolization to hormonally inactive T3 sulfate
D. All of the above

Decreased clearance rather than increased production is the reason for increased rT3.

826. Low T3 state can be induced in normal individuals by?

Harrison's 20th Ed. Chapter 377 Page 2708

A. Exercise
B. Dehydration
C. Fasting
D. Insomnia

Low T3 state is an adaptive phenomenon and can be induced in normal individuals by fasting.

827. Amiodarone contains which of the following elements?

Harrison's 20th Ed. Chapter 377 Page 2708

A. Zinc
B. Iodine
C. Calcium
D. Iron

Amiodarone is structurally related to thyroid hormone & contains 39% iodine by weight.

828. Which of the following statements about amiodarone-induced thyrotoxicosis (AIT) is false?

Harrison's 20th Ed. Chapter 377 Page 2708

A. Type 1 AIT is associated with an underlying thyroid abnormality
B. No intrinsic thyroid abnormalities in Type 2 AIT
C. Increased vascularity in AIT1, decreased vascularity in AIT2
D. None of the above

829. Amiodarone has antiparasite activity against?

Antimicrob Agents Chemother. 2011;55(1):203-10

A. Treponema pallidum
B. Trypanosoma cruzi
C. Babesia duncani
D. Toxoplasma gondii

Amiodarone has a selective antiproliferative effect on T. cruzi.

830. During pregnancy, thyroid hormone requirements are?

Int J Reprod Biomed (Yazd). 2016;14(11):677–86

A. Increased
B. Decreased
C. Same
D. Any of the above

831. During pregnancy, urinary iodide excretion is?

Int J Reprod Biomed (Yazd). 2016;14(11):677–86

A. Increased
B. Decreased
C. Same
D. Any of the above

Thyroid Nodular Disease and Thyroid Cancer

832. Goiter refers to?

Harrison's 20th Ed. Chapter 378 Page 2710

A. Enlarged thyroid gland
B. Enlarged thyroid & ectopic thyroid gland
C. Enlarged thyroid, & ectopic thyroid & parathyroid gland
D. All of the above

Goiter refers to an enlarged thyroid gland.

833. Which of the following can lead to goiter?

Harrison's 20th Ed. Chapter 378 Page 2710

A. Iodine deficiency
B. Autoimmune diseases
C. Nodular diseases
D. All of the above

Biosynthetic defects, iodine deficiency, autoimmune disease, and nodular diseases can lead to goiter.

834. Thyroid nodular disease is characterized by?

Harrison's 20th Ed. Chapter 378 Page 2710

A. Disordered growth of thyroid cells
B. Growth of thyroid cells may be hyperplastic or neoplastic
C. Normal thyroid parenchyma replaced
D. All of the above

835. Which of the following about nodular thyroid disease is false?

Harrison's 20th Ed. Chapter 378 Page 2710

A. By USG, thyroid nodules are present in ~50% of adults
B. Majority of thyroid nodules are <1 cm in diameter
C. May be solitary or multiple, functional or nonfunctional
D. None of the above

Nodular thyroid disease occurs in ~3–7% of adults when assessed by physical examination.

836. Which of the following about diffuse nontoxic goiter is false?

Harrison's 20th Ed. Chapter 378 Page 2710

A. Diffuse enlargement of thyroid
B. Absence of nodules
C. Absence of hyperthyroidism
D. None of the above

When diffuse enlargement of thyroid occurs in the absence of nodules and hyperthyroidism, it is referred to as a diffuse nontoxic goiter or simple goiter or colloid goiter.

837. Which of the following is related to diffuse nontoxic goiter?

Harrison's 20th Ed. Chapter 378 Page 2710

A. Endemic goiter
B. Sporadic goiter
C. Juvenile goiter
D. All of the above

838. Which of the following diffuse goiter is most commonly caused by iodine deficiency?

Harrison's 20th Ed. Chapter 378 Page 2710

A. Endemic goiter
B. Sporadic goiter
C. Juvenile goiter
D. All of the above

Worldwide, diffuse goiter is most commonly caused by iodine deficiency and is termed endemic goiter when it affects >5% of the population.

839. Which of the following statements is false?

Harrison's 20th Ed. Chapter 378 Page 2711

A. Goiter is more common in women than men
B. TSH levels are normal or slightly increased in endemic goiter
C. Iodide has direct actions on thyroid vasculature
D. None of the above

840. Endemic goiter may be caused by?

Harrison's 20th Ed. Chapter 378 Page 2711

A. Exposure to cassava root
B. Exposure to vegetables of the Cruciferae family
C. Exposure to milk where goitrogens are present in grass
D. All of the above

841. Which of the following statements about diffuse goiter is false?

Harrison's 20th Ed. Chapter 378 Page 2711

A. Symmetrically enlarged
B. Nontender
C. Soft thyroid gland without palpable nodules
D. None of the above

842. In goiter, lateral lobe of thyroid has a volume greater than?

Harrison's 20th Ed. Chapter 378 Page 2711

A. Tongue of the individual being examined
B. Thumb of the individual being examined
C. External ear of the individual being examined
D. Both eyes of the individual being examined

Goiter is defined as a lateral lobe with a volume greater than the thumb of the individual being examined.

843. On ultrasound, total thyroid volume exceeding how much is considered abnormal?

Harrison's 20th Ed. Chapter 378 Page 2711

A. 10 mL
B. 20 mL
C. 30 mL
D. 40 mL

On ultrasound, total thyroid volume exceeding 30 mL is considered abnormal.

844. Which of the following is called Pemberton's maneuver?
N Engl J Med 2004;350:1338

A. Elevation of one arm followed by elevation of other arm
B. Abduction of one arm followed by abduction of other arm
C. Elevation of both arms until they touch the side of the head
D. Abduction of both arms

Pemberton's maneuver is elevation of both arms "until they touch the side of the head". It elicits, after a minute or so, congestion of the face, cyanosis, and lastly distress. The observed vascular engorgement and facial congestion indicate impaired venous outflow from the head & neck. Tracheal compromise may accompany it. Tracheal compression or obstruction of the thoracic inlet is more likely with substernal MNGs

845. Which of the following best relates to Pemberton's sign?
J Clin Endocrinol Metab, 2014,99(6):1949-54

A. Apple effect
B. Bubble gum effect
C. Cork effect
D. Dinner table effect

One hypothesis is that Pemberton's sign as a result of arm elevation causing "plugging" and obstructing the thyroid gland and its surrounding structure against bony thoracic inlet or so-called thyroid "cork effect." According to others, the obstruction is due to elevation of the thoracic inlet against the thyroid.

846. Which of the following is true in a case of goiter due to iodine deficiency?
Harrison's 20th Ed. Chapter 378 Page 2711

A. Low total T4
B. Normal T3
C. Normal TSH
D. All of the above

In a case of goiter due to iodine deficiency, a low total T4, with normal T3 and TSH, reflecting enhanced T4 $\rightarrow$ T3 conversion is frequently observed.

847. Which of the following is true in a case of subclinical thyrotoxicosis?
Harrison's 20th Ed. Chapter 378 Page 2711

A. Low TSH
B. Normal free T3
C. Normal free T4
D. All of the above

Low TSH with a normal free T3 & free T4, particularly in older patients, suggests the possibility of thyroid autonomy or undiagnosed Graves' disease, and is termed subclinical thyrotoxicosis. Treatment is increasingly recommended in elderly to reduce the risk of atrial fibrillation & bone loss.

848. Urinary iodine levels are considered low, when its levels are?
Harrison's 20th Ed. Chapter 378 Page 2711

A. < 50 μg/L
B. < 100 μg/L
C. < 150 μg/L
D. < 200 μg/L

Low urinary iodine levels (<50 μg/L) support a diagnosis of iodine deficiency.

849. Which of the following about nontoxic multinodular goiter (MNG) is false?
Harrison's 20th Ed. Chapter 378 Page 2711

A. More common in women than men
B. Increases in prevalence with age
C. More common in iodine-deficient regions
D. Most patients are hypothyroid

Most patients with nontoxic multinodular goiter (MNG) are asymptomatic and euthyroid.

850. Which of the following about nontoxic multinodular goiter (MNG) is false?
Harrison's 20th Ed. Chapter 378 Page 2711

A. Hypercellular / hyperplastic / cystic filled with colloid
B. Fibrosis is extensive
C. Most nodules within MNG are monoclonal in origin
D. TSH is usually not elevated

Most nodules within MNG are polyclonal in origin.

851. Tracheal compression must exceed what % of tracheal diameter before there is a significant airway compromise?
Harrison's 20th Ed. Chapter 378 Page 2711

A. 50%
B. 60%
C. 70%
D. 80%

In nontoxic multinodular goiter, tracheal deviation is common, but compression must usually exceed 70% of the tracheal diameter before there is a significant airway compromise.

852. Which of the following USG finding raises high suspicion for thyroid malignancy?
Harrison's 20th Ed. Chapter 378 Page 2712 Figure 378-1

A. Hypoechoic solid nodule
B. Irregular borders
C. Microcalcifications
D. All of the above

853. Which of the following USG finding indicates low suspicion for thyroid malignancy?
Harrison's 20th Ed. Chapter 378 Page 2712 Figure 378-1

A. Spongiform nodule
B. Microcystic areas
C. Comprising > 50% of nodule volume
D. All of the above

854. Iodine induced hyperthyroidism best relates to?
Harrison's 20th Ed. Chapter 378 Page 2712

A. Wolff-Chaikoff effect
B. Jod-Basedow effect
C. Disulfiram-like effect
D. Gallavardin effect

Jod-Basedow Phenomenon: Iodine induced hyperthyroidism. Wolff-Chaikoff Effect: Iodine induced hypothyroidism. Contrast agents and other iodine-containing substances should be avoided because of the risk of inducing the Jod-Basedow effect, characterized by enhanced thyroid hormone production by autonomous nodules.

855. Which of the following is false about solitary hyperfunctioning thyroid adenomas?

Ann Endocrinol. 2003;64(1):17-22

A. Benign monoclonal tumors
B. Autonomously produce thyroxine (T4) & triiodothyronine (T3)
C. Not influenced by thyrotropin (TSH)
D. None of the above

Solitary hyperfunctioning thyroid adenomas are benign monoclonal tumors characterized by their capacity to grow and produce thyroxine (T4) and triiodothyronine (T3) autonomously, i.e. in the absence of thyrotropin (TSH). Mutations of the TSH receptor (TSH-R) have been found in the majority of solitary hyperfunctioning thyroid adenomas. The rate of development of thyrotoxicosis in patients with hyperfunctioning adenomas who are euthyroid initially is about 4% per year and depends on the size of the adenoma, iodine intake and age of the patient.

856. Which of the following is false about thyroid autonomy?

Genomics 2011;97(2):94-100

A. TSH-independent function & proliferation of thyroid follicles
B. Most frequent cause is TSH receptor mutations
C. Highly prevalent in geographic regions with iodide deficiency
D. None of the above

857. Gene important for thyroid function is?

Genomics 2011;97(2):94-100

A. Tpo
B. Nis
C. Thrsp
D. All of the above

Genes important for thyroid function are Tpo, Nis, Thrsp and Iyd. The iodotyrosine deiodinase (iyd) also known as DEHAL1, facilitates iodide salvage in the thyroid cell thyroid by catalyzing the NADPH-dependent deiodination of mono (L-MIT) and diiodotyrosine (L-DIT). iyd and oncogen junB are upregulated, while sodium-iodide-symporter (Nis) and thyroid peroxidase (Tpo) are downregulated by iodide. Iodine status is a major factor that affects the expression of NIS gene.

858. Low levels of NIS expression is found in?

Front Endocrinol (Lausanne). 2018; 9: 566

A. Non-toxic multinodular goiter (NMNG)
B. Diffuse iodine deficiency goiter (IDG)
C. Solitary malignant thyroid nodules
D. All of the above

Low levels of NIS expression is found in non-toxic multinodular goiter (NMNG), diffuse iodine deficiency goiter (IDG), and solitary malignant thyroid nodules.

859. MBq stands for?

The Journal of Clinical Endocrinology & Metabolism 88(3):975–77

A. Mega Bequeath
B. Mega Bequest
C. Mega Bequep
D. Mega Bequerel

Bequerel (Bq) is a unit of radioactivity, 1 disintegration per second. Mega Bequerel (MBq) is 106 disintegrations per second. Gray (Gy) is a unit of absorbed dose (1 Joule/kg), Rad is a unit of absorbed dose (100 erg/g), Curie (Ci) is a unit of radioactivity ($3.7x10^{10}$ disintegrations per second). 1 MBq=27 Ci, 1 GBq=27 mCi, 1 mCi=37 MBq.

860. Variable affecting the outcome of radioiodine dose is?

The Journal of Clinical Endocrinology & Metabolism 88(3):975–77

A. Age
B. Gender
C. Gland size
D. All of the above

861. Variable affecting the outcome of radioiodine dose is?

The Journal of Clinical Endocrinology & Metabolism 88(3):975–77

A. Severity & duration of underlying autoimmune thyroid stimulus
B. Preceding antithyroid drug therapy
C. Stopping time of antithyroid drug before radioiodine treatment
D. All of the above

There is no single radioiodine dose or treatment method that can reliably accomplish the goal of euthyroidism. Variables affecting outcome include age, gender, gland size, severity & duration of underlying autoimmune thyroid stimulus, radiation delivered to the gland (^{131}I fractional uptake, homogeneity of distribution, and effective half-life) and preceding antithyroid drug therapy and stopping time before radioiodine treatment.

862. What is the dosage of ^{131}I in nontoxic multinodular goiter?

Harrison's 20th Ed. Chapter 378 Page 2712

A. 1.7 MBq per gram of tissue
B. 2.7 MBq per gram of tissue
C. 3.7 MBq per gram of tissue
D. 4.7 MBq per gram of tissue

Dosage of ^{131}I depends on size of goiter & radioiodine uptake and its usually ~3.7 MBq (0.1 mCi) per gram of tissue, corrected for uptake (typical dose 370-1070 MBq [10–29 mCi]).

863. Effectiveness of ^{131}I therapy is increased by concurrent administration of?

Harrison's 20th Ed. Chapter 378 Page 2712

A. Low-dose recombinant T3
B. Low-dose recombinant T4
C. Low-dose recombinant TSH
D. Low-dose recombinant glucocorticoids TSH

Effectiveness of ^{131}I therapy is increased by concurrent administration of low-dose recombinant TSH (0.1 mg IM).

864. Which of the following is a ^{131}I therapy complication while treating nontoxic MNG?

Harrison's 20th Ed. Chapter 378 Page 2712

A. Thyroid swelling and tracheal compression
B. Radiation-induced hypothyroidism
C. Autoimmune thyrotoxicosis
D. All of the above

865. Germline & somatic activating mutations of TSHR have been reported in?

Front Endocrinol (Lausanne). 2018; 9: 566

A. Familial nonautoimmune hyperthyroidism (FNAH)
B. Sporadic congenital nonautoimmune hyperthyroidism (SCNAH)
C. Autonomously functioning thyroid nodules (AFTNs)
D. All of the above

866. Compensated hypothyroidism best relates to?

Front Endocrinol (Lausanne). 2018; 9: 566

A. Euthyroidism with normal serum TSH

B. Euthyroidism with elevated serum TSH

C. Euthyroidism with decreased serum TSH

D. Any of the above

Loss-of-function mutations of TSHR have been found to cause "compensated hypothyroidism" i.e. euthyroidism with elevated serum TSH.

867. TSHR mutation concurrent with which of the following thyroid cancer-related genetic alterations have a high probability of thyroid cancer?

Front Endocrinol (Lausanne). 2018; 9: 566

A. BRAF

B. GNAS

C. RAS

D. All of the above

TSHR mutation concurrent with other thyroid cancer-related genetic alterations like BRAF, GNAS, RAS, TP53, TRK, PAX8/PPARr, and RET/PTC, or TSHR mutations occurring with very high allelic frequency may have a high probability of thyroid cancer.

868. Genetic abnormality known to confer functional autonomy of thyroid is?

Harrison's 20th Ed. Chapter 378 Page 2712

A. Gαq/Gα11 mutations

B. Gsα mutations

C. Giα mutations

D. CaSR mutations

Genetic abnormalities known to confer functional autonomy, such as activating TSH-R or Gsα mutations, are not usually found in the autonomous regions of toxic MNG goiter.

869. Which of the following about thyroid-stimulating hormone (TSH) receptor (TSHR) is false?

Front Endocrinol (Lausanne). 2018; 9: 566

A. Member of the glycoprotein hormone receptors (GPHRs)

B. Member of class A G protein-coupled receptors (GPCRs)

C. Ligand is thyrotropin

D. None of the above

870. Which of the following is the most frequently detected TSH mutation in autonomously functioning thyroid nodules (AFTN)?

Front Endocrinol (Lausanne). 2018; 9: 566

A. M453R

B. M453S

C. M453T

D. M453U

M453T is the most prevalent mutation in tissue samples from known AFTNs. Gain-of-function mutations of TSHR constitutively stimulates TSH-adenylcyclase-cAMP pathway to increase the uptake of iodine by thyrocytes and to produce thyroid hormones.

871. Toxic adenoma best relates to?

Harrison's 20th Ed. Chapter 378 Page 2713

A. Solitary, autonomously functioning thyroid nodule

B. Solitary, non-autonomously functioning thyroid nodule

C. Multiple, autonomously functioning thyroid nodule

D. Multiple, non-autonomously functioning thyroid nodule

A solitary, autonomously functioning thyroid nodule is referred to as toxic adenoma.

872. Which of the following about solitary hyperfunctioning nodule is false?

Harrison's 20th Ed. Chapter 378 Page 2713

A. Thyrotoxicosis when nodule is >3 cm.

B. ↓ TSH level

C. Absence of clinical features suggestive of Graves' disease

D. None of the above

873. Which of the following is the treatment of choice in hyperfunctioning solitary nodule?

Harrison's 20th Ed. Chapter 378 Page 2713

A. Radioiodine ablation

B. Lobectomy

C. US guided percutaneous radiofrequency thermal ablation

D. Antithyroid drugs and beta blockers

Radioiodine ablation is the treatment of choice in hyperfunctioning solitary nodule.

874. In solitary hyperfunctioning nodules, mutations that activate TSH-R reside mainly in?

Harrison's 20th Ed. Chapter 378 Page 2713 Figure 378-2

A. Transmembrane 2

B. Transmembrane 3

C. Transmembrane 4

D. Transmembrane 5

Most patients with solitary hyperfunctioning nodules have acquired somatic, activating mutations in TSH-R. The mutations that activate TSH-R reside mainly in transmembrane 5 and intracellular loop 3.

875. Thyroid adenomas or multinodular goitre are frequent in?

Harrison's 20th Ed. Chapter 378 Page 2713

A. Carney complex

B. von Hippel-Lindau disease

C. McCune Albright syndrome

D. All of the above

Thyroid adenomas or multinodular goitre are frequent in McCune Albright syndrome, which is characterized by pure Gs stimulation.

876. Hereditary toxic thyroid hyperplasia (HTTH) is also called?

Front Endocrinol (Lausanne). 2018; 9: 566

A. Tuttle disease

B. Leclère's disease

C. Fagin disease

D. Haugen disease

Hereditary toxic thyroid hyperplasia (HTTH), called Leclère's disease, is characterized by the following clinical characteristics: autosomal dominant transmission; hyperthyroidism with a variable age of onset (from infancy to adulthood, even within a given family); hyperplastic goiter of variable size, but with a steady growth; absence of clinical or biological stigmata of auto-immunity. Contrary to tissue from Graves' disease patients, HTTH cells continue to grow in the absence of stimulation by TSH or TSAb.

877. Thyroid adenoma composed of oncocytic follicular cells arranged in a follicular pattern is termed as?

Harrison's 20th Ed. Chapter 378 Page 2713

A. Leydig cell adenoma
B. Brunner cell adenoma
C. Hürthle cell adenoma
D. Davis cell adenoma

Thyroid adenoma composed of oncocytic follicular cells arranged in a follicular pattern is termed a Hürthle cell adenoma. Oncocytic cell is also called Hürthle, Askanazy and oxyphilic cells.

878. Which of the following about Hürthle cell is false?

The Oncologist 2011;16:1380–87

A. Oncocyte
B. Epithelial cell with an acidophilic cytoplasm
C. Contains large number of mitochondria
D. None of the above

An oncocyte is simply an epithelial cell with an acidophilic cytoplasm, containing a vast number of mitochondria. They are found throughout body, including kidney, salivary glands, parathyroids, as well as thyroid gland.

879. Large polygonal size (10 –15 µm) size of Hürthle cell is due to increased number of?

The Oncologist 2011;16:1380–87

A. Lysosomes
B. Mitochondria
C. Smooth endoplasmic reticulum (ER)
D. Neurosecretory granules

Hürthle cells (HCs) contain up to 5,000 mitochondria, whereas a typical eosinophil may contain 30.

880. Definition of thyroid spongiform lesions on US requires presence of microcystic areas comprising how much of nodule volume?

Harrison's 20th Ed. Chapter 378 Page 2713

A. > 10%
B. > 20%
C. > 40%
D. > 50%

The definition of thyroid spongiform lesions on ultrasound requires the presence of microcystic areas comprising >50% of the nodule volume.

881. Which of the following is the most common malignancy of the endocrine system?

Harrison's 20th Ed. Chapter 378 Page 2714

A. Parathyroid adenoma
B. Pheochromocytoma
C. Enteropancreatic tumor
D. Thyroid carcinoma

Thyroid carcinoma is the most common malignancy of the endocrine system.

882. Which out of the following thyroid carcinoma is aggressive, responds poorly to treatment, & is associated with a bleak prognosis?

Harrison's 20th Ed. Chapter 378 Page 2714

A. Papillary thyroid cancer (PTC)
B. Follicular thyroid cancer (FTC)
C. Anaplastic thyroid cancer (ATC)
D. Medullary thyroid cancer

Anaplastic thyroid cancer (ATC) is aggressive, responds poorly to treatment, and is associated with a bleak prognosis.

883. Which out of the following malignant thyroid growths has the maximum prevalence?

Harrison's 20th Ed. Chapter 378 Page 2713 Table 378-2

A. Follicular carcinomas
B. Papillary carcinomas
C. Medullary thyroid cancer
D. Lymphomas

Increased incidence of thyroid cancers is predominantly due to small T1 papillary cancer tumors (<2 cm).

884. Which out of the following about thyroid cancer is false?

Harrison's 20th Ed. Chapter 378 Page 2714

A. Prognosis is worse in older persons (>65 years) & in males
B. Thyroid cancer is twice as common in women as men
C. H/o childhood (<18) head or neck irradiation is a risk factor
D. None of the above

885. Which out of the following genetic syndrome is associated with thyroid malignancy?

Harrison's 20th Ed. Chapter 378 Page 2714 Table 378-3

A. Cowden's syndrome
B. Familial polyposis
C. Carney complex
D. All of the above

Genetic syndromes associated with thyroid malignancy include Cowden's syndrome, familial polyposis, Carney complex, PTEN (phosphatase and tensin homolog) hamartoma tumor.

886. Serum Tg level integrates which of the following factors?

N Engl J Med. 2016;375(11):1054-67

A. Mass of differentiated thyroid tissue present
B. Inflammation or injury to thyroid gland with release of Tg
C. Amount of stimulation of TSH receptor
D. All of the above

Serum Tg level integrates three major factors : mass of differentiated thyroid tissue present; any inflammation or injury to thyroid gland causing release of Tg; and amount of stimulation of the TSH receptor (by TSH, hCG or TRAb).

887. Increase in incidence of papillary thyroid carcinomas in recent decades is most in which country?

N Engl J Med. 2016;375(7):614-17

A. Japan
B. South Korea
C. Mongolia
D. Ghana

The largest increase in incidence of PTC in recent decades has been in South Korea. Incidence among 15 - 79 years of age increased from 12.2 cases per 100,000 persons in 1993–1997 to 59.9 cases per 100,000 persons in 2003–2007.

888. Thyroid cancers originate as a consequence of mutations that lead to?

Harrison's 20th Ed. Chapter 378 Page 2715

A. Increased rates of proliferation
B. Impaired apoptosis
C. Enhanced invasion, angiogenesis, and metastasis
D. All of the above

889. Which out of the following mutations is relatively specific for thyroid neoplasia?

Harrison's 20th Ed. Chapter 378 Page 2715

A. PAX8–PPARγ1
B. PAX3–FOXO1
C. LCK –TCRB
D. TAL1–TCTA

Follicular thyroid carcinoma and follicular variants of papillary thyroid carcinoma are associated with mutually exclusive mutations of RAS or of the PAX8–PPARG fusion oncogene.

890. Thyroid gland development is related to which of the following developmental transcription factor?

Harrison's 20th Ed. Chapter 375 Page 2692, N Engl J Med. 2016;375(11):1054-67

A. NKX2-1
B. AP-1
C. NF-κB
D. FOXP3

Germline variants in chromosomes 9q22.33 & 14q13.3 are associated with a high risk of differentiated thyroid carcinoma. The genes encoding FOXE1 and NKX2-1, which are master regulators of thyroid development and differentiated function, are adjacent to these loci.

891. Which out of the following about thyroid cancer is false?

Harrison's 20th Ed. Chapter 378 Page 2715

A. Monoclonal in origin
B. Mutation RET/PTC are specific for thyroid neoplasia
C. Mutation PAX8-PPARγ1 are specific for thyroid neoplasia
D. None of the above

892. Which out of the following thyroid cancer does not arise from endodermal-derived thyroid follicular cells?

Harrison's 20th Ed. Chapter 378 Page 2715

A. Papillary thyroid carcinoma (PTC)
B. Follicular thyroid carcinoma (FTC)
C. Poorly differentiated and anaplastic thyroid carcinomas (ATC)
D. Medullary thyroid carcinoma (MTC)

Medullary thyroid carcinoma is the canonical C-cell tumor.

893. Which out of the following is the most common type of thyroid cancer?

Harrison's 20th Ed. Chapter 378 Page 2715

A. Papillary thyroid carcinoma
B. Follicular thyroid carcinoma
C. Poorly differentiated and anaplastic thyroid carcinomas
D. Medullary thyroid carcinoma

PTC is the most common type of thyroid cancer, accounting for 80–85% of well-differentiated thyroid malignancies.

894. Which out of the following oncoprotein best relates to papillary thyroid carcinoma?

Harrison's 20th Ed. Chapter 378 Page 2715

A. Ki-ras
B. BRAF V600E
C. CagA
D. BCR-ABL1

RAS and BRAF, members of the MAP kinase pathway, which classically mediates the transcription of genes involved in cell proliferation and survival,

895. BRAF V600E mutation has been detected in?

Harrison's 20th Ed. Chapter 69 Page 493

A. Melanomas
B. Thyroid tumors
C. Hairy cell leukemia
D. All of the above

BRAF V600E mutation has been detected in a notable fraction of melanomas, thyroid tumors, and hairy cell leukemia.

896. Which out of the following drugs inhibit the BRAF V600E serine kinase activity?

Harrison's 20th Ed. Chapter 69 Page 493

A. Regorafenib
B. Sorafenib
C. Vemurafenib
D. All of the above

Vemurafenib and dabrafenib, with selective capacity to inhibit the BRAF V600E serine kinase activity.

897. Which of the following about papillary thyroid carcinoma is false?

Harrison's 20th Ed. Chapter 378 Page 2715

A. Most papillary thyroid carcinomas are indolent clinically
B. One of the lowest mutation densities of cancers
C. BRAF V600E mutations is the most common genetic alteration
D. None of the above

898. Which of the following about "noninvasive follicular thyroid neoplasms with papillary-like nuclear features"?

N Engl J Med. 2016;375(11):1054-67

A. Benign entity
B. Encapsulated noninvasive
C. Follicular variants of papillary thyroid carcinoma
D. None of the above

Encapsulated noninvasive follicular variants of papillary thyroid carcinoma have been reclassified as a benign entity and renamed as "noninvasive follicular thyroid neoplasms with papillary-like nuclear features". NIFTP is considered as a pre-cancerous tumor.

899. Papillary thyroid carcinomas have mutually exclusive activating mutations in?

N Engl J Med. 2016;375(11):1054-67

A. BRAF
B. RAS
C. RTK
D. All of the above

Papillary thyroid carcinomas have mutually exclusive activating mutations in BRAF, RAS, and RTK. These mutants activate mitogen-activated protein kinase (MAPK) inhibiting iodide uptake and metabolism. RTKs trigger RAS/MAP kinase pathway. Simultaneous RET, BRAF & RAS mutations rarely occur in same tumor.

900. MTC, when associated with multiple endocrine neoplasia (MEN) type 2, harbors an inherited mutation of?

Harrison's 20th Ed. Chapter 67 Page 457

A. RET gene
B. TRK1 gene
C. CTNNB1 gene
D. All of the above

Multiple endocrine neoplasia type 2, a dominant disorder characterized by pituitary adenomas, medullary carcinoma of thyroid, and pheochromocytoma, is due to gain-of-function mutations in the proto-oncogene RET on chromosome 10.

901. Loss-of-function mutations in the RET gene causes?
Harrison's 20th Ed. Chapter 67 Page 457

A. Progressive systemic sclerosis
B. Hirschsprung's disease
C. Congenital hypothyroidism
D. Ehlers-Danlos syndrome

Loss-of-function mutations in the RET gene cause Hirschsprung's disease.

902. Mutations in which of the following occur in ATCs, but not in PTC or FTC?
Harrison's 20th Ed. Chapter 378 Page 2715

A. TERT
B. BRAF
C. CTNNB1
D. All of the above

Most of the mutations seen in differentiated thyroid cancers have also been detected in ATCs. However, mutations in CTNNB1, which encodes β-catenin, occur in ~two-thirds of ATCs, but not in PTC or FTC.

903. Characteristic cytologic features of nuclei in PTC is?
Harrison's 20th Ed. Chapter 378 Page 2715

A. Orphan Annie-eye nuclei
B. Open-faced nuclei
C. Closed-faced nuclei
D. All of the above

904. Typical nuclear characteristic in papillary thyroid carcinoma is?
Int. J. Med. Sci. 2019;16(3):450-60

A. 'Orphan Annie' nuclei
B. Intranuclear pseudoinclusions (cytoplasmic invaginations)
C. Nuclear grooves (folds in the nuclear membrane)
D. All of the above

Typical nuclear characteristics of PTC are 'Orphan Annie' nuclei, intranuclear pseudoinclusions (due to cytoplasmic invaginations) and nuclear grooves (folds in the nuclear membrane). Or, tumor cells with empty nuclei or those showing just a thin rim of peripheral chromatin. Histologic finding of these cells arranged in either papillary structures versus follicles distinguishes the classic and follicular variants of PTC, respectively.

905. Orphan Annie-eye nuclei are characteristically seen in?
J Oral Maxillofac Pathol. 2013;17(2):154-55

A. Papillary thyroid carcinoma
B. Polymorphous low grade adenocarcinoma
C. Cribriform adenocarcinoma of tongue
D. All of the above

906. Orphan Annie-eye nuclei are characteristically seen in?
J Oral Maxillofac Pathol. 2013;17(2):154-55

A. Hashimoto's disease
B. Grave's disease
C. Nodular goiter
D. All of the above

Orphan Annie-eye nuclei are characteristically seen in papillary thyroid carcinoma, polymorphous low grade adenocarcinoma, cribriform adenocarcinoma of tongue and autoimmune thyroiditis (Hashimoto's disease, Grave's disease, and nodular goiter).

907. Psammoma bodies are observed most commonly in?
Int. J. Med. Sci. 2019;16(3):450-60

A. Papillary thyroid carcinoma (PTC)
B. Meningioma
C. Papillary serous cystadenocarcinoma of ovary
D. All of the above

The presence of psammoma bodies (calcium salt deposits) in a cervical lymph node provides further evidence of PTC. Psammoma bodies (PBs) are concentric lamellated calcified structures, observed most commonly in papillary thyroid carcinoma (PTC), meningioma, papillary serous cystadenocarcinoma of ovary & mesothelioma. PBs represent a process of dystrophic calcification. It may also serve as a barrier against the spread of neoplasm.

908. Which of the following about Psammoma bodies is false?
Int. J. Med. Sci. 2019;16(3):450-60

A. Laminated concentric calcific spherules
B. Reflect necrotic, degenerated papillary structures
C. Psammoma in Greek means "sand"
D. None of the above

Psammoma bodies are laminated concentric calcific spherules.

909. Major pathologic feature of PTC is?
Int. J. Med. Sci. 2019;16(3):450-60

A. Ground-glass, clear nuclei ("Orphan Annie")
B. Nuclear grooves, Papillary fronds with fibrovascular cores
C. Psammoma bodies
D. All of the above

910. Papillary thyroid carcinoma has a propensity to spread via?
Harrison's 20th Ed. Chapter 378 Page 2715

A. Lymphatics
B. Hematogenous
C. Direct
D. Does not spread

Papillary thyroid carcinoma has a propensity to spread via lymphatic system but can metastasize hematogenously as well, particularly to bone and lung. PTC may invade locally within thyroid gland as well as through thyroid capsule and into adjacent structures in the neck.

911. Which of the following about follicular thyroid carcinoma (FTC) is false?
Harrison's 20th Ed. Chapter 378 Page 2715

A. More common in iodine deficient regions
B. Nuclear features of follicular adenomas & carcinomas same
C. Spreads by hematogenous routes
D. None of the above

Follicular thyroid carcinoma is distinguished from follicular adenoma on the basis of capsular invasion, vascular invasion, extrathyroidal tumor extension, lymph node metastases, or systemic metastases. Vascular invasion is the most reliable sign of malignancy.

912. Which of the following about follicular thyroid carcinoma (FTC) is false?
The Oncologist 2011;16:585–93

A. Mostly nonfunctional
B. Usually unifocal
C. Metastasis most to lung, then bone
D. None of the above

Most follicular cancers are nonfunctional. Follicular carcinoma is usually unifocal with a propensity for hematogenous spread to metastasis most commonly to lungs followed by bone.

913. Presence of distant metastases (M1) becomes apparent in which stage of papillary or follicular thyroid cancers?

Harrison's 20th Ed. Chapter 378 Page 2714 Table 378-4

A. Stage III
B. Stage IVA
C. Stage IVB
D. Stage IVC

914. T1b denotes what size and extent of the papillary or follicular thyroid cancer?

Harrison's 20th Ed. Chapter 378 Page 2714 Table 378-4

A. ≤1 cm
B. >1 cm but ≤2 cm
C. >2 cm but ≤4 cm
D. >4 cm

915. Any papillary or follicular thyroid cancer with extension into perithyroidal soft tissue or sternothyroid muscle is labeled as?

Harrison's 20th Ed. Chapter 378 Page 2714 Table 378-4

A. T2
B. T3
C. T4a
D. T4b

916. Any papillary or follicular thyroid cancer with invasion into prevertebral fascia or encasement of carotid artery or mediastinal vessels is labeled as?

Harrison's 20th Ed. Chapter 378 Page 2714 Table 378-4

A. T2
B. T3
C. T4a
D. T4b

917. Any papillary or follicular thyroid cancer with invasion into subcutaneous soft tissues, larynx, trachea, esophagus, or recurrent laryngeal nerve is labeled as?

Harrison's 20th Ed. Chapter 378 Page 2714 Table 378-4

A. T2
B. T3
C. T4a
D. T4b

Thyroid Cancer Classification include: T for size & extent of papillary or follicular thyroid cancer (T1a ≤1 cm; T1b >1 cm but ≤2 cm; T2 >2 cm but ≤4 cm; T3 >4 cm or any tumor with extension into perithyroidal soft tissue or sternothyroid muscle; T4a invasion into subcutaneous soft tissues, larynx, trachea, esophagus, or recurrent laryngeal nerve; T4b invasion into prevertebral fascia or encasement of carotid artery or mediastinal vessels).

918. All well-differentiated thyroid cancers 'beyond' what size should be surgically excised?

Harrison's 20th Ed. Chapter 378 Page 2716

A. T1a
B. T1b
C. T2
D. T3

All well-differentiated thyroid cancers >1cm (T1b or larger) should be surgically excised.

919. Near-total thyroidectomy is appropriate for?

Harrison's 20th Ed. Chapter 378 Page 2716

A. Tumor size >4 cm
B. Clinical evidence of extrathyroidal invasion
C. Presence of metastases
D. All of the above

920. For patients at high risk for recurrence, bilateral surgery are given of radioiodine for?

Harrison's 20th Ed. Chapter 378 Page 2716

A. Remnant ablation
B. Potential treatment of iodine-avid metastases
C. Monitoring of serum Thyroglobulin (Tg) levels
D. All of the above

For patients at high risk for recurrence, bilateral (near total thyroidectomy) allows use of ^{131}I for remnant ablation & potential treatment of iodine-avid metastases, as well as for monitoring of serum Tg levels.

921. What level of TSH should be achieved for those with known metastatic disease in papillary or follicular thyroid cancer?

Harrison's 20th Ed. Chapter 378 Page 2716

A. <0.1 mIU/L
B. 0.1 to 0.5 mIU/L
C. 0.5 to 2.0 mIU/L
D. 2.0 to 4.0 mIU/L

922. What level of TSH should be achieved for those with low risk of recurrence in papillary or follicular thyroid cancer?

Harrison's 20th Ed. Chapter 378 Page 2716

A. <0.1 mIU/L
B. 0.1 to 0.5 mIU/L
C. 0.5 to 2.0 mIU/L
D. 2.0 to 4.0 mIU/L

923. After near-total thyroidectomy, what quantity of thyroid tissue remains in the thyroid bed?

Harrison's 20th Ed. Chapter 378 Page 2716

A. < 1 gm
B. < 3 gm
C. < 5 gm
D. < 8 gm

After near-total thyroidectomy, <1 gm of thyroid tissue remains in the thyroid bed.

924. Radioiodine uptake by well differentiated thyroid cancer is determined primarily by?

Harrison's 20th Ed. Chapter 378 Page 2716

A. Expression of thyroglobulin (Tg)
B. Expression of sodium iodide symporter (NIS)
C. Expression of thyroid peroxidase (TPO)
D. Expression of thyroid-stimulating hormone receptor (TSH-R)

Radioiodine uptake by well differentiated thyroid cancer is determined primarily by expression of NIS basolateral membrane of thyroid follicular cells and is stimulated by TSH, requiring expression of the TSH-R.

925. Which of the following is a thyroid-specific gene?
Harrison's 20th Ed. Chapter 375 Page 2693

A. Thyroglobulin (Tg)
B. Thyroid peroxidase (TPO)
C. Thyroid-stimulating hormone receptor (TSH-R)
D. All of the above

Besides sodium iodide symporter (NIS), Thyroglobulin (Tg), Thyroid peroxidase (TPO) and Thyroid-stimulating hormone receptor (TSH-R) have thyroid-specific gene.

926. Sodium iodide symporter (NIS) is also expressed in?
Harrison's 20th Ed. Chapter 375 Page 2693

A. Salivary glands
B. Lactating breast
C. Placenta
D. All of the above

Sodium iodide symporter (NIS) is highly expressed in thyroid gland, but low levels are present in the salivary glands, lactating breast, and placenta.

927. Recurrence & survival rates are improved from radioiodine therapy in patients of?
Harrison's 20th Ed. Chapter 378 Page 2716

A. T1a
B. T1b
C. T2
D. None of the above

With radioiodine therapy, neither recurrence nor survival rates are improved in patients with T1 tumors (≤2 cm) confined to thyroid and also with larger (>2 cm but <4 cm) low-risk tumors, such as minimally invasive follicular cancer or encapsulated PTC follicular variant.

928. Radioiodine reduces recurrence & may increase survival for?
Harrison's 20th Ed. Chapter 378 Page 2716

A. T1a
B. T1b
C. T2
D. T3

929. Radioiodine reduces recurrence & may increase survival for?
Harrison's 20th Ed. Chapter 378 Page 2716

A. Larger tumors, more aggressive variants of papillary cancer
B. Tumor vascular invasion, extrathyroidal invasion
C. Large-volume lymph node metastases
D. All of the above

Radioiodine therapy reduces recurrence and may increase survival for older patients, and higher risk patients (larger tumors, more aggressive variants of papillary cancer, tumor vascular invasion, extrathyroidal invasion, presence of large-volume lymph node metastases).

930. Radioablation is much more effective when there is minimal remaining?
Harrison's 20th Ed. Chapter 378 Page 2716

A. Normal thyroid tissue
B. Thyroid carcinoma tissue
C. Thyroid metastasis
D. All of the above

Radioablation is much more effective when there is minimal remaining "normal" thyroid tissue.

931. Ideally, what should be the level of serum TSH at the time of ^{131}I therapy?
Harrison's 20th Ed. Chapter 378 Page 2716

A. > 25 mIU/L
B. > 50 mIU/L
C. > 75 mIU/L
D. > 100 mIU/L

Ideally, the serum TSH level should be >25 mIU/L at the time of ^{131}I therapy.

932. For remnant ablation after thyroidectomy for thyroid cancer, which of the following is true?
Harrison's 20th Ed. Chapter 378 Page 2716

A. Thyroid hormone withdrawal better than rhTSH injection
B. rhTSH better than thyroid hormone withdrawal protocol
C. Both approaches have equal success rates
D. All of the above

After thyroidectomy for thyroid cancer, TSH level is raised by either using a thyroid hormone withdrawal protocol or recombinant human TSH injection (rhTSH). Both approaches have equal success in achieving remnant ablation.

933. Dose and schedule of Recombinant human TSH (rhTSH) before administration of ^{131}I is?
Harrison's 20th Ed. Chapter 378 Page 2716

A. 0.9 mg once daily for two consecutive days
B. 1.8 mg once daily for two consecutive days
C. 0.9 mg once daily for five consecutive days
D. 1.8 mg once daily for five consecutive days

934. ^{131}I is given how many hours after the recombinant human TSH (rhTSH) administration?
Harrison's 20th Ed. Chapter 378 Page 2716

A. 24 hours
B. 48 hours
C. 72 hours
D. 100 hours

Recombinant human TSH (rhTSH) is administered as two daily consecutive injections (0.9 mg). ^{131}I is given 24 hours after the second injection.

935. For remnant ablation, what dose of ^{131}I is given after thyroidectomy for thyroid cancer?
Harrison's 20th Ed. Chapter 378 Page 2716

A. 30 mCi
B. 100 mCi
C. 150 mCi
D. 175 mCi

The dose of ^{131}I given after thyroidectomy for thyroid cancer depends on the indication for therapy with lower doses of 1100 MBq (30 mCi) given for remnant ablation but higher doses of up to 5500 MBq (150 mCi) used as adjuvant therapy when residual disease is suspected or present.

936. Which of the following is a sensitive tumor marker of residual/recurrent thyroid cancer after ablation of residual postsurgical thyroid tissue?

Harrison's 20th Ed. Chapter 378 Page 2716

A. Serum thyroglobulin
B. Serum thyroglobulin antibody
C. Serum TPO
D. Serum anti TPO antibody

Serum thyroglobulin is a sensitive tumor marker of residual/recurrent thyroid cancer after ablation of the residual postsurgical thyroid tissue. The specificity of Tg measurement in the follow-up of thyroid cancer is highest after thyroidectomy and adjuvant radioiodine ablation of the thyroid remnants.

937. Vast majority of papillary thyroid cancer (PTC) recurrences are in?

Harrison's 20th Ed. Chapter 378 Page 2716

A. Cervical lymph nodes
B. Mediastinal lymph nodes
C. Axillary lymph nodes
D. All of the above

Neck ultrasound should be performed ~6 months after thyroid ablation because vast majority of PTC recurrences are in cervical lymph nodes. Ultrasound is more sensitive than whole-body scanning (WBS) in this scenario.

938. Low risk of papillary thyroid cancer (PTC) structural recurrence is < 3% at 5 years when?

Harrison's 20th Ed. Chapter 378 Page 2716

A. No clinical evidence of residual disease after ablation
B. Negative cervical sonography
C. Basal Tg < 0.2 ng/mL on levothyroxine
D. All of the above

939. Which of the following is used in addition to ^{131}I to treat gross residual neck disease or specific metastatic lesions?

Harrison's 20th Ed. Chapter 378 Page 2716

A. Peptide radioreceptor therapy (PRRT)
B. External-beam radiotherapy
C. Stereotactic body radiation therapy (SBRT)
D. All of the above

In addition to radioiodine, external beam radiotherapy is used to treat gross residual neck disease or specific metastatic lesions.

940. Which of the following target pathways are known to be active in thyroid cancer?

Harrison's 20th Ed. Chapter 378 Page 2716

A. BRAF
B. EGFR
C. VEGFR
D. All of the above

Target pathways known to be active in thyroid cancer are RAS, BRAF, RET, EGFR, VEGFR, and angiogenesis pathways. Role of kinase inhibitors is under probe.

941. Which of the following best relates to Sorafenib?

Harrison's 20th Ed. Chapter 378 Page 2717

A. JAK1/2 kinase inhibitor
B. Cyclin-dependent kinase inhibitor
C. Bruton's tyrosine kinase inhibitor
D. Multi-kinase inhibitor

Sorafenib blocks up to 40 kinases, including anti-angiogenic (vascular endothelial growth factor receptor [VEGFR], platelet-derived growth factor receptor [PDGFR]), antiproliferative drivers (serine/threonine-protein kinase B-raf [BRAF] and mast/stem cell growth factor receptor [c-Kit]).

942. Which of the following is a multi-kinase Inhibitor?

Harrison's 20th Ed. Chapter 69 Page 494 Table 69-5

A. Pazopanib
B. Sorafenib
C. Regorafenib
D. All of the above

943. Which of the following is a multikinase Inhibitor?

Harrison's 20th Ed. Chapter 69 Page 494 Table 69-5

A. Sunitinib
B. Vandetanib
C. Cabozantinib
D. All of the above

944. Sorafenib best relates to?

Harrison's 20th Ed. Chapter 67 Page 460

A. BRAF
B. RET
C. ALK
D. All of the above

Vemurafenib targets mutations in BRAF, sunitinib & sorafenib target mutations in RET. Sorafenib inhibits c-RAF and is a VEGFR antagonist. The recommended daily dose of sorafenib is 800 mg.

945. Which of the following tyrosine kinase inhibitors has activity against thyroid cancer?

Harrison's 20th Ed. Chapter 68 Page 464

A. Sorafenib
B. Cabozantinib
C. Lenvatinib
D. All of the above

946. Sorafenib has antitumor activity in which of the following malignancies?

Harrison's 20th Ed. Chapter 68 Page 464

A. Renal cell cancer (RCC)
B. Hepatocellular carcinoma (HCC)
C. Differentiated thyroid cancer
D. All of the above

947. Which of the following about anaplastic thyroid cancer is false?

Harrison's 20th Ed. Chapter 378 Page 2717

A. Poorly differentiated
B. Aggressive cancer
C. Poor prognosis
D. None of the above

Most patients with anaplastic thyroid cancer die within 6 months of diagnosis.

948. Which of the following provide survival benefit in patients of anaplastic thyroid cancer?
Harrison's 20th Ed. Chapter 378 Page 2717

A. Radioiodine
B. Chemotherapy (anthracyclines & paclitaxel)
C. External beam radiation therapy
D. Immune checkpoint inhibition therapy

949. Lymphoma in the thyroid gland arises in the background of?
Harrison's 20th Ed. Chapter 378 Page 2717

A. Pernicious anemia
B. Graves' disease
C. Hashimoto's thyroiditis
D. Myasthenia gravis

Lymphoma in the thyroid gland often arises in the background of Hashimoto's thyroiditis.

950. Which of the following is the most common type of lymphoma in thyroid?
Harrison's 20th Ed. Chapter 378 Page 2717

A. Hodgkin's disease
B. Diffuse large-cell lymphoma
C. Cutaneous T cell lymphoma
D. Multiple myeloma

Diffuse large-cell lymphoma is the most common type in thyroid.

951. Lymphoma in the thyroid gland is highly sensitive to?
Harrison's 20th Ed. Chapter 378 Page 2717

A. Radioiodine
B. Chemotherapy (anthracyclines & paclitaxel)
C. External radiation therapy
D. Immune checkpoint inhibition therapy

Lymphoma in the thyroid gland is highly sensitive to external radiation.

952. Which of the following is a familial form of medullary thyroid cancer (MTC)?
Harrison's 20th Ed. Chapter 378 Page 2717

A. MEN 2A
B. MEN 2B
C. Familial MTC without other features of MEN
D. All of the above

953. Which of the following about MTC is false?
Harrison's 20th Ed. Chapter 378 Page 2717

A. MTC is more aggressive in MEN 2B than in MEN 2A
B. Familial MTC (FMTC) is more aggressive than sporadic MTC
C. All patients with MTC should be tested for RET mutations
D. None of the above

954. Which of the following should be excluded before any surgery in MEN patients?
Harrison's 20th Ed. Chapter 378 Page 2717

A. Hyperparathyroidism
B. Pheochromocytoma
C. Paraganglioma
D. All of the above

MTC is found in virtually all patients with MEN 2. Prophylactic thyroidectomy is performed in many carriers of RET mutations. Pheochromocytomas should be excluded before any surgery in MEN patients.

955. Which of the following provides a marker of residual or recurrent disease in MTC?
Harrison's 20th Ed. Chapter 378 Page 2717

A. Thyroglobulin
B. Thyroid-stimulating hormone receptor (TSH-R)
C. Calcitonin
D. All of the above

Elevated serum calcitonin provides a marker of residual or recurrent disease.

956. Palpable thyroid nodules are found in what percentage of adults?
Harrison's 20th Ed. Chapter 378 Page 2717

A. ~ 1%
B. ~ 3%
C. ~ 5%
D. ~ 7%

Palpable thyroid nodules are found in about 5% of adults.

957. Thyroid nodules are more common in?
Harrison's 20th Ed. Chapter 378 Page 2717

A. Iodine-deficient areas
B. Women
C. With aging
D. All of the above

Thyroid nodules are more common in iodine-deficient areas, in women, and with aging.

958. Most palpable thyroid nodules are of what size?
Harrison's 20th Ed. Chapter 378 Page 2717

A. > 1 cm in diameter
B. > 2 cm in diameter
C. > 3 cm in diameter
D. > 4 cm in diameter

Most palpable thyroid nodules are >1 cm in diameter. ~15% of "palpable" thyroid nodules are not confirmed on imaging.

959. CT, thyroid ultrasound reveal thyroid nodules in what percentage of individuals aged >50 years?
Harrison's 20th Ed. Chapter 378 Page 2717

A. ~ 20%
B. ~ 30%
C. ~ 40%
D. ~ 50%

CT, thyroid US & pathologic studies, reveal thyroid nodules in ~50% of individuals aged >50 years.

960. Which of the following statements about thyroid nodules is false?

Harrison's 20th Ed. Chapter 378 Page 2717

A. Most patients with thyroid nodules have normal thyroid function
B. Thyroid function should be assessed by measuring TSH level
C. "Hot" nodule is almost never malignant
D. None of the above

961. Which of the following statements about thyroid nodules is false?

Harrison's 20th Ed. Chapter 378 Page 2717

A. Spongiform nodule has a < 3% chance of cancer
B. 10–20% of solid hypoechoic nodules with smooth borders are malignant
C. FNAC for any thyroid nodule <1 cm is not recommended
D. None of the above

962. FNA biopsy is particularly useful for detecting?

Harrison's 20th Ed. Chapter 378 Page 2717

A. Papillary thyroid cancer (PTC)
B. Follicular thyroid cancer (FTC)
C. Medullary thyroid cancer (MTC)
D. All of the above

FNA biopsy is particularly useful for detecting PTC.

963. Risk of thyroid malignancy in atypia or follicular lesion of unknown significance (AUS/FLUS) is?

Harrison's 20th Ed. Chapter 378 Page 2718 Table 378-5

A. 2–4%
B. 5–15%
C. 15–30%
D. 60– 75%

964. Which of the following system is used for classification for thyroid cytology?

Harrison's 20th Ed. Chapter 378 Page 2718 Table 378-5

A. Veterans
B. Bethesda
C. Chicago
D. Fitzpatrick

965. In Bethesda system, which of the following category was previously labeled as indeterminate?

Harrison's 20th Ed. Chapter 378 Page 2718 Table 378-5

A. Atypia or follicular lesion of undetermined significance
B. Follicular neoplasm
C. Suspicious for malignancy
D. All of the above

Disorders of the Adrenal Cortex

966. Corticosteroid hormone produced by adrenal cortex is?
Harrison's 20th Ed. Chapter 379 Page 2719

A. Glucocorticoids
B. Mineralocorticoids
C. Adrenal androgens
D. All of the above

Corticosteroid hormones produced by adrenal cortex are glucocorticoids, mineralocorticoids & adrenal androgens.

967. Which of the following is produced by adrenal cortex?
Harrison's 20th Ed. Chapter 379 Page 2719

A. Dehydroepiandrosterone
B. Aldosterone
C. Cortisol
D. All of the above

Cortisol is a glucocorticoids, aldosterone is a mineralocorticoids and dehydroepiandrosterone (DHEA) is an adrenal androgen precursors.

968. Glucocorticoids and mineralocorticoids regulate which of the following?
Harrison's 20th Ed. Chapter 379 Page 2719

A. Physiologic stress response
B. Blood pressure
C. Electrolyte homeostasis
D. All of the above

969. Glucocorticoids, mineralocorticoids and sex steroids act through?
Harrison's 20th Ed. Chapter 379 Page 2719

A. Transmembrane receptors
B. Nuclear receptors
C. Transcription factors
D. All of the above

Glucocorticoids & mineralocorticoids act through specific nuclear receptors.

970. Adrenal androgen precursors are converted to sex steroids in?
Harrison's 20th Ed. Chapter 379 Page 2719

A. Adrenal cortex
B. Adrenal medulla
C. Gonads
D. All of the above

Adrenal androgen precursors are converted in the gonads and peripheral target cells to sex steroids.

971. Hormone excess disorders of the adrenal cortex are usually the result of?
Harrison's 20th Ed. Chapter 379 Page 2719

A. Inherited glandular disorders
B. Enzymatic disorders
C. Autoimmune disorders
D. Neoplasia

Hormone excess disorders of the adrenal cortex are usually the result of neoplasia.

972. Adrenal nodules lead to increased production of all except?
Harrison's 20th Ed. Chapter 379 Page 2719

A. Adrenocorticotropic hormone
B. Glucocorticoids
C. Mineralocorticoids
D. Adrenal androgen precursors

Hormone excess leads to increased production of adrenocorticotropic hormone by pituitary or neuroendocrine cells (ectopic ACTH) or increased production of glucocorticoids, mineralocorticoids, or adrenal androgen precursors by adrenal nodules.

973. Which of the following is the cholesterol side-chain cleavage enzyme?
Harrison's 20th Ed. Chapter 379 Page 2719 Figure 379-1

A. CYP11A1
B. CYP11B1
C. CYP17A1
D. CYP21A2

Cholesterol side-chain cleavage is catalyzed by cytochrome P450scc (CYP11A1).

974. Each normal adrenal gland weighs?
Harrison's 20th Ed. Chapter 379 Page 2719

A. 2– 6 gram
B. 6–11 gram
C. 11–18 gram
D. 18–31 gram

Each normal adrenal gland weighs 6-11 gram.

975. Arterial blood supply is from?
Harrison's 20th Ed. Chapter 379 Page 2719

A. Zona glomerulosa to adrenal medulla
B. Adrenal medulla to zona glomerulosa
C. Zona fasciculata to adrenal medulla
D. Adrenal medulla to zona fasciculata

976. Which of the following is located outermost in adrenal gland?
Harrison's 20th Ed. Chapter 379 Page 2719

A. Zona glomerulosa
B. Zona fasciculata
C. Zona reticularis
D. Adrenal medulla

Adrenal glands are located above the kidneys and have their own blood supply. Arterial blood supply is from outside to inside. Initially to subcapsular region, then to outer cortical zona glomerulosa, then to intermediate zona fasciculata, then to inner zona reticularis and eventually to adrenal medulla. Function of these three zones can be remembered by the mnemonic "Salt, Sugar, Sex," as they correlate to the function of hormones produced in each layer of the adrenal cortex. The names of these zones can be remembered as "GFR" for Glomerulosa, Fasciculata and Reticularis.

977. Which of the following statements is false?
Harrison's 20th Ed. Chapter 379 Page 2719

A. Right suprarenal vein drains into inferior vena cava
B. Left suprarenal vein drains into left renal vein
C. Adrenals originate from the urogenital ridge
D. None of the above

978. Chief source of blood to the adrenal glands include?
Harrison's 20th Ed. Chapter 379 Page 2719

A. Superior adrenal arteries
B. Middle adrenal artery
C. Inferior adrenal artery
D. All of the above

979. Which of the following adrenal artery originates directly from the abdominal aorta?
Harrison's 20th Ed. Chapter 379 Page 2719

A. Superior adrenal arteries
B. Middle adrenal artery
C. Inferior adrenal artery
D. All of the above

Superior adrenal arteries are small branches coming from inferior phrenic artery, middle adrenal artery comes directly from abdominal aorta and inferior adrenal artery originates from the renal artery bilaterally.

980. Which of the following about adrenal glands is false?
Harrison's 20th Ed. Chapter 379 Page 2720

A. Adrenals originate from urogenital ridge
B. Sexual differentiation occurs at 7th - 9th week of gestation
C. Left suprarenal vein drains into vena cava
D. SF1 and DAX1 are orphan nuclear receptors

The right suprarenal vein drains directly into the vena cava, while the left suprarenal vein drains into the left renal vein. Adrenals originate from urogenital ridge and separate from gonads and kidneys around sixth week of gestation. By seventh to ninth week of gestation, adrenal cortex starts to produce cortisol and the adrenal sex steroid precursor DHEA.

981. Nuclear receptor steroidogenic factor 1 (SF1) is encoded by which gene?
Harrison's 20th Ed. Chapter 379 Page 2720

A. NR5A1
B. NROB1
C. X-ALD
D. AIRE

982. Nuclear receptor DAX 1 is encoded by which gene?
Harrison's 20th Ed. Chapter 379 Page 2720

A. NR5A1
B. NROB1
C. X-ALD
D. AIRE

Orphan nuclear receptors SF1 (steroidogenic factor 1) is encoded by gene NR5A1 while DAX 1 (dosage-sensitive sex reversal gene 1 is encoded by gene NROB1.

983. Production of which of the following is not under the control of hypothalamic-pituitary-adrenal (HPA) axis?
Harrison's 20th Ed. Chapter 379 Page 2720

A. Glucocorticoids
B. Mineralocorticoids
C. Adrenal androgen precursors
D. All of the above

Production of glucocorticoids and adrenal androgens is under the control of the hypothalamic-pituitary-adrenal (HPA) axis, whereas mineralocorticoids are regulated by the renin-angiotensin-aldosterone (RAA) system.

984. Hypothalamic release of corticotropin releasing hormone (CRH) occurs in response to?
Harrison's 20th Ed. Chapter 379 Page 2720

A. Endogenous or exogenous stress
B. ACTH
C. Sleep
D. Diet

Hypothalamic release of corticotropin releasing hormone (CRH) occurs in response to endogenous or exogenous stress.

985. Size of polypeptide pro-opiomelanocortin (POMC) is?
Harrison's 20th Ed. Chapter 379 Page 2720

A. 141 amino acid
B. 241 amino acid
C. 341 amino acid
D. 441 amino acid

Corticotropin-releasing hormone (CRH) stimulates cleavage of 241-amino acid polypeptide proopiomelanocortin (POMC) by pituitary-specific prohormone convertase (PC1) to produce adrenocorticotropic hormone (ACTH).

986. Size of ACTH peptide is?
Harrison's 20th Ed. Chapter 379 Page 2720

A. 21 amino acid
B. 39 amino acid
C. 76 amino acid
D. 98 amino acid

ACTH peptide contains 39 amino acids but first 24 are sufficient to elicit a physiologic response.

987. Prohormone convertase 1 (PC1) is encoded by which of the following gene?
Endocrine Reviews. 2016;37:347–71

A. NF1
B. PCSK1
C. GNAS1
D. MEN1

Prohormone convertase 1 (PC1), encoded by PCSK1 gene on chromosome 5, is a calcium-dependent serine endoprotease that is involved in the processing of a variety of proneuropeptides and prohormones.

988. Major site of expression of prohormone convertase 1 (PC1) is?
Endocrine Reviews. 2016;37:347–71

A. Pituitary
B. Hypothalamus
C. Endocrine pancreas
D. All of the above

Major sites of expression of prohormone convertase 1 (PC1) are pituitary, hypothalamus & endocrine pancreas, adrenal medulla, thyroid gland, enteroendocrine L and K cells of small intestine.

989. Prohormone convertase 1 (PC1) is crucial for the processing of?
Endocrine Reviews. 2016;37:347–71

A. Pro-opiomelanocortin (POMC)
B. Proinsulin
C. Proglucagon
D. All of the above

PC1 is crucial for the processing of a number of neuropeptides and peptide hormones such as pro-opiomelanocortin (POMC), proinsulin, and proglucagon.

990. Prohormone convertase 1 (PC1) leads to the formation of which of the following from proglucagon in the small intestine?

Endocrine Reviews. 2016;37:347–71

A. Glucagon-like peptide (GLP)-1 and -2
B. Oxyntomodulin
C. Glicentin
D. All of the above

PC1 produce the end-product from the precursor like glucagon-like peptide (GLP)-1 and -2, oxyntomodulin, and glicentin from proglucagon in the small intestine; ACTH & α-MSH from POMC in the anterior lobe of the pituitary gland; insulin from proinsulin in β-cells of the islets of Langerhans in pancreas. β-MSH is a product of PC2 cleavage only.

991. Which of the following is a POMC-derived peptide?

Endocrine Reviews. 2016;37:347–71

A. α-MSH
B. β-MSH
C. ACTH
D. All of the above

992. Which of the following about α-MSH is false?

Endocrine Reviews. 2016;37:347–371

A. Anorexigenic hormone
B. Cleavage product of POMC
C. Binds to melanocortin receptors MCR3 and MCR4
D. None of the above

993. ACTH determines the synthesis of which of the following?

Harrison's 20th Ed. Chapter 379 Page 2720

A. Adrenal cortisol
B. Adrenal mineralocorticoid
C. Adrenal androgen
D. All of the above

ACTH acts as the pivotal regulator of adrenal cortisol synthesis, with additional short-term effects on mineralocorticoid & adrenal androgen synthesis.

994. Circadian rhythm best relates to?

Harrison's 20th Ed. Chapter 379 Page 2720

A. Supraoptic nucleus
B. Suprachiasmatic nucleus
C. Arcuate nucleus
D. Pineal gland

Suprachiasmatic nucleus is the master pacemaker (~ 20,000 neurons) of circadian or biological rhythms (body's master clock). Supraoptic nuclei relate to fluid balance, milk let-down, & parturition. Arcuate nuclei relate to control of anterior pituitary & feeding. Paraventricular nuclei are slave oscillators to suprachiasmatic nucleus and best relate to fluid balance, milk let-down, parturition, autonomic & anterior pituitary control.

995. Which of the following best relates to cell-specific clock genes?

Harrison's 20th Ed. Chapter 475 Page 3504, EMBO Rep. 2018;19(1):18–28

A. TAL1
B. BMAL1
C. PAX3
D. KAL1

At the molecular level, mammalian circadian rhythms are generated by a transcription-translation autoregulatory feedback loop. The central players in this pathway are BMAL1 (brain and muscle ARNT-like1) and CLOCK (Circadian Locomotor Output Cycles Kaput) that are encoded by the genes Arntl and Clock, respectively.

996. Which of the following is used as a peripheral marker of an individual's circadian rhythm?

Harrison's 20th Ed. Chapter 475 Page 3507

A. Dystonin
B. Calcitonin
C. Melatonin
D. Serotonin

Melatonin is one of the most commonly used peripheral markers of an individual's circadian rhythm, reflecting rhythmic function of the suprachiasmatic nucleus (SCN). Circadian rhythms of melatonin can be measured in saliva or plasma, while 6-sulphatoxymelatonin (aMT6S), a metabolite generated from the breakdown of melatonin, can be measured in urine.

997. Which of the following about melatonin is false?

Harrison's 20th Ed. Chapter 475 Page 3504 Table 475-1

A. Hormone
B. Produced by pineal gland
C. Derived from L-tryptophan
D. None of the above

998. Peak levels of adrenal cortisol secretion is in?

Harrison's 20th Ed. Chapter 379 Page 2720

A. Morning
B. Afternoon
C. Evening
D. Night

999. The plasma level of ACTH are lowest at?

Harrison's 20th Ed. Chapter 379 Page 2720

A. Just prior to waking up
B. Just after waking up
C. Before sleeping
D. After meals

Adrenal cortisol secretion exhibits a distinct circadian rhythm, starting to rise in the early morning hours prior to awakening with peak levels in the morning and low levels in the evening. Plasma ACTH peak just prior to waking and a nadir before sleeping.

1000. The time at which the peak of circadian rhythm occur is called?

Harrison's 20th Ed. Chapter 379 Page 2720 Figure 379-2

A. Acrophase
B. Prophase
C. Bathyphase
D. Mesor

Circulating cortisol concentrations, acrophase is ~8:30 AM.

1001. The time at which the trough of circadian rhythm occurs is called?

Harrison's 20th Ed. Chapter 475 Page 3504 Table 475-1

A. Acrophase
B. Prophase
C. Bathyphase
D. Mesor

1002. Which of the following statements is false?

Harrison's 20th Ed. Chapter 379 Page 2720

A. Glucocorticoid excess is diagnosed by dexamethasone suppression test
B. Glucocorticoid deficiency is assessed by ACTH stimulation test
C. Oral or IV sodium loading assesses mineralocorticoid excess
D. None of the above

1003. Which of the following statements about dexamethasone is false?

Harrison's 20th Ed. Chapter 379 Page 2720

A. Potent synthetic glucocorticoid
B. Suppresses CRH
C. Suppresses ACTH
D. None of the above

Dexamethasone is a potent synthetic glucocorticoid that suppresses CRH/ACTH by binding hypothalamic-pituitary glucocorticoid receptors (GRs).

1004. Cortisol excess can be due to?

Harrison's 20th Ed. Chapter 379 Page 2720

A. Autonomous adrenal nodule
B. ACTH-producing pituitary adenoma
C. ACTH-producing ectopic tumors
D. All of the above

1005. How many amino acids of ACTH peptide are sufficient to elicit a physiologic response?

Harrison's 20th Ed. Chapter 379 Page 2720

A. First 6 amino acids
B. First 12 amino acids
C. First 18 amino acids
D. First 24 amino acids

The ACTH peptide contains 39 amino acids but the first 24 are sufficient to elicit a physiologic response.

1006. A normal response in standard ACTH stimulation test is defined as a cortisol level of?

Harrison's 20th Ed. Chapter 379 Page 2720

A. > 5 μg/dL, 30–60 min after cosyntropin stimulation
B. > 10 μg/dL, 30–60 min after cosyntropin stimulation
C. > 15 μg/dL, 30–60 min after cosyntropin stimulation
D. > 20 μg/dL, 30–60 min after cosyntropin stimulation

1007. In standard ACTH stimulation test, blood samples for cortisol are collected at?

Harrison's 20th Ed. Chapter 379 Page 2720

A. 0 minutes
B. 30 minutes
C. 60 minutes
D. All of the above

The standard ACTH stimulation test involves administration of cosyntropin (ACTH 1-24), 0.25 mg IM or IV, and collection of blood samples at 0, 30, and 60 minutes for cortisol. A normal response is defined as a cortisol level > 20 μg/dL 30-60 minutes after cosyntropin stimulation or an increment of >10 μg/dL over baseline.

1008. In insulin tolerance test (ITT), blood samples for which of the following are collected?

Harrison's 20th Ed. Chapter 379 Page 2720

A. Glucose
B. Cortisol
C. Growth hormone
D. All of the above

Insulin tolerance test (ITT) is used to assess adrenal function. Insulin induced hypoglycemia represents a strong stress signal that triggers hypothalamic CRH release and activation of the entire HPA axis.

1009. In insulin tolerance test (ITT), a normal response is defined as?

Harrison's 20th Ed. Chapter 379 Page 2720

A. Cortisol >20 μg/dL and GH >3.1 μg/L
B. Cortisol >20 μg/dL and GH >4.1 μg/L
C. Cortisol >20 μg/dL and GH >5.1 μg/L
D. Cortisol >20 μg/dL and GH >6.1 μg/L

In insulin tolerance test (ITT), a normal response is defined as a cortisol >20 μg/dL and GH >5.1 μg/L.

1010. Which of the following about cosyntropin is false?

Clinical Pharmacology: Advances and Applications 2010:2 77–82

A. Synthetic derivative of adrenocorticotropic hormone (ACTH)
B. Contains the first 24 of 39 amino acids of natural ACTH
C. Also referred to as tetracosactide
D. None of the above

Biologic activity of ACTH resides in the N-terminal portion of the molecule and that the 1–20 amino acid residue is the minimal sequence retaining full activity. C-terminal portion of ACTH molecule and the 22–39 amino acid residues exhibit the greatest degree of antigenicity.

1011. Which of the following may increase cortisol metabolism?

Clinical Pharmacology: Advances and Applications 2010:2 77–82

A. Rifampin
B. Ketoconazole
C. Metyrapone
D. All of the above

Rifampin and phenytoin may increase cortisol metabolism. Metyrapone, etomidate, ketoconazole, megesterol, and mitotate may interfere with cosyntropin function and subsequent response.

1012. Which of the following may increase cortisol metabolism?

Clinical Pharmacology: Advances and Applications 2010:2 77–82

A. Increased melanotropic activity
B. Increased growth hormone secretion
C. Lipogenesis (adipokinetic)
D. All of the above

The extra-adrenal effects, which natural ACTH and cosyntropin have in common, include increased melanotropic activity, increased growth hormone secretion, and lipogenesis.

1013. Cosyntropin produces secretion of?

Clinical Pharmacology: Advances and Applications 2010:2 77–82

A. 17-OH corticosteroids
B. 17- ketosteroids
C. 17- ketogenic steroids
D. All of the above

Cosyntropin produces secretion of 17-OH corticosteroids, 17- ketosteroids &/or 17- ketogenic steroids.

1014. Which of the following disease states respond to ACTH?

Harrison's 20th Ed. Chapter 472 Page 2720 Figure 472-7

A. Esophageal spasm
B. Infantile spasms
C. Porphyria cutanea tarda
D. Biliary cirrhosis

Corticotropin (adrenocorticotropic hormone, ACTH) or its synthetic derivative tetracosactide is the treatment of choice of infantile spasms, including the West syndrome which is a severe epilepsy syndrome composed of the triad of infantile spasms, interictal EEG pattern termed hypsarrhythmia (chaotic, high- to extremely high–voltage, polymorphic delta and theta rhythms with superimposed multifocal spikes and wave discharges), and mental retardation. ACTH causes suppression of excessive secretion of corticotropin-releasing hormone (CRH).

1015. Normal pulsatile, circadian pattern of ACTH release is regulated by?

Harrison's 20th Ed. Chapter 472 Page 2720

A. Corticotropin-releasing hormone
B. Free plasma cortisol concentration
C. Sleep-wake cycle
D. All of the above

Normal pulsatile, circadian pattern of ACTH release is regulated by CRH.

1016. Stress causes which of the following?

Harrison's 20th Ed. Chapter 472 Page 2720

A. Release of CRH
B. Release of AVP
C. Activation of sympathetic nervous system
D. All of the above

Stress (pyrogens, surgery, hypoglycemia, exercise & severe emotional trauma) causes the release of CRH and arginine vasopressin (AVP) and activation of the sympathetic nervous system.

1017. Factors increasing ACTH release include?

Harrison's 20th Ed. Chapter 472 Page 2720

A. Response to eating
B. Vasopressin
C. Angiotensin II
D. All of the above

ACTH & cortisol levels increase in response to eating. ACTH release is regulated by the level of free cortisol in plasma.

1018. Factors decreasing ACTH release include?

Harrison's 20th Ed. Chapter 472 Page 2720

A. β-endorphin
B. Enkephalin
C. Inflammatory cytokines
D. All of the above

1019. The biologic half-life of ACTH in the circulation is?

Harrison's 20th Ed. Chapter 472 Page 2720

A. < 10 minutes
B. < 15 minutes
C. < 20 minutes
D. < 60 minutes

Most protein hormones (ACTH, GH, prolactin, PTH, LH) have relatively short half-lives (<20 minutes), leading to sharp peaks of secretion and decay.

1020. During critical illness, levels of corticosteroid-binding globulin?

N Engl J Med 2003;348:727-34

A. Decrease
B. Increase
C. Remain same
D. All of the above

1021. Suppression of the hypothalamic-pituitary-adrenal axis has been reported with?

N Engl J Med 2003;348:727-34

A. Exogenous corticosteroid therapy for > 3 weeks
B. Medroxyprogesterone
C. Megestrol acetate
D. All of the above

1022. What level of cortisol level best identifies persons with clinical features of corticosteroid insufficiency?

N Engl J Med 2003;348:727-34

A. <15 μg per deciliter
B. <25 μg per deciliter
C. <35 μg per deciliter
D. <45 μg per deciliter

1023. Synthetic peptide consisting of the first 24 amino acids of corticotropin and used in corticotropin stimulation test is?

N Engl J Med 2003;348:727-34

A. Cosyntropin
B. Syntropin
C. Adrenomedulin
D. All of the above

1024. Insulin-tolerance test (ITT) should not be performed in patients with?

Harrison's 20th Ed. Chapter 472 Page 2720

A. Ischemic heart disease
B. Epilepsy
C. Severe cortisol deficiency
D. All of the above

Insulin-tolerance test is contraindicated in patients with coronary disease, cerebrovascular disease or seizure disorders. Short cosyntropin test can be used instead.

1025. Mineralocorticoid production is initiated by?

Harrison's 20th Ed. Chapter 472 Page 2721

A. Release of renin
B. Cleavage of angiotensinogen to angiotensin I
C. Cleavage of angiotensin I to angiotensin II by ACE
D. Angiotensin II activation of angiotensin II receptor type 1

Mineralocorticoid production is initiated by the release of renin from juxtaglomerular cells in kidney, resulting in cleavage of angiotensinogen to angiotensin I in liver. Angiotensin-converting enzyme (ACE) cleaves angiotensin I to angiotensin II, which binds and activates the angiotensin II receptor type 1 (AT1R), resulting in increased adrenal aldosterone production and vasoconstriction.

1026. Which of the following is required for the initiation of steroidogenesis?

Harrison's 20th Ed. Chapter 472 Page 2721

A. CRH stimulation
B. ACTH stimulation
C. POMC stimulation
D. All of the above

1027. Which of the following is an ACTH receptor?

Harrison's 20th Ed. Chapter 472 Page 2721

A. Melanocortin 1 receptor
B. Melanocortin 2 receptor
C. Melanocortin 3 receptor
D. Melanocortin 4 receptor

The ACTH receptor is melanocortin 2 receptor (MC2R).

1028. MC2R (melanocortin 2 receptor) interacts with which of the following to bind ACTH?

Harrison's 20th Ed. Chapter 472 Page 2721

A. MRAP
B. MRBP
C. MRCP
D. MRDP

ACTH stimulation is required for initiation of steroidogenesis. ACTH receptor MC2R (melanocortin 2 receptor) interacts with MC2R-accessory protein (MRAP) and this complex at adrenocortical cell membrane binds to ACTH.

1029. ACTH stimulation best relates to which signaling pathway?

Harrison's 20th Ed. Chapter 472 Page 2721

A. Protein kinase A (PKA) signaling pathway
B. Calcium signaling pathway
C. Kinase signaling pathway
D. Wnt signaling pathway

1030. Which of the following about protein kinase A (PKA) is false?

Harrison's 20th Ed. Chapter 472 Page 2721

A. Inactive PKA is a tetramer
B. It has two regulatory & two catalytic subunits
C. cAMP dissociates the tetramer
D. None of the above

PKA is a cAMP-dependent serine—threonine protein kinase. In its inactive state, it is a tetrameric holoenzyme consisting of a dimer of two regulatory and two catalytic subunits (Cα and Cβ encoded by genes PRKACA and PRKACB, respectively); under physiologic conditions, PKA activity is induced by G-protein–coupled receptors through increased levels of cAMP. On binding of cAMP, the regulatory subunits dissociate from the catalytic subunits, allowing the enzyme to become active.

1031. PKA activation affects steroidogenesis through?

Harrison's 20th Ed. Chapter 472 Page 2721

A. Increase in import of cholesterol esters
B. Breaks cholesterol esters to cholesterol
C. Increases availability & phosphorylation of CREB
D. All of the above

ACTH stimulation generates cyclic AMP (cAMP) which then upregulates protein kinase A (PKA) signaling pathway. PKA activation increases import of cholesterol esters, increases activity of hormone-sensitive lipase, which cleaves cholesterol esters to cholesterol for import into mitochondrion and increases availability & phosphorylation of CREB (cAMP response element binding), a transcription factor that enhances transcription of CYP11A1 and other enzymes required for glucocorticoid synthesis.

1032. Which of the following statements is false?

Harrison's 20th Ed. Chapter 472 Page 2721

A. Mineralocorticoid synthesis occurs in zona glomerulosa
B. Glucocorticoid synthesis occurs in zona fasciculata
C. Adrenal androgen synthesis occurs in zona reticularis
D. None of the above

Adrenal steroidogenesis occurs in a zone-specific manner. Mineralocorticoid synthesis occurs in outer zona glomerulosa, glucocorticoid synthesis in zona fasciculata, and adrenal androgen synthesis in inner zona reticularis.

1033. Cholesterol import into mitochondrion is initiated by the action of?

Harrison's 20th Ed. Chapter 472 Page 2721

A. Phosphorylation of CREB
B. Steroidogenic acute regulatory (StAR) protein
C. CYP11A1
D. All of the above

All steroidogenic pathways require cholesterol import into the mitochondrion, a process initiated by the action of steroidogenic acute regulatory (StAR) protein, which moves cholesterol from outer to inner mitochondrial membrane. CREB acts in the nucleus and makes available CYP11A1 which traverses to the mitochondria.

1034. Which of the following about adrenodoxin (ADX) is false?

Proteins. 2000;40(4):590-612

A. Also called ferredoxin
B. Iron sulfoprotein
C. Found in the mitochondrial matrix
D. None of the above

Adrenodoxin serve as generic electron transfer proteins for all mitochondrial P450s, and not just for those involved in steroidogenesis.

1035. Which of the following about adrenodoxin reductase (AdRed) is false?

Proteins. 2000;40(4):590-612

A. Flavoprotein loosely bound to inner mitochondrial membrane
B. Accepts electrons from NADPH, converting it to NADP+
C. Passes electrons to adrenodoxin (Adx)
D. None of the above

Adrenodoxin reductase (AdRed), a flavoprotein loosely bound to the inner mitochondrial membrane, accepts electrons (e−) from NADPH, converting it to NADP+. These electrons are passed to adrenodoxin (Adx) 1:1, an iron-sulfur protein in solution in mitochondrial matrix that functions as a freely diffusible electron shuttle mechanism. Electrons from charged adrenodoxin are accepted by any available cytochrome P450. The uncharged adrenodoxin may be again bound to adrenodoxin reductase to receive another pair of electrons. For P450scc, three pairs of electrons must be transported to the P450 to convert cholesterol to pregnenolone. The flow of cholesterol into the mitochondria is facilitated by StAR.

1036. Mutations in the CYP11A1 gene result in?

Proteins. 2000;40(4):590-612

A. Adrenal insufficiency
B. MEN2
C. Porphyria
D. All of the above

Mutations in the CYP11A1 gene that result in significantly diminished cholesterol side-chain cleavage activity leading to adrenal insufficiency and XY DSD (sex reversal), phenotypes that are similar to those associated with inactivating mutations in the STARD1 gene.

1037. Through CYP11A1, cholesterol is converted to which of the following?

Harrison's 20th Ed. Chapter 379 Page 2719

A. Pregnenolone
B. 17-hydroxyprogesterone
C. Progesterone
D. 18-hydroxycorticosterone

1038. Which of the following enzyme converts pregnenolone to progesterone?

Harrison's 20th Ed. Chapter 379 Page 2719 Figure 379-1

A. CYP17A1
B. CYP21A2
C. CYP11B1
D. HSD3B2

1039. HSD3B2 is required for which of the following conversions?

Harrison's 20th Ed. Chapter 379 Page 2719 Figure 379-1

A. Pregnenolone to Progesterone
B. 17-hydroxypregnenolone to 17-hydroxyprogesterone
C. DHEA to Androstenedione
D. All of the above

1040. CYP17A1 is required for which of the following conversions?

Harrison's 20th Ed. Chapter 379 Page 2719 Figure 379-1

A. Pregnenolone to 17-hydroxypregnenolone
B. 17-hydroxypregnenolone to DHEA
C. Progesterone to 17-hydroxyprogesterone
D. All of the above

1041. Which of the following enzyme converts progesterone to 17-hydroxyprogesterone?

Harrison's 20th Ed. Chapter 379 Page 2719 Figure 379-1

A. CYP17A1
B. CYP21A2
C. CYP11B1
D. HSD3B2

1042. Which of the following enzyme converts 17-hydroxyprogesterone to 11-deoxycortisol?

Harrison's 20th Ed. Chapter 379 Page 2719 Figure 379-1

A. CYP17A1
B. CYP21A2
C. CYP11B1
D. HSD3B2

1043. Which of the following enzyme converts 17-hydroxyprogesterone to androstenedione?

Harrison's 20th Ed. Chapter 379 Page 2719 Figure 379-1

A. CYP17A1
B. CYP21A2
C. CYP11B1
D. HSD3B2

1044. Which of the following enzyme converts 11-deoxycortisol to cortisol?

Harrison's 20th Ed. Chapter 379 Page 2719 Figure 379-1

A. CYP17A1
B. CYP21A2
C. CYP11B1
D. HSD3B2

1045. Which out of the following is the first molecule in the production of aldosterone?

Harrison's 20th Ed. Chapter 379 Page 2719 Figure 379-1

A. Corticosterone
B. Deoxycorticosterone
C. 18-hydroxycorticosterone
D. Progesterone

1046. Which out of the following is the first molecule in the production of cortisone?

Harrison's 20th Ed. Chapter 379 Page 2719 Figure 379-1

A. Cortisol
B. 11-Deoxycortisol
C. 17-hydroxypregnenolone
D. 17-hydroxyprogesterone

1047. Which out of the following is the first molecule in the production of 5-Dihydrotestosterone?

Harrison's 20th Ed. Chapter 379 Page 2719 Figure 379-1

A. Testosterone
B. Androstenedione
C. DHEA
D. DHEAS

1048. Which out of the following is the first molecule in the production of DHEAS?

Harrison's 20th Ed. Chapter 379 Page 2719 Figure 379-1

A. 17-hydroxypregnenolone
B. Androstenedione
C. DHEA
D. Progesterone

1049. Starting from pregnenolone, which of the following goes through maximum number of conversion steps?

Harrison's 20th Ed. Chapter 379 Page 2719 Figure 379-1

A. 5-Dihydrotestosterone
B. Progesterone
C. DHEAS
D. Aldosterone

1050. Which of the following does not participate in the production of cortisone?

Harrison's 20th Ed. Chapter 379 Page 2719 Figure 379-1

A. 11-Deoxycortisol
B. Deoxycorticosterone
C. 17-hydroxyprogesterone
D. 17-hydroxypregnenolone

1051. Which of the following does not participate in the production of 5-Dihydrotestosterone?

Harrison's 20th Ed. Chapter 379 Page 2719 Figure 379-1

A. Testosterone
B. Androstenedione
C. DHEA
D. DHEAS

1052. Which of the following does not participate in the production of aldosterone?

Harrison's 20th Ed. Chapter 379 Page 2719 Figure 379-1

A. 17-hydroxyprogesterone
B. 17-hydroxypregnenolone
C. 11-Deoxycortisol
D. All of the above

1053. Which of the following participates in the production of aldosterone?

Harrison's 20th Ed. Chapter 379 Page 2719 Figure 379-1

A. Deoxycorticosterone
B. Corticosterone
C. 18-hydroxycorticosterone
D. All of the above

1054. Which of the following has a role in glucocorticoid synthesis?

Harrison's 20th Ed. Chapter 379 Page 2719 Figure 379-1

A. Deoxycorticosterone
B. Corticosterone
C. 18-hydroxycorticosterone
D. All of the above

1055. Glucocorticoid synthesis occurs in?

Harrison's 20th Ed. Chapter 379 Page 2721

A. Zona fasciculata
B. Zona reticularis
C. Zona glomerulosa
D. All of the above

Adrenal steroidogenesis occurs in a zone-specific fashion, with mineralocorticoid synthesis occurring in the outer zona glomerulosa, glucocorticoid synthesis in the zona fasciculata and adrenal androgen synthesis in the inner zona reticularis.

1056. Basic substrate for steroidogenesis is?

Harrison's 20th Ed. Chapter 379 Page 2721

A. Triglycerides
B. Cholesterol
C. Amino acids
D. Polysaccharides

Cholesterol from diet and from endogenous synthesis is the substrate for steroidogenesis. All steroidogenic pathways require cholesterol import into the mitochondrion by a process initiated by the action of steroidogenic acute regulatory protein (StAR) which shuttles cholesterol from the outer to the inner mitochondrial membrane.

1057. Which of the following steroidogenic enzyme is not located in the mitochondrion?

Harrison's 20th Ed. Chapter 379 Page 2721

A. 17α-hydroxylase
B. CYP11A1
C. 11β-hydroxylase
D. CYP11B1

1058. Which of the following steroidogenic enzyme is located in the endoplasmic reticulum membrane?

Harrison's 20th Ed. Chapter 379 Page 2721

A. 17α-hydroxylase (CYP17A1)
B. 21-hydroxylase (CYP21A2)
C. Aromatase (CYP19A1)
D. All of the above

Majority of steroidogenic enzymes are cytochrome P450 (CYP) enzymes. Those located in the mitochondrion are side chain cleavage enzyme, CYP11A1, 11β-hydroxylase (CYP11B1), aldosterone synthase (CYP11B2). Those located in the endoplasmic reticulum membrane are 17α-hydroxylase (CYP17A1), 21-hydroxylase (CYP21A2), and aromatase (CYP19A1).

1059. Which of the following is required for synthesis of glucocorticoids?

Harrison's 20th Ed. Chapter 379 Page 2721

A. Pregnenolone
B. Progesterone
C. 17-hydroxyprogesterone
D. All of the above

1060. Which of the following is required for synthesis of glucocorticoids?

Harrison's 20th Ed. Chapter 379 Page 27211

A. 3β-HSD2
B. CYP17A1
C. CYP21A2
D. All of the above

Glucocorticoid synthesis requires conversion of pregnenolone to progesterone by 3β-HSD2, followed by conversion to 17-hydroxyprogesterone (17OHP) by CYP17A1, further hydroxylation at carbon 21 by CYP21A2, and lastly, 11β-hydroxylation by CYP11B1 to generate active cortisol.

1061. Which of the following steroidogenic enzyme is required for conversion from deoxycorticosterone to aldosterone?

Harrison's 20th Ed. Chapter 379 Page 2721

A. CYP11B1
B. CYP11B2
C. CYP17A1
D. CYP21A2

1062. Which of the following steroidogenic enzyme is not required in mineralocorticoid synthesis?

Harrison's 20th Ed. Chapter 379 Page 2721

A. 3β-HSD2
B. CYP11B2
C. CYP21A2
D. All of the above

Mineralocorticoid synthesis also requires progesterone, which is first converted to deoxycorticosterone (DOC) by CYP21A2 and then converted via corticosterone and 18-hydroxycorticosterone to aldosterone in three steps catalyzed by CYP11B2.

1063. Which of the following is termed as universal sex steroid precursor?

Harrison's 20th Ed. Chapter 379 Page 2721

A. DHEA
B. DHEAS
C. Pregnenolone
D. Progesterone

For adrenal androgen synthesis, pregnenolone undergoes conversion by CYP17A1 to generate the universal sex steroid precursor DHEA. The majority of DHEA is secreted by the adrenal in the form of its sulfate ester, DHEAS, generated by DHEA sulfotransferase (SULT2A1).

1064. Which compound of DHEA is a useful index of adrenal androgen secretion?

Harrison's 20th Ed. Chapter 379 Page 2721

A. Sulfate
B. Phosphate
C. Chloride
D. None of the above

Measurement of the sulfate conjugate of DHEA is a useful index of adrenal androgen secretion, as little DHEA sulfate is formed in gonads. The majority of DHEA is secreted by the adrenal in the form of its sulfate ester, DHEAS, generated by DHEA sulfotransferase (SULT2A1).

1065. Cortisol circulates in the plasma as?

Harrison's 20th Ed. Chapter 379 Page 2721

A. Free cortisol
B. Albumin-bound cortisol
C. Bound to cortisol-binding globulin (CBG)
D. All of the above

Cortisol circulates in blood mainly bound to cortisol-binding globulin (CBG) and to a lesser extent to albumin, with only a minor fraction circulating as free, unbound hormone.

1066. 11β-hydroxysteroid dehydrogenase 1 (11β-HSD 1) is primarily expressed in?

Harrison's 20th Ed. Chapter 379 Page 2722

A. Liver
B. Lung
C. Kidney
D. All of the above

Enzyme that regulates cortisol metabolism is HSD11B1 (11β-hydroxysteroid dehydrogenase type 1). Isoform HSD11B1 is primarily expressed in liver.

1067. Function of HSD11B1 is?

Harrison's 20th Ed. Chapter 379 Page 2722

A. Converting inactive cortisone to active cortisol
B. Converting cortisol to inactive cortisone
C. Promote binding of free cortisol to transcortin
D. Inhibit binding of free cortisol to transcortin

HSD11B1 acts as a reductase, converting inactive cortisone to active glucocorticoid, cortisol.

1068. Function of HSD11B2 is?

Harrison's 20th Ed. Chapter 379 Page 2722

A. Converting cortisone to cortisol
B. Converting cortisol to cortisone
C. Promote binding of free cortisol to transcortin
D. Inhibit binding of free cortisol to transcortin

HSD11B2 (11β-hydroxysteroid dehydrogenase 2) isoform converts cortisol to the inactive metabolite, cortisone.

1069. Which of the following functions as a tissue-specific prereceptor regulator of glucocorticoid action?

Harrison's 20th Ed. Chapter 379 Page 2722

A. 11β-hydroxylase dehydrogenase type 1 (11β-HSD1)
B. 21-hydroxylase (CYP21A2)
C. 3β-HSD2
D. 17α-hydroxylase/17,20-lyase (CYP17A1)

In adipose, liver, muscle and brain, cortisol is generated from cortisone within the cell by enzyme 11β-hydroxylase dehydrogenase type 1 (11β-HSD1) and therefore functions as a tissue-specific prereceptor regulator of glucocorticoid action.

1070. For the conversion of inactive cortisone to active cortisol, 11β-HSD1 requires which of the following?

Harrison's 20th Ed. Chapter 379 Page 2722

A. NADPH
B. H6PDH
C. GSH
D. LDH

For the conversion of inactive cortisone to active cortisol, 11β-HSD1 requires reduced form of nicotinamide adenine dinucleotide phosphate (NADPH), which is provided by the enzyme hexose-6-phosphate dehydrogenase (H6PDH).

1071. Basic structure of steroids is built upon a nucleus with how many rings?

IJCS 2016;4(3):124-32

A. Three-rings
B. Four-rings
C. Five-rings
D. Six-rings

Steroid molecules possess a common chemical skeleton of four fused rings A/B/C, consisting of three cyclohexane phenanthrene rings and a cyclopentane ring, D. This steroid scaffold contains 17 carbon atoms.

1072. Number of carbon atoms in 17-hydroxycorticosteroids is?

IJCS 2016;4(3):124-32

A. 17
B. 18
C. 19
D. 21

Adrenal steroids contain either 19 or 21 carbon atoms. C21 steroids with a hydroxyl group at position 17 are termed 17-hydroxycorticosteroids.

1073. Number of carbon atoms in 17-ketosteroids is?

IJCS 2016;4(3):124-132

A. 17
B. 18
C. 19
D. 20

C19 steroids have methyl groups at C-18 & C-19. C19 steroids with a ketone group at C-17 are termed 17-ketosteroids.

1074. C19 steroids have predominantly?

IJCS 2016;4(3):124-32

A. Androgenic properties
B. Glucocorticoid properties
C. Mineralocorticoid properties
D. All of the above

C19 steroids have predominantly androgenic activity.

1075. Cyclopentanophenanthrene nucleus is a constituent of?

IJCS 2016;4(3):124-32

A. Steroids
B. Insulin
C. Pepsin
D. Growth hormone

1076. Steroids pass through the cell membrane by?
Harrison's 20th Ed. Chapter 379 Page 2722

A. Passive diffusion
B. Active transport
C. Catalytic transport
D. All of the above

Steroids diffuse passively through the cell membrane and bind to intracellular receptors.

1077. Cortisol binds & activates glucocorticoid receptor (GR) in?
Harrison's 20th Ed. Chapter 379 Page 2722

A. Cell membrane
B. Cytoplasm
C. Nucleus
D. All of the above

In the cytosol of target cells, cortisol binds & activates the glucocorticoid receptor (GR).

1078. Which of the following about glucocorticoid receptor (GR) is false?
Harrison's 20th Ed. Chapter 379 Page 2722, Nucleic Acids Research, 2017;45(14):8596–608

A. Ligand regulated transcription factor
B. Unliganded GR are in cytoplasm bound to chaperone proteins
C. Upon binding ligand, translocates to the nucleus
D. None of the above

1079. Which of the following is a part of glucocorticoid receptor (GR) architecture?
Nucleic Acids Research, 2017;45(14):8596–608

A. N-terminal domain (NTD)
B. Zinc finger DNA binding domain (DBD)
C. Ligand-binding domain (LBD)
D. All of the above

GR contains an unstructured N-terminal domain (NTD) containing activation function-1 (AF-1) region; a zinc finger DNA binding domain (DBD); a hinge region; and a ligand-binding domain (LBD).

1080. Cortisol binding and activation of glucocorticoid receptor (GR) relates best with?
Harrison's 20th Ed. Chapter 379 Page 2722

A. Ubiquilin 2
B. Heat shock proteins
C. Senataxin
D. TAR DNA binding protein

1081. Heat shock proteins best relate to?
Front Immunol. 2016;7:171

A. Chaperone
B. Gap junction protein
C. Endosomal trafficking protein
D. Acetyl-CoA-transporter

Heat-shock proteins (HSPs), or stress proteins, also known as chaperones, play crucial roles in folding/unfolding of proteins, assembly of multiprotein complexes, transport/sorting of proteins into correct subcellular compartments, cell-cycle control and signaling, and protection of cells against stress/apoptosis.

1082. Which of the following is a HSP?
Front Immunol. 2016;7:171

A. HSP70, HSP90
B. Calreticulin
C. GP96
D. All of the above

GR-mediated transrepression involves binding of GR to other TFs, such as activator protein-1 (AP-1) and nuclear factor-kappa-light-chain-enhancer of activated B cells (NF-κB), through protein-protein interactions. This mechanism is referred to as tethering.

1083. After binding of glucocorticoid to glucocorticoid receptor (GR) leads to which of the following?
Harrison's 20th Ed. Chapter 379 Page 2722

A. Dissociation of the heat shock proteins (HSP90) from GR
B. Transrepression of NF-κB & activator protein-1 (AP-1)
C. Dimerization of GR
D. All of the above

NF-κB and AP-1 are pro-inflammatory transcription factors that are repressed by cortisol-bound GR. In the cytosol of target cells, cortisol binds and activates glucocorticoid receptor (GR), which results in dissociation of heat shock proteins (HSPs) from the receptor and subsequent dimerization.

1084. Glucocorticoid response elements (GRE) are located in?
Harrison's 20th Ed. Chapter 379 Page 2722

A. Nucleus
B. Mitochondria
C. Endoplasmic reticulum
D. Golgi bodies

Cortisol-bound GR dimers translocate to nucleus and activate glucocorticoid response elements (GRE) in the DNA sequence thereby enhancing transcription of glucocorticoid-regulated genes (GR transactivation).

1085. In which of the following, corticosterone is the major glucocorticoid?
Harrison's 20th Ed. Chapter 379 Page 2723

A. Rodents
B. Dogs
C. Snakes
D. Birds

Corticosterone has weaker glucocorticoid activity than cortisol. In rodents, corticosterone is the major glucocorticoid.

1086. Glucocorticoids block transcription of?
Harrison's 20th Ed. Chapter 307 Page 2128 Table 307-3

A. IL-1
B. TNF-α
C. IFN-γ
D. All of the above

Glucocorticoids block transcription of IL-1, -2, -3, -6, TNF-α, and IFN-γ.

1087. Cortisol is inactivated to cortisone by?
Harrison's 20th Ed. Chapter 379 Page 2723

A. 11β-hydroxysteroid dehydrogenase type 1 (11β-HSD1)
B. 11β-hydroxysteroid dehydrogenase type 2 (11β-HSD2)
C. Nicotinamide adenine dinucleotide (NADH)
D. Serum glucocorticoid-inducible kinase-1 (SGK-1)

1088. Cortisol is inactivated to cortisone in?

Harrison's 20th Ed. Chapter 379 Page 2723

A. Kidney
B. Colon
C. Salivary glands
D. All of the above

Cortisol is inactivated to cortisone by the microsomal enzyme 11β-hydroxysteroid dehydrogenase type 2 (11β-HSD2) mainly in the kidney but also in the colon and salivary glands.

1089. Which of the following exerts mineralocorticoid activity?

Harrison's 20th Ed. Chapter 379 Page 2723

A. Cortisol
B. Aldosterone
C. Deoxycorticosterone (DOC)
D. All of the above

In addition to cortisol and aldosterone, deoxycorticosterone (DOC) also exerts mineralocorticoid activity.

1090. Which of the following is expressed in outer (glomerulosa) cell layer of adrenal cortex?

Harrison's 20th Ed. Chapter 379 Page 2723

A. 17-hydroxylase
B. 21-hydroxylase
C. Aldosterone synthase
D. All of the above

Phenomenon of zonation exists in adrenal cortex in which selective genes express enzymes that form specific hormones. Aldosterone synthase (CYP11B2) for aldosterone synthesis is expressed only in outer (glomerulosa) cell layer. 21- & 17-hydroxylase are expressed in (inner) fasciculata-reticularis cell layers, which form cortisol & androgen biosynthesis, respectively.

1091. Which of the following occurres when angiotensin II binds to the AT1 receptor?

Harrison's 20th Ed. Chapter 379 Page 2723

A. Increased intracellular sodium
B. Increased intracellular calcium
C. Inhibition of calcium ATPase enzymes
D. All of the above

Binding of angiotensin II to AT1 receptor causes glomerulosa cell membrane depolarization by increasing intracellular sodium through inhibition of sodium potassium (Na^+/K^+) ATPase enzymes. This leads to an increase in intracellular calcium by opening of voltage-dependent calcium channels or inhibition of calcium ATPase enzymes. Consequently, calcium signaling pathway is triggered, resulting in upregulation of aldosterone synthase (CYP11B2) transcrip-tion.

1092. Mineralocorticoid receptor (MR) action best relates to?

Harrison's 20th Ed. Chapter 379 Page 2723

A. Serum glucocorticoid-inducible kinase 1 (SGK-1)
B. Nedd4 protein
C. Epithelial Na channel (ENaC)
D. All of the above

1093. Mutant epithelial Na^+ channel (ENaC) best relates to?

Harrison's 20th Ed. Chapter 379 Page 2723

A. TTP-HUS syndrome
B. Liddle's syndrome
C. Type 1 hepatorenal syndrome
D. Fanconi's syndrome

Disruption of NEDD4-2 dependent ENaC targeting results in Liddle's syndrome, a rare autosomal dominant salt-sensitive hypertension.

1094. NEDD4-2 stands for?

J Am Soc Nephrol 2018 ;29:1706–19

A. Neural precursor cell-expressed developmentally down-regulated 4-2
B. Nephrogenic precursor cell-expressed developmentally down-regulated 4-2
C. Neutral precursor cell-expressed developmentally down-regulated 4-2
D. Natural precursor cell-expressed developmentally down-regulated 4-2

When ENaC associates with Nedd4–2, it is ubiquitylated, endocytosed and degraded in proteasomes or lysosomes. In the absence of Nedd4–2, channel internalization and degradation fall, which increases plasma membrane abundance of ENaC, thereby contributing to the salt-sensitive hypertension.

1095. Which of the following about Ubiquitin is false?

J Am Soc Nephrol 2018 ;29:1706–19

A. E1 is ubiquitin-activating enzyme
B. E2 is ubiquitin-conjugating enzyme
C. E3 is ubiquitin-ligase
D. None of the above

Ubiquitination is a process of reversible post-translational modification of proteins. NEDD4 ligases are key mediators in protein trafficking of transmembrane receptors and ion channels. Nedd4–2 is an E3 ubiquitin-protein ligase that associates with transport proteins, causing their ubiquitylation, and then internalization and degradation. Nedd4–2 associates with the β- or γ-subunits of ENaC and SGK1 is a negative regulator Nedd4-2.

1096. Which of the following is an ENaC inhibitor?

J Am Soc Nephrol 2018 ;29:1706–19

A. Rifampin
B. Amiloride
C. Midodrine
D. Streptomycin

Amiloride-induced ENaC blockade eliminates ENaC-mediated Na+ absorption in principal cells, while stimulating HCl secretion by type A intercalated cells.

1097. Which of the following about serum glucocorticoid-inducible kinase 1 (SGK-1) is false?

Int. J. Mol. Sci. 2016, 17, 1307

A. SGK1 is strongly upregulated by mineralocorticoids
B. Aldosterone-induced SGK1 increases ENaC activity
C. SGK1 is a negative regulator Nedd4-2
D. None of the above

Human SGK1 is ubiquitously expressed throughout the whole body. SGK1 is strongly upregulated by mineralocorticoids. Aldosterone-induced SGK1 increases ENaC activity indirectly by reducing ubiquitination of ENaC via phosphorylation and inhibition of the E3 ubiquitin ligase neuronal precursor cell expressed developmentally down-regulated 4-2 (Nedd4-2). SGK1 is a negative regulator Nedd4-2.

Cushing's Syndrome

1098. Which of the following hormone is measured in urine?
Harrison's 20th Ed. Chapter 369 Page 2651

A. 17-hydroxycorticosteroid
B. 5-hydroxyindoleacetic acid
C. Vanillylmandelic acid
D. All of the above

Various hormone measured in urine include 17-hydroxycorticosteroids, 17-ketosteroids, vanillylmandelic acid, metanephrine, catecholamines, 5-hydroxyindoleacetic acid and calcium.

1099. Physiologically active form of cortisol is?
Harrison's 20th Ed. Chapter 369 Page 2651

A. Free cortisol
B. Protein-bound cortisol
C. Cortisol metabolites
D. All of the above

Following its release from the adrenal, cortisol circulates in bloodstream mainly bound to cortisol-binding globulin (CBG) and to a lesser extent to albumin, with only a minor fraction circulating as free, unbound hormone. A 24 hour urine free cortisol measurement largely reflects the amount of unbound cortisol.

1100. What percentage of circulating cortisol is in the free, bioavailable form?
Current Opinion in Critical Care 2007,13:363–69

A. < 5%
B. < 20%
C. < 30%
D. < 40%

Free cortisol is a physiologically active hormone that is not protein-bound. Normally, <5% of circulating cortisol is free. Free cortisol enters cells directly and does not require active transport.

1101. Cortisol-binding system in plasma is?
Endocrinology. 2010;151:649–59

A. Transcortin
B. Adrenocortin
C. Epicortin
D. Anacortin

Glucocorticoid carrier transcortin is also called corticosteroid-binding globulin (CBG).

1102. Property of cortisol-binding globulin (CBG) is ?
Endocrinology. 2010;151:649–59

A. High-affinity, low-capacity
B. Low-affinity, high-capacity
C. High-affinity, high-capacity
D. Low-affinity, low-capacity

CBG (transcortin) is synthesized and secreted from liver. It is a high-affinity binding protein for glucocorticoids.

1103. Property of albumin for cortisol binding is?
Endocrinology. 2010;151:649–59

A. High-affinity, low-capacity
B. Low-affinity, high-capacity
C. High-affinity, high-capacity
D. Low-affinity, low-capacity

Plasma has two cortisol-binding systems. One is a high-affinity, low-capacity α2-globulin termed transcortin or cortisol-binding globulin (CBG) and albumin which is a low-affinity, high-capacity protein.

1104. Cortisol binds to albumin beyond what concentration?
Crit Care. 2006;10:176

A. 5 μg/dL
B. 15 μg/dL
C. 25 μg/dL
D. 45 μg/dL

When concentration of cortisol is > 25 μg/dL, part of excess binds to albumin.

1105. Which of the following statements about cortisol metabolites is false?
Crit Care. 2006;10:176

A. Biologically inactive
B. Bind weakly to circulating plasma proteins
C. Low levels in urine are typical of children with 3β-HSD2 deficiency
D. None of the above

Cortisol metabolites are biologically inactive & bind weakly to circulating plasma proteins.

1106. The daily secretion of cortisol ranges between?
J Clin Endocrinol Metab. 2006;91:3725–45

A. 5 and 10 mg
B. 10 and 15 mg
C. 15 and 30 mg
D. 30 and 60 mg

Daily secretion of cortisol ranges between 15 & 30 mg (8 - 10 mg/m^2), with a pronounced circadian cycle.

1107. Cortisol inactivation occurs mainly in?
Harrison's 20th Ed. Chapter 379 Page 2723

A. Spleen
B. Lung
C. Kidney
D. Skeletal muscles

Cortisol is inactivated to cortisone by the microsomal enzyme 11β-hydroxysteroid dehydrogenase type 2 (11β-HSD2) mainly in the kidney but also in colon, salivary glands and other target tissues.

1108. Average daily secretion of aldosterone ranges between?
J Clin Endocrinol Metab. 2006;91:3725–45

A. 5 and 10 μg
B. 10 and 15 μg
C. 50 and 250 μg
D. 300 and 600 μg

With normal salt intake, average daily secretion of aldosterone is between 50 & 250 μg.

1109. What percentage of circulating aldosterone is normally inactivated during a single passage through liver?
J Clin Endocrinol Metab. 2006;91:3725–45

A. > 10%
B. > 25%
C. > 50%
D. > 75%

During a single passage through liver, >75% of circulating aldosterone is normally inactivated by conjugation with glucuronic acid.

1110. The major androgen secreted by adrenal gland is?
J Clin Endocrinol Metab. 2006;91:3725–45

A. Dehydroepiandrosterone (DHEA)
B. Androstenedione
C. 11β-hydroxyandrostenedione
D. Testosterone

Major androgen secreted by adrenal is dehydroepiandrosterone (DHEA) & its sulfuric acid ester (DHEAS). Smaller amounts of androstenedione, 11β-hydroxyandrostenedione & testosterone are secreted.

1111. In females, almost all urine 17-ketosteroids are derived from?
J Clin Endocrinol Metab. 2006;91:3725–45

A. Ovaries
B. Adrenal
C. Endometrium
D. All of the above

DHEA is the major precursor of urinary 17-ketosteroids. 2/3 of urine 17-ketosteroids in male are derived from adrenal metabolites, remaining 1/3 comes from testicular androgens. In female, almost all urine 17-ketosteroids are derived from the adrenal.

1112. What level of basal DHEAS suggests an adrenal tumor?
Harrison's 20th Ed. Chapter 387 Page 2800

A. > 1000 μg / L
B. > 3000 μg / L
C. > 5000 μg / L
D. > 7000 μg / L

A basal DHEAS level >18.5 μmol / L (>7000 μg / L) suggests an adrenal tumor.

1113. Which of the following is involved in the etiology of hirsutism?
Harrison's 20th Ed. Chapter 387 Page 2800

A. Testosterone
B. Androstenedione
C. Dehydroepiandrosterone (DHEA)
D. All of the above

Principal circulating steroids involved in the etiology of hirsutism are testosterone, androstenedione, dehydroepiandrosterone (DHEA) and its sulfated form (DHEAS).

1114. Which of the following hormones is embedded within larger precursor polypeptides?
Harrison's 20th Ed. Chapter 370 Page 2654

A. ACTH
B. Glucagon
C. PTH
D. All of the above

Many hormones are embedded within larger precursor polypeptides that are proteolytically processed to yield the biologically active hormone. Examples are proopiomelanocortin (POMC) - ACTH, proglucagon - glucagon, proinsulin - insulin and pro-PTH - PTH.

1115. Size of polypeptide proopiomelanocortin (POMC) is?
Harrison's 20th Ed. Chapter 371 Page 2663

A. 141 amino acid
B. 266 amino acid
C. 344 amino acid
D. 448 amino acid

ACTH (39 amino acids) is derived from the POMC precursor protein (266 amino acids).

1116. POMC (Pro-opiomelanocortin) is made in?
Harrison's 20th Ed. Chapter 371 Page 2663

A. Anterior pituitary
B. Posterior pituitary
C. Lymphocytes
D. All of the above

POMC is made in brain, anterior & posterior pituitary and lymphocytes. Development of corticotrope cells, which express the proopiomelanocortin (POMC) gene, requires the T-Pit transcription factor.

1117. Pro-opiomelanocortin (POMC) is a precursor molecule for?
Harrison's 20th Ed. Chapter 371 Page 2663

A. β-Lipotropin
B. Metenkephalin
C. Corticotropin-like intermediate lobe protein (CLIP)
D. All of the above

1118. Pro-opiomelanocortin (POMC) is a precursor molecule for?
Harrison's 20th Ed. Chapter 371 Page 2663

A. ACTH
B. β-Endorphin
C. α-Melanocyte-stimulating hormone
D. All of the above

POMC precursor protein (266 amino acids) that also generates several other peptides, including ACTH, β-lipoprotein, β-endorphin, metencephalin, α-melanocyte stimulating hormone (β-MSH) and corticotropin-like intermediate lobe protein (CLIP).

1119. Which of the following is released in equimolar concentrations with ACTH?
Harrison's 20th Ed. Chapter 371 Page 2663

A. β-Lipotropin
B. β-endorphin
C. Corticotropin-like intermediate lobe protein (CLIP)
D. All of the above

β-lipotropin (β-LPT) is released in equimolar concentrations with ACTH, suggesting that they are cleaved enzymatically from the parent POMC before or during secretory process. β-endorphin levels may or may not correlate with circulating levels of ACTH, depending on the nature of stimulus.

1120. The POMC gene is induced by all except?
Harrison's 20th Ed. Chapter 371 Page 2663

A. CRH
B. Glucocorticoids
C. Arginine vasopressin
D. IL-6

The POMC gene is potently suppressed by glucocorticoids and induced by corticotropin releasing hormone (CRH), arginine vasopressin (AVP), and proinflammatory cytokines, including IL-6 as well as leukemia inhibitory factor.

1121. Size of CRH is?
Harrison's 20th Ed. Chapter 371 Page 2663

A. 41 amino acid
B. 64 amino acid
C. 84 amino acid
D. 98 amino acid

CRH, a 41 - amino-acid hypothalamic peptide synthesized in the paraventricular nucleus as well as in higher brain centers, is the predominant stimulator of ACTH synthesis and release. The CRH receptor is a GPCR that is expressed on the corticotrope and signals to induce POMC transcription.

1122. ACTH -secreting corticotrope cells constitute what percentage of pituitary cell population?

Harrison's 20th Ed. Chapter 371 Page 2663

A. 5%
B. 10%
C. 15%
D. 20%

ACTH secreting corticotrope cells constitute about 20% of the pituitary cell population.

1123. Which of the following about ACTH secretion is false?

Harrison's 20th Ed. Chapter 371 Page 2663

A. Pulsatile
B. Circadian rhythm
C. Circadian rhythmicity determined by variations in secretory pulse amplitude rather than changes in pulse frequency
D. None of the above

ACTH secretion is pulsatile and exhibits a characteristic circadian rhythm, peaking around 6 A.M. and reaching a nadir around midnight. Adrenal glucocorticoid secretion, which is driven by ACTH, follows a parallel diurnal pattern. ACTH circadian rhythmicity is determined by variations in secretory pulse amplitude rather than changes in pulse frequency.

1124. Which of the following is an ACTH-inducing cytokine?

Harrison's 20th Ed. Chapter 371 Page 2663

A. IL–1
B. IL–2
C. IL–6
D. All of the above

ACTH-inducing cytokines (tumor necrosis factor (TNF, IL-1, IL-2, IL-6 and leukemia inhibitory factor) activates hypothalamic CRH and AVP secretion, pituitary POMC gene expression and local pituitary paracrine cytokine networks.

1125. Neuropeptide 'Urocortin' is related to?

Annu Rev Pharmacol Toxicol 2004; 44:525-57

A. ACTH
B. CRH
C. Leptin
D. FSH

Urocortin, a neuropeptide related to CRH, mimics many of the central effects of CRH (appetite suppression, anxiety).

1126. Which of the following is an angiotensin receptor?

Cardiovascular Research. 2010;86(3):401–09

A. AT1a
B. AT1b
C. AT2
D. All of the above

Angiotensin receptors are AT1a, AT1b and AT2.

1127. Renin is a?

Harrison's 20th Ed. Chapter 271 Page 1892

A. Proteolytic enzyme
B. Hormone
C. Prohormone
D. Cytokine

Renin is a proteolytic enzyme produced & stored in granules of juxta-glomerular cells surrounding afferent arterioles of glomeruli in kidney. Active renin cleaves a substrate, angiotensinogen to form an inactive decapeptide, angiotensin 1.

1128. Which of the following about renin is false?

Harrison's 20th Ed. Chapter 271 Page 1892

A. Renin is an aspartyl protease
B. Precursor of renin, prorenin, is enzymatically inactive
C. Renin is synthesized in afferent renal arteriole
D. None of the above

1129. Which of the following is the primary stimuli for renin secretion?

Harrison's 20th Ed. Chapter 271 Page 1892

A. Decreased NaCl transport in macula densa
B. Decreased pressure in renal afferent arteriole
C. Sympathetic nervous system stimulation via β1 adrenoreceptors
D. All of the above

There are three primary stimuli for renin secretion : decreased NaCl transport in distal portion of thick ascending limb of loop of Henle that abuts the corresponding afferent arteriole (macula densa), decreased pressure or stretch within renal afferent arteriole (baroreceptor mechanism) and sympathetic nervous system stimulation of renin secreting cells via β1 adrenoreceptors.

1130. Factor that decreases renin release is?

Harrison's 20th Ed. Chapter 271 Page 1892

A. Atrial natriuretic peptide
B. Increased dietary potassium
C. Angiotensin II
D. All of the above

Increased dietary intake of potassium decreases renin release, whereas decreased potassium intake increases it. Angiotensin II exerts negative feedback control on renin release that is independent of alterations in renal blood flow, blood pressure, or aldosterone secretion. Atrial natriuretic peptides also inhibit renin release.

1131. Which of the following is false?

Harrison's 20th Ed. Chapter 271 Page 1892

A. Angiotensin I is a decapeptide
B. Angiotensin II is an octapeptide
C. Angiotensin III is a heptapeptide
D. None of the above

Angiotensin I is a decapeptide. Angiotensin II is an octapeptide. angiotensin III is a heptapeptide.

1132. Which of the following is false about 'juxtaglomerular cells'?

Harrison's 20th Ed. Chapter 37 Page 237

A. Specialized myoepithelial cells
B. Cuff efferent arterioles
C. Act as pressure transducers
D. Release renin

Juxtaglomerular cells are specialized myoepithelial cells that cuff the afferent arterioles. They may be seen as miniature pressure transducers, sensing renal perfusion pressure & changes in afferent arteriolar perfusion pressures.

1133. Which of the following is false about macula densa cells?

Harrison's 20th Ed. Chapter 271 Page 1892

A. DCT epithelial cells
B. Directly opposed to juxtaglomerular cells
C. Chemoreceptors
D. Monitor potassium load

Macula densa cells are a group of distal convoluted tubular epithelial cells directly opposed to juxtaglomerular cells. They function as chemoreceptors, monitoring sodium (or chloride) load presented to the distal tubule.

1134. Renin acts on?

Harrison's 20th Ed. Chapter 271 Page 1892

A. Angiotensinogen
B. Angiotensin I
C. Angiotensin II
D. All of the above

Once released into circulation, active renin cleaves angiotensinogen to form an inactive decapeptide, angiotensin I. A converting enzyme located in pulmonary circulation converts angiotensin 1 to the active octapeptide angiotensin II by releasing C-terminal histidyl-leucine dipeptide.

1135. Angiotensin-converting enzyme (ACE) is present mostly in?

Int J Mol Med. 2002;9(3):317-25

A. Pulmonary capillary endothelium
B. Basolateral surface of hepatocytes
C. Basolateral surface of principal cells of kidneys
D. Basolateral surface of intestinal epithelial cells

Angiotensin converting enzyme (ACE, kininase II) is an endothelial luminal ectoenzyme. The majority of ACE is found on pulmonary capillary endothelium (PCE). ACE converts Angiotensin I to octapeptide angiotensin II.

1136. Angiotensinogen is synthesized in?

Harrison's 20th Ed. Chapter 271 Page 1892

A. Liver
B. Spleen
C. Skin
D. All of the above

Angiotensinogen, renin, and angiotensin II are also synthesized locally in brain, pituitary, aorta, arteries, heart, adrenal glands, kidneys, adipocytes, leukocytes, ovaries, testes, uterus, spleen, and skin.

1137. Half-life of renin is?

Lancet 1969;I:213

A. 2–4 minutes
B. 5–10 minutes
C. 10– 20 minutes
D. 30–45 minutes

Half-life of renin is 10–20 minutes.

1138. Tissues that have a local renin-angiotensin system & produce angiotensin II include?

Harrison's 20th Ed. Chapter 271 Page 1892

A. Uterus
B. Placenta
C. Vascular tissue
D. All of the above

1139. Tissues that have a local renin-angiotensin system and produce angiotensin II include all except?

Harrison's 20th Ed. Chapter 271 Page 1892

A. Heart
B. Brain
C. Adrenal cortex
D. Pancreas

Angiotensinogen, renin and angiotensin II are also synthesized locally in brain, pituitary, aorta, arteries, heart, adrenal glands, kidneys, adipocytes, leukocytes, ovaries, testes, uterus, spleen and skin.

1140. Which of the following proteases can lead to formation of Angiotensin II?

Harrison's 20th Ed. Chapter 271 Page 1892

A. Tonin
B. Chymase
C. Cathepsins
D. All of the above

Angiotensin II in tissues may be formed by the enzymatic activity of renin or by other proteases like tonin, chymase and cathepsins.

1141. Excess tissue angiotensin II may contribute to?

Harrison's 20th Ed. Chapter 271 Page 1892

A. Atherosclerosis
B. Cardiac hypertrophy
C. Renal failure
D. All of the above

Excess tissue angiotensin II, a mitogen, may contribute to atherosclerosis, cardiac hypertrophy & renal failure.

1142. Escape phenomenon in kidneys pertains to which hormone?

Harrison's 20th Ed. Chapter 303 Page 2098

A. Aldosterone
B. Renin
C. Angiotensin II
D. Potassium

Aldosterone initially causes sodium retention followed by natriuresis to reestablish sodium balance in 3–5 days preventing edema. This process is called escape phenomenon. It signifies an "escape" by renal tubules from the sodium-retaining action of aldosterone. There is no escape from the potassium-losing effects of mineralocorticoids.

1143. Mineralocorticoids are the major determinants of the metabolism of?

Harrison's 20th Ed. Chapter 303 Page 2098

A. Sodium
B. Potassium
C. Chloride
D. All of the above

Mineralocorticoids are the major determinants of potassium metabolism mediated by the binding of aldosterone to MR in epithelial cells (principal cells in renal cortical collecting duct).

1144. Which is the most common cause of cushingoid features?

Harrison's 20th Ed. Chapter 373 Page 2680

A. Pituitary corticotrope adenomas
B. Ectopic tumor ACTH production
C. Iatrogenic hypercortisolism
D. Cortisol-producing adrenal adenomas

Iatrogenic hypercortisolism is the most common cause of cushingoid features. Pituitary corticotrope adenomas account for 70% of patients with endogenous causes of Cushing's syndrome. ACTH-producing adenomas account for about 10–15% of all pituitary tumors. Ectopic tumor ACTH production, cortisol-producing adrenal adenomas, adrenal carcinoma, adrenal hyperplasia and rarely ectopic tumor CRH production account for the other causes.

1145. Cushing's syndrome refers to?

Harrison's 20th Ed. Chapter 379 Page 2723

A. Exogenous ACTH tumor
B. Adrenal tumor
C. Pituitary ACTH-secreting tumor
D. All of the above

Cushing's syndrome includes a constellation of clinical features that result from chronic exposure to excess glucocorticoids "of any etiology". The disorder can be ACTH-dependent (pituitary corticotrope adenoma, ectopic secretion of ACTH by nonpituitary tumor) or ACTH-independent (adrenocortical adenoma, adrenocortical carcinoma, nodular adrenal hyperplasia) as well as iatrogenic (administration of exogenous glucocorticoids).

1146. Cushing's disease refers to?

Harrison's 20th Ed. Chapter 379 Page 2723

A. ACTH-producing pituitary tumor
B. Exogenous ACTH tumor
C. Pituitary ACTH-secreting tumor
D. All of the above

Cushing's disease refers specifically to Cushing's syndrome caused by a pituitary corticotrope adenoma. A key feature of Cushing disease is that ACTH secretion is relatively resistant to glucocorticoid feedback

1147. The first name of Cushing was?

Harrison's 20th Ed. Chapter 379 Page 2723

A. James
B. Scott
C. Harvey
D. Greg

Cushing's syndrome is caused by an ACTH-producing corticotrope adenoma of the pituitary as initially described by Harvey Cushing in 1912.

1148. Cushing's disease more common in boys in which age group?

Harrison's 20th Ed. Chapter 379 Page 2723

A. Infancy
B. Prepubertal
C. Middle age
D. Old age

Cushing's disease more frequently affects women, with the exception of prepubertal cases, where it is more common in boys.

1149. Most common cause of Cushing's syndrome is?

Harrison's 20th Ed. Chapter 379 Page 2723

A. Iatrogenic administration of steroids
B. Adrenal macronodular hyperplasia
C. Adrenal micronodular dysplasia
D. Adrenal neoplasia

The most common cause of Cushing's syndrome is medical use of glucocorticoids for immunosuppression.

1150. Which out of the following is the most common cause of Cushing's syndrome?

Harrison's 20th Ed. Chapter 379 Page 2724 Table 379-1

A. Cushing's disease
B. Ectopic ACTH syndrome
C. Adrenocortical adenoma
D. Adrenocortical carcinoma

1151. Female: male ratio is more in all except?

Harrison's 20th Ed. Chapter 379 Page 2724 Table 379-1

A. Ectopic ACTH syndrome
B. Cushing's disease
C. Adrenocortical adenoma
D. Adrenocortical carcinoma

Female : male ratio is 1 : 1 in ectopic ACTH syndrome while it is 4 : 1 in the rest.

1152. Pituitary corticotrope adenomas can be found in?

Harrison's 20th Ed. Chapter 379 Page 2724

A. Multiple endocrine neoplasia type 1 (MEN 1)
B. Multiple endocrine neoplasia type 2 (MEN 2)
C. Multiple endocrine neoplasia type 3 (MEN 3)
D. Multiple endocrine neoplasia type 4 (MEN 4)

Pituitary corticotrope adenomas can be found in multiple endocrine neoplasia type 1 (MEN 1).

1153. Pituitary adenomas causative of Cushing's disease frequently harbor mutations in?

Harrison's 20th Ed. Chapter 379 Page 2724

A. USP6
B. USP7
C. USP8
D. USP9

Ubiquitin-specific peptidase 8 (USP8) is an endosome-associated deubiquitinase (DUB). USP8 gene on chromosome 15 is recurrently mutated in human pituitary corticotrophin adenomas, causing Cushing disease via up-regulation of EGFR signaling and consequent upregulated expression of ACTH precursor POMC.

1154. Which of the following can secrete ectopic CRH, ectopic ACTH and catecholamines?

Harrison's 20th Ed. Chapter 379 Page 2724

A. Medullary thyroid carcinoma
B. Pheochromocytoma
C. Advanced small-cell lung cancer
D. All of the above

1155. Somatic mutations in which of the following can cause ACTH-independent cortisol producing tumour?

Harrison's 20th Ed. Chapter 379 Page 2724

A. USP8
B. SGK-1
C. PRKACA
D. All of the above

Constitutively activating mutations in the PKA catalytic subunit PRKACA are found as somatic mutations in one-third of cortisol-producing adrenocortical adenomas and, as germline mutations, can also represent a rare cause of macronodular adrenal hyperplasia associated with cortisol excess.

1156. In ACTH-independent macronodular hyperplasia (AIMAH), which of the following receptor is ectopically expressed in the adrenal gland?

Harrison's 20th Ed. Chapter 379 Page 2724

A. Luteinizing hormone
B. Vasopressin
C. Serotonin
D. All of the above

In ACTH-independent macronodular adrenal hyperplasia (AIMAH), adrenal cortisol excess occurs due to ectopic expression of receptors not usually found in adrenals. These include receptors for luteinizing hormone, vasopressin, serotonin, interleukin-1, or gastric inhibitory peptide (GIP). Activation of these receptors results in upregulation of PKA signaling with a subsequent increase in cortisol production.

1157. Which of the following is a cause of ACTH-independent Cushing's syndrome?

Harrison's 20th Ed. Chapter 379 Page 2724

A. ACTH-independent macronodular hyperplasia (AIMAH)
B. Primary pigmented nodular adrenal disease (PPNAD)
C. McCune-Albright syndrome
D. All of the above

Adrenocortical carcinomas may also cause ACTH-independent disease.

1158. Primary pigmented nodular adrenal disease (PPNAD) is best related to which of the following?

Harrison's 20th Ed. Chapter 379 Page 2724

A. Crow-Fukase Syndrome
B. Hirschsprung disease
C. Carney's complex
D. Von Hippel–Lindau syndrome

Mutations in a regulatory subunit of PKA (PRKAR1A) are found in primary pigmented nodular adrenal disease (PPNAD) as part of Carney's complex.

1159. Which of the following is a feature of Carney's complex?

Harrison's 20th Ed. Chapter 379 Page 2724

A. Cardiac myxomas
B. Hyperlentiginosis
C. Sertoli's cell tumors
D. All of the above

Carney's complex is an autosomal dominant multiple neoplasia condition associated with cardiac myxomas, hyperlentiginosis, Sertoli's cell tumors, and PPNAD.

1160. McCune-Albright syndrome is caused by activating mutations in which of the following?

Harrison's 20th Ed. Chapter 379 Page 2724

A. GNAS-1
B. PKA
C. CREB
D. StAR

McCune Albright syndrome is caused by activating mutations in the stimulatory G protein alpha subunit 1, GNAS- 1 (guanine nucleotide binding protein alpha stimulating activity polypeptide 1).

1161. McCune Albright syndrome is associated with which of the following?

Harrison's 20th Ed. Chapter 379 Page 2724

A. Polyostotic fibrous dysplasia
B. Unilateral cafe-au-lait spots
C. Precocious puberty
D. All of the above

McCune Albright syndrome is associated with polyostotic fibrous dysplasia, unilateral cafe-au-lait spots and precocious puberty.

1162. Which of the following is upregulated by cortisol excess?

Harrison's 20th Ed. Chapter 379 Page 2724

A. Gluconeogenesis
B. Lipolysis
C. Protein catabolism
D. All of the above

1163. Which of the following is a mineralocorticoid action in cortisol excess scenario?

Harrison's 20th Ed. Chapter 379 Page 2724

A. Diastolic hypertension
B. Hypokalemia
C. Edema
D. All of the above

1164. Which of the following is a result of interference by cortisol excess with central regulatory systems?

Harrison's 20th Ed. Chapter 379 Page 2724

A. Hypogonadism
B. Amenorrhea
C. Decreased thyroid-stimulating hormone (TSH)
D. All of the above

1165. Location of "buffalo hump" is?

Harrison's 20th Ed. Chapter 379 Page 2725 Table 379-2

A. Neck
B. Interscapular region
C. Over lumbar spine
D. Any of the above

Fat pad on back of neck (dorsocervical) is called "buffalo hump".

1166. Which of the following features of Cushing's syndrome is considered more specific?

Harrison's 20th Ed. Chapter 379 Page 2725

A. Diastolic hypertension
B. Osteoporosis
C. Easy bruising & broad, purplish striae
D. Obesity

1167. Which of the following features of Cushing's syndrome is considered more specific?

Harrison's 20th Ed. Chapter 379 Page 2725

A. Fragility of the skin with easy bruising
B. Broad, purplish striae
C. Proximal myopathy
D. All of the above

1168. Which of the following features of Cushing's syndrome is considered nonspecific?

Harrison's 20th Ed. Chapter 379 Page 2725

A. Hirsutism
B. Depression
C. Obesity
D. All of the above

Signs & symptoms of hypercortisolism (obesity, diastolic hypertension, osteoporosis, diabetes, hirsutism and depression) are nonspecific. More specific features of Cushing's syndrome are fragility of the skin, with easy bruising and broad (>1 cm), purplish striae and signs of proximal myopathy.

1169. Which of the following about clinical features of ectopic ACTH syndrome is false?

Harrison's 20th Ed. Chapter 379 Page 2725

A. Brisk onset & rapid progression of signs & symptoms
B. Hyperpigmentation of knuckles, scars & friction prone areas
C. Severe myopathy
D. None of the above

Hypertension, hypokalemic alkalosis, glucose intolerance and edema are also more pronounced in ectopic ACTH syndrome patients. Serum potassium levels <3.3 mmol/L are evident in ~70% of patients with ectopic ACTH secretion but are seen in < 10% of patients with pituitary-dependent Cushing's syndrome.

1170. Which of the following is associated with Cushing's syndrome?
Harrison's 20th Ed. Chapter 379 Page 2725

A. Deep vein thrombosis
B. Anxiety or depression
C. Increased risk of cardiovascular disease
D. All of the above

1171. Which of the following test is useful for the diagnosis of Cushing's syndrome?
Harrison's 20th Ed. Chapter 379 Page 2726

A. Increased 24-h urinary free cortisol excretion
B. Failure to suppress morning cortisol with dexamethasone
C. Loss of diurnal cortisol secretion
D. All of the above

Diagnosis of Cushing's syndrome is established if results consistently suggest increased 24-hour urinary free cortisol excretion in three separate collections, failure to appropriately suppress morning cortisol after overnight exposure to dexamethasone, and evidence of loss of diurnal cortisol secretion with high levels at midnight, the time of the physiologically lowest secretion.

1172. What value of a 24-hour urinary free cortisol excretion is suggestive of Cushing's syndrome?
Harrison's 20th Ed. Chapter 379 Page 2726 Figure 379-10

A. Twice normal
B. Thrice normal
C. Four times normal
D. Five times normal

24-hour urinary free cortisol excretion thrice normal is suggestive of Cushing's syndrome.

1173. In Cushing's syndrome, after dexamethasone overnight suppression, plasma cortisol remains above?
Harrison's 20th Ed. Chapter 379 Page 2726 Figure 379-10

A. 5 nmol/L
B. 10 nmol/L
C. 25 nmol/L
D. 50 nmol/L

In Cushing's syndrome, after a standard low-dose dexamethasone overnight suppression test (1 mg. at 11 PM), plasma cortisol remains >50 nmol/L at 8 AM. High-dose dexamethasone administration means 2 mg every 6 hour for 48 hours or 8-mg overnight.

1174. In Cushing's syndrome, midnight plasma cortisol remains above?
Harrison's 20th Ed. Chapter 379 Page 2726 Figure 379-10

A. 50 nmol/L
B. 90 nmol/L
C. 110 nmol/L
D. 130 nmol/L

In Cushing's syndrome, midnight plasma cortisol remains >130 nmol/L.

1175. In Cushing's syndrome, midnight salivary cortisol remains above?
Harrison's 20th Ed. Chapter 379 Page 2726 Figure 379-10

A. 1 nmol/L
B. 2.5 nmol/L
C. 4.2 nmol/L
D. 5 nmol/L

In Cushing's syndrome, midnight salivary cortisol remains >5 nmol/L.

1176. Which of the following can affect the outcome of diagnostic tests for Cushing's syndrome?
Harrison's 20th Ed. Chapter 379 Page 2726

A. Antiepileptics
B. Rifampicin
C. Oral contraceptives
D. All of the above

Members of the CYP3A family (CYP3A4, CYP3A5) metabolize the greatest number of drugs in therapeutic use, followed by CYP2D6. Antiepileptics & rifampicin are CYP3A4 inducing drugs. Oral contraceptives raise CBG.

1177. Which of the following is suggestive of Cushing's syndrome?
Harrison's 20th Ed. Chapter 379 Page 2726

A. Urine free cortisol > 50 µg/day
B. Plasma cortisol > 5 µg/dL after standard low-dose dexamethasone suppression test
C. Absence of normal fall of plasma cortisol at midnight
D. All of the above

Laboratory tests for Cushing's syndrome are based on documentation of increased 24-h urinary free cortisol (UFC) excretion, failure to appropriately suppress morning cortisol after overnight exposure to dexamethasone and evidence of loss of diurnal cortisol secretion with high levels at midnight, the time of the physiologically lowest secretion.

1178. Which of the following tests is used for the diagnosis of Cushing's syndrome?
Eur J Endocrinol. 2007;157(3):245-54

A. Midnight serum or salivary cortisol level
B. Dexamethasone-CRH test
C. Desmopressin test
D. All of the above

Tests used for the diagnosis of CS include midnight serum or salivary cortisol, dexamethasone-CRH Test and desmopressin Test.

1179. Which of the following is false about Pseudo-Cushing's states (PCS)?
Eur J Endocrinol. 2007;157(3):245-54

A. Clinical features of Cushing's syndrome
B. Biochemical evidence of hypercortisolism
C. Normal hypothalamic-pituitary-adrenal axis
D. None of the above

PCS are a heterogeneous group of disorders, either physiological or non-physiological, that lead to increased cortisol production and stigmata of hypercortisolism.

1180. Non-physiological condition associated with PCS is?
Eur J Endocrinol. 2007;157(3):245-54

A. Chronic alcoholism
B. Poorly controlled diabetes mellitus
C. Polycystic ovary syndrome (PCOS)
D. All of the above

Non-physiological conditions associated with PCS include chronic alcoholism and alcohol withdrawal syndrome, major depression, poorly controlled diabetes mellitus, polycystic ovary syndrome (PCOS) and obesity. Physiological conditions leading to PCS include surgery associated stress, severe illness, emotional stress, intense aerobic exercise and caloric restriction.

1181. Which of the following about cyclic Cushing's syndrome is false?

Eur J Endocrinol. 2007;157(3):245-54

A. Cortisol excess periods followed by normal cortisol secretion
B. Seen in pituitary corticotroph adenoma
C. Clinical features of Cushing's syndrome
D. None of the above

Cyclic Cushing's syndrome is characterized by repeated episodes of cortisol excess interspersed by periods of normal cortisol secretion. These cycles of hypercortisolism can occur regularly or irregularly with intercyclic phases ranging from days to years. To formally diagnose cyclic CS, three peaks and two troughs of cortisol production should be demonstrated. Most cases originated from a pituitary corticotroph adenoma, followed by ectopic ACTH-producing tumour and an adrenal tumour.

1182. Very high levels of plasma ACTH are found in?

Harrison's 20th Ed. Chapter 379 Page 2726

A. Ectopic ACTH syndrome
B. Adrenocortical adenoma
C. Adrenal hyperplasia
D. Cushing's disease

Very high levels of plasma ACTH are found in some patients with ectopic ACTH syndrome.

1183. Which of the following is best related to computed tomography (CT) scan?

Harrison's 20th Ed. Chapter 379 Page 2727

A. Halmos units
B. Hounsfield units
C. Apostol units
D. Croom units

CT acquires images by passing a thin X-ray beam through the body at many angles to generate cross-sectional images. X-ray transmission measurements are collected by a detector array and digitized into pixels that form an image. The grayscale information in individual pixels is determined by the attenuation of the X-ray beam along its path by tissues of different densities, referenced to the value for water in units known as Hounsfield units.

1184. Which of the following statements is false?

Harrison's 20th Ed. Chapter 379 Page 2727

A. Very high plasma ACTH levels found in ectopic ACTH syndrome
B. Nodules in pituitary or adrenal are a common finding in general population
C. Pituitary corticotrope adenomas fail to enhance following gadolinium administration on T1-weighted MRI images
D. None of the above

1185. Which of the following is the commonest feature of 'Cushing's syndrome'?

Harrison's 20th Ed. Chapter 373 Page 2680 Table 373-7

A. Centripetal obesity
B. Hypertension
C. Hirsutism
D. Proximal myopathy

1186. Which of the following is typical of Cushing's syndrome?

Harrison's 20th Ed. Chapter 373 Page 2680 Table 373-7

A. Moon facies
B. Buffalo hump
C. Truncal obesity
D. All of the above

Hypercortisolism promotes deposition of adipose tissue in upper face (moon facies), interscapular area (buffalo hump), supraclavicular fat pads & mesenteric bed (truncal obesity). Rarely, episternal fatty tumors and mediastinal widening secondary to fat accumulation occur.

1187. Which of the following is a cause of diffuse hyperpigmentation?

Harrison's 20th Ed. Chapter 54 Page 345 Table 54-11

A. Nelson syndrome
B. Ectopic ACTH syndrome
C. Hyperthyroidism
D. All of the above

1188. Ectopic ACTH production causing Cushing's syndrome is mostly seen with?

Harrison's 20th Ed. Chapter 80 Page 603

A. Foregut carcinoids
B. Midgut carcinoids
C. Hindgut carcinoids
D. All of the above

Foregut carcinoids (respiratory tract primarily) are the most common cause of ectopic ACTH syndrome.

1189. Decreased bone mineralization due to use of steroids is particularly pronounced in?

Curr Osteoporos Rep. 2016;14(3):106–13

A. Children
B. Adults
C. Elderly
D. All of the above

Decreased bone mineralization due to use of steroids is particularly pronounced in children.

1190. Normal plasma ACTH level is?

Endocrinol Metab (Seoul). 2015;30(3):297–304

A. 6–76 pg/mL
B. 100–186 pg/mL
C. 190–326 pg/mL
D. 350–496 pg/mL

Normal plasma ACTH levels are 6–76 pg/mL or 1.3 –16.7 pmol/L.

1191. Which of the following is not expressed in pg/mL?

Harrison's 20th Ed. Chapter 379 Page 2727

A. Gastrin
B. AVP
C. 25(OH) vitamin D
D. Testosterone

1192. Which of the following is not expressed in pg/mL?

Harrison's 20th Ed. Chapter 379 Page 2727

A. PTH
B. Glucagon
C. α-fetoprotein
D. NT-proBNP

1193. Ectopic ACTH production accounts for what percentage of cases of Cushing's syndrome?

Harrison's 20th Ed. Chapter 89 Page 664

A. 1–2%

B. 2–6%

C. 6–10%

D. 10–20%

Ectopic ACTH production accounts for 10–20% of cases of Cushing's syndrome.

1194. Which of the following is the most common cause of ectopic ACTH?

Harrison's 20th Ed. Chapter 89 Page 664

A. Islet cell tumor

B. Bronchial carcinoid

C. Pheochromocytoma

D. Small-cell lung cancer (SCLC)

Ectopic ACTH syndrome is common in neuroendocrine tumors. SCLC is the most common cause of ectopic ACTH, followed by bronchial and thymic carcinoids, islet cell tumors & pheochromocytomas.

1195. Which of the following can cause 'Ectopic ACTH syndrome'?

Harrison's 20th Ed. Chapter 89 Page 664

A. Oat cell bronchogenic carcinoma

B. Carcinoid tumors of thymus, pancreas, ovary

C. Medullary carcinoma of thyroid

D. All of the above

Most cases of Ectopic ACTH syndrome are associated with primitive small cell (oat cell) bronchogenic carcinoma, carcinoid tumors of thymus, pancreas, ovary, medullary carcinoma of thyroid, or bronchial adenomas. Rarely, corticotropin-releasing hormone (CRH) is produced by pancreatic islet cell tumors, SCLC, medullary thyroid cancer, carcinoids or prostate cancer. When levels are high enough, CRH can cause pituitary corticotrope hyperplasia and Cushing's syndrome. Tumors that produce CRH sometimes also produce ACTH, raising the possibility of a paracrine mechanism for ACTH production.

1196. Which of the following statements about ectopic ACTH syndrome is false?

Harrison's 20th Ed. Chapter 379 Page 2727

A. Very high plasma ACTH levels

B. Typically resistant to dexamethasone suppression

C. Unresponsive to CRH

D. None of the above

Ectopic sources of ACTH are typically resistant to dexamethasone suppression and unresponsive to CRH.

1197. What ratio of central / peripheral plasma ACTH at baseline after CRH injection is indicative of Cushing's disease?

Harrison's 20th Ed. Chapter 379 Page 2727

A. > 2

B. > 3

C. > 4

D. > 5

1198. What ratio of central / peripheral plasma ACTH at 2–5 minutes after CRH injection is indicative of Cushing's disease?

Harrison's 20th Ed. Chapter 379 Page 2727

A. > 2

B. > 3

C. > 4

D. > 5

By performing bilateral inferior petrosal sinus sampling (IPSS), increased central / peripheral plasma ACTH ratio >2 at baseline and >3 at 2–5 minutes after CRH injection is indicative of Cushing's disease. Ectopic ACTH secreting tumors have a C:P ACTH ratio <2 both in the basal state and following CRH stimulation. A ratio of ≥ 1.4 between the two sinuses (lateralization ratio) is used to predict the site of tumor in patients with Cushing's disease.

1199. Dose of human CRH used in IPSS is?

Harrison's 20th Ed. Chapter 379 Page 2727, North Clin Istanb 2019;6(1):53-58

A. 0.1 µg / kg

B. 0.5 µg / kg

C. 1 µg / kg

D. 1.5 µg / kg

Pituitary veins drains via cavernous sinuses to petrosal sinuses and then jugular bulb. Blood samples for ACTH are obtained in basal state & at 3, 5 and 10 minutes after administration of ovine or human CRH (1 µg/kg, maximum 100 µg) simultaneously from both IPSS and a peripheral vein.

1200. Patients with ectopic ACTH syndrome should undergo blood sampling for?

Harrison's 20th Ed. Chapter 379 Page 2727

A. Fasting gut hormones

B. Chromogranin A

C. Calcitonin

D. All of the above

Patients with ectopic ACTH syndrome should undergo blood sampling for fasting gut hormones, chromogranin A, calcitonin and biochemical exclusion of pheochromocytoma.

1201. Ectopic ACTH production is caused by increased expression of which of the following gene?

Harrison's 20th Ed. Chapter 89 Page 664

A. Proopiomelanocortin (POMC)

B. ACTH

C. Corticotropin-releasing hormone (CRH)

D. All of the above

Ectopic ACTH production is caused by increased expression of the proopiomelanocortin (POMC) gene, which encodes ACTH, along with melanocyte-stimulating hormone (MSH), β-lipotropin & several other peptides.

1202. Metabolic manifestation of ectopic ACTH syndrome is?

Harrison's 20th Ed. Chapter 89 Page 664

A. Fluid retention, hypertension & hypokalemia

B. Metabolic alkalosis

C. Glucose intolerance

D. All of the above

Metabolic manifestations of ectopic ACTH syndrome include fluid retention and hypertension, hypokalemia, metabolic alkalosis, glucose intolerance, and occasionally steroid psychosis.

1203. Which of the following is false about ectopic ACTH syndrome?

Harrison's 20th Ed. Chapter 89 Page 664

A. Caused by nonpituitary tumors secreting ACTH / CRH

B. Bilateral adrenal hyperplasia

C. Typical s/s of Cushing's syndrome present

D. Hypokalemic alkalosis

Ectopic ACTH syndrome is caused by nonpituitary tumors that secrete either ACTH and/or CRH & cause bilateral adrenal hyperplasia. Ectopic production of CRH results in clinical, biochemical, and radiologic features indistinguishable from those caused by hypersecretion of pituitary ACTH. Typical signs & symptoms of Cushing's syndrome may be absent or minimal with ectopic ACTH production & hypokalemic alkalosis is a prominent manifestation. Excess mineralocorticoids produced by ACTH stimulation of the adrenal gland, high levels of cortisol exert activity through the mineralocorticoid receptor, leading to severe hypokalemia.

1204. Which of the following tests is useful in the diagnosis of 'Ectopic ACTH syndrome'?

Harrison's 20th Ed. Chapter 89 Page 664

A. Urine free cortisol level (UFC)
B. Plasma ACTH level
C. High-dose dexamethasone suppression test
D. All of the above

Urine free cortisol levels are typically greater than two to four times normal and the plasma ACTH level is usually >22 pmol/L (>100 pg/mL). A suppressed ACTH level excludes ectopic ACTH syndrome and indicates an ACTH-independent cause of Cushing's syndrome. High-dose dexamethasone fails to suppress ectopic ACTH in ~90% of cases.

1205. Which of the following is used in treatment of Ectopic ACTH syndrome?

Harrison's 20th Ed. Chapter 89 Page 665

A. Ketoconazole
B. Metyrapone
C. Mitotane
D. All of the above

Medical therapy with ketoconazole, metyrapone, mitotane or other agents that block steroid synthesis or action is often the most practical strategy for managing the hypercortisolism associated with ectopic ACTH production. Adrenalectomy is not practical.

1206. Which of the following drugs inhibits the early steps of steroidogenesis?

Harrison's 20th Ed. Chapter 379 Page 2728

A. Metyrapone
B. Ketoconazole
C. Mitotane
D. All of the above

Antimycotic ketoconazole inhibits the early steps of steroidogenesis.

1207. Which of the following drugs inhibits cortisol synthesis at the level of 11β-hydroxylase?

Harrison's 20th Ed. Chapter 379 Page 2728

A. Metyrapone
B. Ketoconazole
C. Mitotane
D. All of the above

Metyrapone inhibits cortisol synthesis at the level of 11β-hydroxylase.

1208. Metyrapone inhibits cortisol synthesis at the level of?

Harrison's 20th Ed. Chapter 379 Page 2728

A. 11β-hydroxylase (CYP11B1)
B. 11β-hydroxysteroid dehydrogenase type 2 (HSD11B2)
C. 17α-hydroxylase (CYP17A1)
D. 21-hydroxylase (CYP21A2)

Metyrapone inhibits cortisol synthesis at the level of 11β-hydroxylase.

1209. Which of the following is a derivative of insecticide o,p'DDD?

Harrison's 20th Ed. Chapter 379 Page 2728

A. Ketoconazole
B. Metyrapone
C. Mitotane
D. All of the above

Mitotane, a derivative of the insecticide o,p'DDD, is an adrenolytic agent.

1210. Which of the following intravenous anesthetic agent is used to lower cortisol?

Harrison's 20th Ed. Chapter 379 Page 2728

A. Ketamine
B. Etomidate
C. Fospropofol
D. Methohexital

Subhypnotic doses of etomidate effectively reduce the high systemic cortisol and aldosterone concentrations associated with Cushing's syndrome with mild sedation as a side-effect.

1211. Which of the following hypercorticolism state shows the best recovery rate after tumour removal?

Harrison's 20th Ed. Chapter 379 Page 2728

A. Ectopic ACTH syndrome
B. Adrenal Cushing's syndrome
C. Cushing's disease
D. All of the above

Ectopic ACTH syndrome shows the best recovery rate (80%) and adrenal Cushing's has the lowest (40%), with Cushing's disease intermediate (60%) after tumour removal.

1212. Which of the following about primary aldosteronism (PA) is false?

Circulation. 2018;138:823–35

A. Most common form of secondary hypertension
B. Inappropriately elevated aldosterone production
C. Low plasma renin
D. None of the above

Primary aldosteronism (PA) is the most common cause of secondary hypertension, with a prevalence of 20% among patients with resistant hypertension, 10% in those with severe hypertension (SBP ≥180, DBP ≥110 mm Hg), and 6% in those with otherwise uncomplicated hypertension. PA is defined as inappropriately elevated aldosterone production in the setting of low plasma renin.

1213. Primary aldosteronism should be routinely implemented in patients with?

Circulation. 2018;138:823–35

A. Hypertension with hypokalemia
B. Resistant hypertension
C. Early-onset hypertension
D. All of the above

Screening for PA should be routinely implemented in patients with resistant hypertension, hypertension with hypokalemia, or early-onset hypertension.

1214. Mineralocorticoid receptor (MR) is highly expressed in?

Circulation. 2018;138:823–35

A. Distal convoluted tubule & cortical collecting duct of kidney
B. Colonic mucosa
C. Eccrine sweat glands
D. All of the above

1215. Mineralocorticoid receptor (MR) is expressed in?
Circulation. 2018;138:823–35

A. Cardiomyocytes
B. Vascular smooth muscle cells
C. Endothelial cells
D. All of the above

1216. Mineralocorticoid receptor (MR) is expressed in?
Circulation. 2018;138:823–35

A. Brown adipose tissue
B. Macrophages
C. Neurons in hippocampus, hypothalamus, and brainstem
D. All of the above

Mineralocorticoid receptor (MR) is highly expressed in epithelial cells lining the distal convoluted tubule & cortical collecting duct of kidney, colonic mucosa & eccrine sweat glands. Also, MR is expressed in cardiomyocytes, vascular smooth muscle cells, endothelial cells, cells within brown adipose tissue, macrophages & neurons in hippocampus, hypothalamus, and brainstem.

1217. Aldosterone production is increased by?
Circulation. 2018;138:823–35

A. Angiotensin II
B. High plasma potassium concentration
C. Adrenocorticotropic hormone
D. All of the above

Renin and aldosterone normally rise and fall in parallel. PA is characterized by an autonomous aldosterone production which is inappropriately high for sodium state and is not regulated by angiotensina II or plasma potassium concentrations.

1218. Mineralocorticoid excess is caused by which of the following?
Harrison's 20th Ed. Chapter 379 Page 2728

A. Bilateral micronodular hyperplasia
B. Adrenocortical carcinoma
C. Glucocorticoid-remediable aldosteronism (GRA)
D. All of the above

Commonest cause of mineralocorticoid excess is primary aldosteronism, reflecting excess production of aldosterone by adrenal zona glomerulosa. Bilateral micronodular hyperplasia, unilateral adrenal adenomas, adrenocortical carcinoma and glucocorticoid-remediable aldosteronism (GRA) cause primary aldosteronism. The clinical hallmark of mineralocorticoid excess is hypokalemic hypertension.

1219. Which of the following is caused by a chimeric gene?
Harrison's 20th Ed. Chapter 379 Page 2728

A. Bilateral micronodular hyperplasia
B. Unilateral adrenal adenomas
C. Adrenocortical carcinoma
D. Glucocorticoid-remediable aldosteronism (GRA)

Glucocorticoid-remediable aldosteronism (GRA) is caused by a chimeric gene resulting from cross-over of promoter sequences between the CYP11B1 (11β-hydroxylase) and CYP11B2 (aldosterone synthase) genes that are involved in glucocorticoid and mineralocorticoid synthesis respectively. Consequently, aldosterone production is regulated by ACTH rather than by renin.

1220. Which of the following is a dexamethasone suppressible hyperaldosteronism?
Harrison's 20th Ed. Chapter 379 Page 2728 Table 379-3

A. Bilateral micronodular hyperplasia
B. Unilateral adrenal adenomas
C. Adrenocortical carcinoma
D. Glucocorticoid-remediable aldosteronism (GRA)

1221. Which of the following about Glucocorticoid remediable aldosteronism (GRA) is false?
Harrison's 20th Ed. Chapter 379 Page 2728

A. Early onset severe familial hypertension
B. Primary aldosteronism
C. Normalization of hypertension with glucocorticoids
D. None of the above

First described in 1996 by Sutherland, familial hyperaldosteronism Type 1 or glucocorticoid remediable aldosteronism (GRA) is rare familial form (autosomal dominant) of primary aldosteronism characterized by a normalization of hypertension with the administration of glucocorticoids (dexamethasone).

1222. Which of the following about Glucocorticoid remediable aldosteronism (GRA) is false?
Harrison's 20th Ed. Chapter 379 Page 2728

A. Low renin hypertension with high aldosterone / renin ratio
B. Failure to suppress aldosterone with salt loading
C. Elevated 18-hydroxycortisol, 18-hydroxycorticosterone, and 18-oxocortisol levels
D. None of the above

GRA is a low renin hypertension characterized by high aldosterone/renin ratio, failure to suppress aldosterone with salt loading, and elevated 18-hydroxycortisol, 18-hydroxycorticosterone, and 18-oxocortisol levels. Histologic studies show specific hyperplasia of zona fasciculata, with concomitant atrophy of zona glomerulosa.

1223. Which of the following can cause hypokalemic hypertension?
Harrison's 20th Ed. Chapter 379 Page 2729

A. Syndrome of apparent mineralocorticoid excess (SAME)
B. Excess licorice ingestion
C. Liddle's syndrome
D. All of the above

1224. Liddle's syndrome best relates to?
Harrison's 20th Ed. Chapter 379 Page 2729

A. Pendrin
B. ENaC
C. Aquaporin-2 (AQP-2)
D. Basolateral aquaporin-3 & aquaporin-4

Autosomal dominant Liddle's syndrome with excess mineralocorticoid activity is caused by mutations in the β or γ subunits of amiloride-sensitive epithelial Na^+ channels (ENaC) that disrupts its interaction with Nedd4 leading to decreased receptor internalization, degradation & constitutively active ENAC manifesting as hypokalemic hypertension.

1225. Which of the following is false about bilateral cortical nodular hyperplasia?
Harrison's 20th Ed. Chapter 379 Page 2728

A. ~80% of patients with primary aldosteronism
B. Hypokalemia less likely
C. Less radiologic evidence for adrenal pathology
D. None of the above

Patients with bilateral hyperplasia are unlikely to have hypokalemia & have lower levels of aldosterone & less radiologic evidence for adrenal pathology. They constitute ~80% of patients with primary aldosteronism. Hypertension associated with idiopathic bilateral nodular hyperplasia does not usually benefit from bilateral adrenalectomy, whereas hypertension associated with aldosterone-producing tumors is usually improved or cured by removal of the adenoma.

1226. Syndrome of apparent mineralocorticoid excess (SAME) is caused by inactivating mutations in which of the following gene?

Harrison's 20th Ed. Chapter 379 Page 2729

A. RET
B. HSD11B2
C. GNAS1
D. PRKAR1A

Syndrome of apparent mineralocorticoid excess (SAME) is caused by inactivating mutations in the HSD11B2 gene resulting in in lack of renal inactivation of cortisol to cortisone leading to excess activation of the MR by cortisol. Severe hypokalemic hypertension in childhood is the characteristic manifestation. An increased free cortisol over free cortisone ratio is suggestive of SAME and can be treated with dexamethasone.

1227. Which of the following about SAME I is false?

Harrison's 20th Ed. Chapter 379 Page 2729

A. Caused by inactivating mutations in HSD11B2 gene
B. Seen in childhood
C. Severe hypokalemic hypertension
D. None of the above

1228. Which of the following about SAME II is false?

Harrison's 20th Ed. Chapter 379 Page 2729

A. Caused by inactivating mutations in HSD11B2 gene
B. Seen in adulthood
C. Normokalemic hypertension
D. None of the above

1229. The clinical hallmark of mineralocorticoid excess is?

Harrison's 20th Ed. Chapter 379 Page 2729

A. Hyponatremia
B. Hypokalemic hypertension
C. Metabolic alkalosis
D. All of the above

The clinical hallmark of mineralocorticoid excess is hypokalemic hypertension. Suppressed renin levels associated with high aldosterone levels strongly suggest a PA diagnosis.

1230. Connshing syndrome best relates to?

Harrison's 20th Ed. Chapter 379 Page 2729

A. ↑ aldosterone and ↓ cortisol
B. ↑ aldosterone and ↑ cortisol
C. ↓ aldosterone and ↓ cortisol
D. ↓ aldosterone and ↑ cortisol

Patients with primary aldosteronism may suffer from concurrent mild autonomous cortisol excess (MACE), termed Connshing syndrome (simultaneous presence of Cushing and Conn syndromes).

1231. Autonomous aldosterone production causes all except?

Harrison's 20th Ed. Chapter 379 Page 2729

A. Increased potassium excretion
B. Increased plasma renin
C. Sodium retention
D. Increased H^+ excretion

Autonomous aldosterone production causes sodium retention, plasma renin supression, HTN, cardiovascular damage, and increased potassium excretion, leading to variable degree of hypokalemia.

1232. Diagnostic screening for mineralocorticoid excess should be done in?

Harrison's 20th Ed. Chapter 379 Page 2729

A. Drug resistant hypertension
B. Hypokalemia
C. Onset of disease before the age of 40 years
D. All of the above

Diagnostic screening for mineralocorticoid excess is not currently recommended for all patients with hypertension and should be done in those who have hypertension associated with drug resistance, hypokalemia, an adrenal mass or onset of disease before the age of 40 years.

1233. Which of the following is mandatory before testing ARR?

Harrison's 20th Ed. Chapter 379 Page 2729

A. Stopping antihypertensive medication
B. Normalized serum potassium
C. Restricted dietary salt intake one week before testing
D. Adequate sleep

Concurrent measurement of plasma renin & aldosterone with subsequent calculation of aldosterone-renin ratio (ARR) is an accepted screening test for PA. Serum potassium needs to be normalized prior to testing.

1234. Which of the following antihypertensive drug must be stopped for at least 4 weeks prior to ARR measurement?

Harrison's 20th Ed. Chapter 379 Page 2729

A. Diuretics
B. ACE inhibitors
C. MR antagonists
D. α1 Blockers

Stopping antihypertensive medication can be risky. For practical purposes, patient can remain on usual antihypertensive medications, with the exception that MR antagonists (spironolactone or eplerenone) need to be stopped at least 4 weeks prior to ARR measurement.

1235. Which of the following can cause false-positive results in ARR testing?

Harrison's 20th Ed. Chapter 379 Page 2729

A. β Blockers
B. ACE inhibitors
C. AT1R blockers
D. Calcium antagonists

1236. Which of the following can cause false-negative results in ARR testing?

Harrison's 20th Ed. Chapter 379 Page 2729

A. β Blockers
B. ACE inhibitors
C. Diuretics
D. Calcium antagonists

1237. Which of the following antihypertensive drug has no effect on ARR?

Harrison's 20th Ed. Chapter 379 Page 2730 Table 379-4

A. α1 Blockers
B. α2 Sympathomimetics
C. Calcium antagonists
D. All of the above

1238. Which of the following antihypertensive drug increases the value of ARR?

Harrison's 20th Ed. Chapter 379 Page 2730 Table 379-4

A. β Blockers
B. ACE inhibitors
C. AT1R blockers
D. All of the above

1239. Which of the following antihypertensive drug decreases renin?

Harrison's 20th Ed. Chapter 379 Page 2730 Table 379-4

A. β Blockers
B. ACE inhibitors
C. AT1R blockers
D. Calcium antagonists

1240. Which of the following antihypertensive drug increases aldosterone?

Harrison's 20th Ed. Chapter 379 Page 2730 Table 379-4

A. β Blockers
B. ACE inhibitors
C. AT1R blockers
D. Calcium antagonists

In premenopausal ovulating women or those using oral contraceptives, false positives can occur during the luteal phase, but only if renin is measured as DRC.

1241. Which of the following antihypertensive medication is recommended while determining ARR?

Arch Endocrinol Metab. 2017;61(3):305-12

A. Verapamil
B. Hydralazine
C. α-1 blockers (doxazosin or prazosin)
D. All of the above

Recommended antihypertensives during ARR estimation are verapamil, hydralazine, and α-1 blockers (doxazosin or prazosin). Clonidine can be added if a fourth medication is needed.

1242. Aldosterone-renin ratio (ARR) screening is positive if the ratio is?

Harrison's 20th Ed. Chapter 379 Page 2729

A. > 150 pmol/L per ng/mL per hour
B. > 350 pmol/L per ng/mL per hour
C. > 550 pmol/L per ng/mL per hour
D. > 750 pmol/L per ng/mL per hour

Aldosterone-renin ratio (ARR) is the most sensitive test that screens for PA. ARR screening is positive if the ratio is >750 pmol / L per ng / mL per hour, with a concurrently high normal or increased aldosterone (>450 pmol/L). ARR involves concurrent measurement of plasma renin and aldosterone.

1243. Minimum aldosterone concentration for determining ARR is?

Arch Endocrinol Metab. 2017;61(3):305-12

A. 6.5 ng/dL
B. 12.5 ng/dL
C. 24.5 ng/dL
D. 32.5 ng/dL

In the presence of low renin levels, the aldosterone-to-renin ratio may be elevated even when aldosterone is not high. Therefore, a minimum aldosterone concentration of 12.5 to 15 ng/dL has been proposed as part of the screening criteria.

1244. What is the relationship between direct renin concentration (DRC) and plasma renin activity (PRA)?

Arch Endocrinol Metab. 2017;61(3):305-12

A. PRA = DRC/2
B. PRA = DRC/8
C. PRA = DRC/12
D. PRA = DRC/16

Relationship between direct renin concentration (DRC) and plasma renin activity (PRA) is PRA = DRC / 12. Most commercial kits measure direct renin concentration; however, the aldosterone-to-renin ratios used in PA screening were determined using PRA.

1245. PA screening is considered positive if?

Arch Endocrinol Metab. 2017;61(3):305-12

A. Aldosterone levels ≥ 12.5 ng/dL
B. Aldosterone/PRA ratio ≥ 30
C. Aldosterone/DRC ratio ≥ 2.5
D. All of the above

If a patient has aldosterone levels ≥ 12.5 ng/dL and aldosterone/PRA (ng/mL/h) ratio ≥ 30 or aldosterone/DRC (mU/L) ratio ≥ 2.5, the PA screening is considered positive. If a patient has aldosterone levels ≥ 20 ng/dL and suppressed PRA or DRC levels, there is no need for further confirmatory testing and computed tomography (CT) scan is advised to investigate PA etiology.

1246. Criteria for the diagnosis of primary aldosteronism include?

Harrison's 20th Ed. Chapter 379 Page 2729

A. Diastolic hypertension without edema
B. Hyposecretion of renin (low PRA levels) that do not increase during volume depletion
C. Hypersecretion of aldosterone that does not suppress in response to volume expansion
D. All of the above

Criteria for the diagnosis of primary aldosteronism are diastolic hypertension without edema, hyposecretion of renin (low PRA levels) that fails to increase appropriately during volume depletion (upright posture, sodium depletion), and hypersecretion of aldosterone that does not suppress appropriately in response to volume expansion.

1247. Which of the following is false about primary aldosteronism?

Harrison's 20th Ed. Chapter 379 Page 2729

A. Hypokalemia
B. Diastolic hypertension
C. No edema
D. None of the above

Hypersecretion of aldosterone causes hypokalemia, diastolic hypertension, headaches, polyuria, polydipsia, left ventricular hypertrophy disproportionate to level of BP. Edema is characteristically absent they exhibit an "escape" phenomenon from the sodium-retaining aspects of mineralocorticoids.

1248. Diagnostic confirmation of mineralocorticoid excess is done by?

Harrison's 20th Ed. Chapter 379 Page 2729

A. Saline infusion test
B. Oral sodium loading test
C. Fludrocortisone suppression test
D. All of the above

1249. Which of the following about saline infusion test is false?

Harrison's 20th Ed. Chapter 379 Page 2729, Arch Endocrinol Metab. 2017;61(3):305-12

A. Infusion of 2 L of 0.9% saline IV over 4 hours in morning
B. Aldosterone levels > 10 ng/dL confirm the diagnosis of PA
C. Aldosterone < 5 ng/dL excludes the diagnosis of PA
D. None of the above

In saline infusion test, failure of aldosterone to suppress <140 pmol/L (5 ng/dL) is indicative of autonomous mineralocorticoid excess.

1250. Which of the following about Furosemide test is false?
Arch Endocrinol Metab. 2017;61(3):305-12

A. 40 mg IV in morning
B. Patient in upright position for 2 hours
C. After 2 hours, PRA < 2 ng/mL/h (or DRC < 24 mU/L) confirms the PA diagnosis
D. None of the above

In Furosemide test, patient receives furosemide 40 mg IV in morning and stays in an upright position for 2 hours. PRA < 2 ng/mL/hour (or DRC < 24 mU/L) confirms the PA diagnosis. Although patients with essential hypertension can present low renin levels, PRA increases above 2 ng/mL/hour after furosemide injection.

1251. Which of the following about Captopril test is false?
Harrison's 20th Ed. Chapter 379 Page 2729, Arch Endocrinol Metab. 2017;61(3):305-12

A. 50 mg of captopril orally after sitting or standing for 1 hour
B. In PA, aldosterone level remains elevated
C. In PA, renin remains suppressed
D. None of the above

In Captopril test, patients receive 50 mg of captopril orally after sitting or standing for at least 1 hour. Plasma aldosterone is normally suppressed by captopril (> 30%). In patients with PA, aldosterone level remains elevated and renin remains suppressed.

1252. Which of the following is difficult to catheterize in adrenal vein sampling (AVS)?
Harrison's 20th Ed. Chapter 379 Page 2729, Arch Endocrinol Metab. 2017;61(3):305-12

A. Right adrenal vein
B. Left adrenal vein
C. Inferior vena cava
D. All of the above

In adrenal vein sampling (AVS), the right adrenal vein may be difficult to catheterize because it is short and enters the inferior vena cava at an acute angle.

1253. Correct positioning of catheter in adrenal vein during AVS procedure is confirmed by?
Harrison's 20th Ed. Chapter 379 Page 2729, Arch Endocrinol Metab. 2017;61(3):305-12

A. Concurrent ACTH measurement
B. Concurrent cortisol measurement
C. Concurrent DHEA measurement
D. All of the above

AVS requires concurrent measurement of cortisol to document correct placement of the catheter in the adrenal veins and should demonstrate a cortisol gradient >3 between the vena cava and each adrenal vein. Cosyntropin infusion maximizes the gradient of cortisol from adrenal vein to inferior vena cava, confirming the successful sampling of the adrenal vein. Lateralization is confirmed by an aldosterone / cortisol ratio that is at least twofold higher on one side than the other.

1254. In primary aldosteronism, which of the following fail to suppress plasma aldosterone?
Harrison's 20th Ed. Chapter 379 Page 2729

A. Captopril
B. Oral sodium
C. Fludrocortisone
D. All of the above

The diagnosis of primary aldosteronism can be confirmed by demonstrating failure to suppress plasma aldosterone to by IV infusion of 2 liters of isotonic saline over 4 hours, an oral NaCl load, fludrocortisone or captopril.

1255. Drug that is of use in primary aldosteronism is?
Harrison's 20th Ed. Chapter 379 Page 2729

A. Spironolactone
B. Eplerenone
C. Amiloride
D. All of the above

1256. Maximum dose of MR antagonist spironolactone is?
Harrison's 20th Ed. Chapter 379 Page 2729

A. 200 mg/day
B. 300 mg/day
C. 400 mg/day
D. 500 mg/day

1257. Maximum dose of MR antagonist eplerenone is?
Harrison's 20th Ed. Chapter 379 Page 2729

A. 200 mg/day
B. 300 mg/day
C. 400 mg/day
D. 500 mg/day

1258. Which of the following is used in the treatment of Glucocorticoid-remediable aldosteronism (GRA)?
Harrison's 20th Ed. Chapter 379 Page 2729

A. Eplerenone
B. Fludrocortisone
C. Dexamethasone
D. Amiloride

Treatment of GRA consists of administering lowest possible dose of dexamethasone to control blood pressure.

1259. Liddle's syndrome patients are very sensitive to which of the following treatment?
Harrison's 20th Ed. Chapter 379 Page 2729

A. Amiloride
B. Dexamethasone
C. Fludrocortisone
D. Eplerenone

Liddle's syndrome patients are very sensitive to amiloride treatment. They not respond to MR antagonist treatment because the defect is due to a constitutively active ENaC.

1260. Which of the following is a finding in nonaldosterone-related mineralocorticoid excess?
Harrison's 20th Ed. Chapter 379 Page 2729

A. Suppressed renin
B. Suppressed aldosterone
C. Hypokalemic hypertension
D. All of the above

1261. Increased free cortisol / free cortisone ratio is suggestive of?
Harrison's 20th Ed. Chapter 379 Page 2730

A. Liddle's syndrome
B. Syndrome of apparent mineralocorticoid excess (SAME)
C. McCune-Albright syndrome
D. All of the above

Increased free cortisol over free cortisone ratio is suggestive of SAME & is treated with dexamethasone.

1262. Urinary steroid metabolite profiling by Gas chromatography / mass spectrometry (GC/MS) is normal in?
Harrison's 20th Ed. Chapter 379 Page 2730

A. Liddle's syndrome
B. CYP11B1 deficiency
C. CYP17A1 deficiency
D. DOC-producing adrenocortical carcinoma

Urinary steroid metabolite profiling by gas chromatography/mass spectrometry (GC/MS) is used for the diagnosis of nonaldosterone-related mineralocorticoid excess. It is is normal in Liddle's syndrome.

1263. Which of the following about Liddle's syndrome is false?
Harrison's 20th Ed. Chapter 379 Page 2730

A. Very sensitive to amiloride treatment
B. Does not respond to MR antagonist treatment
C. Defect is due to a constitutively active ENaC
D. None of the above

1264. What is the prevalence of incidentalomas in the general population?
Harrison's 20th Ed. Chapter 379 Page 2731

A. 0.5–2%
B. 2–5%
C. 5–10%
D. 10–15%

"Incidentalomas" are common with a prevalence of at least 2-5% in the general population. Prevalence increases with age.

1265. Which of the following genetic syndrome has adrenal tumor as one of their features?
Harrison's 20th Ed. Chapter 379 Page 2731

A. MEN 1
B. Carney's complex
C. McCune-Albright syndrome
D. All of the above

Most solitary adrenal tumors are monoclonal neoplasms. MEN 1 (MEN1), MEN 2 (RET), Carney's complex (PRKAR1A) and McCune-Albright (GNAS1) are genetic syndromes that can have adrenal tumors as one of their features.

1266. Which out of the following is the most common cause of a unilateral malignant adrenal mass is?
Harrison's 20th Ed. Chapter 379 Page 2731 Table 379-5

A. Malignant pheochromocytoma
B. Adrenal neuroblastoma
C. Lymphoma
D. Metastasis from another solid tissue tumor

Most common cause of a malignant adrenal mass is metastasis originating from another solid tissue tumor (breast, lung).

1267. Which of the following is a malignant unilateral adrenal mass?
Harrison's 20th Ed. Chapter 379 Page 2731 Table 379-5

A. Adrenocortical adenoma
B. Adrenal neuroblastoma
C. Adrenal ganglioneuroma
D. Adrenal myelolipoma

1268. Which of the following is a indeterminate unilateral adrenal mass?
Harrison's 20th Ed. Chapter 379 Page 2731 Table 379-5

A. Adrenal neuroblastoma
B. Adrenocortical oncocytoma
C. Adrenal hemangioma
D. Adrenal cyst

1269. Which of the following is the most prevalent benign unilateral adrenal mass?
Harrison's 20th Ed. Chapter 379 Page 2731 Table 379-5

A. Endocrine-inactive adrenocortical adenoma
B. Cortisol-producing adrenocortical adenoma
C. Aldosterone-producing adrenocortical adenoma
D. DHEA-producing adrenocortical adenoma

1270. Which of the following is the most prevalent malignant unilateral adrenal mass?
Harrison's 20th Ed. Chapter 379 Page 2731 Table 379-5

A. Adrenocortical carcinoma
B. Malignant pheochromocytoma
C. Primary adrenal lymphoma
D. Metastases in adrenal

1271. Bilateral adrenal enlargement/masses may be caused by?
Harrison's 20th Ed. Chapter 379 Page 2731 Table 379-5

A. Congenital adrenal hyperplasia
B. Amyloidosis
C. Tuberculosis
D. All of the above

Bilateral adrenal enlargement/masses may be caused by congenital adrenal hyperplasia, bilateral macronodular hyperplasia, bilateral hemorrhage, granuloma, amyloidosis, or infiltrative disease including tuberculosis.

1272. Adrenocortical carcinoma is the cause of an adrenal mass in what percentage of patients?
Harrison's 20th Ed. Chapter 379 Page 2731

A. 1%
B. 3%
C. 5%
D. 7%

ACC is the cause of an adrenal mass in 5% of patients.

1273. Which of the following statements is false?
Harrison's 20th Ed. Chapter 379 Page 2731

A. Most solitary adrenal tumors are monoclonal neoplasms
B. Majority of adrenal nodules are endocrine-inactive adrenocortical adenomas
C. Incidentally discovered adrenal masses are called adrenal "incidentalomas"
D. None of the above

1274. Patients with an adrenal mass of what size require a diagnostic evaluation?

Harrison's 20th Ed. Chapter 379 Page 2731

A. > 1 cm
B. > 2 cm
C. > 3 cm
D. > 4 cm

Patients with an adrenal mass >1 cm require a diagnostic evaluation.

1275. Which of the following is secreted by an adrenal mass?

Harrison's 20th Ed. Chapter 379 Page 2731

A. Catecholamine
B. Cortisol
C. Aldosterone
D. Any of the above

1276. Which of the following is most frequently secreted by adrenocortical carcinoma?

Harrison's 20th Ed. Chapter 379 Page 2731

A. Catecholamine
B. Cortisol
C. Aldosterone
D. DHEA

Overproduction of adrenal androgen precursors, DHEA and its sulfate, is rare by an adrenal mass. However, it is most frequently seen in context of ACC, as are increased levels of steroid precursors such as 17-hydroxyprogesterone (17OHP).

1277. Which of the following is the procedure of choice for imaging adrenal glands?

Harrison's 20th Ed. Chapter 379 Page 2731

A. Unenhanced CT
B. Enhanced CT
C. MRI
D. All of the above

Unenhanced CT is the procedure of choice for imaging the adrenal glands.

1278. Which of the following is more likely with increasing diameter of the adrenal mass?

Harrison's 20th Ed. Chapter 379 Page 2731

A. Adrenocortical carcinoma (ACC)
B. Pheochromocytoma
C. Benign adrenal myelolipoma
D. All of the above

1279. Which of the following favor that an adrenal lesion is malignant?

Harrison's 20th Ed. Chapter 379 Page 2731

A. Lobulated and inhomogeneous
B. Size > 4 cm
C. Tumor density on unenhanced CT >20 Hounsfield Units
D. All of the above

1280. Which of the following favor that an adrenal lesion is benign?

Harrison's 20th Ed. Chapter 379 Page 2731

A. Rounded and homogenous
B. Size < 4 cm
C. Tumor density on unenhanced CT <10 Hounsfield Units
D. All of the above

1281. Which of the following may also exhibit lobulated and inhomogeneous features of adrenal gland?

Harrison's 20th Ed. Chapter 379 Page 2731

A. Adrenocortical carcinoma (ACC)
B. Pheochromocytoma
C. Adrenomyelolipoma
D. All of the above

1282. Fine-needle aspiration (FNA) or CT-guided biopsy of an adrenal mass is very rarely indicated for the diagnosis of?

Harrison's 20th Ed. Chapter 379 Page 2731

A. Adrenocortical carcinoma (ACC)
B. Pheochromocytoma
C. Adrenomyelolipoma
D. None of the above

1283. Which of the following tumor-suppressor gene is associated with adrenocortical carcinoma (ACC)?

Harrison's 20th Ed. Chapter 379 Page 2731

A. VHL
B. PRKAR1A
C. TP53
D. RB1

Genes that positively influence growth are known as tumor-suppressor genes. Normal function of tumor-suppressor genes is to restrain cell growth, and this function is lost in cancer. It requires two genetic events to inactivate a tumor-suppressor gene mutation, while only one genetic event is required to activate an oncogene. Tumor-suppressor genes are epigenetically silenced in cancer cells.

1284. Which of the following Li-Fraumeni syndrome is false?

Harrison's 20th Ed. Chapter 87 Page 653

A. Familial cancer syndrome
B. Germline abnormalities of the tumor-suppressor gene p53
C. Increased incidence of soft tissue sarcomas
D. None of the above

Li-Fraumeni syndrome is a familial cancer syndrome in which affected individuals have germline abnormalities of the tumor-suppressor gene p53 and an increased incidence of soft tissue sarcomas and other malignancies, including breast cancer, osteosarcoma, brain tumor, leukemia, and adrenal carcinoma.

1285. Genetic changes identified in ACC include?

Harrison's 20th Ed. Chapter 379 Page 2732

A. TP53 mutation R337H
B. Alterations in the Wnt/β-catenin pathway
C. Insulin-like growth factor 2 (IGF2) overexpression
D. All of the above

1286. Which of the following histopathologic classification is used for adrenocortical carcinoma (ACC)?
Harrison's 20th Ed. Chapter 379 Page 2732

A. Knopp
B. Weiss
C. Schneider
D. Justin

Weiss score for ACC takes into account high nuclear grade; mitotic rate (>5/HPF); atypical mitosis; <25% clear cells; diffuse architecture; and presence of necrosis, venous invasion and invasion of sinusoidal structures and tumor capsule. The presence of three or more elements suggests ACC. Weiss score carries no prognostic value.

1287. Which of the following features of adrenal tumor is indicative of malignancy?
Harrison's 20th Ed. Chapter 379 Page 2732

A. Excess production of glucocorticoids precursors
B. Excess production of adrenal androgen precursors
C. Mixed excess production of several corticosteroid classes
D. All of the above

1288. Metastasis in ACC most frequently occurs to?
Harrison's 20th Ed. Chapter 379 Page 2732

A. Liver
B. Kidney
C. Bone
D. Brain

Metastasis in ACC most frequently occurs to liver and lung.

1289. In ACC, most important prognostic histopathologic parameter is?
Harrison's 20th Ed. Chapter 379 Page 2732

A. FlowJo
B. Ki67
C. CFDA-SE
D. None of the above

The tumor proliferation rate is widely estimated immunohistochemically using the Ki67 antibody MIB-1, which identifies the cells of late G1, S, G2, and M phases. In ACC, most important prognostic histopathologic parameter is the Ki67 proliferation index, with Ki67 <10% indicative of slow to moderate growth velocity, whereas a Ki67 ≥10% is associated with poor prognosis including high risk of recurrence and rapid progression.

1290. Features suggestive of adrenocortical carcinoma (ACC) include all except?
Harrison's 20th Ed. Chapter 379 Page 2732

A. Size > 4–6 cm
B. Soft tissue calcifications visible on CT
C. Tumor inhomogeneity
D. Low unenhanced CT values (<10 HU)

Features suggestive of malignancy include large size (>4–6 cm), irregular margins & tumor inhomogeneity, soft tissue calcifications visible on CT & high unenhanced CT attenuation values (>10 HU).

1291. Principal drug for the treatment of adrenocortical carcinoma (ACC) is?
Harrison's 20th Ed. Chapter 379 Page 2732

A. Mitotane
B. Ketoconazole
C. Mifepristone
D. Metyrapone

Principal drug for treatment of ACC is mitotane (derivative of insecticide o,p'-DDD), isomer of DDT. o,p'-DDD is an inhibitor of adrenal steroid synthesis thus requires glucocorticoid replacement.

1292. In ACC, following removal of the primary tumor, which of the following predict a high risk of recurrence?
Harrison's 20th Ed. Chapter 379 Page 2732

A. Tumor size >8 cm
B. Vascular invasion, capsule invasion or violation
C. Ki67 proliferation index ≥10%
D. All of the above

Patients with confirmed ACC and successful removal of the primary tumor should receive adjuvant treatment with mitotane, particularly in patients with a high risk of recurrence as determined by tumor size >8 cm, histopathologic signs of vascular invasion, capsule invasion or violation, & Ki67 proliferation index ≥10%.

1293. In ACC, which of the following chemotherapeutic agent is useful?
Harrison's 20th Ed. Chapter 379 Page 2732

A. Cisplatin
B. Etoposide
C. Doxorubicin
D. All of the above

In ACC, the established first line chemotherapy regimen is the combination of cisplatin, etoposide, and doxorubicin plus continuing mitotane.

1294. Primary adrenal insufficiency is most commonly caused by?
Harrison's 20th Ed. Chapter 379 Page 2733

A. Autoimmune adrenalitis
B. Congenital adrenal hyperplasia
C. X-linked adrenoleukodystrophy
D. Adrenal metastases

Primary adrenal insufficiency is most commonly caused by autoimmune adrenalitis may occur sporadically (30–40%) or as a manifestation of polyglandular autoimmune syndromes (60–70%).

1295. In adrenal insufficiency, production of which of the following hormone is decreased?
Harrison's 20th Ed. Chapter 379 Page 2733

A. Glucocorticoids
B. Mineralocorticoids
C. Adrenal androgens
D. All of the above

Adrenal insufficiency is the decreased production of adrenocortical hormones (glucocorticoids, mineralocorticoids, and adrenal androgens).

1296. Tertiary adrenal insufficiency is the result of decreased production of?
Harrison's 20th Ed. Chapter 379 Page 2733

A. Cortisol
B. Adrenocorticotropic hormone (ACTH)
C. Corticotropin-releasing hormone (CRH)
D. All of the above

Primary adrenal insufficiency (Addison disease) is caused by a disorder of adrenal glands. Secondary adrenal insufficiency is the result of decreased production of ACTH and tertiary adrenal insufficiency is the result of decreased production of CRH (corticotropin-releasing hormone) by hypothalamus.

1297. Which of the following rarely cause adrenal insufficiency?
Harrison's 20th Ed. Chapter 379 Page 2733

A. Adrenal metastases
B. Tuberculous adrenalitis
C. X-linked adrenoleukodystrophy
D. Sarcoidosis

1298. Adrenals is a frequent site for which of the following chronic granulomatous diseases?
Harrison's 20th Ed. Chapter 379 Page 2734 Table 379-7

A. Tuberculosis
B. Histoplasmosis
C. Coccidioidomycosis
D. All of the above

The adrenal is a frequent site for chronic granulomatous diseases, mainly tuberculosis but also histoplasmosis, coccidioidomycosis & cryptococcosis.

1299. In primary adrenal insufficiency, which of the following also occur with increased frequency?
Harrison's 20th Ed. Chapter 379 Page 2733

A. Hypo- or hyperthyroidism
B. Pernicious anemia
C. Premature ovarian failure
D. All of the above

1300. In primary adrenal insufficiency, which of the following also occur with increased frequency?
Harrison's 20th Ed. Chapter 379 Page 2733

A. Vitiligo
B. Premature ovarian failure
C. Type 1 diabetes mellitus
D. All of the above

In primary adrenal insufficiency, coincident autoimmune disease most frequently includes thyroid autoimmune disease, vitiligo and premature ovarian failure. Less commonly, additional features may include type 1 diabetes and pernicious anemia caused by vitamin B12 deficiency.

1301. Mutant gene in autoimmune polyglandular syndrome 1 is?
Harrison's 20th Ed. Chapter 379 Page 2733

A. PIRE
B. TIRE
C. MIRE
D. AIRE

1302. AIRE gene best relates to?
Harrison's 20th Ed. Chapter 379 Page 2733

A. Epigenetic regulator genes
B. Autoimmune regulator gene
C. Spliceosome pathway genes
D. DNA damage response genes

Autoimmune polyglandular syndrome 1 (APS1), also termed APECED (autoimmune polyendocrinopathy-candidiasis ectodermal dystrophy) is transmitted in an autosomal recessive manner and is caused by mutations in the autoimmune regulator gene AIRE leading to its deficiency.

1303. "C" in APECED gene stands for?
Harrison's 20th Ed. Chapter 379 Page 2733

A. Carcinoma
B. Candidiasis
C. Calcinosis
D. Caif-au-lait

Autoimmune polyglandular syndrome 1 (APS1) is caused by mutations in the autoimmune polyendocrinopathy candidiasis ectodermal dystrophy (APECED) gene located on chromosome 21q22.3.

1304. Which of the following gene regions is involved in immune regulation?
Harrison's 20th Ed. Chapter 379 Page 2733

A. CTLA-4
B. PTPN22
C. CLEC16A
D. All of the above

APS2 is of polygenic inheritance, with confirmed associations with the HLA-DR3 gene region in the major histocompatibility complex and distinct gene regions involved in immune regulation (CTLA-4, PTPN22, CLEC16A).

1305. Autoimmune polyglandular syndrome 1 (APS1) consists of all except?
Harrison's 20th Ed. Chapter 379 Page 2733

A. Parathyroid insufficiency
B. Adrenal insufficiency
C. Chronic mucocutaneous candidiasis
D. Myasthenia gravis

Combination of parathyroid & adrenal insufficiency & chronic mucocutaneous candidiasis constitutes Autoimmune polyglandular syndrome 1 (APS1). APS1 patients invariably develop chronic mucocutaneous candidiasis, usually manifest in childhood, and preceding adrenal insufficiency by years or decades. Pernicious anemia, chronic active hepatitis, alopecia, primary hypothyroidism and premature gonadal failure may also be associated.

1306. Autoimmune polyglandular syndrome 2 (APS2) consists of all except?
Harrison's 20th Ed. Chapter 379 Page 2733

A. Hypothyroidism, hyperthyroidism
B. Chronic mucocutaneous candidiasis
C. Premature ovarian failure
D. Vitiligo

APS2 is of polygenic inheritance, with confirmed associations with the HLA-DR3 gene region in the major histocompatibility complex and distinct gene regions involved in immune regulation (CTLA-4, PTPN22, CLEC16A).

1307. Tall stature is a feature of which of the following causes of primary adrenal insufficiency?
Harrison's 20th Ed. Chapter 379 Page 2734 Table 379-7

A. Autoimmune polyglandular syndrome 1 (APS1)
B. Autoimmune polyglandular syndrome 2 (APS2)
C. Familial glucocorticoid deficiency
D. Triple A syndrome

1308. Progressive external ophthalmoplegia is a feature of which of the following causes of primary adrenal insufficiency?
Harrison's 20th Ed. Chapter 379 Page 2734 Table 379-7

A. Kearns-Sayre syndrome
B. Smith-Lemli-Opitz syndrome
C. Triple A syndrome
D. MIRAGE syndrome

1309. Myelodysplasia is a feature of which of the following causes of primary adrenal insufficiency?
Harrison's 20th Ed. Chapter 379 Page 2734 Table 379-7

A. Kearns-Sayre syndrome
B. Smith-Lemli-Opitz syndrome
C. Triple A syndrome
D. MIRAGE syndrome

1310. Which of the following causes of primary adrenal insufficiency is a cholesterol synthesis disorder?
Harrison's 20th Ed. Chapter 379 Page 2734 Table 379-7

A. Kearns-Sayre syndrome
B. Smith-Lemli-Opitz syndrome
C. Triple A syndrome
D. MIRAGE syndrome

1311. Which of the following mass lesions can affect hypothalamic-pituitary region?
Harrison's 20th Ed. Chapter 379 Page 2735 Table 379-8

A. Craniopharyngioma
B. Meningioma
C. Ependymoma
D. All of the above

1312. Sheehan's syndrome best relates to?
Harrison's 20th Ed. Chapter 379 Page 2735 Table 379-8

A. Autoimmune hypophysitis
B. Pituitary apoplexy / hemorrhage
C. Pituitary irradiation
D. All of the above

1313. Which of the following can cause pituitary infiltration?
Harrison's 20th Ed. Chapter 379 Page 2735 Table 379-8

A. Tuberculosis
B. Actinomycosis
C. Sarcoidosis
D. All of the above

1314. Congenital isolated ACTH deficiency best relates to which of the following gene?
Harrison's 20th Ed. Chapter 379 Page 2735 Table 379-8

A. PROP-1
B. SOX3
C. POMC
D. TBX19

1315. Combined pituitary hormone deficiency (CPHD) best relates to which of the following gene?
Harrison's 20th Ed. Chapter 379 Page 2735 Table 379-8

A. PROP-1
B. T-Pit
C. SF-1
D. All of the above

1316. Red hair pigmentation best relates to?
Harrison's 20th Ed. Chapter 379 Page 2735 Table 379-8

A. POMC
B. SOX3
C. LHX4
D. HESX1

Sequential cleavage of the precursor protein pre–pro–opiomelanocortin (POMC) generates the melanocortin peptides adrenocorticotrophin (ACTH), melanocyte–stimulating hormones (MSH) α, β, and γ as well as the opioid–receptor ligand β–endorphin. Proopiomelanocortin (POMC) deficiency causes early-onset obesity and red hair pigmentation.

1317. Measurement of which of the following is helpful in the diagnosis of X-linked adrenoleukodystrophy?
Harrison's 20th Ed. Chapter 379 Page 2733

A. Sodium
B. Magnesium
C. Long-chain fatty acids
D. Triglycerides

X-linked adrenoleukodystrophy is caused by mutations in the X-ALD gene–encoding the peroxisomal membrane transporter protein ABCD1. Its disruption results in accumulation of very long chain (>24 carbon atoms) fatty acids. Long-chain fatty acids should be measured in the plasma to exclude X-ALD.

1318. X-linked adrenoleukodystrophy manifests as?
Harrison's 20th Ed. Chapter 379 Page 2733

A. Cerebral adrenoleukodystrophy (ALD)
B. Adrenomyeloneuropathy (AMN)
C. Adrenal insufficiency
D. All of the above

1319. Which of the following factors regulate adrenal development and steroidogenesis?
Harrison's 20th Ed. Chapter 379 Page 2734

A. DAX-1
B. MC2R
C. TXNRD2
D. MCM4

1320. Which of the following factors regulate cholesterol synthesis, import and cleavage?
Harrison's 20th Ed. Chapter 379 Page 2734

A. DHCR7
B. StAR
C. CYP11A1
D. All of the above

1321. Which of the following factors regulate elements of the adrenal ACTH response pathway?
Harrison's 20th Ed. Chapter 379 Page 2734

A. SF-1
B. MC2R
C. NNT
D. CDKN1C

Mutations causing primary adrenal insufficiency include factors regulating adrenal development and steroidogenesis (DAX-1, SF-1), cholesterol synthesis, import and cleavage (DHCR7, StAR, CYP11A1), elements of the adrenal ACTH response pathway (MC2R, MRAP), and factors involved in redox regulation (NNT, TXNRD2) and DNA repair (MCM4, CDKN1C).

1322. Which of the following deficiencies is present in primary adrenal insufficiency?

Harrison's 20th Ed. Chapter 379 Page 2734

A. Glucocorticoid & mineralocorticoid secretion are lost in primary adrenal insufficiency (Addison's disease)

B. Glucocorticoid secretion are lost in secondary adrenal insufficiency

C. Adrenal androgen secretion is disrupted in both primary and secondary adrenal insufficiency

D. None of the above

1323. Which of the following deficiencies is present in primary adrenal insufficiency?

Harrison's 20th Ed. Chapter 379 Page 2733

A. Glucocorticoid

B. Mineralocorticoid

C. Adrenal androgen

D. All of the above

In primary adrenal insufficiency (Addison's disease) there is loss of glucocorticoid, mineralocorticoid and adrenal androgen secretion. Secondary adrenal insufficiency is the consequence of dysfunction of the hypothalamic-pituitary component of the HPA axis. In secondary adrenal insufficiency, only glucocorticoid deficiency is present, as the adrenal itself is intact and thus still amenable to regulation by RAA system.

1324. Which of the following is the most frequent presentation in adrenal insufficiency?

Harrison's 20th Ed. Chapter 379 Page 2733

A. Weakness

B. Pigmentation of mucous membranes

C. Salt craving

D. Diarrhea

1325. Which of the following best relates to secondary adrenal insufficiency?

Harrison's 20th Ed. Chapter 379 Page 2734

A. Alabaster-colored pale skin

B. Pellagra-like skin

C. EM-like skin

D. All of the above

In museums, statues and vases are carved from alabaster. Alabaster is usually white and translucent. It appears to be lit from within. In secondary adrenal insufficiency, skin has an alabaster-like paleness due to lack of ACTH secretion.

1326. Which of the following is an early sign of hyperpigmentation in Addison's disease?

Harrison's 20th Ed. Chapter 379 Page 2734

A. Darkening of areolae of nipples

B. Bluish-black patches on mucous membranes

C. Persistent tanning following sun exposure

D. Alabaster-like paleness of skin

Persistent tanning following sun exposure is an early sign in Addison's disease. A distinguishing feature of primary adrenal insufficiency is hyperpigmentation, which is caused by excess of proopiomelanocortin (POMC)-derived peptides and ACTH stimulation of melanocytes. Hyperpigmentation is most pronounced in skin areas exposed to increased friction or shear stress and is increased by sunlight.

1327. Which of the following favors a diagnosis of primary adrenocortical insufficiency?

Harrison's 20th Ed. Chapter 379 Page 2734

A. Dehydration

B. Hyponatremia

C. Hyperkalemia

D. All of the above

Severe dehydration, hyponatremia, and hyperkalemia are characteristic of severe mineralocorticoid insufficiency and favor a diagnosis of primary adrenocortical insufficiency.

1328. Which of the following is a characteristic biochemical feature in primary adrenal insufficiency?

Harrison's 20th Ed. Chapter 379 Page 2734

A. Hyperkalemia

B. Hyponatremia

C. Hypercalcemia

D. Hypomagnesemia

Hyponatremia is a characteristic biochemical feature in primary adrenal insufficiency and is found in 80% of patients at presentation while, hyperkalemia is present in 40% of patients at initial diagnosis. Hyponatremia is caused by mineralocorticoid deficiency but can also occur in secondary adrenal insufficiency due to diminished inhibition of antidiuretic hormone (ADH) release by cortisol, resulting in mild syndrome of inappropriate secretion of antidiuretic hormone (SIADH).

1329. Which of the following is false about primary adrenal insufficiency?

Harrison's 20th Ed. Chapter 379 Page 2737 Figure 379-16

A. High renin

B. High ACTH level

C. Low aldosterone

D. None of the above

1330. Which of the following is false about secondary adrenal insufficiency?

Harrison's 20th Ed. Chapter 379 Page 2737 Figure 379-16

A. Normal renin

B. Low normal ACTH level

C. Normal aldosterone

D. None of the above

Patients with secondary adrenocortical hypofunction are not hyperpigmented, have low ACTH levels, evidence of multiple hormone deficiencies, have near-normal level of aldosterone secretion.

1331. Acute adrenocortical insufficiency may result from?

Harrison's 20th Ed. Chapter 379 Page 2734

A. Meningococcal septicemia

B. Anticoagulant therapy

C. Pregnancy

D. All of the above

1332. Acute adrenocortical insufficiency may result from?

Harrison's 20th Ed. Chapter 379 Page 2734

A. Pseudomonas septicemia

B. Coagulation disorder

C. Rapid withdrawal of steroids

D. All of the above

Acute adrenocortical insufficiency may result from septicemia with Pseudomonas or meningococcemia (Waterhouse-Friderichsen syndrome), anticoagulant therapy or a coagulation disorder, bilateral adrenal hemorrhage in newborn due to birth trauma, during pregnancy, following idiopathic adrenal vein thrombosis, as a complication of venography, rapid withdrawal of steroids from those on chronic steroid therapy, congenital adrenal hyperplasia, those on mitotane, ketoconazole, phenytoin, rifampin.

1333. In rapid ACTH stimulation test, dose of cosyntropin is?

Harrison's 20th Ed. Chapter 379 Page 2734 Figure 379-16

A. 50 μg
B. 150 μg
C. 250 μg
D. 500 μg

In rapid ACTH stimulation test, 250 μg of cosyntropin is given IM or IV.

1334. In rapid ACTH stimulation test, cortisol level at 60 minutes after cosyntropin should be?

Harrison's 20th Ed. Chapter 379 Page 2734

A. > 6 μg/dL
B. > 12 μg/dL
C. > 18 μg/dL
D. > 21 μg/dL

In adrenal insufficiency, upon ACTH stimulation testing, cortisol level at 60 minutes after cosyntropin should be > 21 μg/dL.

1335. Primary & secondary adrenal insufficiency can be distinguished by measuring?

Harrison's 20th Ed. Chapter 379 Page 2734

A. Renin
B. Aldosterone
C. Angiotensin I
D. Angiotensin II

If rapid ACTH stimulation test is abnormal, then primary and secondary adrenal insufficiency can be distinguished by measuring aldosterone levels from the same blood samples. In secondary adrenal insufficiency, the aldosterone increment will be normal (> 5 ng/dL). In primary adrenal insufficiency, plasma ACTH and associated peptides (β-LPT) are elevated.

1336. Which of the following is given in the treatment of adrenal insufficiency?

Harrison's 20th Ed. Chapter 379 Page 2736

A. Hydrocortisone
B. Fludrocortisone
C. DHEA
D. All of the above

Replacement therapy in adrenal insufficiency aims to correct both glucocorticoid & mineralocorticoid deficiencies by hydrocortisone and fludrocortisone respectively. In females with adrenal insufficiency and low androgen levels, DHEA may improve quality of life & bone mineral density.

1337. What proportion of total glucocorticoid dose should be given in morning?

Harrison's 20th Ed. Chapter 379 Page 2736

A. One third
B. One half
C. Two third
D. Three fourth

Dose of hydrocortisone for most adults is 20–30 mg/day. To simulate normal diurnal adrenal rhythm, two-thirds of the dose is taken in morning & remaining one-third is taken in late afternoon.

1338. What is the equipotency dose of dexamethasone for 1 mg of hydrocortisone?

Harrison's 20th Ed. Chapter 379 Page 2736

A. 0.025 mg
B. 0.05 mg
C. 0.1 mg
D. 0.5 mg

There are no well-established dose equivalencies, but as a guide, equipotency can be assumed for 1 mg hydrocortisone, 1.6 mg cortisone acetate, 0.2 mg prednisolone, 0.25 mg prednisone and 0.025 mg dexamethasone.

1339. In adrenal insufficiency, during fever, the dose of hydrocortisone should be?

Harrison's 20th Ed. Chapter 379 Page 2737

A. Remain the same
B. Doubled
C. Tripled
D. Quadrupled

During periods of intercurrent illness (fever), dose of hydrocortisone should be doubled.

1340. 40 mg of hydrocortisone is equivalent to how many micrograms of fludrocortisone?

Harrison's 20th Ed. Chapter 379 Page 2737

A. 25
B. 50
C. 100
D. 150

40 mg hydrocortisone is equivalent to 100 μg of fludrocortisone.

1341. Initial dose of fludrocortisone in primary adrenal insufficiency should be?

Harrison's 20th Ed. Chapter 379 Page 2737

A. 25–50 μg
B. 50–100 μg
C. 100–150 μg
D. 150–200 μg

Mineralocorticoid replacement in primary adrenal insufficiency should be initiated at a dose of 100–150 μg fludrocortisone.

1342. Mineralocorticoid replacement is initiated when daily hydrocortisone dose has been reduced to?

Harrison's 20th Ed. Chapter 379 Page 2736

A. < 25 mg
B. < 50 mg
C. < 75 mg
D. < 100 mg

Mineralocorticoid replacement can be initiated once daily hydrocortisone dose is reduced to < 50 mg as at higher doses hydrocortisone provides sufficient stimulation of MRs.

1343. Which of the following drug has antimineralocorticoid activity?

Harrison's 20th Ed. Chapter 379 Page 2737

A. Spironolactone
B. Progesterone
C. Drospirenone
D. All of the above

Physiologically, progesterone normally exerts antimineralocorticoid activity. Drospirenone, an analogue of spironolactone has both antimineralocorticoid and antiandrogenic activities.

1344. In Addison's disease, mineralocorticoid administration is unnecessary at hydrocortisone doses of?

Harrison's 20th Ed. Chapter 379 Page 2737

A. > 10 mg/day
B. > 40 mg/day
C. > 80 mg/day
D. > 100 mg/day

In Addison's disease, mineralocorticoid administration is unnecessary at hydrocortisone doses of >100 mg/day because of the mineralocorticoid effects of hydrocortisone at such dosages.

1345. Adrenal androgen replacement can be achieved by administration of?

Harrison's 20th Ed. Chapter 379 Page 2738

A. DHEA
B. DHEAS
C. Androstenedione
D. All of the above

1346. Treatment with DHEA is monitored by measurement of?

Harrison's 20th Ed. Chapter 379 Page 2738

A. Androstenedione
B. Testosterone
C. Sex hormone-binding globulin (SHBG)
D. All of the above

Adrenal androgen replacement can be achieved by once-daily administration of 25–50 mg DHEA. Treatment is monitored by measurement of DHEAS, androstenedione, testosterone, and sex hormone–binding globulin (SHBG) 24 h after the last DHEA dose.

1347. Adrenal androgen formation is regulated by?

Lancet 2005; 365: 2125–36

A. ACTH
B. Gonadotropins
C. γ-melanocyte-stimulating hormone
D. β-endorphin

Adrenal androgen formation is regulated by ACTH, not by gonadotropins. Adrenal androgens are suppressed by exogenous glucocorticoids.

1348. Which of the following is the most potent androgen?

Lancet 2005; 365: 2125–36

A. DHEA
B. Androstenedione
C. 11-hydroxyandrostenedione
D. Testosterone

The principal adrenal androgens are DHEA, androstenedione, and 11-hydroxyandrostenedione. Testosterone is a gonadal steroid. DHEA & androstenedione are weak androgens & exert their effects via conversion to potent androgen testosterone in extraglandular tissues.

1349. The plasma level of cortisol is increased by?

Lancet 2005; 365: 2125–36

A. Dietary potassium loading
B. Sodium restriction
C. Upright posture
D. None of the above

Plasma level of aldosterone, but not of cortisol, is increased by dietary potassium loading, sodium restriction or by assumption of upright posture.

1350. Urine 17-ketosteroid values are highest in?

Lancet 2005; 365: 2125–36

A. Infants
B. Young adults
C. Middle age
D. Old age

Urinary 17-KS originate in adrenal gland or gonad. In normal women, 90% of urinary 17-KS is derived from adrenal while in men 60–70% is of adrenal origin. Urine 17-KS is highest in young adults & decline with age.

1351. Rapid ACTH stimulation test is performed?

Lancet 2005; 365: 2125–36

A. Early morning
B. Afternoon
C. Late evening
D. Any time of the day

Rapid ACTH stimulation test can be performed at any time of the day. It involves administration of 25 units (0.25 mg) of cosyntropin IV or IM & measurement of plasma cortisol levels before administration, 30 & 60 minutes after administration.

1352. Criterion for a normal response in "Rapid ACTH stimulation test" is a cortisol level of?

Lancet 2005; 365: 2125–36

A. >8 μg/dL above baseline
B. >12 μg/dL above baseline
C. >16 μg/dL above baseline
D. >18 μg/dL above baseline

Criterion for a normal rapid ACTH stimulation test response is a stimulated cortisol level of >500 nmol/L (>18 μg/dL), and the minimal stimulated normal increment of cortisol is >200 nmol/L (>7 g/dL) above baseline.

1353. Normally, in screening 'overnight dexamethasone suppression test', plasma cortisol level at 8 AM should be?

Lancet 2005; 365: 2125–36

A. < 5 μg/dL
B. < 10 μg/dL
C. < 15 μg/dL
D. < 20 μg/dL

The best screening procedure to test pituitary-adrenal suppressibility is the overnight dexamethasone suppression test. Measurement of plasma cortisol levels at 8 AM following oral administration of 1 mg dexamethasone the previous midnight is done. 8 AM value for plasma cortisol in normal individuals should be <140 nmol/L (5 μg/dL).

1354. During stress, plasma cortisol levels should be constantly maintained at?

Lancet 2005; 365: 2125–36

A. 10 μg/dL
B. 20 μg/dL
C. 30 μg/dL
D. 40 μg/dL

Continuous hydrocortisone infusion maintains plasma cortisol constantly at stress levels of 30 μg/dL.

1355. Which of the following is false in acutely ill patients?

Lancet 2005; 365: 2125–36

A. Cortisol levels rise four- to sixfold
B. Diurnal variation is abolished
C. Unbound fractions of cortisol rises
D. None of the above

During critical illnesses cortisol levels rise 4–6 fold, diurnal variation is abolished & unbound fractions of cortisol rise in circulation & target tissues.

1356. Functional or relative adrenal insufficiency is?

Lancet 2005; 365: 2125–36

A. Adrenal insufficiency on withdrawal of long term steroids
B. Subnormal cortisol production during acute severe illness
C. Failure to take replacement therapy in adrenal insufficiency
D. Ineffective replacement therapy in adrenal insufficiency

Subnormal cortisol production during acute severe illness has been termed "functional" or "relative" adrenal insufficiency.

1357. Following cosystropin, increment of less than what between peak & baseline cortisol levels defines relative adrenal insufficiency?

Lancet 2005; 365: 2125–36

A. < 3 μg/dL
B. < 6 μg/dL
C. < 9 μg/dL
D. < 12 μg/dL

Relative adrenal insufficiency is defined as a <9 μg/dL increment between peak & baseline cortisol levels following administration of 250 μg of cosystropin as an IV bolus.

1358. What value of a random cortisol level is indicative of relative adrenal insufficiency?

Lancet 2005; 365: 2125–36

A. ≤ 5 μg/dL
B. ≤ 10 μg/dL
C. ≤ 15 μg/dL
D. ≤ 20 μg/dL

1359. What value of a random cortisol level excludes the diagnosis of relative adrenal insufficiency?

Lancet 2005; 365: 2125–36

A. > 24 μg/dL
B. > 34 μg/dL
C. > 44 μg/dL
D. > 54 μg/dL

A random cortisol level of <=15 μg/dL is indicative of relative adrenal insufficiency and a random cortisol level >34 g/dL usually excludes the diagnosis of relative adrenal insufficiency.

1360. Isolated aldosterone deficiency occurs in?

Lancet 2005; 365: 2125–36

A. Protracted heparin administration
B. Pretectal disease of nervous system
C. Severe postural hypotension
D. All of the above

Isolated aldosterone deficiency with normal cortisol production occurs in hyporeninism, as an inherited biosynthetic defect, following removal of aldosterone-secreting adenomas, during protracted heparin therapy, in pretectal disease of CNS, and in severe postural hypotension.

1361. Invariably, patients affected by CAH exhibit?

Harrison's 20th Ed. Chapter 379 Page 2738

A. Glucocorticoid deficiency
B. Excess production of mineralocorticoids
C. Deficient production of sex steroids
D. All of the above

Invariably, patients affected by CAH exhibit glucocorticoid deficiency. Depending on the exact step of enzymatic block, they may also have excess production of mineralocorticoids or deficient production of sex steroids.

1362. The most common form of CAH is due to impairment of?

Harrison's 20th Ed. Chapter 379 Page 2738

A. 17-hydroxylase/17,20-lyase (CYP17)
B. 21-hydroxylase (CYP21A2)
C. 11β-hydroxylase (CYP11B1)
D. HSD3B2

Most common form of CAH (90–95% of cases) is a result of impairment of CYP21A2 (21-Hydroxylase).

1363. Which of the following is the nonfunctional pseudogene near 21-hydroxylase gene?

Harrison's 20th Ed. Chapter 456 Page 3355

A. CYP21A1G
B. CYP21A1K
C. CYP21A1P
D. CYP21A1Z

21-hydroxylase gene (CYP21A2) is adjacent to a nonfunctional pseudogene (CYP21A1P). Many of the nucleotide substitutions that are found in CYP21A2 gene in patients with congenital adrenal hyperplasia correspond to sequences that are present in CYP21A1P pseudogene, suggesting gene conversion as one cause of mutagenesis.

1364. Glucocorticoid deficiency, mineralocorticoid excess, adrenal androgen excess is a feature of which variants of CAH?

Harrison's 20th Ed. Chapter 379 Page 2738 Table 379-10

A. 21-Hydroxylase deficiency
B. 11β-Hydroxylase deficiency
C. 17α-Hydroxylase deficiency
D. All of the above

1365. Glucocorticoid deficiency, mineralocorticoid excess, androgen deficiency is a feature of which variants of CAH?

Harrison's 20th Ed. Chapter 379 Page 2738 Table 379-10

A. 21-Hydroxylase deficiency
B. 11β-Hydroxylase deficiency
C. 17α-Hydroxylase deficiency
D. All of the above

1366. Glucocorticoid deficiency, mineralocorticoid deficiency, adrenal androgen excess is a feature of which variants of CAH?

Harrison's 20th Ed. Chapter 379 Page 2738 Table 379-10

A. 21-Hydroxylase deficiency
B. 11β-Hydroxylase deficiency
C. 17α-Hydroxylase deficiency
D. All of the above

1367. CYP17A1 deficiency is characterized by?

Harrison's 20th Ed. Chapter 379 Page 2738 Table 379-10

A. Hypogonadism
B. Hypokalemia
C. Hypertension
D. All of the above

CYP17A1 deficiency is characterized by hypogonadism, hypokalemia, and hypertension. It causes decreased production of cortisol & shunting of precursors into the mineralocorticoid pathway with hypokalemic alkalosis, hypertension, and suppressed plasma renin activity.

1368. CAH best relates to?

Harrison's 20th Ed. Chapter 379 Page 2738

A. Salt-wasting crisis
B. Testicular adrenal rest tumors
C. Increased pituitary ACTH release
D. All of the above

1369. CAH caused by deficiency of 21-hydroxylase is characterized by?

Lancet 2005; 365: 2125–36

A. Cortisol deficiency
B. With or without aldosterone deficiency
C. Androgen excess
D. All of the above

CAH caused by deficiency of 21-hydroxylase is characterised by glucocorticoid deficiency, with or without aldosterone deficiency, and androgen excess.

1370. The highest rates of classic CAH occur in?

Lancet 2005; 365: 2125–36

A. Alaska
B. Brazil
C. Philippines
D. USA

The highest rates of classic CAH occur in two geographically isolated populations—Yupic Eskimos of Alaska (one in 280) & French island of La Réunion (one in 2100). High rates have also been reported in Brazil (one in 7500) and the Philippines (one in 7000).

1371. The 21-hydroxylase gene is located on chromosome?

Lancet 2005; 365: 2125–36

A. 6
B. 8
C. 10
D. 12

21-hydroxylase gene is located on chromosome 6p21·3 within HLA histocompatibility complex. There are two highly homologous 21-hydroxylase genes resulting from ancestral duplication : an active gene, CYP21A2 (CYP21B) & an inactive pseudogene CYP21A1P (CYP21A, CYP21P).

1372. A very high concentration of which of the following is diagnostic of classic 21-hydroxylase deficiency?

Lancet 2005; 365: 2125–36

A. Androstenedione
B. 11-deoxycortisol
C. 17-hydroxyprogesterone
D. Pregnenolone

A very high concentration of 17-hydroxyprogesterone (>242 nmol/L; normal < 3 nmol/L at 3 days in full-term infant) in a randomly timed blood sample is diagnostic of classic 21-hydroxylase deficiency.

1373. What value of stimulated concentration of 17-hydroxyprogesterone is diagnostic of 21-hydroxylase deficiency?

Lancet 2005; 365: 2125–36

A. > 15 nmol/L
B. > 25 nmol/L
C. > 35 nmol/L
D. > 45 nmol/L

A corticotropin stimulated concentration of 17-hydroxyprogesterone higher than 45 nmol/L is diagnostic of 21-hydroxylase deficiency.

1374. "Hypertensive" variant of congenital adrenal hyperplasia (CAH) is due to deficiency of?

Lancet 2005; 365: 2125–36

A. 21-hydroxylase (CYP21A2)
B. 17-hydroxylase/17,20-lyase (CYP17)
C. 11β-hydroxylase (CYP11B1)
D. 3β-HSD2

CYP11B1 deficiency causes a "hypertensive" variant of CAH. Hypertension & hypokalemia occur because of impaired conversion of 11-deoxycorticosterone to corticosterone, resulting in the accumulation of 11-deoxycorticosterone, a potent mineralocorticoid.

1375. 21-Hydroxylase (CYP21A2) deficiency is characterized by?

Harrison's 20th Ed. Chapter 379 Page 2738

A. Decreased glucocorticoid and mineralocorticoid synthesis
B. Increased pituitary ACTH release
C. Increased synthesis of adrenal androgen precursors
D. All of the above

21-Hydroxylase (CYP21A2) deficiency is characterized by decreased glucocorticoid & mineralocorticoid synthesis with diminished negative feedback via HPA axis leading to increased pituitary ACTH release, which drives increased synthesis of adrenal androgen precursors and subsequent androgen excess.

1376. Normal cortisol production rate in children is?

Harrison's 20th Ed. Chapter 379 Page 2738

A. ~ 1–3 mg/m^2 per day
B. ~ 3–6 mg/m^2 per day
C. ~ 6–10 mg/m^2 per day
D. ~ 10–13 mg/m^2 per day

Normal cortisol production rate in children is ~10–13 mg/m^2 per day.

1377. In CAH, levels of which of the following should be regularly monitored and kept within the normal reference range?

Harrison's 20th Ed. Chapter 379 Page 2738

A. Plasma renin
B. Androstenedione
C. Testosterone
D. All of the above

1378. In CAH, prednisone is the drug of choice in all except?

Lancet 2005; 365: 2125–36

A. Infants
B. Children
C. Adolescents
D. Adults

Therapy in CAH is daily administration of glucocorticoids to suppress pituitary ACTH secretion. Prednisone is the drug of choice except in infants, in whom hydrocortisone is usually used.

1379. Chemical adrenalectomy can be done by?

Lancet 2005; 365: 2125–36

A. Ketoconazole
B. Mitotane
C. Metyrapone
D. All of the above

Chemical adrenalectomy can be done with ketoconazole or mitotane or aminoglutethimide or metyrapone or Mifepristone. These are not curative but effective as long as chronically administered in selected patients.

1380. What ratio of serum aldosterone to PRA suggests autonomy of aldosterone secretion?

Lancet 2005; 365: 2125–36

A. > 10
B. > 15
C. > 30
D. > 50

The ratio of plasma aldosterone to plasma renin activity (PA/PRA) is a useful screening test. A ratio > 30: 1 in conjunction with a plasma aldosterone concentration >555 pmol/L (>20 ng/dL) has a sensitivity of 90% and a specificity of 91% for an aldosterone-producing adenoma.

1381. Increased production of aldosterone occurs in secondary aldosteronism in response to?

Lancet 2005; 365: 2125–36

A. Activation of sympathetic system
B. Activation of parasympathetic system
C. Activation of renin-angiotensin system
D. All of the above

In secondary aldosteronism, an appropriately increased production of aldosterone in response to activation of renin-angiotensin system occurs.

1382. Secondary aldosteronism occurs in association with?

Lancet 2005; 365: 2125–36

A. Accelerated phase of hypertension
B. Underlying edema disorder
C. Bartter & Gitelman syndromes
D. All of the above

Secondary aldosteronism occurs with accelerated phase of hypertension or an underlying edema disorder. Secondary hyperaldosteronism occurs without edema or hypertension in Bartter & Gitelman syndromes.

1383. Secondary aldosteronism is a feature of?

Lancet 2005; 365: 2125–36

A. Cirrhosis
B. Nephrotic syndrome
C. Congestive heart failure
D. All of the above

Secondary aldosteronism is present edematous states like cirrhosis, nephrotic syndrome and congestive heart failure. Stimulus for aldosterone release is arterial hypovolemia and/or hypotension.

1384. As compared to essential hypertension, patients with primary aldosteronism have a higher incidence of?

Lancet 2005; 365: 2125–36

A. Left ventricular hypertrophy (LVH)
B. Albuminuria
C. Stroke
D. All of the above

1385. Which of the following is a cause of systolic and diastolic hypertension?

Lancet 2005; 365: 2125–36

A. 17α-hydroxylase deficiency
B. 11β-hydroxylase deficiency
C. 11-hydroxysteroid dehydrogenase deficiency
D. All of the above

Adrenal causes of hypertension are primary aldosteronism, Cushing's syndrome, 17α-hydroxylase deficiency, 11β-hydroxylase deficiency, 11-hydroxysteroid dehydrogenase deficiency (licorice) and pheochromocytoma.

1386. What percentage of adrenal glands are destroyed before adrenal insufficiency appears?

Lancet 2005; 365: 2125–36

A. > 25%
B. > 50%
C. > 75%
D. > 90%

Addison's disease results from progressive destruction of adrenals, which must involve >90% of the glands before adrenal insufficiency appears.

Pheochromocytoma

1387. Which of the following about pheochromocytomas and paragangliomas is false?

Harrison's 20th Ed. Chapter 380 Page 2739

A. Catecholamine-producing tumors
B. Derived from sympathetic nervous system
C. Derived from parasympathetic nervous system
D. None of the above

Pheochromocytomas and paragangliomas (PGPCs) are catecholamine-producing tumors that arise from adrenal medulla, or from extra-adrenal ganglial sympathetic / parasympathetic chains (of chromaffin or non-chromaffin origin), respectively. Extra-adrenal pheochromocytomas are described as paragangliomas.

1388. Pheochromocytoma was first described in 1800 by?

Harrison's 20th Ed. Chapter 380 Page 2739

A. Jeff Kamilaris
B. Duke Stratakis
C. Charles Sugrue
D. Emil Zuckerkandl

Charles Sugrue of Cork (1775-1816) first described the classical medical condition phaeochromocytoma. The histological findings were first reported by Felix Fraenkel and Max Schottelius in 1886.

1389. In pheochromocytoma, mean age at diagnosis is about?

Harrison's 20th Ed. Chapter 380 Page 2740

A. 20 years
B. 30 years
C. 40 years
D. 50 years

In pheochromocytoma, mean age at diagnosis is about 40 years, although the tumors can occur from early childhood until late in life.

1390. The "rule of tens" for pheochromocytomas states?

Harrison's 20th Ed. Chapter 380 Page 2740, Urol Case Rep. 2014;2(4):139–141

A. ~ 10% are bilateral
B. ~ 10% are extraadrenal
C. ~ 10% are malignant
D. All of the above

1391. The "rule of tens" for pheochromocytomas states?

Harrison's 20th Ed. Chapter 380 Page 2740, Urol Case Rep. 2014;2(4):139–141

A. ~ 10% are pediatric
B. ~ 10% are familial
C. ~ 10% are malignant
D. All of the above

The "rule of tens" for pheochromocytomas states that ~10% are bilateral, 10% are extraadrenal & 10% are malignant. These percentages are higher in the inherited syndromes. Pheochromocytomas have been termed the "10% tumor," in which 10% are malignant, 10% are bilateral, 10% are pediatric, 10% are familial, and 10% are extra-adrenal. Also, 10% of pheochromocytomas are found incidentally. 10% have negative activity on MIBG imaging. 10% of subjects with metastatic pheochromocytomas presented with tumors smaller than 5 cm. 98% of pheochromocytomas are located in abdomen, and 90% are found within the adrenal medulla.

1392. Which of the following is part of parasympathetic system?

Harrison's 20th Ed. Chapter 380 Page 2740

A. Glomus tympanicum
B. Glomus jugulare
C. Glomus vagale
D. All of the above

Pheochromocytomas and paragangliomas arise from cells of sympathetic (adrenal medulla or sympathetic trunk) or parasympathetic (carotid body, glomus tympanicum, glomus jugulare, glomus vagale) paraganglia.

1393. Which of the following about paraganglioma is false?

Harrison's 20th Ed. Chapter 380 Page 2740

A. Catecholamine-producing tumors in skull base & neck
B. Tumors arising from parasympathetic nervous system
C. Secrete little or no catecholamines
D. None of the above

Paraganglioma refers to catecholamine-producing tumors in skull base & neck, as well as tumors that arise from parasympathetic nervous system, which may secrete little or no catecholamines. Etiology of most sporadic pheochromocytomas & paragangliomas is unknown.

1394. What percentage of pheochromocytoma are a part of an inherited familial disorder?

Harrison's 20th Ed. Chapter 380 Page 2740

A. ~ 10%
B. ~ 30%
C. ~ 50%
D. ~ 70%

1395. PCPGs can be divided into Cluster I and Cluster II diseases based on?

Cancers 2019,11,436

A. T cell immunoreactivity
B. mRNA-expression signatures
C. DNA ligase
D. Bacteriophage

A 'gene expression signature' can be defined as a single or a combined gene expression alteration with validated specificity in terms of diagnosis, prognosis or prediction of therapeutic response.

1396. Cluster 1 mutations are associated with?

Harrison's 20th Ed. Chapter 380 Page 2740

A. Abnormal activation of kinase signaling pathways
B. Pseudohypoxia & aberrant VEGF signaling
C. Genetic mutations affecting gene translation
D. Genetic mutations affecting protein synthesis

1397. Cluster 2 mutations are associated with all except?

Harrison's 20th Ed. Chapter 380 Page 2740

A. Abnormal activation of kinase signaling pathways
B. Pseudohypoxia & aberrant VEGF signaling
C. Genetic mutations affecting gene translation
D. Genetic mutations affecting protein synthesis

Cluster 1 mutations are associated with pseudohypoxia and aberrant VEGF signaling (VHL, PHD, FH, or SDHx) whereas cluster 2 mutations are associated with abnormal activation of kinase signaling pathways (RET, NF1, TMEM127, MAX, or KIF1Bβ).

1398. Which of the following statements is false?

Harrison's 20th Ed. Chapter 380 Page 2740

A. RET (rearranged during transfection) is a proto-oncogene
B. Succinate dehydrogenase (SDH) is an enzyme of Krebs cycle
C. VHL protein is a component of an ubiquitin E3 ligase
D. None of the above

1399. Germ-line mutations in which of the following can cause inherited pheochromocytoma?

Harrison's 20th Ed. Chapter 380 Page 2740

A. RET
B. VHL
C. NF1
D. All of the above

PCPGs result from genetic abnormalities, mostly disruption/mutation in single disease-related genes. ~25% of patients of pheochromocytoma are inherited due to germ-line mutations in the RET, VHL, NF1, SDHB, SDHC, SDHD, SDHA, SDHAF2, TMEM127 and MAX genes (>20 susceptible genes). Germline mutations may lead to clinical syndromes like von Hippel-Lindau disease, multiple endocrine neoplasia type 2 syndrome, and neurofibromatosis type 1. While, somatic mutations in key oncogenic pathways, such as SDHx, VHL, HIF2A, H-RAS, NF1, RET, or MAX, predispose PCPG formation.

1400. The VHL protein is a component of?

Harrison's 20th Ed. Chapter 380 Page 2740

A. Ubiquitin E3 ligase
B. Mitochondrial kinase
C. Cytosolic kinase
D. All of the above

The VHL protein is a component of a ubiquitin E3 ligase. Von Hippel-Lindau syndrome involves disruption of a ubiquitin E3 ligase termed the VHL tumor suppressor, or VHL gene.

1401. Which of the following diseases is related to E3 ubiquitin protein ligase?

Harrison's 20th Ed. Chapter 417 Page 3043

A. Hallervorden-Spatz disease
B. Wilson's disease
C. Parkinson's Disease
D. Frontotemporal dementia

PARK2 encodes parkin, an E3 ubiquitin protein ligase. Mutations in parkin appear to be the major cause of autosomal recessive Parkinson's disease.

1402. Which of the following disease is labeled as the "great masquerader"?

Harrison's 20th Ed. Chapter 380 Page 2740

A. Pheochromocytoma
B. Pulmonary Embolism
C. Fibromyalgia
D. All of the above

Historically, syphilis and tuberculosis were labeled as the "great masqueraders" as their protean symptoms & potential for multi-organ involvement. In the modern era, pheochromocytoma, pulmonary embolism, fibromyalgia, lupus, sarcoidosis, vasculitis and lymphoma have been labeled as great masqueraders.

1403. Classic triad of pheochromocytoma consists of all except?

Harrison's 20th Ed. Chapter 380 Page 2740

A. Palpitation
B. Hypertension
C. Headache
D. Profuse sweating

Classic triad of pheochromocytoma consists of episodes of palpitations, headaches & profuse sweating (diaphoresis). Association with episodic or sustained hypertension, makes pheochromocytoma a likely diagnosis.

1404. Which of the following is the dominant sign of pheochromocytoma?

Harrison's 20th Ed. Chapter 380 Page 2740

A. Palpitation
B. Hypertension
C. Headache
D. Profuse sweating

1405. In pheochromocytoma, which of the following is the most common symptom?

Lancet 2005;366:665-75

A. Sustained hypertension
B. Paroxysmal hypertension
C. Orthostatic hypotension
D. Flushing

1406. In pheochromocytoma, which of the following is the least common symptom?

Lancet 2005;366:665-75

A. Palpitations
B. Sweating
C. Headache
D. Anxiety

1407. Paroxysmal attacks in pheochromocytoma generally last for?

Harrison's 20th Ed. Chapter 380 Page 2740

A. < 1 hours
B. < 3 hours
C. < 6 hours
D. < 12 hours

Paroxysmal attacks in pheochromocytoma generally last less than an hour.

1408. Paroxysmal attack in pheochromocytoma is precipitated by?

Harrison's 20th Ed. Chapter 380 Page 2740

A. Positional changes
B. Exercise
C. Pregnancy
D. All of the above

1409. Drugs that can induce paroxysmal attacks in pheochromocytoma include?

Harrison's 20th Ed. Chapter 380 Page 2740

A. Opiates
B. Tricyclic antidepressants
C. Metoclopramide
D. All of the above

Paroxysmal attacks in pheochromocytoma are precipitated by surgery, positional changes, exercise, pregnancy, urination (bladder pheochromocytomas) & medications (tricyclic antidepressants, opiates, metoclopramide).

1410. Drugs that can induce paroxysmal attacks in pheochromocytoma include?

Harrison's 20th Ed. Chapter 380 Page 2740

A. Glucagon
B. IV Methyldopa
C. Tricyclic antidepressants
D. All of the above

1411. Which of the following is false about pheochromocytoma?

Harrison's 20th Ed. Chapter 380 Page 2741

A. Pheochromocytomas synthesize catecholamines
B. Pheochromocytomas store catecholamines
C. Pheochromocytoma can be asymptomatic for years
D. None of the above

1412. Plasma and urinary metanephrine measure which metabolite of catecholamines?

Harrison's 20th Ed. Chapter 380 Page 2741

A. E-methylated metabolites
B. S-methylated metabolites
C. L-methylated metabolites
D. O-methylated metabolites

1413. Catecholamine related to pheochromocytoma is?

Harrison's 20th Ed. Chapter 380 Page 2741

A. Norepinephrine
B. Epinephrine
C. Dopamine
D. All of the above

Pheochromocytomas & paragangliomas synthesize and store catecholamines, which include norepinephrine (noradrenaline), epinephrine (adrenaline), and dopamine. Elevated plasma & urinary levels of catecholamines & metanephrines form the cornerstone of diagnosis. Most tumors continuously leak O-methylated metabolites which are detected by measurement of metanephrines.

1414. Diagnosis of pheochromocytoma is highly likely when plasma & urinary levels of catecholamines & metanephrines are?

Harrison's 20th Ed. Chapter 380 Page 2741

A. Two times the upper limit of normal
B. Three times the upper limit of normal
C. Four times the upper limit of normal
D. Five times the upper limit of normal

1415. Which out of the following has maximum sensitivity in the diagnosis of pheochromocytoma?

Harrison's 20th Ed. Chapter 380 Page 2741 Table 380-2

A. Plasma-free metanephrines
B. Plasma catecholamines
C. Urinary catecholamines
D. VMA

1416. Which out of the following has maximum specificity in the diagnosis of pheochromocytoma?

Harrison's 20th Ed. Chapter 380 Page 2741 Table 380-2

A. Plasma-free metanephrines
B. Plasma catecholamines
C. Urinary-fractionated metanephrines
D. Urinary total metanephrines

1417. Which out of the following has maximum sensitivity in the diagnosis of pheochromocytoma?

Harrison's 20th Ed. Chapter 380 Page 2741 Table 380-2

A. 24-h urinary fractionated metanephrines
B. Plasma free metanephrines
C. CT / MRI
D. All of the above

1418. Which out of the following has maximum specificity in the diagnosis of pheochromocytoma?

Harrison's 20th Ed. Chapter 380 Page 2741 Table 380-2

A. Urinary total metanephrines
B. MIBG scintigraphy
C. 18Fluoro-DOPA PET/CT
D. All of the above

1419. Which of the following provides better diagnostic sensitivity in the diagnosis of phaeochromocytomas?

Harrison's 20th Ed. Chapter 380 Page 2741 Table 380-2

A. CT / MRI
B. 18Fluoro-DOPA PET/CT
C. 131I-MIBG
D. Somatostatin receptor scintigraphy

1420. Radioactive tracer used to localize phaeochromocytomas is?

Harrison's 20th Ed. Chapter 380 Page 2741

A. 131I- or 123I-metaiodobenzylguanidine (MIBG)
B. 111In-somatostatin analogues
C. 18F-dopa (or dopamine)
D. All of the above

Pheochromocytoma tumor can be localized by radioactive tracers like ^{131}I- or ^{123}I-metaiodobenzylguanidine (MIBG), ^{111}In-somatostatin analogues, or ^{18}F-dopa (or dopamine) positron-emission tomography (PET) or ^{18}F-fluorodeoxyglucose (FDG) PET. ^{131}I-MIBG is also used in treatment of malignant phaeochromocytoma using 200-mCi doses at monthly intervals, over three to six cycles.

1421. Histologically, which of the following patterns relate to pheochromocytomas & paragangliomas?

Harrison's 20th Ed. Chapter 380 Page 2741

A. Mosaic pattern
B. Trabecular pattern
C. Fiddle-shaped pattern
D. Zellballen pattern

1422. Which of the following is false about "Zellballen" pattern?

Harrison's 20th Ed. Chapter 380 Page 2741

A. Seen histologically in pheochromocytomas & paragangliomas
B. Nests of neuroendocrine chief cells
C. Peripheral glial-like sustentacular cells
D. None of the above

Histologically, clusters and discretely scattered cells, with occasional acinar configuration and fine reddish intracytoplasmic granules are the established facts of a paraganglioma. Cell clusters enveloped by thin vascular channels are called zellballen pattern or "balls of cells" are diagnostic of pheochromocytoma/paraganglioma (adrenal or extra adrenal). Zellballen means "balls of cells" in German.

1423. Which of the following stains is almost always positive in pheochromocytoma?

Harrison's 20th Ed. Chapter 380 Page 2741

A. Beta catenin
B. NapsinA
C. Chromogranin
D. Calretinin

Chromogranin helps differentiate pheochromocytoma (almost always positive) from adrenocortical carcinoma (almost always negative).

1424. Which of the following immunostain highlights sustentacular cells?

Harrison's 20th Ed. Chapter 380 Page 2741

A. Synaptophysin
B. Chromogranin
C. S-100
D. All of the above

1425. Which of the following is considered in the differential diagnosis of pheochromocytoma?

Harrison's 20th Ed. Chapter 380 Page 2741

A. Mastocytosis
B. Carcinoid syndrome
C. Autonomic epilepsy
D. All of the above

In the differential diagnosis of pheochromocytoma, the disorders to be considered include essential hypertension, anxiety attacks, use of cocaine or amphetamines, mastocytosis or carcinoid syndrome, intracranial lesions, clonidine withdrawal, autonomic epilepsy and factitious crises (from use of sympathomimetic amines).

1426. When an asymptomatic adrenal mass is identified, likely diagnoses other than pheochromocytoma include?

Harrison's 20th Ed. Chapter 380 Page 2741

A. Nonfunctioning adrenal adenoma
B. Aldosteronoma
C. Cortisol-producing adenoma
D. All of the above

When an asymptomatic adrenal mass is identified, likely diagnoses other than pheochromocytoma include a nonfunctioning adrenal adenoma, an aldosteronoma and a cortisol-producing adenoma (Cushing's syndrome).

1427. Which of the following is an α-adrenoceptor blocker?

Lancet 2005;366:665–75

A. Prazosin
B. Doxazosin
C. Urapidil
D. All of the above

α-adrenoceptor blockers are phenoxybenzamine, prazosin, doxazosin & urapidil.

1428. In pheochromocytoma, phenoxybenzamine should be administered for at least how many days prior to surgery?

Harrison's 20th Ed. Chapter 380 Page 2743

A. 2 to 5 days
B. 5 to 10 days
C. 10 to 14 days
D. 14 to 21 days

Adequate alpha adrenergic blockade with phenoxybenzamine generally requires 10 - 14 days, with a typical final dose of 20–30 mg three times per day or 0.5–4 mg/kg of body weight. Before surgery, blood pressure should be consistently below 160/90 mm Hg.

1429. Which of the following is useful for control of blood pressure in pheochromocytoma?

Harrison's 20th Ed. Chapter 380 Page 2743

A. Oral phenoxybenzamine
B. Oral prazosin
C. Intravenous phentolamine
D. All of the above

1430. Which of the following antihypertensive is useful for control of blood pressure in pheochromocytoma?

Harrison's 20th Ed. Chapter 380 Page 2743

A. Sodium nitroprusside
B. Calcium channel blockers
C. Angiotensin-converting enzyme inhibitors
D. All of the above

1431. Malignant pheochromocytoma can metastasize to?

Lancet 2005;366:665-75

A. Bones
B. Lungs
C. Liver
D. All of the above

Term malignant pheochromocytoma is restricted to tumors with distant metastases, most commonly to lungs, bone or liver, suggesting a vascular pathway of spread.

1432. Distant metastases occur in which of the following germline mutation pheochromocytoma?

Harrison's 20th Ed. Chapter 380 Page 2743

A. RET
B. VHL
C. SDHD
D. SDHB

Distant metastases occur in carriers of SDHB mutations.

1433. Which of the following features of pheochromocytoma have a higher risk for malignant disease?

Lancet 2005;366:665-75

A. Large size (5 cm)
B. Paragangliomas with SDHB mutations
C. Increased plasma / urinary dopamine and dopa
D. All of the above

Malignant pheochromocytoma is associated with mutation of gene encoding the B subunit of mitochondrial complex II enzyme succinate dehydrogenase enzyme (SDHB). Highest predictive value for its diagnosis includes extra-adrenal tumor location, presence of SDHB mutations, and tumor size.

1434. Averbuch's chemotherapy protocol for treatment of malignant pheochromocytoma consists of all except?

Harrison's 20th Ed. Chapter 380 Page 2743

A. Dacarbazine
B. Methotrexate
C. Cyclophosphamide
D. Vincristine

Averbuch's chemotherapy protocol includes dacarbazine, cyclophosphamide, and vincristine, repeated every 21 days for three to six cycles. Other chemotherapeutic options are sunitinib and temozolomide/thalidomide.

1435. What percentage of patients with a pheochromocytoma or paraganglioma have an inherited syndrome?

Harrison's 20th Ed. Chapter 380 Page 2744

A. ~10%
B. ~30%
C. ~50%
D. ~75%

About 25–33% of patients with a pheochromocytoma or paraganglioma have an inherited syndrome.

1436. Classic features of neurofibromatosis include?

Harrison's 20th Ed. Chapter 86 Page 649

A. Café au lait spots
B. Axillary freckling of skin
C. Lisch nodules of iris
D. All of the above

Classic features of Neurofibromatosis type 1 (NF 1) or Von Recklinghausen's Disease include multiple benign Schwann cell neurofibromas, pigmented café au lait macules (CALM), freckling of non-sun-exposed skin of axilla, Lisch nodules of iris and pseudoarthrosis of the tibia.

1437. Lisch nodules of iris best relates to which of the following?

Harrison's 20th Ed. Chapter 86 Page 649

A. Pigmentation
B. Hamartoma
C. Prolapse
D. Dysplasia

Lisch nodules refers to hamartomas of the iris.

1438. NF1 gene that causes von Recklinghausen's disease is on which chromosome?

Harrison's 20th Ed. Chapter 86 Page 649

A. 6
B. 12
C. 17
D. 18

NF1 gene on chromosome 17 causes von Recklinghausen's disease. NF1 gene is a tumor-suppressor gene & encodes a neurofibromin which modulates signal transduction through the ras GTPase pathway.

1439. Multiple endocrine neoplasia type 2A is characterized by?

Harrison's 20th Ed. Chapter 380 Page 2744

A. Medullary thyroid carcinoma (MTC)
B. Pheochromocytoma
C. Hyperparathyroidism
D. All of the above

MEN2A is characterized by MTC, benign pheochromocytoma & hyperparathyroidism.

1440. Multiple endocrine neoplasia type 2B is characterized by?

Harrison's 20th Ed. Chapter 380 Page 2744

A. Medullary thyroid carcinoma (MTC)
B. Pheochromocytoma
C. Multiple mucosal neuromas
D. All of the above

MEN2B includes MTC, benign pheochromocytoma (~50%) & multiple mucosal neuromas, marfanoid habitus and other developmental disorders. It typically lacks hyperparathyroidism. Both types of MEN 2 are caused by mutations in RET (rearranged in transfection) that encodes a tyrosine kinase.

1441. Which of the following is not a feature of pheochromocytomas in MEN 2?

Harrison's 20th Ed. Chapter 380 Page 2744

A. Benign
B. Located in adrenals
C. MTC may be symptomatic before pheochromocytoma
D. Bilateral

Pheochromocytomas in MEN 2 are benign, located in the adrenals, and bilateral. Pheochromocytoma may be symptomatic before MTC.

1442. Mutations of which of the following genes occurs in MEN2?

Harrison's 20th Ed. Chapter 380 Page 2744

A. TERC
B. SPINK5
C. TRIM37
D. RET

1443. Which of the following is not a feature of MEN type 2A?

Harrison's 20th Ed. Chapter 380 Page 2744

A. Medullary thyroid carcinoma (MTC)
B. Pheochromocytoma
C. Mucosal neuromas
D. Hyperparathyroidism

1444. Which of the following is not a feature of MEN type 2B?

Harrison's 20th Ed. Chapter 380 Page 2744

A. Medullary thyroid carcinoma (MTC)
B. Pheochromocytoma
C. Mucosal neuromas
D. Hyperparathyroidism

1445. Which of the following about pheochromocytoma in MEN 2 is false?

Harrison's 20th Ed. Chapter 380 Page 2744

A. Occurs in ~50%
B. Benign
C. Bilateral
D. All of the above

1446. Mutations of which of the following gene causes paraganglioma syndrome 1 (PGL1)?

Harrison's 20th Ed. Chapter 380 Page 2744

A. SDHA
B. SDHB
C. SDHC
D. SDHD

Succinate dehydrogenase (SDH) is formed by four subunits (A - D). Mutations of SDHB (PGL4), SDHC (PGL3), and SDHD (PGL1) predispose to three of the paraganglioma syndromes.

1447. Which is the most frequent paraganglioma syndrome?

Harrison's 20th Ed. Chapter 380 Page 2744

A. PGL1
B. PGL2
C. PGL3
D. PGL4

1448. Which is the second most frequent paraganglioma syndrome?

Harrison's 20th Ed. Chapter 380 Page 2744

A. PGL1
B. PGL2
C. PGL3
D. PGL4

1449. Adrenal, extra-adrenal abdominal, and thoracic pheochromocytomas are absent in?

Harrison's 20th Ed. Chapter 380 Page 2744

A. PGL1
B. PGL2
C. PGL3
D. PGL4

PGL1 is most frequent, followed by PGL4. PGL3 is rare. Adrenal, extraadrenal abdominal & thoracic pheochromocytomas are components of PGL1, PGL4, and PGL5, are rare in PGL3 and absent in PGL2.

1450. Von Hippel–Lindau disease and pheochromocytoma best relate to which of the following?

Harrison's 20th Ed. Chapter 380 Page 2744

A. Fusion gene mutation
B. Point mutation
C. Transversion
D. Missense mutation

1451. Which of the following is not a feature of Von Hippel–Lindau syndrome?

Harrison's 20th Ed. Chapter 380 Page 2744, Lancet 2005;366:665-675

A. Renal clear-cell carcinoma
B. Retinal hemiangioblastoma
C. Testicular tumour
D. Pancreatic neuroendocrine tumour

VHL is an autosomal dominant disorder that predisposes to retinal & cerebellar hemangioblastomas, which also occur in the brain stem & spinal cord. Other features of VHL are clear cell renal carcinomas, pancreatic neuroendocrine tumors, endolymphatic sac tumors (ELSTs) of the inner ear, cystadenomas of the epididymis & broad ligament, and multiple pancreatic or renal cysts.

1452. Type of mutation in VHL gene in pheochromocytoma is?

Harrison's 20th Ed. Chapter 380 Page 2744

A. Point
B. Missense
C. Transition
D. Frameshift

Patients with pheochromocytoma predominantly have missense mutations in VHL gene. Mutations involving single nucleotides are referred to as point mutations. Substitutions are called transitions if a purine or pyrimidine is replaced by another purine or pyrimidine base. Changes from a purine to a pyrimidine, or vice versa, are called transversions. If the DNA sequence change occurs in a coding region and alters an amino acid, it is called a missense mutation. Polymorphisms are sequence variations that have a frequency of at least 1%. Small nucleotide deletions or insertions cause a shift of the codon reading frame (frameshift). Most commonly, reading frame alterations result in an abnormal protein segment of variable length before termination of translation occurs at a stop codon (nonsense mutation).

1453. Elevation of which of the following strongly suggests MEN 2?

Harrison's 20th Ed. Chapter 380 Page 2746

A. Serum calcitonin
B. Glucagon
C. Secretin
D. Vasoactive intestinal peptide

Elevation of serum calcitonin strongly suggests MEN 2 and should prompt testing for RET mutations.

Diabetes Mellitus: Diagnosis, Classification, and Pathophysiology

1454. Which of the following about diabetes mellitus (DM) is false?
Harrison's 20th Ed. Chapter 396 Page 2850

A. Group of common metabolic disorders
B. Common phenotype is hyperglycemia
C. Caused by interaction of genetics & environmental factors
D. None of the above

1455. In DM, factors contributing to hyperglycemia include?
Harrison's 20th Ed. Chapter 396 Page 2850

A. Reduced insulin secretion
B. Decreased glucose utilization
C. Increased glucose production
D. All of the above

In DM, factors contributing to hyperglycemia include reduced insulin secretion, decreased glucose utilization, and increased glucose production.

1456. In US, DM is the leading cause of?
Harrison's 20th Ed. Chapter 396 Page 2850

A. End-stage renal disease (ESRD)
B. Nontraumatic lower extremity amputations
C. Adult blindness
D. All of the above

1457. Most recent classification of diabetes mellitus is based on?
Harrison's 20th Ed. Chapter 396 Page 2850

A. Pathogenic process leading to hyperglycemia
B. Age of onset
C. Type of therapy
D. All of the above

"Pathogenic process leading to hyperglycemia" is the basis of classification of DM, as opposed to earlier criteria such as age of onset or type of therapy.

1458. Type 2 diabetes mellitus is characterized by all except?
Harrison's 20th Ed. Chapter 396 Page 2850

A. Insulin resistance
B. Impaired insulin secretion
C. Increased hepatic glucose production
D. Autoimmunity against the insulin-producing beta cells

Type 1 DM is the result of autoimmunity against insulin-producing β-cells, resulting in complete or near-total insulin deficiency. Type 2 DM is a heterogeneous group of disorders characterized by variable degrees of insulin resistance, impaired insulin secretion, and increased hepatic glucose production.

1459. Which of the following about type 1 DM is false?
Harrison's 20th Ed. Chapter 396 Page 2850

A. Changes in glucose tolerance are unidirectional
B. Due to autoimmunity against insulin-producing beta cells
C. Complete or near-total insulin deficiency
D. None of the above

Type 1A DM results from autoimmune beta cell destruction causing insulin deficiency. Individuals with type 1B DM lack immunologic markers indicative of an autoimmune destructive process of beta cells. They develop insulin deficiency by unknown mechanisms & are ketosis prone.

1460. Which of the following is not a separate category in the etiologic classification of diabetes mellitus?
Harrison's 20th Ed. Chapter 396 Page 2851 Table 396-1

A. Type 1 diabetes
B. Type 2 diabetes
C. Gestational diabetes mellitus (GDM)
D. Maturity-onset diabetes of the young (MODY)

1461. All of the following viruses can cause DM except?
Harrison's 20th Ed. Chapter 396 Page 2851 Table 396-1

A. Congenital Rubella
B. CMV
C. EBV
D. Coxsackie

Viral infections like congenital rubella, cytomegalovirus and coxsackie have been implicated in pancreatic islet destruction.

1462. All of the following drugs can cause DM except?
Harrison's 20th Ed. Chapter 396 Page 2851 Table 396-1

A. Diazoxide
B. Pyrantel pamoate
C. Pentamidine
D. Phenytoin

1463. Drugs that can cause DM include?
Harrison's 20th Ed. Chapter 396 Page 2851 Table 396-1

A. Nicotinic acid
B. Asparaginase
C. Beta-adrenergic agonists
D. All of the above

1464. Drugs that can cause DM include?
Harrison's 20th Ed. Chapter 396 Page 2851 Table 396-1

A. Thiazides
B. Hydantoins
C. Beta blockers
D. All of the above

1465. Drugs that can cause DM include?
Harrison's 20th Ed. Chapter 396 Page 2851 Table 396-1

A. α-interferon
B. Protease inhibitors
C. Clozapine
D. All of the above

Drugs that can cause DM include glucocorticoids, vacor (a rodenticide), pentamidine, nicotinic acid, diazoxide, β-adrenergic agonists, thiazides, calcineurin and mTOR inhibitors, hydantoins, asparaginase, α-interferon, protease inhibitors, atypical antipsychotics, epinephrine

1466. Syndromes associated with DM are all except?
Harrison's 20th Ed. Chapter 396 Page 2851 Table 396-1

A. Down syndrome
B. Klinefelter syndrome
C. Turner syndrome
D. Cri-du-chat syndrome

Genetic syndromes associated with diabetes are Wolfram's syndrome, Down's syndrome, Klinefelter's syndrome, Turner's syndrome, Friedreich's ataxia, Huntington's chorea, Laurence-Moon-Biedl syndrome, myotonic dystrophy, porphyria, Prader-Willi syndrome, Alström syndrome, Berardinelli-Seip syndrome.

1467. Which of the following is also known as DIDMOAD syndrome?
Harrison's 20th Ed. Chapter 382 Page 2760

A. Alström syndrome
B. Wolfram syndrome
C. Prader-Willi syndrome
D. Down's syndrome

Wolfram syndrome (WS) also known as DIDMOAD, is a neurodegenerative disorder characterized by type I diabetes mellitus (DM), diabetes insipidus (DI), sensorineural deafness (D), bilateral optical atrophy (OA) and neurological signs.

1468. Endocrinopathies associated with DM are all except?
Harrison's 20th Ed. Chapter 396 Page 2851 Table 396-1

A. Somatostatinoma
B. Aldosteronoma
C. Hypothyroidism
D. Pheochromocytoma

Endocrinopathies associated with DM are acromegaly, Cushing's syndrome, glucagonoma, pheochromocytoma, hyperthyroidism, somatostatinoma, aldosteronoma.

1469. Disease of the exocrine pancreas associated with DM is?
Harrison's 20th Ed. Chapter 396 Page 2851 Table 396-1

A. Pancreatic neoplasia
B. Fibrocalculous pancreatopathy
C. Mutations in carboxyl ester lipase
D. All of the above

Diseases of the exocrine pancreas associated with DM are pancreatitis, pancreatectomy, neoplasia, cystic fibrosis, hemochromatosis, fibrocalculous pancreatopathy, mutations in carboxyl ester lipase.

1470. Which of the following is associated with carboxyl ester lipase (CEL)?
Harrison's 20th Ed. Chapter 456 Page 3364 Table 456-6

A. MODY 3
B. MODY 6
C. MODY 8
D. MODY 10

1471. Which of the following about Carboxyl-ester lipase (CEL) is false?
Diabetes 2014;63:259–69

A. Expressed in pancreatic acinar & lactating mammary cells
B. Encodes a digestive enzyme of cholesterol ester digestion
C. CEL-MODY develop pancreatic cysts & diabetes in 40s
D. None of the above

1472. Which of the following is associated with hepatocyte nuclear transcription factor (HNF) 4α?
Harrison's 20th Ed. Chapter 396 Page 2851 Table 396-1

A. MODY 1
B. MODY 2
C. MODY 3
D. MODY 4

1473. Which of the following is associated with hepatocyte nuclear transcription factor (HNF) 1α?
Harrison's 20th Ed. Chapter 396 Page 2851 Table 396-1

A. MODY 1
B. MODY 2
C. MODY 3
D. MODY 4

1474. Which of the following is associated with glucokinase?
Harrison's 20th Ed. Chapter 396 Page 2851 Table 396-1

A. MODY 1
B. MODY 2
C. MODY 3
D. MODY 4

1475. Which of the following is a pancreatic islet regulator/ protein?
Harrison's 20th Ed. Chapter 396 Page 2851 Table 396-1

A. SLC2A2 (GLUT2)
B. GATA4
C. GATA6
D. All of the above

Pancreatic islet regulators/proteins include KLF11, PAX4, BLK, GATA4, GATA6, SLC2A2 (GLUT2), RFX6, GLIS3

1476. Which of the following produces a genetic defect in insulin action?
Harrison's 20th Ed. Chapter 396 Page 2851 Table 396-1

A. Down's syndrome
B. Prader–Willi syndrome
C. Wolfram's syndrome
D. Rabson–Mendenhall syndrome

1477. Which of the following produces a genetic defect in insulin action?
Harrison's 20th Ed. Chapter 396 Page 2851 Table 396-1

A. Lipodystrophy syndromes
B. Leprechaunism
C. Rabson-Mendenhall syndrome
D. All of the above

Genetic defects in insulin action is produced by Type A insulin resistance, Leprechaunism, Rabson-Mendenhall syndrome and Lipodystrophy syndromes.

1478. Mutations in the insulin receptor gene produce?

Diabetologia. 2010;53:2454–55

A. Donohue's syndrome
B. Rabson–Mendenhall syndrome
C. Type A insulin resistance
D. All of the above

These phenotypes are diagnosed at birth or in infancy due to the presence of signs of severe hyperinsulinaemia such as acanthosis nigricans, abnormal dentition, hyperandrogenism and pseudo-acromegaly. Type 2 diabetes develops early in life and its treatment is challenging. Insulin is used in very high doses, but microvascular complications develop early and aggressively.

1479. Maturity onset diabetes of the young (MODY) is characterized by all except?

Harrison's 20th Ed. Chapter 396 Page 2851

A. Autosomal dominant inheritance
B. Autosomal recessive inheritance
C. Early onset hyperglycemia
D. Impairment of insulin secretion

Maturity onset diabetes of the young (MODY) is characterized by autosomal dominant inheritance, early onset of hyperglycemia, and impairment in insulin secretion.

1480. Which of the following is related to viral infection of islets?

Harrison's 20th Ed. Chapter 396 Page 2851

A. Maturity onset diabetes of the young (MODY)
B. Monogenic diabetes
C. Fulminant diabetes
D. Gestational diabetes mellitus (GDM)

A form of acute onset of type 1 diabetes, termed fulminant diabetes, is noted in Japan and may be related to viral infection of islets.

1481. Glucose intolerance developing during which of the following periods is 'not' called gestational diabetes mellitus (GDM)?

Harrison's 20th Ed. Chapter 396 Page 2851

A. First trimester
B. Second trimester
C. Third trimester
D. None of the above

American Diabetes Association (ADA) recommends that diabetes diagnosed within the first trimester be classified as preexisting pregestational diabetes rather than GDM. Glucose intolerance developing during the second or third trimester of pregnancy is classified as gestational diabetes mellitus (GDM).

1482. Which of the following is false about women with GDM?

Harrison's 20th Ed. Chapter 396 Page 2851

A. 1 in 7 pregnancies worldwide affected by glucose intolerance
B. Most GDM revert to normal glucose tolerance postpartum
C. 35–60% of of GDM develop DM in the next 5 years
D. Children of GDM mothers developing type 2 DM later in life

One in seven pregnancies worldwide is affected by either GDM or preexisting DM. Most GDM women revert to normal glucose tolerance postpartum. 35–60% of GDM developing DM in next 10–20 years. Children of GDM mothers have an increased risk of developing metabolic syndrome & type 2 DM later in life.

1483. Which of the following epidemiological figures is correct?

Harrison's 20th Ed. Chapter 396 Page 2851

A. Prevalence of DM in 1985 ~30 million
B. Prevalence of DM in 2017 ~415 million
C. Prevalence of DM in 2040 projected to be ~642 million
D. All of the above

1484. Number of individuals with diabetes in India in 2015 were?

Harrison's 20th Ed. Chapter 396 Page 2851

A. ~ 50 million
B. ~ 60 million
C. ~ 70 million
D. ~ 80 million

Countries with greatest number of individuals with diabetes in 2015 were China (109.6 million), India (73 million), United States (30.3 million), Brazil (14 million), and Russian Federation (9 million).

1485. Which of the following statements about DM is false?

Harrison's 20th Ed. Chapter 396 Page 2852

A. Prevalence of DM increases with age
B. Prevalence of DM is more among men than women
C. DM-related mortality rates are higher in men than women
D. Indigenous populations have a greater incidence DM

The prevalence of diabetes is similar among men and women.

1486. Variability in the prevalence of DM is due to?

Harrison's 20th Ed. Chapter 396 Page 2852

A. Genetic factors
B. Behavioral factors
C. Environmental factors
D. All of the above

1487. Out of the following countries, which one has the highest incidence of type 1 DM?

Harrison's 20th Ed. Chapter 396 Page 2852

A. Japan
B. China
C. Scandinavia
D. United States of America

Scandinavia has the highest incidence of type 1 DM. US, Japan and China have a lower rate.

1488. In the ADA criteria for diagnosis of DM, what is meant by "fasting state"?

Harrison's 20th Ed. Chapter 396 Page 2852 Table 396-2

A. No oral intake since last 8 hours
B. No oral intake for last 12 hours
C. No caloric intake for last 8 hours
D. No caloric intake for last 12 hours

Fasting state is defined as no "caloric" intake for at least 8 hours.

1489. Which of the following is a category of glucose tolerance?

Harrison's 20th Ed. Chapter 396 Page 2852

A. Normal glucose homeostasis
B. Impaired glucose homeostasis
C. Diabetes mellitus
D. All of the above

Glucose tolerance is classified into three broad categories. They are normal glucose homeostasis, impaired glucose homeostasis, or diabetes mellitus.

1490. Glucose tolerance can be assessed by?

Harrison's 20th Ed. Chapter 396 Page 2852

A. Fasting plasma glucose (FPG)
B. Response to oral glucose challenge
C. Hemoglobin A1c (HbA1c)
D. All of the above

Glucose tolerance can be assessed by fasting plasma glucose (FPG), the response to oral glucose challenge, or the hemoglobin A1c (HbA1c).

1491. Which of the following define normal glucose tolerance?

Harrison's 20th Ed. Chapter 396 Page 2852

A. FPG < 100 mg/dL
B. Plasma glucose < 140 mg/dL following oral glucose challenge
C. HbA1c < 5.7%
D. All of the above

1492. Which of the following statements is false about DM?

Harrison's 20th Ed. Chapter 396 Page 2852

A. Diagnostic criteria based on FPG, OGTT & HbA1c differ among individuals
B. DM is defined as level of glycemia at which diabetes-specific complications occur
C. DM is defined as deviation of FPG, OGTT & HbA1c from a population-based mean
D. None of the above

Diagnostic criteria based on FPG, oral glucose tolerance test (OGTT) & HbA1c differ among individuals. DM is defined as the level of glycemia at which diabetes-specific complications occur rather than deviation from a population-based mean.

1493. Which of the following is false about criteria for the diagnosis of diabetes mellitus?

Harrison's 20th Ed. Chapter 396 Page 2852 Table 396-2

A. Random blood glucose ≥ 200 mg/dL
B. Fasting plasma glucose ≥ 126 mg/dL
C. Hemoglobin A1c ≥ 6%
D. 2-hour plasma glucose ≥ 200 mg/dL during OGTT

Criteria for the diagnosis of DM includes symptoms of diabetes + random blood glucose ≥ 200 mg/dL, or fasting plasma glucose ≥ 126 mg/dL, or Hemoglobin A1c ≥ 6.5% or 2-hour plasma glucose ≥ 200 mg/dL during an oral glucose tolerance test.

1494. Impaired fasting glucose (IFG) is labeled when fasting plasma glucose level are between?

Harrison's 20th Ed. Chapter 396 Page 2852

A. 80–125 mg/dL
B. 100–125 mg/dL
C. 125–180 mg/dL
D. 125–200 mg/dL

Impaired fasting glucose (IFG) is defined when fasting plasma glucose level is between 100–125 mg/dL.

1495. After 2 hours of 75-gram oral glucose load, impaired glucose tolerance is defined when plasma glucose levels are between?

Harrison's 20th Ed. Chapter 396 Page 2852

A. 100 & 180 mg/dL
B. 126 & 180 mg/dL
C. 140 & 199 mg/dL
D. 160 & 200 mg/dL

Impaired glucose tolerance (IGT) is defined as plasma glucose levels between 140 and 199 mg/dL, 2 hours after a 75-gram oral glucose load.

1496. Individuals with impaired fasting glucose (IFG) are at increased risk of developing?

Harrison's 20th Ed. Chapter 396 Page 2852

A. Type 1 DM
B. Type 2 DM
C. Pancreatitis
D. Hypothyroidism

1497. Individuals with impaired fasting glucose are at increased risk of developing which of the following condition?

Harrison's 20th Ed. Chapter 396 Page 2852

A. Neuropathy
B. Arthropathy
C. Cardiovascular diseases
D. Renal failure

Individuals with IFG, IGT or HbA1c 5.7–6.4% are at greater risk for developing type 2 DM & cardiovascular disease.

1498. Individuals with IFG, IGT or HbA1c 5.7–6.4% are labeled as?

Harrison's 20th Ed. Chapter 396 Page 2852

A. Prediabetes
B. Increased risk of diabetes
C. Intermediate hyperglycemia
D. Any of the above

1499. Which of the following is not used for the diagnosis of DM and in routine clinical care in DM?

Harrison's 20th Ed. Chapter 396 Page 2852

A. Fasting plasma glucose
B. Oral glucose tolerance test
C. HbA1c
D. All of the above

1500. Oral glucose tolerance test (OGTT) is of use in?

Harrison's 20th Ed. Chapter 396 Page 2853

A. MODY
B. Gestational diabetes
C. Drug induced diabetes
D. All of the above

For the diagnosis of DM, HbA1c or FPG are the most reliable and convenient tests. OGTT, although a valid means for diagnosing DM, is not used in routine clinical care with the exception of pregnancy care and screening for gestational diabetes.

1501. Epidemiologic studies suggest that type 2 DM may be present for how many years before diagnosis?

Harrison's 20th Ed. Chapter 396 Page 2853

A. 3 years
B. 5 years
C. 7 years
D. 10 years

Epidemiologic studies suggest that type 2 DM may be present for up to a decade before diagnosis.

1502. American Diabetes Association (ADA) recommends screening for DM in which of the following?

Harrison's 20th Ed. Chapter 396 Page 2853

A. > 35 years - every three years
B. > 40 years - every three years
C. > 45 years - every three years
D. > 50 years - every year

American Diabetes Association (ADA) recommends screening all individuals >45 years every 3 years.

1503. Which of the following is considered as a risk factor for Type 2 diabetes mellitus?

Harrison's 20th Ed. Chapter 396 Page 2853 Table 396-3

A. Acanthosis nigricans
B. HDL cholesterol level < 35 mg/dL
C. Triglyceride level > 250 mg/dL
D. All of the above

1504. Which of the following is considered as a risk factor for Type 2 diabetes mellitus?

Harrison's 20th Ed. Chapter 396 Page 2853 Table 396-3

A. Polycystic ovary syndrome
B. Hypertension
C. Asian American
D. All of the above

1505. Glucose homeostasis reflects which of the following?

Harrison's 20th Ed. Chapter 396 Page 2853

A. Energy intake from ingested food
B. Hepatic glucose production (gluconeogenesis)
C. Peripheral tissue glucose uptake & utilization
D. All of the above

Glucose homeostasis is determined by a balance between energy intake from ingested food, hepatic glucose production (gluconeogenesis), and peripheral tissue glucose uptake & utilization.

1506. Glucagon stimulates glycogenolysis and gluconeogenesis by?

Harrison's 20th Ed. Chapter 396 Page 2853

A. Pancreas
B. Renal medulla
C. Pulmonary parenchyma
D. Skeletal muscles

Glucagon is secreted by pancreatic alpha cells when blood glucose or insulin levels are low or during exercise. It stimulates glycogenolysis and gluconeogenesis by the liver and renal medulla.

1507. Tissue that uses glucose in an insulin-independent fashion is?

Harrison's 20th Ed. Chapter 396 Page 2853

A. Lung
B. Brain
C. Heart
D. All of the above

Brain uses glucose in an insulin-independent fashion.

1508. Which of the following factors that influence glucose homeostasis is secreted by skeletal myocytes?

Int J Endocrinol. 2018;2018:7816806

A. Irisin
B. Leptin
C. Resistin
D. Adiponectin

Factors secreted by skeletal myocytes (irisin), adipocytes (leptin, resistin, adiponectin) and bone also influence glucose homeostasis.

1509. Which of the following about irisin is false?

Int J Endocrinol. 2018;2018:7816806

A. Exercise induced myokine
B. Secreted mainly in skeletal muscle
C. Product of type I membrane protein cleavage encoded by fibronectin type III domain containing 5 (FNDC5) genes
D. None of the above

Studies show decreased irisin concentrations in T2DM regardless of the time of diagnosis & whether they are undergoing any treatment and even lower concentration in the presence of complications of T2DM. FNDC5 converts to irisin after exercise.

1510. Human irisin has similarity with?

Int J Endocrinol. 2018;2018:7816806

A. Insulin
B. Glucagon
C. Leptin
D. All of the above

Mouse, rat, and human irisin are 100% identical; the rates of similarity are 85% for insulin, 90% for glucagon, and 83% for leptin.

1511. Which of the following about insulin is false?

Harrison's 20th Ed. Chapter 396 Page 2853

A. Anabolic hormone
B. Promotes storage of carbohydrate
C. Promotes fat and protein synthesis
D. None of the above

Insulin is an anabolic hormone that promotes storage of carbohydrate and fat & protein synthesis.

1512. Major portion of postprandial glucose is used by?

Harrison's 20th Ed. Chapter 396 Page 2853

A. Liver
B. Skeletal muscle
C. Brain
D. Adipose tissue

Major portion of postprandial glucose is used by skeletal muscle, an effect of insulin-stimulated glucose uptake. Brain uses glucose in an insulin-independent fashion.

1513. Factors secreted by which of the following influence glucose homeostasis?

Harrison's 20th Ed. Chapter 396 Page 2853

A. Skeletal myocytes
B. Adipocytes
C. Bone
D. All of the above

Factors secreted by skeletal myocytes, adipocytes (leptin, resistin, adiponectin), and bone influence glucose homeostasis.

1514. The human insulin gene is located on?

Proc Natl Acad Sci USA. 2009;106(41):17419–24

A. Short arm of chromosome 11
B. Long arm of chromosome 11
C. Short arm of chromosome 12
D. Long arm of chromosome 12

The human INS gene is a single copy gene located on the short arm of chromosome 11. Insulin receptor belongs to the superfamily of receptor tyrosine kinases (RTKs).

1515. Which of the following conditions is associated with chromosome 11?

Proc Natl Acad Sci USA. 2009;106(41):17419–24

A. Beckwith-Wiedemann syndrome
B. Emanuel syndrome
C. Jacobsen syndrome
D. All of the above

1516. Which of the following conditions is associated with chromosome 11?

Proc Natl Acad Sci USA. 2009;106(41):17419–24

A. Potocki–Shaffer syndrome
B. Russell–Silver syndrome
C. WAGR syndrome
D. All of the above

1517. Which of the following is best related to ATP sensitive potassium channels?

Harrison's 20th Ed. Chapter 396 Page 2853

A. mRNA
B. Pyruvate
C. GLUT 2
D. GLUT 4

1518. 86-amino-acid precursor polypeptide of insulin is called?

Harrison's 20th Ed. Chapter 396 Page 2853

A. C-peptide
B. Preinsulin
C. Proinsulin
D. Preproinsulin

Insulin is initially synthesized as a single-chain 86-amino-acid precursor polypeptide, preproinsulin.

1519. Proteolytic processing of "preproinsulin" results in the formation of?

Harrison's 20th Ed. Chapter 396 Page 2853

A. C peptide
B. Proinsulin
C. Insulin
D. All of the above

In rough ER and Golgi apparatus (GA), proteolytic processing of "preproinsulin" removes amino terminal signal peptide, giving rise to proinsulin.

1520. Which of the following is structurally related to insulin-like growth factors I and II?

Harrison's 20th Ed. Chapter 396 Page 2853

A. Preproinsulin
B. Proinsulin
C. Insulin
D. Glucagon

Proinsulin is structurally related to insulin-like growth factors I and II.

1521. Cleavage of proinsulin generates which of the following?

Harrison's 20th Ed. Chapter 396 Page 2853

A. C peptide
B. A chain of insulin
C. B chain of insulin
D. All of the above

Proinsulin cleavage generates C peptide and A and B chains of insulin.

1522. The A and B chains of insulin contain how many amino acids respectively?

Harrison's 20th Ed. Chapter 396 Page 2853

A. 21 & 30 amino acids
B. 30 & 21 amino acids
C. 21 & 29 amino acids
D. 29 & 21 amino acids

Insulin hormone is a posttranslational 51-residue anabolic globular protein product of preproinsulin that is secreted by the β-cells in the Islets of Langerhans. Insulin gene encodes preproinsulin polypeptide. Insulin contains two chains, A (21 residues) and B (30 residues).

1523. The A and B chains of insulin are connected by which of the following bond?

Harrison's 20th Ed. Chapter 396 Page 2854

A. Hydrogen
B. Amino acid
C. Disulfide
D. Calcium

1524. Number of disulfide bonds in insulin is?

Experimental Diabetes Research. 2012, Article ID 509437

A. 1
B. 2
C. 3
D. 4

A & B chains of insulin contain 21 & 30 amino acids respectively. They are connected by disulfide bonds derived from cysteine residues (A7-B7 and A20-B19). An intra-chain disulfide bond also exists within the A-chain (A6-A11). The sequence of human insulin is identical to that of porcine insulin except for the change of Ala^{B30} to Thr^{B30} in human insulin.

1525. Which of the following statements is false?

Experimental Diabetes Research. 2012, Article ID 509437

A. Preproinsulin is synthesized in the cytoplasm
B. Proinsulin is produced in the endoplasmic reticulum (ER)
C. Conversion of proinsulin to insulin occurs in secretory granules
D. None of the above

As preproinsulin is synthesized in the cytoplasm and cotranslationally translocated into lumen of ER where it is cleaved and proinsulin is produced. Proinsulin undergoes protein folding with three disulfide bonds. Properly folded proinsulin is then delivered to Golgi apparatus and packaged into secretory granules. Conversion of proinsulin to insulin takes place in secretory granules. Mature insulin is released by calcium dependent exocytosis. ER stress due to increased misfolded proinsulin (unfolded protein response (UPR)) induces β cell dysfunction & diabetes.

1526. Conversion of proinsulin to insulin occurs through?

Experimental Diabetes Research. 2012, Article ID 509437

A. Oxidoreductases
B. Transferases
C. Endoproteases
D. Isomerases

1527. Conversion of proinsulin to insulin occurs through?

Experimental Diabetes Research. 2012, Article ID 509437

A. Ligases
B. Exopeptidases
C. Hydrolases
D. All of the above

The conversion of proinsulin to insulin occurs through the joint action of two types of proteases. Trypsin-like endoprotease activity and exopeptidase activity resembling that of carboxypeptidase B to remove the basic residues left after tryptic-like cleavage.

1528. Which of the following has specific receptor on the β-cell?
Experimental Diabetes Research. 2012, Article ID 509437

A. Glucagon
B. Glucagon-like peptide (GLP-1)
C. Cholecystokinin
D. All of the above

Glucagon, glucagon-like peptide (GLP-1), cholecystokinin and gastric inhibitory peptide have specific receptors on the β-cell.

1529. Which of the following is an inhibitor of insulin secretion?
Experimental Diabetes Research. 2012, Article ID 509437

A. Adrenaline
B. Noradrenaline
C. Somatostatin
D. All of the above

Inhibitors of insulin secretion include catecholamines (adrenaline and noradrenaline) which interact with adrenergic receptors on the β-cell membrane , and somatostatin which is secreted by δ-cells of the pancreatic islets.

1530. Which of the following syndromes is related to diabetes mellitus?
Experimental Diabetes Research. 2012, Article ID 509437

A. Fanconi–Bickel syndrome
B. Wolcott–Rallison syndrome
C. Jansen's syndrome
D. DiGeorge syndrome

Wolcott–Rallison syndrome (WRS) is an autosomal recessive disease, characterized by neonatal/ early-onset non-autoimmune insulin-requiring diabetes associated with skeletal dysplasia and growth retardation. PERK is an endoplasmic reticulum (ER) transmembrane protein, which plays a key role in translation control during the unfolded protein response. ER dysfunction is central to the disease processes.

1531. Which of the following bind to the insulin receptor?
Harrison's 20th Ed. Chapter 396 Page 2853

A. Insulin-like growth factor I
B. Insulin-like growth factor II
C. Insulin
D. All of the above

Insulin-like growth factors I and II bind weakly to the insulin receptor.

1532. Other than insulin, β cells also secrete?
Harrison's 20th Ed. Chapter 396 Page 2854

A. Ptyalin
B. Amylin
C. Amylase
D. Lipase

1533. Which of the following is secreted by β cells?
Harrison's 20th Ed. Chapter 396 Page 2854

A. Insulin
B. Amylin
C. C-peptide
D. All of the above

Insulin is stored as microcrystalline arrays of zinc insulin hexamers within specialized glucose-regulated secretory vescicles. Mature insulin molecule & C-peptide are stored together in large dense core vesicles (LDCV) and co-secreted in equimolar concentrations from secretory granules in beta cells. Pancreatic beta cells co-secrete islet amyloid polypeptide (IAPP) or amylin along with insulin. It is a major component of amyloid fibrils found in islets of patients with type 2 diabetes. Its analogue is being used in treating both type 1 and type 2 DM.

1534. Which of the following about C-peptide is false?
Harrison's 20th Ed. Chapter 396 Page 2854

A. Formed from proinsulin
B. Cleared more slowly than insulin
C. Useful marker of insulin secretion
D. None of the above

1535. Transcription of the insulin gene is regulated primarily by which of the following transcription factor?
Experimental Diabetes Research. 2012, Article ID 509437

A. PDX-1
B. BETA/NeuroD
C. RIPE3b1/MafA
D. All of the above

Transcription of the insulin gene is regulated primarily by transcription factors such as PDX-1, BETA/ NeuroD, and RIPE3b1/MafA.

1536. Insulin synthesis is stimulated by glucose levels above?
Harrison's 20th Ed. Chapter 396 Page 2854

A. 30 mg%
B. 40 mg%
C. 50 mg%
D. 70 mg%

Glucose levels > 70 mg/dL stimulate insulin synthesis by enhancing protein translation & processing.

1537. Word insulin is derived from a Latin word "insula" meaning?
Clinical Chemistry 2002;48:2270-88

A. Protected
B. Projected
C. Island
D. High land

1538. Frederick G Banting, who discovered insulin was a?
Clinical Chemistry 2002;48:2270-88

A. Physiologist
B. Biochemist
C. Orthopedic surgeon
D. Physician

Frederick G. Banting (1891–1941) was a Canadian orthopedic surgeon. Charles Best (1899–1978) was a student assistant. J.J.R. Macleod was the head of physiology at the University of Toronto. Success with purification of pancreatic extracts was largely the work of J.B. Collip. Banting and Macleod jointly earned a Nobel Prize in Physiology or Medicine for the discovery of insulin in 1923. Banting shared his winning money with Best and Macleod with Collip. By the end of 1923, insulin came in commercial production at the Eli Lilly laboratories in Indianapolis, USA.

1539. Antidiabetic hormone was named as "insuline" by?
Clinical Chemistry 2002;48:2270-88

A. Minkowski
B. Schafer
C. Collip
D. MacCleod

At the end of the 19 th century Von Mering and Minkowski noted that removal of pancreas led to the development of DM in dogs. In 1916, Schafer first speculated that an antidiabetic hormone, which he named "insuline". Insulin was the first 'peptide' hormone discovered.

1540. Amino-acid sequence of insulin was elucidated by?

Clinical Chemistry 2002;48:2270-88

A. Von Mering
B. Langerhans
C. Sanger
D. Hodgkin

Amino-acid sequence of insulin was elucidated by Sanger in mid 1950's.

1541. Which of the following glucose transporter is the insulin-responsive isoform?

Clinical Chemistry 2002;48:2270-88

A. Na^+ dependent
B. Na^+ independent
C. Ca^{++} dependent
D. Ca^{++} independent

Two major types of glucose transporters into cells are known: Na^+ dependent & Na^+ independent. Only the Na^+ independent transporters possess an insulin-responsive isoform. Na^+ dependent glucose transporter family has been identified in small intestinal epithelium (SGLT1) and renal proximal tubule (SGLT2). They absorb glucose against its concentration gradient by coupling the movement of glucose into these cells with the concomitant movement of Na^+ into the cell with the help of Na^+/K^+-ATPase ion pump.

1542. Which of the following Na^+ independent glucose transporter is in highest concentration in insulin-sensitive tissues?

Clinical Chemistry 2002;48:2270-88

A. GLUT 1
B. GLUT 2
C. GLUT 3
D. GLUT 4

GLUT 4 is the transporter that is in highest concentration in insulin-sensitive tissues, including skeletal muscle, cardiac muscle, and adipose tissue. Upon binding & activation to the insulin receptor (IR), insulin enhances this passive glucose uptake by increasing the number of transporters, from intracellular compartments, into the plasma membrane of target cells.

1543. Glucose is transported into the pancreatic β cells via?

Harrison's 20th Ed. Chapter 396 Page 2854 Figure 396-5

A. GLUT 2
B. GLUT 3
C. GLUT 4
D. GLUT 5

GLUT 2 is expressed on surface of β-cells. Glucose is transported into the β-cell by the GLUT2 glucose transporter. Therefore, insulin positively regulates its own secretion from the β-cell.

1544. "SUR" stands for?

Harrison's 20th Ed. Chapter 396 Page 2854 Figure 396-5

A. Sugar receptor
B. Sulfonylurea receptor
C. Sucrose receptor
D. Sulphar receptor

SUR stands for sulfonylurea receptor & is the binding site for drugs (sulfonylureas, meglitinides) that act as insulin secretagogues. It is an ATP-sensitive K^+ channel.

1545. Sulfonylurea receptor (SUR) best relates to which of the following?

Harrison's 20th Ed. Chapter 396 Page 2854 Figure 396-5

A. ATP-sensitive K^+ channel
B. Cyclic adenosine monophosphate (cAMP)
C. GLUT 2
D. Insulin

1546. Glucose, in addition to stimulating insulin secretion by β-cells also?

Clinical Chemistry 2002;48:2270-88

A. Activates insulin gene transcription
B. Enhances insulin mRNA stability
C. Stimulates insulin mRNA translation
D. All of the above

Glucose, in addition to stimulating insulin secretion by β-cells, also activates insulin gene transcription, enhances insulin mRNA stability, and stimulates its translation. High ambient glucose concentration in the islets promotes insulin biosynthesis and is the primary regulator of secretion. Systemic insulin levels are regulated by secretion rather than by biosynthesis.

1547. Which of the following acts as a rate-limiting step that controls glucose-regulated insulin secretion?

Harrison's 20th Ed. Chapter 396 Page 2854

A. Pyruvate
B. Glucose-6-phosphate
C. Glucokinase
D. All of the above

Glucose phosphorylation by "glucokinase" is the rate-limiting step that controls glucose-regulated insulin secretion.

1548. Which of the following is false about insulin secretion?

Harrison's 20th Ed. Chapter 396 Page 2854

A. Secreted in a pulsatile pattern
B. Meals induce large bursts of insulin secretion
C. About 50% of secreted insulin is degraded by liver
D. None of the above

1549. Greater secretory bursts of insulin secretion occur at what interval?

Harrison's 20th Ed. Chapter 396 Page 2854

A. 5–45 minutes
B. 45–80 minutes
C. 80–150 minutes
D. 150–180 minutes

Insulin is secreted in a pulsatile pattern, with small secretory bursts occurring about every 10 minutes, superimposed upon greater amplitude oscillations of about 80–150 minutes.

1550. Beta cell membrane depolarization that stimulates insulin secretion by opening calcium channels is done by?

Harrison's 20th Ed. Chapter 396 Page 2854

A. Stimulation of ATP-sensitive K^+ channel
B. Inhibition of ATP-sensitive K^+ channel
C. Stimulation of ATP-sensitive Ca^{++} channel
D. Inhibition of ATP-sensitive Ca^{++} channel

Further metabolism of the phosphorylated product of glucose i.e. glucose-6-phosphate generates ATP which leads to inhibition of ATP-sensitive K^+ channel (Kir6.2). This induces beta cell membrane depolarization which opens voltage-dependent calcium channels and causes insulin secretion.

1551. Which of the following glucose transporters is crucial for glucose uptake by skeletal muscle and fat?
Harrison's 20th Ed. Chapter 396 Page 2854

A. GLUT 1
B. GLUT 2
C. GLUT 3
D. GLUT 4

Glucose transporter - GLUT4 is translocated to cell surface following activation of PI-3-kinase pathway which is stimulated by insulin. GLUT4 is crucial for glucose uptake by skeletal muscle & fat.

1552. Major portion of postprandial glucose is utilized by?
Harrison's 20th Ed. Chapter 396 Page 2854

A. Skeletal muscle
B. Liver
C. Adipose tissue
D. Brain

Major portion of postprandial glucose is utilized by skeletal muscle through insulin-stimulation.

1553. Which of the following about incretin hormones is false?
Harrison's 20th Ed. Chapter 396 Page 2854

A. Bind specific receptors on beta cell
B. Stimulate insulin secretion through cyclic AMP production
C. Effect only when blood glucose is above the fasting level
D. None of the above

1554. Which of the following about incretin hormones is false?
Harrison's 20th Ed. Chapter 396 Page 2854

A. Glucagon-like peptide-1 (GLP-1) is an incretin hormone
B. Glucose dependent insulinotropic peptide (GIP) is an incretin hormone
C. Suppress glucagon production and secretion
D. None of the above

1555. Glucagon-like peptide 1 (GLP-1) is released from which cells in the small intestine?
Harrison's 20th Ed. Chapter 396 Page 2854

A. K
B. L
C. M
D. N

Glucagon-like peptide 1 (GLP-1) is the most potent incretin and is released from L cells in the small intestine and stimulates insulin secretion following food ingestion.

1556. What proportion of insulin in portal system is degraded by the liver?
Harrison's 20th Ed. Chapter 396 Page 2854

A. 10%
B. 25%
C. 50%
D. 75%

Once insulin is secreted into the portal venous system, ~50% is degraded by the liver.

1557. Insulin best relates to which of the following?
Harrison's 20th Ed. Chapter 396 Page 2854

A. Tyrosine phosphatase
B. Tyrosine kinase
C. mTOR serine-threonine kinase
D. Histone deacetylase

Insulin in systemic circulation binds to receptors in target sites thereby stimulating intrinsic tyrosine kinase activity, leading to recruitment of intracellular signaling molecules like insulin receptor substrates (IRS).

1558. Activation by insulin of which of the following pathway stimulates translocation of GLUT4 to the cell surface?
Harrison's 20th Ed. Chapter 396 Page 2854

A. Sorbitol pathway
B. Hexosamine pathway
C. PI-3-kinase pathway
D. All of the above

Activation by insulin of the phosphatidylinositol-3'-kinase (PI-3-kinase) pathway stimulates translocation of a facilitative glucose transporter - GLUT4 to the cell surface. This is crucial for glucose uptake by skeletal muscle and fat.

1559. Destruction of pancreatic β cells in Type 1 DM develops as a result of which of the following?
Harrison's 20th Ed. Chapter 396 Page 2854

A. Genetic factors
B. Environmental factors
C. Immunologic factors
D. All of the above

Type 1 DM develops as a result of the synergistic effects of genetic, environmental, and immunologic factors that ultimately destroy the pancreatic beta cells and produce insulin deficiency.

1560. Type 1 DM most commonly develops before what age?
Harrison's 20th Ed. Chapter 396 Page 2854

A. 5 years
B. 10 years
C. 15 years
D. 20 years

Type 1 DM can develop at any age, but most commonly develops before 20 years of age.

1561. What percentage of beta cell mass is destroyed when type 1 diabetes becomes clinically apparent?
Harrison's 20th Ed. Chapter 396 Page 2854

A. 40%
B. 60%
C. 80%
D. 100%

Progressive impairment in insulin release due to gradual decline in beta cell mass results in type 1 diabetes when 70–80% of the beta cell mass is destroyed.

1562. In relation to type 1 DM, honeymoon period is?
Harrison's 20th Ed. Chapter 396 Page 2854

A. Increased insulin requirement after marriage
B. Glycemic control achieved by OHA
C. Insulin requirement is nil or modest
D. Weight gain after insulin treatment

After the initial clinical presentation of type 1 DM, a "honeymoon" phase may ensue during which time glycemic control is achieved with modest doses of insulin or, rarely, insulin is not needed. A "honeymoon" phase may be seen in the first 1 or 2 years after the onset of diabetes and is associated with reduced insulin requirements.

1563. Which of the following about type 1 DM is false?
Harrison's 20th Ed. Chapter 396 Page 2854

A. Most have evidence of islet-directed autoimmunity
B. Mostly, autoantibodies against β cell antigens appear after a triggering event
C. Functional, but insufficient number of β cells exist
D. None of the above

1564. In type 1 DM, stage 1 disease is characterized by the development of?
Harrison's 20th Ed. Chapter 396 Page 2855 Figure 396-6

A. ≥ 1 islet cell autoantibody
B. ≥ 2 islet cell autoantibody
C. ≥ 3 islet cell autoantibody
D. ≥ 4 islet cell autoantibody

1565. In type 1 DM, normoglycemia is found in which stage of the disease?
Harrison's 20th Ed. Chapter 396 Page 2855 Figure 396-6

A. Stage 1 disease
B. Stage 2 disease
C. Stage 3 disease
D. None of the above

1566. In type 1 DM, which of the following is true for stage 2 disease?
Harrison's 20th Ed. Chapter 396 Page 2855 Figure 396-6

A. Normoglycemia
B. Dysglycemia
C. Diabetes range hyperglycemia
D. Any of the above

Stage 1 disease is characterized by the development of ≥ 2 islet cell autoantibodies but maintenance of normoglycemia. Stage 2 disease is defined by continued autoimmunity & development of dysglycemia. Stage 3 is defined by development of hyperglycemia that exceeds diagnostic criteria for the diagnosis of diabetes.

1567. Concordance of type 1 DM in identical twins ranges between?
Harrison's 20th Ed. Chapter 396 Page 2855

A. 10 and 20%
B. 20 and 40%
C. 40 and 60%
D. 60 and 80%

The concordance of type 1 DM in identical twins ranges between 40 and 60%.

1568. Major susceptibility gene for type 1 DM is on chromosome?
Harrison's 20th Ed. Chapter 396 Page 2855

A. 1
B. 5
C. 6
D. 12

The major susceptibility gene for type 1 DM is located in the HLA region on chromosome 6.

1569. Haplotypes most strongly associated with type 1 DM include all except?
Harrison's 20th Ed. Chapter 396 Page 2855

A. DQA1*0301
B. DQA1*0102
C. DQB1*0302
D. DQB1*0201

*Haplotypes DQA1*0301, DQB1*0302 & DQB1*0201 are most strongly associated with type 1 DM.*

1570. Haplotypes most strongly associated with type 1 DM are present in what percentage of children with type 1 DM?
Harrison's 20th Ed. Chapter 396 Page 2855

A. 20%
B. 40%
C. 60%
D. 80%

1571. Haplotypes most strongly associated with type 1 DM are present in what percentage of normal US population?
Harrison's 20th Ed. Chapter 396 Page 2855

A. 0%
B. 2%
C. 5%
D. 10%

*Haplotypes DQA1*0301, DQB1*0302 & DQB1*0201 are most strongly associated with type 1 DM. These haplotypes are present in 40% of children with type 1 DM as compared to 2% of the normal U.S. population and most individuals with predisposing haplotypes do not develop diabetes.*

1572. The strongest single association with type 1 DM is with which haplotype?
Harrison's 20th Ed. Chapter 396 Page 2855

A. DQB1*0202
B. DQB1*0302
C. DQB1*0402
D. DQB1*0602

*Haplotypes that carry DQA1*0501 or DQB1*0302 gene are strongly associated with type 1 diabetes.*

1573. Presence of which haplotype in an individual confers the highest known genetic risk for type 1 diabetes mellitus?
Harrison's 20th Ed. Chapter 396 Page 2855

A. DR3
B. DR4
C. Both DR3 & DR4
D. None of the above

Most individuals with type 1 DM have the HLA DR3 and/or DR4 haplotype. Presence of both DR3 & DR4 haplotypes in one individual confers a 20-fold increased risk for type 1 diabetes.

1574. Which of the following gene is considered "protective" for type 1 diabetes mellitus?
Harrison's 20th Ed. Chapter 396 Page 2855

A. DQB1*0302
B. DQB1*0402
C. DQB1*0502
D. DQB1*0602

*Haplotype DQA1*0102, DQB1*0602 is extremely rare in individuals with type 1 DM & provide protection from type 1 DM. DQB1*0602 is considered "protective" for type 1 diabetes.*

1575. Glucagon is produced by?
Harrison's 20th Ed. Chapter 396 Page 2855

A. Alpha cells
B. Beta cells
C. Delta cells
D. PP cells

1576. Somatostatin is produced by?
Harrison's 20th Ed. Chapter 396 Page 2855

A. Alpha cells
B. Beta cells
C. Delta cells
D. PP cells

1577. Which of the following islet cell type is spared from the autoimmune process?
Harrison's 20th Ed. Chapter 396 Page 2855

A. Alpha cells
B. Delta cells
C. PP cells
D. All of the above

Islet cell type alpha produces glucagon, delta produces somatostatin and PP produces pancreatic polypeptide. All these three though functionally and embryologically similar to beta cells and express most of the same proteins as beta cells, are spared from the autoimmune process.

1578. In type 1A DM, after all beta cells are destroyed, which of the following statements is false?
Harrison's 20th Ed. Chapter 396 Page 2855

A. Inflammatory process abates
B. Islets become atrophic
C. Immunologic markers disappear
D. None of the above

After all beta cells are destroyed in type 1A DM, the inflammatory process abates, the islets become atrophic, and immunologic markers disappear.

1579. In pathogenesis of type 1 DM, all of the following are true except?
Harrison's 20th Ed. Chapter 396 Page 2855

A. Pancreatic islets are infiltrated by lymphocytes
B. All islet cell types are involved
C. Release of TNFα, interferon γ & IL-1 play a role
D. Direct CD8+ mediated cytotoxicity

In type 1 DM, insulitis occurs (lymphocytic infiltration of pancreatic islets). Beta cell death could be due to toxic effects of TNF-α, interferon-γ and IL-1. Formation of nitric oxide metabolites, apoptosis & direct CD8+ T cell cytotoxicity may also contribute.

1580. In pathogenesis of type 1 DM, islet destruction is mediated by?
Harrison's 20th Ed. Chapter 396 Page 2855

A. T lymphocytes
B. B lymphocytes
C. Eosinophils
D. Neutrophils

In pathogenesis of type 1 DM, islet destruction is mediated by T lymphocytes rather than islet autoantibodies.

1581. Pancreatic islet molecules targeted in autoimmune process in type 1 DM are all except?
Harrison's 20th Ed. Chapter 396 Page 2855

A. Insulin
B. Glutamic acid decarboxylase (GAD)
C. Integrin
D. ZnT-8

Pancreatic islet molecules targeted by autoimmune process include insulin, glutamic acid decarboxylase (GAD), ICA-512/IA-2, and phogrin (insulin secretory granule protein). Pancreatic islet molecules targeted by the autoimmune process include insulin, glutamic acid decarboxylase (GAD), ICA-512/IA-2 (homology with tyrosine phosphatases), and a beta cell–specific zinc transporter (ZnT-8).

1582. Which of the following autoantigens is not found is type I DM?
Harrison's 20th Ed. Chapter 396 Page 2855

A. GAD-65
B. GLUR
C. ICA-512 / IA-2
D. ZnT-8

Islet cell autoantibodies (ICAs) are directed at pancreatic islet molecules such as GAD, insulin, IA-2/ ICA-512, and ZnT-8. ICAs serve as a marker of autoimmune process of type 1 DM.

1583. Which of the following viruses may act as an environmental trigger in genetically susceptible individuals for type 1 DM?
Harrison's 20th Ed. Chapter 396 Page 2856

A. Coxsackie
B. Rubella
C. Enteroviruses
D. All of the above

1584. Which of the following may act as an environmental trigger in genetically susceptible individuals for type 1 DM?
Harrison's 20th Ed. Chapter 396 Page 2856

A. Bovine milk proteins
B. Nitrosourea compounds
C. Vitamin D deficiency
D. All of the above

1585. Molecular mimicry between microbial proteins & host tissues has been reported in?
Harrison's 20th Ed. Chapter 396 Page 2856

A. Type 1 diabetes mellitus
B. Rheumatoid arthritis
C. Multiple sclerosis
D. All of the above

Molecular mimicry between microbial proteins & host tissues is reported in rheumatic fever, type 1 diabetes mellitus, rheumatoid arthritis, GBS, celiac disease & multiple sclerosis.

1586. In type 2 DM, which of the following is true?
Harrison's 20th Ed. Chapter 396 Page 2856

A. Insulin resistance precedes insulin secretory defects
B. Insulin secretory defects precede insulin resistance
C. Insulin resistance simultaneous with insulin secretory defects
D. Any of the above

In type 2 DM, insulin resistance precedes insulin secretory defects and diabetes develops only if insulin secretion becomes inadequate.

1587. Concordance of type 2 DM in identical twins is between?
Harrison's 20th Ed. Chapter 396 Page 2856

A. 10 –30%
B. 30–50%
C. 50–70%
D. 70–90%

The concordance of type 2 DM in identical twins is between 70 and 90%.

1588. If both parents have type 2 DM, risk of developing diabetes is?
Harrison's 20th Ed. Chapter 396 Page 2856

A. ~ 10%
B. ~ 20%
C. ~ 30%
D. ~ 40%

Individuals with both parents having type 2 DM, the risk approaches 40%.

1589. Type 2 DM is characterized by?
Harrison's 20th Ed. Chapter 396 Page 2856

A. Impaired insulin secretion
B. Insulin resistance
C. Excessive hepatic glucose production
D. All of the above

1590. Type 2 DM is characterized by?
Harrison's 20th Ed. Chapter 396 Page 2856

A. Abnormal fat metabolism
B. Systemic low-grade inflammation
C. Obesity
D. All of the above

Type 2 DM is characterized by impaired insulin secretion, insulin resistance, excessive hepatic glucose production, abnormal fat metabolism, and systemic low-grade inflammation. Visceral or central obesity is very common in type 2 DM.

1591. In type 2 DM, which of the following is false?
Harrison's 20th Ed. Chapter 396 Page 2856

A. IGT is characterized by elevations in postprandial glucose
B. ↑ in hepatic glucose production leads to fasting hyperglycemia
C. Glucagon augments hepatic glucose production
D. None of the above

1592. In type 2 DM, which of the following is false?
Harrison's 20th Ed. Chapter 396 Page 2856

A. IR impairs glucose utilization by insulin-sensitive tissues
B. Glucose metabolism in insulin-independent tissues is also altered in type 2 DM
C. ↑ed hepatic glucose output causes increased FPG levels
D. ↓ed peripheral glucose utilization causes postprandial hyperglycemia

Glucose metabolism in insulin-independent tissues is not altered in type 2 DM. Increased hepatic glucose output predominantly accounts for increased FPG levels, whereas decreased peripheral glucose usage results in postprandial hyperglycemia.

1593. Which of the following play predominant role in insulin resistance?
Harrison's 20th Ed. Chapter 396 Page 2856

A. Prereceptor defects
B. Receptor defects
C.` Postreceptor defects
D. All of the above

Postreceptor defects play the predominant role in insulin resistance. Although insulin receptor levels and tyrosine kinase activity in skeletal muscle are reduced in T2DM, these are not a primary defect.

1594. Adipocytes secrete which of the following?
Harrison's 20th Ed. Chapter 396 Page 2857

A. Leptin
B. Resistin
C. Adiponectin
D. All of the above

Adipocytes secrete adipokines like nonesterified free fatty acids, retinol-binding protein 4, leptin, TNF-α, resistin, IL-6 and adiponectin.

1595. Which of the following about Brown adipose tissue (BAT) is false?
Biochem. J. (2013) 453, 167–78

A. Thermogenesis
B. Extensive neuronal and vascular connections
C. Abundant mitochondria
D. None of the above

BAT (brown adipose tissue) has an inherent capacity to convert excess food energy into thermal energy. Brown adipocytes have abundant mitochondria and uniquely express UCP1 (uncoupling protein-1). UCP1 dissipates proton gradient of inner mitochondrial membrane that is formed as a result of oxidative phosphorylation of nutrients. This process, also known as thermogenesis, generates heat (non-shivering thermogenesis) instead of ATP.

1596. Elevated levels of free fatty acids can cause which of the following?
Harrison's 20th Ed. Chapter 396 Page 2857

A. Impair glucose utilization in skeletal muscle
B. Promote glucose production by liver
C. Impair beta cell function
D. All of the above

Elevated levels of free fatty acids can impair glucose utilization in skeletal muscle, promote glucose production by liver and impair beta cell function.

1597. Which of the following is an insulin-sensitizing peptide?
Harrison's 20th Ed. Chapter 396 Page 2857

A. Leptin
B. Resistin
C. Adiponectin
D. All of the above

Production by adipocytes of adiponectin, an insulin-sensitizing peptide, is reduced in obesity, and this may contribute to hepatic insulin resistance.

1598. Overall β cell function is reduced by how much at the onset of type 2 DM?
Harrison's 20th Ed. Chapter 396 Page 2857

A. 20%
B. 30%
C. 40%
D. 50%

Overall beta cell function is reduced by ~ 50% at the onset of type 2 DM.

1599. β cell mass is decreased by how much in individuals with long-standing type 2 DM?

Harrison's 20th Ed. Chapter 396 Page 2857

A. 20%
B. 30%
C. 40%
D. 50%

Beta cell mass is decreased by ~ 50% in individuals with long-standing type 2 DM.

1600. "Glucose toxicity" refers to?

Harrison's 20th Ed. Chapter 396 Page 2857

A. Acute hyperglycemia impairing islet function
B. Chronic hyperglycemia impairing islet function
C. Seizures in hyperglycemia
D. All of the above

Chronic hyperglycemia paradoxically impairs islet function (glucose toxicity) and leads to a worsening of hyperglycemia.

1601. All can cause islet cell dysfunction except?

Harrison's 20th Ed. Chapter 396 Page 2857

A. Hyperglycemia
B. Hypoglycemia
C. Hyperlipidemia
D. Islet cell autoantibodies

1602. Which of the following can worsen islet function?

Harrison's 20th Ed. Chapter 396 Page 2857

A. Chronic hyperglycemia
B. Elevation of free fatty acid levels
C. Dietary fat
D. All of the above

Chronic hyperglycemia impairs islet function ("glucose toxicity") so does elevation of free fatty acid levels ("lipotoxicity") and dietary fat.

1603. In type 2 DM, which of the following occurs in the liver?

Harrison's 20th Ed. Chapter 396 Page 2857

A. Gluconeogenesis leading to fasting hyperglycemia
B. Decreased glycogen storage in postprandial state
C. Increased VLDL-triglyceride synthesis due to lipolysis and free fatty acid flux from adipocytes
D. None of the above

1604. Which of the following is not part of the constellation of metabolic derangements in metabolic syndrome?

Harrison's 20th Ed. Chapter 396 Page 2857

A. Hypertension
B. Cerebrovascular disease
C. Central or visceral obesity
D. IGT / IFG

Metabolic syndrome, insulin resistance syndrome, and syndrome X is a constellation of metabolic derangements that includes insulin resistance, hypertension, dyslipidemia (↓ HDL & ↑ triglycerides), central or visceral obesity, type 2 DM or IGT / IFG, and accelerated cardiovascular disease.

1605. "Ominous octet" that leads to hyperglycemia includes?

Diabetes. 2009;58(4):773-95

A. Reduced insulin secretion from pancreatic β-cells
B. Elevated glucagon secretion from pancreatic α cells
C. Increased production of glucose in liver
D. All of the above

1606. "Ominous octet" that leads to hyperglycemia includes?

Diabetes. 2009;58(4):773-95

A. Neurotransmitter dysfunction & insulin resistance in brain
B. Enhanced lipolysis
C. Increased renal glucose reabsorption
D. All of the above

An "ominous octet" that leads to hyperglycemia, which occur in isolation or in combination, has been proposed for eight pathophysiological mechanisms underlying T2DM. These include (i) reduced insulin secretion from pancreatic β-cells, (ii) elevated glucagon secretion from pancreatic α cells, (iii) increased production of glucose in liver, (iv) neurotransmitter dysfunction and insulin resistance in the brain, (v) enhanced lipolysis, (vi) increased renal glucose reabsorption, (vii) reduced incretin effect in the small intestine, and (viii) impaired or diminished glucose uptake in peripheral tissues such as skeletal muscle, liver, and adipose tissue.

1607. Which of the following is a feature of severe insulin resistance in adults?

Harrison's 20th Ed. Chapter 396 Page 2857

A. Women
B. Severe hyperinsulinemia
C. Hyperandrogenism
D. All of the above

1608. Which of the following is a feature of polycystic ovary syndrome (PCOS)?

Harrison's 20th Ed. Chapter 396 Page 2857

A. Affects premenopausal women
B. Chronic anovulation
C. Hyperandrogenism
D. All of the above

PCOS affects premenopausal women & is characterized by chronic anovulation, hyperandrogenism with insulin resistance that increases the risk for type 2 DM, independent of the effects of obesity.

1609. All are proved to delay or prevent DM except?

Harrison's 20th Ed. Chapter 396 Page 2857

A. Life style modification
B. Metformin
C. Ramipril
D. Atorvastatin

1610. All are proved to delay or prevent DM except?

Harrison's 20th Ed. Chapter 396 Page 2857

A. Acarbose
B. Metformin
C. NSAIDs
D. Orlistat

Diabetes Prevention Program (DPP) demonstrated that metformin prevented or delayed diabetes by 31% compared to placebo. α-glucosidase inhibitors, metformin, thiazolidinediones, GLP-1 receptor pathway modifiers, and orlistat prevent or delay type 2 DM, but are not FDA approved for this purpose. Ramipril and pravastatin reduced the number of new cases of diabetes.

1611. All are risk factors for type 2 DM except?

Harrison's 20th Ed. Chapter 396 Page 2858

A. Hypertension
B. Acanthosis nigricans
C. PCOD
D. Ataxia telangiectasia

1612. All of the following are true about MODY except?
Harrison's 20th Ed. Chapter 396 Page 2858

A. Monogenic
B. Autosomal dominant
C. MODY 4 is due to mutation in IPF-1
D. MODY 1 is due to mutation in glucokinase gene

MODY 2 is due to mutations in the glucokinase gene. MODY 4 is a rare variant caused by mutations in insulin promoter factor (IPF) 1. Six different variants of MODY have been identified so far, and all are transmitted as autosomal dominant disorders.

1613. Hepatocyte nuclear transcription factor (HNF) is expressed in?
Harrison's 20th Ed. Chapter 396 Page 2858

A. Liver
B. Pancreatic islets
C. Kidney
D. All of the above

HNF are expressed in liver, pancreatic islets and kidney. Therefore, patients may also have renal absorption abnormalities and renal cysts.

1614. MODY 1 is caused by mutations in?
Harrison's 20th Ed. Chapter 396 Page 2858

A. HNF-4 alpha
B. HNF-1 alpha
C. HNF-1 beta
D. All of the above

MODY 1, MODY 3, and MODY 5 are caused by mutations in the hepatocyte nuclear transcription factors (HNF) 4alpha, HNF-1alpha, and HNF-1beta, respectively.

1615. Mutations in which of the following is the most common cause of pancreatic agenesis?
Harrison's 20th Ed. Chapter 396 Page 2858

A. Mutations in transcription factor GATA3
B. Mutations in transcription factor GATA6
C. Mutations in hepatocyte nuclear transcription factor
D. Mutations in Runt-related transcription factor 2

Mutations in the transcription factor GATA6 are the most common cause of pancreatic agenesis.

1616. Mutations in which of the following causes diabetes and deafness?
Harrison's 20th Ed. Chapter 396 Page 2858

A. Mutations in glucokinase gene
B. Mutations in mitochondrial DNA
C. Mutations in pancreatic and duodenal homeobox 1
D. Mutations in ATP-sensitive potassium channel subunits

Mutations in mitochondrial DNA are associated with diabetes and deafness.

1617. MIDY stands for?
Harrison's 20th Ed. Chapter 396 Page 2858

A. Mutant induced Diabetes of young
B. Mutant induced Diabetes of Youth
C. Mutant Ips-gene-induced Diabetes of Youth
D. Mutant Ins-gene-induced Diabetes of Youth

Mutations in the coding sequence of insulin gene that interfere with proinsulin folding, processing, and bioactivity are designated as Mutant Ins-gene-induced Diabetes of Youth (MIDYs).

1618. Complications due to chronic hyperglycemia in DM begin to appear during which decade of hyperglycemia?
Harrison's 20th Ed. Chapter 396 Page 2858

A. First decade
B. Second decade
C. Third decade
D. Fourth decade

Symptoms & signs of DM and its complications may be secondary to acute hyperglycemia and may occur at any stage of the disease. Those related to chronic hyperglycemia begin to appear during the second decade of hyperglycemia.

1619. What level of blood pressure is considered hypertension in individuals with diabetes?
Harrison's 20th Ed. Chapter 396 Page 2858

A. >130 / 80 mm Hg
B. >140 / 80 mm Hg
C. >130 / 90 mm Hg
D. >140 / 90 mm Hg

Blood pressure > 130 / 80 mm Hg is considered hypertension in individuals with diabetes.

1620. Testing for loss of protective sensation (LOPS) is done by?
Harrison's 20th Ed. Chapter 396 Page 2858

A. Monofilament testing
B. Ankle reflexes
C. Vibration perception threshold
D. All of the above

Testing for loss of protective sensation (LOPS) is done by monofilament testing, vibration, pinprick, ankle reflexes or vibration perception threshold (using a biothesiometer).

1621. Type 1 DM patients have an increased risk of which of the following diseases?
Harrison's 20th Ed. Chapter 396 Page 2859

A. Adrenal insufficiency
B. Pernicious anemia
C. Celiac disease
D. All of the above

Type 1 DM have an increased risk of autoimmune disorders such as autoimmune–thyroid disease, adrenal insufficiency, pernicious anemia, celiac disease and vitiligo.

1622. Latent autoimmune diabetes of the adult is best related to which of the following?
Harrison's 20th Ed. Chapter 396 Page 2859

A. PCOS
B. Diabetic ketoacidosis
C. GAD antibodies
D. GlyR antibodies

Latent autoimmune diabetes of the adult is the term applied to those 5–10% of phenotypic type 2 DM do not have absolute insulin deficiency but have autoimmune markers (GAD & other ICA autoantibodies) suggestive of type 1 DM.

1623. Which of the following is false about monogenic forms of diabetes?
Harrison's 20th Ed. Chapter 396 Page 2859

A. Onset of diabetes at <30 years of age
B. Autosomal pattern of diabetes inheritance
C. Lack of nearly complete insulin deficiency
D. None of the above

Monogenic forms of diabetes should be considered in those with diabetes onset at <30 years of age, an autosomal pattern of diabetes inheritance and lack of nearly complete insulin deficiency.

Diabetes Mellitus: Management and Therapies

1624. Goal of therapy for type 1 or type 2 diabetes mellitus is?
Harrison's 20th Ed. Chapter 397 Page 2859

A. To eliminate symptoms related to hyperglycemia
B. To eliminate long-term micro- and macrovascular complications
C. To allow patient to achieve as normal a lifestyle as possible
D. All of the above

Goals of therapy for type 1 or type 2 diabetes mellitus are to eliminate symptoms related to hyperglycemia, to reduce or eliminate the long-term microvascular & macrovascular complications of DM, and to allow the patient to achieve as normal a lifestyle as possible.

1625. Symptoms of diabetes usually resolve when the plasma glucose is less than?
Harrison's 20th Ed. Chapter 397 Page 2859

A. 250 mg/dL
B. 200 mg/dL
C. 180 mg/dL
D. 120 mg/dL

Symptoms of diabetes usually resolve when the plasma glucose is <11.1 mmol/L or <200 mg/dL.

1626. Clinically significant hypoglycemia is defined as a plasma glucose of?
Harrison's 20th Ed. Chapter 397 Page 2859

A. 32 mg/dL
B. 54 mg/dL
C. 60 mg/dL
D. 70 mg/dL

Clinically significant hypoglycemia is defined as a plasma glucose of <3.0 mmol/L or 54 mg/dL.

1627. Guidelines for a well-developed service base is called?
Harrison's 20th Ed. Chapter 397 Page 2859

A. Recommended care
B. Limited care
C. Comprehensive care
D. Inclusive care

As resources available for diabetes care vary widely throughout world, International Diabetes Federation (IDF) issued guidelines for "recommended care" i.e. a well-developed service base & with health care funding systems consuming a significant part of their national wealth), "limited care" i.e. health care settings with very limited resources, and "comprehensive care" i.e. health care settings with considerable resources.

1628. Under treatment goals for adults with diabetes, level of preprandial capillary plasma glucose should be?
Harrison's 20th Ed. Chapter 397 Page 2860 Table 397-2

A. Between 70 and 110 mg/dL
B. Between 70 and 126 mg/dL
C. Between 80 and 126 mg/dL
D. Between 80 and 130 mg/dL

1629. Under treatment goals for adults with diabetes, level of postprandial capillary plasma glucose should be?
Harrison's 20th Ed. Chapter 397 Page 2860 Table 397-2

A. < 140 mg/dL
B. < 160 mg/dL
C. < 180 mg/dL
D. < 200 mg/dL

1630. Under treatment goals for adults with diabetes, level of HbA1c should be?
Harrison's 20th Ed. Chapter 397 Page 2860 Table 397-2

A. < 6.0%
B. < 6.5%
C. < 7.0%
D. < 7.5%

1631. Under treatment goals for adults with diabetes, level of blood pressure should be?
Harrison's 20th Ed. Chapter 397 Page 2860 Table 397-2

A. < 110/70 mm Hg
B. < 120/80 mm Hg
C. < 130/90 mm Hg
D. < 140/90 mm Hg

BP goal of <130 / 80 mm Hg may be appropriate for younger individuals or individuals with cardiovascular risk factors.

1632. Which of the following is considered as the primary goal out of the following treatment goals for adults with diabetes?
Harrison's 20th Ed. Chapter 397 Page 2860 Table 397-2

A. Preprandial capillary plasma glucose
B. Postprandial capillary plasma glucose
C. HbA1c
D. Blood pressure

HbA1c is considered as the primary treatment goal for adults with diabetes.

1633. A diabetes educator is which of the following health care professional?
Harrison's 20th Ed. Chapter 397 Page 2860

A. Nurse
B. Dietician
C. Pharmacist
D. All of the above

A certified diabetes educator is a health care professional (nurse, dietician, or pharmacist) with specialized patient education skills.

1634. Primary measures of Medical nutrition therapy (MNT) is directed at?
Harrison's 20th Ed. Chapter 397 Page 2860

A. Preventing or delaying onset of T2 DM in high-risk individuals
B. Improving glycemic control
C. Managing diabetes-related complications
D. All of the above

1635. Secondary measures of Medical nutrition therapy (MNT) is directed at?

Harrison's 20th Ed. Chapter 397 Page 2860

A. Preventing or delaying onset of T2 DM in high-risk individuals
B. Improving glycemic control
C. Managing diabetes-related complications
D. All of the above

1636. Tertiary measures of Medical nutrition therapy (MNT) is directed at?

Harrison's 20th Ed. Chapter 397 Page 2860

A. Preventing or delaying onset of T2 DM in high-risk individuals
B. Improving glycemic control
C. Managing diabetes-related complications
D. All of the above

Primary measures of MNT are directed at preventing or delaying the onset of type 2 DM in high-risk individuals. Secondary measures of MNT are directed at improving glycemic control. Tertiary measures of MNT are directed at managing diabetes-related complications (cardiovascular disease, nephropathy).

1637. Which of the following is an indicator of diet quality?

Int. J. Mol. Sci. 2018, 19, 3662

A. Dietary total antioxidant capacity (TAC)
B. Glycemic index (GI)
C. Glycemic load (GL)
D. All of the above

Dietary total antioxidant capacity (TAC) is associated with insulin resistance and oxidative stress (OS). OS is recognized as a contributor to the pathogenesis of obesity, type 2 diabetes, atherosclerosis, and nonalcoholic fatty liver disease (NAFLD). OS is defined as a disturbance in the balance between production of reactive oxygen species (free radicals) and antioxidant defense system in body cells, has been related to insulin resistance (IR), a pathological condition where a normal or elevated insulin level produces an attenuated biological response.

1638. What is the glycemic index (GI) of glucose?

Am J Clin Nutr 2002;76:5–56

A. 0
B. 25
C. 50
D. 100

1639. Glycemic load (GL) is calculated by the formula?

Am J Clin Nutr 2002;76:5–56

A. (Glycemic index × dietary carbohydrate content) ÷ 100
B. (Glycemic index ÷ dietary carbohydrate content) ÷ 100
C. (Glycemic index + dietary carbohydrate content) ÷ 100
D. (Glycemic index – dietary carbohydrate content) ÷ 100

Glycemic index (GI) is a tool to measure how individual foods are expected to impact blood sugar levels. The number is a comparison between individual foods and glucose. Reference food glucose is given a value of 100. Glycemic load (GL) is an equation that takes into account the planned portion size of a food as well as the glycemic index of that food. Glycemic Load = GI/100 multiplied by the net grams of planned carbohydrate. Some research laboratories continue to use white bread as the reference food.

1640. Foods are considered to be of high glycemic index, if the GI value is?

Nutrients 2018, 10, 1361

A. ≥ 50
B. ≥ 70
C. ≥ 100
D. ≥ 120

1641. Foods are considered to be of low glycemic index, if the GI value is?

Nutrients 2018, 10, 1361

A. ≤ 100
B. ≤ 70
C. ≤ 55
D. ≤ 35

1642. Foods are considered to be of low glycemic load, if the GL value is?

Nutrients 2018, 10, 1361

A. ≤ 10
B. ≤ 20
C. ≤ 30
D. ≤ 40

1643. Foods are considered to be of high glycemic load, if the GL value is?

Nutrients 2018, 10, 1361

A. ≥ 5
B. ≥ 10
C. ≥ 15
D. ≥ 20

Foods have been classified by GI into low (GI ≤ 55), medium (GI 56–69), and high (GI ≥ 70) categories, and classified by GL as being low (GL ≤ 10), medium (GL 11–19), and high (GL ≥ 20).

1644. There are no Glycemic Index values given for?

Am J Clin Nutr 2002;76:5–56

A. Eggs, meat, poultry, fish
B. Avocados, salad vegetables
C. Cheese
D. All of the above

There are no Glycemic Index values given for meat, poultry, fish, avocados, salad vegetables, cheese, or eggs because these foods contain little or no carbohydrate.

1645. Which of the following is a satiety related hormone?

Nutrients 2018, 10, 1361

A. Peptide tyrosine-tyrosine (PYY)
B. Amylin
C. Oxyntomodulin
D. All of the above

1646. Which of the following is a satiety related hormone?

Nutrients 2018, 10, 1361

A. Insulin
B. Leptin
C. Ghrelin
D. All of the above

Regulation of satiety is a complex mechanism dependent on satiety related hormones such as insulin, leptin, ghrelin, cholecystokinin (CCK), glucagon-like peptide 1 (GLP-1), peptide tyrosine-tyrosine (PYY), enterostatin, amylin, and oxyntomodulin.

1647. Medical nutrition therapy (MNT) recommends supplementation of diet in diabetic patients with?

Harrison's 20th Ed. Chapter 397 Page 2860

A. Vitamin C
B. Vitamin E
C. Chromium
D. None of the above

Currently, evidence does not support supplementation of diet with vitamins, antioxidants (vitamin C and E) or micronutrients (chromium) in patients with diabetes.

1648. In diabetics, ADA recommends moderate aerobic physical activity of?

Harrison's 20th Ed. Chapter 397 Page 2861

A. 60 minutes per week
B. 120 minutes per week
C. 150 minutes per week
D. 180 minutes per week

In diabetics, ADA recommends 150 minutes per week, distributed over at least 3 days, of moderate aerobic physical activity with no gaps longer than 2 days.

1649. Which of the following is a relative contraindication to vigorous exercise in DM?

Harrison's 20th Ed. Chapter 397 Page 2861

A. Microalbuminuria
B. Untreated proliferative retinopathy
C. Loss of protective sensation (LOPS)
D. Fatty liver

Untreated proliferative retinopathy is a relative contraindication to vigorous exercise as it may lead to vitreous hemorrhage or retinal detachment.

1650. Negative psychological reactions related to emotional burdens in diabetics is called?

Harrison's 20th Ed. Chapter 397 Page 2861

A. Diabetes rack
B. Diabetes distress
C. Diabetes anguish
D. Diabetes misery

Diabetes distress refers to an emotional state where people experience feelings like stress, guilt, or denial that arise from living with diabetes and the burden of self-management. But, it does not meet the qualifications for major depressive disorder (MDD).

1651. Which of the following is used for screening of diabetes distress?

Diabetes Ther.2017;8(1):1–7

A. DDS 11
B. DDS 17
C. DDS 23
D. DDS 31

The DDS17 is a validated survey instrument that assesses diabetes-related emotional distress. Older version was called the Problems Areas in Diabetes Questionnaire (PAID) which had 20 variables. Shorter surveys have been developed including PAID-5 and PAID-1.

1652. HbA1c reflects average glycemic control over previous?

Harrison's 20th Ed. Chapter 397 Page 2861

A. 1–2 months
B. 2–3 months
C. 3–4 months
D. 4–5 months

HbA1c reflects average glycemic control over previous 2-3 months because erythrocytes have an average life span of 120 days. Glycemic level in the preceding month contributes ~50% to the HbA1c value.

1653. Amounts of blood obtained from the fingertip puncture for blood glucose estimation is?

Harrison's 20th Ed. Chapter 397 Page 2861

A. 3–10 μL
B. 10–18 μL
C. 18–30 μL
D. 30–50 μL

Amounts of blood obtained from the fingertip puncture for blood glucose estimation is 3 - 10 μL.

1654. Current continuous glucose monitoring (CGM) systems measure glucose in?

Harrison's 20th Ed. Chapter 397 Page 2861

A. Plasma
B. Whole blood
C. Interstitial fluid
D. Lymph

Current continuous glucose monitoring (CGM) systems measure the glucose in interstitial fluid, which is in equilibrium with the blood glucose.

1655. HbA1c as a biomarker for monitoring the levels of glucose among diabetic patients was first proposed by?

Biomark Insights. 2016;11:95-104

A. Koenig
B. Huisman
C. Rahbar
D. Bunn

Historically, HbA1c was first isolated by Huisman in 1958 and characterized by Bookchin and Gallop in 1968, as a glycoprotein. Elevated levels of HbA1c in diabetic patients were reported by Rahbar in 1969. Bunn identified the pathway leading to the formation of HbA1c in 1975. Using the HbA1c as a biomarker for monitoring the levels of glucose among diabetic patients was first proposed by Koenig in 1976.

1656. Normal adult hemoglobin consists of?

Biomark Insights. 2016;11:95-104

A. HbA (α2β2)
B. HbA2 (α2δ2)
C. HbF (α2γ2)
D. All of the above

Normal adult hemoglobin consists predominantly of HbA (α2β2), HbA2 (α2δ2), and HbF (α2γ2) in the composition of 97%, 2.5%, and 0.5%, respectively.

1657. What percentage of total HbA is termed HbA1?

Biomark Insights. 2016;11:95-104

A. ~ 2%
B. ~ 6%
C. ~ 14%
D. ~ 26%

1658. HbA1 is made up of which of the following fractions?

Biomark Insights. 2016;11:95-104

A. HbA1a1, HbA1a2
B. HbA1b
C. HbA1c
D. All of the above

About 6% of total HbA is termed HbA1, which in turn is made up of HbA1a1, HbA1a2, HbA1b, and HbA1c fractions, defined by their electrophoretic and chromatographic properties.

1659. HbA1c constitutes what percentage of the total HbA fraction?

Biomark Insights. 2016;11:95-104

A. ~ 2%
B. ~ 3%
C. ~ 4%
D. ~ 5%

HbA1c is the most abundant of HbA1 fractions and in health comprises ~5% of the total HbA fraction.

1660. Glycation of hemoglobin occurs by nonenzymatic reaction between glucose & N-terminal end of which chain?
Biomark Insights. 2016;11:95-104

A. α
B. β
C. γ
D. δ

The glycation of hemoglobin occurs by nonenzymatic reaction between glucose and N-terminal end of β-chain, which forms a Schiff base. HbA1c is formed when glucose attaches to N-terminal valine of the β-chain of hemoglobin. If the glucose attaches to proteins in the plasma, fructosamine or glycated albumin results.

1661. HbA1c is best related to?
Biomark Insights. 2016;11:95-104

A. Schiff base
B. Gomori base
C. Wolff base
D. Glomb base

Schiff base formed from nonenzymatic reaction between glucose & N-terminal end of β-chain undergoes rearrangement through Maillard reaction. Schiff base is converted into Amadori products, of which the best known is HbA1c.

1662. Advanced glycated end products (AGEs) best relate to?
Diabetes Care 2016;39:1299–1306

A. Nerodori products
B. Sinodori products
C. Klodori products
D. Amadori products

In the primary step of glycated hemoglobin formation, hemoglobin and blood glucose interact to form an unstable Schiff base (aldimine, pre-HbA1c) in a reversible reaction. In the secondary step, which is irreversible, aldimine is gradually converted into the stable ketoamine form (Fructosamine) through Amadori rearrangement. The major sites of hemoglobin glycosylation, in the order of prevalence, are β-Val-1, β-Lys-66, and α-Lys-61. Stable Amadori products can undergo further modifications to form AGEs.

1663. The most common cross-linked AGE is?
Diabetes Care 2016;39:1299–1306

A. Glucoseline
B. Glucosenet
C. Glucoseset
D. Glucosepane

The most common cross-linked AGE is glucosepane. It do not return to normal, even when hyperglycemia is corrected. Clinically important AGEs include pentosidine, CML, CEL, & 3-deoxyglucosone. AGEs activate the receptor for AGE (RAGE) resulting in the production of proinflammatory cytokines and increased oxidative stress. . Proteolysis of RAGE leads to a truncated soluble form of RAGE (sRAGE) which is found in serum and can be measured.

1664. Which of the following is an inhibitor of AGE formation?
Diabetes Care 2016;39:1299–1306

A. Aspirin
B. Aminoguanidine
C. Iodobenzylguanidine
D. All of the above

Inhibitor of AGE formation, aminoguanidine (Pimagedine) is a hydrazine derivative that reduces glycation. It is a scavenger of reactive carbonyl groups that mediate advanced carbonyl reactions. It can prevent the formation of glycoxidation & lipoxidation products and can interrupt vicious cycles of oxidative damage.

1665. Which of the following is false about HbA1C?
Diabetes Care 2016;39:1299–1306, Harrison's 20th Ed. Chapter 397 Page 2862

A. HbA1c levels ↑ by ~0.1% per decade >30 years of age
B. More stringent glycemic control (≤6%) is not beneficial
C. HbA1c is dependent on the erythrocyte (RBC) lifespan
D. None of the above

1666. Which of the following is false about HbA1C?
Harrison's 20th Ed. Chapter 397 Page 2861

A. Primary predictor of long-term complications of DM
B. Recent intercurrent illnesses do not impact HbA1c
C. HbA1c and SMBG are complementary
D. None of the above

1667. In standardized assays, HbA1C of 6% approximates what level of mean plasma glucose value?
Harrison's 20th Ed. Chapter 397 Page 2862

A. 105 mg/dL
B. 114 mg/dL
C. 126 mg/dL
D. 135 mg/dL

In standardized assays, HbA1C approximates the following mean plasma glucose values: 6% = 7.0 mmol/L (126 mg/dL), 7% = 8.6 mmol/L (154 mg/dL), 8% = 10.2 mmol/L (183 mg/dL), 9% = 11.8 mmol/L (212 mg/dL), 10% = 13.4 mmol/L (240 mg/dL), 11% = 14.9 mmol/L (269 mg/dL) and 12% = 16.5 mmol/L (298 mg/dL).

1668. What is the normal range of HbA1c in people without diabetes?
Diabetes Care. 2008;31(8):1473-78

A. 0% to 2%
B. 2% to 4%
C. 4% to 6%
D. 6% to 8%

The normal range of HbA1c is 4% to 6% in people without diabetes.

1669. Which of the formula is correct to calculate estimated average blood glucose from HbA1c values?
Diabetes Care. 2008;31(8):1473-78

A. BG (mg/dL) = [HbA1C (%) × 28.7] – 44.7
B. BG (mg/dL) = [HbA1C (%) × 28.7] – 45.7
C. BG (mg/dL) = [HbA1C (%) × 28.7] – 46.7
D. BG (mg/dL) = [HbA1C (%) × 28.7] – 47.7

Estimated Average Blood Glucose (eAG) (mg/dL) = [HbA1C (%) x 28.7] – 46.7.

1670. Which of the formula is correct to calculate mean blood glucose (MBG) from HbA1c values in DCCT study?
Acta Inform Med. 2016;24(4):233–38

A. MBG = (HbA1c% × 35.6) – 75.3
B. MBG = (HbA1c% × 35.6) – 76.3
C. MBG = (HbA1c% × 35.6) – 77.3
D. MBG = (HbA1c% × 35.6) – 78.3

1671. Which of the formula is correct to calculate mean blood glucose (MBG) from HbA1c values in UKPDS trial?
Acta Inform Med. 2016;24(4):233–38

A. MBG = (HbA1c% × 34) – 100
B. MBG = (HbA1c% × 35) – 100
C. MBG = (HbA1c% × 36) – 100
D. MBG = (HbA1c% × 37) – 100

1672. Nathan's formula to calculate mean blood glucose (MBG) from HbA1c values is?

Acta Inform Med. 2016;24(4):233–238

A. MBG = (HbA1c% × 33.3) – 83
B. MBG = (HbA1c% × 33.3) – 84
C. MBG = (HbA1c% × 33.3) – 85
D. MBG = (HbA1c% × 33.3) – 86

1673. A 1% rise in HbA1C translates into how much increase in mean glucose level?

Diabetes Care. 2008;31(8):1473-78

A. 15 mg/dL
B. 25 mg/dL
C. 35 mg/dL
D. 45 mg/dL

A 1% rise in the A1C translates into a 35 mg/dL increase in the mean glucose level. Each 1 percent reduction in the HbA1c reduces the risk of complications by up to 30%.

1674. In patients who have achieved glycemic goal, ADA recommends measurement of the HbA1C how frequently?

Harrison's 20th Ed. Chapter 397 Page 2862

A. Once per year
B. Twice per year
C. Thrice per year
D. Four times per year

In patients who have achieved glycemic goal, ADA recommends HbA1C estimation twice a year.

1675. Which disease may interfere with the HbA1C result?

Harrison's 20th Ed. Chapter 397 Page 2862

A. Hemoglobinopathies
B. Transfusions
C. Uremia
D. All of the above

Hemoglobinopathies, anemias, reticulocytosis, transfusions & uremia may interfere with HbA1C result.

1676. Which other glycated compound can be measured for determining glycemic control?

Harrison's 20th Ed. Chapter 397 Page 2862

A. Albumin
B. Globulin
C. Ketone
D. All of the above

Degree of glycation of albumin, or measurement of 1,5-anhydroglucitol can be used as an alternative indicator of glycemic control when HbA1c is inaccurate. Fructosamine assay (measuring glycated albumin) reflects glycemic status over prior 2 weeks.

1677. 1,5-Anhydroglucitol (1,5-AG) structurally resembles which of the following?

Harrison's 20th Ed. Chapter 397 Page 2862, Endocrine. 2013;43(1):33-40

A. Glucose
B. Glycated hemoglobin (HbA1c)
C. Fructosamine
D. All of the above

1,5-Anhydroglucitol (1,5-AG) structurally resembles glucose. 1,5-AG level is reflective of short-term glucose status, postprandial hyperglycemia, and glycemic variability which are not captured by HbA1c assay. It is utilized as a marker of glycemic control and in contrast to HbA1c & Fructosamine (FA) whose levels are higher in uncontrolled diabetes, levels of 1,5 AG are lower. 1,5 AG is more sensitive than HbA1c and FA in response to short-term anti glycemic therapy and its levels were reduced in patients with T2DM.

1678. Which of the following about 1,5-Anhydroglucitol (1,5-AG) is false?

Endocrine. 2013;43(1):33-40

A. Dietary monosaccharide similar to glucose
B. Freely filtered in the renal glomerulus
C. Competes with glucose for reabsorption in renal tubules
D. None of the above

Lower concentrations of 1,5-AG correlate with more frequent hyperglycemic episodes, most commonly postprandial hyperglycemia, and reflect trends over a 1 to 2 week timeline.

1679. What measure of oral glucose is equivalent to 75 gram of anhydrous glucose?

Journal of diabetes and its complications. 2019;33:231-35

A. 62.5 gram
B. 72.5 gram
C. 82.5 gram
D. 92.5 gram

82.5 gram of oral glucose is equivalent to 75 gram of anhydrous glucose.

1680. Which other glycated compound can be measured for determining glycemic control?

Diabetes Care 2016;39:1299–1306

A. Fructosamine
B. Glycated albumin
C. Advanced glycation end products (AGEs)
D. All of the above

Other glycated proteins that have been evaluated in clinical studies of the management and diagnosis of patients with diabetes include fructosamine, glycated albumin & advanced glycation end products (AGEs). All glycated serum proteins are fructosamines, and since albumin is the most abundant serum protein, measurement of fructosamine is thought to largely reflect the concentration of glycated albumin.

1681. Nonglycemic factor that may influence interpretation of HbA1c is?

Diabetes Care 2016;39:1299–1306

A. Physiological (age, race)
B. Chronic renal failure
C. Iron-deficiency anemia
D. All of the above

Nonglycemic factors that may influence interpretation of HbA1c are physiological (age, race), chronic renal failure, iron-deficiency anemia, erythrocyte life span, glycation "phenotypes", drugs (dapsone, antiretroviral), vitamin C and vitamin E.

1682. Nonglycemic factor that may interfere with HbA1c measurement is?

Diabetes Care 2016;39:1299–1306

A. Uremia
B. Hemoglobin variants
C. Opiates, bilirubin, triglyceride, alcohol
D. All of the above

1683. Which of the following statements about glycemic control is false?

Harrison's 20th Ed. Chapter 397 Page 2862

A. Normalization of plasma glucose for long periods of time is extremely difficult
B. Improvement in glycemic control lowers risk of diabetes-specific microvascular complications
C. Target for glycemic control must be individualized
D. None of the above

1684. A higher HbA1c goal is appropriate for?

Harrison's 20th Ed. Chapter 397 Page 2862

A. Very young
B. Very old
C. Individuals with limited life span or comorbid conditions
D. All of the above

A higher HbA1c goal may be appropriate for the very young or old or in individuals with limited life span or comorbid conditions.

1685. Which of the following clinical trials has examined glycemic control in type 2 DM?

Harrison's 20th Ed. Chapter 397 Page 2862

A. ACCORD
B. ADVANCE
C. VADT
D. All of the above

Action to Control Cardiovascular Risk in Diabetes [ACCORD], Action in Diabetes and Vascular Disease: Preterax and Diamicron MR Controlled Evaluation [ADVANCE], Veterans Affairs Diabetes Trial [VADT] have examined glycemic control in type 2 DM along with UKPDS.

1686. Which of the following insulin is formulated as U-200 (200 units/mL)?

Harrison's 20th Ed. Chapter 397 Page 2863

A. Regular insulin
B. Short-acting
C. Long-acting
D. All of the above

1687. Which of the following insulin is formulated as U-300 (300 units/mL)?

Harrison's 20th Ed. Chapter 397 Page 2863

A. Regular insulin
B. Short-acting
C. Long-acting
D. All of the above

1688. Plasma glucose values are higher than whole blood values by?

Diabetes Metab J. 2016;40(5):365-66

A. 2–5%
B. 5–10%
C. 10–15%
D. 15–20%

Plasma glucose values are 10–15% higher than whole blood values when the hematocrit is normal. Postprandial capillary blood glucose levels are higher than venous blood glucose levels by up to 20%. Measurement of glucose in serum is not recommended for the diagnosis of diabetes.

1689. After sample collection, concentration of glucose decreases at a rate of?

Diabetes Metab J. 2016;40(5):365-66

A. 1% to 3% per hour
B. 3% to 5% per hour
C. 5% to 7% per hour
D. 7% to 9% per hour

After sample collection, concentration of glucose decreases due to glycolysis by erythrocyte, white blood cells, and platelet, which degrades glucose at a rate of 5% to 7% per hour.

1690. Which of the following insulin has the native insulin amino acid sequence?

Harrison's 20th Ed. Chapter 397 Page 2863

A. Insulin glulisine
B. Insulin glargine
C. Neutral protamine Hagedorn (NPH) insulin
D. Insulin detemir

Regular and NPH insulin have the native insulin amino acid sequence.

1691. Which of the following is preferred over regular insulin for prandial coverage?

Harrison's 20th Ed. Chapter 397 Page 2863

A. Aspart
B. Lispro
C. Glulisine
D. All of the above

Insulin aspart, lispro or glulisine is preferred over regular insulin for prandial coverage.

1692. Which of the following insulins has the longest duration of action?

Harrison's 20th Ed. Chapter 397 Page 2863

A. Insulin glargine
B. NPH insulin
C. Insulin detemir
D. Insulin degludec

Because of modification & extension of carboxy-terminal terminus of B chain, insulin degludec forms multihexamers in subcutaneous tissue and binds albumin, prolonging its duration of action (>42 hours).

1693. Which of the following insulins has a minimal peak activity?

Harrison's 20th Ed. Chapter 397 Page 2863 Table 397-4

A. Degludec
B. Determir
C. Glargine
D. All of the above

Degludec, determir, and glargine have minimal peak activity.

1694. Basal insulin is provided by which of the following insulins?

Harrison's 20th Ed. Chapter 397 Page 2863

A. Insulin glargine
B. Aspart
C. Lispro
D. Glulisine

Long-acting insulins (NPH, glargine, detemir, degludec) supply basal insulin, whereas regular, aspart, or lispro provides prandial insulin.

1695. Mixing of intermediate and short-acting insulin formulations alters the insulin absorption profile of?

Harrison's 20th Ed. Chapter 397 Page 2863

A. Short-acting insulin
B. Intermediate acting insulin
C. Both of the above
D. None of the above

Mixing of intermediate and short-acting insulin formulations may alter the insulin absorption profile especially of the short-acting insulins.

1696. Which of the following insulins should not be mixed with other insulins?

Harrison's 20th Ed. Chapter 397 Page 2863

A. Glargine
B. Detemir
C. Degludec
D. All of the above

Do not mix insulin glargine, detemir, or degludec with other insulins.

1697. Short-acting insulin analogues should be injected how many minutes before a meal?

Harrison's 20th Ed. Chapter 397 Page 2863

A. < 10 minutes
B. < 15 minutes
C. < 20 minutes
D. < 30 minutes

1698. Regular insulin should be injected how many minutes before a meal?

Harrison's 20th Ed. Chapter 397 Page 2863

A. < 10 minutes
B. < 15 minutes
C. < 20 minutes
D. < 30 minutes

Short-acting insulin analogues should be injected just before (<10 minutes) and regular insulin 30–45 minutes prior to a meal.

1699. Which of the following insulin is used in the insulin infusion device?

Harrison's 20th Ed. Chapter 397 Page 2864 Figure 397-1

A. Glulisine
B. Lispro
C. Aspart
D. All of the above

Glulisine, lispro, or insulin aspart is used in the insulin infusion device.

1700. Which of the following insulin regimen reproduces the precise insulin secretory pattern of the pancreatic islet?

Harrison's 20th Ed. Chapter 397 Page 2864

A. Short + Intermediate
B. Short + long
C. Intermediate + long
D. None of the above

No insulin regimen reproduces the precise insulin secretory pattern of the pancreatic islet.

1701. Daily requirement of insulin in individuals with type 1 DM is?

Harrison's 20th Ed. Chapter 397 Page 2864

A. 0.1–0.4 U/kg per day
B. 0.4–1 U/kg per day
C. 1.1–1.8 U/kg per day
D. 1.8–2.1 U/kg per day

1702. What percentage of insulin requirement in type 1 DM patients is given as basal insulin?

Harrison's 20th Ed. Chapter 397 Page 2864

A. 25%
B. 33%
C. 50%
D. 75%

In general, individuals with type 1 DM require 0.4–1 U/kg per day of insulin divided into multiple doses, with ~50% of the insulin given as basal insulin.

1703. For preprandial insulin dose in type 1 DM patient, insulin-to-carbohydrate ratio commonly is?

Harrison's 20th Ed. Chapter 397 Page 2864

A. 1 unit for 5–10 gram of carbohydrate
B. 1 unit for 10–15 gram of carbohydrate
C. 1 unit for 15–20 gram of carbohydrate
D. 1 unit for 20–25 gram of carbohydrate

For preprandial insulin dose in type 1 DM patient, insulin-to-carbohydrate ratio of 1 unit / 10–15 gram of carbohydrate is useful. To this insulin, add correcting insulin dose based on preprandial blood glucose (1 unit of insulin for every 50 mg/dL) over the preprandial glucose target. Also alternatively, body weight in kg × blood glucose – desired glucose in mg/dL]/1500.

1704. Morning hyperglycemia is best related to?

Harrison's 20th Ed. Chapter 397 Page 2864

A. Somogyi effect
B. Dawn phenomenon
C. "Saw-tooth" phenomenon
D. "Second-wind" phenomenon

Dawn phenomenon differs from the Somogyi effect in that it is not preceded by an episode of hypoglycemia. Due to a surge in hormone levels in morning, diabetes patients suffer from dawn phenomenon (or dawn effect), an abnormally high morning increase in blood glucose due to impaired response in insulin secretion. The Somogyi effect is the development of rebound hyperglycemia after an episode of hypoglycemia, often induced by excess insulin or inadequate calorie intake with insulin therapy.

1705. Dawn phenomenon is also called?

N Engl J Med 1985; 312:1473-79

A. Liver bump
B. Liver pump
C. Liver hump
D. Liver dump

Liver dump occurs when liver dumps glucose into blood stream. Morning hyperglycemia in diabetic individuals may be caused by the Somogyi effect, dawn phenomenon, or poor blood glucose control. Dawn Phenomenon is different from Chronic Somogyi Rebound, because it is not brought on by nocturnal hypoglycemia. The confirmation of the dawn phenomenon is the normal or high plasma glucose level during the nocturnal plasma glucose measurement. In turn, low plasma glucose concentration at this time suggests the presence of the Somogyi effect.

1706. Which of the following hormones play a role in Dawn phenomenon?

N Engl J Med 1985; 312:1473-79

A. Norepinephrine and epinephrine
B. Growth hormone
C. Glucagon
D. All of the above

Nocturnal surges in growth hormone secretion are predominantly responsible for the dawn phenomenon in DM patients.

1707. 1% increase in HbA1c can be associated with how much increase in risk of cardiovascular complications?

Diabetes Care. 2010;33(5):983-90

A. 1–2%
B. 5–10%
C. 15–20%
D. 25–30%

1% increase in HbA1c can be associated with a 15–20% increased risk of cardiovascular complications.

1708. 0.8% reduction in HbA1c produces a cardiovascular death risk reduction of?

J. Intern. Med. 2010;268(5):471-82

A. 15%
B. 25%
C. 35%
D. 45%

0.8% reduction in A1c could produce a cardiovascular death risk reduction as high as 45%.

1709. Fasting glucose is primarily determined by?

Harrison's 20th Ed. Chapter 397 Page 2864

A. Prior evening long-acting insulin
B. Morning short acting insulin
C. Morning long-acting insulin
D. Pre-supper short-acting insulin

1710. Prelunch glucose glucose is primarily determined by?

Harrison's 20th Ed. Chapter 397 Page 2864

A. Prior evening long-acting insulin
B. Morning short acting insulin
C. Morning long-acting insulin
D. Pre-supper short-acting insulin

1711. Presupper glucose glucose is primarily determined by?

Harrison's 20th Ed. Chapter 397 Page 2864

A. Prior evening long-acting insulin
B. Morning short acting insulin
C. Morning long-acting insulin
D. Pre-supper short-acting insulin

Fasting glucose is primarily determined by the prior evening long-acting insulin, pre-lunch glucose is a function of morning short-acting insulin, pre-supper glucose is a function of morning long-acting insulin and bedtime glucose is a function of the pre-supper, short-acting insulin.

1712. Which of the following insulins is used in continuous subcutaneous insulin infusion (CSII)?

Harrison's 20th Ed. Chapter 397 Page 2865

A. NPH
B. Ultralente
C. Glargine
D. Lispro

Most physicians use lispro, glulisine, or insulin aspart in CSII.

1713. Which of the following is an analogue of amylin?

Harrison's 20th Ed. Chapter 397 Page 2865

A. Liraglutide
B. Exenatide
C. Canagliflozin
D. Pramlintide

Pramlintide is an analogue of amylin. In type 1 DM, pramlintide is started as a 15 μg SC injection before each meal and titrated up to a maximum of 30-60 μg as tolerated. In type 2 DM, pramlintide is started as a 60 μg SC injection before each meal and may be titrated up to a maximum of 120 μg.

1714. Which of the following about Pramlintide is false?

Harrison's 20th Ed. Chapter 397 Page 2865

A. Analogue of amylin
B. Slows gastric emptying
C. Suppresses glucagon
D. Alter insulin levels

Pramlintide reduces postprandial glycemic excursions in type 1 & type 2 DM on insulin. It does not alter insulin levels. It delays gastric emptying, decreases postprandial glucagon release, and modulates appetite through its actions mainly via central effects (area postrema).

1715. Which out of the following modalities for treatment of DM produces highest HbA1c% reduction?

Harrison's 20th Ed. Chapter 397 Page 2866 Table 397-5

A. Medical nutrition therapy and physical activity
B. GLP-1 receptor agonists
C. Amylin agonists
D. Nonsulfonylurea insulin secretagogues

1716. Which out of the following modalities for treatment of DM produces highest HbA1c% reduction?

Harrison's 20th Ed. Chapter 397 Page 2866 Table 397-5

A. α-Glucosidase inhibitors
B. Biguanides
C. Dipeptidyl peptidase IV inhibitors
D. Thiazolidinediones

1717. Which out of the following modalities for treatment of DM produces least HbA1c% reduction?

Harrison's 20th Ed. Chapter 397 Page 2866 Table 397-5

A. GLP-1 receptor agonists
B. Amylin agonists
C. Thiazolidinediones
D. Sodium-glucose cotransporter 2 inhibitors

Glucose-lowering agents are subdivided into agents that increase insulin secretion, reduce glucose production, increase insulin sensitivity, enhance GLP-1 action, or promote urinary excretion of glucose.

1718. Oral glucose lowering agents that is effective in type 1 DM is?

Harrison's 20th Ed. Chapter 397 Page 2865

A. Sulfonylureas
B. Biguanides
C. Thiazolidinediones
D. Amylin agonists

Oral glucose lowering agents with the exception of α-glucosidase inhibitors and an amylin analogue - Pramlintide are ineffective in type 1 DM.

1719. Weight gain does not occur with which of the following drugs for type 2 DM?

Harrison's 20th Ed. Chapter 397 Page 2865

A. Insulin
B. Insulin secretagogues
C. Thiazolidinediones
D. Metformin

Metformin reduces fasting plasma glucose and insulin levels, improves the lipid profile, and promotes modest weight loss.

1720. Which of the following about metformin is false?

N Engl J Med 2014;371:1547-48

A. Concentrated in enterocytes and hepatocytes
B. Circulates essentially unbound
C. Eliminated unchanged by the kidneys
D. None of the above

In humans, metformin is absorbed through the upper small intestine, is concentrated in enterocytes and hepatocytes, circulates essentially unbound, and is eliminated, unchanged, by kidneys.

1721. Metformin is best related to which of the following processes?

N Engl J Med 2014;371:1547-48

A. Glycolysis
B. Gluconeogenesis
C. Glycogenesis
D. All of the above

At the whole-body level, metformin itself does not affect insulin sensitivity in muscle or adipose tissue but consistently reduces endogenous glucose production by inhibiting gluconeogenesis.

1722. Which of the following is a mechanisms of action of metformin?

N Engl J Med 2014;371:1547-48

A. Delayed intestinal glucose absorption
B. Enhanced release of glucagon-like peptide 1
C. Inhibition of glucagon signaling
D. All of the above

Proposed mechanisms of action have included delayed intestinal glucose absorption, enhanced release of glucagon-like peptide 1, augmented lactate production by enterocytes, and activation of AMP activated protein kinase in hepatocytes consequent to decreased energy charge, as well as inhibition of glucagon signaling, glycolytic enzymes, transcription of gluconeogenic enzymes, or mitochondrial complex I (which is made up of NADH and a reductase).

1723. Which of the following is related to the action of Metformin?

N Engl J Med 2014;371:1547-48

A. Mitochondrion specific isoform of glycerophosphate dehydrogenase (mGPD)
B. Dihydroxyacetone phosphate (DHAP)
C. Glycerol-3-phosphate (G3P)
D. All of the above

Metformin suppresses gluconeogenesis by inhibiting a mitochondrion specific isoform of glycerophosphate dehydrogenase (mGPD) which decelerates dihydroxyacetone phosphate (DHAP) – glycerophosphate shuttle (glycerophosphate is also called glycerol-3-phosphate [G3P]). Therefore, ratios of G3P to DHAP, NADH to NAD, and lactate to pyruvate all increase in the cytoplasm. Gluconeogenesis decreases, and therefore secretion of glucose by the hepatocyte decreases, and excess levels of glycerol and lactate are released into the plasma.

1724. Metformin best relates to which of the following?

Front. Endocrinol. 2017;8:6

A. Lotus corniculatus
B. Galega officinalis
C. Trigonella foenum-graecum
D. Trifolium pretense

Galega officinalis, a herbaceous plant, was found to contain guanidine, galegine, and biguanide, which decreased blood glucose levels. It is also known as Goat's rue, French lilac, or Italian fitch.

1725. Half-life of metformin is?

Front. Endocrinol. 2017;8:6

A. ~ 5 hours
B. ~ 8 hours
C. ~ 12 hours
D. ~ 18 hours

Half-life of metformin is ~ 5 hours.

1726. The primary route of elimination of metformin is via?

Front. Endocrinol. 2017;8:6

A. Liver
B. Kidney
C. Lung
D. Intestine

The primary route of elimination of metformin is via kidney.

1727. The major toxicity of metformin is?

Harrison's 20th Ed. Chapter 397 Page 2865

A. Aganulocytosis
B. Lactic acidosis
C. Seizure
D. Hypoxemia

The major toxicity of metformin is lactic acidosis.

1728. Levels of which of the following is lower during metformin treatment?

Harrison's 20th Ed. Chapter 397 Page 2865

A. Iron
B. Vitamin B12
C. Vitamin C
D. All of the above

Vitamin B12 levels are ~30% lower during metformin treatment. Long-term therapy with metformin can reversibly reduce intestinal absorption of vitamin B12 and folate, but rarely leads to macrocytic anemia.

1729. Which of the following is a biguanide?

J Res Med Sci. 2014;19(7):658–64

A. Metformin
B. Proguanil
C. Chlorproguanil
D. All of the above

Some biguanides like Proguanil & Chlorproguanil are also used as antimalarial drugs. Biguanides stimulate adenosine monophosphate kinase (AMPK) resulting in the inhibition of key enzymes involved in gluconeogenesis and glycogen synthesis in the liver. Phenformin & buformin are also biguanides.

1730. Drug interaction between metformin and which of the following drugs results in increase in metformin blood levels?

J Res Med Sci. 2014;19(7):658–64

A. Pioglitazone
B. Cimetidine
C. Atorvastatin
D. Clopidogrel

Potential drug interaction exists between metformin and cimetidine, resulting in an increase in metformin blood levels.

1731. Metformin should not be used in patients with?
Harrison's 20th Ed. Chapter 397 Page 2865

A. Renal insufficiency
B. Liver disease
C. Severe hypoxemia
D. All of the above

Metformin should not be used in patients with renal insufficiency, any form of acidosis, unstable congestive heart failure (CHF), liver disease or severe hypoxemia.

1732. Which of the following drugs should be withheld well before intravenous contrast administration?
Harrison's 20th Ed. Chapter 397 Page 2865

A. Pioglitazone
B. Metformin
C. Acarbose
D. Glipizide

1733. Maximum dose of metformin is?
Harrison's 20th Ed. Chapter 397 Page 2865

A. 500 mg daily
B. 1000 mg daily
C. 1500 mg daily
D. 2000 mg daily

1734. Which of the following about metformin is false?
Harrison's 20th Ed. Chapter 397 Page 2865

A. Metformin is effective as monotherapy
B. Long-term use reduces microvascular complications
C. Metallic taste is a side effect
D. None of the above

1735. Which of the following is a first generation sulfonylurea?
Harrison's 20th Ed. Chapter 397 Page 2865

A. Chlorpropamide
B. Tolazamide
C. Tolbutamide
D. All of the above

First-generation sulfonylureas have longer half-lives, higher risk of hypoglycemia & slower onset of action.

1736. Which of the following interact with ATP-sensitive potassium channel (K_{ATP}) on the beta cell?
Harrison's 20th Ed. Chapter 397 Page 2865

A. Glimepiride
B. Glipizide
C. Glyburide
D. All of the above

Insulin secretagogues stimulate insulin secretion by interacting with ATP-sensitive potassium channel on the beta cell (K_{ATP}).

1737. Which of the following interact with ATP-sensitive potassium channel (K_{ATP}) on the beta cell?
Harrison's 20th Ed. Chapter 397 Page 2865

A. Repaglinide
B. Nateglinide
C. Mitiglinide
D. All of the above

Repaglinide, nateglinide and mitiglinide are not sulfonylureas but also interact with the ATP-sensitive potassium channel (K_{ATP}).

1738. Which of the following has a low affinity for ATP-sensitive potassium channel isoform present in myocardium and brain?
Harrison's 20th Ed. Chapter 397 Page 2865

A. Glimepiride
B. Glipizide
C. Gliclazide
D. All of the above

A related isoform of ATP-sensitive potassium channels is present in myocardium and brain. Sulfonylureas except glyburide have a low affinity for this isoform.

1739. Which of the following cause weight gain?
Harrison's 20th Ed. Chapter 397 Page 2866

A. Insulin
B. Sulfonylureas
C. Thiazolidinedione
D. All of the above

1740. Which of the following cause weight loss?
Harrison's 20th Ed. Chapter 397 Page 2866

A. Metformin
B. Incretins
C. Sodium-glucose cotransporter 2 inhibitors
D. All of the above

Insulin, sulfonylureas, and thiazolidinedione all cause weight gain. Metformin, incretins, and sodium-glucose cotransporter 2 inhibitors are weight neutral or can help with weight loss.

1741. Which of the following is false about incretin effect?
Harrison's 20th Ed. Chapter 397 Page 2867

A. Amplification of insulin secretion from pancreas more when glucose is ingested orally than when given intravenously
C. Suppression of glucagon secretion
C. Slowing of gastric emptying
D. None of the above

The incretin effect refers to the amplification of insulin secretion that occurs when glucose is ingested orally as opposed to infused intravenously in amounts that result in identical glucose excursions. In healthy subjects, incretin effect accounts for ~70% of total amount of insulin released in response to an oral glucose load.

1742. Which of the following is a gut hormone?
Front. Endocrinol. 2018;9:387

A. Glucose-dependent insulinotropic polypeptide (GIP)
B. Glucagon-like peptide 1 (GLP-1)
C. Peptide tyrosyl-tyrosyl (PYY)
D. All of the above

Any gut hormone which under physiological circumstances stimulates or contributes to stimulation of the secretion of pancreatic hormones [insulin, glucagon, PP (pancreatic polypeptide), and pancreatic somatostatin] is an incretin. These hormones are secreted by endocrine cells located in epithelium of the small intestine.

1743. Which of the following is true for "incretin" hormones?
Harrison's 20th Ed. Chapter 397 Page 2867

A. Hormones produced in the small intestine
B. Produced during a meal that enter vasculature
C. Trigger insulin release by pancreatic beta cells
D. All of the above

Incretin hormones potentiate glucose-induced insulin secretion. Glucagon-like peptide-1 (GLP-1) is produced from the proglucagon gene in L cells of small intestine and secreted in response to nutrients. GIP is produced from the K cells of small intestine.

1744. 'Incretin effect' refers to?
Harrison's 20th Ed. Chapter 397 Page 2867

A. Plasma insulin response to glucose taken orally is more than when administered intravenously
B. Plasma insulin response to glucose administered intravenously is more than when taken orally
C. Over response to insulin
D. Under response to insulin

1745. Which of the following is true for "incretin" hormones?
Harrison's 20th Ed. Chapter 397 Page 2867

A. Decrease insulin secretion
B. Increase insulin secretion
C. Prevents insulin degradation
D. Augments insulin degradation

The incretins are hormones that work to augment glucose-stimulated insulin secretion. There are two main incretin hormones in humans, GIP (glucose-dependent insulinotropic peptide; also known as gastric inhibitory peptide) and GLP-1 (glucagon-like peptide-1). GLP-1 inhibits glucagon secretion and delays stomach emptying. Both hormones are secreted by endocrine L cells located in the epithelium of small intestine. Glucose in small intestine stimulates incretin release. Incretins are carried through the circulation to their target tissue like pancreatic beta cells. Incretin stimulation of beta cells causes them to secrete more insulin in response to the same amount of blood glucose.

1746. Which of the following is a short-acting GLP-1 receptor agonist?
Harrison's 20th Ed. Chapter 397 Page 2867

A. Liraglutide
B. Exanatide
C. Albiglutide
D. Dulaglutide

Short-acting GLP-1 receptor agonists are exanatide and lixisenatide. Long-acting GLP-1 receptor agonists include liraglutide, exenatide, albiglutide, dulaglutide, and lixisenatide. Exenatide is resistant to DPP-4 degradation.

1747. Exenatide was originally isolated from?
Harrison's 20th Ed. Chapter 397 Page 2867, Toxicon. 2012;59(4):464-71

A. Snake venom
B. Lizard venom
C. Spider venom
D. Scorpion venom

Incretin mimetic Exenatide is a peptide GLP-1 receptor agonist that was originally isolated from Gila monster (lizard) venom. It is resistant to degradation by DPP-4, the major protease that breaks down GIP and GLP-1.

1748. Which of the following is present in the saliva of Gila monster?
Harrison's 20th Ed. Chapter 397 Page 2867

A. Exendin-1
B. Exendin-2
C. Exendin-3
D. Exendin-4

Exendin-4 mimetic Exenatide is a synthetic version of a peptide initially identified in saliva of the Gila monster (exendin-4). Exendin-4 is an agonist for GLP-1 receptor present in the venom of Heloderma suspectum or Gila monster, a venomous lizard indigenous to the Southwestern United States.

1749. GLP-1 receptors are found in?
Harrison's 20th Ed. Chapter 397 Page 2867

A. Islets of Langerhans
B. Gastrointestinal tract
C. Brain
D. All of the above

GLP-1 receptors are found in islets, gastrointestinal tract and the brain.

1750. Which of the following is an action on GLP-1 receptor agonists?
Harrison's 20th Ed. Chapter 397 Page 2867

A. Increase glucose-stimulated insulin secretion
B. Suppress glucagon
C. Slow gastric emptying
D. All of the above

GLP-1 receptor agonists not only increases insulin secretion but increases β-cell proliferation and survival, reduces β-cell apoptosis, suppresses glucagon secretion, delays gastric emptying & suppresses appetite

1751. Use of GLP-1 receptor agonists is contraindicated in individuals with?
Harrison's 20th Ed. Chapter 397 Page 2867

A. Carcinoma breast
B. Ischemic heart disease
C. Ischemic stroke
D. Medullary carcinoma of the thyroid

1752. Use of GLP-1 receptor agonists is contraindicated in individuals with?
Harrison's 20th Ed. Chapter 397 Page 2867

A. Medullary carcinoma of thyroid
B. Multiple endocrine neoplasia
C. Pancreatic disease
D. All of the above

Because of an increased risk of thyroid C-cell tumors in rodents, use of GLP-1 receptor agonists is contraindicated in individuals with medullary carcinoma of thyroid or multiple endocrine neoplasia, or pancreatic disease.

1753. The major protease that breaks down GIP and GLP-1 is?
Harrison's 20th Ed. Chapter 397 Page 2867

A. Dipeptidyl peptidase (DPP) 1
B. Dipeptidyl peptidase (DPP) 2
C. Dipeptidyl peptidase (DPP) 3
D. Dipeptidyl peptidase (DPP) 4

1754. DPP-IV is expressed on the cell surface of?
Harrison's 20th Ed. Chapter 397 Page 2867

A. Pneumatocytes
B. Pancreatic β cells
C. Endothelial cells
D. Astrocytes

Dipeptidyl peptidase 4 (DPP-IV), which is widely expressed on the cell surface of endothelial cells and some lymphocytes, degrades a wide range of peptides and is not GLP-1 specific. DPP 4 is a cell-surface and circulating-peptidase enzyme and is also known as CD26 (a T-cell activating antigen).

1755. Which of the following is false about DPP-IV inhibitors?
Harrison's 20th Ed. Chapter 397 Page 2867

A. Preferential effect on postprandial blood glucose
B. Promotes insulin secretion in absence of hypoglycemia
C. Avoided in patients with pancreatic disease
D. None of the above

1756. DPP-IV inhibitors should be avoided in patients with?
Harrison's 20th Ed. Chapter 397 Page 2867

A. Heavy alcohol use
B. Severely elevated serum triglycerides
C. Hypercalcemia
D. All of the above

1757. Dipeptidyl peptidase-4 (DPP- 4) inhibitors best relate to which of the following?
Harrison's 20th Ed. Chapter 397 Page 2867

A. Glinides
B. Gliptins
C. Flozins
D. Diones

1758. Dipeptidyl peptidase-4 (DPP- 4) inhibitors best relate to which of the following?
Harrison's 20th Ed. Chapter 397 Page 2867

A. Serine protease enzyme
B. Cysteine protease enzyme
C. Threonine protease enzyme
D. Aspartic protease enzyme

1759. Which of the following statements is false?
Harrison's 20th Ed. Chapter 397 Page 2867

A. GLP-1 receptor agonists are incretin mimetics
B. DPP-4 inhibitors are incretin enhancers
C. DPP-4 inhibitors are competitive reversible inhibitors of DPP-4
D. None of the above

DPP-4 inhibitors include sitagliptin, vildagliptin, saxagliptin, linagliptin, alogliptin, anagliptin, teneligliptin, trelagliptin, omarigliptin, evogliptin, and gemigliptin. Peptidomimetic DPP-4 inhibitors include sitagliptin, gemigliptin, teneligliptin, vildagliptin, saxagliptin, and anagliptin. Non-peptidomimetic DPP-4 inhibitors include alogliptin and linagliptin.

1760. Which of the following is a common adverse reaction with gliptins?
Harrison's 20th Ed. Chapter 397 Page 2867

A. Nasopharyngitis
B. Upper respiratory tract infection
C. Headache
D. All of the above

The three most commonly reported adverse reactions in clinical trials with gliptins were nasopharyngitis, upper respiratory tract infection, and headache.

1761. Which of the following is false about α-Glucosidase inhibitors?
Harrison's 20th Ed. Chapter 397 Page 2867

A. Reduce postprandial hyperglycemia
B. Delay glucose absorption
C. Do not affect glucose utilization
D. Enhances insulin secretion

α-Glucosidase inhibitors reduce postprandial hyperglycemia by delaying glucose absorption; they do not affect glucose utilization or insulin secretion. α-Glucosidase inhibitors like Acarbose, miglitol and voglibose specifically inhibit α-glucosidases in the brush border of the small intestine.

1762. α-Glucosidase inhibitors should be used with caution with?
Harrison's 20th Ed. Chapter 397 Page 2867

A. Bile acid resins
B. Antacids
C. Sulfonylureas
D. All of the above

1763. Absorption of which of the following is possible when α-Glucosidase inhibitors are given?
Harrison's 20th Ed. Chapter 397 Page 2867

A. Glucose
B. Sucrose
C. Maltose
D. All of the above

Absorption of complex carbohydrates is retarded in those taking α-Glucosidase inhibitors. If hypoglycemia occurs, patient should consume glucose.

1764. α-Glucosidase inhibitors should not be used in individuals with?
Harrison's 20th Ed. Chapter 397 Page 2867

A. Inflammatory bowel disease
B. Gastroparesis
C. Serum creatinine > 2 mg/dL
D. All of the above

a-Glucosidase inhibitors should not be used in individuals with inflammatory bowel disease, gastroparesis or a serum creatinine > 2 mg/dL.

1765. PPAR-γ nuclear receptor forms a heterodimer with?
Harrison's 20th Ed. Chapter 397 Page 2867

A. Pregnane X receptor
B. Retinoid X receptor
C. Farnesoid X receptor
D. Retinoic acid receptor

Peroxisome proliferator-activated receptor γ (PPAR-γ) nuclear receptor forms a heterodimer with the retinoid X receptor.

1766. "PPAR" stands for?
Harrison's 20th Ed. Chapter 397 Page 2867

A. Peroxisome-protein-activated receptor
B. Peroxisome-proliferator-activated receptor
C. Peroxisome-producer-activated receptor
D. Peroxisome-promoter-activated receptor

Peroxisome-proliferator-activated receptors (PPARs) are a subfamily of 48-member nuclear-receptor superfamily & regulate gene expression in response to ligand binding. Peroxisome-proliferator-activated receptor g (PPARg) is a transcription factor activated by thiazolidinediones (TZDs).

1767. PPAR-γ is found at highest levels in?
Harrison's 20th Ed. Chapter 397 Page 2867

A. Adipocytes
B. Liver
C. Skeletal muscles
D. Pancreas

PPARg is a transcription factor that is activated by certain fatty acids, prostanoids & thiazolidinediones. Whereas the isoform PPARg1 is expressed in most tissues, PPARg2 is specific for adipose tissue, where it has a key role in regulation of normal adipocyte differentiation & proliferation as well as fatty acid uptake & storage.

1768. Which of the following is a PPARα agonist?
N Engl J Med 2004;351:1106-18

A. Fenofibrate
B. Bezafibrate
C. Gemfibrozil
D. All of the above

Fibrates like fenofibrate, bezafibrate, ciprofibrate & gemfibrozil act as full or partial PPARα agonists.

1769. PPARδ is expressed in which of the following tissues?
N Engl J Med 2004;351:1106-18

A. Skin
B. Brain
C. Adipose tissue
D. All of the above

Highest expression of PPARδ is in the skin, brain, and adipose tissue.

1770. Expression of PPARγ is lowest in which of the following tissues?
N Engl J Med 2004;351:1106-18

A. Adipose tissue
B. Pancreatic beta cells
C. Skeletal muscle
D. Macrophages

PPARγ is expressed most abundantly in adipose tissue but is also found in pancreatic β cells, vascular endothelium, and macrophages. Its expression is low in tissues that express predominantly PPARα such as the liver, the heart, and skeletal muscle.

1771. Major toxicity of Troglitazone is?
Harrison's 20th Ed. Chapter 397 Page 2867

A. Blood dyscrasias
B. Hepatotoxicity
C. Cardiac arrhythmias
D. All of the above

Troglitazone was withdrawn from U.S. market after reports of hepatotoxicity and an association with an idiosyncratic liver reaction that sometimes led to hepatic failure.

1772. PPAR-γ receptor agonists are responsible for?
Harrison's 20th Ed. Chapter 397 Page 2867

A. Promotion of adipocyte differentiation
B. Reduction of hepatic fat accumulation
C. Promotion of fatty acid storage
D. All of the above

PPAR-γ receptor agonists regulate a large number of genes, promote adipocyte differentiation, reduce hepatic fat accumulation, and promote fatty acid storage.

1773. Thiazolidinediones promote a redistribution of fat from?
Harrison's 20th Ed. Chapter 397 Page 2867

A. Central to peripheral locations
B. Peripheral to central locations
C. Upper to lower locations
D. Lower to upper locations

Thiazolidinediones promote a redistribution of fat from central to peripheral locations.

1774. The prototype of thiazolidinediones class of drugs is?
Harrison's 20th Ed. Chapter 397 Page 2867

A. Rosiglitazone
B. Pioglitazone
C. Troglitazone
D. Balaglitazone

The prototype of thiazolidinediones class of drugs is troglitazone.

1775. Which of the following is false about Rosiglitazone?
Harrison's 20th Ed. Chapter 397 Page 2867

A. Raises low-density lipoprotein (LDL)
B. Raises high-density lipoprotein (HDL)
C. Raises triglycerides
D. None of the above

1776. Which of the following is false about Pioglitazone?
Harrison's 20th Ed. Chapter 397 Page 2867

A. Raises HDL
B. Raises LDL
C. Lowers triglycerides
D. None of the above

Rosiglitazone raises low-density lipoprotein (LDL), high-density lipoprotein (HDL), and triglycerides slightly. Pioglitazone raises HDL to a greater degree and LDL a lesser degree but lowers triglycerides.

1777. Thiazolidinediones are associated with which of the following?
Harrison's 20th Ed. Chapter 397 Page 2867

A. Weight gain
B. Reduction in hematocrit
C. Increase in plasma volume
D. All of the above

Thiazolidinediones are associated with weight gain, a reduction in hematocrit and an increase in plasma volume.

1778. Thiazolidinediones are associated with which of the following?
Harrison's 20th Ed. Chapter 397 Page 2867

A. Worsening of diabetic macular edema
B. Increased risk of fractures in women
C. Induces ovulation in premenopausal women with PCOS
D. All of the above

Thiazolidinediones may worsen diabetic macular edema. An increased risk of fractures has also been noted in women taking these agents. Thiazolidinediones induce ovulation in premenopausal women with polycystic ovary syndrome. Safety of thiazolidinediones in pregnancy is not established.

1779. Pioglitazone increases the risk of?
Harrison's 20th Ed. Chapter 397 Page 2867

A. Cataract
B. Bladder cancer
C. Peripheral arterial disease
D. Dementia

Because of a possible increased risk of bladder cancer, pioglitazone is part of an ongoing FDA safety review.

1780. Which of the following metabolic abnormalities are linked to Diabetes mellitus Type 2?
N Engl J Med 2012;366:1319-27

A. Inflammation
B. Hypercoagulation
C. Endothelial cell dysfunction
D. All of the above

Commonly associated metabolic abnormalities include hypertension, dyslipidemia, inflammation, hypercoagulation, and endothelial cell dysfunction.

1781. In type 2 diabetes, which of the following factors does not contribute to the hyperglycemic state?

N Engl J Med 2012;366:1319-27

A. Increased Glucagon Secretion
B. Impaired Incretin Effect
C. Increased Amylin Secretion
D. Increased Hepatic Glucose Production

1782. In type 2 diabetes, Beta-cell failure is mediated by?

N Engl J Med 2012;366:1319-27

A. Genetic factors
B. Glucotoxicity
C. Lipotoxicity
D. All of the above

In type 2 diabetes, Beta-cell failure is mediated by genetic factors and exposure to chronically elevated levels of blood glucose (glucotoxicity) and free fatty acids (lipotoxicity).

1783. Plasma glucose level of 200 mg per deciliter is equivalent to?

N Engl J Med 2012;366:1319-27

A. 9.1 mmol per liter
B. 10.1 mmol per liter
C. 11.1 mmol per liter
D. 12.1 mmol per liter

Plasma glucose level of 200 mg per deciliter is equivalent to 11.1 mmol per liter.

1784. Control of glycemia delays which of the following complications of diabetes?

N Engl J Med 2012;366:1319-27

A. Nephropathy
B. Retinopathy
C. Neuropathy
D. All of the above

Control of glycemia in type 1 & 2 diabetes delays the onset and slows the progression of microvascular complications, including nephropathy, retinopathy, and neuropathy.

1785. In general, the glycated hemoglobin level should be checked how frequently?

N Engl J Med 2012;366:1319-27

A. At least monthly
B. At least three monthly
C. At least twice yearly
D. At least once yearly

In general, the glycated hemoglobin level should be checked at least twice yearly.

1786. American Diabetes Association recommends what amount of saturated fat in a diabetic diet?

N Engl J Med 2012;366:1319-27

A. Less than 3% saturated fat
B. Less than 5% saturated fat
C. Less than 7% saturated fat
D. Less than 9% saturated fat

In Diabetes, American Diabetes Association (ADA) recommends a balanced diet rich in fiber, whole grains, and legumes, and that contains <7% saturated fat and reduced trans fats. Foods with a high glycemic index need to be avoided.

1787. Diabetic patients should perform moderate-intensity aerobic exercise per week for?

N Engl J Med 2012;366:1319-27

A. At least 90 minutes
B. At least 120 minutes
C. At least 150 minutes
D. At least 180 minutes

Diabetic patients should be encouraged to engage in at least 150 minutes of moderate-intensity aerobic exercise per week.

1788. Which of the following hypoglycemic agents improve insulin sensitivity?

N Engl J Med 2012;366:1319-27

A. Metformin
B. Pioglitazone
C. Rosiglitazone
D. All of the above

1789. Which of the following about Metformin is false?

N Engl J Med 2012;366:1319-27

A. Rarely causes hypoglycemia
B. Acts by stimulating AMP-activated protein kinase
C. Reduces hepatic glucose production
D. Causes weight gain

Metformin improves insulin sensitivity. Acts by stimulating AMP-activated protein kinase and reduces hepatic glucose production. It does not cause weight gain and may result in a slight weight loss, and it rarely causes hypoglycemia.

1790. Which of the following about Thiazolidinediones is false?

N Engl J Med 2012;366:1319-27

A. Peroxisome proliferator–activated receptor alpha activators
B. Enhances insulin sensitivity in peripheral tissues
C. Reduce hepatic glucose production
D. Rosiglitazone increases risk of myocardial infarction

Thiazolidinediones (pioglitazone and rosiglitazone) are peroxisome proliferator–activated receptor?activators that enhance insulin sensitivity in peripheral tissues and reduce hepatic glucose production. Use of rosiglitazone increases risk of myocardial infarction. Pioglitazone was associated with a reduction in the secondary composite cardiovascular disease outcome but also with increased risks of edema and heart failure.

1791. Agents that increase circulating insulin levels include all except?

N Engl J Med 2012;366:1319-27

A. Sitagliptin
B. Repaglinide
C. Pioglitazone
D. Exenatide

Agents that increase circulating insulin levels include exogenous insulin that acts by activating plasma-membrane receptors, stimulating glucose uptake by responsive tissues and decreasing hepatic glucose production. Sulfonylureas (glipizide etc.) stimulate insulin release by closure of specific potassium channels on beta cells. Meglitinides (repaglinide etc.) have actions similar to those of sulfonylureas but have a short duration of action (hours) and are most effective preprandially. GLP-1–receptor agonists (exenatide & liraglutide) are injectable agents that are structurally similar to endogenous GLP-1 and activate GLP-1 receptors. Dipeptidyl peptidase IV (DPP-IV) inhibitors (sitagliptin) are oral agents that inhibit the degradation of GLP-1 and result in modest elevations of circulating GLP-1 levels.

1792. Which of the following is not used as an injectable agent in treatment of diabetes?

N Engl J Med 2012;366:1319-27

A. Sitagliptin
B. Pramlintide
C. Exenatide
D. Insulin

Alpha-glucosidase inhibitors (acarbose) interfere with the digestion of glucose polymers, thereby decreasing carbohydrate absorption. Bile acid sequestrant colesevelam reduces hepatic glucose production and increases incretin levels by unknown mechanisms; it also reduces LDL cholesterol levels. The dopamine agonist bromocriptine activates D2 dopamine receptors and increases insulin sensitivity by unknown mechanisms; a rapid-release form was approved by the FDA for this indication. Pramlintide, an amylin mimetic, is an injectable agent that stimulates receptors for amylin. It suppresses glucagon secretion, delays gastric emptying, and decreases appetite.

1793. Which of the following is useful in the treatment of diabetes?

N Engl J Med 2012;366:1319-27

A. Colesevelam
B. Bromocriptine
C. Pramlintide
D. All of the above

1794. Factor that can influence the Hemoglobin A1c level is?

Cleveland clinic J of Med 2011;78:380

A. Iron deficiency anemia
B. Blood transfusions
C. Renal failure
D. All of the above

Many factors can influence the hemoglobin A1c level, such as anemia, iron deficiency, blood transfusions, hemolytic anemia, and renal failure.

1795. Type 2 diabetes is characterized by?

Cleveland clinic J of Med 2013;80(11):683

A. Insulin resistance
B. Decreased beta-cell function
C. Progressive beta-cell decline
D. All of the above

Type 2 diabetes is characterized by insulin resistance, decreased beta-cell function, and progressive beta-cell decline.

1796. Which of the following is not an antihyperglycemic agent?

Cleveland clinic J of Med 2013;80(11):683

A. Amylin analogues
B. Dopamine agonists
C. Dobutamine agonists
D. Alpha-glucosidase inhibitors

Available antihyperglycemic groups include metformin, sulfonylureas, meglitinides, alpha-glucosidase inhibitors, thiazolidinediones, gliptins, glucagon-like peptide-1 agonists, amylin analogues, colesevelam, dopamine agonists, and insulin.

1797. Antihyperglycemics act on which of the following?

Cleveland clinic J of Med 2013;80(11):683

A. Pancreas
B. Gut
C. Muscle
D. All of the above

Most of the available antihyperglycemics target liver, pancreas, gut, and muscle to improve insulin sensitivity, reduce insulin resistance, or stimulate insulin secretion.

1798. Sodium-glucose cotransporters relate best with?

Cleveland clinic J of Med 2013;80(11):683

A. Membrane protein
B. Tubular protein
C. Glomerular protein
D. Ductal protein

Membrane proteins called sodium-glucose cotransporters reabsorb glucose at the proximal tubule and return it into the peripheral circulation. Glucose enters the tubular epithelial cell with sodium by passive cotransport via the sodium glucose cotransporters, and then exits on the other side via the glucose transporter GLUT in the basolateral membrane.

1799. Which of the following sodium-glucose transporters act in early segment of proximal tubule of kidney to reabsorbs glucose?

Cleveland clinic J of Med 2013;80(11):683

A. SGLT2
B. SGLT3
C. SGLT4
D. SGLT5

Sodium-glucose transporters SGLT1 and SGLT2 act in the proximal tubule of kidney. SGLT2 is found only in the proximal tubule and reabsorbs most of the glucose (90%) in early segment of proximal tubule, while SLGT1 reabsorbs the remaining glucose at the distal end.

1800. SGLT1 is found mainly in?

Harrison's 20th Ed. Chapter 397 Page 2867, Cleveland clinic J of Med 2013;80(11):683

A. Proximal tubule of kidney
B. Distal tubule of kidney
C. Gastrointestinal tract
D. Pancreas

SGLT1 is found mainly in the gastrointestinal tract.

1801. Which of the following is up-regulated in patients with type 2 diabetes?

Cleveland clinic J of Med 2013;80(11):683

A. SGLT2
B. SGLT3
C. SGLT4
D. SGLT5

Patients with type 2 diabetes have a higher capacity for glucose reabsorption in the proximal tubule as a result of the up-regulation of SGLT2.

1802. Which of the following is the first SGLT2 inhibitor used for the treatment of type 2 diabetes?

Cleveland clinic J of Med 2013;80(11):683

A. Sitagliptin
B. Colesevelam
C. Canagliflozin
D. Rifampin

Canagliflozin is a Sodium-Glucose Co-Transporter 2 Inhibitor. It blocks reabsorption of glucose in the proximal tubule, lowers renal threshold for glucose and increases urinary glucose excretion thereby lowering the serum glucose level in patients with hyperglycemia. This mechanism of action is insulin-independent. Canagliflozin is the first SGLT2 inhibitor to be approved in the United States. Dapagliflozin was the first SGLT2 inhibitor approved in Europe. Empagliflozin and Ipragliflozin are awaiting approval.

1803. Canagliflozin is not indicated for patients with?
Cleveland clinic J of Med 2013;80(11):683

A. Type 1 diabetes
B. Type 2 diabetes with ketonuria
C. End-stage renal disease
D. All of the above

Canagliflozin is not indicated for patients with type 1 diabetes, type 2 diabetes with ketonuria, or end-stage renal disease (estimated GFR< 45 mL/min or receiving dialysis), pregnant women and patients under 18 years of age.

1804. Euglycemic DKA best relates with?
Harrison's 20th Ed. Chapter 397 Page 2868

A. Sitagliptin
B. Pioglitazone
C. Canagliflozin
D. Insulin

1805. Which of the following about SGLT2 inhibitors is false?
Harrison's 20th Ed. Chapter 397 Page 2868

A. Should not be prescribed in type 1 DM
B. Increase glucagon secretion by stimulating alpha cell
C. Glucose-lowering effect is insulin independent
D. None of the above

1806. SGLT2 inhibitors have the potential to cause?
Harrison's 20th Ed. Chapter 397 Page 2868

A. Urinary and genital mycotic infections
B. Bladder cancer
C. Leg and foot amputation and bone fractures
D. All of the above

1807. Empagliflozin & canagliflozin reduces?
Harrison's 20th Ed. Chapter 397 Page 2868

A. CVD events and all cause CV mortality in T2DM
B. Risk for nephropathy
C. Rate of hospitalization for CHF
D. All of the above

1808. Which of the following is a bile acid sequestrant (BAS)?
Harrison's 20th Ed. Chapter 397 Page 2868

A. Colesevelam
B. Colestimide
C. Colestipol
D. All of the above

Bile acid metabolism is abnormal in type 2 DM. Cholestyramine and colestipol are first-generation BAS. Second-generation BASs include colesevelam and colestimide (also called colestilan).

1809. Colesevelam was first introduced as?
Harrison's 20th Ed. Chapter 397 Page 2868

A. Antihistaminic
B. Diuretic
C. LDLc-lowering drug
D. Anti-inflammatory

Colesevelam was first introduced as an LDLc-lowering drug in 2000.

1810. Bile acid sequestrant (BAS) are contraindicated in ?
Harrison's 20th Ed. Chapter 397 Page 2868

A. Hypercholesterolemia
B. Hypertriglyceridemia
C. Type 2 DM
D. All of the above

Bile acid–binding resins increase plasma triglycerides and should be used with caution in patients with hypertriglyceridemia.

1811. Which of the following is approved for use in T2DM?
Harrison's 20th Ed. Chapter 397 Page 2868

A. Bosentan
B. Bromocriptine
C. Reboxetine
D. Quinagolide

Quick-release Bromocriptine mesylate was approved by FDA in 2009, for treatment of type 2 diabetes. Bromocriptine is thought to act on circadian neuronal activities in hypothalamus, to reset an abnormally elevated hypothalamic drive for increased plasma glucose, free fatty acids, and triglycerides in insulin-resistant patients.

1812. In which of the following situations, insulin is considered as initial therapy in type 2 DM?
Harrison's 20th Ed. Chapter 397 Page 2868

A. In acutely ill hospitalized patients
B. Lean individuals or those with severe weight loss
C. Individuals with underlying renal or hepatic disease
D. All of the above

1813. Insulin therapy in type 2 DM is initiated with?
Harrison's 20th Ed. Chapter 397 Page 2868

A. Single dose of long-acting insulin at bedtime
B. Premeal doses of short-acting insulin
C. Long-acting insulin + short-acting insulin
D. Any of the above

Insulin therapy is ultimately required by a substantial number of individuals with type 2 DM. insulin is usually initiated in a single dose of long-acting insulin (0.2 - 0.4 U/kg per day), given in the evening (NPH) or just before bedtime (NPH, glargine, detemir or degludec).

1814. The insulin dose is adjusted with increments of?
Harrison's 20th Ed. Chapter 397 Page 2868

A. 5%
B. 10%
C. 15%
D. 20%

The insulin dose may be adjusted in 10% increments as dictated by SMBG results.

1815. Patients are considered to have severe hyperglycemia when their FPG is more than?
Harrison's 20th Ed. Chapter 397 Page 2868

A. 200 mg/dL
B. 250 mg/dL
C. 300 mg/dL
D. 350 mg/dL

Patients are considered to have mild hyperglycemia when their FPG is between 126–199 mg/dL), moderate hyperglycemia when FPG is between 200–250 mg/dL and severe hyperglycemia when FPG is between > 250 mg/dL. Mild hyperglycemia is responsive to a single, oral glucose lowering agent, while those with moderate hyperglycemia will require >1 oral agent or insulin. Patients with severe hyperglycemia are unlikely to achieve normoglycemia with oral therapy.

1816. Which of the following is a 'long acting' insulin analogue?
Harrison's 20th Ed. Chapter 397 Page 2868

A. Insulin detemir
B. Insulin glulisine
C. Insulin lispro
D. Insulin aspart

1817. Which of the following drugs is used as monotherapy for type 2 DM?
Harrison's 20th Ed. Chapter 397 Page 2868

A. Metformin
B. α-glucosidase inhibitors
C. Thiazolidinediones
D. All of the above

Insulin secretagogues, biguanides, α-glucosidase inhibitors, thiazolidinediones, GLP-1 receptor agonists, DPP-IV inhibitors, SLGT2 inhibitors & insulin are approved for monotherapy of type 2 DM.

1818. Which of the following drugs does not directly cause hypoglycemia?
Harrison's 20th Ed. Chapter 397 Page 2868

A. Biguanides
B. α glucosidase inhibitors
C. Thiazolidinediones
D. All of the above

Biguanides, α-glucosidase inhibitors, thiazolidinediones, GLP-1 receptor agonists, DPP-IV inhibitors and SLGT2 inhibitors do not directly cause hypoglycemia.

1819. Antihyperglycemic drugs that begin to lower plasma glucose immediately are all except?
Harrison's 20th Ed. Chapter 397 Page 2868

A. GLP-1 receptor agonists
B. DPP-IV inhibitors
C. Thiazolidinediones
D. α-glucosidase inhibitors

Insulin secretagogues, GLP-1 receptor agonists, DPP-IV inhibitors, α-glucosidase inhibitors, & SLGT2 inhibitors begin to lower plasma glucose immediately, whereas glucose-lowering effects of biguanides and thiazolidinediones are delayed by weeks.

1820. Durability of glycemic control is less for which of the following?
Harrison's 20th Ed. Chapter 397 Page 2868

A. Sulfonylureas
B. Metformin
C. Thiazolidinediones
D. All of the above

Durability of glycemic control is less for sulfonylureas as compared to metformin or thiazolidinediones.

1821. Which of the following drugs target insulin resistance in type 2 DM?
Harrison's 20th Ed. Chapter 397 Page 2868

A. α-glucosidase inhibitors
B. GLP-1 receptor agonists
C. DPP-IV inhibitors
D. Thiazolidinediones

1822. Which of the following is a professional society for the study of diabetes mellitus?
Harrison's 20th Ed. Chapter 397 Page 2868

A. EASD
B. IDF
C. AACE
D. All of the above

1823. Which of the following has a beneficial cardiovascular effect in type 2 DM and CVD, or at high-risk of CVD?
Harrison's 20th Ed. Chapter 397 Page 2869

A. Empagliflozin
B. Canagliflozin
C. Liraglutide
D. All of the above

Empagliflozin, canagliflozin, and liraglutide have a beneficial cardiovascular effect in type 2 DM and CVD individuals, or who are at high-risk of CVD,

1824. Which of the following is a new therapy under development for type 2 DM?
Harrison's 20th Ed. Chapter 397 Page 2869

A. Activators of glucokinase
B. Inhibitors of 11 β-hydroxysteroid dehydrogenase-1
C. GPR40 agonists
D. All of the above

New therapies under development for type 2 DM include activators of glucokinase, inhibitors of 11 b-hydroxysteroid dehydrogenase-1, GPR40 agonists, monoclonal antibodies to reduce inflammation and salsalate.

1825. GPR40 is also known as?
Curr Drug Targets. 2016;17(11):1292-300

A. FFA receptor 1
B. FFA receptor 2
C. FFA receptor 3
D. FFA receptor 4

G protein-coupled receptor 40/Free fatty acid receptor 1 (GPR40/FFAR1) is primarily expressed in pancreatic β-cells and is activated by medium-chain and long-chain free fatty acids (FFAs). GPR40 agonists (fasiglifam) augment glucose dependent insulin secretion (GDIS) from pancreatic β-cells. GPR40 is not expressed in the liver.

1826. Which of the following is GPR40 / FFAR1 agonist?
Drug Saf. 2018;41(6):625-40

A. Fasiglifam
B. Pramlintide
C. Rimonabant
D. Contrave

Fasiglifam (TAK-875) is a G protein-coupled receptor 40 agonist. Clinical development of fasiglifam was halted due to these liver safety concerns.

1827. Which of the following is an allosteric activator of glucokinase?
J Med Chem. 2012;55(16):7021-36

A. Epitizide
B. Piragliatin
C. Indoramin
D. Moxonidine

Piragliatin, an allosteric activator of glucokinase (GK). Piragliatin, a glucokinase activator (GKA) was found to lower pre- and postprandial glucose levels, improve the insulin secretory profile, increase β-cell sensitivity to glucose, and decrease hepatic glucose output in patients with T2D.

1828. Which of the following is known to have an impact on glucose metabolism & useful in treatment of T2DM?

Harrison's 20th Ed. Chapter 397 Page 2869

A. Inhibitors of sarcosine dehydrogenase
B. Inhibitors of dihydroorotate dehydrogenase
C. Inhibitors of 11 β-hydroxysteroid dehydrogenase-1
D. Inhibitors of dihydropyrimidine dehydrogenase

Increased glucocorticoid activity at peripheral tissues plays a role in the pathogenesis of metabolic syndrome & T2DM. Intracellular cortisol concentrations are determined by plasma levels & also by the activity of 11β-hydroxysteroid dehydrogenase type 1 (11β-HSD1) which catalyzes the conversion of inactive cortisone to active cortisol. 11β-HSD1 is a bidirectional enzyme that interconverts hormonally inactive cortisone to cortisol. Major immediate effect of 11β-HSD1 inhibition in patients with diabetes relate to reduced glucocorticoid-mediated hepatic glucose output.

1829. Which of the following elements potentiate action of insulin?

Harrison's 20th Ed. Chapter 326 Page 2319

A. Zinc
B. Copper
C. Chromium
D. Selenium

Chromium potentiates action of insulin in those with impaired glucose tolerance by increasing insulin receptor mediated signaling, although its usefulness in treating type 2 diabetes is uncertain. Rich food sources of chromium include yeast, meat & grain products.

1830. Which of the following differentiates hyperglycemic hyperosmolar state (HHS) from diabetic ketoacidosis (DKA)?

Harrison's 20th Ed. Chapter 397 Page 2870

A. Plasma ketones
B. Anion gap
C. Serum bicarbonate
D. All of the above

Diabetic ketoacidosis is characterized by a serum glucose level >250 mg/dL, pH <7.3, serum bicarbonate level <18 mEq/L, elevated serum ketone level, and dehydration.

1831. Which of the following differentiates hyperglycemic hyperosmolar state (HHS) from diabetic ketoacidosis (DKA)?

Harrison's 20th Ed. Chapter 397 Page 2870

A. Arterial pH
B. Osmolality
C. Arterial PCO_2
D. All of the above

1832. Plasma glucose of 250 mg/dL is equivalent to how many mmol/L?

Harrison's 20th Ed. Chapter 397 Page 2870

A. 11.9 mmol/L
B. 12.9 mmol/L
C. 13.9 mmol/L
D. 14.9 mmol/L

1833. Which of the following about hyperglycemic hyperosmolar state (HHS) is false?

Harrison's 20th Ed. Chapter 397 Page 2870

A. Primarily seen in elderly individuals with type 2 DM
B. No nausea, vomiting, and abdominal pain
C. No Kussmaul respirations
D. None of the above

1834. Fruity odor of breath in hyperglycemia is due to?

Harrison's 20th Ed. Chapter 397 Page 2870

A. Acetoacetate
B. Beta-hydroxybutyrate
C. Acetone
D. All of the above

Diabetes causes intense lipolysis, which aggravates beta-oxidation process and results in increased NADH/NAD⁺ ratios. Main ketone bodies are acetoacetate, beta-hydroxybutyrate, and acetone, and these are used as energy supply for human body, especially for brain. Acetoacetate is produced from acetyl-CoA during lipolysis, then is metabolized to acetone & betahydroxybutyrate through decarboxylation and reduction, respectively. Acetoacetate & beta-hydroxybutyrate can be metabolized back to acetyl-CoA in extra-hepatic tissues, while the acetone is mainly eliminated via urine and/or exhalation. Acetone is more abundant in breath as it is much more volatile than the other two ketone bodies.

1835. Which of the following is a new potential biomarker in diabetic breathomics?

RSC Adv., 2017, 7, 17480

A. Isocyanate
B. Isopropanol
C. Sorbitol
D. Diethylene

Breathomics refers to the metabolomic study of exhaled breath and focuses on health-related breath biomarkers. Isopropanol (IPA) was postulated to be a reduction product of acetone (ACE) through reverse reaction of alcohol dehydrogenase (ADH). High levels of acetone in liver results in increased production of isopropanol, especially in the presence of elevated NADH/NAD⁺ ratios.

1836. Which of the following is a classic sign of DKA?

Harrison's 20th Ed. Chapter 397 Page 2870

A. Abdominal tenderness
B. Kussmaul respiration
C. Tachycardia
D. Dehydration/hypotension

Kussmaul respirations and a fruity odor on patient's breath (secondary to metabolic acidosis & increased acetone) are classic signs of diabetic ketoacidosis.

1837. Cerebral edema in DKA is seen most frequently in?

Harrison's 20th Ed. Chapter 397 Page 2870

A. Children
B. Adults
C. Elderly
D. All of the above

Cerebral edema, an extremely serious nonmetabolic complication of DKA, is seen most frequently in children as DKA is resolving.

1838. Which of the following is a factor that precipitates DKA?

Harrison's 20th Ed. Chapter 397 Page 2870 Table 397-7

A. Mesenteric infarction
B. Pregnancy
C. Cocaine
D. All of the above

Events that can precipitate DKA include inadequate insulin administration, infection (pneumonia/UTI/gastroenteritis/sepsis), infarction (cerebral, coronary, mesenteric, peripheral), cocaine and pregnancy.

1839. In DKA, levels of which of the following is increased?

Harrison's 20th Ed. Chapter 397 Page 2870

A. Glucagon
B. Cortisol
C. Growth hormone
D. All of the above

DKA results from relative or absolute insulin deficiency combined with counterregulatory hormone excess (glucagon, catecholamines, cortisol and growth hormone).

1840. In liver, decreased ratio of insulin to glucagon promotes which of the following?

Harrison's 20th Ed. Chapter 397 Page 2870

A. Gluconeogenesis
B. Glycogenolysis
C. Ketone body formation
D. All of the above

The decreased ratio of insulin to glucagon promotes gluconeogenesis, glycogenolysis, and ketone body formation in liver. There is an increase in substrate delivery from fat and muscle (free fatty acid, amino acids) to the liver.

1841. Which of the following occur in DKA?

Harrison's 20th Ed. Chapter 397 Page 2870

A. Reduced hepatic level of fructose-2,6-bisphosphate
B. Decreased activity of pyruvate kinase
C. Increased activity of phosphoenolpyruvate carboxykinase
D. All of the above

Combination of insulin deficiency & hyperglycemia reduces hepatic level of fructose-2,6-bisphosphate, which alters activity of phosphofructokinase & fructose-1,6-biphosphatase. Glucagon excess decreases activity of pyruvate kinase, whereas insulin deficiency increases the activity of phosphoenolpyruvate carboxykinase.

1842. Ketonemia is defined as a ketone level more than?

Am Fam Physician. 2013;87(5):337-46

A. 0.12 mmol/L
B. 0.22 mmol/L
C. 0.32 mmol/L
D. 0.42 mmol/L

Ketonemia is defined as a ketone level > 0.42 mmol/L.

1843. In liver normally, free fatty acids from lipolysis are converted to?

Harrison's 20th Ed. Chapter 397 Page 2870

A. Pyruvate
B. Glycogen
C. Very low-density lipoprotein (VLDL)
D. High-density lipoprotein (HDL)

Lipolysis is defined as the hydrolytic cleavage of ester bonds in triglycerides (TGs), resulting in the generation of fatty acids (FAs) and glycerol. Normally, free fatty acids from lipolysis are converted to very low-density lipoprotein (VLDL) in the liver. The increased FFA increase VLDL-triglyceride production. VLDL clearance is also reduced because activity of insulin-sensitive lipoprotein lipase in muscle and fat is decreased.

1844. Which of the following is a major lipase controlling lipolysis?

The Journal of biological chemistry. 2003;278(50):50428–34

A. Adipose triglyceride lipase (ATGL)
B. Hormone-sensitive lipase (HSL)
C. Monoacylglycerol lipase (MAGL)
D. All of the above

Three major lipases controlling lipolysis are adipose triacylglycerol lipase (converts triacylglycerol to diacylglycerol and one free fatty acid), HSL (converts diacylglycerol to monoacylglycerol and one free fatty acid) and monoacylglycerol lipase (converts monoacylglycerol to glycerol and one free fatty acid).

1845. Enzyme mediating increased ketone body formation in DKA is?

Harrison's 20th Ed. Chapter 397 Page 2870

A. HMG CoA reductase
B. CPT - I
C. CPT - II
D. Acyl CoA transferase

In DKA, hyperglucagonemia alters hepatic metabolism to favor ketone body formation, through activation of enzyme carnitine palmitoyltransferase I. This enzyme is crucial for regulating fatty acid transport into the mitochondria, where beta oxidation and conversion to ketone bodies occur. CPT1 is a key factor to regulate fatty acids beta-oxidation. It is also an energy sensor to meet body energy needs by regulating fatty acids oxidation process.

1846. Which of the following about carnitine palmitoyltransferase I is false?

The Journal of biological chemistry. 2003;278(50):50428–34

A. Located at the outer membrane of mitochondria
B. Is the rate-limiting enzyme in fat oxidation
C. Catalyzes the exchange of CoA bound to LCFAs for carnitine
D. None of the above

1847. Which isoform of CPT1 is expressed in liver and kidney?

The Journal of biological chemistry. 2003;278(50):50428–434

A. CPT1A
B. CPT1B
C. CPT1C
D. All of the above

Carnitine palmitoyltransferase 1 (CPT1) enzyme exists in three different isoforms: CPT1A is expressed in liver and kidney, CPT1B in cardiac and skeletal muscle, and CPT1C in the brain. CPT1A is the key regulatory enzyme of hepatic long-chain fatty acid β-oxidation. CPT1A decreases gluconeogenesis while CPT1B increases the glucose uptake by peripheral tissues.

1848. CPT1 is tightly regulated by?

The Journal of biological chemistry. 2003;278(50):50428–34

A. Malonyl-CoA
B. HMG-CoA
C. Succinyl-CoA
D. Acetyl-CoA

CPT1 is tightly regulated by its physiological inhibitor malonyl-CoA, first intermediate in FA biosynthesis.

1849. Which of the following cannot cross the mitochondrial membranes by simple diffusion?

The Journal of biological chemistry. 2003;278(50):50428–34

A. Short-chain fatty acids
B. Medium-chain fatty acids
C. Long-chain fatty acids
D. All of the above

Mitochondrial β-oxidation of long-chain fatty acids is a major source of energy production, especially during fasting, illness, or sustained exercise. Contrary to medium- and short-chain fatty acids that can cross mitochondrial membranes by simple diffusion, long-chain fatty acids are imported into mitochondrial matrix by the carnitine palmitoyltransferase (CPT) system.

1850. Overexpression of CPTI is associated with tumor progression in?

The Journal of biological chemistry. 2003;278(50):50428–34

A. Breast cancer
B. Gastric cancer
C. Prostate cancer
D. All of the above

Overexpression of CPTI is associated with tumor progression in breast, gastric, & prostate cancer.

1851. Which of the following is emerging as a modality to treat diabetes?

J Mol Genet Med 2016;10(4):238

A. CPT1A inhibitors
B. Malonyl-CoA analogues
C. Glycidic acid analogues
D. All of the above

1852. Which of the following drugs has antihyperglycemic potential?

J Mol Genet Med 2016;10(4):238

A. Elomoxir
B. Teglicar
C. ST1326
D. All of the above

1853. At physiologic pH, ketoacids are neutralized by bicarbonate?

Harrison's 20th Ed. Chapter 397 Page 2870

A. Albumin
B. Bicarbonate
C. Potassium
D. All of the above

At physiologic pH, ketone bodies exist as ketoacids, which are neutralized by bicarbonate.

1854. DKA is characterized by?

Harrison's 20th Ed. Chapter 397 Page 2871

A. Serum glucose > 250 mg/dL
B. Serum bicarbonate <15 mmol/L
C. Increased anion gap
D. All of the above

DKA is characterized by hyperglycemia (serum glucose > 250 mg/dL), ketosis, metabolic acidosis (serum bicarbonate <15 mmol/L) and increased anion gap.

1855. Which of the following is observed in DKA?

Harrison's 20th Ed. Chapter 397 Page 2871

A. Leukocytosis
B. Elevated blood urea nitrogen and serum creatinine
C. Hypertriglyceridemia and hyperlipoproteinemia
D. All of the above

1856. In DKA, the elevated amylase is usually of which origin?

Harrison's 20th Ed. Chapter 397 Page 2871

A. Salivary
B. Gastric
C. Pancreatic
D. All of the above

In DKA the amylase is usually of salivary origin and thus is not diagnostic of pancreatitis.

1857. In DKA, elevation in serum amylase is due to?

Harrison's 20th Ed. Chapter 397 Page 2871

A. Acute pancreatitis
B. Acidemia
C. Infection
D. All of the above

1858. In DKA, interference from which of the following may falsely elevate serum creatinine measurement?

Harrison's 20th Ed. Chapter 397 Page 2871

A. Acetoacetate
B. Hypertriglyceridemia
C. Hyperglycemia
D. Blood Urea

Interference from acetoacetate may falsely elevate the serum creatinine measurement in DKA.

1859. For every 100 mg/dL rise in serum glucose, serum sodium is reduced by?

Harrison's 20th Ed. Chapter 397 Page 2871

A. 1.0 meq/L
B. 1.2 meq/L
C. 1.4 meq/L
D. 1.6 meq/L

For every 100 mg/dL rise in serum glucose, serum sodium is reduced by 1.6 mmol/L.

1860. Formula for serum sodium correction in DKA is?

Am Fam Physician. 2013;87(5):337-346, Ann Intern Med. 2010;152(1):ITC1-1–ITC1-15

A. Na + 0.014 (glucose – 100)
B. Na + 0.015 (glucose – 100)
C. Na + 0.016 (glucose – 100)
D. Na + 0.017 (glucose – 100)

In DKA, hyperglycemia causes pseudohyponatremia.

1861. Serum osmolality is calculated by which of the following formula?

Harrison's 20th Ed. Chapter 397 Page 2871

A. [2 × (S. Na^+ + K^+) + P. glucose (mg/dL)/18 + BUN/2.8]
B. [3 × (S. Na^+ + K^+) + P. glucose (mg/dL)/18 + BUN/2.8]
C. [4 × (S. Na^+ + K^+) + P. glucose (mg/dL)/18 + BUN/2.8]
D. [5 × (S. Na^+ + K^+) + P. glucose (mg/dL)/18 + BUN/2.8]

Serum osmolality is calculated by [2 × (serum sodium + serum potassium) + plasma glucose (mg/dL)/18 + BUN/2.8]

1862. Which of the following is not a precipitating event in DKA?

Harrison's 20th Ed. Chapter 397 Page 2870 Table 397-7

A. Cerebral infarction
B. Cocaine
C. Pregnancy
D. Hypothyroidism

Precipitating events in DKA are inadequate insulin administration, infection, infarction (cerebral, coronary, mesenteric, peripheral), cocaine & pregnancy.

1863. Nitroprusside reaction does not detect which of the following?
Harrison's 20th Ed. Chapter 397 Page 2871

A. Acetoacetate
B. Acetone
C. Beta-hydroxybutyrate
D. All of the above

Acetoacetate is preferentially detected by the commonly used nitroprusside ketosis detection reagent. Nitroprusside reaction only detects acetoacetate and acetone and not beta-hydroxybutyrate.

1864. Which of the following drug may cause false-positive reactions in the nitroprusside test used to detect urine ketones?
Harrison's 20th Ed. Chapter 397 Page 2871

A. Captopril
B. Atorvastatin
C. Aspirin
D. All of the above

1865. Which of the following drug may cause false-positive reactions in the nitroprusside test used to detect urine ketones?
Harrison's 20th Ed. Chapter 397 Page 2871

A. Penicillamine
B. Azithromycin
C. Cephalosporin
D. All of the above

Captopril or penicillamine may cause false-positive nitroprusside test used to detect urine ketones.

1866. In DKA, fluid deficit is?
Harrison's 20th Ed. Chapter 397 Page 2871

A. 1–2 Liters
B. 2–3 Liters
C. 3–5 Liters
D. 5–7 Liters

In DKA, fluid deficit is 3–5 Liters.

1867. Which of the following intravenous solution is preferred for initial use in DKA to reduce hyperchloremia?
Harrison's 20th Ed. Chapter 397 Page 2871

A. 0.45% saline
B. Normal saline
C. Lactated Ringer's IV solution
D. Any of the above

Initial use of lactated Ringer's IV solution reduces hyperchloremia that occurs with normal saline.

1868. In DKA, IV short-acting regular insulin is begun in the dose of?
Harrison's 20th Ed. Chapter 397 Page 2871

A. 0.01 units/kg per hour
B. 0.05 units/kg per hour
C. 0.1 units/kg per hour
D. 0.15 units/kg per hour

After an initial bolus of IV (0.1 units/kg) short-acting regular insulin, 0.1 units/kg of regular insulin per hour must be continued till acidosis resolves and the patient is metabolically stable. Then, the insulin infusion rate can be decreased to 0.02–0.1 units/kg per hour.

1869. In DKA, with insulin therapy, hyperglycemia improves due to?
Harrison's 20th Ed. Chapter 397 Page 2871

A. Insulin-mediated glucose disposal
B. Reduced hepatic glucose release
C. Rehydration
D. All of the above

Hyperglycemia usually improves at a rate of 50 to 100 mg/dL per hour as a result of insulin-mediated glucose disposal, reduced hepatic glucose release, and rehydration.

1870. In DKA, following insulin therapy, the decline in plasma glucose within the first 1 to 2 hours is mostly related to?
Harrison's 20th Ed. Chapter 397 Page 2872

A. Insulin-mediated glucose disposal
B. Reduced hepatic glucose release
C. Volume expansion
D. All of the above

The decline in the plasma glucose within the first 1 to 2 hours may be more rapid and is mostly related to volume expansion.

1871. With insulin, ketoacidosis resolves due to?
Harrison's 20th Ed. Chapter 397 Page 2872

A. Increased peripheral ketone body use
B. Suppression of hepatic ketone body formation
C. Bicarbonate regeneration
D. All of the above

With insulin, ketoacidosis begins to resolve due to reduced lipolysis, increased peripheral ketone body use, suppression of hepatic ketone body formation, and increased bicarbonate regeneration.

1872. With insulin therapy in DKA, which of the following resolves faster?
Harrison's 20th Ed. Chapter 397 Page 2872

A. Acidosis
B. Ketosis
C. Hyperglycemia
D. All of the above

In DKA, following insulin therapy, acidosis and ketosis resolve more slowly than hyperglycemia.

1873. Which of the following statements is false?
Harrison's 20th Ed. Chapter 397 Page 2872

A. As ketoacidosis improves, β-hydroxybutyrate is converted to acetoacetate
B. Ketone levels increase in nitroprusside reaction
C. Hyperchloremic acidosis follows successful treatment
D. None of the above

1874. Estimated deficit of potassium stores in DKA is?
Harrison's 20th Ed. Chapter 397 Page 2872

A. 1–3 meq/kg
B. 3–5 meq/kg
C. 5–7 meq/kg
D. 7–9 meq/kg

Estimated deficit of potassium stores in DKA is 3–5 meq/kg.

1875. In DKA, treatment with insulin & fluids may lead to hypokalemia due to?

Harrison's 20th Ed. Chapter 397 Page 2872

A. Insulin-mediated potassium transport into cells
B. Correction of acidosis promotes potassium entry into cells
C. Urinary loss of potassium salts of organic acids
D. All of the above

1876. In DKA, which salt of potassium should be avoided for replacement?

Harrison's 20th Ed. Chapter 397 Page 2872

A. Chloride
B. Phosphate
C. Acetate
D. Any of the above

To reduce the amount of chloride administered, potassium phosphate or acetate can be substituted for the chloride salt.

1877. In DKA, bicarbonate replacement is avoided because rapid reversal of acidosis may?

Harrison's 20th Ed. Chapter 397 Page 2872

A. Impair cardiac function
B. Reduce tissue oxygenation
C. Promote hypokalemia
D. All of the above

In DKA, bicarbonate use increases risk of cerebral edema.

1878. Which of the following may develop in DKA?

Harrison's 20th Ed. Chapter 397 Page 2872

A. Hypokalemia
B. Hypophosphatemia
C. Hypomagnesemia
D. All of the above

1879. In DKA, insulin should not be administered until potassium level is?

Harrison's 20th Ed. Chapter 397 Page 2871 Table 397-8

A. > 3.0 meq/L
B. > 3.1 meq/L
C. > 3.2 meq/L
D. > 3.3 meq/L

In DKA, insulin should not be administered until potassium level is >3.3 meq/L.

1880. During treatment of DKA, very large changes occur in the serum levels of all except?

Harrison's 20th Ed. Chapter 397 Page 2871 Table 397-8

A. Sodium
B. Potassium
C. Chloride
D. Magnesium

1881. Total-body stores which of the following elements is not reduced in DKA?

Harrison's 20th Ed. Chapter 397 Page 2871 Table 397-8

A. Sodium
B. Chloride
C. Calcium
D. Magnesium

Total-body stores of sodium, potassium, chloride, phosphorous & magnesium are reduced in DKA.

1882. In treatment of DKA, glucose should be added to 0.45% saline infusion when plasma glucose level is around?

Harrison's 20th Ed. Chapter 397 Page 2871 Table 397-8

A. 100 mg/dL
B. 150 mg/dL
C. 200 mg/dL
D. 250 mg/dL

When plasma glucose reaches 250 mg/dL, glucose should be added to 0.45% saline infusion to maintain plasma glucose in 200 to 250 mg/dL range & insulin infusion should be continued.

1883. In hyperglycemic hyperosmolar state (HHS), the blood glucose level is usually above?

Harrison's 20th Ed. Chapter 397 Page 2870 Table 397-6

A. 300 mg%
B. 400 mg%
C. 500 mg%
D. 600 mg%

The most notable laboratory features in HHS are marked hyperglycemia, hyperosmolality and prerenal azotemia.

1884. All are features of hyperglycemic hyperosmolar state except?

Harrison's 20th Ed. Chapter 397 Page 2870 Table 397-6

A. Normal Na^+, K^+, Cl^-
B. Glucose between 600–1200 mg%
C. Normal PCO_2
D. pH < 7.3

In contrast to DKA, acidosis and ketonemia are absent or mild.

1885. Which of the following symptom is absent in HHS?

Harrison's 20th Ed. Chapter 397 Page 2872

A. Nausea, vomiting
B. Abdominal pain
C. Kussmaul respiration
D. All of the above

In HHS, nausea, vomiting, abdominal pain & Kussmaul respirations, characteristic of DKA, are absent.

1886. As compared to DKA, lower levels of which of the following is found in HHS?

Harrison's 20th Ed. Chapter 397 Page 2872

A. Counter-regulatory hormones
B. Free fatty acids
C. Ketone bodies
D. All of the above

The absence of ketosis in HHS is not understood.

1887. In HHS, moderate ketonuria, if present, is secondary to?
Harrison's 20th Ed. Chapter 397 Page 2872

A. Starvation
B. Infection
C. Oliguria
D. All of the above

In HHS, moderate ketonuria, if present, is secondary to starvation.

1888. Which of the following statements is false?
Harrison's 20th Ed. Chapter 397 Page 2872

A. Dehydration in HHS > DKA
B. HHS patient is usually young
C. Mortality higher in HHS than DKA
D. HHS patient have more mental status changes than DKA

Typical patient of HHS is an elderly type 2 DM individual, with a several week history of polyuria, weight loss & diminished oral intake that culminates in mental confusion, lethargy, or coma. In HHS, fluid losses & dehydration are more pronounced than in DKA. HHS has a substantially higher mortality than DKA.

1889. In HHS, the calculated free water deficit averages?
Harrison's 20th Ed. Chapter 397 Page 2872

A. 3–4 Liters
B. 4–6 Liters
C. 6–8 Liters
D. 9–10 Liters

In HHS, the calculated free water deficit averages 9–10 Liters which should be reversed over the next 1–2 days.

1890. Which of the following statements is false?
Harrison's 20th Ed. Chapter 397 Page 2874

A. Total parenteral nutrition increases insulin requirements
B. Glucocorticoids increase insulin resistance
C. Pregnancy is associated with marked insulin resistance
D. None of the above

1891. Glucocorticoids produce hyperglycemia due to?
Harrison's 20th Ed. Chapter 397 Page 2874

A. Decreased glucose utilization
B. Increase hepatic glucose production
C. Impaired insulin secretion
D. All of the above

Glucocorticoids increase insulin resistance, decrease glucose utilization, increase hepatic glucose production, and impair insulin secretion.

1892. Which of the following about steroid-induced diabetes is false?
Harrison's 20th Ed. Chapter 397 Page 2874

A. Dose-related
B. Reversible
C. Most pronounced in the postprandial period
D. None of the above

1893. Which of the following statements is false?
Harrison's 20th Ed. Chapter 397 Page 2874

A. HbA1c target in pregnancy is < 6.5%
B. High glucose levels are teratogenic to fetus
C. Insulin crosses placenta
D. Macrosomia is due to anabolic effects of insulin

Pregnancy is associated with marked insulin resistance. Glucose at high levels is a teratogen to developing fetus, readily crosses placenta. Insulin does not cross placenta. Anabolic & growth effects of insulin results in macrosomia.

1894. Gestational diabetes mellitus (GDM) occurs in what percentage of pregnancies?
Harrison's 20th Ed. Chapter 397 Page 2874

A. 2%
B. 4%
C. 5%
D. 7%

Gestational diabetes occurs in approximately 7% of pregnancies.

1895. Newborns of pregnant women with gestational diabetes are at increased risk of?
Harrison's 20th Ed. Chapter 397 Page 2874

A. Hypoglycemia
B. Hyperbilirubinemia
C. Polycythemia
D. All of the above

Pregnant women with gestational diabetes are at increased risk of stillbirth, preeclampsia and delivery of infants who are large for their gestational age with resulting birth lacerations, shoulder dystocia, and birth trauma including brachial plexus injury. These fetuses are at risk of hypoglycemia, hyperbilirubinemia and polycythemia.

1896. In women with high risk of GDM, screening for glucose intolerance must be done between?
Harrison's 20th Ed. Chapter 397 Page 2874

A. 3 & 12 weeks of pregnancy
B. 12 & 24 weeks of pregnancy
C. 24 & 28 weeks of pregnancy
D. 28 & 36 weeks of pregnancy

Current recommendations advise screening for glucose intolerance between weeks 24 and 28 of pregnancy in women with high risk for GDM.

1897. Most crucial period of glycemic control during pregnancy is?
Harrison's 20th Ed. Chapter 397 Page 2874

A. Soon after fertilization
B. Around 3 months
C. Around 7 months
D. Intrapartum

Most crucial period of glycemic control is soon after fertilization. The risk of fetal malformations is increased 4 to 10 times in individuals with uncontrolled DM at the time of conception.

1898. Gestational diabetes is best treated with?
Harrison's 20th Ed. Chapter 397 Page 2874

A. Insulin
B. Metformin
C. Sulfonylurea
D. Any of the above

Therapy for GDM involves MNT & insulin, if hyperglycemia persists. Oral glucose-lowering agents have not been approved for use during pregnancy. More data on safety & efficacy of glyburide for management of gestational diabetes are needed before it supplants insulin as treatment agent of choice.

1899. Which of the following statements is false?
Harrison's 20th Ed. Chapter 466 Page 3442

A. Women are more sensitive to insulin than men
B. Prevalence of type 2 DM is similar in men & women
C. Women with DM have a greater risk for MI than men
D. Women with DM have less LVH than men

1900. Supplementation of which of the following in pregnancy with diabetes mellitus reduces risk of fetal neural tube defects?
Harrison's 20th Ed. Chapter 466 Page 3442

A. Iron
B. Calcium
C. Folate
D. Vitamin B12

Folate supplementation reduces the incidence of fetal neural tube defects, which occur with greater frequency in fetuses of diabetic mothers.

1901. Leprechaunism is related to?
Harrison's 20th Ed. Chapter 397 Page 2875

A. General anesthesia
B. Lipodystrophy
C. Bulimia
D. All of the above

Lipodystrophy, or the loss of subcutaneous fat tissue, may be generalized in the genetic condition leprechaunism.

1902. Generalized lipodystrophy is associated with deficiency of?
Harrison's 20th Ed. Chapter 397 Page 2875

A. Leptin
B. Ghrelin
C. Neuropeptide Y
D. All of the above

1903. Generalized lipodystrophy is accompanied by?
Harrison's 20th Ed. Chapter 397 Page 2875

A. Acanthosis nigricans
B. Hepatic steatosis
C. Severe hypertriglyceridemia
D. All of the above

Generalized lipodystrophy is associated with leptin deficiency and severe insulin resistance and is accompanied by acanthosis nigricans, hepatic steatosis, and severe hypertriglyceridemia.

Diabetes Mellitus: Complications

1904. Which of the following investigated effects of multifactorial risk-factor control in T2DM?

N Engl J Med 2018;379:633-44

A. Steno-1 Study
B. Steno-2 Study
C. Steno-3 Study
D. Steno-4 Study

The Steno-2 Study investigated effects of multifactorial risk-factor control and showed long-lasting reductions in risks of death and cardiovascular events among T2DM patients in whom these risks were reduced. The risk factors considered to be the strongest predictors for cardiovascular outcomes and death include low physical activity, smoking, and glycated hemoglobin, systolic blood-pressure, and LDL cholesterol levels outside target ranges.

1905. Which of the following is a microvascular chronic complication of DM?

Harrison's 20th Ed. Chapter 398 Page 2875 Table 398-1

A. Macular edema
B. Glaucoma
C. Cataracts
D. Periodontal disease

Macular edema is a microvascular chronic complication of diabetes mellitus.

1906. Which of the following is not a diabetes-specific complication?

Harrison's 20th Ed. Chapter 398 Page 2875

A. Retinopathy
B. Neuropathy
C. Nephropathy
D. Coronary heart disease

Microvascular complications (retinopathy, neuropathy, nephropathy) are diabetes-specific whereas macrovascular complications (coronary heart disease, peripheral arterial disease, cerebrovascular disease) are similar to those in nondiabetics but occur at greater frequency in individuals with diabetes.

1907. Which of the following is a macrovascular complication of diabetes?

Harrison's 20th Ed. Chapter 398 Page 2875

A. Coronary heart disease (CHD)
B. Peripheral arterial disease (PAD)
C. Cerebrovascular disease
D. All of the above

1908. Which of the following is a nonvascular complication of diabetes?

Harrison's 20th Ed. Chapter 398 Page 2875

A. Infections
B. Skin changes
C. Hearing loss
D. All of the above

Nonvascular complications of DM include infections, skin changes, and hearing loss.

1909. Which of the following is a complication of diabetes?

Harrison's 20th Ed. Chapter 398 Page 2875

A. Pachydermoperiostosis
B. Cheiroarthropathy
C. Spondyloarthropathy
D. Jaccoud's arthropathy

Cheiroarthropathy refers to thickened skin & reduced joint mobility.

1910. Coronary heart disease (CHD) & mortality rate are how many times greater in patients with type 2 DM?

Harrison's 20th Ed. Chapter 398 Page 2875

A. 1–2 times
B. 2–4 times
C. 4–6 times
D. 6–8 times

CHD events and mortality rate are two to four times greater in patients with type 2 DM.

1911. CHD & mortality rate in T2DM correlate with?

Harrison's 20th Ed. Chapter 398 Page 2875

A. Fasting plasma glucose levels
B. Postprandial plasma glucose levels
C. Hemoglobin A1c (HbA1c)
D. All of the above

CHD events and mortality rate in patients with type 2 DM correlate with fasting & postprandial plasma glucose levels as well the hemoglobin A1c (HbA1c).

1912. The redox potential is zero for?

J Am Chem Soc. 2008 Mar 19; 130(11): 3371–81

A. Oxygen
B. Hydrogen
C. Nitrogen
D. Helium

The redox potential is a measure (in volts) of the affinity of a substance for electrons, its electro-negativity compared with hydrogen (which is set at 0).

1913. In the Diabetes Control and Complications Trial (DCCT), which of the following complication showed maximum reduction with improved glycemic control?

Harrison's 20th Ed. Chapter 398 Page 2876

A. Retinopathy
B. Microalbuminuria
C. Clinical nephropathy
D. Neuropathy

DCCT demonstrated that improvement of glycemic control reduced nonproliferative & proliferative retinopathy (47%), microalbuminuria (39%), clinical nephropathy (54%) & neuropathy (60%).

1914. Which of the following complications of diabetes did not reduce after intensive therapy in DCCT + EDIC trial?

Harrison's 20th Ed. Chapter 398 Page 2876

A. Autonomic neuropathy
B. Bladder and sexual dysfunction
C. Cardiac autonomic neuropathy
D. Cognitive function

In the intensive therapy group, difference in cognitive function was not observed either during the DCCT phase or during follow-up EDIC phase. autonomic neuropathy, bladder and sexual dysfunction, and cardiac autonomic neuropathy were reduced.

1915. Which of the following trial was not for the study of chronic complications of diabetes mellitus?

Harrison's 20th Ed. Chapter 398 Page 2876

A. Diabetes Control and Complications Trial (DCCT)
B. Tuskegee Study
C. Kumamoto study
D. United Kingdom Prospective Diabetes Study (UKPDS)

Tuskegee Study (1932–1972) was a prospective study of 431 African-American men with seropositive latent syphilis of >3 years' duration.

1916. UKPDS results show that with each % point reduction in HbA1c, there is reduction in T2DM microvascular complications of?

Harrison's 20th Ed. Chapter 398 Page 2876

A. 13%
B. 23%
C. 35%
D. 52%

The UKPDS demonstrated that each percentage point reduction in HbA1c was associated with a 35% reduction in T2DM microvascular complications.

1917. Positive impact of a period of improved glycemic control on CVD is termed as?

Harrison's 20th Ed. Chapter 398 Page 2876

A. Bequest effect
B. Legacy effect
C. Patrimony effect
D. Heritage effect

1918. Positive impact of a period of improved glycemic control on CVD is termed as?

Harrison's 20th Ed. Chapter 398 Page 2876

A. Amalgam memory
B. Conflation memory
C. Blend memory
D. Metabolic memory

The positive impact of a period of improved glycemic control on CVD is termed a legacy effect or metabolic memory.

1919. Which of the following statements about diabetes-related complications is false?

Harrison's 20th Ed. Chapter 398 Page 2876

A. Duration & degree of hyperglycemia correlate with complication
B. Blood pressure control is critical, especially in type 2 DM
C. Not all DM individuals develop diabetes-related complications
D. None of the above

1920. Which of the following statements about diabetes-related complications is false?

Harrison's 20th Ed. Chapter 398 Page 2876

A. Genetic susceptibility essential for developing retinopathy
B. Genetic susceptibility essential for developing nephropathy
C. Intensive glycemic control is beneficial in all forms of DM
D. None of the above

1921. Hyperglycemia influences gene expression through?

Harrison's 20th Ed. Chapter 398 Page 2876

A. Somatic mutations
B. Epigenetic changes
C. Mosaicism
D. Insertions and deletions

Hyperglycemia leads to epigenetic changes that influence gene expression in affected cells.

1922. Which of the following is effect of hyperglycemia?

Harrison's 20th Ed. Chapter 398 Page 2876

A. Increases glucose metabolism via the sorbitol pathway
B. Increases formation of diacylglycerol & PKC activation
C. Increases the flux through hexosamine pathway
D. All of the above

1923. "AGE" stands for?

Harrison's 20th Ed. Chapter 398 Page 2876

A. Activated glycosylation end products
B. Anti glycosylation end products
C. Advanced glycosylation end products
D. Associated glycosylation end products

Increased intracellular glucose leads to the formation of advanced glycosylation end products (AGEs) via the nonenzymatic glycosylaton of intra- and extracellular proteins.

1924. Which of the following is an advanced glycosylation end product?

Harrison's 20th Ed. Chapter 398 Page 2876

A. Pentosidine
B. Glucosepane
C. Carboxymethyllysine
D. All of the above

Chronic hyperglycemia leads to formation of advanced glycosylation end products (AGEs) like pentosidine, glucosepane, and carboxymethyllysine.

1925. Intracellular glucose is converted to sorbitol by which enzyme?

Harrison's 20th Ed. Chapter 398 Page 2877

A. Aldose reductase
B. Phosphofructokinase
C. Fructose-1,6-bisphosphatase
D. Phosphoenolpyruvate carboxykinase

Intracellular glucose is predominantly metabolized by phosphorylation and subsequent glycolysis, but when increased, some glucose is converted to sorbitol by the enzyme aldose reductase (polyol pathway).

1926. Which of the following vascular endothelial growth factor is increased locally in diabetic proliferative retinopathy?

Harrison's 20th Ed. Chapter 398 Page 2877

A. VEGF-A
B. VEGF-C
C. VEGF-D
D. All of the above

Growth factor vascular endothelial growth factor A (VEGF-A) is increased locally in diabetic proliferative retinopathy.

1927. In T2DM, which of the following accumulate in tissues?
Harrison's 20th Ed. Chapter 398 Page 2877

A. Triglycerides
B. Diacylglycerol
C. Ceramides
D. All of the above

1928. Individuals with DM are how much more likely to become legally blind than individuals without DM?
Harrison's 20th Ed. Chapter 398 Page 2877

A. 5 times
B. 10 times
C. 15 times
D. 25 times

Individuals with DM are 25 times more likely to become legally blind than individuals without DM.

1929. Which of the following is a feature of nonproliferative diabetic retinopathy?
Harrison's 20th Ed. Chapter 398 Page 2877

A. Retinal vascular microaneurysms
B. Blot hemorrhages
C. Cotton-wool spots
D. All of the above

Nonproliferative diabetic retinopathy usually appears late in the first decade or early in the second decade of the disease and is marked by retinal vascular microaneurysms, blot hemorrhages and cotton-wool spots.

1930. Which of the following can lead to retinal ischemia?
Harrison's 20th Ed. Chapter 398 Page 2877

A. Loss of retinal pericytes
B. Increased retinal vascular permeability
C. Abnormal retinal microvasculature
D. All of the above

The pathophysiologic mechanisms in nonproliferative retinopathy include loss of retinal pericytes, increased retinal vascular permeability, alterations in retinal blood flow, and abnormal retinal microvasculature, all of which can lead to retinal ischemia.

1931. Which of the following is the hallmark of "proliferative" diabetic retinopathy?
Harrison's 20th Ed. Chapter 398 Page 2877

A. Retinal vascular microaneurysms
B. Blot hemorrhages
C. Neovascularization
D. Cotton wool spots

1932. Neovascularization in proliferative diabetic retinopathy occurs in response to?
Harrison's 20th Ed. Chapter 398 Page 2877

A. Hyperglycemia
B. Ketoacidosis
C. Hyperlipidemia
D. Retinal hypoxemia

Appearance of neovascularization in response to retinal hypoxia is the hallmark of proliferative diabetic retinopathy.

1933. Which of the following is false about neovascular vessels in diabetic retinopathy?
Harrison's 20th Ed. Chapter 398 Page 2877

A. Appear near the optic nerve and/or macula
B. Rupture easily leading to vitreous hemorrhage
C. Not all nonproliferative retinopathy go on to develop proliferative retinopathy
D. None of the above

1934. Individuals who have had DM for >20 years, what is the probability of detecting nonproliferative retinopathy?
Harrison's 20th Ed. Chapter 398 Page 2877

A. 25%
B. 50%
C. 75%
D. 100%

Nonproliferative retinopathy is found in almost all individuals who have had DM for >20 years.

1935. The earliest clinical signs of diabetic retinopathy is?
N Engl J Med 2004;350:48-58

A. Dot intraretinal hemorrhages
B. Cotton-wool spots
C. Neovascular glaucoma
D. Diabetic macular edema

1936. Lesion that occurs early in histopathology of diabetic retinopathy is?
N Engl J Med 2004;350:48-58

A. Selective loss of pericytes from retinal capillaries
B. Loss of capillary endothelial cells
C. Proliferation of capillary endothelial cells
D. None of the above

The pathophysiologic mechanisms invoked in nonproliferative retinopathy include loss of retinal pericytes, increased retinal vascular permeability, alterations in retinal blood flow and abnormal retinal microvasculatur. All of these lead to retinal ischemia.

1937. During the first 6 to 12 months of improved glycemic control, established diabetic retinopathy?
Harrison's 20th Ed. Chapter 398 Page 2877

A. Improves
B. Remains the same
C. Worsens
D. Any of the above

During the first 6 to 12 months of improved glycemic control, established diabetic retinopathy may transiently worsen.

1938. Which of the following reduces the progression of diabetic retinopathy?
Harrison's 20th Ed. Chapter 398 Page 2877

A. Aspirin
B. Fenofibrate
C. Omega-3 fatty acids
D. All of the above

Fenofibrate reduces the progression of diabetic retinopathy.

1939. Which of the following is considered as gold standard therapy for proliferative diabetic retinopathy (PDR)?

Harrison's 20th Ed. Chapter 398 Page 2877

A. Laser photocoagulation
B. Anti-VEGF therapy
C. triamcinolone acetonide (IVTA)
D. Intravitreal Microplasmin

Laser photocoagulation is considered gold standard therapy for PDR with anti-VEGF agents used as its adjunct treatment to reduce the adverse effects.

1940. Which of the following is an Anti-VEGF agent?

Journal of Ophthalmology. 2018, Article ID 1694187

A. Ranibizumab
B. Bevacizumab
C. Aflibercept
D. All of the above

1941. Individuals with diabetic nephropathy commonly have which of the following?

Harrison's 20th Ed. Chapter 398 Page 2878

A. Diabetic retinopathy
B. Diabetic neuropathy
C. Diabetic dermopathy
D. All of the above

Individuals with diabetic nephropathy commonly have diabetic retinopathy.

1942. Which of the following soluble factors is involved in the pathogenesis of diabetic nephropathy?

Harrison's 20th Ed. Chapter 398 Page 2878

A. Angiotensin II
B. Endothelin
C. Advanced glycation end products (AGEs)
D. All of the above

Chronic hyperglycemia leads to diabetic nephropathy, and the soluble factors involved are growth factors, angiotensin II, endothelin, advanced glycation end products [AGEs].

1943. Which of the following hemodynamic alterations in renal microcirculation leads to diabetic nephropathy?

Harrison's 20th Ed. Chapter 398 Page 2878

A. Glomerular hyperfiltration
B. Glomerular hyperperfusion
C. Increased glomerular capillary pressure
D. All of the above

Chronic hyperglycemia leads to diabetic nephropathy, and the hemodynamic alterations in renal microcirculation involved are glomerular hyperfiltration or hyperperfusion, increased glomerular capillary pressure.

1944. Which of the following structural changes in the glomerulus leads to diabetic nephropathy?

Harrison's 20th Ed. Chapter 398 Page 2878

A. Increased extracellular matrix
B. Basement membrane thickening
C. Mesangial expansion
D. All of the above

Chronic hyperglycemia leads to diabetic nephropathy, and the structural changes in the glomerulus involved are increased extracellular matrix, basement membrane thickening, mesangial expansion & fibrosis.

1945. Which of the following accelerates the decline in renal function in individuals with diabetic nephropathy?

Harrison's 20th Ed. Chapter 398 Page 2878

A. Alcohol
B. Smoking
C. Emotional stress
D. All of the above

Smoking accelerates the decline in renal function in individuals with diabetic nephropathy.

1946. What percentage of patients with diabetes develop diabetic nephropathy?

Harrison's 20th Ed. Chapter 398 Page 2878

A. 5–10%
B. 10–20%
C. 20–40%
D. 40–60%

20 - 40% of patients with diabetes develop diabetic nephropathy.

1947. Diabetic kidney disease refers to albuminuria and reduced GFR of?

Harrison's 20th Ed. Chapter 398 Page 2878

A. < 90 mL/min/1.73 m^2
B. < 60 mL/min/1.73 m^2
C. < 30 mL/min/1.73 m^2
D. < 15 mL/min/1.73 m^2

Diabetic kidney disease refers to albuminuria and reduced GFR (<60 mL/min/1.73 m^2).

1948. Once marked albuminuria and reduction in GFR occurs, which of the following pathologic changes is reversible?

Harrison's 20th Ed. Chapter 398 Page 2878

A. Thickening of the glomerular basement membrane
B. Glomerular hypertrophy
C. Mesangial volume expansion
D. None of the above

In diabetic nephropathy, once there is marked albuminuria and a reduction in GFR, the pathologic changes are irreversible.

1949. Which of the following is false about T2DM?

Harrison's 20th Ed. Chapter 398 Page 2878

A. Albuminuria may be present when T2DM is diagnosed
B. Albuminuria less predictive of diabetic kidney disease
C. Hypertension more commonly accompanies albuminuria
D. None of the above

Screening for albuminuria should commence 5 years after the onset of type 1 DM and then annually, and at the time of diagnosis of type 2 DM.

1950. Screening for albuminuria annually should be performed in?

Harrison's 20th Ed. Chapter 398 Page 2878 Figure 398-4

A. Type 1 diabetes of ≥ 5 years
B. In patients with type 2 diabetes
C. During pregnancy
D. All of the above

Screening for microalbuminuria should be performed in patients with type 1 diabetes for >=5 years, in patients with type 2 diabetes and during pregnancy.

1951. Non-diabetes-related condition that may increase / cause albuminuria is?
Harrison's 20th Ed. Chapter 398 Page 2878 Figure 398-4

A. Severe hyperglycemia
B. Severe hypertension
C. Vigorous exercise
D. All of the above

1952. Non-diabetes-related condition that may increase / cause albuminuria is?
Harrison's 20th Ed. Chapter 398 Page 2878 Figure 398-4

A. Urinary tract infection
B. Hematuria
C. Heart failure
D. All of the above

Nondiabetes-related conditions that might increase / cause albuminuria are urinary tract infection, hematuria, heart failure, febrile illness, severe hyperglycemia, severe hypertension, and vigorous exercise.

1953. Which of the following renal tubular acidosis may occur in type 1 or 2 DM?
Harrison's 20th Ed. Chapter 398 Page 2878

A. Type I
B. Type II
C. Type III
D. Type IV

Type IV renal tubular acidosis (hyporeninemic hypoaldosteronism) may occur in type 1 or 2 DM.

1954. In a 24 hour collected urine sample, microalbuminuria is defined as?
Harrison's 20th Ed. Chapter 398 Page 2878

A. 10 to 100 mg/day
B. 20 to 200 mg/day
C. 30 to 299 mg/day
D. 40 to 400 mg/day

1955. In a spot urine collection, microalbuminuria is defined as?
Harrison's 20th Ed. Chapter 398 Page 2878

A. 10 to 100 μg/mg creatinine
B. 20 to 200 μg/mg creatinine
C. 30 to 299 μg/mg creatinine
D. 40 to 400 μg/mg creatinine

Microalbuminuria is defined as 30 to 299 mg/day in a 24-hour collection or 30 to 299 μg/mg creatinine in a spot collection.

1956. Interventions effective in slowing progression from microalbuminuria to overt nephropathy include all except?
Harrison's 20th Ed. Chapter 398 Page 2878

A. Strict blood pressure control
B. Administration of ACE inhibitors or ARBs
C. Administration of beta blockers
D. Treatment of dyslipidemia

Interventions effective in slowing progression from microalbuminuria to overt nephropathy include near normalization of glycemia, strict blood pressure control, administration of ACE inhibitors or ARBs and treatment of dyslipidemia.

1957. In type 1 DM, preferred drug for blood pressure control is?
Harrison's 20th Ed. Chapter 398 Page 2879

A. ACE inhibitors
B. ARBs
C. Beta blockers
D. Calcium channel blockers

1958. In type 2 DM, preferred drug for blood pressure control is?
Harrison's 20th Ed. Chapter 398 Page 2879

A. Diuretics
B. ARBs
C. Beta blockers
D. Calcium channel blockers

Drug-specific benefit in diabetic nephropathy, independent of blood pressure control, has been shown for ACE inhibitors in type 1 DM and ARBs in type 2 DM. ACE inhibitors (in types 1 and 2 DM) and ARBs (in type 2 DM) slow the progression of diabetic renal disease.

1959. The ADA suggests what quantity of protein intake in individuals with diabetic kidney disease?
Harrison's 20th Ed. Chapter 398 Page 2879

A. 0.6 mg/kg of body weight/day
B. 0.8 mg/kg of body weight/day
C. 1.0 mg/kg of body weight/day
D. 1.2 mg/kg of body weight/day

ADA suggests a protein intake of 0.8 mg/kg of body weight/day in individuals with diabetic kidney disease.

1960. Leading cause of death in diabetic individuals on dialysis is?
Harrison's 20th Ed. Chapter 398 Page 2879

A. Atherosclerosis
B. Infection
C. Dyselectrolytemia
D. Suicide

Atherosclerosis is the leading cause of death in diabetic individuals on dialysis.

1961. In diabetic nephropathy, referral for transplant evaluation should be made when GFR approaches?
Harrison's 20th Ed. Chapter 398 Page 2879

A. 10 mL/min per 1.73 m^2
B. 20 mL/min per 1.73 m^2
C. 30 mL/min per 1.73 m^2
D. 40 mL/min per 1.73 m^2

Referral for transplant evaluation should be made when the GFR approaches 20 mL/min per 1.73 m^2.

1962. Diabetic neuropathy occurs in what percentage of individuals with long-standing type 1 and type 2 DM?
Harrison's 20th Ed. Chapter 398 Page 2879

A. ~ 25%
B. ~ 50%
C. ~ 75%
D. ~ 100%

Diabetic neuropathy occurs in ~50% of individuals with long-standing type 1 and type 2 DM.

1963. Diabetic neuropathy manifests as?
Harrison's 20th Ed. Chapter 398 Page 2879

A. Diffuse neuropathy
B. Mononeuropathy
C. Radiculopathy / polyradiculopathy
D. Any of the above

1964. Which of the following is also associated with diabetic peripheral neuropathy?
Harrison's 20th Ed. Chapter 398 Page 2879

A. CVD
B. Hypertension
C. Elevated triglycerides
D. All of the above

1965. Which of the following is a risk factor for diabetic neuropathy?
Harrison's 20th Ed. Chapter 398 Page 2879

A. Age
B. Body mass index (BMI)
C. Race
D. All of the above

Apart from duration of diabetes and glycemic control, additional risk factors for diabetic neuropathy are body mass index (BMI) and smoking.

1966. Which of the following nerve fibers are lost in diabetic neuropathy?
Harrison's 20th Ed. Chapter 398 Page 2879

A. Myelinated
B. Unmyelinated
C. Myelinated + unmyelinated
D. All of the above

Both myelinated and unmyelinated nerve fibers are lost in diabetic neuropathy.

1967. The most common form of diabetic neuropathy is?
Harrison's 20th Ed. Chapter 398 Page 2879

A. Distal symmetric polyneuropathy
B. Diabetic polyradiculopathy
C. Mononeuropathy
D. Mononeuropathy multiplex

The most common form of diabetic neuropathy is distal symmetric polyneuropathy (DSPN).

1968. Which of the following about pain of DSPN is false?
Harrison's 20th Ed. Chapter 398 Page 2879

A. Typically involves the lower extremities
B. Present at rest
C. Worsens at night
D. None of the above

1969. Painful diabetic neuropathy is called acute if the duration is?
Harrison's 20th Ed. Chapter 398 Page 2879

A. < 1 month
B. < 3 months
C. < 9 months
D. < 12 months

Acute (<12 months) form of painful diabetic neuropathy is sometimes treatment-related, occurring in the context of improved glycemic control.

1970. As diabetic neuropathy progresses, the pain?
Harrison's 20th Ed. Chapter 398 Page 2879

A. Decreases
B. Increases
C. Remains the same
D. Any of the above

As diabetic neuropathy progresses, the pain subsides & eventually disappears, but a sensory deficit persists and motor defects may develop.

1971. Which of the following is a feature of DSPN?
Harrison's 20th Ed. Chapter 398 Page 2879

A. Muscular atrophy or foot drop
B. Loss of ankle deep-tendon reflexes
C. Abnormal position sense
D. All of the above

In DSPN, physical examination often reveals proprioceptive sensory loss, loss of ankle deep-tendon reflexes, abnormal position sense, and muscular atrophy or foot drop.

1972. DM-related autonomic neuropathy involves which of the following?
Harrison's 20th Ed. Chapter 398 Page 2879

A. Cholinergic system
B. Noradrenergic system
C. Peptidergic system
D. All of the above

1973. Cardiovascular autonomic neuropathy, is reflected by?
Harrison's 20th Ed. Chapter 398 Page 2879

A. Decreased heart rate variability
B. Resting tachycardia
C. Orthostatic hypotension
D. All of the above

Cardiovascular autonomic neuropathy is reflected by decreased heart rate variability, resting tachycardia and orthostatic hypotension. It is associated with an increase in CVD.

1974. Which of the following is a feature of autonomic neuropathy?
Harrison's 20th Ed. Chapter 398 Page 2879

A. Hyperhidrosis of the upper extremities
B. Anhidrosis of lower extremities
C. Foot ulcers
D. All of the above

1975. Which of the following is due to autonomic neuropathy?
Harrison's 20th Ed. Chapter 398 Page 2879

A. Gastroparesis
B. Bladder-emptying abnormalities
C. Hypoglycemia unawareness
D. All of the above

1976. Involvement of which of the following cranial nerves is most common in DM?
Harrison's 20th Ed. Chapter 398 Page 2879

A. II
B. III
C. VI
D. VII

Involvement of the third cranial nerve is most common in DM and manifests as diplopia.

1977. Which of the following diabetic neuropathy is usually self-limited and resolve over 6–12 months?

Harrison's 20th Ed. Chapter 398 Page 2879

A. Autonomic neuropathy
B. Distal symmetric polyneuropathy (DSPN)
C. Mononeuropathy
D. Polyradiculopathy

Diabetic polyradiculopathies are usually self-limited and resolve over 6–12 months.

1978. Which of the following drug is used for pain associated with diabetic neuropathy?

Harrison's 20th Ed. Chapter 398 Page 2879

A. Venlafaxine
B. Duloxetine
C. Mirtazapine
D. Vortioxetine

Duloxetine & pregabalin have been approved by USFDA for pain associated with diabetic neuropathy.

1979. Which of the following is a centrally acting opioid?

Harrison's 20th Ed. Chapter 398 Page 2879

A. Alvimopan
B. Methylnaltrexone
C. Tapentadol
D. All of the above

Tapentadol is a FDA-approved centrally acting opioid useful in diabetic neuropathy, but not as a first line therapy due to addiction potential.

1980. Which of the following antiepileptic drug is useful in the treatment of chronic, painful diabetic neuropathy?

Harrison's 20th Ed. Chapter 398 Page 2880

A. Gabapentin
B. Venlafaxine
C. Carbamazepine
D. All of the above

Chronic, painful diabetic neuropathy may respond to duloxetine, pregabalin, tricyclic antidepressants, gabapentin, venlafaxine, carbamazepine, tramadol, and topical capsaicin.

1981. Which of the following drug is most useful in orthostatic hypotension due to diabetic autonomic neuropathy?

Harrison's 20th Ed. Chapter 398 Page 2880

A. Midodrine
B. Clonidine
C. Octreotide
D. All of the above

Orthostatic hypotension due to diabetic autonomic neuropathy may respond to midodrine and droxidopa.

1982. Dysfunction in which of the following is important in the development of gastroparesis?

Harrison's 20th Ed. Chapter 398 Page 2880

A. Parasympathetic
B. Sympathetic
C. Parasympathetic + sympathetic
D. Any of the above

Parasympathetic dysfunction secondary to chronic hyperglycemia is important in the development of gastroparesis.

1983. Which of the following is a feature of DM-related GI autonomic neuropathy?

Harrison's 20th Ed. Chapter 398 Page 2880

A. Postprandial abdominal bloating / early satiety
B. Nocturnal diarrhea alternating with constipation
C. Gastroparesis
D. All of the above

1984. Symptoms of diabetic cystopathy begin with?

Harrison's 20th Ed. Chapter 398 Page 2880

A. Inability to sense a full bladder & failure to void completely
B. Urinary hesitancy
C. Incontinence
D. Recurrent urinary tract infections.

Symptoms of diabetic cystopathy begin with an inability to sense a full bladder & failure to void completely. As bladder contractility worsens, bladder capacity & postvoid residual increase, leading to symptoms of urinary hesitancy, decreased voiding frequency, incontinence, and recurrent urinary tract infections.

1985. One of the earliest sign of diabetic neuropathy is?

Harrison's 20th Ed. Chapter 398 Page 2880

A. Erectile dysfunction
B. Gastroparesis
C. Anhidrosis of the lower extremities
D. Distal sensory loss

1986. Which of the following is very common in DM?

Harrison's 20th Ed. Chapter 398 Page 2880

A. Anorgasmia
B. Retrograde ejaculation
C. Painful ejaculation
D. Sperm-free ejaculation

Erectile dysfunction and retrograde ejaculation are very common in DM and may be one of the earliest signs of diabetic neuropathy.

1987. Which of the following may minimize symptoms of diabetic gastroparesis (DGp)?

Harrison's 20th Ed. Chapter 398 Page 2880

A. Smaller & more frequent meals
B. Low fat meal
C. Low fiber meal
D. All of the above

Diabetic gastroparesis is defined as delayed or disordered gastric emptying with associated upper gastrointestinal (GI) symptoms in the absence of any mechanical obstruction or ulceration. Smaller & more frequent meals, low in fat and fiber may minimize symptoms of gastroparesis.

1988. Which of the following medication slows gastric emptying?

Harrison's 20th Ed. Chapter 398 Page 2880

A. Biguanides
B. Sulphonylureas
C. GLP-1-receptor agonists
D. SGLT2 inhibitors

Opioids & GLP-1-receptor agonists slow gastric emptying. Amylin analog (pramlinitide) & calcineurin inhibitors also delay gastric emptying.

1989. Which of the following is considered in the differential diagnosis of diabetic gastroparesis (DGp)?

Diabetes Ther. 2018;9 (Suppl 1):S1-S42

A. Rumination syndrome
B. Anorexia nervosa and bulimia
C. Cyclic vomiting syndrome
D. All of the above

1990. Drugs that improve symptoms of gastroparesis in DM include all except?

Diabetes Ther. 2018;9 (Suppl 1):S1-S42

A. Domperidone
B. Loperamide
C. Metoclopramide
D. Erythromycin

Drugs that promote gastric emptying include dopamine agonists (metoclopramide, domperidone), bethanechol. Erythromycin interacts with motilin receptor and may promote gastric emptying. Diabetic diarrhea is treated symptomatically with loperamide and may respond to octreotide.

1991. Which of the following is increased in individuals with DM?

Harrison's 20th Ed. Chapter 398 Page 2880

A. Coronary artery disease
B. Cerebrovascular disease
C. Peripheral artery disease
D. All of the above

1992. Which of the following statements is correct for cardiovascular death rate among men and women in type 2 DM?

Harrison's 20th Ed. Chapter 398 Page 2880

A. More in men than women
B. More in women than men
C. Equal in men and women
D. Any of the above

After controlling for all known cardiovascular risk factors, type 2 DM increases the cardiovascular death rate twofold in men and fourfold in women.

1993. Elevated HbA1C is predictive of?

Harrison's 20th Ed. Chapter 398 Page 2880

A. Diabetes risk
B. CHD risk
C. Stroke risk
D. All of the above

Elevated HbA1C is predictive of diabetes risk, & also risk of CHD, stroke, and all-cause mortality.

1994. Which of the following glucose lowering therapy has cardiovascular benefit?

Harrison's 20th Ed. Chapter 398 Page 2880

A. Sitagliptin
B. Canagliflozin
C. Pramlintide
D. Rosiglitazone

1995. Which of the following glucose lowering therapy has cardiovascular benefit?

Harrison's 20th Ed. Chapter 398 Page 2880

A. Metformin
B. Acarbose
C. Mitiglinide
D. Liraglutide

Empagliflozin, canagliflozin and liraglutide reduce CVD events & all cause cardiovascular mortality in patients with type 2 DM and established CVD, the risk for nephropathy, and the rate of hospitalization for CHF.

1996. Most common pattern of dyslipidemia in DM is?

Harrison's 20th Ed. Chapter 398 Page 2881

A. Increased LDLc and reduced HDLc
B. Increased VLDLc and reduced HDLc
C. Increased LDLc and increased Tg
D. Increased Tg and reduced HDLc

Most common pattern of dyslipidemia is hypertriglyceridemia & reduced HDL cholesterol levels.

1997. Which of the following best relates to DM?

Harrison's 20th Ed. Chapter 398 Page 2881

A. Triglyceride-rich lipoproteins
B. Small dense LDL
C. Chylomicron remnants
D. All of the above

DM itself does not increase levels of low-density lipoprotein (LDL), but small dense LDL particles found in type 2 DM are more atherogenic because they are more easily glycated and susceptible to oxidation.

1998. In DM, if triglycerides remain high (>500 mg/dL), treatment with which of the following reduces the risk of pancreatitis?

Harrison's 20th Ed. Chapter 398 Page 2881

A. Egg yolks
B. Fish oil
C. Vitamin E
D. Selenium

In DM, if triglycerides remain high (>500 mg/dL), treatment with fish oil and fibrate drugs may reduce the risk of pancreatitis.

1999. Statin usage is associated with a mild increase in the risk of developing?

Harrison's 20th Ed. Chapter 398 Page 2881

A. Hypertension
B. Type 2 DM
C. Asthma
D. Gallstones

Statin usage is associated with a mild increase in the risk of developing type 2 DM.

2000. Which of the following is a PCSDK9 inhibitor?

Harrison's 20th Ed. Chapter 400 Page 2899 Table 400-5, World J Cardiol 2017;9(2):76-91

A. Abaloparatide
B. Denosumab
C. Evolocumab
D. Romosozumab

FDA approved two novel medications - Evolocumab and Alirocumab for low-density lipoprotein cholesterol reduction: . These agents target and inactivate proprotein convertase subtilsinkexin type 9 (PCSK9), a hepatic protease that attaches and internalizes LDL receptors into lysosomes hence promoting their destruction. By preventing LDL receptor destruction, LDL-C levels can be lowered 50–60% above that achieved by statin therapy alone.

2001. In the treatment of hypertriglyceridemia, which of the following should not be used?

Harrison's 20th Ed. Chapter 397 Page 2868

A. HMG CoA reductase inhibitors
B. Bile acid binding resins
C. Fibric acid derivative
D. All of the above

Bile acid binding resins should not be used if hypertriglyceridemia is present.

2002. Hypertension can accelerate which of the following complications of DM?

Harrison's 20th Ed. Chapter 398 Page 2881

A. Cardiovascular disease
B. Nephropathy
C. Retinopathy
D. All of the above

Hypertension can accelerate other complications of DM, particularly CVD, nephropathy, and retinopathy.

2003. All patients with diabetes and hypertension should be treated with?

Harrison's 20th Ed. Chapter 398 Page 2881

A. ACE inhibitor or ARB
B. Beta blockers
C. Thiazide diuretics
D. Calcium channel blockers

2004. In T2DM, when BP is not readily controlled, which of the following should be considered?

Harrison's 20th Ed. Chapter 398 Page 2881

A. Pheochromocytoma
B. Cushing's syndrome
C. Renovascular hypertension
D. All of the above

In T2DM, when BP is not readily controlled, possibility of renovascular hypertension should be considered.

2005. Which of the following structural changes in the foot occur in DM?

Harrison's 20th Ed. Chapter 398 Page 2881

A. Hammer toe
B. Claw toe deformity
C. Charcot joint
D. All of the above

Structural changes in the foot in DM can be hammer toe, claw toe deformity, prominent metatarsal heads, Charcot joint, callus & thickened nails.

2006. In T2DM, foot ulcer is most common at?

Harrison's 20th Ed. Chapter 398 Page 2881

A. Little toe
B. Metatarsophalangeal area
C. Distal phalanxes
D. Calcaneus

In T2DM foot ulcers are most common at great toe or metatarsophalangeal areas.

2007. In DM, risk factor for foot ulcers or amputation include all except?

Harrison's 20th Ed. Chapter 398 Page 2881

A. Female sex
B. Diabetes for >10 years
C. Visual impairment
D. Diabetic nephropathy

In DM, risk factors for foot ulcers or amputation include male sex, diabetes for >10 years, peripheral neuropathy, abnormal structure of foot, PAD, smoking, history of previous ulcer or amputation, visual impairment, poor glycemic control, and diabetic nephropathy, especially dialysis.

2008. All of the following drugs are glucose-neutral except?

Harrison's 20th Ed. Chapter 398 Page 2882

A. ACE inhibitors
B. Beta blockers
C. Calcium channel blockers
D. Central adrenergic antagonists

ACE inhibitors, calcium channel blockers, α-adrenergic blockers, central adrenergic antagonists & vasodilators are glucose- and lipid-neutral. β-blockers & thiazide diuretics increase insulin resistance.

2009. Which of the following infections occur almost exclusively in diabetics?

Harrison's 20th Ed. Chapter 398 Page 2882

A. Rhinocerebral mucormycosis
B. Emphysematous infections of gall bladder & urinary tract
C. "Malignant" or invasive otitis externa
D. All of the above

Rare infections like rhinocerebral mucormycosis, emphysematous infections of gall bladder & urinary tract, and "malignant" or invasive otitis externa (usually secondary to P. aeruginosa infection in the soft tissue surrounding the external auditory canal) are seen almost exclusively in diabetics.

2010. The most common skin manifestations of DM is?

Harrison's 20th Ed. Chapter 398 Page 2882

A. Xerosis
B. Lichenoid eruption
C. Poikiloderma
D. Milia

The most common skin manifestations of DM are xerosis and pruritus.

2011. Diabetic dermopathy is referred to as?

Harrison's 20th Ed. Chapter 398 Page 2882

A. Velvety plaques
B. Pigmented pretibial papules
C. Scleredema
D. Necrobiosis lipoidica diabeticorum

Diabetic dermopathy, also called pigmented pretibial papules, or "diabetic skin spots" begins as an erythematous macule or papule that evolves into an area of circular hyperpigmentation.

2012. Emphysematous pyelonephritis is most common in which of the following diseases?

Harrison's 20th Ed. Chapter 398 Page 2882

A. HIV
B. Diabetes
C. Tuberculosis
D. All of the above

Emphysematous pyelonephritis & cystitis almost always occur in diabetic patients, often with urinary obstruction & chronic infection.

2013. Which of the following occurs at increased frequency in individuals with type 1 DM?

Harrison's 20th Ed. Chapter 398 Page 2882

A. Vitiligo
B. Alopecia
C. Mucocutaneous candidiasis
D. All of the above

Vitiligo occurs at increased frequency in individuals with type 1 DM.

2014. Which of the following about acanthosis nigricans is false?

Harrison's 20th Ed. Chapter 398 Page 2882

A. Hyperpigmented velvety plaques
B. Seen on neck, axilla, or extensor surfaces
C. Feature of severe insulin resistance
D. None of the above

2015. Acanthosis nigricans diminishes with?

Harrison's 20th Ed. Chapter 394 Page 2843

A. Stress removal
B. Weight loss
C. Sunlight avoidance
D. All of the above

Acanthosis nigricans reflects the severity of underlying insulin resistance and diminishes with weight loss.

2016. Which of the following relates to diabetes mellitus?

Harrison's 20th Ed. Chapter 398 Page 2882

A. Granuloma annulare
B. Lichen planus
C. Scleredema
D. All of the above

2017. Skin tags are also called?

Harrison's 20th Ed. Chapter 54 Page 346

A. Acrodermon
B. Acrochordon
C. Acrochondron
D. Acrochiron

Skin tags are also called acrochordons.

2018. Acanthosis nigricans may be a reflection of?

Harrison's 20th Ed. Chapter 54 Page 346

A. Acromegaly
B. Cushing's syndrome
C. Polycystic ovary syndrome
D. All of the above

Acanthosis nigricans is associated with obesity & insulin resistance, and it may be a reflection of an endocrinopathy such as acromegaly, Cushing's syndrome, polycystic ovary syndrome.

2019. Acanthosis nigricans may be a reflection of an internal malignancy related to?

Harrison's 20th Ed. Chapter 54 Page 346

A. Lung
B. Liver
C. Gastrointestinal tract
D. Pancreas

Acanthosis nigricans can be a reflection of internal malignancy, most commonly of gastrointestinal tract.

2020. Which of the following drugs can cause involuntary weight loss?

Harrison's 20th Ed. Chapter 43 Page 271 Table 43-1

A. Serotonin reuptake inhibitors
B. Metformin
C. ACE inhibitors
D. All of the above

Medications that can cause weight loss are antibiotics, nonsteroidal anti-inflammatory drugs, serotonin reuptake inhibitors, metformin, levodopa and ACE inhibitors.

2021. Acanthosis nigricans is associated with?

Harrison's 20th Ed. Chapter 54 Page 346

A. Acromegaly
B. Cushing's syndrome
C. Stein-Leventhal syndrome
D. All of the above

Acanthosis nigricans is associated with obesity and insulin resistance. It may reflect an endocrinopathy such as acromegaly, Cushing's syndrome, polycystic ovary syndrome, or insulin-resistant diabetes mellitus (type A, type B, and lipoatrophic forms).

2022. Which of the following is false about necrobiosis lipoidica?

Harrison's 20th Ed. Chapter 54 Page 351

A. Found on thigh
B. Obliterative endarteritis
C. Telangiectasias
D. Erythematous border

Lesions of necrobiosis lipoidica are found primarily on the shins (90%). Features include central yellow color, atrophy, telangiectasias, and erythematous border. Biopsy shows necrobiosis of collagen, granulomatous inflammation and obliterative endarteritis.

2023. Which of the following is false about 'Prayer hand deformity'?

Cureus 2018;10(6):e2772

A. Type 1 diabetes mellitus
B. Digital sclerosis
C. Contractures
D. None of the above

Patients with insulin-dependent diabetes mellitus may develop digital sclerosis & contractures (prayer hand deformity). Diabetic hand syndrome includes limited joint mobility (LJM) (diabetic cheiroarthropathy), Dupuytren's contracture, stenosing tenosynovitis (trigger finger), carpal tunnel syndrome (CTS), Charcot neuroarthropathy, reflex sympathetic dystrophy and a variety of hand infections.

2024. Most frequent cause of neuropathic joint disease is?

Harrison's 20th Ed. Chapter 367 Page 2642

A. Leprosy
B. Meningomyelocele
C. Diabetes mellitus
D. Amyloidosis

Diabetes mellitus is the most frequent cause of neuropathic joint disease (Charcot joint).

2025. Joint most commonly affected in diabetes mellitus is?

Harrison's 20th Ed. Chapter 367 Page 2642

A. Knee, hip & ankle
B. Glenohumeral joint
C. Elbow & wrist
D. Tarsal & tarsometatarsal joint

Neuropathic arthritis is encountered most often in patients with diabetes mellitus, with an incidence of ~0.5%. The tarsal and tarsometatarsal joints are most often affected, with the metatarsophalangeal and talotibial joints next most commonly involved. The knees and spine are occasionally involved.

2026. Which of the following describes "Rocker foot"?

Harrison's 20th Ed. Chapter 367 Page 2642

A. Calluses over metatarsal heads
B. Convexity of sole
C. Osteophyte protrusion from top of foot
D. All of the above

Downward collapse of the tarsal bones leads to convexity of the sole, referred to as a "rocker foot."

2027. Lisfranc fracture-dislocation is related to?

Harrison's 20th Ed. Chapter 367 Page 2642

A. Knee, hip & ankle
B. Glenohumeral joint
C. Elbow & wrist
D. Tarsometatarsal joint

Lisfranc fracture-dislocation refers to describe the destructive changes at tarsometatarsal joints.

2028. Which of the following tests is not useful in differentiating neuropathic joint disease from osteomyelitis?

Harrison's 20th Ed. Chapter 367 Page 2642

A. MRI
B. Indium 111 labeled white blood cells
C. Indium 111 labeled immunoglobulin G
D. Technetium bone scan

2029. Somatostatinoma syndrome consists of all except?

Harrison's 20th Ed. Chapter 80 Page 609

A. Diabetes mellitus
B. Gallbladder disease
C. Hyperchlorhydria
D. Diarrhea & steatorrhea

Somatostatinoma syndrome is due to an NET that secretes excessive amounts of somatostatin causing diabetes mellitus, gallbladder disease, diarrhea, and steatorrhea.

2030. Systemic conditions that can be associated with pruritus include?

Harrison's 20th Ed. Chapter 52 Page 325 Table 52-3

A. Chronic renal disease
B. Thyroid disease
C. Polycythemia vera
D. All of the above

Systemic conditions that can be associated with pruritus include chronic renal disease, cholestasis, pregnancy, malignancy, thyroid disease, polycythemia vera, and delusions of parasitosis.

Hypoglycemia

2031. For diagnosis of hypoglycemia, Whipple's triad consists of all except?

Harrison's 20th Ed. Chapter 399 Page 2883

A. History of diabetes mellitus
B. Hypoglycemic symptoms
C. Low plasma glucose level
D. Relief of symptoms after plasma glucose level is raised

Whipple's triad for diagnosis of hypoglycemia includes symptoms consistent with hypoglycemia, low plasma glucose concentration and relief of symptoms after plasma glucose level is raised.

2032. Lower limit of fasting plasma glucose concentration normally is?

Harrison's 20th Ed. Chapter 399 Page 2883

A. ~40 mg/dL
B. ~50 mg/dL
C. ~60 mg/dL
D. ~70 mg/dL

2033. Lower venous glucose levels occur normally during?

Harrison's 20th Ed. Chapter 399 Page 2883

A. Late after a meal
B. During pregnancy
C. During prolonged fasting
D. All of the above

Lower limit of fasting plasma glucose concentration is normally ~70 mg/dL (~3.9 mmol/L), but lower venous glucose levels occur normally, late after a meal, during pregnancy & during prolonged fasting (>24 hours).

2034. Hypoglycemia should be considered in any patient with?

Harrison's 20th Ed. Chapter 399 Page 2883

A. Episodes of confusion
B. Altered level of consciousness
C. Seizure
D. All of the above

Hypoglycemia should be considered in any patient with episodes of confusion, an altered level of consciousness, or a seizure.

2035. Nesidioblastosis best relates with?

Harrison's 20th Ed. Chapter 399 Page 2883 Table 399-1

A. Disorders of Gluconeogenesis and fatty acid oxidation
B. Insulin secretagogue
C. Functional β-cell disorders
D. Insulin autoimmune hypoglycemia

2036. Which of the following critical illness can lead to hypoglycemia?

Harrison's 20th Ed. Chapter 399 Page 2883 Table 399-1

A. Hepatic failure
B. Renal failure
C. Cardiac failure
D. All of the above

2037. Which of the following hormone deficiency can lead to hypoglycemia?

Harrison's 20th Ed. Chapter 399 Page 2883 Table 399-1

A. Cortisol deficiency
B. Growth hormone deficiency
C. Glucagon deficiency
D. All of the above

2038. In fasting state, plasma glucose concentrations are normally maintained within?

Harrison's 20th Ed. Chapter 399 Page 2883

A. 50–110 mg/dL
B. 50–126 mg/dL
C. 70–110 mg/dL
D. 70–126 mg/dL

In the fasting state, plasma glucose concentrations are normally maintained within 70–110 mg/dL (3.9 –6.1 mmol/L).

2039. Between meals and during fasting, plasma glucose levels are maintained by?

Harrison's 20th Ed. Chapter 399 Page 2883

A. Endogenous glucose production
B. Hepatic glycogenolysis
C. Hepatic (and renal) gluconeogenesis
D. All of the above

Between meals and during fasting, plasma glucose levels are maintained by endogenous glucose production, hepatic glycogenolysis and hepatic (and renal) gluconeogenesis.

2040. Hepatic glycogen stores are sufficient to maintain plasma glucose levels for?

Harrison's 20th Ed. Chapter 399 Page 2883

A. 4 hours
B. 8 hours
C. 12 hours
D. 18 hours

Hepatic glycogen stores are sufficient to maintain plasma glucose levels for ~8 hours.

2041. Precursors required for gluconeogenesis include?

Harrison's 20th Ed. Chapter 399 Page 2883

A. Lactate
B. Pyruvate
C. Acetyl CoA
D. All of the above

Muscle provides lactate, pyruvate, alanine, glutamine and other amino acids. Triglycerides in adipose tissue are broken down into glycerol. Free fatty acids generate acetyl CoA for gluconeogenesis.

2042. In hypoglycemia, which of the following is the first physiologic response to falling plasma glucose levels?

Harrison's 20th Ed. Chapter 399 Page 2883

A. Decreased Insulin
B. Increased Glucagon
C. Increased Epinephrine
D. Increased Cortisol

Decrease in insulin secretion is the first defense against hypoglycemia.

2043. In hypoglycemia, which of the following is the second defense against hypoglycemia?

Harrison's 20th Ed. Chapter 399 Page 2884 Table 399-2

A. Decreased Insulin
B. Increased Glucagon
C. Increased Epinephrine
D. Increased Cortisol

Glucagon is the primary glucose counterregulatory factor and the second defense against hypoglycemia.

2044. In hypoglycemia, which of the following is the third defense against hypoglycemia?

Harrison's 20th Ed. Chapter 399 Page 2884 Table 399-2

A. Decreased Insulin
B. Increased Glucagon
C. Increased Epinephrine
D. Increased Cortisol

Epinephrine is the third defense against hypoglycemia. It is of critical value when glucagon is deficient.

2045. Symptoms of hypoglycemia appear at a glycemic threshold of?

Harrison's 20th Ed. Chapter 399 Page 2884 Table 399-2

A. < 50 mg/dL
B. 50–55 mg/dL
C. 65–70 mg/dL
D. 80–85 mg/dL

2046. Insulin production decreases at a glycemic threshold of?

Harrison's 20th Ed. Chapter 399 Page 2884 Table 399-2

A. < 50 mg/dL
B. 50–55 mg/dL
C. 65–70 mg/dL
D. 80–85 mg/dL

2047. Glucagon, epinephrine, cortisol and growth hormone production increases at a glycemic threshold of?

Harrison's 20th Ed. Chapter 399 Page 2884 Table 399-2

A. < 50 mg/dL
B. 50–55 mg/dL
C. 65–70 mg/dL
D. 80–85 mg/dL

2048. Decreased cognition occurs at a glycemic threshold of?

Harrison's 20th Ed. Chapter 399 Page 2884 Table 399-2

A. < 50 mg/dL
B. 50–55 mg/dL
C. 65–70 mg/dL
D. 80–85 mg/dL

2049. Rate of glucose disappearance by the brain is not altered by?

Harrison's 20th Ed. Chapter 399 Page 2884 Table 399-2

A. Insulin
B. Glucagon
C. Epinephrine
D. All of the above

Rate of glucose disappearance by brain is not altered by insulin, glucagon, epinephrine, cortisol or growth hormone.

2050. Which of the following plays no role in defense against acute hypoglycemia?

Harrison's 20th Ed. Chapter 399 Page 2883

A. Glucagon
B. Adrenomedullary epinephrine
C. Cortisol
D. All of the above

When hypoglycemia is prolonged beyond ~4 hours, cortisol & growth hormone also support glucose production and restrict glucose utilization to a limited extent (~20% compared to epinephrine). Thus, cortisol and growth hormone play no role in defense against acute hypoglycemia.

2051. What is the primary mechanism of action of glucagon in treatment of hypoglycemia?

Harrison's 20th Ed. Chapter 399 Page 2884

A. Stimulates hepatic glycogenolysis
B. Stimulates gluconeogenesis
C. Reduces glucose utilization in peripheral tissues
D. All of the above

Glucagon primarily acts by stimulating hepatic glycogenolysis.

2052. Neuroglycopenic symptoms of hypoglycemia include all except?

Harrison's 20th Ed. Chapter 399 Page 2884

A. Fatigue
B. Hunger
C. Seizure
D. Loss of consciousness

Neuroglycopenic symptoms are a direct result of CNS neuronal glucose deprivation that include behavioral changes, confusion, fatigue, seizure, loss of consciousness & cardiac arrhythmias. Hypoglycemia-induced autonomic responses include adrenergic symptoms like palpitations, tremor, and anxiety while cholinergic symptoms are sweating, hunger, and paresthesia.

2053. Cholinergic symptoms of hypoglycemia include all except?

Harrison's 20th Ed. Chapter 399 Page 2884

A. Sweating
B. Palpitations
C. Hunger
D. Paresthesias

Cholinergic symptoms of hypoglycemia, mediated by acetylcholine released from sympathetic postganglionic neurons are sweating, hunger and paresthesias. Adrenergic symptoms, mediated by norepinephrine released from sympathetic postganglionic neurons and epinephrine released from the adrenal medullae are palpitations, tremor and anxiety.

2054. Hypoglycemia activates which of the following responses?

Harrison's 20th Ed. Chapter 399 Page 2884

A. Pro-inflammatory responses
B. Pro-coagulant responses
C. Pro-atherothrombotic responses
D. All of the above

Hypoglycemia activates pro-inflammatory, pro-coagulant and pro-atherothrombotic responses in T1DM, T2DM, and non-diabetic individuals.

2055. What percentage of people with T1DM die as a result of hypoglycemia?

Harrison's 20th Ed. Chapter 399 Page 2885

A. 1–3%
B. 3–5%
C. 6–10%
D. 12–18%

An estimated 6–10% of people with T1DM die as a result of hypoglycemia.

2056. Which of the following can cause hypoglycemia in T2DM?

Harrison's 20th Ed. Chapter 399 Page 2885

A. Insulin
B. Sulfonylureas
C. Glinides
D. All of the above

2057. Which of the following do not cause hypoglycemia in T2DM?

Harrison's 20th Ed. Chapter 399 Page 2885

A. Glucagon-like peptide 1 (GLP-1) receptor agonists
B. Dipeptidyl peptidase IV (DPP-IV) inhibitors
C. α-glucosidase inhibitors do not cause hypoglycemia.
D. All of the above

Insulin, sulfonylureas, or glinides can cause hypoglycemia in T2DM. Metformin, thiazolidinediones, α-glucosidase inhibitors, glucagon-like peptide 1 (GLP-1) receptor agonists, and dipeptidyl peptidase IV (DPP-IV) inhibitors do not cause hypoglycemia.

2058. In which of the following situtations, sensitivity to insulin is increased?

Harrison's 20th Ed. Chapter 399 Page 2885

A. In the middle of the night
B. Late after exercise
C. Weight loss
D. All of the above

Sensitivity to insulin is increased with improved glycemic control, in the middle of the night, late after exercise, or with increased fitness or weight loss.

2059. Hypoglycemia following alcohol ingestion is due to?

Harrison's 20th Ed. Chapter 399 Page 2885

A. Insulin sensitivity is increased
B. Influx of exogenous glucose is reduced
C. Endogenous glucose production is reduced
D. Insulin clearance is reduced

Endogenous glucose production is reduced following alcohol ingestion. Ethanol blocks gluconeogenesis but not glycogenolysis.

2060. Insulin clearance is reduced in?

Harrison's 20th Ed. Chapter 399 Page 2885

A. Sepsis
B. Renal failure
C. Insulinoma
D. Exercise

2061. Clinical syndrome of defective glucose counterregulation includes which of the following?

Harrison's 20th Ed. Chapter 399 Page 2885

A. Absent decrements in insulin
B. Absent increments in glucagon
C. Attenuated increment in epinephrine
D. All of the above

The clinical syndrome of defective glucose counterregulation includes absent decrements in insulin, absent increments in glucagon and the attenuated increment in epinephrine. This functional and potentially reversible disorder is distinct from classic diabetic autonomic neuropathy—a structural and irreversible disorder.

2062. Clinical syndrome of hypoglycemia unawareness best relates to?

Harrison's 20th Ed. Chapter 399 Page 2885

A. Absent decrements in insulin
B. Absent increments in glucagon
C. Attenuated sympathoadrenal response
D. All of the above

The attenuated sympathoadrenal response to hypoglycemia causes the clinical syndrome of hypoglycemia unawareness. Affected patients are at a 6x increased risk of severe iatrogenic hypoglycemia during intensive glycemic therapy of diabetes.

2063. GLUT is best described as a?

N Engl J Med 1999;341:248

A. Transmembrane protein
B. Nuclear protein
C. Cytoplasmic protein
D. Mitochondrial protein

Group of glucose transporters (GLUT) consists of five homologous trans-membrane proteins, GLUT-1, 2, 3, 4, and 5 that are encoded by distinct genes.

2064. Which of the following GLUT is an insulin-responsive glucose transporter?

N Engl J Med 1999;341:248

A. GLUT-1
B. GLUT-2
C. GLUT-3
D. GLUT-4

GLUT-4 is the main insulin-responsive glucose transporter, located primarily in muscle cells & adipocytes.

2065. Which of the following GLUT is a fructose transporter?

N Engl J Med 1999;341:248

A. GLUT-2
B. GLUT-3
C. GLUT-4
D. GLUT-5

GLUT-5 is distributed in small intestine, sperm, kidney, brain, adipose cells and muscle. It is characteristically a fructose transporter and has a very low affinity for glucose.

2066. Which of the following GLUT is found in placenta?

N Engl J Med 1999;341:248

A. GLUT-1
B. GLUT-2
C. GLUT-3
D. GLUT-4

GLUT-3 is distributed in neurons and placenta. It is a high-affinity glucose transporter.

2067. Blood-to-brain glucose transport is facilitated by?
N Engl J Med 2004;350:2272-9

A. GLUT-1
B. GLUT-2
C. GLUT-3
D. GLUT-4

Mutations in GLUT-1 are associated with intractable seizures resulting from a reduction in glucose transport across the blood–brain barrier.

2068. Fanconi–Bickel syndrome is caused by mutations in which of the following glucose transporters?
N Engl J Med 1999;341:248

A. GLUT-1
B. GLUT-2
C. GLUT-3
D. GLUT-4

GLUT-2 mutations cause the rare, autosomal recessive Fanconi - Bickel syndrome characterized by hepatic & renal glycogen accumulation, nephropathy & impaired utilization of glucose & galactose.

2069. Falling arterial glucose concentrations are sensed by?
N Engl J Med 2004;350:2272-9

A. Brain
B. Hepatic portal vein
C. Carotid body
D. All of the above

2070. Which of the following is true about syndrome of hypoglycemia unawareness?
N Engl J Med 2004;350:2272-9

A. Attenuated sympathetic neural response
B. Attenuated adrenomedullary response
C. Loss of neurogenic warning symptoms
D. All of the above

Periods of relative or absolute therapeutic insulin excess leading to falling glucose concentrations, with absent counterregulatory glucagon responses, reduced autonomic responses, reduced epinephrine responses cause hypoglycemia unawareness.

2071. Which of the following is a feature of hypoglycemia-associated autonomic failure (HAAF)?
Harrison's 20th Ed. Chapter 399 Page 2885

A. Result of recent antecedent iatrogenic hypoglycemia
B. Functional
C. Potentially reversible
D. All of the above

2072. Syndrome of hypoglycemia unawareness can be reversed by?
Harrison's 20th Ed. Chapter 399 Page 2886

A. >1 week of scrupulous avoidance of hypoglycemia
B. >1 week of scrupulous avoidance of hyperglycemia
C. >2 weeks of scrupulous avoidance of hypoglycemia
D. >2 weeks of scrupulous avoidance of hyperglycemia

Syndrome of hypoglycemia unawareness can be reversed by 2–3 weeks of scrupulous avoidance of hypoglycemia.

2073. Which of the following clinical trials investigated potential benefits of tight glucose control?
Harrison's 20th Ed. Chapter 399 Page 2886

A. NICE-SUGAR study
B. ADVANCE and ACCORD studies
C. Veterans Affairs Diabetes Trial (VADT)
D. All of the above

2074. Severe hypoglycemia can & does occur at HbA1c values of?
Harrison's 20th Ed. Chapter 399 Page 2886

A. 2–4%
B. 4–6%
C. 6–8%
D. 8–10%

Severe hypoglycemia can & does occur at HbA1c values of 8–10% in both T1DM and T2DM.

2075. Glycemic maintenance goals have been modified to lie between?
Harrison's 20th Ed. Chapter 399 Page 2886

A. 80 and 100 mg/dL
B. 100 and 126 mg/dL
C. 126 and 140 mg/dL
D. 140 and 180 mg/dL

Glycemic maintenance goals have been modified to lie between 140 and 180 mg/dL.

2076. Which of the following therapeutic interventions reduces hypoglycemia?
Harrison's 20th Ed. Chapter 399 Page 2886

A. Whole-organ pancreatic transplantation
B. Islet-cell pancreatic transplantation
C. Stem cell-derived β-cells transplantation
D. All of the above

2077. A reasonable therapeutic goal of HbA1c level should be?
Harrison's 20th Ed. Chapter 399 Page 2886

A. That reduces microvascular disease
B. That does not cause severe hypoglycemia
C. That preserves awareness of hypoglycemia
D. All of the above

2078. Intervention that stimulate counterregulatory responses in hypoglycemia include?
Harrison's 20th Ed. Chapter 399 Page 2886

A. Selective serotonin-reuptake inhibitors
B. β-adrenergic receptor antagonists
C. Opiate receptor antagonists
D. All of the above

Interventions to stimulate counterregulatory responses like selective serotonin-reuptake inhibitors, β-adrenergic receptor antagonists, opiate receptor antagonists, and fructose are experimental.

2079. Use of which of the following drugs can cause hypoglycemia?
Harrison's 20th Ed. Chapter 399 Page 2886

A. Pentamidine
B. Quinine
C. Salicylates
D. All of the above

2080. Use of which of the following drugs can cause hypoglycemia?
Harrison's 20th Ed. Chapter 399 Page 2886

A. Angiotensin-converting enzyme inhibitors
B. Quinolone antibiotics
C. Beta-adrenergic receptor antagonists
D. All of the above

Drugs associated with hypoglycemia include angiotensin-converting enzyme inhibitors, angiotensin receptor antagonists, beta-adrenergic receptor antagonists, quinolone antibiotics, indomethacin, quinine and sulfonamides. Pentamidine is toxic to the pancreatic beta cell. Initially it causes insulin release with hypoglycemia, and later predisposes to diabetes mellitus. Quinine stimulates insulin secretion. Salicylates and sulfonamides can cause hypoglycemia.

2081. Which of the following is a cause of fasting hypoglycemia?
Harrison's 20th Ed. Chapter 399 Page 2886

A. Ethanol use
B. Sepsis
C. Renal failure
D. All of the above

Apart from insulin and sulfonylureas, ethanol use, sepsis and renal failure are causes of fasting hypoglycemia. In sepsis, endogenous glucose production is impaired due to hepatic hypoperfusion, and cytokine induced glucose utilization is increased.

2082. Which of the following tissues is rich in macrophages?
Harrison's 20th Ed. Chapter 399 Page 2887

A. Liver
B. Spleen
C. Lung
D. All of the above

2083. Brain can utilize which of the following substrates?
Harrison's 20th Ed. Chapter 399 Page 2887

A. Lactate
B. Pyruvate
C. Ketone bodies
D. All of the above

2084. Non-islet cell tumor hypoglycemia (NICTH) is also called?
Harrison's 20th Ed. Chapter 399 Page 2887

A. Fasting hypoglycemia
B. Alternate hypoglycemia
C. Atypical hypoglycemia
D. Fugal hypoglycemia

Fasting hypoglycemia is also termed as non - islet cell tumor hypoglycemia.

2085. Fasting hypoglycemia occurs with which of the following?
Harrison's 20th Ed. Chapter 399 Page 2887

A. Hepatoma
B. Adrenocortical tumors
C. Carcinoids
D. All of the above

2086. Which of the following best relates to fasting hypoglycemia?
Harrison's 20th Ed. Chapter 399 Page 2887

A. Small IGF-I
B. Small IGF-II
C. Big IGF-I
D. Big IGF-II

Hepatoma, adrenocortical tumors and carcinoids can cause fasting hypoglycemia (non-islet cell tumor hypoglycemia) due to overproduction of an incompletely processed form of insulinomimetic compound - insulin-like growth factor (IGF) II ("big IGF-II") that does not complex normally with circulating binding proteins and thus more readily gains access to target tissues.

2087. Hypoglycemia due to endogenous hyperinsulinism can be caused by?
Harrison's 20th Ed. Chapter 399 Page 2887

A. Primary β-cell disorder
B. Antibody to insulin or to insulin receptor
C. Ectopic insulin secretion
D. All of the above

2088. Endogenous hyperinsulinism is diagnosed by?
Harrison's 20th Ed. Chapter 399 Page 2887

A. Fasting plasma insulin ≥ 3 μU/mL
B. Fasting plasma C-peptide ≥ 0.6 ng/mL
C. Fasting plasma glucose ≤ 55 mg/dL
D. All of the above

Despite of hypoglycemia, plasma insulin & C-peptide levels are high in endogenous hyperinsulinism. Insulinoma - an insulin secreting pancreatic islet β-cell tumor is the prototypical cause of endogenous hyperinsulinism. Critical diagnostic findings are a plasma insulin concentration ≥3 μU/mL, plasma C-peptide concentration ≥0.6 ng/mL and a plasma proinsulin concentration ≥5.0 pmol/L when the plasma glucose concentration is <55 mg/dL with symptoms of hypoglycemia. A low plasma β-hydroxybutyrate concentration (≤2.7 mmol/L) and an increment in plasma glucose level of >25 mg/dL after IV administration of glucagon (1 mg) indicate increased insulin (or IGF) actions.

2089. Condition in which patients with fasting endogenous hyperinsulinemic hypoglycemia have diffuse islet involvement with β-cell hypertrophy is called?
Harrison's 20th Ed. Chapter 399 Page 2887

A. Nesidioblastosis
B. Aviablastosis
C. Progblastosis
D. Mutblastosis

Some patients with fasting endogenous hyperinsulinemic hypoglycemia have diffuse islet involvement with b-cell hypertrophy and sometimes hyperplasia. This pattern is commonly referred to as nesidioblastosis.

2090. Noninsulinoma pancreatogenous hypoglycemia best relates to?
Harrison's 20th Ed. Chapter 399 Page 2887

A. Fasting hypoglycemia
B. Postprandial hypoglycemia
C. Diabetic ketoacidosis
D. IGF-II

2091. Which of the following statements about insulinomas is false?
Harrison's 20th Ed. Chapter 399 Page 2887

A. > 90% of insulinomas are benign
B. > 99% are within the substance of pancreas
C. CT or MRI detects ~ 70–80% of insulinomas
D. None of the above

2092. Which of the following inhibits insulin release from pancreas?
Harrison's 20th Ed. Chapter 399 Page 2887

A. Furosemide
B. Thiazide
C. Ethacrynic acid
D. Diazoxide

Diazoxide has a hyperglycemic effect due to inhibition of insulin release from pancreas, as well as an extrapancreatic (catecholamine-induced) effect.

2093. Factitious hypoglycemia due to self-ingestion of sulfonylurea is best diagnosed by?

Harrison's 20th Ed. Chapter 399 Page 2888

A. High plasma insulin level
B. High plasma C-peptide level
C. High plasma sulfonylurea level
D. All of the above

Sulfonylureas stimulate endogenous insulin and can be best detected by measuring drug levels in plasma or urine. Ingestion of an insulin secretagogue causes hypoglycemia with increased C-peptide levels, whereas exogenous insulin causes hypoglycemia with low C-peptide levels reflecting suppression of insulin secretion.

2094. Pseudohypoglycemia may be due to?

Harrison's 20th Ed. Chapter 399 Page 2888

A. Myeloproliferative diseases
B. Leukemoid reactions
C. Colony stimulating factor treatment
D. All of the above

Hypoglycemia can be artifactual; hyperleukocytosis from leukemia, myeloproliferative diseases, leukemoid reactions, or colony stimulating factor treatment can increase glucose consumption in the test tube after blood is drawn, leading to pseudohypoglycemia.

2095. Which of the following statements about postprandial (reactive) hypoglycemia is false?

Harrison's 20th Ed. Chapter 399 Page 2888

A. Occurs only after meals
B. Self-limited
C. Alimentary hypoglycemia
D. None of the above

Postprandial (reactive) hypoglycemia occurs only after meals and is self-limited. Causes include enzymatic defects in carbohydrate metabolism like hereditary fructose intolerance and galactosemia, post gastric surgery (alimentary hypoglycemia).

2096. Which of the following might help in the treatment of postprandial (reactive) hypoglycemia?

Harrison's 20th Ed. Chapter 399 Page 2888

A. Metformin
B. α-glucosidase inhibitor
C. Glucagon
D. All of the above

Alpha-glucosidase inhibitor delays carbohydrate digestion and glucose absorption from intestine and may be useful in reactive hypoglycemia.

2097. Monocarboxylate transporter 1 best relates to?

Harrison's 20th Ed. Chapter 399 Page 2888

A. Exercise-induced hypoglycemia
B. Postprandial Hypoglycemia
C. Fasting Hypoglycemia
D. Factitious hypoglycemia

Exercise-induced hypoglycemia follows exercise. It results in hyperinsulinemia caused by increased activity of monocarboxylate transporter 1 in beta cells.

2098. Somogyi effect is best understood as?

Joslin's Diabetes mellitus 13th Ed. 499

A. Post hyperglycemic hypoglycemia
B. Post hypoglycemic hyperglycemia
C. Nocturnal hypoglycemia
D. All of the above

2099. In urgent treatment of hypoglycemia, what should be the reasonable initial dose of oral glucose?

Harrison's 20th Ed. Chapter 399 Page 2888

A. 10 gram
B. 20 gram
C. 30 gram
D. 40 gram

Reasonable initial dose of oral glucose is 20 grams for urgent oral treatment of hypoglycemia.

2100. Which of the following statements is false?

Harrison's 20th Ed. Chapter 399 Page 2888

A. Glucagon stimulates insulin secretion
B. Glucagon is ineffective in glycogen-depleted individuals
C. Octreotide suppresses insulin secretion
D. None of the above

2101. Bilateral nontender parotid enlargement occurs with all except?

Harrison's 20th Ed. Chapter 32 Page 2888

A. Bulimia
B. Diabetes mellitus
C. Cirrhosis
D. Thyroxine

Bilateral nontender parotid enlargement occurs with diabetes mellitus, cirrhosis, bulimia, HIV/AIDS, and drugs (e.g., iodide, propylthiouracil).

2102. Which of the following is not a cause of bilateral parotid gland enlargement?

Harrison's 20th Ed. Chapter 354 Page Table 354-3

A. Hypopituitarism
B. Diabetes mellitus
C. Chronic pancreatitis
D. Hepatic cirrhosis

Bilateral parotid gland enlargement is due to viral infections, sarcoidosis, IgG4 syndrome, Sjogren's syndrome, diabetes mellitus, hyperlipoproteinemias, chronic pancreatitis, hepatic cirrhosis, acromegaly, gonadal hypofunction.

ANSWERS

1. C
2. B
3. D
4. A
5. D
6. D
7. D
8. D
9. D
10. D
11. B
12. D
13. C
14. B
15. D
16. D
17. D
18. D
19. D
20. C
21. C
22. B
23. C
24. D
25. A
26. D
27. D
28. D
29. A
30. A
31. D
32. A
33. B
34. C
35. D
36. C
37. A
38. C
39. B
40. B
41. D
42. D
43. A
44. D
45. B
46. A
47. D
48. B
49. D
50. D
51. D
52. D
53. C
54. D
55. D
56. C
57. D
58. B
59. D
60. D
61. D
62. D
63. C
64. D
65. D
66. A
67. B
68. D
69. D
70. C
71. B
72. C
73. D
74. C
75. A
76. B
77. C
78. D
79. B
80. D
81. D
82. D
83. C
84. D
85. D
86. D
87. D
88. C
89. D
90. B
91. B
92. D
93. D
94. A
95. D
96. D
97. D
98. C
99. D
100. D
101. D
102. D
103. D
104. D
105. D
106. D
107. D
108. C
109. D
110. D
111. D
112. D
113. C
114. C
115. A
116. C
117. B
118. B
119. C
120. D
121. A
122. A
123. A
124. A
125. D
126. B
127. B
128. D
129. A
130. D
131. D
132. D
133. C
134. C
135. B
136. B
137. D
138. D
139. D
140. B
141. C
142. B
143. D
144. D
145. C
146. B
147. D
148. D
149. D
150. B
151. D
152. D
153. D
154. B
155. B
156. B
157. A
158. C
159. D
160. D
161. D
162. D
163. B
164. C
165. A
166. A
167. D
168. D
169. A
170. C
171. B
172. D
173. D
174. D
175. C
176. B
177. D
178. B
179. C
180. C
181. D
182. B
183. C
184. D
185. C
186. C
187. C
188. D
189. D
190. C
191. D
192. D
193. D
194. D
195. D
196. D
197. D
198. D
199. D
200. A
201. D
202. B
203. D
204. C
205. A
206. B
207. A
208. D
209. C
210. B
211. D
212. D
213. D
214. A
215. B
216. B
217. C
218. D
219. C
220. C
221. B
222. B
223. A
224. D
225. D
226. D
227. D
228. D
229. D
230. A
231. A
232. A
233. C
234. C

ANSWERS

235. A
236. A
237. D
238. D
239. D
240. D
241. C
242. D
243. C
244. D
245. C
246. C
247. C
248. A
249. D
250. D
251. A
252. A
253. B
254. D
255. C
256. D
257. D
258. D
259. C
260. D
261. D
262. D
263. D
264. D
265. B
266. B
267. C
268. D
269. C
270. B
271. D
272. D
273. D
274. D
275. D
276. A
277. B
278. C
279. A
280. D
281. D
282. A
283. D
284. A
285. B
286. D
287. C
288. B
289. C
290. D
291. B
292. A
293. C
294. D
295. D
296. B
297. D
298. D
299. A
300. D
301. B
302. B
303. A
304. C
305. D
306. D
307. A
308. D
309. C
310. D
311. B
312. B
313. A
314. C
315. B
316. D
317. D
318. C
319. D
320. A
321. D
322. D
323. C
324. D
325. D
326. C
327. D
328. D
329. D
330. D
331. B
332. D
333. B
334. D
335. C
336. B
337. D
338. D
339. D
340. A
341. C
342. D
343. D
344. D
345. C
346. B
347. B
348. B
349. C
350. C
351. D
352. D
353. A
354. D
355. C
356. D
357. B
358. C
359. D
360. C
361. B
362. B
363. C
364. D
365. D
366. A
367. C
368. B
369. C
370. B
371. D
372. D
373. D
374. D
375. D
376. C
377. B
378. B
379. D
380. B
381. C
382. A
383. A
384. A
385. D
386. A
387. C
388. C
389. B
390. C
391. D
392. A
393. C
394. B
395. A
396. A
397. A
398. B
399. A
400. C
401. B
402. D
403. D
404. D
405. D
406. A
407. C
408. A
409. B
410. D
411. C
412. D
413. D
414. B
415. D
416. C
417. D
418. C
419. D
420. D
421. C
422. A
423. C
424. D
425. D
426. D
427. D
428. D
429. D
430. D
431. D
432. A
433. B
434. D
435. D
436. D
437. C
438. D
439. A
440. D
441. B
442. D
443. D
444. D
445. C
446. A
447. D
448. C
449. D
450. D
451. D
452. D
453. D
454. B
455. A
456. A
457. D
458. B
459. D
460. B
461. D
462. D
463. C
464. D
465. B
466. A
467. D
468. C

ANSWERS

469. D
470. B
471. A
472. A
473. A
474. A
475. C
476. C
477. D
478. B
479. D
480. C
481. D
482. B
483. D
484. D
485. D
486. D
487. D
488. B
489. A
490. C
491. B
492. C
493. D
494. B
495. D
496. D
497. B
498. B
499. D
500. B
501. D
502. B
503. D
504. D
505. A
506. B
507. C
508. D
509. D
510. C
511. A
512. C
513. C
514. C
515. D
516. D
517. B
518. B
519. C
520. C
521. D
522. D
523. C
524. B
525. D
526. A
527. D
528. D
529. D
530. D
531. B
532. D
533. D
534. A
535. D
536. A
537. D
538. D
539. D
540. D
541. D
542. A
543. C
544. B
545. C
546. D
547. D
548. A
549. D
550. D
551. A
552. C
553. D
554. D
555. C
556. A
557. B
558. B
559. D
560. D
561. D
562. B
563. D
564. D
565. A
566. D
567. D
568. C
569. A
570. B
571. D
572. B
573. A
574. C
575. C
576. A
577. A
578. C
579. D
580. D
581. D
582. B
583. B
584. D
585. D
586. D
587. D
588. D
589. C
590. C
591. D
592. D
593. D
594. D
595. D
596. C
597. B
598. D
599. C
600. D
601. C
602. C
603. A
604. A
605. D
606. D
607. A
608. A
609. D
610. D
611. B
612. A
613. C
614. A
615. C
616. C
617. D
618. C
619. C
620. C
621. D
622. B
623. D
624. A
625. A
626. D
627. D
628. D
629. D
630. A
631. A
632. D
633. B
634. A
635. A
636. B
637. C
638. D
639. D
640. C
641. D
642. B
643. A
644. D
645. D
646. D
647. D
648. C
649. C
650. B
651. D
652. D
653. D
654. D
655. A
656. C
657. D
658. B
659. C
660. D
661. A
662. B
663. D
664. D
665. A
666. D
667. A
668. D
669. D
670. D
671. D
672. D
673. B
674. D
675. D
676. D
677. D
678. D
679. B
680. D
681. C
682. D
683. A
684. D
685. A
686. B
687. A
688. D
689. B
690. C
691. B
692. D
693. D
694. C
695. A
696. A
697. B
698. A
699. D
700. D
701. D
702. D

ANSWERS

703. D
704. D
705. C
706. B
707. D
708. D
709. C
710. C
711. D
712. A
713. D
714. D
715. D
716. D
717. D
718. B
719. D
720. D
721. D
722. D
723. B
724. C
725. B
726. A
727. D
728. D
729. D
730. B
731. D
732. B
733. C
734. A
735. C
736. B
737. D
738. A
739. D
740. D
741. D
742. D
743. D
744. A
745. B
746. D
747. C
748. C
749. A
750. D
751. D
752. C
753. D
754. D
755. D
756. D
757. D
758. D
759. D
760. C
761. D
762. B
763. D
764. D
765. D
766. C
767. D
768. B
769. B
770. B
771. B
772. D
773. A
774. A
775. B
776. D
777. D
778. B
779. B
780. D
781. A
782. A
783. C
784. B
785. C
786. C
787. A
788. D
789. A
790. A
791. D
792. D
793. D
794. D
795. D
796. C
797. B
798. B
799. D
800. D
801. A
802. B
803. C
804. B
805. B
806. D
807. D
808. B
809. D
810. A
811. A
812. D
813. B
814. B
815. B
816. A
817. A
818. D
819. C
820. B
821. D
822. D
823. C
824. D
825. A
826. C
827. B
828. D
829. B
830. A
831. A
832. A
833. D
834. D
835. D
836. D
837. D
838. A
839. D
840. D
841. D
842. B
843. C
844. C
845. C
846. D
847. D
848. A
849. D
850. C
851. C
852. D
853. D
854. B
855. D
856. D
857. D
858. D
859. D
860. D
861. D
862. C
863. C
864. D
865. D
866. B
867. D
868. B
869. D
870. C
871. A
872. D
873. A
874. D
875. C
876. B
877. C
878. D
879. B
880. D
881. D
882. C
883. B
884. D
885. D
886. D
887. B
888. D
889. A
890. A
891. D
892. D
893. A
894. B
895. D
896. C
897. D
898. D
899. D
900. A
901. B
902. C
903. A
904. D
905. D
906. D
907. D
908. D
909. D
910. A
911. D
912. D
913. D
914. B
915. B
916. D
917. C
918. B
919. D
920. D
921. A
922. C
923. A
924. B
925. D
926. D
927. D
928. D
929. D
930. A
931. A
932. C
933. A
934. A
935. A
936. A

ANSWERS

937. A
938. D
939. B
940. D
941. D
942. D
943. D
944. B
945. D
946. D
947. D
948. D
949. C
950. B
951. C
952. D
953. D
954. B
955. C
956. C
957. D
958. A
959. D
960. D
961. D
962. A
963. B
964. B
965. D
966. D
967. D
968. D
969. B
970. C
971. D
972. A
973. A
974. B
975. A
976. A
977. D
978. D
979. B
980. C
981. A
982. B
983. B
984. A
985. B
986. B
987. B
988. D
989. D
990. D
991. D
992. D
993. D
994. B
995. B
996. C
997. D
998. A
999. C
1000. A
1001. C
1002. D
1003. D
1004. D
1005. D
1006. D
1007. D
1008. D
1009. C
1010. D
1011. A
1012. D
1013. D
1014. B
1015. A
1016. D
1017. D
1018. D
1019. C
1020. A
1021. D
1022. A
1023. A
1024. D
1025. A
1026. B
1027. B
1028. A
1029. A
1030. D
1031. D
1032. D
1033. B
1034. D
1035. D
1036. A
1037. A
1038. D
1039. D
1040. D
1041. A
1042. B
1043. A
1044. C
1045. D
1046. C
1047. C
1048. A
1049. D
1050. B
1051. D
1052. D
1053. D
1054. D
1055. A
1056. B
1057. A
1058. D
1059. D
1060. D
1061. B
1062. D
1063. A
1064. A
1065. D
1066. A
1067. A
1068. B
1069. A
1070. A
1071. B
1072. D
1073. C
1074. A
1075. A
1076. A
1077. B
1078. D
1079. D
1080. B
1081. A
1082. D
1083. D
1084. A
1085. A
1086. D
1087. B
1088. D
1089. D
1090. C
1091. D
1092. D
1093. B
1094. A
1095. D
1096. B
1097. D
1098. D
1099. A
1100. A
1101. A
1102. A
1103. B
1104. C
1105. D
1106. C
1107. C
1108. C
1109. D
1110. A
1111. B
1112. D
1113. D
1114. D
1115. B
1116. D
1117. D
1118. D
1119. A
1120. B
1121. A
1122. D
1123. D
1124. D
1125. B
1126. D
1127. A
1128. D
1129. D
1130. D
1131. D
1132. B
1133. D
1134. A
1135. A
1136. D
1137. C
1138. D
1139. D
1140. D
1141. D
1142. A
1143. B
1144. C
1145. D
1146. A
1147. C
1148. B
1149. A
1150. A
1151. A
1152. A
1153. C
1154. B
1155. C
1156. D
1157. D
1158. C
1159. D
1160. A
1161. D
1162. D
1163. D
1164. D
1165. A
1166. C
1167. D
1168. D
1169. D
1170. D

ANSWERS

1171. D
1172. B
1173. D
1174. D
1175. D
1176. D
1177. D
1178. D
1179. D
1180. D
1181. D
1182. A
1183. B
1184. D
1185. A
1186. D
1187. D
1188. A
1189. A
1190. A
1191. C
1192. C
1193. D
1194. D
1195. D
1196. D
1197. A
1198. B
1199. C
1200. D
1201. A
1202. D
1203. C
1204. B
1205. D
1206. B
1207. A
1208. A
1209. C
1210. B
1211. A
1212. D
1213. D
1214. D
1215. D
1216. D
1217. D
1218. D
1219. D
1220. D
1221. D
1222. D
1223. D
1224. B
1225. D
1226. B
1227. D
1228. D
1229. B
1230. B
1231. B
1232. D
1233. B
1234. C
1235. A
1236. B
1237. D
1238. A
1239. A
1240. A
1241. D
1242. D
1243. B
1244. C
1245. D
1246. D
1247. D
1248. D
1249. D
1250. D
1251. D
1252. A
1253. B
1254. D
1255. D
1256. C
1257. A
1258. C
1259. A
1260. D
1261. B
1262. A
1263. D
1264. B
1265. D
1266. D
1267. B
1268. B
1269. A
1270. A
1271. D
1272. C
1273. D
1274. A
1275. D
1276. D
1277. A
1278. D
1279. D
1280. D
1281. D
1282. D
1283. C
1284. D
1285. D
1286. B
1287. D
1288. A
1289. B
1290. D
1291. A
1292. D
1293. D
1294. A
1295. D
1296. C
1297. A
1298. D
1299. D
1300. D
1301. D
1302. B
1303. B
1304. D
1305. D
1306. B
1307. C
1308. A
1309. D
1310. B
1311. D
1312. B
1313. D
1314. D
1315. A
1316. A
1317. C
1318. D
1319. A
1320. D
1321. B
1322. D
1323. D
1324. A
1325. A
1326. C
1327. D
1328. B
1329. D
1330. D
1331. D
1332. D
1333. C
1334. D
1335. B
1336. D
1337. B
1338. A
1339. B
1340. C
1341. C
1342. B
1343. D
1344. D
1345. A
1346. D
1347. A
1348. D
1349. D
1350. B
1351. D
1352. D
1353. A
1354. C
1355. D
1356. B
1357. C
1358. C
1359. B
1360. D
1361. A
1362. B
1363. C
1364. B
1365. C
1366. A
1367. D
1368. D
1369. D
1370. A
1371. A
1372. C
1373. D
1374. C
1375. D
1376. D
1377. D
1378. A
1379. D
1380. C
1381. C
1382. D
1383. D
1384. D
1385. D
1386. D
1387. D
1388. C
1389. C
1390. D
1391. D
1392. D
1393. D
1394. B
1395. B
1396. B
1397. B
1398. D
1399. D
1400. A
1401. C
1402. D
1403. B
1404. B

ANSWERS

1405. A
1406. D
1407. A
1408. D
1409. D
1410. C
1411. D
1412. D
1413. D
1414. B
1415. A
1416. D
1417. D
1418. D
1419. A
1420. D
1421. D
1422. D
1423. C
1424. C
1425. D
1426. D
1427. D
1428. C
1429. D
1430. D
1431. D
1432. D
1433. D
1434. B
1435. B
1436. D
1437. B
1438. C
1439. D
1440. D
1441. C
1442. D
1443. C
1444. D
1445. D
1446. D
1447. A
1448. D
1449. B
1450. D
1451. C
1452. B
1453. A
1454. D
1455. D
1456. D
1457. A
1458. D
1459. D
1460. D
1461. C
1462. A,B & C
1463. D
1464. D
1465. D
1466. D
1467. B
1468. C
1469. D
1470. C
1471. D
1472. A
1473. C
1474. B
1475. D
1476. D
1477. D
1478. D
1479. B
1480. C
1481. A
1482. C
1483. D
1484. C
1485. B
1486. D
1487. C
1488. C
1489. D
1490. D
1491. D
1492. C
1493. C
1494. B
1495. C
1496. B
1497. C
1498. D
1499. B
1500. B
1501. D
1502. C
1503. D
1504. D
1505. D
1506. B
1507. B
1508. A
1509. D
1510. D
1511. D
1512. B
1513. D
1514. A
1515. D
1516. D
1517. B
1518. D
1519. B
1520. B
1521. D
1522. A
1523. C
1524. C
1525. D
1526. C
1527. B
1528. D
1529. D
1530. B
1531. D
1532. B
1533. D
1534. D
1535. D
1536. D
1537. C
1538. C
1539. B
1540. C
1541. B
1542. D
1543. A
1544. B
1545. A
1546. D
1547. C
1548. D
1549. C
1550. B
1551. D
1552. A
1553. D
1554. D
1555. B
1556. C
1557. B
1558. C
1559. D
1560. D
1561. C
1562. C
1563. D
1564. B
1565. A
1566. B
1567. C
1568. C
1569. B
1570. B
1571. B
1572. B
1573. C
1574. D
1575. A
1576. C
1577. D
1578. D
1579. B
1580. A
1581. C
1582. B
1583. D
1584. D
1585. D
1586. A
1587. D
1588. D
1589. D
1590. D
1591. D
1592. B
1593. C`
1594. D
1595. D
1596. D
1597. C
1598. D
1599. D
1600. B
1601. B
1602. D
1603. D
1604. B
1605. D
1606. D
1607. D
1608. D
1609. D
1610. C
1611. D
1612. D
1613. D
1614. A
1615. B
1616. B
1617. D
1618. B
1619. A
1620. D
1621. D
1622. C
1623. D
1624. D
1625. B
1626. B
1627. A
1628. D
1629. C
1630. C
1631. D
1632. C
1633. D
1634. A
1635. B
1636. C
1637. D

ANSWERS

1638. D
1639. A
1640. B
1641. C
1642. A
1643. A, D
1644. D
1645. D
1646. D
1647. D
1648. C
1649. B
1650. B
1651. B
1652. B
1653. A
1654. C
1655. A
1656. D
1657. B
1658. D
1659. D
1660. B
1661. A
1662. D
1663. D
1664. B
1665. D
1666. D
1667. C
1668. C
1669. C
1670. C
1671. C
1672. D
1673. C
1674. B
1675. D
1676. A
1677. A
1678. D
1679. C
1680. D
1681. D
1682. D
1683. D
1684. D
1685. D
1686. B
1687. C
1688. C
1689. C
1690. C
1691. D
1692. D
1693. D
1694. A
1695. A
1696. D
1697. A
1698. D
1699. D
1700. D
1701. B
1702. C
1703. B
1704. B
1705. D
1706. D
1707. C
1708. D
1709. A
1710. B
1711. C
1712. D
1713. D
1714. D
1715. A
1716. B
1717. B
1718. D
1719. D
1720. D
1721. B
1722. D
1723. D
1724. B
1725. A
1726. B
1727. B
1728. B
1729. D
1730. B
1731. D
1732. B
1733. D
1734. D
1735. D
1736. D
1737. D
1738. D
1739. D
1740. D
1741. D
1742. D
1743. D
1744. A
1745. B
1746. B
1747. B
1748. D
1749. D
1750. D
1751. D
1752. D
1753. D
1754. C
1755. D
1756. D
1757. B
1758. A
1759. D
1760. D
1761. D
1762. D
1763. A
1764. D
1765. B
1766. B
1767. A
1768. D
1769. D
1770. C
1771. B
1772. D
1773. A
1774. C
1775. D
1776. D
1777. D
1778. D
1779. B
1780. D
1781. C
1782. D
1783. C
1784. D
1785. C
1786. C
1787. C
1788. D
1789. D
1790. A
1791. C
1792. A
1793. D
1794. D
1795. D
1796. C
1797. D
1798. A
1799. A
1800. C
1801. A
1802. C
1803. D
1804. C
1805. D
1806. D
1807. D
1808. D
1809. C
1810. B
1811. B
1812. D
1813. A
1814. B
1815. B
1816. A
1817. D
1818. D
1819. C
1820. A
1821. D
1822. D
1823. D
1824. D
1825. A
1826. A
1827. B
1828. C
1829. C
1830. D
1831. D
1832. C
1833. D
1834. C
1835. B
1836. B
1837. A
1838. D
1839. D
1840. D
1841. D
1842. D
1843. C
1844. D
1845. B
1846. D
1847. A
1848. A
1849. C
1850. D
1851. D
1852. D
1853. B
1854. D
1855. D
1856. A
1857. B
1858. A
1859. D
1860. C
1861. A
1862. D
1863. C
1864. A
1865. A
1866. C
1867. C
1868. C
1869. D
1870. C
1871. D

ANSWERS

1872. C
1873. D
1874. B
1875. D
1876. A
1877. D
1878. D
1879. D
1880. A
1881. C
1882. D
1883. D
1884. D
1885. D
1886. D
1887. A
1888. B
1889. D
1890. D
1891. D
1892. D
1893. C
1894. D
1895. D
1896. C
1897. A
1898. A
1899. D
1900. C
1901. B
1902. A
1903. D
1904. B
1905. A
1906. D
1907. D
1908. D
1909. B
1910. B
1911. D
1912. B
1913. D
1914. D
1915. B
1916. C
1917. B
1918. D
1919. D
1920. D
1921. B
1922. D
1923. C
1924. D
1925. A
1926. A
1927. D
1928. D
1929. D
1930. D
1931. C
1932. D
1933. D
1934. D
1935. A
1936. A
1937. C
1938. B
1939. A
1940. D
1941. A
1942. D
1943. D
1944. D
1945. B
1946. C
1947. B
1948. D
1949. D
1950. D
1951. D
1952. D
1953. D
1954. C
1955. C
1956. C
1957. A
1958. B
1959. B
1960. A
1961. B
1962. B
1963. D
1964. D
1965. B
1966. C
1967. A
1968. D
1969. D
1970. A
1971. D
1972. D
1973. D
1974. D
1975. D
1976. B
1977. D
1978. B
1979. C
1980. D
1981. A
1982. A
1983. D
1984. A
1985. A
1986. B
1987. D
1988. C
1989. D
1990. B
1991. D
1992. B
1993. D
1994. B
1995. D
1996. D
1997. B
1998. B
1999. B
2000. C
2001. B
2002. D
2003. A
2004. C
2005. D
2006. B
2007. A
2008. B
2009. D
2010. A
2011. B
2012. B
2013. A
2014. D
2015. B
2016. D
2017. B
2018. D
2019. C
2020. D
2021. D
2022. A
2023. D
2024. C
2025. D
2026. B
2027. D
2028. D
2029. C
2030. D
2031. A
2032. D
2033. D
2034. D
2035. C
2036. D
2037. D
2038. C
2039. D
2040. B
2041. D
2042. A
2043. B
2044. C
2045. B
2046. D
2047. C
2048. A
2049. D
2050. C
2051. A
2052. B
2053. B
2054. D
2055. C
2056. D
2057. D
2058. D
2059. C
2060. B
2061. D
2062. C
2063. A
2064. D
2065. D
2066. C
2067. A
2068. B
2069. D
2070. D
2071. D
2072. C
2073. D
2074. D
2075. D
2076. D
2077. D
2078. D
2079. D
2080. D
2081. D
2082. D
2083. D
2084. A
2085. D
2086. D
2087. D
2088. D
2089. A
2090. B
2091. D
2092. D
2093. C
2094. D
2095. D
2096. B
2097. A
2098. B
2099. B
2100. D
2101. D
2102. A

Neurology 7

NEUROLOGY

Neurologic Causes of Weakness and Paralysis

1. Motor system dysfunction leads to?
Harrison's 20th Ed. Chapter 21, Page 135

A. Weakness or paralysis
B. Ataxia
C. Abnormal movements
D. All of the above

2. Normal motor function involves integrated muscle activity that is modulated by?
Harrison's 20th Ed. Chapter 21, Page 135

A. Red nucleus
B. Brainstem reticular formation
C. Lateral vestibular nucleus
D. All of the above

Normal motor function involves integrated muscle activity that is modulated by activity of cerebral cortex, basal ganglia, cerebellum, red nucleus, brainstem reticular formation, lateral vestibular nucleus and spinal cord.

3. Which of the following statements is false?
Harrison's 20th Ed. Chapter 21, Page 135

A. Myopathic weakness is most marked in proximal muscles
B. UMN lesion cause weakness in extensors and abductors of upper limb
C. UMN lesion cause weakness in flexors of lower limb
D. None of the above

4. Which of the following is related to muscle tone?
Harrison's 20th Ed. Chapter 21, Page 135

A. Spasticity
B. Rigidity
C. Paratonia (or gegenhalten)
D. All of the above

5. Tone is the resistance of a muscle to?
Harrison's 20th Ed. Chapter 21, Page 135

A. Active stretch
B. Passive stretch
C. Gravitational stretch
D. Anti-gravity stretch

Tone is the resistance of a muscle to passive stretch.

6. Increased muscle tone is found in?
Harrison's 20th Ed. Chapter 21, Page 135

A. Spasticity
B. Rigidity
C. Paratonia
D. All of the above

7. Which of the following is false about spasticity?
Harrison's 20th Ed. Chapter 21, Page 135

A. Associated with disease of upper motor neurons
B. Velocity-dependent
C. Affects antigravity muscles
D. None of the above

Tone is the resistance of a muscle to passive stretch. Spasticity is the increase in tone associated with disease of upper motor neurons. It is velocity-dependent, has a sudden release after reaching a maximum ("clasp-knife" phenomenon), and predominantly affects antigravity muscles (upper-limb flexors & lower-limb extensors).

8. Which of the following is false about rigidity?
Harrison's 20th Ed. Chapter 21, Page 135

A. Hypertonia present throughout the range of motion
B. Affects flexors & extensors equally
C. Occurs with certain extrapyramidal disorders
D. None of the above

9. Which of the following about 'Spasticity' is false?
Harrison's 20th Ed. Chapter 21, Page 135

A. Velocity-dependent
B. Sudden release at maximum
C. Affects antigravity muscles
D. None of the above

Spasticity refers to an increase in tone associated with disease of upper motor neurons. Spasticity is velocity-dependent, has a sudden release after reaching a maximum and predominantly affects the antigravity muscles (upper-limb flexors and lower-limb extensors).

10. Which of the following is false about paratonia?
Harrison's 20th Ed. Chapter 21, Page 135

A. Present throughout the range of motion
B. Affects flexors & extensors equally
C. Results from disease of the frontal lobes
D. None of the above

11. Which of the following about 'Paratonia' is false?
Harrison's 20th Ed. Chapter 21, Page 135

A. Also called gegenhalten
B. Increased tone varies irregularly
C. Present throughout range of motion
D. None of the above

12. Which of the following about 'Paratonia' is false?
Harrison's 20th Ed. Chapter 21, Page 135

A. Increased muscle tone
B. Affects flexors & extensors equally
C. Results from disease of frontal lobes
D. None of the above

Paratonia (gegenhalten) is increased tone that varies irregularly related to the degree of relaxation. It is present throughout the range of motion and affects flexors & extensors equally. Results from disease of frontal lobes.

13. Paratonic rigidity or gegenhalten results from disease of?
Harrison's 20th Ed. Chapter 21, Page 135

A. Frontal lobes
B. Temporal lobes
C. Parietal lobes
D. Occipital lobes

Paratonia (or gegenhalten) is increased tone that varies irregularly in a manner that may seem related to the degree of relaxation, is present throughout the range of motion, and affects flexors and extensors equally; it usually results from disease of the frontal lobes.

14. Which of the following about 'flaccidity' is false?
Harrison's 20th Ed. Chapter 21, Page 135

A. Weakness
B. Decreased tone
C. Disorder of motor unit
D. None of the above

Weakness with decreased tone is called flaccidity. It occurs with disorders of motor units which consists of a single lower motor neuron and all of the muscle fibers that are innervated by it.

15. Which of the following is false about fasciculation?
Harrison's 20th Ed. Chapter 21, Page 135

A. Visible twitch
B. Palpable twitch
C. Spontaneous discharge of a motor unit
D. None of the above

Fasciculations are visible or palpable twitch within a muscle due to spontaneous discharge of a motor unit.

16. Which of the following statements is false?
Harrison's 20th Ed. Chapter 21, Page 135

A. Distal weakness is likely to be neuropathic
B. Symmetric proximal weakness is likely to be myopathic
C. Fasciculations indicate that weakness is myopathic
D. Early atrophy indicate that weakness is neuropathic

Fasciculations & early atrophy indicate that weakness is neuropathic.

17. Which of the following is false about UMN lesions?
Harrison's 20th Ed. Chapter 21, Page 136

A. Distal muscle groups are affected more severely
B. Axial movements are spared
C. Rapid repetitive movements are slowed & coarse
D. Normal rhythmicity is disturbed

Rapid repetitive movements are slowed and coarse, however, normal rhythmicity is maintained.

18. Which of the following is false about upper motor neuron weakness?
Harrison's 20th Ed. Chapter 21, Page 136

A. Proximal muscle groups affected more than distal
B. Axial movements spared
C. Affects ability to perform rapid repetitive movements
D. Normal movement rhythmicity is maintained

In UMN lesions, distal muscle groups are affected more severely than proximal ones.

19. With corticobulbar involvement, which of the following is affected?
Harrison's 20th Ed. Chapter 21, Page 136

A. Pharyngeal muscles
B. Jaw muscles
C. Tongue muscles
D. Upper facial muscles

With corticobulbar involvement, weakness occurs in the lower face & tongue. Typically, extraocular, upper facial, pharyngeal & jaw muscles are spared.

20. Pseudobulbar palsy consists of all except?
Harrison's 20th Ed. Chapter 21, Page 136

A. Dysarthria
B. Dysphagia
C. Dystonia
D. Dysphonia

Bilateral corticobulbar lesions produce a pseudobulbar palsy which consists of dysarthria, dysphagia, dysphonia, bilateral facial weakness and a brisk jaw jerk.

21. Upper motor neurons have their cell bodies in which layer of the primary motor cortex?
Harrison's 20th Ed. Chapter 21, Page 136 Figure 21-1

A. 3
B. 4
C. 5
D. 6

Upper motor neurons have their cell bodies in layer V of the primary motor cortex which consists of the precentral gyrus, or Brodmann's area 4 and the premotor & supplemental motor cortex area 6.

22. What percentage of corticospinal axons remain ipsilateral in the anterior spinal cord?
Harrison's 20th Ed. Chapter 21, Page 136 Figure 21-1

A. 2–10%
B. 5–20%
C. 10–30%
D. 20–50%

At cervicomedullary junction, most corticospinal axons decussate into contralateral corticospinal tract of the lateral spinal cord, but 10–30% remain ipsilateral in the anterior spinal cord.

23. What proportion of pyramidal axons do not decussate and remain ipsilateral?
Harrison's 20th Ed. Chapter 21, Page 136 Figure 21-1

A. 2–10%
B. 5–15%
C. 10–30%
D. 20–35%

At cervicomedullary junction, most pyramidal axons decussate into contralateral corticospinal tract of lateral spinal cord, but 10–30% remain ipsilateral in anterior spinal cord.

24. Corticospinal neurons innervate most densely the lower motor neurons of which of the following?
Harrison's 20th Ed. Chapter 21, Page 136 Figure 21-1

A. Tongue
B. Extra-ocular muscles
C. Hand muscles
D. Muscles of facial expression

Corticospinal neurons innervate most densely the lower motor neurons of hand muscles.

25. Which of the following originates predominantly in the red nucleus?
Harrison's 20th Ed. Chapter 21, Page 136 Figure 21-1

A. Ventromedial bulbospinal pathways
B. Ventrolateral bulbospinal pathways
C. Posteromedial bulbospinal pathways
D. Posterolateral bulbospinal pathways

The descending ventromedial bulbospinal pathways consists of tectospinal pathway, vestibulospinal pathway and the reticulospinal pathway. The descending ventrolateral bulbospinal pathways originates predominantly in the red nucleus (rubrospinal pathway).

26. Which of the following facilitates distal limb muscles?

Harrison's 20th Ed. Chapter 21, Page 136 Figure 21-1

A. Tectospinal pathway
B. Vestibulospinal pathway
C. Reticulospinal pathway
D. Rubrospinal pathway

Pathways that influence axial & proximal muscles are tectospinal pathway, vestibulospinal pathway and reticulospinal pathway. Pathway that facilitates distal limb muscles is rubrospinal pathway.

27. Descending ventromedial bulbospinal pathways include?

Harrison's 20th Ed. Chapter 21, Page 136 Figure 21-1

A. Tectospinal pathway
B. Vestibulospinal pathway
C. Reticulospinal pathway
D. All of the above

Descending ventromedial bulbospinal pathways include tectospinal, vestibulospinal, and reticulospinal pathways. These pathways influence axial & proximal muscles and are involved in the maintenance of posture and integrated movements of the limbs and trunk.

28. All of the following are part of descending ventromedial bulbospinal pathways except?

Harrison's 20th Ed. Chapter 21, Page 136 Figure 21-1

A. Tectospinal pathway
B. Vestibulospinal pathway
C. Reticulospinal pathway
D. Rubrospinal pathway

Descending ventrolateral bulbospinal pathways, which originate predominantly in red nucleus (rubrospinal pathway), facilitate distal limb muscles. Bulbospinal system is also called extrapyramidal upper motor neuron system.

29. Which of the following is false about lower motor neuron weakness?

Harrison's 20th Ed. Chapter 21, Page 136 Figure 21-2

A. Due to loss of α neurons
B. Due to loss of γ motor neurons
C. Absent tendon stretch reflex suggests involvement of spindle afferent fibers
D. Fasciculations signify anterior horn cell disease

Loss of γ-motor neurons does not cause weakness but decreases muscle tone and attenuates the stretch reflexes elicited on examination.

30. Which of the following is false about motor neurons?

Harrison's 20th Ed. Chapter 21, Page 136 Figure 21-2

A. α motor neurons innervate extrafusal muscle fibers
B. γ motor neurons innervate intrafusal muscle fibers
C. α motor neuron receives direct excitatory input from corticomotoneurons & primary muscle spindle afferents
D. α motor neurons receive direct excitation from Renshaw cell interneurons

α-motor neurons receive direct inhibition from Renshaw cell interneurons.

31. Motor neurons receive excitatory input from?

Harrison's 20th Ed. Chapter 21, Page 136 Figure 21-2

A. Descending upper motor neuron pathways
B. Segmental sensory inputs
C. Interneurons
D. All of the above

32. Which of the following is false about myopathic weakness?

Harrison's 20th Ed. Chapter 21, Page 137

A. Due to disorders of muscle fibers
B. Due to defect in neuromuscular junctions
C. In EMG, size of each motor unit action potential is reduced
D. Distribution of weakness is distal

Distribution of myopathic weakness is typically proximal. Lower motor neuron weakness is most profound distally.

33. Which of the following about Pronator Drift is false?

N Engl J Med. 2013;369:16 e20

A. Indicates subtle upper motor neuron disorder
B. May be seen in inborn errors of metabolism
C. Performed with outstretched upper limbs with palms facing upward
D. None of the above

In the presence of an upper motor neuron lesion, the supinator muscles in the upper limb are weaker than the pronator muscles, and as a result, the arm drifts downward and the palm turns toward the floor.

34. Fatigable weakness is suggestive of disorders of?

Harrison's 20th Ed. Chapter 21, Page 137

A. Neuromuscular junction weakness
B. Myopathic weakness
C. Psychogenic weakness
D. All of the above

Fatigable weakness indicates towards disorders of neuromuscular junction, which cause functional loss of muscle fibers due to failure of their repeated activation.

35. Most lesions that produce hemiparesis are?

Harrison's 20th Ed. Chapter 21, Page 137

A. Above the foramen magnum
B. In the upper cervical cord
C. In the lower cervical cord
D. Any of the above

Most lesions that produce hemiparesis are above the foramen magnum.

36. In hemiparesis, simultaneous language disorder point to a lesion in ?

Harrison's 20th Ed. Chapter 21, Page 137

A. Cerebral cortical lesion
B. Subcortical hemispheric lesion
C. Brainstem lesion
D. Any of the above

In hemiparesis, simultaneous language disorder point to a cortical lesion.

37. A "pure motor" hemiparesis of face, arm & leg is due to a lesion in?

Harrison's 20th Ed. Chapter 21, Page 137

A. Posterior limb of the internal capsule
B. Cerebral peduncle in the midbrain
C. Upper pons
D. Any of the above

38. Hemiparesis due to a cortical lesion is suggested by all except?

Harrison's 20th Ed. Chapter 21, Page 137

A. "Pure motor" hemiparesis
B. Disorders of visual-spatial integration
C. Apraxia
D. Seizures

Language disorders point to a cortical lesion. Homonymous visual field defects are due to either a cortical or a subcortical hemispheric lesion.

39. Chronic hemiparesis that evolves over months is due to?

Harrison's 20th Ed. Chapter 21, Page 137

A. Sarcoidosis
B. Primary central nervous system (CNS) lymphoma
C. Chronic subdural hematoma
D. All of the above

Chronic hemiparesis that evolves over months is due to a neoplasm/vascular malformation, chronic subdural hematoma, or a degenerative disease.

40. In the workup of a patient with proximal or distal weakness, the first investigation out of the following is?

Harrison's 20th Ed. Chapter 21, Page 137 Figure 21-3

A. Computed tomography (CT)
B. Magnetic resonance imaging (MRI)
C. Electromyography (EMG) & Nerve conduction studies (NCS)
D. Myelography

41. Disease of cerebral hemispheres that produces acute paraparesis is?

Harrison's 20th Ed. Chapter 21, Page 137

A. Anterior cerebral artery ischemia
B. Superior sagittal sinus or cortical venous thrombosis
C. Acute hydrocephalus
D. All of the above

42. Diseases of the cerebral hemispheres that produce acute paraparesis include?

Harrison's 20th Ed. Chapter 21, Page 137

A. Unpaired anterior cerebral artery ischemia
B. Superior sagittal sinus or cortical venous thrombosis
C. Acute hydrocephalus
D. All of the above

If hemispheric signs are present in a patient with subacute or chronic spastic paraparesis, a parasagittal meningioma or chronic hydrocephalus is likely.

43. Paraparesis can arise due to?

Harrison's 20th Ed. Chapter 21, Page 137

A. Anterior horn cell disorders
B. Cauda equina syndrome
C. Peripheral neuropathies
D. Any of the above

44. Acute paraparesis can be due to which of the following diseases of cerebral hemispheres?

Harrison's 20th Ed. Chapter 21, Page 137

A. Superior sagittal sinus thrombosis
B. Cortical venous thrombosis
C. Acute hydrocephalus
D. Any of the above

45. Acute monoparesis due to focal cortical ischemia is characterized by?

Harrison's 20th Ed. Chapter 21, Page 138

A. Weakness is predominantly distal
B. Weakness affects non-antigravity muscles
C. Not associated with sensory impairment or pain
D. All of the above

46. Weakness limited to respiratory muscles is due to?

Harrison's 20th Ed. Chapter 21, Page 138

A. Motor neuron disease
B. Myasthenia gravis
C. Polymyositis/dermatomyositis
D. All of the above

47. Which of the following is a cause of episodic generalized weakness?

Harrison's 20th Ed. Chapter 21, Page 138

A. Myasthenia gravis
B. Lambert-Eaton myasthenic syndrome
C. Multiple sclerosis
D. All of the above

48. Which of the following is false about 'Tetany'?

DeJong's The Neurologic Examination, 7th Ed. Page Page 766

A. Tingling around mouth
B. Manifestation of hypocalcemia
C. Manifestation of respiratory alkalosis
D. None of the above

49. Muscular rigidity may occur in?

DeJong's The Neurologic Examination, 7th Ed. Page Page 473

A. Epilepsy
B. Tetany
C. Tetanus
D. All of the above

Muscular rigidity may also occur in epilepsy, tetany, and tetanus.

50. Which of the following is a sign of tetany?

DeJong's The Neurologic Examination, 7th Ed. Page 767

A. Chvostek's sign
B. Trousseau's sign
C. Hochsinger's sign
D. All of the above

In Hochsinger's sign, when pressure on inner aspect of biceps muscle is applied, spasm and contraction of hand occurs in tetany. It is a variant of Trousseau sign.

51. Which of the following is a sign of tetany?

DeJong's The Neurologic Examination, 7th Ed. Page 767

A. Schultze's sign
B. Kashida's thermic sign
C. Escherich's sign
D. All of the above

52. Characteristics of dystonia include all except?

DeJong's The Neurologic Examination, 7th Ed. Page 767

A. Ill sustained muscle contractions
B. Repetitive twisting movements
C. Abnormal posture
D. Often has a genetic basis

Dystonia is a disorder characterized by sustained muscle contractions, resulting in repetitive twisting movements and abnormal posture. It often has a genetic basis.

53. Which of the following is labeled as the "Fifth vital sign"?

Harrison's 20th Ed. Chapter 9, Page 51

A. Pain assessment
B. Skin hue
C. Cooperation of patient
D. Colour of nails

Numbness, Tingling, and Sensory Loss

54. Which of the following is not a positive sensory symptom?
Harrison's 20th Ed. Chapter 22, Page 139

A. Tingling
B. Numbness
C. Burning
D. Pricking

Loss of sensory function (diminished or absent feeling) is termed negative phenomena experienced as numbness and abnormal finding on sensory examination.

55. Hyperesthesia means pain or increased sensitivity in response to?
Harrison's 20th Ed. Chapter 22, Page 139

A. Touch
B. Pain
C. Warm or cold stimuli
D. All of the above

Hyperesthesia means pain or increased sensitivity in response to touch.

56. Allodynia refers to?
Harrison's 20th Ed. Chapter 22, Page 139

A. Pain on imagination
B. Fear of pain
C. Painful response to nonpainful stimulus
D. Nonpainful response to painful stimulus

Painful response to nonpainful stimulus is termed allodynia. Like, elicitation of a painful sensation by application of a vibrating tuning fork.

57. Hyperpathia includes which of the following?
Harrison's 20th Ed. Chapter 22, Page 139

A. Hyperesthesia
B. Allodynia
C. Hyperalgesia
D. All of the above

Hyperpathia, a broad term, encompasses all the phenomena described by hyperesthesia, allodynia, and hyperalgesia. With hyperpathia, the threshold for a sensory stimulus is increased and perception is delayed, but once felt, is unduly painful.

58. Sense of vibration is tested with a tuning fork that vibrates at?
Harrison's 20th Ed. Chapter 22, Page 139

A. 128 Hz
B. 256 Hz
C. 512 Hz
D. Any of the above

Sense of vibration is tested with a tuning fork that vibrates at 128 Hz.

59. Cortical sensation are tested by?
Harrison's 20th Ed. Chapter 22, Page 139

A. Two-point discrimination
B. Bilateral simultaneous stimulation
C. Graphesthesia
D. All of the above

Commonly used tests of cortical function are two-point discrimination, touch localization, bilateral simultaneous stimulation & tests for graphesthesia and stereognosis.

60. Normal individuals can distinguish separation of points by what minimum distance in 2-PD test?
Harrison's 20th Ed. Chapter 22, Page 139

A. 1 mm
B. 3 mm
C. 5 mm
D. 7 mm

Normal individuals can distinguish separation of points by 3 mm distance in two-point discrimination test.

61. Which of the following is false about small-fiber polyneuropathy?
Harrison's 20th Ed. Chapter 22, Page 139

A. Burning, painful dysesthesias
B. Sparing of proprioception
C. Sparing of motor function
D. Absent tendon reflexes

62. Which of the following is false about large-fiber polyneuropathy?
Harrison's 20th Ed. Chapter 22, Page 139

A. Vibration & position sense deficits
B. Imbalance
C. Absent tendon reflexes
D. None of the above

Small-fiber polyneuropathies are characterized by burning, painful dysesthesias with reduced pinprick & thermal sensation but sparing of proprioception, motor function & deep tendon reflexes. Large-fiber polyneuropathies are characterized by vibration & position sense deficits, imbalance, absent tendon reflexes & variable motor dysfunction but preservation of most cutaneous sensation.

63. Which of the following is the prototypical positive symptom?
Harrison's 20th Ed. Chapter 22, Page 139

A. Raw feelings
B. Burning
C. Tingling (pins and needles)
D. Itch

The prototypical positive symptom is tingling (pins & needles). Other positive sensory phenomena include itch & altered sensations that are described as pricking, band like, lightning-like shooting feelings (lancinations), aching, knife like, twisting, drawing, pulling, tightening, burning, searing, electrical, or raw feelings. Positive phenomena represent excessive activity in sensory pathways.

64. Term hyperpathia includes which of the following?
Harrison's 20th Ed. Chapter 22, Page 139

A. Hyperesthesia
B. Allodynia
C. Hyperalgesia
D. All of the above

Term hyperpathia encompasses all phenomena described by hyperesthesia, allodynia & hyperalgesia.

65. Sensory ataxia includes which of the following?
Harrison's 20th Ed. Chapter 22, Page 139

A. Imbalance, particularly with eyes closed or in dark
B. Clumsiness of precision movements
C. Unsteadiness of gait
D. All of the above

66. Continuous involuntary movements of outstretched hands & fingers with eyes closed is called?

Harrison's 20th Ed. Chapter 21, Page 139

A. Alogia
B. Spooning
C. Punding
D. Pseudoathetosis

Pseudoathetosis refers to continuous involuntary movements of the outstretched hands & fingers, particularly with eyes closed.

67. Which of the following cutaneous receptor highly developed in the finger pads?

DeJong's The Neurologic Examination, 7th Ed. Page 526

A. Merkel cell endings
B. Meissner's corpuscles
C. Pacinian corpuscles
D. Ruffini endings

68. Fibers below which level are grouped together in fasciculus gracilis?

DeJong's The Neurologic Examination, 7th Ed. Page 528

A. About C8
B. About T4
C. About T8
D. About T12

All the fibers below about T8 are grouped together in the fasciculus gracilis. Analogous fibers above T8 form the fasciculus cuneatus.

69. Sense of vibration is tested with an oscillating tuning fork that vibrates at?

Harrison's 20th Ed. Chapter 22, Page 140

A. 128 Hz
B. 256 Hz
C. 512 Hz
D. Any of the above

Sense of vibration is tested with an oscillating tuning fork that vibrates at 128 Hz.

70. Which of the following statements is false?

Harrison's 20th Ed. Chapter 22, Page 140

A. Vibration is tested over bony points, beginning distally
B. Examiner may serve as control
C. Interside comparison are important
D. None of the above

71. In two-point discrimination test on fingertips, a normal person can distinguish what distance of separation of points?

Harrison's 20th Ed. Chapter 22, Page 141, DeJong's The Neurologic Examination, 7th Ed. Page 542

A. About 2 mm
B. About 3 mm
C. About 4 mm
D. About 5 mm

In two-point discrimination test on fingertips, a normal individual can distinguish about 3 mm. separation of points. Normal two-point discrimination is about 1 mm on the tip of the tongue, 2 to 3 mm on the lips, 2 to 4 mm on the fingertips, 4 to 6 mm on the dorsum of fingers, 8 to 12 mm on the palm, 20 to 30 mm on the back of the hand, and 30 to 40 mm on the dorsum of the foot.

72. Which of the following can be used to demonstrate a sensory level on trunk in myelopathy?

DeJong's The Neurologic Examination, 7th Ed. Page 542

A. Stereognosis
B. Graphesthesia
C. Two-point discrimination
D. All of the above

Two-point discrimination may also be used to demonstrate a sensory level on the trunk in myelopathy.

73. Which of the following is true about small-fiber polyneuropathies?

Harrison's 20th Ed. Chapter 22, Page 142

A. Reduced proprioception
B. Reduced thermal sensation
C. Variable motor dysfunction
D. Absent deep tendon reflexes

Small-fiber polyneuropathies are characterized by burning, painful dysesthesias with reduced pinprick and thermal sensation but with sparing of proprioception, motor function, and deep tendon reflexes.

74. Large-fiber polyneuropathies are characterized by all except?

Harrison's 20th Ed. Chapter 22, Page 142

A. Vibration and position sense deficits
B. Absent tendon reflexes
C. Variable motor dysfunction
D. Cutaneous sensation dysfunction

Large-fiber polyneuropathies are characterized by vibration & position sense deficits, imbalance, absent tendon reflexes, and variable motor dysfunction but preservation of most cutaneous sensation.

75. Sensory neuronopathy (or ganglionopathy) is best related to?

Harrison's 20th Ed. Chapter 22, Page 142

A. Leprosy
B. Sjögren's syndrome
C. Vitamin B12 deficiency
D. Isoniazid

Sensory neuronopathy (or ganglionopathy) is characterized by pain & numbness that progress to sensory ataxia and impairment of all sensory modalities with time. It is usually paraneoplastic or idiopathic in origin or related to an autoimmune disease, particularly Sjögren's syndrome.

76. In Déjerine-Roussy syndrome, the lesion is in?

Harrison's 20th Ed. Chapter 22, Page 142

A. Spinal cord
B. Brainstem
C. Thalamus
D. Cortex

Lesions affecting thalamic VPL nucleus or adjacent white matter, produce a syndrome of persistent, unrelenting unilateral thalamic pain, called Déjerine-Roussy syndrome.

77. In pseudothalamic syndrome, the lesion is in?

Harrison's 20th Ed. Chapter 22, Page 142

A. Spinal cord
B. Brainstem
C. Thalamus
D. Cortex

Anterior parietal infarction presents as a pseudothalamic syndrome with contralateral loss of primary sensation from head to toe.

78. The principal symptom of focal sensory seizures is?

Harrison's 20th Ed. Chapter 22, Page 142

A. Sense of warmth
B. Tingling
C. A sense of movement without detectable motion
D. Rushing feeling

The principal symptom of focal sensory seizures is tingling.

79. Which of the following nucleus of thalamus is related to sensory pathway?

DeJong's The Neurologic Examination, 7th Ed. Page 524

A. Lateral geniculate nucleus
B. Medial geniculate nucleus
C. Ventral posterolateral nucleus
D. Ventral anterior nucleus

80. Which of the following is a classic sign of tabes dorsalis?

DeJong's The Neurologic Examination, 7th Ed. Page 537

A. Abadie's sign
B. Biernacki's sign
C. Pitres' sign
D. All of the above

Abadie's sign is the absence of pain on squeezing the Achilles tendon. Biernacki's sign is the absence of pain on pressure on the ulnar nerve. Pitres' sign is loss of pain squeezing testicles. All these are classic signs of tabes dorsalis.

81. General visceral afferent fibers are found in all of the following cranial nerves except?

DeJong's The Neurologic Examination, 7th Ed. Page 539

A. V
B. VII
C. IX
D. X

General visceral afferent fibers are found in cranial nerves VII, IX, and X and in the thoracolumbar and sacral autonomic nerves.

82. Finger agnosia occurs most commonly as part of?

DeJong's The Neurologic Examination, 7th Ed. Page 543

A. Gerstmann's syndrome
B. Central cord syndrome
C. Brown-Séquard syndrome
D. Wallenberg's syndrome

Finger agnosia occurs most commonly as part of Gerstmann's syndrome (finger agnosia, agraphia, acalculia, and right-left disorientation).

83. Which of the following is a cause of dissociated sensory loss?

DeJong's The Neurologic Examination, 7th Ed. Page 545

A. Anterior spinal artery stroke
B. Syringomyelia
C. Wallenberg's syndrome
D. All of the above

Patients with Brown-Séquard syndrome have extreme dissociation of modalities, with loss of pain & temperature on one side of body and loss of touch, pressure, position & vibration on the other side of body.

84. Which of the following is false about Brown-Séquard syndrome?

DeJong's The Neurologic Examination, 7th Ed. Page 545

A. Hemisection of the spinal cord
B. Absent pain & temperature sensation contralaterally
C. Loss of proprioceptive sensation & power ipsilaterally
D. None of the above

Hemisection of spinal cord produces Brown-Séquard syndrome, with absent pain & temperature sensation contralaterally & loss of proprioceptive sensation & power ipsilaterally below the lesion.

85. Which of the following does not cause large fiber sensory neuropathy?

DeJong's The Neurologic Examination, 7th Ed. Page 550

A. Uremia
B. Amyloidosis
C. Sjögren's syndrome
D. Vitamin B12 deficiency

86. Which of the following causes small fiber sensory neuropathy?

DeJong's The Neurologic Examination, 7th Ed. Page 550

A. Amyloidosis
B. Hereditary sensory autonomic neuropathy
C. Diabetes mellitus
D. All of the above

Large fiber sensory neuropathies include uremia, Sjögren's syndrome, vitamin B12 deficiency, toxins (pyridoxine, cisplatin, metronidazole) & some cases of diabetes (pseudotabes). Small fiber neuropathies include amyloidosis, hereditary sensory autonomic neuropathy, and some cases of diabetes mellitus (pseudosyringomyelia).

87. In generalized peripheral neuropathies, which of the following is affected first?

DeJong's The Neurologic Examination, 7th Ed. Page 549

A. Pain
B. Vibration
C. Cold
D. Heat

In generalized peripheral neuropathies, vibration is often the first modality affected.

88. During recovery, which of the following sensation returns first?

DeJong's The Neurologic Examination, 7th Ed. Page 552

A. Tactile
B. Pain
C. Pressure
D. Heat

The pattern of sensory return with recovering spinal lesions, pressure sensation returns first and its recovery is usually the most complete, followed, in turn, by tactile, pain, cold, and heat sensibilities.

89. Which of the following sensory loss occurs in syringomyelia?

DeJong's The Neurologic Examination, 7th Ed. Page 552

A. Pinprick & temperature
B. Light touch
C. Position sense
D. Vibration

In syringomyelia there is a dissociated sensory loss with impairment of pinprick & temperature appreciation. Light touch, position sense and vibration appreciation are preserved.

90. Which of the following is related to Lhermitte's sign?

DeJong's The Neurologic Examination, 7th Ed. Page 552

A. Flexion of the neck

B. Electric shock like sensation

C. Radiation down the back & into the legs

D. All of the above

In Lhermitte's sign, flexion of neck leads to an electric shock like sensation that radiates down the back and into the legs. It is seen in patients with a cervical lesion affecting posterior columns like multiple sclerosis, cervical spondylosis or recent irradiation to the cervical region. Vitamin B12 deficiency syndrome & Cisplatin toxicity can also cause it.

91. Pansensory loss contralaterally is produced by a lesion in?

DeJong's The Neurologic Examination, 7th Ed. Page 552

A. Cervical spinal cord

B. Thalamus

C. Tegmentum of pons & midbrain

D. Lateral medulla

A lesion in tegmentum of pons & midbrain, where lemniscal & spinothalamic tracts merge, causes pansensory loss contralaterally.

Gait Disorders, Imbalance, and Falls

92. Sensory information for postural control is primarily generated by?

Harrison's 20th Ed. Chapter 23, Page 143

A. Visual system
B. Vestibular system
C. Proprioceptive receptors in the muscle spindles & joints
D. All of the above

Loss of two of the above three pathways is sufficient to compromise standing balance.

93. Gait that results from avoidance of pain associated with weight-bearing is called?

Harrison's 20th Ed. Chapter 23, Page 143

A. Antalgic gait
B. Steppage gait
C. Scissoring gait
D. Functional gait

94. Which of the following is the commonest etiology of gait disorders?

Harrison's 20th Ed. Chapter 23, Page 143 Table 23-1

A. Parkinsonism
B. Cerebellar degeneration
C. Multiple infarcts
D. Sensory deficits

95. Which of the following is a feature of cautious gait?

Harrison's 20th Ed. Chapter 23, Page 144

A. Abbreviated stride
B. Widened base
C. Lowered center of mass
D. All of the above

96. Which of the following is a stiff-legged gait?

Harrison's 20th Ed. Chapter 23, Page 144

A. Dystonia
B. Stiff-person syndrome
C. Spastic gait
D. All of the above

97. Freezing of gait is seen in?

Harrison's 20th Ed. Chapter 23, Page 144

A. Progressive supranuclear palsy (PSP)
B. Multiple-system atrophy
C. Corticobasal degeneration
D. All of the above

Freezing gait is a feature of Parkinson's disease, progressive supranuclear palsy, multiple system atrophy, corticobasal degeneration, and primary pallidal degeneration.

98. Pill-rolling tremor is a characteristic feature of?

Harrison's 20th Ed. Chapter 23, Page 144

A. Progressive supranuclear palsy
B. Multiple system atrophy
C. Corticobasal degeneration
D. Parkinson's disease

99. Pill-rolling tremor of Parkinson's disease is seen in?

Harrison's 20th Ed. Chapter 23, Page 144

A. Progressive supranuclear palsy (PSP)
B. Multiple-system atrophy
C. Corticobasal degeneration
D. None of the above

100. Which of the following about progressive supranuclear palsy (PSP) is false?

Harrison's 20th Ed. Chapter 23, Page 144

A. Gait more erect compared to stooped posture of Parkinson's
B. No pill-rolling tremor
C. Falls within the first year
D. None of the above

101. Gait with a dancing quality is a feature of?

Harrison's 20th Ed. Chapter 23, Page 144

A. Tardive dyskinesia
B. Huntington's disease
C. Stiff-Person syndrome
D. Psychogenic cause

In Huntington's disease, unpredictable occurrence of choreic movements gives gait a dancing quality.

102. "Higher level gait disorder" refers to?

Harrison's 20th Ed. Chapter 23, Page 144

A. Sensory ataxia
B. Cerebellar ataxia
C. Frontal gait disorder
D. All of the above

Frontal gait disorder is also known as higher level gait disorder.

103. Term "gait apraxia" refers to?

Harrison's 20th Ed. Chapter 23, Page 144

A. Cautious gait
B. Cerebellar gait ataxia
C. Frontal gait disorder
D. Sensory ataxia

104. Which of the following terms is used to describe frontal gait disorders?

Harrison's 20th Ed. Chapter 23, Page 144

A. "Slipping clutch" syndrome
B. Gait ignition failure
C. Lower-body parkinsonism
D. All of the above

105. The lesion in frontal gait disorder is in?

Harrison's 20th Ed. Chapter 23, Page 144

A. Locus coeruleus
B. Periaqueductal gray
C. Centrum ovale
D. Substantia nigra pars compacta

Vascular small-vessel disease is the most common cause of frontal gait disorder. The lesion is in subcortical region in deep frontal white matter & centrum ovale.

106. Which of the following is a feature of normal pressure (communicating) hydrocephalus?

Harrison's 20th Ed. Chapter 23, Page 144

A. Gait disorder
B. Mental changes
C. Incontinence
D. All of the above

107. Which of the following is an early feature of cerebellar gait ataxia?

Harrison's 20th Ed. Chapter 23, Page 144

A. Lateral instability of the trunk
B. Erratic foot placement
C. Difficulty maintaining balance when turning
D. Wide base of support

Cerebellar gait ataxia is characterized by a wide base of support, lateral instability of trunk, erratic foot placement, decompensation of balance when attempting to walk on a narrow base, difficulty maintaining balance when turning (early feature), and unable to walk tandem heel to toe. Patients with cerebellar ataxia do not complain of dizziness. Neurologic examination reveals cerebellar signs.

108. Which of the following is false about sensory ataxia?

Harrison's 20th Ed. Chapter 23, Page 145 Table 23-2

A. Narrow base, looks down
B. Normal initiation
C. Regular stride with path deviation
D. None of the above

109. Steppage gait best relates to?

Harrison's 20th Ed. Chapter 23, Page 145

A. Neuromuscular disease
B. Cerebellar gait ataxia
C. Sensory ataxia
D. Functional disorders

110. "Astasia-abasia" best relates to?

Harrison's 20th Ed. Chapter 23, Page 145

A. Cautious gait
B. Cerebellar gait ataxia
C. Functional gait disorder
D. Sensory ataxia

Hysterical gait disorders with odd gyrations of posture & wastage of muscular energy (astasia-abasia), extreme slow motion & dramatic fluctuations over time are seen in somatoform disorders & conversion reaction.

111. Gait disorder associated with urinary urgency & incontinence, point towards the diagnosis of?

Harrison's 20th Ed. Chapter 23, Page 145

A. Cerebellar gait ataxia
B. Sensory ataxia
C. Functional disorders
D. Hydrocephalus

Gait disorder may be associated with urinary urgency & incontinence, particularly in patients with cervical spine disease or hydrocephalus.

112. For assessment of a gait disorder, which of the following must be noted?

Harrison's 20th Ed. Chapter 23, Page 145

A. Cadence (steps per minute)
B. Velocity and stride length
C. Watching the patient rise from a chair
D. All of the above

113. Which of the following favour diagnosis of a vestibular disorder?

Harrison's 20th Ed. Chapter 23, Page 145

A. Vertigo
B. Nystagmus
C. Impaired standing balance
D. All of the above

114. Which of the following is the most common risk factor for falls in older persons?

Harrison's 20th Ed. Chapter 23, Page 146 Table 23-3

A. History of falls
B. Visual deficit
C. Cognitive impairment
D. Muscle weakness

115. Which of the following are at high risk for falls?

Harrison's 20th Ed. Chapter 23, Page 146

A. Polypharmacy (use of ≥ 4 prescription medications)
B. Patients with a history of falls
C. Those requiring >12 seconds to complete TUG test
D. All of the above

The Timed Up & Go ("TUG") test involves timing a patient as they stand up from a chair, walk 10 feet, turn, then sit down. Patients with a history of falls, or those requiring >12 seconds to complete the TUG test, are high risk for falls.

116. Which of the following is a cause of drop attacks and collapsing falls?

Harrison's 20th Ed. Chapter 23, Page 146

A. Syncope or orthostatic hypotension
B. Atonic seizures
C. Myoclonus
D. All of the above

117. Thalamic astasia relates best with?

Harrison's 20th Ed. Chapter 23, Page 146

A. Toppling falls
B. Drop attacks and collapsing falls
C. Falls due to gait freezing
D. Falls related to sensory loss

118. Toppling falls relates best with?

Harrison's 20th Ed. Chapter 23, Page 146

A. Syncope
B. Progressive supranuclear palsy (PSP)
C. Parkinson's disease
D. Acute obstructive hydrocephalus

Toppling falls are an early feature of PSP..

Confusion and Delirium

119. In confusion, which of the following is reduced?
Harrison's 20th Ed. Chapter 24, Page 147

A. Comprehension
B. Coherence
C. Capacity to reason
D. All of the above

120. Which of the following terms are used to describe patients with delirium?
Harrison's 20th Ed. Chapter 24, Page 147

A. Encephalopathy
B. Acute brain failure
C. Acute confusional state
D. All of the above

121. Cognitive domain includes which of the following?
Harrison's 20th Ed. Chapter 24, Page 147

A. Memory
B. Executive function
C. Visuospatial tasks
D. All of the above

Cognitive domains include memory, executive function, visuospatial tasks and language.

122. Which of the following about delirium is false?
Harrison's 20th Ed. Chapter 24, Page 147

A. Hallmark of delirium is a deficit of attention
B. Fluctuates over hours or days
C. It is a clinical diagnosis that is made only at bedside
D. None of the above

123. Which of the following is a feature of hyperactive subtype of delirium?
Harrison's 20th Ed. Chapter 24, Page 147

A. Hallucinations
B. Agitation, and hyperarousal
C. Life-threatening autonomic instability
D. All of the above

Severe alcohol withdrawal (delirium tremens) is the classic example of hyperactive subtype of delirium.

124. Most consistently identified risk factor for delirium is?
Harrison's 20th Ed. Chapter 24, Page 147

A. Preexisting hearing & visual impairment
B. Baseline cognitive dysfunction
C. Malnutrition
D. Medication

Two most consistently identified risk factors for delirium are older age & baseline cognitive dysfunction.

125. Patients with which of the following diseases clinically resembles hyperactive delirium?
Harrison's 20th Ed. Chapter 24, Page 148

A. Alzheimer's disease
B. Dementia with Lewy bodies
C. Parkinson's disease dementia
D. All of the above

Dementia with Lewy bodies (DLB) is characterized by a fluctuating course, prominent visual hallucinations, parkinsonism & attentional deficit that clinically resembles hyperactive delirium. They are vulnerable to delirium.

126. Which of the following is a screening tool for identifying patients with delirium?
Harrison's 20th Ed. Chapter 24, Page 147

A. Confusion Assessment Method (CAM)
B. Nursing Delirium Screening Scale (NuDESC)
C. Organic Brain Syndrome Scale
D. All of the above

127. Presence of which of the following helps in diagnosis of delirium?
Harrison's 20th Ed. Chapter 24, Page 147

A. Acute onset of confusion and fluctuating course
B. Inattention accompanied by disorganized thinking
C. Inattention accompanied by altered level of consciousness
D. All of the above

128. Which of the following best relates to delirium?
Harrison's 20th Ed. Chapter 24, Page 148

A. Sundowning
B. Fast-working
C. Mock sun
D. Rainbow

In delirium, fluctuations may occur over hours or days and may worsen at night. This is called sundowning. It is typical but not essential for the diagnosis of delirium.

129. Which of the following is essential in history taking of a delirium patient?
Harrison's 20th Ed. Chapter 24, Page 149

A. Patient's baseline cognitive function
B. Time course of the present illness
C. Current medications
D. All of the above

130. Which of the following is false about "Digit span forward" test?
Harrison's 20th Ed. Chapter 24, Page 149

A. Test of attention
B. Normal capacity is six numbers
C. Asking patient to repeat digits in same order told
D. None of the above

131. Which of the following is false about "Digit span backward" test?
Harrison's 20th Ed. Chapter 24, Page 149

A. Test of working memory
B. Normal capacity is five numbers
C. Asking patient to repeat digits in reverse order
D. None of the above

Most common bedside test of working memory involves asking patients to repeat a series of digits orally, with the clinician gradually increasing the number of to-be-retained digits. Asking the patient to repeat digits in the same order as they were delivered is called digit span forward which is a test of attention. Clinician may also ask the patient to repeat digits in reverse order. This is called digit span backward which is a test of working memory. Capacity for digit span forward is typically six numbers, while normal adults can generally repeat five digits backward.

132. Deficiency of which of the following can cause delirium?

Harrison's 20th Ed. Chapter 24, Page 150 Table 24-2

A. Vitamin B12
B. Thiamine
C. Niacin
D. All of the above

133. Which of the following can cause delirium?

Harrison's 20th Ed. Chapter 24, Page 150 Table 24-2

A. Anticholinergic drugs
B. Narcotics
C. Benzodiazepines
D. All of the above

134. Which of the following is a drug of abuse?

Harrison's 20th Ed. Chapter 24, Page 149

A. γ-hydroxybutyrate (GHB)
B. Phencyclidine (PCP)
C. Bath salts
D. All of the above

135. Which of the following sedatives is less likely to lead to delirium in critically ill patients?

Harrison's 20th Ed. Chapter 24, Page 151

A. Dexmedetomidine
B. Propofol
C. Fentanyl
D. Midazolam

136. Which of the following drug may be effective for delirium prevention?

Harrison's 20th Ed. Chapter 24, Page 151

A. Agomelatine
B. Luzindole
C. Ramelteon
D. Prazosin

Melatonin and its agonist ramelteon have shown beneficial results for delirium prevention.

Dementia

137. Which of the following does not appear in the definition of dementia?

Harrison's 20th Ed. Chapter 25, Page 152

A. Acquired
B. Deterioration in cognitive abilities
C. Impairment in activities of daily living
D. Co-morbid diseases

It is defined as an acquired deterioration in cognitive abilities that impairs the successful performance of activities of daily living. The common forms of dementia are progressive.

138. Which of the following is most commonly affected in dementia?

Harrison's 20th Ed. Chapter 25, Page 152

A. Visuospatial ability
B. Calculation
C. Episodic memory
D. Language

Episodic memory is the most common cognitive ability lost with dementia. Other mental faculties like language, visuospatial, praxis, calculation, judgment, and problem-solving abilities are also affected. Neuropsychiatric and social deficits may also develop in dementia syndromes resulting in depression, withdrawal, hallucinations, delusions, agitation, insomnia, and disinhibition.

139. Clinical course of dementia may be static in which of the following?

Harrison's 20th Ed. Chapter 25, Page 152

A. Alzheimer's disease
B. Anoxic encephalopathy
C. Dementia with Lewy bodies
D. Frontotemporal dementia

Clinical course of dementia may be slowly progressive (Alzheimer's disease), static (anoxic encephalopathy) or may fluctuate from day to day or minute to minute (dementia with Lewy bodies).

140. Memory loss is not typically a presenting feature in?

Harrison's 20th Ed. Chapter 25, Page 152

A. Alzheimer's disease
B. Anoxic encephalopathy
C. Dementia with Lewy bodies
D. Frontotemporal dementia

Memory loss is not typically a presenting feature in Frontotemporal dementia (FTD). They are more likely to present with difficulties with judgment, mood, executive control, movement, and behavior.

141. Behavior and mood are modulated by which of the following pathway?

Harrison's 20th Ed. Chapter 25, Page 152

A. Noradrenergic pathway
B. Serotonergic pathway
C. Dopaminergic pathway
D. All of the above

142. Which of the following pathways is critical for attention & memory functions?

Harrison's 20th Ed. Chapter 25, Page 152

A. Noradrenergic pathway
B. Serotonergic pathway
C. Dopaminergic pathway
D. Cholinergic pathway

Behavior and mood are modulated by noradrenergic, serotonergic, and dopaminergic pathways, while cholinergic signaling is critical for attention and memory functions.

143. Pathological process in Alzheimer's disease (AD) begins in?

Harrison's 20th Ed. Chapter 25, Page 152

A. Entorhinal cortex
B. Hippocampus
C. Posterior temporal neocortex
D. Parietal neocortex

AD begins in entorhinal cortex of the medial temporal lobe, then involves hippocampus, posterior temporal & parietal neocortex and eventually causes a relatively diffuse degeneration throughout cerebral cortex.

144. Dorsolateral prefrontal cortex has connections with?

Harrison's 20th Ed. Chapter 25, Page 152

A. Central band of caudate nucleus
B. Ventromedial caudate nucleus
C. Nucleus accumbens
D. All of the above

Dorsolateral prefrontal cortex has connections through frontal-striatal pathways with a central band of caudate nucleus. Lesions here result in executive dysfunction, manifesting as poor organization and planning, decreased cognitive flexibility & impaired working memory. Lateral orbital frontal cortex connects with ventromedial caudate, and lesions cause impulsiveness, distractibility, and disinhibition. Anterior cingulate cortex and adjacent medial prefrontal cortex project to nucleus accumbens and interruption here produces apathy, poverty of speech, emotional blunting, or even akinetic mutism.

145. The striatum comprises of all except?

Harrison's 20th Ed. Chapter 25, Page 152

A. Caudate nucleus
B. Putamen
C. Globus pallidus
D. Nucleus accumbens

The striatum comprises of caudate, putamen and nucleus accumbens.

146. Which of the following is the single strongest risk factor for dementia?

Harrison's 20th Ed. Chapter 25, Page 152

A. Race/ethnicity
B. Geographical location
C. Intoxications
D. Age

The single strongest risk factor for dementia is increasing age.

147. After Alzheimer disease, which of the following is the most common cause of dementia?

Harrison's 20th Ed. Chapter 25, Page 153

A. Vascular dementia
B. Multiple system atrophy
C. Parkinson disease dementia
D. Frontotemporal dementia

Vascular disease is considered the second most frequent cause for dementia after Alzheimer disease.

148. In patients aged <65 years, which of the following is the most common cause of dementia?

Harrison's 20th Ed. Chapter 25, Page 153

A. Vascular dementia
B. Multiple system atrophy
C. Parkinson disease dementia
D. Frontotemporal dementia

In patients aged <65 years, Frontotemporal dementia (FTD) is the most common cause of dementia.

149. Binswanger's syndrome best relates to?

Harrison's 20th Ed. Chapter 25, Page 152 Table 25-1

A. Alcoholism
B. Encephalopathy
C. Head trauma
D. Diffuse white matter disease

150. Pseudodementia is best related to?

Harrison's 20th Ed. Chapter 25, Page 152 Table 25-1

A. Depression
B. Schizophrenia
C. Conversion reaction
D. HIV

Severely depressed or anxious individuals may appear demented, a phenomenon called pseudodementia. Dementia associated with depression (pseudodementia), schizophrenia, and conversion reaction are potentially reversible while that with HIV is not.

151. Which of the following is not a potentially reversible dementia?

Harrison's 20th Ed. Chapter 25, Page 152 Table 25-1

A. Depression
B. Normal-pressure hydrocephalus
C. HIV
D. Alcoholism

The three most common potentially reversible dementias are depression, normal pressure hydrocephalus (NPH), alcohol dependence. Others include subacute combined degeneration, pellagra, adrenal insufficiency and Cushing's syndrome, due to drug, medication, and narcotic poisoning.

152. Which of the following is false about "Benign forgetfulness of the elderly"?

Harrison's 20th Ed. Chapter 25, Page 153, JMAJ 2001;44(6):274-278

A. Not so progressive
B. Does not impair productive daily functioning
C. Revised Hasegawa's Dementia Scale (HDS-R) useful
D. None of the above

"Benign forgetfulness of the elderly" or "benign senescent forgetfulness" or benign senescent amnesia (BSA) implies that changes in memory functions are part of "normal" aging and not associated with central nervous system pathology. Features of BSA include nonprogressive, partial disturbance of episodic memory or word amnesia, with no disorientation, no disturbance of judgement or abstract thinking, aware of memory decline, and mild and not affecting daily life. In contrast, features of AD include progressive, disturbance of memory in general (first-delayed recall), with disorientation (first-temporal disorientation), reduction of all intellectual capabilities, unaware of memory decline, and affecting daily life.

153. Factors that predict progression from MCI to an AD dementia include?

Harrison's 20th Ed. Chapter 25, Page 153

A. Apolipoprotein ε4 (Apo ε4) allele
B. Low cerebrospinal fluid Aβ
C. Elevated tau on PET imaging
D. All of the above

Factors that predict progression from MCI to an AD dementia include a prominent memory deficit, family history of dementia, presence of apolipoprotein ε4 (Apo ε4) allele, small hippocampal volumes, an AD-like signature of cortical atrophy, low cerebrospinal fluid Aβ, & elevated tau or evidence of brain amyloid deposition on positron emission tomography (PET) imaging.

154. Which of the following can predict progression from mild cognitive impairment (MCI) to Alzheimer's disease (AD)?

Harrison's 20th Ed. Chapter 25, Page 153

A. Diffuse white matter disease
B. Ventricular system dilatation
C. Hippocampal atrophy
D. Subdural effusion

In neuroimaging studies, factors that predict progression from MCI to AD include a memory deficit >1.5 SD from normal, family history of dementia, presence of an apolipoprotein ε4 (Apo ε4) and small hippocampal volumes + posterior-predominant cortical atrophy.

155. Major degenerative dementias include?

Harrison's 20th Ed. Chapter 25, Page 153

A. Alzheimer's disease
B. Creutzfeldt-Jakob disease
C. Dementia with Lewy bodies
D. All of the above

Major degenerative dementias include AD, DLB, FTD, HD & prion diseases like CJD.

156. Which of the following specific protein is abnormal aggregated in frontotemporal dementia?

Harrison's 20th Ed. Chapter 25, Page 153 Table 25-2

A. Tau
B. TDP-43
C. FUS
D. All of the above

157. FUS refers to?

Harrison's 20th Ed. Chapter 25, Page 153

A. Fused in sarcoplasm
B. Fused in synuclein
C. Fused in sarcoma
D. Fused in specimen

158. Which of the following specific protein is abnormal aggregated in Alzheimer's disease?

Harrison's 20th Ed. Chapter 25, Page 153 Table 25-2

A. Aβ
B. α-Synuclein
C. PrP^{SC}
D. All of the above

159. α-Synuclein best relates to?

Harrison's 20th Ed. Chapter 25, Page 153 Table 25-2

A. Alzheimer's disease
B. Creutzfeldt-Jakob disease
C. Dementia with Lewy bodies
D. Frontotemporal dementia

Lewy bodies are α-Synuclein neuronal inclusions, found in Dementia with Lewy bodies (DLB).

160. The major degenerative dementias can be distinguished by?

Harrison's 20th Ed. Chapter 25, Page 153

A. Initial or first symptoms
B. Neuroimaging features
C. Neurologic findings
D. All of the above

The major degenerative dementias can be distinguished by the initial symptoms, neuropsychological, neuropsychiatric, neurologic findings and neuroimaging features.

161. Which of the following suggests FTD and not AD?

Harrison's 20th Ed. Chapter 25, Page 153

A. Personality change
B. Disinhibition
C. Weight gain or compulsive eating
D. All of the above

Personality change, disinhibition & weight gain or compulsive eating suggest FTD and not AD. FTD is also suggested by prominent apathy, compulsivity, loss of empathy for others, or progressive loss of speech fluency or single word comprehension and by a relative sparing of memory & visuo-spatial abilities.

162. The diagnosis of DLB is suggested by?

Harrison's 20th Ed. Chapter 25, Page 153

A. Early visual hallucinations
B. Parkinsonism
C. Capgras syndrome
D. All of the above

Diagnosis of DLB is suggested by early visual hallucinations, parkinsonism, proneness to delirium or sensitivity to psychoactive medications, rapid eye movement (REM) behavior disorder (RBD) or Capgras syndrome, the delusion that a familiar person has been replaced by an impostor.

163. Rapid progression of dementia with motor rigidity & myoclonus suggests?

Harrison's 20th Ed. Chapter 25, Page 153

A. Alzheimer's disease
B. Frontotemporal dementia
C. Cortical basal degeneration
D. Creutzfeldt-Jakob disease

Rapid progression of dementia in association with diffuse motor rigidity, akinetic-mute state & startle-sensitive myoclonus suggests CJD.

164. Rapid progression of the dementia with motor rigidity & myoclonus suggests which of the following?

Harrison's 20th Ed. Chapter 25, Page 153

A. Alzheimer's disease
B. Prion disease
C. Frontotemporal dementia
D. Parkinson's disease

Rapid progression of dementia with motor rigidity & myoclonus suggests a prion disease.

165. Gait disturbance is common in?

Harrison's 20th Ed. Chapter 25, Page 153

A. Vascular dementia
B. PD/DLB
C. NPH
D. Any of the above

Gait disturbance is common in vascular dementia, PD/DLB, or NPH.

166. Dementia in a patient with a history of recurrent head trauma suggests?

Harrison's 20th Ed. Chapter 25, Page 153

A. Chronic subdural hematoma
B. Chronic traumatic encephalopathy
C. NPH
D. Any of the above

Dementia in a patient with a history of recurrent head trauma suggests chronic subdural hematoma, chronic traumatic encephalopathy, intracranial hypotension, or NPH.

167. Which of the following statements is false?

Harrison's 20th Ed. Chapter 25, Page 154

A. Typical AD spares motor systems until later in the course
B. FTD patients may mimic amyotrophic lateral sclerosis (ALS)
C. DLB often starts with visual hallucinations or dementia
D. None of the above

168. Which of the following is a feature of Corticobasal syndrome (CBS)?

Harrison's 20th Ed. Chapter 25, Page 154

A. Dystonia
B. Myoclonus
C. Alien limb phenomena
D. All of the above

Features of Corticobasal syndrome (CBS) include asymmetric akinesia & rigidity, dystonia, myoclonus, alien limb phenomena, pyramidal signs, prefrontal deficits (nonfluent aphasia with or without motor speech impairment), executive dysfunction, apraxia, or a behavioral disorder.

169. Unexplained falls is a feature of?

Harrison's 20th Ed. Chapter 25, Page 154

A. Alzheimer's disease
B. Frontotemporal dementia
C. Cortical basal degeneration
D. Progressive supranuclear palsy

Progressive supranuclear palsy (PSP) is associated with unexplained falls, axial rigidity, dysphagia, and vertical gaze deficits.

170. CJD is suggested by the presence of?

Harrison's 20th Ed. Chapter 25, Page 154

A. Diffuse rigidity
B. Akinetic-mute state
C. Startle-sensitive myoclonus
D. All of the above

CJD is suggested by the presence of diffuse rigidity, akinetic-mute state & prominent startle-sensitive myoclonus.

171. Dementia with peripheral neuropathy suggests?

Harrison's 20th Ed. Chapter 25, Page 154

A. Vitamin B12 deficiency
B. Thyroid dysfunction
C. Lyme disease
D. All of the above

Dementia with a peripheral neuropathy suggests vitamin B12 deficiency, heavy metal intoxication, thyroid dysfunction, Lyme disease, or vasculitis.

172. Brief screening tools used to detect dementia & follow progression include?

Harrison's 20th Ed. Chapter 25, Page 155

A. Mini-Mental State Examination (MMSE)
B. Montreal Cognitive Assessment (MOCA)
C. Cognistat
D. All of the above

Brief screening tools that can be used to identify dementia and follow its progression include Mini-Mental State Examination (MMSE), the Montreal Cognitive Assessment (MOCA), and Cognistat.

173. In Mini-Mental Status Examination (MMSE), scoring is done out of?

Harrison's 20th Ed. Chapter 25, Page 155

A. 20
B. 30
C. 40
D. 50

Mini-mental status examination (MMSE) is a brief screening tool to confirm the presence of cognitive impairment & to follow progression of dementia. It is a 30-point test of cognitive function.

174. MMSE contains tests for?

Harrison's 20th Ed. Chapter 25, Page 155

A. Orientation
B. Working memory
C. Episodic memory
D. All of the above

MMSE contains tests of orientation, working memory (spell world backwards), episodic memory (orientation & 3-word recall), language comprehension, naming, and figure copying.

175. MMSE is named after?

Harrison's 20th Ed. Chapter 25, Page 155

A. Samuels
B. Blumenthal
C. Campbell
D. Folstein

Folstein mini-mental status examination (MMSE) is an easy, standardized screening examination of cognitive function especially working and episodic memory. The test is 85% sensitive and 85% specific for the diagnosis of dementia.

176. Mini-Mental Status Examination (MMSE) provides information regarding?

Harrison's 20th Ed. Chapter 25, Page 155

A. Orientation
B. Language
C. Visuospatial skills
D. All of the above

Mini-Mental Status Examination (MMSE) can provide information regarding orientation, language, and visuospatial skills.

177. Capgras syndrome is best related to?

Harrison's 20th Ed. Chapter 25, Page 154 Table 25-4

A. Alzheimer's disease
B. Cortical basal degeneration
C. Creutzfeldt-Jakob disease
D. Dementia with Lewy bodies

178. Posterior parietal atrophy on imaging is seen in?

Harrison's 20th Ed. Chapter 25, Page 154 Table 25-4

A. Alzheimer's disease
B. Cortical basal degeneration
C. Creutzfeldt-Jakob disease
D. Dementia with Lewy bodies

179. Cortical ribboning and basal ganglia or thalamus hyperintensity on imaging is seen in?

Harrison's 20th Ed. Chapter 25, Page 154 Table 25-4

A. Alzheimer's disease
B. Cortical basal degeneration
C. Creutzfeldt-Jakob disease
D. Dementia with Lewy bodies

180. Which of the following is a cholinesterase inhibitor?

Harrison's 20th Ed. Chapter 25, Page 157

A. Ropinirole
B. Galantamine
C. Clomipramine
D. Doxylamine

181. Which of the following is not a cholinesterase inhibitor?

Harrison's 20th Ed. Chapter 25, Page 157

A. Donepezil
B. Rivastigmine
C. Galantamine
D. All of the above

Clomipramine is a tricyclic antidepressant, pramipexole and ropinirole are agonists of dopamine D2/3 receptors while doxylamine is an antihistaminic.

182. Which of the following drugs is useful in moderate to severe Alzheimer's disease?

Harrison's 20th Ed. Chapter 25, Page 157

A. Memantine
B. Amifostine
C. Trientine
D. All of the above

Memantine acts by blocking overexcited N-methyl-D-aspartate (NMDA) glutamate receptors.

Aphasia, Memory Loss, Hemispatial Neglect, Frontal Syndromes, and Other Cerebral Disorders

183. Cerebral cortex of human brain contains approximately how many neurons?

Harrison's 20th Ed. Chapter 26, Page 157

A. 5 billion
B. 10 billion
C. 20 billion
D. 50 billion

184. Cerebral cortex of human brain has an area of?

Harrison's 20th Ed. Chapter 26, Page 157

A. 0.5 m^2
B. 1.5 m^2
C. 2.5 m^2
D. 3.5 m^2

Human cerebral cortex contains ~20 billion neurons spread over an area of 2.5 m^2.

185. Primary sensory & motor areas constitute what percentage of cerebral cortex?

Harrison's 20th Ed. Chapter 26, Page 157

A. 10%
B. 15%
C. 20%
D. 25%

Primary sensory & motor areas constitute 10% of the cerebral cortex.

186. Which of the following is part of association cortex?

Harrison's 20th Ed. Chapter 26, Page 157

A. Heteromodal area
B. Paralimbic area
C. Limbic area
D. All of the above

Modality-selective, heteromodal, paralimbic, and limbic areas collectively known as the association cortex.

187. In the brain, there are no centers for?

Harrison's 20th Ed. Chapter 26, Page 157

A. Hearing words
B. Perceiving space
C. Storing memories
D. All of the above

In the brain, there are no centers for "hearing words," "perceiving space," or "storing memories."

188. Which of the following large-scale neural network is meant for face & object recognition?

Harrison's 20th Ed. Chapter 26, Page 157

A. Perisylvian network
B. Parietofrontal network
C. Occipitotemporal network
D. Prefrontal network

Five anatomically defined large scale networks perform cognitive and behavioral functions in human brain. They are a left-dominant perisylvian network for language, a right-dominant parietofrontal network for spatial orientation, occipitotemporal network for face and object recognition, limbic network for retentive memory and prefrontal network for the executive control of cognition and compartment.

189. Which of the following Brodmann area corresponds to the primary auditory cortex?

Harrison's 20th Ed. Chapter 26, Page 158 Figure 26-1

A. 33–34
B. 36–37
C. 39–40
D. 41–42

190. Which of the following Brodmann area corresponds to primary motor cortex?

Harrison's 20th Ed. Chapter 26, Page 158 Figure 26-1

A. 1
B. 2
C. 3
D. 4

191. Which of the following Brodmann area corresponds to primary somatosensory cortex?

Harrison's 20th Ed. Chapter 26, Page 158 Figure 26-1

A. 1–3
B. 2–4
C. 3–5
D. 4–6

192. Which of the following Brodmann area corresponds to primary visual cortex?

Harrison's 20th Ed. Chapter 26, Page 158 Figure 26-1

A. 11
B. 13
C. 17
D. 21

193. Wernicke's area is located in?

Harrison's 20th Ed. Chapter 26, Page 158

A. Anterior temporal lobe
B. Parietotemporal junction
C. Inferior frontal gyrus
D. Superior frontal gyrus

Broca's area is situated in the inferior frontal gyrus. Wernicke's area is located at the parietotemporal junction.

194. 'Recovery from aphasia will be best for the language most used' refers to?

DeJong's The Neurologic Examination, 7th Ed. Page 98

A. Pitres' law
B. Hering's law
C. Alexander's law
D. Brodmann law

Pitres' law states that recovery from aphasia will be best for the language most used.

195. Which of the following is the single most common finding in aphasic patients?

Harrison's 20th Ed. Chapter 26, Page 158

A. Anomia
B. Apraxia
C. Aphemia
D. Alexia

A deficit of naming, called anomia, is the single most common finding in aphasic patients.

196. Anomia refers to?

Harrison's 20th Ed. Chapter 26, Page 158

A. Naming with the wrong word
B. Deficit of naming
C. Naming a different object
D. Any of the above

Deficit of naming or anomia is the single most common finding in aphasic patients. Naming with the wrong word is called paraphasia that can be semantic or phonemic.

197. Inability to read aloud or comprehend single words and simple sentences is called?

Harrison's 20th Ed. Chapter 26, Page 158

A. Alexia
B. Agraphia
C. Anomia
D. Paraphasia

Alexia means an inability to read aloud or comprehend written words & sentences. Agraphia (or dysgraphia) means an acquired deficit in spelling or grammar of written language.

198. Which of the following is impaired in Wernicke's aphasia?

Harrison's 20th Ed. Chapter 26, Page 158 Table 26-1

A. Comprehension
B. Repetition of spoken language
C. Naming
D. All of the above

Comprehension, repetition of spoken language and naming are impaired in Wernicke's aphasia. Fluency is preserved or increased.

199. Which of the following is preserved in Broca's aphasia?

Harrison's 20th Ed. Chapter 26, Page 158 Table 26-1

A. Comprehension
B. Repetition of spoken language
C. Naming
D. Fluency

200. Which of the following is considered as "minimal dysfunction" syndrome of the language network?

Harrison's 20th Ed. Chapter 26, Page 160

A. Anomic aphasia
B. Isolation aphasia
C. Wernicke's aphasia
D. Conduction aphasia

201. Anomic aphasia is the single most common language disturbance seen in?

Harrison's 20th Ed. Chapter 26, Page 160

A. Head trauma
B. Metabolic encephalopathy
C. Alzheimer's disease
D. All of the above

Anomic aphasia is the single most common language disturbance seen in head trauma, metabolic encephalopathy, and Alzheimer's disease.

202. Which of the following results when superior temporal gyrus is damaged?

Harrison's 20th Ed. Chapter 26, Page 160

A. Isolation aphasia
B. Anomic aphasia
C. Pure word deafness
D. Pure alexia without agraphia

203. Fluency is severely impaired in?

Harrison's 20th Ed. Chapter 26, Page 160

A. Aphemia
B. Alexia
C. Anomia
D. Wernicke's aphasia

Aphemia is an acute onset of severely impaired fluency.

204. Apraxia refers to?

Harrison's 20th Ed. Chapter 26, Page 160

A. Repetition of spoken language
B. Disorder of initiating skilled/learned movement
C. Impaired comprehension
D. No purposeful speech

205. In apraxia, complex motor deficit is attributed to?

Harrison's 20th Ed. Chapter 26, Page 160

A. Pyramidal dysfunction
B. Extrapyramidal dysfunction
C. Cerebellar dysfunction
D. None of the above

Apraxia refers to a complex motor deficit that cannot be attributed to pyramidal, extrapyramidal, cerebellar, or sensory dysfunction. It is a disorder of planning & initiating a skilled or learned movement unrelated to a significant motor or sensory deficit.

206. Alien hand syndrome best relates to?

Harrison's 20th Ed. Chapter 26, Page 160

A. Sympathetic dyspraxia
B. Ideational apraxia
C. Ideomotor apraxia
D. Limb-kinetic apraxia

207. Gerstmann's Syndrome includes all except?

Harrison's 20th Ed. Chapter 26, Page 160

A. Acalculia
B. Aphasia
C. Right-left confusion
D. Finger anomia

Gerstmann tetrad comprises of acalculia, alexia, finger anomia and right-left confusion. Pure Gerstmann syndrome is without aphasia.

208. In isolated Gerstmann's syndrome, the damage is in?
Harrison's 20th Ed. Chapter 26, Page 160

A. Superior parietal lobule in dominant hemisphere
B. Inferior parietal lobule in dominant hemisphere
C. Superior parietal lobule in non-dominant hemisphere
D. Inferior parietal lobule in non-dominant hemisphere

Isolated Gerstmann's syndrome results from damage to inferior parietal lobule (angular gyrus) in the left hemisphere.

209. Statements uttered in a monotone are termed?
Harrison's 20th Ed. Chapter 26, Page 160

A. Primary progressive aphasia (PPA)
B. Anomic aphasia
C. Aprosodia
D. Prosopagnosia

210. Which of the following is a subtype of primary progressive aphasia (PPA)?
Harrison's 20th Ed. Chapter 26, Page 161

A. Agrammatic
B. Semantic
C. Logopenic
D. All of the above

211. Which of the following PPAs is not seen with CVAs?
Harrison's 20th Ed. Chapter 26, Page 161

A. Agrammatic
B. Semantic
C. Logopenic
D. All of the above

212. Which symptom can occur in Bálint's syndrome?
Harrison's 20th Ed. Chapter 26, Page 162

A. Optic ataxia
B. Oculomotor apaxia
C. Simultagnosia
D. All of the above

Bálint's syndrome is a state of severe spatial disorientation involving deficits in orderly visuomotor scanning of the environment (oculomotor apraxia) and in accurate manual reaching toward visual targets (optic ataxia) and simultanagnosia and reflects an inability to integrate visual information in the center of gaze with more peripheral information.

213. Bálint's syndrome may result from?
Harrison's 20th Ed. Chapter 26, Page 162

A. Hypoglycemia
B. Sagittal sinus thrombosis
C. Atypical forms of Alzheimer's disease
D. All of the above

214. Face recognition deficit is termed as?
Harrison's 20th Ed. Chapter 26, Page 162

A. Primary progressive aphasia (PPA)
B. Apperceptive agnosia
C. Aprosodia
D. Prosopagnosia

Face & object recognition deficits are known as prosopagnosia & visual object agnosia. Lesions in prosopagnosia & visual object agnosia consist of bilateral infarctions in the territory of posterior cerebral arteries.

215. Which of the following artery is involved in lesions in prosopagnosia?
Harrison's 20th Ed. Chapter 26, Page 163

A. Anterior cerebral artery
B. Middle cerebral artery
C. Posterior cerebral artery
D. Internal carotid artery

The characteristic lesions in prosopagnosia & visual object agnosia of acute onset consist of bilateral infarctions in the territory of posterior cerebral arteries that involve fusiform gyrus.

216. Combination of progressive associative agnosia & fluent aphasia with word comprehension impairment is known as?
Harrison's 20th Ed. Chapter 26, Page 163

A. Amnestic dementia
B. Behavioral variant of frontotemporal dementia (bvFTD)
C. Semantic dementia
D. Semantic PPA

217. Which of the following is not included in paralimbic area?
Harrison's 20th Ed. Chapter 26, Page 164

A. Hippocampus
B. Hypothalamus
C. Amygdala
D. Entorhinal cortex

Limbic system is a distributed network consisting of limbic & paralimbic areas (hippocampus, amygdala & entorhinal cortex), anterior & medial nuclei of thalamus, medial & basal parts of striatum, and hypothalamus.

218. Which of the following functions is related to limbic system?
Harrison's 20th Ed. Chapter 26, Page 164

A. Coordination of emotion
B. Autonomic tone
C. Endocrine function
D. All of the above

Functions related to limbic system include coordination of emotion, motivation, autonomic tone, endocrine function and declarative (explicit) memory for recent episodes & experiences.

219. Cause of transient global amnesia is?
Harrison's 20th Ed. Chapter 26, Page 165

A. Migraine
B. Temporal lobe seizures
C. TIA in the posterior cerebral territory
D. All of the above

220. Which of the following is best related to visuospatial disorientation?
N Engl J Med. 2005;352:692-9

A. Optic ataxia
B. Ocular apraxia
C. Simultanagnosia
D. All of the above

Bilateral parietal lesions produce Bálint's syndrome, which is characterized by impaired eye-hand coordination (optic ataxia), difficulty initiating voluntary eye movements (ocular apraxia), and visuospatial disorientation (simultanagnosia).

221. Which of the following is not a major type of memory?
N Engl J Med. 2005;352:692-9

A. Working
B. Sequential
C. Episodic
D. Remote

Memory is divided into three major types - working, episodic, and remote.

222. Working memory lasts for what duration?
N Engl J Med. 2005;352:692-9

A. < 5 seconds
B. < 10 seconds
C. < 20 seconds
D. < 30 seconds

Working memory lasts for <30 seconds.

223. Which of the following types of memory is tested by asking the patient to recall digits backwards?
N Engl J Med. 2005;352:692-9

A. Working
B. Episodic
C. Remote
D. All of the above

Working memory is highly vulnerable to distraction, requiring attention and vigilance for its maintenance. It is tested by asking the patient to recall digits backwards.

224. Which of the following types of memory is tested by asking the patient to recall three words after 3 to 5 minutes?
N Engl J Med. 2005;352:692-9

A. Working
B. Episodic
C. Remote
D. All of the above

Episodic memory is tested by asking a patient to recall three words after 3 to 5 minutes.

225. Hippocampal complex is critical for which of the following types of memory?
N Engl J Med. 2005;352:692-9

A. Working
B. Episodic
C. Remote
D. All of the above

Hippocampal complex is critical for episodic memory, and physiologic changes in synapses in this brain region accompany new episodic memories.

226. More permanent stores of words, dates, historic facts or names require which of the following?
N Engl J Med. 2005;352:692-9

A. Hippocampal complex
B. Left anterior temporal cortex
C. Prefrontal lobe
D. Parietal lobe

More permanent stores of words, dates, facts or names require left anterior temporal cortex.

227. Most common cognitive deficits that follow seizures, hypoglycemia, hypoxia is?
N Engl J Med. 2005;352:692-9

A. Working memory deficits
B. Episodic memory deficits
C. Remote memory deficits
D. None of the above

Hippocampal complex is vulnerable to metabolic insults such as seizures, hypoglycemia, hypoxia, and neurodegenerative processes, which explains why episodic memory deficits are the most common cognitive deficits that follow these disorders.

228. The process of memory retrieval requires which of the following cerebral lobes?
N Engl J Med. 2005;352:692-9

A. Frontal lobe
B. Temporal lobe
C. Parietal lobe
D. All of the above

The process of memory encoding is dependent upon frontal lobes and hippocampal complex, while the process of retrieval requires frontal lobes.

229. Memory function includes which of the following?
N Engl J Med. 2005;352:692-9

A. Registration (encoding or acquisition)
B. Retention (storage or consolidation)
C. Retrieval (decoding or recall)
D. All of the above

Memory function includes registration (encoding or acquisition), retention (storage or consolidation), stabilization (consolidation), and retrieval (decoding or recall).

230. The basal ganglia, cerebellum, and supplementary motor area are critical for?
N Engl J Med. 2005;352:692-9

A. Episodic memory
B. Semantic memory
C. Procedural memory
D. Working memory

Procedural (implicit) memory involves centers outside the hippocampus such as amygdala, basal ganglia, cerebellum, and sensory cortex.

231. The medial temporal lobes, including the hippocampus and parahippocampus, are critical for?
N Engl J Med. 2005;352:692-9

A. Episodic memory
B. Semantic memory
C. Procedural memory
D. Working memory

Episodic memory requires dorsomedial nucleus of thalamus and medial temporal lobes.

232. Which of the following is damaged in Korsakoff's syndrome due to thiamine deficiency?
N Engl J Med. 2005;352:692-9

A. Dorsomedial nucleus of thalamus
B. Medial temporal lobes
C. Amygdala
D. Basal ganglia

Dorsomedial nucleus of thalamus is damaged in Korsakoff's syndrome due to thiamine deficiency resulting in loss of episodic memory.

233. Inferolateral temporal lobes are critical for?

N Engl J Med. 2005;352:692-9

A. Episodic memory
B. Semantic memory
C. Procedural memory
D. Working memory

234. Prefrontal cortex, Broca's area, Wernicke's area are critical for?

N Engl J Med. 2005;352:692-9

A. Episodic memory
B. Semantic memory
C. Procedural memory
D. Phonologic working memory

235. Prefrontal cortex, visual-association areas are critical for?

N Engl J Med. 2005;352:692-9

A. Episodic memory
B. Semantic memory
C. Procedural memory
D. Spatial working memory

236. Which memory is involved in remembering unchanging facts, principles & rules (number of days in a week)?

N Engl J Med. 2005;352:692-9

A. Semantic memory
B. Declarative (explicit) memory
C. Procedural (implicit) memory
D. All of the above

Semantic memory contains unchanging facts, principles, associations, and rules (number of days in a week). Injury to anterior temporal neocortex leads to loss of semantic memory.

237. Which kind of memory is involved in remembering facts about the world and past personal events?

N Engl J Med. 2005;352:692-9

A. Semantic memory
B. Declarative (explicit) memory
C. Procedural (implicit) memory
D. All of the above

Declarative (explicit) memory refers to facts about world & past personal events that must be consciously retrieved to be remembered. Episodic is prototypical declarative explicit memory.

238. Which kind of memory is involved in learning and retaining a skill or procedure like riding a bicycle, getting dressed, or driving a car?

N Engl J Med. 2005;352:692-9

A. Semantic memory
B. Declarative (explicit) memory
C. Procedural (implicit) memory
D. All of the above

Procedural (implicit) memory is involved in learning and retaining a skill or procedure such as riding a bicycle, getting dressed, or driving a car. Abilities stored in procedural memory become automatic and do not require conscious implementation.

239. Executive memory function is highly dependent upon which of the following?

N Engl J Med. 2005;352:692-9

A. Working
B. Episodic
C. Remote
D. All of the above

Executive function refers to mental activity involved in planning, initiating, and regulating behavior. It is highly dependent upon working memory.

240. Which of the following is not a part of the components of medial temporal lobe memory system?

Harrison's 20th Ed. Chapter 423 Page 3109

A. Hippocampus
B. Amgdala
C. Entorhinal region
D. Perirhinal region

Components of medial temporal lobe memory system include hippocampus and adjacent cortex, including the entorhinal, perirhinal, and parahippocampal regions.

241. In AD, the early deficits involve which class of memory?

Harrison's 20th Ed. Chapter 25 Page 155

A. Working memory
B. Episodic memory
C. Executive function
D. Language

In AD the early deficits involve verbal or visual episodic memory, category generation ("name as many animals as you can in one minute"), and visuoconstructive ability. Tasks requiring patient to recall a long list of words or a series of pictures after a predetermined delay will demonstrate deficits.

242. An autosomal dominant family history of dementia can be found in which of the following?

Harrison's 20th Ed. Chapter 25 Page 154

A. Huntington's disease
B. Alzheimer's disease
C. Frontotemporal dementia
D. All of the above

An autosomal dominant family history is found in HD and in familial forms of AD, FTD, DLB, or prion disorders.

243. Early presence of visual hallucinations is a feature of which of the following dementias?

Harrison's 20th Ed. Chapter 426 Page 3119

A. Creutzfeldt-Jakob disease
B. Schizophrenia
C. Frontotemporal dementia
D. Dementia with Lewy bodies

Diagnosis of DLB is suggested by early presence of visual hallucinations, parkinsonism, delirium, rapid-eye-movement (REM) sleep disorder or Capgras syndrome (delusion that a familiar person has been replaced by an impostor).

244. Capgras syndrome is an early feature in which of the following degenerative diseases?

Harrison's 20th Ed. Chapter 25 Page 153

A. Alzheimer's disease
B. Creutzfeldt-Jakob disease
C. Frontotemporal dementia
D. Dementia with Lewy bodies

Capgras syndrome—delusion that a familiar person has been replaced by an impostor, is an early feature of Dementia with Lewy bodies.

245. Early prominent gait disturbance is a feature of?

Harrison's 20th Ed. Chapter 423 Page 3109

A. Alzheimer's disease
B. Dementia with Lewy bodies
C. Creutzfeldt-Jakob disease
D. Vascular dementia

Early prominent gait disturbance with only mild memory loss suggests vascular dementia. Gait disturbance is common in vascular dementia, PD/DLB, or normal-pressure hydrocephalus (NPH).

246. On neuroimaging studies, extensive white matter abnormalities correlate best with?

Harrison's 20th Ed. Chapter 425 Page 3118

A. Alzheimer's disease
B. Frontotemporal dementia
C. Vascular etiology
D. Creutzfeldt-Jakob disease

On neuroimaging studies, extensive white matter abnormalities correlate best with a vascular etiology for dementia.

247. In amyloid imaging of brain for diagnosis of Alzheimer's disease (AD), which of the following is used?

Harrison's 20th Ed. Chapter 25 Page 156

A. Pittsburgh Compound-A
B. Pittsburgh Compound-B
C. Pittsburgh Compound-C
D. Pittsburgh Compound-D

Amyloid imaging with radioligands like Pittsburgh Compound-B (PiB), 18F-AV-45 and tau PET tracers, such as 18F-T807 and T808 help in detecting brain amyloid associated with amyloid angiopathy or neuritic plaques of AD.

248. EEG is helpful in the diagnosis of which of the following?

Harrison's 20th Ed. Chapter 25 Page 156

A. Alzheimer's disease
B. Frontotemporal dementia
C. Cortical basal degeneration
D. Creutzfeldt-Jakob disease

Electroencephalogram (EEG) is rarely helpful except in CJD (repetitive bursts of diffuse high-amplitude sharp waves, or "periodic complexes").

249. Which of the following is the major source of cholinergic input to the cerebral cortex?

Harrison's 20th Ed. Chapter 423 Page 3109

A. Globus pallidus
B. Thalamus
C. Nucleus accumbens
D. Nucleus basalis of Meynert

Nucleus basalis of Meynert is the major source of cholinergic input to the cerebral cortex.

250. Agents useful for reducing the signs of dementia include?

N Engl J Med. 2004;351:56-67

A. Donepezil
B. Rivastigmine
C. Galantamine
D. All of the above

251. Which of the following drugs used in management of dementia is not a cholinesterase inhibitor?

N Engl J Med. 2004;351:56-67

A. Donepezil
B. Rivastigmine
C. Galantamine
D. Memantine

252. Which of the following drugs used in the management of dementia is a NMDA-receptor antagonist?

N Engl J Med. 2004;351:56-67

A. Donepezil
B. Rivastigmine
C. Galantamine
D. Memantine

253. Ribot's law states that?

N Engl J Med. 2005;352:692-9

A. Events just before ictus are most vulnerable to dissolution
B. Remote memories are most resistant
C. A+B
D. None of the above

254. The most common clinical disorder disrupting semantic memory is?

N Engl J Med. 2005;352:692-9

A. Alzheimer's disease
B. Parkinsons's disease
C. Multiple sclerosis
D. Progressive supranuclear palsy

255. Disorders affecting procedural memory include all except?

N Engl J Med. 2005;352:692-9

A. Alzheimer's disease
B. Parkinsons's disease
C. Huntington's disease
D. Olivopontocerebellar degeneration

256. After Alzheimer disease, which of the following is the most common cause of dementia?

Cleveland Clinic Journal of Medicine 2014;81(4):243

A. Vascular dementia
B. Multiple system atrophy
C. Parkinson disease dementia
D. Frontotemporal dementia

After Alzheimer disease, vascular dementia is the most common dementia, accounting for ~ 20%–30% of cases.

257. Which of the following is used as a bedside tool to differentiate Alzheimer dementia from vascular dementia?

Cleveland Clinic Journal of Medicine 2014;81(4):243

A. Trail making test
B. Folstein mini-mental state examination
C. Hachinski ischemic score
D. Montreal cognitive assessment

The Hachinski ischemic score is a good bedside tool to help differentiate Alzheimer dementia from vascular dementia.

258. Executive dysfunction may be identified by which of the following?

Cleveland Clinic Journal of Medicine 2014;81(4):243

A. St. Louis University mental status examination
B. Folstein mini-mental state examination
C. Montreal cognitive assessment
D. All of the above

Executive dysfunction may be identified using the Trail making test or Executive Interview (EXIT25). Office-based tools like Folstein mini-mental state examination, Montreal cognitive assessment, or St. Louis University mental status examination may also uncover these deficits.

259. Out of the following, which is the most common neurodegenerative dementia in the elderly?

Cleveland Clinic Journal of Medicine 2014;81(4):243

A. Progressive supranuclear palsy
B. Frontotemporal dementia
C. Corticobasal degeneration
D. Dementia with Lewy bodies

After Alzheimer disease and Vascular dementias, Dementia with Lewy bodies is the next most common neurodegenerative dementia in the elderly.

260. Which of the following is a less common feature of Dementia with Lewy bodies?

Cleveland Clinic Journal of Medicine 2014;81(4):243

A. Progressive loss of cognitive function
B. Prominent visual hallucinations
C. Autonomic failure
D. Parkinsonism

Progressive loss of cognitive function, prominent visual hallucinations and parkinsonism (bradykinesia, masked facies & rigidity. Resting tremor is less common. Dementia occurs before or concurrently with parkinsonism) are characteristic features of Dementia with Lewy bodies, progression of which usually occurs over years but can be more rapid than in Alzheimer disease.

261. McKeith consensus criteria is the gold standard for diagnosing which of the following?

Cleveland Clinic Journal of Medicine 2014;81(4):243

A. Progressive supranuclear palsy
B. Frontotemporal dementia
C. Corticobasal degeneration
D. Dementia with Lewy bodies

McKeith criteria is the gold standard for diagnosing probable Lewy body dementia, based on clinical and imaging features.

262. Which of the following about progressive supranuclear palsy is false?

Cleveland Clinic Journal of Medicine 2014;81(4):243

A. Sporadic atypical parkinsonian disorder
B. Onset between age 50 and 70
C. Accumulation of tau protein aggregates in basal ganglia
D. None of the above

Progressive supranuclear palsy is a sporadic atypical parkinsonian disorder with onset between age 50 and 70 and gradual progression. Familial cases are infrequent. Histologically, PSP is characterized by accumulation of tau protein aggregates in basal ganglia, brainstem, and cerebral cortex.

263. Degenerative process in progressive supranuclear palsy involves which of the following neurons?

Cleveland Clinic Journal of Medicine 2014;81(4):243

A. Dopaminergic neurons
B. Cholinergic neurons
C. Gamma-aminobutyric acid (GABA) neurons
D. All of the above

Degenerative process in progressive supranuclear palsy involves dopaminergic, cholinergic, and gamma-aminobutyric acid (GABA)-ergic neurons.

264. Which of the following is not a feature of progressive supranuclear palsy?

Cleveland Clinic Journal of Medicine 2014;81(4):243

A. Vertical gaze palsy
B. Gait and balance impairment
C. Limb rigidity is more prominent than axial rigidity
D. Cognitive impairment

The hallmark of progressive supranuclear palsy is vertical gaze palsy. Earliest symptom is gait & balance impairment (falls usually backward). Axial (especially neck) rigidity is more prominent than limb rigidity. Retrocollis (the head is drawn back) occurs in <25% of patients.

265. Which of the following signs is related to progressive supranuclear palsy?

DeJong's The Neurologic Examination, 7th Ed. Page 253

A. Negro's sign
B. Myerson's sign
C. Omega sign
D. Hanes sign

In progressive supranuclear palsy, omega sign refers to a characteristic facial dystonia with knitting of the brows and widening of the palpebral fissures.

266. "Leonine facies" is a feature of which of the following?

Cleveland Clinic Journal of Medicine 2014;81(4):243

A. Progressive supranuclear palsy
B. Frontotemporal dementia
C. Corticobasal degeneration
D. Dementia with Lewy bodies

In PSP, gaze abnormality combined with rare blinking & facial dystonia form the classic facial expression of astonishment called "leonine facies." The face is stiff and deeply furrowed, with a look of surprise.

267. 'Hummingbird sign' and "morning glory flower" on MRI is a feature of which of the following?

Cleveland Clinic Journal of Medicine 2014;81(4):243

A. Progressive supranuclear palsy
B. Frontotemporal dementia
C. Corticobasal degeneration
D. Dementia with Lewy bodies

In PSP, brain MRI shows atrophy of brainstem, particularly midbrain. Thinning of superior part of midbrain & dilation of third ventricle ("hummingbird sign" on sagittal sections or "morning glory flower" on axial sections) support the diagnosis and differentiate it from Parkinson disease and other atypical parkinsonian disorders.

268. 'Hot cross bun' sign on MRI is a feature of which of the following?

Cleveland Clinic Journal of Medicine 2014;81(4):243

A. Multiple system atrophy
B. Frontotemporal dementia
C. Corticobasal degeneration
D. Dementia with Lewy bodies

In MSA, Brain MRI shows atrophy of putamen (hypointensity of putamen with a hyperintense rim). Pons atrophy may also be present, revealing a "hot cross bun" sign in axial images.

269. Rapid-eye-movement sleep behavior disorders are infrequent in which of the following?

Cleveland Clinic Journal of Medicine 2014;81(4):243

A. Parkinson disease
B. Multiple system atrophy
C. Progressive supranuclear palsy
D. Lewy body dementia

Rapid-eye-movement sleep behavior disorders are infrequent in PSP, unlike in Parkinson disease, multiple system atrophy, and Lewy body dementia.

270. Which of the following clinical features is least common in corticobasal degeneration?

Cleveland Clinic Journal of Medicine 2014;81(4):243

A. Dementia
B. Parkinsonism
C. Higher cortical dysfunction
D. Gait disorder

In corticobasal degeneration, the frequency of clinical features is : parkinsonism (100%), higher cortical dysfunction (93%), dyspraxia (82%), gait disorder (80%), unilateral limb dystonia (71%), tremor (55%), and dementia (25%).

271. MRI of which of the following diseases may show asymmetric cortical atrophy especially in posterior frontal and parietal lobes?

Cleveland Clinic Journal of Medicine 2014;81(4):243

A. Progressive supranuclear palsy
B. Frontotemporal dementia
C. Corticobasal degeneration
D. Dementia with Lewy bodies

In CBD, MRI may be normal initially. As the disease progresses, asymmetric cortical atrophy may be seen, especially in the posterior frontal and parietal lobes.

272. Which of the following is not a prominent feature of Multiple system atrophy (MSA)?

Cleveland Clinic Journal of Medicine 2014;81(4):243

A. Psychiatric symptoms
B. Parkinsonism
C. Cerebellar signs
D. Pyramidal tract dysfunction

Multiple system atrophy is characterized by sporadic parkinsonism, cerebellar signs (involving balance and coordination), pyramidal tract dysfunction, and autonomic insufficiency in varying combinations. In contrast to dementia with Lewy bodies, psychiatric symptoms are not a major feature, except possibly depression.

273. In Parkinson disease dementia, volume of which of the following is reduced?

Cleveland Clinic Journal of Medicine 2014;81(4):243

A. Temporal
B. Occipital
C. Subcortical areas
D. All of the above

In Parkinson disease dementia, reduced volume extends to temporal, occipital, and subcortical areas.

274. In patients with Parkinson disease dementia, which of the following drugs is effective?

Cleveland Clinic Journal of Medicine 2014;81(4):243

A. Selective serotonin reuptake inhibitors
B. Midodrine
C. Memantine
D. Rivastigmine

Acetylcholinesterase inhibitor rivastigmine (FDA-approved) has a positive impact on global assessment, cognitive function, behavioral disturbance, and activities of daily living rating scales in patients with Parkinson disease dementia.

275. Behavioral & language changes accompany which of the following forms of dementia?

Cleveland Clinic Journal of Medicine 2014;81(4):243

A. Alzheimer disease
B. Vascular dementia
C. Primary progressive aphasia
D. All of the above

Behavioral & language changes accompany Alzheimer disease, vascular dementia, primary progressive aphasia.

276. Which of the following is not a feature of the classic triad of normal-pressure hydrocephalus?

Cleveland Clinic Journal of Medicine 2014;81(4):243

A. Gait impairment
B. Cognitive impairment
C. Progressive aphasia
D. Urinary frequency or incontinence

Normal-pressure hydrocephalus is characterized by the classic triad of gait impairment, cognitive impairment, and urinary frequency or incontinence.

277. Degree of enlargement of cerebral ventricles is calculated by?

Cleveland Clinic Journal of Medicine 2014;81(4):243

A. Armstrong ratio
B. Litvan ratio
C. Evans ratio
D. Cooper ratio

In 1942, William Evans calculated degree of enlargement of cerebral ventricles and defined its normal limits. He defined & computed a ratio of transverse diameter of the anterior horns to the greatest internal diameter of the skull in the sagittal direction. This index was for children and the normal range was 0.20 to 0.25, and that a ratio of 0.25 to 0.30 represents early ventricular enlargement while values above 0.30 define ventricular enlargement.

278. Which of the following is a rapidly progressive dementia?

Cleveland Clinic Journal of Medicine 2014;81(4):243

A. Hashimoto encephalopathy
B. Paraneoplastic limbic encephalitis
C. Creutzfeldt-Jakob disease
D. All of the above

279. Which of the following is true for Creutzfeldt-Jakob disease?

Cleveland Clinic Journal of Medicine 2014;81(4):243

A. EEG positive for periodic sharp-wave complexes
B. CSF with a positive 14-3-3 protein assay
C. MRI with high signal abnormalities in caudate nucleus & putamen
D. All of the above

For the diagnosis of Creutzfeldt-Jakob disease, two of the following must be present : Myoclonus (muscle twitching), Pyramidal or extrapyramidal findings, Visual or cerebellar deficits and Akinetic mutism (patient appears alert but is unresponsive). In addition, one of the above three tests must be positive.

280. Progression of which of the following neurodegenerative dementias is sudden, stepwise?

Cleveland Clinic Journal of Medicine 2014;81(4):243

A. Vascular dementia
B. Multiple system atrophy
C. Parkinson disease dementia
D. Frontotemporal dementia

281. Progression of which of the following neurodegenerative dementias is gradual with fluctuation in cognition?

Cleveland Clinic Journal of Medicine 2014;81(4):243

A. Vascular dementia
B. Multiple system atrophy
C. Parkinson disease dementia
D. Dementia with Lewy bodies

282. Visual hallucinations is a typical feature of which of the following neurodegenerative dementias?

Cleveland Clinic Journal of Medicine 2014;81(4):243

A. Vascular dementia
B. Multiple system atrophy
C. Parkinson disease dementia
D. Dementia with Lewy bodies

Disorders of the Eye

283. About how many rods are present in human retina?
Harrison's 20th Ed. Chapter 28, Page 177

A. 10 million
B. 50 million
C. 75 million
D. 100 million

284. About how many cones are present in human retina?
Harrison's 20th Ed. Chapter 28, Page 177

A. 1 million
B. 3 million
C. 5 million
D. 10 million

285. Which of the following statements about vision is false?
Harrison's 20th Ed. Chapter 28, Page 177

A. Rods operate in dim (scotopic) illumination
B. Cones function under daylight (photopic) conditions
C. Rods specialized for color perception
D. Fovea is packed exclusively with cones

The cone system is specialized for color perception and high spatial resolution.

286. Which of the following statements is false?
Harrison's 20th Ed. Chapter 28, Page 28, 177

A. Rods operate in scotopic illumination
B. Cones function under photopic conditions
C. Cone system is specialized for color perception
D. Rod system is specialized for high spatial resolution

Rods operate in dim (scotopic) illumination. Cones function under daylight (photopic) conditions. Cone system is specialized for color perception & high spatial resolution.

287. How many fibers are present in each optic nerve?
Harrison's 20th Ed. Chapter 28, Page, 177

A. 1 million
B. 2 million
C. 3 million
D. 4 million

288. How many ganglion cells are present in each retina?
Harrison's 20th Ed. Chapter 28, Page, 177

A. One million
B. Five million
C. Ten million
D. Twenty million

After processing of photoreceptor responses, the flow of sensory information converges on a final common pathway, i.e. ganglion cells. There are a million ganglion cells in each retina and hence a million fibers in each optic nerve.

289. The majority of cones are within?
Harrison's 20th Ed. Chapter 28, Page 177

A. Macula
B. Optic disc
C. Peripheral retina
D. Evenly distributed all over retina

Majority of cones are within macula which is that portion of retina that serves the central 10° of vision. Fovea is In the middle of macula and is packed exclusively with cones.

290. Which cell in the inner nuclear layer of retina is activated when photoreceptors hyperpolarize in response to light?
Harrison's 20th Ed. Chapter 28, Page 177

A. Bipolar cells
B. Amacrine cells
C. Horizontal cells
D. All of the above

Photoreceptors hyperpolarize in response to light, activating bipolar, amacrine & horizontal cells in the inner nuclear layer of retina.

291. Majority of ganglion cell axons synapse on cells in?
Harrison's 20th Ed. Chapter 28, Page 177

A. Medical geniculate body
B. Lateral geniculate body
C. Edinger-Westphal nuclei
D. Primary visual cortex

Majority of ganglion cell axons synapse on cells in the lateral geniculate body, a thalamic relay station. Cells in lateral geniculate body project in turn to the primary visual cortex.

292. Melanopsin is best related to?
Harrison's 20th Ed. Chapter 28, Page 177

A. Pupillary constriction
B. Visual orientation
C. Eye movements
D. Gaze stabilization

Ganglion cells that mediate pupillary constriction and circadian rhythms are light sensitive owing to a novel visual pigment, melanopsin.

293. Pupil responses are mediated by input to?
Harrison's 20th Ed. Chapter 28, Page 177

A. Superior colliculus
B. Pretectal olivary nuclei
C. Suprachiasmatic nucleus
D. All of the above

Pupil responses are mediated by input to pretectal olivary nuclei in the midbrain which send their output to the Edinger-Westphal nuclei, which in turn provide parasympathetic innervation to the iris sphincter via an interneuron in the ciliary ganglion.

294. Circadian rhythms are timed by a retinal projection to?
Harrison's 20th Ed. Chapter 28, Page 177

A. Superior colliculus
B. Pretectal olivary nuclei
C. Suprachiasmatic nucleus
D. All of the above

Circadian rhythms are timed by a retinal projection to the suprachiasmatic nucleus.

295. Visual orientation & eye movements are served by retinal input to?

Harrison's 20th Ed. Chapter 28, Page 177

A. Superior colliculus
B. Pretectal olivary nuclei
C. Suprachiasmatic nucleus
D. All of the above

Visual orientation & eye movements are served by retinal input to superior colliculus.

296. Brainstem accessory optic system is best related to?

Harrison's 20th Ed. Chapter 28, Page 177

A. Pupillary constriction
B. Visual orientation
C. Eye movements
D. Gaze stabilization and optokinetic reflexes

Gaze stabilization & optokinetic reflexes are governed by a group of small retinal targets known collectively as brainstem accessory optic system.

297. Phenomenon by which eyes maintain targets of visual interest on the fovea is called?

Harrison's 20th Ed. Chapter 28, Page 177

A. Acculization
B. Focussation
C. Foveation
D. Maculization

Eyes maintain targets of visual interest on fovea. This activity is called foveation.

298. Each eye is moved by how many extraocular muscles?

Harrison's 20th Ed. Chapter 28, Page 177

A. 4
B. 5
C. 6
D. 8

299. Which of the following control brainstem eye movement centers?

Harrison's 20th Ed. Chapter 28, Page 177

A. Frontal cortex
B. Temporal cortex
C. Cingulate gyrus
D. Limbic system

Large regions of frontal and parietooccipital cortex control brainstem ocular motor nuclei eye movement centers by providing descending supranuclear input.

300. Bell's reflex refers to?

Harrison's 19th Ed. 2647

A. Elevation & adduction of eyes on attempted lid closure
B. Elevation & abduction of eyes on attempted lid closure
C. Depression & adduction of eyes on attempted lid closure
D. Depression & abduction of eyes on attempted lid closure

Bell's reflex, also called palpebral oculogyric reflex, refers to elevation & abduction of eyes on attempted lid closure.

301. Term used to describe parallel rays from infinity focused perfectly on the retina is?

Harrison's 20th Ed. Chapter 28, Page 178

A. Emmetropia
B. Immetropia
C. Ammetropia
D. Smmetropia

In emmetropia, parallel rays from infinity are focused perfectly on retina.

302. To test acuity, Rosenbaum card is held at what distance from the patient?

Harrison's 20th Ed. Chapter 28, Page 178

A. 9 inches
B. 12 inches
C. 14 inches
D. 18 inches

The Snellen chart is used to test acuity at a distance of 6 meters (20 feet). A scale version of Snellen chart called Rosenbaum card is held at 36 cm or 14 inches from the patient.

303. Legal blindness is defined as a best corrected acuity of?

Harrison's 20th Ed. Chapter 28, Page 178

A. 6/20
B. 6/30
C. 6/40
D. 6/60

Legal blindness is defined by Internal Revenue Service as a best corrected acuity of 6/60 (20/200) or less in the better eye or a binocular visual field subtending 20° or less.

304. Patients with which of the following disorders should avoid driving?

Harrison's 20th Ed. Chapter 28, Page 178

A. Bitemporal hemianopia
B. Homonymous hemianopia
C. Junctional scotoma
D. All of the above

Patients with a homonymous hemianopia should not drive.

305. In abbreviation PERRLA, "A" stands for?

Harrison's 20th Ed. Chapter 28, Page 178

A. Absent
B. Asymmetric
C. Accommodation
D. Alignment

Abbreviation PERRLA stands for pupils equal, round, and reactive to light and accommodation.

306. Light-near dissociation occurs with?

Harrison's 20th Ed. Chapter 28, Page 178

A. Neurosyphilis
B. Parinaud's syndrome
C. Adie's tonic pupil
D. All of the above

Light-near dissociation occurs with neurosyphilis (Argyll Robertson pupil), with lesions of dorsal midbrain (Parinaud's syndrome), and after aberrant regeneration (oculomotor nerve palsy, Adie's tonic pupil).

307. Marcus Gunn pupil is best related to?

Harrison's 20th Ed. Chapter 28, Page 178

A. Neurosyphilis
B. Cataract
C. Oculomotor nerve palsy
D. Retrobulbar optic neuritis

Direct pupillary response is weaker than the consensual pupillary response evoked by shining a light into the other eye. This relative afferent pupillary defect is called Marcus Gunn pupil elicited with the swinging flashlight test. It is an extremely useful sign in retrobulbar optic neuritis and other optic nerve diseases.

308. Tonic pupils is associated with?

Harrison's 20th Ed. Chapter 28, Page 178

A. Shy-Drager syndrome
B. Diabetes mellitus
C. Amyloidosis
D. All of the above

309. Marcus Gunn pupil indicates?

Harrison's 20th Ed. Chapter 28, Page 178

A. Retrobulbar optic neuritis
B. Herpes zoster infection
C. Diabetes mellitus
D. All of the above

An eye with no light perception has no pupillary response to direct light stimulation. If the retina or optic nerve is only partially injured, direct pupillary response will be weaker than consensual pupillary response evoked by shining a light into other eye. This relative afferent pupillary defect (Marcus Gunn pupil) can be elicited with the swinging flashlight test. It is an extremely useful sign in retrobulbar optic neuritis & optic nerve diseases.

310. Which of the following is not a feature of Horner's syndrome?

Harrison's 20th Ed. Chapter 28, Page 178

A. Miosis
B. Ipsilateral ptosis
C. Anisocoria
D. Anhidrosis

Horner's syndrome is a triad of miosis, ipsilateral ptosis & anhidrosis. Anhidrosis is an inconstant feature. Brainstem stroke, carotid dissection & neoplasm impinging on the sympathetic chain cause of Horner's syndrome, but most cases are idiopathic.

311. Which of the following feature of Horner's syndrome is inconstant?

Harrison's 20th Ed. Chapter 28, Page 192

A. Miosis
B. Ipsilateral ptosis
C. Anhidrosis
D. All of the above

312. In Adie's syndrome, a tonic pupil occurs in conjunction with?

Harrison's 20th Ed. Chapter 28, Page 178

A. Weak or absent tendon reflexes in lower extremities
B. Weak or absent tendon reflexes in upper extremities
C. Xerophthalmia
D. Strabismus

Adie's syndrome is a benign disorder in which tonic pupil occurs in conjunction with weak or absent tendon reflexes in lower extremities. It is assumed to represent a mild dysautonomia mostly seen in healthy young women.

313. Tonic pupils are associated with?

Harrison's 20th Ed. Chapter 28, Page 178

A. Shy-Drager syndrome
B. Diabetes
C. Amyloidosis
D. All of the above

Tonic pupils are associated with Shy-Drager syndrome, segmental hypohidrosis, diabetes, amyloidosis or incidentally in an otherwise completely normal, asymptomatic individual..

314. Gardener's pupil best relates to?

Harrison's 20th Ed. Chapter 28, Page 179

A. Narcotic use
B. Exposure to tropane alkaloids contained in plants
C. Perforating injury of eye
D. Adhesions (synechia)

Gardener's pupil refers to mydriasis induced by exposure to tropane alkaloids, contained in plants like deadly nightshade, jimsonweed, or angel's trumpet.

315. Retina does not contain cones for which of the following colour?

Harrison's 20th Ed. Chapter 28, Page 179

A. Red
B. Yellow
C. Green
D. Blue

For colour vision, retina contains three classes of cones, with visual pigments of differing peak spectral sensitivity. Red (560 nm), green (530 nm), and blue (430 nm).

316. In retina, which of the following is not a class of cones?

Harrison's 20th Ed. Chapter 28, Page 179

A. Red
B. Green
C. Yellow
D. Blue

317. Which of the following is false about colour vision?

Harrison's 20th Ed. Chapter 28, Page 179

A. Red & green cone pigments are encoded on X chromosome
B. Blue cone pigment is encoded on chromosome 7
C. Mutations of blue cone pigment are common
D. Ishihara color plates is used to detect red-green color blindness

318. Blue cone pigment is encoded on chromosome?

Harrison's 20th Ed. Chapter 28, Page 179

A. 5
B. 6
C. 7
D. 8

Red & green cone pigments are encoded on X chromosome, while blue cone pigment is on chromosome 7. Mutations of the blue cone pigment are exceedingly rare.

319. Ishihara color plates are used to detect?

Harrison's 20th Ed. Chapter 28, Page 179

A. Red color blindness
B. Green color blindness
C. Blue color blindness
D. Red-green color blindness

Ishihara color plates can be used to detect red-green color blindness.

320. Which of the following statements about colour blindness is false?

Harrison's 20th Ed. Chapter 28, Page 179

A. Mutations of blue cone pigment are exceedingly rare
B. Mutations of red & green pigments cause congenital X-linked color blindness
C. Only male children must be screened
D. None of the above

321. Acquired defects in color vision can result from?

Harrison's 20th Ed. Chapter 28, Page 179

A. Disease of macula
B. Disease of optic nerve
C. Bilateral strokes involving occipital lobe
D. All of the above

322. Vision can be impaired by all except?

Harrison's 20th Ed. Chapter 28, Page 179

A. Colour blindness
B. Damage to Optic chiasma
C. Damage to Optic tract
D. Damage to Occipital lobes

Vision can be impaired by damage to the visual system anywhere from the eyes to the occipital lobes. Anomalous trichromats and dichromats have 6/6 (20/20) visual acuity. Also, a unilateral postchiasmal lesion leaves the visual acuity in each eye unaffected.

323. Dimension of central binocular field is?

Harrison's 20th Ed. Chapter 28, Page 180 Figure 28-3

A. 40°
B. 80°
C. 120°
D. 160°

Visual fields overlap partially, creating 120° of central binocular field flanked by a 40° monocular crescent on either side.

324. Arcuate scotomas shaped like a Turkish scimitar result from?

Harrison's 20th Ed. Chapter 28, Page 181

A. Ischemic optic neuropathy
B. Glaucoma
C. Optic disc drusen
D. All of the above

Glaucoma selectively destroys axons that enter superotemporal or inferotemporal poles of optic disc, resulting in arcuate scotomas shaped like a Turkish scimitar, which emanate from the blind spot & curve around fixation to end flat against the horizontal meridian. Arcuate or nerve fiber layer scotomas also result from optic neuritis, ischemic optic neuropathy, optic disc drusen, and branch retinal artery or vein occlusion.

325. In visual field analysis, which of the following indicates that lesion anterior to the optic chiasm?

Harrison's 20th Ed. Chapter 28, Page 181

A. Scotoma is confined to one eye
B. Cecocentral scotoma
C. Arcuate or nerve fiber layer scotomas
D. All of the above

326. Homonymous hemianopia is produced by a postchiasmal lesion in?

Harrison's 20th Ed. Chapter 28, Page 181

A. Optic tract
B. Lateral geniculate body
C. Optic radiations
D. Any of the above

A postchiasmal lesion anywhere in the optic tract, lateral geniculate body, optic radiations, or visual cortex can produce a homonymous hemianopia (temporal hemifield defect in contralateral eye and a matching nasal hemifield defect in ipsilateral eye).

327. Damage to the optic radiations in the temporal lobe (Meyer's loop) produces?

Harrison's 20th Ed. Chapter 28, Page 181

A. Bitemporal hemianopia
B. Superior quadrantic homonymous hemianopia
C. Inferior quadrantic homonymous hemianopia
D. Total homonymous hemianopia

Symmetric compression of optic chiasm by a pituitary adenoma, meningioma, craniopharyngioma, glioma, or aneurysm results in a bitemporal hemianopia. Damage to the optic radiations in the temporal lobe (Meyer's loop) produces a superior quadrantic homonymous hemianopia, whereas injury to the optic radiations in the parietal lobe results in an inferior quadrantic homonymous hemianopia. Occlusion of posterior cerebral artery supplying occipital lobe causes total homonymous hemianopia.

328. Cortical blindness is distinguished from bilateral prechiasmal visual loss by?

Harrison's 20th Ed. Chapter 28, Page 181

A. Normal visual acuity
B. Normal color vision
C. Normal pupillary responses
D. All of the above

Cortical blindness is distinguished from bilateral prechiasmal visual loss by normal pupillary responses and normal optic fundi.

329. Hutchinson's sign is best related to?

Harrison's 20th Ed. Chapter 28, Page 182

A. Herpes simplex
B. Herpes zoster
C. Sarcoidosis
D. Sjögren's syndrome

Hutchinson's sign refers to vesicles forming on tip of the nose, reflecting nasociliary (V1) nerve involvement due to Herpes Zoster. Vesicles may precede the development of sight-threatening ophthalmic herpes zoster.

330. Hutchinson pupil best relates to?

DeJong's The Neurologic Examination, 7th Ed. Page 750

A. Mastication muscles
B. Macula lutea
C. Uncal herniation
D. Seizures

Hutchinson pupil refers to third nerve palsy due to uncal herniation presenting as unilaterally dilated pupil, unreactive to light, in the setting of coma.

331. Law of equal innervation is known by the name of?

DeJong's The Neurologic Examination, 7th Ed. Page 204

A. Pitres' law
B. Hering's law
C. Alexander's law
D. Brodmann law

Hering's law, or the law of equal innervation, states that the same amount of innervation goes to an extraocular muscle and to its yoked fellow.

332. Which of the following is a cause of scleritis?

Harrison's 20th Ed. Chapter 28, Page 182

A. Rheumatoid arthritis
B. Lupus erythematosus
C. Polyarteritis nodosa
D. All of the above

Scleritis is associated with connective tissue diseases like rheumatoid arthritis, lupus erythematosus, polyarteritis nodosa, granulomatosis with polyangiitis, or relapsing polychondritis.

333. Which of the following can cause panuveitis?

Harrison's 20th Ed. Chapter 28, Page 182

A. Sarcoidosis
B. Behçet's disease
C. Inflammatory bowel disease
D. All of the above

334. Chronic inflammation occurs in which of the following structures in intermediate uveitis?

Harrison's 20th Ed. Chapter 28, Page 182

A. Anterior vitreous
B. Ciliary body
C. Peripheral retina
D. All of the above

Term "intermediate uveitis" describes inflammation of anterior vitreous, ciliary body & peripheral retina, which may or may not be associated with infection or systemic disease. Term "pars planitis" refers to a subset of intermediate uveitis associated with snowbank & snowball formation in the absence of an infectious or systemic disease.

335. Which of the following is a cause of Roth's spots?

Harrison's 20th Ed. Chapter 28, Page 183

A. Subacute bacterial endocarditis
B. Leukemia
C. Diabetes
D. All of the above

Roth's spots are white-centered retinal hemorrhages. They are pathognomonic for subacute bacterial endocarditis (SABE), but they also appear in leukemia, diabetes.

336. Amaurosis in Greek language means?

Neurology. 1989;39(12):1622-4

A. Fake
B. Dangerous
C. Dark
D. Slow

Amaurosis in Greek means darkening, dark, or obscure.

337. Fugax in Latin language means?

Neurology. 1989;39(12):1622-4

A. Below the ground
B. Water
C. Fleeting
D. Sleep

Latin meaning of fugax is fleeting.

338. Amaurosis Fugax is best related to?

Harrison's 20th Ed. Chapter 28, Page 183

A. Multiple sclerosis
B. Schizophrenia
C. Transient ischemic attack of retina
D. All of the above

Amaurosis Fugax or refers to a transient ischemic attack of the retina. Interruption of blood flow to retina for more than a few seconds, mostly by an embolus, results in transient monocular blindness. Emboli are composed of cholesterol (Hollenhorst plaque), calcium, or platelet-fibrin debris mostly coming from an atherosclerotic plaque in carotid artery or aorta.

339. Retinal arterial occlusion occurs in which of the following?

Harrison's 20th Ed. Chapter 28, Page 183

A. Retinal migraine
B. Pregnancy
C. Blood dyscrasias
D. All of the above

340. Susac's syndrome consists of?

American Journal of Neuroradiology. 2004;25(3):351-352

A. Encephalopathy
B. Branch retinal artery occlusions
C. Hearing loss
D. All of the above

Susac's syndrome refers to clinical triad of encephalopathy, branch retinal artery occlusions & hearing loss.

341. Cotton-wool spots in optic fundus refer to?

Harrison's 20th Ed. Chapter 28, Page 184

A. Sclerosis of retinal arterioles
B. Splinter hemorrhages
C. Focal infarcts of the nerve fiber layer of retina
D. Leakage of lipid & fluid into the macula

342. Hard exudate in optic fundus refer to?

Harrison's 20th Ed. Chapter 28, Page 184

A. Sclerosis of retinal arterioles
B. Splinter hemorrhages
C. Focal infarcts of the nerve fiber layer of retina
D. Leakage of lipid & fluid into the macula

Marked systemic hypertension causes sclerosis of retinal arterioles, splinter hemorrhages, focal infarcts of the nerve fiber layer of retina (cotton-wool spots), & leakage of lipid and fluid (hard exudate) into the macula.

343. "Blood and thunder" appearance in optical fundus is best related to?

Harrison's 20th Ed. Chapter 28, Page 184

A. Marked systemic hypertension
B. Retinal arterial occlusion
C. Central retinal vein occlusion
D. Optic neuritis

In central retinal vein occlusion due to frank obstruction may result in extensive retinal bleeding ("blood and thunder" appearance of optical fundus), infarction, and visual loss.

344. Which of the following is false about anterior ischemic optic neuropathy (AION)?

Harrison's 20th Ed. Chapter 28, Page 184

A. Decreased blood flow through posterior ciliary arteries
B. Causes painless & sudden monocular visual loss
C. Consists of two forms: arteritic and nonarteritic
D. None of the above

345. Risk factor for nonarteritic form of AION is?

Harrison's 20th Ed. Chapter 28, Page 184

A. Diabetes
B. Renal failure
C. Hypertension
D. All of the above

Erectile dysfunction drugs may cause AION. AION in one eye increases the likelihood of AION in the other eye. Glucocorticoids should not be prescribed in nonarteritic AION.

346. Which of the following occurs in conjunction with giant cell (temporal) arteritis?

Harrison's 20th Ed. Chapter 28, Page 184

A. Anterior ischemic optic neuropathy (AION)
B. Posterior ischemic optic neuropathy
C. Optic neuritis
D. Toxic optic neuropathy

~5% of patients, especially those >age 60, develop the arteritic form of AION in conjunction with giant cell (temporal) arteritis that causes insufficient blood flow through the posterior ciliary arteries that supply the optic disc. High doses of glucocorticoids or Tocilizumab is useful.

347. Acute visual loss, induced by the combination of severe anemia and hypotension is best related to?

Harrison's 20th Ed. Chapter 28, Page 185

A. Anterior ischemic optic neuropathy (AION)
B. Posterior ischemic optic neuropathy
C. Optic Neuritis
D. Leber's hereditary optic neuropathy

Posterior ischemic optic neuropathy causes acute visual loss, induced by the combination of severe anemia and hypotension.

348. Phrase "the doctor sees nothing, and the patient sees nothing" is best related to?

Harrison's 20th Ed. Chapter 28, Page 185 Figure 28-10

A. Anterior ischemic optic neuropathy (AION)
B. Posterior ischemic optic neuropathy
C. Retrobulbar optic neuritis
D. Leber's hereditary optic neuropathy

349. Which of the following is false about Optic Neuritis?

Harrison's 20th Ed. Chapter 28, Page 185

A. Ocular pain with eye movements
B. Female preponderance
C. Gradual recovery of vision after a single episode
D. None of the above

Virtually all patients experience a gradual recovery of vision after a single episode of optic neuritis, even without treatment.

350. Clinically definite multiple sclerosis develops after optic neuritis in?

Harrison's 20th Ed. Chapter 28, Page 185

A. 25%
B. 50%
C. 75%
D. 100%

Clinically definite multiple sclerosis develops after optic neuritis in 50% cases.

351. Leber's optic neuropathy is caused by a point mutation at codon?

Harrison's 20th Ed. Chapter 28, Page 185

A. 11776
B. 11777
C. 11778
D. 11779

Leber's Hereditary Optic Neuropathy is caused by a point mutation at codon 11778 in the mitochondrial gene encoding nicotinamide adenine dinucleotide dehydrogenase (NADH) subunit 4. These mitochondrial mutations are inherited from the mother by all her children, but usually only sons develop symptoms.

352. Toxic Optic Neuropathy results from exposure to?

Harrison's 20th Ed. Chapter 28, Page 185

A. Ethambutol
B. Methyl alcohol
C. Carbon monoxide
D. All of the above

Toxic Optic Neuropathy results in acute visual loss with bilateral optic disc swelling and central or cecocentral scotomas due to exposure to ethambutol, methyl alcohol (moonshine), ethylene glycol (antifreeze), or carbon monoxide. Other potential offending drugs or toxins are disulfiram, ethchlorvynol, chloramphenicol, amiodarone, monoclonal anti-CD3 antibody, ciprofloxacin, digitalis, streptomycin, lead, arsenic, thallium, d-penicillamine, isoniazid, emetine, and sulfonamides. Deficiency states induced by starvation, malabsorption, or alcoholism can lead to insidious visual loss.

353. Optic atrophy refers to?

Harrison's 20th Ed. Chapter 28, Page 185 Figure 28-11

A. Optic disc pallor
B. Arteriolar narrowing
C. Nerve fiber layer destruction
D. All of the above

Optic atrophy is not a specific diagnosis but refers to the combination of optic disc pallor, arteriolar narrowing & nerve fiber layer destruction produced by various eye diseases, especially optic neuropathies.

354. Which of the following is false about papilledema?

Harrison's 20th Ed. Chapter 28, Page 185

A. Optic disc edema
B. Optic disc swelling
C. Due to raised intracranial pressure
D. Visual acuity is not affected

Papilledema refers to bilateral optic disc swelling due to raised intracranial pressure. Other forms of optic disc swelling like optic neuritis or ischemic optic neuropathy are called "optic disc edema."

355. Which of the following is false regarding 'Papilledema'?

Harrison's 20th Ed. Chapter 28, Page 185

A. Bilateral optic disc swelling
B. Due to raised intracranial pressure
C. Transient visual obscuration
D. Visual acuity is generally affected by papilledema

356. Which of the following is a classic symptom of papilledema?

Harrison's 20th Ed. Chapter 28, Page 185

A. Central or cecocentral scotoma
B. Transient visual obscurations
C. Loss of color perception
D. All of the above

Transient visual obscurations are a classic symptom of papilledema. Obscurations follow abrupt shifts in posture or happen spontaneously.

357. Papilledema is a feature of?

Harrison's 20th Ed. Chapter 28, Page 185

A. High-altitude cerebral edema (HACE)
B. Brain leukostasis
C. POEMS syndrome
D. All of the above

358. Papilledema is a feature of?

Harrison's 20th Ed. Chapter 28, Page 185

A. Cat-scratch disease
B. Hypoparathyroidism
C. Acute toxicity of vitamin A
D. All of the above

359. Papilledema is a feature of?

Harrison's 20th Ed. Chapter 28, Page 185

A. Cerebral malaria
B. Malignant hypertension
C. Chronic hypocalcemia
D. All of the above

360. In papilledema, the earliest change is?

DeJong's The Neurologic Examination, 7th Ed. Page 170

A. Pallor of the temporal portion of the disc
B. Loss of previously observed spontaneous venous pulsations
C. Disc margins stand out distinctly
D. All of the above

In papilledema, the earliest change is loss of previously observed spontaneous venous pulsations (SVPs). It is an old saying that when the patient sees (normal vision) and the doctor sees (observes disc abnormalities), it is papilledema; when patient doesn't see (impaired vision) and the doctor sees (observes disc abnormalities), it is papillitis; when the patient doesn't see (has impaired vision) and the doctor doesn't see (observes no disc abnormality), it is retrobulbar neuritis.

361. "Champagne cork" disc best relates to?

DeJong's The Neurologic Examination, 7th Ed. Page 170

A. Anterior ischemic optic neuropathy (AION)
B. Optic neuritis
C. Papilledema
D. Optic disc drusen

In chronic papilledema, hemorrhages & exudates resolve. What is left is a markedly swollen "champagne cork" disc bulging up from the plane of retina.

362. Which of the following best relates to optic disc drusen?

Harrison's 20th Ed. Chapter 28, Page 186 Figure 28-13

A. Refractile deposits within the substance of optic nerve head
B. Fulminant papilledema
C. Optic nerve fiber layer destruction
D. Optic pallor

Optic disc drusen are refractile calcified, mulberry-like deposits of unknown etiology within the optic disc, giving rise to "pseudopapilledema."

363. Which of the following is false about optic disc drusen?

Harrison's 20th Ed. Chapter 28, Page 186

A. Innocuous in nature
B. Unrelated to drusen of the retina
C. B-ultrasound is the most sensitive way to detect them
D. None of the above

364. Fragile neovascular vessels that proliferate on surface of retina are seen in?

Harrison's 20th Ed. Chapter 28, Page 186

A. Diabetes
B. Sickle cell anemia
C. Ischemic ocular diseases
D. All of the above

Fragile neovascular vessels that proliferate on the surface of the retina in diabetes, sickle cell anemia, and other ischemic ocular diseases.

365. Retinal detachment can produce which of the following symptoms?

Harrison's 20th Ed. Chapter 28, Page 186

A. Floaters
B. Flashing lights
C. Scotoma in peripheral visual field corresponding to detachment
D. All of the above

366. In most eyes, retinal detachment starts with a?

Harrison's 20th Ed. Chapter 28, Page 186

A. Hole in the peripheral retina
B. Flap in the peripheral retina
C. Tear in the peripheral retina
D. Any of the above

In most eyes, retinal detachment starts with a hole, flap, or tear in the peripheral retina (rhegmatogenous retinal detachment). Patients with peripheral retinal thinning (lattice degeneration) are vulnerable to this process.

367. Which of the following is false about scintillating scotomas of migraine?

Harrison's 20th Ed. Chapter 28, Page 187

A. Remain visible in the dark
B. Remain visible with the eyes closed
C. Headache develops afer visual symptoms recede
D. None of the above

368. Which of the following is a sign of brainstem ischemia?

Harrison's 20th Ed. Chapter 28, Page 187

A. Diplopia
B. Vertigo
C. Dysarthria
D. All of the above

Signs of brainstem ischemia are diplopia, vertigo, numbness, weakness, and dysarthria.

369. Which of the following is a cause of hemianopic cortical visual loss?

Harrison's 20th Ed. Chapter 28, Page 187

A. Occipital lobe stroke
B. Lobar hemorrhage
C. Arteriovenous malformation
D. All of the above

In a case of occipital lobe stroke due to thrombotic occlusion of vertebrobasilar system, embolus, or dissection, the only finding on examination is a homonymous visual field defect that stops abruptly at the "vertical meridian". Lobar hemorrhage, tumor, abscess, and arteriovenous malformation are other common causes of hemianopic cortical visual loss.

370. Formation of cataract occurs more rapidly in patients with a history of?

Harrison's 20th Ed. Chapter 28, Page 187

A. Uveitis
B. Diabetes mellitus
C. Vitrectomy
D. All of the above

371. Genetic disease leading to the formation of cataract is?

Harrison's 20th Ed. Chapter 28, Page 187

A. Myotonic dystrophy
B. Neurofibromatosis type 2
C. Galactosemia
D. All of the above

372. In glaucoma, axons entering which of the following aspects of optic disc are damaged first?

Harrison's 20th Ed. Chapter 28, Page 187

A. Inferotemporal
B. Inferonasal
C. Superonasal
D. Any of the above

In glaucoma, axons entering inferotemporal and superotemporal aspects of optic disc are damaged first, producing typical nerve fiber bundle or arcuate scotomas on perimetric testing.

373. Which of the following condition is caused due to variants in the gene for complement factor H?

Harrison's 20th Ed. Chapter 28, Page 188

A. Retinal detachment
B. Cataract
C. Glaucoma
D. Macular degeneration

Susceptibility to macular degeneration is associated with variants in the gene for complement factor H, an inhibitor of alternative complement pathway.

374. Which of the following is useful in macular degeneration?

Harrison's 20th Ed. Chapter 28, Page 188

A. Bevacizumab
B. Ranibizumab
C. Aflibercept
D. All of the above

Exudative macular degeneration can be treated with intraocular injection of antagonists to vascular endothelial growth factor. Bevacizumab, ranibizumab, or aflibercept is administered by direct injection into the vitreous cavity. These antibodies cause the regression of neovascular membranes by blocking the action of vascular endothelial growth factor.

375. Bone spicules in the peripheral retina best relate to?

Harrison's 20th Ed. Chapter 28, Page 188

A. Central serous chorioretinopathy
B. Diabetic retinopathy
C. Melanoma of the choroid
D. Retinitis pigmentosa

In retinitis pigmentosa, irregular black deposits of clumped pigment are seen in the peripheral retina. These are called bone spicules because of their resemblance to the spicules of cancellous bone.

376. Retinitis pigmentosa is due to a mutation in the gene for?

Harrison's 20th Ed. Chapter 28, Page 188

A. Peripherin
B. Tyrosinase (TYR)
C. Gene for transcription factor C/EBPα
D. Gene for Gsα subunit

Retinitis pigmentosa is due to a mutation in the gene for rhodopsin or in the gene for peripherin.

377. Which of the following is false about retinitis pigmentosa?

Harrison's 20th Ed. Chapter 28, Page 188

A. Progressive night blindness
B. Visual field constriction with a ring scotoma
C. Abnormal electroretinogram (ERG)
D. None of the above

378. Treatment with which of the following drugs causes retinopathy that resembles that of retinitis pigmentosa?

Harrison's 20th Ed. Chapter 28, Page 188

A. Chloroquine
B. Hydroxychloroquine
C. Thioridazine
D. All of the above

379. Retinitis pigmentosa occur in association with?

Harrison's 20th Ed. Chapter 28, Page 188

A. Bassen-Kornzweig disease
B. Kearns-Sayre syndrome
C. Refsum's disease
D. All of the above

380. Which is the most common primary tumor of the eye?

Harrison's 20th Ed. Chapter 28, Page 189

A. Retinoblastoma
B. Melanoma
C. Hemangioblastoma
D. Astrocytic hamartoma

381. Which of the following is not a cause of enophthalmos?

Harrison's 20th Ed. Chapter 28, Page 189

A. Horner's syndrome
B. Fracture of the orbital floor
C. Space-occupying lesion in the orbit
D. All of the above

382. Protrusion of the globe in orbital inflammation is due particularly to engorgement of which extraocular muscle?

Harrison's 20th Ed. Chapter 28, Page 189

A. Medial rectus
B. Lateral rectus
C. Superior rectus
D. All of the above

Orbital inflammation & engorgement of extraocular muscles, particularly medial rectus and inferior rectus, account for the protrusion of the globe.

383. Which of the following is a cause of myogenic ptosis?

Harrison's 20th Ed. Chapter 28, Page 190

A. Myasthenia gravis
B. Kearns-Sayre syndrome
C. Myotonic dystrophy
D. All of the above

384. Which of the following is not a feature of Kearns-Sayre syndrome?

Harrison's 20th Ed. Chapter 28, Page 190

A. Frontal balding
B. Retinal pigmentary changes
C. Abnormalities of cardiac conduction
D. "Ragged-red fibers" on peripheral muscle biopsy

In Kearns-Sayre syndrome, retinal pigmentary changes and abnormalities of cardiac conduction develop along with characteristic "ragged-red fibers" on peripheral muscle biopsy. In autosomal dominant myotonic dystrophy, ptosis, ophthalmoparesis, cataract, pigmentary retinopathy, muscle wasting, myotonia, frontal balding, and cardiac abnormalities are seen.

385. Which of the following in not a feature of myasthenia gravis?

Harrison's 20th Ed. Chapter 28, Page 190

A. Muscle wasting
B. Diplopia
C. Pupils are always normal
D. Fluctuating ptosis

Fluctuating ptosis that worsens late in the day is typical of myasthenia gravis.

386. Which of the following is not innervated by oculomotor nerve?

Harrison's 20th Ed. Chapter 28, Page 191

A. Levator palpebrae superioris
B. Inferior oblique
C. Superior oblique
D. Iris sphincter

Third cranial nerve innervates medial, inferior, and superior recti; inferior oblique; levator palpebrae superioris; and iris sphincter. Lateral rectus and superior oblique muscles are not supplied by third cranial nerve. Abducens or the sixth cranial nerve innervates lateral rectus muscle. Trochlear or the fourth cranial nerve innervates the contralateral superior oblique.

387. Total palsy of the oculomotor nerve causes all except?

Harrison's 20th Ed. Chapter 28, Page 191

A. Ptosis
B. Dilated pupil
C. Eye is "down and out"
D. Eye is "down and in"

Total palsy of oculomotor nerve causes ptosis, dilated pupil, and leaves the eye "down and out" because of the unopposed action of lateral rectus and superior oblique muscles.

388. Total palsy of oculomotor nerve leaves the eye?

Harrison's 20th Ed. Chapter 28, Page 191

A. Down and in
B. Down and out
C. Up and in
D. Up and out

389. Which of the following is false about III nerve palsy?

Harrison's 20th Ed. Chapter 28, Page 191

A. Nothnagel's syndrome is ipsilateral III palsy and contralateral cerebellar ataxia
B. Benedikt's syndrome is ipsilateral III nerve palsy and contralateral tremor, chorea, and athetosis
C. Weber's syndrome is ipsilateral III nerve palsy with contralateral hemiparesis
D. None of the above

Nothnagel's syndrome is also called ophthalmoplegia-ataxia syndrome. It is a variant of Parinaud's syndrome, with uni- or bilateral III nerve palsy & ataxia accompanied by vertical gaze deficits & other neurologic signs.

390. Which of the following is not a midbrain syndrome?

DeJong's The Neurologic Examination, 7th Ed. Page 337

A. Millard-Gubler syndrome
B. Weber's syndrome
C. Claude's syndrome
D. Benedikt's syndrome

Millard-Gubler syndrome, Foville syndrome & Raymond's syndrome are pontine syndromes. The three midbrain syndromes are Weber's syndrome, Claude's syndrome & Benedikt's syndrome. Benedikt's is essentially Weber's + Claude's. Parinaud's and Nothnagel's syndrome are also due to lesion in the midbrain.

391. Which of the following is a syndrome of the medulla?

DeJong's The Neurologic Examination, 7th Ed. Page 337

A. Avellis's syndrome
B. Jackson's syndrome
C. Schmidt's syndrome
D. All of the above

The two primary medullary syndromes are the lateral medullary syndrome (Wallenberg) and the medial medullary syndrome (Dejerine). Other syndromes of the medulla include Avellis's, Jackson's, Schmidt's, Céstan-Chenais, and Babinski-Nageotte.

392. Which of the following is called hemimedullary syndrome?

DeJong's The Neurologic Examination, 7th Ed. Page 340

A. Babinski-Nageotte syndrome
B. Céstan-Chenais syndrome
C. Dejerine's syndrome
D. Schmidt's syndrome

393. Injury to the red nucleus causes which of the following?

Harrison's 20th Ed. Chapter 28, Page 191

A. Nothnagel's syndrome
B. Benedikt's syndrome
C. Weber's syndrome
D. All of the above

394. Injury to the superior cerebellar peduncle causes which of the following?

Harrison's 20th Ed. Chapter 28, Page 191

A. Nothnagel's syndrome
B. Benedikt's syndrome
C. Weber's syndrome
D. All of the above

395. Injury to the superior cerebral peduncle causes which of the following?

Harrison's 20th Ed. Chapter 28, Page 191

A. Nothnagel's syndrome
B. Benedikt's syndrome
C. Weber's syndrome
D. All of the above

396. Ipsilateral oculomotor palsy is a feature of?
Harrison's 20th Ed. Chapter 28, Page 191

A. Nothnagel's syndrome
B. Benedikt's syndrome
C. Weber's syndrome
D. All of the above

397. Contralateral tremor, chorea, and athetosis is a feature of?
Harrison's 20th Ed. Chapter 28, Page 191

A. Nothnagel's syndrome
B. Benedikt's syndrome
C. Weber's syndrome
D. All of the above

In Nothnagel's syndrome, injury to the superior cerebellar peduncle causes ipsilateral oculomotor palsy and contralateral cerebellar ataxia. In Benedikt's syndrome, injury to the red nucleus results in ipsilateral oculomotor palsy and contralateral tremor, chorea, and athetosis. Claude's syndrome incorporates features of both of these syndromes, by injury to both the red nucleus and the superior cerebellar peduncle. In Weber's syndrome, injury to the cerebral peduncle causes ipsilateral oculomotor palsy with contralateral hemiparesis.

398. Which of the following cranial nerves has "head tilt test" as a cardinal diagnostic feature?
Harrison's 20th Ed. Chapter 28, Page 191

A. Oculomotor nerve
B. Trochlear nerve
C. Abducens nerve
D. All of the above

Trochlear nerve or fourth cranial nerve originates in midbrain and innervates the contralateral superior oblique. Its action is to depress and intort the eyeball. Its palsy results in hypertropia & excyclotorsion with patients complaining of vertical diplopia, especially upon reading or looking down which is exacerbated by tilting head toward the side with the muscle palsy & alleviated by tilting it away. This "head tilt test" is a cardinal diagnostic feature of trochlear nerve palsy.

399. Isolated trochlear nerve palsy results from all of the following causes except?
Harrison's 20th Ed. Chapter 28, Page 191

A. Aneurysm
B. Meningitis
C. Tumor
D. Infarction

Isolated trochlear nerve palsy does not result from aneurysm.

400. Which of the following is false about Trochlear Nerve?
Harrison's 20th Ed. Chapter 28, Page 191

A. Palsy results in hypertropia
B. Palsy results in excyclotorsion
C. Head tilt test is diagnostic
D. None of the above

401. Isolated trochlear nerve palsy occurs due to all except?
Harrison's 20th Ed. Chapter 28, Page 191

A. Infarction
B. Herniation
C. Aneurysm
D. Tumour

402. Foville's syndrome includes all except?
Harrison's 20th Ed. Chapter 28, Page 191

A. Lateral gaze palsy
B. Ipsilateral facial palsy
C. Contralateral hemiparesis
D. Contralateral hemianesthesia

403. Which of the following is false about Millard-Gubler syndrome?
Harrison's 20th Ed. Chapter 28, Page 191

A. Due to ventral pontine injury
B. Lateral gaze palsy
C. Ipsilateral facial palsy
D. Contralateral hemiparesis

404. Which of the following is false about Gradenigo's syndrome?
Harrison's 20th Ed. Chapter 28, Page 191

A. Mastoiditis
B. Deafness
C. Ipsilateral abducens palsy
D. None of the above

405. Which of the following can produce ophthalmoplegia?
Harrison's 20th Ed. Chapter 28, Page 191

A. Lambert-Eaton myasthenic syndrome
B. Giant cell (temporal) arteritis
C. Miller Fisher syndrome
D. All of the above

406. Most common cause of internuclear ophthalmoplegia is?
Harrison's 20th Ed. Chapter 28, Page 191

A. Multiple sclerosis
B. Intracranial tumor
C. Stroke
D. Concussion trauma

407. Which of the following is false for Parinaud's syndrome?
Harrison's 20th Ed. Chapter 28, Page 191

A. Also known as dorsal midbrain syndrome
B. Supranuclear vertical gaze disorder
C. Hydrocephalus from aqueductal stenosis
D. None of the above

408. Which of the following has no relation with Parinaud's syndrome?
Harrison's 20th Ed. Chapter 28, Page 191

A. Pineal region tumors
B. Beevor's sign
C. Setting sun sign
D. Collier's sign

409. Lateral gaze palsy, ipsilateral facial palsy, and contralateral hemiparesis are features of?

Harrison's 20th Ed. Chapter 28, Page 191

A. Foville's syndrome
B. Millard-Gubler syndrome
C. Gradenigo's syndrome
D. Tolosa-Hunt syndrome

Foville's syndrome occurs as a result of dorsal pontine injury damaging abducens nucleus. It includes lateral gaze palsy, ipsilateral facial palsy, and contralateral hemiparesis incurred by damage to descending corticospinal fibers. Abducens nucleus contains interneurons that project via medial longitudinal fasciculus to the medial rectus subnucleus of the contralateral oculomotor complex. Therefore, abducens nuclear lesion produces a complete lateral gaze palsy from weakness of both the ipsilateral lateral rectus and the contralateral medial rectus.

410. Injury to which of the following leads to Millard-Gubler syndrome?

Harrison's 20th Ed. Chapter 28, Page 191

A. Dorsal pons
B. Ventral pons
C. Medial longitudinal fasciculus
D. Paramedian pontine reticular formation

Millard-Gubler syndrome consists of lateral rectus weakness only, instead of gaze palsy as abducens fascicle is injured rather than the nucleus from ventral pontine injury.

411. Gradenigo's syndrome relates best with which of the following?

Harrison's 20th Ed. Chapter 28, Page 191

A. Subacute sclerosing panencephalitis (SSPE)
B. Progressive multifocal leukoencephalopathy
C. Transverse sinus thrombosis
D. Pituitary adenoma

Headache and earache are the most frequent symptoms of transverse sinus thrombosis. A transverse sinus thrombosis may also present with otitis media, sixth nerve palsy, and retroorbital or facial pain (Gradenigo's syndrome). Sigmoid sinus and internal jugular vein thrombosis may present with neck pain.

412. Which of the following is a cause of abducens palsy?

Harrison's 20th Ed. Chapter 28, Page 191

A. Raised intracranial pressure
B. After lumbar puncture
C. Spontaneous dural cerebrospinal fluid leak
D. All of the above

Unilateral or bilateral abducens palsy is a classic sign of raised intracranial pressure, probably related to rostral-caudal displacement of brainstem. Low intracranial pressure after lumbar puncture, spinal anesthesia, or spontaneous dural cerebrospinal fluid leak may also cause abducens palsy.

413. Which of the intracranial locations can produce multiple ocular motor nerve palsies?

Harrison's 20th Ed. Chapter 28, Page 192

A. Cavernous sinus
B. Superior orbital fissure
C. Orbital apex
D. All of the above

Lesions at cavernous sinus, superior orbital fissure, and orbital apex can produce multiple ocular motor nerve palsies as all three ocular motor nerves are in close proximity.

414. Name of the law that states "jerk nystagmus increases with gaze in the direction of the fast phase" is?

DeJong's The Neurologic Examination, 7th Ed. Page 221

A. Pitres' law
B. Hering's law
C. Alexander's law
D. Brodmann law

Hering's law, or the law of equal innervation, states that the same amount of innervation goes to an extraocular muscle and to its yoked fellow.

415. Nystagmus occurs due to?

Harrison's 20th Ed. Chapter 28, Page 192

A. Vestibular stimulation
B. Optokinetic stimulation
C. Congenital sensory nystagmus
D. All of the above

416. Congenital sensory nystagmus may be due to?

Harrison's 20th Ed. Chapter 28, Page 192

A. Albinism
B. Leber's congenital amaurosis
C. Bilateral cataract
D. All of the above

417. Vestibular nystagmus results from dysfunction of?

Harrison's 20th Ed. Chapter 28, Page 192

A. Labyrinth
B. Vestibular nerve
C. Vestibular nucleus in the brainstem
D. All of the above

418. Downbeat nystagmus results from all except?

Harrison's 20th Ed. Chapter 28, Page 192

A. Chiari malformation
B. Lithium or anticonvulsant intoxication
C. Damage to the pontine tegmentum
D. Alcoholism

Downbeat nystagmus results from lesions near the craniocervical junction, brainstem or cerebellar stroke, lithium or anticonvulsant intoxication, alcoholism & multiple sclerosis. Upbeat nystagmus is associated with damage to pontine tegmentum from stroke, demyelination, or tumor.

419. Saccadomania or dancing eyes best relate to?

Harrison's 20th Ed. Chapter 28, Page 193

A. Opsoclonus
B. Rebound nystagmus
C. Seesaw nystagmus
D. Ocular bobbing

Ocular flutter & opsoclonus are types of saccadic intrusions, spontaneous saccades away from fixation. They may be confused with nystagmus.

420. Which of the following best relates to positional nystagmus?

DeJong's The Neurologic Examination, 7th Ed. Page 294

A. Wartenberg pendulum test
B. Hoover's test
C. Wada test
D. Dix-Hallpike test

421. Who was the inventor of the ophthalmoscope?

DeJong's The Neurologic Examination, 7th Ed. Page 208

A. Helmholtz
B. Welch
C. Allyn
D. Purkinje

Helmholtz was the inventor of ophthalmoscope.

Pathobiology of Neurologic Diseases

422. Neuropil consists of?
Harrison's 20th Ed. Chapter 443, Page 3260

A. Axons
B. Dendrites
C. Glial cell processes
D. All of the above

423. What proportion of 23,000 genes encoded in human genome are expressed in human nervous system?
Harrison's 20th Ed. Chapter 417 Page 3039

A. ~ one-fourth
B. ~ one-third
C. ~ one-half
D. ~ three-fourth

Over one-third of 23,000 genes encoded in human genome are expressed in human nervous system.

424. Each mature brain is composed of how many neurons?
Harrison's 20th Ed. Chapter 417 Page 3039

A. 10 million
B. 100 million
C. 10 billion
D. 100 billion

425. Each mature brain is composed of how many synapses?
Harrison's 20th Ed. Chapter 417 Page 3039

A. $\sim 10^{10}$
B. $\sim 10^{15}$
C. $\sim 10^{20}$
D. $\sim 10^{25}$

Each mature brain is composed of 100 billion neurons, several million miles of axons and dendrites, and $>10^{15}$ synapses.

426. Which of the following is false about myelin?
Harrison's 20th Ed. Chapter 416, Page 3030

A. It speeds impulse conduction
B. Single oligodendrocyte ensheaths multiple CNS axons
C. Each Schwann cell myelinates a single PNS axon
D. It is a protein-rich material

Myelin is a lipid-rich material formed by a spiraling process of the membrane of myelinating cell around the axon.

427. Which of the following about myelin is false?
Harrison's 20th Ed. Chapter 417 Page 3039

A. Lipid-rich insulating substance that surrounds axons
B. Speeds impulse conduction
C. Single oligodendrocyte ensheaths multiple axons in CNS
D. None of the above

428. Which of the following about oligodendrocyte precursor cells (OPCs) is false?
Harrison's 20th Ed. Chapter 417 Page 3039

A. Highly motile cells
B. Migrate along inner surface of endothelial cells
C. Migration regulated by Wnt pathway signaling
D. None of the above

429. Which of the following regulate oligodendrocyte differentiation and myelination?
Harrison's 20th Ed. Chapter 417 Page 3039

A. LINGO-1
B. PSA-NCAM
C. Chrm1
D. All of the above

Oligodendrocyte differentiation & myelination is inhibited by LINGO-1, PSA-NCAM, hyaluronan, Nogo-A, Wnt pathway, notch signaling, and M1 muscarinic receptor Chrm1. Retinoic acid receptor RXRγ have an excitatory influence.

430. Which of the following is a remyelinating agent?
Harrison's 20th Ed. Chapter 417 Page 3039

A. Prilocaine
B. Polidocanol
C. Clemastine
D. Chlorprothixene

Antihistamine clemastine, that works via binding to Chrm1 muscarinic receptor, has shown efficacy as a remyelinating agent in patients with chronic optic neuropathy due to MS.

431. Brain microglia secrete which of the following?
Harrison's 20th Ed. Chapter 417 Page 3040

A. Glial-derived neurotrophic factor (GDNF)
B. Brain derived neurotrophic factor (BDNF)
C. Ciliary neurotrophic factor
D. All of the above

432. Which of the function of microglial cell?
Harrison's 20th Ed. Chapter 417 Page 3040

A. Synaptic pruning
B. Clearing cellular debris & protein
C. Promotion of learning and memory
D. All of the above

433. Which of the following about microglia is false?
Harrison's 20th Ed. Chapter 417 Page 3040

A. Located throughout the brain parenchyma
B. Downregulate inflammatory responses & promote tissue repair
C. Activated microglia promote formation of β-amyloid
D. None of the above

434. Astrocytes secrete which of the following?
Harrison's 20th Ed. Chapter 417 Page 3041

A. Apolipoprotein E
B. Thrombospondins
C. Glypicans
D. All of the above

Astrocytes influence synapses by secreting factors (apolipoprotein E, thrombospondins & glypicans) that regulate development, maintenance, and pruning of presynaptic & postsynaptic structures.

435. Which of the following is secreted by activated microglia?

Harrison's 20th Ed. Chapter 417 Page 3041

A. IL-1a
B. TNF
C. C1q
D. All of the above

Activated microglia secrete IL-1a, TNF, and C1q, that induces astrocytes to transform to A1 type which actively participate in the injury process.

436. Glymphatic system best relates to?

Harrison's 20th Ed. Chapter 417 Page 3042

A. Aquaporin-4 water channels
B. Sleep
C. Cervical lymph nodes
D. All of the above

437. Which of the following is a protein involved in protection from oxidative stress?

Harrison's 20th Ed. Chapter 417 Page 3043

A. α-synuclein
B. Parkin
C. PINK1
D. DJ-1

PINK1 is a mitochondrial kinase. DJ-1 is a protein involved in protection from oxidative stress. Parkin is a ubiquitin ligase.

438. Superoxide dismutase mutations are associated with?

Harrison's 20th Ed. Chapter 417 Page 3043

A. Huntington's disease (HD)
B. Familial amyotrophic lateral sclerosis (ALS)
C. Frontotemporal dementia (FTD)
D. Progressive supranuclear palsy (PSP)

439. TAR DNA binding protein 43 (TDP-43) is associated with?

Harrison's 20th Ed. Chapter 417 Page 3043

A. Huntington's disease (HD)
B. Familial amyotrophic lateral sclerosis (ALS)
C. Frontotemporal dementia (FTD)
D. Progressive supranuclear palsy (PSP)

440. Mitochondrial dysfunction is strongly linked to the pathogenesis of?

Harrison's 20th Ed. Chapter 417 Page 3043

A. Gerstmann-Sträussler-Scheinker disease (GSS)
B. Huntington's disease (HD)
C. Creutzfeldt-Jakob disease (CJD)
D. Friedreich's ataxia

441. Autophagy is impaired in?

Harrison's 20th Ed. Chapter 417 Page 3043

A. AD
B. PD
C. HD
D. All of the above

442. Which of the following induces autophagy?

Harrison's 20th Ed. Chapter 417 Page 3043

A. Rapamycin
B. Sorafenib
C. Piaglitazone
D. Metformin

Rapamycin is a selective inhibitor of TORC1 (target of rapamycin complex 1). Resveratrol, rapamycin, spermidine, and metformin have been shown to delay aging in experimental animal models.

Headache

443. Which cranial structure is pain-insensitive?
Harrison's 20th Ed. Chapter 13, Page 85

A. Scalp
B. Choroid plexus
C. Dural sinuses
D. Falx cerebri

444. Which cranial structure is pain-sensitive?
Harrison's 20th Ed. Chapter 13, Page 85

A. Ventricular ependyma
B. Choroid plexus
C. Pial veins
D. Falx cerebri

Pain-producing cranial structures include scalp, middle meningeal artery, dural sinuses, falx cerebri and proximal segments of large pial arteries. Ventricular ependyma, choroid plexus, pial veins, and much of the brain parenchyma are not pain-producing.

445. Which of the following is a type of primary headache?
Harrison's 20th Ed. Chapter 13, Page 85 Table 13-1

A. Migraine
B. Tension-type
C. Cluster
D. All of the above

446. Which of the following is not a type of primary headache?
Harrison's 20th Ed. Chapter 13, Page 85 Table 13-1

A. Idiopathic stabbing
B. Exertional
C. Systemic infection
D. Tension-type

Primary headaches are those in which headache and its associated features are the disorder in itself, whereas secondary headaches are those caused by exogenous disorders. Examples of primary headache are migraine, tension-type, cluster, idiopathic stabbing & exertional. Examples of secondary headache are systemic infection, head injury, vascular disorders, subarachnoid hemorrhage & brain tumor.

447. Of the following cause of primary headache, which one is the most common?
Harrison's 20th Ed. Chapter 13, Page 85 Table 13-1

A. Migraine
B. Tension-type
C. Cluster
D. Exertional

Relative frequency of various types of primary headache is migraine 16%, tension-type 69%, cluster 0.1%, idiopathic stabbing 2% and exertional 1%.

448. Of the following cause of secondary headache, which one is the most common?
Harrison's 20th Ed. Chapter 13, Page 85 Table 13-1

A. Systemic infection
B. Vascular disorders
C. Subarachnoid hemorrhage
D. Brain tumor

Relative frequency of various types of secondary headache is systemic infection 63%, head injury 4%, vascular disorders 1%, subarachnoid hemorrhage <1% and brain tumor 0.1%.

449. Which of the following is a part of the trigeminocervical complex?
Harrison's 20th Ed. Chapter 13, Page 85

A. Trigeminal nucleus caudalis
B. Dorsal horns of C1
C. Dorsal horns of C2
D. All of the above

Caudal portion of trigeminal nucleus along with first & second cervical nerve roots is called the trigeminocervical complex.

450. Which of the following is a cranial autonomic symptom?
Harrison's 20th Ed. Chapter 13, Page 85

A. Lacrimation
B. Rhinorrhea
C. Ptosis
D. All of the above

Cranial autonomic symptoms include lacrimation, conjunctival injection, nasal congestion, rhinorrhea, periorbital swelling, aural fullness, and ptosis. These are prominent in trigeminal autonomic cephalalgias (TACs), including cluster headache and paroxysmal hemicrania, and may be seen in migraine.

451. Which of the following symptoms suggest that the headache has a serious underlying disorder?
Harrison's 20th Ed. Chapter 13, Page 86 Table 13-2

A. Pain induced by bending, lifting, cough
B. Pain that disturbs sleep or presents upon awakening
C. Vomiting that precedes headache
D. All of the above

Features that suggest headache has a serious underlying disorder include sudden-onset headache, first severe headache, "worst" headache ever, vomiting that precedes headache, subacute worsening over days or weeks, pain induced by bending, lifting or cough, pain that disturbs sleep or presents immediately upon awakening, known systemic illness, onset after age 55 years, fever or unexplained systemic signs, abnormal neurologic examination and pain associated with local tenderness (region of temporal artery).

452. Which of the following is not a vascular headache?
Harrison's 20th Ed. Chapter 13, Page 85

A. Migraine
B. Cluster headache
C. Tension-type headache
D. All of the above

Migraine & other primary headache types are not vascular headaches. Migraine is a brain disorder.

453. Acute, severe headache with stiff neck but without fever suggests?
Harrison's 20th Ed. Chapter 13, Page 86

A. Cerebral metastases
B. Carcinomatous meningitis
C. Subarachnoid hemorrhage
D. Posterior fossa mass

Acute, severe headache (maximal in <5 minutes, lasting >5 minutes) with stiff neck but without fever suggests subarachnoid hemorrhage.

454. Vomiting that precedes the appearance of headache by weeks is highly characteristic of?

Harrison's 20th Ed. Chapter 13, Page 86

A. Meningitis
B. Subarachnoid hemorrhage
C. Posterior fossa brain tumors
D. Temporal arteritis

Vomiting that precedes appearance of headache by weeks is highly characteristic of posterior fossa brain tumors.

455. Head pain appearing abruptly after bending, lifting or coughing can be due to?

Harrison's 20th Ed. Chapter 13, Page 86

A. Posterior fossa mass
B. Chiari malformation
C. Low cerebrospinal fluid (CSF) volume
D. All of the above

Head pain appearing abruptly after bending, lifting or coughing can be due to posterior fossa mass, Chiari malformation or low cerebrospinal fluid (CSF) volume.

456. Jaw claudication is a feature of?

Harrison's 20th Ed. Chapter 13, Page 86, 676, 3072

A. Vinca alkaloid use
B. Temporal (giant cell) arteritis
C. Occlusion of common carotid artery
D. All of the above

457. Giant cell arteritis is closely associated with?

Harrison's 20th Ed. Chapter 356, Page 2583

A. Granulomatosis with polyangiitis (Wegener's)
B. Eosinophilic granulomatosis with polyangiitis (Churg-Strauss)
C. Polymyalgia rheumatica
D. Polyarteritis nodosa

Giant cell arteritis is closely associated with polymyalgia rheumatica (40–50%).

458. Which of the following is a feature of temporal arteritis?

Harrison's 20th Ed. Chapter 13, Page 86

A. Head pain is infrequently throbbing
B. Scalp tenderness is present
C. Head pain is worse at night & aggravated by exposure to cold
D. All of the above

459. Chronic daily headache (CDH) means headache for how many days per month?

Harrison's 20th Ed. Chapter 13, Page 87

A. 3 days per month
B. 7 days per month
C. 10 days per month
D. 15 days per month

Chronic daily headache (CDH) or near-daily headache could be suspected when a patient experiences headache on 15 days or more per month. It affects ~4% of adults & encompasses different headache syndromes, both primary and secondary.

460. Which of the following is a secondary cause of Daily or Near-Daily Headache?

Harrison's 20th Ed. Chapter 13, Page 87 Table 13-3

A. Giant cell arteritis
B. Sarcoidosis
C. Behçet's syndrome
D. All of the above

461. In "Coat-hanger headache", the pain is in?

Harrison's 20th Ed. Chapter 18, Page 126

A. Suboccipital region
B. Posterior cervical region
C. Shoulder region
D. All of the above

462. Which of the following is the cause of "coat-hanger headache"?

Harrison's 20th Ed. Chapter 18, Page 126

A. Neck muscle spasm
B. Neck muscle tear
C. Neck muscle ischemia
D. Neck muscle inflammation

"Coat-hanger headache" is most likely due to neck muscle ischemia in a patient of orthostatic hypotension.

463. Which of the following is a feature of new daily persistent headache (NDPH)?

Harrison's 20th Ed. Chapter 422, Page 3107

A. Headache on most if not all days
B. Ipsilateral conjunctival injection and lacrimation
C. Very frequent short-lasting attacks
D. Periodicity

464. Which of the following is false about post-lumbar puncture headache?

Harrison's 20th Ed. Chapter 13, Page 88

A. Usually begins within 48 hours
B. Incidence is between 10 and 30%
C. Is dramatically positional
D. Aggravated by abdominal compression

465. Which of the following is false about lumbar puncture headache?

Harrison's 20th Ed. Chapter 13, Page 88

A. Worsened by head shaking
B. Worsened by jugular vein compression
C. Location is bitemporal
D. Epidural blood patch is an effective treatment

466. Which of the following is not a feature of lumbar puncture headache?

Harrison's 20th Ed. Chapter 13, Page 88

A. Dramatically positional
B. Begins when the patient sits or stands upright
C. Relief by abdominal compression
D. Relief by jugular vein compression

Low CSF volume headache is positional (recumbency improves headache within minutes), occipitofrontal, begins within 48 hours following lumbar puncture, but may be delayed for up to 12 days (incidence 10–30%) & caffeine, abdominal binder & oral theophylline provide temporary relief. Symptoms result from low CSF volume rather than low CSF pressure.

467. Headache on rising in the morning or nocturnal headache is characteristic of?

Harrison's 20th Ed. Chapter 13, Page 88

A. Obstructive sleep apnea
B. Poorly controlled hypertension
C. Raised CSF pressure headache
D. All of the above

468. Sleep disruption and early morning headaches that improve during the day are characteristics of?

Harrison's 20th Ed. Chapter 13, Page 88

A. Migraine
B. Cluster headache
C. Brain tumors
D. Unruptured aneurysms

469. Headaches that build up over hours, maintained for several hours to days, relieved by sleep are sugestive of?

Harrison's 20th Ed. Chapter 13, Page 88

A. Migraine
B. Cluster headache
C. Brain tumors
D. Unruptured aneurysms

470. Headache in the absence of any exogenous cause is a feature of?

Harrison's 20th Ed. Chapter 13, Page 88

A. Migraine
B. Tension-type headache
C. Trigeminal autonomic cephalalgias
D. All of the above

Migraine and Other Primary Headache Disorders

471. Prevalence of migraine increases steeply at?

N Engl J Med. 2017;377:553-61

A. 10 to 14 years of age
B. 20 to 24 years of age
C. 30 to 34 years of age
D. 40 to 44 years of age

Although migraine may begin early in childhood, but its prevalence increases steeply at 10 to 14 years of age. Prevalence continues to increase until 35 to 39 years of age, after which it gradually decreases, particularly among women after menopause.

472. Migraine is associated with an increased risk of?

N Engl J Med. 2017;377:553-61

A. Asthma
B. Stroke
C. Anxiety and depression
D. All of the above

Migraine is associated with increased risks of asthma, stroke, anxiety & depression, & other pain disorders. Although, it is exceedingly rare for cerebral ischemia or infarction to occur during a migraine attack.

473. Which of the following is a common premonitory symptom in migraine?

N Engl J Med. 2017;377:553-61

A. Eye lid twitching
B. Itching
C. Sneezing
D. Yawning

Yawning, mood change, light sensitivity, neck pain, and fatigue are common premonitory symptoms typical of a migraine attack.

474. Which of the following is an infrequent phase in a migraine attack?

Harrison's 20th Ed. Chapter 422, Page 3096, N Engl J Med. 2017;377:553-61

A. Aura
B. Premonitory (prodrome)
C. Headache phase
D. Postdrome

A migraine attack has three phases—premonitory (prodrome), headache phase and postdrome. ~20–25% of migraine patients have a fourth, aura phase. Aura symptoms may include visual disturbances (wavy lines or bright or dark spots), or sensory changes (numbness or tingling), language dysfunction, and vertigo.

475. Which of the following is a paroxysmal disorder?

DeJong's The Neurologic Examination, 7th Ed. Page 791

A. Migraine
B. Periodic paralysis
C. Narcolepsy
D. All of the above

Some disorders occur episodically in patients who are otherwise well and have no abnormalities on neurologic examination between attacks (paroxysmal disorders). They include migraine, seizures, episodic ataxias, certain movement disorders, narcolepsy, and periodic paralysis.

476. Which of the following is not a category of migraine?

DeJong's The Neurologic Examination, 7th Ed. Page 792

A. Classic migraine
B. Contemporary migraine
C. Common migraine
D. Complicated migraine

Migraine is a very common cause of recurrent headaches. It is divided into two large categories: with aura (classic migraine) and without aura (common migraine). When the neurologic dysfunction (with or without headache) is unusually severe or prolonged, becoming the most prominent part of migraine episode, the condition is called complicated migraine.

477. What percentage of patients have migraine without aura?

DeJong's The Neurologic Examination, 7th Ed. Page 792

A. 25%
B. 55%
C. 75%
D. 85%

~ 85% of patients have migraine without aura.

478. Which of the following is not a feature of prodromal phase of a migraine attack?

Harrison's 20th Ed. Chapter 422, Page 3096

A. Cutaneous allodynia
B. Polyuria
C. Yawning
D. Cognitive dysfunction

Cutaneous allodynia refers to the experience of normal touch as uncomfortable.

479. Which of the following is not a feature of headache phase of a migraine attack?

Harrison's 20th Ed. Chapter 422, Page 3096

A. Photophobia
B. Phonophobia
C. Palinopsia
D. Allodynia

Features of the premonitory (prodromal) phase of migraine include yawning, tiredness, cognitive dysfunction, mood change, neck discomfort, polyuria, and food cravings. Headache phase follows with features like nausea, photophobia, phonophobia and allodynia. During postdrome phase, the patient feels tired/weary, has problems concentrating, and has mild neck discomfort.

480. Which of the following can be a cause of hyperosmia?

DeJong's The Neurologic Examination, 7th Ed. Page 142

A. Functional
B. Substance abuse
C. Migraine
D. All of the above

Hyperosmia is usually functional, but it can occur with certain types of substance abuse and in migraine.

481. To be called as suffering from chronic migraine, episodes of migraine on how many days per month must a patient have?

Harrison's 20th Ed. Chapter 422, Page 3096

A. Two or more days per month
B. Four or more days per month
C. Six or more days per month
D. Eight or more days per month

Patients with episodes of migraine on eight or more days per month and with at least 15 total days of headache per month are considered to have chronic migraine.

482. Status migrainosus refers to a migraine attack that lasts longer than?

DeJong's The Neurologic Examination, 7th Ed. Page 793

A. 12 hours
B. 24 hours
C. 48 hours
D. 72 hours

Status migrainosus refers to a migraine attack that lasts longer than 72 hours despite treatment.

483. Which of the following is not included in the simplified diagnostic criteria for migraine?

Harrison's 20th Ed. Chapter 422, Page 3100 Table 422-3

A. Photophobia
B. Phonophobia
C. Allodynia
D. Throbbing, unilateral headache

Although migraine headache is characteristically severe, unilateral, and throbbing, it may also be moderate, bilateral, and constant in quality. The features of migraine other than headache, particularly sensitivity to light and sound, nausea, and interference with the ability to function, may be more useful in diagnosis than the character of the headache.

484. Out of the following, which is the commonest symptom accompanying severe migraine?

Harrison's 20th Ed. Chapter 422, Page 3098 Table 422-2

A. Photophobia
B. Scalp tenderness
C. Vomiting
D. Vertigo

485. Out of the following, which of the following is the most frequent symptoms accompanying severe migraine?

Harrison's 20th Ed. Chapter 422, Page 3098 Table 422-2

A. Photophobia
B. Vomiting
C. Fortification spectra
D. Light headedness

486. In which patient of headache should we apply the simplified diagnostic criteria for migraine?

Harrison's 20th Ed. Chapter 422, Page 3100 Table 422-3

A. Repeated attacks of headache lasting 4–72 hours
B. Patients of headache with a normal physical examination
C. In whom there is no other reasonable cause for headache
D. All of the above

International Headache Society Classification.

487. Which of the following is a type of complicated migraine?

DeJong's The Neurologic Examination, 7th Ed. Page 792

A. Hemiplegic migraine
B. Ophthalmoplegic migraine
C. Basilar artery migraine
D. All of the above

488. Which of the following episodic syndromes may be associated with migraine?

Harrison's 20th Ed. Chapter 422, Page 3097 Table 422-1

A. Cyclical vomiting syndrome
B. Abdominal migraine
C. Benign paroxysmal vertigo
D. All of the above

Primary Headache Disorders, Modified from International Classification of Headache Disorders-III-Beta (Headache Classification Committee of the International Headache Society, 2018).

489. Which of the following is a feature of visual snow syndrome?

Harrison's 20th Ed. Chapter 422, Page 3096, Brain 2014;137(5): 1419–1428

A. Palinopsia
B. Nyctalopia
C. Entoptic phenomena
D. All of the above

Diagnosis of visual snow syndrome (continuous perception of tiny flickering dots in the entire field of vision) can be confirmed if the symptoms have lasted longer than three months & person has two of the following additional symptoms: sensitivity to light (photophobia), seeing image of an object after it has moved (palinopsia), impaired night vision (nyctalopia) or seeing small floating objects (entoptic phenomena). Most people with visual snow syndrome have normal vision tests and normal brain images. Differential diagnosis includes migraine visual aura.

490. In acephalgic migraine, which of the following is least prominent?

Harrison's 20th Ed. Chapter 422, Page 3096

A. Recurrent neurologic symptoms
B. Nausea or vomiting
C. Headache
D. Vertigo

Patients with acephalgic migraine ((typical aura without headache) have recurrent neurologic symptoms, with nausea or vomiting, but with little or no headache. Vertigo may be prominent.

491. Migraine activators (triggers) include all except?

Harrison's 20th Ed. Chapter 422, Page 3096

A. Red wine
B. Menstruation
C. Pregnancy
D. Lack of sleep

492. Migraine deactivators include all except?

Harrison's 20th Ed. Chapter 422, Page 3096

A. Sleep
B. Pregnancy
C. Exhiliration
D. Hunger

Triggers include glare, bright lights, sounds, or other afferent stimulation; hunger, excess stress, physical exertion, stormy weather or barometric pressure changes, hormonal fluctuations during menses, lack of or excess sleep & alcohol or other chemical stimulation such as with nitrates.

493. Which of the following medication can exacerbate migraine?

N Engl J Med. 2017;377:553-61

A. Nasal decongestants
B. Selective serotonin-reuptake inhibitor antidepressants
C. Proton-pump inhibitors
D. All of the above

Multiple medications can exacerbate migraine, including oral contraceptives, postmenopausal hormone therapy, nasal decongestants, selective serotonin-reuptake inhibitor antidepressants, and proton-pump inhibitors.

494. Sensory sensitivity in migraine is due to dysfunction of monoaminergic sensory control systems located in?

Harrison's 20th Ed. Chapter 422, Page 3096

A. Hypothalamus
B. Thalamus
C. Putamen
D. Globus pallidus

Sensory sensitivity, characteristic of migraine, is probably due to dysfunction of monoaminergic sensory control systems located in brainstem & hypothalamus.

495. Key pain input in migraine is from?

Harrison's 20th Ed. Chapter 422, Page 3098 Figure 422-1

A. Meningeal vessels
B. Pia mater
C. Arachnoid mater
D. All of the above

496. Neurons of trigeminocervical complex (TCC) synapse on neurons in thalamus through which tract?

Harrison's 20th Ed. Chapter 422, Page 3098 Figure 422-1

A. Thalamocapsular tract
B. Thalamogeniculate tract
C. Quintothalamic tract
D. All of the above

497. Modulation of trigeminovascular nociceptive input come from?

Harrison's 20th Ed. Chapter 422, Page 3098 Figure 422-1

A. Dorsal raphe nucleus
B. Locus coeruleus
C. Nucleus raphe magnus
D. All of the above

Key pathway for pain in migraine is trigeminovascular input from meningeal vessels. It then passes through trigeminal ganglion & synapses on second-order neurons in trigeminocervical complex (TCC). These neurons in turn project in quintothalamic tract and, after decussating in brainstem, synapse on neurons in thalamus. Important modulation of trigeminovascular nociceptive input comes from dorsal raphe nucleus, locus coeruleus and nucleus raphe magnus.

498. Which of the following is related to migraine?

Harrison's 20th Ed. Chapter 422, Page 3096

A. Gepants
B. Ditans
C. Triptans
D. All of the above

Activation of cells in the trigeminal nucleus results in the release of vasoactive neuropeptides particularly calcitonin gene-related peptide (CGRP) at vascular terminations of the trigeminal nerve and within the trigeminal nucleus. CGRP receptor antagonists called gepants are effective in the acute treatment of migraine as are monoclonal antibodies to CGRP. Exclusive agonists of 5-HT1F receptor are called ditans.

499. Migraine is associated with the release of?

N Engl J Med. 2017;377:553-61

A. Neurotensin
B. Substance P
C. Calcitonin gene-related peptide (CGRP)
D. Cholecystokinin

Migraine is associated with the release of neurotransmitters & neuromodulators, including neuropeptides calcitonin gene-related peptide (CGRP) & pituitary adenylate cyclase-activating peptide (PACAP).

500. MIDAS stands for?

Harrison's 20th Ed. Chapter 422, Page 3098

A. Migraine Disease Assessment Score
B. Migraine Disability Assessment Score
C. Migraine Drug Assessment Score
D. Migraine Diagnosis Assessment Score

MIDAS stands for Migraine Disability Assessment Score meant to assess the extent of a patient's disease and disability.

501. MIDAS questionnaire assesses migraine disability based on how many questions?

Harrison's 20th Ed. Chapter 422, Page 3100 Figure 422-4

A. 5
B. 8
C. 10
D. 12

502. Severe migraine disability is labeled when MIDAS score is?

Harrison's 20th Ed. Chapter 422, Page 3100 Figure 422-4

A. > 5
B. > 10
C. > 15
D. > 20

For questions 1–5, add the total number of days to arrive at the score. If MIDAS Score is 6 or more, consultation with doctor is needed.

503. MIDAS questionnaire asks about events that happened during last how many months?

Harrison's 20th Ed. Chapter 422, Page 3100 Figure 422-4

A. 1 month
B. 3 months
C. 6 months
D. 12 months

504. Drugs used for prophylactic treatment of migraine include all except?

Harrison's 20th Ed. Chapter 422, Page 3103

A. Amitriptyline
B. Sodium valproate
C. Metoclopramide
D. Cyproheptadine

Drugs that have been approved by the FDA for the prophylactic treatment of migraine include propranolol, timolol, sodium valproate, topiramate, methysergide, amitriptyline, nortriptyline, flunarizine, phenelzine, gabapentin and cyproheptadine.

505. Drugs effective in treatment of migraine are?
Harrison's 20th Ed. Chapter 422, Page 3101 Table 422-4

A. Nonsteroidal anti-inflammatory agents
B. 5-HT$_{1B/1D}$ receptor agonists
C. Dopamine receptor antagonists
D. All of the above

Drugs effective in the treatment of migraine are nonsteroidal anti-inflammatory agents, 5HT$_{1B/1D}$ receptor agonists and dopamine receptor antagonists.

506. Triptans are least potent agonist of which of the following?
Harrison's 20th Ed. Chapter 422, Page 3096

A. 5-HT$_{1A}$ receptor
B. 5-HT$_{1B}$ receptor
C. 5-HT$_{1D}$ receptor
D. 5-HT$_{1F}$ receptor

Triptans are potent agonists of 5-HT$_{1B}$, 5-HT$_{1D}$, and 5-HT$_{1F}$ receptors and are less potent at the 5-HT$_{1A}$ receptor.

507. Antimigraine efficacy of the triptans is due to their ability to stimulate?
Harrison's 20th Ed. Chapter 422, Page 3096

A. 5-HT$_{1A}$ receptors
B. 5-HT$_{1B}$ receptors
C. 5-HT$_{1C}$ receptors
D. 5-HT$_{1E}$ receptors

Antimigraine efficacy of triptans relates to their ability to stimulate 5-HT$_{1B/1D}$ receptors, which are located on both blood vessels and nerve terminals.

508. Which of the following about triptans is false?
Harrison's 20th Ed. Chapter 422, Page 3096

A. Potent agonists of 5-HT$_{1B}$ & 5-HT$_{1D}$ receptors
B. Arrest nerve signaling in nociceptive pathways of trigeminovascular system
C. Promote cranial vasoconstriction
D. None of the above

509. Which of the following about ditans is false?
Harrison's 20th Ed. Chapter 422, Page 3096

A. Exclusive agonists of 5-HT$_{1F}$ receptor
B. Act only at neural & not vascular targets
C. Effective in acute migraine
D. None of the above

510. Which of the following about migraineurs is false?
Harrison's 20th Ed. Chapter 422, Page 3096, 131

A. Dopamine receptor hypersensitivity
B. Sensitive to environmental & sensory stimuli
C. Experience more prolonged periods of disequilibrium
D. None of the above

511. Which of the following gene has been incriminated in the causation of Familial hemiplegic migraine (FHM)?
Harrison's 20th Ed. Chapter 422, Page 3096

A. tRNAL$^{eu(UUR)}$
B. CACNA1A
C. DRD2
D. All of the above

Mutations involving the Cav2.1 (P/Q) type voltage-gated calcium channel CACNA1A gene cause familial hemiplegic migraine 1 (FHM 1). Mutations in Na^{+}-K^{+}ATPase ATP1A2 gene causes FHM 2. Mutations in neuronal voltage-gated sodium channel SCN1A cause FHM 3.

512. In PET examination in migraine patients, activation of which of the following area is fundamental to expression of migraine?
Harrison's 20th Ed. Chapter 422, Page 3099 Figure 422-2

A. Hypothalamic
B. Dorsal midbrain
C. Dorsolateral pontine
D. Thalamus

When seen in Positron emission tomography (PET) imaging in migraine patients, activation of dorsolateral pontine area, which includes noradrenergic locus coeruleus, is fundamental to the expression of migraine.

513. Which of the following is a 5-HT$_{1F}$ receptor agonist?
Harrison's 20th Ed. Chapter 422, Page 3100

A. Rimegepant
B. Ubrogepant
C. Lasmiditan
D. All of the above

Two new classes of therapeutic agents for migraine treatment, CGRP receptor antagonists (rimegepant & ubrogepant), and 5-HT$_{1F}$ receptor agonist (lasmiditan), should soon be available.

514. Which of the following is most efficacious amongst triptans?
Harrison's 20th Ed. Chapter 422, Page 3100

A. Frovatriptan
B. Naratriptan
C. Almotriptan
D. Rizatriptan

Rizatriptan & eletriptan are the most efficacious of the triptans.

515. Which of the following about 5HT$_{1B/1D}$ receptor agonists is false?
Harrison's 20th Ed. Chapter 422, Page 3101

A. Not effective in migraine with aura
B. Contraindicated in patients with a h/o cardiovascular & cerebrovascular disease
C. Recurrence of headache common
D. None of the above

516. Which of the following triptan is documented porphyrinogenic and unsafe in porphyria?
Harrison's 20th Ed. Chapter 422, Page 2991 Table 409-4

A. Rizatriptan
B. Sumatriptan
C. Zolmitriptan
D. All of the above

Triptans available for treatment of migraine include sumatriptan, almotriptan, eletriptan, frovatriptan, naratriptan, rizatriptan, and zolmitriptan.

517. Which of the following drugs for treatment of acute migraine can be administered by nasal route?
Harrison's 20th Ed. Chapter 422, Page 3101 Table 422-4

A. Dihydroergotamine
B. Sumatriptan
C. Zolmitriptan
D. All of the above

518. Route of administration of sumatriptan is?
Harrison's 20th Ed. Chapter 422, Page 3101 Table 422-4

A. Oral
B. Nasal
C. Subcuteneous
D. All of the above

519. In migraine, use of which of the following may decrease the likelihood of a response to triptans in future?
Harrison's 20th Ed. Chapter 422, Page 3102

A. Isometheptene
B. Meperidine
C. Prochlorperazine
D. Dihydroergotamine

There is evidence that use of opioids may decrease the likelihood of a response to triptans in future.

520. Methysergide may cause retroperitoneal or cardiac valvular fibrosis when used for more than?
Harrison's 20th Ed. Chapter 422, Page 3103

A. 3 months
B. 6 months
C. 9 months
D. 12 months

Methysergide may cause retroperitoneal or cardiac valvular fibrosis when it is used for > 6 months. Risk of fibrosis is about 1:1500 and is likely to reverse after drug is stopped.

521. For instituting prophylactic treatment of migraine, what should be the frequency of attacks?
Harrison's 20th Ed. Chapter 422, Page 3103

A. At least three attacks per day
B. At least three attacks per week
C. At least three attacks per month
D. At least three attacks per year

522. Drugs used for prophylactic treatment of migraine include all except?
Harrison's 20th Ed. Chapter 422, Page 3103

A. Timolol
B. Sodium valproate
C. Methysergide
D. Sumatriptan

Antihypertensive agents (betaadrenergic blockers & candesartan), anticonvulsant agents (topiramate & divalproex sodium), and tricyclic antidepressants (amitriptyline & nortriptyline) are standard preventive therapies for migraine.

523. Which of the following is useful for prevention of chronic migraine?
N Engl J Med. 2017;377:553-61

A. Coenzyme Q10
B. Melatonin
C. Petasites
D. OnabotulinumtoxinA

OnabotulinumtoxinA is a Food and Drug Administration (FDA) approved therapy for prevention of chronic migraine, defined as headache occurring on more than 15 days per month, with migraine features on at least 8 of those days.

524. Which of the following drug is useful in patients of migraine who are obese?
N Engl J Med. 2017;377:553-61

A. Divalproex sodium
B. Topiramate
C. Candesartan
D. Nortriptyline

525. Electrical stimulation of which part of brain results in migraine-like headache?
Harrison's 20th Ed. Chapter 422, Page 3103

A. Temporal lobe
B. Midbrain in the region of dorsal raphe
C. Putamen
D. Globus pallidum

526. Which of the following is a monoclonal antibody to CGRP receptor?
Harrison's 20th Ed. Chapter 422, Page 3103

A. Erenumab
B. Eptinezumab
C. Fremanezumab
D. Galcanezumab

Monoclonal antibodies to the CGRP receptor (erenumab) or to the peptide (eptinezumab, fremanezumab & galcanezumab) are effective and well tolerated in migraine. They can be used as preventive agents.

527. Chronic head-pain syndrome best relates to?
Harrison's 20th Ed. Chapter 422, Page 3103

A. Migraine
B. Tension-type headache (TTH)
C. Cluster headache
D. All of the above

Term tension-type headache (TTH) is commonly used to describe a chronic head-pain syndrome characterized by bilateral tight, band like discomfort.

528. Which of the following is an accompanying feature of tension-type headache?
Harrison's 20th Ed. Chapter 422, Page 3103

A. Nausea, vomiting
B. Photophobia, phonophobia
C. Aggravation with movement
D. None of the above

TTH patients have headaches without accompanying features like nausea, vomiting, photophobia, phonophobia, osmophobia, throbbing & aggravation with movement.

529. For chronic TTH, which is the only proven treatment?
Harrison's 20th Ed. Chapter 422, Page 3104

A. Amitriptyline
B. Selective serotonin reuptake inhibitors
C. Benzodiazepines
D. Acupuncture

For chronic TTH, amitriptyline is the only proven treatment.

530. Trigeminal autonomic cephalalgias include all except?
Harrison's 20th Ed. Chapter 422, Page 3104

A. Cluster headache
B. Migraine
C. Paroxysmal hemicrania
D. SUNCT

Trigeminal autonomic cephalalgias (TACs) includes cluster headache, paroxysmal hemicrania & SUNCT (short-lasting unilateral neuralgiform headache attacks with conjunctival injection & tearing). TAC features are short-lasting attacks of head pain with cranial autonomic symptoms (lacrimation, conjunctival injection, or nasal congestion).

531. Short-lasting headaches without prominent cranial autonomic syndromes include?
Harrison's 20th Ed. Chapter 422, Page 3104

A. Trigeminal neuralgia
B. Primary stabbing headache
C. Hypnic headache
D. All of the above

Short-lasting headaches without prominent cranial autonomic syndromes are trigeminal neuralgia, primary stabbing headache & hypnic headache.

532. Which of the following is false about cluster headache?
Harrison's 20th Ed. Chapter 422, Page 3104

A. Men are affected more than women
B. Ipsilateral autonomic features
C. Propranolol and amitriptyline are ineffective
D. Lithium is not beneficial

533. Which of the following is false about cluster headache?
Harrison's 20th Ed. Chapter 422, Page 3104

A. Pain is strictly unilateral
B. Pain affects the same side in subsequent episodes
C. Certain foods or emotional factors precipitate pain
D. On-off vulnerability to alcohol

534. Which of the following is false about cluster headache?
Lancet 2005; 366: 843–55

A. Circadian rhythmicity of painful attacks
B. Autonomic symptoms
C. Severe unilateral pain
D. Hypothalamic dysfunction has no role in acute attacks

535. Which of the following is most useful during acute attack of cluster headache?
Lancet 2005; 366: 843–55

A. 100% oxygen inhalation
B. Valsalva manuevre
C. Hyperventilation
D. All of the above

536. Which of the following is a feature of cluster headache?
Harrison's 20th Ed. Chapter 422, Page 3104

A. Periodicity
B. Unilateral pain
C. A pain-free interval
D. All of the above

537. Drugs used for preventive treatment of cluster headache include all except?
Harrison's 20th Ed. Chapter 422, Page 3105

A. Prednisone
B. Lithium
C. Cyproheptadine
D. Methysergide

Oral glucocorticoids, methysergide, lithium are useful for chronic form of cluster headache.

538. Which of the following is a feature of paroxysmal hemicrania?
Harrison's 20th Ed. Chapter 422, Page 3105

A. Very frequent short-lasting attacks
B. Equal male: female ratio
C. Excellent response to indomethacin
D. All of the above

539. Which of the following is a feature of SUNCT?
Harrison's 20th Ed. Chapter 422, Page 3106

A. Ipsilateral conjunctival injection and lacrimation
B. Lack of refractory period to triggering
C. Lack of response to indomethacin
D. All of the above

540. Secondary SUNCT is seen in?
Harrison's 20th Ed. Chapter 422, Page 3106

A. Anterior communicating artery aneurysm
B. Post head injury
C. Posterior fossa or pituitary lesions
D. Hypertension

SUNCT (short-lasting unilateral neuralgiform headache attacks with conjunctival injection and tearing) can be seen with posterior fossa or pituitary lesions.

541. Most effective treatment for prevention of SUNCT is?
Harrison's 20th Ed. Chapter 422, Page 3106

A. Prednisone
B. Lamotrigine
C. Cyproheptadine
D. Lithium

Most effective treatment for prevention of SUNCT is lamotrigine. Topiramate, gabapentin and carbamazepine offer modest benefit.

542. "Fortification spectrum" is characteristic of?
Harrison's 20th Ed. Chapter 422, Page 187

A. Cluster headache
B. Migraine
C. Pseudotumour cerebri
D. Giant cell arteritis

In classic Migraine a visual aura lasting about 20 minutes occurs in both eyes (open or closed) with a small central disturbance in the field of vision marching toward the periphery leaving a transient scotoma. The expanding border of migraine scotoma has a scintillating, dancing or zigzag edge resembling the bastions of a fortified city, hence the term fortification spectra. It can be confused with amaurosis fugax (briefer and occurs in only one eye).

543. Which of the following best relates to migraine?
DeJong's The Neurologic Examination, 7th Ed. Page 164

A. Quadrantopsia
B. Teichopsias
C. Achromatopsia
D. Metamorphopsia

Scintillating scotomas of migraine are called teichopsias.

544. Which of the following is false about Bickerstaff migraine?

Lancet 1961a;1:15-7

A. Episodes begin with total blindness

B. Symptoms (vertigo, ataxia) persist for 20–30 minutes

C. Occurs only in males

D. Full recovery after the episode is the rule

Basilar-type migraine, basilar migraine, basilar artery migraine, and Bickerstaff migraine is now referred to as migraine with brainstem aura. According to the ICHD-3 beta, there must be at least 2 of the following non-ischemic "brainstem" symptoms present: dysarthria, vertigo, tinnitus, impaired hearing, double vision, ataxia, and decreased level consciousness.

545. Lower-half headache or facial migraine is called?

American Journal of Neuroradiology. 2000;21(4):766-769

A. Basilar migraine

B. Carotidynia

C. Raeder's syndrome

D. Ophthalmoplegic migraine

546. Common precipitant of carotidynia attacks is?

American Journal of Neuroradiology. 2000;21(4):766-769

A. Cervical spondylosis

B. Dental trauma

C. Hypertension

D. All of the above

Carotidynia or Fay syndrome was described by Fay in 1927 as an atypical neuralgia in neck & face. It was classified by the International Headache Society in 1988 as an idiopathic neck pain syndrome associated with tenderness over the carotid bifurcation without structural abnormality. Carotydinia was removed as a pathological entity from the second International Headache Society classification in 2004.

Coma

547. Which of the following is a feature of coma?
Harrison's 20th Ed. Chapter 300, Page 2068

A. Deep sleep like state
B. Eyes closed
C. Patient cannot be aroused
D. All of the above

Coma is defined as a deep sleep like state, with eyes closed and the patient cannot be aroused. Stupor refers to a state where in patient can be transiently awakened by vigorous stimuli, accompanied by motor behavior of avoidance or withdrawal from uncomfortable or aggravating stimuli. Drowsiness simulates light sleep & is characterized by easy arousal and persistence of alertness for brief periods. Stupor and drowsiness are usually accompanied by some degree of confusion.

548. At bedside, which of the following term is not ambiguous and is preferred?
Harrison's 20th Ed. Chapter 300, Page 2068

A. Lethargy
B. Drowsiness
C. Semicoma
D. Obtundation

At bedside, stupor, drowsiness and coma are precise narrative descriptions of the level of arousal and of the type of responses evoked by various stimuli and are preferable to ambiguous terms such as lethargy, semicoma, or obtundation.

549. Which of the following is false about vegetative state?
Harrison's 20th Ed. Chapter 300, Page 2068

A. Awake-appearing but nonresponsive state
B. Respiratory and autonomic functions are retained
C. Yawning, swallowing, limb & head movements persist
D. None of the above

A vegetative state signifies an awake-appearing but nonresponsive state often in a patient who has come out of coma. The eyelids may open periodically, giving the appearance of wakefulness. Respiratory & autonomic functions are retained. Yawning, coughing, swallowing, and limb & head movements persist, often meaningless.

550. Which of the following is false about minimally conscious state?
Harrison's 20th Ed. Chapter 300, Page 2068

A. Patient displays rudimentary vocal or motor behaviors
B. Patient displays response to touch, visual stimuli, or command
C. Cerebral hypoperfusion & head trauma are common causes
D. None of the above

551. Persistent vegetative state is the term used when prognosis for regaining mental faculties is almost nil after being in a vegetative state for?
Harrison's 20th Ed. Chapter 300, Page 2068

A. Three months
B. Six months
C. Nine months
D. One year

Patients in the minimally conscious state carry a better prognosis for some recovery compared to those in a persistent vegetative state.

552. Which of the following is false about akinetic mutism?
Harrison's 20th Ed. Chapter 300, Page 2069

A. Partially or fully awake state
B. Patient is able to form impressions and think
C. Patient remains virtually immobile and mute
D. None of the above

Akinetic mutism refers to a partially or fully awake state wherein the patient is able to form impressions & think, as demonstrated by later recounting of events, but remains virtually immobile & mute.

553. Akinetic mutism results from damage in?
Harrison's 20th Ed. Chapter 300, Page 2069

A. Ventral pons
B. Medial thalamic nuclei
C. Temporal lobe
D. Any of the above

Akinetic mutism results from damage in regions of medial thalamic nuclei or frontal lobes (particularly orbitofrontal surfaces) or from extreme hydrocephalus.

554. Abulia describes a milder form of?
Harrison's 20th Ed. Chapter 300, Page 2069

A. Parkinsonism
B. Akinetic mutism
C. Catatonia
D. Locked-in state

Abulia is a milder form of akinetic mutism characterized by mental & physical slowness with diminished ability to initiate activity. It is usually the result of damage to frontal lobes and its connections.

555. Which of the following occurs as part of a major psychosis?
Harrison's 20th Ed. Chapter 300, Page 2069

A. Akinetic mutism
B. Abulia
C. Catatonia
D. Locked-in state

Catatonia occurs as part of a major psychosis (schizophrenia or major depression).

556. Catatonia is differentiated from akinetic mutism by?
Harrison's 20th Ed. Chapter 300, Page 2069

A. Level of awakening
B. Babinski signs
C. Blinking
D. Mobility

Catatonia is differentiated from akinetic mutism by clinical evidence of cerebral damage such as Babinski signs and hypertonicity of the limbs present in akinetic mutism.

557. "Waxy flexibility" is a feature of which of the following?
Harrison's 20th Ed. Chapter 300, Page 2069

A. Abulia
B. Akinetic mutism
C. Catatonia
D. Locked-in state

In catatonia, the patient retains the posture in which they have been placed by the examiner ("waxy flexibility," or catalepsy).

558. "Locked-in state" results from damage in?
Harrison's 20th Ed. Chapter 300, Page 2069

A. Ventral pons
B. Medial thalamic nuclei
C. Temporal lobe
D. Any of the above

"Locked-in state" results from an infarction or hemorrhage of ventral pons that transects all descending motor (corticospinal and corticobulbar) pathways.

559. "Locked-in state" like condition may be seen in?
Harrison's 20th Ed. Chapter 300, Page 2069

A. Guillain-Barré syndrome
B. Critical illness neuropathy
C. Pharmacologic neuromuscular blockade
D. Any of the above

These are awake but de-efferented states.

560. The principal cause of coma is?
Harrison's 20th Ed. Chapter 300, Page 2069

A. Lesions that damage substantial portion of RAS
B. Destruction of large portions of both cerebral hemispheres
C. Suppression of thalamocerebral function by drugs, toxins, hypoglycemia, anoxia, azotemia, or hepatic failure
D. All of the above

Principal causes of coma are lesions that damage the reticular activating system (RAS) or its projections, destruction of large portions of both cerebral hemispheres and suppression of reticulo-cerebral function by drugs, toxins, or metabolic derangements such as hypoglycemia, anoxia, azotemia, or hepatic failure.

561. Metabolic derangement that can lead to suppression of reticulocerebral function is?
Harrison's 20th Ed. Chapter 300, Page 2069

A. Hypoglycemia
B. Uremia
C. Hepatic failure
D. All of the above

Metabolic derangements that can lead to suppression of reticulocerebral function are hypoglycemia, anoxia, uremia, and hepatic failure.

562. Which of the following is false about brain herniation?
Harrison's 20th Ed. Chapter 300, Page 2069

A. Displacement of brain tissue into a contiguous compartment
B. Displacement of brain tissue by an overlying or adjacent mass
C. "False localizing" signs
D. None of the above

563. Brain herniation can be?
Harrison's 20th Ed. Chapter 300, Page 2069 Figure 300-1

A. Transfalcial
B. Uncal
C. Foraminal
D. All of the above

Brain herniations can be of the following types : uncal, central, transfalcial and foraminal.

564. Which is the most common form of brain herniation?
Harrison's 20th Ed. Chapter 300, Page 2069

A. Transfalcial
B. Foraminal herniation
C. Transtentorial herniation
D. Any of the above

The most common form of herniation is transtentorial herniation, in which brain tissue is displaced from supratentorial to infratentorial compartment through tentorial opening.

565. Uncus refers to which of the following?
Harrison's 20th Ed. Chapter 300, Page 2069

A. Lingual gyrus
B. Cingulate gyrus
C. Anterior medial temporal gyrus
D. Parahippocampal gyrus

Uncus refers to anterior medial temporal gyrus.

566. Kernohan-Woltman sign best relates to?
Harrison's 20th Ed. Chapter 300, Page 2069

A. Hypoglycemia
B. Central fever
C. Transtentorial herniation
D. Epileptic coma

Transtentorial herniation refers to part of brain being displaced from supratentorial to infratentorial compartment through the tentorial opening. Consequent lateral displacement of midbrain may compress the opposite cerebral peduncle against the tentorial edge, thus eliciting Kernohan-Woltman sign.

567. Kernohan-Woltman sign refers to?
Harrison's 20th Ed. Chapter 300, Page 2069

A. Contralateral pupillary dilatation in brain mass lesion
B. Waxing and waning levels of consciousness
C. Hemiparesis contralateral to original hemiparesis
D. Bilateral nystagmus

Kernohan-Woltman sign refers to a Babinski response and hemiparesis contralateral to the original hemiparesis due to compression of the opposite cerebral peduncle.

568. Brain herniation can cause which of the following?
Harrison's 20th Ed. Chapter 300, Page 2069

A. Cranial nerve palsy
B. Compression of anterior and posterior cerebral arteries
C. Hydrocephalus
D. All of the above

569. Coma results due to damage in reticular activating system (RAS) at the level of?
Harrison's 20th Ed. Chapter 300, Page 2069

A. Medulla oblongata
B. Pons
C. Lower midbrain
D. Upper midbrain

Coma results due to damage in reticular activating system (RAS) at the level of upper midbrain or its projections.

570. Which of the following finding suggests that the lesion is in the upper brainstem?
Harrison's 20th Ed. Chapter 300, Page 2069

A. Pupillary enlargement
B. Loss of light reaction
C. Loss of vertical and adduction movements of eyes
D. All of the above

Pupillary enlargement with loss of light reaction and loss of vertical and adduction movements of the eyes suggests that the lesion is in the upper brainstem. On the other hand, if pupillary light reaction and eye movements are intact, the lesion is more widespread or the cause of coma is metabolic suppression of the cerebral hemispheres.

571. The term 'coma dépassé' means?
N Engl J Med. 2001;344:1215

A. Hysteria
B. Irreversible coma
C. Coma during pregnancy
D. Coma in children

In 1959, Mollaret & Goulon introduced the term coma dépassé (irreversible coma) in 23 comatose patients who lost consciousness, brainstem reflexes & respiration & whose EEGs were flat.

572. As brain death occurs, which is the last part of brain to cease to function?
N Engl J Med. 2001;344:1216

A. Cerebral cortex
B. Midbrain
C. Pons
D. Medulla oblongata

As brain death occurs, patients lose their reflexes in a rostral-to-caudal direction, and medulla oblongata is the last part of brain to cease to function.

573. Misdiagnosis of brain death is possible in?
N Engl J Med. 2001;344:1215

A. Locked-in syndrome
B. Hypothermia
C. Drug intoxication
D. All of the above

Misdiagnosis of brain death is possible in locked-in syndrome, hypothermia or drug intoxication.

574. In the tests to confirm brain death, "hollow-skull sign" is a finding in which of the following?
N Engl J Med. 2001;344:1215

A. EEG
B. Dynamic radionuclide brain scan
C. Cerebral angiography
D. Transcranial Doppler measurements

When brain death has occurred, a dynamic radionuclide brain scan shows no intracranial filling - the so called hollow-skull sign.

575. Which part of brain is damaged in "locked-in syndrome"?
N Engl J Med. 2001;344:1215

A. Medulla oblongata
B. Pons
C. Midbrain
D. Thalamus

The locked-in syndrome (pseudocoma) is a consequence of destruction of base of pons mostly caused by acute embolus to basilar artery. Patient cannot move limbs, grimace, or swallow (damaged corticospinal & corticobulbar tracts), but upper rostral mesencephalic structures involved in voluntary blinking and vertical eye movements remain intact. Consciousness persists because tegmentum, with the reticular formation, is not affected.

576. Cingulate gyrus is likely to be involved in which of the following brain herniations?
Harrison's 20th Ed. Chapter 300, Page 2070

A. Temporal transtentorial herniation
B. Central transtentorial herniation
C. Transfalcial herniation
D. Foraminal herniation

In transfalcial herniation, the cingulate gyrus is displaced under the falx and across the midline.

577. Cerebellar tonsils are likely to be involved in which of the following brain herniations?
Harrison's 20th Ed. Chapter 300, Page 2070

A. Temporal transtentorial herniation
B. Central transtentorial herniation
C. Transfalcial herniation
D. Foraminal herniation

In foraminal herniation, cerebellar tonsils move downward into foramen magnum, causing compression of medulla that may result in respiratory arrest and death.

578. Drowsiness occurs when horizontal displacement of the pineal calcification occurs by?
Harrison's 20th Ed. Chapter 300, Page 2070

A. 1 to 3 mm
B. 3 to 5 mm
C. 6 to 8 mm
D. > 9 mm

579. Stupor occurs when horizontal displacement of the pineal calcification occurs by?
Harrison's 20th Ed. Chapter 300, Page 2070

A. 1 to 3 mm
B. 3 to 5 mm
C. 6 to 8 mm
D. > 9 mm

580. Coma occurs when horizontal displacement of the pineal calcification occurs by?
Harrison's 20th Ed. Chapter 300, Page 2070

A. 1 to 3 mm
B. 3 to 5 mm
C. 6 to 8 mm
D. > 9 mm

On CT/MRI, horizontal displacement of pineal calcification of 3 to 5 mm is associated with drowsiness, 6 to 8 mm with stupor, and >9 mm with coma, in acutely appearing masses.

581. Cerebral blood flow is principally influenced by all except?
Harrison's 20th Ed. Chapter 300, Page 2070

A. Systemic blood pressure
B. pH
C. PCO_2
D. PO_2

CBF is strongly influenced by systemic blood pressure, pH and PCO_2. CBF increases with hypercapnia and acidosis and decreases with hypocapnia and alkalosis.

582. In adults, volume of CSF within ventricles and surrounding the brain and spinal cord is about?

Harrison's 20th Ed. Chapter 300, Page 2075

A. 50 mL
B. 100 mL
C. 150 mL
D. 200 mL

583. Brain volume is normally about?

DeJong's The Neurologic Examination, 7th Ed. Page 740

A. 1000 mL
B. 1200 mL
C. 1400 mL
D. 1600 mL

Brain volume is normally approximately 1400 mL.

584. Monro-Kellie hypothesis best relates to?

DeJong's The Neurologic Examination, 7th Ed. Page 741

A. Intracranial pressure
B. Intracranial volume
C. Intraocular pressure
D. Intraocular volume

Monro-Kellie hypothesis refers to the fact that because cranium cannot expand, and brain cannot be significantly compressed, when volume of one of the compartments increases (blood, brain & CSF), volume in the other compartments must undergo a compensatory decrease.

585. Cerebral blood volume is about?

Harrison's 20th Ed. Chapter 300, Page 2075

A. 50 mL
B. 100 mL
C. 150 mL
D. 200 mL

About 150 mL of CSF is present within the ventricles and surrounding the brain and spinal cord. Cerebral blood volume is also ~150 mL.

586. Cerebral blood flow (CBF) in gray matter is about?

Harrison's 20th Ed. Chapter 300, Page 2070

A. 25 mL per 100 gram/minute
B. 50 mL per 100 gram/minute
C. 75 mL per 100 gram/minute
D. 100 mL per 100 gram/minute

587. Cerebral blood flow (CBF) in white matter is about?

Harrison's 20th Ed. Chapter 300, Page 2070

A. 10 mL per 100 gram/minute
B. 20 mL per 100 gram/minute
C. 30 mL per 100 gram/minute
D. 40 mL per 100 gram/minute

588. Mean cerebral blood flow (CBF) is about?

Harrison's 20th Ed. Chapter 300, Page 2070

A. 25 mL per 100 gram/minute
B. 35 mL per 100 gram/minute
C. 45 mL per 100 gram/minute
D. 55 mL per 100 gram/minute

589. Oxygen consumption of brain tissue is?

Harrison's 20th Ed. Chapter 300, Page 2070

A. 1.5 mL per 100 gram/minute
B. 2.5 mL per 100 gram/minute
C. 3.5 mL per 100 gram/minute
D. 4.5 mL per 100 gram/minute

590. Glucose utilization of brain tissue is?

Harrison's 20th Ed. Chapter 300, Page 2070

A. 1 mg per 100 gram/minute
B. 3 mg per 100 gram/minute
C. 5 mg per 100 gram/minute
D. 7 mg per 100 gram/minute

591. After the cessation of blood flow, brain stores of glucose provide energy for approximately?

Harrison's 20th Ed. Chapter 300, Page 2070

A. 1 minute
B. 2 minutes
C. 3 minutes
D. 4 minutes

592. After the cessation of cerebral blood flow, oxygen stores last for approximately?

Harrison's 20th Ed. Chapter 300, Page 2070

A. 3 to 5 seconds
B. 8 to 10 seconds
C. 12 to 15 seconds
D. 20 to 30 seconds

Cerebral neurons are fully dependent on cerebral blood flow (CBF) and the related delivery of oxygen and glucose. CBF approximates 75 mL per 100 gram/minute in gray matter and 30 mL per 100 gram/minute in white matter (mean of 55 mL per 100 gram/minute). Oxygen consumption is 3.5 mL per 100 gram/minute, and glucose utilization is 5 mg per 100 gram/minute. Brain stores of glucose provide energy for ~2 minutes after blood flow is interrupted, and oxygen stores last 8 to 10 seconds after cessation of blood flow.

593. Normal CSF pressure is?

Harrison's 20th Ed. Chapter 300, Page 2075

A. 20–70 mm H_2O
B. 80–120 mm H_2O
C. 50–180 mm H_2O
D. 120–280 mm H_2O

594. Normal CSF osmolarity is?

Harrison's 20th Ed. Chapter 300, Page 2075

A. 280–285 mOsm/L
B. 285–292 mOsm/L
C. 292–297 mOsm/L
D. 298–302 mOsm/L

595. Normal CSF pH is?

Harrison's 20th Ed. Chapter 300, Page 2075

A. 7.31–7.34
B. 7.34–7.37
C. 7.37–7.40
D. 7.40–7.44

596. Which receptor for PGE2 in brain is essential for fever?
Harrison's 20th Ed. 103

A. EP-1
B. EP-2
C. EP-3
D. EP-4

Elevation of PGE2 in brain starts the process of raising hypothalamic set point for core temperature. Out of the 4 receptors for PGE2, EP-3 is essential for fever.

597. In metabolic disorders, most neuronal damage is caused by which of the following?
Harrison's 20th Ed. Chapter 300, Page 2070

A. Hypoglycemia
B. Hyponatremia
C. Hypoxia-ischemia
D. All of the above

Hypoxia-ischemia causes most neuronal destruction. Other metabolic disorders like hypoglycemia, hyponatremia, hyperosmolarity, hypercapnia, hypercalcemia, and hepatic and renal failure cause only minor neuropathologic changes.

598. Which of the following changes occur in hepatic encephalopathy (HE)?
Harrison's 20th Ed. Chapter 300, Page 2070

A. Increased synthesis of glutamine in astrocytes
B. Increases in inhibitory neurotransmitter GABA
C. Synthesis of putative "false" neurotransmitters
D. All of the above

In hepatic encephalopathy (HE), high ammonia concentrations lead to increased synthesis of glutamine in astrocytes with osmotic swelling, mitochondrial energy failure, production of reactive nitrogen & oxygen species, increases in inhibitory neurotransmitter GABA, and synthesis of putative "false" neurotransmitters.

599. Which of the following is typical of chronic hepatic encephalopathy (HE)?
Harrison's 20th Ed. Chapter 300, Page 2070

A. Development of diffuse astrocytosis
B. Depletion of catecholamines
C. Increases in brain calcium
D. All of the above

Over a period of time, development of a diffuse astrocytosis is typical of chronic HE.

600. Which of the following does not contribute to the development of uremic encephalopathy?
Harrison's 20th Ed. Chapter 300, Page 2070

A. Urea
B. Creatinine
C. Guanidine
D. Calcium

601. Which of the following occur in uremic encephalopathy?
Harrison's 20th Ed. Chapter 300, Page 2070

A. Accumulation of creatinine and guanidine
B. Depletion of catecholamines
C. Increases in brain calcium
D. All of the above

Contributors to uremic encephalopathy include accumulation of neurotoxic substances (creatinine, guanidine), depletion of catecholamines, altered glutamate & GABA tone, increases in brain calcium, inflammation with disruption of blood brain barrier.

602. Sodium below what level is associated with coma and convulsions?
Harrison's 20th Ed. Chapter 300, Page 2070

A. 125 mmol/L
B. 121 mmol/L
C. 119 mmol/L
D. 115 mmol/L

Sodium levels <125 mmol/L induce confusion & <119 mmol/L are associated with coma & convulsions.

603. In hyperosmolar coma, the serum osmolarity is generally more than?
Harrison's 20th Ed. Chapter 300, Page 2070

A. >280 mOsmol/L
B. >300 mOsmol/L
C. >320 mOsmol/L
D. >350 mOsmol/L

In hyperosmolar coma, the serum osmolarity is generally >350 moSmol/L.

604. Disorder that occlude small blood vessels throughout the brain causing bihemispheral damage is?
Harrison's 20th Ed. Chapter 300, Page 2070

A. Cerebral malaria
B. Thrombotic thrombocytopenic purpura
C. Hyperviscosity
D. All of the above

Disorders that occlude small blood vessels throughout the brain causing bihemispheral damage are cerebral malaria, thrombotic thrombocytopenic purpura, and hyperviscosity.

605. In coma, which of the following is not included initially in determining severity and nature of coma?
Harrison's 20th Ed. Chapter 300, Page 2070

A. Vital signs
B. Funduscopy
C. Nuchal rigidity
D. Respiratory patterns

606. Which of the following is the least likely cause of fever in coma?
Harrison's 20th Ed. Chapter 300, Page 2071

A. Heat stroke
B. Neuroleptic malignant syndrome
C. Central fever
D. Anticholinergic drug intoxication

607. Hypothermia in coma is observed in?
Harrison's 20th Ed. Chapter 300, Page 2071

A. Phenothiazine intoxication
B. Hypoglycemia
C. Extreme hypothyroidism
D. All of the above

Hypothermia in coma is observed with alcohol, barbiturate, sedative, or phenothiazine intoxication; hypoglycemia; peripheral circulatory failure; or extreme hypothyroidism.

608. Hypothermia itself causes coma only when the temperature is?

Harrison's 20th Ed. Chapter 300, Page 2071

A. <34°C
B. <33°C
C. <32°C
D. <31°C

Hypothermia itself causes coma only when the temperature is <31°C (87.8°F), regardless of the underlying etiology.

609. Marked hypertension in coma suggests?

Harrison's 20th Ed. Chapter 300, Page 2071

A. Cerebral hemorrhage
B. Large cerebral infarction
C. Head injury
D. All of the above

Marked hypertension suggests hypertensive encephalopathy, cerebral hemorrhage, large cerebral infarction, or head injury.

610. Cushing response best relates to?

Harrison's 20th Ed. Chapter 300, Page 2071

A. Hypertension
B. Cyanosis
C. Convulsion
D. Hypothermia

Cushing response refers to marked hypertension in a case of coma that may be secondary to a rapid rise in intracranial pressure (ICP), most often after cerebral hemorrhage or head injury.

611. Hypotension is characteristic of coma due to?

Harrison's 20th Ed. Chapter 300, Page 2071

A. Profound hypothyroidism
B. Sepsis
C. Alcohol intoxication
D. All of the above

Hypotension is characteristic of coma from alcohol or barbiturate intoxication, internal hemorrhage, myocardial infarction, sepsis, profound hypothyroidism, or Addisonian crisis.

612. On funduscopic examination, subhyaloid hemorrhage suggests?

Harrison's 20th Ed. Chapter 300, Page 2071

A. Meningococcemia
B. Subarachnoid hemorrhage
C. Bleeding diathesis
D. All of the above

Subhyaloid hemorrhages on funduscopic examination indicate subarachnoid hemorrhage.

613. Cutaneous petechiae in coma suggest?

Harrison's 20th Ed. Chapter 300, Page 2071

A. Thrombotic thrombocytopenic purpura
B. Meningococcemia
C. Bleeding diathesis associated with an ICH
D. All of the above

Cutaneous petechiae suggest thrombotic thrombocytopenic purpura, meningococcemia, or a bleeding diathesis associated with an intracerebral hemorrhage.

614. Multifocal myoclonus indicates which of the following?

Harrison's 20th Ed. Chapter 300, Page 2071

A. Uremia
B. Haloperidol intoxication
C. Prion disease
D. Any of the above

Multifocal myoclonus almost always indicates a metabolic disorder (uremia, anoxia), drug intoxication (lithium or haloperidol), or a prion disease.

615. In a drowsy and confused patient, bilateral asterixis is a certain sign of?

Harrison's 20th Ed. Chapter 300, Page 2071

A. Drug intoxication
B. Cerebral malaria
C. Septicemia
D. Head injury

In a drowsy and confused patient, bilateral asterixis is a certain sign of metabolic encephalopathy or drug intoxication.

616. Bilateral damage rostral to the midbrain produces which of the following?

Harrison's 20th Ed. Chapter 300, Page 2071

A. Extension of elbows and wrists with pronation of arm
B. Flexion of elbows and wrists with supination of arm
C. Arm extension with leg flexion
D. Arm extension with flaccid legs

617. Bilateral damage to motor tracts in midbrain or caudal diencephalon produces which of the following?

Harrison's 20th Ed. Chapter 300, Page 2071

A. Extension of elbows and wrists with pronation of arm
B. Flexion of elbows and wrists with supination of arm
C. Arm extension with leg flexion
D. Arm extension with flaccid legs

Flexion of elbows and wrists and supination of arm (decortication) suggests bilateral damage rostral to the midbrain, whereas extension of elbows and wrists with pronation (decerebration) indicates damage to motor tracts in midbrain or caudal diencephalon.

618. Combination of arm extension with leg flexion or flaccid legs is associated with lesions in?

Harrison's 20th Ed. Chapter 300, Page 2071

A. Basal ganglia
B. Midbrain
C. Pons
D. Medulla oblongata

Combination of arm extension with leg flexion or flaccid legs is associated with lesions in pons.

619. Which of the following stimuli is useful in eliciting abduction withdrawal movements of limbs?

Harrison's 20th Ed. Chapter 300, Page 2071

A. Tickling the nostrils with a cotton wisp
B. Pressure on the knuckles or bony prominences
C. Pinprick stimulation
D. Pinching the skin

Abduction-avoidance movement of a limb is usually purposeful and denotes an intact corticospinal system. Posturing in response to noxious stimuli indicates severe damage to corticospinal system.

620. Which of the following is not a brainstem reflex?
Harrison's 20th Ed. Chapter 300, Page 2071

A. Pupillary responses to light
B. Spontaneous and elicited eye movements
C. Corneal responses
D. Jaw jerk

Brainstem reflexes include pupillary responses to light, spontaneous and elicited eye movements, corneal responses, and respiratory pattern. As a rule, if these brainstem activities, particularly pupillary reactions and eye movements, are preserved, coma is due to bilateral hemispheral disease.

621. Normally reactive and round pupils of midsize excludes?
Harrison's 20th Ed. Chapter 300, Page 2072

A. Midbrain damage
B. Pontine damage
C. Temporal lobe damage
D. Occipital lobe damage

In coma, normally reactive & round pupils of midsize (2.5–5 mm) essentially excludes midbrain damage, either primary or secondary to compression.

622. Reaction to light is difficult to appreciate in pupils?
Harrison's 20th Ed. Chapter 300, Page 2072

A. < 2 mm in diameter
B. < 3 mm in diameter
C. < 4 mm in diameter
D. < 5 mm in diameter

Reaction to light is often difficult to appreciate in pupils <2 mm in diameter.

623. A transitional sign that accompanies early midbrain–third nerve compression is?
Harrison's 20th Ed. Chapter 300, Page 2072

A. Pupil > 6 mm is diameter
B. Oval and slightly eccentric pupil
C. Unilateral miosis
D. Reactive and bilaterally small

In coma, an oval & slightly eccentric pupil is a transitional sign that accompanies early midbrain–third nerve compression.

624. Bilaterally dilated and unreactive pupils indicate?
Harrison's 20th Ed. Chapter 300, Page 2072

A. Severe cortical damage
B. Severe thalamic damage
C. Severe midbrain damage
D. Severe pontine damage

In coma, bilaterally dilated & unreactive pupils, indicates severe midbrain damage, usually from compression by a supratentorial mass.

625. Which of the following causes fixed pupils in drug induced coma?
DeJong's The Neurologic Examination, 7th Ed. Page 199

A. Digoxin
B. Glutethimide
C. Piperidine
D. Methyprylon

Glutethimide intoxication causes fixed pupils in drug induced coma, has fortunately become rare.

626. Reactive pupils are smaller in size in which of the following?
Harrison's 20th Ed. Chapter 300, Page 2072

A. Metabolic encephalopathies
B. Hydrocephalus
C. Thalamic hemorrhage
D. All of the above

627. Reactive pupils are smaller in size in which of the following?
Harrison's 20th Ed. Chapter 300, Page 2072

A. Narcotic overdose
B. Barbiturate overdose
C. Pontine hemorrhage
D. All of the above

628. Cause of misleading pupillary enlargement is?
Harrison's 20th Ed. Chapter 300, Page 2072

A. Nebulizer treatments
B. Direct ocular trauma
C. Use of drugs with anticholinergic activity
D. All of the above

Ingestion of drugs with anticholinergic activity, use of mydriatic eye drops, nebulizer treatments, and direct ocular trauma can cause misleading pupillary enlargement. Horizontal divergence of eyes at rest is normal in drowsiness.

629. Unilateral miosis in coma is due to lesion in?
Harrison's 20th Ed. Chapter 300, Page 2072

A. Lower brainstem (medulla)
B. Sympathetic efferents originating in posterior hypothalamus
C. Medial longitudinal fasciculus (MLF)
D. Any of the above

630. Eyes turn down & inward with which of the following lesion?
Harrison's 20th Ed. Chapter 300, Page 2072

A. Frontal lobe lesions
B. Thalamic lesions
C. Pontine lesions
D. Medullary lesions

Eyes turn down & inward with thalamic hemorrhage & upper midbrain lesions.

631. Which of the following statements about eyes in a state of coma is correct?
Harrison's 20th Ed. Chapter 300, Page 2072

A. Eyes look toward hemispheral lesion & away from brainstem lesion
B. Eyes look away from hemispheral lesion & toward a brainstem lesion
C. Eyes look away from hemispheral or a brainstem lesion
D. Eyes look towards hemispheral or a brainstem lesion

Conjugate horizontal ocular deviation to one side indicates damage to pons on the opposite side or to frontal lobe on the same side. The rule therefore is "eyes look toward a hemispheral lesion and away from a brainstem lesion". "Wrong-way eyes" refers to eyes that may on a rare occasion turn paradoxically away from the side of a deep hemispheral lesion.

632. "Ocular bobbing" is diagnostic of?

Harrison's 20th Ed. Chapter 300, Page 2072

A. Bilateral occipital infarct
B. Bilateral pontine damage
C. Bilateral temporal lobe infarct
D. Cerebellar damage

"Ocular bobbing" describes a brisk downward and slow upward movement of the eyes associated with loss of horizontal eye movements and is diagnostic of bilateral pontine damage, usually from thrombosis of the basilar artery.

633. "Ocular dipping" is diagnostic of?

Harrison's 20th Ed. Chapter 300, Page 2072

A. Diffuse cortical anoxic damage
B. ICSOL
C. SAH
D. Tubercular meningitis

"Ocular dipping" is a slower, arrhythmic downward movement followed by a faster upward movement in patients with normal reflex horizontal gaze indicating diffuse cortical anoxic damage.

634. "Doll's eye" oculocephalic reflex is indicative of which of the following?

Harrison's 20th Ed. Chapter 300, Page 2072

A. Reduced cortical influence on brainstem & damaged brainstem pathways
B. Reduced cortical influence on brainstem & intact brainstem pathways
C. Normal cortical influence on brainstem & damaged brainstem pathways
D. Normal cortical influence on brainstem & intact brainstem pathways

The oculocephalic reflexes, elicited by moving the head from side to side or vertically and observing eye movements in the direction opposite to the head movement, depend on the integrity of the ocular motor nuclei and their interconnecting tracts that extend from the midbrain to the pons and medulla. The movements, called somewhat inappropriately "doll's eyes" (which refers more accurately to the reflex elevation of the eyelids with flexion of the neck), are normally suppressed in the awake patient. The ability to elicit them therefore indicates both reduced cortical influence on the brainstem and intact brainstem pathways, indicating that coma is caused by a lesion or dysfunction in the cerebral hemispheres. Oculovestibular & oculocephalic reflexes provide essentially the same information.

635. Midbrain and third nerve function are tested by?

Harrison's 20th Ed. Chapter 300, Page 2071, Figure 300-3

A. Pupillary reaction to light
B. Spontaneous and reflex eye movements
C. Corneal responses
D. Respiratory & pharyngeal responses

636. Pontine function is tested by?

Harrison's 20th Ed. Chapter 300, Page 2071, Figure 300-3

A. Pupillary reaction to light
B. Spontaneous and reflex eye movements
C. Respiratory responses
D. Pharyngeal responses

637. Pontine function is tested by?

Harrison's 20th Ed. Chapter 300, Page 2071, Figure 300-3

A. Spontaneous eye movements
B. Reflex eye movements
C. Corneal responses
D. All of the above

638. Medullary function is tested by?

Harrison's 20th Ed. Chapter 300, Page 2071, Figure 300-3

A. Pupillary reaction to light
B. Spontaneous and reflex eye movements
C. Corneal responses
D. Respiratory & pharyngeal responses

In coma, midbrain & third nerve function are tested by pupillary reaction to light, pontine function by spontaneous & reflex eye movements & corneal responses, and medullary function by respiratory and pharyngeal responses.

639. Reflex conjugate, horizontal eye movements are dependent on?

Harrison's 20th Ed. Chapter 300, Page 2071, Figure 300-3

A. Medial longitudinal fasciculus (MLF)
B. Superior colliculus
C. Cerebellum
D. Temporal radiation

Reflex conjugate, horizontal eye movements are dependent on medial longitudinal fasciculus (MLF) that interconnects sixth & contralateral third nerve nuclei.

640. Acronym "COWS" that refers to "cold water opposite, warm water same" is for which of the following?

Harrison's 20th Ed. Chapter 300, Page 2072

A. Tonic deviation of head
B. Tonic deviation of both eyes
C. Direction of nystagmus
D. All of the above

Head rotation (oculocephalic reflex) or caloric stimulation of the labyrinths (oculovestibular reflex) elicits contraversive eye movements. Oculovestibular test is performed by irrigating the external auditory canal with cool water in order to induce convection currents in labyrinths. After a brief latency, result is tonic deviation of both eyes to the side of cool-water irrigation and nystagmus in the opposite direction. (Acronym "COWS" refers to direction of nystagmus - "cold water opposite, warm water same.") Loss of induced conjugate ocular movements indicates brainstem damage.

641. Presence of corrective nystagmus indicates which of the following?

Harrison's 20th Ed. Chapter 300, Page 2072

A. Frontal lobes are functioning
B. Frontal lobes are connected to the brainstem
C. Functional or hysterical coma is likely
D. All of the above

Presence of corrective nystagmus indicates that the frontal lobes are functioning and connected to the brainstem; thus functional or hysterical coma is likely.

642. Corneal reflex depends on the integrity of pontine pathways between?

Harrison's 20th Ed. Chapter 300, Page 2072

A. Fifth and same sided seventh cranial nerve
B. Fifth and opposite sided seventh cranial nerve
C. Fifth and both seventh cranial nerves
D. Any of the above

Corneal reflex depends on the integrity of pontine pathways between fifth (afferent) & both seventh (efferent) cranial nerves.

643. Corneal reflex in conjunction with reflex eye movements is a useful test of?

Harrison's 20th Ed. Chapter 300, Page 2072

A. Midbrain function
B. Pontine function
C. Medullary function
D. All of the above

Corneal reflex in conjunction with reflex eye movements is a useful test of pontine function.

644. When CNS-depressant drugs are given, which of these is the first to disappear?

Harrison's 20th Ed. Chapter 300, Page 2072

A. Corneal responses
B. Reflex eye movements
C. Non-reactivity of pupils to light
D. Any of the above

CNS-depressant drugs diminish or eliminate the corneal responses soon after reflex eye movements are paralyzed but before the pupils become unreactive to light.

645. Agonal gasps are the result of damage to?

Harrison's 20th Ed. Chapter 300, Page 2072

A. Cortex
B. Midbrain
C. Pons
D. Medulla

Agonal gasps are the result of lower brainstem (medullary) damage and are recognized as the terminal respiratory pattern of severe brain damage.

646. Which of the following abnormalities of respiration may be seen in coma?

DeJong's The Neurologic Examination, 7th Ed. Page 38

A. Cheyne - Stokes breathing
B. Biot breathing
C. Kussmaul breathing
D. All of the above

Abnormalities of respiration, such as Cheyne-Stokes, Biot, or Kussmaul breathing may be seen in coma and other neurologic disorders.

647. Which of the following respiratory pattern is seen in ponto-mesencephalic lesions?

Harrison's 20th Ed. Chapter 300, Page 2072

A. Shallow, slow, regular
B. Cheyne-Stokes respiration
C. Kussmaul breathing
D. Tachypnea

Kussmaul or rapid, deep breathing is usually seen in metabolic acidosis but may also occur with pontomesencephalic lesions.

648. Cheyne-Stokes respiration in its classic cyclic form is seen in which of the following conditions?

Harrison's 20th Ed. Chapter 300, Page 2072

A. Light coma
B. Deep coma
C. Sleep
D. Awake state

Cheyne-Stokes respiration in its classic cyclic form signifies bihemispheral damage or metabolic suppression and commonly accompanies light coma.

649. Tachypnea occurs in which of the following conditions?

Harrison's 20th Ed. Chapter 300, Page 2072

A. Tuberculosis of CNS
B. Lymphoma of CNS
C. Fungal infection of CNS
D. All of the above

Tachypnea occurs with lymphoma of the CNS.

650. In nonhabituated patients, what level of ethanol causes impaired mental activity?

Harrison's 20th Ed. Chapter 300, Page 2072

A. 0.2 gram/dL
B. 0.3 gram/dL
C. 0.4 gram/dL
D. 0.5 gram/dL

651. In nonhabituated patients, what level of ethanol is associated with stupor?

Harrison's 20th Ed. Chapter 300, Page 2072

A. 0.2 gram/dL
B. 0.3 gram/dL
C. 0.4 gram/dL
D. 0.5 gram/dL

In nonhabituated patients, generally an ethanol level of 43 mmol/L (0.2 gram/dL) causes impaired mental activity and a level of >65 mmol/L (0.3 gram/dL) is associated with stupor.

652. Most cases of coma (and confusion) are due to?

Harrison's 20th Ed. Chapter 300, Page 2072, DeJong's The Neurologic Examination, 7th Ed. Page 748

A. Hemorrhage
B. Tumor
C. Metabolic or toxic origin
D. Hydrocephalus

Most cases of coma (and confusion) are metabolic or toxic in origin. With rare exception, metabolic encephalopathies are characterized by reactive pupils and a symmetric neurologic examination. Any asymmetry in motor or sensory responses and any pupillary or eye movement abnormality should prompt an immediate, vigorous search for structural disease.

653. Which of the score is used to assess level of coma?

DeJong's The Neurologic Examination, 7th Ed. Page 749

A. FOUR score
B. ACDU
C. AVPU
D. All of the above

The FOUR (Full Outline of UnResponsiveness) score has four components (eye, motor, brainstem, and respiration). Other coma scales are the Innsbruck, Glasgow-Liege, reaction level, coma recovery, ACDU (Alert, Confused, Drowsy, Unresponsive), and AVPU (Alert, responds to Voice, responds to Pain, Unresponsive).

654. Coma must be distinguished from?

DeJong's The Neurologic Examination, 7th Ed. Page 749

A. Persistent vegetative state (PVS)
B. Locked-in syndrome
C. Mutism
D. All of the above

655. Which of the following reflex is related to brain death?
DeJong's The Neurologic Examination, 7th Ed. Page 759

A. Lazarus reflex
B. Galant reflex
C. Churchill Cope reflex
D. Bezold-Jarisch reflex

The Lazarus reflex is a reflex movement in brain-dead. Patient briefly raise their arms & drop them crossed on their chests. The phenomenon is named after the Biblical figure Lazarus of Bethany, whom Jesus raised from the dead in the Gospel of John.

656. In a case of coma, which of the following may not be detected by CT scan?
Harrison's 20th Ed. Chapter 300, Page 2072

A. Acute brainstem infarction
B. Sagittal sinus thrombosis
C. Encephalitis
D. All of the above

Bilateral hemisphere infarction, acute brainstem infarction, encephalitis, meningitis, mechanical shearing of axons (closed head trauma), sagittal sinus thrombosis, and subdural hematoma isodense to adjacent brain may not be detected.

657. In coma, EEG is useful in which of the following conditions?
Harrison's 20th Ed. Chapter 300, Page 2072

A. Clinically unrecognized seizure
B. Herpesvirus encephalitis
C. Prion (Creutzfeldt-Jakob) disease
D. All of the above

The EEG is useful in metabolic or drug-induced states and is diagnostic when coma is due to clinically unrecognized seizure, to herpesvirus encephalitis, or to prion (Creutzfeldt-Jakob) disease.

658. Which of the following is typical of metabolic coma?
Harrison's 20th Ed. Chapter 300, Page 2073

A. Delta or triphasic waves in the frontal regions
B. Widespread fast beta activity
C. Widespread variable 8- to 12-Hz activity
D. Normal alpha activity

Predominant high-voltage slowing (delta or triphasic waves) in the frontal regions is typical of metabolic coma.

659. Which of the following is typical of coma due to sedative drugs (diazepines, barbiturates)?
Harrison's 20th Ed. Chapter 300, Page 2073

A. Delta or triphasic waves in the frontal regions
B. Widespread fast beta activity
C. Widespread variable 8- to 12-Hz activity
D. Normal alpha activity

Widespread fast beta activity implies sedative drugs (diazepines, barbiturates) as a cause of coma.

660. Alpha coma results from?
Harrison's 20th Ed. Chapter 300, Page 2073

A. Hyperventilation
B. Hypoglycemia
C. Pontine damage
D. Subdural hematoma

Alpha coma results from pontine or diffuse cortical damage and is associated with a poor prognosis.

661. Which of the following is typical of locked-in syndrome?
Harrison's 20th Ed. Chapter 300, Page 2073

A. Delta or triphasic waves in the frontal regions
B. Widespread fast beta activity
C. Widespread variable 8- to 12-Hz activity
D. Normal alpha activity

Normal alpha activity on EEG is found in locked-in syndrome, hysteria or catatonia.

662. Which of the following condition causes sudden coma?
Harrison's 20th Ed. Chapter 300, Page 2073

A. Acute hydrocephalus
B. Basilar artery embolism
C. Cerebral infarction
D. Encephalitis

Conditions that cause sudden coma include drug ingestion, cerebral hemorrhage, trauma, cardiac arrest, epilepsy, or basilar artery embolism.

663. Gaze paresis is a feature of which cerebrovascular disease?
Harrison's 20th Ed. Chapter 300, Page 2073

A. Thalamic hemorrhage
B. Pontine hemorrhage
C. Cerebellar hemorrhage
D. Subarachnoid hemorrhage

Occipital headache, vomiting, gaze paresis, and inability to stand are features of cerebellar hemorrhage.

664. Asymmetric limb paresis is a feature of which cerebrovascular disease?
Harrison's 20th Ed. Chapter 300, Page 2073

A. Basilar artery thrombosis
B. Infarction in middle cerebral artery territory
C. Acute hydrocephalus
D. Subarachnoid hemorrhage

665. Neurologic prodrome or warning spells are a feature of which of the following?
Harrison's 20th Ed. Chapter 300, Page 2073

A. Basilar artery thrombosis
B. Infarction in middle cerebral artery territory
C. Acute hydrocephalus
D. Subarachnoid hemorrhage

Neurologic prodrome or warning spells, diplopia, dysarthria, vomiting, eye movement and corneal response abnormalities, and asymmetric limb paresis are features of basilar artery thrombosis.

666. Hyperventilation and excessive sweating are a feature of which cerebrovascular disease?
Harrison's 20th Ed. Chapter 300, Page 2073

A. Thalamic hemorrhage
B. Pontine hemorrhage
C. Cerebellar hemorrhage
D. Subarachnoid hemorrhage

Sudden onset, pinpoint pupils, loss of reflex eye movements and corneal responses, ocular bobbing, posturing, hyperventilation, and excessive sweating are features of pontine hemorrhage.

667. Vomiting is a feature of which of the following?
Harrison's 20th Ed. Chapter 300, Page 2073

A. Thalamic hemorrhage
B. Cerebellar hemorrhage
C. Subarachnoid hemorrhage
D. All of the above

668. Precipitous coma after headache and vomiting is a feature of which of the following?

Harrison's 20th Ed. Chapter 300, Page 2073

A. Thalamic hemorrhage
B. Pontine hemorrhage
C. Cerebellar hemorrhage
D. Subarachnoid hemorrhage

Precipitous coma after headache and vomiting is a feature of subarachnoid hemorrhage.

669. Acute hydrocephalus accompanies particularly which of the following?

Harrison's 20th Ed. Chapter 300, Page 2073

A. Thalamic hemorrhage
B. Pontine hemorrhage
C. Cerebellar hemorrhage
D. Subarachnoid hemorrhage

The syndrome of acute hydrocephalus accompanies particularly subarachnoid hemorrhage.

670. Which of the following diseases cause meningeal irritation?

Harrison's 20th Ed. Chapter 300, Page 2073, Table 300-1

A. Fat embolism
B. Cholesterol embolism
C. Carcinomatous meningitis
D. All of the above

Fat embolism, cholesterol embolism, carcinomatous and lymphomatous meningitis cause meningeal irritation with or without fever, and with an excess of WBCs or RBCs in CSF, usually without focal or lateralizing cerebral or brainstem signs. CT or MRI shows no mass lesion.

671. Which of the following diseases cause focal brainstem or lateralizing cerebral signs?

Harrison's 20th Ed. Chapter 300, Page 2073, Table 300-1

A. Herpes simplex encephalitis
B. Thrombotic thrombocytopenic purpura
C. Pituitary apoplexy
D. All of the above

672. Cellular content of the CSF is not normal in which of the following?

Harrison's 20th Ed. Chapter 300, Page 2073, Table 300-1

A. Malaria
B. Fat embolism
C. Typhoid fever
D. Eclampsia

673. Which of the following is a feature of brain death?

Harrison's 20th Ed. Chapter 300, Page 2073

A. Heart rate unresponsive to atropine
B. Diabetes insipidus
C. Absent Babinski signs
D. All of the above

674. In a valid apnea testing, PCO_2 should be at least?

Harrison's 20th Ed. Chapter 300, Page 2073

A. 30–40 mm Hg
B. 40–50 mm Hg
C. 50–60 mm Hg
D. 60–70 mm Hg

To confirm brain death, apnea is confirmed if no respiratory effort is observed in the presence of a sufficiently elevated PCO_2 i.e. 50-60 mm Hg.

675. A "coma cocktail," consists of all except?

DeJong's The Neurologic Examination, 7th Ed. Page 746

A. Dextrose
B. Flumazenil
C. Cobalamin
D. Naloxone

A "coma cocktail," consisting of dextrose, flumazenil, naloxone, and thiamine, is sometimes used in the initial management of the comatose patient.

Severe Acute Encephalopathies and Critical Care Weakness

676. Encephalopathy is a general term describing brain dysfunction that is ?

Harrison's 20th Ed. Chapter 301, Page 2074

A. Diffuse
B. Global
C. Multi-focal
D. Any of the above

677. Which of the following is false about vasogenic brain edema?

Harrison's 20th Ed. Chapter 301, Page 2074

A. Abnormal permeability of blood-brain barrier (BBB)
B. Influx of fluid & solutes into brain
C. Caused by ischemia, trauma, infection & metabolic derangements
D. None of the above

678. Which of the following is false about cytotoxic brain edema?

Harrison's 20th Ed. Chapter 301, Page 2074

A. Due to cellular swelling & membrane breakdown
B. Caused by head trauma & stroke
C. Leads to necrotic cell death & tissue infarction
D. None of the above

679. Release of which of the following leads to influx of calcium & sodium ions?

Harrison's 20th Ed. Chapter 301, Page 2074

A. Dopamine
B. Serotonin
C. Histamine
D. Glutamate

Ischemic cascade is initiated when delivery of substrates like oxygen & glucose is inadequate to sustain brain cellular functions. Release of excitatory amino acids like glutamate leads to influx of calcium & sodium ions, which disrupt cellular homeostasis.

680. Which of the following is related to ischemic cascade?

Harrison's 20th Ed. Chapter 301, Page 2074

A. Increased intracellular calcium concentration
B. Activation of proteases & lipases
C. Lipid peroxidation & free radical–mediated cell membrane injury
D. All of the above

681. Events that can cause "secondary brain insults" include all except?

Harrison's 20th Ed. Chapter 301, Page 2075

A. Systemic hypertension
B. Hypoxia
C. Seizures
D. Hyperglycemia

Systemic hypotension & hypoxia reduce substrate delivery to vulnerable brain tissue (penumbra). Fever, seizures & hyperglycemia can increase cellular metabolism. Clinically these events are known as secondary brain insults because they lead to exacerbation of the primary brain injury.

682. Which of the following about penumbra is false?

Harrison's 20th Ed. Chapter 301, Page 2075

A. Ischemic but reversibly dysfunctional tissue surrounding a core area of infarction
B. Can be imaged by perfusion imaging using MRI or CT
C. Immediate goal of treatment is to optimize cerebral perfusion in ischemic penumbra
D. None of the above

683. In MRI, which of the following provides an estimate of ischemic penumbra?

Harrison's 20th Ed. Chapter 301, Page 2075

A. Perfusion defect
B. Diffusion deficit
C. Diffusion-perfusion mismatch
D. All of the above

The discrepancy between the region of poor perfusion and diffusion deficit is called diffusion-perfusion mismatch and is a measure of ischemic penumbra.

684. Which of the following about apoptosis is false?

Harrison's 20th Ed. Chapter 301, Page 2075

A. Programmed cell death
B. Occurs without cerebral edema
C. Not seen on brain imaging
D. None of the above

685. Cerebral perfusion pressure (CPP) is defined as?

Harrison's 20th Ed. Chapter 301, Page 2075

A. Systolic blood pressure – intracranial pressure
B. Diastolic blood pressure – intracranial pressure
C. Mean arterial pressure – intracranial pressure
D. Mean arterial pressure (MAP) + intracranial pressure

Cerebral perfusion pressure (CPP) is defined as the mean systemic arterial pressure (MAP) minus the intracranial pressure (ICP).

686. Which of the following is responsible for autoregulation of cerebral blood flow?

Harrison's 20th Ed. Chapter 301, Page 2075

A. Stems of ACA, MCA, PCA
B. Circle of Willis
C. Microcirculation
D. All of the above

Cerebral blood flow (CBF) remains relatively constant over a wide range of blood pressures due to physiologic autoregulation that occur in microcirculation or by vessels below the resolution of those seen on angiography.

687. Cerebral blood flow is principally influenced by all except?

Harrison's 20th Ed. Chapter 301, Page 2075

A. Systemic blood pressure
B. pH
C. PCO_2
D. PO_2

CBF is strongly influenced by systemic blood pressure, pH and PCO_2. CBF increases with hypercapnia and acidosis and decreases with hypocapnia and alkalosis.

688. Which of the following statements is false?
Harrison's 20th Ed. Chapter 301, Page 2075

A. CBF increases with hypercapnia & acidosis
B. CBF decreases with hypocapnia and alkalosis
C. CBF becoming pressure-dependent is ominous
D. None of the above

689. Volume of CSF within ventricles and surrounding the brain and spinal cord is about?
Harrison's 20th Ed. Chapter 301, Page 2075

A. 50 mL
B. 100 mL
C. 150 mL
D. 200 mL

690. Cerebral blood volume is about?
Harrison's 20th Ed. Chapter 301, Page 2075

A. 50 mL
B. 100 mL
C. 150 mL
D. 200 mL

About 150 mL of CSF is present within the ventricles and surrounding the brain and spinal cord. Cerebral blood volume is also ~150 mL.

691. To avoid secondary ischemic brain injury, intracranial pressure should be maintained at?
Harrison's 20th Ed. Chapter 301, Page 2077

A. < 5 mm Hg
B. < 10 mm Hg
C. < 15 mm Hg
D. < 20 mm Hg

In general, ICP should be maintained at <20 mm Hg.

692. To avoid secondary ischemic brain injury, cerebral perfusion pressure (CPP) should be maintained at?
Harrison's 20th Ed. Chapter 301, Page 2077

A. ≥ 40 mm Hg
B. ≥ 50 mm Hg
C. ≥ 60 mm Hg
D. ≥ 70 mm Hg

In treatment of SAH, cerebral perfusion pressure should be maintained at ≥ 60 mm Hg.

693. Which of the following is an early sign of elevated ICP?
Harrison's 20th Ed. Chapter 301, Page 2077

A. Drowsiness and a diminished level of consciousness
B. Unilateral pupillary changes
C. Coma
D. All of the above

Early signs of elevated ICP include drowsiness and a diminished level of consciousness while coma and unilateral pupillary changes are late signs.

694. Which of the following has been shown to improve outcome in patients with elevated ICP?
Harrison's 20th Ed. Chapter 301, Page 2078

A. Intubation and hyperventilation to $PaCO_2$ 30–35 mm Hg
B. High dose barbiturates ("pentobarb coma")
C. Decompressive hemicraniectomy
D. Hypothermia to 33°C

695. "Histotoxic hypoxia" is produced by?
Harrison's 20th Ed. Chapter 301, Page 2078

A. Shock
B. Asphyxiation
C. Carbon monoxide poisoning
D. Any of the above

Carbon monoxide & cyanide poisoning are termed histotoxic hypoxia because they cause a direct impairment of the respiratory chain.

696. Which of the following reflexes pertain to brainstem function?
Harrison's 20th Ed. Chapter 301, Page 2078

A. Oculocephalic (doll's eyes) reflex
B. Oculovestibular (caloric) reflex
C. Corneal reflex
D. All of the above

697. Selective persistent memory deficits after brief cardiac arrest is due to injury to?
Harrison's 20th Ed. Chapter 301, Page 2078

A. Cerebral cortex
B. Basal ganglia
C. Hippocampus
D. Hypothalamus

Selective persistent memory deficits after brief cardiac arrest is due to injury to hippocampal CA1 neurons which are vulnerable to even brief episodes of hypoxia-ischemia.

698. Which of the following convey a poor prognosis after a severe hypoxic-ischemic insult?
Harrison's 20th Ed. Chapter 301, Page 2078

A. Myoclonic status epilepticus
B. Absence of pupillary light reflex day 3 after injury
C. Bilateral absence of N20 somatosensory evoked response
D. All of the above

Absence of pupillary light reflex or absence of a motor response to pain on day 3 following injury, bilateral absence of early cortical somatosensory evoked response (SSEPs) and myoclonic status epilepticus within 24 hours after a primary circulatory arrest convey a poor prognosis.

699. Neuron-specific enolase (NSE) has relevance in which of the following conditions?
Harrison's 20th Ed. Chapter 301, Page 2078

A. Creutzfeldt-Jakob disease (CJD)
B. Small-cell cancer of the lung
C. Gastrointestinal neuroendocrine tumors (Carcinoids)
D. All of the above

Elevations of CSF neuron-specific enolase & tau occur in CJD but lack specificity for diagnosis. Plasma NSE levels are also used as a marker of GI-NETs (carcinoids). A very elevated serum level (>33 μg/L) of biochemical marker neuron-specific enolase (NSE) within first 3 days is indicative of brain damage after resuscitation from cardiac arrest & predicts a poor outcome.

700. Which of the following about watershed distribution of brain is false?
Harrison's 20th Ed. Chapter 301, Page 2078

A. Most metastases develop at watershed areas of brain
B. Balint's syndrome results from infarctions in watershed areas between distal PCA & MCA territories
C. Watershed infarcts occurs at distal territories between major cerebral arteries in low flow states
D. None of the above

701. Which of the following CNS injuries may occur following open heart or coronary artery bypass grafting (CABG) surgery?
Harrison's 20th Ed. Chapter 301, Page 2079

A. Acute encephalopathy
B. Stroke
C. Chronic syndrome of cognitive impairment
D. All of the above

702. Which of the following is preferred to reduce delirium & shorten the duration of mechanical ventilation in critically ill patients requiring sedation?
Harrison's 20th Ed. Chapter 301, Page 2079

A. Haloperidol
B. Lorazepam
C. Midazolam
D. Dexmedetomidine

In critically ill patients requiring sedation, use of the centrally acting α2 agonist dexmedetomidine reduces delirium & shortens the duration of mechanical ventilation.

703. Biomarkers of blood brain barrier (BBB) dysfunction include?
Harrison's 20th Ed. Chapter 301, Page 2080

A. S-100β
B. Plasma-soluble prion protein (PrPc)
C. Ubiquitin carboxyl-terminal hydrolase isoenzyme L1 (UCHL1)
D. All of the above

704. Which of the following about osmotic demyelination syndrome is false?
Harrison's 20th Ed. Chapter 301, Page 2080

A. Demyelination without inflammation in base of pons
B. Relative sparing of axons & nerve cells
C. Presents as quadriplegia & pseudobulbar palsy
D. None of the above

Previously called central pontine myelinolysis.

705. Which of the following is a feature of acute Wernicke's disease?
Harrison's 20th Ed. Chapter 301, Page 2080

A. Global confusion
B. Impairment of eye movements
C. Gait ataxia
D. All of the above

Characteristic clinical triad of acute Wernicke's disease is ophthalmoplegia, ataxia & global confusion.

706. Ocular motor abnormalities in acute Wernicke's disease include?
Harrison's 20th Ed. Chapter 301, Page 2080

A. Horizontal nystagmus on lateral gaze
B. Lateral rectus palsy
C. Conjugate gaze palsies
D. All of the above

Ocular motor abnormalities in acute Wernicke's disease include horizontal nystagmus on lateral gaze, usually bilateral lateral rectus palsy, conjugate gaze palsies, and rarely ptosis. Pupils are usually spared. Horizontal nystagmus may persist even after treatment.

707. Gait ataxia in acute Wernicke's disease results from?
Harrison's 20th Ed. Chapter 301, Page 2080

A. Polyneuropathy
B. Cerebellar involvement
C. Vestibular paresis
D. All of the above

Gait ataxia results from a combination of polyneuropathy, cerebellar involvement & vestibular paresis.

708. Feature of amnestic syndrome (Korsakoff's syndrome) is?
Harrison's 20th Ed. Chapter 301, Page 2081

A. Gaps in memory
B. Confabulation
C. Disordered temporal sequencing
D. All of the above

Damage to medial thalamic nuclei & mammillary bodies occur in Korsakoff's syndrome. Mammillary body atrophy may be visible on MRI in the chronic phase. Amnestic defect is related to lesions in dorsal medial nuclei of thalamus.

709. Thiamine is a cofactor of which of the following enzymes?
Harrison's 20th Ed. Chapter 301, Page 2081

A. Transketolase
B. Pyruvate dehydrogenase
C. α-ketoglutarate dehydrogenase
D. All of the above

Thiamine is a cofactor of transketolase, pyruvate dehydrogenase, and α-ketoglutarate dehydrogenase and others. Thiamine deficiency leads to glutamate accumulation due to impairment of α-ketoglutarate dehydrogenase activity resulting in excitotoxic cell damage. Glucose infusions may precipitate Wernicke's Zdisease.

710. Which of the following about posterior reversible encephalopathy syndrome (PRES) is false?
Harrison's 20th Ed. Chapter 301, Page 2081

A. Pathogenesis of hyperperfusion due to endothelial dysfunction
B. Vasogenic edema
C. Affects posterior rather than anterior portions of brain
D. None of the above

711. Which of the following can lead to posterior reversible encephalopathy syndrome (PRES)?
Harrison's 20th Ed. Chapter 301, Page 2082 Table 301-3

A. Cyclosporine
B. Tacrolimus
C. Methotrexate
D. All of the above

712. Which of the following can lead to posterior reversible encephalopathy syndrome (PRES)?
Harrison's 20th Ed. Chapter 301, Page 2082 Table 301-3

A. HELLP syndrome
B. Hemolytic-uremic syndrome (HUS)
C. Cocaine use
D. All of the above

713. Clinical presentation of posterior reversible encephalopathy syndrome include?
Harrison's 20th Ed. Chapter 301, Page 2081

A. Prominent headaches
B. Seizures
C. Focal neurologic deficits
D. All of the above

714. Typical focal deficit in hyperperfusion states is?
Harrison's 20th Ed. Chapter 301, Page 2081

A. Glaucoma
B. Cortical visual loss
C. Posterior Uveitis
D. Amaurosis Fugax

Typical focal deficit in hyperperfusion states is cortical visual loss, given the tendency of the process to involve the occipital lobes. Increased capillary pressure or endothelial dysfunction play a role in its pathophysiology. The rapidity of rise, rather than absolute value of pressure, is the most important risk factor.

715. Most common peripheral nervous system (PNS) complication related to critical illness is?
Harrison's 20th Ed. Chapter 301, Page 2083

A. Critical illness polyneuropathy
B. Critical illness myopathy
C. Guillain-Barré syndrome
D. Myasthenia gravis

716. Medication that impairs neuromuscular transmission is?
Harrison's 20th Ed. Chapter 301, Page 2083

A. Aminoglycosides
B. Beta-blocking agents
C. Cisatracurium
D. All of the above

717. Risk factors for prolonged action of neuromuscular blocking agents include?
Harrison's 20th Ed. Chapter 301, Page 2083

A. Female sex
B. Metabolic acidosis
C. Renal failure
D. All of the above

718. Which of the following about cachectic myopathy is false?
Harrison's 20th Ed. Chapter 301, Page 2083

A. Serum creatine kinase levels normal
B. Electromyography (EMG) normal
C. Muscle biopsy shows type II fiber atrophy
D. None of the above

719. Which of the following about acute necrotizing intensive care myopathy is false?
Harrison's 20th Ed. Chapter 301, Page 2083

A. Elevations in serum creatine kinase
B. Elevations in urine myoglobin
C. Both EMG & muscle biopsy may be normal initially
D. None of the above

720. Which of the following about thick-filament myopathy is false?
Harrison's 20th Ed. Chapter 301, Page 2083

A. Occurs in the setting of glucocorticoid & nd-NMBA use
B. Actual myopathy with muscle damage
C. Invariably improves & most patients return to normal
D. None of the above

721. Amaurosis Fugax is best related to?
Harrison's 20th Ed. Chapter 28, Page 183

A. Cluster headache
B. Transient ischemic attack of retina
C. Hysterical conversion reaction
D. All of the above

Amaurosis fugax or a transient ischemic attack of the retina or transient monocular blindness, occurs from emboli to central retinal artery of one eye indicating carotid stenosis or local ophthalmic artery disease as the cause.

722. Amaurosis Fugax is the result of?
Harrison's 20th Ed. Chapter 28, Page 183

A. Trauma
B. Emboli
C. Vascular spasm
D. Any of the above

Amaurosis fugax usually results from an embolus stuck in a retinal arteriole. Complete occlusion of the central retinal artery produces arrest of blood flow and a milky retina with a cherry-red fovea.

723. Emboli causing amaurosis fugax are composed of?
Harrison's 20th Ed. Chapter 28, Page 183

A. Cholesterol
B. Calcium
C. Platelet-fibrin debris
D. Any of the above

Emboli causing amaurosis fugax are composed of cholesterol (Hollenhorst plaque), calcium, or platelet-fibrin debris. Most common source is atherosclerotic plaque in carotid artery or aorta.

724. Which of the following statements about amaurosis fugax is false?
Harrison's 20th Ed. Chapter 28, Page 183, 187

A. Briefer duration than migraine
B. Occurs in both eyes
C. Not followed by headache
D. Associated with antiphospholipid antibody syndrome

Amaurosis fugax refers to a transient ischemic attack of retina and occurs in only one eye (painless monocular loss of vision). It can be a part of high-altitude neurologic events.

725. Which of the following is false about Charcot-Bouchard miliary aneurysm?
Angiology. 2018;69(1):17-30

A. Aneurysms of brain blood vessels of <300 μm diameter
B. Located in brainstem
C. Associated with chronic hypertension
D. None of the above

Charcot-Bouchard miliary aneurysms (French physicians Jean-Martin Charcot and Charles-Joseph Bouchard) are aneurysms of brain small blood vessels (<300 μm diameter). While, saccular aneurysms (berry aneurysms) occur in larger-sized blood vessels. Charcot-Bouchard aneurysms are most often located in the brainstem and are associated with chronic hypertension.

726. Hypothesis of homunculus organization of fibers in internal capsule means?
Brain. 2017;140:3055-3061

A. Sensory & motor fibers have same orientation
B. Sensory & motor fibers have different orientation
C. Adjacent regions on cortex correspond on adjacent areas on body surface
D. None of the above

Homunculus means 'little man' in Latin, first described by Penfield and Boldrey, 1937. Functional mapping & lesion studies have shown that primary motor & somatosensory cortices are so arranged that adjacent regions on cortex correspond on adjacent areas on body surface. In somatotropic representations, arms are always medial to legs except in primary sensiromotor cortex & in posterior columns.

727. Which of the following tracts is not present in the posterior limb of internal capsule?

DeJong's The Neurologic Examination, 7th Ed. Page 59

A. Cortico-pontine

B. Superior thalamic radiation

C. Anterior thalamic radiation

D. Corticospinal tract

Anterior thalamic radiation is part of anterior limb of internal capsule.

728. Genu of the internal capsule is at the level of?

DeJong's The Neurologic Examination, 7th Ed. Page 59

A. Foremen of Lushka

B. Foramen of Magendie

C. Foramen of Monro

D. Foramen magnum

729. Hippocampus-fornix-anterior thalamus-cingulate gyrus-cingulum bundle-perihippocampal cortex-hippocampus - this circuit is called?

DeJong's The Neurologic Examination, 7th Ed. Page 51

A. Papez's circuit

B. Hafez's circuit

C. Parkinson's circuit

D. Peter's circuit

Structures of limbic lobe are connected in Papez circuit (cigulate gyrus → parahippocampal gyrus → hippocampus → fornix → mammillary body → anterior nucleus of thalamus → cingulate gyrus).

Neuroimaging in Neurologic Disorders

730. Which of the following investigation is recommended in meningeal disease?

Harrison's 20th Ed. Chapter 416, Page 3030 Table 416-1

A. CT (noncontrast)
B. CT contrast
C. MRI
D. MRI with contrast

731. Which of the following investigation is recommended in myelopathy?

Harrison's 20th Ed. Chapter 416, Page 3030 Table 416-1

A. CT (noncontrast)
B. CT contrast
C. MRI
D. MRI with contrast

732. MRI + contrast is the investigation of choice for all of the following except?

Harrison's 20th Ed. Chapter 416, Page 3030 Table 416-1

A. Neoplasm (primary or metastatic)
B. White matter disorders
C. Infection/abscess
D. Immunosuppressed with focal findings

733. Which of the following is the most sensitive technique for detecting acute ischemic stroke of brain?

Harrison's 20th Ed. Chapter 416, Page 3030

A. CT angiography (CTA)
B. Perfusion CT (pCT)
C. MR angiography (MRA)
D. Diffusion MR

Diffusion MR is the most sensitive technique for detecting acute ischemic stroke of brain or spinal cord, encephalitis, abscesses and prion diseases.

734. In normal CNS, which of the following structure lacks blood-brain barrier (BBB)?

Harrison's 20th Ed. Chapter 416, Page 3031

A. Pituitary gland
B. Choroid plexus
C. Dura
D. All of the above

In normal CNS, the pituitary gland, choroid plexus, and dura lack blood-brain barrier (BBB) and enhance after contrast administration.

735. In a routine brain CT study, radiation dose is normally about?

Harrison's 20th Ed. Chapter 416, Page 3031

A. 0.2 to 1 mSv
B. 2 to 5 mSv
C. 6 to 12 mSv
D. 22 to 50 mSv

In a routine brain CT study, radiation dose is normally between 2 and 5 mSv (millisievert).

736. Rise in serum creatinine of at least 1 mg/dL within how many hours of contrast administration defines contrast nephropathy?

Harrison's 20th Ed. Chapter 416, Page 3031

A. 6 hours
B. 12 hours
C. 24 hours
D. 48 hours

737. Risk factors for contrast nephropathy include all except?

Harrison's 20th Ed. Chapter 416, Page 3031

A. Solitary kidney
B. Diabetes mellitus
C. Hypertension
D. Advanced age (>80 years)

Risk factors for contrast nephropathy include advanced age (>80 years), preexisting renal disease (serum creatinine exceeding 2 mg/dL), solitary kidney, diabetes mellitus, dehydration, paraproteinemia, concurrent use of nephrotoxic medication or chemotherapeutic agents, and high contrast dose.

738. What is the eGFR threshold below which iodinated contrast should not be given?

Harrison's 20th Ed. Chapter 416, Page 3033

A. 90 mL/min/1.73 meter^2
B. 75 mL/min/1.73 meter^2
C. 60 mL/min/1.73 meter^2
D. 30 mL/min/1.73 meter^2

The American College of Radiology suggests using an estimated glomerular filtration rate (eGFR) of 30 mL/min/1.73 meter^2 as a threshold below which iodinated contrast should not be given without serious consideration of the potential for contrast nephropathy.

739. Use of which of the following may reduce the incidence of contrast nephropathy?

Harrison's 20th Ed. Chapter 416, Page 3033

A. Acetylcysteine
B. Oxygen inhalation
C. Osmolar diuretics
D. Loop diuretics

Apart from hydration and reduction in dose of contrast media, use of bicarbonate & acetylcysteine may reduce the incidence of contrast nephropathy.

740. Severe allergic reactions occur in what proportion of patients receiving nonionic media?

Harrison's 20th Ed. Chapter 416, Page 3033

A. 0.04%
B. 0.12%
C. 0.18%
D. 0.24%

Severe allergic reactions occur in 0.04% of patients receiving nonionic media, sixfold lower than with ionic media.

741. Which of the following is not related to magnetic resonance imaging (MRI)?

Harrison's 20th Ed. Chapter 416, Page 3033

A. Hydrogen protons in biologic tissues
B. Dynamic magnetic field
C. Static magnetic field
D. Radiofrequency (Rf) waves

MRI is a complex interaction between hydrogen protons in biologic tissues, a static magnetic field (the magnet), and energy (echo) in the form of radiofrequency (Rf) waves of a specific frequency.

742. T2W images are more sensitive than T1W images to all of the following except?

Harrison's 20th Ed. Chapter 416, Page 3034

A. Edema
B. Fat-containing structures
C. Demyelination
D. Infarction

T2-weighted (T2W) images are more sensitive than T1-weighted (T1W) images to edema, demyelination, infarction, and chronic hemorrhage, while T1W imaging is more sensitive to subacute hemorrhage and fat-containing structures.

743. MRI involves imaging of?

N Engl J Med. 1993; 328:708-716

A. Electron
B. Proton
C. Neutron
D. All of the above

MRI involves imaging of the proton which is the positively charged spinning nucleus of hydrogen atoms found in abundance in tissues containing water, proteins, lipids & other macromolecules. Protons align with or against the direction of the magnetic field.

744. Which of the following is related to MRI?

N Engl J Med. 1993; 328:708-716

A. Larmor or resonance frequency
B. Body coil
C. Pulse sequence
D. All of the above

745. Which of the following is an MRI image?

N Engl J Med. 1993; 328:708-716

A. T1-weighted
B. T2-weighted
C. Proton-density-weighted
D. All of the above

746. In MRI, the degree of weighting depends on?

N Engl J Med. 1993; 328:708-716

A. Pulse sequence
B. Repetition time
C. Echo time
D. All of the above

747. Which of the following statements is false?

N Engl J Med. 1993; 328:708-716

A. Fluids appear dark in T1-weighted images
B. Fluids appear bright in proton-density-weighted images
C. Fluids appear bright in T2-weighted images
D. None of the above

748. Which of the following statements about gadolinium is false?

Harrison's 20th Ed. Chapter 416, Page 3034

A. Heavy-metal element
B. Paramagnetic substance
C. Chelated to DTPA
D. Approximate dose 2 mL/kg IV

Approximate dose of gadolinium is 0.2 mL/kg body weight administered intravenously. Gadolinium has the greatest ability to capture thermal neutrons.

749. Gadolinium is produced from which of the following minerals?

N Engl J Med. 2007;357:720-722

A. Ilmenite
B. Zircon
C. Monazite
D. Sillimanite

Gadolinium is produced both from monazite and bastnäsite.

750. Which of the following countries has deposits of monazite sands?

N Engl J Med. 2007;357:720-722

A. India
B. Brazil
C. South Africa
D. All of the above

751. Symbol of Gadolinium is?

N Engl J Med. 2007;357:720-722

A. Ga
B. Gd
C. Gl
D. Gm

Symbol of Gadolinium is Gd with atomic number 64 and atomic weight of 157.25.

752. Which of the following is best related to gadolinium contrast agents?

Harrison's 20th Ed. Chapter 416, Page 3035

A. Nephrogenic diabetes insipidus (NDI)
B. Nephrogenic Syndrome of Inappropriate Antidiuresis
C. Nephrogenic systemic fibrosis (NSF)
D. Nephrotic syndrome

Patients with renal insufficiency exposed to gadolinium contrast agents may develop a rare complication - nephrogenic systemic fibrosis (NSF) between 5 and 75 days following exposure.

753. Nephrogenic systemic fibrosis (NSF) involves which of the following parts of the body most?

Cleveland Clinic Journal of Medicine 2008;75(2):95-111

A. Upper extremities
B. Between ankles and thighs
C. Trunk
D. Face

754. Nephrogenic systemic fibrosis (NSF) involves which of the following parts of the body least?

Cleveland Clinic Journal of Medicine 2008;75(2):95-111

A. Upper extremities
B. Between ankles and thighs
C. Trunk
D. Face

NSF typically presents between ankles and the thighs (symmetric, progresses to involve the entire lower extremities). Upper extremity involvement occurs frequently, but usually with lower extremity disease. Trunk is involved less commonly than legs and arms. The face is typically spared.

755. Which of the following is a laboratory biomarker for NSF?

Cleveland Clinic Journal of Medicine 2008;75(2):95-111

A. Anti nuclear antibodies
B. Rheumatoid factor
C. Anti-SCL70 antibodies
D. None of the above

There is no laboratory biomarker for NSF.

756. Which of the following is characteristic and pathognomonic of NSF?

Cleveland Clinic Journal of Medicine 2008;75(2):95-111

A. Proliferation of dermal spindle cells
B. Thick collagen bundles with surrounding clefts
C. Immunohistochemically CD34 reactivity in fibroblast-like cells
D. Absence of mucin and elastic fibers

A characteristic and almost pathognomonic staining profile is the immunohistochemical identification of CD34 reactivity in the fibroblast-like cells. Cells expressing CD34 are normally found in the umbilical cord, the bone marrow (as pluripotential hematopoietic stem cells), and in the vascular endothelium.

757. Disorder that causes thickening & hardening of skin of extremities & trunk is?

Cleveland Clinic Journal of Medicine 2008;75(2):95-111

A. Systemic sclerosis
B. Scleromyxedema
C. Eosinophilic fasciitis
D. All of the above

Besides NSF, other disorders that can cause thickening & hardening of skin of extremities & trunk include systemic sclerosis or scleroderma, scleromyxedema, and eosinophilic fasciitis.

758. Most frequently used radionuclide moiety in Positron Emission Tomography (PET) is?

Harrison's 20th Ed. Chapter 416, Page 3037

A. 2-[^{16}F]fluoro-2-deoxy-d-glucose
B. 2-[^{17}F]fluoro-2-deoxy-d-glucose
C. 2-[^{18}F]fluoro-2-deoxy-d-glucose
D. 2-[^{19}F]fluoro-2-deoxy-d-glucose

In Positron Emission Tomography (PET), the most frequently used moiety is 2-[^{18}F]fluoro-2-deoxy-d-glucose (FDG), an analogue of glucose. It is taken up by cells competitively with 2-deoxyglucose.

Seizures and Epilepsy

759. Seizure is derived from a Latin word "sacire" that means?
Harrison's 20th Ed. Chapter 418, Page 3050

A. "to invade"
B. "to destroy"
C. "to silence"
D. "to take possession of"

Seizure is derived from Latin word "sacire" meaning "to take possession of".

760. What percentage of population will have at least one seizure in lifetime?
Harrison's 20th Ed. Chapter 418, Page 3050

A. ~1–3%
B. ~3–5%
C. ~5–10%
D. ~10–15%

761. Highest incidence of seizure is in which of the following age groups?
Harrison's 20th Ed. Chapter 418, Page 3050

A. Infancy
B. Early childhood & late adulthood
C. Middle age
D. Old age

~5–10% percentage of population will have at least one seizure in lifetime and the highest incidence is in early childhood and late adulthood.

762. Which of the following is false about epilepsy?
Harrison's 20th Ed. Chapter 418, Page 3050

A. Single seizure
B. Acute
C. No correctable or avoidable circumstance
D. All of the above

Epilepsy is a clinical phenomenon & is said to be present when a person has recurrent seizures due to a chronic, underlying process. A person with a single seizure or recurrent seizures due to correctable or avoidable circumstances, does not have epilepsy. By definition, epilepsy is two or more unprovoked seizures.

763. What is the prevalence of epilepsy?
Harrison's 20th Ed. Chapter 418, Page 3050

A. 2 – 6 persons per 1000
B. 3 – 9 persons per 1000
C. 4 – 20 persons per 1000
D. 5 – 30 persons per 1000

The prevalence of epilepsy is estimated at 5 - 30 persons per 1000.

764. In which year did the International League Against Epilepsy (ILAE) classify seizure disorders?
Harrison's 20th Ed. Chapter 418, Page 3050 , Harrison's 19th Ed. 2542

A. 1965
B. 1978
C. 1981
D. 1995

In 1981, the International League against Epilepsy (ILAE) classification is based on clinical features of seizures and associated EEG findings. Etiology or cellular substrate are not considered. ILAE (2005-2009) has updated approach to classify seizures. ILAE Commission on Classification and Terminology provided an updated approach to classification of seizures in 2017.

765. Which of the following term is no longer used in classification of seizures?
Harrison's 20th Ed. Chapter 418, Page 3050

A. Partial seizures
B. Focal onset seizures
C. Generalized onset seizures
D. Unknown Onset seizures

In the new classification system (International League against Epilepsy (ILAE) Commission on Classification and Terminology, 2017), term partial seizures is no longer used and subcategories of "simple focal seizures" and "complex focal seizures" have been eliminated.

766. Focal seizures are associated with?
Harrison's 20th Ed. Chapter 418, Page 3051

A. Structural abnormalities of brain
B. Cellular abnormalities
C. Biochemical abnormalities
D. All of the above

Focal seizures are associated with structural abnormalities of brain, there are exception though.

767. Generalized seizures are associated with?
Harrison's 20th Ed. Chapter 418, Page 3051

A. Cellular abnormality
B. Biochemical abnormality
C. Structural abnormality
D. Any of the above

Generalized seizures may result from cellular, biochemical, or structural abnormalities.

768. Main difference between simple partial and complex partial seizure is?
Harrison's 20th Ed. Chapter 418, Page 3051

A. Unilateral or bilateral
B. Focal or generalized
C. Consciousness or unconsciousness
D. Absence or presence of aura

If consciousness is fully preserved during seizure, it was termed simple partial seizure. If consciousness is impaired, the seizure was termed complex partial seizure.

769. Motor manifestations of focal seizures can be all except?
Harrison's 20th Ed. Chapter 418, Page 3051

A. Tonic
B. Clonic
C. Myoclonic
D. Atonic

770. Nonmotor manifestations of focal seizures can be?
Harrison's 20th Ed. Chapter 418, Page 3051

A. Sensory
B. Autonomic
C. Emotional
D. All of the above

Focal seizures can have motor manifestations (tonic, clonic, or myoclonic movements) or nonmotor manifestations (sensory, autonomic, or emotional symptoms).

771. Which of the following is a feature of focal motor seizure?
Harrison's 20th Ed. Chapter 418, Page 3051

A. Jacksonian march
B. Todd's paralysis
C. Epilepsia partialis continua
D. All of the above

In focal motor seizures, after initiation from a restricted region, abnormal discharges may spread to other wider areas. This is called a "Jacksonian march". Following focal motor seizure, patient may have localized paresis in the involved region for minutes to many hours (Todd's paralysis). Focal motor seizure may continue for hours or days (epilepsia partialis continua).

772. Which of the following is often refractory to medical therapy?
Harrison's 20th Ed. Chapter 418, Page 3051

A. Jacksonian march
B. Todd's paralysis
C. Epilepsia partialis continua
D. All of the above

Focal motor seizure may continue for hours or days. Epilepsia partialis continua is the term applied to this condition. It is often refractory to medical therapy.

773. Which of the following is false about auras?
Harrison's 20th Ed. Chapter 418, Page 3051

A. Subjective
B. "Internal" events
C. Not directly observable by someone else
D. None of the above

Subjective, "internal" events that are not directly observable by someone else are referred to as auras.

774. Which of the following about focal seizures with dyscognitive features is false?
Harrison's 20th Ed. Chapter 418, Page 3051

A. Begins with an aura
B. Behavioral arrest denotes beginning of ictal phase
C. Reterograde amnesia
D. Automatisms

Focal seizures with dyscognitive features are characterized by focal seizure activity with transient unconsciousness, beginning with an aura which are subjective, internal events that are not directly observable by others. Behavioral arrest or motionless stare denotes beginning of ictal phase which marks the onset of the period of amnesia & automatisms. Following seizure anterograde amnesia, confusion or postictal aphasia may be present. Automatisms are involuntary, automatic behaviors that have a wide range of manifestations.

775. In seizure, retrograde component of amnesia may dominate in?
Harrison's 20th Ed. Chapter 418, Page 164

A. Absence seizure
B. Temporal lobe epilepsy
C. Myoclonic seizure
D. Febrile seizure

Occasionally associated with temporal lobe epilepsy or herpes simplex encephalitis, the retrograde component of amnesia may dominate.

776. Which of the following is false about seizures that may occur exclusively during sleep?
Harrison's 20th Ed. Chapter 418, Page 170

A. Mimic a primary sleep disorder
B. Typically occur during episodes of NREM sleep
C. May occur as generalized tonic-clonic movements
D. None of the above

777. A focal seizure that evolves into a generalized seizure frequently arise from?
Harrison's 20th Ed. Chapter 418, Page 3051

A. Frontal lobe
B. Temporal lobe
C. Parietal lobe
D. Occipital lobe

A focal seizure that evolves into a generalized seizure frequently arises from a region in frontal lobe. But, may happen with focal seizures occurring elsewhere in the brain.

778. Which of the following is false about typical absence seizures?
Harrison's 20th Ed. Chapter 418, Page 3051

A. Sudden, brief loss of consciousness with loss of postural control
B. Typically lasts for only seconds
C. Consciousness returns as suddenly as it was lost
D. No postictal confusion

Absence seizures are characterized by sudden, brief lapses of consciousness "without" loss of postural control. Patients stare & cease normal activity for a few seconds, return immediately to normal & have no memory of the event or no postictal confusion.

779. Which of the following occurs as bilateral motor sign in typical absence seizures?
Harrison's 20th Ed. Chapter 418, Page 3051

A. Small-amplitude, clonic movements of hands
B. Large-amplitude, clonic movements of hands
C. Small-amplitude, tonic movements of hands
D. Large-amplitude, tonic movements of hands

Absence seizures are usually accompanied by subtle, bilateral motor signs such as rapid blinking of eyelids, chewing movements, or small-amplitude, clonic movements of hands.

780. Which of the following is false about typical absence seizures?
Harrison's 20th Ed. Chapter 418, Page 3052

A. Usually begin in childhood (4 to 8 yrs)
B. EEG shows generalized, symmetric, 3-Hz spike-&-wave
C. EEG discharge begin & end suddenly on an abnormal background
D. Hyperventilation provokes EEG discharges & seizures

The EEG hallmark of typical absence seizures is a generalized, symmetric, 3-Hz spike-and-wave discharge that begins and ends suddenly, superimposed on a "normal" EEG background. Hyperventilation provokes these EEG discharges.

781. Which of the following will trigger a seizure in most patients with untreated typical absence seizures?
Harrison's 20th Ed. Chapter 418, Page 3052

A. Exercise
B. Hyperventilation
C. Breath holding
D. Lack of sleep

Hyperventilation for 3 minutes will trigger a seizure in most patients with untreated absence seizures.

782. Absence seizures were also called?

Epilepsy Currents, 2013;13(3):135–140

A. Narcolepsy
B. Cataplexy
C. Pyknolepsy
D. All of the above

The term "absence" was first used to describe seizures in 1705 and was reported as pyknolepsy ("heaped up, closely packed, aggregated attacks") in the early 20th century. Childhood absence epilepsy (CAE), also known as pyknolepsy, is an idiopathic generalized epilepsy which occurs in otherwise normal children.

783. What percentage of patients of typical absence seizures will have a spontaneous remission during adolescence?

Harrison's 17th Ed. 2499

A. ~ 10–20%
B. ~ 30–40%
C. ~ 50–60%
D. ~ 60–70%

~ 60-70% patients of absence seizures have a spontaneous remission during adolescence.

784. In atypical absence seizures, EEG finding of generalized, spike-and-wave pattern has a frequency of?

Harrison's 20th Ed. Chapter 418, Page 3052

A. <= 4.0 per second
B. <= 3.5 per second
C. <= 3.0 per second
D. <= 2.5 per second

EEG in atypical absence seizures shows a generalized, slow spike-and-wave pattern with a frequency of <= 2.5 per second, as well as other abnormal EEG activity.

785. When compared to typical absence seizures, patients with atypical absence seizures have?

Harrison's 20th Ed. Chapter 418, Page 3052

A. Lapse of consciousness of longer duration
B. Less abrupt onset and cessation
C. Less responsive to anticonvulsants
D. All of the above

786. The most common seizure type resulting from metabolic derangements is?

Harrison's 20th Ed. Chapter 418, Page 3052

A. Absence seizures
B. Myoclonic seizures
C. Grand Mal seizures
D. Atonic seizures

Grand Mal seizures are the main seizure type in ~10% of all persons with epilepsy. They are also the most common seizure type resulting from metabolic derangements.

787. "Ictal cry" is related to tonic contraction of which of the following?

Harrison's 20th Ed. Chapter 418, Page 3052

A. Muscles of inspiration and larynx
B. Muscles of expiration and larynx
C. Muscles of inspiration and pharynx
D. Muscles of expiration and pharynx

Tonic contraction of muscles of expiration and larynx at the onset will produce a loud moan or "Ictal cry".

788. Ictal cry is observed in which phase of Grand Mal seizure?

Harrison's 20th Ed. Chapter 418, Page 3052

A. Preictal phase
B. Ictal phase
C. Postictal phase
D. Any of the above

Initial phase of Grand Mal seizure is tonic contraction of muscles throughout the body. Tonic contraction of muscles of expiration and larynx at the onset produces a loud moan or "ictal cry".

789. During tonic phase of Grand Mal seizure, which of the following does not occur?

Harrison's 20th Ed. Chapter 418, Page 3052

A. Increase in heart rate
B. Increase in blood pressure
C. Impaired respiration
D. Constriction of pupils

A marked enhancement of sympathetic tone during ictal phase of Grand Mal seizure leads to increases in heart rate, blood pressure, and pupillary size. Respiration is impaired.

790. In Grand Mal seizure, initial tonic phase evolves into clonic phase after?

Harrison's 20th Ed. Chapter 418, Page 3052

A. 10–20 seconds
B. 30–60 seconds
C. 60–120 seconds
D. 120–180 seconds

In Grand Mal seizure, initial tonic phase evolves into clonic phase after 10 - 20 seconds. Ictal phase usually lasts no more than 1 minute.

791. Postictal phase in Grand Mal seizures is characterized by all except?

Harrison's 20th Ed. Chapter 418, Page 3052

A. Irritability
B. Bladder or bowel incontinence
C. Muscular flaccidity
D. Excessive salivation

Postictal phase in Grand Mal seizures is characterized by unresponsiveness, muscular flaccidity, excessive salivation and bladder or bowel incontinence.

792. Which of the following is typical of EEG of clonic phase of Grand Mal seizure?

Harrison's 20th Ed. Chapter 418, Page 3052

A. High-amplitude activity interrupted by slow waves
B. High-amplitude activity interrupted by fast waves
C. Low-amplitude activity interrupted by slow waves
D. Low-amplitude activity interrupted by fast waves

EEG during the tonic phase of Grand Mal seizure shows a progressive increase in generalized low-voltage fast activity, followed by generalized high-amplitude, polyspike discharges. In clonic phase, high-amplitude activity is typically interrupted by slow waves to create a spike-and-slow-wave pattern.

793. Which of the following is false about atonic seizures?

Harrison's 20th Ed. Chapter 418, Page 3052

A. Sudden loss of postural muscle tone
B. Consciousness is briefly impaired
C. Significant postictal confusion
D. Seen in association with known epilepsy syndromes

Atonic seizures are characterized by sudden loss of postural muscle tone lasting 1-2 seconds. Consciousness is briefly impaired, but there is usually no postictal confusion. Atonic seizures are usually seen in association with known epilepsy syndromes.

794. Myoclonic seizure is a type of?

Harrison's 20th Ed. Chapter 418, Page 3052

A. Focal seizure
B. Generalized seizure
C. Focal, generalised or unclear seizure
D. Any of the above

795. Pathologic myoclonus is mostly seen in association with?

Harrison's 20th Ed. Chapter 418, Page 3052

A. Metabolic disorders
B. Degenerative CNS diseases
C. Anoxic brain injury
D. All of the above

Pathologic myoclonus is commonly seen with metabolic disorders, degenerative CNS diseases or anoxic brain injury.

796. Myoclonic seizures are caused by?

Harrison's 20th Ed. Chapter 418, Page 3052

A. Cortical dysfunction
B. Subcortical dysfunction
C. Spinal dysfunction
D. Any of the above

Myoclonic seizures are considered to be true epileptic events becacuse they are caused by cortical (versus subcortical or spinal) dysfunction.

797. Which of the following is false about myoclonic jerks associated with syncope?

Harrison's 20th Ed. Chapter 418, Page 128

A. May be multifocal or generalized
B. Typically arrhythmic
C. Short duration (<30 seconds)
D. None of the above

Whereas tonic-clonic movements are the hallmark of a generalized seizure, myoclonic & other movements may occur in ~90% of syncopal episodes. Myoclonic jerks associated with syncope may be multifocal or generalized. They are typically arrhythmic and of short duration (<30 seconds).

798. Which of the following is false about autonomic epilepsy?

Harrison's 20th Ed. Chapter 418, Page 128

A. Cardiovascular
B. Gastrointestinal
C. Pulmonary
D. All of the above

Autonomic manifestations of seizures (autonomic epilepsy or seizures have cardiovascular, gastrointestinal, pulmonary, urogenital, pupillary, and cutaneous manifestations that are similar to the premonitory features of syncope.

799. Which of the following differentiates seizure from syncope?

Harrison's 20th Ed. Chapter 418, Page 128

A. Seizures are rarely provoked by emotions or pain
B. Loss of consciousness in seizure is longer with postictal drowsiness & disorientation
C. Fecal incontinence occurs very rarely with syncope
D. All of the above

Loss of consciousness in seizure usually lasts >5 minutes and has postictal drowsiness & disorientation, whereas reorientation occurs almost immediately after a syncopal event. Muscle aches last longer and are more severe following a seizure. Seizures, unlike syncope, are rarely provoked by emotions or pain. Incontinence of urine may occur with seizures & syncope, but fecal incontinence occurs very rarely with syncope.

800. Tornado epilepsy best relates to?

DeJong's The Neurologic Examination, 7th Ed. Page 73

A. Sleep
B. Vertigo
C. Vision
D. Hearing

Tornado epilepsy refers to vertigo due to involvement of the vestibular cortex in a seizure discharge.

801. Giant slow waves relate best with which of the following?

Harrison's 20th Ed. Chapter 418, Page 3052

A. Atonic seizures
B. Myoclonic seizure
C. Epileptic spasms
D. Atypical absence seizures

EEG in epileptic spasms which if an unclassifiable seizure disorder shows hypsarrhythmias (diffuse, giant slow waves with a chaotic background of irregular, multifocal spikes and sharp waves).

802. "Electrodecremental response" in EEG is a feature of?

Harrison's 20th Ed. Chapter 418, Page 3052

A. Atonic seizures
B. Myoclonic seizure
C. Epileptic spasms
D. Atypical absence seizures

"Electrodecremental response" or a marked suppression of EEG background is a feature of epileptic spasms.

803. Rhomboid pattern seen in electromyogram is a feature of?

Harrison's 20th Ed. Chapter 418, Page 3052

A. Atonic seizures
B. Myoclonic seizure
C. Epileptic spasms
D. Atypical absence seizures

804. Which of the following is an epilepsy syndrome?

Harrison's 20th Ed. Chapter 418, Page 3052

A. Juvenile myoclonic epilepsy (JME)
B. Lennox-Gastaut syndrome
C. Mesial temporal lobe epilepsy (MTLE)
D. All of the above

805. Which of the following gene for various epilepsy syndromes is associated with severe mental retardation?

Harrison's 20th Ed. Chapter 418, Page 3053 Table 418-2

A. CHRNA4
B. KCNQ2
C. SCN1B
D. Doublecortin

Doublecortin (Xq21-24), expressed primarily in frontal lobes directly regulates microtubule polymerization and bundling. X-linked dominant classic lissencephaly is associated with severe mental retardation and seizures in males, subcortical band heterotopia with more subtle findings in females.

806. Gene associated with autosomal dominant nocturnal frontal lobe epilepsy (ADNFLE) is?

Harrison's 20th Ed. Chapter 418, Page 3053 Table 418-2

A. CHRNA4
B. KCNQ2
C. SCN1A
D. LGI1

807. Gene associated with autosomal dominant partial epilepsy with auditory features (ADPEAF) is?
Harrison's 20th Ed. Chapter 418, Page 3053 Table 418-2

A. CHRNA4
B. KCNQ2
C. SCN1A
D. LGI1

808. Gene associated with benign familial neonatal seizures is?
Harrison's 20th Ed. Chapter 418, Page 3053 Table 418-2

A. CHRNA4
B. KCNQ2
C. SCN1A
D. LGI1

809. Gene associated with benign familial neonatal seizures is?
Harrison's 20th Ed. Chapter 418, Page 3053 Table 418-2

A. CHRNA4
B. KCNQ2
C. SCN1A
D. LGI1

810. Gene associated with autosomal dominant familial focal epilepsy with variable foci (FFEVF) is?
Harrison's 20th Ed. Chapter 418, Page 3053 Table 418-2

A. CSTB
B. DEPDC5
C. EPM2A
D. LGI1

811. Gene associated with Unverricht-Lundborg disease is?
Harrison's 20th Ed. Chapter 418, Page 3053 Table 418-2

A. CSTB
B. DEPDC5
C. EPM2A
D. LGI1

812. Seizures in Juvenile myoclonic epilepsy (JME) are most frequent in?
Harrison's 20th Ed. Chapter 418, Page 3052, N Engl J Med. 1999;340:1565

A. Morning
B. Afternoon
C. Evening
D. Night

Syndrome of JME, also known as Janz syndrome, accounts for ~7% of all cases of epilepsy. It is characterized by onset of myoclonic seizures, generalized tonic-clonic seizures, & absence seizures in adolescents (12 - 18 years) who have normal intellectual function, with EEG findings of rapid, generalized spike-wave & polyspike-wave discharges. They are most frequent in morning after awakening and can be provoked by sleep deprivation. Consciousness is preserved.

813. Which of the following statements about Lennox-Gastaut syndrome is true?
Harrison's 20th Ed. Chapter 418, Page 3052

A. Multiple seizure types
B. EEG shows slow (<3 Hz) spike-&-wave discharges
C. Impaired cognitive function
D. All of the above

Triad of Lennox-Gastaut syndrome includes multiple seizure types, slow (<3 Hz) spike-and-wave discharges on EEG and impaired cognitive function.

814. Seizure types in Lennox-Gastaut syndrome include all except?
Harrison's 20th Ed. Chapter 418, Page 3052

A. Generalized tonic-clonic
B. Atonic
C. Myoclonic
D. Atypical absence seizures

In children with Lennox-Gastaut syndrome, multiple seizure types include generalized tonic-clonic, atonic and atypical absence seizures.

815. Which of the following is a feature of epilepsia partialis continua?
N Engl J Med. 2014;371:1737-46

A. Continuous muscular clonic twitching affecting limited part of body
B. Consciousness is preserved
C. Involves the face, arms, or both
D. All of the above

Epilepsia partialis continua is defined as almost continuous (at least 1 hour) regular or irregular muscular clonic twitching affecting a limited part of the body. Consciousness is typically preserved, and the twitching most commonly involves the face, arms, or both occurring at least once every 10 seconds, typically in isolation or in clusters of 1 to 2 Hz.

816. Epilepsia Partialis Continua is seen in?
N Engl J Med. 2014;371:1737-46

A. Rasmussen's encephalitis
B. Cerebral venous sinus thrombosis
C. Hyponatremia
D. All of the above

Differential Diagnosis of Epilepsia Partialis Continua include nonprogressive causes (Vascular causes (stroke, cerebral venous sinus thrombosis), Metabolic causes (hyperosmolar hyperglycemic nonketotic syndrome, hyponatremia), Neoplasm (central nervous system neoplasm or hematologic neoplasm), Infectious or immunologic causes (human immunodeficiency virus, encephalitis), Cortical dysplasia, Mitochondrial causes or inborn error of metabolism, Perinatal central nervous system injury, Cryptogenic causes. Progressive cause include Rasmussen's encephalitis.

817. Which of the following about Rasmussen's encephalitis is false?
N Engl J Med. 2014;371:1737-46

A. Epilepsia partialis continua
B. Hemiparesis
C. Seizures are typically refractory to medication
D. None of the above

Rasmussen's encephalitis, which was first described in 1958 by Dr. Theodore Rasmussen, is a progressive neurologic disease of unknown cause. Patients typically present in childhood with focal-onset seizures, which then progress over a period of months to refractory epilepsy with progressive hemiparesis. Epilepsia partialis continua develops in approximately 50 to 90% of persons with Rasmussen's encephalitis, and fixed hemiparesis typically occurs within 2 to 3 years after the onset of seizures. Seizures are typically refractory to medication, as was the case with this patient, but glucocorticoids and intravenous immune globulin can be effective in controlling seizures. Various other immunosuppressive medications have been tried, but the most effective therapy remains hemispherectomy.

818. Most common syndrome associated with focal seizures with dyscognitive features is?
Harrison's 20th Ed. Chapter 418, Page 3053

A. Mesial temporal lobe epilepsy (MTLE)
B. Lennox-Gastaut syndrome
C. Juvenile myoclonic epilepsy (JME)
D. All of the above

Mesial temporal lobe epilepsy (MTLE) is the most common syndrome associated with focal seizures with dyscognitive features. Formerly it was known as "psychomotor epilepsy" (Gibbs et al, 1940).

819. In mesial temporal lobe epilepsy (MTLE), the characteristic MRI finding is?

Harrison's 20th Ed. Chapter 418, Page 3053

A. Hippocampal calcification
B. Hippocampal sclerosis
C. Increased signal intensity in fronto-temporal region
D. Normal MRI

On high-resolution MRI, characteristic & essential finding of MTLE is hippocampal sclerosis.

820. In mesial temporal lobe epilepsy (MTLE), the MRI finding include all except?

Harrison's 20th Ed. Chapter 418, Page 3054 Table 418-3

A. Small hippocampus
B. Small temporal lobe
C. Small temporal horn
D. Hippocampal sclerosis

MRI findings in Mesial Temporal Lobe Epilepsy Syndrome include small hippocampus, small temporal lobe, enlarged temporal horn and hippocampal sclerosis.

821. Which of the following is an MRI finding of hippocampal sclerosis?

Harrison's 20th Ed. Chapter 418, Page 3054 Table 418-1

A. Abnormal high signal intensity
B. Blurring of internal laminar architecture
C. Reduced size of hippocampus
D. All of the above

This triad of imaging findings is consistent with hippocampal sclerosis includes abnormal high signal intensity, blurring of internal laminar architecture and reduced size of hippocampus.

822. Word Hippocampus best relates to?

American Journal of Roentgenology. 1998;171:1139-46

A. Hippopotamus
B. Seahorse
C. Hippocrates
D. Snail

Hippocampus means "Seahorse".

823. Which of the following is a part of hippocampus?

American Journal of Roentgenology. 1998;171:1139-46

A. Subiculum
B. Ammon's horn
C. Dentate gyrus
D. All of the above

824. Which of the following is a part of Ammon's horn?

American Journal of Roentgenology. 1998;171:1139-46

A. CA1
B. CA2
C. CA3
D. All of the above

Hippocampus consists of 3 major regions: subiculum, hippocampus proper (Ammon's horn) & dentate gyrus. Hippocampus & dentate gyrus have a three layered cortex. Subiculum is the transition zone from the three to six layered cortex. Important regions of hippocampus proper include CA1, CA2, CA3.

825. Intracranial amobarbital or Wada test is performed for?

Harrison's 20th Ed. Chapter 418, Page 3054 Table 418-3

A. Circulation adequacy of cerebral hemispheres
B. IQ level
C. Cerebral functions are localized to which hemisphere
D. Sleep pattern

Named after Canadian neurologist Juhn A. Wada (University of British Columbia), this test is used to establish which cerebral functions are localized to which hemisphere. It is also known as the "intracarotid sodium amobarbital procedure" (ISAP) and is performed prior to ablative surgery for epilepsy and prior to tumor resection. The aim is to determine which side of the brain is responsible for certain vital cognitive functions, namely speech and memory. Sodium amobarbital is injected into one cerebral hemisphere at a time. Material-specific memory deficits on intracranial amobarbital (Wada) test is a feature of MTLE.

826. Which of the following is an idiopathic epilepsy associated with identified gene mutations?

Harrison's 20th Ed. Chapter 418, Page 3054 Table 418-2

A. Generalized epilepsy with febrile seizures plus (GEFS+)
B. Benign familial neonatal convulsions (BFNC)
C. Autosomal dominant partial epilepsy with auditory features
D. All of the above

ADNFLE, BFNC, GEFS+, ADPEAF and FFEVF are idiopathic epilepsies associated with identified gene mutations.

827. Which of the following about Generalized epilepsy with febrile seizures plus (GEFS+) is false?

Harrison's 20th Ed. Chapter 418, Page 3054 Table 418-2

A. Autosomal dominant inheritance
B. Presents with febrile seizures
C. May have variable seizure types not associated with fever
D. Autosomal recessive inheritance

"Generalized epilepsy with febrile seizures plus" is a genetic syndrome consisting of febrile seizures plus at least one other type of seizure (absence, myoclonic, atonic, or afebrile generalized tonic–clonic seizures). It has autosomal dominant inheritance.

828. Dravet's syndrome best relates to which of the following?

Harrison's 20th Ed. Chapter 418, Page 3054 Table 418-2

A. Myoclonic epilepsies due to storage diseases
B. Severe myoclonic epilepsy in infancy
C. Febrile convulsions
D. Early cryptogenic focal epilepsy

829. Which of the following gene is associated with Generalized epilepsy with febrile seizures plus (GEFS+)?

Harrison's 20th Ed. Chapter 418, Page 3054 Table 418-2

A. CHRNA4
B. SCN1A
C. KCNQ2
D. LGI1

In Generalized epilepsy with febrile seizures plus (GEFS+), mutation occurs in the SCN1A gene for the voltage-gated sodium channel which modifies gating and inactivation properties of the channel. Mutations in other sodium channel subunits (SCN2A) and GABAA receptor subunit (GABRG2 and GABRA1) have been reported.

830. Which of the following about benign familial neonatal convulsions (BFNC) is false?

Harrison's 20th Ed. Chapter 418, Page 3054 Table 418-2

A. Autosomal dominant inheritance
B. Onset in first week of life
C. Mutations in KCNQ2 (20q13.3)
D. None of the above

BFNC has autosomal dominant inheritance with onset in 1st week of life. Infants are normal with no neurologic or metabolic abnormality. Mutations have been identified in KCNQ2, gene for potassium channels on chromosomes 20q.

831. Gene responsible for progressive myoclonus epilepsy (PME) or Unverricht-Lundborg disease is?

Harrison's 20th Ed. Chapter 418, Page 3054 Table 418-2

A. LGI1
B. EPM2A
C. CSTB
D. SCN1B

Progressive myoclonus epilepsy (PME) (Unverricht-Lundborg disease) has autosomal recessive inheritance with age of onset between 6-15 years presenting as myoclonic seizures, ataxia and progressive cognitive decline. CSTB mutation causes PME.

832. Gene responsible for Autosomal dominant familial focal epilepsy with variable foci (FFEVF) is?

Harrison's 20th Ed. Chapter 418, Page 3054 Table 418-2

A. LGI1
B. EPM2A
C. CSTB
D. DEPDC5

833. Which of the following is false about progressive myoclonus epilepsy (Lafora's disease)?

Harrison's 20th Ed. Chapter 418, Page 3054 Table 418-2

A. Autosomal recessive inheritance
B. Age of onset - 6 to 19 years
C. Polyglucosan intracellular inclusion bodies
D. Gene mution in SCN1B

Gene mution occurs in EPM2A (6q24). The protein tyrosine phosphatase (PTP) - Laforin influences glycogen metabolism.

834. Gene responsible for autosomal dominant nocturnal frontal lobe epilepsy (ADNFLE) is?

Harrison's 20th Ed. Chapter 418, Page 3054 Table 418-2

A. CHRNA4
B. EPM2A
C. CSTB
D. SCN1B

Autosomal dominant nocturnal frontal lobe epilepsy (ADNFLE) occurs during childhood & presents as brief, nighttime seizures with prominent motor movements. Gene responsible is CHRNA4 (20q13.2).

835. Which of the following about autosomal dominant partial epilepsy with auditory features (ADPEAF) is false?

Harrison's 20th Ed. Chapter 418, Page 3054 Table 418-2

A. Type of idiopathic lateral temporal lobe epilepsy
B. Age of onset usually between 10 and 25 years
C. Gene mutation in LGI1 (10q24)
D. None of the above

836. Episodic dyscontrol syndrome is also called?

Archives of Disease in Childhood 2010;95:841-842

A. Rage attacks
B. Time attacks
C. Ground attacks
D. Wall attacks

837. West syndrome includes?

DeJong's The Neurologic Examination, 7th Ed. Page 504, Lancet 1841;1:724-725

A. Infantile spasms
B. Mental retardation
C. Hypsarrhythmic EEG
D. All of the above

West syndrome is a triad of infantile spasms, mental retardation & hypsarrhythmic EEG pattern (electroclinical epileptic syndrome). The syndrome is called 'West syndrome' after Dr. West, who first described the condition in his 4-month-old son in 1841. This type of epilepsy occurs in about one in 2,500-3,000 children.

838. Characteristics of Landau-Kleffner syndrome include?

Neurology 1957;7:523-530

A. Auditory agnosia or "word deafness"
B. Normal hearing
C. Abnormal electrical brain activity
D. All of the above

A childhood disorder, in LKS there occurs gradual or sudden loss of ability to understand and use spoken language (auditory agnosia or "word deafness"). All children with LKS have abnormal EEG and may have epileptic seizures usually at night. Hearing tests show normal hearing.

839. Which of the following factor is important in the genesis of seizures and epilepsy?

Harrison's 20th Ed. Chapter 418, Page 3054

A. Endogenous factors
B. Epileptogenic factors
C. Precipitating factors
D. All of the above

Seizures & epilepsy result from a dynamic interplay between endogenous factors, epileptogenic factors and precipitating factors.

840. Which of the following schistosomes causes Jacksonian epilepsy?

Harrison's 20th Ed. Chapter 216, Page 1639

A. S. japonicum
B. S. mansoni
C. S. haematobium
D. S. mekongi

S. japonicum is associated with granulomatous lesions in brain, causing epileptic seizures, encephalopathy with headache, visual impairment, motor deficit & ataxia.

841. Which of the following schistosomes is associated with transverse myelitis?

Harrison's 20th Ed. Chapter 216, Page 1552

A. S. japonicum
B. S. intercalatum
C. S. haematobium
D. S. mekongi

842. Which of the following schistosomes is associated with transverse myelitis?

Harrison's 20th Ed. Chapter 216, Page 1552

A. S. japonicum
B. S. mansoni
C. S. intercalatum
D. S. mekongi

843. Which of the following schistosomes presents with urinary manifestations?

Harrison's 20th Ed. Chapter 216, Page 1552

A. S. japonicum
B. S. haematobium
C. S. intercalatum
D. S. mekongi

CNS schistosomiasis presents as Jacksonian epilepsy due to S. japonicum infection. S. mansoni & S. haematobium infections have been associated with transverse myelitis. S. haematobium infection leads to dysuria, frequency and hematuria.

844. Which of the following is false about seizures due to inborn errors of metabolism?

Harrison's 20th Ed. Chapter 418, Page 3054

A. Occur once regular feeding begins
B. Occur typically 2 - 3 days after birth
C. Idiosyncratic side effect to Valproic acid common
D. None of the above

Seizures due to inborn errors of metabolism usually present once regular feeding begins, typically 2-3 days after birth.

845. Pyridoxine deficiency causes seizures during?

Harrison's 20th Ed. Chapter 418, Page 3054

A. Neonatal period (<1 month)
B. Infants and children (>1 month and <12 years)
C. Adolescents (12–18 years)
D. Young adults (18–35 years)

Pyridoxine (vitamin B6) deficiency is an important cause of neonatal seizures.

846. Febrile seizures have a peak incidence between?

Harrison's 20th Ed. Chapter 418, Page 3054

A. 1 and 3 months
B. 3 and 9 months
C. 9 and 18 months
D. 18 and 24 months

Febrile seizures usually occur between 3 months and 5 years of age and have a peak incidence between 18 and 24 months.

847. Febrile seizure is likely to occur during?

Harrison's 20th Ed. Chapter 418, Page 3054

A. Rising phase of temperature curve
B. Peak of temperature curve
C. Declining phase of temperature curve
D. Any of the above

Febrile seizure is likely to occur during rising phase of the temperature curve i.e. during 1st day.

848. Which of the following is false about simple febrile seizure?

Harrison's 20th Ed. Chapter 418, Page 3054

A. Single, isolated event
B. Brief in duration
C. Symmetric in appearance
D. None of the above

A simple febrile seizure is a single, isolated event, brief in duration and symmetric in appearance. Simple febrile seizures are not associated with an increase in risk of developing epilepsy subsequently.

849. Which of the following is false about complex febrile seizures?

Harrison's 20th Ed. Chapter 418, Page 3054

A. Duration > 15 minutes
B. Repeated seizure activity
C. Not associated with increased risk of developing epilepsy
D. Focal features

Complex febrile seizures are characterized by repeated seizure activity, duration >15 minutes, or by focal features. Recurrences are more likely when febrile seizure occurs in first year of life. Complex febrile seizures have a risk of 2–5% of developing epilepsy subsequently.

850. Mild head injury is defined as a concussion with amnesia or loss of consciousness of?

Harrison's 20th Ed. Chapter 418, Page 3055

A. < 30 minutes
B. < 45 minutes
C. < 60 minutes
D. .< 90 minutes

Mild head injury is defined as a concussion with amnesia or loss of consciousness of <30 minutes.

851. Primary epilepsy syndromes present during which of the following age groups?

Harrison's 20th Ed. Chapter 418, Page 3055 Table 418-4

A. Neonatal period (<1 month)
B. Infants and children (>1 month and <12 years)
C. Adolescents (12–18 years)
D. Young adults (18–35 years)

852. Seizure disorder due to brain tumor is seen in which of the following age groups?

Harrison's 20th Ed. Chapter 418, Page 3055 Table 418-4

A. Adolescents (12–18 years)
B. Young adults (18–35 years)
C. Older adults (> 35 years)
D. All of the above

853. Hypocalcemia or hypomagnesemia are a cause of seizure disorder in which of the following age groups?

Harrison's 20th Ed. Chapter 418, Page 3055 Table 418-4

A. Neonatal period (<1 month)
B. Infants and children (>1 month and <12 years)
C. Adolescents (12–18 years)
D. Young adults (18–35 years)

854. Which of the following anti-tubercular drug cause epilepsy?

Harrison's 20th Ed. Chapter 418, Page 3056 Table 418-5

A. Isoniazid
B. Rifampin
C. Pyrazinamide
D. Ethambutol

855. Which of the following analgesics can cause epilepsy?

Harrison's 20th Ed. Chapter 418, Page 3056 Table 418-5

A. Aspirin
B. Diclofenac sodium
C. Tramadol
D. Nimusilide

856. Which of the following antimicrobial/antiviral can cause epilepsy?

Harrison's 20th Ed. Chapter 418, Page 3056 Table 418-5

A. Quinolones
B. Acyclovir
C. Ganciclovir
D. All of the above

857. Which of the following antimalarials can cause seizure?

Harrison's 20th Ed. Chapter 418, Page 3056 Table 418-5

A. Mefloquine
B. Quinine
C. Artemether
D. Halofantrine

Antimalarials - chloroquine and mefloquine can cause seizure.

858. Acute seizure in older adults is mostly due to?

Harrison's 20th Ed. Chapter 418, Page 3055

A. Embolic stroke
B. Hemorrhagic stroke
C. Thrombotic stroke
D. All of the above

Acute seizures occurring at the time of stroke are seen more often with embolic rather than hemorrhagic or thrombotic stroke. Chronic seizures are associated with all forms of stroke.

859. Diseases due to ion-channel mutations "channelopathies" include?

N Engl J Med. 2003;349:1257-66

A. Episodic ataxia
B. Familial hemiplegic migraine
C. Long-QT syndrome
D. All of the above

Ion-channel mutations "channelopathies" are characterized by paroxysmal episodes of neurologic or cardiac dysfunction, include episodic ataxia, periodic paralysis, familial hemiplegic migraine, and the long-QT syndrome.

860. The initial bursting activity in seizure is caused by?

Harrison's 20th Ed. Chapter 418, Page 3055

A. Influx of extracellular calcium (Ca^{2+})
B. Opening of voltage-dependent sodium (Na^+) channels
C. Gamma-aminobutyric acid (GABA) receptors
D. All of the above

861. Hyperpolarizing after potential during seizure is mediated by?

Harrison's 20th Ed. Chapter 418, Page 3055

A. Influx of extracellular calcium (Ca^{2+})
B. Opening of voltage-dependent sodium (Na^+) channels
C. Gamma-aminobutyric acid (GABA) receptors
D. All of the above

The initiation phase of focal seizure activity is characterized by two concurrent events in an aggregate of neurons: (1) high-frequency bursts of action potentials and (2) hypersynchronization. The bursting activity is caused by a relatively long-lasting depolarization of the neuronal membrane due to influx of extracellular calcium (Ca^{2+}), which leads to the opening of voltage-dependent sodium (Na^+) channels, influx of Na^+, and generation of repetitive action potentials. This is followed by a hyperpolarizing after potential mediated by gamma-aminobutyric acid (GABA) receptors or potassium (K^+) channels, depending on cell type.

862. Which of the following is a co-agonist of glutamate at the NMDA receptor?

Harrison's 20th Ed. Chapter 418, Page 3055

A. Tyrosine
B. Glycine
C. L-tryptophan
D. Arginine

Glycine is a co-agonist of glutamate at the (N-methyl D-aspartate) NMDA receptor. NMDA glutaminergic receptors are excitatory.

863. Which of the following is an analogue of glutamate?

Harrison's 20th Ed. Chapter 418, Page 3056

A. Glunamic acid
B. Tranaxemic acid
C. Tritoin acid
D. Domoic acid

Domoic acid is an analogue of glutamate (principal excitatory neurotransmitter in brain), causes profound seizures via direct activation of excitatory amino acid receptors throughout CNS.

864. Which of the following about gamma-aminobutyric acid (GABA) is false?

Harrison's 20th Ed. Chapter 418, Page 3056

A. GABA is an inhibitory neurotransmitter in adult CNS
B. $GABA_A$ receptors are located postsynaptically
C. $GABA_B$ receptors are located presynaptically
D. None of the above

865. Which of the following is a precipitant of epilepsy?

Harrison's 20th Ed. Chapter 418, Page 3056

A. Psychological or physical stress
B. Sleep deprivation
C. Hormonal changes with menstrual cycle
D. All of the above

Precipitating factors of epilepsy include sleep deprivation, fever, hypoxia, systemic diseases, electrolyte or metabolic derangements, acute infection, drugs that lower the seizure threshold, or alcohol or illicit drug use/withdrawal.

866. Pronator drift is an indicator of?

Harrison's 20th Ed. Chapter 418, Page 3027

A. Lower motor neuron weakness
B. Upper motor neuron weakness
C. Muscle wasting
D. Sensory neuropathy

Pronator drift is a pathologic sign and indicates UMN type weakness. Person is asked to extend arms by 90 degrees, supinate forearms, close eyes and hold the position. If a forearm pronates then the person is said to have pronator drift on that side.

867. Antiepileptic drug that acts by potentiation of GABA receptor function is?

Harrison's 20th Ed. Chapter 418, Page 3057

A. Phenytoin
B. Lamotrigine
C. Benzodiazepine
D. Valproic acid

868. Antiepileptic drug that acts by increasing the availability of GABA is?

Harrison's 20th Ed. Chapter 418, Page 3057

A. Phenytoin
B. Lamotrigine
C. Benzodiazepine
D. Valproic acid

869. Antiepileptic drug that acts by increasing the availability of GABA is?

Harrison's 20th Ed. Chapter 418, Page 3057

A. Tiagabine
B. Valproic acid
C. Gabapentin
D. All of the above

870. Antiepileptic drug that acts by decreasing glutamate release is?

Harrison's 20th Ed. Chapter 418, Page 3057

A. Phenytoin
B. Lamotrigine
C. Benzodiazepine
D. Valproic acid

871. Antiepileptic drug that acts by inhibiting voltage-gated Ca++ channels is?

Harrison's 20th Ed. Chapter 418, Page 3057

A. Phenytoin
B. Lamotrigine
C. Benzodiazepine
D. Valproic acid

Antiepileptic drugs that act by inhibiting Na+ dependent action potentials are phenytoin, carbamazepine, lamotrigine, topiramate, zonisamide, lacosamide & rufinamide. One that acts by inhibiting voltage-gated Ca^{++} channels are phenytoin, gabapentin & pregabalin while lamotrigine, topiramate & felbamate act by decreasing glutamate release. Ezogabine acts by facilitating opening of potassium channels. Benzodiazepines & barbiturates potentiate GABA receptor function, while valproic acid, gabapentin & tiagabine increase availability of GABA. Ethosuximide & valproic acid act by inhibiting T-type Ca^{++} channels in thalamic neurons.

872. Which of the following is a glutamate receptor?

Front. Mol. Neurosci. 2018;11:217

A. AMPA
B. Kainate (Ka)
C. NMDA
D. All of the above

Major excitatory neurotransmitter is amino acid glutamate. Glutamate receptors are postsynaptic. Ionotropic subclasses are alpha-amino-2,3-dihydro-5-methyl-3-oxo-4-isoxazolepropanoic acid (AMPA), kainate receptors (Ka) & N-methyl-D-aspartate (NMDA). These allow ion influx upon activation by glutamate.

873. Antagonists to which of the following glutamate receptor suppresses seizure activity?

Front. Mol. Neurosci. 2018;11:217

A. AMPA
B. Kainate (Ka)
C. NMDA
D. All of the above

NMDA, AMPA & kainate agonists induce seizure activity, whereas their antagonists suppress seizure activity.

874. Which of the following is a $GABA_B$ agonist?

Front. Mol. Neurosci. 2018;11:217

A. Baclofen
B. Barbiturate
C. Benzodiazepine
D. All of the above

$GABA_A$ receptor agonists are barbiturates and benzodiazepines. They suppress seizure activity. $GABA_B$ receptors agonist is baclofen and exacerbates hyperexcitability and seizures.

875. In an individual known to have epilepsy, initial routine interictal EEG may be normal up to what percentage of time?

Harrison's 20th Ed. Chapter 418, Page 3059

A. 10%
B. 30%
C. 60%
D. 75%

In an individual known to have epilepsy, the initial routine interictal EEG may be normal up to 60% of the time.

876. Which of the following investigation can be useful to localize potential seizure foci?

Harrison's 20th Ed. Chapter 418, Page 3059

A. EEG
B. Magnetoencephalography (MEG)
C. Magnetic source image (MSI)
D. MRI

Magnetic source image (MSI) can be useful to localize potential seizure foci.

877. Which of the following about EEG is false?

Harrison's 20th Ed. Chapter 418, Page 3059

A. Presence of epileptiform activity is not specific for epilepsy
B. In epileptic, initial interictal EEG is normal in ~ 60%
C. A normal EEG implies a better prognosis
D. None of the above

878. Which of the following is useful in the evaluation of a patient with epilepsy?

Harrison's 20th Ed. Chapter 418, Page 3059

A. FLAIR
B. SPECT
C. PET
D. All of the above

FLAIR has increased sensitivity for detection of abnormalities of cortical architecture. Positron emission tomography (PET) & single photon emission computed tomography (SPECT) are used to evaluate patients with medically refractory seizures.

879. FLAIR stands for?

Harrison's 20th Ed. Chapter 418, Page 3059

A. Fluid-attenuated inversion radiation
B. Fluid-augmented inversion radiography
C. Fluid-attenuated inversion radiography
D. Fluid-attenuated inversion recovery

880. Estimation of which of the following helps to distinguish between organic and psychogenic seizures?

Harrison's 20th Ed. Chapter 418, Page 3061

A. Serum insulin levels
B. Serum growth hormone levels
C. Serum prolactin levels
D. Serum vasopressin levels

Most generalized seizures and some focal seizures are accompanied by rises in serum prolactin during the immediate 30 minute postictal period, whereas psychogenic seizures are not. Peripheral WBC count also increase significantly after a generalized seizure.

881. "Reflex epilepsy" best relates to?

Harrison's 20th Ed. Chapter 418, Page 3061

A. Alcohol intake
B. Sleep deprivation
C. Specific music or an individual's voice
D. Physical exertion

Seizures that are induced by highly specific stimuli such as a video game monitor, music, or an individual's voice are categorized as "reflex epilepsy".

882. Risk factors associated with recurrent seizures include?

Harrison's 20th Ed. Chapter 418, Page 3061

A. Abnormal neurologic examination
B. Seizures presenting as status epilepticus
C. Abnormal EEG
D. All of the above

Risk factors associated with recurrent seizures include an abnormal neurologic examination, seizures presenting as status epilepticus, postictal Todd's paralysis, strong family history of seizures, an abnormal EEG.

883. In EEG, rhythmic activity of vertically oriented pyramidal cells of cerebral cortex normally recorded represents?

Harrison's 20th Ed. Chapter 418, Page 3057

A. Presynaptic potentials
B. Postsynaptic potentials
C. Difference of Pre- and Postsynaptic potentials
D. None of the above

The rhythmic activity normally recorded represents the postsynaptic potentials of vertically oriented pyramidal cells of the cerebral cortex and is characterized by its frequency..

884. In EEG, which of the following rhythm is faster than alpha rhythm?

Harrison's 20th Ed. Chapter 418, Page 3057

A. Beta
B. Theta
C. Delta
D. All of the above

EEG waveforms are divided into four major frequency bands: delta (0–3⁺ Hz), theta (4–7⁺ Hz), alpha (8–13 Hz), and beta (>14 Hz). They are named in Greek order of historical discovery rather than low to high frequency numbers Muscle artifact is high amplitude irregular activity, usually in the frequency range of about 20–50 Hz.

885. Out of the following, which is the slowest frequency in EEG?

Harrison's 20th Ed. Chapter 418, Page 3057

A. Alpha
B. Beta
C. Theta
D. Delta

886. "Posterior dominant rhythm" is also called?

Harrison's 20th Ed. Chapter 418, Page 3057

A. Alpha rhythm
B. Beta rhythm
C. Theta rhythm
D. Delta rhythm

A symmetrical rhythm is observed over the posterior head regions during relaxed wakefulness with eyes closed, that undergoes amplitude attenuation with eye opening or mental alerting activities. It is called the posterior dominant rhythm or alpha rhythm, as in adults it has a frequency of 8–13 Hz. Alpha rhythm is also called Berger rhythm.

887. Which rhythm produces an underlying undulation of EEG?

Harrison's 20th Ed. Chapter 418, Page 3057

A. Alpha rhythm
B. Beta rhythm
C. Theta rhythm
D. Delta rhythm

Delta activity produces an underlying undulation of EEG. Riding on top of delta activity may be frequencies in the other bands, such as components of alpha & high frequency "jittery" activity in the beta range.

888. In EEG, calibration marker shows what level of voltage as standard?

Britton JW. American Epilepsy Society; 2016

A. 1 microvolt
B. 10 microvolt
C. 100 microvolt
D. 1000 microvolt

Each EEG channel is a record of voltage over time. The calibration marker shows one second and 100-microvolt standards.

889. Normal EEG background voltages are in the range of?

Britton JW. American Epilepsy Society; 2016

A. 10–20 microvolts
B. 20–50 microvolts
C. 30–100 microvolts
D. 40–150 microvolts

Normal EEG background voltages are in the range of 30–100 microvolts.

890. Which of the following about alpha rhythm is false?

Britton JW. American Epilepsy Society; 2016

A. Most prominent when subject is quietly relaxed with eyes closed, but not asleep
B. Waxing and waning
C. Higher on right side of the brain
D. None of the above

Alpha rhythm is 8 and 12 Hz, waxing and waning, with a posterior maximum, (parieto-occipital). It can spread into any electrodes of 10–20 system except Fp1 & Fp2. It is most prominent when subject is quietly relaxed with eyes closed, but not asleep. Alpha rhythm usually is higher on right side of brain.

891. Which of the following medication increase β activity in EEG?

Britton JW. American Epilepsy Society; 2016

A. Barbiturates
B. Benzodiazepines
C. Chloral hydrate
D. All of the above

Beta activity is a fast rhythm of 13 per second and greater, is visualized on the EEG as a "jitteriness" of the trace. Barbiturates, benzodiazepines and chloral hydrate increase beta activity.

892. In EEG, which of the following signifies an encephalopathy?

Britton JW. American Epilepsy Society; 2016

A. Localized slow frequency
B. Localized fast frequency
C. Diffuse slow frequency
D. Diffuse fast frequency

Alterations of brain function results in abnormal slow frequency activity in EEG. Diffuse slow activity signifies an encephalopathy.

893. In EEG, which of the following suggest epileptiform activity?

Britton JW. American Epilepsy Society; 2016

A. Spikes
B. Sharp waves
C. Spike-wave complexes
D. Any of the above

Epileptiform activity characteristic of epilepsy includes spikes, sharp waves and spike-wave complexes.

894. Each EEG electrode can detect synchronous activity generated by how much area of surface cerebral cortex?

Britton JW. American Epilepsy Society; 2016

A. ~ 3 sq. cm.
B. ~ 6 sq. cm.
C. ~ 9 sq. cm.
D. ~ 12 sq. cm.

Each EEG electrode can detect synchronous activity generated by ~ 6 sq. cm. of cortex.

895. Usually, EEG is performed after how many hours after a seizure episode?

N Engl J Med. 2001;344:1146

A. 6 hours
B. 12 hours
C. 24 hours
D. 48 hours

896. EEG should include recordings during?

N Engl J Med. 2001;344:1146

A. Sleep
B. Photic stimulation
C. Hyperventilation
D. All of the above

It is customary to perform EEG 48 hours or more after a suspected seizure, because EEG shortly after a seizure may give misleading findings. To provoke abnormalities, EEG should be recorded during sleep, sleep deprivation, photic stimulation, and hyperventilation (Activating procedures).

897. Electrocerebral silence is observed in?

Britton JW. American Epilepsy Society; 2016

A. Irreversible brain damage
B. Hypothermia
C. Drug overdose
D. All of the above

In electrocerebral silence, there is a reduction in amplitude of EEG until activity cannot be detected. It happens in irreversible brain damage, hypothermic patients or with drug overdose.

898. In visual evoked potentials (VEPs), the component of major clinical importance is?

J Neurol Neurosurg Psychiatry 2005;76(Suppl II):ii16–ii22

A. P100 response
B. P200 response
C. P300 response
D. P400 response

Visual evoked potentials (VEPs) are elicited by monocular stimulation with a reversing checkerboard pattern and are recorded from the occipital region in the midline and on either side of scalp. The component of major clinical importance is P100 response, a positive peak having a latency of approximately 100 ms.

899. VEPs are most useful in detecting dysfunction of visual pathways at the level?

J Neurol Neurosurg Psychiatry 2005;76(Suppl II):ii16–ii22

A. Anterior to optic chiasm
B. Optic chiasm
C. Optic radiation
D. Visual cortex

VEPs are most useful in detecting dysfunction of the visual pathways anterior to the optic chiasm. In acute severe optic neuritis, P100 is frequently lost or grossly attenuated and as clinical recovery occurs and visual acuity improves, P100 is restored. VEP findings are helpful in indicating previous or subclinical optic neuritis. In cortical blindness, VEPs may be normal. Multifocal VEP is likely to be more sensitive than routine VEP.

900. Which of the following statements is false about EEG?

Britton JW. American Epilepsy Society; 2016

A. Normal EEG shows posteriorly situated 8-13 Hz a rhythm
B. Alpha rhythm attenuates with eye opening
C. Right-sided placements are indicated by even numbers, left-sided placements by odd numbers
D. Midline placements are indicated by M

Right-sided electrode placements are indicated by even numbers, left-sided placements by odd numbers, and midline placements by Z.

901. Delta activity in EEG is seen in which stage of Hepatic Encephalopathy?

Harrison's 20th Ed. Chapter 300, Page 2073

A. Stage I
B. Stage II
C. Stage III
D. Stage IV

Hepatic encephalopathy is associated with triphasic or δ waves.

902. In EEG, periodic lateralized epileptiform discharges (PLEDs) is typical of?

Britton JW. American Epilepsy Society; 2016

A. Subacute sclerosing panencephalitis (SSPE)
B. Herpes simplex encephalitis
C. Jakob-Creutzfeldt disease
D. Hepatic encephalopathy

In EEG, periodic lateralized epileptiform discharges (PLEDs) is typical of herpes simplex encephalitis.

903. The specific order of electrode pairs is called?

Britton JW. American Epilepsy Society; 2016

A. Montage
B. Prelage
C. Consure
D. Primark

The specific order of electrode pairs is called a montage.

904. Which of the following statements about therapeutic range of antiepileptic drugs is false?

Harrison's 20th Ed. Chapter 418, Page 3061 Table 418-8

A.	Carbamazepine	15 - 20 μg/ml
B.	Valproic acid	50 - 100 μg/ml
C.	Phenytoin	10 - 20 μg/ml
D.	Phenobarbital	15 - 40 μg/ml

Therapeutic range of Carbamazepine is 4–10 μg/ml. Ethosuximide 40–100 μg/ml, Primidone 5–12 μg/ml, Lamotrigine 3–14 μg/ml, Levetiracetam 5–30 μg/ml, Gabapentin 2–20 μg/ml.

905. Which of the following is the first-line medication in focal seizures?

Harrison's 20th Ed. Chapter 418, Page 3061 Table 418-8

A. Valproic acid
B. Lamotrigine
C. Topiramate
D. Ethosuximide

906. Which of the following is the first-line medication in typical absence seizures?

Harrison's 20th Ed. Chapter 418, Page 3061 Table 418-8

A. Valproic acid
B. Levetiracetam
C. Carbamazepine
D. Phenytoin

907. Which of the following is the first-line medication in atypical absence seizures?

Harrison's 20th Ed. Chapter 418, Page 3061 Table 418-8

A. Valproic acid
B. Phenytoin
C. Carbamazepine
D. Ethosuximide

908. Which of the following is the first-line medication in myoclonic seizures?

Harrison's 20th Ed. Chapter 418, Page 3061 Table 418-8

A. Valproic acid
B. Phenytoin
C. Carbamazepine
D. Ethosuximide

909. Which of the following is not a first-line medication in seizures?

Harrison's 20th Ed. Chapter 418, Page 3061 Table 418-8

A. Valproic acid
B. Lamotrigine
C. Carbamazepine
D. Gabapentin

910. Which of the following anti-epileptic drugs is preferred in Lennox-Gastaut syndrome?

Harrison's 20th Ed. Chapter 418, Page 3062 Table 418-9

A. Phenobarbital
B. Valproic acid
C. Gabapentin
D. Lamotrigine

Anti-epileptic drugs useful in Lennox-Gastaut syndrome include Lamotrigine, Topiramate, Felbamate, Rufinamide. Corpus callosotomy has been shown to be effective for disabling tonic or atonic seizures, usually when they are part of a mixed-seizure syndrome (e.g., Lennox-Gastaut syndrome).

911. Which of the following anti-epileptic drugs does not have significant drug interactions?

Harrison's 20th Ed. Chapter 418, Page 3062 Table 418-9

A. Phenobarbital
B. Valproic acid
C. Gabapentin
D. Lamotrigine

912. Which of the following anti-epileptic medications have enzyme-inducing effects?

Harrison's 20th Ed. Chapter 418, Page 3062 Table 418-9

A. Phenytoin
B. Phenobarbital
C. Primidone
D. All of the above

Enzyme-inducing anti-epileptic drugs (phenytoin, carbamazepine, oxcarbazepine, topiramate, phenobarbital, and primidone) cause a transient and reversible deficiency of vitamin K–dependent clotting factors in about 50% of newborn infants.

913. Carbamazepine and phenytoin are contraindicated in which of the following epilepsies?

N Engl J Med. 1999;340:1565

A. Juvenile myoclonic epilepsy (JME)
B. Absence seizures
C. Myoclonic seizures
D. All of the above

Carbamazepine, oxcarbazepine, and phenytoin can worsen certain types of generalized seizures, including absence, myoclonic, tonic, and atonic seizures.

914. Which of the following is an adverse effect of carbamazepine?

Harrison's 20th Ed. Chapter 418, Page 3062 Table 418-9

A. Leukopenia
B. Aplastic anemia
C. Hepatotoxicity
D. All of the above

Carbamazepine can cause leukopenia, aplastic anemia, or hepatotoxicity

915. Treatment of choice for juvenile myoclonic epilepsy is?

N Engl J Med. 1999;340:1565

A. Valproic acid
B. Lamotrigine
C. Acetazolamide
D. Topiramate

Valproic acid is the treatment of choice for juvenile myoclonic epilepsy, but lamotrigine, clonazepam, acetazolamide, primidone & topiramate are useful.

916. Which of the following anti-epileptic medications rarely cause skin rashes?

Harrison's 20th Ed. Chapter 418, Page 3062 Table 418-9

A. Gabapentin
B. Divalproex sodium
C. Levetiracetam
D. All of the above

917. Which of the following anti-epileptic drug causes skin rashes?

Harrison's 20th Ed. Chapter 418, Page 3062 Table 418-9

A. Gabapentin
B. Divalproex sodium
C. Levetiracetam
D. Lamotrigine

Lamotrigine causes skin rash during initiation of therapy. This can be extremely severe and lead to Stevens-Johnson syndrome if unrecognized and if the medication is not discontinued immediately.

918. What percentage of patients with epilepsy do not respond to treatment with a single antiepileptic drug?

Harrison's 20th Ed. Chapter 418, Page 3065

A. ~ one-fourth
B. ~ one-third
C. ~ one-half
D. ~ two-third

About one-third of epileptic patients do not respond to treatment with a single antiepileptic drug.

919. Most recurrences of epilepsy occur how many months after discontinuing therapy?

Harrison's 20th Ed. Chapter 418, Page 3065

A. 3 months
B. 4 months
C. 5 months
D. 6 months

Most recurrences occur in the first 3 months after discontinuing therapy.

920. Most common surgical procedure for patients with temporal lobe epilepsy involves resection of?

Harrison's 20th Ed. Chapter 418, Page 3065

A. Anteromedial temporal lobe
B. Anterolateral temporal lobe
C. Posteromedial temporal lobe
D. Posterolateral temporal lobe

Most common surgical procedure for temporal lobe epilepsy is resection of anteromedial temporal lobe.

921. One of the most specific signs of a metabolic encephalopathy is?

Harrison's 20th Ed. Chapter 300, Page 2071

A. Bilateral asterixis
B. Confusion
C. Seizure
D. Vomiting

Bilateral asterixis, a negative myoclonus, is a certain sign of metabolic encephalopathy or drug intoxication.

922. Asterixis can be found in?

Harrison's 20th Ed. Chapter 300, Page 2071

A. Any tonically held posture
B. Tonically held tongue
C. Voluntary limb motion
D. All of the above

923. In an awake patient of uremic encephalopathy, the typical movement abnormality is?

Harrison's 20th Ed. Chapter 300, Page 2071

A. Myoclonic jerking and tremor
B. Partial seizure
C. Primary generalized seizure
D. Absence seizure

924. Which of the following statements about status epilepticus is false?

Harrison's 20th Ed. Chapter 418, Page 3066

A. Continuous seizures
B. Repetitive, discrete seizures
C. Impaired consciousness in the interictal period
D. May be nonconvulsive

Status epilepticus refers to continuous seizures or repetitive, discrete seizures with impaired consciousness in the interictal period. Its subtypes include generalized convulsive status epilepticus (GCSE) and nonconvulsive status epilepticus (persistent absence seizures or focal seizures).

925. In generalized convulsive status epilepticus (GCSE), which of the following leads to irreversible neuronal injury?

Harrison's 20th Ed. Chapter 418, Page 3066

A. Cardiorespiratory dysfunction
B. Hyperthermia
C. Metabolic derangements
D. All of the above

926. Which of the following is the first medicine that is recommended for generalized tonic-clonic status epilepticus in adults?

Harrison's 20th Ed. Chapter 418, Page 3067 Figure 418-5

A. Lorazepam
B. Fosphenytoin
C. Valproate
D. Phenobarbital

Lorazepam is recommended for generalized tonic-clonic status epilepticus in adults in doses of 0.1 - 0.15 mg/kg IV over 1 - 2 minutes to be repeated once if no response is obtained after 5 minutes.

927. Which of the following drugs should be given concomitantly with lorazepam in management of status epilepticus?

Harrison's 20th Ed. Chapter 418, Page 3066

A. Carbamazepine
B. Fosphenytoin
C. Valproate
D. Phenobarbital

Lorazepam is the most effective benzodiazepine for treating status epilepticus. Phenytoin or fosphenytoin should be given concomitantly since Lorazepam has a short half-life. Other drugs, like gabapentin, carbamazepine and phenobarbital should be reserved for patients with contraindications to phenytoin (allergy or pregnancy) or ongoing seizures despite phenytoin.

928. Nonconvulsive status epilepticus best relates to?

Harrison's 20th Ed. Chapter 418, Page 3066

A. Hysterical conversion reaction
B. Epileptic coma
C. Sleep
D. Excessive exercise

Epileptic coma refers to generalized electrical seizures are associated with coma, even in the absence of motor convulsions (nonconvulsive status epilepticus).

929. Which of the following is false about "Sudden unexpected death in epileptic patients (SUDEP)?

Harrison's 20th Ed. Chapter 418, Page 3066

A. Affects young people with convulsive seizures
B. Tends to occur at night
C. May result from brainstem-mediated effects of seizures on cardiac rhythms or pulmonary function
D. None of the above

Sudden unexpected death in epileptic patients (SUDEP) affects young people with convulsive seizures and tends to occur at night. It may result from brainstem-mediated effects of seizures on cardiac rhythms or pulmonary function.

930. Which of the following drug is effective as adjunctive therapy in catamenial epilepsy?

Harrison's 20th Ed. Chapter 418, Page 3067

A. Prednisolone
B. Beta blockers
C. Medroxyprogesterone
D. Diuretics

There may be an increase in seizure frequency around menses due to effects of estrogen or progesterone on neuronal excitability or changes in antiepileptic drug levels due to altered protein binding. Natural progestins or intramuscular medroxyprogesterone may be of benefit to a subset of women.

931. During pregnancy, seizure frequency decreases in what percentage of women?

Harrison's 20th Ed. Chapter 418, Page 3067

A. 10%
B. 20%
C. 30%
D. 40%

During pregnancy, seizure frequency will remain unchanged in ~50% of women, increase in 30%, and decrease in 20%.

932. Which of the following anti-epileptic medications can significantly antagonize effects of oral contraceptives?

Harrison's 20th Ed. Chapter 418, Page 3068

A. Carbamazepine
B. Phenytoin
C. Topiramate
D. All of the above

Carbamazepine, phenytoin, phenobarbital, and topiramate can significantly antagonize the effects of oral contraceptives via enzyme induction.

933. Ratio of drug concentration in breast milk relative to serum is maximum with which of the following antiepileptic drug?

Harrison's 20th Ed. Chapter 418, Page 3068

A. Levetiracetam
B. Phenobarbital
C. Carbamazepine
D. Phenytoin

934. Ratio of drug concentration in breast milk relative to serum is minimum with which of the following antiepileptic drug?

Harrison's 20th Ed. Chapter 418, Page 3068

A. Valproic acid
B. Phenobarbital
C. Carbamazepine
D. Phenytoin

Ratio of drug concentration in breast milk relative to serum is 300% for levetiracetam, ~80% for ethosuximide, 40–60% for phenobarbital, 40% for carbamazepine, 15% for phenytoin, and 5% for valproic acid.

935. Neonatal unconjugated hyperbilirubinemia & resultant clinical jaundice affect what percentage of newborns?

N Engl J Med. 2013;369:2021-30

A. Approximately 35%
B. Approximately 55%
C. Approximately 70%
D. Approximately 85%

Neonatal unconjugated hyperbilirubinemia & resultant clinical jaundice affect up to approximately 85% of newborns.

936. Which out of the following best relates to kernicterus?

N Engl J Med. 2013;369:2021-30

A. Acute bilirubin encephalopathy
B. Chronic bilirubin encephalopathy
C. Hyperoxic brain injury
D. None of the above

937. Which of the following is a feature of Kernicterus?

N Engl J Med. 2013;369:2021-30

A. Extrapyramidal movement disorders
B. Auditory neuropathy spectrum disorders
C. Oculomotor pareses
D. All of the above

938. In Kernicterus, bilirubin-induced neuropathology is seen in which of the following?

N Engl J Med. 2013;369:2021-30

A. Globus pallidus
B. Hippocampal CA2 neurons
C. Cerebellar Purkinje's cells
D. All of the above

Kernicterus or chronic bilirubin encephalopathy is a permanent disabling neurologic condition that is classically characterized by the extrapyramidal movement disorders of dystonia, choreoathetosis, or both; hearing loss due to auditory neuropathy spectrum disorders; and oculomotor pareses. These central nervous system (CNS) sequelae reflect the regional CNS topography of bilirubin-induced neuropathology, which involves the globus pallidus, subthalamic nucleus, brainstem nuclei, hippocampal CA2 neurons, and cerebellar Purkinje's cells.

939. Medical condition that increases risk of severe hyperbilirubinemia or bilirubin neurotoxicity is?

N Engl J Med. 2013;369:2021-30

A. Glucose-6-phosphate dehydrogenase deficiency
B. Rh isoimmunization
C. Sepsis
D. All of the above

Medical conditions that increase the risk of severe hyperbilirubinemia or bilirubin neurotoxicity, such as glucose-6-phosphate dehydrogenase deficiency, Rh isoimmunization, and sepsis.

940. Phenobarbital increases bilirubin clearance by activating the phenobarbital enhancer module in promoter sequence of?

N Engl J Med. 2013;369:2021-30

A. MRP2
B. UGT1A1
C. FIC1
D. BSEP

Phenobarbital increases bilirubin clearance by activating the phenobarbital enhancer module in the promoter sequence of bilirubin-UDP-glucuronosyltransferase (UGT1A1), which enhances bilirubin conjugation.

941. Which of the following has protective effect against bilirubin-induced neuromotor dysfunction?

N Engl J Med. 2013;369:2021-30

A. Ciprofloxacin
B. Rifampin
C. Minocycline
D. Atorvastatin

Minocycline has protective effect against bilirubin-induced neuromotor dysfunction, cerebellar hypoplasia & auditory-pathway abnormalities in Gunn rat pups.

Cerebrovascular Diseases

942. By definition, neurologic signs and symptoms of transient ischemic attack (TIA) last for less than?

Harrison's 20th Ed. Chapter 419, Page 3068

A. < 1 hour

B. < 6 hours

C. < 12 hours

D. < 24 hours

Typically the neurologic signs and symptoms of a TIA last for 5 to 15 minutes but, by definition, must last for <24 hours, without evidence of brain infarction on brain imaging.

943. A generalized reduction in cerebral blood flow due to systemic hypotension produces?

Harrison's 20th Ed. Chapter 419, Page 3068

A. Syncope

B. Transient ischemic attack

C. Hypoxic-ischemic encephalopathy

D. Any of the above

A generalized reduction in cerebral blood flow due to systemic hypotension (cardiac arrhythmia, myocardial infarction or hemorrhagic shock) usually produces syncope.

944. Focal brain ischemia or infarction is usually caused by?

Harrison's 20th Ed. Chapter 419, Page 3068

A. Thrombosis of cerebral vessels

B. Emboli from a proximal arterial source

C. Emboli from the heart

D. All of the above

Focal brain ischemia or infarction is caused by thrombosis of cerebral vessels or by emboli from a proximal arterial source or heart.

945. Neurologic symptoms in intracranial hemorrhage is caused by?

Harrison's 20th Ed. Chapter 419, Page 3068

A. Mass effect on neural structures

B. From the toxic effects of blood itself

C. By increasing intracranial pressure

D. All of the above

Intracranial hemorrhage is caused by bleeding directly into or around the brain. It leads to neurologic symptoms by producing a mass effect on neural structures, from the toxic effects of blood itself, or by increasing intracranial pressure.

946. Acute stroke may begins as which of the following?

Harrison's 20th Ed. Chapter 419, Page 3068

A. Sudden severe headache

B. Change in vision

C. Change in gait

D. Any of the above

947. What percentage of ischemic stroke patients have hemiparesis?

Harrison's 20th Ed. Chapter 419, Page 3068

A. 30%

B. 50%

C. 85%

D. 100%

Acute stroke has a sudden onset of loss of sensory and/or motor function on one side of the body (nearly 85% of ischemic stroke patients have hemiparesis), change in vision, gait or ability to speak or understand; or a sudden severe headache.

948. In the acronym FAST, "S" stands for?

Harrison's 20th Ed. Chapter 419, Page 3068

A. Stroke

B. Sensory deficit

C. Speech abnormality

D. Sleep

In the acronym FAST about common physical symptoms of stroke & its treatment, F stands for Facial weakness, A for Arm weakness, S for Speech abnormality and T for Time.

949. Conditions that may mimic stroke include?

Harrison's 20th Ed. Chapter 419, Page 3069, N Engl J Med. 2000;343:710

A. Seizure

B. Metabolic encephalopathy

C. Migraine

D. All of the above

Causes of sudden-onset neurologic symptoms that may mimic stroke include hypoglycemia, seizure, intracranial tumor, (acephalgic) migraine, hypertensive encephalopathy and metabolic encephalopathy.

950. Intracranial tumor may present with acute neurologic symptoms due to?

Harrison's 20th Ed. Chapter 419, Page 3069

A. Hemorrhage

B. Seizure

C. Hydrocephalus

D. Any of the above

Intracranial tumor may present with acute neurologic symptoms due to hemorrhage, seizure or hydrocephalus.

951. Which of the following is a stroke syndrome?

Harrison's 20th Ed. Chapter 419, Page 3069

A. Large-vessel stroke within the anterior circulation

B. Large-vessel stroke within the posterior circulation

C. Small-vessel disease of anterior/posterior circulation

D. All of the above

Stroke syndromes are divided into large vessel stroke within anterior circulation, large-vessel stroke within posterior circulation and small-vessel disease of either vascular bed. Internal carotid artery & its branches comprise the anterior circulation of brain.

952. Occlusion of proximal MCA is most often due to?

Harrison's 20th Ed. Chapter 419, Page 3069

A. Embolus

B. Intracranial atherothrombosis

C. Vasospasm

D. None of the above

Occlusion of proximal MCA or one of its major branches is mostly due to embolus (artery-to-artery, cardiac, or of unknown source) rather than intracranial atherothrombosis.

953. Collateral formation via which of the following prevents MCA stenosis from becoming symptomatic?

Harrison's 20th Ed. Chapter 419, Page 3069

A. Deep penetrating arterioles
B. Venous sinuses
C. Leptomeningeal vessels
D. All of the above

Collateral formation via leptomeningeal vessels prevents MCA stenosis from becoming symptomatic.

954. Cortical branches of MCA supply which of the following?

Harrison's 20th Ed. Chapter 419, Page 3069

A. Frontal pole
B. Lower temporal pole convolution
C. Occipital pole convolution
D. None of the above

Cortical branches of MCA supply the lateral surface of hemisphere except for frontal pole and a strip along the superomedial border of frontal and parietal lobes (supplied by ACA), and lower temporal and occipital pole convolutions (supplied by PCA).

955. Lenticulostriate arteries from proximal MCA (M1 segment) supply all except?

Harrison's 20th Ed. Chapter 419, Page 3069

A. Putamen
B. Outer globus pallidus
C. Anterior limb of internal capsule
D. Body of caudate nucleus

Proximal MCA (M1 segment) gives rise to penetrating lenticulostriate arteries that supply putamen, outer globus pallidus, posterior limb of internal capsule, adjacent corona radiata & most of caudate nucleus.

956. Temporal cortex is supplied by?

Harrison's 20th Ed. Chapter 419, Page 3069

A. Inferior division of MCA
B. Superior division of MCA
C. ACA
D. PCA

MCA divides into superior & inferior divisions (M2 branches) in sylvian fissure. Branches of the inferior division supply inferior parietal and temporal cortex, and superior division supply the frontal and superior parietal cortex.

957. In a right handed person, occlusion of right MCA leads to all except?

Harrison's 20th Ed. Chapter 419, Page 3069

A. Global aphasia
B. Anosognosia
C. Constructional apraxia
D. Dysarthria

Global aphasia occurs when the dominant hemisphere is involved. When nondominant hemisphere is affected, anosognosia, constructional apraxia, and neglect are found. Contralateral hemiplegia, hemianesthesia, homonymous hemianopia occur in both instances. Dysarthria is common because of facial weakness.

958. Which of the following is a partial syndrome?

Harrison's 20th Ed. Chapter 419, Page 3071

A. Brachial syndrome
B. Broca aphasia
C. Frontal opercular syndrome
D. All of the above

959. Which of the following artery supplying dominant hemisphere is occluded in Wernicke's aphasia without weakness?

Harrison's 20th Ed. Chapter 419, Page 3071

A. Stem of MCA
B. Penetrating lenticulostriate arteries of MCA
C. Proximal superior division of MCA
D. Inferior division of MCA

If a fluent (Wernicke's) aphasia occurs without weakness, inferior division of MCA supplying posterior part (temporal cortex) of dominant hemisphere is probably involved.

960. Which of the following artery supplying the nondominant hemisphere is occluded in a case of hemineglect or spatial agnosia without weakness?

Harrison's 20th Ed. Chapter 419, Page 3071

A. Stem of MCA
B. Penetrating lenticulostriate arteries of MCA
C. Proximal superior division of MCA
D. Inferior division of MCA

Hemineglect or spatial agnosia without weakness indicates that the inferior division of MCA in the nondominant hemisphere is occluded.

961. Which of the following artery is occluded in a case of pure motor stroke contralateral to the lesion?

Harrison's 20th Ed. Chapter 419, Page 3071

A. Stem of MCA
B. Penetrating lenticulostriate arteries of MCA
C. Proximal superior division of MCA
D. Inferior division of MCA

Occlusion of a lenticulostriate vessel of MCA produces lacunar stroke within the internal capsule producing pure motor stroke or sensory-motor stroke contralateral to the lesion.

962. Lacunar infarction affecting which of the following areas produces very few clinical signs?

Harrison's 20th Ed. Chapter 419, Page 3071

A. Genu of internal capsule
B. Posterior limb of internal capsule
C. Globus pallidus and putamen
D. All of the above

Lacunar infarction affecting the globus pallidus and putamen often produce few clinical signs, but parkinsonism and hemiballismus occur.

963. Anterior cerebral artery (ACA) arises from the Internal carotid artery at the level of?

Journal of Neurosurgery 2000;93(6): 1084-1088, JMS 2018;1(1):5-9

A. Anterior clinoid process
B. Optic chiasma
C. Optic nerve
D. Olfactory trigone

Term Heubner's artery was first used in 1909 by Aitken, after Heubner's classical description of the vessel in 1872. Classically, RAH travels back on its parent ACA and passes above the carotid bifurcation and middle cerebral artery into the medial part of sylvian fissure before entering the anterior perforated substance. Anatomical variations are frequent.

964. "Recurrent artery of Heubner" supplies which part of internal capsule?

Journal of Neurosurgery 2000;93(6): 1084-1088, JMS 2018;1(1):5-9

A. Anterior limb
B. Genu
C. Posterior limb
D. Retrolentiform part

Lenticulostriate recurrent artery of Heubner (RAH) supplies blood to medial portion of orbitofrontal cortex, anterior portion of caudate nucleus, anterior third of putamen, external segment of globus pallidus, and anterior crus of internal capsule. RAH also supplies olfactory region, anterior hypothalamus, nucleus accumbens, parts of uncinate fasciculus, diagonal band of Broca, and the basal nucleus of Meynert.

965. "Recurrent artery of Heubner" is a branch of?

Journal of Neurosurgery 2000;93(6): 1084-1088, JMS 2018;1(1):5-9

A. Internal carotid artery
B. Anterior cerebral artery
C. Middle cerebral artery
D. Posterior cerebral artery

966. Which of the following is called Heubner's disease?

Journal of Neurosurgery 2000;93(6): 1084-1088, JMS 2018;1(1):5-9

A. Carcinomatous meningitis
B. Primary central nervous system vasculitis
C. Syphilitic endarteritis
D. Necrotizing arteritis

Johann Otto Leonhardt Heubner (1843-1926) described lenticulostriate recurrent artery in 1872. It can be damaged with improper clip placement during repair of aneurysms near the anterior communicating artery. He also described syphilitic endarteritis (Heubner's disease).

967. "Arteria termatica of Wilder" best relates to?

Neurology Asia 2013; 18(3):249–259

A. Internal carotid artery
B. Anterior cerebral artery
C. Middle cerebral artery
D. Posterior cerebral artery

Wilder was the first to describe fusion of both A2 segments to form a single artery & introduced the term arteria termatica of Wilder in 1885. Also known as the unpaired pericallosal stem artery, unpaired anterior cerebral artery, common anterior cerebral trunk & azygos pericallosal artery.

968. Which of the following is not supplied by the deep penetrating branches of the A1 segment of ACA?

Harrison's 20th Ed. Chapter 419, Page 3071

A. Anterior limb of internal capsule
B. Amygdala
C. Body of caudate nucleus
D. Anterior hypothalamus

The A1 segment of anterior cerebral artery (ACA) gives rise to deep penetrating branches that supply the anterior limb of internal capsule, anterior perforate substance, amygdala, anterior hypothalamus, and inferior part of the head of caudate nucleus.

969. Occlusion of a single A2 segment of anterior cerebral artery (ACA) results in which of the following?

Harrison's 20th Ed. Chapter 419, Page 3071

A. Abulia
B. Bilateral pyramidal signs with paraparesis
C. Urinary incontinence
D. All of the above

Occlusion of a single A2 segment of ACA results in profound abulia, bilateral pyramidal signs with paraparesis and urinary incontinence.

970. Anterior choroidal artery arises from?

Harrison's 20th Ed. Chapter 419, Page 3071

A. Internal carotid artery
B. Middle cerebral artery
C. Anterior cerebral artery
D. Posterior cerebral artery

Anterior choroidal artery arises from ICA & supplies posterior limb of internal capsule & white matter posterolateral to it, through which geniculocalcarine fibers pass partly.

971. Complete syndrome of anterior choroidal artery occlusion consists of?

Harrison's 20th Ed. Chapter 419, Page 3071

A. Contralateral hemiplegia
B. Hemianesthesia
C. Homonymous hemianopia
D. All of the above

The complete syndrome of anterior choroidal artery occlusion consists of contralateral hemiplegia, hemianesthesia and homonymous hemianopia.

972. Anterior choroidal strokes are usually the result of?

Harrison's 20th Ed. Chapter 419, Page 3071

A. Embolus
B. In situ Thrombosis
C. Vasospasm
D. None of the above

Anterior choroidal strokes are usually the result of in situ thrombosis, and iatrogenic occlusion during surgical clipping of aneurysms of ICA.

973. "Fetal posterior cerebral artery" refers to?

Harrison's 20th Ed. Chapter 419, Page 3072

A. Single PCA
B. Absent PCA
C. PCA arising from internal carotid artery (ICA)
D. PCA arising from MCA

Anatomic configuration of PCA arising from ICA is called fetal posterior cerebral artery (20%).

974. Bilateral common carotid artery occlusions at their origin may occur in?

Harrison's 20th Ed. Chapter 419, Page 3072

A. Temporal arteritis
B. Takayasu's arteritis
C. Kawasaki disease
D. Polyarteritis nodosa

Bilateral common carotid artery occlusions at their origin may occur in Takayasu's arteritis.

975. The vertebral arteries join to form the basilar artery at?

Harrison's 20th Ed. Chapter 419, Page 3072

A. Foramen magnum
B. Lower medulla oblongata
C. Pontomedullary junction
D. Interpeduncular fossa

Vertebral arteries join to form basilar artery at the pontomedullary junction.

976. Basilar artery divides into two posterior cerebral arteries at?

Harrison's 20th Ed. Chapter 419, Page 3072

A. Foramen magnum
B. Lower medulla oblongata
C. Pontomedullary junction
D. Interpeduncular fossa

Basilar artery divides into two posterior cerebral arteries in the interpeduncular fossa.

977. Posterior circulation supplies which of the following?

Harrison's 20th Ed. Chapter 419, Page 3072

A. Hippocampus
B. Medial temporal lobes
C. Occipital lobes
D. All of the above

The posterior circulation is composed of the paired vertebral arteries, the basilar artery, and the paired posterior cerebral arteries. It supplies the cerebellum, medulla, pons, midbrain, subthalamus, thalamus, hippocampus, and medial temporal and occipital lobes.

978. The artery of Percheron arises from?
Harrison's 20th Ed. Chapter 419, Page 3072

A. Anterior cerebral artery
B. Posterior cerebral artery
C. Vertebral artery
D. Basilar artery

Thalamogeniculate, Percheron and posterior choroidal arteries are the penetrating branches of the proximal P1 segment of PCA.

979. Occlusion of artery of Percheron produces?
Harrison's 20th Ed. Chapter 419, Page 3073

A. Paresis of upward gaze
B. Drowsiness
C. Abulia
D. All of the above

Occlusion of artery of Percheron produces paresis of upward gaze, drowsiness & abulia.

980. Which of the following is a penetrating artery of P1 segment of PCA?
Harrison's 20th Ed. Chapter 419, Page 3072

A. Thalamogeniculate artery
B. Percheron artery
C. Posterior choroidal artery
D. All of the above

981. P1 syndrome produces which of the following signs?
Harrison's 20th Ed. Chapter 419, Page 3072

A. Midbrain signs
B. Subthalamic signs
C. Thalamic signs
D. All of the above

P1 syndrome is due to disease of proximal P1 segment of PCA or its penetrating branches namely thalamogeniculate, Percheron, and posterior choroidal arteries. It is diagnosed by various midbrain, subthalamic, and thalamic signs.

982. Involvement of subthalamic nucleus is best related to?
Harrison's 20th Ed. Chapter 419, Page 3073

A. Upward gaze
B. Drowsiness
C. Hemiballismus
D. Abulia

If the subthalamic nucleus is involved, contralateral hemiballismus may occur.

983. Weber's syndrome results due to occlusion of?
Harrison's 20th Ed. Chapter 419, Page 3073

A. Anterior cerebral artery
B. Middle cerebral artery
C. Posterior cerebral artery
D. Basilar artery

984. Claude's syndrome results due to occlusion of?
Harrison's 20th Ed. Chapter 419, Page 3073

A. Anterior cerebral artery
B. Middle cerebral artery
C. Posterior cerebral artery
D. Basilar artery

985. In Claude's syndrome, ataxia is due to involvement of?
Harrison's 20th Ed. Chapter 419, Page 3073

A. Cerebellum
B. Superior cerebellar peduncle
C. Red nucleus
D. All of the above

III nerve palsy with contralateral ataxia is called Claude's syndrome. Ataxia is due to involvement of red nucleus or dentatorubrothalamic tract.

986. In Weber's syndrome, hemiplegia is due to involvement of?
Harrison's 20th Ed. Chapter 419, Page 3073

A. Internal capsule
B. Cerebral peduncle
C. Corpus callosum
D. Pyramidal decussation

III nerve palsy with contralateral hemiplegia is called Weber's syndrome. Hemiplegia is localized to the cerebral peduncle. Hermann Weber, German physician, 1863.

987. Complete oculomotor nerve lesion results in all except?
Harrison's 20th Ed. Chapter 419, Page 3073

A. Ipsilateral ptosis
B. Pupillary dilatation
C. Loss of pupillary & accommodation reflexes
D. Medical deviation of the eye

Complete oculomotor (III) nerve lesion results in ipsilateral ptosis, pupillary dilatation, loss of pupillary and accommodation reflexes and 'lateral' deviation of the eye. III CN supplies all extra-ocular muscles except lateral rectus and superior oblique.

988. Brown's tendon sheath syndrome simulates which of the following?
DeJong's The Neurologic Examination, 7th Ed. Page 211

A. Superior oblique palsy
B. Inferior oblique palsy
C. Superior rectus palsy
D. Inferior rectus palsy

Brown's tendon sheath syndrome, most often congenital, is limitation of free movement of superior oblique tendon through the trochlea. Restriction of movement causes an impairment of upgaze in adduction simulating inferior oblique palsy.

989. Edinger-Westphal nucleus located in?
Harrison's 20th Ed. Chapter 419, Page 3073

A. Upper mid-brain
B. Lower mid-brain
C. Pons
D. Medulla oblongata

990. Fascicles from III CN nuclei run forward & laterally through?
Harrison's 20th Ed. Chapter 419, Page 3073

A. Substantia nigra
B. Red nuclei
C. Dentate nuclei
D. Olivary nuclei

III cranial nerve nuclei are located in midbrain. They consist of Edinger-Westphal nucleus located in upper mid-brain supplying fibers to pupils and motor nucleus located in lower mid-brain supplying extra-ocular muscles, except lateral rectus and superior oblique. Fascicles from the III CN nuclei run forward & laterally through red nuclei and converge at the inter-peduncular fossa. Lesion of lower mid-brain affects extraocular muscles but spares pupils, whereas lesions involving both upper & lower parts of mid-brain are associated with pupillary dilatation.

991. Lower branch of occulomotor nerve supplies all of the following extraocular muscles except?

Harrison's 20th Ed. Chapter 419, Page 3073

A. Medial rectus
B. Levator palpebrae superioris
C. Inferior rectus
D. Inferior oblique

After emerging from mid-brain, III CN lies between posterior cerebral artery and the superior cerebellar artery. It runs forward parallel to the posterior communicating artery and enters the orbit through the superior orbital fissure, dividing into an upper and a lower branch. The upper branch supplies the levator palpebrae superioris and superior rectus muscles. The lower branch supplies three muscles: the medial rectus, the inferior rectus, and the inferior oblique muscle. The nerve to the inferior oblique muscle conveys the preganglionic parasympathetic fibers to the ciliary ganglion from which the post-ganglionic parasympathetic fibers arise to supply the ciliary muscle and the muscles of the iris (pupilloconstrictor fibers).

992. Hemiballismus is due to damage to which of the following?

Harrison's 20th Ed. Chapter 419, Page 3073

A. Substantia nigra
B. Red nucleus
C. Thalamus
D. Subthalamic nucleus

If the subthalamic nucleus is involved, contralateral hemiballismus may occur.

993. Which of the following is false about "Thalamic Dejerine-Roussy syndrome"?

Harrison's 20th Ed. Chapter 419, Page 3073

A. Contralateral hemisensory loss
B. Agonizing pain in affected area later
C. Responds poorly to analgesics
D. None of the above

Thalamic Dejerine-Roussy syndrome consists of contralateral hemisensory loss followed later by agonizing, searing or burning pain in the affected areas. Symptoms are persistent and respond poorly to analgesics. May respond to carbamazepine or gabapentin.

994. Occlusion of the posterior cerebral artery can produce which of the following?

Harrison's 20th Ed. Chapter 419, Page 3073

A. Peduncular hallucinosis
B. Contralateral homonymous hemianopia, macular sparing
C. Acute disturbance in memory
D. All of the above

All the above presentations occur due to occlusion of distal PCA causing infarction of hippocampus, medial temporal & occipital lobes. Peduncular hallucinosis means visual hallucinations of brightly colored scenes & objects. Because memory has bilateral representation, this defect clears soon.

995. Anton's syndrome results due to occlusion of?

Harrison's 20th Ed. Chapter 419, Page 3074

A. Bilateral occlusion of distal ACA
B. Bilateral occlusion of distal MCA
C. Bilateral occlusion of distal PCA
D. Bilateral occlusion of vertebral artery

Anton's syndrome is due to bilateral infarction in the distal PCAs. It produces cortical blindness with preserved pupillary light reaction.

996. In Anton's syndrome, patient is often unaware of?

Harrison's 20th Ed. Chapter 419, Page 3074

A. Smell
B. Hearing
C. Blindness
D. Colour vision

In Anton's syndrome, patient is unaware of blindness. Bilateral infarction in distal PCAs produces cortical blindness (blindness with preserved pupillary light reaction).

997. "Gun-barrel" vision is best related to?

Harrison's 20th Ed. Chapter 419, Page 3074

A. Anton's syndrome
B. Balint's syndrome
C. Claude's syndrome
D. Wallenberg's syndrome

In Anton's syndrome, rarely, only peripheral vision is lost and central vision is spared, resulting in "gun-barrel" vision.

998. Which symptom can occur in Balint's syndrome?

Harrison's 20th Ed. Chapter 419, Page 3074

A. Optic ataxia
B. Oculomotor apaxia
C. Asimultanagnosia
D. All of the above

Balint's syndrome is a disorder of the orderly visual scanning of the environment, usually resulting from infarctions secondary to low flow in "watershed" between distal PCA & MCA territories. There occurs persistence of a visual image for several minutes despite gazing at another scene (palinopsia) or an inability to synthesize whole of an image (asimultanagnosia).

999. Experiencing persistence of a visual image for several minutes despite gazing at another scene is called?

Harrison's 20th Ed. Chapter 419, Page 3074

A. Optic ataxia
B. Ocular ataxia
C. Simultagnosia
D. Palinopia

In palinopia, patients experience persistence of a visual image for several minutes despite gazing at another scene.

1000. Embolic occlusion of the top of basilar artery can produce which of the following?

Harrison's 20th Ed. Chapter 419, Page 3074

A. Ptosis
B. Pupillary asymmetry
C. Lack of reaction to light
D. All of the above

Embolic occlusion of the top of the basilar artery can produce any or all of the central or peripheral territory symptoms. The hallmark is the sudden onset of bilateral signs, ptosis, pupillary asymmetry or lack of reaction to light and somnolence.

1001. The vertebral artery enters into the transverse cervical vertebral foramen at?

Harrison's 20th Ed. Chapter 419, Page 3074

A. C7
B. C6
C. C4
D. C3

The first (V1) segment of vertebral artery extends from its origin to its entrance into the sixth or fifth transverse vertebral foramen.

1002. Branches from which segment of vertebral artery supply brainstem and cerebellum?

Harrison's 20th Ed. Chapter 419, Page 3074

A. 1
B. 2
C. 3
D. 4

Fourth (V4) segment of vertebral artery courses upward from foramen magnum to join the other vertebral artery and forms the basilar artery. Only the fourth segment gives rise to branches that supply the brainstem and cerebellum.

1003. Which segment of the vertebral artery pierce the dura at the foramen magnum?

Harrison's 20th Ed. Chapter 419, Page 3074

A. 1
B. 2
C. 3
D. 4

Third segment of vertebral artery (V3) passes through transverse foramen end circles around the arch of the atlas to pierce dura at foramen magnum.

1004. Which of the following statements about vertebral artery is false?

Harrison's 20th Ed. Chapter 419, Page 3075

A. Arises from innominate artery on right side
B. Consists of four segments
C. Atherothrombotic lesion has predilection for V3 segment
D. None of the above

Atherothrombotic lesions have a predilection for V1 & V4 segments of vertebral artery.

1005. Which of the following conditions affect the second & third segments of vertebral artery?

Harrison's 20th Ed. Chapter 419, Page 3075

A. Dissection
B. Fibromuscular dysplasia
C. Encroachment by osteophytic spurs
D. All of the above

Atheromatous disease rarely narrows second & third segments of vertebral artery, but this region is vulnerable to dissection, fibromuscular dysplasia and encroachment by osteophytic spurs within the vertebral foramina.

1006. Vertebral artery receives collateral blood supply from which of the following?

Harrison's 20th Ed. Chapter 419, Page 3075

A. Ascending cervical arteries
B. Thyrocervical arteries
C. Occipital arteries
D. All of the above

Vertebral artery receives collateral blood supply from the ascending cervical, thyrocervical or occipital arteries which is usually sufficient to prevent low-flow TIAs or stroke.

1007. "Subclavian steal" is best related to?

Harrison's 20th Ed. Chapter 419, Page 3075

A. Raynauds phenomenon
B. Posterior circulation TIA
C. Upper limb clubbing
D. All of the above

If the subclavian artery is occluded proximal to the origin of vertebral artery, there is reversal in the direction of blood flow in the ipsilateral vertebral artery. Exercise of the ipsilateral arm may increase demand on vertebral flow, producing posterior circulation TIAs, or "subclavian steal."

1008. In medial medullary syndrome, which of the following structures is involved?

Harrison's 20th Ed. Chapter 419, Page 3073 Figure 419-7

A. Ipsilateral twelfth nerve
B. Contralateral pyramidal tract
C. Contralateral medial lemniscus
D. All of the above

Medial medullary syndrome is due to occlusion of vertebral artery or branch of vertebral or lower basilar artery. Paralysis with atrophy of half tongue due to ipsilateral XII nerve occurs. On the opposite side, due to involvement of pyramidal tract & medial lemniscus, paralysis of arm & leg, impaired tactile & proprioceptive sense over half the body occur. Face is spared.

1009. Occlusion of which of the following artery is responsible for producing lateral medullary syndrome?

Harrison's 20th Ed. Chapter 419, Page 3073 Figure 419-7

A. Vertebral
B. Posterior inferior cerebellar
C. Superior lateral medullary artery
D. All of the above

Occlusion of any of the five vessels is responsible for producing lateral medullary syndrome. They are vertebral, posterior inferior cerebellar (PICA), superior, middle or inferior lateral medullary arteries.

1010. Which of the following is false for lateral medullary syndrome?

Harrison's 20th Ed. Chapter 419, Page 3073 Figure 419-7

A. Falling to side of lesion
B. Horner's syndrome
C. Impaired touch over opposite half of face
D. Loss of taste

Due to damage to descending tract and nucleus of fifth nerve, pain, numbness, impaired sensation over half the face occurs on the side of lesion.

1011. Which of the following is false for lateral medullary syndrome?

Harrison's 20th Ed. Chapter 419, Page 3073 Figure 419-7

A. Oscillopsia
B. Nystagmus
C. Strabismus
D. Dysphagia

Due to damage to vestibular nucleus, nystagmus, diplopia, oscillopsia, vertigo, nausea & vomiting occur in lateral medullary syndrome. Dysphagia, hoarseness, paralysis of palate & vocal cord, diminished gag reflex occur due to damage to issuing fibers of IX & X nerves.

1012. Loss of taste in lateral medullary syndrome is due to lesion in?

Harrison's 20th Ed. Chapter 419, Page 3073 Figure 419-7

A. Nucleus of fifth nerve
B. Vestibular nucleus
C. Nucleus and tractus solitarius
D. Cuneate and gracile nuclei

Loss of taste in lateral medullary syndrome is due to lesion in nucleus & tractus solitarius on side of lesion.

1013. Nystagmus, diplopia, oscillopsia, vertigo, nausea, vomiting in lateral medullary syndrome is due to lesion in?

Harrison's 20th Ed. Chapter 419, Page 3073 Figure 419-7

A. Descending sympathetic tract
B. Cerebellar hemisphere
C. Vestibular nucleus
D. Spinocerebellar tract

Nystagmus, diplopia, oscillopsia, vertigo, nausea, vomiting in lateral medullary syndrome is due to lesion in Vestibular nucleus.

1014. Numbness of ipsilateral arm, trunk, or leg in lateral medullary syndrome is due to lesion in?

Harrison's 20th Ed. Chapter 419, Page 3073 Figure 419-7

A. Nucleus of fifth nerve
B. Vestibular nucleus
C. Nucleus and tractus solitarius
D. Cuneate and gracile nuclei

Numbness of ipsilateral arm, trunk, or leg in lateral medullary syndrome is due to lesion in cuneate and gracile nuclei.

1015. Which of the following is not a part of lateral medullary (or Wallenberg's) syndrome?

Harrison's 20th Ed. Chapter 419, Page 3073 Figure 419-7

A. Vertigo
B. Numbness of ipsilateral face
C. Numbness of contralateral limbs
D. Contralateral Horner's syndrome

Horner's syndrome (miosis, ptosis, decreased sweating) occurs on side of lesion in lateral medullary syndrome due to damage to descending sympathetic tract.

1016. Which of the following is not a feature of vertebral artery occlusion?

Harrison's 20th Ed. Chapter 419, Page 3075

A. Vertigo
B. Diplopia
C. Quadriparesis
D. Hemiparesis

Embolic occlusion or thrombosis of a V4 segment causes ischemia of the lateral medulla. The constellation of vertigo, numbness of the ipsilateral face and contralateral limbs, diplopia, hoarseness, dysarthria, dysphagia, and ipsilateral Horner's syndrome is called the lateral medullary (or Wallenberg's) syndrome. Hemiparesis is not a feature of vertebral artery occlusion. However, quadriparesis may result from occlusion of the anterior spinal artery.

1017. Which of the following can occur in cerebellar infarction?

Harrison's 20th Ed. Chapter 419, Page 3076

A. Headache
B. Neck stiffness
C. Unilateral dysmetria
D. All of the above

Headache, neck stiffness and unilateral dysmetria favor cerebellar infarction.

1018. Which of the following are branches of the basilar artery?

Harrison's 20th Ed. Chapter 419, Page 3076

A. Paramedian
B. Short circumferential
C. Long circumferential
D. All of the above

Branches of the basilar artery supply the base of pons and superior cerebellum. The three groups are paramedian (7- 10 in number supplying a wedge of pons on either side of midline), short circumferential (5-7 in number supplying lateral two-thirds of pons & middle & superior cerebellar peduncles) and bilateral long circumferential (superior cerebellar & anterior inferior cerebellar arteries coursing around pons to supply the cerebellar hemispheres).

1019. Occlusion of which of the following leads to "Top of the basilar" syndromes?

Harrison's 20th Ed. Chapter 419, Page 3076

A. Proximal basilar artery
B. Both vertebral arteries
C. Distal basilar artery
D. Any of the above

Atheromatous lesions can occur anywhere along the basilar trunk but are most frequent in the proximal basilar & distal vertebral segments. Clinical picture varies depending on the retrograde collateral flow from posterior communicating arteries. Atherothrombosis may also occlude distal portion of basilar artery (emboli from heart or proximal vertebral or basilar segments) and lead to "top of the basilar" syndromes.

1020. Which of the following can occur upon complete basilar occlusion?

Harrison's 20th Ed. Chapter 419, Page 3076

A. Bilateral long tract signs (sensory & motor)
B. Signs of cranial nerve dysfunction
C. Signs of cerebellar dysfunction
D. All of the above

1021. Corticobulbar and corticospinal tracts are damaged bilaterally due to occlusion of?

Harrison's 20th Ed. Chapter 419, Page 3076

A. Vertebral artery
B. Basilar artery
C. Anterior inferior cerebellar artery
D. Superior cerebellar artery

Basilar artery or lone vertebral artery occlusion can damage corticobulbar and corticospinal tracts bilaterally. Complete basilar occlusion leads to a constellation of bilateral long tract signs (sensory and motor) with signs of cranial nerve and cerebellar dysfunction.

1022. "Locked-in" state of preserved consciousness with quadriplegia and cranial nerve signs suggests?

Harrison's 20th Ed. Chapter 419, Page 3076

A. Complete pontine & upper midbrain infarction
B. Complete pontine & lower midbrain infarction
C. Complete pontine & medulla oblongata infarction
D. Any of the above

"Locked-in" state of preserved consciousness with quadriplegia and cranial nerve signs suggests complete pontine and lower midbrain infarction. Atherothrombotic occlusion of basilar artery with infarction causes bilateral brainstem signs, gaze paresis or internuclear ophthalmoplegia with ipsilateral hemiparesis, or unequivocal signs of bilateral pontine disease.

1023. TIAs in the proximal basilar distribution produces which of the following?

Harrison's 20th Ed. Chapter 419, Page 3077

A. Vertigo
B. Diplopia
C. Facial or circumoral numbness
D. All of the above

TIAs in the proximal basilar distribution produces vertigo, diplopia, dysarthria, facial or circumoral numbness and hemisensory symptoms.

1024. Constellation of bilateral long tract signs with signs of cranial nerve and cerebellar dysfunction is suggestive of?

Harrison's 20th Ed. Chapter 419, Page 3073 Figure 419-7

A. Complete basilar artery occlusion
B. Complete posterior cerebral artery occlusion
C. Complete middle cerebral artery occlusion
D. Complete anterior cerebral artery occlusion

Constellation of bilateral long tract signs (sensory and motor) with signs of cranial nerve and cerebellar dysfunction is suggestive of complete basilar artery occlusion.

1025. Which of the following syndromes occur due to occlusion of vertebral artery?

Harrison's 20th Ed. Chapter 419, Page 3073 Figure 419-7

A. Medial medullary syndrome
B. Lateral medullary syndrome
C. Total unilateral medullary syndrome
D. All of the above

Occlusion of vertebral artery can produce medial and lateral and total unilateral medullary syndrome. The last one being a combination of medial and lateral syndromes.

1026. Lateral pontomedullary syndrome is due to occlusion of which of the following vessel?

Harrison's 20th Ed. Chapter 419, Page 3073 Figure 419-7

A. Vertebral artery
B. Basilar artery
C. Anterior inferior cerebellar artery
D. Superior cerebellar artery

Lateral pontomedullary syndrome is due to occlusion of vertebral artery. It is a combination of lateral medullary and lateral inferior pontine syndrome.

1027. Which of the following syndromes occur due to occlusion of anterior inferior cerebellar artery?

Harrison's 20th Ed. Chapter 419, Page 3074 Figure 419-8

A. Medial medullary syndrome
B. Medial inferior pontine syndrome
C. Lateral inferior pontine syndrome
D. All of the above

Occlusion of anterior inferior cerebellar artery produces lateral inferior pontine syndrome.

1028. Which of the following syndrome occurs due to occlusion of superior cerebellar artery?

Harrison's 20th Ed. Chapter 419, Page 3076 Figure 419-10

A. Lateral midpontine syndrome
B. Medial superior pontine syndrome
C. Lateral superior pontine syndrome
D. Total unilateral medullary syndrome

Lateral superior pontine syndrome occurs due to occlusion of superior cerebellar artery - a branch of basilar artery.

1029. Horner's syndrome is produced by occlusion of which of the following arteries?

Harrison's 20th Ed. Chapter 419, Page 3077

A. Anterior inferior cerebellar artery
B. Superior cerebellar artery
C. Vertebral artery
D. All of the above

In lateral medullary syndrome due to occlusion of vertebral artery, Horner's syndrome occurs due to damage to descending sympathetic tract. Lateral inferior pontine syndrome due to occlusion of anterior inferior cerebellar artery produces Horner's syndrome. Lateral superior pontine syndrome due to occlusion of superior cerebellar artery sometimes produces Horner's syndrome.

1030. Deafness is produced by occlusion of which of the following arteries?

Harrison's 20th Ed. Chapter 419, Page 3077

A. Anterior inferior cerebellar artery
B. Upper basilar artery
C. Anterior cerebral artery
D. Any of the above

1031. Which of the following is a common presentation in both medial midbrain syndrome and lateral midbrain syndrome?

Harrison's 20th Ed. Chapter 419, Page 3077 Figure 419-11

A. Paralysis of face, arm and leg
B. Hemiataxia
C. Tremor
D. Eye "down and out" on side of lesion

1032. Which of the following is not reliably detected by CT radiographic images?

Harrison's 20th Ed. Chapter 419, Page 3078

A. Cerebral infarction for first 24 to 48 hours
B. Ischemic strokes in posterior fossa
C. Small cortical infarcts
D. All of the above

Cerebral infarction infarct may not be seen reliably for 24 to 48 hours. Also, CT may fail to show small ischemic strokes in posterior fossa and small infarcts on cortical surface.

1033. "Insular ribbon sign" is an earliest indicator of?

Harrison's 16th Ed. 2386

A. Meningitis
B. Subarachnoid hemorrhage
C. Cerebral infarction
D. All of the above

"Insular ribbon sign" is caused by edema within insular cortex and basal ganglia and is an earliest indicator of cerebral infarction in MCA territory.

1034. Which of the following is used to visualize extra- or intracranial arterial dissection?

Harrison's 20th Ed. Chapter 419, Page 3078

A. MR angiography
B. MRI with fat saturation
C. MRI with IV gadolinium contrast
D. All of the above

MRI with fat saturation is used to visualize extra- or intracranial arterial dissection as it images clotted blood within dissected vessel wall.

1035. Which of the following statements is false?

Harrison's 20th Ed. Chapter 419, Page 3079

A. Transcranial Doppler (TCD) can measure success of thrombolysis following rtP A administration
B. CT perfusion imaging increases sensitivity for detecting ischemic penumbra
C. MR perfusion studies can measure ischemic penumbra
D. None of the above

Ischemic Stroke

1036. A fall in cerebral blood flow to zero causes death of brain tissue within?
Harrison's 20th Ed. Chapter 420, Page 3079

A. 30 seconds to 1 minute
B. 1 to 4 minutes
C. 4 to 10 minutes
D. 10 to 15 minutes

A fall in cerebral blood flow to zero causes death of brain tissue within 4 to 10 minutes.

1037. When cerebral blood flow falls to <16 to 18 mL/100 gram per minute, how long would it take for brain infarction?
Harrison's 20th Ed. Chapter 420, Page 3079

A. 1 hour
B. 2 hours
C. 3 hours
D. 4 hours

When cerebral blood flow falls to <16–18 mL/100 gram/minute, brain infarction occurs in 1 hour.

1038. Decrease in cerebral blood flow to what extent causes cerebral ischemia without infarction?
Harrison's 20th Ed. Chapter 420, Page 3079

A. < 50 mL/I00 grams tissue per minute
B. < 40 mL/I00 grams tissue per minute
C. < 30 mL/I00 grams tissue per minute
D. < 20 mL/I00 grams tissue per minute

Cerebral blood flow of < 20 mL/I00 grams tissue per minute causes ischemia without infarction unless prolonged for several hours or days.

1039. Location of "Ischemic penumbra" is?
Harrison's 20th Ed. Chapter 420, Page 3079

A. Center of the core region of infarction
B. Within the core region of infarction
C. Surrounding the core region of infarction
D. Any of the above

Tissue surrounding the core region of infarction is ischemic but reversibly dysfunctional and is called as the ischemic penumbra.

1040. Which of the following is false about ischemic penumbra?
Harrison's 20th Ed. Chapter 420, Page 3079

A. Ischemic tissue around core region of infarction
B. Reversibly dysfunctional
C. Imaged by perfusion-diffusion imaging with MRI or CT
D. None of the above

In ischemic penumbra, cellular death occurs by apoptosis days to weeks later. Saving the ischemic penumbra is the goal of revascularization therapies.

1041. If no improvement in cerebral flow occurs, what will happen to ischemic penumbra?
Harrison's 20th Ed. Chapter 420, Page 3079

A. Will improve
B. Will infarct
C. Will continue to remain the same
D. Any of the above

The ischemic penumbra will eventually infarct if no change in flow occurs.

1042. In ischemic penumbra, mechanism of cell death is?
Harrison's 20th Ed. Chapter 420, Page 3079

A. Apoptosis
B. Necrotic
C. Mechanical
D. Toxicity due to free radicals

In Ischemic penumbra, apoptotic cellular death occurs days to weeks later.

1043. Cerebral ischemia produces necrosis due to?
Harrison's 20th Ed. Chapter 420, Page 3079

A. Lack of oxygen & glucose
B. Excess extracellular glutamate
C. Generation of free radicals
D. All of the above

1044. Which of the following dramatically worsens brain injury during ischemia?
Harrison's 20th Ed. Chapter 420, Page 3079

A. Fever
B. Headache
C. Seizure
D. Vomiting

1045. Which of the following worsens brain injury during ischemia?
Harrison's 20th Ed. Chapter 420, Page 3079

A. Fever
B. Hyperglycemia
C. Hypovolemia
D. All of the above

Fever dramatically worsens brain injury during ischemia as does hyperglycemia. Hypovolemia should be avoided as it contributes to hypotension and worsening infarction.

1046. Which of the following favour the diagnosis of cerebral hemorrhage rather than ischemia?
Harrison's 20th Ed. Chapter 420, Page 3080

A. Lower initial blood pressure
B. Higher initial blood pressure
C. Fluctuating blood pressure
D. Any of the above

1047. Which of the following favour the diagnosis of cerebral hemorrhage rather than ischemia?
Harrison's 20th Ed. Chapter 420, Page 3080

A. A more depressed level of consciousness
B. Higher initial blood pressure
C. Worsening of symptoms after onset
D. Any of the above

A more depressed level of consciousness, higher initial blood pressure, or worsening of symptoms after onset favor hemorrhage, and a deficit that is maximal at onset or remits suggests ischemia.

1048. BP should not be lowered acutely in acute ischemic stroke because it affects blood flow in?

Harrison's 20th Ed. Chapter 420, Page 3080

A. Cerebral arteries
B. Cerebral veins
C. Collateral channels
D. All of the above

Because collateral blood flow within the ischemic brain is blood pressure dependent, blood pressure should not be lowered acutely.

1049. In acute ischemic stroke, BP should be lowered if it is?

Harrison's 20th Ed. Chapter 420, Page 3080

A. > 140/90 mm Hg
B. > 150/100 mm Hg
C. > 165/110 mm Hg
D. > 185/110 mm Hg

1050. In acute ischemic stroke, BP should be lowered if?

Harrison's 20th Ed. Chapter 420, Page 3080

A. Malignant hypertension is present
B. Concomitant myocardial ischemia present
C. Thrombolytic therapy is planned
D. All of the above

In acute ischemic stroke, BP should be lowered if there is malignant hypertension, concomitant myocardial ischemia or if BP is >185/110 mm Hg or if thrombolytic therapy is anticipated. Routine lowering of blood pressure worsens outcome.

1051. In acute ischemic stroke, serum glucose should be kept at?

Harrison's 20th Ed. Chapter 420, Page 3080

A. < 100 mg/dL
B. < 120 mg/dL
C. < 160 mg/dL
D. < 180 mg/dL

Serum glucose should be monitored and kept at < 180 mg/dL using an insulin infusion if necessary, and above 60 mg/dL.

1052. In acute ischemic stroke, what percentage of patients develop cerebral edema to cause obtundation or brain herniation?

Harrison's 20th Ed. Chapter 420, Page 3080

A. 0.5 to 1%
B. 1 to 2%
C. 2 to 4%
D. 5 to 10%

5 to 10% of patients develop enough cerebral edema to cause obtundation or brain herniation.

1053. In acute ischemic stroke, cerebral edema peaks on?

Harrison's 20th Ed. Chapter 420, Page 3080

A. Day 1
B. Day 2–3
C. Day 4–5
D. Day 5–6

In acute ischemic stroke, cerebral edema peaks on day 2 - 3 & cause mass effect for ~10 days.

1054. Which of the following point towards the diagnosis of cerebellar infarction?

Harrison's 20th Ed. Chapter 420, Page 3080

A. Vertigo
B. Vomiting
C. Head or neck pain
D. All of the above

Cerebellar infarction due to vertebral artery dissection mimics labyrinthitis because of prominent vertigo and vomiting. Head or neck pain favour the diagnosis.

1055. The time of acute ischemic stroke onset is defined as?

Harrison's 20th Ed. Chapter 420, Page 3081

A. Time the patient's symptoms began
B. Time the patient was last seen as normal
C. Time to bed in those who awaken with stroke
D. All of the above

Time of stroke onset is defined as the time patient's symptoms began or time patient was last seen as normal. A patient who awakens with stroke has the onset defined as when they went to bed.

1056. Which of the following investigation is necessary prior to IV rtPA therapy?

Harrison's 20th Ed. Chapter 420, Page 3081

A. Brain imaging
B. Blood glucose
C. PTT/International normalized ratio (INR)
D. All of the above

Only brain imaging, blood glucose and perhaps PTT/international normalized ratio (INR) are necessary prior to IV rtPA therapy.

1057. In acute ischemic stroke, rtPA is approved in US for which of the following time window?

Harrison's 20th Ed. Chapter 420, Page 3081

A. 0 to 1 hour
B. 0 to 3 hours
C. 0 to 6 hours
D. 0 to 12 hours

In acute ischemic stroke, rtPA is approved in the 3 to 4.5 hours time window in Europe and Canada, but is still only approved for 0–3 hours in United States and Canada.

1058. Following administration of rtPA, no other antithrombotic treatment must be given for?

Harrison's 20th Ed. Chapter 420, Page 3081 Table 420-1

A. 6 hours
B. 12 hours
C. 24 hours
D. 48 hours

Following administration of rtPA, no other antithrombotic treatment must be given for 24 hours.

1059. The established dose of rtPA to be administered within 3 hours of acute ischemic stroke is?

Harrison's 20th Ed. Chapter 420, Page 3081 Table 420-1

A. 0.1 mg/kg
B. 0.3 mg/kg
C. 0.9 mg/kg
D. 1.2 mg/kg

The National Institute of Neurological Disorders and Stroke (NINDS) recombinant tPA (rtPA) Stroke Study used IV rtPA (0.9 mg/kg to a 90-mg max; 10% as a bolus, then the remainder over 60 min) in patients with ischemic stroke within 3 hours of onset.

1060. Which of the following studied the value of thrombolytics via an intraarterial route in acute ischemic stroke?

Harrison's 20th Ed. Chapter 420, Page 3081

A. PROACT II
B. ECASS
C. ATLANTIS
D. NINDS

Prolyse in Acute Cerebral Thromboembolism (PROACT) II trial found benefit for intraarterial pro-urokinase for acute middle cerebral artery (MCA) occlusions up to 6th hour following onset of stroke. Intraarterial administration of a thrombolytic agent for acute ischemic stroke (AIS) is not approved by U.S. FDA.

1061. In Chinese Acute Stroke Trial (CAST), dose of aspirin was?

Harrison's 20th Ed. Chapter 420, Page 3082

A. 75 mg/day
B. 160 mg/day
C. 300 mg/day
D. 625 mg/day

In CAST, patients with ischemic stroke received 160 mg/day of aspirin for up to 4 weeks. In International Stroke Trial (IST), dose of aspirin was 300 mg/day.

1062. Neuroprotection is the concept related to?

Harrison's 20th Ed. Chapter 420, Page 3082

A. Preventing reinfarction
B. Prolonging brain's tolerance to ischemia
C. Checking the risk factors
D. All of the above

Neuroprotection refers to providing a treatment that prolongs brain's tolerance to ischemia.

1063. What percentage of strokes remain unexplained despite extensive evaluation?

Harrison's 20th Ed. Chapter 420, Page 3082

A. 5%
B. 20%
C. 30%
D. 50%

Nearly 30% of strokes remain unexplained despite extensive evaluation.

1064. Emboli in 'Hollenhorst plaque' are composed of?

Harrison's 20th Ed. Chapter 420, Page 3082

A. Cholesterol
B. Calcium
C. Platelet-fibrin debris
D. Bacteria

American ophthalmologist Dr Robert Hollenhorst (1913-2008) who first described Hollenhorst plaque as a cholesterol embolus that originated from an atheromatous plaque in a more proximal vessel, usually internal carotid artery. It is a sign of severe atherosclerosis & is seen in a blood vessel of retina on ophthalmoscopy as a bright, glistening, refractile plaque at bifurcation of a retinal arteriole. These may break up & move, and may not be present at subsequent visits.

1065. What proportion of all ischemic strokes are due to cardioembolism?

Harrison's 20th Ed. Chapter 420, Page 3082

A. ~ 10%
B. ~ 20%
C. ~ 30%
D. ~ 40%

Cardioembolism is responsible for ~20% of all ischemic strokes.

1066. Sudden onset of neurologic dysfunction in embolic stroke is usually maximum at?

Harrison's 20th Ed. Chapter 420, Page 3082

A. Onset
B. At 12 hours
C. At 24 hours
D. At 48 hours

Embolic strokes tend to be sudden in onset, with maximum neurologic deficit at the onset.

1067. Which of the following vessels is infrequently involved in embolization from heart?

Harrison's 20th Ed. Chapter 420, Page 3082

A. Anterior cerebral artery (ACA)
B. Middle cerebral artery (MCA)
C. Posterior cerebral artery (PCA)
D. Branches of posterior cerebral artery

Emboli from heart most often lodge in MCA, the PCA, or one of their branches. Anterior cerebral artery (ACA) territory is involved infrequently.

1068. Emboli of what size are large enough to occlude stem of MCA?

Harrison's 20th Ed. Chapter 420, Page 3082

A. 0.5–1 mm
B. 1–2 mm
C. 2–3 mm
D. 3–4 mm

Emboli of the size of 3 - 4 mm are large enough to occlude stem of MCA.

1069. Which of the following is the most common cause of cerebral cardioembolism?

Harrison's 20th Ed. Chapter 420, Page 3082

A. Rheumatic heart disease with atrial fibrillation
B. Nonrheumatic atrial fibrillation
C. Recent MI
D. Mitral valve prolapse

Nonrheumatic atrial fibrillation is the most common cause of cerebral embolism. Others are mural thrombus, myocardial infarction, dilated cardiomyopathy, mitral stenosis, mechanical valve, bacterial endocarditis. Mitral valve prolapse is not a source of emboli unless prolapse is severe.

1070. Patients with atrial fibrillation have an average annual risk of stroke of?

Harrison's 20th Ed. Chapter 420, Page 3082

A. ~ 1%
B. ~ 5%
C. ~ 10%
D. ~ 15%

Patients with atrial fibrillation have an average annual risk of stroke of ~ 5%.

1071. CHA_2DS_2-VASc score is calculating risk of stroke in?

Harrison's 20th Ed. Chapter 420, Page 3085 Table 420-3

A. Nonvalvular atrial fibrillation
B. Mitral valve prolapse
C. Patent foramen ovale
D. Mechanical heart value

1072. Maximum points in CHA_2DS_2-VASc score is for?
Harrison's 20th Ed. Chapter 420, Page 3085 Table 420-3

A. Diabetes mellitus
B. Hypertension
C. Congestive heart failure
D. Stroke or TIA

CHA_2DS_2-VASc score is a calculator for anticoagulation for atrial fibrillation. It is calculated by summing of points for age >75 years (2), hypertension (1), congestive heart failure (1), diabetes (1), and stroke or TIA (2). Anticoagulation is recommended for a score of ≥2.

1073. Which of the following location of recent transmural myocardial infarction is mostly the source of cerebral emboli?
Harrison's 20th Ed. Chapter 420, Page 3083

A. Anteroapical ventricular wall
B. Inferior ventricular wall
C. Posterior ventricular wall
D. Lateral ventricular wall

Recent transmural MI involving anteroapical ventricular wall is a source of cerebral emboli.

1074. Which of the following is usually not a source of cerebral emboli?
Harrison's 20th Ed. Chapter 420, Page 3083

A. Prosthetic valves
B. Mitral valve prolapse
C. Ischemic cardiomyopathy
D. Myocardial infarction

Mitral valve prolapse is usually not a source of cerebral emboli unless the prolapse is severe.

1075. Patent foramen ovale (PFO) is present in what percentage of the general population?
Harrison's 20th Ed. Chapter 420, Page 3083

A. ~ 1%
B. ~ 5%
C. ~ 10%
D. ~ 15%

Patent foramen ovale (PFO) are present in ~15% of the general population. Besides venous clot, fat, tumor emboli, bacterial endocarditis, IV air and amniotic fluid emboli at childbirth may be responsible for paradoxical embolization. Risk is elevated in the presence of a coexisting atrial septal aneurysm. However, there is no evidence for percutaneous PFO closure for stroke prevention.

1076. Most common source of artery-to-artery embolic stroke is?
Harrison's 20th Ed. Chapter 420, Page 3083

A. Aortic arch
B. Common carotid bifurcation
C. Common carotid
D. Vertebral arteries

Common carotid bifurcation and proximal internal carotid artery atherosclerosis is the most common source of artery-to-artery embolus.

1077. What proportion of all ischemic strokes are due to carotid atherosclerosis?
Harrison's 20th Ed. Chapter 420, Page 3083

A. ~ 10%
B. ~ 20%
C. ~ 30%
D. ~ 40%

10% of ischemic stroke are due to carotid atherosclerosis.

1078. Which of the following degrees of arterial narrowing is at lower risk of stroke?
Harrison's 20th Ed. Chapter 420, Page 3083

A. 50%
B. 75%
C. 90%
D. Near occlusion

Greater degrees of arterial narrowing are generally associated with a higher risk of stroke. Those with near occlusions are at lower risk of stroke.

1079. Which of the following is associated with dissections of the internal carotid or vertebral arteries?
Harrison's 20th Ed. Chapter 420, Page 3085

A. Marfan's disease
B. Cystic medial necrosis
C. Fibromuscular dysplasia
D. All of the above

Ehlers-Danlos type IV, Marfan's disease, cystic medial necrosis, and fibromuscular dysplasia are associated with dissections of the internal carotid or vertebral arteries.

1080. What proportion of all strokes are due to small-vessel disease?
Harrison's 20th Ed. Chapter 420, Page 3085

A. ~ 10%
B. ~ 20%
C. ~ 30%
D. ~ 40%

Small-vessel strokes account for ~20% of all strokes.

1081. The underlying pathology in lacunar stroke is?
Harrison's 20th Ed. Chapter 420, Page 3085

A. Congenital anomaly
B. Embolism
C. Lipohyalinosis
D. All of the above

Lacunar infarction refers to infarction following atherothrombotic or lipohyalinotic occlusion of a small artery in the brain. Lipohyalinosis appears as an eosinophilic deposit in the connective tissue of the vessel wall.

1082. In lacunar infarction, what size of a small artery is occluded in brain?
Harrison's 20th Ed. Chapter 420, Page 3085

A. 10 to 100 μm
B. 20 to 200 μm
C. 30 to 300 μm
D. 40 to 400 μm

Lacunar infarction refers to infarction following atherothrombotic or lipohyalinotic occlusion of a small artery (30 to 300 μm) in brain. These vessels are too small to be visualized on CT angiography.

1083. "Lacune" in Latin means?
Harrison's 20th Ed. Chapter 420, Page 3085

A. Deficit
B. Lake
C. River
D. Stone

Lacunes in Latin mean "lake". Clinically, lacunae are "small, deep cerebral infarcts".

1084. Lacunar infarcts range in size from?

Harrison's 20th Ed. Chapter 420, Page 3085

A. 1 mm to 5 mm
B. 1 mm to 10 mm
C. 2 mm to 10 mm
D. 3 mm to 20 mm

Lacunar infarcts range in size from 3 mm to 20 mm.

1085. The principal risk factor for lacunar infarcts is?

Harrison's 20th Ed. Chapter 420, Page 3085

A. Hypertension
B. Diabetes mellitus
C. Cigarette smoking
D. Stress

Hypertension and age are the principal risk factors for lacunar infarcts.

1086. Which of the following is not a lacunar syndrome?

Harrison's 20th Ed. Chapter 420, Page 3085

A. Pure motor hemiparesis due to infarct in posterior limb of the internal capsule or pons
B. Pure sensory stroke due to infarct in ventral thalamus
C. Ataxic hemiparesis due to infarct in ventral pons or internal capsule
D. Dysarthria and clumsy hand due to infarction in medulla

Lacunar syndrome dysarthria and a clumsy hand or arm due to infarction in the ventral pons or in the genu of the internal capsule.

1087. Lenticulostriate arteries originate from?

Harrison's 20th Ed. Chapter 420, Page 3086 Figure 420-3

A. Anterior cerebral arteries
B. Middle cerebral arteries
C. Vertebral arteries
D. All of the above

In the anterior circulation, small penetrating arteries called "lenticulostriates" arise from the proximal portion of anterior & middle cerebral arteries to supply deep subcortical structures. In the posterior circulation, similar arteries arise directly from vertebral & basilar arteries to supply brainstem.

1088. Which of the following increases risk of venous thrombosis and arterial thrombosis?

Harrison's 20th Ed. Chapter 420, Page 3085

A. Antiphospholipid syndrome
B. Systemic malignancy
C. Homocysteinemia
D. Factor V Leiden mutation

Besides increasing risk of venous thrombosis, Protein S deficiency and homocysteinemia may cause arterial thromboses as well.

1089. Which of the following can be a cause of embolic stroke?

Harrison's 20th Ed. Chapter 420, Page 3085

A. Polycythemia vera
B. Libman-Sacks endocarditis
C. Nephrotic syndrome
D. Sickle cell anemia

Systemic lupus erythematosus with Libman-Sacks endocarditis can be a cause of embolic stroke.

1090. Cerebral veins contain how much of the total cerebral blood volume?

Semin Cerebrovasc Dis Stroke. 2004;4:2-17

A. 30%
B. 50%
C. 70%
D. 90%

Cerebral veins contain 70% of the total cerebral blood volume.

1091. Veins that connect superior sagittal sinus with the scalp veins are called?

Semin Cerebrovasc Dis Stroke. 2004;4:2-17

A. Representative veins
B. Envoy veins
C. Emissary veins
D. Messenger veins

Superior sagittal sinus (SSS) drains major part of the cortex. It also receives diploic veins, themselves connected to scalp veins by emissary veins, which explains the occurrence of SSS thrombosis after scalp infection or minor head trauma.

1092. Lateral sinuses (LS) drain blood from which of the following?

Semin Cerebrovasc Dis Stroke. 2004;4:2-17

A. Cerebellum
B. Brainstem
C. Posterior part of cerebral hemispheres
D. All of the above

The lateral sinuses (LS) drain blood from the cerebellum, brainstem, and posterior part of the cerebral hemispheres. They also receive some of the diploic veins and some small veins from the middle ear, another classic source of septic thrombosis.

1093. Which of the following is a feature of superficial cerebral veins or cortical veins?

Semin Cerebrovasc Dis Stroke. 2004;4:2-17

A. Thin walls
B. No muscle fibers
C. No valves
D. All of the above

The superficial cerebral veins or cortical veins have thin walls, no muscle fibers, and no valves, thereby permitting both dilation & reversal of the direction of blood flow when the sinus into which they drain is occluded.

1094. Which of the following drain into cavernous sinuses?

Semin Cerebrovasc Dis Stroke. 2004;4:2-17

A. Superior and inferior ophthalmic veins
B. Sphenoparietal sinus
C. Middle cerebral vein
D. All of the above

Cavernous sinuses drain the blood flow from the orbits through the superior & inferior ophthalmic veins, and from the anterior part of the base of brain by the sphenoparietal sinus and the middle cerebral vein.

1095. The cavernous sinuses empty into which of the following?

Semin Cerebrovasc Dis Stroke. 2004;4:2-17

A. Superior petrosal sinus
B. Straight sinus
C. Great vein of Galen
D. Superior sagittal sinus

The cavernous sinuses empty into both the superior and the inferior petrosal sinuses and ultimately into the internal jugular veins.

1096. Thrombosis of which of the following venous sinuses mostly manifests as cranial nerve palsies?

Semin Cerebrovasc Dis Stroke. 2004;4:2-17

A. Petrosal sinuses
B. Straight sinus
C. Superior sagittal sinus
D. Transverse sinus

Because of the close relationship of the petrosal sinuses to cranial nerves, thrombosis of petrosal sinuses (with or without thrombosis of transverse sinus) may produce cranial nerve palsies, especially cranial nerves III, V, VI, VII, and VIII. Thrombosis of the petrosal sinuses is characterized mainly by a fifth nerve palsy for the superior petrosal sinus and by a sixth nerve palsy for the inferior sinus.

1097. Which of the following statements about thrombosis of cerebral venous sinuses is false?

N Engl J Med. 2005;352:1791-8

A. In most patients, thrombosis occurs in > one sinus
B. Hypoplasia & atresia of transverse sinuses frequent
C. A prothrombotic risk factor or a direct cause is identified in ~ 85% of patients
D. None of the above

1098. Most common pattern of clinical presentation of CVT is?

Semin Cerebrovasc Dis Stroke. 2004;4:2-17

A. Focal deficits
B. Isolated intracranial hypertension
C. Subacute diffuse encephalopathy
D. Acute painful ophthalmoplegia

The most common pattern of clinical presentations of CVT (~75%) is characterized by the presence of focal signs such as focal deficits or partial seizures. Any neurological symptoms such as aphasia, hemiparesis, hemianopsia, and amnesia can occur with CVT. CVT can be totally asymptomatic.

1099. The most frequent but least specific symptom of sinus thrombosis is?

N Engl J Med. 2005;352:1791-8

A. Severe headache
B. Ophthalmoplegia
C. Focal deficits
D. Partial seizures

The most frequent but least specific symptom of sinus thrombosis is severe headache, which is present in >90% of adult patients.

1100. Classic picture of deep cerebral venous thrombosis is?

Semin Cerebrovasc Dis Stroke. 2004;4:2-17

A. Intracranial hypertension
B. Progressive cerebellar incoordination & cranial N. palsies
C. Acute coma, decerebration & extrapyramidal hypertonia
D. Partial seizures

Classic picture of deep cerebral venous thrombosis is that of an acute coma with decerebration and extrapyramidal hypertonia leading to death within a few days, or complicated by akinetic mutism and dementia when resolving. Thrombosis of the deep venous system, the straight sinus and its branches, causes centrally located, often bilateral thalamic lesions, with behavioral symptoms such as delirium, amnesia, and mutism, which can be the only manifestation of sinus thrombosis. Thalamic edema is the imaging hallmark.

1101. Venous sinus thrombosis pertains to which of the following?

Harrison's 20th Ed. Chapter 420, Page 3085

A. Thrombosis of lateral sinus
B. Thrombosis of sagittal sinus
C. Thrombosis of small cortical veins
D. All of the above

Thrombosis of lateral or sagittal sinus or of small cortical veins fall under the category of venous sinus thrombosis.

1102. Which of the following mutation carries a high risk of venous sinus thrombosis in women who take oral contraceptives?

Harrison's 20th Ed. Chapter 420, Page 3085

A. Thrombin G20210 mutation
B. Prothrombin G20210 mutation
C. Antiprothrombin G20210 mutation
D. Antithrombin G20210 mutation

1103. Venous sinus thrombosis as a complication of which of the following?

Harrison's 20th Ed. Chapter 420, Page 3085

A. Syphilis
B. Inflammatory bowel disease
C. Rheumatoid arthritis
D. Pancreatic carcinoma

Women who take oral contraceptives and have the prothrombin G20210 mutation are at a high risk for sinus thrombosis. Also, it occurs as a complication of pregnancy and postpartum period, inflammatory bowel disease, intracranial infections (meningitis), and dehydration. It is also seen with increased incidence in patients with laboratory-confirmed thrombophilia including polycythemia, sickle cell anemia, deficiencies of proteins C and S, factor V Leiden mutation (resistance to activated protein C), antithrombin III deficiency, and homocysteinemia. Some patients with CVT carry more than one congenital thrombophilia factors. Extensive etiologic and complete coagulation work-up should be systematically performed in patients of CVT.

1104. Which of the following investigation is normal in patients with venous sinus thrombosis?

Harrison's 20th Ed. Chapter 420, Page 3085

A. CT
B. MR-venography
C. CT-venography
D. Conventional X-ray angiography

CT imaging is normal in patients with venous sinus thrombosis unless an intracranial venous hemorrhage has occurred, but the venous sinus occlusion is readily visualized using MR- or CT-venography or conventional X-ray angiography.

1105. Which of the following is the brain CT finding in a case of superior sagittal sinus thrombosis?

Semin Cerebrovasc Dis Stroke. 2004;4:2-17

A. Dense triangle sign
B. Empty delta sign
C. Cord sign
D. All of the above

Brain CT findings in CVT include the "dense triangle sign" (occlusion of SSS by fresh clot on noncontrast CT), the "empty delta sign" (filling of collateral veins in SSS wall after contrast injection, contrasting with the nonenhancement of clot inside the thrombosed sinus), and the "cord sign" (visualization of a thrombosed cortical vein on noncontrast CT). The same radiologic signs have been described on MRI. Normal brain CT scan does not rule out CVT.

1106. Use of which of the following has no proven value in intracranial hypertension management in CVT?

Semin Cerebrovasc Dis Stroke. 2004;4:2-17

A. Acetazolamide
B. Glycerol
C. Mannitol
D. Corticosteroids

Intracranial hypertension is common in CVT and should be treated immediately. Definitive treatment is establishing reperfusion of the venous structures (Heparin, Intravenous thrombolysis, thrombectomy). Elevating head of the bed by 30° improves venous drainage. Good pain control and thermal regulation, acetazolamide, glycerol, or mannitol, surgical ventricular drainage, and surgical decompression are useful. Corticosteroids should be avoided. They increase the risk of systemic infections and are of no proven value in CVT. Moreover, there is concern about their thrombogenic risk.

1107. Recurrent sinus thrombosis within one year occurs in what percentage of patients?

N Engl J Med. 2005;352:1791-8

A. 2%
B. 4%
C. 6%
D. 8%

Recurrent sinus thrombosis occurs in 2% of patients and ~4% of patients have an extracranial thrombotic event within one year.

1108. Usually, vitamin K antagonists are given for what length of time after a first episode of sinus thrombosis?

N Engl J Med. 2005;352:1791-8

A. Six months
B. One year
C. Five years
D. Life long

Optimal duration of oral anticoagulant treatment after the acute phase is unknown. Usually, vitamin K antagonists are given for six months after a first episode of sinus thrombosis, or longer in the presence of predisposing factors, with a target INR of 2.5.

1109. Anticoagulation in patients with venous sinus thrombosis is often continued indefinitely if?

Harrison's 20th Ed. Chapter 420, Page 3085

A. Hypercoagulable state is found
B. Thrombophilia is diagnosed
C. Patient has a h/o coma
D. Patient has a h/o seizure

Intravenous heparin reduces morbidity & mortality, regardless of the presence of intracranial hemorrhage. If an underlying hypercoagulable state is not found, vitamin K antagonists (VKAs) are given for 3–6 months then switch over to aspirin. Anticoagulation is often continued indefinitely if thrombophilia is diagnosed.

1110. Mortality after treatment with anticoagulant drugs in patients of cerebral venous sinus thrombosis (CVST) is?

J Neurol Neurosurg Psychiatry 2001;70:105 - 108

A. 2% to 5%
B. 5% to 10%
C. 10% to 15%
D. 15% to 20%

Treatment with anticoagulant drugs leads to a moderate benefit for patients with CVST compared with placebo treatment, but mortality after treatment with anticoagulant drugs is still 5% to 10%.

1111. Sickle cell anemia (SS disease) is a common cause of stroke in?

Harrison's 20th Ed. Chapter 420, Page 3085

A. Infants
B. Children
C. Adults
D. Old

Sickle cell anemia (SS disease) is a common cause of stroke in children.

1112. Which of the following is a common cause of stroke in children?

Harrison's 20th Ed. Chapter 420, Page 3085

A. Temporal (giant cell) arteritis
B. Hypercoagulable disorders
C. Fibromuscular dysplasia
D. Sickle cell anemia

Sickle cell anemia (SS disease) is a common cause of stroke in children.

1113. Which of the following investigation is useful in predicting stroke in childhood in SS disease carriers?

Harrison's 20th Ed. Chapter 420, Page 3085

A. MR-venography
B. CT-venography
C. Conventional X-ray angiography
D. Transcranial Doppler ultrasonography

Documenting high-velocity blood flow within MCAs using transcranial Doppler ultrasonography can predict the chances of stroke in childhood in SS disease carriers.

1114. Which of the following diseases affects cervical arteries and occurs mainly in women?

Harrison's 20th Ed. Chapter 420, Page 3085

A. Temporal (giant cell) arteritis
B. Fibromuscular dysplasia
C. Moyamoya disease
D. Binswanger's disease

Fibromuscular dysplasia affects the cervical arteries & occurs mainly in women. Carotid or vertebral arteries show multiple rings of segmental narrowing alternating with dilatation. Involvement of the renal arteries is common and may cause hypertension.

1115. Which of the following about fibromuscular dysplasia is false?

Harrison's 20th Ed. Chapter 420, Page 3085

A. Affects carotid or vertebral arteries
B. Occurs mainly in women
C. Involvement of renal arteries is common
D. None of the above

1116. Which of the following is false about Temporal (giant cell) arteritis?

Harrison's 20th Ed. Chapter 420, Page 3086

A. Affects elderly persons
B. Affects internal & external carotid system
C. May cause blindness
D. Rarely causes stroke

Temporal (giant cell) arteritis rarely causes stroke as internal carotid artery is usually not inflamed.

1117. Which is the most common form of vasculitis that affects the carotid artery?

Harrison's 20th Ed. Chapter 420, Page 3086

A. Temporal arteritis
B. Takayasu's arteritis
C. Kawasaki disease
D. Polyarteritis nodosa

1118. Moyamoya disease results from progressive stenosis and occlusion of?

Harrison's 20th Ed. Chapter 420, Page 3086

A. Distal Basilar artery
B. Distal vertebral artery
C. Distal internal carotid artery
D. None of the above

Moyamoya disease is an occlusive disease involving large intracranial arteries, especially distal internal carotid artery and stem of middle and anterior cerebral arteries.

1119. 'Moyamoya' in Japanese language means?
Harrison's 20th Ed. Chapter 420, Page 3087

A. Cotton ball
B. Pin head
C. Puff of smoke
D. Needle

Lenticulostriate arteries (anterior circulation) develop a rich collateral circulation around the occlusive lesion, which on conventional X-ray angiography appears like a "puff of smoke" (moyamoya in Japanese).

1120. In Moyamoya disease, vascular inflammation is?
Harrison's 20th Ed. Chapter 420, Page 3087

A. Absent
B. Mild
C. Moderate
D. Severe

In Moyamoya disease, vascular inflammation is absent.

1121. Posterior reversible encephalopathy syndrome (PRES) can occur with?
Harrison's 20th Ed. Chapter 420, Page 3087

A. Head injury
B. Seizure
C. Eclampsia
D. Any of the above

Posterior reversible encephalopathy syndrome (PRES) can occur with head injury, seizure, migraine, sympathomimetic drug use, eclampsia and in the postpartum period.

1122. Reversible cerebral vasoconstriction syndrome (RCVS) closely resembles which of the following?
Harrison's 20th Ed. Chapter 420, Page 3087

A. Migraine
B. Amaurosis Fugax
C. Subarachnoid hemorrhage
D. Benign positional vertigo

Reversible cerebral vasoconstriction syndrome (RCVS) typically presents with sudden, severe headache closely mimicking SAH. Patients may experience ischemic infarction and intracerebral hemorrhage and typically have new-onset severe hypertension.

1123. CADASIL is due to mutations in which gene?
Harrison's 20th Ed. Chapter 420, Page 3087

A. Notch-1
B. Notch-2
C. Notch-3
D. Notch-4

CADASIL is caused by mutations in Notch-3 gene. Notch-3 is a member of a highly conserved gene family characterized by epidermal growth factor repeats in its extracellular domain.

1124. Which of the following is categorized under monogenic disorders as a cause of stroke?
Harrison's 20th Ed. Chapter 420, Page 3087

A. CADASIL
B. CARASIL
C. HERNS
D. All of the above

Stroke due to monogenic disorders represent <1% of all stroke patients. They are cerebral autosomal-dominant arteriopathy with subcortical infarcts and leukoencephalopathy (CADASIL), cerebral autosomal-recessive arteriosclerosis with subcortical infarcts and leukoencephalopathy (CARASIL), hereditary endotheliopathy with retinopathy, nephropathy, and stroke (HERNS), Fabry disease, pseudoxanthoma elasticum, Neurofibromatosis type 1, familial MoyaMoya disease, Ehlers-Danlos syndrome type IV, Marfan syndrome.

1125. Which of the following is false about CADASIL?
Harrison's 20th Ed. Chapter 420, Page 3087

A. Onset is in IV or V decade of life
B. Autosomal recessive condition
C. Presents as small-vessel strokes, progressive dementia
D. Extensive symmetric white matter changes in MRI

CADASIL (cerebral autosomal dominant arteriopathy with subcortical infarcts and leukoencephalopathy) is an autosomal dominant inherited disorder.

1126. Which of the following is a monogenic ischemic stroke syndrome?
Harrison's 20th Ed. Chapter 420, Page 3087

A. Moyamoya disease
B. Binswanger's disease
C. CADASIL
D. None of the above

CADASIL (cerebral autosomal dominant arteriopathy with subcortical infarcts and leukoencephalopathy) is a monogenic ischemic stroke syndrome. Genetic testing is available. Other monogenic ischemic stroke syndromes include cerebral autosomal recessive arteriopathy with subcortical infarcts and leukoencephalopathy (CARASIL) and hereditary endotheliopathy, retinopathy, nephropathy, and stroke (HERNS).

1127. In Greek, word "mitos" means?
N Engl J Med. 2013;369:2236-51

A. Lamp
B. Thread
C. Tail
D. Baloon

Word mitochondrion is derived from Greek words mitos (meaning thread) and chondrion (meaning granule).

1128. Which of the following is a mitochondrial syndrome?
N Engl J Med. 2013;369:2236-51

A. Joubert syndrome
B. Senior-Loken syndrome
C. Leigh's disease
D. Caroli's syndrome

Mitochondrial syndromes include MELAS syndrome (mitochondrial encephalomyopathy, lactic acidosis, and strokelike episodes caused by mutation of mitochondrial transfer RNAs), and Leigh's disease (caused by mutations in genes related to oxidative phosphorylation).

1129. Which of the following disorders can mimic multiple sclerosis?
Harrison's 20th Ed. Page 3194 Table 436-4

A. Acute disseminated encephalomyelitis (ADEM)
B. Mitochondrial encephalopathy with lactic acidosis and stroke (MELAS)
C. Cerebral autosomal dominant arteriopathy, subcortical infarcts, and leukoencephalopathy (CADASIL)
D. All of the above

1130. Chronic progressive subcortical arteriosclerotic leukoencephalopathy is called?
Harrison's 20th Ed. Chapter 420, Page 3087

A. Moyamoya disease
B. Binswanger's disease
C. CADASIL
D. None of the above

Binswanger's disease is also called chronic progressive subcortical encephalopathy. It is one of the most common causes of dementia. The term Binswanger's disease should be used with caution, because it does not clearly identify a single entity.

1131. Small-vessel strokes, progressive dementia, and extensive symmetric white matter changes in MRI is suggestive of which of the following?

Harrison's 20th Ed. Chapter 420, Page 3087

A. Moyamoya disease
B. Binswanger's disease
C. CADASIL
D. None of the above

CADASIL (cerebral autosomal dominant arteriopathy with subcortical infarcts and leukoencephalopathy) is an inherited disorder that presents as small-vessel strokes, progressive dementia, and extensive symmetric white matter changes visualized by MRI in the fourth or fifth decade of life. It is caused by one of several mutations in Notch-3 gene.

1132. In CADASIL, which of the following is a prominent manifestation?

Harrison's 20th Ed. Chapter 420, Page 3087

A. Transient blindness
B. Migraine with aura
C. Vertigo
D. Amnesia

In CADASIL, ~40% of patients have migraine with aura.

1133. Which of the following mutation is associated with multiple small vessel strokes with hemorrhagic transformation?

Harrison's 20th Ed. Chapter 420, Page 3087

A. COL4A1
B. COL4A2
C. COL4A3
D. COL4A4

COL4A1 mutation is associated with multiple small vessel strokes with hemorrhagic transformation.

1134. In the first 3 months after TIA, risk of stroke is?

Harrison's 20th Ed. Chapter 420, Page 3087

A. ~ 10–15%
B. ~ 20–35%
C. ~ 40–60%
D. ~ 60–85%

Risk of stroke after TIA is ~10–15% in first 3 months, with most events occurring in first 2 days.

1135. Most neurologic events occur within what duration after a TIA?

Harrison's 20th Ed. Chapter 420, Page 3087

A. First 2 days
B. First 7 days
C. First 15 days
D. First 30 days

Most neurologic events occur in first 2 days after TIA. Risk of stroke is ~10% in first 3 months.

1136. Which of the following estimates risk of stroke following TIA?

Harrison's 20th Ed. Chapter 420, Page 3087 Table 420-5

A. ABCD2 Score
B. SAPS II Score
C. IPI score
D. Modified Child-Pugh classification

APACHE (acute physiology and chronic health evaluation) system and SAPS (simplified acute physiology score) system are severity-of-illness (SOI) scoring systems. International Prognostic Index (IPI) is for NHL. Modified Child-Pugh classification is a staging system for cirrhosis.

1137. Which of the following is not a part of ABCD2 Scoring system for TIA?

Harrison's 20th Ed. Chapter 420, Page 3087 Table 420-5

A. Age
B. Sex
C. Hypertension
D. Diabetes

ABCD2 Scoring system for TIA includes age, blood pressure (SBP & DBP), clinical symptoms (unilateral weakness, speech disturbance without weakness), duration and diabetes. 2 points are for unilateral weakness and duration >60 minutes each, rest have one point.

1138. Which of the following leads to poor metabolism of clopidogrel into its active form?

Harrison's 20th Ed. Chapter 420, Page 3087

A. Decreased CYP2D6 activity
B. Decreased CYP2C19 activity
C. Decreased CYP2C9 activity
D. All of the above

Failure to respond to the combination of aspirin & clopidogrel is linked to carriage of a common CYP2C19 polymorphism (common in Asians) that leads to poor metabolism of clopidogrel into its active form (clopidogrel hypometabolism).

1139. Which of the following is the most significant of the modifiable risk factors to reduce the burden of stroke?

Harrison's 20th Ed. Chapter 420, Page 3088

A. Hypertension
B. Older age
C. Diabetes mellitus
D. Dyslipidemia

1140. The average duration of a TIA is?

Harrison's 20th Ed. Chapter 420, Page 3088

A. ~ 1 minute
B. ~ 12 minutes
C. ~ 35 minutes
D. ~ 56 minutes

The average duration of a TIA is ~12 minutes.

1141. Brain infarction occurs in what percentage of TIAs even when neurologic signs and symptoms are absent?

Harrison's 18th Ed. 3280

A. 1–5%
B. 3–20%
C. 10–20%
D. 15–50%

Even in absence of neurologic signs & symptoms, infarcts of brain occur in 15 - 50% of TIAs.

1142. Systolic Blood Pressure Intervention Trial (SPRINT), recommends that all hypertension should be treated to a target of?

Harrison's 20th Ed. Chapter 420, Page 3088

A. < 120/80 mm Hg
B. < 130/80 mm Hg
C. < 140/90 mm Hg
D. < 150/90 mm Hg

1143. SPRINT trial suggests that lowering SBP to <120 mm Hg reduces stroke & heart attack by?

Harrison's 20th Ed. Chapter 420, Page 3088

A. 13%
B. 23%
C. 33%
D. 43%

SPRINT trial suggests that lowering systolic blood pressure to <120 mm Hg reduces stroke & heart attack by 43% compared to systolic blood pressure <140 mm Hg, without an increased risk of syncope or falls.

1144. Out of the following, which drug is of least importance in reducing the risk of stroke in hypertensives with TIA?

Harrison's 20th Ed. Chapter 420, Page 3088

A. Thiazide diuretics
B. Calcium channel blockers
C. Angiotensin-converting enzyme inhibitors
D. Angiotensin receptor blockers

Lowering BP to normotensive levels reduces risk of stroke in hypertensives with TIA. Drugs of value are thiazide diuretics, ACE inhibitors &ARBs. Statins reduce it by 16–30%. In diabetics, pioglitazone is effective.

1145. Which of the following is related to the trial 'SPARCL'?

Harrison's 20th Ed. Chapter 420, Page 3088

A. Aspirin
B. Pioglitazone
C. Atorvastatin
D. Clopidogrel

1146. Which of the following is false about Stroke Prevention by Aggressive Reduction in Cholesterol Levels (SPARCL) trial?

Harrison's 20th Ed. Chapter 420, Page 3088

A. Done on patients with recent stroke or TIA
B. Secondary stroke reduction
C. Dose of atorvastatin used was 80 mg/day
D. None of the above

SPARCL (Stroke Prevention by Aggressive Reduction in Cholesterol Levels) trial showed benefit in secondary stroke reduction for patients with recent stroke or TIA who were prescribed atorvastatin, 80 mg/day.

1147. Which of the following is a primary prevention trial advocating use of statins to reduce the risk of stroke?

Harrison's 20th Ed. Chapter 420, Page 3088

A. SPARCL
B. CAPRIE
C. JUPITER
D. MATCH

Justification for the Use of Statins in Prevention: An Intervention Trial Evaluating Rosuvastatin (JUPITER) was a primary prevention trial. It found that patients with low LDL (<130 mg/dL) caused by elevated C-reactive protein benefitted by daily use of rosuvastatin. Primary stroke occurrence was reduced by 51% with no increase in rates of intracranial hemorrhage.

1148. Which of the following platelet antiaggregation agents is least preferred to prevent atherothrombotic events?

Harrison's 20th Ed. Chapter 420, Page 3088

A. Aspirin
B. Clopidogrel
C. Dipyridamole
D. Ticlopidine

Though Ticlopidine is more effective than aspirin, it has been abandoned because of its adverse effects like diarrhea, skin rash, neutropenia and thrombotic thrombocytopenic purpura (TTP).

1149. Which of the following about aspirin is false?

Harrison's 20th Ed. Chapter 420, Page 3088

A. Aspirin acetylates platelet cyclooxygenase
B. Irreversibly inhibits formation of thromboxane A2 in platelets
C. Action lasts for the usual 8 day life of platelets
D. None of the above

1150. Which of the following about aspirin is false?

Harrison's 20th Ed. Chapter 420, Page 3088

A. Inhibits formation in endothelial cells of prostacyclin
B. Inhibition of prostacyclin is transient
C. Higher doses of aspirin are not more effective than lower doses
D. None of the above

1151. Which of the following about Clopidogrel is false?

Harrison's 20th Ed. Chapter 420, Page 3088

A. Clopidogrel is a prodrug
B. Thienopyridine derivative
C. Blocks adenosine diphosphate (ADP) receptor on platelets
D. None of the above

Thienopyridine derivatives include clopidogrel & prasugrel.

1152. Which of the following is an ADP receptor?

Harrison's 20th Ed. Chapter 113, Page 840

A. P2X1
B. P2Y1
C. P2Y12
D. All of the above

ADP receptors include P2X1, P2Y1, and P2Y12.

1153. Which of the following is an inhibitor of ADP P2Y12 receptor?

Harrison's 20th Ed. Chapter 114, Page 845 Figure 114-3

A. Clopidogrel
B. Prasugrel
C. Ticagrelor
D. All of the above

Clopidogrel & prasugrel irreversibly block ADP receptor on platelet surface P2Y12., Cangrelor & ticagrelor are reversible inhibitors of P2Y12.

1154. Which of the following is responsible for bioactivation of clopidogrel?

Harrison's 20th Ed. Chapter 113, Page 841

A. CYP2C9
B. DPYD
C. CYP2D6
D. CYP2C19

CYP2C19 is responsible for bioactivation of antiplatelet drug clopidogrel. Omeprazole phenocopy this effect by inhibiting CYP2C19. Loss-of-function polymorphisms in CYP2C19 is the strongest individual variable affecting pharmacokinetics & antiplatelet response to clopidogrel.

1155. Which of the following is an antiplatelet drug?

Harrison's 20th Ed. Chapter 420, Page 844

A. Cangrelor
B. Ticagrelor
C. Vorapaxar
D. All of the above

1156. Which of the following drug was studied in the CAPRIE, MATCH and CHARISMA trials?
Harrison's 20th Ed. Chapter 420, Page 3088

A. Ticlopidine
B. Dipyridamole
C. Clopidogrel & Aspirin
D. Statins

These three trials concluded that use of clopidogrel in combination with aspirin is not recommended for stroke prevention. But, may be beneficial in acute period.

1157. Which of the following trials was done for cerebral small-vessel disease?
Harrison's 20th Ed. Chapter 420, Page 3088, N Engl J Med. 2012;367:817-25

A. SPS3 trial
B. CHARISMA
C. CURRENT–OASIS 7
D. CURE

The Secondary Prevention of Small Subcortical Strokes (SPS3) trial investigators concluded that among patients with recent lacunar strokes, addition of clopidogrel to aspirin did not significantly reduce risk of recurrent stroke & did significantly increase the risk of bleeding & death.

1158. Which of the following drug was studied in the ESPS II, ESPRIT and PRoFESS trials?
Harrison's 20th Ed. Chapter 420, Page 3088

A. Ticlopidine & Aspirin
B. Dipyridamole & Aspirin
C. Clopidogrel & Aspirin
D. Statins & Aspirin

Dipyridamole with aspirin combination drug was studied in three trials.

1159. Which of the following about Dipyridamole is false?
Harrison's 20th Ed. Chapter 420, Page 3088

A. Inhibits uptake of adenosine by vascular endothelium
B. Potentiates antiaggregatory effects of prostacyclin
C. Its erratic absorption depends on stomach pH
D. None of the above

Antiplatelet agent Dipyridamole inhibits uptake of adenosine by vascular endothelium. Consequently, accumulated adenosine acts as an inhibitor of platelet aggregation. It also potentiates the antiaggregatory effects of prostacyclin. Dipyridamole is erratically absorbed depending on stomach pH.

1160. Which of the following is the principal side effect of dipyridamole?
Harrison's 20th Ed. Chapter 420, Page 3088

A. Diarrhea
B. Headache
C. Skin rash
D. Neutropenia

The principal side effect of dipyridamole is headache.

1161. What is the overall 'relative' reduction in risk of all vascular events with antiplatelet agents?
Harrison's 20th Ed. Chapter 420, Page 3088

A. 5%
B. 10%
C. 18%
D. 25%

Antiplatelet agents produce an overall relative reduction in risk of nonfatal stroke of about 25–30% and of all vascular events of about 25%.

1162. Individuals with a 10–15% risk of vascular events per year have a reduction to how much with use of antiplatelet agents?
Harrison's 20th Ed. Chapter 420, Page 3088

A. ~ 1.5–5%
B. ~ 7.5–11%
C. ~ 14.5–21%
D. ~ 27.5–41%

Individuals with a 10–15% risk of vascular events per year experience a reduction in stroke to ~ 7.5–11% with use of antiplatelet agents.

1163. How much is the average annual risk of another stroke in a patient who has experienced atherothrombotic stroke or TIA?
Harrison's 20th Ed. Chapter 420, Page 3089

A. 3–6%
B. 8–10%
C. 12–20%
D. 28–40%

Every patient who has experienced atherothrombotic stroke or TIA should take antiplatelet agent regularly, because average annual risk of another stroke is 8–10%.

1164. In chronic nonvalvular, nonrheumatic AF (NVAF), anticoagulation with warfarin reduces risk of cerebral embolism by?
Harrison's 20th Ed. Chapter 420, Page 3089

A. ~ 17%
B. ~ 27%
C. ~ 47%
D. ~ 67%

In chronic nonvalvular, nonrheumatic atrial fibrillation (NVAF), warfarin (a vitamin K antagonist - VKA) reduces the risk of cerebral embolism by ~67% both for primary & secondary prevention of stroke or TIA. The risk of a major bleeding complication is 1–3% per year.

1165. Which of the following agents was used in ARISTOTLE trial?
Harrison's 20th Ed. Chapter 420, Page 3089

A. Apixaban
B. Aspirin
C. Atorvastatin
D. Abciximab

In Apixaban for Reduction in Stroke and Other Thromboembolic Events in Atrial Fibrillation (ARISTOTLE) trial, patients were randomized between apixaban, 5 mg twice daily, and dose-adjusted warfarin (INR 2-3).

1166. Which of the following agents was used in ROCKET-AF trial?
Harrison's 20th Ed. Chapter 420, Page 3089

A. Rivaroxaban
B. Ramipril
C. Rosuvastatin
D. Recombinant tPA

Rivaroxaban Once Daily Oral Direct Factor Xa Inhibition Compared with Vitamin K Antagonism for Prevention of Stroke and Embolism Trial in Atrial Fibrillation (ROCKET-AF).

1167. Which of the following statements is false?
Harrison's 20th Ed. Chapter 420, Page 3089

A. Intermittent AF carries the same risk of stroke as chronic AF
B. Dabigatran requires no blood monitoring to titrate its dose
C. Dabigatran is less effective than warfarin in patients with prosthetic heart valve implantation
D. None of the above

1168. In ACTIVE-A trial, which of the following drugs was not used?
Harrison's 20th Ed. Chapter 420, Page 3089

A. Clopidogrel
B. Aspirin
C. Ticlopidine
D. Irbesartan

In Atrial Fibrillation Clopidogrel Trial with Irbesartan for Prevention of Vascular Events (ACTIVE-A) trial, patients who cannot take anticoagulants, clopidogrel plus aspirin was compared to aspirin alone.

1169. NASCET and ECST trials advocate carotid endarterectomy when carotid artery stenosis is more than?
Harrison's 20th Ed. Chapter 420, Page 3090

A. 30%
B. 50%
C. 70%
D. 90%

North American Symptomatic Carotid Endarterectomy Trial (NASCET) & European Carotid Surgery Trial (ECST) showed benefit for carotid endarterectomy when stenosis of ≥70%.

1170. Carotid endarterectomy is most beneficial within how many weeks of symptom onset?
Harrison's 20th Ed. Chapter 420, Page 3090

A. 2 weeks
B. 4 weeks
C. 6 weeks
D. 8 weeks

1171. Carotid endarterectomy is most beneficial in?
Harrison's 20th Ed. Chapter 420, Page 3090

A. Men
B. Those >75 years
C. When performed within 2 weeks of symptom onset
D. All of the above

Carotid endarterectomy is most beneficial when performed within 2 weeks of symptom onset. Benefits more men than women and those >75 years.

1172. Which of the following trails does not address carotid endarterectomy?
Harrison's 20th Ed. Chapter 420, Page 3090

A. ACAS
B. ECST
C. WARSS
D. NASCET

Warfarin-Aspirin Reinfarction Stroke Study (WARSS) study found no benefit of warfarin sodium over aspirin for secondary prevention of stroke. Similarly, Warfarin-Aspirin Symptomatic Intracranial Disease (WASID) study demonstrated no benefit of warfarin over aspirin in patients with symptomatic intracranial atherosclerosis. North American Symptomatic Carotid Endarterectomy Trial (NASCET) and the European Carotid Surgery Trial (ECST) showed a substantial benefit for surgery in patients with a symptomatic carotid stenosis of ≥ 70%. ECST found harm for patients with stenosis <30% treated surgically. Meta-analysis of NASCET and ECST trials showed that endarterectomy is most beneficial when performed within 2 weeks of symptom onset, in patients >75 years, and men appear to benefit more than women.

1173. What is the annual stroke rate in the natural history of asymptomatic carotid stenosis?
Harrison's 20th Ed. Chapter 420, Page 3090

A. ~ 1%
B. ~ 2%
C. ~ 3%
D. ~ 4%

1174. What is the annual stroke rate in the natural history of symptomatic carotid stenosis?
Harrison's 20th Ed. Chapter 420, Page 3090

A. ~ 10%
B. ~ 11%
C. ~ 12%
D. ~ 13%

The natural history of asymptomatic carotid stenosis is ~2% per year stroke rate, while symptomatic patients experience a 13% per year risk of stroke.

1175. SAPPHIRE, CREST, and ICSS pertain to which of the following?
Harrison's 20th Ed. Chapter 420, Page 3090

A. Anticoagulation in stroke
B. Use of atherothrombotics in TIA/stroke
C. Carotid artery stenting and angioplasty
D. Extracranial-to-intracranial (EC-IC) bypass surgery

Stenting and Angioplasty with Protection in Patients at High Risk for Endarterectomy (SAPPHIRE) trial was done in high risk patients with symptomatic carotid stenosis >50% or asymptomatic stenosis >80% by either stenting combined with a distal emboli-protection device or endarterectomy. Carotid Revascularization Endarterectomy versus Stenting Trial (CREST) and International Carotid Stenting (ICSS) trial also studied symptomatic patients treated with stents or endarterectomy.

1176. Which of the following has been found to be dramatically harmful in stroke treatment?
Harrison's 20th Ed. Chapter 420, Page 3091

A. Extracranial-to-intracranial (EC-IC) bypass surgery
B. Intracranial stenting of intracranial atherosclerosis
C. Balloon angioplasty coupled with stenting
D. Carotid endarterectomy

Intracranial stenting of intracranial atherosclerosis was found to be dramatically harmful as compared to aspirin in Stenting and Aggressive Medical Management for Preventing Recurrent Stroke in Intracranial Stenosis (SAMMPRIS) trial.

Intracranial Hemorrhage

1177. Bleeding into subdural and epidural spaces is principally produced by?

Harrison's 20th Ed. Chapter 421, Page 3091

A. Trauma
B. Coagulation disorders
C. Hypertension
D. Cocaine use

Bleeding into subdural and epidural spaces is principally produced by trauma.

1178. Subarachnoid hemorrhage results from?

Harrison's 20th Ed. Chapter 421, Page 3091

A. Trauma
B. Rupture of intracranial aneurysm
C. Arteriovenous malformation (AVM)
D. Any of the above

SAH results from trauma or the rupture of an intracranial aneurysm or arteriovenous malformation (AVM).

1179. Which of the following clinical trial addresses effect of acute blood pressure lowering on ICH functional outcome?

Harrison's 20th Ed. Chapter 421, Page 3091

A. INTERACT2
B. STICH
C. ARUBA
D. WASID

INTERACT2 trial is a large phase 3 clinical trial to address the effect of acute blood pressure lowering on ICH functional outcome.

1180. Which of the following is a clinical trial designed similarly to INTERACT2?

Harrison's 20th Ed. Chapter 421, Page 3091

A. ATACH2
B. STAR-D
C. TACT
D. HYVET

1181. In intraparenchymal hemorrhage, mean arterial blood pressure should be?

Harrison's 20th Ed. Chapter 421, Page 3091

A. < 160 mm Hg
B. < 150 mm Hg
C. < 140 mm Hg
D. < 130 mm Hg

1182. In patients with spontaneous ICH whose initial SBP was 150 – 220 mm Hg, systolic blood pressure can be safely lowered acutely and rapidly to?

Harrison's 20th Ed. Chapter 421, Page 3091

A. < 110 mm Hg
B. < 120 mm Hg
C. < 130 mm Hg
D. < 140 mm Hg

Systolic blood pressure (SBP) can be safely lowered acutely and rapidly to < 140 mm Hg in patients with spontaneous ICH whose initial SBP was 150 - 220 mm Hg (INTERACT2).

1183. In intraparenchymal hemorrhage, cerebral perfusion pressure should be maintained above?

Harrison's 20th Ed. Chapter 421, Page 3091

A. 20–40 mm Hg
B. 40–50 mm Hg
C. 50–70 mm Hg
D. 70–80 mm Hg

Current recommendation in hypertensive patients of intraparenchymal hemorrhage is to maintain the cerebral perfusion pressure (mean arterial pressure [MAP] minus ICP) at 50–70 mm Hg.

1184. Which of the following drugs is useful in lowering blood pressure in intraparenchymal hemorrhage?

Harrison's 20th Ed. Chapter 421, Page 3092

A. Nicardipine
B. Labetalol
C. Esmolol
D. All of the above

Intraparenchymal hemorrhage is exacerbated by acutely elevated BP & should be lowered to a mean arterial BP of <130 mm Hg by nonvasodilating IV drugs like nicardipine, labetalol or esmolol.

1185. Intraparenchymal hemorrhage accounts for what proportion of all strokes?

Harrison's 20th Ed. Chapter 421, Page 3092

A. ~ 1%
B. ~ 5%
C. ~ 10%
D. ~ 15%

1186. Out of the following hemorrhagic stroke subtypes, which has the maximum frequency of occurrence?

Harrison's 20th Ed. Chapter 421, Page 3092

A. Intraparenchymal
B. Subdural
C. Epidural
D. Subarachnoid

Intraparenchymal hemorrhage is the most common type of intracranial hemorrhage. It accounts for ~10% of all strokes and is associated with a 35–45% case fatality rate within the first month. Hypertension, coagulopathy, sympathomimetic drugs (cocaine, methamphetamine), and cerebral amyloid angiopathy (CAA) cause most of intraparenchymal hemorrhages.

1187. Which of the following is the most important cause of intraparenchymal hemorrhage in the young?

Harrison's 20th Ed. Chapter 421, Page 3092

A. Hypertension
B. Cerebral amyloid angiopathy
C. Cocaine use
D. Heavy alcohol consumption

Advanced age & heavy alcohol consumption increase risk of intraparenchymal hemorrhage. Cocaine & methamphetamine use is one of the most important cause in young (<45 years).

1188. Which of the following is associated with cocaine use?
Harrison's 20th Ed. Chapter 421, Page 3092

A. Intracerebral hemorrhage (ICH)
B. Ischemic stroke (IS)
C. Subarachnoid hemorrhage (SAH)
D. All of the above

Intracerebral hemorrhage, ischemic stroke, and SAH are all associated with cocaine use.

1189. Hypertensive intraparenchymal hemorrhage is due to spontaneous rupture of?
Harrison's 20th Ed. Chapter 421, Page 3092

A. Penetrating artery
B. Bifurcation of artery
C. Aneurysm of artery
D. Any of the above

Hypertensive intraparenchymal hemorrhage usually results from spontaneous rupture of a small penetrating artery deep in the brain.

1190. Which of the following is not a common site for hypertensive intraparenchymal hemorrhage?
Harrison's 20th Ed. Chapter 421, Page 3092

A. Basal ganglia
B. Cerebellum
C. Pons
D. Medulla oblongata

The most common sites of hypertensive intraparenchymal hemorrhage are basal ganglia (esp. putamen), thalamus, cerebellum and pons.

1191. Out of the following, which is the most common site for hypertensive intraparenchymal hemorrhage?
Harrison's 20th Ed. Chapter 421, Page 3092

A. Thalamus
B. Putamen
C. Caudate nucleus
D. Globus pallidus

Putamen is the most common site for hypertensive intraparenchymal hemorrhage.

1192. In hypertensive intraparenchymal hemorrhage, if blood dissects into the ventricular space, the morbidity?
Harrison's 20th Ed. Chapter 421, Page 3092

A. Remains the same
B. Increases
C. Decreases
D. Any of the above

In hypertensive intraparenchymal hemorrhage, blood may dissect into the ventricular space which substantially 'increases' morbidity and may cause hydrocephalus.

1193. Most hypertensive intraparenchymal hemorrhages develop over what period of time?
Harrison's 20th Ed. Chapter 421, Page 3092

A. 1 to 10 minutes
B. 10 to 30 minutes
C. 30 to 90 minutes
D. 90 to 180 minutes

Most hypertensive intraparenchymal hemorrhages develop over 30 to 90 minutes.

1194. Which of the following statements about intracerebral hemorrhages is false?
Harrison's 20th Ed. Chapter 421, Page 3092

A. Almost always occur in awake state
B. Abrupt onset of focal neurologic deficit
C. Seizures are common
D. Focal deficit worsens steadily over 30 to 90 minutes

Intracerebral hemorrhages almost always occur in awake state. Hemorrhage presents as abrupt onset of focal neurologic deficit. Seizures are uncommon. Focal deficit worsens steadily over 30–90 minutes with a diminishing level of consciousness & signs of raised ICP (headache/vomiting).

1195. In hypertensive putaminal hemorrhage, the eyes deviate towards which side?
Harrison's 20th Ed. Chapter 421, Page 3092

A. Away from the side of hemiparesis
B. Towards the side of hemiparesis
C. Remain in the center
D. Rotate upwards

In putaminal hypertensive hemorrhage, contralateral hemiparesis is the sentinel sign. Eyes deviate away from the side of hemiparesis.

1196. In hypertensive intraparenchymal hemorrhage, if there is a downward & inward deviation of eyes, the location of hemorrhage is in?
Harrison's 20th Ed. Chapter 421, Page 3092

A. Putamen
B. Thalamus
C. Pons
D. Cerebellum

Thalamic hemorrhages may extend inferiorly into upper midbrain and cause deviation of eyes downward and inward.

1197. In thalamic hemorrhage, which of the following sensory modality is affected?
Harrison's 20th Ed. Chapter 421, Page 3092

A. Exteroceptive
B. Proprioceptive
C. Cortical
D. All of the above

Thalamic hemorrhages also produce contralateral hemiplegia due to involvement of adjacent internal capsule. Prominent sensory deficit involving all modalities is usually present.

1198. Which of the following is true in thalamic hemorrhage?
Harrison's 20th Ed. Chapter 421, Page 3092

A. Unequal pupils with absence of light reaction
B. Absence of convergence
C. Ipsilateral Horner's syndrome
D. All of the above

Thalamic hemorrhages by extension inferiorly into upper midbrain may lead to homonymous visual field defect, unequal pupils with absence of light reaction, skew deviation with eye opposite hemorrhage displaced downward & medially, ipsilateral Horner's syndrome, absence of convergence, paralysis of vertical gaze, and retraction nystagmus.

1199. Contralateral pain3 syndrome is also called?
Harrison's 20th Ed. Chapter 421, Page 3092

A. Cogan's syndrome
B. Brugada syndrome
C. Wallenberg's syndrome
D. Déjérine-Roussy syndrome

Thalamic Déjérine-Roussy syndrome consists of contralateral hemisensory loss followed later by persistent agonizing, searing, or burning pain in the affected areas. It is responds poorly to analgesics. Carbamazepine, gabapentin or tricyclic antidepressants may be beneficial.

1200. In hypertensive intraparenchymal hemorrhage, if there is impairment of doll's head or oculocephalic maneuver, the location of hemorrhage is in?

Harrison's 20th Ed. Chapter 421, Page 3092

A. Putamen
B. Thalamus
C. Pons
D. Cerebellum

In pontine hemorrhages, there is impairment of reflex horizontal eye movements evoked by head turning (doll's head or oculocephalic maneuver).

1201. Which of the following is a feature of pontine hemorrhages?

Harrison's 20th Ed. Chapter 421, Page 3092

A. Hyperpnea
B. Severe hypertension
C. Hyperhidrosis
D. All of the above

1202. Excessive sweating (hyperhidrosis) is a feature of which of the following CVAs?

Harrison's 20th Ed. Chapter 421, Page 3092

A. Basal ganglia hemorrhage
B. Thalamic hemorrhage
C. Pontine hemorrhage
D. Cerebellar hemorrhage

Presentation of pontine hemorrhage include sudden onset, pinpoint pupils (1 mm) reactive to light, loss of reflex eye movements and corneal responses, ocular bobbing, posturing, hyperventilation, severe hypertension and excessive sweating.

1203. Decerebrate rigidity is most frequent which of the following hypertensive intraparenchymal hemorrhage?

Harrison's 20th Ed. Chapter 421, Page 3092

A. Basal ganglia hemorrhage
B. Thalamic hemorrhage
C. Pontine hemorrhage
D. Cerebellar hemorrhage

In pontine hemorrhages, deep coma with quadriplegia usually occurs over a few minutes with prominent decerebrate rigidity.

1204. Cerebellar hemorrhages are characterized by?

Harrison's 20th Ed. Chapter 421, Page 3092

A. Occipital headache
B. Repeated vomiting
C. Ataxia of gait
D. All of the above

Cerebellar hemorrhages develop over several hours & are characterized by occipital headache, repeated vomiting, and ataxia of gait.

1205. In mild cases of cerebellar hemorrhage, there may be no other neurologic sign other than?

Harrison's 20th Ed. Chapter 421, Page 3092

A. Gait ataxia
B. Occipital headache
C. Repeated vomiting
D. Seizure

In mild cases of cerebellar hemorrhage, there may be no other neurologic signs other than gait ataxia.

1206. Which of the following about cerebellar hemorrhage is false?

Harrison's 20th Ed. Chapter 421, Page 3092

A. Forced deviation of eyes to opposite side
B. Paresis of conjugate lateral gaze toward side of hemorrhage
C. Usually develop over several hours
D. None of the above

In cerebellar hemorrhage, dizziness or vertigo may be prominent. There is paresis of conjugate lateral gaze toward the side of hemorrhage, forced deviation of eyes to opposite side, or an ipsilateral sixth nerve palsy.

1207. Which of the following lobar hemorrhage causes arm weakness?

Harrison's 20th Ed. Chapter 421, Page 3093

A. Occipital hemorrhage
B. Left temporal hemorrhage
C. Parietal hemorrhage
D. Frontal hemorrhage

Major neurologic deficit with occipital hemorrhage is hemianopia, with left temporal hemorrhage, it is aphasia and delirium, with parietal hemorrhage, it is a hemisensory loss and with frontal hemorrhage, it is arm weakness.

1208. Which of the following is uncommon in lobar hemorrhages?

Harrison's 20th Ed. Chapter 421, Page 3093

A. Focal headaches
B. Vomiting
C. Drowsiness
D. Stiff neck

Most patients with lobar hemorrhages have focal headaches and more than half vomit or are drowsy. Stiff neck and seizures are uncommon.

1209. Which of the following is mainly affected in cerebral amyloid angiopathy?

Harrison's 20th Ed. Chapter 421, Page 3093

A. Arterioles
B. Venules
C. Capillaries
D. All of the above

1210. Cerebral amyloid angiopathy affects mainly?

Harrison's 20th Ed. Chapter 421, Page 3093

A. Children
B. Adults
C. Elderly
D. All of the above

Cerebral amyloid angiopathy is a disease of the elderly in which arteriolar degeneration occurs and amyloid is deposited in the walls of the cerebral arteries.

1211. Cerebral amyloid angiopathy cause which of the following?

Harrison's 20th Ed. Chapter 421, Page 3093

A. Intraparenchymal hemorrhage
B. Lobar hemorrhage
C. Cerebellar hemorrhage
D. Subarachnoid hemorrhage

Cerebral amyloid angiopathy causes both single and recurrent lobar hemorrhages and is the most common cause of lobar hemorrhage in elderly.

1212. Intracranial hemorrhages associated with anticoagulant therapy occur in?

Harrison's 20th Ed. Chapter 421, Page 3093

A. Lobar hemorrhage
B. Thalamic hemorrhage
C. Pontine hemorrhage
D. Any location

Intracranial hemorrhages associated with anticoagulant therapy & hematologic disorders can occur at any location (lobar or subdural) and may present as multiple intracerebral hemorrhages. Skin and mucous membrane bleeding is usually evident and offers a diagnostic clue.

1213. Which of the following hematologic disorders can cause ICH?

Harrison's 20th Ed. Chapter 421, Page 3093

A. Leukemia
B. Aplastic anemia
C. Thrombocytopenic purpura
D. All of the above

ICH associated with hematologic disorders like leukemia, aplastic anemia and thrombocytopenic purpura. Any site is possible and may present as multiple ICHs.

1214. Which of the following is a cause of stroke in young?

Harrison's 20th Ed. Chapter 421, Page 3093

A. Cocaine use
B. Moyamoya disease
C. Dissection of the internal carotid or vertebral arteries
D. All of the above

1215. Which of the following is associated with stimulant use?

Harrison's 20th Ed. Chapter 421, Page 3093

A. ICH
B. Ischemic stroke
C. Subarachnoid hemorrhage (SAH)
D. All of the above

Cocaine enhances sympathetic activity causing acute, sometimes severe, hypertension, and this may lead to hemorrhage. Over 50% of stimulant-related intracranial hemorrhages are intracerebral & rest are subarachnoid when a saccular aneurysm is usually identified. Acute hypertension causes aneurysmal rupture.

1216. Which of the following worsens the prognosis in intracerebral hemorrhage?

Harrison's 20th Ed. Chapter 421, Page 3093

A. Extension into the ventricular system
B. Advanced age
C. Location within the posterior fossa
D. All of the above

Extension into ventricular system, advanced age, location within posterior fossa & depressed level of consciousness at initial presentation worsens prognosis in intracerebral hemorrhage.

1217. Which of the following metastatic tumors is associated with ICH?

Harrison's 20th Ed. Chapter 421, Page 3093

A. Choriocarcinoma
B. Renal cell carcinoma
C. Bronchogenic carcinoma
D. All of the above

Choriocarcinoma, malignant melanoma, renal cell carcinoma and bronchogenic carcinoma are among the most common metastatic tumors associated with ICH.

1218. What volume of supratentorial hematomas due to hypertensive intracerebral hemorrhage have a good prognosis?

Harrison's 20th Ed. Chapter 421, Page 3094

A. < 30 mL
B. < 60 mL
C. < 90 mL
D. < 120 mL

1219. What volume of supratentorial hematomas due to hypertensive intracerebral hemorrhage have a poor prognosis?

Harrison's 20th Ed. Chapter 421, Page 3094

A. > 10 mL
B. > 25 mL
C. > 40 mL
D. > 60 mL

Volume and location of hematoma determine prognosis. Supratentorial hematomas due to hypertensive intracerebral hemorrhage with volumes <30 mL have a good prognosis 30 to 60 mL, an intermediate prognosis and >60 mL, a poor prognosis during initial hospitalization.

1220. What diameter of cerebellar hematoma will require surgical evacuation?

Harrison's 20th Ed. Chapter 421, Page 3094

A. > 0.5 cm
B. > 1.5 cm
C. > 2 cm
D. > 3 cm

Most cerebellar hematomas >3 cm in diameter require surgical evacuation.

1221. Reversible posterior leukoencephalopathy best relates to which of the following?

Harrison's 20th Ed. Chapter 421, Page 3093

A. Hypertensive encephalopathy
B. Intracranial hemorrhages due to anticoagulant therapy
C. Head injury
D. Primary intraventricular hemorrhage

MRI brain imaging shows a pattern of typically posterior (occipital > frontal) brain edema that is reversible and termed reversible posterior leukoencephalopathy.

1222. Hemorrhages into the spinal cord are usually the result of?

Harrison's 20th Ed. Chapter 421, Page 3093

A. AVM
B. Cavernous malformation
C. Metastatic tumor
D. All of the above

Hemorrhages into spinal cord are the result of an AVM, cavernous malformation or metastatic tumor.

1223. Spot sign best relates to?

Harrison's 20th Ed. Chapter 421, Page 3094

A. Subdural hematoma
B. Intraventricular leak
C. Ongoing bleeding within a hematoma
D. Hemangioma

CT angiography (CTA) or postcontrast CT imaging may reveal one or more small areas of enhancement within a hematoma. This "spot sign" represents ongoing bleeding. Presence of a spot sign is associated with an increased risk of hematoma expansion, increased mortality and lower likelihood of favorable functional outcome.

1224. Which is the agent of first choice in reversing warfarin induced coagulopathy in intracerebral hemorrhage?

Harrison's 20th Ed. Chapter 421, Page 3094

A. Prothrombin complex concentrate infusion
B. Fresh-frozen plasma
C. Vitamin K
D. Any of the above

Agent of first choice in reversing warfarin induced coagulopathy in intracerebral hemorrhage is prothrombin complex concentrate (PCCs). Fresh frozen plasma (FFP) is an alternative.

1225. Which of the following is an effective antidote to oral thrombin inhibitor dabigatran?

Harrison's 20th Ed. Chapter 421, Page 3094

A. Vitamin K
B. Prothrombin complex concentrates (PCC)
C. Fresh frozen plasma
D. None of the above

There is no effective antidote to ICH associated with oral thrombin inhibitor dabigatran. PCC may partially reverse the effects of oral factor Xa inhibitors and are reasonable to administer if available.

1226. Which of the following is a monoclonal antibody to dabigatran?

Harrison's 20th Ed. Chapter 421, Page 3094

A. Andexanet alfa
B. Idarucizumab
C. Ciraparantag
D. All of the above

Idarucizumab is a monoclonal antibody to dabigatran and is a specific reversal agent for dabigatran. It binds dabigatran with high affinity to form a 1:1 complex that is then cleared by kidneys. Idarucizumab is given as an intravenous bolus of 5 gram.

1227. Which of the following is a universal anti-Xa antidote?

Harrison's 20th Ed. Chapter 273, Page 1915

A. Eptinezumab
B. Fremanezumab
C. Andexanet
D. Galcanezumab

Andexanet is a universal anti-Xa antidote for betrixaban, rivaroxaban, apixaban, and edoxaban.

1228. Which of the following is not helpful for the edema from intracerebral hematoma?

Harrison's 20th Ed. Chapter 421, Page 3094

A. Glucocorticoids
B. Osmotic agents
C. Induced hyperventilation
D. Ventriculostomy

Glucocorticoids are not helpful for the edema from intracerebral hematoma.

1229. Largest AVMs are most frequently found in?

Harrison's 20th Ed. Chapter 421, Page 3095

A. Anterior half of hemispheres
B. Posterior half of hemispheres
C. Brainstem
D. Spinal cord

AVMs occur in all parts of cerebral hemispheres, brainstem & spinal cord. The largest ones are mostly located in posterior half of the hemispheres, commonly forming a wedge-shaped lesion extending from cortex to the ventricle.

1230. Bleeding, headache and seizures due to AVMs are most common between the ages of?

Harrison's 20th Ed. Chapter 421, Page 3095

A. 1 and 10 years
B. 10 and 30 years
C. 30 and 50 years
D. 50 and 75 years

Bleeding, headache and seizures due to AVMs are most common between the ages of 10 & 30 years.

1231. Which of the following is a familial AVM?

Harrison's 20th Ed. Chapter 421, Page 3095

A. Sagging brain syndrome
B. Osler-Rendu-Weber syndrome
C. Posterior cortical atrophy syndrome
D. Capgras' syndrome

Familial AVM may be a part of the autosomal dominant syndrome of hereditary hemorrhagic telangiectasia called Osler-Rendu-Weber syndrome. It is due to mutations in either endoglin or activin receptor-like kinase 1, both involved in transforming growth factor (TGF) signaling & angiogenesis.

1232. Which of the following statements about AVM bleed is false?

Harrison's 20th Ed. Chapter 421, Page 3095

A. Hemorrhage is mainly intraparenchymal
B. Symptomatic cerebral vasospasm is rare
C. Smaller lesions have a higher hemorrhage rate
D. MRI is gold standard for evaluating anatomy of AVM

Hemorrhage is mainly intraparenchymal. Symptomatic cerebral vasospasm is rare. Smaller lesions have a higher hemorrhage rate. Conventional X-ray angiography is the gold standard for evaluating precise anatomy of AVM.

1233. Which of the following increases risk of AVM rupture?

Harrison's 20th Ed. Chapter 421, Page 3095

A. Presence of deep venous drainage
B. Presence of venous outflow stenosis
C. Presence of intranidal aneurysms
D. All of the above

Paradoxically, smaller AVM lesions have a higher hemorrhage rate.

1234. Which of the following is a common location of capillary telangiectasias in brain?

Harrison's 20th Ed. Chapter 421, Page 3095

A. Pons
B. Mid brain
C. Medulla oblongata
D. Cerebellum

Capillary telangiectasias are true capillary malformations located typically in pons and deep cerebral white matter as in hereditary hemorrhagic telangiectasia (Osler-Rendu-Weber) syndrome. Bleeding rarely produces mass effect or significant symptoms.

1235. Intracranial hemorrhage located usually in brainstem is due to which of the following?

Harrison's 20th Ed. Chapter 421, Page 3092 Table 421-1

A. Hypertensive hemorrhage
B. Cocaine abuse
C. Capillary telangiectasias
D. Arteriovenous malformation

Capillary telangiectasias are true capillary malformations in normal brain structure. Pons & deep cerebral white matter are typical locations. Hereditary hemorrhagic telangiectasia (Osler-Rendu-Weber) syndrome is an example.

1236. Lobar intracranial Hemorrhage is due to?
Harrison's 20th Ed. Chapter 421, Page 3092 Table 421-1

A. Metastatic brain tumor
B. Amyloid angiopathy
C. Arteriovenous malformation
D. All of the above

1237. Which of the following is not an acquired vascular lesions?
Harrison's 20th Ed. Chapter 421, Page 3095

A. Dural arteriovenous fistulas
B. Cavernous angiomas
C. Capillary telangiectasias
D. None of the above

Capillary telangiectasias are true capillary malformations. Dural AV fistulas are acquired connections from a dural artery to dural sinus. Cavernous angiomas are tufts of capillary sinusoids in deep hemispheric white matter & brainstem with no normal intervening neural structures.

1238. Which of the following gene is responsible in causing cavernous angiomas?
Harrison's 20th Ed. Chapter 421, Page 3095, N Engl J Med. 2002;347:1711

A. NOTCH3
B. APP
C. BRI
D. KRIT1

KRIT1, CCM2 and PDCD10 have been identified as genes causing cavernous angiomas. KRIT1 and CCM2 have a role in blood vessel formation. PDCD10 is an apoptotic gene.

1239. Pulse-synchronous cephalic bruit ("pulsatile tinnitus") is a feature of?
Harrison's 20th Ed. Chapter 421, Page 3095

A. Dural arteriovenous fistulas
B. Cavernous angiomas
C. Capillary telangiectasias
D. All of the above

1240. Which of the following genes can cause autosomal dominant amyloid angiopathies?
N Engl J Med. 2002;347:1711

A. APP
B. CST3
C. BRI
D. All of the above

APP, CST3, BRI genes cause autosomal dominant amyloid angiopathies.

1241. Primary class of antibody that is associated with antiphospholipid antibody syndrome is?
Harrison's 20th Ed. Chapter 350, Page 2526

A. Anticardiolipin antibodies (aCL)
B. Lupus anticoagulant (LA)
C. Antibodies against β2GP1 (anti-β2GPI)
D. All of the above

1242. Thrombotic events associated with antiphospholipid antibodies include?
Harrison's 20th Ed. Chapter 350, Page 2526

A. Deep vein thrombosis (DVT)
B. Pulmonary embolus
C. Placental vascular thrombosis
D. All of the above

1243. The lupus anticoagulants prolong which of the following coagulation test results?
Disease-a-Month. 2003;49:696-741

A. Activated partial thromboplastin time (aPTT)
B. Prothrombin time
C. Dilute Russell viper venom time (dRVVT)
D. All of the above

1244. Which of these is a natural anticoagulant?
Disease-a-Month. 2003;49:696-741

A. Beta2-Gp1
B. Activated protein C
C. Annexin V
D. All of the above

1245. Sneddon syndrome consists of?
Disease-a-Month. 2003;49:696-741

A. Stroke
B. Livido reticularis
C. Hypertension
D. All of the above

1246. Obstetric complications in antiphospholipid syndrome are usually seen at?
Disease-a-Month. 2003;49:696-741

A. 10 or more weeks of gestation
B. 8 or more weeks of gestation
C. 6 or more weeks of gestation
D. 4 or more weeks of gestation

1247. Which of the following is the preferred test for diagnosis of antiphospholipid antibody?
Disease-a-Month. 2003;49:696-741

A. aPTT
B. KCT
C. dRVVT
D. Bleeding time

1248. Antiphospholipid syndrome is a disorder characterized by?
Disease-a-Month. 2003;49:696-741

A. Recurrent arterial thrombosis
B. Spontaneous abortions
C. Thrombocytopenia
D. All of the above

Subarachnoid Hemorrhage

1249. Which of the following is false about idiopathic SAHs localized to perimesencephalic cisterns?
Harrison's 20th Ed. Chapter 302, Page 2084

A. Benign
B. Venous or capillary source
C. Angiography is unrevealing
D. None of the above

Some idiopathic SAHs are localized to perimesencephalic cisterns and are benign with a venous or capillary source. Angiography is unrevealing.

1250. Which of the following is the most common cause of SAH?
Harrison's 20th Ed. Chapter 302, Page 2084

A. Rupture of a saccular aneurysm
B. Bleeding from a vascular anomaly
C. Extension into subarachnoid space from a primary intracerebral hemorrhage
D. Idiopathic

After head trauma, the most common cause of SAH is rupture of a saccular aneurysm.

1251. What percentage of adults harbor intracranial aneurysms?
Harrison's 20th Ed. Chapter 302, Page 2084

A. 1%
B. 2%
C. 3%
D. 4%

Autopsy & angiography studies show that ~2% of adults harbor intracranial aneurysms.

1252. In SAH, the mortality rate over the first month is?
Harrison's 20th Ed. Chapter 302, Page 2084

A. ~ 15%
B. ~ 25%
C. ~ 35%
D. ~ 45%

SAH patients who arrive alive at hospital, the mortality rate over the next month is ~ 45%.

1253. In SAH, the rate of rebleeding in the first month is about?
Harrison's 20th Ed. Chapter 302, Page 2084

A. 20%
B. 30%
C. 40%
D. 50%

In SAH, if the patient survives but aneurysm is not obliterated, the rate of rebleeding is about 20% in first 2 weeks, 30% in first month.

1254. Annual risk of rupture for aneurysms ≥10 mm in size is?
Harrison's 20th Ed. Chapter 302, Page 2084

A. ~ 0.1–0.5%
B. ~ 0.5–1%
C. ~ 1.0–1.5%
D. ~ 1.5–2%

Annual risk of rupture for aneurysms <10 mm size is ~0.1%, for aneurysms ≥10 mm in size it is ~ 0.5–1%.

1255. An aneurysm is termed 'Giant' when its diameter is?
Harrison's 20th Ed. Chapter 302, Page 2084

A. > 0.5 cm
B. > 1.0 cm
C. > 1.5 cm
D. > 2.5 cm

Berry aneurysms >2.5 cm in diameter are called giant aneurysms, and account for 5% of cases.

1256. Most common location of an intracranial aneurysm is?
Harrison's 20th Ed. Chapter 302, Page 2084

A. Anterior communicating artery
B. Posterior communicating artery
C. Terminal internal carotid artery
D. Vertebral artery

1257. Most common location of an intracranial aneurysm is?
Harrison's 20th Ed. Chapter 302, Page 2084

A. Anterior communicating artery
B. MCA bifurcation
C. Posterior communicating artery
D. Middle of basilar artery

1258. Most common location of an intracranial aneurysm is?
Harrison's 20th Ed. Chapter 302, Page 2084

A. Anterior communicating artery
B. Posterior communicating artery
C. Top of basilar artery
D. Middle of basilar artery

The three most common locations of berry aneurysms are the terminal internal carotid artery, MCA bifurcation, and top of basilar artery. Their risk of rupture is ~6% in the first year.

1259. Mycotic aneurysms are best related to?
Harrison's 20th Ed. Chapter 302, Page 2084

A. Hypertension
B. Diabetes mellitus
C. Bacterial endocarditis
D. Trauma

Mycotic aneurysms are usually located distal to the first bifurcation of major arteries of the circle of Willis. Most result from infected emboli due to bacterial endocarditis.

1260. Mycotic aneurysms are usually located distal to which bifurcation of major arteries of circle of Willis?
Harrison's 20th Ed. Chapter 302, Page 2084

A. 1st
B. 2nd
C. 3rd
D. 4th

Mycotic aneurysms due to infected emboli are usually located distal to the first bifurcation of major arteries of the circle of Willis.

1261. Anterior circulation accounts for what percentage of all intracranial aneurysms?
Harrison's 20th Ed. Chapter 302, Page 2084

A. 25%
B. 45%
C. 65%
D. 85%

~85% of aneurysms occur in the anterior circulation, mostly on the circle of Willis.

1262. What percentage of all intracranial aneurysms are multiple?
Harrison's 20th Ed. Chapter 302, Page 2084

A. 5%
B. 10%
C. 20%
D. 40%

~20% of patients have multiple aneurysms, many at mirror sites bilaterally.

1263. Which of the following characteristics of a berry aneurysm make it at greater risk of rupture?
Harrison's 20th Ed. Chapter 302, Page 2084

A. >7 mm in diameter
B. At the top of basilar artery
C. At the origin of posterior communicating artery
D. Any of the above

Those >7 mm in diameter and those at the top of the basilar artery and at the origin of the posterior communicating artery are at greater risk of rupture.

1264. The site of rupture of a berry aneurysm is?
Harrison's 20th Ed. Chapter 302, Page 2084

A. Base of the neck
B. Top of the neck
C. Dome
D. Any of the above

The site of rupture of a berry aneurysm most often is the dome. As an aneurysm develops, it typically forms a neck with a dome. Arterial internal elastic lamina disappears at the base of neck. Media thins & connective tissue replaces smooth-muscle cells. Most often, the dome is the site of rupture.

1265. Patients first complaint upon regaining consciousness in SAH is?
Harrison's 20th Ed. Chapter 302, Page 2084

A. Blurred vision
B. Headache
C. Thirst
D. Nausea

Most patients first complain of headache upon regaining consciousness.

1266. The location of headache in SAH is?
Harrison's 20th Ed. Chapter 302, Page 2084

A. Frontal
B. Occipital
C. Temporal
D. Generalized

In SAH, headache is sudden, usually generalized, often with neck stiffness and vomiting.

1267. Which of the following is a feature of headache in SAH?
Harrison's 20th Ed. Chapter 302, Page 2084

A. Sudden onset
B. Severe headache associated with exertion
C. A change in the patient's usual headache pattern
D. All of the above

1268. Which of the following is a feature of aneurysmal rupture SAH?
Harrison's 20th Ed. Chapter 302, Page 2084

A. Sudden headache
B. Absence of focal neurologic symptoms
C. Generalized headache with neck stiffness and vomiting
D. All of the above

1269. Common deficits that result due to middle cerebral bifurcation aneurysmal rupture include all except?
Harrison's 20th Ed. Chapter 302, Page 2084

A. Hemiparesis
B. Aphasia
C. Abulia
D. Acalculia

ACA or MCA bifurcation aneurysms may rupture into adjacent brain or subdural space and form a hematoma large enough to produce mass effect resulting in hemiparesis, aphasia and abulia.

1270. III cranial nerve palsy, with pupillary dilatation, loss of ipsilateral light reflex and focal pain above or behind the eye suggests what location of an aneurysm?
Harrison's 20th Ed. Chapter 302, Page 2084

A. Posterior communicating artery aneurysm
B. Aneurysm in the cavernous sinus
C. Anterior cerebral artery aneurysm
D. Anterior inferior cerebellar artery aneurysm

1271. VI cranial nerve palsy suggests what location of an aneurysm?
Harrison's 20th Ed. Chapter 302, Page 2084

A. Posterior communicating artery aneurysm
B. Aneurysm in the cavernous sinus
C. Anterior cerebral artery aneurysm
D. Anterior inferior cerebellar artery aneurysm

1272. Occipital and posterior cervical pain suggests what location of an aneurysm?
Harrison's 20th Ed. Chapter 302, Page 2084

A. Posterior communicating artery aneurysm
B. Aneurysm in the cavernous sinus
C. Anterior cerebral artery aneurysm
D. Anterior inferior cerebellar artery aneurysm

1273. Visual field defects suggests what location of an aneurysm?
Harrison's 20th Ed. Chapter 302, Page 2084

A. Posterior communicating artery aneurysm
B. Aneurysm in the cavernous sinus
C. Anterior cerebral artery aneurysm
D. Anterior inferior cerebellar artery aneurysm

1274. Occipital and posterior cervical pain suggests what location of an aneurysm?

Harrison's 20th Ed. Chapter 302, Page 2084

A. Posterior communicating artery aneurysm
B. Aneurysm in the cavernous sinus
C. Anterior cerebral artery aneurysm
D. Posterior inferior cerebellar artery aneurysm

1275. Pain in or behind the eye and in the low temple suggests what location of an aneurysm?

Harrison's 20th Ed. Chapter 302, Page 2084

A. Posterior communicating artery aneurysm
B. Aneurysm in the cavernous sinus
C. Anterior cerebral artery aneurysm
D. MCA aneurysm

III cranial nerve palsy associated with pupillary dilatation, loss of ipsilateral light reflex and focal pain above or behind the eye, may occur with an expanding aneurysm at the junction of posterior communicating artery and internal carotid artery. VI cranial nerve palsy may indicate an aneurysm in cavernous sinus, and visual field defects can occur with an anterior cerebral artery aneurysm. Occipital and posterior cervical pain may signal a posterior inferior cerebellar artery or anterior inferior cerebellar artery aneurysm. Pain in or behind the eye and in the low temple can occur with an expanding MCA aneurysm.

1276. 'Sentinel bleed' is the term used for small aneurysmal rupture into?

Harrison's 20th Ed. Chapter 302, Page 2085

A. Subarachnoid space
B. White matter
C. Gray matter
D. Thalamus

Aneurysms with small ruptures & leaks of blood into subarachnoid space are sentinel bleeds. "Sentinel" or "warning" headache is a sudden, severe headache that resolves & that is retrospectively identified to have occurred days to weeks before the SAH.

1277. 'Wide-neck aneurysms' are those in which the ratio of neck diameter to that of the largest dome is?

N Engl J Med. 2006;354:387-96

A. > 0.2
B. > 0.3
C. > 0.4
D. > 0.5

1278. In a case of SAH who also has third-nerve palsy, which artery is possibly involved?

N Engl J Med. 2006;354:387-96

A. Anterior communicating artery
B. Posterior communicating artery
C. Anterior cerebral artery
D. Middle cerebral artery

1279. In a case of SAH who also has bilateral weakness in legs or abulia, which artery is possibly involved?

N Engl J Med. 2006;354:387-96

A. Anterior communicating artery
B. Posterior communicating artery
C. Anterior cerebral artery
D. Middle cerebral artery

1280. In a case of SAH who also has aphasia, hemiparesis, or visuospatial neglect, which artery is possibly involved?

N Engl J Med. 2006;354:387-96

A. Anterior communicating artery
B. Posterior communicating artery
C. Anterior cerebral artery
D. Middle cerebral artery

1281. In a case of SAH who also has retinal and subhyaloid hemorrhage, which artery is possibly involved?

N Engl J Med. 2006;354:387-96

A. Anterior communicating artery
B. Posterior communicating artery
C. Anterior cerebral artery
D. Any of the above

1282. Clinical scale of Hunt and Hess is used in?

Harrison's 20th Ed. Chapter 302, Page 2085, N Engl J Med. 2006;354:387-96

A. Bacterial meningitis
B. HIV dementia
C. Subarachnoid hemorrhage
D. Multiple sclerosis

Initial clinical manifestations of SAH can be graded by Hunt-Hess or World Federation of Neurosurgical Societies (WFNS) classification.

1283. Which of the following grading systems is related to SAH?

CCJM 2015;82(3):177-192

A. Hunt and Hess
B. World Federation of Neurological Surgeons (WFNS)
C. Fisher or its modified version
D. All of the above

Different grading systems used for SAH are based on the findings on initial neurologic examination and on initial noncontrast CT (thickness of blood and intraventricular hemorrhage) are those developed by Hunt and Hess and by the World Federation of Neurological Surgeons (WFNS), and the CT grading scales (Fisher or its modified version).

1284. Which of the following is not a cause of delayed neurologic deficit in SAH?

Harrison's 20th Ed. Chapter 302, Page 2085

A. Infection
B. Hydrocephalus
C. Vasospasm
D. Hyponatremia

There are four major causes of delayed neurologic deficits in SAH. They are rerupture, hydrocephalus, vasospasm, and hyponatremia.

1285. Peak incidence of rerupture of an untreated aneurysm following SAH is within?

Harrison's 20th Ed. Chapter 302, Page 2085

A. 1 day
B. 3 days
C. 7 days
D. 14 days

Incidence of rerupture of an untreated aneurysm in the first month following SAH is ~30% with the peak in the first 7 days. Rerupture is associated with a 50% mortality rate and poor outcome.

1286. Chronic hydrocephalus after SAH manifests as?
Harrison's 20th Ed. Chapter 302, Page 2085

A. Gait difficulty
B. Incontinence
C. Impaired mentation
D. All of the above

Hydrocephalus is the most common early neurologic complication after aneurysmal subarachnoid hemorrhage, with an overall incidence of 50%. Chronic hydrocephalus may develop weeks to months after SAH and manifest as gait difficulty, incontinence, or impaired mentation.

1287. Delayed vasospasm in SAH is due to?
Harrison's 20th Ed. Chapter 302, Page 2085

A. Hypertension
B. Hyperviscosity
C. Clotted blood & its breakdown products on artery
D. All of the above

Delayed vasospasm is due to direct effects of clotted blood & its breakdown products on arteries within subarachnoid space.

1288. Signs of cerebral ischemia due to vasospasm following SAH is most often on which day?
Harrison's 20th Ed. Chapter 302, Page 2085

A. Day 1
B. Day 3
C. Day 7
D. Day 14

Signs of cerebral ischemia appear 4 to 14 days after SAH, most often at 7 days.

1289. In most cases of SAH, focal vasospasm is preceded by?
Harrison's 20th Ed. Chapter 302, Page 2085

A. Headache
B. Seizure
C. Decline in mental status
D. Vomiting

In most SAH cases, focal vasospasm is preceded by decline in mental status.

1290. Hyponatremia following SAH is due to?
Harrison's 20th Ed. Chapter 302, Page 2085

A. Inappropriate secretion of vasopressin
B. Secretion of atrial natriuretic factors
C. Secretion of brain natriuretic factors
D. All of the above

Hyponatremia following SAH or "cerebral salt-wasting syndrome" develop in first 2 weeks due to inappropriate secretion of vasopressin & secretion of atrial and brain natriuretic peptides. It should not be treated with free-water restriction as this may increase risk of stroke. It clears over 1 to 2 weeks.

1291. Xanthochromic CSF in SAH usually lasts for?
Harrison's 20th Ed. Chapter 302, Page 2085

A. 1 to 4 days
B. 1 to 2 weeks
C. 1 to 3 weeks
D. 1 to 4 weeks

Xanthochromic CSF in SAH is due to lysis of RBCs & subsequent conversion of hemoglobin to bilirubin which stains spinal fluid yellow within 6 to 12 hours. It peaks in intensity at 48 hours and lasts for 1 to 4 weeks.

1292. Incidence of symptomatic vasospasm in MCA & ACA is high when early CT scans show subarachnoid clots of what size in basal cisterns?
Harrison's 20th Ed. Chapter 302, Page 2086

A. > 2 x 3 mm
B. > 3 x 3 mm
C. > 4 x 3 mm
D. > 5 x 3 mm

1293. Incidence of symptomatic vasospasm in MCA & ACA is high when early CT scans show blood layer of what thickness in the cerebral fissures?
Harrison's 20th Ed. Chapter 302, Page 2086

A. > 0.1 mm
B. > 0.25 mm
C. > 0.6 mm
D. > 1 mm

High incidence of symptomatic vasospasm in MCA & ACA is observed when early CT scans show subarachnoid clots >5 x 3 mm in basal cisterns or layers of blood >1 mm thick in cerebral fissures. CT scans less reliably predict vasospasm in vertebral, basilar or posterior cerebral arteries.

1294. Secondary to intracranial hemorrhage, which of the following ECG finding is unusual?
Harrison's 20th Ed. Chapter 302, Page 2086

A. Prolonged QRS complex
B. Increased QT interval
C. "Peaked" or deeply inverted symmetric T waves
D. Serious ventricular dysrhythmias

Prolonged QRS, increased QT interval & prominent "peaked" or deeply inverted symmetric T waves occur secondary to intracranial hemorrhage. Serious ventricular dysrhythmias are unusual.

1295. Echocardiography in a case of SAH reveals relative sparing of?
Harrison's 20th Ed. Chapter 302, Page 2086

A. Apex
B. Inferior wall
C. Anterior wall
D. Posterior wall

In SAH, echocardiography shows regional wall motion abnormalities (RWMA) that follow distribution of sympathetic nerves rather than major coronary arteries, with relative sparing of ventricular wall apex.

1296. In endovascular treatment of aneurysms, coils are made of?
Harrison's 20th Ed. Chapter 302, Page 2086, N Engl J Med. 2006;354:387-96

A. Platinum
B. Silver
C. Gold
D. Steel

Newer endovascular technique involves placing platinum coils within aneurysm via a femoral artery catheter to enhance thrombosis & over time is walled-off from circulation.

1297. Intracranial hypertension following aneurysmal rupture occurs secondary to all except?
Harrison's 20th Ed. Chapter 302, Page 2086

A. Subarachnoid blood
B. Parenchymal hematoma
C. Systemic hypertension
D. Loss of vascular autoregulation

Intracranial hypertension following aneurysmal rupture occurs secondary to subarachnoid blood, parenchymal hematoma, acute hydrocephalus, or loss of vascular autoregulation.

1298. Which of the following are poor prognostic signs in SAH?
Harrison's 20th Ed. Chapter 302, Page 2086

A. High ICP refractory to treatment
B. Rerupture of untreated aneurysm in 1st month of SAH
C. Vasospasm causing symptomatic ischemia & infarction
D. All of the above

High ICP refractory to treatment is a poor prognostic sign. Rerupture is associated with a 60% mortality and poor outcome. Vasospasm following SAH causes symptomatic ischemia and infarction and is a major cause of delayed morbidity and death.

1299. In treatment of SAH, intracranial pressure should be maintained at?
Harrison's 20th Ed. Chapter 302, Page 2077

A. < 5 mm Hg
B. < 10 mm Hg
C. < 15 mm Hg
D. < 20 mm Hg

In general, ICP should be maintained at <20 mm Hg.

1300. In treatment of SAH, cerebral perfusion pressure (CPP) should be maintained at?
Harrison's 20th Ed. Chapter 302, Page 2086

A. 30–40 mm Hg
B. 40–50 mm Hg
C. 50–60 mm Hg
D. 60–70 mm Hg

In treatment of SAH, cerebral perfusion pressure should be maintained at 60–70 mm Hg.

1301. Which of the following drugs is most suited to lower raised blood pressure in patients with acute SAH?
Harrison's 20th Ed. Chapter 302, Page 2086

A. Nifedipine
B. Amlodipine
C. Nicardipine
D. Any of the above

1302. Which of the following drugs is most suited to lower raised blood pressure in patients with acute SAH?
Harrison's 20th Ed. Chapter 302, Page 2086

A. Labetalol
B. Esmolol
C. Nicardipine
D. Any of the above

Patients with acute SAH should have blood pressure lowered to a normal range with nonvasodilating agents such as nicardipine, labetalol, or esmolol.

1303. "Triple-H" therapy in SAH refers to all except?
Cleveland Clinic Journal of Medicine. 2015;82(3):177-192

A. Hypertension
B. Hemodilution
C. Hypervolemia
D. Hyperventilation

"Triple-H" therapy in SAH includes hypertension, hemodilution and hypervolemia and is achieved by volume expansion. However, clinical data supporting this intervention, to prevent delayed cerebral ischemia due to vasospasm, have been called into question.

1304. In SAH, if symptomatic vasospasm persists despite optimal medical therapy, which drug is then used?
Harrison's 20th Ed. Chapter 302, Page 2086

A. Intravenous nitroglycerine
B. Intra-arterial papaverine
C. EACA
D. Intravenous phenylephrine

If symptomatic vasospasm persists despite optimal medical therapy, intra-arterial vasodilators & percutaneous transluminal angioplasty are considered. Vasodilators like verapamil & nicardipine do not last > 8-24 hours. Intra-arterial papaverine is an effective vasodilator, but neurotoxic.

1305. Which of the following drugs is preferred for reducing vasospasm in SAH?
Harrison's 20th Ed. Chapter 302, Page 2086

A. Nifedipine
B. Amlodipine
C. Nicardipine
D. Nimodipine

1306. Which of the following is a complication of correction of marked hyponatremia of several days' duration?
Harrison's 20th Ed. Chapter 302, Page 2086

A. Cortical venous thrombosis
B. Hydrocephalus
C. Osmotic demyelination syndrome
D. All of the above

Care must be taken not to correct serum sodium too quickly in patients with marked hyponatremia of several days' duration as osmotic demyelination syndrome may occur.

1307. "Pentobarb coma" refers to?
Harrison's 20th Ed. Chapter 302, Page 2077

A. Coma due to accidental ingestion of barbiturates
B. Coma due to barbiturates given for induction of anesthesia
C. High-dose barbiturates for refractory elevated ICP
D. Any of the above

High-dose barbiturate therapy for refractory elevated ICP is termed "pentobarb coma".

1308. Emergent treatment of elevated ICP is most quickly achieved by which of the following?
Harrison's 20th Ed. Chapter 302, Page 2077

A. Ventriculostomy
B. Hyperventilation
C. High-dose barbiturates
D. Hypothermia

Emergent treatment of elevated ICP is most quickly achieved by intubation and hyperventilation to bring $PaCO_2$ level to 30–35 mm Hg.

1309. Heritable connective-tissue disorders associated with presence of intracranial aneurysm & subarachnoid hemorrhage include?
N Engl J Med. 2006;354:387-96

A. Polycystic kidney disease
B. Ehlers–Danlos syndrome (type IV)
C. Pseudoxanthoma elasticum
D. All of the above

Alzheimer's Disease

1310. Alois Alzheimer belonged to which nation?

JAMA. 1969;208(6):1017-1018

A. Spain
B. Germany
C. Poland
D. Sweden

Alzheimer's disease (AD) was first described by German psychiatrist Alois Alzheimer (14 June 1864 - 19 December 1915) in a patient at Frankfurt asylum named Mrs. Auguste Deter.

1311. Which of the following President of United States of America suffered from Alzheimer's disease?

A. Richard Nixon
B. Lyndon B Johnson
C. Gerald Ford
D. Ronald Reagan

1312. Cognitive changes of AD characteristically begin with?

Harrison's 20th Ed. Chapter 423, Page 3108

A. Memory impairment
B. Language deficit
C. Visuospatial deficit
D. Any of the above

Cognitive changes of AD follow a characteristic pattern, beginning with memory impairment and going on to language and visuospatial deficits, followed by executive dysfunction.

1313. The nonmemory complaints in a patient of AD include?

Harrison's 20th Ed. Chapter 423, Page 3108

A. Word -finding difficulty
B. Organizational difficulty
C. Navigational difficulty
D. All of the above

~ 20% of patients with AD patients present with non-memory complaints like word finding, organizational or navigational difficulty.

1314. Which of the following can be a primary manifestations of AD?

Harrison's 20th Ed. Chapter 423, Page 3108

A. Posterior cortical atrophy syndrome
B. Progressive "logopenic" aphasia
C. Asymmetric akinetic rigid-dystonic syndrome
D. All of the above

Upstream visual processing dysfunction (referred to as posterior cortical atrophy syndrome), a progressive "logopenic" aphasia, an asymmetric akinetic rigid-dystonic ("corticobasal") syndrome or a dysexecutive "frontal variant" of AD are the primary manifestations of AD for years before progressing to involve memory and other cognitive domains.

1315. Term mild cognitive impairment (MCI) is applied when memory loss falls how many standard deviations below normal on standardized memory tests?

Harrison's 20th Ed. Chapter 423, Page 3108

A. 0.5
B. 1.0
C. 1.5
D. 2.0

Term mild cognitive impairment (MCI) is applied when memory loss falls 1.5 standard deviations below normal on standardized memory tests.

1316. What percentage of mild cognitive impairment individuals will progress to Alzheimer's disease (AD) in 4 years?

Harrison's 20th Ed. Chapter 423, Page 3108

A. ~ 20%
B. ~ 30%
C. ~ 40%
D. ~ 50%

Approximately 50% of patients with mild cognitive impairment (MCI) will progress to AD over 4 years (roughly 12% per year).

1317. "Prodromal AD" refers to a person with?

Harrison's 20th Ed. Chapter 423, Page 3108

A. Amyloid imaging positive with PET
B. Low cerebrospinal Ab42
C. Mildly elevated cerebrospinal tau
D. All of the above

"Prodromal AD" refers to a person with biomarker evidence of AD (amyloid imaging positive with positron emission tomography or low cerebrospinal Ab42 and mildly elevated tau) in the absence of symptoms.

1318. In the middle and later stages of AD, which of the following remains intact?

Harrison's 20th Ed. Chapter 423, Page 3108

A. Social graces
B. Routine behavior
C. Superficial conversation
D. All of the above

In middle stages of AD, social graces, routine behavior & superficial conversation remain surprisingly intact, even in the later stages of AD illness.

1319. In AD, which of the following in language becomes impaired first?

Harrison's 20th Ed. Chapter 423, Page 3108

A. Naming
B. Comprehension
C. Fluency
D. Any of the above

In AD, language becomes impaired. It affects naming first, then comprehension, and finally fluency.

1320. In AD, which of the following is the first to become impaired?

Harrison's 20th Ed. Chapter 423, Page 3108

A. Word-finding difficulties
B. Naming
C. Loss of judgment and reasoning
D. Fluency

Word-finding difficulties & circumlocution is evident in early stages, even when naming & fluency are intact. Apraxia emerges, and patients have trouble performing learned sequential motor tasks. Visuospatial deficits interfere with dressing, eating or even walking and patients fail to solve simple puzzles or copy geometric figures. Simple calculations and clock reading become difficult in parallel.

1321. Which of the following develop in the late stages of AD?

Harrison's 20th Ed. Chapter 423, Page 3108

A. Loss of judgment and reasoning
B. Shuflling gait with generalized muscle rigidity
C. Capgras' syndrome
D. All of the above

1322. Which of the following is rare in AD?

Harrison's 20th Ed. Chapter 423, Page 3108

A. Hyperactive tendon reflexes
B. Myoclonic jerks
C. Resting tremor
D. Delusion

Patients of AD often look parkinsonian but rarely have a high-amplitude, low-frequency rhythmic, resting tremor. Hyperactive tendon reflexes and myoclonic jerks develop in the end stages of AD.

1323. Of the following, which is the most common cause of death in AD?

Harrison's 20th Ed. Chapter 423, Page 3108

A. Secondary infections
B. Pulmonary emboli
C. Heart disease
D. Aspiration

Aspiration is the most common cause of death in AD. Others include malnutrition, secondary infections, pulmonary emboli, and heart disease.

1324. The typical duration of Alzheimer's disease is?

Harrison's 20th Ed. Chapter 423, Page 3108

A. 2–3 years
B. 4–6 years
C. 6–8 years
D. 8–10 years

The typical duration of AD is 8 to 10 years, but the course can range from 1 to 25 years.

1325. Neuroimaging studies in AD may show atrophy in?

Harrison's 20th Ed. Chapter 423, Page 3108

A. Medial temporal lobes
B. Lateral and medial parietal lobes
C. Lateral frontal cortex
D. All of the above

As AD progresses, posterior predominant cortical atrophy becomes apparent, along with atrophy of medial temporal memory structures. In typical amnestic AD, neuroimaging studies (CT & MRI) show atrophy that begins in medial temporal lobes before spreading to lateral and medial parietal lobes and lateral frontal cortex.

1326. On neuroimaging studies (CT and MRI), which of the following is a single specific finding for the diagnosis of AD?

Harrison's 20th Ed. Chapter 423, Page 3108

A. Posterior-predominant cortical atrophy
B. Atrophy of medial temporal memory structures
C. Hydrocephalus
D. None of the above

Neuroimaging studies (CT & MRI) do not show a single specific pattern with AD and may be normal early in the disease.

1327. Which of the following PET finding is required for entry into treatment trials for AD?

Harrison's 20th Ed. Chapter 423, Page 3109

A. Amyloid positivity
B. Temporal-parietal hypometabolism
C. Temporal-parietal hypoperfusion
D. Lower activity of FDG in the parietal lobes

Amyloid binding with PET is typical for AD and amyloid PET positivity is becoming required for entry into treatment trials for AD.

1328. At autopsy, AD is misdiagnosed with?

Harrison's 20th Ed. Chapter 423, Page 3109

A. Frontotemporal lobar degeneration (FTLD)
B. DLB
C. Hippocampal sclerosis of elderly
D. All of the above

1329. Early prominent gait disturbance with only mild memory loss suggests?

Harrison's 20th Ed. Chapter 423, Page 3109

A. Vascular dementia
B. Parkinson's disease (PD)
C. Dementia with Lewy bodies (DLB)
D. Creutzfeldt-Jacob disease (CJD)

Early prominent gait disturbance with only mild memory loss suggests vascular dementia or, rarely, NPH.

1330. Resting tremor with stooped posture, bradykinesia and masked facies suggests?

Harrison's 20th Ed. Chapter 423, Page 3109

A. Vascular dementia
B. Parkinson's disease (PD)
C. Alzheimer's disease (AD)
D. Creutzfeldt-Jacob disease (CJD)

Resting tremor with stooped posture, bradykinesia and masked facies suggest PD or DLB.

1331. Which of the following features suggests Dementia with Lewy bodies?

Harrison's 20th Ed. Chapter 423, Page 3109

A. Early appearance of parkinsonian features
B. Visual hallucinations
C. Delusional misidentification
D. All of the above

Early appearance of parkinsonian features in association with fluctuating alertness, visual hallucinations or delusional misidentification suggests DLB.

1332. Which of the following features suggests CJD?

Harrison's 20th Ed. Chapter 423, Page 3109

A. Rapid progression over a few weeks or months
B. Rigidity
C. Myoclonus
D. All of the above

Rapid progression over a few weeks or months associated with rigidity and myoclonus suggests CJD.

1333. Which of the following features suggests frontotemporal dementia (FTD)?

Harrison's 20th Ed. Chapter 423, Page 3109

A. Prominent behavioral changes
B. Intact navigation
C. Focal anterior-predominant atrophy
D. All of the above

Prominent behavioral changes with intact navigation and focal anterior-predominant atrophy on brain imaging are typical of FTD.

1334. Which of the following clinical features of Alzheimer's disease occurs in the later phases of the disease?

N Engl J Med. 2004;351:56-67

A. Amnesic type of memory impairment
B. Deterioration of language
C. Visuospatial deficits
D. Gait disturbances

1335. Which of the following is a genetic disorder associated with dementia?

Harrison's 20th Ed. Chapter 423, Page 3109

A. Frontotemporal dementia (FTD)
B. Huntington's disease (HD)
C. Prion disease
D. All of the above

A positive family history of dementia suggests either one of the familial forms of AD or one of the other genetic disorders associated with dementia, such as FTD, HD, prion disease or rare hereditary ataxias.

1336. Risk factors for AD are?

Harrison's 20th Ed. Chapter 423, Page 3109

A. Old age
B. Positive family history
C. Female gender
D. All of the above

Risk factors for AD are old age, positive family history, female gender, past history of head trauma with concussion, very low educational attainment, exposure to aluminum, mercury & viruses, elevated homocysteine & cholesterol levels, hypertension, diminished serum folic acid, low levels of exercise, low dietary intake of fruits, vegetables, red wine & diabetes. Use of NSAID's & capacity to express complex written language in early adulthood reduces risk of AD.

1337. Most severe pathology in Alzheimer's disease is found in?

Harrison's 20th Ed. Chapter 423, Page 3109

A. Hippocampus
B. Lateral temporal cortex
C. Nucleus basalis of Meynert
D. All of the above

Most severe pathology is found in medial temporal lobe (entorhinal/perirhinal cortex and hippocampus), lateral temporal cortex and nucleus basalis of Meynert (lateral septum), the last being a major source of cholinergic input to cerebral cortex.

1338. Which of the following statements is true about microscopic findings in Alzheimer's disease?

Harrison's 20th Ed. Chapter 423, Page 3109

A. Neuritic plaques contain Ab amyloid
B. Silver staining neurofibrillary tangles in cytoplasm
C. Aβ amyloid in arterial walls of cerebral blood vessels
D. All of the above

In AD, microscopic examination of brain shows neuritic plaques containing Aβ amyloid, silver-staining neurofibrillary tangles (NFTs) in neuronal cytoplasm, and accumulation of Aβ amyloid in arterial walls of cerebral arterioles (amyloid angiopathy).

1339. In Alzheimer's disease, the neuritic plaque contains?

Harrison's 20th Ed. Chapter 423, Page 3109

A. Aβ amyloid
B. Apo ε4
C. α antichymotrypsin
D. All of the above

Neuritic plaques contain a central core that includes Aβ amyloid, proteoglycans, Apo ε4 and α-antichymotrypsin.

1340. Which of the following statements is true about Aβ amyloid in Alzheimer's disease?

Harrison's 20th Ed. Chapter 423, Page 3109

A. Neuritic plaques contains Aβ amyloid
B. It is a protein of 39–42 amino acids
C. Derived proteolytically from amyloid precursor protein
D. All of the above

Aβ amyloid is a protein of 39-42 amino acids that is derived proteolytically from a larger transmembrane protein, amyloid precursor protein (APP).

1341. Amyloid precursor protein (APP) is catabolized by?

Harrison's 20th Ed. Chapter 423, Page 3110 Figure 423-2

A. α secretase
B. β secretase
C. γ secretase
D. All of the above

Amyloid precursor protein (APP) is catabolized by α, β and γ secretases.

1342. Ab peptide results from cleavage of amyloid precursor protein (APP) by?

Harrison's 20th Ed. Chapter 423, Page 3110 Figure 423-2

A. β secretase
B. δ secretase
C. ε secretase
D. All of the above

Aβ peptide results from cleavage of APP by β-and γ-secretases.

1343. Which of the following products of Amyloid precursor protein (APP) is neurotoxic?

Harrison's 20th Ed. Chapter 423, Page 3110 Figure 423-2

A. Aβ42
B. Aβ40
C. P3
D. All of the above

A key initial step is the digestion of APP by either β secretase (BASE) or α secretase (ADAM10 or ADAM17 [TACE]), producing smaller nontoxic products. Cleavage of APP by α and β secretases results in two products i.e. α secretase product and β secretase product. γ secretase acts on α secretase product to produce nontoxic P3 peptide. Similarly, γ secretase acts on β secretase product to produce nontoxic Aβ40 and toxic Aβ42 peptide. Excess production of Aβ42 is a key initiator of cellular damage in Alzheimer's disease. Therapeutics for AD have focussed on attempts to reduce accumulation of Aβ42 by antagonizing β or γ secretases, promoting α secretase, or clearing Aβ42 that has already formed by use of specific antibodies.

1344. In familial early-onset Alzheimer's disease, increased production of which peptide is most neurotoxic?

Harrison's 20th Ed. Chapter 423, Page 3109, N Engl J Med. 2003;349:1056-63

A. Aβ36
B. Aβ38
C. Aβ40
D. Aβ42

Soluble amyloid fibrils (oligomers) lead to dysfunction of neural cells in AD. Misfolded Aβ42 molecules may be the most toxic form of this protein. Accumulation of oligomers eventually leads to formation of neuritic plaques.

1345. In Alzheimer's disease, neuritic plaque is surrounded by?

Harrison's 20th Ed. Chapter 423, Page 3109

A. Dystrophic, tau-immunoreactive neurites
B. Activated microglia
C. Macrophages
D. All of the above

In AD, neuritic plaque core is surrounded by debris of degenerating neurons, microglia & macrophages.

1346. In Alzheimer's disease, amyloid angiopathy may lead to?

Harrison's 20th Ed. Chapter 423, Page 3109

A. Microhemorrhages
B. Large lobar hemorrhages
C. Ischemic infarctions
D. All of the above

Accumulation of Aβ amyloid in cerebral arterioles, termed amyloid angiopathy, can lead to microhemorrhages, large lobar hemorrhages, or ischemic infarctions.

1347. Neurofibrillary tangles (NFTs) in Alzheimer's disease is characterized by all except?

Harrison's 20th Ed. Chapter 423, Page 3109

A. Found in neuronal cytoplasm
B. Paired helical & twisted neurofilaments
C. Represent abnormally phosphorylated tau protein
D. Gold staining

NFTs are silver-staining, twisted neurofilaments in neuronal cytoplasm that represent abnormally phosphorylated tau protein and appear as paired helical filaments by electron microscopy.

1348. Tau protein is characterized by all except?

Harrison's 20th Ed. Chapter 423, Page 3109

A. It is a microtubule associated protein
B. Functions to assemble and stabilize microtubules
C. In Alzheimer's disease, it is hypophosphorylated
D. Progressive supranuclear palsy may represent a tau pathologic process

Tau (t) is a microtubule-associated protein that assembles & stabilizes microtubules that convey cell organelles, glycoproteins through neuron. A 'hyperphosphorylated' state of tau impairs its capacity to bind to microtubules.

1349. Tau protein has pathological significance in which of the following disorders?

Harrison's 20th Ed. Chapter 423, Page 3111

A. Alzheimer's disease
B. Frontotemporal dementia
C. Progressive supranuclear palsy
D. All of the above

Tau plays a major role in the pathogenesis of FTD, PSP and Cortical Basal Degeneration (CBD).

1350. In Alzheimer's disease, which of the following neurotransmitters in cerebral cortex is decreased?

Harrison's 20th Ed. Chapter 423, Page 3109

A. Acetylcholine
B. Norepinephrine
C. Serotonin
D. All of the above

AD is associated with decreased levels of acetylcholine, its synthetic enzyme choline acetyltransferase and nicotinic cholinergic receptors in cerebral cortex due to degeneration of cholinergic neurons in nucleus basalis of Meynert. There is also reduction in norepinephrine levels in brainstem nuclei like locus coeruleus.

1351. APP gene implicated in the pathogenesis of Alzheimer's disease is present on which chromosome?

Harrison's 20th Ed. Chapter 423, Page 3109

A. Chromosome 9
B. Chromosome 11
C. Chromosome 18
D. Chromosome 21

APP gene implicated in the pathogenesis of Alzheimer's disease is present on chromosome 21.

1352. Adults with which of the following consistently develop typical neuropathologic hallmarks of AD?

Harrison's 20th Ed. Chapter 423, Page 3109

A. Klienfelter syndrome
B. Turner syndrome
C. Down's syndrome (trisomy 21)
D. All of the above

Adults with trisomy 21 (Down's syndrome) consistently develop the typical neuropathologic hallmarks of AD if they survive beyond age 40.

1353. Presenilin-1 (PSEN-1) gene implicated in the pathogenesis of Alzheimer's disease is present on which chromosome?

Harrison's 20th Ed. Chapter 423, Page 3110

A. Chromosome 9
B. Chromosome 11
C. Chromosome 14
D. Chromosome 21

Presenilin-1 (PSEN-1) gene implicated in the pathogenesis of Alzheimer's disease is present on chromosome 14 and encodes a presenilin-1 protein called S182.

1354. Presenilin-2 (PSEN-2) gene implicated in the pathogenesis of Alzheimer's disease is present on which chromosome?

Harrison's 20th Ed. Chapter 423, Page 3110

A. Chromosome 1
B. Chromosome 11
C. Chromosome 14
D. Chromosome 21

Presenilin-2 (PSEN-2) gene implicated in the pathogenesis of Alzheimer's disease is present on chromosome 1 and encodes presenilin-2 protein called STM2 (seven transmembrane domains).

1355. Which of the following about S182 & STM2 is false?

Harrison's 20th Ed. Chapter 423, Page 3110

A. Cytoplasmic neuronal proteins
B. Widely expressed throughout nervous system
C. Homologous to cell-trafficking protein - sel 12
D. None of the above

S182 and STM2 are cytoplasmic neuronal proteins, widely expressed in the nervous system and are homologous to a cell-trafficking protein - sel 12 found in the nematode Caenorhabditis elegans.

1356. Mutations in which of the following gene causes early age-of-onset Familial Alzheimer's disease (FAD)?

Harrison's 20th Ed. Chapter 423, Page 3110

A. APP
B. Presenilin-1 (PS-1)
C. Presenilin-2 (PS-2)
D. Apo e gene

Mutations in Presenilin-1 (PS-1) gene cause an early-onset AD (onset before age 60) transmitted in an autosomal dominant, highly penetrant fashion.

1357. Apo ε gene implicated in the pathogenesis of Alzheimer's disease is present on which chromosome?

Harrison's 20th Ed. Chapter 423, Page 3110

A. Chromosome 1
B. Chromosome 11
C. Chromosome 19
D. Chromosome 21

Apo ε gene implicated in the pathogenesis of Alzheimer's disease is present on chromosome 19.

1358. Gene implicated in pathogenesis of Alzheimer's disease is?
Harrison's 20th Ed. Chapter 423, Page 3110

A. APP
B. Presenilin-1 (PSEN-1) & Presenilin-2 (PSEN-2)
C. Apo ε gene
D. All of the above

AD genes include APP, Presenilin-1 (PSEN-1), Presenilin-2 (PSEN-2) and Apo ε gene.

1359. Mutations in which gene is the most common cause of late-onset familial & sporadic forms of Alzheimer's disease?
Harrison's 20th Ed. Chapter 423, Page 3110

A. APP
B. Presenilin-1 (PS-1)
C. Presenilin-2 (PS-2)
D. Apo ε gene

Apo ε gene on chromosome 19 leads to late onset familial and sporadic forms of AD.

1360. Age of onset of sporadic & familial forms of AD is modulated by which allelic variants of apolipoprotein e?
Harrison's 20th Ed. Chapter 423, Page 3110, N Engl J Med. 2001;344:1516

A. ε 2
B. ε 3
C. ε 4
D. All of the above

Apo e4 allele has a strong association with sporadic and late-onset familial cases of AD. Apo ε4 remains the single most important biologic marker associated with risk for AD.

1361. For Alzheimer's disease, which allelic variant of apolipoprotein ε is protective?
Harrison's 20th Ed. Chapter 423, Page 3111

A. ε 2
B. ε 3
C. ε 4
D. All of the above

There is evidence that the Apo ε2 allele may be "protective" against Alzheimer's disease.

1362. Carrying of which APO ε allele nearly doubles the lifetime risk of Alzheimer's disease?
N Engl J Med. 2003;349:1056-63

A. APO ε2
B. APO ε3
C. APO ε4
D. None of the above

Apo ε4 allele is an important risk factor for AD.

1363. Apo ε4 allele associated with which of the following diseases?
Harrison's 20th Ed. Chapter 423, Page 3111

A. AD
B. FTD
C. DLB
D. CJD

Apo ε4 allele is not associated with FTD, DLB, or CJD.

1364. Which of the following gene is implicated in AD pathogenesis?
Harrison's 20th Ed. Chapter 423, Page 3111

A. Clusterin (CLU)
B. Phosphatidylinositol-binding clathrin assembly protein (PICALM)
C. Complement component (3b/4b) receptor 1 (CR1)
D. All of the above

Recent genome-wide association studies have implicated the clusterin (CLU), phosphatidylinositol-binding clathrin assembly protein (PICALM), and complement component (3b/4b) receptor 1 (CR1) genes in AD pathogenesis. CLU may play a role in synapse turnover, PICALM participates in clathrin-mediated endocytosis & CR1 may be involved in amyloid clearance through complement pathway.

1365. Polycystic lipomembranous osteodysplasia with sclerosing leukoencephalopathy (PLOSL) is also called?
Neurol India. 2018;66:538-41

A. Nasu–Hakola disease
B. Motohashi-Shinohara disease
C. Akai-Tateishi disease
D. Nakamagoe-Shioya disease

PLOSL or Nasu–Hakola disease is an autosomal recessive disease due to mutations in TYROBP and TREM2 that are expressed in microglia & osteoclasts (both derived from monocyte–macrophage lineage). There occurs delayed differentiation of osteoclasts & microgliosis, resulting in an imbalance of bone-remodeling capability leading to bony cysts formation. Inflammatory & immunological imbalance in brain result in brain atrophy and dementia.

1366. TREM stands for?
N Engl J Med. 2013;368:182

A. Triggering receptor expressed on myeloma cells
B. Triggering receptor expressed on macrophage cells
C. Triggering receptor expressed on myeloid cells
D. Triggering receptor expressed on monocyte cells

1367. Which of the following about TREM2 is false?
N Engl J Med. 2013;368:182

A. TREM2 is a member of immunoglobulin family
B. TREM2 is an innate immune receptor
C. TREM2 signals through TYROBP
D. None of the above

TREM2 is an innate immune receptor expressed on cell membrane of a subset of myeloid cells like immature dendritic cells, osteoclasts, tissue macrophages & microglia. TREM2 is a member of immunoglobulin family and acts as a phagocytic receptor of bacteria. It recognizes anionic lipopolysaccharides in cell wall of bacteria and signals through a transmembrane adapter protein called TYROBP (also called DAP12). When a bacterium binds to TREM2 on macrophages, activation of the signaling pathway triggers the phagocytic uptake of bacteria and the release of reactive oxygen species (ROS). Heterozygous rare variants in TREM2 are associated with a significant increase in the risk of Alzheimer's disease.

1368. Which of the under mentioned drug for Alzheimer's disease is a cholinesterase inhibitor?
Harrison's 20th Ed. Chapter 423, Page 3111

A. Galantamine
B. Donepezil
C. Rivastigmine
D. All of the above

Pharmacologic action of donepezil, rivastigmine, and galantamine is inhibition of cholinesterase primarily acetylcholinesterase, with a resulting increase in cerebral acetylcholine levels.

1369. Which of the following drug has been discarded due to hepatotoxicity?
Harrison's 20th Ed. Chapter 423, Page 3111

A. Donepezil
B. Rivastigmine
C. Tacrine
D. Galantamine

1370. Which of the following acts on N-methyl-D-aspartate (NMDA) channels?

Harrison's 20th Ed. Chapter 423, Page 3111

A. Donepezil
B. Rivastigmine
C. Memantine
D. Galantamine

Memantine acts by blocking overexcited N-methyl-D-aspartate (NMDA) channels. It is used along with cholinesterase inhibitors and is not approved for mild AD.

1371. Which of the following drugs is contraindicated in patients with Parkinson's disease?

N Engl J Med. 2003;349:1056-63

A. Galantamine
B. Donepezil
C. Rivastigmine
D. Haloperidol

1372. Which of the following drugs is associated with an increased risk of stroke?

N Engl J Med. 2003;349:1056-63

A. Galantamine
B. Donepezil
C. Rivastigmine
D. Risperidone

1373. Tarenflurbil and Semagacestat are?

Harrison's 20th Ed. Chapter 423, Page 3111

A. Estrogen analogues
B. Vaccines
C. Gamma secretase inhibitors
D. HMG-CoA reductase inhibitors

Tarenflurbil and Semagacestat are gamma secretase inhibitors. Their use is being explored in AD treatment with a hypothesis that they would diminish the production of Aβ42.

1374. EEG studies are most useful for the diagnosis of?

N Engl J Med. 2001;344:1516, Harrison's 17th Ed. 2542

A. Alzheimer's disease
B. Frontotemporal dementia
C. Parkinson's disease
D. Creutzfeldt - Jakob disease

Abnormal periodic EEG discharges & cortical/basal ganglia abnormalities on diffusion-weighted MRI are unique diagnostic features of CJD.

1375. "Leukoaraiosis" refers to?

Harrison's 20th Ed. Chapter 423, Page 3087

A. White skin tags
B. White lines around umbilicus
C. Diffuse white matter disease
D. White nails

Leukoaraiosis or subcortical arteriosclerotic leukoencephalopathy or Binswanger's disease is a diffuse white matter disease which presents with dementia with lacunar infarctions found on MRI. Term Binswanger's disease should be used with caution, because it does not clearly identify a single entity.

Frontotemporal Dementia

1376. Which of the following statements about frontotemporal dementia (FTD) is false?

Harrison's 20th Ed. Chapter 424, Page 3115

A. Begins in fifth to seventh decade
B. Family history of dementia is common
C. Behavioral symptoms predominate in early stages
D. None of the above

FTD begins in V to VII decades. Unlike AD, behavioral symptoms predominate in early stages of FTD.

1377. Primary progressive aphasia is related to?

Harrison's 20th Ed. Chapter 424, Page 3115

A. FTD
B. PSP
C. CBD
D. Motor neuron disease

The left-hemisphere presentation of FTD is called primary progressive aphasia with nonfluent and semantic variants.

1378. Which of the following clinical variant is seen in familial and sporadic FTD?

Harrison's 20th Ed. Chapter 424, Page 3115

A. Behavioral variant
B. Semantic variant
C. Nonfluent/agrammatic variant
D. All of the above

Three core clinical syndromes seen in familial and sporadic FTD are behavioral variant (bvFTD), semantic variant and nonfluent/agrammatic variant. The last two are forms of primary progressive aphasia (PPA).

1379. Which of the following FTD variant may be most often accompanied by motor neuron disease (MND)?

Harrison's 20th Ed. Chapter 424, Page 3115

A. Behavioral variant (bvFTD)
B. Semantic variant (svPPA)
C. Nonfluent/agrammatic variant (nfvPPA)
D. All of the above

Most often bvFTD, but other two can be accompanied by motor neuron disease (MND), and is called FTD-MND.

1380. Which of the following is considered part of the FTLD clinical spectrum?

Harrison's 20th Ed. Chapter 424, Page 3115

A. Corticobasal syndrome (CBS)
B. Progressive supranuclear palsy syndrome (PSP-S)
C. Primary progressive aphasia (PPA)
D. All of the above

1381. Degeneration in which of the following areas of brain predicts bvFTD?

Harrison's 20th Ed. Chapter 424, Page 3115 Figure 424-1

A. Anterior cingulate atrophy
B. Frontoinsular atrophy
C. Orbital & dorsolateral prefrontal cortex atrophy
D. All of the above

Right hemisphere-predominant or symmetric anterior cingulate/medial prefrontal, orbital and anterior insular degeneration predicts bvFTD. Patients with nonfluent/agrammatic PPA show left (dominant) frontal opercular, dorsalinsula and precentral gyrus degeneration, whereas left anterior temporal (temporopolar) atrophy presents with semantic variant PPA.

1382. Which of the following statements about frontotemporal dementia is false?

Harrison's 20th Ed. Chapter 424, Page 3115 Figure 424-1

A. Memory and visuospatial skills relatively spared
B. Cholinergic system is relatively spared
C. Marked atrophy of temporal and/or frontal lobes
D. None of the above

Visuoconstructive ability, arithmetic calculations and navigation may remain normal late in any FTD syndrome. Distinguishing anatomic hallmark of FTD is a focal atrophy of frontal, insular, and/or temporal cortex. Cholinergic system is spared in FTD.

1383. In FTD, mutations occur in which of the following genes?

Harrison's 20th Ed. Chapter 424, Page 3115

A. C9ORF72
B. MAPT
C. GRN
D. All of the above

The most common autosomal dominantly inherited mutations causing FTD involve the C9ORF72 on chromosome 9, GRN on chromosome 17, altering progranulin protein gene and MAPT onchromosome 17, causing loss of function in tau molecule genes. Both MAPT & GRN mutations are associated with parkinsonian features. Mutations in valosin-containing protein (VCP, chromosome 9), TANK binding kinase 1 (TBK-1), T cell-restricted intracellular antigen-1 (TIA1), and charged multivesicular body protein 2b (CHMP2b, chromosome 3) genes also lead to autosomal dominant familial FTD.

1384. In ALS, mutations occur in which of the following genes?

Harrison's 20th Ed. Chapter 424, Page 3115

A. C9ORF72
B. TARDBP
C. MAPT
D. GRN

Mutations in the TARDBP (encoding TDP-43) and FUS (encoding fused in sarcoma [FUS]) genes cause familial ALS, sometimes in association with an FTD syndrome.

1385. TDP-43 stands for?

Harrison's 20th Ed. Chapter 424, Page 3043

A. TAR DNA binding protein 43
B. TAR depleted protein 43
C. TAR dense protein 43
D. TAR divided protein 43

TDP-43 stands for TAR DNA binding protein 413.

1386. Most common genetic cause of familial or sporadic FTD is?

Harrison's 20th Ed. Chapter 424, Page 3115

A. Trinucleotide expansions
B. Pentanucleotide expansions
C. Hexanucleotide expansions
D. Heptanucleotide expansions

Hexanucleotide (GGGGCC) expansions in the noncoding portion of C90RF72 represent the most common genetic cause of familial or sporadic FTD (usually presenting as bvFTD with or without MND) and amyotrophic lateral sclerosis (ALS) leading to reduced C90RF72 mRNA expression, nuclear mRNA foci containing transcribed portions of the expansion and other mRNAs, neuronal cytoplasmic inclusions containing dipeptide repeat proteins translated from the repeat mRNA and transactive response DNA-binding protein of 43 kDa (TDP-43) neuronal cytoplasmic and glial inclusions.

1387. Progranulin binds to which of the following?
Harrison's 20th Ed. Chapter 424, Page 3115

A. NMDA receptor
B. Tumor necrosis factor (TNF) receptors
C. Interleukin (IL) 7 receptor (CD 127)
D. ACh receptor

Progranulin is a growth factor that binds to tumor necrosis factor (TNF) receptors and participates in tissue repair and tumor growth.

1388. The gross pathologic hallmark of FTLD is a focal atrophy of?
Harrison's 20th Ed. Chapter 424, Page 3115

A. Frontal cortex
B. Insular cortex
C. Temporal cortex
D. Any of the above

Gross pathologic hallmark of FTLD is a focal atrophy of frontal, insular and/or temporal cortex. Atrophy often begins focally in one hemisphere before spreading to anatomically interconnected regions, including basal ganglia.

1389. Microscopic findings seen across all patients with FTLD include which of the following?
Harrison's 20th Ed. Chapter 424, Page 3115

A. Gliosis
B. Microvacuolation
C. Neuronal loss
D. All of the above

Microscopic findings seen across all patients with FTLD include gliosis, microvacuolation and neuronal loss. Protein composition of neuronal & glial inclusions contain either tau or TDP-43 in ~90% of patients (FTLD-TDP), remaining ~10% showing inclusions containing FUS (FTLD-FUS).

1390. Frontotemporal lobar degeneration pathology is divided according to presence of which inclusions in neurons & glia?
Harrison's 20th Ed. Chapter 424, Page 3116 Figure 424-2

A. Tau
B. TDP-43
C. FUS
D. All of the above

Frontotemporal dementia syndromes have in common the underlying frontotemporal lobar degeneration pathology. It can be divided according to the presence of tau, TDP-43, or FUS-containing inclusions in neurons and glia.

1391. Which of the following is not a member of FTLD-tau category?
Harrison's 20th Ed. Chapter 424, Page 3116 Figure 424-2

A. Pick's disease
B. Corticobasal degeneration (CBD)
C. Neuronal intermediate filament inclusion disease (NIFID)
D. Progressive supranuclear palsy (PSP)

1392. Which of the following is not a member of FTLD-FUS category?
Harrison's 20th Ed. Chapter 424, Page 3116 Figure 424-2

A. Neuronal intermediate filament inclusion disease (NIFID)
B. Basophilic inclusion body disease (BIBD)
C. Atypical frontotemporal lobar degeneration with ubiquitin-positive inclusions (aFTLD-U)
D. Frontotemporal dementia with parkinsonism linked to chromosome 17 (FTDP-17)

1393. Which of the following best relates to Pick bodies?
Harrison's 20th Ed. Chapter 424, Page 3116

A. Astrocytic plaque
B. Intraneuronal cytoplasmic inclusions
C. Ballooned neurons
D. All of the above

Pick's disease is characterized by selective involvement of anterior frontal & temporal neocortex and pathologically by intraneuronal cytoplasmic inclusions (Pick bodies) which are argyrophilic, staining positively with the Bielschowsky silver method (but not with the Gallyas method) and also with immunostaining for hyperphosphorylated tau.

1394. According to immunohistochemistry, tufted astrocyte is characteristic of?
Harrison's 20th Ed. Chapter 424, Page 3117 Figure 424-3

A. Pick's disease
B. Progressive supranuclear palsy
C. Corticobasal degeneration
D. FTLD-TDP, type A

1395. According to immunohistochemistry, astrocytic plaque is characteristic of?
Harrison's 20th Ed. Chapter 424, Page 3117 Figure 424-3

A. Pick's disease
B. Progressive supranuclear palsy
C. Corticobasal degeneration
D. FTLD-TDP, type A

1396. Which of the following drugs is effective in FTD?
Harrison's 20th Ed. Chapter 424, Page 3116

A. L-dopa
B. Selegiline
C. Pramipexole
D. None of the above

Treatment is symptomatic and there are currently no therapies known to slow progression or improve symptoms.

1397. Which of the following is also called Richardson syndrome?
Harrison's 20th Ed. Chapter 424, Page 3116

A. Corticobasal syndrome (CBS)
B. Frontotemporal dementia syndrome
C. Progressive supranuclear palsy syndrome (PSP-S)
D. Frontotemporal dementia with motor neuron disease

Progressive supranuclear palsy syndrome (PSP-S) is also known as Steele-Richardson-Olszewski syndrome or Richardson syndrome.

1398. Which of the following structures of brain is involved in PSP-S?
Harrison's 20th Ed. Chapter 424, Page 3116

A. Brainstem
B. Basal ganglia
C. Diencephalon
D. All of the above

PSP-S is a degenerative disorder that involves the brainstem, basal ganglia, diencephalon and selected areas of cortex.

1399. PSP begins with which of the following?
Harrison's 20th Ed. Chapter 424, Page 3116

A. Frequent falls
B. Symmetrical axial rigidity
C. Dementia
D. Seizure

Clinically, PSP-S begins with unexplained falls (frequently backwards) and executive or subtle personality changes (mental rigidity, impulsivity or apathy). Frequent unexplained falls are common secondary to a combination of axial rigidity, inability to look down, and bad judgment.

1400. Which of the following diseases cause ophthalmoparesis?
Harrison's 20th Ed. Chapter 424, Page 3116, 3156, 3279, 1055

A. Myotonic dystrophy
B. Metronidazole therapy
C. Machado-Joseph disease
D. All of the above

Besides PSP, Wernicke's syndrome, Myotonic dystrophy, Machado-Joseph disease, SCA7 and prolonged Metronidazole therapy can cause ophthalmoparesis.

1401. Which of the following diseases can cause supranuclear ophthalmoplegia?
Harrison's 20th Ed. Chapter 424, Page 1225

A. Whipple's disease
B. Multiple sclerosis
C. Wernicke's encephalopathy
D. All of the above

1402. Which of the following controls vertical gaze?
Harrison's 20th Ed. Chapter 424, Page 192

A. Nucleus basalis of Meynert
B. Nucleus locus coeruleus
C. Nucleus of Cajal
D. Nucleus of the solitary tract (NTS)

Vertical gaze is controlled at the level of midbrain. Lesions of rostral interstitial nucleus of medial longitudinal fasciculus and interstitial nucleus of Cajal cause supranuclear paresis of upgaze, downgaze or all vertical eye movements.

1403. Which of the following is an ocular finding in PSP?
Harrison's 20th Ed. Chapter 424, Page 3116

A. Slow ocular saccades
B. Eyelid apraxia
C. Impairment of downward gaze
D. All of the above

Progressive oculomotor syndrome in PSP begins with square wave jerks, followed by slowed saccades (vertical worse than horizontal) before resulting in progressive supranuclear ophthalmoparesis. In PSP, oculomotor disorder is supranuclear because oculocephalic reflexes (vertical doll's head maneuver) are preserved.

1404. "Hummingbird sign" on MRI is typical of which of the following?
Harrison's 20th Ed. Chapter 427, Page 3122

A. Corticobasal syndrome (CBS)
B. Frontotemporal dementia syndrome
C. Progressive supranuclear palsy syndrome (PSP-S)
D. Frontotemporal dementia with motor neuron disease

MRI may reveal a characteristic atrophy of the midbrain with relative preservation of the pons, the "hummingbird sign" on midsagittal images.

1405. Globose tangles best relate to?
Harrison's 20th Ed. Chapter 424, Page 3116

A. HD
B. PSP
C. CBD
D. AD

In PSP, accumulation of hyperphosphorylated 4-repeat tau is seen within neurons and glia. Neuronal inclusions often take the form of NFTs, which may be large, spherical ("globose") and coarse in brainstem, cerebellar dentate and diencephalic neurons.

1406. PSP is characterized by degeneration of which of the following?
Harrison's 20th Ed. Chapter 424, Page 3116

A. Substantia nigra
B. Globus pallidus
C. Subthalamic nucleus
D. All of the above

In PSP, the most prominent involvement (degeneration) is in subthalamic nucleus, globus pallidus, substantia nigra, locus coeruleus, periaqueductal gray, tectum, oculomotor nuclei and dentate nucleus of cerebellum.

1407. Which of the following is a neuropathological feature in PSP?
Harrison's 20th Ed. Chapter 424, Page 3117

A. Tufted astrocytes
B. Thorny astrocytes
C. Coiled oligodendroglial inclusions ("coiled bodies")
D. All of the above

PSP is associated with prominent tau-positive glial pathologies, such as tufted astrocytes, thorny astrocytes and coiled oligodendroglial inclusions ("coiled bodies").

1408. In PSP, neurofibrillary tangles are histochemically positive for which of the following?
Harrison's 20th Ed. Chapter 424, Page 3117

A. Tau
B. Amyloid
C. α-synuclein
D. All of the above

Pathologically, PSP is characterized by deposition of neurofibrillary tangles histochemically positive for tau and negative for amyloid or α-synuclein.

1409. "Alien hand" phenomenon is a feature of?
Harrison's 20th Ed. Chapter 424, Page 3117

A. PSP
B. DLB
C. CBS
D. AD

In corticobasal syndrome (CBS), apraxia of one arm and hand is called the alien hand. The limb exhibits unintended motor actions like grasping, groping, drifting or undoing.

1410. Corticobasal syndrome (CBS) can be due to?
Harrison's 20th Ed. Chapter 424, Page 3117

A. CBD
B. PSP
C. FTLD-TDP
D. All of the above

CBS refers to the clinical syndrome while CBD refers to a specific histopathologic FTLD-tau entity. CBS can be due to CBD, PSP, FTLD-TDP or even AD.

1411. Severe tauopathy burden in subcortical white matter is pathognomonic of?
Harrison's 20th Ed. Chapter 424, Page 3117

A. PSP
B. DLB
C. CBD
D. AD

In CBD, microscopic features include ballooned & achromatic tau-positive neurons, astrocytic plaques and dystrophic glial tau pathomorphologies that overlap with those seen in PSP. Most specifically, CBD features a severe tauopathy burden in the subcortical white matter, consisting of threads and oligodendroglial coiled bodies.

1412. Which of the following is a characteristic feature of dementia with Lewy Bodies (DLB)?

Harrison's 20th Ed. Chapter 424, Page 3117

A. Seizure
B. Symmetrical axial rigidity
C. Visual hallucinations
D. Auditory hallucinations

DLB is characterized by visual hallucinations, parkinsonism, fluctuating alertness, falls and REM sleep behavior disorder (RBD).

1413. Often, the first manifestation of illness in PDD and DLB is?

Harrison's 20th Ed. Chapter 424, Page 3117

A. Blindness
B. Seizure
C. Loss of memory
D. Delirium

PDD and DLB are highly sensitive to metabolic perturbations, and in some patients, the first manifestation of illness is a delirium, often precipitated by an infection, new medicine or other systemic disturbance. In DLB, there is relative preservation of memory.

1414. In DLB, Lewy bodies are found in?

Harrison's 20th Ed. Chapter 424, Page 3117

A. Cingulate gyrus
B. Amygdala
C. Substantia nigra
D. All of the above

Key neuropathologic feature of DLB is the presence of Lewy bodies in specific brainstem nuclei, substantia nigra, amygdala, cingulate gyrus and ultimately neocortex.

1415. Which of the following about Lewy bodies is false?

Harrison's 20th Ed. Chapter 424, Page 3117

A. Intraneuronal cytoplasmic inclusions
B. Stain with periodic acid–Schiff (PAS) & ubiquitin
C. Composed of straight neurofilaments 7 to 20 nm long
D. None of the above

Lewy bodies are intraneuronal cytoplasmic inclusions that stain with periodic acid-Schiff (PAS) & ubiquitin. They are composed of straight neurofilaments 7–20 nm long with surrounding amorphous material.

1416. In idiopathic PD, Lewy bodies are typically found in?

Harrison's 20th Ed. Chapter 424, Page 3117

A. Substantia nigra
B. Amygdala
C. Cingulate gyrus
D. All of the above

Lewy bodies are typically found in the substantia nigra of patients with idiopathic PD, where they can be readily seen with hematoxylin-and-eosin staining.

1417. Which of the following is a rapidly progressive dementing condition?

Harrison's 20th Ed. Chapter 423, Page 3112

A. Hashimoto's encephalopathy
B. Viral or bacterial encephalitides
C. Creutzfeldt-Jakob disease
D. All of the above

Besides Creutzfeldt-Jakob disease (CJD), viral or bacterial encephalitides, Hashimoto's encephalopathy, central nervous system (CNS) vasculitis, lymphoma, or paraneoplastic/autoimmune syndromes are other rapidly progressive dementing conditions.

1418. George Huntington belonged to which country?

A. Great Britain
B. America
C. Australia
D. Canada

Huntington's disease (HD) was described by George Huntington, an American physician in 1872. Huntington's gene is single, causal gene and an accurate genetic test for HD is available.

1419. Huntington's disease (HD) is caused by mutations in the Huntington's gene on the?

Harrison's 20th Ed. Chapter 428, Page 3137

A. Short arm of chromosome 4
B. Long arm of chromosome 4
C. Short arm of chromosome 5
D. Long arm of chromosome 5

HD is caused by mutations in the Huntington's gene on the short arm of chromosome 4.

1420. "Huntingtin" is a?

Harrison's 20th Ed. Chapter 428, Page 3137

A. Cell membrane protein
B. Cytoplasmic protein
C. Nuclear protein
D. Nuclear membrane protein

Huntingtin gene (HTT) encodes the highly conserved cytoplasmic protein huntingtin which is present in all neurons.

1421. Chorea is a characteristic feature of which of the following?

Harrison's 20th Ed. Chapter 423, Page 3112

A. Dementia with Lewy Bodies (DLB)
B. Huntington's disease (HD)
C. Cortical basal degeneration (CBD)
D. Creutzfeldt-Jakob disease (CJD)

HD is an autosomal dominant, degenerative brain disorder characterized by chorea, behavioral disturbance & frontal executive disorder in IV or V decade. Memory is frequently not impaired.

1422. In Huntington's disease (HD), which of the following is predominantly atrophied?

Harrison's 20th Ed. Chapter 423, Page 3112

A. Striatum
B. Cerebellum
C. Hippocampus
D. Mamillary bodies

Neuropathology of HD consists of widespread cerebral atrophy with prominent involvement of striatum and cerebral cortex.

1423. Which of the following is not a feature of normal-pressure hydrocephalus (NPH)?

Harrison's 20th Ed. Chapter 423, Page 3112

A. Abnormal gait
B. Dementia
C. Chorea
D. Urinary incontinence

Clinical triad of normal-pressure hydrocephalus (NPH) includes abnormal gait (ataxic or apractic), mild to moderate dementia and urinary incontinence.

1424. Cortical atrophy is not a feature of?

Harrison's 20th Ed. Chapter 423, Page 3112

A. AD
B. FTD
C. NPH
D. CJD

In NPH, neuroimaging shows enlarged lateral ventricles (hydrocephalus) with little or no cortical atrophy with a patent aqueduct of Sylvius suggesting communicating hydrocephalus.

1425. Which of the following is not a MRI feature of normal-pressure hydrocephalus?

Harrison's 20th Ed. Chapter 423, Page 3112

A. Stretching of corpus callosum
B. Elevation of the floor of third ventricle
C. Enlargement of the aqueduct
D. Dilation of the lateral ventricle

MRI feature of normal-pressure hydrocephalus (NPH) include dilation of lateral ventricle, stretching of corpus callosum, depression of the floor of third ventricle, enlargement of the patent aqueduct (communicating hydrocephalus).

1426. Which of the following is a feature of gait abnormality in NPH?

Harrison's 20th Ed. Chapter 423, Page 3112

A. External hip rotation
B. Low foot clearance
C. Short strides
D. All of the above

Characteristic "magnetic" gait with external hip rotation, low foot clearance and short strides, along with prominent truncal sway or instability, favors NPH.

1427. Dementia & seizures in Marchiafava-Bignami disease is related to?

Harrison's 20th Ed. Chapter 423, Page 3112

A. Male
B. Italian
C. Drinkers of red wine
D. All of the above

1428. Which of the following degenerates in Marchiafava-Bignami disease?

Harrison's 20th Ed. Chapter 423, Page 3112

A. Caudate nucleus
B. Thalamus
C. Corpus callosum
D. Substantia nigra

Marchiafava-Bignami disease consists of dementia and seizures with degeneration of corpus callosum in male Italian drinkers of red wine.

1429. Which of the following is not related to Wernicke's encephalopathy?

Harrison's 20th Ed. Chapter 423, Page 3113

A. Confusion
B. Seizure
C. Ataxia
D. Diplopia

Clinical presentation of Wernicke's encephalopathy include confusion, ataxia, & diplopia due to ophthalmoplegia.

1430. Thiamine deficiency damages which of the following?

Harrison's 20th Ed. Chapter 423, Page 3113

A. Thalamus
B. Mammillary bodies
C. Midline cerebellum
D. All of the above

Thiamine (vitamin B1) deficiency damages thalamus, mammillary bodies, midline cerebellum, periaqueductal grey matter of midbrain, peripheral nerves and trochlear & abducens nuclei.

1431. In Thiamine deficiency, damage to which of the following correlates most closely with memory loss?

Harrison's 20th Ed. Chapter 423, Page 3113

A. Dorsomedial thalamus
B. Mammillary bodies
C. Midline cerebellum
D. Periaqueductal grey matter of midbrain

In thiamine deficiency, damage to dorsomedial thalamus correlates most closely with memory loss.

1432. Which of the following is related to Korsakoff's psychosis?

Harrison's 20th Ed. Chapter 423, Page 3113

A. Prolonged untreated thiamine deficiency
B. Irreversible dementia
C. Amnestic syndrome
D. All of the above

Prolonged untreated thiamine deficiency results in irreversible dementia/amnestic syndrome (Korsakoff's psychosis) or even death.

1433. In Vitamin B_{12} deficiency, damage occurs to?

Harrison's 20th Ed. Chapter 423, Page 3113

A. Posterior columns
B. Corticospinal tracts
C. Peripheral nerves
D. All of the above

In Vitamin B_{12} deficiency, damage occur to posterior columns, corticospinal tracts, peripheral nerves and cerebral myelinated fibers (dementia).

1434. In Vitamin B_{12} deficiency, neurologic damage is related to?

Harrison's 20th Ed. Chapter 423, Page 3113

A. Inhibition of δ-aminolevulinic acid dehydrase
B. Deficiency of S-adenosyl methionine
C. Elevated plasma levels of Aβ amyloid
D. All of the above

Mechanism of neurologic damage in Vitamin B_{12} deficiency is related to deficiency of S-adenosyl methionine which is required for methylation of myelin phospholipids.

1435. Limbic encephalitis best relates to?

Harrison's 20th Ed. Chapter 423, Page 3113

A. Primary neoplasms of CNS
B. Metastatic neoplasms of CNS
C. Paraneoplastic syndrome
D. Isolated vasculitis of CNS

A paraneoplastic syndrome of dementia associated with occult carcinoma (small cell lung cancer) is termed limbic encephalitis in which confusion, agitation, seizures, poor memory, emotional changes, and frank dementia may occur.

1436. Which of the following chronic metal exposure can lead to choreoathetosis?

Harrison's 20th Ed. Chapter 423, Page 3113

A. Chronic mercury poisoning
B. Aluminum poisoning
C. Chronic arsenic intoxication
D. Chronic lead poisoning

Chronic mercury poisoning produces dementia, peripheral neuropathy, ataxia, and tremulousness that may progress to choreoathetosis.

1437. Mees' lines are best related to?

Harrison's 20th Ed. Chapter 423, Page 3113

A. Chronic mercury poisoning
B. Aluminum poisoning
C. Chronic arsenic intoxication
D. Chronic lead poisoning

Mees' lines are transverse white lines of the fingernails seen in chronic arsenic intoxication.

1438. Which of the following chronic metal exposure can lead to myoclonic jerks?

Harrison's 20th Ed. Chapter 423, Page 3113

A. Chronic mercury poisoning
B. Aluminum poisoning
C. Chronic arsenic intoxication
D. Chronic lead poisoning

Dialysis dementia syndrome due to aluminum overexposure is associated with confusion, aphasia, memory loss, agitation, and, later, lethargy and stupor. Speech arrest and myoclonic jerks are common and associated with severe and generalized EEG changes.

1439. "Dementia pugilistica" is related to which of the following?

Harrison's 20th Ed. Chapter 423, Page 3113

A. Nonconvulsive seizure disorder
B. Transient global amnesia (TGA)
C. Chronic metal exposure
D. Recurrent head trauma in professional boxers

Recurrent head trauma in professional boxers may lead to dementia, called the "punch drunk" syndrome or dementia pugilistica.

1440. In Transient global amnesia (TGA), which of the following memory types is lost?

Harrison's 20th Ed. Chapter 423, Page 3113

A. Working
B. Episodic
C. Remote
D. All of the above

Transient global amnesia is characterized by sudden onset of a severe episodic memory deficit in the setting of an emotional stimulus or physical exertion, in persons over age 50 years.

1441. Along with dementia, myoclonus is a feature of which of the following disease?

Harrison's 20th Ed. Chapter 423, Page 3113

A. Neuronal cerebrolipofuscinoses
B. Creutzfeldt - Jakob disease
C. Corticobasal degeneration (CBD)
D. All of the above

Vascular Dementia

1442. Which of the following can disrupt structural cognitive networks in Vascular cognitive impairment and vascular dementia (VCI-VaD)?

Harrison's 20th Ed. Chapter 425, Page 3118

A. Chronic progressive white matter degeneration
B. Disrupted cerebrovascular autoregulation
C. Blood brain barrier dysfunction
D. All of the above

Microinfarcts, microbleeds, macroinfarcts, large hemorrhages, chronic progressive white matter degeneration, altered cerebral hemodynamics, disrupted cerebrovascular autoregulation, neurovascular decoupling (loss of normal hemodynamic responses to neural activity), and blood brain barrier dysfunction can disrupt structural cognitive networks in Vascular cognitive impairment and vascular dementia (VCI-VaD).

1443. On neuroimaging, by the age of 70 years, what proportion of population has white matter disease & lesions?

Harrison's 20th Ed. Chapter 425, Page 3118

A. 30%
B. 50%
C. 70%
D. 90%

By the age of 70 years, 70% of the population has white matter disease & lesions on neuroimaging, with small infarcts (lacunar infarcts) found in 11–24% of the population.

1444. Which of the following statements is false?

Harrison's 20th Ed. Chapter 425, Page 3118

A. Hemorrhages account for ~20% of all strokes
B. Ischemic strokes compose 80% of all strokes
C. Chronic cerebral small vessel disease (SVD) has the strongest association with cognitive impairment
D. None of the above

SVD typically causes occlusion of deep-penetrating arterioles and disease of draining venules, causing damage to subcortical structures such as the basal ganglia, thalami, and white matter tracts.

1445. Average volume of lacunes is?

Harrison's 20th Ed. Chapter 425, Page 3118

A. 2 mm
B. 4 mm
C. 6 mm
D. 8 mm

Lacunes average 2 mm in volume, but can range from 0.2 to 15 mm.

1446. Which of the following about small vessel disease (SVD) is false?

Harrison's 20th Ed. Chapter 425, Page 3118

A. Sporadic
B. CADASIL is a genetic SVD-related VaD syndrome
C. SVD accounts for 36–67% of all VaDs
D. None of the above

1447. Which of the following abnormality is associated with SVD?

Harrison's 20th Ed. Chapter 425, Page 3118

A. Blood-brain-barrier compromise
B. Chronic cerebral hypoperfusion
C. Hippocampal atrophy & sclerosis
D. All of the above

SVD is associated with blood-brain-barrier (BBB) compromise, acculmulating white matter disease, and a state of chronic cerebral hypoperfusion, hippocampal atrophy & sclerosis.

1448. Which of the following increase the risk of dementia?

Harrison's 20th Ed. Chapter 425, Page 3118

A. White matter hyperintensities (WMH)
B. Cortical microinfarcts
C. Enlarged Virchow-Robin spaces (eVRS)
D. All of the above

Neuroimaging markers of SVD include white matter hyperintensities (WMH) of presumed vascular origin, microbleeds, cortical microinfarcts and enlarged Virchow-Robin spaces (eVRS). They increase the risk of dementia.

1449. Subcortical arteriosclerotic encephalopathy is also called?

Harrison's 20th Ed. Chapter 425, Page 3118

A. Lewy body disease
B. Binswanger's disease
C. Huntington's disease
D. Prion disease

Binswanger's disease is also called subcortical arteriosclerotic encephalopathy. It is considered a prototypical clinical syndrome of vascular cognitive impairment (VCI) and a pathologically homogenous subgroup.

1450. Which of the following neuroimaging technique is used for assessment of blood brain barrier integrity?

Harrison's 20th Ed. Chapter 425, Page 3118

A. Functional MRI (fMRI)
B. Magnetic resonance angiography (MRA)
C. Magnetic resonance venography (MRV)
D. Dynamic contrast-enhanced MRI (DCE-MRI)

Novel neuroimaging technique for assessment of blood brain barrier integrity is dynamic contrast-enhanced MRI (DCE-MRI).

1451. Which of the following about Binswanger's disease is false?

Harrison's 20th Ed. Chapter 425, Page 3118

A. Progressive confluent subcortical & periventricular white matter disease
B. Extensive demyelination & destruction of white matter with relative sparing of subcortical U fibers
C. Gradual accumulation of focal neurological deficits
D. None of the above

Subcortical U-fibers have a relatively slower rate of myelin turnover and are spared in Binswanger's disease & Neuromyelitis Optica (NMO). Multiple sclerosis (MS) & progressive multifocal leukoencephalopathy (PML) typically demonstrate early U-fiber involvement.

1452. Subcortical U fibers are involved in which of the following?

Harrison's 20th Ed. Chapter 425, Page 3118

A. CADASIL
B. Multiple sclerosis (MS)
C. Acute Disseminated Encephalomyelitis (ADEM)
D. All of the above

1453. Infarct in which of the following locations results in marked cognitive dysfunction & dementia?

Harrison's 20th Ed. Chapter 425, Page 3118

A. Thalamus
B. Basal ganglia
C. Angular gyrus
D. All of the above

A strategically placed infarct, usually in the thalamus, basal ganglia or angular gyrus can also result in marked cognitive dysfunction & dementia.

1454. Occlusion of which of the following artery can lead to bilateral infarction of dorsomedial nucleus & mammillothalamic tracts?

Harrison's 20th Ed. Chapter 425, Page 3118

A. Recurrent artery of Heubner
B. Artery of Percheron (AOP)
C. Artery of Adamkiewicz
D. Marginal artery of Drummond

Single paramedian artery (artery of Percheron) supplies both anteromedial thalamic regions, and its occlusion results in altered mental status, vertical gaze palsy, and memory impairment.

Dementia with Lewy Bodies

1455. Lewy body and Lewy neurite pathology most often begins in?

Harrison's 20th Ed. Chapter 426, Page 3119

A. Enteric and autonomic nervous systems
B. Optic nerve
C. Somatic nerves
D. All of the above

Lewy body & Lewy neurite pathology begins in the enteric & autonomic nervous systems before ascending through the brainstem to substantia nigra, limbic system, and ultimately cerebral cortex. Disease may also begin in the olfactory bulb & spread inward through olfactory system connections.

1456. "Neurons release the same neurotransmitters at all of their synapses" is called?

Proc. R. Soc. Med.28. ; 1935: 319-332

A. Bloch's law
B. Bell - Magendie law
C. Bunsen - Roscoe law
D. Dale's principle

Formulated by Henry Dale (1875 - 1968), British neurophysiologist in the 1940's, the original hypothesis was that each neuron releases only one type of neurotransmitter.

1457. DLB is a progressive dementia syndrome characterised by?

Harrison's 20th Ed. Chapter 426, Page 3119

A. Spontaneous parkinsonism
B. Visual hallucinations
C. Fluctuating cognition
D. All of the above

1458. DLB syndrome is characterized by?

Harrison's 20th Ed. Chapter 426, Page 3119

A. Neuroleptic sensitivity
B. Hyposmia
C. Rapid eye movement (REM) sleep behavior disorder (RBD)
D. All of the above

DLB syndrome is characterized by visual hallucinations, parkinsonism, fluctuating alertness, neuroleptic sensitivity, rapid eye movement (REM) sleep behavior disorder (RBD), and often hyposmia and excessive daytime sleepiness. The side-effects of neuroleptics (drowsiness, parkinsonism, and falls) are more prominent in dementia with Lewy bodies (DLB).

1459. Which of the following best relates to DLB syndrome?

Harrison's 20th Ed. Chapter 426, Page 3119

A. Déjà entendu
B. Jamais vu
C. Reduplicative paramnesia
D. Cryptomnesia

Reduplicative paramnesia (RP) is a subset of delusional misidentification syndromes. It is marked by a delusional belief that a place or location has been duplicated, existing in two or more places simultaneously, or that it has been 'relocated' to another site.

1460. Which of the following symptoms referable to brainstem pathology may accompany or precede DLB?

Harrison's 20th Ed. Chapter 426, Page 3119

A. Constipation
B. Orthostatic lightheadedness
C. Depression/anxiety
D. All of the above

Both PDD & DLB may be accompanied or preceded by symptoms referable to brainstem pathology below substantia nigra including constipation, orthostatic lightheadedness, depression/anxiety and RBD.

1461. Which of the following is false about DLB and PDD?

Harrison's 20th Ed. Chapter 426, Page 3119

A. Highly sensitive to metabolic disturbances
B. Marked day-to-day variation in cognitive functioning
C. Relative preservation of episodic memory
D. None of the above

1462. In Lewy body disease (LBD), Lewy bodies and Lewy neurites are found in?

Harrison's 20th Ed. Chapter 426, Page 3119

A. Substantia nigra
B. Amygdala
C. Cingulate gyrus
D. All of the above

Presence of Lewy bodies & Lewy neurites is the key neuropathological feature in Lewy body disease (LBD). They are present throughout specific brainstem nuclei, substantia nigra, amygdala, cingulate gyrus and ultimately, the neocortex causing profound cholinergic deficit.

1463. Patients with DLB are extremely sensitive to which of the following medications?

Harrison's 20th Ed. Chapter 426, Page 3119

A. Oral anticoagulant medication
B. Antiplatelet medication
C. Dopaminergic medication
D. All of the above

Patients with DLB are extremely sensitive to dopaminergic medications and atypical antipsychotics.

Parkinson's Disease

1464. Paralysis agitans was described in Ayurveda (Charaka Samhita) centuries ago by the name of?

N Engl J Med. 1998;339:1049

A. Adhyashana
B. Kampavata
C. Jatharagni
D. Shalmali

Paralysis agitans described by James Parkinson is an independent description of Kampavata (Kampa:tremor, Vata:metabolic derangement predisposing to neurologic and mental diseases) described in Ayurveda (Charaka Samhita) centuries ago. Several preparations containing Mucuna pruriens (Kapikachu) were descrided for treatment of patients with Kampavata. The major active compound present in Mucuna pruriens is levodopa.

1465. The first name of Parkinson was?

Harrison's 20th Ed. Chapter 427, Page 3120

A. John
B. James
C. Jack
D. George

Parkinson disease was first described by English physician James Parkinson in 1817.

1466. Corpus Luysii is the name given to?

Principles of Neurology, Adams RD, 5th Ed. 57

A. Claustrum
B. Subthalamic nucleus
C. Globus pallidus
D. Substantia nigra

Corpus Luysii is the name given to subthalamic nucleus (STN) which is the only glutamatergic nucleus in the "basal ganglia".

1467. Which of the following is commonest neurodegenerative disease?

Harrison's 20th Ed. Chapter 427, Page 3120

A. Alzheimer's disease (AD)
B. Parkinson's disease (PD)
C. Wilson's disease (WD)
D. SCA 3 (spinocerebellar ataxia)

Parkinson's disease (PD) is the second commonest neurodegenerative disease, exceeded only by Alzheimer's disease (AD).

1468. In patients under the age of 65 years, which of the following is the most common cause of dementia?

Harrison's 20th Ed. Chapter 427, Page 153

A. Frontotemporal lobar degeneration
B. Multisystem atrophy
C. Parkinson's disease
D. Huntington's disease

In patients under the age of 65 years, FTD rivals AD as the most common cause of dementia.

1469. Which of the following is not included in the cardinal features of PD?

Harrison's 20th Ed. Chapter 427, Page 3120

A. Rest tremor
B. Masked facies (hypomimia)
C. Bradykinesia
D. Gait dysfunction with postural instability

Cardinal features of PD include rest tremor, rigidity, bradykinesia and gait impairment with postural instability. Nondopaminergic features (as they do not fully respond to dopaminergic therapy) include freezing of gait, speech difficulty, autonomic disturbances, sensory alterations, mood disorders, sleep dysfunction, cognitive impairment, and dementia.

1470. The whistle-smile sign is also called?

DeJong's The Neurologic Examination, 7th Ed. Page 253

A. Levine's sign
B. Comet sign
C. Hanes sign
D. Gower sign

Because of their paucity of facial expression, patients with Parkinson's disease may fail to smile after being asked to whistle—the whistle-smile (Hanes) sign.

1471. Non-motor features of PD include all except?

Harrison's 20th Ed. Chapter 427, Page 3120 Table 427-1

A. Sleep disturbances
B. Cognitive impairment
C. Loss of taste
D. Loss of smell

Non-motor aspects of PD include depression and anxiety, cognitive impairment, sleep disturbances, sensory abnormalities and pain, loss of smell (anosmia) and disturbances of autonomic function.

1472. Clinicopathologic correlation is better if which of the following is included to define Parkinson's Disease?

Harrison's 20th Ed. Chapter 427, Page 3120

A. Rest tremor
B. Asymmetry of motor impairment
C. Good response to levodopa
D. All of the above

Clinicopathologic correlation studies have determined that parkinsonism associated with rest tremor, asymmetry of motor impairment, and a good response to levodopa is more likely to predict the correct pathologic diagnosis of PD (International Parkinson's Disease and Movement Disorder Society (MDS)).

1473. Decreased smell function is among the first signs of which of the following diseases?

Harrison's 20th Ed. Chapter 25, Page 153

A. Wilson's disease
B. Parkinson's disease
C. Progressive supranuclear palsy
D. All of the above

1474. Decreased smell function is found in which of the following diseases?

Harrison's 20th Ed. Chapter 29, Page 194, 197

A. iRBD
B. Parkinson's disease
C. Alzheimer's disease
D. All of the above

Decreased smell function is among the first signs, if not the first sign, of such neurodegenerative diseases as Parkinson's disease (PD) and Alzheimer's disease (AD), signifying their "presymptomatic" phase. Olfactory impairment in PD often predates the clinical diagnosis by at least 4 years. Others include Huntington's disease, Down's syndrome, parkinsonism-dementia complex of Guam, dementia with Lewy bodies (DLB), multiple system atrophy, corticobasal degeneration, frontotemporal dementia, multiple sclerosis (MS) and idiopathic rapid eye movement (REM) behavioral sleep disorder (iRBD). Smell loss is minimal or nonexistent in progressive supranuclear palsy and MPTP-induced parkinsonism.

1475. Pathological hallmark feature of PD is?
Harrison's 20th Ed. Chapter 427, Page 3120

A. Degeneration of dopaminergic neurons in SNc
B. Reduced striatal dopamine
C. Intracytoplasmic proteinaceous inclusions (Lewy bodies)
D. All of the above

Pathologically, the hallmark features of PD are degeneration of dopaminergic neurons in the substantia nigra pars compacta (SNc), reduced striatal dopamine, and intracytoplasmic proteinaceous inclusions known as Lewy bodies. There is relative sparing of caudate nucleus.

1476. Cholinergic neurons are present in?
Harrison's 20th Ed. Chapter 427, Page 3120

A. Locus coeruleus (LC)
B. Nucleus basalis of Meynert (NBM)
C. Raphe nuclei of the brainstem
D. All of the above

1477. Norepinephrine neurons are present in?
Harrison's 20th Ed. Chapter 427, Page 3120

A. Locus coeruleus (LC)
B. Nucleus basalis of Meynert (NBM)
C. Raphe nuclei of the brainstem
D. All of the above

Cholinergic neurons are present in nucleus basalis of Meynert (NBM). Norepinephrine neurons are present in locus coeruleus (LC) and serotonin neurons in raphe nuclei of the brainstem, and neurons of the olfactory system, cerebral hemispheres, spinal cord, and peripheral autonomic nervous system.

1478. Pathological changes in PD (Lewy body pathology) begin in?
Harrison's 20th Ed. Chapter 427, Page 3120

A. Peripheral autonomic nervous system
B. Olfactory system
C. Dorsal motor nucleus of vagus nerve in lower brainstem
D. All of the above

In PD, pathology begins in peripheral autonomic nervous system, olfactory system & dorsomotor nucleus of vagus nerve in lower brainstem, and then spreads in a sequential manner to affect the upper brainstem and cerebral hemispheres. Thus, dopamine neurons are affected in midstage disease (Braak staging).

1479. Which of the following is mostly responsible for signs of parkinsonism?
Harrison's 20th Ed. Chapter 427, Page 3120

A. Decreased traffic in indirect striato-pallidal pathway
B. Increased traffic in direct striato-nigral pathway
C. Decreased ability of thalamus to activate frontal cortex
D. All of the above

Striatal dopamine denervation results in increased traffic in indirect striato-pallidal pathway and decreased traffic in direct pathway. Downstream consequence of this is increased activity in striatal outflow stemming from the increased activity of STN and ultimately GPi/SNr neurons. Because striatal outflow is inhibitory to the thalamus (GABA), there is a decrease in the ability of thalamus to activate frontal cortex leading to signs of parkinsonism.

1480. Which of the following is not a component of basal ganglia?
Harrison's 20th Ed. Chapter 427, Page 3120

A. Striatum (putamen & caudate nucleus)
B. Subthalamic nucleus (STN)
C. Globus pallidus pars externa (GPe)
D. Claustrum

Basal ganglia are subcortical nuclei that include striatum (putamen & caudate nucleus), subthalamic nucleus (STN), globus pallidus pars externa (GPe), globus pallidus pars interna (GPi) & SNc. Symptom complex of Parkinsonism reflect damage to different components of basal ganglia.

1481. Which of the following is the revised criteria for the clinical diagnosis of PD?
Harrison's 20th Ed. Chapter 427, Page 3120

A. UK brain bank criteria
B. UK brain store criteria
C. UK brain support criteria
D. UK brain diagnosis criteria

UK brain bank criteria is the revised criteria for the clinical diagnosis of PD.

1482. In PD, metabolic imaging (PET/SPECT) shows which of the following?
Harrison's 20th Ed. Chapter 427, Page 3121

A. Reduced uptake in posterior putamen
B. Increased activity in GPi
C. Decreased activity in thalamus
D. All of the above

Imaging of brain dopamine system in PD with positron emission tomography (PET) or single-photon emission computed tomography (SPECT) shows reduced uptake of striatal dopaminergic markers, particularly in posterior putamen, increased activity in the GPi with decreased activity in thalamus.

1483. Commonest cause of familial PD is due to mutations of?
Harrison's 20th Ed. Chapter 427, Page 3121

A. LRRK1 gene
B. LRRK2 gene
C. LRRK3 gene
D. LRRK4 gene

Mutations of LRRK2 (leucine rich repeat kinase 2) gene are the commonest cause of familial PD and are responsible for ~1% of typical sporadic cases of the disease.

1484. Familial Parkinson's disease is associated with mutations in which of the following genes?
Harrison's 20th Ed. Chapter 427, Page 3043

A. PINK1
B. DJ-1
C. Parkin
D. All of the above

Familial Parkinson's disease is associated with mutations in leucine rich repeat kinase 2 (LRRK2, α-synuclein, parkin, PINK1 and DJ-1. PINK1 is a mitochondrial kinase and DJ- 1 is a protein involved in protection from oxidative stress. Parkin, which causes autosomal recessive early-onset Parkinson's disease, is a ubiquitin ligase.

1485. Atypical parkinsonism group of neurodegenerative conditions include?
Harrison's 20th Ed. Chapter 427, Page 3122

A. Multiple System Atrophy (MSA)
B. Progressive Supranuclear Palsy (PSP)
C. Corticobasal syndrome (CBS)
D. All of the above

1486. Diagnosis of atypical Parkinsonism is favoured by all except?
Harrison's 20th Ed. Chapter 427, Page 3122

A. Early speech impairment
B. Early gait impairment
C. Absence of rest tremor
D. Asymmetry

Atypical Parkinsonism is characterized by early speech and gait impairment, absence of rest tremor, no asymmetry, poor or no response to levodopa, and an aggressive clinical course. Pathologically, neurodegeneration occurs without Lewy bodies. Metabolic imaging of basal ganglia/thalamus network shows decreased activity in GPi with increased activity in thalamus, reverse of what is seen in PD.

1487. Manifestations of multiple-system atrophy (MSA) include all except?

Harrison's 20th Ed. Chapter 427, Page 3122

A. Parkinsonian features
B. Cerebellar features
C. Sensory features
D. Autonomic features

Multiple-system atrophy (MSA) manifests as a combination of parkinsonian, cerebellar, and autonomic features. When parkinsonian features are predominant, term MSA-p is used and when cerebellar features are predominant, term MSA-c is used.

1488. Degeneration of which of the following is found in MSA?

Harrison's 20th Ed. Chapter 427, Page 3122

A. SNc
B. Striatum
C. Inferior olivary nuclei
D. All of the above

1489. Glial cytoplasmic inclusions (GCIs) characteristic of MSA stain positive for?

Harrison's 20th Ed. Chapter 427, Page 3122

A. Tau
B. α-synuclein
C. UCHL-1
D. Parkin

Pathologically, MSA is characterized by degeneration of SNc, striatum, cerebellum & inferior olivary nuclei coupled with characteristic glial cytoplasmic inclusions (GCIs) that stain for α-synuclein.

1490. "Hot cross buns" sign relates to which of the following?

Harrison's 20th Ed. Chapter 427, Page 3122

A. MSA
B. PSP
C. Corticobasal ganglionic degeneration
D. All of the above

The pontine "hot cross buns" sign is a MRI feature of MSA-c.

1491. PSP is characterized by?

Harrison's 20th Ed. Chapter 427, Page 3122

A. Slow ocular saccades
B. Eyelid apraxia
C. Restricted vertical eye movements
D. All of the above

1492. Which of the following eye movements is impaired in PSP?

Harrison's 20th Ed. Chapter 427, Page 3122

A. Upward gaze
B. Downward gaze
C. Lateral gaze
D. Medial gaze

PSP is a form of atypical parkinsonism, characterized by slow ocular saccades, eyelid apraxia & restricted vertical eye movements particularly impairment of downward gaze.

1493. Which of the following is associated with PSP?

Harrison's 20th Ed. Chapter 427, Page 3122

A. Hyperextension of neck with early gait disturbance & falls
B. Swallowing difficulty & cognitive impairment
C. Little or no response to levodopa therapy
D. All of the above

In PSP (Richardson), hyperextension of neck with early gait disturbance & falls occurs. Speech & swallowing difficulty and cognitive impairment become obvious in later stages. There is usually little or no response to levodopa. In the "Parkinson" form of PSP, resemblence to PD is observed in early stages including a positive response to levodopa. The gait of PSP is typically more erect compared with stooped posture of typical Parkinson's disease, and toppling falls within the first year also suggest the possibility of PSP.

1494. "Hummingbird sign" on mid sagittal MRI images relates to which of the following?

Harrison's 20th Ed. Chapter 427, Page 3122

A. MSA
B. PSP
C. Corticobasal ganglionic degeneration
D. All of the above

The "hummingbird sign" on mid sagittal MRI images is a feature of progressive supranuclear palsy (PSP) and is due to atrophy of midbrain with relative preservation of pons.

1495. Pathologically, PSP is characterized by?

Harrison's 20th Ed. Chapter 427, Page 3122

A. Degeneration of SNc, striatum, STN, midline thalamic nuclei & pallidum
B. Neurofibrillary tangles
C. Inclusions positive for tau protein
D. All of the above

Pathologically, PSP is characterized by degeneration of SNc, striatum, STN, midline thalamic nuclei & pallidum, along with neurofibrillary tangles & inclusions that stain positive for tau protein.

1496. Corticobasal syndrome (CBS) presents with?

Harrison's 20th Ed. Chapter 427, Page 3123

A. Asymmetric dystonic contractions
B. Clumsiness of one hand
C. Apraxia, agnosia, focal limb myoclonus, or alien limb phenomenon
D. All of the above

CBS, least common of the three atypical parkinsonisms, presents with both cortical & basal ganglia features. These include asymmetric dystonic contractions & clumsiness of one hand along with cortical sensory disturbances like apraxia, agnosia, focal limb myoclonus, or alien limb phenomenon (where the limb assumes a position in space without patient being aware of the position or recognizing that limb belongs to him/her). Dementia may occur at any stage of the disease.

1497. Carbon monoxide or manganese damage which of the following?

Harrison's 20th Ed. Chapter 427, Page 3123

A. Substantia nigra
B. Subthalamic nucleus (STN)
C. Globus pallidus
D. All of the above

Carbon monoxide or manganese damage globus pallidus & presentation resembles atypical parkinsonism.

1498. Most common cause of secondary parkinsonism is?

Harrison's 20th Ed. Chapter 427, Page 3123

A. Calcium channel blockers (flunarizine, cinnarizine)
B. Amiodarone
C. Lithium
D. Dopamine-blocking agents like neuroleptics

Dopamine-blocking agents like neuroleptics are the most common cause of secondary parkinsonism. Metoclopramide is neuroleptic agent also.

1499. Which of the following is false about Dopa-Responsive Dystonia?
Harrison's 20th Ed. Chapter 427, Page 3123

A. Due to impaired production of dopa & dopamine in brain
B. No abnormalities on FD-PET, no neurodegeneration
C. Responds to levodopa
D. None of the above

Dopa-Responsive Dystonia should be considered in dystonia individuals aged <20 years who present with a clinical picture resembling PD. It is due to a mutation in GTP-Cyclohydrolase 1 gene leading to impaired production of dopa & dopamine. It responds to levodopa and is not associated with abnormalities on fluoro-dopa positron emission tomography (FD-PET). There is no evidence of neurodegeneration.

1500. Parkinsonism can be seen as a feature of?
Harrison's 20th Ed. Chapter 427, Page 3123

A. Wilson's disease
B. Huntington's disease
C. Hallervorden-Spatz disease
D. All of the above

Parkinsonism is a feature of Wilson's disease, Huntington's disease (Westphal variant), dopa-responsive dystonia and pantothenate kinase (PANK)–associated neurodegeneration (formerly called Hallervorden Spatz disease).

1501. Which of the following is the cause of PD in majority?
Harrison's 20th Ed. Chapter 427, Page 3123

A. Sporadic
B. Genetic
C. Cerebrovascular disease
D. Drugs

Most PD cases occur sporadically (85–90%) and are of unknown cause. Gene mutations are the only known causes of PD in younger-onset patients.

1502. Which of the following is a primary autonomic degenerative disorder?
Harrison's 20th Ed. Chapter 18, Page 126

A. Multiple system atrophy (Shy-Drager syndrome)
B. Dementia with Lewy bodies
C. Pure autonomic failure
D. All of the above

1503. α-synuclein, aggregates predominantly in the cytoplasm of neurons in all of the following except?
Harrison's 20th Ed. Chapter 18, Page 126

A. Parkinson's disease
B. Dementia with Lewy bodies
C. Pure autonomic failure
D. Multiple system atrophy

1504. Which of the following is a Lewy body disorder?
Harrison's 20th Ed. Chapter 18, Page 126

A. Parkinson's disease
B. Dementia with Lewy bodies
C. Pure autonomic failure
D. All of the above

Primary autonomic degenerative disorders are multiple system atrophy (Shy-Drager syndrome), Parkinson's disease, dementia with Lewy bodies, and pure autonomic failure. These are also called "synucleinopathies" due to the presence of α-synuclein that aggregates predominantly in cytoplasm of neurons in Lewy body disorders (Parkinson's disease, dementia with Lewy bodies & pure autonomic failure) and in the glia in multiple system atrophy (MSA).

1505. Peak age of onset of Sporodic Parkinson's disease (PD) is in which decade of life?
Harrison's 20th Ed. Chapter 427, Page 3123

A. 50s
B. 60s
C. 70s
D. 80s

Most cases of PD begin after the age of 60 years and the incidence increases up to the age of ~80 years (range is 35 to 85 years) and the course of the illness ranges between 10 and 25 years.

1506. Factors linked to a reduced incidence of PD include all except?
Harrison's 20th Ed. Chapter 427, Page 3123

A. Coffee drinking
B. Smoking
C. Use of NSAIDs
D. Alcohol use

Factors linked to a reduced incidence of PD include coffee drinking, smoking, use of nonsteroidal anti-inflammatory drugs, and estrogen replacement in postmenopausal women.

1507. Environmental risk factors for PD include all except?
Harrison's 20th Ed. Chapter 427, Page 3123

A. Exposure to pesticides
B. Consumption of well water
C. Rural living
D. Urban living

Risk factors include a positive family history, male gender, head injury, exposure to pesticides, consumption of well water, and rural living.

1508. Which of the following neurotoxin produces parkinsonism?
Harrison's 20th Ed. Chapter 427, Page 3123

A. Apamin
B. Botulinum
C. MPTP
D. Tetanospasmin

MPTP (1-methyl-4-phenyl-1,2,5,6-tetrahydropyridine) is a byproduct of the illicit manufacture of a heroin-like drug, causes a PD-like syndrome in addicts. MPTP is transported to CNS, where it is metabolized to form MPP⁺, a mitochondrial toxin that is selectively taken up by, and damages, dopamine neurons. MPTP toxicity can be prevented by coadministration of a MAO-B inhibitor that blocks its conversion to the toxic pyridinium ion MPP⁺.

1509. Toxins that can produce secondary Parkinsonism include all except?
Harrison's 20th Ed. Chapter 427, Page 3121 Table 427-2

A. 1-Methyl-1,2,4,6 tetrahydropyridine (MPTP)
B. Manganese
C. Cyanide
D. Carbon dioxide

1510. Toxins that can produce secondary PD include all except?
Harrison's 20th Ed. Chapter 427, Page 3121 Table 427-2

A. Methanol
B. Ethanol
C. Carbon monoxide
D. Carbon disulfide

1-Methyl-1,2,4,6 tetrahydropyridine (MPTP), Manganese, Cyanide, Methanol, Carbon monoxide, Carbon disulfide, Hexane produce parkinsonism.

1511. Drug that can cause secondary parkinsonism is?
Harrison's 20th Ed. Chapter 427, Page 3123

A. Amiodarone
B. Lithium
C. Cinnarizine
D. All of the above

Drugs that can cause secondary parkinsonism include metoclopramide, flunarizine, cinnarizine, tetrabenazine, amiodarone, and lithium.

1512. Drugs that can produce secondary PD include all except?

Harrison's 20th Ed. Chapter 427, Page 3123

A. Metoclopramide
B. Reserpine
C. Methyldopa
D. Clonidine

1513. Drugs that can produce secondary PD include all except?

Harrison's 20th Ed. Chapter 427, Page 3123

A. Lithium carbonate
B. Valproic acid
C. Phenytoin
D. Fluoxetine

Drugs that can produce secondary PD include neuroleptics (typical antipsychotics), some atypical antipsychotics, antiemetics (compazine, metoclopramide), dopamine-depleting agents (reserpine, tetrabenazine), alpha methyldopa, lithium carbonate, valproic acid, fluoxetine.

1514. Mutations in which of the following gene numerically represent the most important risk factor for the development of PD?

Harrison's 20th Ed. Chapter 427, Page 3125

A. Glucocerebrosidase
B. α-glucosidase
C. α-galactosidase A
D. Hexosaminidase A

Mutations in the glucocerebrosidase (GBA) gene associated with Gaucher's disease numerically represent the most important risk factor for the development of PD. There is a reciprocal interaction between glucocerebrosidase and α-synuclein. In sporadic PD, glucocerebrosidase concentrations & enzymatic activity are reduced in substantia nigra. α-synuclein is degraded by chaperone-mediated & macro autophagy. α-synuclein inhibits activity of glucocerebrosidase, therefore there is bidirectional feedback between α-synuclein & glucocerebrosidase.

1515. Autophagy is impaired in which of the following diseases?

Harrison's 20th Ed. Chapter 417, Page 3044

A. Alzheimer's disease
B. Parkinson's disease
C. Huntington's disease
D. All of the above

Autophagy is the degradation of cystolic components in lysosomes. Autophagy plays an important role in degradation of protein aggregates in neurodegenerative diseases and it is impaired in AD, Parkinson's disease and Huntington's disease.

1516. Which of the following drug induces autophagy?

Harrison's 20th Ed. Chapter 417, Page 3044

A. Resveratrol
B. Spermidine
C. Rapamycin
D. Metformin

Rapamycin induces autophagy.

1517. As a cause of PD, which LRRK2 mutation is the commonest?

Harrison's 20th Ed. Chapter 427, Page 3125

A. p.G2017S
B. p.G2018S
C. p.G2019S
D. p.G2020S

Seven different LRRK2 mutations have been linked to PD, with p.G2019S being the commonest.

1518. The protein LRRK2 is also called?

Brain.2005;128(12):2786-96

A. Kardarin
B. Mardarin
C. Dardarin
D. Pardarin

The protein LRRK2 is also called "dardarin" from the Basque term "dardara" which means "to tremble."

1519. Confirmed genes responsible for the autosomal dominant form of PD are?

Harrison's 20th Ed. Chapter 427, Page 3124 Table 427-4

A. SNCA (PARK1)
B. LRRK2 (PARK8)
C. VPS35 (PARK17)
D. All of the above

1520. Phenotype of LRRK2 p.G2019S mutations is distinguished from that of sporadic PD by?

Harrison's 20th Ed. Chapter 427, Page 3125

A. Mask like face
B. Leg tremor
C. Frequent falls
D. Dementia

Phenotype of LRRK2 p.G2019S mutations is indistinguishable from that of sporadic PD, although tremor appears to be more common, and leg tremor may be a useful diagnostic clue. In G2019S mutation, glycine to serine substitution (G2019S) occurs within the protein kinase domain encoded by exon 41.

1521. Which of the following gene leads to an autosomal dominant form of PD?

Harrison's 20th Ed. Chapter 427, Page 3124 Table 427-4

A. SNCA (PARK1)
B. LRRK2 (PARK8)
C. VPS35 (PARK17)
D. All of the above

1522. Which of the following gene leads to an autosomal recessive form of PD?

Harrison's 20th Ed. Chapter 427, Page 3124 Table 427-4

A. PARK-Parkin (PARK2)
B. PARK-PINK1 (PARK6)
C. PARK-DJ1 (PARK7)
D. All of the above

1523. Which of the following about Kufor-Rakeb syndrome (KRS) is false?

Harrison's 20th Ed. Chapter 427, Page 3124 Table 427-4

A. Autosomal-recessive form of juvenile-onset PD
B. Caused by ATP13A2 gene mutations
C. Supranuclear upgaze paresis, facial-faucial-finger minimyoclonus
D. None of the above

Kufor-Rakeb syndrome (KRS; PARK 9) is a rare autosomal-recessive form of nigro-striatal-pallidal-pyramidal neurodegeneration caused by ATP13A2 gene mutations presenting as juvenile-onset Parkinson's disease (PD). Rapidly progressive symptoms of parkinsonism, spasticity, supranuclear upgaze paresis, facial-faucial-finger minimyoclonus, visual hallucinations, oculogyric dystonic spasms, and dementia, usually noted between 12 & 16 years, leads to severe motor handicap.

1524. Which of the following genes is mutated in PARK7 Parkinson's disease?

Harrison's 20th Ed. Chapter 427, Page 3124 Table 427-4

A. PINK1
B. DJ-1
C. Parkin
D. UCHL- 1

1525. Which of the following about PD due to mutations in Parkin & PINK1 is false?

Harrison's 20th Ed. Chapter 427, Page 3125

A. Autosomal recessive and early-onset PD
B. Commonly complicated by dystonia
C. Lewy bodies are typically absent
D. None of the above

1526. Which of the following is false for familial Parkinson's disease?

Harrison's 20th Ed. Chapter 427, Page 3125

A. Mutations in a-synuclein and ubiquitin carboxy-terminal hydroxylase L1 (UCH-L1)
B. Characteristic histopathologic feature is Lewy body
C. Lewy body is eosinophilic cytoplasmic inclusion that contains neurofilaments and α-synuclein
D. None of the above

1527. Which of the following about basal ganglia is false?

Harrison's 20th Ed. Chapter 427, Page 3125

A. Striatum is the major input region of basal ganglia and receives its major input from cortex
B. GPi & SNr are the major output regions
C. Output of basal ganglia provides inhibitory (GABAergic) tone to thalamic & brainstem neurons
D. None of the above

1528. Glutamate is the neurotransmitter for which of the following pathways?

Harrison's 20th Ed. Chapter 427, Page 3126 Figure 427-5

A. Globus pallidus externa—subthalamic nucleus
B. Substantia nigra compacta—striatum
C. Subthalamic nucleus—Substantia nigra reticulata
D. Globus pallidus interna—thalamus

1529. Gamma aminobutyric acid (GABA) is the neurotransmitter for which of the following pathways?

Harrison's 20th Ed. Chapter 427, Page 3126 Figure 427-5

A. Globus pallidus externa—subthalamic nucleus
B. Striatum—Globus pallidus interna
C. Globus pallidus interna—thalamus
D. All of the above

1530. Which of the following pathways is excitatory?

Harrison's 20th Ed. Chapter 427, Page 3126 Figure 427-5

A. Globus pallidus externa—subthalamic nucleus
B. Striatum—Globus pallidus externa
C. Globus pallidus interna—thalamus
D. Subthalamic nucleus—Globus pallidus interna

1531. Which of the following pathways is inhibitory?

Harrison's 20th Ed. Chapter 427, Page 3126 Figure 427-5

A. Globus pallidus externa—subthalamic nucleus
B. Striatum—Globus pallidus externa
C. Globus pallidus interna—thalamus
D. All of the above

1532. Which of the following is false in PD?

Harrison's 20th Ed. Chapter 427, Page 3125

A. Increased firing of neurons in STN
B. Increased firing of neurons in GPi
C. Excessive inhibition of thalamus
D. None of the above

In PD, dopamine denervation causes increased firing of neurons in STN & GPi, resulting in excessive inhibition of thalamus with consequent reduced activation of cortical motor systems & development of parkinsonian features.

1533. Which of the following is most frequently present in patients with true PD?

Harrison's 20th Ed. Chapter 427, Page 3125

A. Rest tremor
B. Rigidity
C. Bradykinesia
D. Masked facies

Three cardinal signs of PD are rest tremor, rigidity & bradykinesia. Tremor is present in 85% of patients with true PD and diagnosis of PD is difficult if tremor is absent.

1534. Most disabling motor feature of PD is?

Harrison's 20th Ed. Chapter 427, Page 3125

A. Rest tremor
B. Rigidity
C. Bradykinesia
D. Stooped posture

The most disabling motor feature of PD is bradykinesia.

1535. Which of the following is false about 'rest tremor' in PD?

Harrison's 20th Ed. Chapter 427, Page 3125

A. Frequency of 4 to 6 Hz
B. Appear bilaterally, first distally
C. May appear in lips, tongue and jaw
D. Spares head and neck

Rest tremor, at a frequency of 4 to 6 Hz, typically appears unilaterally, first distally, involving the digits and wrist with a "pill-rolling" character. Tremor usually spreads proximally, ipsilaterally, and occasionally to the leg before crossing to the other side. It may appear later in lips, tongue and jaw but spares the head and neck.

1536. Testing for postural instability in PD is done by?

Harrison's 20th Ed. Chapter 427, Page 147

A. Swing test
B. Push test
C. Pull test
D. Lift test

In advanced PD, postural instability is one of the most disabling feature. It can be tested in office with the "pull test". A Tai Chi exercise program has been demonstrated to reduce the risk of falls and injury in patients with Parkinson's disease.

1537. Term used to describe gait in PD is?

Harrison's 20th Ed. Chapter 427, Page 146

A. Pigeon gait
B. Antalgic gait
C. Scissor gait
D. Festinating gait

Festinating gait is a classic sign of parkinsonism due to a combination of flexed posture and loss of postural reflexes. The patient accelerates to "catch up" with body's center of gravity. In Parkinson's disease, the fall due to freezing of gait. Feet stick to floor & center of mass keeps moving, resulting in a disequilibrium & a forward fall. Gait freezing can also occur as the patient attempts to turn & change direction.

1538. In Latin "festino" means?

A. "to fall"
B. "to freeze"
C. "to hurry"
D. "to swing"

In Latin "festino" means "to hurry".

1539. Manifestation that may be present long before the onset of motor signs in PD include?

Harrison's 20th Ed. Chapter 427, Page 3120, 3131

A. Anosmia
B. Depression
C. Sleep disorders
D. All of the above

1540. Which of the following symptom precedes onset of PD?

Harrison's 20th Ed. Chapter 427, Page 154, 3131

A. Rapid eye movement - behavioral disorder (RBD)
B. Micrographia
C. Hypophonia
D. All of the above

Epidemiologic studies suggest that clinical symptoms reflecting this nondopaminergic degeneration, such as constipation, anosmia, rapid eye movement (REM) behavior sleep disorder, restless legs and rapid eye movement–behavioral disorder (RBD) and cardiac denervation can precede the onset of the classic motor features of PD.

1541. Cardiac postganglionic adrenergic innervation is markedly impaired in?

Harrison's 20th Ed. Chapter 427, Page 3163

A. Multiple system atrophy (MSA)
B. Parkinson's disease (PD)
C. Guillain Barre syndrome
D. Diabetes Mellitus

Cardiac postganglionic adrenergic innervation, measured by uptake of fluorodopamine on positron emission tomography, is markedly impaired in the dysautonomia of Parkinson's disease (PD) but is usually normal in MSA.

1542. Neurogenic dysphagia results from?

Harrison's 20th Ed. Chapter 427, Page 251

A. Cerebrovascular accidents
B. Parkinson's disease
C. Amyotrophic lateral sclerosis
D. All of the above

1543. Constipation is common in?

Harrison's 20th Ed. Chapter 427, Page 269, 3131

A. Parkinson's disease
B. Multiple sclerosis
C. Diabetic neuropathy
D. All of the above

1544. 'Early appearance of hallucinations' favours which of the following diagnosis?

DeJong's The Neurologic Examination, 7th Ed. Page 488

A. Parkinson's disease
B. Wilson's disease
C. Cortical dementia with Lewy bodies (DLB)
D. Alzheimer's disease

In DLB, parkinsonian features are compounded by early appearance of hallucinations or drug-induced hallucinations and disturbances in arousal and behavior.

1545. 'Early imbalance & falls' favours the diagnosis of?

DeJong's The Neurologic Examination, 7th Ed. Page 488

A. Parkinson's disease
B. Progressive supranuclear palsy (PSP)
C. Cortical dementia with Lewy bodies (DLB)
D. Multiple system atrophy (MSA)

The development of early imbalance and falls suggests progressive supranuclear palsy (PSP).

1546. 'Early urinary incontinence, orthostatic hypotension, and dysarthria' favours which of the following diagnosis?

DeJong's The Neurologic Examination, 7th Ed. Page 488

A. Parkinson's disease
B. Progressive supranuclear palsy (PSP)
C. Cortical dementia with Lewy bodies (DLB)
D. Multiple system atrophy (MSA)

The development of early urinary incontinence, orthostatic hypotension and dysarthria suggest multiple system atrophy (MSA).

1547. Parkinsonian symptoms develop when striatal dopamine depletion reaches how much of normal?

Harrison's 20th Ed. Chapter 427, Page 3122

A. 10 to 30%
B. 30 to 50%
C. 50 to 70%
D. 70 to 90%

Symptoms develop when striatal dopamine depletion reaches 50 to 70% of normal.

1548. Which of the following symptoms respond poorly to therapy in PD?

Harrison's 20th Ed. Chapter 427, Page 3129

A. Bradykinesia
B. Abnormal posture
C. Balance difficulties
D. Rigidity

1549. Which of the following symptoms respond poorly to therapy in PD?

Harrison's 20th Ed. Chapter 427, Page 3129

A. Cognitive symptoms
B. Abnormal posture
C. Tremor
D. Rigidity

Cognitive symptoms, hypophonia, autonomic dysfunction & balance difficulties respond poorly to symptomatic therapy. While, bradykinesia, tremor, rigidity & abnormal posture respond well.

1550. Dopamine agonists act directly on which of the following postsynaptic dopamine receptor?

Harrison's 17th Ed. 2554

A. D1 type
B. D2 type
C. D3 type
D. D4 type

Dopamine agonists readily cross the blood-brain barrier and act directly on postsynaptic dopamine receptors - primarily D2 type.

1551. Which of the following statements is false?

Harrison's 20th Ed. Chapter 427, Page 3126

A. Levodopa is a dopamine precursor
B. Dopamine does not cross blood-brain barrier (BBB)
C. Domperidone is a peripheral dopamine-blocking agent
D. None of the above

1552. Which of the following area of the brain is not protected by the blood-brain barrier (BBB)?

Harrison's 20th Ed. Chapter 427, Page 3126, J Neuroinflammation 2010;7:70

A. Posterior pituitary gland
B. Pineal gland
C. Area postrema
D. All of the above

Four areas of brain are not protected by the blood-brain barrier. These areas include posterior pituitary gland, pineal gland, median eminence of hypothalamus and area postrema. Area postrema (a paired circumventricular organ & vomiting center in medulla) is not covered by BBB because it senses toxins in blood that other parts of brain are protected from. Area postrema triggers nausea & vomiting to prevent further ingestion of toxins.

1553. "No on" effect refers to?

Harrison's 20th Ed. Chapter 427, Page 3126

A. Loss of benefit following an individual dose
B. Delay in turning on the response
C. No response at all to a given dose
D. None of the above

With continued levodopa therapy, duration of benefit following an individual dose becomes progressively shorter. This loss of benefit is known as "wearing off effect". Patients may experience a delay in turning on (delayed-on) or no response at all to a given dose (no-on).

1554. Which of the following is false for Dyskinesias in PD?

Harrison's 20th Ed. Chapter 427, Page 3126

A. Choreiform and dystonic movements
B. Occur as a peak dose effect
C. Occur at the beginning or end of the dose
D. None of the above

Dyskinesias refer to choreiform and dystonic movements that can occur as a peak dose effect or at the beginning or end of the dose (diphasic dyskinesias).

1555. Nature of dyskinesia due to levodopa therapy is?

Harrison's 20th Ed. Chapter 427, Page 3126

A. Choreiform
B. Dystonia
C. Myoclonus
D. Any of the above

Nature of dyskinesia due to levodopa therapy can be choreiform in nature but can manifest as dystonic movements, myoclonus or other movement disorders predominantly involving the lower extremities, relieved by increasing the dose of levodopa. Dyskinesias tend to occur at the time of levodopa peak plasma concentration and maximal clinical benefit (peak-dose dyskinesia). "Diphasic dyskinesias" occur as the levodopa dose begins to take effect and again as it wears off.

1556. Which of the following is false about levodopa-induced motor complications?

Harrison's 20th Ed. Chapter 427, Page 3127

A. More likely to occur in females
B. More likely to occur in younger individuals with more severe disease
C. More likely to occur with higher doses of levodopa
D. None of the above

Levodopa-induced motor complications are more likely to occur in female, younger individuals with more severe disease and with the use of higher doses (mg/kg) of levodopa.

1557. Punding refers to?

Harrison's 20th Ed. Chapter 427, Page 3127

A. Hypersexuality
B. Meaningless assembly & disassembly of objects
C. Phobic cry
D. Craving for levodopa

PD patients taking high doses of levodopa can develop purposeless, stereotyped behaviors such as the meaningless assembly and disassembly or collection and sorting of objects. This is known as punding. This term is taken from Swedish description of meaningless behaviors seen in chronic amphetamine users.

1558. Dopamine dysregulation syndrome refers to?

Harrison's 20th Ed. Chapter 427, Page 3127

A. Hypersexuality
B. Meaningless assembly & disassembly of objects
C. Phobic cry
D. Craving for levodopa

In dopamine dysregulation syndrome, patients have a craving for levodopa and take frequent and unnecessary doses of the drug in an addictive manner.

1559. Levodopa can be combined with?

Harrison's 20th Ed. Chapter 427, Page 3127

A. Carbidopa
B. Benserazide
C. Entacapone
D. All of the above

To prevent peripheral metabolism of levodopa to dopamine & development of nausea & vomiting due to activation of dopamine receptors in area postrema, levodopa is used in combination with peripheral decarboxylase inhibitor (carbidopa or benserazide) or COMT inhibitor (tolcapone or entacapone).

1560. Which of the following statements about Levodopa is false?

Harrison's 20th Ed. Chapter 427, Page 3127

A. Is a precursor of dopamine
B. It is not metabolized centrally by dopa-decarboxylase
C. It is metabolized peripherally by dopa-decarboxylase
D. It is metabolized by COMT & MAO

Levodopa is a precursor of dopamine and is metabolized centrally & peripherally by dopa-decarboxylase, catechol-O-methyltransferase (COMT) and monoamine oxidase. Inhibitors of monoamine oxidase type B (MAO-B) block central dopamine metabolism & increase synaptic concentrations of the neurotransmitter.

1561. Which of the following is not a 'Dopamine agonist'?
Harrison's 20th Ed. Chapter 427, Page 3127

A. Levodopa
B. Pergolide
C. Bromocriptine
D. Pramipexole

Levodopa is a precursor of dopamine.

1562. Which of the following dopamine agonist is an ergot derivative?
Harrison's 20th Ed. Chapter 427, Page 3127

A. Bromocriptine
B. Pergolide
C. Cabergoline
D. All of the above

1563. Which of the following dopamine agonist is a nonergot derivative?
Harrison's 20th Ed. Chapter 427, Page 3127

A. Pramipexole
B. Ropinirole
C. Rotigotine
D. All of the above

Dopamine agonists include ergot alkaloids like bromocriptine, cabergoline, lisuride and pergolide and second generation non-ergot alkaloids like pramipexole, ropinirole and rotigotine.

1564. Which of the following antiparkinsonian drug is associated with valvular disease?
Harrison's 20th Ed. Chapter 427, Page 3127

A. Levodopa
B. Pergolide
C. Pramipexole
D. Rotigotine

Pergolide is associated with asymptomatic valvular disease on chronic administration.

1565. Which of the following is administered as a transdermal patch?
Harrison's 20th Ed. Chapter 427, Page 3127

A. Pramipexole
B. Ropinirole
C. Rotigotine
D. Levodopa

Rotigotine is administered as a once-daily transdermal patch.

1566. Which of the following is used as a rescue agent for treatment of severe "off" episodes?
Harrison's 20th Ed. Chapter 427, Page 3127

A. Apomorphine
B. Ropinirole
C. Pramipexole
D. Levodopa

Apomorphine is a dopamine agonist but must be administered parenterally (SC/continuous infusion) and is used as a rescue agent for the treatment of severe "off" episodes.

1567. Which of the following is an impulse-control disorder?
Harrison's 20th Ed. Chapter 427, Page 3127

A. Pathologic gambling
B. Hypersexuality
C. Compulsive eating
D. All of the above

1568. What amount of carbidopa is necessary to block peripheral levodopa decarboxylation into dopamine?
Harrison's 17th Ed. 2556

A. 10 mg/day
B. 25 mg/day
C. 50 mg/day
D. 75 mg/day

Mostly, 75 mg/day of carbidopa is necessary to block peripheral levodopa decarboxylation into dopamine.

1569. MAO is responsible for the deactivation of?
Cleveland Clinic Journal of Medicine 2010:77;860

A. Norepinephrine
B. 5-hydroxytryptamine
C. Dopamine
D. All of the above

Intramitochondrial enzyme MAO is responsible for the deactivation of norepinephrine, 5-hydroxytryptamine, and dopamine.

1570. With MAO inhibitors, tyramine-induced hypertensive crisis is named as?
Harrison's 20th Ed. Chapter 427, Page 3128

A. Alcohol effect
B. Diet effect
C. Cheese effect
D. Wine effect

Inhibition of MAO-A prevents metabolism of tyramine in gut, leading to a potentially fatal hypertensive reaction known as a "cheese effect" as it can be precipitated by foods rich in tyramine (some cheeses, aged meats & red wine).

1571. Which of the following is a monoamine oxidase (MAO) B inhibitor?
Harrison's 20th Ed. Chapter 427, Page 3128

A. Pramipexole
B. Pergolide
C. Selegiline
D. Entacapone

Selegiline & rasagiline are selective & irreversible monoamine oxidase (MAO) B inhibitor that block central dopamine metabolism & increase its synaptic concentration. They do not functionally inhibit MAO-A.

1572. Which of the following is a monoamine oxidase (MAO) inhibitor?
Harrison's 20th Ed. Chapter 427, Page 1563

A. Furazolidone
B. Cycloserine
C. Clarithromycin
D. Amikacin

Furazolidone inhibits monoamine oxidase (MAO) gradually over several days.

1573. Which of the following is a monoamine oxidase (MAO) inhibitor?
Harrison's 20th Ed. Chapter 427, Page 1055

A. Linezolid
B. Rifapentine
C. Clarithromycin
D. Capreomycin

Linezolid is a weak MAO inhibitor and can be associated with the serotonin syndrome when given concomitantly with serotonergic drugs (SSRI). Iproniazid was the first antidepressant introduced and is a MAOI anti-tuberculous drug.

1574. Which of the following is a reversible MAO-B inhibitor?
Harrison's 20th Ed. Chapter 427, Page 3128

A. Glycinamide
B. Safinamide
C. N-acetylprocainamide (NAPA)
D. Dichlorphenamide

1575. Which of the following is not a MAO inhibitor?
Harrison's 20th Ed. Chapter 427, Page 3308 Table 450-4

A. Isocarboxazid
B. Phenelzine
C. Tetrabenazine
D. Tranylcypromine

MAO inhibitors include selegiline, isocarboxazid, phenelzine and tranylcypromine. The last three are irreversible enzyme inhibitors that binds to MAO covalently, destroying its function forever.

1576. MAO catabolizes which of the following?
Cleveland Clinic Journal of Medicine 2010:77;860

A. Norepinephrine
B. Serotonin
C. Dopamine
D. All of the above

MAO is a flavin-containing enzyme critical for regulating neurotransmitter levels by catabolizing endogenous monoamines (NE, serotonin & dopamine) & exogenous amines (dietary tyramine). MAO exists in two subtypes, A & B. MAO-A preferentially metabolizes serotonin (5-HT) & NE. MAO-B preferentially metabolizes trace amines, including phenethylamine. MAO-A & MAO-B metabolize DA & tyramine.

1577. Which of the following have only MAO-B?
Cleveland Clinic Journal of Medicine 2010:77;860

A. Intestine
B. Brain
C. Platelets
D. Liver

MAO-A is the major enzyme outside of brain, with the exception of platelets and lymphocytes, which have only MAO-B. Ratio of MAO-A to MAO-B in human brain is 25%:75%, whereas in liver, ratio is 50%:50%, in intestine, ratio is 80%:20% & in peripheral adrenergic neurons, ratio is 90%:10%.

1578. Which of the following is a selective MAO-A inhibitor?
Cleveland Clinic Journal of Medicine 2010:77;860

A. Phenelzine
B. Isocarboxazid
C. Clorgyline
D. Moclobemide

Nonselective MAO inhibitors are phenelzine, isocarboxazid & tranylcypromine. Selegiline is selective for MAO-B. Clorgyline is selective for MAO-A. Moclobemide is a reversible MAO inhibitor.

1579. Which of the following is a Catechol O-methyltransferase (COMT) inhibitor?
Harrison's 20th Ed. Chapter 427, Page 3128

A. Selegiline
B. Entacapone
C. Bromocriptine
D. Pergolide

Entacapone and tolcapone are catechol-O-methyl transferase (COMT) inhibitors. They augment the effects of levodopa by blocking peripheral enzymatic degradation of levodopa and dopamine.

1580. Which of the following is a long-acting, once daily COMT inhibitor?
Harrison's 20th Ed. Chapter 427, Page 3128

A. Tolcapone
B. Entacapone
C. Opicapone
D. All of the above

1581. Discoloration of urine can be due to which of the following drugs?
Harrison's 20th Ed. Chapter 427, Page 3128

A. Selegiline
B. Entacapone
C. Bromocriptine
D. Pergolide

Though not of clinical concern, discoloration of urine can be seen with both COMT inhibitors (tolcapone and entacapone) due to accumulation of a metabolite.

1582. Which of the following is a side effect of tolcapone?
Harrison's 20th Ed. Chapter 427, Page 3128

A. Severe diarrhea
B. Hepatic toxicity
C. Discoloration of urine
D. All of the above

1583. Which of the following clinical studies relate to treatment of PD?
Harrison's 20th Ed. Chapter 427, Page 3128

A. DATATOP study
B. ADAGIO study
C. STRIDE-PD study
D. All of the above

1584. The only oral agent that reduces dyskinesia while improving parkinsonian features is?
Harrison's 20th Ed. Chapter 427, Page 3128

A. Selegiline
B. Amantadine
C. Bromocriptine
D. Pergolide

Amantadine, an antiviral agent, is the only oral agent that reduces dyskinesia while improving parkinsonian features.

1585. Livedo reticularis is the side effect of?
Harrison's 20th Ed. Chapter 427, Page 3128

A. Selegiline
B. Amantadine
C. Bromocriptine
D. Pergolide

Amantadine is a weak NMDA-receptor antagonist. Its side effects are livido reticularis, weight gain, and impaired cognitive function.

1586. Which of the following about Amantadine is false?
Harrison's 20th Ed. Chapter 427, Page 3128

A. Withdrawal-like symptoms on discontinuation
B. Antiviral agent

C. Potent anti-dyskinesia agent
D. None of the above

1587. Which of the following anticonvulsant has antiparkinsonian effects?

Harrison's 20th Ed. Chapter 427, Page 3128

A. Oxcarbazepine
B. Tiagabine
C. Felbamate
D. Zonisamide

1588. Which of the following is a A_{2A} antagonist?

Harrison's 20th Ed. Chapter 427, Page 3129

A. Rolofylline
B. Istradefylline
C. Pentifylline
D. Pentoxifylline

The A_{2A} antagonist Istradefylline is approved in Japan.

1589. Which of the following drugs has neuroprotective function in PD?

Harrison's 20th Ed. Chapter 427, Page 3129

A. Levodopa
B. Bromocryptine
C. Selegiline
D. Amantadine

Selegiline in addition to a mild symptomatic effect has a neuroprotective function. High doses of coenzyme Q_{10}, intrastriatal infusion of neurotrophic factors and exercise may be beneficial.

1590. Which of the following drugs have the potential of a neuroprotective therapy in PD?

Harrison's 20th Ed. Chapter 427, Page 3129

A. Rasagiline
B. Pramipexole
C. Ropinirole
D. All of the above

Rasagiline, selegiline, pramipexole, ropinirole & coenzyme Q_{10} are promising neuroprotection or disease modification agents in PD.

1591. Deep brain stimulation (DBS) for PD primarily targets which of the following?

Harrison's 20th Ed. Chapter 427, Page 3129

A. Ventrolateral thalamus
B. Subthalamic nucleus (STN)
C. Substantia nigra, pars compacta
D. Motor cortex

DBS for PD primarily targets subthalamic nucleus (STN) or internal segment of globus pallidus (GPi). GPi stimulation may be associated with a reduced frequency of depression.

1592. Trophic factors with beneficial effects on dopamine neurons include?

Harrison's 20th Ed. Chapter 427, Page 3130

A. Ciliary neurotrophic factor (CNTF)
B. Brain-derived neurotrophic factor (BDNF)
C. Neurturin
D. All of the above

Trophic factors that have beneficial effects on dopamine neurons in laboratory studies include Glial-derived neurotrophic factor (GDNF) and neurturin.

1593. In gene therapy for PD, which of the following is used as viral vector?

Harrison's 20th Ed. Chapter 427, Page 3130

A. AAV1
B. AAV2
C. AAV3
D. AAV4

Gene therapy involves viral vector delivery of DNA of a therapeutic protein to specific target regions. The AAV2 virus is used as viral vector as it does not cause inflammatory response, is not incorporated into host genome, and is associated with long-lasting transgene expression.

1594. Which of the following may be helpful for both depression & PD motor features?

Harrison's 20th Ed. Chapter 427, Page 3130

A. Selegiline
B. Rasagiline
C. Pramipexole
D. Ropinirole

1595. In patients of PD with psychotic symptoms, which of the following drug is preferred?

Harrison's 20th Ed. Chapter 427, Page 3130

A. Quetiapine
B. Clozapine
C. Risperidone
D. Olanzapine

Quetiapine is recommended because it lacks the risk of agranulocytosis associated with clozapine. Risperidone, olanzapine and aripiprazole are not well tolerated by most patients with PD due to a higher incidence of drug-induced parkinsonism (DIP) and akathisia.

1596. Which of the following in PD patients is a harbinger of a developing dementia?

Harrison's 20th Ed. Chapter 427, Page 3130

A. Panic attacks
B. Sweating
C. Constipation
D. Hallucinations

Hallucinations in PD patients are often a harbinger of a developing dementia. In contrast to AD, hallucinations are typically visual, formed and nonthreatening.

1597. Which atypical neuroleptic is also an inverse agonist of serotonin 5-HT2A receptor?

Harrison's 20th Ed. Chapter 427, Page 3130

A. Pimavanserin
B. Quetiapine
C. Clozapine
D. All of the above

Atypical neuroleptic Pimavanserin is also an inverse agonist of the serotonin 5-HT2A receptor.

1598. Cause of neuropsychiatric symptoms in PD can be?

Harrison's 20th Ed. Chapter 427, Page 3130

A. Accompanying Alzheimer's disease (AD)
B. Accompanying cortical dementia with Lewy bodies (DLB)
C. Side effect of pharmacotherapy
D. All of the above

Neuropsychiatric symptoms of later stages of PD may be direct result of PD or accompanying Alzheimer's disease, cortical dementia with Lewy bodies or as a side effect of its drugs.

1599. In dementia in PD (PDD), which of the following is relatively spared?

Harrison's 20th Ed. Chapter 427, Page 3130

A. Language
B. Memory
C. Calculation
D. All of the above

In contrast to AD, PDD primarily affects executive functions & attention, with relative sparing of language, memory, and calculation domains.

1600. To preserve or regain cognitive functions in PD, which of the following drug is withdrawn first?

Harrison's 20th Ed. Chapter 427, Page 3130

A. Anticholinergics
B. Dopamine agonists
C. COMT inhibitors
D. MAO-B inhibitors

To preserve or regain cognitive functions in PD, drugs are discontinued in the following sequence: anticholinergics, amantadine, dopamine agonists, COMT inhibitors, and MAO-B inhibitors. Patients are managed with lowest dose of standard levodopa.

1601. Which of the following drugs reduce the rate of deterioration of cognitive function in PD?

Harrison's 20th Ed. Chapter 427, Page 3130

A. Memantine
B. Rivastigmine
C. Donepezil
D. All of the above

Anticholinesterase agents (memantine, rivastigmine & donepezil) reduce the rate of deterioration of cognitive function and can improve attention in PD.

1602. Which of the following is typical of REM behavior disorder (RBD)?

Harrison's 20th Ed. Chapter 427, Page 3131

A. Violent movements & vocalizations during REM sleep
B. Orthostatic hypotension & fainting on awakening
C. Visual hallucinations
D. All of the above

REM behavior disorder (RBD) is a syndrome comprised of violent movements and vocalizations during REM sleep possibly representing acting out of dreams due to a failure of normal inhibition of motor movements that typically accompanies REM sleep.

Tremor, Chorea, and Other Movement Disorders

1603. Which of the following best relate to hyperkinetic movement disorders?
Harrison's 20th Ed. Chapter 428, Page 3132

A. Voluntary
B. Involuntary
C. Seizure
D. Passive

Hyperkinetic movement disorders are characterized by involuntary movements occurring in isolation or in combination, unaccompanied by weakness.

1604. Which of the following is not a kind of tremor?
Harrison's 20th Ed. Chapter 428, Page 3132

A. Rest tremor
B. Kinetic tremor
C. Akinetic tremor
D. Postural tremor

Tremor consists of alternating contractions of agonist & antagonist muscles in an oscillating, rhythmic manner. It can be most prominent at rest (rest tremor), on assuming a posture (postural tremor), on actively reaching for a target (kinetic tremor) or on carrying out a movement (action tremor).

1605. PD is characterized by which of the following tremor?
Harrison's 20th Ed. Chapter 428, Page 3132

A. Rest tremor
B. Kinetic tremor
C. Postural tremor
D. All of the above

1606. Essential tremor (ET) is characterized by which of the following tremor?
Harrison's 20th Ed. Chapter 428, Page 3132

A. Rest tremor
B. Kinetic tremor
C. Postural tremor
D. All of the above

1607. Cerebellar disease is characterized by which of the following tremor?
Harrison's 20th Ed. Chapter 428, Page 3132

A. Rest tremor
B. Kinetic tremor
C. Postural tremor
D. All of the above

PD is characterized by a resting tremor, essential tremor (ET) by a postural tremor, and cerebellar disease by an intention or kinetic tremor associated with hypotonia & past pointing.

1608. Which of the following about physiologic tremor is false?
Harrison's 20th Ed. Chapter 428, Page 3133

A. High-frequency (10 - 12 Hz)
B. Postural or action tremor
C. Affecting the upper extremities
D. None of the above

1609. Enhanced physiologic tremor (EPT) can be seen with the use of?
Harrison's 20th Ed. Chapter 428, Page 3133

A. Valproate
B. Lithium
C. Alcohol
D. All of the above

Enhanced physiologic tremors (EPT) are mild, high-frequency, postural or action tremors usually of no clinical consequence seen in anxiety, fatigue, hyperthyroidism, electrolyte abnormalities, valproate, lithium, smoking, caffeine or alcohol.

1610. Which of the following is the most common movement disorder?
Harrison's 20th Ed. Chapter 428, Page 3133

A. Myoclonus
B. Tic
C. Essential tremor (ET)
D. Dystonia

ET is the most common movement disorder, affecting ~5% of the population.

1611. Which of the following is not a feature of essential tremor?
Harrison's 20th Ed. Chapter 428, Page 3133

A. Bilaterality
B. Frequency of 6 to 10 Hz
C. Postural dependency
D. Aggravation with alcohol

Essential tremor (ET) presentation includes bilaterality, higher frequency (6 to 10 Hz), and postural dependency and significant relief with alcohol.

1612. Which part of body is affected most in essential tremor (ET)?
Harrison's 20th Ed. Chapter 428, Page 3133

A. Arms
B. Head
C. Legs
D. Tongue

Essential tremor (ET) is the most common movement disorder characterized by 6- to 10-Hz postural & kinetic tremor affecting the upper extremities mostly. Tremor involves head in ~30%, voice in ~20%, tongue in ~20%, face/jaw in ~10%, and lower limbs in ~10% of cases. Multiple body parts are involved in ~50% of cases.

1613. Which of the following about ET is false?
Harrison's 20th Ed. Chapter 428, Page 3133

A. Bilateral & symmetric
B. Improved by alcohol & worsened by stress
C. Patients have relatively large handwriting
D. None of the above

1614. All of the following can aggravate essential tremors except?
Harrison's 20th Ed. Chapter 428, Page 3133

A. Valproic acid
B. Tricyclic antidepressants
C. Alcohol
D. Serotonin reuptake blockers

Alcohol consumption reduces ET. Stress and drugs that can aggravate any tremor include valproic acid, lithium, beta-adrenergic agonists, methylxanthines, thyroxin, glucocorticoids, tricyclic antidepressants, and serotonin reuptake blockers.

1615. Drugs that have usefulness in treatment of essential tremors include all except?

Harrison's 20th Ed. Chapter 428, Page 3133

A. Primidone
B. Propranolol
C. Valproic acid
D. Gabapentin

Primidone and propranolol are the first-line treatments for ET. Additional useful medications, with or without the primary agents, include benzodiazepines, gabapentin, topiramate, and botulinum toxin injections to affected muscle groups. Surgical therapies targeting the VIM nucleus of the thalamus can be very effective for severe and drug-resistant cases.

1616. Criteria for Essential Tremor of the International Parkinson and Movement Disorder Society (2017) includes all except?

N Engl J Med. 2018;378:1802-10

A. Bilateral upper-limb action tremor
B. Duration of at least 5 years
C. With or without tremor in head, voice, or lower limbs
D. Absence of other neurologic signs

According to International Parkinson and Movement Disorder Society (2017), criteria for isolated tremor syndrome include bilateral upper-limb action tremor, duration of at least 3 years, with or without tremor in other locations (head, voice, or lower limbs) and absence of other neurologic signs, such as dystonia, ataxia, or parkinsonism.

1617. Criteria for Essential Tremor plus of the International Parkinson and Movement Disorder Society (2017) includes characteristics of essential tremor with?

N Engl J Med. 2018;378:1802-10

A. Impaired tandem gait
B. Questionable dystonic posturing
C. Memory impairment
D. Any of the above

According to International Parkinson and Movement Disorder Society (2017), besides characteristics of essential tremor, criteria for essential tremor plus includes additional neurologic signs of uncertain clinical significance such as impaired tandem gait, questionable dystonic posturing, memory impairment, or other mild neurologic signs that do not suffice to make an additional syndrome classification or diagnosis. Essential tremor with additional tremor at rest should be classified as essential tremor plus.

1618. Association with which of the following gene is found in patients with young-onset ET?

N Engl J Med. 2018;378:1802-10

A. PLOD1 gene
B. LINGO1 gene
C. COL1A1 gene
D. TNXB gene

Association with LINGO1 gene is found in patients with young-onset ET.

1619. Which of the following about LINGO1 protein is false?

N Engl J Med. 2018;378:1802-10

A. Inhibits cell differentiation during development
B. Inhibits axonal regeneration
C. Inhibits synaptic plasticity
D. None of the above

1620. Which of the following is noted in the cerebellum of persons with essential tremor?

N Engl J Med. 2018;378:1802-10

A. Decreased levels of N-acetylaspartate on Magnetic resonance spectroscopy
B. Increased LINGO1 levels
C. γ-aminobutyric acid (GABA) dysfunction
D. All of the above

In ET, cerebellar metabolism is high at rest, increases with arm extension & decreases with administration of ethanol. Cellular bursts in cerebellar receiving zone of thalamus (ventral intermediate nucleus, VIM) correlate strongly with tremor itself.

1621. Which of the following is included in "Essential tremor plus"?

N Engl J Med. 2018;378:1802-10

A. Impaired tandem gait
B. Questionable dystonic posturing
C. Impaired memory
D. Any of the above

In "Essential tremor plus" additional "soft" or mild neurologic signs of uncertain clinical significance like impaired tandem gait, questionable dystonic posturing, or impaired memory are included.

1622. Which of the following is best related to essential tremor?

N Engl J Med. 2018;378:1802-10

A. Killian's triangle
B. Triangle of Koch
C. Guillain–Mollaret triangle
D. Calot triangle

The Guillain–Mollaret triangle comprises of the ipsilateral red nucleus in midbrain, inferior olive in medulla and contralateral dentate nucleus in cerebellum. Together, these form the dentato-rubro-olivary pathway. Pathology in this triangle disinhibits (and so activates) inferior olivary nucleus.

1623. Which of the following about essential tremor is false?

N Engl J Med. 2018;378:1802-10

A. Often familial, with autosomal dominant pattern
B. Related to gene that encodes LINGO1
C. Rhythmic activity in cortico–ponto–cerebello–thalamo–cortical loop
D. None of the above

Pathophysiology of essential tremor almost certainly involves rhythmic activity in the cortico-ponto-cerebello-thalamo-cortical loop.

1624. Swollen axons of Purkinje's cells are called?

N Engl J Med. 2018;378:1802-10

A. Missiles
B. Torpedoes
C. Gun barrels
D. Cannons

Swollen axons of Purkinje's cells seen in pathological studies are called Torpedoes.

1625. Potential tremor-inducing drugs include all except?

N Engl J Med. 2018;378:1802-10

A. Valproate
B. Sympatholytic agents
C. Selective serotonin-reuptake inhibitors
D. Lithium and toxins like mercury, lead, or manganese.

Potential tremor-inducing drugs include valproate, selective serotonin-reuptake inhibitors, sympathomimetic agents, or lithium and toxins like mercury, lead, or manganese.

1626. Differential diagnoses of isolated tremor syndromes without other neurologic signs include?

N Engl J Med. 2018;378:1802-10

A. Enhanced physiologic tremor
B. Isolated focal tremors
C. Orthostatic tremors
D. All of the above

Differential diagnoses of isolated tremor syndromes without other neurologic signs include enhanced physiologic tremor, isolated focal tremors (isolated tremors of head, voice, or palate), and orthostatic tremors.

1627. Tremor syndromes with prominent additional neurologic signs include?

N Engl J Med. 2018;378:1802-10

A. Dystonic tremors
B. Holmes tremor
C. Myorhythmia
D. All of the above

Tremor syndromes with prominent additional neurologic signs include dystonic tremors, tremors combined with parkinsonism, intention tremor syndromes, Holmes tremor (combined low-frequency rest, posture, and intention tremor due to lesions in the cerebellar outflow tract), & myorhythmia.

1628. Which of the following about Holmes tremor is false?

N Engl J Med. 2018;378:1802-10

A. Resting, postural & intention tremor
B. Caused by lesions in brainstem, thalamus and cerebellum
C. Stereotactic thalamotomy & DBS in VIM effective
D. None of the above

1629. Primidone is metabolized to phenobarbital and?

N Engl J Med. 2018;378:1802-10

A. Phenylpropanolamine
B. Phenylhydrazine
C. L-dihydroxyphenylserine
D. Phenylethylmalonamide

Primidone is metabolized to phenylethylmalonamide (PEMA) and phenobarbital.

1630. Rating scale assessment of essential tremor is?

N Engl J Med. 2018;378:1802-10

A. WHIGET scale
B. TETRAS
C. Fahn-Tolosa-Marin scale
D. All of the above

The Essential Tremor Rating Assessment Scale (TETRAS) was developed by the Tremor Research Group to quantify essential tremor severity & its impact on activities of daily living.

1631. Which of the following statements is false about dystonia?

Harrison's 20th Ed. Chapter 428, Page 3133

A. Co-contraction of agonist and antagonist muscles
B. Appear during attempted voluntary movement
C. Exacerbated by stress and fatigue
D. None of the above

Co-contraction of agonist and antagonist muscles is a fundamental feature of dystonia and characteristically present during attempted voluntary movement. Dystonia is exacerbated by stress and fatigue and attenuated by sensory inputs [touching affected body part or sensory trick (geste antagoniste)]. The geste antagoniste sign is a legacy of Paris Neurological School. The term was introduced by Meige & Feindel in their 1902 book on tics while mentioning Brissaud, who first described this sign in 1893.

1632. Most of the genetic forms of dystonia belong to which phenotypic group?

Harrison's 20th Ed. Chapter 428, Page 3133

A. Isolated dystonia
B. Combined dystonia
C. Complex dystonia
D. Any of the above

When dystonia is the only disease manifestation with the exception of tremor, its grouped in "isolated dystonia". When dystonia co-occurs with another movement disorder like parkinsonism or myoclonus, its grouped in "combined dystonia" and when dystonia is only one of several clinical manifestations and may be a less prominent or even inconsistent feature, it is in the "complex dystonia" phenotypic group.

1633. Which of the following is a clinical phenotype of focal dystonia?

Harrison's 20th Ed. Chapter 428, Page 3134

A. Spasmodic dysphonia
B. Blepharospasm
C. Oromandibular dystonia (OMD)
D. All of the above

Focal dystonia can be focal, multifocal or segmental. The major clinical phenotypes of focal dystonia are cervical dystonia, blepharospasm, oromandibular dystonia (OMD), spasmodic dysphonia and limb dystonia.

1634. Which of the following is a combination of oromandibular dystonia (OMD) and blepharospasm?

Harrison's 20th Ed. Chapter 428, Page 3134

A. Dopa responsive dystonia (DRD)
B. Idiopathic torsion dystonia (ITD)
C. Meige's syndrome
D. Lubag form of dystonia-parkinsonism

1635. Which of the following best relates to Meige's syndrome?

Harrison's 20th Ed. Chapter 428, Page 3134

A. Cervical dystonia
B. Limb dystonia
C. Oromandibular dystonia (OMD)
D. Spasmodic dysphonia

Meige's syndrome is a combination of OMD and blepharospasm that predominantly affects women aged >60 years.

1636. Which of the following is a focal dystonia?

Harrison's 20th Ed. Chapter 428, Page 3134

A. Blepharospasm
B. Torticollis
C. Laterocollis
D. All of the above

Most common forms of dystonia are in adults - blepharospasm, cervical dystonias (torticollis, laterocollis, anterocollis, retrocollis), oromandibular dystonia, spasmodic dysphonia.

1637. Which of the following is the least common dystonia?

Harrison's 20th Ed. Chapter 428, Page 3134

A. Cervical dystonia
B. Oromandibular dystonia (OMD)
C. Blepharospasm
D. Spasmodic dysphonia

Frequency of focal dystonias is cervical dystonia (~50%), blepharospasm (~20%), Focal hand or leg dystonia (~5%), spasmodic dysphonia (~2%), musician's dystonia (~3%), or OMD (~1%).

1638. Which of the following is a gene for isolated dystonia?

Harrison's 20th Ed. Chapter 428, Page 3134

A. TOR1A
B. THAP1
C. ANO3
D. All of the above

Well established genes for isolated dystonia are TOR1A, THAP1, ANO3, GNAL and KMT2B.

1639. Which of the following is called Dopa-responsive dystonia (DRD)?

Harrison's 20th Ed. Chapter 428, Page 3134

A. Boerhaave syndrome
B. Segawa syndrome
C. Reye's syndrome
D. Sweet syndrome

Dopa-responsive dystonia (DRD is also called Segawa syndrome).

1640. Segawa syndrome is caused by mutations in which of the following gene?

Harrison's 20th Ed. Chapter 428, Page 3134

A. TAF1 gene
B. ATP1A3 gene
C. SGCE gene
D. GCH1 gene

Segawa syndrome is caused by mutations in GCH1 gene (GTP cyclohydrolase-1) that encodes for the rate-limiting enzyme in biosynthesis of dopamine via the biopterin pathway without nigral cell loss.

1641. Any patient suspected of having a childhood-onset dystonia should receive a trial of?

Harrison's 20th Ed. Chapter 428, Page 3134

A. Valproate
B. Lithium
C. Levodopa
D. Serotonin reuptake blockers

Any patient suspected of having a childhood-onset dystonia should receive a trial of levodopa to exclude Dopa responsive dystonia (DRD) or the Segawa variant (DYT5).

1642. Dystonia frequently accompanied by psychiatric disturbances goes in favour of?

Harrison's 20th Ed. Chapter 428, Page 3134

A. Idiopathic torsion dystonia (ITD)
B. Myoclonic dystonia
C. X-linked dystonia-parkinsonism (Lubag)
D. Dopa responsive dystonia (DRD)

Myoclonic dystonia results from mutations in SGCE gene (sarcoglycan epsilon) which codes for the ε member of sarcoglycan family. It typically manifests as a combination of dystonia and action-induced, alcohol-responsive myoclonic jerks predominantly involving the upper body half, frequently accompanied by psychiatric disturbances such as depression, anxiety-related disorders, and alcohol dependence.

1643. Which of the following is an X-linked recessive dystonia parkinsonism?

Harrison's 20th Ed. Chapter 428, Page 3134

A. Huntington's disease
B. X-linked dystonia-parkinsonism (Lubag)
C. Leigh's disease
D. All of the above

X-linked dystonia-parkinsonism (Lubag) affects Filipino men originating principally from the Panay Island. Retrotransposon insertion in TAF1 (TATA-Box Binding Protein Associated Factor 1) gene is the most likely cause of disease.

1644. Which of the following is a complex dystonia?

Harrison's 20th Ed. Chapter 428, Page 3134

A. Wilson's disease (WD)
B. Huntington's disease (HD)
C. Lesh Nyhan syndrome
D. All of the above

In complex dystonias, dystonia is one part (usually non-dominant neurologic feature) of a syndrome with multiple different manifestations. Wilson's disease (WD), Huntington's disease (HD) & Lesh Nyhan syndrome belong to complex dystonias.

1645. Most effective treatment for generalized primary dystonia is?

Harrison's 20th Ed. Chapter 428, Page 3135

A. Primidone
B. Propranolol
C. Valproic acid
D. Anticholinergic drugs

Anticholinergic drugs are the most effective forms of treatment for generalized primary dystonia.

1646. Dystonic storm can occur in response to?

Harrison's 20th Ed. Chapter 428, Page 3136

A. Anticholinergic drug overdose
B. Inadequate anticholinergic drug dose
C. Stress situation
D. All of the above

1647. George Huntington belonged to which country?

Harrison's 20th Ed. Chapter 428, Page 3136

A. Great Britain
B. America
C. Australia
D. Canada

Huntington's disease (HD) was described by George Huntington, an American physician in 1872. Huntington's gene is single, causal gene and an accurate genetic test for HD is available.

1648. Which of the following is most characteristic feature of HD?

Harrison's 20th Ed. Chapter 428, Page 3136

A. Gait disturbance
B. Chorea
C. Oculomotor abnormalities
D. Myoclonus

HD is characterized by rapid, nonpatterned, semi-purposeful, involuntary choreiform movements. Dysarthria, gait disturbance, and oculomotor abnormalities are common features. As disease progresses, chorea is reduced & dystonia, rigidity, bradykinesia, myoclonus, and spasticity emerge.

1649. Westphal variant of Huntington's disease (HD) relates to which of the following?

Harrison's 20th Ed. Chapter 428, Page 3136

A. Alzheimer's disease
B. Parkinsonian syndrome
C. Orthostatic hypotension
D. Dementia

HD can present as an akinetic-rigid or parkinsonian syndrome (Westphal variant).

1650. Which of the following is a typical MRI finding in Huntington's Disease (HD)?

Harrison's 20th Ed. Chapter 428, Page 3136

A. Atrophy of the thalamus
B. Progressive atrophy of head of the caudate nucleus
C. Iron accumulation in striatum
D. Atrophy of the midbrain

HD predominantly strikes striatum. Progressive atrophy of head of the caudate nucleus and consequent enlargement of lateral ventricles is seen in MRI. Putamen can be equally or even more severely affected.

1651. Huntington's disease (HD) is caused by mutations in the Huntington's gene on the?

Harrison's 20th Ed. Chapter 428, Page 3137

A. Short arm of chromosome 4
B. Long arm of chromosome 4
C. Short arm of chromosome 5
D. Long arm of chromosome 5

HD is caused by mutations in the Huntington's gene on the short arm of chromosome 4. Alleles from normal individuals have between 12 and 37 CAG repeats. HD is caused by an increase in the number of polyglutamine (CAG) repeats (>40) in the coding sequence of the huntingtin gene. The larger the number of repeats, the earlier the disease is manifest.

1652. Phenomenon referred to as 'anticipation' is relevant to which of the following?

Harrison's 20th Ed. Chapter 428, Page 3137

A. Huntington's disease (HD)
B. Wilson's disease
C. Tourette's syndrome (TS)
D. Restless legs syndrome

In Huntington's disease, acceleration of disease process occur, particularly in males, with subsequent generations having larger numbers of repeats & earlier age of disease onset, a phenomenon referred to as anticipation.

1653. Which of the following about huntingtin is false?

Harrison's 20th Ed. Chapter 428, Page 3137

A. Cytoplasmic protein
B. Widely distributed in neurons
C. Function is not known
D. None of the above

1654. Which of the following drug is useful in the treatment of Huntington's disease?

Harrison's 20th Ed. Chapter 428, Page 3137

A. Levodopa
B. Trihexyphenidyl
C. Tetrabenazine
D. All of the above

Tetrabenazine is a presynaptic dopamine depleting agent & is approved for the treatment of chorea.

1655. Which of the following HD-like (HDL) disorders is an autosomal dominant condition?

Harrison's 20th Ed. Chapter 428, Page 3137

A. HDL-1
B. HDL-2
C. HDL-4
D. All of the above

HD-like (HDL) disorders 1, 2 and 4 are inherited autosomal dominant conditions that typically present in adulthood and closely mimic HD.

1656. Which of the following is a prion disease?

Harrison's 20th Ed. Chapter 428, Page 3137

A. HD-like (HDL) disorders 1
B. α-Synuclein Parkinson's disease (PD)
C. Creutzfeldt-Jakob disease (CJD)
D. All of the above

1657. Which of the following HD-like (HDL) disorders 1 is related to PRNP gene?

Harrison's 20th Ed. Chapter 428, Page 3137

A. HDL-1
B. HDL-2
C. HDL-4
D. All of the above

HDL-1, a prion disease, is due to expansion of an octapeptide repeat in PRNP, the gene encoding the prion protein. Patients exhibit personality change in third or fourth decade, followed by chorea, rigidity, myoclonus, ataxia & epilepsy.

1658. Which of the following HD-like (HDL) disorders 1 is related to acanthocytosis?

Harrison's 20th Ed. Chapter 428, Page 3137

A. HDL-1
B. HDL-2
C. HDL-4
D. All of the above

HDL-2 manifests in the third or fourth decade with chorea, dystonia or parkinsonism and dementia and acanthocytosis.

1659. Which of the following HD-like (HDL) disorders 1 is related to junctophilin-3 (JPH3) gene?

Harrison's 20th Ed. Chapter 428, Page 3137

A. HDL-1
B. HDL-2
C. HDL-4
D. All of the above

HDL-2 is caused by an abnormally expanded CTG/CAG trinucleotide repeat expansion in the junctophilin-3 (JPH3) gene.

1660. Which of the following HD-like (HDL) disorders is related to TBP gene?

Harrison's 20th Ed. Chapter 428, Page 3137

A. HDL-1
B. HDL-2
C. HDL-4
D. All of the above

HDL-4, the most common HDL, is caused by expansion of trinucleotide repeats in TBP, the gene that encodes the TATA box binding protein involved in regulating transcription.

1661. Which of the following HD-like (HDL) disorders 1 is identical to spinocerebellar ataxia (SCA) 17?

Harrison's 20th Ed. Chapter 428, Page 3137

A. HDL-1
B. HDL-2
C. HDL-4
D. All of the above

HDL-4 is identical to spinocerebellar ataxia (SCA) 17 and most patients present primarily with ataxia rather than chorea.

1662. Mutations in which of the following gene causes Chorea-acanthocytosis (neuroacanthocytosis)?

Harrison's 20th Ed. Chapter 428, Page 3137

A. TCF7L2
B. PRC1
C. VPS13C
D. VPS13A

Chorea-acanthocytosis (neuroacanthocytosis) is a progressive and fatal autosomal recessive disorder characterized by chorea with red cell abnormalities on peripheral blood smear (acanthocytes). Chorea can be severe with self mutilating behavior, dystonia, tics, seizures and polyneuropathy. Mutations in VPS13A gene encoding chorein is documented.

1663. Sydenham's choreas responds to which of the following?

Harrison's 20th Ed. Chapter 428, Page 3137

A. Dopamine-blocking agents
B. Valproic acid
C. Carbamazepine
D. All of the above

Sydenham's chorea (St. Vitus' dance) is of acute onset and responds to dopamine-blocking agents, valproic acid, and carbamazepine. Chorea may recur in later life, particularly in association with pregnancy (chorea gravidarum) or treatment with sex hormones.

1664. Chorea may be associated with which of the following?

Harrison's 20th Ed. Chapter 428, Page 3137

A. Cryptococcal encephalitis
B. Progressive rubella panencephalitis
C. Herpes simplex virus encephalitis
D. Limbic encephalitis

Chorea may be associated with NMDA receptor antibody-positive encephalitis following herpes simplex virus encephalitis.

1665. Most common systemic disorder that causes chorea is?

Harrison's 20th Ed. Chapter 428, Page 3137

A. Hyperthyroidism
B. HIV disease
C. Systemic lupus erythematosus (SLE)
D. Polycythemia rubra vera

Systemic lupus erythematosus is the most common systemic disorder that causes chorea. Choreas can also be seen with hyperthyroidism, Sjögren's syndrome, HIV disease, metabolic alterations, polycythemia rubra vera, with many medications (anticonvulsants, cocaine, CNS stimulants, estrogens, lithium) and paraneoplastic syndromes associated with anti-CRMP-5 or anti-Hu antibodies.

1666. Which of the following is X-linked disorder?

Harrison's 20th Ed. Chapter 456, Page 3361

A. Rett's syndrome
B. Danon's disease
C. Hunter disease (MPS II)
D. All of the above

1667. Which of the following is X-linked disorder?

Harrison's 20th Ed. Chapter 456, Page 3361

A. Fabry disease
B. Alport's syndrome
C. Ehlers-Danlos syndrome Type V
D. All of the above

1668. Which of the following is X-linked disorder?

Harrison's 20th Ed. Chapter 456, Page 3361

A. Dent's disease
B. IPEX syndrome
C. Wiskott-Aldrich syndrome (WAS)
D. All of the above

1669. Which of the following is X-linked disorder?

Harrison's 20th Ed. Chapter 428, Page 3361

A. Adrenomyeloneuropathy
B. Kennedy's syndrome
C. McLeod syndrome
D. All of the above

1670. Disorder having excess brain iron accumulation on MRI is?

Harrison's 20th Ed. Chapter 428, Page 3141

A. Autosomal dominant neuroferritinopathy
B. Hallervorden-Spatz disease
C. Neuroacanthocytosis
D. Aceruloplasminemia

Neurodegenerative diseases with brain iron accumulation (NBIA) manifesting with chorea include autosomal dominant neuroferritinopathy, autosomal recessive pantothenate-kinase-associated neurodegeneration (PKAN; Hallervorden-Spatz disease), and aceruloplasminemia. Iron accumulation in globus pallidus provides on MRI the characteristic "eye of the tiger" appearance.

1671. Which of the following best relates to hemiballismus?

Harrison's 20th Ed. Chapter 428, Page 3138

A. Chorea
B. Athetosis
C. Choreoathetosis
D. Any of the above

Hemiballismus is a violent form of chorea composed of wild, flinging, large-amplitude movements of proximal limb muscles on one side of the body.

1672. Which of the following is a violent form of chorea?

Harrison's 20th Ed. Chapter 428, Page 3138

A. Hemiballismus
B. Monoballism
C. Paraballism
D. All of the above

In hemiballismus proximal limb muscles are predominantly affected. These movements may affect just one limb (monoballism) or, more exceptionally, both upper or lower limbs (paraballism).

1673. In hemiballismus, most often the lesion is in?

Harrison's 20th Ed. Chapter 428, Page 3138

A. Globus pallidus
B. Cerebellum
C. Subthalamic nucleus
D. Pedunculopontine nucleus

Most common cause of hemiballismus is a lesion (infarct or hemorrhage) of subthalamic nucleus (STN), but cases can also be seen with lesions in the putamen, thalamus and parietal cortex.

1674. Phonic (or vocal) tic with expression of obscene words is called?

Harrison's 20th Ed. Chapter 428, Page 3138

A. Grunting
B. Echolalia
C. Palilalia
D. Coprolalia

1675. Which of the following is a kind of vocal tic?
Harrison's 20th Ed. Chapter 428, Page 3138

A. Echolalia
B. Palilalia
C. Coprolalia
D. All of the above

Vocal tics include grunting, echolalia (repeating other people's words), palilalia (repeating one's own words), and coprolalia (expression of obscene words).

1676. Tics may present in adulthood with?
Harrison's 20th Ed. Chapter 428, Page 3138

A. PD
B. HD
C. Levodopa therapy
D. All of the above

Tics may present in adulthood and can also be seen with PD, HD, trauma, dystonia, drugs (levodopa, neuroleptics) and toxins.

1677. Which of the following is a neurobehavioral disorder?
Harrison's 20th Ed. Chapter 428, Page 3138

A. Essential tremor (ET)
B. Wilson's disease
C. Huntington's disease (HD)
D. Tourette's syndrome (TS)

Tourette's syndrome (TS) is a neurobehavioral disorder named after French neurologist Georges Gilles de la Tourette.

1678. Associated behavioral disturbance with Tourette's syndrome (TS) include?
Harrison's 20th Ed. Chapter 428, Page 3138

A. Anxiety, depression
B. Attention deficit hyperactivity disorder
C. Obsessive-compulsive disorder
D. All of the above

Associated behavioral disturbances with Tourette's syndrome (TS) include anxiety, depression, attention deficit hyperactivity disorder, and obsessive-compulsive disorder.

1679. Which of the following gene is implicated in Tourette's syndrome?
Harrison's 20th Ed. Chapter 428, Page 3138

A. VPS13A
B. BHC2
C. C9Orf
D. None of the above

TS is considered as a genetic disorder, but no specific gene mutation has been identified. The risk of a family with one affected child having a second is about 25%.

1680. PANDAS is best related to?
Harrison's 20th Ed. Chapter 428, Page 3138

A. Trauma
B. β-hemolytic streptococcal infection
C. Obsessive-compulsive disorder
D. Levodopa

PANDAS refers to pediatric autoimmune neuropsychiatric disorder associated with streptococcal infection.

1681. Effective medication in treatment of Tourette's syndrome is?
Harrison's 20th Ed. Chapter 428, Page 3138

A. Clonidine
B. Guanfacine
C. Olanzapine
D. All of the above

Clonidine, Guanfacine, Atypical neuroleptics (risperidone, olanzapine, ziprasidone) and classical neuroleptics (haloperidol, fluphenazine, or pimozide) are useful in treatment of TS.

1682. Which of the following about myoclonus is false?
Harrison's 20th Ed. Chapter 428, Page 3138

A. Rapid, jerky movement of <100 msec duration
B. Asterixis is a negative myoclonus
C. Interferes with normal movement
D. Suppressible

Myoclonus is a rapid, jerky movement of <100 msec. duration due to single or repetitive muscle discharges. It occur spontaneously, in association with voluntary movement (action myoclonus) or in response to an external stimulus (reflex or startle myoclonus).

1683. Myoclonic jerks can be?
Harrison's 20th Ed. Chapter 428, Page 3138

A. Focal
B. Multifocal
C. Generalized
D. Any of the above

Myoclonic jerks can be focal, multifocal, segmental or generalized and can occur spontaneously, in association with voluntary movement (action myoclonus) or in response to an external stimulus (reflex or startle myoclonus).

1684. Which of the following is an example of negative myoclonus?
Harrison's 20th Ed. Chapter 428, Page 3138

A. Tic
B. Dystonia
C. Asterixis
D. Hypnagogic jerks

Negative myoclonus consists of a brief loss of muscle activity (asterixis in hepatic failure). Myoclonic jerks differ from tics in that they interfere with normal movement and are not suppressible.

1685. Myoclonus can be seen in association with pathology in?
Harrison's 20th Ed. Chapter 428, Page 3138

A. Cortical region
B. Subcortical region
C. Spinal cord region
D. All of the above

Myoclonus can be seen in association with pathology in cortical, subcortical, brainstem or spinal cord regions and associated with hypoxemic damage, encephalopathy, and neurodegeneration.

1686. Reversible myoclonus can be seen with which of the following?
Harrison's 20th Ed. Chapter 428, Page 3138

A. Renal failure
B. Electrolyte imbalance
C. Hypocalcemia
D. All of the above

Reversible myoclonus can be seen with metabolic disturbances (renal failure, electrolyte imbalance, hypocalcemia), toxins and many medications.

1687. Which of the following is false about essential myoclonus?
Harrison's 20th Ed. Chapter 428, Page 3138

A. Focal
B. Very brief lightning-like movements
C. Alcohol sensitive
D. Benign familial condition

Essential myoclonus is a relatively benign familial condition characterized by multifocal, very brief, lightning-like movements that are frequently alcohol sensitive.

1688. Which of the following is useful in the treatment of myoclonus?
Harrison's 20th Ed. Chapter 428, Page 3139

A. Valproic acid
B. Piracetam
C. Levetiracetam
D. All of the above

Treatment primarily consists of treating the underlying condition or removing offending agent. Valproic acid, piracetam, clonazepam, primidone and levetiracetam may be effective.

1689. Which of the following is an example of Dystonia?
Harrison's 20th Ed. Chapter 428, Page 3139

A. Blepharospasm
B. Torticollis
C. Oromandibular dystonia
D. All of the above

Dystonia is the most common acute hyperkinetic drug reaction. It is typically generalized in children and focal in adults like blepharospasm, torticollis, or oromandibular dystonia.

1690. Which of the following about tardive dyskinesia (TD) is false?
Harrison's 20th Ed. Chapter 428, Page 3139

A. Choreiform movements
B. Mouth, lips, and tongue mostly involved
C. Valbenazine helpful in refractory cases
D. None of the above

Valbenazine is an ester of tetrabenazine useful in the treatment of tardive dyskinesia. It acts as a vesicular monoamine transporter type 2 (VMAT-2) inhibitor & blocks storage of dopamine.

1691. Use of metoclopramide for more than how many weeks increases the risk of tardive dyskinesia (TD)?
Harrison's 20th Ed. Chapter 428, Page 3139

A. 2 weeks
B. 4 weeks
C. 6 weeks
D. 12 weeks

FDA has warned that use of metoclopramide for more than 12 weeks increases the risk of TD.

1692. Which of the following may occur after chronic neuroleptic exposure?
Harrison's 20th Ed. Chapter 428, Page 3139

A. Tardive akathisia
B. Tardive TS
C. Tardive tremor syndrome
D. All of the above

1693. Levels of which of the following is markedly elevated in neuroleptic malignant syndrome (NMS)?
Harrison's 20th Ed. Chapter 428, Page 3139

A. Creatine kinase
B. Lactic dehydrogenase
C. Lactic acid
D. All of the above

Neuroleptic malignant syndrome (NMS) is characterized by muscle rigidity, elevated temperature, altered mental status, hyperthermia, tachycardia, labile blood pressure, renal failure, and markedly elevated creatine kinase levels. Myoclonus is not a feature of NMS but of serotonin syndrome.

1694. Myoclonus can result with the use of which of the following drugs?
Harrison's 20th Ed. Chapter 428, Page 3139

A. Phenytoin
B. Fluoxetine
C. Buspirone
D. All of the above

Drugs can be associated with parkinsonism & hyperkinetic movement disorders like phenytoin (chorea, dystonia, tremor, myoclonus), carbamazepine (tics and dystonia), tricyclic antidepressants (dyskinesias, tremor, myoclonus), fluoxetine (myoclonus, chorea, dystonia), oral contraceptives (dyskinesia), adrenergics (tremor), buspirone (akathisia, dyskinesias, myoclonus), and digoxin, cimetidine, diazoxide, lithium, methadone, and fentanyl (dyskinesias).

1695. Which of the following is a paroxysmal dyskinesia?
Harrison's 20th Ed. Chapter 428, Page 3140

A. Paroxysmal kinesigenic dyskinesia (PKD)
B. Paroxysmal nonkinesigenic dyskinesias (PNKD)
C. Paroxysmal exertion-induced dyskinesia (PED)
D. All of the above

1696. Which of the following gene is associated with paroxysmal PED?
Harrison's 20th Ed. Chapter 428, Page 3140

A. SLC2A1
B. SLC2A2
C. SLC2A3
D. SLC2A4

1697. Restless Legs Syndrome was first described by?
Harrison's 20th Ed. Chapter 428, Page 3140

A. Christopher Ross
B. Micheal Emre
C. Thomas Willis
D. James Hardy

Restless legs syndrome (RLS) is a neurologic disorder and was first described in seventeenth century by English physician Thomas Willis.

1698. The restless legs syndrome (RLS) is also known as?
N Engl J Med. 2003;348:2103-9

A. Earley's syndrome
B. Hening's syndrome
C. Wetter's syndrome
D. Ekbom's syndrome

The restless legs syndrome (RLS) is also known as Ekbom's syndrome (Ekbom KA. Restless legs syndrome. Acta Med. Scand 1945;158(suppl):1–123).

1699. Which of the following is not a core symptom required for diagnosis of RLS?

Harrison's 20th Ed. Chapter 428, Page 3140

A. Urge to move the legs
B. Symptoms begin or worsen with rest
C. Partial or complete relief by movement
D. Worsening during daytime

According to International RLS Study Group (1995), the four core symptoms required for diagnosis of RLS are an urge to move the legs, symptoms begin or worsen with rest, partial or complete relief by movement and worsening during the evening or night. Paresthesias secondary to peripheral neuropathy persist with activity.

1700. Which of the following is false about periodic leg movements (PLMs) associated with RLS?

Harrison's 20th Ed. Chapter 428, Page 3140, N Engl J Med. 2003;348:2103-9

A. Occur during sleep
B. Brief involuntary movements
C. Recur every 5–90 seconds
D. None of the above

RLS is usually associated with semirhythmic leg movements during sleep that are referred to as periodic limb movements of sleep.

1701. Periodic leg movements can be observed in which of the following conditions?

N Engl J Med. 2003;348:2103-9

A. Sleep apnea
B. Spinal cord lesions
C. Stroke
D. All of the above

Periodic leg movements that are apparent on polysomnography. Apart from RLS, they are observed in sleep apnea, neurodegenerative diseases, spinal cord lesions, stroke, narcolepsy, and with treatment with antidepressant or neuroleptic agents.

1702. Which of the following description best relate to RLS?

BMJ 2012;344:e3056

A. Tearing of the skin
B. Legs immersed in ice cold water
C. Insects crawling under the skin
D. Tight rope around the legs

Urge to move legs is typical of RLS accompanied by abnormal sensations described as burning, tingling, aching, or "insects crawling under the skin".

1703. Which of the following description best relate to RLS?

N Engl J Med. 2003;348:2103-9

A. "Creepy-crawly" sensation
B. "Like ants marching in my legs"
C. "Like soda water in the veins"
D. All of the above

The sensation in RLS may be described as a muscle ache or tension. Other patients describe a "creepy-crawly" sensation or a feeling "like ants marching in my legs" or "like soda water in the veins."

1704. Which of the following about primary restless legs syndrome is false?

Harrison's 20th Ed. Chapter 428, Page 3140

A. Genetic with autosomal dominant pattern of inheritance
B. Mean age of onset is 27 years
C. Neurologic examination is normal
D. None of the above

1705. Which of the following about restless legs syndrome is false?

BMJ 2012;344:e3056

A. More prevalent in women than in men
B. Prevalence increases with age
C. Most common movement disorder in pregnancy
D. None of the above

1706. Secondary RLS may be associated with?

Harrison's 20th Ed. Chapter 428, Page 3140

A. Pregnancy
B. Peripheral neuropathy
C. Renal failure
D. All of the above

Secondary RLS may be associated with pregnancy, anemia, ferritin deficiency, renal failure, and peripheral neuropathy.

1707. Factor that may exacerbate RLS symptoms is?

Cleveland Clinic Journal of Medicine. 2005;72 (9):773

A. Cold & heat
B. Fatigue
C. Stress
D. All of the above

Factors other than immobility that may exacerbate RLS include cold, heat, fatigue & stress.

1708. Secondary RLS may be associated with?

Harrison's 20th Ed. Chapter 428, Page 3140, BMJ 2012;344:e3056

A. Ferritin deficiency
B. Renal failure
C. Peripheral neuropathy
D. All of the above

Secondary RLS may be associated with pregnancy, anemia, ferritin deficiency, renal failure, and peripheral neuropathy. Restless legs syndrome may also be associated with cardiovascular disease, obesity, diabetes, rheumatological disorders, radiculopathy, Parkinson's disease, multiple sclerosis, Charcot-Marie-Tooth disease, and spinal cord lesions.

1709. RLS has been reported to occur with which of the following?

N Engl J Med. 2003;348:2103-9

A. During pregnancy
B. In patients undergoing dialysis
C. Iron deficiency
D. All of the above

1710. Restless legs syndrome (RLS) is related to which of the following?

Harrison's 20th Ed. Chapter 428, Page 3140

A. Iron metabolism
B. Copper metabolism
C. Zinc metabolism
D. Magnesium metabolism

Pathogenesis of RLS probably involves disordered dopamine function (peripheral or central), in association with an abnormality of iron metabolism. Low serum ferritin (<50 µg/L) favours its diagnosis. Serum ferritin correlates inversely with symptom severity. Iron is an essential cofactor for tyrosine hydroxylase and seems to have a crucial role in dopamine metabolism.

1711. Severity of RLS can be exacerbated by?

BMJ 2012;344:e3056

A. Dopamine agonists
B. Serotonergic antidepressants
C. Anticonvulsants
D. Opiates

RLS is characterised by upregulation of dopaminergic transmission, with postsynaptic desensitisation. Dopamine agonists (pramipexole, ropinirole & rotigotine), Levodopa, anticonvulsants, analgesics, gabapentin and opiates can be effective in RLS. Symptoms can be exacerbated by sleep deprivation, caffeine, alcohol, serotonergic antidepressants (selective serotonin reuptake inhibitors and serotonin noradrenaline reuptake inhibitors), and pregnancy.

1712. Treatment of choice for RLS is with?

Harrison's 20th Ed. Chapter 428, Page 3140

A. Opioids
B. Benzodiazepines
C. Pramipexole
D. Gabapentin

Symptoms of RLS are exquisitely sensitive to dopaminergic drugs (pramipexole or ropinirole), which are the treatments of choice. Opioids, benzodiazepines, and gabapentin may also be of therapeutic value.

1713. Vesper's curse best relates to?

Cleveland Clinic Journal of Medicine. 2005;72 (9):773

A. Congestive heart failure + Lumbar spinal stenosis
B. Congestive heart failure + OSA
C. Congestive heart failure + Parkinsonism
D. Congestive heart failure + Blindness

Vesper's curse refers to lumbosacral and associated leg pain and paresthesias arousing patients from a sound sleep occurring in patients with congestive heart failure in association with lumbar spinal stenosis. An increase in right atrial filling pressure reflected in elevated paraspinal venous volumes within the reduced confines of a stenotic lumbar spine is believed to be the precipitating cause of this syndrome.

1714. Polymorphism in which of the following genes has been linked to RLS?

Harrison's 20th Ed. Chapter 428, Page 174

A. BTBD9
B. MEIS1
C. PTPRD
D. All of the above

Polymorphisms in BTBD9, MEIS1, MAP2K5/LBXCOR and PTPRD genes have been linked to RLS.

1715. Which of the following conditions may have a common pathophysiology as of RLS?

Harrison's 20th Ed. Chapter 428, Page 174

A. Somnambulism
B. Sleep enuresis
C. Periodic limb movement disorder (PLMD)
D. REM sleep behavior disorder (RBD)

Most patients with restless legs also experience PLMD, although the reverse is not the case.

1716. Wilson's disease is caused by mutations in?

Harrison's 20th Ed. Chapter 428, Page 3140

A. ATP5B gene
B. ATP6B gene
C. ATP7B gene
D. ATP8B gene

Wilson's disease is caused by mutations in the ATP7B gene encoding a P-type ATPase.

1717. What was the first name of Wilson who described Wilson's disease?

Harrison's 20th Ed. Chapter 428, Page 3140

A. Camelo
B. Hebert
C. Charles
D. Kinnier

Wilson's disease was first described by English neurologist Kinnier Wilson at the beginning of twentieth century. At around the same time, German physicians Kayser & Fleischer separately noted the characteristic association of corneal pigmentation with hepatic and neurologic features.

1718. Which of the following in Wilson's disease can manifest alone?

Harrison's 20th Ed. Chapter 428, Page 3140

A. Neurologic disorders
B. Psychiatric disorders
C. Liver disorders
D. Any of the above

Wilson's disease (WD) is an autosomal recessive inherited disorder of copper metabolism that may manifest with neurologic, psychiatric, and liver disorders, alone or in combination. About half of WD patients (esp. younger patients) manifest with liver abnormalities.

1719. Which of the following marks the onset of neurologic manifestations in WD?

Harrison's 20th Ed. Chapter 428, Page 3140

A. Bradykinesia
B. Tremor
C. Dystonia
D. Dysarthria

Neurologic onset usually manifests in the second decade with tremor and rigidity. Tremor is usually in upper limbs, bilateral, and asymmetric.

1720. Kayser-Fleischer (KF) rings are seen in nearly what proportion of WD patients with hepatic presentations?

Harrison's 20th Ed. Chapter 428, Page 3140

A. 20%
B. 40%
C. 80%
D. 100%

Kayser-Fleischer (KF) rings are seen in 80% of WD patients with hepatic presentations.

1721. Kayser-Fleischer (KF) rings are seen in nearly what proportion of WD patients with neurologic features?

Harrison's 20th Ed. Chapter 428, Page 3140

A. 20%
B. 40%
C. 80%
D. 100%

Kayser-Fleischer (KF) rings are seen in nearly all WD patients with neurologic features. It is very rare for WD patients with neurologic features not to have KF rings.

1722. Which of the following statements about Kayser-Fleischer (KF) rings is false?

Harrison's 20th Ed. Chapter 428, Page 3140

A. Represent deposition of copper in Descemet's membrane
B. Grayish discoloration of the peripheral cornea
C. Best detected by slit-lamp examination
D. None of the above

Kayser-Fleischer rings (KF rings) represent the deposition of copper in Descemet's membrane producing grayish discoloration of peripheral cornea. They are best detected by slit-lamp examination.

1723. The neuropathologic lesion in WD is in?
Harrison's 20th Ed. Chapter 428, Page 3140

A. Substantia nigra
B. Striatum
C. Globus pallidus
D. Thalamus

Neuropathologic examination is characterized by neurodegeneration and astrogliosis in the basal ganglia, particularly in the striatum.

1724. In WD, which of the following is false?
Harrison's 20th Ed. Chapter 428, Page 3141

A. Low levels of blood copper
B. Low levels of blood ceruloplasmin
C. High levels of urinary copper
D. None of the above

In WD, low levels of blood copper and ceruloplasmin and high levels of urinary copper are found but normal levels do not exclude the diagnosis.

1725. In WD, MRI shows symmetric hyperintensity on T2-weighted images in?
Harrison's 20th Ed. Chapter 428, Page 3141

A. Putamen
B. Caudate
C. Globus pallidus
D. All of the above

In WD, MRI shows symmetric hyperintensity on T2-weighted images in putamen, caudate & pallidum.

1726. Which of the following is the gold standard for the diagnosis of WD?
Harrison's 20th Ed. Chapter 428, Page 3141

A. Kayser-Fleischer (KF) rings
B. Generalized atrophy on CT brain scan
C. Hyperintensity of putamen on T2-weighted MRI images
D. High copper levels in liver biopsy

Liver biopsy with demonstration of high copper levels is the gold standard for diagnosis of WD.

1727. Which of the following blocks the absorption of copper?
Harrison's 20th Ed. Chapter 428, Page 3141

A. Penicillamine
B. Tetrathiomolybdate
C. Trientine
D. Zinc

Tetrathiomolybdate blocks absorption of copper. Penicillamine increases copper excretion. Trientine & zinc are useful drugs for maintenance therapy.

1728. Which of the following statements about Penicillamine is false?
Harrison's 20th Ed. Chapter 428, Page 3141

A. Worsens symptoms in initial stages of therapy
B. Increases copper excretion
C. Should be coadministered with pyridoxine
D. None of the above

1729. What time after therapy, KF rings may disappear?
Harrison's 20th Ed. Chapter 428, Page 3141

A. 6 months
B. 1 year
C. 2 years
D. Never disappear

KF rings tend to decrease after 3–6 months of therapy and disappear by 2 years.

1730. In neurodegeneration with brain iron accumulation (NBIA), the iron accumulates in?
Harrison's 20th Ed. Chapter 428, Page 3141

A. Pineal gland
B. Basal ganglia
C. Corpus callosum
D. Cerebral cortex

Neurodegeneration with brain iron accumulation (NBIA) represents a group of inherited disorders characterized by iron accumulation in the basal ganglia.

1731. NBIA can manifest as which of the following?
Harrison's 20th Ed. Chapter 428, Page 3141

A. Parkinsonism
B. Neuropsychiatric abnormalities
C. Retinal degeneration
D. Any of the above

NBIA can manifest as a progressive neurologic disorder that may manifest as parkinsonism, dystonia, neuropsychiatric abnormalities, retinal degeneration, cognitive disorders and cerebellar dysfunction.

1732. Most common form of NBIA is?
Harrison's 20th Ed. Chapter 428, Page 3141

A. Restless legs syndrome
B. Wilson's disease
C. Pantothenate kinase-associated neurodegeneration
D. Machado-Joseph disease

1733. "Eye of the tiger" sign in MRI best relates with?
Harrison's 20th Ed. Chapter 428, Page 3141

A. Restless legs syndrome
B. Wilson's disease
C. Hallervorden-Spatz disease
D. Machado-Joseph disease

Pantothenate kinase-associated neurodegeneration (PKAN) known earlier as Hallervorden-Spatz disease (HSD) is the most common form of NBIA. It is caused by a mutation in PANK2 gene. Onset is in early childhood & manifests as a combination of dystonia, parkinsonism & spasticity. MRI shows a characteristic low signal abnormality in center of globus pallidus on T2-weighted scans known as the "eye of the tiger" sign caused by iron accumulation. Systemic & CSF iron levels, as well as plasma ferritin, transferrin, and ceruloplasmin, all are normal.

1734. The most common psychogenic movement disorder is?
Harrison's 20th Ed. Chapter 428, Page 3141

A. Tremor affecting the upper limbs
B. Tremor affecting the lower limbs
C. Tremor affecting the lips & tongue
D. Tremor affecting the body

Tremor affecting the upper limbs is the most common psychogenic movement disorder.

1735. Astasia-abasia is best related to?
Harrison's 20th Ed. Chapter 428, Page 3141

A. Parkinsonism
B. Cerebellar degeneration
C. Psychogenic movement disorder
D. Nystagmus

Astasia-abasia refers to odd gyrations of posture with wastage of muscular energy, extreme slow motion, and dramatic fluctuations over time observed in patients with somatoform disorders and conversion reaction with no underlying pathology.

Amyotrophic Lateral Sclerosis and Other Motor Neuron Diseases

1736. Lou Gehrig's disease is the other name of?

N Engl J Med. 2001;344:1688

A. Amyotrophic lateral sclerosis
B. Myasthenia gravis
C. Multiple sclerosis
D. Subacute combined degeneration of cord

ALS is often called Lou Gehrig's disease after Lou Gehrig (1903-1941), a hall-of-fame baseball player for New York Yankees who suffered with ALS. People in England and Australia call ALS as Motor Neurone Disease (MND). The French refer to it as Maladie de Charcot, after the French doctor Jean-Martin Charcot, who first wrote about ALS in 1869.

1737. Which of the following is the most common form of progressive motor neuron disease?

Harrison's 20th Ed. Chapter 429, Page 3141

A. Amyotrophic lateral sclerosis
B. Primary lateral sclerosis
C. Progressive muscular atrophy
D. Familial spastic paraplegia

Amyotrophic lateral sclerosis (ALS) is the most common form of progressive motor neuron disease.

1738. Which of the following is the most devastating of the neurodegenerative disorders?

Harrison's 20th Ed. Chapter 429, Page 3141

A. Amyotrophic lateral sclerosis
B. Primary lateral sclerosis
C. Progressive muscular atrophy
D. Familial spastic paraplegia

Amyotrophic lateral sclerosis is a neurodegenerative disease & is the most devastating of the neurodegenerative disorders.

1739. Which of the following is involved in motor neuron degenerative disorders?

Harrison's 20th Ed. Chapter 429, Page 3142

A. Anterior horn cells in spinal cord
B. Brainstem nuclei innervating bulbar muscles
C. Corticospinal motor neurons
D. All of the above

Pathologic hallmark of motor neuron degenerative disorders is death of lower motor neurons. These include anterior horn cells in spinal cord, brainstem nuclei innervating bulbar muscles, upper or corticospinal motor neurons originating in layer five of motor cortex and descending via the pyramidal tract to synapse with lower motor neurons, either directly or indirectly via interneurons. Characteristically, in ALS, upper or lower motor neurons both will eventually be involved.

1740. Acute sporadic motor neuron diseases include?

Harrison's 20th Ed. Chapter 429, Page 3143 Table 429-2

A. Poliomyelitis
B. Herpes zoster
C. Coxsackie virus
D. All of the above

Acute sporadic motor neuron diseases include Poliomyelitis, Herpes zoster, West Nile virus and Coxsackie virus.

1741. Chronic sporadic motor neuron disease with predominant involvement of upper motor neurons is?

Harrison's 20th Ed. Chapter 429, Page 3143 Table 429-2

A. Amyotrophic lateral sclerosis
B. Multifocal motor neuropathy with conduction block
C. Motor neuropathy with paraproteinemia
D. Primary lateral sclerosis

Chronic sporadic MND with predominant involvement of UMN is primary lateral sclerosis. Upper and lower motor neuron are involved in Amyotrophic lateral sclerosis (ALS).

1742. Chronic sporadic motor neuron disease with predominant involvement of lower motor neurons are?

Harrison's 20th Ed. Chapter 429, Page 3143 Table 429-2

A. Multifocal motor neuropathy with conduction block
B. Motor neuropathy with paraproteinemia or cancer
C. Motor-predominant peripheral neuropathies
D. All of the above

In Amyotrophic lateral sclerosis, both upper & lower motor neurons are involved. In Primary lateral sclerosis, predominantly upper motor neurons are involved. In Multifocal motor neuropathy with conduction block, Motor neuropathy with paraproteinemia or cancer and Motor-predominant peripheral neuropathies, predominantly lower motor neurons are affected.

1743. Disease that affect lower motor neurons of spinal cord is?

Harrison's 20th Ed. Chapter 429, Page 3142

A. Pseudobulbar palsy
B. Primary lateral sclerosis (PLS)
C. Familial spastic paraplegia (FSP)
D. Progressive muscular atrophy

In spinal muscular atrophy (SMA), also called progressive muscular atrophy, the lower motor neurons of spinal cord are most severely involved.

1744. Diseases that affect only upper motor neurons innervating the brainstem and spinal cord are?

Harrison's 20th Ed. Chapter 429, Page 3142

A. Pseudobulbar palsy
B. Primary lateral sclerosis (PLS)
C. Familial spastic paraplegia (FSP)
D. All of the above

Pseudobulbar palsy, primary lateral sclerosis (PLS), and familial spastic paraplegia (FSP) affect only upper motor neurons innervating the brainstem and spinal cord.

1745. Lipofuscin accumulation in motor neurons is seen in which of the following diseases?

Harrison's 20th Ed. Chapter 429, Page 3142

A. Amyotrophic lateral sclerosis
B. Spinal muscular atrophy (SMA)
C. Primary lateral sclerosis (PLS)
D. All of the above

Lipofuscin, the age pigment, gets accumulated in motor neurons in ALS, pseudobulbar palsy, primary lateral sclerosis (PLS), familial spastic paraplegia (FSP), bulbar palsy and spinal muscular atrophy (SMA).

1746. Which of the following is a marker for degeneration?
Harrison's 20th Ed. Chapter 429, Page 3142

A. Phosphorylated tau
B. β-amyloid
C. Ubiquitin
D. α-synuclein

Ubiquitin is a marker for degeneration.

1747. In sporadic and familial amyotrophic lateral sclerosis, the affected neurons ultrastructurally demonstrate which of the following?
Harrison's 20th Ed. Chapter 429, Page 3142

A. Ubiquitin (+)ve aggregates associated with protein TDP41
B. Ubiquitin (+)ve aggregates associated with protein TDP42
C. Ubiquitin (+)ve aggregates associated with protein TDP43
D. Ubiquitin (+)ve aggregates associated with protein TDP44

In sporadic & familial ALS, affected neurons demonstrate ubiquitin-positive aggregates, typically associated with protein TDP43 along with proliferation of astroglia and microglia that are inevitable accompaniment of all degenerative processes in the central nervous system (CNS).

1748. In amyotrophic lateral sclerosis, the structures that are left intact include?
Harrison's 20th Ed. Chapter 429, Page 3142

A. Sensory apparatus
B. Centers for control & coordination of movement
C. Centers for cognitive processes
D. All of the above

A remarkable feature of ALS is the selectivity of neuronal cell death. Entire sensory apparatus, regulatory mechanisms for the control and coordination of movement and the components of brain that are needed for cognitive processes remain intact.

1749. Until late in the disease, ALS spares neurons that innervate?
N Engl J Med. 2017;377:162-72

A. Diaphragm muscles
B. Sphincter muscles
C. Tongue muscles
D. Neck muscles

ALS typically begins in limbs. ~ One third of cases are bulbar causing difficulty chewing, speaking, or swallowing. Until late in the disease, ALS spares neurons that innervate eye & sphincter muscles (bladder).

1750. In amyotrophic lateral sclerosis, the structures that are left intact include?
Harrison's 20th Ed. Chapter 429, Page 3142

A. Motor neurons for ocular motility
B. Parasympathetic neurons in sacral spinal cord
C. Sensory apparatus
D. All of the above

In ALS, within motor system, there is selectivity of involvement. Motor neurons required for ocular motility remain unaffected, as do the parasympathetic neurons in the sacral spinal cord (the nucleus of Onufrowicz, or Onuf) that innervate the sphincters of the bowel and bladder.

1751. Which of the following is affected in the very late stages of the ALS?
Harrison's 20th Ed. Chapter 429, Page 3142

A. Sensory functions
B. Ocular motility
C. Cognitive functions
D. Bowel and bladder functions

Even in the late stages of the illness, sensory, bowel and bladder, and cognitive functions are preserved. Even when there is severe brainstem disease, ocular motility is spared until the very late stages of theillness.

1752. In ALS, the cause leading to death is?
Harrison's 20th Ed. Chapter 429, Page 3143

A. Infections
B. Depression and suicide
C. Respiratory paralysis
D. Cardiovascular event

In ALS, the cause leading to death is respiratory paralysis.

1753. In ALS, the median survival is from?
Harrison's 20th Ed. Chapter 429, Page 3143

A. 3 months to 12 months
B. 1 to 3 years
C. 3 to 5 years
D. 6 to 8 years

In ALS, the median survival is from 3 to 5 years.

1754. Which of the following is a risk factor for ALS?
Harrison's 20th Ed. Chapter 429, Page 3143

A. Exposure to pesticides & insecticides
B. Smoking
C. Service in the military
D. All of the above

The strongest risk factor for ALS is military service.

1755. Familial ALS (FALS) is due to mutations in which of the following genes?
Harrison's 20th Ed. Chapter 429, Page 3143

A. Gene encoding protein C90rf72
B. Gene encoding cytosolic enzyme SOD1
C. Gene encoding RNA binding proteins TDP43
D. Any of the above

Familial ALS (FALS) is inherited as autosomal dominant trait. It is due to mutations in multiple genes, including those encoding the protein C90rf72 (open reading frame 72 on chromosome 9), cytosolic enzyme SOD1 (superoxide dismutase), the RNA binding proteins TDP43 (encoded by the TAR DNA binding protein gene) and FUS/TLS (fused in sarcoma/translocated in liposarcoma).

1756. Familial ALS (FALS) is most commonly due to mutations in which of the following genes?
Harrison's 20th Ed. Chapter 429, Page 3143

A. Gene encoding protein C90rf72
B. Gene encoding cytosolic enzyme SOD1
C. Gene encoding RNA binding proteins TDP43
D. Gene encoding proteins optineuron, TBK1 & profilin-1

Most common cause of FALS is mutation in C90rf72 (~45–50%). Mutations in SOD1 account for 20% of cases of FALS, whereas TDP43 and FUS/TLS each represent about 5% of familial cases. Minority of cases (~1–2%) are caused by mutations in genes encoding proteins optineuron, TBK1 and profilin-1.

1757. Which of the following gene is implicated in childhood onset motor neuron disease?

Harrison's 20th Ed. Chapter 429, Page 3143

A. Alsin
B. Senataxin
C. Dynactin
D. All of the above

Predominantly lower motor neuron disease with early hoarseness due to laryngeal dysfunction is due to mutations in the gene encoding cellular accessory motor protein dynactin. Mutations in senataxin, a helicase, cause an early adult-onset, slowly evolving ALS variant. Slowly disabling degenerative, predominantly upper motor neuron disease that starts in first decade is caused by mutations in a gene that expresses a novel signaling molecule with properties of a guanine exchange factor, termed alsin.

1758. Which of the following is not a feature of ALS?

Harrison's 20th Ed. Chapter 429, Page 3143

A. Absence of pain or of sensory changes
B. Normal bowel and bladder function
C. Normal roentgenographic studies of spine
D. Raised proteins in cerebrospinal fluid (CSF)

Absence of pain or of sensory changes, normal bowel & bladder function, normal roentgenographic studies of the spine, and normal cerebrospinal fluid (CSF), all favor ALS.

1759. Involuntary excess in weeping or laughing (pseudobulbar affect) is a feature of?

Harrison's 20th Ed. Chapter 429, Page 3143

A. Multifocal motor neuropathy with conduction block
B. Amyotrophic lateral sclerosis
C. Kennedy's disease
D. Adult Tay-Sachs disease

In ALS, degeneration of corticobulbar projections innervating brainstem results in dysarthria and exaggeration of motor expressions of emotion which leads to involuntary excess in weeping or laughing (pseudobulbar affect).

1760. Which of the following antibiotics has neuroprotective properties?

N Engl J Med. 2003;348:1365-75

A. Azithromycin
B. Minocycline
C. Spiramycin
D. Vancomycin

Minocycline is a second-generation tetracycline with neuroprotective properties. Minocycline inhibits ischemia-induced up-regulation of nitric oxide synthase, caspase 1, and reactive microgliosis. Neuroprotection by minocycline has been observed in Huntington's disease, ALS, brain injury, Parkinson's disease, and multiple sclerosis.

1761. Differential diagnosis of amyotrophic lateral sclerosis is?

Harrison's 20th Ed. Chapter 429, Page 3146

A. Compression of cervical spinal cord
B. Thyrotoxicosis
C. Chronic lead poisoning
D. All of the above

D/D of ALS includes cervical spinal cord compression, cervicomedullary junction tumors, cervical or foramen magnum tumors, cervical spondylosis, chronic lead poisoning, thyrotoxicosis, hexosaminidase A, or alpha-glucosidase deficiency, multifocal motor neuropathy with conduction block (MMCB), Lyme disease.

1762. Fasciculations may be taken as benign, if?

Harrison's 20th Ed. Chapter 429, Page 3146

A. There is absence of weakness
B. There is absence of atrophy
C. There is no denervation phenomena electrophysiologically.
D. All of the above

1763. Amyotrophic lateral sclerosis may develop concurrently with which of the following?

Harrison's 20th Ed. Chapter 429, Page 3146

A. Parkinsonism
B. Frontotemporal dementia
C. Chronic traumatic encephalopathy
D. All of the above

1764. The most commonly mutated gene in ALS is?

N Engl J Med. 2017;377:162-72

A. NOD2
B. NLRP3
C. C9ORF72
D. CERCR1

1765. Which of the following genes are involved in RNA processing, transport and metabolism?

Harrison's 20th Ed. Chapter 429, Page 3146

A. C9orf73
B. TDP43
C. FUS
D. All of the above

Genes involved in RNA processing, transport and metabolism are C90rf73, TDP43 and FUS.

1766. Which of the following is an intronic repeat disorder?

Harrison's 20th Ed. Chapter 429, Page 3146

A. Amyotrophic lateral sclerosis
B. Myotonic dystrophy
C. Spinocerebellar atrophy type 8
D. All of the above

1767. Mutations in gene encoding which of the following protein cause an aggressive, infantile motor neuron disease?

Harrison's 20th Ed. Chapter 429, Page 3146

A. Tyrosine phosphatase non-receptor 22
B. GLE1
C. Lymphoid tyrosine phosphatase
D. Cryopyrin

1768. Riluzole - a glutamate antagonist is useful in treatment of?

Harrison's 20th Ed. Chapter 429, Page 3146

A. Amyotrophic lateral sclerosis
B. Multiple sclerosis
C. Subacute combined degeneration of cord
D. Myasthenia gravis

Riluzole is approved for ALS. Riluzole reduces excitotoxicity by diminishing glutamate release.

1769. Which of the following drug is useful in the treatment of amyotrophic lateral sclerosis?

Harrison's 20th Ed. Chapter 429, Page 3146

A. Nusinersen
B. Edaravone
C. IV immunoglobulin
D. All of the above

1770. Disease in which peripheral motor neurons are affected without involvement of corticospinal motor system is?

Harrison's 20th Ed. Chapter 429, Page 3146

A. X-Linked spinobulbar muscular atrophy (Kennedy's disease)
B. Adult Tay-Sachs disease
C. Spinal muscular atrophy
D. All of the above

Diseases in which peripheral motor neurons are affected without involvement of corticospinal motor system include X-Linked spinobulbar muscular atrophy (Kennedy's disease), adult tay-sachs disease, spinal muscular atrophy, Multifocal Motor Neuropathy with Conduction Block, Fazio-Londe syndrome, Machado-Joseph disease and olivopontocerebellar degenerations.

1771. Which of the following is false for Kennedy's Disease?

Harrison's 20th Ed. Chapter 429, Page 3147

A. X-linked spinobulbar muscular atrophy
B. Lower motor neuron disorder
C. Gynecomastia and reduced fertility
D. None of the above

Azoospermia & male-factor infertility occurs in association with mild loss of function mutations in androgen receptor. Trinucleotide (CAG) repeat expansion, from a mean of 22 repeats to greater than 40 repeats, within a highly polymorphic region of androgen receptor is associated with spinal & bulbar muscular atrophy (Kennedy disease). These patients may show evidence of partial androgen insensitivity in adolescence or adulthood (gynecomastia).

1772. Which of the following diseases is caused by deficiency of enzyme β-hexosaminidase (hex A)?

Harrison's 20th Ed. Chapter 429, Page 3147

A. Familial spastic paraplegia
B. Werdnig-Hoffmann disease
C. Adult Tay-Sachs disease
D. Kugelberg-Welander disease

1773. Which of the following is false about Adult Tay-Sachs Disease?

Harrison's 20th Ed. Chapter 429, Page 3147

A. Very slowly progressive
B. Dysarthria
C. Cerebellar atrophy
D. None of the above

1774. Intraneuronal inclusions "Bunina bodies" are a pathognomonic feature of?

N Engl J Med. 2001;344:1688

A. Motor neuron disease
B. Multiple sclerosis
C. Subacute combined degeneration of cord
D. Myasthenia gravis

1775. Which of the following is false about spinal muscular atrophy?

Harrison's 20th Ed. Chapter 429, Page 3147

A. Genetic lower motor neuron disease
B. Early onset
C. Locus on chromosome 5
D. None of the above

Spinal muscular atrophy (SMA) maps to a locus on chromosome 5 encoding a putative motor neuron survival protein (SMN, for survival motor neuron) that is important in the formation & trafficking of RNA complexes across nuclear membrane.

1776. Which of the following is false about spinal muscular atrophy?

Harrison's 20th Ed. Chapter 429, Page 3147

A. Extensive loss of large motor neurons
B. Evidence of denervation atrophy on muscle biopsy
C. Electrophysiologic evidence of denervation
D. None of the above

1777. Werdnig-Hoffmann Disease is the name given to?

Harrison's 20th Ed. Chapter 429, Page 3147

A. SMA I
B. SMA II
C. SMA III
D. None of the above

1778. Kugelberg-Welander disease is the name given to?

Harrison's 20th Ed. Chapter 429, Page 3147

A. SMA I
B. SMA II
C. SMA III
D. None of the above

1779. Which out of the following carries the worst prognosis?

Harrison's 20th Ed. Chapter 429, Page 3147

A. SMA I
B. SMA II
C. SMA III
D. None of the above

Infantile SMA or SMA I is known as Werdnig-Hoffmann disease with earliest onset & most rapidly fatal course. Chronic childhood SMA (SMA II) begins later in childhood & evolves with slowly progressive course. Juvenile SMA (SMA III or Kugelberg-Welander disease) manifests in late childhood & has a slow course. EP studies distinguish SMA III from myopathic syndromes.

1780. Which of the following drug is useful in the treatment of spinal muscular atrophy?

Harrison's 20th Ed. Chapter 429, Page 3146

A. Nusinersen
B. Edaravone
C. IV immunoglobulin
D. All of the above

1781. Which of the following is false about 'Multifocal Motor Neuropathy with Conduction Block' (MMCB)?

Harrison's 20th Ed. Chapter 429, Page 3147

A. Elevated serum titers of mono- & polyclonal antibodies to ganglioside GM1
B. No corticospinal tract signs
C. Respond to intravenous immunoglobulin therapy
D. None of the above

1782. Multifocal motor neuropathy with conduction block (MMCB) evolves in association with which of the following?

Harrison's 20th Ed. Chapter 429, Page 3146

A. Tuberculosis
B. Lymphoma
C. Syphilis
D. All of the above

MMCB is a diffuse, lower motor axonal neuropathy mimicking ALS which sometimes evolves in association with lymphoma or multiple myeloma.

1783. Which of the following is true for Fazio-Londe syndrome?

Harrison's 20th Ed. Chapter 429, Page 3147

A. ALS variant
B. Juvenile onset
C. Involves musculature innervated by brainstem mainly
D. All of the above

Fazio-Londe syndrome is an ALS variant of juvenile onset that involves mainly the musculature innervated by the brainstem.

1784. Which of the following about primary lateral sclerosis is false?

Harrison's 20th Ed. Chapter 429, Page 3147

A. Affects adults in mid to late life
B. Combined involvement of corticospinal & corticobulbar tracts
C. Progressive spastic weakness of limbs, dysarthria & dysphagia
D. None of the above

1785. Which of the following is absent in primary lateral sclerosis?

Harrison's 20th Ed. Chapter 429, Page 3147

A. Fasciculations
B. Amyotrophy
C. Sensory changes
D. All of the above

In primary lateral sclerosis, fasciculations, amyotrophy, and sensory changes are absent. Neither electromyography nor muscle biopsy shows denervation. There occurs a selective loss of large pyramidal cells in precentral gyrus & degeneration of corticospinal & corticobulbar projections. Peripheral motor neurons & other neuronal systems are spared.

1786. Which of the following is false for Hereditary Spastic Paraplegia (HSP) in adults?

Harrison's 20th Ed. Chapter 429, Page 3147

A. X-linked transmission
B. Presents in third or fourth decade
C. Progressive spastic weakness in lower extremities
D. Long survival

In its pure form, most adult-onset HSP are transmitted as an autosomal dominant trait. HSP has long survival because respiratory function is spared.

1787. Which of the following is false for Hereditary Spastic Paraplegia (HSP)?

Harrison's 20th Ed. Chapter 429, Page 3147

A. Sexual function preserved
B. Spastin and atlastin gene mutations common
C. Degeneration of corticospinal tracts
D. None of the above

In HSP, sexual function tends to be preserved. Gene implicated is spastin & atlastin in dominantly inherited and childhood-onset dominant HSP respectively. Degeneration of corticospinal tracts (dying-back or distal axonopathy) occurs in HSP, most severe at more caudal levels in spinal cord. Posterior column (vibration & position) abnormalities and disturbance of bowel & bladder function happen.

1788. Which of the following is a disorder of CNS myelin?

Harrison's 20th Ed. Chapter 429, Page 3147

A. Fragile X syndrome
B. Pelizaeus-Merzbacher syndrome
C. Prader-Willi syndrome
D. Rett syndrome

Pelizaeus-Merzbacher disease is a widespread dysmyelinating disorder of CNS myelin caused by mutations in the gene for proteolipid protein (PLP) that normally promotes extracellular compaction between adjacent myelin lamellae.

Prion Diseases

1789. Scrapie agent is synonym of?
Harrison's 20th Ed. Chapter 430, Page 3148

A. Amyloid
B. Prion
C. Myelin
D. None of the above

Prions cause scrapie in sheep & goats & Creutzfeldt-Jakob disease in humans. Prions are abnormal proteins that propagate & cause disease by altering the structure of a normal cell protein.

1790. Prions play a key role in which of the following illnesses?
Harrison's 20th Ed. Chapter 430, Page 3148

A. Creutzfeldt-Jakob disease (CJD)
B. Alzheimer's disease (AD)
C. Parkinson's disease (PD)
D. All of the above

Prions play a key role in Alzheimer's disease (AD) and Parkinson's disease (PD).

1791. Which of the following about prions is false?
Harrison's 20th Ed. Chapter 430, Page 3148

A. Infectious proteins
B. Self-propagating
C. Lacks nucleic acid
D. None of the above

Prions are the only known 'transmissible pathogens' that are devoid of nucleic acid (RNA or DNA).

1792. Which of the following is a prion protein?
Harrison's 20th Ed. Chapter 430, Page 3148

A. PrP^{Sc}
B. α-synuclein
C. Aβ
D. All of the above

Creutzfeldt-Jakob disease (CJD) is caused by accumulation of PrP^{Sc} prions. α-synuclein prions cause multiple system atrophy (MSA), Aβ prions contribute to AD, α-synuclein prions to PD & tau prions to some types of frontotemporal dementia (FTD).

1793. Most CJD patients are between the age of?
Harrison's 20th Ed. Chapter 430, Page 3148

A. 20 & 35 years
B. 35 & 45 years
C. 50 & 75 years
D. 75 & 90 years

Most CJD patients are between 50 & 75 years of age. CJD is relentlessly progressive & generally causes death within 9 months of onset.

1794. The fundamental event underlying prion diseases is?
Harrison's 20th Ed. Chapter 430, Page 3148

A. α-to-β structural transition in PrP
B. α-to-β structural transition in PrP^{SC}
C. α-to-γ structural transition in PrP
D. α-to-γ structural transition in PrP^{SC}

α-to-β structural transition in prion protein (PrP^{C}) is the fundamental event underlying prion diseases

1795. Prion diseases may manifest as?
Harrison's 20th Ed. Chapter 430, Page 3148

A. Infectious disorders
B. Genetic disorders
C. Sporadic disorders
D. All of the above

Prion diseases manifest as infectious, genetic & sporadic disorders. No other single etiology illness present with such wide spectrum clinical manifestations.

1796. Disease causing isoform of prion is?
Harrison's 20th Ed. Chapter 430, Page 3149 Table 430-1

A. PrP^{C}
B. PrP^{D}
C. PrP^{Sc}
D. PrP^{Sd}

Prions reproduce by binding to normal, cellular isoform of prion protein (PrP^{C}) & stimulating conversion of PrP^{C} into disease-causing isoform (PrP^{Sc}).

1797. Which of the following statements about prions is false?
Harrison's 20th Ed. Chapter 430, Page 3148

A. Devoid of nucleic acid
B. Prion diseases result from accumulation of PrP^{Sc}
C. Pathologic hallmarks of CJD are spongiform degeneration and astrocytic gliosis
D. CSF is always abnormal in CJD

In CJD, CSF is nearly always normal but may show protein elevation & rarely mild pleocytosis.

1798. Which of the following is the precursor of PrP^{Sc}?
Harrison's 20th Ed. Chapter 430, Page 3149 Table 430-1

A. PrP 27-30
B. PrP^{C}
C. PrP^{D}
D. PRNP

PrP^{C} is the precursor of PrP^{Sc}

1799. Which of the following retains prion infectivity and polymerizes into amyloid?
Harrison's 20th Ed. Chapter 430, Page 3149 Table 430-1

A. PrP 27-30
B. PrP^{C}
C. PrP^{D}
D. PRNP

PrP 27-30 retains prion infectivity and polymerizes into amyloid.

1800. In humans, PrP gene (PRNP) is located on?
Harrison's 20th Ed. Chapter 430, Page 3149 Table 430-1

A. Short arm of chromosome 12
B. Short arm of chromosome 14
C. Short arm of chromosome 16
D. Short arm of chromosome 20

In humans, PrP gene is designated PRNP and is located on the short arm of chromosome 20.

1801. Which of the following about prions is false?
Harrison's 20th Ed. Chapter 430, Page 3148

A. Prions reproduce by binding to PrP^C
B. PrP^C is rich in a helix & has little β structure
C. PrP^{Sc} has less a helix & high amount of β structure
D. PrP 27-30 is a fragment of PrP^C

PrP 27-30 is a fragment of PrP^{Sc}, generated by truncation of the NH2-terminus by limited digestion with proteinase K.

1802. Which is the most common prion disorder in humans?
Harrison's 20th Ed. Chapter 430, Page 3148

A. Sporadic CJD (sCJD)
B. Familial CJD (fCJD)
C. Gerstmann-Straussler-Scheinker disease (GSS)
D. Fatal familial insomnia (FFI)

Sporadic CJD is the most common prion disorder in humans (~85%).

1803. Inherited prion disease caused by mutations in PrP gene is?
Harrison's 20th Ed. Chapter 430, Page 3148

A. Familial CJD (fCJD)
B. Gerstmann-Straussler-Scheinker disease (GSS)
C. Fatal familial insomnia (FFI)
D. All of the above

fCJD, GSS disease & FFI are dominantly inherited prion diseases caused by mutations in PrP gene.

1804. Iatrogenic CJD can be caused by?
Harrison's 20th Ed. Chapter 430, Page 3151

A. Corneal transplantation
B. Contaminated EEG electrode implantation
C. Implantation of duramater grafts
D. All of the above

Accidental transmission of CJD to humans can occur with corneal transplantation, contaminated EEG electrode implantation, duramater/pericardium graft Transmission of CJD prions from contaminated human growth hormone (hGH) preparations derived from human pituitaries has been responsible for fatal cerebellar disorders with dementia.

1805. Which of the following is a prion disease endemic in deer & elk in regions of North America?
Harrison's 20th Ed. Chapter 430, Page 3149

A. Mink encephalopathy
B. Bovine spongiform encephalopathy (BSE)
C. Chronic wasting disease (CWD)
D. Kuru

Chronic wasting disease (CWD) is a prion disease endemic in deer and elk in regions of North America. In contrast to other prion diseases, CWD is highly communicable. Feces from asymptomatic, infected cervids contain prions that are responsible for the spread of CWD.

1806. Which of the following about PrP prion diseases is false?
Harrison's 20th Ed. Chapter 430, Page 3149

A. Aberrant metabolism of PrP
B. PrP isoforms are encoded by a chromosomal gene
C. Epigenetically heritable
D. None of the above

1807. Pathologic hallmarks of Creutzfeldt-Jakob disease (CJD) is?
Harrison's 20th Ed. Chapter 430, Page 3151

A. Spongiform degeneration
B. Astrocytic gliosis
C. Lack of inflammatory response
D. All of the above

Pathologic hallmarks of CJD are spongiform degeneration, astrocytic gliosis & lack of inflammatory response.

1808. "Florid plaques" is characteristic feature of?
Harrison's 20th Ed. Chapter 430, Page 3152

A. sCJD (Creutzfeldt-Jakob disease)
B. fCJD
C. vCJD
D. iCJD

Presence of "florid plaques" is a characteristic feature of vCJD. These are composed of a central core of PrP amyloid, surrounded by vacuoles in a pattern suggesting petals on a flower.

1809. Most patients with CJD present with?
Harrison's 20th Ed. Chapter 430, Page 3152

A. Deficits in higher cortical function
B. Cerebellar gait & coordination deficits
C. Extrapyramidal dysfunction
D. Visual impairment

Most patients with CJD present with deficits in higher cortical function.

1810. Dementia with myoclonus is seen in?
Harrison's 20th Ed. Chapter 430, Page 3152

A. Alzheimer's disease (AD)
B. Unverricht-Lundborg disease
C. Creutzfeldt-Jakob disease (CJD)
D. All of the above

Dementia with myoclonus can be due to Alzheimer's disease (AD), dementia with Lewy bodies, corticobasal degeneration, cryptococcal encephalitis, or myoclonic epilepsy disorder—Unverricht-Lundborg disease.

1811. Which of the following about myoclonus in CJD is false?
Harrison's 20th Ed. Chapter 430, Page 3152

A. Persists during sleep
B. Elicited by loud sounds & bright lights
C. Occur later in the course of CJD
D. None of the above

In CJD, myoclonus is neither specific nor confined to CJD and tends to occur later in the course. Myoclonus persists during sleep, is elicited by loud sounds or bright lights.

1812. Most patients with CJD survive for what length of time after onset of clinical signs & symptoms?
Harrison's 20th Ed. Chapter 430, Page 3152

A. 6–12 months
B. 12–24 months
C. 24–48 months
D. 48–60 months

Most patients with CJD survive for 6–12 months after the onset of clinical signs and symptoms. Some live for up to 5 years.

1813. Clinical abnormalities in CJD involve?
Harrison's 20th Ed. Chapter 430, Page 3152

A. CNS
B. PNS
C. ANS
D. All of the above

Clinical abnormalities in CJD are confined to the CNS.

1814. Which of the following is a finding in CJD?

Harrison's 20th Ed. Chapter 430, Page 3152

A. Fever
B. Leukocytosis
C. Pleocytosis in CSF
D. None of the above

Fever, elevated ESR, leukocytosis, or pleocytosis in CSF point towards another etiology to explain patient's CNS dysfunction.

1815. Which of the following is the typical MRI finding in Creutzfeldt-Jakob disease?

Harrison's 20th Ed. Chapter 430, Page 3152

A. Insular ribon
B. Basal ganglia hypointensity
C. Cortical ribboning
D. All of the above

On FLAIR sequences and diffusion-weighted imaging, ~90% of CJD patients show increased intensity in basal ganglia and cortical ribboning. This pattern is not seen with other neurodegenerative disorders but is seen infrequently with viral encephalitis, paraneoplastic syndromes or seizures.

1816. Ataxia is a prominent & presenting feature in?

Harrison's 20th Ed. Chapter 430, Page 3152

A. Familial CJD (fCJD)
B. Gerstmann-Straussler-Scheinker disease (GSS)
C. Fatal familial insomnia (FFI)
D. Sporadic Creutzfeldt-Jakob disease (sCJD)

Ataxia is a prominent & presenting feature in GSS disease, with dementia occurring late in the disease course. Early ataxia & visual hallucinations with a prominent psychiatric prodrome point towards vCJD.

1817. Insomnia & dysautonomia are a feature of?

Harrison's 20th Ed. Chapter 430, Page 3152

A. Familial CJD (fCJD)
B. Gerstmann-Straussler-Scheinker disease (GSS)
C. Fatal familial insomnia (FFI)
D. vCJD

FFI is characterized by insomnia & dysautonomia. Dementia occurs in terminal phase of illness.

1818. Prominent psychiatric prodrome is a feature of?

Harrison's 20th Ed. Chapter 430, Page 3152

A. Familial CJD (fCJD)
B. Gerstmann-Straussler-Scheinker disease (GSS)
C. Fatal familial insomnia (FFI)
D. Variant CJD (vCJD)

1819. Most common disorder to be mistaken for CJD is?

Harrison's 20th Ed. Chapter 430, Page 3152

A. AD
B. FTD
C. Progressive supranuclear palsy
D. Dementia with Lewy bodies

Dementia with Lewy bodies is the most common disorder mistaken for CJD. Absence of abnormalities on diffusion-weighted & fluid-attenuated inversion recovery (FLAIR) magnetic resonance imaging (MRI) almost always distinguishes other dementing conditions from CJD.

1820. Which of the following is false for Hashimoto's encephalopathy?

Harrison's 20th Ed. Chapter 430, Page 3152

A. Subacute progressive encephalopathy
B. Tonic-clonic seizures
C. Periodic triphasic complexes on EEG
D. Fluctuations in severity

Myoclonus & periodic triphasic complexes on EEG, high titers of antithyroglobulin or antithyroid peroxidase (antimicrosomal) antibodies and improvement with glucocorticoid therapy point towards Hashimoto's encephalopathy.

1821. On FLAIR sequences & diffusion-weighted imaging MRI, which of the following suggests sCJD?

Harrison's 20th Ed. Chapter 430, Page 3152

A. Entorhinal cortex & hippocampal atrophy
B. Frontal, insular, and/or temporal atrophy
C. Cortical ribboning
D. Posterior parietal atrophy

In diffusion/ fluid-attenuate inversion recovery MRI, cortical ribboning & increased intensity in the basal ganglia distinguishing sCJD from most other conditions. Markedly abnormal periodic complexes on EEG (repetitive, high-voltage, triphasic & polyphasic sharp discharges) provide further aid. Entorhinal cortex & hippocampal atrophy suggests AD, frontal, insular, and/or temporal atrophy suggests FTD, posterior parietal atrophy suggests DLB.

1822. In CJD, levels of which of the following is elevated in CSF?

Harrison's 20th Ed. Chapter 430, Page 3153

A. Neuron-specific enolase
B. Tau
C. Stress protein 14-3-3
D. All of the above

1823. Stress protein 14-3-3 is elevated in the CSF of?

Harrison's 20th Ed. Chapter 430, Page 3152

A. Herpes simplex virus encephalitis
B. Multi-infarct dementia
C. Stroke
D. All of the above

1824. Stress protein 14-3-3 is elevated in the CSF of all except?

Harrison's 20th Ed. Chapter 430, Page 3152

A. Herpes simplex virus encephalitis
B. Multi-infarct dementia
C. AD
D. CJD

1825. Which of the following about CJD is true?

Harrison's 20th Ed. Chapter 430, Page 3153

A. Contagious
B. Communicable
C. Transmissible
D. Vulnerable to common inactivation procedures

CJD is not contagious or communicable but it is transmissible.

1826. Sterilization for Creutzfeldt-Jakob disease (CJD) contaminated materials is done by?

Harrison's 20th Ed. Chapter 430, Page 3153

A. Hcl

B. NaOH

C. $NaHCO_3$

D. HNO_3

Prions are extremely resistant to common inactivation procedures. Autoclaving at 134°C for 5 hours or treatment with 2 N NaOH for several hours is recommended for sterilization of prions.

1827. Besides PrP, which of the following proteins can become prions?

Harrison's 20th Ed. Chapter 430, Page 3153

A. Amyloid beta (Aβ)

B. Huntingtin

C. α-synuclein

D. All of the above

Besides PrP, proteins like amyloid beta (Aβ), tau, α-synuclein & huntingtin can all become prions.

Ataxic Disorders

1828. Symptoms and signs of ataxia consist of?

Harrison's 20th Ed. Chapter 431, Page 3154

A. Gait impairment
B. Visual blurring due to nystagmus
C. Tremor with movement
D. All of the above

Symptoms & signs of ataxia consist of gait impairment, unclear or scanning speech, visual blurring due to nystagmus, hand incoordination & tremor with movement.

1829. Ataxia is due to involvement of?

Harrison's 20th Ed. Chapter 431, Page 3154

A. Cerebellum
B. Spinocerebellar pathway
C. Fronto-ponto-cerebellar pathway
D. All of the above

Ataxia is due to involvement of cerebellum & its afferent and efferent pathways, including spinocerebellar pathways, and frontopontocerebellar pathway originating in the rostral frontal lobe.

1830. Which of the following about true cerebellar ataxia is false?

Harrison's 20th Ed. Chapter 431, Page 3154

A. It is devoid of vertiginous complaints
B. It is an unsteady gait due to imbalance
C. Not associated with vestibular nerve or labyrinthine disease
D. None of the above

True cerebellar ataxia is clearly an unsteady gait due to imbalance and is different from ataxia associated with vestibular nerve or labyrinthine disease. Ataxia associated with vestibular nerve or labyrinthine disease results in a gait disorder associated with significant degrees of dizziness, light-headedness or perception of movement which are absent in true cerebellar ataxia.

1831. Sensory information for postural control is primarily generated by?

Harrison's 20th Ed. Chapter 431, Page 3154

A. Visual system
B. Vestibular system
C. Proprioceptive receptors in muscle spindles & joints
D. All of the above

Sensory information for postural control is primarily generated by visual system, vestibular system and by proprioceptive receptors in the muscle spindles and joints. Loss of two of the three pathways is compromises standing balance. Clinically, gait disorder must be viewed as the product of a neurologic deficit and a functional adaptation.

1832. Bilateral ataxia with symmetric involvement suggests which of the following?

Harrison's 20th Ed. Chapter 431, Page 3154

A. Genetic etiology
B. Metabolic etiology
C. Toxic etiology
D. Any of the above

A gradual & progressive increase in ataxic symptoms with bilateral & symmetric involvement suggests a genetic, metabolic, immune or toxic etiology.

1833. Acute & reversible ataxias are caused by?

Harrison's 20th Ed. Chapter 431, Page 3154

A. Intoxication with alcohol
B. Phenytoin
C. Lithium
D. All of the above

Acute & reversible ataxias are caused by intoxication with alcohol, phenytoin, lithium, barbiturates. Other agents include toluene exposure, gasoline sniffing, glue sniffing, spray painting, or exposure to methyl mercury or bismuth , treatment with cytotoxic chemotherapeutic drugs like fluorouracil & paclitaxel.

1834. "As if walking on a slippery surface" best relates to?

Harrison's 20th Ed. Chapter 23, Page 144

A. Cautious gait
B. Stiff-legged gait
C. Freezing gait
D. Frontal dait disorder

Cautious gait refers to describe a patient who walks with an abbreviated stride & lowered center of mass, as if walking on a slippery surface. This disorder is both common and nonspecific.

1835. Which of the following is the commonest etiology of gait disorders?

Harrison's 20th Ed. Chapter 431, Page 23 Table 23-1

A. Sensory deficits
B. Parkinsonism
C. Cerebellar degeneration
D. Psychogenic

1836. Stiff-legged gait category includes which of the following?

Harrison's 20th Ed. Chapter 23, Page 144

A. Spastic gait
B. Dystonia
C. Stiff-Person syndrome
D. All of the above

1837. Causes of freezing gait include?

Harrison's 20th Ed. Chapter 23, Page 144

A. Parkinson's disease
B. Progressive supranuclear palsy
C. Corticobasal degeneration
D. All of the above

Difficulty with gait initiation leads to a freezing gait seen in PD, progressive supranuclear palsy, multiple system atrophy, corticobasal degeneration & primary pallidal degeneration.

1838. Pill-rolling tremor is specific for?

Harrison's 20th Ed. Chapter 23, Page 144

A. Parkinson's disease
B. Progressive supranuclear palsy
C. Corticobasal degeneration
D. All of the above

Patients of PSP, MSA and CBD frequently present with axial stiffness, postural instability, and a shuffling gait but lack the characteristic pill-rolling tremor of Parkinson's disease.

1839. "Gait apraxia" is characteristic of?

Harrison's 20th Ed. Chapter 23, Page 144

A. Sensory ataxia
B. Cerebellar gait ataxia
C. Frontal gait disorder
D. Psychogenic gait disorder

Frontal gait disorder or "gait apraxia" features wide base of support, short stride, shuffling along floor and difficulty with starts & turns.

1840. Which of the following relate to frontal gait disorders?

Harrison's 20th Ed. Chapter 23, Page 144

A. Gait apraxia
B. "Slipping clutch" syndrome
C. Lower body parkinsonism
D. All of the above

Difficulty with gait initiation is referred to as "slipping clutch" syndrome & lower body parkinsonism.

1841. Cerebellar gait ataxia is characterized by all except?

Harrison's 20th Ed. Chapter 23, Page 144

A. Unable to walk tandem heel to toe
B. Difficulty in maintaining balance when turning
C. Narrow base of support
D. Falls is a late event

Cerebellar gait ataxia is characterized by a wide base of support, erratic foot placement, difficulty in maintaining balance on turning (an early feature) and tandem gait. Falls in daily life is a late event.

1842. Sensory ataxia is characterized by?

Harrison's 20th Ed. Chapter 23, Page 144

A. Stance destabilized by eye closure
B. Look down at their feet when walking
C. Joint position & vibration sense diminished in lower limbs
D. All of the above

In sensory ataxia, stance is destabilized by eye closure. Patient looks down at their feet when walking and do poorly in dark. Joint position & vibration sense is diminished in lower limbs.

1843. Which of the following is a feature of vestibular disorder?

Harrison's 20th Ed. Chapter 23, Page 144

A. Vertigo
B. Nystagmus
C. Poor balance
D. All of the above

Feature of vestibular disorders are vertigo (subjective appreciation or illusion of movement), nystagmus (vestibulo-oculomotor sign) & poor balance (impairment of vestibulo-spinal function).

1844. Symptoms & signs of true cerebellar ataxia consist of all except?

Harrison's 20th Ed. Chapter 23, Page 144

A. Gait impairment
B. Hand incoordination
C. Romberg sign
D. Tremor with movement

Ataxia due to vestibular nerve or labyrinthine disease results in gait disorder associated with dizziness, light-headedness or perception of movement. Cerebellar ataxia presents as gait impairment, scanning speech, visual blurring due to nystagmus, hand incoordination and tremor with movement. True cerebellar ataxia is devoid of vertiginous complaints. In sensory ataxia, imbalance worsens when visual input is removed (Romberg sign).

1845. Symptoms & signs of true cerebellar ataxia consist of all except?

Harrison's 20th Ed. Chapter 23, Page 144

A. Nystagmus
B. Scanning speech
C. Dizziness
D. Tremor with movement

Patients with hereditary ataxia or alcoholic cerebellar degeneration do not complain of dizziness.

1846. True cerebellar ataxia result from the involvement of?

Harrison's 20th Ed. Chapter 23, Page 144

A. Cerebellum
B. Spinocerebellar pathway
C. Frontopontocerebellar pathway
D. All of the above

True cerebellar ataxia result from involvement of cerebellum, spinocerebellar pathways and frontopontocerebellar pathway from rostral frontal lobe. True cerebellar ataxia is devoid of vertiginous complaints (dizziness, light-headedness or the perception of movement) and is clearly an unsteady gait due to imbalance.

1847. Which of the following may lead to development of ataxia of gait?

Harrison's 20th Ed. Chapter 431, Page 3154

A. B1 deficiency
B. B12 deficiency
C. Hyponatremia
D. All of the above

Subacute development of ataxia of gait may be due to vitamin B1 and B12 deficiency and hyponatremia.

1848. Anti-Tr autoantibody is related to which of the following?

Harrison's 20th Ed. Chapter 431, Page 3154

A. Breast cancer
B. Ovarian cancer
C. Small-cell lung cancer
D. Hodgkin's disease

Paraneoplastic cerebellar ataxia may present with various tumor states. Autoantibodies related to breast and ovarian cancers is anti-Yo, with small-cell lung cancer is anti-PQ type voltage-gated calcium channel, and with Hodgkin's disease is anti-Tr.

1849. Paraneoplastic Opsoclonus-Myoclonus Syndrome is related to which of the following?

Harrison's 20th Ed. Chapter 90, Page 672

A. Breast cancer
B. Lung cancer
C. Neuroblastoma
D. All of the above

Opsoclonus is a disorder of eye movement characterized by involuntary, chaotic saccades that occur in all directions of gaze frequently associated with myoclonus & ataxia. When the cause of opsoclonus-myoclonus is paraneoplastic, tumors involved are usually cancer of lung and breast in adults, neuroblastoma in children and ovarian teratoma in adolescents and young women.

1850. Patients with which of the following disorder fall over backwards?

Harrison's 20th Ed. Chapter 23, Page 144

A. Progressive supranuclear palsy
B. Cerebellar pathology
C. Lesions of the vestibular system
D. Patients with somatosensory deficits

Patients with cerebellar pathology may lean & topple toward side of lesion. Patients with lesions of vestibular system have lateral pulsion & toppling falls. Patients with progressive supranuclear palsy fall over backwards. Gait freezing in Parkinson's disease results in a forward fall.

1851. Which of the following is not a cause of symmetric ataxia?

Harrison's 20th Ed. Chapter 431, Page 3154 Table 431-1

A. Inherited ataxia
B. Hypothyroidism
C. Multiple sclerosis
D. Meningovascular syphilis

Demyelinating disease multiple sclerosis presents with focal and ipsilateral cerebellar signs of subacute duration (days to weeks).

1852. Paraneoplastic cerebellar ataxia is associated with?

Harrison's 20th Ed. Chapter 431, Page 3154

A. Breast cancer
B. Small-cell lung cancer
C. Hodgkin's disease
D. All of the above

Paraneoplastic cerebellar ataxia is associated with breast and ovarian cancers (anti-Yo), small-cell lung cancer (anti-PQ type voltage-gated calcium channel), and Hodgkin's disease (anti-Tr).

1853. Which of the following is best related to congenital cyst of the posterior fossa?

Harrison's 20th Ed. Chapter 431, Page 3155

A. Haw River syndrome
B. Bassen-Kornzweig syndrome
C. Chiari malformation
D. Dandy-Walker syndrome

1854. Which of the findings dominate presentation of inherited ataxias?

Harrison's 20th Ed. Chapter 431, Page 3155

A. Optic nerves & retina
B. Peripheral nerves
C. Cerebellar
D. Spinal cord

Findings of cerebellar disease dominate the clinical picture of inherited ataxias. There may also be characteristic changes in the basal ganglia, brainstem, spinal cord, optic nerves, retina and peripheral nerves.

1855. Which of the following is caused by an untranslated pentanucleotide repeat?

Harrison's 20th Ed. Chapter 431, Page 3155

A. SCA6
B. SCA7
C. SCA10
D. SCA17

Autosomal spinocerebellar ataxias (SCAs) include SCA types 1 through SCA28, dentatorubropallidoluysian atrophy (DRPLA) & episodic ataxia (EA) types 1 and 2. SCA1, SCA2, SCA3 [Machado-Joseph disease (MJD)], SCA6, SCA7, and SCA17 are caused by CAG triplet repeat expansions in different genes. SCA8 is due to an untranslated CTG repeat expansion, SCA12 is linked to an untranslated CAG repeat, and SCA10 is caused by an untranslated pentanucleotide repeat.

1856. Ataxins are?

Harrison's 20th Ed. Chapter 431, Page 3155

A. Expanded polyserine proteins
B. Expanded polyglutamine proteins
C. Expanded polyarginine proteins
D. Expanded polyleucine proteins

CAG encodes glutamine & expanded CAG triplet repeat expansions in SCA's result in expanded polyglutamine proteins, termed ataxins, that produce a toxic gain of function with autosomal dominant inheritance.

1857. About what number of glutamines due to expanded polyglutamine ataxins are potentially toxic to neurons?

Harrison's 20th Ed. Chapter 431, Page 3155

A. 10
B. 20
C. 30
D. 40

Expanded polyglutamine ataxins with more than ~40 glutamines are potentially toxic to neurons. They impair neuronal functions, alter efficiency of ubiquitin-proteosome system of protein turnover and induce neuronal apoptosis.

1858. Which of the following is a CAG repeat disease?

Harrison's 20th Ed. Chapter 431, Page 3155

A. Machado-Joseph disease (MJD)
B. Huntington's disease
C. Dentatorubral-pallidoluysian atrophy (DRPLA)
D. All of the above

Besides Machado-Joseph Disease (MJD), other CAG repeat diseases include Huntington's disease, dentatorubral-pallidoluysian atrophy (DRPLA) and X-chromosomal Spinobulbar Muscular Atrophy (SBMA or Kennedy's Disease). Other triplet repeat expansions diseases include Fragile X-syndrome (FRAXA) - CGG repeat, Fragile X-syndrome (FRAXE)–GCC repeat, Dystrophia myotonica (DM)–CTG repeat and Friedreich ataxia (FRDA1)–GAA repeat.

1859. Which of the following about increase in number of "nucleotide repeats" is false?

Harrison's 20th Ed. Chapter 431, Page 3155

A. Length correlates with severity of disease
B. Repeat length increases from one generation to next
C. Leads to anticipation
D. None of the above

Nucleotide repeat expansion disorders are associated with an increase in number of nucleotide repeats above a threshold. Repeats alter gene regulatory sequences and tends to further expand during cell division. Length of nucleotide repeat correlates with severity of disease. Repeat length increases from one generation to the next, and disease manifests severely and at an earlier age - phenomenon called anticipation.

1860. Dynamic mutation refers to?

Harrison's 20th Ed. Chapter 456, Page 3356

A. Decreasingly severe phenotype in next generation
B. Increasingly severe phenotype in next generation
C. Decreasingly severe genotype in next generation
D. Increasingly severe genotype in next generation

In subsequent generations, expanded repeat may increase further in length & result in an increasingly severe phenotype - dynamic mutation.

1861. Which of the following Trinucleotide Repeat Disorders has autosomal recessive inheritance?

Harrison's 20th Ed. Chapter 456, Page 3363 Table 456-5

A. Spinocerebellar ataxia type 1 (SCA1)
B. Machado Joseph disease (MJD)
C. Dentorubral pallidoluysiane atrophy (DRPLA)
D. Friedreich ataxia (FRDA1)

Friedreich ataxia (FRDA1) is GAA repeat autosomal recessive congenital ataxia.

1862. Which of the following was also called olivopontocerebellar atrophy?

Harrison's 20th Ed. Chapter 431, Page 3155

A. Spinocerebellar ataxia 1
B. Spinocerebellar ataxia 2
C. Spinocerebellar ataxia 3
D. Spinocerebellar ataxia 6

SCA1 was previously referred to as olivopontocerebellar atrophy.

1863. Which clinical phenotype of spinocerebellar ataxia has been described in patients from India?

Harrison's 20th Ed. Chapter 431, Page 3156

A. Spinocerebellar ataxia 1
B. Spinocerebellar ataxia 2
C. Spinocerebellar ataxia 6
D. Spinocerebellar ataxia 7

Clinical phenotype of spinocerebellar ataxia (SCA2) has been described in patients from Cuba and India.

1864. Which out of the following is the most common inherited autosomal dominant ataxia?

Harrison's 20th Ed. Chapter 431, Page 3156

A. Spinocerebellar ataxia 1
B. Spinocerebellar ataxia 2
C. Spinocerebellar ataxia 3
D. Spinocerebellar ataxia 6

In most populations, Machado-Joseph Disease (MJD) or spinocerebellar ataxias 3 is the most common autosomal dominant ataxia.

1865. Amyotrophic lateral sclerosis - parkinsonism - dystonia type presentation is in which clinical type of MJD?

Harrison's 20th Ed. Chapter 431, Page 3156

A. Type I MJD
B. Type II MJD
C. Type III MJD
D. None of the above

1866. Ataxic type presentation is seen in which type of MJD?

Harrison's 20th Ed. Chapter 431, Page 3156

A. Type I MJD
B. Type II MJD
C. Type III MJD
D. None of the above

1867. Ataxic-amyotrophic type presentation is seen in which clinical type of MJD?

Harrison's 20th Ed. Chapter 431, Page 3156

A. Type I MJD
B. Type II MJD
C. Type III MJD
D. None of the above

1868. Which is the most common clinical type of MJD?

Harrison's 20th Ed. Chapter 431, Page 3156

A. Type I MJD
B. Type II MJD
C. Type III MJD
D. All of the above

MJD is of three clinical types. Type I MJD - amyotrophic lateral sclerosis–parkinsonism–dystonia type), type II MJD - ataxic type, Type III MJD - ataxic-amyotrophic type. Type II is the most common form of MJD.

1869. The mean age of onset of symptoms in MJD is?

Harrison's 20th Ed. Chapter 431, Page 3156

A. 5 years
B. 10 years
C. 15 years
D. 25 years

The mean age of onset of symptoms in MJD is 25 years.

1870. Patients retain full intellectual function in which clinical type of MJD?

Harrison's 20th Ed. Chapter 431, Page 3156

A. Type I MJD
B. Type II MJD
C. Type III MJD
D. All of the above

Usually, MJD patients retain full intellectual function.

1871. Which of the following is spared in Machado-Joseph Disease (MJD)?

Harrison's 20th Ed. Chapter 431, Page 3156

A. Inferior olives
B. Corpus striatum
C. Pars compacta of substantia nigra
D. Dentate nucleus of cerebellum

Sparing of the inferior olives distinguishes MJD from other dominantly inherited ataxias.

1872. Which of the following spinocerebellar ataxias (SCAs) has pure cerebellar presentation?

Harrison's 20th Ed. Chapter 431, Page 3156

A. SCA1
B. SCA2
C. SCA3
D. SCA5

SCA5 (autosomal dominant type 5) maps to chromosome 11 & presentation includes ataxia & dysarthria.

1873. 'Retinal pigmentary degeneration' occurs in which of the following spinocerebellar ataxias (SCAs)?

Harrison's 20th Ed. Chapter 431, Page 3156

A. SCA1
B. SCA2
C. Machado-Joseph disease
D. SCA7

SCA7 is distinguished from all other SCAs by the presence of retinal pigmentary degeneration.

1874. The color blindness in SCA7 is for which colour?

Harrison's 20th Ed. Chapter 431, Page 3156

A. Red-yellow
B. Green-yellow
C. Blue-yellow
D. Any of the above

In SCA7, visual abnormalities first appear as blue-yellow color blindness and proceed to frank visual loss with macular degeneration.

1875. Haw River syndrome relates to which of the following?
Harrison's 20th Ed. Chapter 431, Page 3156

A. Machado-Joseph disease
B. Dentatorubropallidoluysian atrophy (DRPLA)
C. Friedreich's ataxia
D. Episodic ataxia

Haw River Syndrome (HRS) is an autosomal dominant neurodegenerative disease that has affected five generations of an African-American family in rural North Carolina. It represents a unique spectrum of multiple system degenerations resembling Huntington's disease, spinocerebellar atrophy and dentatorubropallidoluysian atrophy (DRPLA), a neurodegenerative disease that is primarily reported in Japan. Cardinal features in adults are ataxia, choreoathetosis & dementia. Cardinal features in children are mental retardation, behavioral changes, myoclonus, and epilepsy. ATN1 (DRPLA) is the only gene associated with DRPLA.

1876. Gene related to dentatorubropallidoluysian atrophy is?
Harrison's 20th Ed. Chapter 431, Page 3156

A. Dentatin
B. Quadrupin
C. Simplin
D. Atrophin

DRPLA is due to unstable CAG triplet repeats in the open reading frame of a gene "atrophin" located on chromosome 12p12-ter.

1877. Which of the following spinocerebellar ataxias (SCAs) has presentation similar to Huntington disease (HD)?
Harrison's 20th Ed. Chapter 431, Page 3156

A. SCA1
B. SCA2
C. SCA3
D. SCA17

SCAs & HD show broad phenotypic overlap including ataxia, spasticity, Parkinsonian features, dystonia, chorea, dementia & mood disorders. Later three symptoms in a hereditary context should favor a genetic test for HD. Similar phenotypes have been observed in SCA17.

1878. Episodic ataxia episodes are precipitated by?
Harrison's 20th Ed. Chapter 431, Page 3156

A. Hunger
B. Exercise
C. Sleep
D. Meals

Episodes of ataxia in EA 1 & 2, with gait imbalance & slurring of speech, occur spontaneously or are precipitated by sudden movement, excitement, stress, exercise, or excessive fatigue.

1879. Myokymia best relates to which of the following?
Harrison's 20th Ed. Chapter 431, Page 3156

A. Impaired muscle relaxation
B. Groups of fasciculations
C. Prolonged muscle contraction
D. Localized muscle pain

Myokymia refers to groups of fasciculations associated with continuous undulations of muscle.

1880. In episodic ataxia, symptoms and episodic attacks of ataxia responsive to?
Harrison's 20th Ed. Chapter 431, Page 3156

A. Lithium
B. Atypical antipsychotic drugs
C. Acetazolamide
D. Electroconvulsive therapy (ECT)

Symptoms & episodic attacks of episodic ataxia type 1 & 2 are responsive to acetazolamide (AZM) or anticonvulsants.

1881. Which of the following is not a potassium ion channelopathy?
J Neurol Neurosurg Psychiatry 2015;0:1–12

A. Episodic ataxia-1
B. Episodic ataxia-2
C. Benign neonatal familial convulsions
D. Jervell & Lange-Nielsen syndrome

Episodic ataxia-2 is a calcium ion channelopathy.

1882. Which of the following is not a sodium ion channelo-pathy?
J Neurol Neurosurg Psychiatry 2015;0:1–12

A. Paramyotonia congenita
B. Hyperkalemic periodic paralysis
C. Hypokalemic periodic paralysis
D. Generalized epilepsy with febrile convulsions plus

1883. Which of the following is not a calcium ion channelopathy?
J Neurol Neurosurg Psychiatry 2015;0:1–12

A. Episodic ataxia-2
B. Spinocerebellar ataxia-6
C. Familial hemiplegic migraine
D. Autosomal dominant progressive deafness

1884. Neurologic genetic disorders inherited in Mendelian autosomal dominant mutations include all except?
http://omim.org/

A. Huntington's disease (HD)
B. Familial Alzheimer's disease
C. Amyotrophic lateral sclerosis (ALS)
D. Friedreich's ataxia (FA)

1885. Neurologic genetic disorders inherited in Mendelian autosomal dominant mutations include all except?
http://omim.org/

A. Dystrophia myotonica (DM)
B. Ataxia telangiectasia
C. Charcot-Marie-Tooth disease 1A (CMT 1A)
D. Familial hyperkalemic periodic paralysis (HYPP)

1886. Neurologic genetic disorders inherited in Mendelian autosomal dominant mutations include all except?
http://omim.org/

A. Spinocerebellar ataxia (SCA)
B. Tuberous sclerosis
C. Wilson's disease
D. Charcot-Marie-Tooth disease 1A (CMT 1A)

1887. Neurologic genetic disorders inherited as Mendelian autosomal recessive include all except?
http://omim.org/

A. Friedreich's ataxia (FA)
B. Wilson's disease
C. Tuberous sclerosis
D. Ataxia telangiectasia

1888. Neurologic genetic disorders inherited as X-linked recessive traits include all except?

http://omim.org/

A. Duchenne muscular dystrophy (DMD)
B. Spinobulbar muscular atrophy (SBMA)
C. Fragile X syndrome
D. Friedreich's ataxia (FA)

1889. What was the nationality of Nicholaus Friedreich, after whom Friedreich's ataxia has been named?

A. British
B. French
C. German
D. Spanish

Friedreich's ataxia is named after the German physician Nicholaus Friedreich, who first described the condition in 1860s.

1890. Most common form of inherited ataxia is?

Harrison's 20th Ed. Chapter 431, Page 3157

A. Machado-Joseph Disease (MJD)
B. Friedreich's ataxia
C. Dentatorubropallidoluysian atrophy (DRPLA)
D. Episodic ataxia

Friedreich's Ataxia is the most common form of inherited ataxia, comprising half of all hereditary ataxias.

1891. Primary site of pathology in Friedreich's ataxia is?

Harrison's 20th Ed. Chapter 431, Page 3157

A. Spinal cord
B. Dorsal root ganglion cells
C. Peripheral nerves
D. All of the above

Primary pathology in Friedreich's ataxia is in spinal cord (sclerosis and degeneration in spinocerebellar tracts, lateral corticospinal tracts and posterior columns), dorsal root ganglion cells and peripheral nerves (loss of large myelinated fibers).

1892. Which of the following about Friedreich's ataxia is false?

Harrison's 20th Ed. Chapter 431, Page 3157

A. Presents before 25 years of age
B. Lower extremities more severely involved than upper
C. Flexor plantar responses
D. Absence of deep tendon reflexes

Friedreich's ataxia presents before 25 years of age. Lower extremities are more severely involved than upper. Extensor plantar responses (with normal tone in trunk & extremities), absence of deep tendon reflexes are found. Loss of vibratory & proprioceptive sensation occurs.

1893. Which of the following about Friedreich's ataxia is false?

Harrison's 20th Ed. Chapter 431, Page 3157

A. Cardiac involvement occurs in 90% of patients
B. High incidence of diabetes mellitus
C. Severe mental retardation
D. Musculoskeletal deformities are common

1894. Musculoskeletal deformities in Friedreich's ataxia are?

Harrison's 20th Ed. Chapter 431, Page 3157

A. Pes cavus
B. Pes equinovarus
C. Scoliosis
D. All of the above

Cardiomegaly, symmetric hypertrophy, murmurs & conduction defects reported in ~90% of patients. Diabetes mellitus is found in 20%. Pes cavus, pes equinovarus and progressive scoliosis common. Mental retardation is uncommon.

1895. Which of the following is a presentation of Friedreich's ataxia?

Harrison's 20th Ed. Chapter 431, Page 3157

A. Progressive staggering gait
B. Frequent falling
C. Titubation
D. All of the above

Friedreich's ataxia presents with progressive staggering gait, frequent falling and titubation. Dysarthria may be the presenting symptom. Progressive scoliosis, foot deformity, nystagmus or cardiopathy is the initial sign at times.

1896. Which of the following is a finding in Friedreich's ataxia?

Harrison's 20th Ed. Chapter 431, Page 3157

A. Nystagmus & loss of fast saccadic eye movements
B. Truncal titubation
C. Dysmetria and ataxia of trunk & limb movements
D. All of the above

Neurologic examination in Friedreich's ataxia may show nystagmus, loss of fast saccadic eye movements, truncal titubation, dysarthria, dysmetria, and ataxia of trunk & limb movements.

1897. The median age of death in Friedreich's ataxia is?

Harrison's 20th Ed. Chapter 431, Page 3157

A. 25 years
B. 35 years
C. 45 years
D. 55 years

The median age of death in Friedreich's ataxia is 35 years.

1898. In Friedreich's ataxia, sclerosis & degeneration occur in?

Harrison's 20th Ed. Chapter 431, Page 3157

A. Spinocerebellar tracts
B. Lateral corticospinal tracts
C. Posterior columns
D. All of the above

1899. In Friedreich's ataxia, which of the following is most extensively involved?

Harrison's 20th Ed. Chapter 431, Page 3157

A. Cerebral cortex
B. Peripheral nerves
C. Dorsal root ganglion cells
D. Cerebellum

The peripheral nerves are extensively involved in Friedreich's ataxia, with loss of large myelinated fibers.

1900. Which of the following is a large-fiber sensory neuropathy?

Harrison's 20th Ed. Chapter 431, Page 3157

A. Friedreich's ataxia
B. Lepromatous leprosy
C. Diabetes mellitus
D. Antiretroviral therapy neuropathy

1901. Which of the following diseases is due to genetic abnormalities of DNA mismatch/repair?

Harrison's 20th Ed. Chapter 431, Page 3350

A. Bloom's syndrome
B. Ataxia telangiectasia
C. Hereditary nonpolyposis colon cancer (HNPCC)
D. All of the above

Genetic abnormalities of DNA mismatch/repair include xeroderma pigmentosum, Bloom's syndrome, ataxia telangiectasia, and hereditary nonpolyposis colon cancer (HNPCC). They strongly predispose to neoplasia because of the rapid acquisition of additional mutations.

1902. Classic form of Friedreich's ataxia is mapped to chromosome?

Harrison's 20th Ed. Chapter 431, Page 3157

A. 4
B. 5
C. 6
D. 9

Friedreich's ataxia is an autosomal recessive congenital ataxia and is caused by a mutation in gene FXN (formerly known as X25) that codes for frataxin, located on chromosome 9q13-q21.1.

1903. Genes for which of the following are on chromosome 9?

Harrison's 20th Ed. Chapter 431, Page 3157

A. ABL oncogene
B. JAK2 gene
C. C9ORF72
D. All of the above

1904. Mutant gene in classic form of Friedreich's ataxia is?

Harrison's 20th Ed. Chapter 431, Page 3157

A. Frataxin
B. Ataxin 1
C. Ataxin 2
D. All of the above

The classic form of Friedreich's ataxia is mapped to 9q13-q21.1. Mutant gene frataxin contains expanded GAA triplet repeats in the first intron. Because the defect is located on an intron (which is removed from the mRNA transcript between transcription and translation), this mutation does not result in the production of abnormal frataxin proteins. Instead, the mutation causes gene silencing (i.e., the mutation decreases the transcription of the gene) through induction of a heterochromatin structure. In Friedreich's ataxia, patients have 200 - 900 GAA repeats (normal 7–22). Altered protein is called frataxin.

1905. Which of the following about Friedreich's ataxia is false?

Harrison's 20th Ed. Chapter 431, Page 3157

A. Frataxin is a mitochondrial protein for iron homeostasis
B. Excess oxidized intramitochondrial iron
C. Iron chelators and antioxidants are potentially harmful
D. None of the above

Frataxin mRNA and frataxin protein are low in Friedreich's ataxia. Frataxin is a mitochondrial protein involved in iron homeostasis. Mitochondrial iron accumulation due to loss of the iron transporter coded by the mutant frataxin gene results in oxidized intramitochondrial iron resulting in oxidation of cellular components & irreversible cell injury. Iron chelators and antioxidants are potentially harmful.

1906. Which of the following MRI finding is typical of Friedreich's ataxia?

Harrison's 20th Ed. Chapter 431, Page 3157

A. Brainstem atrophy
B. Cerebellar artophy
C. Spinal cord atrophy
D. Obstructive hydrocephalus

Neuroimaging reveals thinning of the cervical spinal cord.

1907. Which of the following drugs is of use in Friedreich's ataxia?

Harrison's 20th Ed. Chapter 431, Page 3158

A. Desferrioxamine
B. Idebenone
C. Ascorbic acid
D. All of the above

Idebenone, a short-chain analogue of coenzyme Q10 and a free-radical scavenger, can improve myocardial hypertrophy when used at an early stage reduces progression of cerebellar manifestation.

1908. Which of the following is a feature of Bassen-Kornzweig syndrome?

Harrison's 20th Ed. Chapter 431, Page 3157

A. Diabetes mellitus
B. Cardiomyopathy
C. Abetalipoproteinemia
D. Hypothyroidism

Bassen-Kornzweig syndrome is an autosomal recessive disorder in which a person is unable to fully absorb dietary fats through intestines. It is caused by a defect in microsomal triglyceride transfer protein (MTP) gene. Defects in MTP result in impairment of formation and secretion of VLDL in liver (abetalipoproteinemia). This defect results in a deficiency of delivery of vitamin E to tissues, including the central & peripheral nervous system, as VLDL is the transport molecule for vitamin E.

1909. Which of the following is false regarding ataxia with vitamin E deficiency (AVED)?

Harrison's 20th Ed. Chapter 431, Page 3157

A. Due to mutations in gene for a tocopherol transfer protein
B. Autosomal recessive
C. Chromosomal localization is on 8q13
D. None of the above

AVED is due to mutations in the gene for alpha-tocopherol transfer protein (a TTP). These patients have an impaired ability to bind vitamin E into the VLDL produced and secreted by the liver, resulting in a deficiency of vitamin E in peripheral tissues.

1910. Ataxia Telangiectasia is also known as?

Neurology. 2018;91(4):175-179

A. Louis-Bar syndrome
B. Nijmegen breakage syndrome (NBS1)
C. Lou Gehrig's disease
D. Pott's disease

Other names for ataxia-telangiectasia are A-T, Ataxia Telangiectasia Syndrome, ATM, Louis-Bar syndrome, Telangiectasia, cerebello-oculocutaneous.

1911. Gene responsible for Ataxia Telangiectasia is found on which chromosome?

Harrison's 20th Ed. Chapter 431, Page 3157

A. Chromosome 11
B. Chromosome 12
C. Chromosome 13
D. Chromosome 14

Ataxia Telangiectasia is inherited as an autosomal recessive disorder and offending gene is found on the long arm of chromosome 11 at 11q22-23. It controls the production of a phosphatidylinositol-3-kinase-like enzyme involved in cellular responses to stress, DNA damage and cell cycle control.

1912. Full name of ATM - the gene for Ataxia Telangiectasia is?
Harrison's 20th Ed. Chapter 68, Page 462

A. Ataxia-telangiectasia mutated kinase
B. Ataxia-telangiectasia manifested kinase
C. Ataxia-telangiectasia morphed kinase
D. Ataxia-telangiectasia magnified kinase

Ataxia-telangiectasia gene - ATM is on chromosome 11 and ATM stands for ataxia-telangiectasia mutated kinase. ATM encodes a protein that is predominantly confined to nucleus of cells and that remains constant throughout all stages of the cell cycle and participate in cell's responses to genomic damage. ATM gene is homologous to genes involved in DNA repair & control of cell cycle checkpoints. Mutations in the ATM gene give rise to defects in meiosis as well as increasing susceptibility to damage from ionizing radiation.

1913. ATM (ataxia-telangiectasia) carries an increased risk of?
Harrison's 20th Ed. Chapter 431, Page 3157

A. Breast cancer
B. Lymphoma
C. Acute T cell leukemias
D. All of the above

ATM (ataxia-telangiectasia) gene carries an increased risk of breast cancer, lymphoma and pancreatic cancer and there is an increased incidence of lymphomas, Hodgkin's disease, acute T cell leukemias, and breast cancer.

1914. A variant of AT - AT-like disease is caused by mutation in?
Harrison's 20th Ed. Chapter 344, Page 2494

A. IKBKAP gene
B. MRE11 gene
C. TRK-fused gene (TFG)
D. Serine palmitoyltransferase long-chain base 1 (SPTLC1) gene

1915. Inherited disease with defective DNA repair is?
Harrison's 20th Ed. Chapter 100, Page 740

A. Fanconi anemia
B. Bloom syndrome
C. Ataxia telangiectasia
D. All of the above

Inherited diseases with defective DNA repair are Fanconi anemia, Bloom syndrome and ataxia telangiectasia. They are also associated with AML.

1916. Mutation of which of the following gene causes a variant of AT (AT-like disease)?
Harrison's 20th Ed. Chapter 344, Page 2494

A. SBDS
B. MRE11
C. CHD7
D. STAT5b

A variant of AT (AT-like disease) is caused by mutation of the MRE11 gene.

1917. AT causes which of the following?
Harrison's 20th Ed. Chapter 344, Page 2494

A. Low IgA
B. IgG2 deficiency
C. Low antibody production
D. All of the above

AT causes a B cell immunodeficiency (low IgA, IgG2 deficiency, and low antibody production) that often requires immunoglobulin replacement therapy. Also, AT is associated with a progressive T cell immunodeficiency.

1918. Which of the following is false about Ataxia Telangiectasia?
Harrison's 20th Ed. Chapter 431, Page 3157

A. Present in first decade of life
B. Progressive telangiectatic lesions with deficits in cerebellar function & nystagmus
C. High incidence of recurrent pulmonary infections and neoplasms of lymphatic and reticuloendothelial system
D. None of the above

1919. In Ataxia Telangiectasia (AT), the most consistent defect of the lymphoid system is?
Harrison's 20th Ed. Chapter 431, Page 3157

A. Poorly developed or absent thymus gland
B. Generalised lymphadenopathy
C. Splenomegaly
D. Lymphedema

Poorly developed or absent thymus gland is the most consistent defect of the lymphoid system.

1920. Telangiectasia in Ataxia telangiectasia usually occur on?
Harrison's 20th Ed. Chapter 431, Page 3157

A. Bulbar conjunctiva
B. Nail bed
C. Intracranial
D. All of the above

Telangiectasia in AT usually occur on the white portion of eye (bulbar conjunctiva) but may also be found on the ears, neck and extremities.

1921. Neurologic manifestation in AT is?
Harrison's 20th Ed. Chapter 431, Page 3157

A. Truncal and limb ataxia
B. Extensor plantar responses & areflexia
C. Myoclonic jerks
D. All of the above

1922. Neuropathologic change seen in ataxia telangiectasia is?
Harrison's 20th Ed. Chapter 431, Page 3157

A. Loss of Purkinje, granule & basket cells in cerebellar cortex and loss of neurons in the deep cerebellar nuclei
B. Loss of anterior horn neurons in spinal cord
C. Loss of dorsal root ganglion cells
D. All of the above

The most striking neuropathologic change in AT is loss of Purkinje, granule, and basket cells in cerebellar cortex as well as of neurons in the deep cerebellar nuclei.

1923. Which of the following laboratory tests is useful in the diagnosis of Ataxia Telangiectasia?
Harrison's 20th Ed. Chapter 431, Page 3157

A. Cryofibrinogen
B. Ceruloplasmin level in blood
C. Alpha-fetoprotein level in blood
D. Apolipoprotein A-1

Alpha-fetoprotein levels in the blood are elevated (> 10 ng/ml) in >95% of patients of AT. AFP is produced only during fetal development. Immunoglobulin deficiency is noted.

1924. Which of the following statements about Ataxia-telangiectasia is false?

Harrison's 20th Ed. Chapter 431, Page 3157

A. Affected child has normal intelligence

B. Hypersensitivity to ionizing radiation

C. Predisposition to malignancy

D. None of the above

AT causes large telangiectatic lesions of face, cerebellar ataxia, immunologic defects & hypersensitivity to ionizing radiation. Affected child has normal or above normal intelligence. Insulin-resistant diabetes mellitus associated with anti-insulin antibodies occurs in patients with ataxia-telangiectasia.

1925. Hereditary forms of mitochondrial cytopathies include?

Harrison's 20th Ed. Chapter 431, Page 3251

A. Kearns-Sayre syndrome

B. Myoclonus epilepsy with ragged red fibers (MERRF)

C. Mitochondrial encephalopathy with lactic acidosis and stroke-like episodes (MELAS)

D. All of the above

Since mtDNA is transmitted exclusively by the mother, mitochondrial cytopathies show maternal inheritance and can be excluded when paternal transmission of the disease occurs in the family.

Disorders of the Autonomic Nervous System

1926. Autonomic nervous system (ANS) regulates which of the following?

Harrison's 20th Ed. Chapter 432, Page 3158

A. Sleep function
B. Glandular function
C. Pupillary function
D. All of the above

Autonomic nervous system (ANS) innervates the entire neuraxis & influences all organ systems. It regulates blood pressure, heart rate, sleep, glandular, pupillary, bladder & bowel function.

1927. Connections between cerebral cortex and autonomic centers occurs in?

Harrison's 20th Ed. Chapter 432, Page 3158

A. Cerebral cortex
B. Brainstem
C. Spinal cord
D. All of the above

Connections between cerebral cortex & autonomic centers in brainstem coordinate autonomic outflow with higher mental functions.

1928. Preganglionic neurons of parasympathetic nervous system leave the central nervous system in all except?

Harrison's 20th Ed. Chapter 432, Page 3158

A. Third cranial nerve
B. Sixth cranial nerve
C. Seventh cranial nerve
D. Tenth cranial nerve

1929. Preganglionic neurons of parasympathetic nervous system leave the central nervous system in all except?

Harrison's 20th Ed. Chapter 432, Page 3158

A. Tenth cranial nerve
B. Eleventh cranial nerve
C. Second sacral nerve
D. Third sacral nerve

Preganglionic neurons of PNS leave CNS in third, seventh, ninth & tenth cranial nerves as well as the second & third sacral nerves.

1930. Preganglionic neurons of sympathetic nervous system exit the spinal cord between?

Harrison's 20th Ed. Chapter 432, Page 3158

A. T1 and L1 segments
B. T1 and L2 segments
C. T1 and L3 segments
D. T1 and L4 segments

Preganglionic neurons of sympathetic nervous system exit spinal cord between first thoracic and the second lumbar segments.

1931. Acetylcholine is the neurotransmitter for all except?

Harrison's 20th Ed. Chapter 432, Page 3158

A. Preganglionic parasympathetic ANS
B. Preganglionic sympathetic ANS
C. Postganglionic parasympathetic ANS
D. Postganglionic sympathetic ANS

1932. Norepinephrine (NE) is the neurotransmitter for?

Harrison's 20th Ed. Chapter 432, Page 3158

A. Preganglionic parasympathetic ANS
B. Preganglionic sympathetic ANS
C. Postganglionic parasympathetic ANS
D. Postganglionic sympathetic ANS

Acetylcholine (ACh) is the preganglionic neurotransmitter for both divisions of ANS as well as postganglionic neurotransmitter of parasympathetic neurons. Norepinephrine (NE) is the neurotransmitter of postganglionic sympathetic neurons, except for cholinergic neurons innervating eccrine sweat glands.

1933. Which of the following statements is false?

Harrison's 20th Ed. Chapter 432, Page 3158

A. Autonomic preganglionic fibers are thinly myelinated
B. Postganglionic neurons (outside CNS) give rise to postganglionic unmyelinated autonomic nerves
C. Responses to sympathetic & parasympathetic stimulation are antagonistic
D. None of the above

1934. With sympathetic activation, which of the following does not occur?

Harrison's 20th Ed. Chapter 432, Page 3159 Table 432-1

A. Increased bowel motility
B. Increased bladder sphincter tone
C. Sweating
D. Ejaculation, orgasm

1935. With parasympathetic activation, which of the following does not occur?

Harrison's 20th Ed. Chapter 432, Page 3159 Table 432-1

A. Increased bowel motility
B. Penile erection
C. Tearing
D. Sweating

1936. Which of the following is regulated by autonomic circuits?

Harrison's 20th Ed. Chapter 432, Page 3158

A. Sleep
B. Pupils
C. Bowel & bladder function
D. All of the above

1937. Which of the following is part of enteric nervous system?

Harrison's 20th Ed. Chapter 432, Page 3159

A. Meissner's plexus
B. Auerbach's plexus
C. Cajal's plexus
D. All of the above

1938. Which of the following about enteric nervous system is false?
Harrison's 20th Ed. Chapter 432, Page 3159

A. Parasympathetic control of GI system is by craniospinal nerves
B. Sympathetic control of GI system is by thoracolumbar region
C. Number of enteric nervous system cells almost equal number of cells in spinal cord
D. None of the above

Parasympathetic control of GI system is by craniospinal nerves (vagus & S2-S4 nerves). Sympathetic control is by thoracolumbar region. Enteric nervous system comprises of Meissner's (submucosal), Auerbach's (myenteric), Cajal's (deep muscular), mucosal & submucosal plexuses.

1939. Most consistent & severe orthostatic hypotension (OH) is caused by lesion in?
Harrison's 20th Ed. Chapter 432, Page 3159

A. Lesions of the afferent limb of baroreflex arc
B. Lesions of the CNS processing centers
C. Lesions of the efferent limb of reflex arcs
D. All of the above

1940. OH is defined as, within 3 minutes of standing up, a sustained drop in SBP and DBP of?
Harrison's 20th Ed. Chapter 432, Page 3159

A. ≥ 20 and ≥ 20 mm Hg respectively
B. ≥ 20 and ≥ 10 mm Hg respectively
C. ≥ 10 and ≥ 10 mm Hg respectively
D. ≥ 10 and ≥ 5 mm Hg respectively

OH is defined as a sustained drop in systolic (≥20 mm Hg) or diastolic (≥10 mm Hg) BP within three minutes of standing.

1941. Which of the following statements about autonomic control of urinary bladder is false?
Harrison's 20th Ed. Chapter 432, Page 3159

A. Upper motor neuron lesion leads to spastic bladder
B. Lower motor neuron lesion leads to flaccid bladder
C. Bladder volume is a useful test for distinguishing between UMN and LMN bladder dysfunction
D. None of the above

Brain & spinal cord disease above lumbar level results in UMN or spastic bladder. PNS disease results in LMN flaccid bladder (large volumes, urinary frequency & overflow incontinence). Measurement of post-void residual bladder volume is useful test to distinguish between UMN & LMN bladder dysfunction.

1942. Most disabling feature of autonomic dysfunction is?
Harrison's 20th Ed. Chapter 432, Page 3160

A. Orthostatic or postural hypotension
B. Progressively severe constipation
C. Loss of sweat function
D. Impotence

When orthostatic or postural hypotension (OH) is specifically due to dysfunction of ANS, it is referred to as neurogenic OH.

1943. OH can cause which of the following symptom?
Harrison's 20th Ed. Chapter 432, Page 3160

A. Diaphoresis
B. Diminished hearing
C. Shortness of breath
D. All of the above

Symptom spectrum of OH is wide. It includes dimming or loss of vision, light headedness, diaphoresis, diminished hearing, pallor, weakness and shortness of breath.

1944. OH can cause which of the following?
Harrison's 20th Ed. Chapter 432, Page 3160

A. Heart rate that is fixed regardless of posture
B. Postprandial hypotension
C. Excessively high nocturnal BP
D. All of the above

Manifestations of impaired baroreflexes are supine hypertension, a heart rate that is fixed regardless of posture, postprandial hypotension, and an excessively high nocturnal BP.

1945. Which of the following statements about OH is false?
Harrison's 20th Ed. Chapter 432, Page 3161

A. Most common causes of OH are not neurologic in origin
B. Neurogenic OH is aggravated/precipitated by autonomic stressors
C. In non-neurogenic OH, BP drop is leads to a compensatory increase in heart rate of >15 beats/minute.
D. None of the above

1946. Which of the following is an autonomic stressor?
Harrison's 20th Ed. Chapter 432, Page 3161

A. Meal
B. Hot bath
C. Exercise
D. All of the above

Autonomic stressors are a meal, hot bath or exercise. Lack of sweating after a hot bath, during exercise, or on a hot day can suggest sudomotor failure.

1947. Drugs that can cause Orthostatic hypotension (OH) include all except?
Harrison's 20th Ed. Chapter 432, Page 3161

A. Diuretics
B. Phenothiazines
C. Beta adrenergic blockers
D. Calcium channel blockers

1948. Drugs that can cause Orthostatic hypotension (OH) include all except?
Harrison's 20th Ed. Chapter 432, Page 3161

A. Insulin
B. Glucagon
C. Barbiturates
D. Ethanol

Drugs that may cause OH are diuretics, antihypertensives, antidepressants, phenothiazines, ethanol, narcotics, insulin, dopamine agonists, barbiturates & calcium channel blocking agents.

1949. Disorders of autonomic function should be considered in patients with which of the following symptom?
Harrison's 20th Ed. Chapter 432, Page 3161

A. Altered sweating
B. Gastroparesis
C. Impotence
D. All of the above

Disorders of autonomic function should be considered in patients with altered sweating (hyperhidrosis or hypohidrosis), gastroparesis (bloating, nausea, vomiting of old food), impotence, constipation or bladder disturbances (urinary frequency, hesitancy or incontinence).

1950. Which of the following is a non-neurogenic cause of OH?
Harrison's 20th Ed. Chapter 432, Page 3161

A. Constipation
B. Hypovolemia
C. Urinary incontinence
D. All of the above

Hypovolemia is a non-neurogenic cause of OH.

1951. Heart rate variation with deep breathing (respiratory sinus arrhythmia) is abolished by administration of?
Harrison's 20th Ed. Chapter 432, Page 3162

A. Atropine
B. Digoxin
C. Beta blockers
D. All of the above

HRDB or Heart rate variation with deep breathing (respiratory sinus arrhythmia) is abolished by atropine but is unaffected by sympathetic blockade (propranolol).

1952. Valsalva response is tested in which position?
Harrison's 20th Ed. Chapter 432, Page 3162

A. Supine
B. Sitting
C. Standing
D. Any of the above

Valsalva response is tested in the supine position.

1953. In Valsalva maneuver, a constant expiratory pressure of how much is maintained for 15 seconds?
Harrison's 20th Ed. Chapter 432, Page 3162

A. 10 mm Hg
B. 20 mm Hg
C. 30 mm Hg
D. 40 mm Hg

Valsalva maneuver assesses the integrity of baroreflex control of heart rate (parasympathetic) & BP (adrenergic). With subject supine, a constant expiratory pressure of 40 mmHg is maintained for 15 seconds while measuring changes in heart rate and beat-to-beat BP.

1954. Fall in BP occurs in which phase of Valsalva maneuver?
Harrison's 20th Ed. Chapter 432, Page 3162

A. Phase I
B. Early phase II
C. Late phase II
D. All of the above

Out of four phases of Valsalva maneuver response, phases I & III are mechanical & related to changes in intrathoracic & intraabdominal pressure. In early phase II, reduced venous return results in a fall in stroke volume and BP, counteracted by a combination of reflex tachycardia and increased total peripheral resistance. Increased total peripheral resistance arrests the BP drop ~5–8 seconds after the onset of maneuver. Late phase II begins with a progressive rise in BP towards or above baseline. Venous return and cardiac output return to normal in phase IV. Persistent peripheral arteriolar vasoconstriction and increased cardiac adrenergic tone results in a temporary BP overshoot and phase IV bradycardia (mediated by baroreceptor reflex).

1955. The 'Valsalva ratio' is defined as?
Harrison's 20th Ed. Chapter 432, Page 3162

A. Maximum phase 1 tachycardia divided by minimum phase 4 bradycardia
B. Maximum phase 2 tachycardia divided by minimum phase 4 bradycardia
C. Maximum phase 3 tachycardia divided by minimum phase 4 bradycardia
D. Maximum phase 4 tachycardia divided by minimum phase 4 bradycardia

Autonomic function during the Valsalva maneuver can be measured using beat-to-beat blood pressure or heart rate changes. Valsalva ratio is defined as the maximum phase II tachycardia divided by minimum phase IV bradycardia. The ratio reflects cardiovagal function.

1956. Sweating is induced by release of acetylcholine from?
Harrison's 20th Ed. Chapter 432, Page 3162

A. Preganglionic parasympathetic ANS
B. Preganglionic sympathetic ANS
C. Postganglionic parasympathetic ANS
D. Postganglionic sympathetic ANS

Sweating is induced by release of acetylcholine (ACh) from sympathetic postganglionic fibers.

1957. Which of the following is a test for sweating?
Harrison's 20th Ed. Chapter 432, Page 3162

A. Quantitative sudomotor axon reflex test (QSART)
B. Thermoregulatory sweat test (TST)
C. Measurement of galvanic skin responses
D. All of the above

1958. A reduced or absent response in 'Quantitative sudomotor axon reflex test (QSART)' indicates?
Harrison's 20th Ed. Chapter 432, Page 3162

A. Lesion of preganglionic sudomotor axon
B. Lesion of postganglionic sudomotor axon
C. Lesion of pre & postganglionic sudomotor axon
D. None of the above

A reduced or absent response indicates a lesion of the postganglionic sudomotor axon.

1959. If both QSART and TST are absent, the lesion is in?
Harrison's 20th Ed. Chapter 432, Page 3162

A. Preganglionic sudomotor axon
B. Postganglionic sudomotor axon
C. Pre & postganglionic sudomotor axon
D. None of the above

A postganglionic lesion is present if both QSART and TST show absent sweating.

1960. If QSART is intact but TST shows anhidrosis, lesion is in?
Harrison's 20th Ed. Chapter 432, Page 3162

A. Preganglionic sudomotor axon
B. Postganglionic sudomotor axon
C. Pre & postganglionic sudomotor axon
D. None of the above

In a preganglionic lesion, QSART is intact but TST shows anhidrosis.

1961. Which of the following is a primary autonomic degenerative disorder?
Harrison's 20th Ed. Chapter 432, Page 126

A. Multiple system atrophy
B. Parkinson's disease
C. Dementia with Lewy bodies
D. All of the above

Primary autonomic degenerative disorders are multiple system atrophy (Shy-Drager syndrome), Parkinson's disease, dementia with Lewy bodies and pure autonomic failure. These are grouped together as "synucleinopathies" due to the presence of alpha-synuclein, a small protein that precipitates predominantly in the cytoplasm of neurons in the Lewy body disorders (Parkinson's disease, dementia with Lewy bodies and pure autonomic failure) and in the glia in multiple system atrophy.

1962. Which of the following is a small-fiber peripheral neuropathy?

Harrison's 20th Ed. Chapter 432, Page 126

A. Diabetes mellitus
B. Amyloid
C. Hereditary sensory and autonomic neuropathies (HSAN)
D. All of the above

Small-fiber peripheral neuropathies are those seen in diabetes mellitus, amyloid, immune-mediated neuropathies, hereditary sensory and autonomic neuropathies (HSAN; particularly HSAN type III, familial dysautonomia).

1963. Multiple system atrophy (MSA) relates best to which of the following?

Harrison's 20th Ed. Chapter 432, Page 3162

A. Horner's syndrome
B. Wernicke-Korsakoff syndrome
C. Shy-Drager syndrome
D. Shapiro's syndrome

Multiple system atrophy (MSA) comprises of autonomic failure (OH and/or a neurogenic bladder) combined with either striatonigral degeneration (Shy-Drager syndrome) or sporadic olivopontocerebellar atrophy.

1964. Parkinsonism seen in multiple system atrophy features which of the following?

Harrison's 20th Ed. Chapter 432, Page 3163

A. No rest tremor
B. Not responsive to levodopa
C. Levodopa-induced dyskinesia uncommon
D. All of the above

1965. Autonomic dysfunction is a common feature in?

Harrison's 20th Ed. Chapter 432, Page 3163

A. Dementia with Lewy bodies (DLB)
B. Multiple system atrophy (MSA)
C. Parkinson's disease
D. All of the above

Autonomic dysfunction is a feature in dementia with Lewy bodies, MSA & Parkinson's disease.

1966. Autonomic dysreflexia is common in patients with traumatic spinal cord lesion above which level?

Harrison's 20th Ed. Chapter 432, Page 3163

A. T3
B. T6
C. T12
D. L2

Markedly increased autonomic discharge or autonomic dysreflexia is common in patients with traumatic spinal cord lesion above the T6 level.

1967. Neuromuscular junction disorders accompanied by autonomic involvement include?

Harrison's 20th Ed. Chapter 432, Page 3163

A. Porphyria
B. Botulism
C. Chronic alcoholism
D. Guillain-Barré syndrome

Peripheral neuropathies as in diabetes mellitus, amyloidosis, chronic alcoholism, porphyria, and Guillain-Barré syndrome lead to chronic autonomic insufficiency. Neuromuscular junction disorders with autonomic involvement include botulism and Lambert-Eaton syndrome.

1968. Autonomic neuropathy typically begins how many years after the onset of diabetes mellitus?

Harrison's 20th Ed. Chapter 432, Page 3163

A. ~ 5
B. ~ 7
C. ~ 10
D. ~ 14

Autonomic neuropathy typically begins ~10 years after the onset of DM.

1969. Autonomic dysfunction occurs in which of the following porphyria?

Harrison's 20th Ed. Chapter 432, Page 3163

A. Acute intermittent porphyria
B. Variegate porphyria
C. Hereditary coproporphyria
D. All of the above

Autonomic dysfunction is most extensively documented in acute intermittent porphyria but can also occur with variegate porphyria and hereditary coproporphyria.

1970. Autoantibodies against which of the following is present in autoimmune autonomic ganglionopathy (AAG)?

Harrison's 20th Ed. Chapter 432, Page 3164

A. A_3 AChR
B. B_3 AChR
C. C_3 AChR
D. D_3 AChR

Autoantibodies against ganglionic ACh receptor (A_3 AChR) are present in the serum of patients of autoimmune autonomic ganglionopathy (AAG).

1971. Paraneoplastic AAG is associated with?

Harrison's 20th Ed. Chapter 432, Page 3164

A. Adenocarcinoma or small-cell carcinoma of lung
B. Lymphoma
C. Thymoma
D. All of the above

1972. Botulinum toxin blocks release of which of the following?

Harrison's 20th Ed. Chapter 432, Page 3164

A. Norepinephrine
B. Acetylcholine
C. Serotonin
D. All of the above

Botulinum toxin binds presynaptically to cholinergic nerve terminals and after uptake into cytosol blocks ACh release.

1973. Pure Autonomic Failure (PAF) consists of?

Harrison's 20th Ed. Chapter 432, Page 3164

A. Postural hypotension
B. Impotence & bladder dysfunction
C. Impaired sweating
D. All of the above

1974. Which of the following statements about Pure Autonomic Failure (PAF) is false?

Harrison's 20th Ed. Chapter 432, Page 3164

A. Involvement of postganglionic sympathetic neurons
B. Low supine plasma NE levels
C. Noradrenergic supersensitivity
D. None of the above

In Pure Autonomic Failure (PAF) there is primary involvement of postganglionic sympathetic neurons that results in low supine plasma NE levels & noradrenergic supersensitivity.

1975. Which of the following is false about Postural Orthostatic Tachycardia Syndrome (POTS)?

Harrison's 20th Ed. Chapter 432, Page 3164

A. Symptomatic orthostatic hypotension
B. Increase in heart rate of > 30 beats/min with standing
C. Women affected five times more often than men
D. Occurs between 15 and 50 years of age

POTS is characterized by symptomatic orthostatic intolerance (not OH) and by either an increase in heart rate to >120 beats/minute or an increase of 30 beats/minute with standing that subsides on sitting or lying down. Women are affected approximately five times more often than men, and most develop the syndrome between the ages of 15 and 50.

1976. Which of the following is a presyncopal symptom?

Harrison's 20th Ed. Chapter 432, Page 3164

A. Lightheadedness
B. Weakness
C. Blurred vision
D. All of the above

1977. Which of the following is a symptom of autonomic overactivity?

Harrison's 20th Ed. Chapter 432, Page 3164

A. Palpitations
B. Tremulousness
C. Nausea
D. All of the above

1978. Hereditary sensory and autonomic neuropathy I (HSAN I) is best related to which of the following?

Harrison's 20th Ed. Chapter 432, Page 3164

A. Dermatan sulfate
B. Sphingomyelin
C. Glucosyl ceramide
D. Heparan sulfate

SPTLC is an enzyme in the regulation of ceramide. Cells from HSAN I patients affected by mutation of SPTLC1 gene produce higher-than-normal levels of glucosyl ceramide triggering apoptosis.

1979. The defective gene in HSAN I is?

Harrison's 20th Ed. Chapter 432, Page 3164

A. SPTLC1
B. SPTLC2
C. SPTLC3
D. SPTLC4

SPTLC is a key enzyme in the regulation of ceramide. Most common responsible gene for HSAN I is SPTLC1 on chromosome 9q.

1980. The defective gene in HSAN III is?

Harrison's 20th Ed. Chapter 432, Page 3164

A. IKBKAP
B. SPTLC2
C. SPTLC3
D. SPTLC4

The defective gene in HSAN III (Riley-Day syndrome or familial dysautonomia) is IKBKAP.

1981. Cause of autonomic storm is?

Harrison's 20th Ed. Chapter 432, Page 3165

A. Brain and spinal cord injury
B. Autonomic neuropathy
C. Pheochromocytoma
D. All of the above

Acute autonomic syndrome may be either acute autonomic failure (acute AAN syndrome) or a state of sympathetic overactivity. Autonomic storm is an acute state of sustained sympathetic surge. Causes are brain & spinal cord injury, toxins & drugs, autonomic neuropathy, and pheochromocytoma.

1982. Which of the following is the most common cause of autonomic storm?

Harrison's 20th Ed. Chapter 432, Page 3165

A. Brain injury
B. Pheochromocytoma
C. Cocaine
D. Tetanus

Brain injury is the most common cause of autonomic storm and typically follows severe head trauma and postresuscitation encephalopathy anoxic-ischemic brain injury.

1983. Massive catecholaminergic surge in autonomic storm can cause which of the following?

Harrison's 20th Ed. Chapter 432, Page 3165

A. Seizures
B. Neurogenic pulmonary edema
C. Myocardial injury
D. All of the above

Massive catecholaminergic surge in autonomic storm can cause seizures, neurogenic pulmonary edema and myocardial injury.

1984. Drug that can produce autonomic storm is?

Harrison's 20th Ed. Chapter 432, Page 3165

A. Phenylpropanolamine
B. Cocaine
C. Amphetamine
D. All of the above

Drugs and toxins that can produce autonomic storm include phenylpropanolamine, cocaine, amphetamine & tricyclic antidepressants, tetanus and botulinum.

1985. Neuroleptic malignant syndrome is seen in psychotic patients treated with?

Harrison's 20th Ed. Chapter 432, Page 3165

A. Amphetamine
B. Phenylpropanolamine
C. Phenothiazine
D. Any of the above

1986. Which of the following is a feature of neuroleptic malignant syndrome?

Harrison's 20th Ed. Chapter 432, Page 3165

A. Muscle rigidity
B. Hyperthermia
C. Hypertension
D. All of the above

Neuroleptic malignant syndrome features muscle rigidity, hyperthermia & hypertension in psychotic patients treated with phenothiazines.

1987. Which of the following drug is effective in chronic and milder autonomic storm?

Harrison's 20th Ed. Chapter 432, Page 3165

A. Morphine sulphate
B. Labetalol
C. Clonidine
D. All of the above

For chronic and milder autonomic storm, propranolol and/or clonidine can be effective.

1988. Allodynia refers to?

Harrison's 20th Ed. Chapter 432, Page 3165

A. Perception of nonpainful stimulus as painful
B. Exaggerated pain response to a painful stimulus
C. Spontaneous pain
D. All of the above

Allodynia refers to the perception of a nonpainful stimulus as painful while hyperpathia refers to an exaggerated pain response to a painful stimulus.

1989. Which of the following must be present for the diagnosis of complex regional pain syndrome (CRPS)?

Harrison's 20th Ed. Chapter 432, Page 3165

A. Vasomotor dysfunction
B. Sudomotor abnormalities
C. Focal edema
D. Any of the above

Pain is the primary clinical feature of CRPS. Vasomotor dysfunction, sudomotor abnormalities, or focal edema may occur alone or in combination but must be present for diagnosis.

1990. CRPS type II develops after?

Harrison's 20th Ed. Chapter 432, Page 3165

A. Injury to a specific peripheral nerve
B. Myocardial infarction
C. Stroke
D. Limb injury

CRPS type I is a regional pain syndrome that usually develops after tissue trauma (myocardial infarction, minor shoulder or limb injury, stroke). CRPS type II is a regional pain syndrome that develops after injury to a specific peripheral nerve, usually a major nerve trunk.

1991. In the treatment of orthostatic hypotension, enough intake of salt & fluids should produce a urine voiding volume between?

Harrison's 20th Ed. Chapter 432, Page 3165

A. 0.5 & 1.0 Liters
B. 1.0 & 1.5 Liters
C. 1.5 & 2.5 Liters
D. 2.5 & 3.5 Liters

In the treatment of orthostatic hypotension, aim is to consume salt & fluids to produce a voiding volume between 1.5 and 2.5 liters of urine (containing > 170 meq/L of Na+) per day.

1992. Which of the following best relates to treatment of orthostatic hypotension?

Harrison's 20th Ed. Chapter 432, Page 3165

A. Modena treatment
B. Bouillon treatment
C. Mercuro treatment
D. Mancini treatment

Bouillon treatment refers to increasing intake of salt and fluids for transient worsening of OH.

1993. Which of the following drugs is useful in the treatment of orthostatic hypotension?

Harrison's 20th Ed. Chapter 432, Page 3165

A. Midodrine
B. Droxidopa
C. Pyridostigmine
D. All of the above

1994. Which of the following drugs is useful in the treatment of orthostatic hypotension?

Harrison's 20th Ed. Chapter 432, Page 3165

A. Fludrocortisone
B. Atomoxetine and yohimbine
C. Octreotide
D. All of the above

Atomoxetine blocks NE reuptake transporter and yohimbine blocks α2 receptors that mediate the sympathetic feedback loop for downregulation of BP in response to atomoxetine.

Trigeminal Neuralgia, Bell's Palsy, and Other Cranial Nerve Disorders

1995. Trigeminal neuralgia (TN) is also called?
Asian Pac. J. Health Sci., 2015;2(1):108-118

A. Prosopalgia
B. Fothergill's disease
C. Tic-douloureux
D. All of the above

Trigeminal neuralgia (TN) is also known as Tic Douloureux, Fothergill's Disease, Suicide Disease or Prosopalgia. John Fothergill (1712-1780) gave the first full & accurate description of trigeminal neuralgia in 1773. Early descriptions of trigeminal neuralgia (Fothergill's disease) can be found in the writings of Galen, Aretaeus of Cappadocia (born circa AD 81), and in the 11th century by Avicenna ("tortura oris").

1996. Which of the following about Trigeminal nerve is false?
Harrison's 20th Ed. Chapter 433, Page 3166

A. Trigeminal nerve is the largest of the cranial nerves.
B. Trigeminal nerve is predominantly sensory
C. Its motor innervation is exclusively in mandibular V3 division
D. None of the above

1997. Which of the following is best related to trigeminal ganglion?
DeJong's The Neurologic Examination, 7th Ed. Page 132

A. Uhthoff 's phenomenon
B. Möbius' syndrome
C. Meckel's cave
D. Cave of septum pellucidum

Trigeminal ganglion lies just beside pons in a depression in the petrous ridge, called Meckel's cave. A large sensory and a smaller motor root join the ganglion to the pons.

1998. Which of the following is false about trigeminal ganglion?
DeJong's The Neurologic Examination, 7th Ed. Page 228

A. Largest ganglion in the peripheral nervous system
B. Named after JL Gasser, also called semilunar ganglion
C. Analogous to a dorsal root ganglion
D. None of the above

Trigeminal or gasserian ganglion is crescent shaped, convex anterolaterally, and is also known as semilunar ganglion. It lies just lateral to internal carotid artery and posterior part of the cavernous sinus. It is analogous to a dorsal root ganglion and contains unipolar sensory neurons, whose central processes enter lateral pons through large sensory root that pass beneath tentorium to connect concave side of ganglion to the brainstem.

1999. Which of the following is related to trigeminal motor dysfunction?
DeJong's The Neurologic Examination, 7th Ed. Page 42

A. Nystagmus
B. Hearing loss
C. Tongue for atrophy/fasciculations
D. Jaw drop

Trigeminal motor function is ascertained by the patient's jaw drop prior to examining mouth and throat. When pterygoids are unilaterally weak, the jaw invariably deviates toward the weak side on opening. It is a sensitive indicator of trigeminal motor root pathology.

2000. Trigeminal motor fibers innervate which of the following muscles?
DeJong's The Neurologic Examination, 7th Ed. Page 135

A. Masseter
B. Temporalis
C. Pterygoids
D. All of the above

Trigeminal motor fibers innervate the masseter, temporalis, and pterygoids (medial & lateral).

2001. Which of the following muscles originate from the skull base?
DeJong's The Neurologic Examination, 7th Ed. Page 227

A. Masseter
B. Temporalis
C. Pterygoids
D. All of the above

2002. Trigeminal nerve supplies which of the following muscles?
DeJong's The Neurologic Examination, 7th Ed. Page 227

A. Anterior belly of digastric
B. Tensor veli palatini
C. Tensor tympani
D. All of the above

Trigeminal (fifth cranial) nerve supplies the mylohyoid, anterior belly of the digastric, tensor veli palatini, and tensor tympani muscles.

2003. Motor part of trigeminal (fifth cranial) nerve innervates which of the following muscle?
Harrison's 20th Ed. Chapter 433, Page 3166

A. Orbicularis oculi
B. Posterior auricular
C. Pterygoid
D. Sternocleidomastoid

The trigeminal (fifth cranial) nerve supplies sensation to the skin of face and anterior half of the head. Its motor part innervates the masseter & pterygoid masticatory muscles as well as the tensor tympani of the middle ear.

2004. Mandibular sensory fibers of trigeminal nerve enter the skull through?
DeJong's The Neurologic Examination, 7th Ed. Page 135

A. Superior orbital fissure
B. Foramen ovale
C. Foramen rotundum
D. Meckel's cave

Ophthalmic division of trigeminal nerve fibers enter skull via superior orbital fissure, and maxillary fibers enter through the foramen rotundum. Both pass through cavernous sinus before joining the gasserian ganglion. Mandibular fibers enter through ovale. Sensory fibers terminate in the principal sensory nucleus in the pons and in the nucleus of the spinal tract, which extends from pons to upper cervical spinal cord.

2005. Motor and principal sensory nuclei of trigeminal nerve are located in?
DeJong's The Neurologic Examination, 7th Ed. Page 227

A. Upper pons
B. Mid pons
C. Lower pons
D. Midbrain

Motor and principal sensory nuclei of trigeminal nerve are located in midpons. The spinal tract & nucleus extend from pons down into upper cervical spinal cord. Trigeminal nuclear structures thus extend from rostral midbrain to rostral spinal cord.

2006. Sensory portion of trigeminal nerve innervates which of the following?

DeJong's The Neurologic Examination, 7th Ed. Page 227

A. Nasal cavities
B. Intracranial dura
C. Cerebral vasculature
D. All of the above

Sensory portion of trigeminal nerve innervates face, teeth, oral & nasal cavities, scalp back to the vertex, intracranial dura & cerebral vasculature, It provides proprioceptive information for muscles of mastication.

2007. Trigeminal neuralgia is rare in which distribution of fifth nerve?

Harrison's 20th Ed. Chapter 433, Page 3166

A. Ophthalmic division
B. Maxillary division
C. Mandibular division
D. None of the above

Trigeminal neuralgia is characterized by excruciating paroxysms of pain in lips, gums, cheek, or chin and, very rarely, in the distribution of the ophthalmic division of the fifth nerve.

2008. Which of the following is the largest of the cranial nerves?

Harrison's 20th Ed. Chapter 433, Page 3166

A. Optic nerve
B. Trigeminal nerve
C. Facial nerve
D. Vestibulocochlear nerve

Trigeminal nerve is the largest of the cranial nerves. Ophthalmic is the smallest of the three divisions while mandibular division is the largest.

2009. Which of the following division of the fifth cranial nerve exits through foramen ovale?

Harrison's 20th Ed. Chapter 433, Page 3166

A. Ophthalmic division
B. Maxillary division
C. Mandibular division
D. None of the above

V1 & V2 traverse the cavernous sinus to exit in the superior orbital fissure and foramen rotundum, located above and below the eye socket respectively. V3 exits through foramen ovale.

2010. Motor innervation of trigeminal nerve is exclusively carried in which division?

Harrison's 20th Ed. Chapter 433, Page 3166

A. Ophthalmic division
B. Maxillary division
C. Mandibular division
D. None of the above

The trigeminal nerve is predominantly sensory and motor innervation is exclusively carried in V3.

2011. Angle of the jaw is innervated by?

DeJong's The Neurologic Examination, 7th Ed. Page 232

A. Greater auricular nerve
B. Auriculotemporal nerve
C. Buccal nerve
D. Lingual nerve

Angle of the jaw is innervated by the greater auricular nerve (C2-3). The three divisions of trigeminal nerve arise from trigeminal ganglion. Each division has a meningeal branch. Terminal branches of V1 are frontal, lacrimal, and nasociliary nerves. Terminal branches of maxillary division are infraorbital, zygomatic, superior alveolar, and pterygopalatine. Terminal branches of mandibular division are buccal, lingual, inferior alveolar, and auriculotemporal.

2012. Trigeminal nerve supplies filaments to which of the ganglia in head?

DeJong's The Neurologic Examination, 7th Ed. Page 232

A. Ciliary
B. Otic
C. Submaxillary
D. All of the above

Trigeminal nerve supplies filaments to 4 ganglia in head—ciliary, sphenopalatine, otic & submaxillary.

2013. Trigeminal nerve is ensheathed by oligodendrocyte-derived myelin for how many millimeters after exit from brainstem?

Harrison's 20th Ed. Chapter 433, Page 3167

A. 2 mm
B. 5 mm
C. 7 mm
D. 11 mm

Trigeminal nerve is ensheathed by oligodendrocyte-derived, rather than Schwann cell-derived, myelin for up to 7 mm after it leaves the brainstem. This may explain high frequency of trigeminal neuralgia in multiple sclerosis which is a disorder of oligodendrocyte myelin.

2014. "Inverse masticatory muscle activity" has been reported in?

DeJong's The Neurologic Examination, 7th Ed. Page 227

A. Syringomyelia
B. Syringobulbia
C. Herpes zoster
D. Encephalitis

"Inverse masticatory muscle activity" has been reported in syringobulbia.

2015. Which cranial nerve carries the efferent limb of jaw jerk reflex?

DeJong's The Neurologic Examination, 7th Ed. Page 235

A. Oculomotor
B. Trigeminal
C. Trochlear
D. Facial

Efferent limb of the jaw jerk is also trigeminal.

2016. Which of the following is a test for trigeminal nerve?

DeJong's The Neurologic Examination, 7th Ed. Page 235, 238

A. Sternutatory reflex
B. Corneal reflex
C. Jaw reflex
D. All of the above

Sternutatory reflex refers to stimulation of nasal mucous membrane with cotton or similar objects. Normally, it causes wrinkling of nose, eye closure & often a forceful exhalation resembling a feeble sneeze, as the nose tries to rid itself of the foreign object. The afferent limb of reflex arc is carried through CN V1, the efferent limb over CNs V, VII, IX, X, and the motor nerves of the cervical and thoracic spinal cord.

2017. Which of the following is a cause of jaw drop?

DeJong's The Neurologic Examination, 7th Ed. Page 238

A. Myasthenia gravis
B. ALS
C. Kennedy's disease
D. All of the above

2018. Which of the following is a cause of trismus?
DeJong's The Neurologic Examination, 7th Ed. Page 239

A. Tetanus
B. Foix-Chavany-Marie syndrome
C. Tetany
D. All of the above

Trismus is marked spasm of the muscles of mastication. It is a classical manifestation of tetanus. It can also occur in encephalitis, rabies, acute dystonic reactions due to neuroleptic medications, tetany, Foix-Chavany-Marie syndrome, polymyositis. Trismus may be psychogenic.

2019. In trigeminal neuralgia, pain lasts for about?
Harrison's 20th Ed. Chapter 433, Page 3167

A. Few seconds to a minute or two
B. Five to ten minutes
C. Half an hour to six hours
D. Twenty four to forty eight hours

In trigeminal neuralgia, pain seldom lasts more than a few seconds or a minute or two. Onset is typically sudden, and bouts tend to persist for weeks or months before remitting spontaneously. Remissions may be long-lasting, but in most patients the disorder ultimately recurs.

2020. Which of the following is related to trigeminal nerve?
DeJong's The Neurologic Examination, 7th Ed. Page 230

A. Balaclava helmet distribution
B. "Onion skin" somatotopic organization
C. Numb chin syndrome
D. All of the above

"Onion skin" somatotopic organization refers to the face being represented as concentric rings from perioral region to preauricular region. Because of "onion skin" somatotopic organization, there is occasionally sparing, less frequently selective involvement of the perioral region compared to the posterior face (balaclava helmet distribution).

2021. In trigeminal neuralgia, trigger zones are least frequent in?
Harrison's 20th Ed. Chapter 433, Page 3167

A. Face
B. Forehead
C. Lips
D. Tongue

Characteristic feature of Trigeminal neuralgia is the presence of trigger zones, typically on the face, lips, or tongue.

2022. In trigeminal neuralgia, objective signs of sensory loss are found in?
Harrison's 20th Ed. Chapter 433, Page 3167

A. Ophthalmic division
B. Maxillary division
C. Mandibular division
D. None of the above

An essential feature of trigeminal neuralgia is that objective signs of sensory loss cannot be demonstrated on examination.

2023. Which of the following artery causes compression of the trigeminal nerve root to cause trigeminal neuralgia?
Harrison's 20th Ed. Chapter 433, Page 3167

A. Superior cerebellar artery
B. Middle cerebral artery
C. Anterior choroidal artery
D. Posterior cerebral artery

Compression of trigeminal nerve root by superior cerebellar artery, anterior inferior cerebellar artery or a tortuous vein causes trigeminal neuralgia in most patients.

2024. Reason of prevalence of trigeminal neuralgia in later life is?
Harrison's 20th Ed. Chapter 433, Page 3167

A. Age-related brain sagging
B. Increased vascular thickness
C. Increased vascular tortuosity
D. All of the above

Age-related brain sagging, increased vascular thickness and tortuosity lead to increased propensity of vascular compression, and this explains the prevalence of trigeminal neuralgia in later life.

2025. Mass lesion that can cause trigeminal neuralgia is?
Harrison's 20th Ed. Chapter 433, Page 3167

A. Aneurysms
B. Neurofibromas & meningiomas
C. Acoustic schwannomas
D. All of the above

2026. Which of the following is characteristic of pain of trigeminal neuralgia?
Harrison's 20th Ed. Chapter 433, Page 3167

A. Superficial stabbing quality
B. Paroxysmal & lancinating
C. Occurs both day and night
D. All of the above

2027. When cluster headache is associated with trigeminal neuralgia, the syndrome is known as?
Harrison's 20th Ed. Chapter 433, Page 3168

A. Glossopharyngeal neuralgia
B. Tic Douloureux
C. Cluster-tic
D. PH-tic syndrome

When cluster headache is associated with trigeminal neuralgia, syndrome is known as cluster-tic.

2028. Which of the following point towards trigeminal neuralgia being related to multiple sclerosis?
Harrison's 20th Ed. Chapter 433, Page 3168, 3189

A. Onset in a young adult
B. Bilateral symptoms
C. Objective sensory loss
D. All of the above

Most cases of trigeminal neuralgia are not MS-related. Atypical features such as onset in a young adult, bilateral symptoms, objective sensory loss, or nonparoxysmal pain should raise concerns that MS could be responsible.

2029. Which of the following about Acute herpes zoster of the trigeminal nerve is false?
DeJong's The Neurologic Examination, 7th Ed. Page 241

A. Affects ophthalmic division (V1) in 80% of cases
B. Cutaneous scarring is common
C. Pain without a cutaneous eruption is called zoster sine zoster
D. None of the above

Acute herpes zoster of trigeminal nerve is extremely painful. It is usually seen in elderly or immunocompromised patients, and affects ophthalmic division (V1) in 80% of cases, causing pain & vesicles over forehead, eyelid & cornea (herpes ophthalmicus). Cutaneous scarring is common. Ophthalmic involvement may lead to keratitis, corneal ulcerations, residual corneal scarring, and sometimes blindness. Zoster may affect any of the trigeminal divisions, and there may be motor involvement. Rarely, trigeminal HZ may be complicated by encephalitis or a syndrome of delayed contralateral hemiparesis due to arteritis. Pain without a cutaneous eruption is referred to as zoster sine zoster or zoster sine herpete.

2030. Pain persisting for how many months after acute HZ eruption is labeled as postherpetic neuralgia (PHN)?

DeJong's The Neurologic Examination, 7th Ed. Page 241

A. 1 month
B. 3 months
C. 6 months
D. 12 months

Pain persisting for more than 3 months after acute HZ eruption is labeled as postherpetic neuralgia (PHN). It is typically dysesthetic with a burning component, constant but with superimposed paroxysms of lacinating pain that may be provoked by touching certain spots within the affected area. It develops in only 10% of those <60, but in 40% of those >60 years.

2031. Roger's sign best relates to?

DeJong's The Neurologic Examination, 7th Ed. Page 241

A. Numb cheek syndrome
B. Numb chin syndrome
C. Trigeminal sensory neuropathy (TSN)
D. Trumpet player's neuropathy

The numb chin syndrome refers to hypesthesia/paresthesias involving lower lip & chin, in the distribution of mental nerve (chin neuropathy, Roger's sign). The numb chin or cheek syndrome can be the presenting manifestation of cancer.

2032. Which of the following drugs are used in cases of trigeminal neuralgia?

Harrison's 20th Ed. Chapter 433, Page 3168

A. Carbamazepine
B. Phenytoin
C. Baclofen
D. All of the above

Drug therapy for trigeminal neuralgia include carbamazepine, oxcarbazepine, lamotrigine, phenytoin and baclofen.

2033. Which of the following is the most important side effect of carbamazepine?

Harrison's 20th Ed. Chapter 433, Page 3168

A. Alopecia
B. Tremor
C. Agranulocytosis
D. Neutrophilia

Therapeutic blood level for carbamazepine is 4 - 12 μg/mL. Carbamazepine, but not oxcarbazepine, induces hepatic metabolism of other medications. Other rare side effects of Carbamazepine are hyponatremia, agranulocytosis, Stevens-Johnson syndrome.

2034. Which of the following is the most widely used procedure in treating trigeminal neuralgia?

Harrison's 20th Ed. Chapter 433, Page 3168

A. Radiofrequency thermal rhizotomy
B. Injection of glycerol in Meckel's cave
C. Microvascular decompression
D. Gamma knife radiosurgery

If drug treatment fails, in surgical therapy, the most widely used method is currently microvascular decompression to relieve pressure on the trigeminal nerve as it exits the pons. This procedure requires a suboccipital craniotomy.

2035. Gasserian ganglion lesions causing trigeminal nerve disorders include all except?

Harrison's 20th Ed. Chapter 433, Page 3168 Table 433-1

A. Trigeminal neuroma
B. Herpes zoster
C. Sarcoidosis
D. Infection

2036. Peripheral trigeminal nerve lesion can be due to?

Harrison's 20th Ed. Chapter 433, Page 3168 Table 433-1

A. Guillain-Barré syndrome
B. Sjögren's syndrome
C. Collagen-vascular diseases
D. All of the above

2037. Which of the following can cause trismus?

Harrison's 20th Ed. Chapter 433, Page 3169

A. Ludwig's angina
B. Phenothiazine
C. Tetanus
D. All of the above

2038. Mental neuropathy is best related to?

Harrison's 20th Ed. Chapter 433, Page 3169

A. Multiple sclerosis
B. Herpes zoster
C. Leprosy
D. Systemic malignancy

Mental neuropathy refers to an isolated sensory loss over chin. It can be the only manifestation of systemic malignancy.

2039. Which of the following about seventh cranial nerve is false?

Harrison's 20th Ed. Chapter 433, Page 3169

A. Supplies all the muscles concerned with facial expression
B. Sensory component is called nervus intermedius
C. Conveys taste sensation from posterior 1/3 of tongue
D. Conveys sensations from anterior wall of external auditory canal

2040. Who's name is best related to phenomenon of neurobiotaxis?

J Anat. 1929;63(Pt 3):396

A. Kappers
B. Marsot
C. Rorick
D. Sumner

CU Ariens Kappers name is closely associated with the phenomenon of neurobiotaxis.

2041. The facial nerve innervates which of the following muscles?

DeJong's The Neurologic Examination, 7th Ed. Page 247

A. Buccinator
B. Platysma
C. Posterior belly of the digastric
D. All of the above

Predominantly motor, the facial nerve innervates muscles of facial expression and muscles of scalp, ear, and buccinator, platysma, stapedius, stylohyoid, and posterior belly of the digastric.

2042. Which of the following is not a component of facial nerve?

DeJong's The Neurologic Examination, 7th Ed. Page 247

A. Motor
B. Sensory
C. Sympathetic
D. Parasympathetic

2043. Facial nerve carries parasympathetic secretory fibers to?
DeJong's The Neurologic Examination, 7th Ed. Page 247

A. Submandibular salivary glands
B. Sublingual salivary glands
C. Lacrimal gland
D. All of the above

Facial nerve carries parasympathetic secretory fibers to submandibular & sublingual salivary glands, lacrimal gland and to mucous membranes of oral & nasal cavities.

2044. Sensory functions of facial nerve include?
DeJong's The Neurologic Examination, 7th Ed. Page 247

A. Taste from anterior two-thirds of tongue
B. Exteroceptive sensation from eardrum
C. Exteroceptive sensation from external auditory canal
D. All of the above

Sensory functions of facial nerve include taste from anterior two-thirds of tongue, exteroceptive sensation from eardrum & external auditory canal.

2045. After its exit from pons, the first branch of facial nerve is?
DeJong's The Neurologic Examination, 7th Ed. Page 247

A. Greater (superficial) petrosal nerve
B. Nerve to the stapedius
C. Chorda tympani
D. Posterior auricular nerve

2046. After its exit from pons, the second branch of facial nerve is?
DeJong's The Neurologic Examination, 7th Ed. Page 256

A. Greater (superficial) petrosal nerve
B. Nerve to the stapedius
C. Chorda tympani
D. Posterior auricular nerve

Facial nerve, from its exit from pons gives branches in the following order : greater (superficial) petrosal nerve, nerve to the stapedius, & chorda tympani, after which facial nerve continues to facial muscles. The mnemonic tear-hear-taste-face helps to recall the sequence.

2047. Which of the following best relates to facial nerve?
DeJong's The Neurologic Examination, 7th Ed. Page 247

A. Pes equinus
B. Pes anserinus
C. Pes cavus
D. Pes planus

2048. Which of the following is related to peripheral facial paralysis?
Harrison's 20th Ed. Chapter 433, Page 3169, DeJong's The Neurologic Examination, 7th Ed. Page 261

A. Marin Amat sign
B. Jaw-winking
C. Facial spasms
D. All of the above

Aberrant regeneration is common after Bell's palsy and after traumatic nerve injury. Axons destined for one muscle regrow to innervate another, so that there is abnormal twitching of face outside the area of intended movement. On blinking or winking, corner of the mouth may twitch. Automatic closure of one eye on opening the mouth is termed as Marin Amat sign, or inverted or reversed Gunn phenomenon (inverse jaw winking). It is a trigeminofacial associated movement.

2049. Which of the following is related to the aberrant regeneration of injured facial nerve?
DeJong's The Neurologic Examination, 7th Ed. Page 261

A. Syndrome of crocodile tears
B. Frey auriculotemporal syndrome
C. Chorda tympani syndrome
D. All of the above

Aberrant regeneration may involve autonomic and taste fibers. Syndrome of crocodile tears is a gustatory-lacrimal reflex, characterized by tearing when eating due to misdirection of salivary axons to lacrimal gland. Frey auriculotemporal syndrome is similar, but with sweating & flushing over cheek rather than lacrimation. In chorda tympani syndrome, there is unilateral swelling & flushing of submental region after eating.

2050. Which of the following is a risk factor for Bell's palsy?
Harrison's 20th Ed. Chapter 433, Page 3169

A. Hypertension
B. Diabetes
C. Migraine
D. All of the above

Most common form of facial paralysis is Bell's palsy & its risk factors are pregnancy & diabetes mellitus.

2051. The annual incidence of Bell's palsy is?
Harrison's 20th Ed. Chapter 433, Page 3169

A. 1 in 60 persons in a lifetime
B. 1 in 600 persons in a lifetime
C. 1 in 6000 persons in a lifetime
D. 1 in 60000 persons in a lifetime

The annual incidence of Bell's palsy is ~25 per 100,000 annually, or about 1 in 60 persons in a lifetime.

2052. In Bell's palsy, maximal weakness is attained by?
Harrison's 20th Ed. Chapter 433, Page 3169

A. 6 hours
B. 12 hours
C. 24 hours
D. 48 hours

The onset of Bell's palsy is abrupt and maximal weakness occurs by 48 hours as a general rule.

2053. Which of the following may precede Bell's palsy for a day or two?
Harrison's 20th Ed. Chapter 433, Page 3169

A. Excessive lacrimations
B. Facial muscle twitching
C. Pain behind the ear
D. Transient blindness

Pain behind the ear may precede Bell's palsy for a day or two.

2054. Which of the following may be present in Bell's palsy?
Harrison's 20th Ed. Chapter 433, Page 3169

A. Loss of taste sensation unilaterally
B. Hyperacusis
C. Mild cerebrospinal fluid lymphocytosis
D. All of the above

2055. Tear production may be quantitated with?
DeJong's The Neurologic Examination, 7th Ed. Page 256, 656

A. Dix-Hallpike test
B. Unterberger-Fukuda stepping test
C. Schwabach test
D. Schirmer test

Tear production may be quantitated with the Schirmer test. Schirmer test, done by placing a strip of sterile filter paper in the lower conjunctival sac and measuring the degree of wetting over 5 minutes.

2056. Which of the following best relates to peripheral facial palsy?
DeJong's The Neurologic Examination, 7th Ed. Page 256

A. Misoplegia
B. Iridoplegia
C. Prosopoplegia
D. Diplegia

With peripheral facial palsy, there is flaccid weakness of all the muscles of facial expression on the involved side, both upper & lower face. This is called prosopoplegia.

2057. Which of the following best relates to peripheral facial palsy?
DeJong's The Neurologic Examination, 7th Ed. Page 257

A. Levator sign of Dutemps and Céstan
B. Bell's phenomenon
C. Negro's sign
D. All of the above

To elicit the levator sign of Dutemps and Céstan, patient is asked to look down, then close the eyes slowly. Because the function of levator palpebrae superioris is no longer counteracted by orbicularis oculi, the upper lid on paralyzed side moves upward slightly. Negro's sign refers to the eyeball on the paralyzed side that deviates outward & elevates more than the normal one when the patient raises the eyes.

2058. Which of the following best relates to peripheral facial palsy?
DeJong's The Neurologic Examination, 7th Ed. Page 257

A. Battle's sign
B. Bergara-Wartenberg sign
C. Marin Amat sign
D. Bon-bon sign

Bergara-Wartenberg sign is a sensitive sign of upper facial weakness. It is loss of the fine vibrations palpable with thumbs or fingertips resting lightly on eyelids as the patient tries to close the eyes as tightly as possible.

2059. Which of the following best relates to peripheral facial palsy?
DeJong's The Neurologic Examination, 7th Ed. Page 260

A. Mona Lisa syndrome
B. Pierre Robin syndrome
C. Löfgren syndrome
D. Wildervanck syndrome

Mona Lisa was pregnant shortly before the famous painting of Leonardo da Vinci was created (1503-1506). It is speculated that Mona Lisa's famous smile is caused by facial muscle contracture and/or synkinesis after Bell's palsy with incomplete nerve regeneration. The risk of facial palsy is three times greater during pregnancy, especially in the third trimester or in the first postpartum week.

2060. Which of the following symptom accompanies Bell's palsy commonly?
DeJong's The Neurologic Examination, 7th Ed. Page 260

A. Increased tearing
B. Pain in or around the ear
C. Taste abnormalities
D. All of the above

The most common symptoms accompanying Bell's palsy are increased tearing, pain in or around the ear, and taste abnormalities.

2061. What percentage of patients of Bell's palsy recover within a few weeks or months?
Harrison's 20th Ed. Chapter 433, Page 3169

A. ~ 40%
B. ~ 60%
C. ~ 80%
D. ~ 100%

~80% of patients of Bell's palsy recover within a few weeks or months.

2062. Electromyography (EMG) evidence of denervation after how many days indicates axonal degeneration in Bell's palsy?
Harrison's 20th Ed. Chapter 433, Page 3169

A. 7 days
B. 10 days
C. 14 days
D. 21 days

In Bell's palsy, EMG evidence of denervation after 10 days indicates that axonal degeneration has taken place and there will be a long delay (3 months) before regeneration occurs, and that it may be incomplete.

2063. In Bell's palsy, recurrences are reported in what percentage of cases?
Harrison's 20th Ed. Chapter 433, Page 3169

A. ~ 2%
B. ~ 5%
C. ~ 7%
D. ~ 9%

In Bell's palsy, recurrences are reported in ~7% of cases.

2064. Which of the following statements about causation of Bell's palsy is false?
Harrison's 20th Ed. Chapter 433, Page 3169, N Engl J Med. 2004;351:1323-31

A. HSV-1 is the cause of most cases of Bell's palsy
B. HSV-1 DNA appear to be specific to Bell's palsy
C. Disease probably reflects virus reactivation from latency in geniculate ganglion, rather than primary infection
D. None of the above

2065. Which of the following is implicated in the causation of Bell's palsy?
Harrison's 20th Ed. Chapter 433, Page 3169

A. Herpes simplex virus type 1
B. Varicella-zoster virus
C. Borrelia burgdorferi
D. All of the above

2066. Which of the following is implicated in Bell's palsy among recipients of inactivated intranasal influenza vaccine?
Harrison's 20th Ed. Chapter 433, Page 3169

A. Reactivation of HSV-1
B. Trauma
C. Escherichia coli enterotoxin
D. All of the above

An increased incidence of Bell's palsy among recipients of inactivated intranasal influenza vaccine resulted from the Escherichia coli enterotoxin used as adjuvant or reactivation of latent virus.

2067. Poor prognostic factors in a case of Bell's palsy are all except?
N Engl J Med. 2004;351:1323-31

A. Older age
B. Hypertension
C. Diabetes mellitus
D. Impairment of taste

2068. Poor prognostic factors in a case of Bell's palsy are all except?
N Engl J Med. 2004;351:1323-31

A. Hypertension
B. Pain other than in the ear
C. Anemia
D. Complete facial weakness

2069. For how many days, electrical studies reveal no changes in involved facial muscles in Bell's palsy?
N Engl J Med. 2004;351:1323-31

A. 1 day
B. 2 days
C. 3 days
D. 4 days

2070. Which of the following is a cause of peripheral facial palsy?
DeJong's The Neurologic Examination, 7th Ed. Page 262

A. Möbius' syndrome
B. Kennedy's syndrome
C. Acute attack of paralytic poliomyelitis
D. All of the above

2071. Causes of acquired peripheral facial weakness include all except?
N Engl J Med. 2004;351:1323-31

A. Diabetes mellitus
B. Hypothyroidism
C. Hypertension
D. HIV infection

2072. Causes of acquired peripheral facial weakness include all except?
N Engl J Med. 2004;351:1323-31

A. Lyme disease
B. Ramsay Hunt syndrome
C. Sarcoidosis
D. Rheumatoid arthritis

2073. Causes of acquired peripheral facial weakness include all except?
N Engl J Med. 2004;351:1323-31

A. Sjögren 's syndrome
B. Parotid-nerve tumors
C. Eclampsia
D. Dental trauma

2074. Causes of acquired peripheral facial weakness include?
N Engl J Med. 2004;351:1323-31

A. Amyloidosis
B. Recipients of inactivated intranasal influenza vaccine
C. Eclampsia
D. All of the above

2075. Recurrent or bilateral facial palsy is found in?
N Engl J Med. 2004;351:1323-31

A. Lymphoma
B. Sarcoidosis
C. Lyme disease
D. All of the above

2076. Recurrent or bilateral facial palsy is found in all except?
N Engl J Med. 2004;351:1323-31

A. Myasthenia gravis
B. Lesions at base of brain
C. Guillain-Barré syndrome
D. Ramsay Hunt syndrome in immunocompetent people

Facial palsy is often bilateral in sarcoidosis and in Guillain-Barre syndrome.

2077. Ramsay Hunt syndrome best relates to?
Harrison's 20th Ed. Chapter 433, Page 3169

A. Escherichia coli enterotoxin
B. Herpes zoster
C. Borrelia burgdorferi
D. Leprosy

Ramsay Hunt syndrome is caused by reactivation of herpes zoster in the geniculate ganglion, consists of a severe facial palsy associated with a vesicular eruption in the external auditory canal and sometimes in pharynx and other parts of the cranial integument. Often eighth cranial nerve is affected as well.

2078. The Melkersson-Rosenthal syndrome consists of?
Harrison's 20th Ed. Chapter 433, Page 3170

A. Recurrent facial paralysis
B. Facial (labial) edema
C. Plication of tongue
D. All of the above

Melkersson-Rosenthal syndrome is characterized by recurrent attacks of facial palsy, nonpitting facial and lip edema, and a congenitally furrowed and fissured tongue (lingua plicata, scrotal tongue).

2079. Which of the following is the cause of Melkersson-Rosenthal syndrome?
Harrison's 20th Ed. Chapter 433, Page 3170

A. Leprosy
B. Herpes zoster
C. Borrelia burgdorferi
D. None of the above

Melkersson-Rosenthal syndrome consists of recurrent facial paralysis. Recurrent and eventually permanent facial (labial) edema and plication of the tongue. Its cause is unknown.

2080. Parry-Romberg syndrome best relates to?
DeJong's The Neurologic Examination, 7th Ed. Page 265

A. Facial myokymia
B. Blepharospasm
C. Facial hemiatrophy
D. Bilateral facial weakness

In facial hemiatrophy (progressive facial hemiatrophy, Parry-Romberg syndrome, Wartenberg syndrome), there is either congenital failure of development or a progressive atrophy of skin, subcutaneous fat & musculature of one half of face. It may be a form of localized scleroderma.

2081. Which of the following is false about supranuclear facial palsy?
Harrison's 20th Ed. Chapter 433, Page 3170

A. Lower facial muscles involved more than upper facial muscles
B. Dissociation of emotional & voluntary facial movements
C. Paralysis of arm & leg or aphasia may be present
D. None of the above

In supranuclear facial palsy, frontalis & orbicularis oculi muscles of forehead are involved less than those of the lower part of face, because upper facial muscles are innervated by corticobulbar pathways from both motor cortices, whereas the lower facial muscles are innervated only by the opposite hemisphere.

2082. Which of the following is false about Millard-Gubler syndrome?
DeJong's The Neurologic Examination, 7th Ed. Page 262

A. Ipsilateral peripheral facial palsy (PFP)
B. Contralateral hemiparesis
C. Lesion is in pons
D. None of the above

Millard-Gubler syndrome is ipsilateral PFP and contralateral hemiparesis, which may be due to pontine stroke, hemorrhage, or tumor.

2083. Foville syndrome consists of?
DeJong's The Neurologic Examination, 7th Ed. Page 262

A. Ipsilateral peripheral facial palsy (PFP)
B. Horizontal gaze palsy
C. Contralateral hemiparesis
D. All of the above

Foville syndrome is ipsilateral PFP and horizontal gaze palsy with contralateral hemiparesis.

2084. Eight-and-a-Half syndrome is the combination of?
DeJong's The Neurologic Examination, 7th Ed. Page 262

A. Ipsilateral lower motor neuron VIth and VIIth nerve palsy
B. Inter-nuclear ophthalmoplegia
C. Ipsilateral gaze paralysis
D. All of the above

Eight-and-a-half syndrome is characterized by internuclear ophthalmoplegia, horizontal gaze paresis and ipsilateral lower motor neuron seventh cranial nerve palsy, a combination of one-and-a-half syndrome with lower motor neuron seventh cranial nerve palsy. Eight-and-a-Half syndrome is caused by a lesion (vascular or demyelinating) in the dorsal tegmentum of the caudal pons involving ipsilateral paramedian pontine reticular formation (PPRF) or abducens nucleus and medial longitudinal fasciculus (MLF), as well as the nucleus and fasciculus of the facial nerve.

2085. Which of the following is a common site for hemorrhagic stroke?
DeJong's The Neurologic Examination, 7th Ed. Page 262

A. Pons
B. Putamen & thalamus
C. Cerebellum
D. All of the above

Pons is one of the most common sites for hemorrhagic stroke apart from putamen, thalamus and cerebellum.

2086. In MRI, diffuse smooth linear enhancement of facial nerve can be seen in?
Harrison's 20th Ed. Chapter 433, Page 3170 Figure 433-3

A. Lyme disease
B. Sarcoidosis
C. Perineural malignant spread
D. All of the above

2087. Which of the following statements about central weakness of the unilateral lower facial area is false?
N Engl J Med. 2004;351:1323-31

A. Lesion above level of contralateral facial nucleus
B. Facial nucleus innervating lower face receives fibers from ipsilateral cerebral hemisphere
C. Facial nucleus innervating upper face receives fibers from both cerebral hemispheres
D. Unilateral lesion in cortex produces contralateral voluntary central-type facial paralysis and contralateral hemiplegia

2088. Which of the following about facial palsy is false?
N Engl J Med. 2004;351:1323-31

A. Hyperacusis results from paralysis of stapedius muscle
B. Lesions proximal to geniculate ganglion have permanent loss of taste and are unable to produce tears
C. Aberrant regeneration of nerve fibres is the cause of syndrome of crocodile tears
D. None of the above

2089. Which of the following about facial nerve is false?
N Engl J Med. 2004;351:1323-31

A. Facial nerve is predominantly motor
B. Facial nucleus is located in caudal pons
C. Facial nerve encircles nucleus of sixth cranial nerve
D. Facial nerve exits in midpons

2090. Which of the following about facial nerve is false?
N Engl J Med. 2004;351:1323-31

A. 8th nerve, motor root of 7th nerve, and nervus intermedius enter internal auditory meatus
B. Sensory cells located in geniculate ganglion continue distally as chorda tympani nerve
C. Peripheral fibers of nervus intermedius portion of facial nerve initiate salivary, lacrimal, and mucous secretion
D. None of the above

2091. Locate the lesion if there is contralateral central facial weakness, lacrimation, salivation, and taste are intact, contralateral hemiparesis and spasticity?
N Engl J Med. 2004;351:1323-31

A. Cortex, subcortical region
B. Pons
C. Cerebellopontine angle
D. All of the above

2092. Locate the lesion if there is ipsilateral peripheral facial weakness; lacrimation, salivation, and taste intact; contralateral hemiparesis, sensory loss, ataxia, nystagmus, ipsilateral abducens palsy, ophthalmoparesis?
N Engl J Med. 2004;351:1323-31

A. Cortex, subcortical region
B. Pons
C. Cerebellopontine angle
D. All of the above

2093. Locate the lesion if there is ipsilateral peripheral facial weakness; lacrimation, salivation, and taste intact; tinnitus, facial numbness, ataxia, nystagmus?

N Engl J Med. 2004;351:1323-31

A. Cortex, subcortical region
B. Pons
C. Cerebellopontine angle
D. All of the above

2094. Locate the lesion if there is ipsilateral peripheral facial weakness; lacrimation, salivation, and taste likely to be involved; tinnitus, nystagmus, hearing loss?

N Engl J Med. 2004;351:1323-31

A. Cortex, subcortical region
B. Pons
C. Cerebellopontine angle
D. Facial nerve in internal auditory canal proximal to or involving geniculate ganglion

2095. Locate the lesion if there is ipsilateral peripheral facial weakness; lacrimation intact but salivation and taste impaired; tinnitus, nystagmus, hearing loss?

N Engl J Med. 2004;351:1323-31

A. Pons
B. Facial nerve in stylomastoid foramen
C. Facial nerve in internal auditory canal proximal to or involving geniculate ganglion
D. Facial nerve distal to internal auditory canal and geniculate ganglion

2096. Locate the lesion if there is ipsilateral peripheral facial weakness; lacrimation, salivation, and taste intact?

N Engl J Med. 2004;351:1323-31

A. Cerebellopontine angle
B. Facial nerve in internal auditory canal proximal to or involving geniculate ganglion
C. Facial nerve distal to internal auditory canal & geniculate ganglion
D. Facial nerve in stylomastoid foramen

2097. House Brackmann grading system is used for assessing?

N Engl J Med. 2004;351:1323-31

A. Facial muscle function
B. Parotid function
C. Hearing function
D. Salivary function

The House-Brackmann scale, Burres-Fisch index and facial nerve function index may be useful to try to quantitate the degree of weakness.

2098. Facial nerve is compressed at its narrowest point, which is?

N Engl J Med. 2004;351:1323-31

A. Entrance to meatal foramen
B. Middle of internal auditory canal
C. Exit point of internal auditory canal
D. Exit point of facial nerve from pons

2099. Which of the following is useful in treatment of Bell's palsy?

Harrison's 20th Ed. Chapter 433, Page 3170

A. Glucocorticoids
B. IV Ig
C. Plasmapharesis
D. All of the above

Antiviral agents valacyclovir (1000 mg daily for 5-7 days) or acyclovir (400 mg five times daily for 10 days) with glucocorticoids (prednisone 60-80 mg daily for first 5 days, then tapered over next 5 days) might be marginally better than prednisolone alone especially in patients with severe clinical presentations.

2100. Decompression surgery should not be performed?

N Engl J Med. 2004;351:1323-31

A. 7 days after the onset of paralysis
B. 14 days after the onset of paralysis
C. 21 days after the onset of paralysis
D. 28 days after the onset of paralysis

2101. Which of the following may be caused by multiple sclerosis or follow Guillain-Barré syndrome?

Harrison's 20th Ed. Chapter 433, Page 3170

A. Blepharospasm
B. Facial myokymia
C. Hemifacial spasm
D. Facial hemiatrophy

Facial myokymia may be caused by MS, MJD, EA1, neuromyotonia (Isaacs' syndrome) or follow GBS. Facial myokymia consists of either persistent rapid flickering contractions of the facial musculature (especially the lower portion of the orbicularis oculus) or a contraction that slowly spreads across the face. It results from lesions of the corticobulbar tracts or brainstem course of the facial nerve.

2102. Which of the following disorders is associated with pregnancy?

Harrison's 20th Ed. Chapter 433, Page 3444

A. Bell's palsy
B. Carpal tunnel syndrome
C. Meralgia paresthetica
D. All of the above

Bell's palsy (idiopathic facial paralysis) is about three fold more likely to occur during the third trimester and immediate postpartum period than in the general population.

2103. Glossopharyngeal Neuralgia may be due to involvement of which of the following cranial nerves?

Harrison's 20th Ed. Chapter 433, Page 3170

A. X
B. XI
C. XII
D. All of the above

2104. Which of the following is false about Glossopharyngeal Neuralgia?

Harrison's 20th Ed. Chapter 433, Page 3170

A. Involves IX & portions of X cranial nerves
B. Pain may radiate from throat to ear
C. Spasms of pain may be initiated by swallowing or coughing
D. None of the above

Glossopharyngeal neuralgia though uncommon resembles trigeminal neuralgia & involves IX & sometimes portions of vagus cranial nerves. Pain is intense & paroxysmal, originates on one side of throat (tonsillar fossa) and may radiate to the ear (tympanic branch of IX). Spasms of pain may be initiated by swallowing or coughing. There is no motor or sensory deficit.

2105. Which of the following cranial nerves is not involved in pontocerebellar angle syndrome?

Harrison's 20th Ed. Chapter 433, Page 3171 Table 433-2

A. V
B. VII
C. VIII
D. XII

V, VII, VIII and sometimes IX are involved in pontocerebellar angle syndrome.

2106. Which of the following cranial nerves is not involved in jugular foramen syndrome?

Harrison's 20th Ed. Chapter 433, Page 3171 Table 433-2

A. IX
B. X
C. XI
D. XII

IX, X XI cranial nerves are involved in jugular foramen syndrome. Hoarseness due to vocal cord paralysis, difficulty in swallowing, deviation of the soft palate to the intact side, anesthesia of posterior wall of pharynx, and weakness of upper part of trapezius & sternocleidomastoid muscles make up jugular foramen syndrome.

2107. Multiple cranial neuropathy can be caused by?

Harrison's 20th Ed. Chapter 433, Page 3171

A. Wegener's granulomatosis
B. Behcet's disease
C. Sarcoidosis
D. All of the above

2108. Multiple cranial neuropathy can be caused by?

Harrison's 20th Ed. Chapter 433, Page 3171

A. Diabetes mellitus
B. Meningitis
C. Enlarging saccular aneurysms
D. All of the above

2109. Which of the following is true for Tolosa-Hunt syndrome?

Harrison's 20th Ed. Chapter 433, Page 3172

A. Aneurysm of carotid artery
B. Carotid-cavernous fistula
C. Idiopathic granulomatous disorder
D. Meningioma

Tolosa-Hunt syndrome is an idiopathic granulomatous disorder that responds to glucocorticoids.

Diseases of the Spinal Cord

2110. What is the length of adult spinal cord?

Harrison's 20th Ed. Chapter 434, Page 3173

A. ~ 34 cm
B. ~ 40 cm
C. ~ 46 cm
D. ~ 52 cm

Adult spinal cord is ~46 cm (18 inches) long, oval in shape and enlarged in cervical & lumbar regions, where neurons that innervate upper & lower extremities, respectively, are located.

2111. The spinal cord has how many segments?

Harrison's 20th Ed. Chapter 434, Page 3173

A. 30
B. 31
C. 32
D. 33

Spinal cord has 31 segments, each defined by exiting ventral motor root & entering dorsal sensory root.

2112. Lumbar spinal cord segments correspond to which vertebral body?

Harrison's 20th Ed. Chapter 434, Page 3173 Table 434-2

A. T8-T10
B. T10 - T12
C. T12 - L1
D. L1

2113. Sacral spinal cord segments correspond to which vertebral body?

Harrison's 20th Ed. Chapter 434, Page 3173 Table 434-2

A. T11
B. T12
C. T12 - L1
D. L1

Upper cervical - same as cord level, lower cervical - 1 level higher, upper thoracic - 2 levels higher, lower thoracic - 2 to 3 levels higher, lumbar - T10 to T12 and sacral - T12 to L1.

2114. Uppermost level of a spinal cord lesion can be localized by?

Harrison's 20th Ed. Chapter 434, Page 3173

A. Sensory level
B. Segmental signs
C. Band of altered sensation
D. All of the above

2115. Intervertebral disks are responsible for what percentage of spinal column length?

Harrison's 20th Ed. Chapter 14, Page 89

A. 10%
B. 15%
C. 20%
D. 25%

Intervertebral disks are composed of a central gelatinous nucleus pulposus surrounded by a tough cartilaginous ring, the annulus fibrosis. Disks are responsible for 25% of spinal column length.

2116. Intervertebral disks are largest in?

Harrison's 20th Ed. Chapter 14, Page 89

A. Cervical region
B. Thoracic region
C. Sacral region
D. None of the above

Intervertebral disks are largest in cervical & lumbar regions where movements of spine are greatest.

2117. Each vertebral arch gives rise to how many processes?

Harrison's 20th Ed. Chapter 14, Page 89

A. 3
B. 5
C. 7
D. 9

Seven processes arise from each vertebral arch—paired pedicles, paired laminae, paired transverse processes and one spinous process.

2118. Uncinate process is best related to?

Harrison's 20th Ed. Chapter 14, Page 89

A. Cervical vertebral body
B. Thoracic vertebral body
C. Lumbar vertebral body
D. Sacral vertebral body

Beginning at C3 level, each cervical (and first thoracic) vertebral body projects a lateral bony process upward called the uncinate process which articulates with the cervical vertebral body above via uncovertebral joint.

2119. Pain-sensitive structures in spine include all except?

Harrison's 20th Ed. Chapter 14, Page 89

A. Periosteum of vertebrae
B. Nucleus pulposus of intervertebral disk
C. Annulus fibrosus of intervertebral disk
D. Dura

Pain-sensitive structures in the spine include the periosteum of the vertebrae, dura, facet joints, annulus fibrosus of the intervertebral disk, epidural veins, and longitudinal ligaments. The nucleus pulposus of the intervertebral disk is not pain-sensitive.

2120. Activation of agonist muscle is accompanied by inhibition of antagonist muscle refers to?

DeJong's The Neurologic Examination, 7th Ed. Page 559

A. Sherrington's law
B. Pitres' law
C. Alexander's law
D. Hering's law

Sherrington's law of reciprocal innervation describes the balance between the contraction of the agonist and the inhibition of the antagonist. When extensors of a limb are contracted, the flexors are relaxed.

2121. Patrick's test is used to demonstrate pain due to?

Anesth Analg 2005;101:1440-53

A. Lumbar spine disease
B. Hip disease
C. Knee disease
D. Ankle disease

Patrick's test or FABER test (Flexion, ABduction and External Rotation) refers to elicitation of hip pain by internal and external rotation at the hip with the knee and hip in flexion.

2122. Gaenslen's test is used to demonstrate pain due to?

Anesth Analg 2005;101:1440-53

A. Lumbar spine disease
B. Hip disease
C. Knee disease
D. Ankle disease

2123. Yeoman's test is used to demonstrate pain due to?

Anesth Analg 2005;101:1440-53

A. Lumbar spine disease
B. Hip disease
C. Knee disease
D. Sacroiliitis

2124. Gillett test is used to demonstrate pain due to?

Anesth Analg 2005;101:1440-53

A. Lumbar spine disease
B. Hip disease
C. Knee disease
D. Sacroiliitis

2125. Pain is referred to which of the following in diseases affecting upper lumbar spine?

Harrison's 20th Ed. Chapter 14, Page 90

A. Lumbar region
B. Groin
C. Anterior thighs
D. All of the above

2126. Pain is referred to which of the following in diseases affecting lower lumbar spine?

Harrison's 20th Ed. Chapter 14, Page 90

A. Buttocks
B. Posterior thighs
C. Calves
D. All of the above

Diseases affecting upper lumbar spine refer pain to lumbar region, groin, or anterior thighs. Diseases affecting lower lumbar spine produce pain referred to buttocks, posterior thighs, calves, or feet.

2127. Which of the following may elicit or worsen radiating pain?

Harrison's 20th Ed. Chapter 14, Page 90

A. Coughing
B. Sneezing
C. Voluntary contraction of abdominal muscles
D. All of the above

Coughing, sneezing or voluntary contraction of abdominal muscles like lifting heavy objects or straining at stool may elicit or worsen the radiating pain.

2128. Characteristic of pain that favors the diagnosis of radiculopathy is?

Harrison's 20th Ed. Chapter 14, Page 90

A. Gnawing
B. Burning
C. Compressing
D. Tearing

Burning or electric quality of pain favors radiculopathy rather than referred pain.

2129. In supine position, passive flexion of extended leg at the hip stretches which of the following?

Harrison's 20th Ed. Chapter 14, Page 90

A. L5 nerve root
B. S1 nerve root
C. Sciatic nerve
D. All of the above

With the patient lying flat, passive flexion of the extended leg at the hip stretches the L5 and S1 nerve roots and the sciatic nerve.

2130. Reverse SLR sign stretches which of the following?

Harrison's 20th Ed. Chapter 14, Page 90

A. L2-L4 nerve roots
B. Lumbosacral plexus
C. Femoral nerve
D. All of the above

Reverse SLR stretches L2-L4 nerve roots, lumbosacral plexus and femoral nerve.

2131. Ely test refers to?

DeJong's The Neurologic Examination, 7th Ed. Page 698

A. SLR
B. Reverse SLR
C. Crossed SLR
D. All of the above

Femoral stretch or Ely test refers to reverse SLR. It is a root stretch test and is useful in evaluation of high lumbar radiculopathy.

2132. Ely test is performed with patient in which position?

DeJong's The Neurologic Examination, 7th Ed. Page 698

A. Supine
B. Prone
C. Sitting
D. Standing

2133. Lasègue test refers to?

DeJong's The Neurologic Examination, 7th Ed. Page 697

A. SLR
B. Reverse SLR
C. Crossed SLR
D. All of the above

SLR or Lasègue test is performed by slowly raising the symptomatic leg with the knee extended. Nerve roots get tense between ~30° and 70°, and pain increases. Pain at <30° raises the question of nonorganicity, and some discomfort & tightness beyond 70° is routine and insignificant.

2134. Fajersztajn's sign refers to?

DeJong's The Neurologic Examination, 7th Ed. Page 697

A. SLR
B. Reverse SLR
C. Crossed SLR
D. All of the above

In crossed SLR, raising the good leg produces pain in the symptomatic leg (Fajersztajn's sign). If positive, the likelihood of a root lesion is very high.

2135. Which of the following is related to accentuation of Lasègue's sign (SLR)?

DeJong's The Neurologic Examination, 7th Ed. Page 697

A. Bonnet phenomenon
B. Bragard's sign
C. Sicard's sign
D. All of the above

In SLR, pain may be more severe, or elicited sooner, if test is carried out with thigh & leg in a position of adduction & internal rotation (Bonnet phenomenon). SLR can be enhanced by passively dorsiflexing the patient's foot (Bragard's sign) or great toe (Sicard's sign) at the elevation angle at which the increased root tension begins to produce pain.

2136. O'Connell's test is performed with patient in which position?

DeJong's The Neurologic Examination, 7th Ed. Page 698

A. Supine
B. Prone
C. Sitting
D. Standing

In O'Connell's test, SLR is first done on the sound limb, and angle of flexion & site of pain are recorded. Then, SLR is done on affected limb, and angle & site of pain again noted. Then, both thighs are flexed simultaneously, with knees extended. Angle of flexion permitted may be greater than that allowed when either the affected limb or the sound limb is flexed alone. If at this point, lowering of the sound limb may result in a marked exacerbation of pain in the affected limb.

2137. Bechterew's test is performed with patient in which position?

DeJong's The Neurologic Examination, 7th Ed. Page 698

A. Supine
B. Prone
C. Sitting
D. Standing

Bechterew's test refers to the observation that in sitting position, patient may be able to extend leg alone without pain, but extending both together causes radicular pain.

2138. Which of the following is typical of herniation of the nucleus pulposus (HNP)?

DeJong's The Neurologic Examination, 7th Ed. Page 700

A. Pain worse on sitting
B. Pain lessened with standing
C. Positive SLR
D. All of the above

In HNP, pain may worsen with cough, sneeze, or Valsalva.

2139. Most common lumbosacral radiculopathy (LSR) involve?

DeJong's The Neurologic Examination, 7th Ed. Page 700

A. L2
B. L3
C. L4
D. L5

Most commonly, LSRs involve either L5 or S1. Upper lumbar radiculopathies are rare.

2140. Involvement of which of the following is critical in distinguishing between L5 radiculopathy & peroneal nerve palsy?

DeJong's The Neurologic Examination, 7th Ed. Page 700

A. Tibialis anterior
B. Tibialis posterior
C. Extensor hallucis longus
D. Extensor digitorum longus

Involvement of tibialis posterior is critical in distinguishing between L5 radiculopathy & peroneal nerve palsy.

2141. In S1 lesions, weakness manifests primarily in the?

DeJong's The Neurologic Examination, 7th Ed. Page 700

A. Gastrosoleus
B. Extensor hallucis longus
C. Extensor digitorum longus
D. Gluteus maximus

In S1 lesions, weakness manifests primarily in the gastrosoleus.

2142. Breakaway weakness refers to?

Harrison's 20th Ed. Chapter 14, Page 92

A. Inability to generate maximum power in other half of body
B. Inability to generate maximum power similar to examiner
C. Fluctuations in maximum power during muscle testing
D. None of the above

Breakaway weakness is defined as fluctuations in maximum power generated during muscle testing.

2143. Lumbar spinal stenosis can be caused by?

Harrison's 20th Ed. Chapter 14, Page 94

A. Acromegaly
B. Renal osteodystrophy
C. Hypoparathyroidism
D. All of the above

Lumbar spinal stenosis can be caused by epidural lipomatosis, osteoporosis, acromegaly, renal osteodystrophy, hypoparathyroidism, and Paget's disease.

2144. Which of the following is false about Tethered cord syndrome?

Harrison's 20th Ed. Chapter 14, Page 96

A. Presents as progressive cauda equina disorder
B. Perineal or perianal pain
C. Low-lying conus (below L1-L2)
D. Long and thickened filum terminale

Tethered cord syndrome presents as a progressive cauda equina disorder or myelopathy in a young adult who complains of perineal or perianal pain. Neuroimaging studies show a low-lying conus (below L1-L2) and a short & thickened filum terminale.

2145. Which of the following spinal root value innervates axilla?

Harrison's 20th Ed. Chapter 14, Page 100 Table 14-4

A. C8
B. T1
C. T2
D. T3

2146. Spurling's sign relates to?

Harrison's 20th Ed. Chapter 14, Page 100

A. Extension & lateral rotation of neck
B. Flexion & lateral rotation of neck
C. Extreme extension of neck
D. Extreme flexion of neck

Extension & lateral rotation of neck narrows ipsilateral intervertebral foramen resulting in radicular symptoms (Spurling's sign).

2147. Cervical angina syndrome relates best with?

Harrison's 20th Ed. Chapter 14, Page 100

A. Vertebrobasilar syndrome
B. Coronary artery ischemia
C. Subclavian steal syndrome
D. All of the above

Cervical angina syndrome refers to pain in neck that is due to coronary artery ischemia.

2148. Horner's syndrome accompanies cervical cord lesion at?
Harrison's 20th Ed. Chapter 434, Page 3173

A. C5
B. C6
C. C7
D. Any cervical level

Horner's syndrome (miosis, ptosis & facial hypohidrosis) may accompany cervical cord lesion at any level.

2149. Which cervical root lesion is most common?
DeJong's The Neurologic Examination, 7th Ed. Page 695

A. C5
B. C6
C. C7
D. C8

In the cervical spine, C7 root lesions are the most common, followed by C6, C5 and C8 lesions. Involvement of the upper cervical roots is rare.

2150. Weakness of triceps & pronator teres is pathognomonic of lesion at?
DeJong's The Neurologic Examination, 7th Ed. Page 696

A. C5
B. C6
C. C7
D. C8

Weakness of triceps & pronator teres is pathognomonic of C7 lesions, since C7 is their only common innervation.

2151. Lesions at C7 produce all except?
Harrison's 20th Ed. Chapter 434, Page 3173

A. Weakness in finger extensors
B. Weakness in wrist extensors
C. Weakness in brachioradialis
D. Weakness in triceps

At C7 lesion, weakness is found only in finger and wrist extensors and triceps.

2152. Lesions at C8 produces?
Harrison's 20th Ed. Chapter 434, Page 3173

A. Weakness in finger and wrist flexors
B. Weakness in finger extensors
C. Weakness in wrist extensors
D. Weakness in supination

At C8, finger and wrist flexion are impaired.

2153. Sensory dermatome at the level of nipples is?
Harrison's 20th Ed. Chapter 434, Page 3173

A. T2
B. T3
C. T4
D. T5

Dermatome at nipples is T4 and at umbilicus is T10.

2154. Beevor's sign is positive in spinal cord lesion at?
Harrison's 20th Ed. Chapter 434, Page 3173

A. T7 - T8
B. T8 - T9
C. T9 - T10
D. T11 - T12

Lesions at T9-T10 paralyze the lower, but not the upper abdominal muscles, resulting in upward movement of the umbilicus when the abdominal wall contracts (Beevor's sign).

2155. Lesions at L2 - L4 cause all except?
Harrison's 20th Ed. Chapter 434, Page 3173

A. Weakness of flexion of thigh
B. Weakness of abduction of thigh
C. Weakness of leg extension at knee
D. Absent patellar reflex

Lesions at L2 - L4 spinal cord levels paralyze flexion & adduction of thigh, weaken leg extension at knee and abolish the patellar reflex.

2156. Lesions at L5-S1 cause all except?
Harrison's 20th Ed. Chapter 434, Page 3173

A. Paralyze movements of foot and ankle
B. Weakness of flexion at knee
C. Weakness of flexion of thigh
D. Absent ankle jerk

Lesions at L5 - S1 paralyse movements of the foot & ankle, flexion at knee, and extension of thigh and abolish the ankle jerks (S1).

2157. Conus medullaris comprises of?
Harrison's 20th Ed. Chapter 434, Page 3173

A. Lower lumbar + sacral + coccygeal segments
B. Sacral + coccygeal segments
C. Lower sacral + coccygeal segments
D. None of the above

Conus medullaris is the tapered caudal termination of the spinal cord, comprising of the lower sacral and single coccygeal segments.

2158. The conus syndrome is characterized by all except?
Harrison's 20th Ed. Chapter 434, Page 3173

A. Bilateral saddle anesthesia
B. Asymmetric leg weakness
C. Bladder and bowel dysfunction
D. Impotence

2159. The conus syndrome is characterized by all except?
Harrison's 20th Ed. Chapter 434, Page 3173

A. Absent bulbocavernosus reflex
B. Absent anal reflex
C. Asymmetric sensory loss in leg
D. Bilateral saddle anesthesia

2160. The root value of bulbocavernosus reflex is?
Harrison's 20th Ed. Chapter 434, Page 3173

A. S1 - S2
B. S2 - S4
C. S3 - S5
D. S4 - S5

2161. The root value of anal reflex is?

Harrison's 20th Ed. Chapter 434, Page 3173

A. S1 - S2
B. S2 - S4
C. S3 - S5
D. S4 - S5

Conus syndrome consists of bilateral saddle anesthesia (S3-S5), prominent bladder & bowel dysfunction (urinary retention & incontinence with lax anal tone), and impotence. Bulbocavernosus (S2-S4) & anal (S4-S5) reflexes are absent. Muscle strength is largely preserved.

2162. Cauda equina lesion is characterized by all except?

Harrison's 20th Ed. Chapter 434, Page 3173

A. Radicular pain
B. Asymmetric leg weakness
C. Variable areflexia in lower extremities
D. Bladder and bowel dysfunction

Lesions of cauda equina are characterized by low back & radicular pain, asymmetric leg weakness & sensory loss, variable areflexia in the lower extremities & relative sparing of bowel & bladder function.

2163. Which of the following is false about cauda equina syndrome?

Harrison's 20th Ed. Chapter 434, Page 3173

A. Sphincters are affected
B. Hip flexion is spared
C. Sensation over anterolateral thighs is spared
D. None of the above

2164. In spinal cord, sacral fibres are placed laterally in all except?

Harrison's 20th Ed. Chapter 434, Page 3174 Figure 434-1

A. Ventral spinothalamic tract
B. Lateral spinothalamic tract
C. Lateral corticospinal tract
D. Posterior column

2165. In spinal posterior columns, fibres from which part of the body are nearest midline?

Harrison's 20th Ed. Chapter 434, Page 3174 Figure 434-1

A. Cervical
B. Thoracic
C. Lumbar
D. Sacral

2166. In lateral spinothalamic tracts, fibres from which part of the body are nearest midline?

Harrison's 20th Ed. Chapter 434, Page 3174 Figure 434-1

A. Cervical
B. Thoracic
C. Lumbar
D. Sacral

2167. In lateral corticospinal tracts, fibres from which part of the body are nearest midline?

Harrison's 20th Ed. Chapter 434, Page 3174 Figure 434-1

A. Cervical
B. Thoracic
C. Lumbar
D. Sacral

2168. Which of the following motor neurons in anterior horn of spinal cord are placed anteriorly?

Harrison's 20th Ed. Chapter 434, Page 3174 Figure 434-1

A. Proximal
B. Distal
C. Flexors
D. Extensors

2169. Brown-Sequard hemicord syndrome features all except?

Harrison's 20th Ed. Chapter 434, Page 3173

A. Ipsilateral weakness
B. Ipsilateral loss of joint position & vibratory sensation
C. Contralateral loss of pain & temperature sensation
D. Bilateral segmental signs

2170. Brown-Sequard syndrome is characterized by?

Harrison's 20th Ed. Chapter 434, Page 3174

A. Absence of cranial nerve signs
B. Ipsilateral loss of propioception
C. Contralateral loss pain & temperature
D. All of the above

Brown-Sequard hemicord syndrome consists of ipsilateral weakness (corticospinal tract) and loss of joint position and vibratory sense (posterior column), with contralateral loss of pain and temperature sense (spinothalamic tract) one or two levels below the lesion. Segmental signs, such as radicular pain, muscle atrophy, or loss of a deep tendon reflex, are unilateral.

2171. Central cord syndrome results from all except?

Harrison's 20th Ed. Chapter 434, Page 3174

A. Spinal trauma
B. Infection
C. Syringomyelia
D. Intrinsic cord tumors

Central cord syndrome is due to damage to gray matter nerve cells & crossing spinothalamic tracts near the central spinal canal. Trauma, syringomyelia, tumors & intrinsic cord tumors cause central cord syndrome.

2172. Dissociated sensory loss in central cord syndrome means?

Harrison's 20th Ed. Chapter 434, Page 3174

A. Loss of JPS & vibration sense with preservation of pain & temperature sense
B. Loss of pain & temperature sense with preservation of JPS & vibration sense
C. Loss of pain sense with preservation of temperature sense
D. Loss of temperature sense with preservation of pain sense

In cervical cord, central cord syndrome produces arm weakness out of proportion to leg weakness and "dissociated" sensory loss (loss of pain & temperature sense with preservation of light touch, joint position, and vibration sense over shoulders, lower neck & upper trunk.

2173. Which of the following is false about anterior spinal artery syndrome?

Harrison's 20th Ed. Chapter 434, Page 3174

A. Due to occlusion of anterior spinal artery
B. Motor, sensory & autonomic functions are lost below the level of lesion
C. Preserved vibration & position sensation
D. None of the above

Anterior spinal artery syndrome is due to infarction of spinal cord due to its occlusion or diminished flow. Destruction spares posterior columns. Motor, sensory and autonomic functions are lost below the level of lesion, Vibration and position sensation are retained.

2174. "Around the clock" pattern of weakness is seen in?
Harrison's 20th Ed. Chapter 434, Page 3174

A. Central cord syndrome
B. Anterior spinal artery syndrome
C. Foramen magnum syndrome
D. All of the above

Compressive lesions near foramen magnum produce weakness of ipsilateral shoulder & arm followed by weakness of ipsilateral leg, then contralateral leg, & finally contralateral arm, an "around the clock" pattern that may begin in any of four limbs. Typical sub-occipital pain spreading to neck & shoulders is present.

2175. Which of the following features does not favour the diagnosis of extramedullary lesions?
Harrison's 20th Ed. Chapter 434, Page 3174

A. Radicular pain
B. Early sacral sensory loss
C. Sparing of sensation in perineal & sacral areas
D. Spastic weakness in legs

Prominent radicular pain with early sacral sensory loss (lateral spinothalamic tract) & spastic weakness in legs (corticospinal tract) with incontinence indicate extramedullary lesions. Extradural masses are generally malignant while intradural masses are generally benign. Therefore, a long duration of symptoms favors an intradural origin.

2176. Which of the following features favours the diagnosis of intramedullary lesions?
Harrison's 20th Ed. Chapter 434, Page 3174

A. Radicular pain
B. Early corticospinal tract signs
C. Sparing of sensation in perineal & sacral areas
D. Spastic weakness in legs

Intramedullary lesions produce poorly localized burning pain & spare sensation in perineal and sacral areas ("sacral sparing"), due to laminated configuration of spinothalamic tract with sacral fibers outermost. Corticospinal tract signs appear later.

2177. Which of the following features favours noncompressive myelopathy?
Harrison's 20th Ed. Chapter 434, Page 3175

A. Neck or back pain preceding paralysis
B. Bladder disturbances preceding paralysis
C. Sensory symptoms preceding paralysis
D. Myelopathy without antecedent symptoms

Epidural compression causes warning signs of neck or back pain, bladder disturbances and sensory symptoms that precede development of paralysis. Noncompressive etiologies produce myelopathy without antecedent symptoms.

2178. Which of the following malignant tumors usually do not metastasize to "thoracic" spinal cord?
Harrison's 20th Ed. Chapter 434, Page 3175

A. Breast
B. Kidney
C. Ovary
D. Lymphoma

Almost any malignant tumor can metastasize to spinal column with breast, lung, prostate, kidney, lymphoma & myeloma being frequent because of high proportion of bone marrow in axial skeleton. Thoracic cord is most commonly involved. Metastases from prostate & ovarian cancer occur disproportionately in sacral & lumbar vertebrae.

2179. Batson's plexus is composed of?
Harrison's 20th Ed. Chapter 434, Page 3175

A. Nerves
B. Arteries
C. Veins
D. Capillaries

Batson's plexus is a network of veins along the anterior epidural space.

2180. Pain in neoplastic epidural compressive myelopathy worsens with?
Harrison's 20th Ed. Chapter 434, Page 3175

A. Movement
B. Coughing
C. Sneezing
D. All of the above

Pain in neoplastic epidural compressive myelopathy typically worsens with movement, coughing or sneezing & awakens patients at night.

2181. Which of the following segment of spine is uncommonly involved by spondylosis?
Harrison's 20th Ed. Chapter 434, Page 3175

A. Cervical spine
B. Thoracic spine
C. Lumbar spine
D. Sacral spine

2182. Which of the following is false about intradural mass lesions?
Harrison's 20th Ed. Chapter 434, Page 3175

A. Slow-growing & benign
B. Initial symptom is radicular pain
C. Asymmetric, progressive spinal cord syndrome
D. None of the above

Most intradural mass lesions are slow-growing & benign. Symptoms usually begin with radicular sensory symptoms followed by an asymmetric, progressive spinal cord syndrome.

2183. Intradural neurofibromas typically arise near?
Harrison's 20th Ed. Chapter 434, Page 3176

A. Anterior root
B. Posterior root
C. Radicle
D. Any of the above

Intradural neurofibromas typically arise near the posterior root.

2184. Which of the following is a primary intramedullary tumor?
Harrison's 20th Ed. Chapter 434, Page 3176

A. Ependymomas
B. Hemangioblastomas
C. Low-grade astrocytoma
D. All of the above

Primary intramedullary tumors of spinal cord include ependymomas, hemangioblastomas, or low-grade astrocytomas in adults. They present as central cord or hemicord syndromes, mostly in cervical region.

2185. Clinical triad of spinal epidural abscess consists of all except?
Harrison's 20th Ed. Chapter 434, Page 3176

A. Midline dorsal pain
B. Fever
C. Progressive limb weakness
D. Sensory loss

Clinical triad of spinal epidural abscess consists of midline dorsal pain, fever & progressive limb weakness.

2186. Which of the following about spinal epidural abscess is false?

Harrison's 20th Ed. Chapter 434, Page 3176

A. Infections of skin is a risk factor

B. Commonly due to hematogenous spread

C. *Streptococcus* aureus most common causative bacteria

D. Lumbar puncture is not recommended

Most cases of spinal epidural abscess are due to Staphylococcus aureus. Gram-negative bacilli, streptococcus, anaerobes, fungi and tuberculosis are other important causes.

2187. The spinal cord is supplied by how many arteries?

Harrison's 20th Ed. Chapter 434, Page 3177

A. 1

B. 2

C. 3

D. 4

Spinal cord is supplied by 3 arteries—single anterior spinal artery & paired posterior spinal arteries.

2188. Which of the following about blood supply of spinal cord is false?

Harrison's 20th Ed. Chapter 434, Page 3177

A. Anterior spinal artery originates in paired branches of vertebral arteries at cranciocervical junction

B. Anterior spinal artery is fed by additional radicular vessels C6, upper thoracic and at T11-L2 level

C. Anterior spinal artery supplies anterior three-fourths of cord

D. Posterior spinal arteries supply the posterior columns

Anterior spinal artery supplies the anterior two-thirds of cord.

2189. Anterior spinal artery feeder - Artery of Adamkiewicz arises at?

Harrison's 20th Ed. Chapter 434, Page 3177

A. C6

B. T4 - T5

C. T11 - L2

D. L4 - L5

Anterior spinal artery is fed by radicular vessels that arise at C6, at an upper thoracic level, and most consistently, at T11 - L2 (artery of Adamkiewicz).

2190. Posterior spinal arteries become less distinct below?

Harrison's 20th Ed. Chapter 434, Page 3177

A. Midcervical level

B. Midthoracic level

C. Midlumbar level

D. Midsacral level

Posterior spinal arteries supply posterior columns & become less distinct below midthoracic level.

2191. With systemic hypotension, greatest ischemic risk of cord infarction is at the level of?

Harrison's 20th Ed. Chapter 434, Page 3177

A. C6

B. T3 - T4

C. T11 - L2

D. L5 - S1

With systemic hypotension, greatest ischemic risk is at T3-T4 and also at boundary zones between anterior & posterior spinal artery territories.

2192. Which of the following is not a feature of anterior cord syndrome?

Harrison's 20th Ed. Chapter 434, Page 3177

A. Paraplegia or quadriplegia

B. Loss of pain & temperature sense

C. Sparing of vibration & position sense

D. Preservation of sphincter control

Anterior cord syndrome is due to acute infarction in the territory of anterior spinal artery that presents as paraplegia or quadriplegia, dissociated sensory loss affecting pain & temperature sense but sparing vibration & position sense, and loss of sphincter control. Sharp midline or radiating back pain localized to the area of ischemia is frequent.

2193. Spinal cord infarction is associated with?

Harrison's 20th Ed. Chapter 434, Page 3177

A. Aortic atherosclerosis

B. Dissecting aortic aneurysm

C. Hypotension from any cause

D. All of the above

Spinal cord infarction results from aortic atherosclerosis, dissecting aortic aneurysm, vertebral artery occlusion or dissection in neck, profound hypotension from any cause, cardiogenic emboli, vasculitis related to collagen vascular disease, and surgical interruption of aortic aneurysms.

2194. Presentation of surfer's myelopathy resembles which of the following?

Harrison's 20th Ed. Chapter 434, Page 3177

A. Anterior cord syndrome

B. Brown-Sequard hemicord syndrome

C. Central cord syndrome

D. Foramen magnum syndrome

A surfer's myelopathy usually occurs in thoracic region. It is caused by prolonged back extension due to lifting upper body off the board while waiting for waves. It typically manifests as anterior cord syndrome.

2195. Recurrent episodes of myelitis are usually due to?

Harrison's 20th Ed. Chapter 434, Page 3177

A. SLE

B. Sarcoid

C. Infection with HSV- 2

D. All of the above

Recurrent episodes of myelitis are due to immune-mediated disease like SLE and sarcoid or to infection with HSV type 2.

2196. Which of the following is a demyelinating condition?

Harrison's 20th Ed. Chapter 434, Page 3177

A. Multiple sclerosis (MS)

B. Neuromyelitis optica (NMO)

C. Postinfectious myelitis

D. All of the above

2197. Acute myelitis in multiple sclerosis presents most commonly as?

Harrison's 20th Ed. Chapter 434, Page 3178

A. Transverse myelopathy

B. Partial cord syndrome

C. Anterior cord syndrome

D. Central cord syndrome

MS may present with acute myelitis and is among the most common causes of partial cord syndrome. MS attacks rarely cause a transverse myelopathy.

2198. Which of the following about neuromyelitis optica (NMO) is false?

Harrison's 20th Ed. Chapter 434, Page 3178

A. Immune-mediated demyelinating disorder
B. Longitudinally extensive severe myelopathy
C. Associated with optic neuritis
D. None of the above

NMO is an immune-mediated demyelinating disorder associated with a severe myelopathy that is typically longitudinally extensive (lesion spans ≥3 vertebral segments) and optic neuritis (often bilateral & may precede or follow myelitis). Brainstem, hypothalamic or focal cerebral white matter involvement may occur. Recurrent myelitis without optic nerve involvement can also occur in NMO.

2199. Neuromyelitis optica (NMO) is associated with?

Harrison's 20th Ed. Chapter 434, Page 3178

A. Antiphospholipid antibodies
B. SLE
C. Connective tissue diseases
D. All of the above

NMO is also associated with SLE, antiphospholipid antibodies and with other connective tissue diseases.

2200. Which of the laboratory findings are observed in NMO?

Harrison's 20th Ed. Chapter 434, Page 3178

A. Oligoclonal bands in CSF absent
B. Serum autoantibodies against aquaporin-4 present
C. Autoantibodies against myelin oligodendrocyte glycoprotein (MOG) may be found
D. All of the above

2201. Which of the following about neuromyelitis optica is false?

European Journal of Neurology 2010,17:1019–1032

A. Also called Devic's disease
B. Idiopathic immune-mediated inflammatory demyelinating disease
C. Predominantly involves spinal cord and optic nerves
D. None of the above

Association between optic neuritis (ON) & spinal cord impairment was first described by Sir Clifford Albutt in 1870. In 1894, Eugene Devic and his student Fernand Gault proposed the nature of the pathological process and named the syndrome as neuromyelitis optica.

2202. Endocrinopathies associated with NMO include?

European Journal of Neurology 2010,17:1019–1032

A. Amenorrhea, galactorrhea
B. Diabetes insipidus
C. Hypothyroidism, hyperphagia (class IV)
D. All of the above

Endocrinopathies associated with NMO include amenorrhea, galactorrhea, diabetes insipidus, hypothyroidism or hyperphagia (class IV).

2203. Cardinal clinical feature of neuromyelitis optica is?

Harrison's 20th Ed. Chapter 434, Page 3178

A. Longitudinally extensive transverse myelitis
B. Optic neuritis—unilateral or bilateral
C. Repeated relapses
D. All of the above

Complete transverse myelitis is typical of NMO & partial transverse myelitis syndromes is indicative of MS.

2204. Which of the following is false about NMO-IgG autoantibody?

Harrison's 20th Ed. Chapter 434, Page 3178

A. Target antigen is AQP4 water-pump channel
B. AQP4 is an integral protein of astrocytic plasma membranes
C. AQP4 is highly concentrated in astrocyte foot processes
D. None of the above

2205. Immune-mediated disorders causing acute transverse myelopathies (ATM) include?

Harrison's 20th Ed. Chapter 434, Page 3178

A. SLE
B. Sjogren's syndrome
C. Behcet's syndrome
D. All of the above

Immune-mediated myelitides include SLE, Sjögren's syndrome, antiphospholipid antibody syndrome, mixed connective tissue disease, Behçet's syndrome and vasculitis related to polyarteritis nodosa, perinuclear antineutrophilic cytoplasmic (p-ANCA) antibodies, primary central nervous system vasculitis and sarcoidosis.

2206. Antiphospholipid antibodies are found in which of the following immune-mediated disorders?

Harrison's 20th Ed. Chapter 434, Page 3178

A. SLE
B. Sjogren's syndrome
C. Behcet's syndrome
D. RA

Myelitis occurs in SLE associated with antiphospholipid antibodies.

2207. In which of the following myelopathies, a large edematous swelling of spinal cord mimicing tumor is observed?

Harrison's 20th Ed. Chapter 434, Page 3178

A. SLE
B. Sarcoidosis
C. Sjogren's syndrome
D. Behcet's syndrome

In sarcoid myelopathy, an edematous swelling of spinal cord may mimic tumor.

2208. Typical neurologic manifestation of sarcoidosis is?

Harrison's 20th Ed. Chapter 434, Page 3178

A. Cranial neuropathy
B. Hypothalamic involvement
C. Meningeal enhancement visualized by MRI
D. All of the above

Typical neurologic manifestation of sarcoidos are cranial neuropathy, hypothalamic involvement or meningeal enhancement visualized by MRI.

2209. Recurrent sacral myelitis which mimic multiple sclerosis is due to?

Harrison's 20th Ed. Chapter 434, Page 3178

A. HSV - 2
B. Herpes zoster
C. Epstein-Barr virus (EBV)
D. Cytomegalovirus (CMV)

HSV-2 causes recurrent sacral myelitis along with outbreaks of genital herpes mimicking MS.

2210. Which of the following about Elsberg's syndrome is false?
Harrison's 20th Ed. Chapter 434, Page 3179

A. HSV-2
B. Recurrent sacral cauda equina neuritis
C. Genital herpes
D. None of the above

HSV-2 produces a syndrome of recurrent sacral cauda equina neuritis in association with outbreaks of genital herpes (Elsberg's syndrome).

2211. A polio-like syndrome can also be caused by which of the following?
Harrison's 20th Ed. Chapter 434, Page 3179

A. Enterovirus 71 & coxsackie
B. Japanese encephalitis virus
C. West Nile virus
D. All of the above

Prototype of viral myelitis is poliomyelitis. A polio-like syndrome can also be caused by enteroviruses (enterovirus 71 & coxsackie), Japanese encephalitis virus and flaviviruses like West Nile virus.

2212. Which of the following can cause myelitis?
Harrison's 20th Ed. Chapter 434, Page 3179

A. Treponema pallidum
B. Borrelia burgdorferi
C. Listeria monocytogenes
D. All of the above

Borrelia burgdorferi (Lyme disease), Listeria monocytogenes, Mycobacterium tuberculosis, and Treponema pallidum (syphilis) can cause myelitis.

2213. Which of the following can cause myelitis?
Harrison's 20th Ed. Chapter 434, Page 3179

A. Schistosomiasis
B. Toxoplasmosis
C. Cysticercosis
D. All of the above

2214. Acyclovir is useful in treatment of myelitis caused by which of the following viruses?
Harrison's 20th Ed. Chapter 434, Page 3179

A. Herpes zoster
B. HSV
C. EBV
D. All of the above

Herpes zoster, HSV & EBV myelitis are treated with IV acyclovir or oral valacyclovir for 10 - 14 days.

2215. Ganciclovir plus foscarnet is indicated for the treatment of?
Harrison's 20th Ed. Chapter 434, Page 3179

A. Herpes zoster
B. HSV
C. EBV
D. CMV

CMV myelitis is treated with ganciclovir plus foscarnet or cidofovir.

2216. Which of the following is not a type of chronic myelopathy?
Harrison's 20th Ed. Chapter 434, Page 3179

A. Syringomyelia
B. Tabes dorsalis
C. HSV myelitis
D. Subacute combined degeneration of cord

2217. Foix-Alajouanine syndrome best relates with?
Harrison's 20th Ed. Chapter 434, Page 3179

A. Dural arteriovenous malformations
B. Progressive thoracic myelopathy
C. Paraparesis
D. All of the above

Foix-Alajouanine syndrome or subacute necrotic myelopathy refers to a progressive thoracic myelopathy with paraparesis developing over weeks or months, characterized by dural arteriovenous malformation (dAVF) of spinal cord, mostly lower thoracic & lumbar in location.

2218. Which of the following about Klippel-Trenaunay-Weber syndrome (KTWS) is false?
Journal of Vascular Surgery: Venous and Lymphatic Disorders 2017;5(4):587

A. Port-wine stain ((nevus flammeus)
B. Varicose veins
C. Bony & soft tissue hypertrophy involving an extremity
D. None of the above

Klippel-Trenaunay-Weber syndrome (KTWS) is characterized by a triad of cutaneous capillary malformations (port-wine stain), varicose veins, and bony and soft tissue hypertrophy involving an extremity.

2219. Differential diagnosis of Klippel-Trenaunay-Weber syndrome include?
Journal of Vascular Surgery: Venous and Lymphatic Disorders 2017;5(4):587

A. Sturge-Weber syndrome
B. Triploid syndrome
C. Proteus syndrome
D. All of the above

Differential diagnosis for patients being considered for KTS includes Sturge-Weber syndrome, Parkes Weber syndrome, lymphatic filariasis, Beckwith Wiedemann syndrome, Russell-Silver syndrome, congenital hemidysplasia with ichthyosiform erythroderma and limb defects (CHILD) syndrome, neurofibromatosis 1, triploid syndrome and Proteus syndrome.

2220. Which of the following disorders is associated with lymphedema?
Harrison's 20th Ed. Chapter 276, Page 1934

A. Neurofibromatosis type 1
B. Noonan's syndrome
C. Yellow nail syndrome
D. All of the above

Disorders associated with lymphedema include Klippel-Trénaunay syndrome, Parkes-Weber syndrome, Noonan's syndrome, yellow nail syndrome, intestinal lymphangiectasia syndrome, lymphangiomyomatosis, and neurofibromatosis type 1.

2221. Tropical spastic paraparesis best relates to?
Harrison's 20th Ed. Chapter 434, Page 3179

A. Human T cell lymphotropic virus-1 (HTLV-1)
B. Epstein-Barr Virus (EBV)
C. *Helicobacter pylori*
D. *Campylobacter jejuni*

2222. Syrinx cavities are caused by all except?
Harrison's 20th Ed. Chapter 434, Page 3180

A. Syringomyelia
B. Trauma
C. Myelitis
D. Chronic arachnoiditis due to tuberculosis

Syringomyelia is a developmental cavity of the cervical cord. Syrinx cavities are acquired cavitations of spinal cord in areas of necrosis. They may be due trauma, myelitis, necrotic spinal cord tumors and chronic arachnoiditis due to tuberculosis.

2223. Which of the following is false about syringomyelia?
Harrison's 20th Ed. Chapter 434, Page 3180

A. Acquired or developmental
B. Symptoms begin in adolescence or early adulthood
C. Associated with Chiari type 1 malformations
D. None of the above

2224. Which of the following is false about syringomyelia?
Harrison's 20th Ed. Chapter 434, Page 3180

A. Dissociated sensory loss in upper limbs
B. Areflexic weakness in upper limbs
C. Spasticity and weakness of the legs
D. None of the above

Dissociated sensory loss can reflect spinothalamic tract involvement in spinal cord (bilateral spinothalamic tract involvement occurs in syringomyelia). There occurs impairment of pinprick & temperature appreciation but relative preservation of light touch, position sense & vibration appreciation.

2225. Which of the following is related to the sensory deficit in syringomyelia?
Harrison's 20th Ed. Chapter 434, Page 3180

A. Poisson distribution
B. Limb-girdle distribution
C. Cape distribution
D. Tibial distribution

In syringomyelia, cape distribution refers to the sensory deficit has a distribution that is "suspended" over nape of the neck, shoulders and upper arms or in the hands. This central cord syndrome initially produces signs & symptoms caused by dysfunction of crossing spinothalamic tract fibers that pass through anterior white commissure at that level. As the lesion expands to anterior gray matter of spinal cord, it may destroy anterior horn cells, causing weakness & wasting of muscles (LMN signs) at the involved levels.

2226. Which of the following is related to the sensory deficit in syringomyelia?
Harrison's 20th Ed. Chapter 434, Page 3180

A. Sparing the face
B. Sacral sparing
C. Pupil-sparing oculomotor palsy
D. Bladder-sparing

In syringomyelia, further enlargement of central lesion leads to involvement of spinothalamic tracts. As spinothalamic tract fibers from sacral areas are most distant from the center of spinal cord, the saddle area is spared ("sacral sparing").

2227. Syringobulbia causes which of the following?
Harrison's 20th Ed. Chapter 434, Page 3180

A. Horizontal or vertical nystagmus
B. Palatal or vocal cord paralysis
C. Tongue weakness with atrophy
D. All of the above

Syringobulbia causes palatal or vocal cord paralysis, dysarthria, horizontal or vertical nystagmus, episodic dizziness or vertigo, and tongue weakness with atrophy.

2228. Which of the following is false about chronic myelopathy of multiple sclerosis?
Harrison's 20th Ed. Chapter 434, Page 3181

A. Bilateral
B. Asymmetric
C. Motor, sensory, and bladder/bowel disturbances
D. None of the above

In chronic progressive myelopathy of MS, involvement is typically bilateral but asymmetric & produces motor, sensory & bladder/bowel disturbances.

2229. Which of the following drugs is effective in patients with primary progressive MS?
Harrison's 20th Ed. Chapter 434, Page 3181

A. Natalizumab
B. Alemtuzumab
C. Ocrelizumab
D. All of the above

Treatment with ocrelizumab, an anti-CD20 B-cell monoclonal antibody, is effective in patients with primary progressive MS.

2230. Which of the following is false about subacute combined degeneration of cord?
Harrison's 20th Ed. Chapter 434, Page 3181

A. Loss of deep tendon reflexes
B. Babinski sign
C. Romberg's sign
D. None of the above

2231. Which of the following is false about subacute combined degeneration of cord?
Harrison's 20th Ed. Chapter 434, Page 3181

A. Macrocytic red blood cells
B. Elevated serum levels of homocysteine
C. Elevated serum levels of methylmalonic acid
D. None of the above

2232. Which of the following condition is virtually identical to subacute combined degeneration?
Harrison's 20th Ed. Chapter 434, Page 3181

A. Adrenomyeloneuropathy
B. Tabes dorsalis
C. Familial spastic paraplegia
D. Hypocupric myelopathy

Hypocupric myelopathy is virtually identical to subacute combined degeneration except there is no neuropathy. Serum levels of B12 are normal, serum copper & ceruloplasmin levels are low.

2233. Which of the following is a copper-binding protein?
Harrison's 20th Ed. Chapter 434, Page 3181

A. Rubinstein
B. Lectin
C. Metallothionein
D. Haptocorrin

Metallothionein is a copper-binding protein.

2234. Which of the following condition producing myelopathy identical to subacute combined degeneration?

Harrison's 20th Ed. Chapter 434, Page 3181

A. Adrenomyeloneuropathy
B. Tabes dorsalis
C. Familial spastic paraplegia
D. Nitrous oxide inhalation

Nitrous oxide inhalation producing a myelopathy identical to subacute combined degeneration.

2235. Which of the following is false about tabes dorsalis?

Harrison's 20th Ed. Chapter 434, Page 3181

A. Fleeting & repetitive lancinating pains in legs
B. Ataxia
C. Acute abdominal pain with vomiting
D. None of the above

2236. Which of the following is false about tabes dorsalis?

Harrison's 20th Ed. Chapter 434, Page 3181

A. Loss of deep tenson reflexes in legs
B. Impaired position & vibratory sense
C. Romberg's sign
D. None of the above

2237. Which of the following polyradiculopathy may simulate tabes dorsalis?

Harrison's 20th Ed. Chapter 434, Page 3181

A. Non-Hodgkin's lymphoma
B. EBV polyradiculopathy
C. CMV polyradiculopathy
D. Diabetic polyradiculopathy

2238. Which of the following is false about adrenomyeloneuropathy?

Harrison's 20th Ed. Chapter 434, Page 3181

A. Mixed motor & sensory neuropathy
B. Flaccid paraplegia
C. Elevated levels of very long chain fatty acids
D. Adrenal insufficiency

Adrenomyeloneuropathy is associated with a mixed motor & sensory neuropathy with spastic paraplegia in adults associated with elevated circulating levels of very long chain fatty acids and adrenal insufficiency. The responsible gene encodes ADLP.

2239. Which of the following is false about Tethered cord syndrome?

Harrison's 20th Ed. Chapter 434, Page 3181

A. Developmental disorder of lower spinal cord & nerve roots
B. A dimple, hair patch, or sinus tract on skin overlying lower back
C. Diastematomyelia
D. None of the above

2240. Lathyrism is due to ingestion of faulty?

Harrison's 20th Ed. Chapter 434, Page 3181

A. Peas
B. Chick peas
C. Soyabean
D. Barley

Lathyrism due to ingestion of chick peas containing the excitotoxin β-N-oxalylaminoalanine (BOAA).

2241. The prospects for recovery from an acute destructive spinal cord lesion fade after?

Harrison's 20th Ed. Chapter 434, Page 3182

A. ~ 1 month
B. ~ 3 months
C. ~ 6 months
D. ~ 12 months

The prospects for recovery from an acute destructive spinal cord lesion fade after ~6 months.

2242. Which of the following is a feature of quadriplegic fever?

Harrison's 20th Ed. Chapter 434, Page 3182

A. Loss of normal thermoregulation
B. Inability to maintain normal body temperature
C. Recurrent fever
D. None of the above

2243. Which of the following is an α2 adrenergic agonist?

Harrison's 20th Ed. Chapter 434, Page 3182

A. Dantrolene
B. Tizanidine
C. Terazosin hydrochloride
D. Oxybutynin

Tizanidine is an α2 adrenergic agonist that increases presynaptic inhibition of motor neurons.

2244. In cervical radiculopathy, weakness of deltoid, supraspinatus & infraspinatus muscles signify lesion in which root?

N Engl J Med. 2005;353:392-9

A. C5
B. C6
C. C7
D. C8

2245. In cervical radiculopathy, weakness of biceps, brachioradialis, wrist extensor muscles signify lesion in the root?

N Engl J Med. 2005;353:392-9

A. C5
B. C6
C. C7
D. C8

2246. In cervical radiculopathy, weakness of triceps, wrist flexor, finger extensor muscles signify lesion in the root?

N Engl J Med. 2005;353:392-9

A. C5
B. C6
C. C7
D. C8

2247. In cervical radiculopathy, weakness of thumb flexors, abductors, intrinsic hand muscles signify lesion in the root?

N Engl J Med. 2005;353:392-9

A. C5
B. C6
C. C7
D. C8

2248. In cervical radiculopathy, sensory loss over lateral upper arm signifies lesion in the root?

N Engl J Med. 2005;353:392-9

A. C5
B. C6
C. C7
D. C8

2249. In cervical radiculopathy, sensory loss over thumb and index finger signifies lesion in the root?

N Engl J Med. 2005;353:392-9

A. C5
B. C6
C. C7
D. C8

2250. In cervical radiculopathy, sensory loss over posterior forearm and third finger signifies lesion in the root?

N Engl J Med. 2005;353:392-9

A. C5
B. C6
C. C7
D. C8

2251. In cervical radiculopathy, sensory loss over fifth finger signifies lesion in the root?

N Engl J Med. 2005;353:392-9

A. C5
B. C6
C. C7
D. C8

2252. In cervical radiculopathy, loss of supinator reflex signifies lesion in the root?

N Engl J Med. 2005;353:392-9

A. C5
B. C6
C. C7
D. C8

2253. In cervical radiculopathy, loss of biceps reflex signifies lesion in the root?

N Engl J Med. 2005;353:392-9

A. C5
B. C6
C. C7
D. C8

2254. In cervical radiculopathy, loss of triceps reflex signifies lesion in the root?

N Engl J Med. 2005;353:392-9

A. C5
B. C6
C. C7
D. C8

2255. In cervical radiculopathy, pain in the region of medial scapular border, lateral upper arm to elbow signifies lesion in the root?

N Engl J Med. 2005;353:392-9

A. C5
B. C6
C. C7
D. C8

2256. In cervical radiculopathy, pain in the region of lateral forearm, thumb and index finger signifies lesion in the root?

N Engl J Med. 2005;353:392-9

A. C5
B. C6
C. C7
D. C8

2257. In cervical radiculopathy, pain in the region of medial scapula, posterior arm, dorsum of forearm & third finger signifies lesion in the root?

N Engl J Med. 2005;353:392-9

A. C5
B. C6
C. C7
D. C8

2258. In cervical radiculopathy, pain in the region of shoulder, ulnar side of forearm, fifth finger signifies lesion in the root?

N Engl J Med. 2005;353:392-9

A. C5
B. C6
C. C7
D. C8

2259. Spurling maneuver is?

N Engl J Med. 2005;353:392-9

A. Foraminal compression test in cervical radiculopathy
B. Opposite of Valsalva maneuver
C. Other name of hyperventilation
D. Breath holding test

2260. Parsonage-Turner syndrome refers to?

N Engl J Med. 2005;353:392-9

A. Acute brachial-plexus neuritis
B. Peripheral entrapment neuropathies
C. Disorders of the rotator cuff and shoulder
D. Referred somatic pain from the neck

2261. Differential diagnosis of cervical radiculopathy include?

N Engl J Med. 2005;353:392-9

A. Peripheral entrapment neuropathies
B. Disorders of rotator cuff & shoulder
C. Acute brachial-plexus neuritis
D. All of the above

2262. Differential diagnosis of cervical radiculopathy include?

N Engl J Med. 2005;353:392-9

A. Thoracic outlet syndrome
B. Herpes zoster
C. Pancoast syndrome
D. All of the above

2263. Tinel's sign and Phalen's maneuver best relate to?

N Engl J Med. 2005;353:392-9

A. Thoracic outlet syndrome
B. Acute brachial-plexus neuritis
C. Carpal tunnel syndrome
D. Pancoast syndrome

2264. Hypoesthesia and weakness in medial three digits and opponens pollicis occurs in?

N Engl J Med. 2005;353:392-9

A. Median nerve entrapment
B. Ulnar nerve entrapment
C. Thoracic outlet syndrome
D. Pancoast syndrome

2265. Hypoesthesia and weakness in the fourth and fifth digits and thumb adductor occurs in?

N Engl J Med. 2005;353:392-9

A. Median nerve entrapment
B. Ulnar nerve entrapment
C. Thoracic outlet syndrome
D. Pancoast syndrome

2266. Which of the following statements about Roo's test is false?

N Engl J Med. 2005;353:392-9

A. It is a kind of provocation test
B. Used for diagnosis of thoracic outlet syndrome
C. Done by rapid flexion and extension of fingers while the arms are abducted at 90° and externally rotated 90°
D. Intermittent paresthesia, most commonly in C5 region

2267. Which of the following is false about paraplegia in extension?

Proc. Rom. Acad., Series B, 2013;15(3):197-215

A. Cause is lesion in pyramidal tracts
B. Clonus present
C. Mass reflex present
D. Position of lower limbs is extended

Paraplegia in extension has following feature : cause is lesion in pyramidal tracts, hypertonia is more in extensors, position of lower limbs is extended, deep reflexes are exaggerated, clonus is present, mass reflex is absent and bladder precipitancy is apparent.

2268. Which of the following is false about paraplegia in flexion?

Proc. Rom. Acad., Series B, 2013;15(3):197-215

A. Cause is lesion in pyramidal tracts and extrapyramidal
B. Clonus present
C. Mass reflex may be present
D. Position of lower limbs is in flexion

Paraplegia in flexion has following feature : cause is lesion in pyramidal and extrapyramidal tracts, hypertonia is more in flexors, position of lower limbs is flexed, deep reflexes are less exaggerated, clonus is absent, mass reflex may be present and automatic bladder is apparent.

2269. Which of the following about central cord syndrome is false?

Proc. Rom. Acad., Series B, 2013;15(3):197-215

A. Occurs almost exclusively in cervical region
B. Due to hyperextension pathogenic mechanism
C. Also known as "inverse paraplegia"
D. None of the above

Central cord syndrome occurs almost exclusively in the cervical region, usually by a hyperextension pathogenic mechanism. It produces localized sensitivity alteration for pain and temperature, with tendon reflex weakness. If the lesion enlarges - greater motor loss in the upper limbs than in lower ones occurs. It is therefore also known as "inverse paraplegia". Sacral sparing is noted.

2270. Which of the following about lateral (Brown-Sequard) syndrome is false?

Proc. Rom. Acad., Series B, 2013;15(3):197-215

A. Ipsilateral proprioceptive loss
B. Ipsilateral motor weakness
C. Controlateral loss of touch, pain and temperature
D. None of the above

In lateral (Brown-Sequard) syndrome, the lesion (e.g. stab wound - injury on a lateral side/hemi-section) produces greater ipsilateral proprioceptive, vibration, light touch sensitivity (posterior column impairment), paresthesias and motor weakness, possible reflex changes, and controlateral loss of sensitivity to touch, pain and temperature.

2271. Which of the following about anterior (ventral) cord syndrome is false?

Proc. Rom. Acad., Series B, 2013;15(3):197-215

A. Frequently occurs after a hyperflexion injury
B. Preserved proprioception
C. Variable loss of motor function, urinary continence
D. None of the above

In anterior (ventral) cord syndrome, the lesion, frequently occurs after a hyperflexion injury. It produces a variable loss of motor function, urinary continence, sensitivity to pain and temperature perception with preserved proprioception.

2272. Which of the following about posterior (dorsal) cord syndrome is false?

Proc. Rom. Acad., Series B, 2013;15(3):197-215

A. Lesion is often nontraumatic
B. Loss of two points discrimination
C. Ataxia
D. None of the above

In posterior (dorsal) cord syndrome, the lesion is more often nontraumatic. It produces loss of two points discrimination (epicritic sensitivity) and of proprioception, associated with ataxia, paresthesias and possibly urinary incontinece. Sensitivity for pain, and light touch, as well as motor function, remain intact.

2273. Which of the following about transverse/transsection (total) cord syndrome is false?

Proc. Rom. Acad., Series B, 2013;15(3):197-215

A. Complete loss of sensory modalities
B. Complete loss of motor functions
C. Complete loss of autonomic modalities
D. None of the above

In transverse/transsection (total) cord syndrome, the lesion results from a crush, and also possibly secondary to hemorrhagic or infectious, insults. It produces complete interruption/loss of any spinal cord control (sensory, motor, also autonomic) in terms of efficient functionality below the lesion level.

2274. "Osinski reflex" is best related to?

Proc. Rom. Acad., Series B, 2013;15(3):197-215

A. Anal reflex
B. Bulbo-cavernosus reflex
C. Cremasteric reflex
D. Anterior abdominal reflex

2275. Which of the following about conus medullaris syndrome is false?

Proc. Rom. Acad., Series B, 2013;15(3):197-215

A. Injury occurs between T11 and L2
B. Results in neurological impairments of bladder & bowel
C. Results in sexual impairment
D. None of the above

In conus medullaris syndrome, the lesion is due to injury of the distal cord (conus), typically between T11 and L2. It results in neurological impairments of bladder, bowel, sexual and lower limbs functionality (mild/ symmetrical). The affected segments may occasionally show preserved reflexes (e.g. bulbo-cavernosus or "Osinski reflex", perianal wink/ano-cutaneous reflex related to micturition). If still absent after the spinal shock has passed, this proves the irreversibility of damage to such neural structures.

2276. Which of the following about cauda equina syndrome is false?

Proc. Rom. Acad., Series B, 2013;15(3):197-215

A. Injury occurs to lumbar-sacral nerve roots
B. Results in neurological impairments of bladder & bowel
C. Results in sexual impairment
D. None of the above

In cauda equina syndrome, injury to the lumbar-sacral (2 or more of its 18) nerve roots within the spinal canal, result in neurological impairments of bladder, bowel, sexual function and/or lower limbs. If there are affected mainly high and/or medium levels (L1-S1), the main symptoms consist in low back pain and somatic sensitive, motor, reflex and/or trophic deficits, whereas insults in the lowest ones (S2-S4) affect the sacral and perineum dermatomes, including with sphincters and/or sexual functions. The prognostic is better.

2277. Which dermatome is represented in apex of the axilla?

Proc. Rom. Acad., Series B, 2013;15(3):197-215

A. T1
B. T2
C. T3
D. T4

Root value at various locations on the body are : C2 – Occipital protuberance, C3 – Supraclavicular fossa, C4 – Top of the acromioclavicular joint, C5 – Lateral side of the antecubital fossa, C6 – Thumb, C7 – Middle finger, C8 – Little finger, T1 – Medial (ulnar) side of the antecubital fossa, T2 – Apex of the axilla, T3 – Third intercostal space, T4 – Fourth ICS (nipple line), T5 – Fifth ICS (midway between T4 and T6), T6 – Sixth IS (level of xiphisternum), T7 – Seventh IS (midway between T6 and T8), T8 – Eighth ICS (midway between T6 and T10), T9 – Ninth IS (midway between T8 and T10), T10 – Tenth ICS (umbilicus), T11 – Eleventh IS (midway between T10 and T12), T12 – Inguinal ligament at mid-point, L1 – Half the distance between T12 and L2, L2 – Mid-anterior thigh, L3 – Medial femoral condyle, L4 – Medial malleolus, L5 – Dorsum of the foot at the third metatarsal phalangeal joint, S1 – Lateral heel, S2 – Popliteal fossa in the mid-line, S3 – Ischial tuberosity, S4 – 5 Perianal area.

2278. Which of the following is a cause of pure motor paraplegia without sensory loss?

Proc. Rom. Acad., Series B, 2013;15(3):197-215

A. Hereditary spastic paraplegia
B. Lathyrism
C. Amyotrophic lateral sclerosis
D. All of the above

Causes of pure motor paraplegia without sensory loss are Hereditary spastic paraplegia, Lathyrism, Amyotrophic lateral sclerosis, Fluorosis, Guillain-Barre syndrome.

2279. Which of the following is a cause of cord compression at multiple levels?

Proc. Rom. Acad., Series B, 2013;15(3):197-215

A. Arachnoiditis
B. Neurofibromatosis
C. Spondylosis—cervical and lumbar level
D. All of the above

Causes of cord compression at multiple levels are Arachnoiditis, Multiple secondaries, Multiple sclerosis, Neurofibramatosis, Spondylosis—cervical and lumbar level.

2280. Which of the following is false about mass reflex?

Proc. Rom. Acad., Series B, 2013;15(3):197-215

A. Stimulation below level of lesion produces flexion reflexes of the lower limb
B. Evacuation of bowel & bladder
C. Sweating of skin below the level of lesion
D. None of the above

In mass reflex occurs in severe injury of spinal cord wherein stimulation below the level of lesion produces flexion reflexes of the lower limbs, evacuation of bowel & bladder and sweating of the skin below the level of lesion.

2281. Which of the following mediates reflex head & neck movements in response to visual & vestibular stimuli?

DeJong's The Neurologic Examination, 7th Ed. Page 130 Table 11.3

A. Corticobulbar tract
B. Rubrospinal tract
C. Medical longitudinal fasciculus
D. All of the above

Descending Medical longitudinal fasciculus (MLF) contains vestibulospinal and reticulospinal fibers, mediates reflex head and neck movements in response to visual and vestibular stimuli.

2282. Which of the following is a trigeminal mediated reflex?

DeJong's The Neurologic Examination, 7th Ed. Page 236

A. Zygomatic reflex
B. Head retraction
C. Nasal reflex of Bechterew
D. All of the above

Various trigeminal mediated reflexes are : Head retraction (A sharp tap with the reflex hammer just below the nose with the head bent slightly forward produces a quick, involuntary backward jerk of the head. Present in bilateral corticospinal lesions rostral to the cervical spine, e.g. amyotrophic lateral sclerosis (ALS). Not present in normals.), Zygomatic reflex (A modification of the jaw jerk. Percussion over the zygoma produces ipsilateral deviation of the mandible. Seen only with supranuclear lesions.), Oculosensory or oculopupillary reflex (Constriction of the pupil, or dilation followed by constriction, in response to a painful stimulus directed toward the eye or its adnexa.), Corneo-oculogyric reflex (Contralateral or upward deviation of the eyes in response to stimulation of the conjunctive or cornea, with associated contraction of the orbicularis.), Corneomandibular reflex (Stimulation of cornea causes contralateral movement of the mandible. May be an associated movement rather than a true reflex. Indicates supranuclear interruption of the ipsilateral corticotrigeminal tract. Said to be the only eye sign in ALS.), Nasal reflex of Bechterew (Similar to sternutatory reflex. Tickling of the nasal mucosa causes contraction of the ipsilateral facial muscles.), Trigeminobrachial reflex (Contralateral flexion and supination of the forearm after stimulation in the distribution of CN V), Trigeminocervical reflex (Contralateral head turn after stimulation in the distribution of CN V).

2283. Which of the following is a facial reflex?

DeJong's The Neurologic Examination, 7th Ed. Page 254

A. McCarthy's reflex
B. Myerson's sign
C. Chvostek's sign
D. All of the above

Transverse Myelitis

2284. Which of the following does not relate well with transverse myelitis?

N Engl J Med. 2010;363:564-72

A. Inflammatory disorder
B. Acute
C. Subacute
D. Chronic

Transverse myelitis is a heterogeneous group of acute or subacute inflammatory disorders with motor, sensory and autonomic (bladder, bowel, and sexual) spinal cord dysfunction.

2285. Transverse myelitis syndrome "most often" occurs due to?

N Engl J Med. 2010;363:564-72

A. Autoimmune phenomenon after infection or vaccination
B. Direct infection
C. Underlying systemic autoimmune disease
D. Acquired demyelinating disease

Transverse myelitis syndrome most often occurs as an autoimmune phenomenon after an infection or vaccination or as a result of a direct infection, an underlying systemic autoimmune disease, acquired demyelinating disease (multiple sclerosis) or idiopathic (15–30%)

2286. In transverse myelitis, most of the recovery occurs over?

N Engl J Med. 2010;363:564-72

A. First 3 months after the event
B. First 6 months after the event
C. First 12 months after the event
D. First 18 months after the event

Most of the recovery in transverse myelitis cases occurs in the first 3 months after the event. Although, improvement may continue for a year or longer.

2287. Pathological hallmark of transverse myelitis within the spinal cord is?

N Engl J Med. 2010;363:564-72

A. Focal collections of neutrophils
B. Focal collections of lymphocytes & monocytes
C. Focal collections of eosinophils
D. Focal collections of basophils

In spinal cord, pathological hallmark of transverse myelitis is the presence of focal collections of lymphocytes and monocytes, with varying degrees of demyelination, axonal injury and astroglial and microglial activation.

2288. Prognosis in transverse myelitis associated with multiple sclerosis is?

N Engl J Med. 2010;363:564-72

A. Good
B. Bad
C. Worse
D. Worst

Transverse myelitis associated with multiple sclerosis may have a substantial or even complete recovery. Transverse myelitis or neuromyelitis optica associated with other diseases usually have clinically significant residual neurologic deficits.

2289. "Spinal shock" consists of all except?

N Engl J Med. 2010;363:564-72

A. Areflexia
B. Sensory loss
C. Severe weakness
D. Hypotonia

"Spinal shock" refers to a combination of severe weakness, hypotonia and areflexia. It is the only recognized predictor of a poor outcome in transverse myelitis.

2290. Which of the following best distinguishes myelopathy from cerebral lesions and peripheral neuropathies?

N Engl J Med. 2010;363:564-72

A. Seizure
B. Sensory level
C. Babinski signs
D. Course of illness

A well-defined truncal sensory level, below which the sensation of pain & temperature is altered or lost, distinguishes myelopathy from cerebral lesions & peripheral neuropathies.

2291. Which of the following is responsible for the Lhermitte's sign in transverse myelitis?

N Engl J Med. 2010;363:564-72

A. Demyelination
B. Axonal injury
C. Astroglial activation
D. Microglial activation

Demyelination is responsible for the Lhermitte's sign that refers to the paresthesias that radiate down the spine or limbs with neck flexion. Demyelination is responsible for the paroxysmal tonic spasms i.e.involuntary dystonic contractions of limb or trunk muscles.

2292. Which of the following is false about idiopathic transverse myelitis?

N Engl J Med. 2010;363:564-72

A. No cerebrospinal fluid abnormalities
B. No MRI abnormalities
C. No identifiable underlying cause
D. None of the above

Patients with possible idiopathic transverse myelitis have clinical events consistent with transverse myelitis but that are not associated with cerebrospinal fluid abnormalities or abnormalities detected on MRI and that have no identifiable underlying cause.

2293. Presentation in transverse myelitis include?

N Engl J Med. 2010;363:564-72

A. Sensory spinal cord dysfunction
B. Motor spinal cord dysfunction
C. Autonomic spinal cord dysfunction
D. All of the above

Diagnostic criteria for transverse myelitis include bilateral (not necessarily symmetric) sensorimotor and autonomic spinal cord dysfunction.

2294. In transverse myelitis, clinical deficits progress to nadir between?
N Engl J Med. 2010;363:564-72

A. 4 hours and 7 days after symptom onset
B. 4 hours and 14 days after symptom onset
C. 4 hours and 21 days after symptom onset
D. 4 hours and 28 days after symptom onset

Progression to nadir of clinical deficits between 4 hours and 21 days after symptom onset is characteristic of transverse myelitis.

2295. Which of the following is true for MRI findings characteristic of myelitis?
N Engl J Med. 2010;363:564-72

A. More than one intrinsic cord lesions
B. Intrinsic cord lesions span at least two vertebral segments
C. Lesions enhance with intravenous gadolinium
D. All of the above

MRI finding of more than one intrinsic cord lesion is characteristic of myelitis. In acute phase, lesions enhance with intravenous gadolinium administration. Lesions in idiopathic transverse myelitis usually span at least two vertebral segments. Normal MRI should prompt a reconsideration of the diagnosis of myelopathy in favor of other disorders of the central or peripheral nervous system.

2296. Serum autoantibodies like antinuclear antibody or extractable nuclear antigen are present in?
N Engl J Med. 2010;363:564-72

A. Multiple sclerosis
B. Neuromyelitis optica
C. Systemic lupus erythematosus
D. All of the above

Serum autoantibodies like antinuclear antibody or extractable nuclear antigen may be present in patients with multiple sclerosis or neuromyelitis optica, systemic lupus erythematosus.

2297. MRI findings in multiple sclerosis include?
N Engl J Med. 2010;363:564-72

A. Short lesions spanning less than two vertebral segments
B. Lesions located in the periphery of the cord
C. Concomitant MRI evidence of demyelinating brain lesions
D. All of the above

Multiple sclerosis is associated with short lesions, spanning fewer than two vertebral segments, located in the periphery of the cord, affecting mainly white matter ("partial" transverse myelitis), and concomitant MRI evidence of demyelinating brain lesions.

2298. MRI findings in Neuromyelitis optica include?
N Engl J Med. 2010;363:564-72

A. Longitudinally extensive lesions spanning three or more vertebral segments
B. Symmetric lesions
C. Lesions situated centrally within the cord
D. All of the above

Neuromyelitis optica is strongly associated with longitudinally extensive transverse myelitis, defined by a lesion that spans three or more vertebral segments on MRI. Such lesions tend to be symmetric and situated centrally within the cord (involving both gray and white matter) and may extend into the brain stem, causing nausea, vomiting, and hiccups.

2299. Serum autoantibody marker NMO-IgG targets?
N Engl J Med. 2010;363:564-72

A. Beta2GPI
B. aCL
C. Astrocytic water channel, aquaporin-4
D. Anti-LKM3

Neuromyelitis optica is specifically associated with the serum autoantibody marker NMO-IgG, which targets the astrocytic water channel, aquaporin-4.

2300. Which of the following is not a monophasic syndrome?
N Engl J Med. 2010;363:564-72

A. Postinfectious transverse myelitis
B. Postvaccination transverse myelitis
C. Idiopathic transverse myelitis
D. Multiple sclerosis

Postinfectious, postvaccination and idiopathic forms of transverse myelitis are usually monophasic syndromes, whereas multiple sclerosis and neuromyelitis optica.spectrum disorders are relapsing diseases that are associated with a high risk of future attacks of transverse myelitis and other neurologic events.

2301. What happens to the IgG index in transverse myelitis?
N Engl J Med. 2010;363:564-72

A. Normal
B. Decreased
C. Increased
D. Any of the above

IgG index is a measure of intrathecal synthesis of immunoglobulin and is calculated by the following formula - (CSF IgG ÷ serum IgG) ÷ (CSF albumin ÷ serum albumin).

Multiple Sclerosis

2302. Which of the following is false about demyelinating disorders?

Harrison's 20th Ed. Chapter 436, Page 3188

A. Immune-mediated preferential destruction of CNS myelin
B. Peripheral nervous system (PNS) is spared
C. No evidence of associated systemic illness
D. None of the above

Demyelinating disorders are immune-mediated conditions characterized by preferential destruction of central nervous system (CNS) myelin. The peripheral nervous system (PNS) is spared, and most patients have no evidence of an associated systemic illness.

2303. Which about Multiple sclerosis (MS) is false?

Harrison's 20th Ed. Chapter 436, Page 3188

A. Onset of MS may be abrupt or insidious
B. Symptoms may be severe or trivial
C. Course can be relapsing or progressive
D. None of the above

2304. Triad in multiple sclerosis (MS) includes all except?

Harrison's 20th Ed. Chapter 436, Page 3188

A. Chronic inflammation
B. Demyelination
C. Remyelination
D. Gliosis

Multiple sclerosis is characterized by a triad of chronic inflammation, demyelination, and gliosis (scarring) with neuronal loss specially in advanced cases. Demyelination is the pathological hallmark. Relative sparing of axons is typical of MS. Lesions of MS typically occur at different times and in different CNS locations (i.e., disseminated in time and space).

2305. Which out of the following is the most common initial symptoms of MS?

Harrison's 20th Ed. Chapter 436, Page 3188 Table 436-1

A. Paresthesias
B. Diplopia
C. Ataxia
D. Vertigo

2306. Which out of the following is the most common initial symptoms of MS?

Harrison's 20th Ed. Chapter 436, Page 3188 Table 436-1

A. Sensory loss
B. Diplopia
C. Optic neuritis
D. Bladder dysfunction

2307. Which of the following about sensory symptoms in MS is false?

Harrison's 20th Ed. Chapter 436, Page 3188

A. Paresthesias
B. Hypesthesia
C. Sensory level
D. None of the above

Sensory symptoms in MS include paresthesias, hypesthesia, unpleasant sensations, bandlike sensation of tightness around torso.

2308. In MS, optic neuritis (ON) is least likely to present as?

Harrison's 20th Ed. Chapter 436, Page 3188

A. Diminished visual acuity
B. Dimness
C. Decreased color perception
D. Complete loss of light perception

Optic neuritis (ON) presents as diminished visual acuity, dimness, or decreased color perception (desaturation) in the central field of vision. Rarely, there is complete loss of light perception.

2309. In MS, which of the following statements is false?

Harrison's 20th Ed. Chapter 436, Page 3188

A. Visual symptoms are generally bilateral
B. Periorbital pain precedes or accompanies visual loss
C. Afferent pupillary defect is usually present
D. Uveitis is uncommon

Visual symptoms are generally monocular but may be bilateral. Periorbital pain often precedes or accompanies visual loss. Afferent pupillary defect is usually present. Funduscopic examination may be normal or reveal optic disc swelling (papillitis). Pallor of optic disc (optic atrophy) commonly follows ON. Uveitis is uncommon.

2310. Which of the following is uncommon in MS?

Harrison's 20th Ed. Chapter 436, Page 3188

A. Hearing loss
B. Uveitis
C. Complete loss of light perception
D. All of the above

2311. Which of the following is characteristic of MS?

Harrison's 20th Ed. Chapter 436, Page 3188

A. Movement-induced muscle spasms
B. Exercise-induced weakness of limbs
C. Monocular visual loss
D. Acquired pendular nystagmus

Exercise-induced weakness of limbs is characteristic of MS. Weakness is of UMN type accompanied by spasticity, hyperreflexia & Babinski signs.

2312. In MS, facial weakness is characterised by?

Harrison's 20th Ed. Chapter 436, Page 3188

A. Resembles idiopathic Bell's palsy
B. Not associated with ipsilateral loss of taste sensation
C. Not associated with retroauricular pain
D. All of the above

Facial weakness due to a MS lesion in pons resembles idiopathic Bell's palsy but is not associated with ipsilateral loss of taste or retroauricular pain.

2313. Which of the following is strongly suggestive of MS?

Harrison's 20th Ed. Chapter 436, Page 3188

A. Horizontal gaze palsy
B. Bilateral internuclear ophthalmoplegia (INO)
C. "One and a half" syndrome
D. Acquired pendular nystagmus

Bilateral internuclear ophthalmoplegia (INO) is particularly suggestive of MS. Other gaze disturbances include horizontal gaze palsy, "one and a half" syndrome (horizontal gaze palsy + an INO) & acquired pendular nystagmus.

2314. Visual blurring in MS may result from?

Harrison's 20th Ed. Chapter 436, Page 3188

A. Keratitis
B. Diplopia
C. Uveitis
D. Retinitis

Visual blurring in MS may result from optic neuritis (ON) or diplopia (double vision).

2315. Ataxia in MS usually manifests as?

Harrison's 20th Ed. Chapter 436, Page 3188

A. Cerebellar tremors
B. Hyperthyroid tremors
C. Episodic ataxia
D. Gait apraxia

Ataxia usually manifests as cerebellar tremors. It involves head and trunk or voice, producing a characteristic cerebellar dysarthria (scanning speech).

2316. In MS, paroxysmal symptoms are due to?

Harrison's 20th Ed. Chapter 436, Page 3188

A. Plaque rupture
B. Spontaneous discharges
C. Neovascularization
D. Disruption in blood-brain barrier

In MS, paroxysmal symptoms are due to spontaneous discharges arising at the edges of demyelinated plaques & spreading to adjacent white matter tracts.

2317. In MS, which of the following is false about paroxysmal symptoms?

Harrison's 20th Ed. Chapter 436, Page 3188

A. Brief duration (10 secopnds to 2 minutes), self-limited
B. High frequency (5–40 episodes per day)
C. No change in consciousness or background EEG
D. None of the above

2318. In MS, paroxysmal symptoms may be precipitated by?

Harrison's 20th Ed. Chapter 436, Page 3188

A. Sleep
B. Anxiety
C. Hyperventilation
D. Hunger

In MS, paroxysmal symptoms may be precipitated by hyperventilation or movement.

2319. Which of the following is false about Lhermitte's symptom?

Harrison's 20th Ed. Chapter 436, Page 3189

A. Electric shock-like sensation
B. Evoked by neck flexion
C. Radiates down the back into legs
D. None of the above

Lhermitte's symptom is an electric shock like sensation, typically induced by flexion of neck, that radiates down the back into legs. Lhermitte's symptom can also occur with compression of cervical spinal cord (cervical spondylosis), radiation-associated myelopathy (6 - 12 weeks after treatment) & Vitamin B12 deficiency syndrome.

2320. In MS, 'Uhthoff's symptom' is related to?

Harrison's 20th Ed. Chapter 436, Page 3189

A. Facial myokymia
B. Visual symptoms
C. Heat sensitivity
D. Movement

Heat sensitivity refers to neurologic symptoms produced by elevation of body's core temperature. Unilateral visual blurring may occur during a hot shower or with physical exercise (Uhthoff's symptom).

2321. Symptoms of bladder dysfunction are present in what percentage of MS patients?

Harrison's 20th Ed. Chapter 436, Page 3189

A. 50%
B. 65%
C. 75%
D. 90%

Bladder dysfunction is present in >90% of MS patients.

2322. Which of the following was once thought to be characteristic of MS?

Harrison's 20th Ed. Chapter 436, Page 3189

A. Euphoria
B. Impaired attention
C. Memory loss
D. Slowed information processing

Euphoria (elevated mood) was once thought to be characteristic of MS but is actually uncommon, occurring in <20% of patients.

2323. In MS, fatigue can be exacerbated by?

Harrison's 20th Ed. Chapter 436, Page 3189

A. Elevated temperatures
B. Depression
C. Sleep disturbances
D. All of the above

90% of patients of MS experience fatigue which is exacerbated by elevated temperatures, depression, or sleep disturbances.

2324. At onset, which of the following is the commonest clinical type of MS?

Harrison's 20th Ed. Chapter 436, Page 3189

A. Relapsing MS (RMS)
B. Secondary progressive MS (SPMS)
C. Primary progressive MS (PPMS)
D. All of the above

Relapsing or bout onset MS (RMS) accounts for 90% of MS cases.

2325. Secondary progressive MS (SPMS) always begins as?

Harrison's 20th Ed. Chapter 436, Page 3189

A. Relapsing MS (RMS)
B. Secondary progressive MS (SPMS)
C. Primary progressive MS (PPMS)
D. Any of the above

Secondary progressive MS (SPMS) always begins as RRMS.

2326. For a patient with RMS, the risk of developing SPMS is?

Harrison's 20th Ed. Chapter 436, Page 3189

A. ~ 1% each year
B. ~ 2% each year
C. ~ 3% each year
D. ~ 4% each year

For a patient with RMS, the risk of developing SPMS is ~2% each year, meaning thereby that great majority of RMS ultimately evolves into SPMS.

2327. Which of the following clinical type of MS experience relapses more?

Harrison's 20th Ed. Chapter 436, Page 3189

A. Relapsing MS (RMS)
B. Secondary progressive MS (SPMS)
C. Primary progressive MS (PPMS)
D. All of the above

Patients with SPMS or PPMS will occasionally experience relapses, far less often than in RMS though.

2328. Which of the following clinical type of MS has a more favorable prognosis?

Harrison's 20th Ed. Chapter 436, Page 3189

A. Relapsing MS (RMS)
B. Secondary progressive MS (SPMS)
C. Primary progressive MS (PPMS)
D. All of the above

Relapsing MS (RMS) is characterized by discrete attacks that evolve over days to weeks with complete recovery over weeks to months. Between attacks, patients are neurologically stable.

2329. Which of the following is false about multiple sclerosis?

Harrison's 20th Ed. Chapter 436, Page 3189

A. Thrice more common in women than men
B. Age of onset is between 20 and 40 years
C. Prevalence decreases at higher latitudes
D. ~10% cases begin <18 years of age

Prevalence rates of MS increase at higher latitudes.

2330. Highest known prevalence for MS is in?

Harrison's 20th Ed. Chapter 436, Page 3189

A. Middle east
B. Orkney Islands
C. Tasmania
D. Fiji

Highest known prevalence for MS is in Orkney Islands (Scotland) (250 per 100,000).

2331. Deficiency of which of the following vitamins is associated with an increase in MS risk?

Harrison's 20th Ed. Chapter 436, Page 3190

A. A
B. D
C. E
D. C

Vitamin D deficiency is associated with an increase in MS risk. Ongoing deficiency may increase the relapse rate in established MS.

2332. Well-established risk factor for MS is?

Harrison's 20th Ed. Chapter 436, Page 3190

A. Vitamin D deficiency
B. Exposure to Epstein-Barr virus (EBV) after early childhood
C. Cigarette smoking
D. All of the above

Well-established risk factors for MS include vitamin D deficiency, exposure to Epstein-Barr virus (EBV) after early childhood and cigarette smoking.

2333. Which of the following races are inherently at higher risk for MS?

Harrison's 20th Ed. Chapter 436, Page 3190

A. Whites
B. Africans
C. Asians
D. All of the above

Whites are inherently at higher risk for MS than Africans or Asians.

2334. Risk of developing MS is highest?

Harrison's 20th Ed. Chapter 436, Page 3190 Table 436-2

A. If an identical twin has MS
B. If a sibling has MS
C. If a parent has MS
D. If a spouse has MS

Risk of developing MS is highest if an identical twin has MS (1 in 3).

2335. If no one in the family has MS, what is the risk of developing MS?

Harrison's 20th Ed. Chapter 436, Page 3190 Table 436-2

A. 1 in 1000
B. 1 in 5000
C. 1 in 10000
D. 1 in 100000

2336. Which of the following is the strongest MS susceptibility region in the genome?

Harrison's 20th Ed. Chapter 436, Page 3190

A. HLA-DRB1 gene in class II region of MHC
B. HLA-DRB2 gene in class II region of MHC
C. HLA-DRB3 gene in class II region of MHC
D. HLA-DRB4 gene in class II region of MHC

The strongest susceptibility signal in genome-wide studies maps to HLA-DRB1 gene in the class II region of the major histocompatibility complex (MHC).

2337. Genes for which of the following have a role in adaptive immune system?

Harrison's 20th Ed. Chapter 436, Page 3190

A. Interleukin (IL) 7 receptor (CD127)
B. IL-2 receptor (CD25)
C. T cell costimulatory molecule LFA-3 (CD58)
D. All of the above

2338. New MS lesions begin with?

Harrison's 20th Ed. Chapter 436, Page 3190

A. Astrocytic proliferation
B. Disruption of blood-brain barrier (BBB)
C. Perivenular cuffing by inflammatory mononuclear cells
D. Infiltration of nervous system by B lymphocytes

New MS lesions begin with perivenular cuffing by inflammatory mononuclear cells, predominantly T cells and macrophages,

2339. Which of the following about MS is false?

Harrison's 20th Ed. Chapter 436, Page 3190

A. Susceptibility to MS is polygenic
B. Proinflammatory autoimmune response against a component of CNS myelin
C. No disruption of the BBB
D. Demyelination

At sites of inflammation in MS lesions, blood-brain barrier (BBB) is disrupted, but unlike vasculitis, the vessel wall is preserved.

2340. "Shadow plaques" refer to?

Harrison's 20th Ed. Chapter 436, Page 3190

A. Astrocytic proliferation (gliotic areas)
B. Remyelination of surviving naked axons
C. Aggregates of T and B cells
D. Any of the above

Surviving oligodendrocytes partially remyelinate surviving naked axons, producing "shadow plaques".

2341. 'Sclerosis' in MS best relates to?

Harrison's 20th Ed. Chapter 436, Page 3190

A. Axonal destruction
B. Astrocytic proliferation (gliosis)
C. Demyelination
D. All of the above

In MS, term sclerosis refers to the prominent astrocytic proliferation leading to gliotic plaques that have a rubbery or hardened texture at autopsy.

2342. In MS, "dirty white matter" refers to?

Harrison's 20th Ed. Chapter 436, Page 3190

A. Prominent astrocytic proliferation
B. Subpial cortical demyelination and neurodegeneration
C. Diffuse low-grade inflammation with microglial proliferation
D. Ectopic clusters of lymphocytic aggregates in white matter

In MS, "dirty white matter" refers to a diffuse low-grade inflammation with microglial proliferation seen across large areas of white matter, associated with reduced myelin staining & axonal injury.

2343. Nerve conduction in myelinated axons occurs in a saltatory manner at a velocity of?

Harrison's 20th Ed. Chapter 436, Page 3190

A. ~ 50 meters / second
B. ~ 70 meters / second
C. ~ 90 meters / second
D. ~ 110 meters / second

Nerve conduction in myelinated axons occurs in saltatory manner at a velocity of ~70 meter per second. In unmyelinated nerves, continuous propagation occurs at ~1 meter per second.

2344. Which of the following is best related to pathophysiology of MS?

Harrison's 20th Ed. Chapter 436, Page 3190

A. Redistribution of potassium channels along naked axon
B. Redistribution of sodium channels along naked axon
C. Redistribution of calcium channels along naked axon
D. Redistribution of chloride channels along naked axon

In MS, due to demyelination, conduction blocks occur. Axons that are normally buried underneath the myelin sheath are exposed. Thereafter, resting axon membrane becomes hyperpolarized due to exposure of voltage-dependent potassium channels. Sodium channels are concentrated at the nodes of Ranvier. With demyelination sodium channels redistribute along the naked axon allowing slow, rather than saltatory, continuous propagation of nerve action potentials through the demyelinated segment.

2345. In northern hemisphere, babies born in which month are significantly more likely to develop MS?

Eur Neurol 2016;76:202-209

A. February
B. May
C. September
D. December

In northern hemisphere, babies born in May are significantly more likely to develop MS than those born in November. This is called "month-of-birth effect". Opposite is true for southern hemisphere.

2346. For diagnosis of MS, symptoms must last for?

Harrison's 20th Ed. Chapter 436, Page 3191

A. 1 day
B. 3 days
C. 5 days
D. 7 days

2347. For diagnosis of MS, symptom episodes must be separated by?

Harrison's 20th Ed. Chapter 436, Page 3191

A. 1 week
B. 2 weeks
C. 3 weeks
D. 4 weeks

Diagnostic criteria for clinically definite MS require documentation of ≥2 episodes of symptoms and ≥2 signs that relate to pathology in anatomically noncontiguous white matter tracts of CNS. Also, symptoms must last for >24 hours and occur as distinct episodes that are separated by a month or more. Abnormal MRI or evoked potentials (EPs) could be considered as a sign.

2348. MS-typical region of CNS involvement is?

Harrison's 20th Ed. Chapter 436, Page 3192 Table 436-3

A. Periventricular
B. Juxtacortical, infratentorial
C. Spinal cord
D. All of the above

As MRI evidence for diagnosis of MS, ≥1 T2 lesion in at least 2 out of 4 MS-typical regions of the CNS, i.e. periventricular, juxtacortical, infratentorial, or spinal cord. Also, simultaneous presence of asymptomatic gadolinium-enhancing and nonenhancing lesions at any time or a new T2 and/or gadolinium-enhancing lesion(s) on follow-up MRI, irrespective of its timing with reference to a baseline scan.

2349. On MRI in MS, characteristic abnormalities are found in what percentage of patients?

Harrison's 20th Ed. Chapter 436, Page 3191

A. > 65%
B. > 75%
C. > 85%
D. > 95%

On MRI in MS, characteristic abnormalities are found in >95% of patients, although >90% of lesions visualized by MRI are asymptomatic.

2350. On MRI in MS, which of the following is the characteristic abnormality?

Harrison's 20th Ed. Chapter 436, Page 3191

A. Posterior brain edema
B. Dawson's fingers
C. Spot sign
D. Mammillary body atrophy

2351. Which of the following statements about MS is false?

Harrison's 20th Ed. Chapter 436, Page 3191

A. Early in MS, most disease activity is clinically silent
B. >90% of lesions visualized by MRI are asymptomatic
C. Patients with benign MS, 15 years after onset are likely to maintain their benign course
D. None of the above

2352. Which of the following does not favour the diagnosis of MS?

Harrison's 20th Ed. Chapter 436, Page 3192

A. Mild CSF pleocytosis (> 5 cells/μL)
B. CSF protein concentration of > 100 mg/dL
C. Lesions in the anterior corpus callosum
D. Dawson's fingers

Pleocytosis of >75 cells/μL, presence of polymorphonuclear leukocytes, or a protein concentration of >100 mg/dL in CSF should raise doubts about MS. Lesions in the anterior corpus callosum are frequent in MS and rare in vascular disease. Dawson's fingers refers to lesions as seen in MRI that are oriented perpendicular to ventricular surface, and corresponding to pathologic pattern of perivenous demyelination.

2353. Which of the following ratio is used to calculate CSF IgG index?

Harrison's 20th Ed. Chapter 436, Page 3192

A. IgG to albumin in CSF divided by IgG to albumin in serum
B. IgG to albumin in serum divided by IgG to albumin in CSF
C. IgG to globulin in CSF divided by IgG to globulin in serum
D. IgG to globulin in serum divided by IgG to globulin in CSF

CSF IgG index is the ratio of IgG to albumin in CSF divided by IgG to albumin in serum. Also calculated as CSF IgG index = (CSF IgG x serum albumin) / (CSF albumin x serum IgG).

2354. Which of the following is a marker of axonal integrity?

Harrison's 19th Ed. 2665

A. Propionyl-CoA carboxylase
B. Argininosuccinate lyase
C. N-acetyl aspartate
D. N-Acetylglutamate synthase

N-acetyl aspartate, which is a marker of axonal integrity. Proton magnetic resonance spectroscopic imaging (MRSI) can quantitate it.

2355. Which of the following is uncommon in MS?

Harrison's 20th Ed. Chapter 436, Page 3192

A. Aphasia
B. Seizures
C. Chorea
D. All of the above

Uncommon or rare symptoms in MS are aphasia, parkinsonism, chorea, isolated dementia, severe muscular atrophy, peripheral neuropathy, episodic loss of consciousness, fever, headache, seizures, or coma.

2356. Disorders that can mimic multiple sclerosis are all except?

Harrison's 20th Ed. Chapter 436, Page 3194 Table 436-4

A. Vitamin B12 deficiency
B. Syphilis
C. Sarcoid
D. HSV-1 encephalitis

Disorders that can mimic multiple sclerosis are acute disseminated encephalomyelitis (ADEM), Antiphospholipid antibody syndrome (APLA), Behçet's disease, Cerebral autosomal dominant arteriopathy, subcortical infarcts, and leukoencephalopathy (CADASIL), Congenital leukodystrophies (adrenoleukodystrophy, metachromatic leukodystrophy), HIV infection, Ischemic optic neuropathy, Lyme disease, Mitochondrial encephalopathy with lactic acidosis and stroke (MELAS), Neoplasms (lymphoma, glioma, meningioma), Sarcoid, Sjögren's syndrome, Stroke & ischemic cerebrovascular disease, Syphilis, Systemic lupus erythematosus, Tropical spastic paraparesis (HTLV I/II infection), Vascular malformations, Vasculitis, Vitamin B12 deficiency.

2357. Clinical features that have a more favorable prognosis in MS include all except?

Harrison's 20th Ed. Chapter 436, Page 3194

A. Optic neuritis or sensory symptoms at onset
B. Pyramidal symptoms
C. Women
D. Age < 40 years at onset

Clinical features that point towards favorable prognosis in MS are ON or sensory symptoms at onset, <2 relapses in 1st year of illness & minimal impairment after 5 years. Those with truncal ataxia, action tremor, pyramidal symptoms or progressive disease are likely to be disabled.

2358. Likelihood of having benign MS is about?

Harrison's 20th Ed. Chapter 436, Page 3193

A. 2%
B. 5%
C. 10%
D. 20%

In benign variant of MS, patients never develop neurologic disability & maintain a benign course. Likelihood of having benign MS is <10%.

2359. Pregnant MS patients experience fewer attacks than expected during?

Harrison's 20th Ed. Chapter 436, Page 3193

A. First trimester
B. Second trimester
C. Third trimester
D. First 3 months postpartum

Pregnant MS patients experience fewer attacks than expected during gestation especially in the last trimester but more attacks than expected in the first 3 months postpartum.

2360. Kurtzke Expanded Disability Status Score (EDSS) is used for?

Harrison's 20th Ed. Chapter 436, Page 3194

A. Parkinson disease
B. Multiple sclerosis
C. Alzheimer's disease
D. Creutzfeldt-Jakob disease

2361. Most patients with Kurtzke Expanded Disability Status Score (EDSS) scores < 3.5 have?

Harrison's 20th Ed. Chapter 436, Page 3194

A. Relapsing/remitting MS (RRMS)
B. Secondary progressive MS (SPMS)
C. Primary progressive MS (PPMS)
D. Progressive/relapsing MS (PRMS)

Kurtzke Expanded Disability Status Score (EDSS) is a measure of neurologic impairment in MS. Most patients with EDSS scores <3.5 have RRMS and are generally not disabled. Patients with EDSS scores >5.5 have progressive MS (SPMS or PPMS), are gait-impaired and occupationally disabled.

2362. Which of the following is used to manage first attacks or acute exacerbations of MS?

Harrison's 20th Ed. Chapter 436, Page 3194

A. Glucocorticoids
B. Mitoxantrone
C. Glatiramer acetate
D. All of the above

Glucocorticoids are used to manage first attacks or acute exacerbations of MS. A 2-3 week course provides short-term clinical benefit. Mild attacks are managed with physical & occupational therapy. Plasma exchange may benefit patients with fulminant attacks of demyelination that are unresponsive to glucocorticoids.

2363. Disease modifying therapies for RMS include?
Harrison's 20th Ed. Chapter 436, Page 3194

A. IFN β1a
B. Mitoxantrone (MTX)
C. Glatiramer acetate (GA)
D. All of the above

Disease-Modifying Therapies for Relapsing Forms of MS (RMS, SPMS with Exacerbations) include IFN-β-1a, IFN-β-1b, glatiramer acetate, natalizumab, ocrelizumab, fingolimod, dimethylfumarate, teriflunomide, mitoxantrone and alemtuzumab.

2364. Which of the following is the mode of action of Interferon β?
Harrison's 20th Ed. Chapter 436, Page 3194

A. Downregulating expression of MHC molecules on APCs
B. Reducing proinflammatory & raising regulatory cytokine levels
C. Inhibiting T-cell proliferation
D. All of the above

Interferon β (IFN-β) is a class I interferon with antiviral properties. Efficacy in MS results from immunomodulatory properties i.e.downregulating expression of MHC molecules on antigen-presenting cells, reducing proinflammatory & increasing regulatory cytokine levels, inhibiting T-cell proliferation and limiting trafficking of inflammatory cells in CNS.

2365. Glatiramer acetate is composed of which of the following amino acids?
Harrison's 20th Ed. Chapter 436, Page 3194

A. L-glutamic acid
B. L-lysine
C. L-tyrosine
D. All of the above

2366. Which of the following is the mechanism of action of Glatiramer acetate?
Harrison's 20th Ed. Chapter 436, Page 3195

A. Induction of antigen-specific suppressor T cells
B. Binding to MHC molecules and displacing bound MBP
C. Altering balance between proinflammatory & regulatory cytokines
D. All of the above

Glatiramer acetate is a synthetic polypeptide composed of four amino acids (L-glutamic acid, L-lysine, L-alanine and L-tyrosine). It acts by induction of antigen-specific suppressor T cells, binding to MHC molecules thereby displacing bound MBP or altering balance between proinflammatory & regulatory cytokines.

2367. Which of the following is a side effect of Fingolimod?
Harrison's 20th Ed. Chapter 436, Page 3196

A. I° & 2° heart block, bradycardia & QT prolongation
B. Macular edema
C. Disseminated varicella-zoster virus & cryptococcal infections
D. All of the above

2368. Risk of progressive multifocal leukoencephalopathy (PML) is associated with?
Harrison's 20th Ed. Chapter 436, Page 3196

A. Mitoxantrone
B. Fingolimod
C. Dimethyl Fumarate (DMF)
D. Glatiramer acetate

Dimethyl Fumarate (DMF) is a small molecule and a Krebs cycle metabolite. Its use carries a risk of developing progressive multifocal leukoencephalopathy (PML).

2369. Which of the following about Natalizumab is false?
Harrison's 20th Ed. Chapter 436, Page 3197

A. Monoclonal antibody against α4 subunit of α4β1 integrin
B. Its use carries a risk of progressive multifocal leukoencephalopathy (PML)
C. Recommended only for JC antibody—negative patients
D. None of the above

2370. Which of the following about Ocrelizumab is false?
Harrison's 20th Ed. Chapter 436, Page 3197

A. Monoclonal antibody against CD20 on surface of mature B cell
B. IV methylprednisolone is given prior to each infusion
C. Carries a nonzero risk of PML
D. None of the above

2371. Which of the following about Teriflunomide is false?
Harrison's 20th Ed. Chapter 436, Page 3197

A. Cytostatic rather than cytotoxic
B. Can remain in the bloodstream for 2 years
C. Active metabolite of leflunomide
D. None of the above

2372. Which of the following drugs used in MS can cause malignancies?
Harrison's 20th Ed. Chapter 436, Page 3197

A. Mitoxantrone Hydrochloride
B. Teriflunomide
C. Ocrelizumab
D. Natalizumab

Mitoxantrone Hydrochloride use carries a risk of acute leukemia.

2373. Which of the following drugs used in MS can cause malignancies?
Harrison's 20th Ed. Chapter 436, Page 3197

A. Alemtuzumab
B. Teriflunomide
C. Ocrelizumab
D. Natalizumab

2374. Which of the following drugs used in MS can cause cardiomyopathy & irreversible congestive heart failure?
Harrison's 20th Ed. Chapter 436, Page 3197

A. Mitoxantrone Hydrochloride
B. Teriflunomide
C. Ocrelizumab
D. Natalizumab

2375. Which of the following drugs used in MS can cause toxic epidermal necrolysis or Stevens-Johnson syndrome?
Harrison's 20th Ed. Chapter 436, Page 3197

A. Mitoxantrone Hydrochloride
B. Teriflunomide
C. Ocrelizumab
D. Natalizumab

2376. Worsening RMS is defined as?

Harrison's 20th Ed. Chapter 436, Page 3197

A. Neurologic status abnormal between MS attacks
B. Worsening CSF IgG index
C. MRI lesions >3 mm in diameter
D. Involvement of more sites of CNS

Rapidly worsening MS is defined as patients whose neurologic status remains significantly abnormal between MS attacks.

2377. Which of the following drugs is used for patients with progressive disability in MS?

Harrison's 20th Ed. Chapter 436, Page 3194

A. Glucocorticoid
B. Plasma exchange
C. Mitoxantrone
D. Glatiramer acetate

Mitoxantrone is an immune suppressant generally reserved for patients with progressive disability who have failed other treatments. Mitoxantrone should not be used as a first-line agent in either RRMS or relapsing SPMS.

2378. Untreated patients of MS should be followed with?

Harrison's 20th Ed. Chapter 436, Page 3199

A. Objective clinical CNS examination
B. Evoked potential testing
C. Kurtzke expanded disability status score (EDSS)
D. Periodic brain MRI scans

Untreated patients are followed closely with periodic brain MRI scans.

2379. In MS, initiating treatment can be delayed if?

Harrison's 20th Ed. Chapter 436, Page 3194

A. Neurologic examinations are normal
B. Single attack or a low attack frequency
C. Low burden of disease as assessed by brain MRI
D. All of the above

In MS, initial treatment may be delayed in patients with normal neurologic examinations, a single attack or a low attack frequency and (3) a low burden of disease as assessed by brain MRI.

2380. Which of the following is the first-line therapy for RMS?

Harrison's 20th Ed. Chapter 436, Page 3194

A. IFN β
B. IV Ig
C. Mitoxantrone
D. Natalizumab

Relapsing forms of MS are treated with IFN-β or glatiramer acetate as first-line therapy.

2381. Which of the following is administered by IV infusion?

Harrison's 20th Ed. Chapter 436, Page 3194

A. IFN-β-1a
B. IFN-β-1b
C. Glatiramer acetate
D. Natalizumab

IFN-β-1a (IM), IFN-β-1b (SC), Glatiramer acetate (SC), Natalizumab (IV infusion).

2382. Which of the following is administered orally?

Harrison's 20th Ed. Chapter 436, Page 3194

A. IFN-β-1a
B. Mitoxantrone
C. Glatiramer acetate
D. Fingolimod

Fingolimod and Dimethyl Fumarate (DMF) are administered orally.

2383. Mitoxantrone is indicated for use in?

Harrison's 20th Ed. Chapter 436, Page 3198

A. SPMS
B. PRMS
C. Worsening RRMS
D. All of the above

Mitoxantrone is indicated in SPMS, PRMS, and worsening RRMS.

2384. Which of the following therapies is effective in treating PPMS?

Harrison's 20th Ed. Chapter 436, Page 3198

A. Glucocorticoids
B. IFN β1a
C. Glatiramer acetate
D. None of the above

No currently available therapies have shown any promise for treating PPMS at this time.

2385. In Marburg's variant of multiple sclerosis, the course of disease is?

Harrison's 20th Ed. Chapter 436, Page 3200

A. Hyperacute
B. Subacute
C. Fulminant
D. Chronic

Acute MS (Marburg's variant) is a fulminant demyelinating process that in some cases progresses inexorably to death within 1–2 years.

2386. Which of the following about Marburg's variant of multiple sclerosis is false?

Harrison's 20th Ed. Chapter 436, Page 3200

A. There are no remissions
B. Does not follow infection or vaccination
C. Death occurs within 1–2 years
D. None of the above

2387. Which of the following is a fulminant demyelinating syndrome?

Harrison's 20th Ed. Chapter 436, Page 3200

A. Weston-Hurst syndrome
B. Balo's concentric sclerosis
C. Acute hemorrhagic leukoencephalitis
D. All of the above

Balo's concentric sclerosis is a fulminant demyelinating syndrome characterized by concentric brain or spinal cord lesions with alternating spheres of demyelination and remyelination.

2388. Which of the following about multiple sclerosis is false?

N Engl J Med. 2006;354:942-55

A. Plaque is a chronic inflammatory, demyelinating lesion
B. Plaque lesions develop in white matter
C. Primary targets are myelin sheath & oligodendrocyte
D. Gray matter lesions are known to occur

2389. Which of the following about acute lesions of multiple sclerosis is false?

N Engl J Med. 2006;354:942-55

A. Indistinct margin, hypercellularity, intense perivascular infiltration, loss of myelin and oligodendrocytes
B. Widespread axonal damage, plasma cells, myelin-laden macrophages
C. Hypertrophic astrocytes
D. Astroglial scarring

2390. Most explosive form of acute disseminated encephalomyelitis (ADEM) is called?

Harrison's 20th Ed. Chapter 436, Page 3200

A. Mitochondrial encephalopathy
B Acute hemorrhagic leukoencephalitis
C. Tropical spastic paraparesis
D. Metachromatic leukodystrophy

Acute hemorrhagic leukoencephalitis is the most explosive form of ADEM. Lesions are vasculitic & hemorrhagic & the clinical course is devastating.

2391. Which of the following is false about acute disseminated encephalomyelitis (ADEM)?

Harrison's 20th Ed. Chapter 436, Page 3200

A. Polyphasic course
B. Postvaccinal encephalomyelitis
C. Postinfectious encephalomyelitis
D. Perivenular inflammation & demyelination

ADEM has a monophasic course & is associated with antecedent immunization (postvaccinal encephalomyelitis) or infection (postinfectious encephalomyelitis). Hallmark of ADEM is presence of widely scattered small foci of perivenular inflammation & demyelination.

2392. ADEM can follow infections with all except?

Harrison's 20th Ed. Chapter 436, Page 3200

A. Measles
B. Varicella
C. Mycoplasma
D. Legionella

2393. ADEM can follow infections with all except?

Harrison's 20th Ed. Chapter 436, Page 3200

A. Rubella
B. Hepatitis B
C. Mumps
D. Infectious mononucleosis virus

Postvaccinal encephalomyelitis may follow administration of smallpox vaccine & rabies vaccine. Postinfectious encephalomyelitis is associated with infection with measles virus, varicella (chickenpox), rubella, mumps, influenza, parainfluenza, infectious mononucleosis viruses and Mycoplasma.

2394. Which CNS antigens correlates with development of ADEM?

Harrison's 20th Ed. Chapter 436, Page 3200

A. Vascular cell adhesion molecule (VCAM)
B. Myelin basic protein (MBP)
C. Bruton's tyrosine kinase (BTK)
D. Stromal-cell derived factor (SDF)

All forms of ADEM result from a cross-reactive immune response to infectious agent or vaccine that triggers an inflammatory demyelinating response. Autoantibodies to MBP and to other myelin antigens have been detected in the CSF from many patients with ADEM.

2395. Cerebellar involvement in ADEM is common in infections due to?

Harrison's 20th Ed. Chapter 436, Page 3200

A. Measles
B. Varicella
C. Mycoplasma
D. Mumps

In ADEM due to chickenpox, cerebellar involvement is often conspicuous.

2396. ADEM is differentiated from MS by?

Harrison's 20th Ed. Chapter 436, Page 3200

A. Simultaneous onset of disseminated symptoms & signs
B. Drowsiness or coma
C. Seizures
D. All of the above

2397. ADEM is differentiated from MS by?

Harrison's 20th Ed. Chapter 436, Page 3200

A. Bilateral involvement of optic nerve
B. Complete transverse myelopathy
C. Monophasic course
D. All of the above

Features that suggest ADEM rather than MS are monophasic course, simultaneous onset of disseminated symptoms & signs, meningismus, drowsiness, coma, seizures, bilateral optic nerve involvement, complete transverse myelopathy.

Neuromyelitis Optica

2398. Devic's disease refers to which of the following?
Harrison's 20th Ed. Chapter 437, Page 3202

A. Acute disseminated encephalomyelitis (ADEM)
B. Isolated dementia
C. Neuromyelitis optica (NMO)
D. Mitochondrial encephalopathy

Neuromyelitis optica (NMO) is also called Devic's disease. Eugène Devic (1858-1930) was a French physician who described clinical pathological features of "acute neuromyelitis optica" (NMO) in 1894.

2399. Which of the following is a limited form of NMO?
Neurology 2015;85:177–189

A. Bilateral recurrent optic neuritis (BRON)
B. Opticospinal MS
C. ON or LETM associated with systemic autoimmune disease
D. All of the above

2400. Which of the following about NMO Spectrum Disorder (NMOSD) is false?
Harrison's 20th Ed. Chapter 437, Page 3202, Neurology 2015;85:177–189

A. Term NMO spectrum disorders (NMOSD) introduced in 2007
B. Incorporates NMO individuals with partial forms
C. Incorporates NMO individuals with involvement of additional structures in CNS
D. None of the above

2401. Which of the following about NMO is false?
Harrison's 20th Ed. Chapter 437, Page 3202

A. More frequent in women than men (>3:1)
B. ON can be bilateral & produces severe visual loss
C. Myelitis can be severe, transverse & typically longitudinally extensive involving ≥3 contiguous vertebral segments
D. None of the above

2402. Which of the following about NMO is false?
Harrison's 20th Ed. Chapter 437, Page 3202

A. Typically progressive symptoms do not occur
B. Astrocytopathy with inflammation
C. Absence of staining of AQP4 by immunohistochemistry
D. None of the above

2403. In neuromyelitis optica, which of the following is involved?
Harrison's 20th Ed. Chapter 437, Page 3202

A. Brainstem
B. Cerebellum
C. Cognitive functions
D. None of the above

In contrast to MS, patients with NMO do not experience brainstem, cerebellar & cognitive involvement, & the brain MRI is typically normal. Over three or more spinal cord segments are involved.

2404. Which is the best available detection method for AQP4-IgG?
Harrison's 20th Ed. Chapter 437, Page 3202 Table 437-1

A. Direct assay
B. Cell-based assay
C. Hybridization assay
D. Heterophile agglutination assay

2405. Which of the following is a chemosensitive vomiting center in brain?
Harrison's 20th Ed. Chapter 437, Page 3202 Table 437-1

A. Habenular trigone
B. Pretectal area
C. Arcuate nucleus
D. Area postrema

Area postrema (AP), located in dorsal medulla, is the chemosensitive vomiting center and has high AQP-4 expression. AP is highly vascularized and lacks blood-brain-barrier, potentially increasing its exposure to blood-borne AQP-4 IgG. AP syndrome with unexplained hiccups, nausea & vomiting is clinical characteristic for NMOSDs and may occur concurrently with a myelitis episode.

2406. Which of the following about longitudinal extensive transverse myelitis (LETM) is false?
Harrison's 20th Ed. Chapter 437, Page 3202

A. LETM is defined as a spinal cord lesion that extends ≥3 contiguous vertebral segments as seen on MRI of spine
B. LETM is a characteristic feature of neuromyelitis optica
C. LETM can also occur in multiple sclerosis, sarcoidosis or Sjögren syndrome
D. None of the above

2407. Autoantibody against which of the following is seen in neuromyelitis optica?
Harrison's 20th Ed. Chapter 437, Page 3202

A. Aquaporin-1
B. Aquaporin-2
C. Aquaporin-3
D. Aquaporin-4

A highly specific autoantibody directed against water channel protein aquaporin-4 is seen in >70% patients of NMO. Aquaporin-4 (AQP4) is localized to foot processes of astrocytes in close apposition to endothelial surfaces, as well as at paranodal regions near nodes of Ranvier.

2408. Levels of which of the following is elevated during acute attacks of myelitis in NMO?
Harrison's 20th Ed. Chapter 437, Page 3203

A. CSF levels of interleukin-6
B. CSF levels of Glial fibrillary acidic protein (GFAP)
C. Levels of AQP4 antibodies
D. All of the above

During acute attacks of myelitis in NMO, CSF levels of interleukin-6 (IL-6) and glial fibrillary acidic protein (GFAP) levels are markedly elevated. Proinflammatory T-lymphocytes of Th17 type recognize an immunodominant epitope of AQP4 and may contribute to its pathogenesis.

2409. The course of NMO is monophasic in what percentage of patients?
Harrison's 20th Ed. Chapter 437, Page 3203

A. 10%
B. 20%
C. 40%
D. 50%

NMO is typically a recurrent disease. Its course is monophasic in <10% of patients. AQP-4 antibodies negative patients are more likely to have a monophasic course.

2410. The highest reported prevalence of NMO is from?
Harrison's 20th Ed. Chapter 437, Page 3203, Multiple Sclerosis Journal 2017;18:1-8

A. Rio de Janeiro
B. Martinique
C. Buenos Aires
D. Caracas

The highest reported prevalence is from Martinique, a region in Latin America (LATAM).

2411. What percentage of NMO patients have a systemic autoimmune disorder?
Harrison's 20th Ed. Chapter 437, Page 3204

A. ~ 10%
B. ~ 20%
C. ~ 30%
D. ~ 40%

Up to 40% of NMO patients have a systemic autoimmune disorder, such as SLE, Sjögren's syndrome, perinuclear antineutrophil cytoplasmic antibody (p-ANCA)-associated vasculitis, myasthenia gravis, Hashimoto's thyroiditis, or mixed connective tissue disease.

2412. Onset of NMO may be associated with acute infection with?
Harrison's 20th Ed. Chapter 437, Page 3204

A. Varicella zoster virus
B. Epstein-Barr virus
C. HIV
D. Any of the above

Onset of NMO may be associated with acute infection with varicella zoster virus, Epstein-Barr virus, HIV, or tuberculosis. Rare cases appear to be paraneoplastic & associated with breast, lung, or other cancers.

2413. In NMO, prophylaxis against relapses is done with which of the following medicines?
Harrison's 20th Ed. Chapter 437, Page 3204

A. Mycophenolate mofetil
B. Rituximab
C. Glucocorticoids plus azathioprine
D. Any of the above

2414. Which is the first line of treatment for acute attacks of NMO?
Harrison's 20th Ed. Chapter 437, Page 3204

A. Plasma exchange
B. High-dose glucocorticoids
C. Interferon beta
D. Alemtuzumab

2415. Which of the following drugs is ineffective & paradoxically increases the risk of NMO relapses?
Harrison's 20th Ed. Chapter 437, Page 3204

A. Interferon beta
B. Glatiramer acetate
C. Fingolimod
D. Natalizumab

Interferon beta is ineffective and paradoxically increases the risk of NMO relapses. Glatiramer acetate, fingolimod, natalizumab & alemtuzumab are ineffective.

2416. Clinical feature that distinguishes ON associated with anti-MOG antibodies from NMO or MS is?
Harrison's 20th Ed. Chapter 437, Page 3204

A. Cerebrospinal fluid (CSF) pleocytosis
B. Papillitis
C. Hiccups
D. Nausea or vomiting

Clinical feature that distinguishes ON associated with anti-MOG antibodies from NMO or MS is the presence of papillitis seen by funduscopy or orbital MRI.

Peripheral Neuropathy

2417. Peripheral nerves are composed of which of the following elements?

Harrison's 20th Ed. Chapter 438, Page 3204

A. Sensory
B. Motor
C. Autonomic
D. All of the above

Peripheral nerves are composed of sensory, motor and autonomic elements.

2418. Which of the following is not a major class of nerves?

Harrison's 20th Ed. Chapter 438, Page 3204

A. Large myelinated
B. Large unmyelinated
C. Small myelinated
D. Small unmyelinated

Nerves can be subdivided into three major classes: large myelinated (6 to 12 μm), small myelinated (2 to 6 μm), and small unmyelinated (0.2 to 2.0 μm). Small myelinated fibers are about three times more numerous than large myelinated axons.

2419. Motor axons conduct impulses at the speed of about?

Harrison's 20th Ed. Chapter 438, Page 3204

A. 25 m/sec
B. 50 m/sec
C. 75 m/sec
D. 100 m/sec

Motor axons are usually large myelinated fibers & conduct impulses at ~ 50 m/sec. Conduction is most efficient when the ratio of axon diameter to total fiber diameter is 0.5 to 0.7.

2420. Sensory fibers are of which type?

Harrison's 20th Ed. Chapter 438, Page 3204

A. Large-diameter myelinated
B. Small-diameter myelinated
C. Small-diameter unmyelinated
D. Any of the above

Sensory fibers may be any of the three types namely, large myelinated, small myelinated or small unmyelinated.

2421. Remak cell best relates to?

DeJong's The Neurologic Examination, 7th Ed. Page 369

A. Schwann cell
B. Neurofilaments
C. Neurotubules
D. All of the above

In unmyelinated axons, a single Schwann cell, sometimes called Remak cell, sends out processes to support several adjacent axons, providing a cytoplasmic coat with minimal myelin.

2422. Large fiber neuropathies spare which of the following?

DeJong's The Neurologic Examination, 7th Ed. Page 369

A. Pain and temperature sensation
B. Proprioception
C. Strength
D. Reflexes

2423. Small fiber neuropathies affect which of the following?

DeJong's The Neurologic Examination, 7th Ed. Page 369

A. Pain
B. Temperature
C. Autonomic function
D. All of the above

Large fiber neuropathies affect strength, reflexes, and proprioception with relative sparing of pain & temperature sensation. Small fiber neuropathies primarily affect pain, temperature & autonomic function.

2424. Proprioception & vibratory sensation are conducted to the brain by?

Harrison's 20th Ed. Chapter 438, Page 3204

A. Large-diameter sensory fibers
B. Smaller-diameter myelinated fibers
C. Smaller-diameter unmyelinated fibers
D. All of the above

Large-diameter sensory fibers conduct proprioception and vibratory sensation to the brain, while the smaller-diameter myelinated and unmyelinated fibers transmit pain and temperature sensation.

2425. Which of the following is a peripheral neuropathy?

Harrison's 20th Ed. Chapter 438, Page 3204

A. Neuronopathy or ganglionopathy
B. Myelinopathy
C. Axonopathy
D. All of the above

Peripheral neuropathies are classified into those that primarily affect the cell body (neuronopathy or ganglionopathy), myelin (myelinopathy) and the axon (axonopathy).

2426. Which of the following is a possibility in symmetric proximal and distal weakness with sensory loss?

Harrison's 20th Ed. Chapter 438, Page 3206 Table 438-2

A. Chronic inflammatory demyelinating polyneuropathy (CIDP)
B. Charcot-Marie-Tooth disease
C. Spinal muscular atrophy (SMA)
D. Diabetes mellitus

In the scenario of symmetric proximal and distal weakness with sensory loss, inflammatory demyelinating polyneuropathy (GBS and CIDP) are a possibility.

2427. Which of the following is a possibility in symmetric distal sensory loss with or without distal weakness?

Harrison's 20th Ed. Chapter 438, Page 3206 Table 438-2

A. Chronic inflammatory demyelinating polyneuropathy (CIDP)
B. Guillain-Barré syndrome
C. Spinal muscular atrophy (SMA)
D. Diabetes mellitus

In the scenario of symmetric distal sensory loss with or without distal weakness, cryptogenic or idiopathic sensory polyneuropathy (CSPN), diabetes mellitus and other metabolic disorders, drugs, toxins, familial (HSAN), CMT, amyloidosis and others are a possibility.

2428. Which of the following is a possibility in asymmetric distal weakness with sensory loss with involvement of multiple nerves?
Harrison's 20th Ed. Chapter 438, Page 3206 Table 438-2

A. Multifocal CIDP
B. Sarcoidosis
C. Hereditary neuropathy with liability to pressure palsies
D. All of the above

Asymmetric distal weakness with sensory loss with involvement of multiple nerves may occur in multifocal CIDP, vasculitis, cryoglobulinemia, amyloidosis, sarcoid, infectious (leprosy, Lyme, hepatitis B, C or E, HIV, CMV), hereditary neuropathy with liability to pressure palsies (HNPP), tumor infiltration

2429. Which of the following is a possibility in asymmetric proximal and distal weakness with sensory loss?
Harrison's 20th Ed. Chapter 438, Page 3206 Table 438-2

A. Diabetes mellitus
B. Meningeal carcinomatosis
C. Hereditary neuropathy with liability to pressure palsies
D. All of the above

Asymmetric proximal and distal weakness with sensory loss can be seen in polyradiculopathy or plexopathy due to diabetes mellitus, meningeal carcinomatosis or lymphomatosis, hereditary plexopathy (HNPP, HNA), idiopathic.

2430. Which of the following is a possibility in asymmetric distal weakness (UMN) without sensory loss?
Harrison's 20th Ed. Chapter 438, Page 3206 Table 438-2

A. Diabetes mellitus
B. Multifocal motor neuropathy
C. Motor neuron disease
D. Progressive muscular atrophy

Asymmetric distal weakness without sensory loss with upper motor neuron findings is seen in motor neuron disease. Those without upper motor neuron findings is seen in progressive muscular atrophy, juvenile monomelic amyotrophy (Hirayama disease), multifocal motor neuropathy, multifocal acquired motor axonopathy.

2431. Which of the following is a possibility in symmetric sensory loss and distal areflexia with upper motor neuron findings?
Harrison's 20th Ed. Chapter 438, Page 3206 Table 438-2

A. Vitamin B12 deficiency
B. Vitamin E deficiency
C. Copper deficiency
D. All of the above

Symmetric sensory loss and distal areflexia with upper motor neuron findings is seen in Vitamin B12, vitamin E, and copper deficiency with combined system degeneration with peripheral neuropathy, hereditary leukodystrophies (adrenomyeloneuropathy).

2432. Which of the following is a possibility in symmetric weakness without sensory loss?
Harrison's 20th Ed. Chapter 438, Page 3206 Table 438-2

A. Guillain-Barré syndrome
B. Spinal muscular atrophy
C. Diabetes mellitus
D. Chronic inflammatory demyelinating polyneuropathy (CIDP)

Symmetric weakness without sensory loss with proximal and distal weakness is seen in spinal muscular atrophy and with distal weakness seen in hereditary motor neuropathy ("distal" SMA) or atypical CMT.

2433. If the patient has only weakness without any evidence of sensory or autonomic dysfunction, the diagnosis can be?
Harrison's 20th Ed. Chapter 438, Page 3204

A. Motor neuropathy
B. Neuromuscular junction abnormality
C. Myopathy
D. Any of the above

If the patient has only weakness without any evidence of sensory or autonomic dysfunction, a motor neuropathy, neuromuscular junction abnormality, or myopathy can be the cause.

2434. Heat intolerance is a symptom due to which of the following abnormalities?
Harrison's 20th Ed. Chapter 438, Page 3205

A. Motor
B. Sensory
C. Autonomic
D. All of the above

Symptoms of autonomic neuropathy are fainting spells or orthostatic lightheadedness (orthostatic fall in blood pressure without an appropriate increase in heart rate), heat intolerance or any bowel, bladder, or sexual dysfunction.

2435. Majority of neuropathies are predominantly?
Harrison's 20th Ed. Chapter 438, Page 3205

A. Motor
B. Sensory
C. Autonomic
D. Combined

Majority of neuropathies are predominantly sensory in nature.

2436. Symmetric proximal and distal weakness is the hallmark of?
Harrison's 20th Ed. Chapter 438, Page 3205

A. Charcot-Marie-Tooth disease
B. Guillain-Barré syndrome (GBS)
C. Motor neuron disease
D. Diabetes mellitus

Symmetric proximal & distal weakness is the hallmark of acquired immune demyelinating polyneuropathies, both acute form (AIDP) also known as Guillain-Barré syndrome (GBS) and the chronic inflammatory demyelinating polyneuropathy (CIDP).

2437. Sharp and lancinating (epicritic pain), relayed by?
Harrison's 20th Ed. Chapter 438, Page 3206

A. A-delta fibers
B. B-delta fibers
C. C-delta fibers
D. D-delta fibers

Neuropathic pain can be burning, dull and poorly localized (protopathic pain, presumably transmitted by polymodal C nociceptor fibers or sharp and lancinating (epicritic pain), relayed by A-delta fibers.

2438. Most likely cause of small-fiber neuropathies is?
Harrison's 20th Ed. Chapter 438, Page 3206

A. Hepatitis B
B. Motor neuron disease
C. Sjogren's syndrome
D. Diabetes mellitus

Most likely cause of small-fiber neuropathies is diabetes mellitus or glucose intolerance.

2439. Which of the following is the cause of combined system degeneration with neuropathy?

Harrison's 20th Ed. Chapter 438, Page 3206

A. Vitamin B12 deficiency
B. Copper deficiency
C. HIV infection
D. All of the above

Symmetric distal sensory neuropathy, with symmetric upper motor neuron involvement, suggests combined system degeneration with neuropathy as seen in vitamin B12 deficiency, copper deficiency, HIV infection, severe hepatic disease & adrenomyeloneuropathy.

2440. Which of the following neuropathies does not present acutely or subacutely?

Harrison's 20th Ed. Chapter 438, Page 3206

A. GBS
B. Diabetes
C. Lyme disease
D. Porphyria

Neuropathies with acute and subacute presentations include GBS, vasculitis, and radiculopathies related to diabetes or Lyme disease. A relapsing course is seen in CIDP and porphyria.

2441. Fixatives containing which element can lead to copper deficiency?

Harrison's 20th Ed. Chapter 438, Page 3206

A. Aluminium
B. Lead
C. Zinc
D. Nickel

Fixatives that contain zinc that can lead to copper deficiency.

2442. Which of the following is not a EDx finding in axonal neuropathy?

Harrison's 20th Ed. Chapter 438, Page 3207

A. Low-amplitude potentials
B. Absence of fibrillations
C. Relatively preserved distal latencies
D. Relatively preserved conduction velocities

Nerve conduction studies (NCS) are helpful in differentiating between axonal degeneration or segmental demyelination. Low-amplitude potentials with relatively preserved distal latencies, conduction velocities, and late potentials, along with fibrillations suggest an axonal neuropathy. Relatively preserved amplitudes, slow conduction velocities, prolonged distal latencies and late potentials, and absence of fibrillations imply a primary demyelinating neuropathy.

2443. Laboratory workup in a suspected case of vasculitis includes?

Harrison's 20th Ed. Chapter 438, Page 3208

A. Cryoglobulins
B. Western blot for Lyme disease
C. Cytomegalovirus (CMV) titer
D. All of the above

Laboratory workup in a suspected case of vasculitis includes antineutrophil cytoplasmic antibodies (ANCA), cryoglobulins, hepatitis serology, Western blot for Lyme disease, HIV, and cytomegalovirus (CMV) titer.

2444. Which of the following tests is done to detect a monoclonal gammopathy?

Harrison's 20th Ed. Chapter 438, Page 3208

A. Serum protein electrophoresis (SPEP)
B. Serum-free light chains
C. Serum kappa / lambda ratio
D. All of the above

2445. Severe painful sensorimotor & autonomic neuropathy and alopecia point towards?

Harrison's 20th Ed. Chapter 438, Page 3207

A. Arsenic toxicity
B. Thallium toxicity
C. Lead toxicity
D. Zinc toxicity

2446. Severe painful sensorimotor neuropathy with or without gastrointestinal disturbance & Mee's lines point towards?

Harrison's 20th Ed. Chapter 438, Page 3207

A. Arsenic toxicity
B. Thallium toxicity
C. Lead toxicity
D. Zinc toxicity

2447. Wrist or finger extensor weakness and anemia with basophilic stippling of blood cells point towards?

Harrison's 20th Ed. Chapter 438, Page 3207

A. Arsenic toxicity
B. Thallium toxicity
C. Lead toxicity
D. Zinc toxicity

Severe painful sensorimotor and autonomic neuropathy and alopecia—thallium toxicity. Severe painful sensorimotor neuropathy with or without gastrointestinal disturbance and Mee's lines—arsenic toxicity and wrist or finger extensor weakness and anemia with basophilic stippling of blood cells—lead toxicity.

2448. Most common cause of sensory ganglionopathies is?

Harrison's 20th Ed. Chapter 438, Page 3207

A. Porphyria
B. Diabetes mellitus
C. Vitamin B12 deficiency
D. Sjögren syndrome

Most common causes of sensory ganglionopathies presenting as severe sensory ataxia are Sjögren syndrome and paraneoplastic neuropathy.

2449. Which of the following investigation is done in patients with neuropathy due to Sjögren's syndrome?

Harrison's 20th Ed. Chapter 438, Page 3207

A. ANA
B. SS-A/Ro antibodies in serum
C. SS-B/La antibodies in serum
D. All of the above

Patients with neuropathy due to Sjögren's syndrome may have ANAs, SS-A/Ro, and SS-B/La antibodies in the serum, but most do not.

2450. Anti-Hu antibodies are 'most commonly' seen in patients with?

Harrison's 20th Ed. Chapter 438, Page 3207

A. Breast cancer
B. Ovarian cancer
C. Lymphoma
D. Small-cell carcinoma of the lung

Antineuronal nuclear antibodies—anti-Hu antibodies are most commonly seen in patients with small-cell carcinoma of the lung but are seen also in breast, ovarian, lymphoma, and other cancers.

2451. Which of the following is an onconeuronal antibody?
Harrison's 20th Ed. Chapter 90, Page 994, 669 Table 90-3

A. Anti-Hu
B. Anti-Amphiphysin
C. Anti-CRMP5
D. All of the above

Onconeuronal antibodies are anti-Hu, anti-Yo, anti-Ma2, anti-amphiphysin, anti-CRMP5, anti-CV2.

2452. Most commonly biopsied nerve is?
Harrison's 20th Ed. Chapter 438, Page 3208

A. Superficial peroneal nerve
B. Common peroneal nerve
C. Sural nerve
D. Superficial lateral cuteneous nerve

Nerve biopsies should be done only if NCS studies are abnormal. Sural nerve is most commonly biopsied because it is a pure sensory nerve and biopsy will not result in loss of motor function.

2453. Which of the following about skin biopsies in a case of neutopathy is false?
Harrison's 20th Ed. Chapter 438, Page 3208

A. Used to diagnose a small-fiber neuropathy
B. Useful when NCS is normal
C. Useful when routine nerve biopsies are normal
D. None of the above

2454. In mnemonic DANG THERAPIST, which is helpful in recalling common causes of peripheral neuropathy, "S" stands for?

A. Syphilis
B. Sepsis
C. Sarcoid
D. Secondaries

The mnemonic DANG THERAPIST for common causes of peripheral neuropathy Diabetes mellitus, Alcohol, Nutritional (B12 deficiency), Guillain-Barre syndrome, Toxins (Pb, As, Zn, Hg), Hematologic (paraproteins), Endocrine (hypothyroid), Rheumatologic (SLE, rheumatoid arthritis, vasculitis), Amyloid, Porphyria, Infectious (syphilis, HIV), Sarcoid, Tumor (paraneoplastic neuropathy).

2455. Which of the following is the most common type of hereditary neuropathy?
Harrison's 20th Ed. Chapter 438, Page 3208

A. Charcot-Marie-Tooth (CMT) disease
B. Hereditary neuropathy with liability to pressure palsies
C. Hereditary neuralgic amyotrophy
D. Hereditary sensory and autonomic neuropathy

Charcot-Marie-Tooth (CMT) disease is the most common type of hereditary neuropathy. CMT used to be called peroneal muscular atrophy. It was also referred to as hereditary motor/sensory neuropathy (HMSN).

2456. Various subtypes of CMT are classified according to?
Harrison's 20th Ed. Chapter 438, Page 3208

A. Predominant pathology
B. Nerve conduction velocities
C. Inheritance pattern
D. All of the above

Various subtypes of CMT are classified according to the nerve conduction velocities and predominant pathology (demyelination or axonal degeneration), inheritance pattern (autosomal dominant, recessive, or X-linked), and the specific mutated genes.

2457. In CMT1, motor conduction velocities in the arms are slowed to?
Harrison's 20th Ed. Chapter 438, Page 3208

A. < 38 m/sec
B. < 48 m/sec
C. < 58 m/sec
D. < 68 m/sec

By definition, motor conduction velocities in the arms are slowed to < 38 m/sec in CMT1 and are greater than 38 m/sec in CMT2.

2458. Transmission of Charcot-Marie-Tooth (CMT) neuropathy diseases is?
Harrison's 20th Ed. Chapter 438, Page 3208

A. Autosomal dominant
B. Autosomal recessive
C. X-linked
D. All of the above

CMT is usually transmitted as autosomal dominant trait, as X-linked-dominant CMT in ~10%. Rare autosomal recessive forms (CMT4) have an early onset & are more severe than dominant types.

2459. Inheritance of CMT1 is?
Harrison's 20th Ed. Chapter 438, Page 3208

A. Autosomal dominant
B. Autosomal recessive
C. X-linked
D. Any of the above

Inheritance of CMT1 is autosomal dominant.

2460. Which of the following is false about Charcot-Marie-Tooth Disease (CMT)?
Harrison's 20th Ed. Chapter 438, Page 3208

A. Heritable neuromuscular disorder
B. Chronic distal sensory and motor neuropathy
C. CMT does not reduce the life span
D. None of the above

CMT is the most common heritable neuromuscular disorder. It is a chronic distal sensory & motor neuropathy. Pes cavus & hammer toes indicate that neuropathy dates from early life. CMT does not reduce life span & rarely involves respiratory muscles.

2461. Which of the following about Charcot–Marie–Tooth disease is false?
Harrison's 20th Ed. Chapter 438, Page 3208

A. CMT1 and 2 are autosomal dominant
B. CMT1 is a demyelinating polyneuropathy
C. CMT2 is an axonal polyneuropathy
D. None of the above

Charcot–Marie–Tooth disease type 1 is most common inherited demyelinating sensorimotor neuropathy, followed by type 2. Both are autosomal dominant. Type 1 is a demyelinating polyneuropathy, whereas type 2 is an axonal sensory polyneuropathy.

2462. Which of the following is an autosomal recessive neuropathy?
Harrison's 20th Ed. Chapter 438, Page 3208

A. CMT1
B. CMT2
C. CMT3
D. CMT4

CMT1, CMT2 and CMT3 have autosomal dominant inheritance (with a few exceptions). CMT4 (genetically heterogenic) is an autosomal recessive neuropathy.

2463. The ratio of occurrence of CMT1:CMT2 is approximately?

Harrison's 20th Ed. Chapter 438, Page 3208

A. 1:1
B. 2:1
C. 3:1
D. 4:1

CMT1 is the most common form of hereditary neuropathy. The ratio of CMT1:CMT2 is ~2:1.

2464. CMT1 is which form of CMT?

Harrison's 20th Ed. Chapter 438, Page 3208

A. Demyelinating
B. Axonal
C. Intermediate
D. Any of the above

2465. CMT2 is which form of CMT?

Harrison's 20th Ed. Chapter 438, Page 3208

A. Demyelinating
B. Axonal
C. Intermediate
D. Any of the above

Demyelinating forms of CMT are classified as CMT1, and axonal forms as CMT2. Nerve conduction velocities (NCVs) intermediate between CMT1 & CMT2 are classified as "intermediate CMT" and most of these are X-linked.

2466. Which of the following physical finding favours diagnosis of CMT?

Harrison's 20th Ed. Chapter 438, Page 3208

A. Inverted champagne bottle appearance of legs
B. Hammer toes
C. High arched feet (pes cavus)
D. All of the above

Wasting & weakness of distal muscles of legs lead to inverted champagne bottle like appearance. Hammer toes & pes cavus are common & indicate onset of CMT in early life.

2467. Which of the following manifestation prompts suspicion of CMT1?

Harrison's 20th Ed. Chapter 438, Page 3208

A. Bed sore
B. Numbness or tingling
C. Footdrop
D. Frequent falls

CMT1 usually present in the first to third decade of life with distal leg weakness (footdrop). People with CMT generally do not complain of numbness or tingling, which helps in distinguishing CMT from acquired forms of neuropathy in which sensory symptoms usually predominate.

2468. Which of the following manifestation prompts suspicion of CMT1?

Harrison's 20th Ed. Chapter 438, Page 3208

A. Reduced sensation to all modalities
B. Reduced muscle stretch reflexes
C. Atrophy of muscles below knee
D. All of the above

In CMT1, reduced sensation to all modalities is apparent on examination. Muscle stretch reflexes are absent or reduced. Atrophy of muscles below knee (particularly anterior compartment), leads to inverted champagne bottle legs.

2469. In CMT1, characteristic nerve biopsy appearance is?

Harrison's 20th Ed. Chapter 438, Page 3208

A. Mulberry appearance
B. Cabbage appearance
C. Potato peel appearance
D. Onion bulb appearance

Nerve biopsies show evidence of repeated demyelination & remyelination. Supernumerary, concentrically arranged, Schwann cells attempting to remyelinate axons give a characteristic "onion bulb" appearance.

2470. The most common form of CMT1 is?

Harrison's 20th Ed. Chapter 438, Page 3208

A. 1A subtype
B. 2A subtype
C. 2B subtype
D. 2C subtype

CMT1A is the most common subtype of CMT1, representing 70% of cases.

2471. CMT 1A subtype is caused by?

Harrison's 20th Ed. Chapter 438, Page 3208

A. Duplication of PMP22 gene
B. Deletion in PMP22
C. Translocation in PMP22
D. All of the above

CMT1A is caused by a 1.5-megabase (Mb) duplication within peripheral myelin protein-22 (PMP-22) gene containing chromosome 17p11.2-12 resulting in patients having three copies of the PMP-22 gene rather than two.

2472. Charcot-Marie-Tooth disease (CMT) type 1B is caused by mutations in gene for?

Harrison's 20th Ed. Chapter 438, Page 3208

A. Proteolipid protein (PLP)
B. MPZ
C. Myelin oligodendrocyte glycoprotein (MOG)
D. Myelin basic protein (MBP)

CMT1B is due to a mutation in the myelin protein zero (MPZ, or P0) gene.

2473. CMT2 is caused by mutations for which gene?

Harrison's 20th Ed. Chapter 438, Page 3208

A. Alpha-galactosidase gene
B. ATP-binding cassette transporter 1 (ABC1) gene
C. Mitofusin 2 (MFN2) gene
D. Transthyretin (TTR) gene

Most common cause of CMT2 is a mutation in the gene for mitofusin 2 (MFN2) which is localized to the outer mitochondrial membrane, where it regulates the mitochondrial network architecture by fusion of mitochondria.

2474. Diagnosis of CMT is favoured by which of the following observation?

Harrison's 20th Ed. Chapter 438, Page 3208

A. Early age of onset
B. Positive family history
C. Long standing symptoms
D. All of the above

Diagnosis of CMT is favoured by an early age of onset, positive family history, and long standing symptoms. If EDx findings indicate a demyelinating process, diagnosis of CMT can be made with confidence.

2475. Which of the following is associated with pes cavus?
Harrison's 20th Ed. Chapter 438, Page 3208, 2975, 3157

A. CMT1x
B. Friedreich's ataxia
C. Plantar fasciitis
D. All of the above

Pes cavus is associated with CMT1x, Friedreich's ataxia, Nemaline myopathy, Central core disease and Plantar fasciitis.

2476. Which of the following is false about Schmidt-Lanterman incisures?
The Journal of Neuroscience. 2005;25(13):3259 -3269

A. Noncompacted regions of myelin
B. Contains cytoplasm
C. Transport metabolic substances across myelin sheath
D. None of the above

Schwann cells form myelin sheath around peripheral nerve axons as either highly compacted membrane or noncompacted cytoplasmic regions (Schmidt-Lanterman incisures or SLI). SLI are important for transport of metabolic substances across myelin sheath and for metabolic maintenance & longitudinal growth of sheath.

2477. When NCV is faster than seen in CMT1 but slower than in CMT2, the condition is termed as?
Harrison's 20th Ed. Chapter 438, Page 3208

A. CMT3
B. CMT4
C. Intermediate CMT (iCMT)
D. Dominant-intermediate CMT (CMTDI)

In dominant-intermediate CMTs (CMTDIs), NCVs are faster than seen in CMT1 (>38 m/s) but slower than in CMT2.

2478. Palpably thickened nerves in CMT1 is due to increase in?
Harrison's 20th Ed. Chapter 438, Page 3208

A. Hyaline
B. Mucopolysaccharides
C. Collagen
D. Glycogen

In CMT1, increased collagen between layers of supernumerary Schwann cells leads to palpably thickened nerves.

2479. Which of the following appears in infancy & is associated with severe demyelination or hypomyelination?
Harrison's 20th Ed. Chapter 438, Page 3208

A. CMT1
B. CMT2
C. CMT3
D. CMT4

CMT3 is an autosomal dominant neuropathy that appears in infancy and is associated with severe demyelination or hypomyelination.

2480. Which of the following type of CMT have an onset later in life?
Harrison's 20th Ed. Chapter 438, Page 3208

A. CMT1
B. CMT2
C. CMT3
D. CMT4

2481. Which of the following is false about myelin?
Harrison's 20th Ed. Chapter 417 Page 3039

A. It speeds impulse conduction
B. Single oligodendrocyte ensheaths multiple CNS axons
C. Each Schwann cell myelinates a single PNS axon
D. It is a protein-rich material

Myelin is a lipid-rich material formed by a spiraling process of the membrane of myelinating cell around the axon.

2482. Pelizaeus Merzbacher disease is caused by mutations in gene for?
Harrison's 20th Ed. Chapter 429 Page 3148

A. Proteolipid protein (PLP)
B. P0 protein
C. Myelin oligodendrocyte glycoprotein (MOG)
D. Myelin basic protein (MBP)

Pelizaeus-Merzbacher syndrome is a dysmyelinating X-linked allelic disorder of CNS, caused by mutations in gene for proteolipid protein (PLP) that promotes extracellular compaction between adjacent myelin lamellae.

2483. Protein restricted to CNS myelin is which of the following?
Harrison's 19th Ed. 444e-4

A. Proteolipid protein (PLP)
B. P_0
C. PMP_{22}
D. GM_1

2484. Protein restricted to PNS myelin is which of the following?
Harrison's 19th Ed. 444e-4

A. Proteolipid protein (PLP)
B. P_0
C. Myelin oligodendrocyte glycoprotein (MOG)
D. GM_1

2485. Protein in both CNS & PNS myelin is?
Harrison's 19th Ed. 444e-4

A. Proteolipid protein (PLP)
B. P_0
C. Myelin oligodendrocyte glycoprotein (MOG)
D. GM_1

2486. DéJerine-Sottas disease is also called?
Harrison's 20th Ed. Chapter 438, Page 3208

A. CMT Type 1
B. CMT Type 2
C. CMT Type 3
D. CMT Type 4

CMT3 was originally described by Deéjerine and Sottas as a hereditary demyelinating sensorimotor polyneuropathy presenting in infancy or early childhood.

2487. DéJerine-Sottas syndrome is similar to?
Harrison's 20th Ed. Chapter 438, Page 3209 Table 438-4

A. CMT2A
B. CMT2B
C. Congenital hypomyelinating neuropathy (CHN)
D. Roussy-Levy Syndrome

DéJerine-Sottas syndrome & congenital hypomyelinating neuropathy are indistinguishable. Nerve biopsy can distinguish them.

2488. DéJerine-Sottas syndrome is caused by mutations of?
Harrison's 20th Ed. Chapter 438, Page 3208

A. PMP22
B. Myelin protein zero (MPZ)
C. Early growth response gene (ERG2)
D. All of the above

Most cases of CMT3 are caused by point mutations in the genes for PMP-22, MPZ, or ERG-2, which are also the genes responsible for CMT1.

2489. Which of the following CMT is extremely rare?
Harrison's 20th Ed. Chapter 438, Page 3208

A. CMT1
B. CMT2
C. CMT3
D. CMT4

CMT4 is extremely rare & is characterized by a severe, childhood-onset sensorimotor polyneuropathy.

2490. Gap junctions consist of membrane-spanning proteins called?
Harrison's 20th Ed. Chapter 438, Page 3210

A. Spannins
B. Membranins
C. Connexins
D. All of the above

Connexins are gap junction structural proteins that are important in cell-to-cell communication. Gap junctions provide direct neuron-neuron electrical conduction and also create openings for the diffusion of ions and metabolites between cells. Gap junctions membrane-spanning proteins, expressed by Schwann cells are connexins, that pair across adjacent cells.

2491. Mutation of which gene of gap junction protein is responsible for X-linked Charcot-Marie-Tooth disease?
Harrison's 20th Ed. Chapter 438, Page 3208

A. Connexin 26
B. Connexin 32
C. Connexin 42
D. Connexin 48

Mutations in connexin 32 are responsible for X-linked form of CMT disease (CMT1X). Mutated gene is GJB1. Connexin 32 is found in both central and peripheral nervous systems.

2492. Connexins have a role in which of the following conditions?
Harrison's 20th Ed. Chapter 438, Page 3208

A. Hereditary hearing impairment (HHI)
B. Angiogenic endothelium
C. Re-entrant cardiac arrhythmias
D. All of the above

2493. Which of the following is false about CMT1X?
Harrison's 20th Ed. Chapter 438, Page 3208, Eur J Neurol. 2015;22:406–9

A. Severe in males than in females
B. NCS shows both demyelination & axonal degeneration
C. Caused by mutations in connexin 32 gene (GJB1)
D. None of the above

Molecular genetic testing of GJB1 (Cx32) detects ~90% of cases of X-linked CMTX1. Affected males pass the abnormal gene to all of their daughters & none of their sons i.e. no male-to-male inheritance. Penetrance is complete in males with GJB1 pathogenic variants. Females who are carriers are at a 50% risk of passing the pathogenic gene to each offspring.

2494. Clinical presentation of CMTX1 can overlap with?
Harrison's 20th Ed. Chapter 438, Page 3208

A. CMT1
B. CMT2
C. Hereditary neuropathy with liability to pressure palsies
D. All of the above

2495. Which of the following is a clinical feature of CMTX1?
Harrison's 20th Ed. Chapter 438, Page 3208

A. Bilateral foot drop
B. Symmetrical atrophy of muscles below knee (stork leg appearance)
C. Absent tendon reflexes in both upper & lower extremities
D. All of the above

The typical CMTX1 affected adult has bilateral foot drop, symmetrical atrophy of muscles below knee (stork leg appearance), pes cavus, atrophy of intrinsic hand muscles, especially thenar muscles of thumb, & absent tendon reflexes in both upper & lower extremities. Proximal muscles usually remain strong. Mild to moderate sensory deficits of position, vibration & pain/temperature occur in feet.

2496. Which of the following is an X-linked disorder?
Harrison's 20th Ed. Chapter 438, Page 3210

A. CMT1X
B. Adrenomyeloneuropathy
C. Pelizeaus-Merzbacher disease
D. All of the above

2497. Cowchock syndrome relates best with?
Eur J Neurol. 2015;22:406–9

A. CMTX1
B. CMTX2
C. CMTX3
D. CMTX4

CMTX4 is also called Cowchock syndrome. It presents as peripheral neuropathy with deafness and intellectual disability.

2498. Which of the following is called tomaculous neuropathy?
J Neurol Sci 1975;25:415-418

A. DéJerine-Sottas Syndrome (DSS)
B. Hereditary neuropathy with liability to pressure palsies
C. Roussy-Levy syndrome
D. Congenital hypomyelinating neuropathy (CHN)

Autosomal dominant disorder hereditary neuropathy with liability to pressure palsies (HNPP) is also called tomaculous neuropathy. Tomaculae are sausage-shaped bodies that indicate segmental demyelination. The first published description of HNPP was in 1947 by De Jong.

2499. HNPP is an autosomal dominant disorder related to?
Harrison's 20th Ed. Chapter 438, Page 3210

A. CMT1A
B. CMT1B
C. CMT1X
D. DéJerine-Sottas Syndrome (DSS)

Hereditary neuropathy with liability to pressure palsies (HNPP) is an autosomal dominant disorder related to CMT1A.

2500. Which of the following about HNPP is false?

Harrison's 20th Ed. Chapter 438, Page 3210

A. Affected individuals have only one copy of PMP-22 gene
B. Weakness in distribution of single peripheral nerves
C. Symptoms precipitated by trivial compression of nerve
D. None of the above

CMT1A is associated with duplication in chromosome 17p11.2 resulting in an extra copy of PMP-22 gene, whereas in HNPP, affected individuals have only one copy of the PMP-22 gene.

2501. Which of the following about HNPP is false?

Harrison's 20th Ed. Chapter 438, Page 3210

A. Painless motor weakness that recovers early
B. Presence of familiar history facilitates early diagnosis
C. Molecular studies are decisive
D. None of the above

Painless acute or subacute mononeuropathy is the classical phenotype of HNPP. It presents as a focal sensory & motor neuropathy in the territory of a single nerve or brachial plexus.

2502. Which of the following have overlapping clinical features?

Harrison's 20th Ed. Chapter 438, Page 3210

A. CMT1A
B. Hereditary neuralgic amyotrophy (HNA)
C. Hereditary neuropathy with liability to pressure palsies
D. All of the above

2503. Most commonly involved nerve in HNPP is?

Harrison's 20th Ed. Chapter 438, Page 3210, Case Rep Neurol 2014;6:281–286

A. Peroneal
B. Ulnar
C. Radial
D. Median

HNPP presents as recurrent focal entrapment neuropathy (numbness & weakness) most frequently is peroneal then ulnar, radial & median nerves.

2504. Electrodiagnostic findings in HNPP include?

Harrison's 20th Ed. Chapter 438, Page 3210

A. Prolongation of distal latencies
B. Conduction block / slowing at entrapment sites
C. Short terminal latency index (TLI)
D. All of the above

2505. Hereditary neuralgic amyotrophy (HNA) is caused by mutations in?

Harrison's 20th Ed. Chapter 438, Page 3210

A. Septin 9 (SEPT9)
B. ATP-binding cassette transporter 1 (ABC1) gene
C. Mitofusin 2 (MFN2) gene
D. Transthyretin (TTR) gene

HNA is caused by mutations in septin 9 (SEPT9). Septins may be important in formation of the neuronal cytoskeleton and have a role in cell division (cytokinesis). It is also called hereditary brachial plexus neuropathy.

2506. Which of the following is best related to hereditary neuralgic amyotrophy (HNA)?

Harrison's 20th Ed. Chapter 438, Page 3210

A. Lumbosacral plexus
B. Brachial plexus
C. Charcot joints
D. Deep dermal ulcerations

HNA is an autosomal dominant disorder characterized by recurrent attacks of pain, weakness, and sensory loss in the distribution of brachial plexus. The lumbosacral plexus, lower cranial nerves, phrenic nerve, autonomic nervous system or a combination of these may also be involved. Attacks may occur in postpartum period, following surgery or at other times of stress.

2507. Symptoms of which of the following disorders can be similar to those of HNA?

Harrison's 20th Ed. Chapter 438, Page 3210

A. Congenital hypomyelinating neuropathy (CHN)
B. Parsonage-Turner syndrome (PTS)
C. Roussy-Levy syndrome
D. Fabry's disease

Parsonage-Turner syndrome (PTS) is also known as idiopathic neuralgic amyotrophy. as with HNA, PTS mainly involves the brachial plexus. Unlike HNA, PTS usually occurs in a older age group (~40 years). The distinctive facial features found in some individuals with HNA do not occur in PTS.

2508. Apart from demyelinating CMT, what else characterizes Roussy-Levy syndrome?

A. Action tremor
B. Deafness
C. Blindness
D. Spina bifida

Roussy-Levy syndrome is a combination of demyelinating CMT with postural and action tremor.

2509. SPTLC is a key enzyme in the regulation of?

Harrison's 20th Ed. Chapter 438, Page 3164

A. Salicylamide
B. Globotriaosylceramide
C. Ceramide
D. Pyroglutamyl histidylprolinamide

Five hereditary sensory and autonomic neuropathies (HSANs) exist, designated HSAN I–V. The most important autonomic variants are HSAN I and HSAN III. HSAN I is dominantly inherited and manifests as a distal small-fiber neuropathy (burning feet syndrome) associated with sensory loss & foot ulcers. The responsible gene on chromosome 9q, is SPTLC1. SPTLC is a key enzyme in the regulation of ceramide. Cells from HSAN I patients with the mutation produce higher-than-normal levels of glucosyl ceramide. HSAN III (Riley-Day syndrome; familial dysautonomia) is an autosomal recessive disorder and is less prevalent than HSAN I. Decreased tearing, hyperhidrosis, reduced sensitivity to pain, areflexia, absent fungiform papillae on tongue, and labile BP may be present. Individuals with HSAN III have afferent baroreflex failure that causes the classic episodic abdominal crises and blood pressure surges in response to emotional stimuli. Pathologic examination of nerves reveals a loss of sympathetic, parasympathetic, and sensory neurons. The defective gene, IKBKAP, prevents normal transcription of important molecules in neural development.

2510. Riley-Day syndrome is also called?

Harrison's 20th Ed. Chapter 438, Page 3164

A. HSAN 1
B. HSAN 2
C. HSAN 3
D. HSAN 4

Hereditary sensory neuropathies (HSN) are also called hereditary sensory & autonomic neuropathies (HSANs). Out of five subtypes, HSAN 1 is most common. HSAN 3 is also called Riley-Day syndrome. Both are autonomic variants of HSAN.

2511. Hereditary sensory and autonomic neuropathy 1A (HSAN1A) is caused by mutations in?

Harrison's 20th Ed. Chapter 438, Page 3210

A. Septin 9 (SEPT9)
B. Serine palmitoyltransferase long-chain base 1 (SPTLC1)
C. Mitofusin 2 (MFN2)
D. Transthyretin (TTR)

HSAN1A is caused by mutations in serine palmitoyltransferase long-chain base 1 (SPTLC1) gene on chromosome 9q.

2512. Hereditary sensory and autonomic neuropathy III (HSAN III) is caused by mutations in?

Harrison's 20th Ed. Chapter 438, Page 3164

A. Septin 9 (SEPT9)
B. IKBKAP
C. Mitofusin 2 (MFN2)
D. Transthyretin (TTR)

The defective gene in HSAN III is IKBKAP. It prevents normal transcription of important molecules in neural development.

2513. Which of the following is a feature of HSAN1?

Harrison's 20th Ed. Chapter 438, Page 3210

A. Deep dermal ulcerations
B. Recurrent osteomyelitis
C. Gross foot and hand deformities
D. All of the above

HSAN1 is associated with degeneration of small myelinated & unmyelinated nerve fibers leading to severe loss of pain & temperature sensation, deep dermal ulcerations, recurrent osteomyelitis, Charcot joints, bone loss, gross foot and hand deformities, and amputated digits. Autonomic neuropathy is not a prominent feature.

2514. Fabry's disease is also called?

Harrison's 20th Ed. Chapter 438, Page 3210

A. Globoid cell leukodystrophy
B. Pediculus humanus corporis
C. Angiokeratoma corporis diffusum
D. Cerebrotendinous xanthomatosis

2515. Which of the following about Fabry disease is false?

Harrison's 20th Ed. Chapter 438, Page 3210

A. X-linked dominant disorder
B. Reddish-purple maculopapular lesions (Angiokeratomas)
C. Premature atherosclerosis
D. None of the above

Premature atherosclerosis (hypertension, renal failure, cardiac disease & stroke) lead to death by fifth decade of life and overshadow the neuropathy manifesting as burning or lancinating pain in hands & feet.

2516. Affected organs in Fabry disease include which of the following?

Harrison's 20th Ed. Chapter 308, Page 2146

A. Endothelium
B. Heart
C. Brain
D. All of the above

Affected organs include the vascular endothelium, heart, brain and kidneys.

2517. Classically, Fabry's disease presents in childhood in males with?

Harrison's 20th Ed. Chapter 308, Page 2146

A. Acroparesthesias
B. Angiokeratoma
C. Hypohidrosis
D. All of the above

Classically, Fabry's disease presents in childhood in males with acroparesthesias, angiokeratoma and hypohidrosis.

2518. Which of the following is related to Fabry's disease?

Harrison's 20th Ed. Chapter 308, Page 2146

A. Zebra bodies
B. Maltese cross
C. Cornea verticillata
D. All of the above

Renal biopsy reveals small clear vacuoles containing globotriaosylceramide in glomeruli, parietal and tubular epithelia. These vacuoles of electron-dense materials in parallel arrays (zebra bodies) are easily seen on electron microscopy. Urinalysis in Fabry's disease may reveal oval fat bodies and birefringent glycolipid globules under polarized light called Maltese cross.

2519. Manifestations of Fabry disease include all except?

Harrison's 20th Ed. Chapter 411, Page 3007

A. Angiokeratomas (telangiectatic skin lesions)
B. Hyperhidrosis
C. Corneal and lenticular opacities
D. Acroparesthesia

Fabry's disease manifests with angiokeratomas (telangiectatic skin lesions), hypohidrosis, corneal and lenticular opacities, acroparesthesia and small-vessel disease of kidney, heart, and brain.

2520. Angiokeratomas in Fabry's disease are best seen in?

Harrison's 20th Ed. Chapter 438, Page 3210, 3007

A. Between umbilicus and knees
B. Nape of the neck
C. FIngers of hand
D. Nose

Angiokeratomas in Fabry's disease are punctate, dark red to blue-black, flat or slightly raised, and usually symmetric. They do not blanch with pressure. They are most dense between umbilicus and knees "bathing suit area" (umbilicus, scrotum, inguinal region and perineum).

2521. Red papules like those seen in angiokeratomas of Fabry disease are seen in?

Harrison's 20th Ed. Chapter 54, Page 350, Table 54-15

A. Cutaneous polyarteritis nodosa
B. Bacillary angiomatosis
C. Lupus pernio
D. Urticaria pigmentosa

2522. Which of the following is related to Fabry disease?

Harrison's 20th Ed. Chapter 54, Page 351

A. Lattice corneal dystrophy
B. Keratoconus
C. Cornea verticillata
D. Corneal beading

Associated findings in Fabry disease include chronic renal disease, peripheral neuropathy & corneal opacities (cornea verticillata).

2523. Which of the following best relates to Fabry disease?

Harrison's 20th Ed. Chapter 411, Page 3007

A. GALA mutations
B. GBA1 mutations
C. LIPA mutations
D. GUSB mutations

Fabry disease results from mutations in GALA (cytogenetic location: Xq22.1) which encodes α-galactosidase A. The GLA gene provides instructions for making an enzyme called alpha-galactosidase A which is active in lysosomes. Alpha-galactosidase A breaks down globotriaosylceramide. Alterations in GLA gene produce an abnormal version of enzyme that is unable to break down globotriaosylceramide effectively. As a result, globotriaosylceramide builds up in body's cells, particularly cells lining blood vessels in the skin and cells in the kidneys, heart & nervous system, damaging the cells. Other names of GALA are AGAL_HUMAN, Agalsidase alfa, Alpha-D-galactosidase A, alpha-D-galactoside galactohydrolase, Alpha-galactosidase, alpha-Galactosidase A, ceramidetrihexosidase, GALA, galactosidase alpha, Melibiase.

2524. Which of the following about angiokeratomas in Fabry disease is false?

Harrison's 20th Ed. Chapter 411, Page 3007

A. Punctate, dark red to blue-black
B. Symmetric
C. Do not blanch with pressure
D. None of the above

Angiokeratomas are punctate, dark red to blue-black, flat or slightly raised, and usually symmetric; they do not blanch with pressure.

2525. Which of the following may occur in Fabry disease?

Harrison's 20th Ed. Chapter 411, Page 3007

A. Isosthenuria
B. Idiopathic hypertrophic myocardiopathy
C. Leg lymphedema without hypoproteinemia
D. All of the above

2526. Fabry disease is caused by mutations in?

Harrison's 20th Ed. Chapter 308, Page 2146

A. Alpha-galactosidase A gene
B. ATP-binding cassette transporter 1 (ABC1) gene
C. Mitofusin 2 (MFN2) gene
D. Transthyretin (TTR) gene

Fabry's disease is an X-linked inborn error of globotriaosylceramide metabolism secondary to deficient lysosomal α-galactosidase A activity, resulting in excessive intracellular storage of globotriaosylceramide.

2527. Accumulation in nerves and blood vessels of which of the following occurs Fabry disease?

Harrison's 20th Ed. Chapter 411, Page 3007

A. Aspartyl glucosamine
B. Galactosylsphingosine
C. Ceramide trihexoside (Globotriaosylceramide)
D. Glycogen

Fabry disease is caused by mutations in alpha-galactosidase A gene that leads to accumulation of ceramide trihexoside in nerves and blood vessels. Fabry's disease is an X-linked inborn error of globotriaosylceramide metabolism secondary to deficient lysosomal α-galactosidase A activity resulting in excessive intracellular storage of globotriaosylceramide.

2528. Accessory pathways (APs) are associated with which of the following?

Harrison's 20th Ed. Chapter 244, Page 1739

A. Ebstein's anomaly
B. Danon's disease
C. Fabry's disease
D. All of the above

Accessory pathways (APs) are associated with Ebstein's anomaly of tricuspid valve & forms of hypertrophic cardiomyopathy including PRKAG2 mutations, Danon's disease and Fabry's disease. APs are associated with various arrhythmias including narrow-complex PSVT, wide-complex tachycardias & sudden death.

2529. Which of the following is a heritable form of CKD?

Harrison's 20th Ed. Chapter 305, Page 2119

A. Alport disease
B. Fabry disease
C. Cystinosis
D. All of the above

Heritable form of CKD are Alport or Fabry disease, cystinosis.

2530. Which of the following is a lysosomal storage disease?

Harrison's 20th Ed. Chapter 411, Page 3003

A. Tay-Sachs disease
B. Pompe disease
C. Fabry disease
D. All of the above

There are more than 50 different lysosomal storage diseases (LSDs), classified according to the nature of the stored material. These include Tay-Sachs disease, Fabry disease, Gaucher disease, Niemann-Pick disease, lysosomal acid lipase deficiencies, the mucopolysaccharidoses and Pompe disease.

2531. Which of the following lysosomal storage diseases is X-linked?

Harrison's 20th Ed. Chapter 411, Page 3004 Table 411-1

A. Hunter (mucopolysaccharidosis type II) disease
B. Danon disease
C. Fabry disease
D. All of the above

All LSDs are inherited as autosomal recessive disorders except for Hunter (mucopolysaccharidosis type II), Danon and Fabry diseases, which are X-linked.

2532. Footdrop is a prominent feature of?

Harrison's 20th Ed. Chapter 438, Page 3210

A. Facioscapulohumeral muscular dystrophy (FSH)
B. Peroneal neuropathy
C. CMT1
D. All of the above

Footdrop is a prominent feature of Refsum disease, myotonic dystrophy type 1 (DM1), Facioscapulohumeral muscular dystrophy (FSH), Type 1 lepra reaction, Udd, and Markesbery-Griggs type distal myopathies.

2533. Adrenoleukodystrophy (ALD) & adrenomyeloneuropathy (AMN) are caused by mutations in?

Harrison's 20th Ed. Chapter 438, Page 3211

A. Alpha-galactosidase A gene
B. ATP-binding cassette transporter 1 (ABC1) gene
C. Mitofusin 2 (MFN2) gene
D. Transthyretin (TTR) gene

2534. Level in urine of very long chain fatty acid (VLCFA) is increased in which of the following?

Harrison's 20th Ed. Chapter 438, Page 3211

A. Fabry's disease
B. Refsum disease
C. Adrenoleukodystrophy & adrenomyeloneuropathy
D. All of the above

Very long chain fatty acid (VLCFA) levels (C24, C25 and C26) are increased in the urine of patients of Adrenoleukodystrophy (ALD) & adrenomyeloneuropathy (AMN). Demonstration of increased plasma VLCFA such as hexacosanoic acid (C26:0) levels is the most frequently used diagnostic assay.

2535. Which of the following is a major phenotype of adrenoleukodystrophy (ALD)?

Arch Neurol. 2005;62(7):1073-1080

A. Rapidly progressive cerebral ALD (CERALD)
B. Adrenomyeloneuropathy (AMN)
C. Addison-only phenotype
D. All of the above

There are 4 major phenotypes of ALD: (1) rapidly progressive cerebral ALD (CERALD) phenotypes, which are most common in childhood and are associated with inflammatory demyelination; (2) adrenomyeloneuropathy (AMN), a slowly progressive noninflammatory distal axonopathy that involves the spinal cord long tracts; (3) Addison-only phenotype of primary adrenocortical insufficiency without demonstrable neurological deficit; and (4) asymptomatic status without clinically evident neurological or endocrine abnormality.

2536. Which of the following represents Lorenzo's oil (LO)?
Arch Neurol. 2005;62(7):1073-1080

A. 1-O-alkyl-2-acyl-sn-glyceryl-3-phosphorylcholine
B. 4:1 glyceryl trioleate - glyceryl trierucate
C. Acyl-monoserine lactone
D. None of the above

2537. Lorenzo's Oil contains?
N Engl J Med. 1993;328:1126-1127

A. 20% erucic acid and 80% oleic acid
B. 40% erucic acid and 60% oleic acid
C. 50% erucic acid and 50% oleic acid
D. 80% erucic acid and 20% oleic acid

Lorenzo's Oil contains 20 percent erucic acid (22:1) and 80 percent oleic acid (18:1).

2538. VLCFA levels are increased in?
Ann Neurol. 1999;45:100-110

A. Zellweger syndrome (cerebrohepatorenal syndrome)
B. Neonatal adrenoleukodystrophy
C. Infantile Refsum's disease
D. All of the above

VLCFA levels are increased in patients homozygous for Zellweger syndrome (cerebrohepatorenal syndrome), neonatal adrenoleukodystrophy, infantile Refsum's disease, and in patients with deficiencies of peroxisomal acyl-coenzyme A oxidase, bifunctional enzyme, and 3-oxoacyl-coenzyme A thiolase.

2539. Diets supplemented with Lorenzo's oil is of use in which of the following?
Harrison's 20th Ed. Chapter 438, Page 3211

A. Fabry's disease
B. Refsum disease
C. Adrenoleukodystrophy & adrenomyeloneuropathy
D. All of the above

Diets low in VLCFAs and supplemented with Lorenzo's oil (erucic & oleic acids) reduce levels of VLCFAs and increase the levels of C22 in serum, fibroblasts and liver.

2540. Refsum disease is caused by accumulation of which of the following in the central & peripheral nervous systems?
Harrison's 20th Ed. Chapter 438, Page 3211

A. Formic acid
B. Glycolic acid
C. Oxalic acid
D. Phytanic acid

Refsum disease (autosomal recessive) is caused by mutations in the gene that encodes for phytanoyl-CoA alpha-hydroxylase (PAHX). This mutations lead to elevation of serum phytanic acid levels and accumulation of phytanic acid in central and peripheral nervous systems. Refsum disease is treated by removing phytanic precursors (phytols: fish oils, dairy products, and ruminant fats) from diet.

2541. The classic tetrad of Refsum disease include all except?
Harrison's 20th Ed. Chapter 438, Page 3211

A. Peripheral neuropathy
B. Retinitis pigmentosa
C. Cerebellar ataxia
D. Normal CSF protein concentration

The classic tetrad of Refsum disease include peripheral neuropathy, retinitis pigmentosa, cerebellar ataxia, and elevated CSF protein concentration.

2542. Presentation of Refsum disease include?
Harrison's 20th Ed. Chapter 438, Page 3211

A. Anosmia
B. Sensorineural deafness
C. Ichthyosis
D. All of the above

Features of Refsum disease include sensorimotor demyelinating neuropathy, sensorineural deafness, cerebellar ataxia, anosmia, retinitis pigmentosa, ichthyosis, syndactyly, shortening of the fourth toe, cardiac conduction abnormalities, cardiomyopathy and cataracts.

2543. Retinitis pigmentosa occurs in association with which of the following diseases?
Harrison's 20th Ed. Chapter 28, Page 188

A. Olivopontocerebellar degeneration
B. Bassen-Kornzweig disease
C. Bardet-Biedl syndrome
D. All of the above

Retinitis pigmentosa occur in association with rare hereditary systemic diseases like olivopontocerebellar degeneration, Bassen-Kornzweig disease, Kearns-Sayre syndrome, Bardet-Biedl syndrome, Refsum's disease, Cranioectodermal dysplasia (Sensenbrenner syndrome), Senior-Loken syndrome, Leigh disease, NARP (neuropathy, ataxia, and retinitis pigmentosa), Usher's syndrome (retinitis pigmentosa and hearing loss), abetalipoproteinemia.

2544. Severe deficiency of which of the following occurs in Tangier Disease (TD)?
Harrison's 20th Ed. Chapter 438, Page 3211

A. High-density lipoproteins (HDL)
B. Low-density lipoproteins (HDL)
C. Very low-density lipoproteins (HDL)
D. Triglycerides

Tangier disease is caused by mutations in the ATP-binding cassette transporter 1 (ABC1) gene, which leads to markedly reduced levels of high-density lipoprotein (HDL) cholesterol levels while triacylglycerol levels are increased.

2545. Presentation of Tangier disease resembles those of?
Harrison's 20th Ed. Chapter 438, Page 3211

A. Guillain-Barré syndrome
B. Syringomyelia
C. Multiple sclerosis
D. Amyotrophic lateral sclerosis

Tangier disease is a rare autosomal recessive disorder that can present as asymmetric multiple mononeuropathies, slowly progressive symmetric polyneuropathy predominantly in legs, and a pseudo-syringomyelia pattern with dissociated sensory loss (i.e. abnormal pain/temperature perception but preserved position/vibration in the arms.

2546. Which of the following is characteristic of Tangier disease?
Harrison's 20th Ed. Chapter 234, Page 1667, 2899

A. Orange tonsils
B. Howship's lacunae
C. Lenticonus
D. Strawberry gums

2547. Which of the following about Tangier disease is false?
Harrison's 20th Ed. Chapter 400, Page 2899

A. Very low levels of HDL-C
B. Low plasma levels of LDL-C
C. Low plasma levels of apoA-I
D. All of the above

2548. Which of the following forms of porphyria are associated with peripheral neuropathy?
Harrison's 20th Ed. Chapter 438, Page 3211

A. Acute intermittent porphyria (AIP)
B. Hereditary coproporphyria (HCP)
C. Variegate porphyria (VP)
D. All of the above

Three forms of porphyria are associated with peripheral neuropathy - acute intermittent porphyria (AIP), hereditary coproporphyria (HCP), and variegate porphyria (VP).

2549. Photosensitive rash is not seen with which of the following porphyrias?
Harrison's 20th Ed. Chapter 438, Page 3211

A. Acute intermittent porphyria (AIP)
B. Hereditary coproporphyria (HCP)
C. Variegate porphyria (VP)
D. All of the above

A photosensitive rash is seen with HCP and VP but not in AIP.

2550. Which of the following tests is useful in porphyria?
Harrison's 20th Ed. Chapter 438, Page 3211

A. Increased urinary excretion of aminolevulinic acid
B. Increased urinary excretion of porphobilinogen
C. Increased urinary excretion of coproporphyrinogen
D. All of the above

Accumulation of intermediary precursors of heme like d-aminolevulinic acid, porphobilinogen, uroporphobilinogen, coproporphyrinogen and protoporphyrinogen is found in urine of patients of porphyria.

2551. Which of the following is decreased in axonal degeneration in motor nerve conduction studies?
Harrison's 20th Ed. Chapter 438, Page 3211

A. F wave
B. Conduction velocity
C. CMAP amplitude
D. Distal latency

The primary abnormalities on EDx are marked reductions in compound motor action potential (CMAP) amplitudes and signs of active axonal degeneration on needle EMG.

2552. Mutations in which of the following genes is responsible for familial amyloid neuropathy?
Harrison's 20th Ed. Chapter 438, Page 3212

A. Transthyretin (FAP 1 & 2)
B. Apolipoprotein A1 (FAP 3)
C. Gelsolin
D. All of the above

Familial amyloid polyneuropathy (FAP) is phenotypically and genetically heterogeneous and is caused by mutations in the genes for transthyretin (TTR), apolipoprotein A1, or gelsolin. The majority of patients with FAP have mutations in the TTR gene.

2553. Which of the following modalities halts disease progression in familial amyloid neuropathy (FAP)?
Harrison's 20th Ed. Chapter 438, Page 3212

A. Plasmapheresis
B. Liver transplantation
C. Kidney transplantation
D. IVIg

Because the liver produces much of the body's TTR, liver transplantation has been used to treat FAP related to TTR mutations. Liver transplantation halts disease progression of FAP.

2554. Which of the following about TTR-related FAP is false?
Harrison's 20th Ed. Chapter 438, Page 3212

A. Carpal tunnel syndrome (CTS) is common
B. Autonomic involvement can be severe
C. Liver transplantation beneficial
D. None of the above

2555. Which of the following about Gelsolin-related amyloidosis (Finnish type) is false?
Harrison's 20th Ed. Chapter 438, Page 3212

A. Lattice corneal dystrophy
B. Multiple cranial neuropathies
C. Autonomic dysfunction does not occur
D. None of the above

2556. Which of the following drugs is beneficial in familial amyloid neuropathy (FAP)?
Harrison's 20th Ed. Chapter 438, Page 3212

A. Paroxetine
B. Nacetyl cysteine
C. Epigallocatechin gallate
D. Tafamidis meglumine

Tafamidis meglumine & diflunisal which prevent misfolding & deposition of mutated TTR, appear to slow the rate of deterioration patients with TTR-related FAP.

2557. AL amyloidosis occurs in?
Harrison's 20th Ed. Chapter 438, Page 3212

A. Multiple myeloma (MM)
B. Waldenström's macroglobulinemia
C. Lymphoma
D. All of the above

AL amyloidosis occurs with multiple myeloma (MM), Waldenström's macroglobulinemia, lymphoma, other plasmacytomas, or lymphoproliferative disorders, or idiopathic.

2558. Presence of which of the following is a risk factors for diabetic neuropathy?
Harrison's 20th Ed. Chapter 438, Page 3212

A. Long-standing, poorly controlled DM
B. Presence of retinopathy
C. Presence of nephropathy
D. All of the above

Risk factors for the development of diabetic neuropathy include long-standing, poorly controlled DM and presence of retinopathy & nephropathy.

2559. Which of the following is the most common form of diabetic neuropathy?
Harrison's 20th Ed. Chapter 438, Page 3212

A. Diabetic truncal radiculoneuropathy (DTRN)
B. Diabetic lumbosacral radiculoplexus neuropathy
C. Oculomotor (III or VI nerve) neuropathy
D. Diabetic sensorimotor polyneuropathy (DSPN)

Diabetic Distal Symmetric Sensory and Sensorimotor Polyneuropathy (DSPN) is the most common form of diabetic neuropathy. Other types of polyneuropathy include autonomic neuropathy, diabetic neuropathic cachexia, polyradiculoneuropathies, cranial neuropathies & other mononeuropathies.

2560. Sensory loss in DSPN begins in?

Harrison's 20th Ed. Chapter 438, Page 3212

A. Nose
B. Fingers
C. Toes
D. Buttocks

DSPN manifests as sensory loss beginning in the toes that gradually progresses over time up the legs and into the fingers and arms.

2561. Which of the following nerves are involved in diabetic sensorimotor polyneuropathy (DSPN)?

Harrison's 20th Ed. Chapter 438, Page 3212

A. Small- and large-fiber sensory
B. Autonomic
C. Motor
D. All of the above

DSPN is a mixed neuropathy with small- & large-fiber sensory, autonomic, & motor nerve involvement in various combinations. Sensory & autonomic symptoms are more prominent than motor.

2562. Which of the following has relevance in the pathogenesis of diabetic sensorimotor polyneuropathy (DSPN)?

Diabetes. 1983;32(11):988-992

A. Myo-inositol
B. Betaine
C. Glutamine
D. All of the above

DSPN could be caused by an increased neuronal glucose conversion to sorbitol by aldose reductase using NADPH as a coenzyme. Sorbitol decreases levels of myo-inositol and phosphoinositides, leading to a decrease in diacylglycerol, protein kinase C, and Na+, K+, ATPase activity. This sequence of events leads to axonal loss & demyelination.

2563. Diabetic autonomic neuropathy is typically seen in combination with?

Harrison's 20th Ed. Chapter 438, Page 3212

A. DSPN
B. Diabetic neuropathic cachexia
C. Polyradiculoneuropathies
D. Cranial neuropathies

Autonomic neuropathy is typically seen in combination with DSPN.

2564. Initial presentation in diabetic amyotrophy or Bruns-Garland Syndrome is?

Harrison's 20th Ed. Chapter 438, Page 3212

A. Pain
B. Sensory loss
C. Muscle weakness
D. Diplopia

Typically, patients of diabetic radiculoplexus neuropathy present with severe pain in low back, hip, and thigh in one leg. Atrophy & weakness of proximal & distal muscles in the affected leg become apparent within a few days or weeks. Neuropathy is often accompanied by severe weight loss.

2565. Asymmetric abrupt-onset diabetic neuropathy is?

Harrison's 20th Ed. Chapter 438, Page 3212

A. Diabetic truncal radiculoneuropathy (DTRN)
B. Diabetic lumbosacral radiculoplexus neuropathy
C. Cranial neuropathy
D. All of the above

Asymmetric abrupt-onset diabetic neuropathies include diabetic truncal radiculoneuropathy (DTRN), diabetic lumbosacral radiculoplexus neuropathy (DLSRPN) & oculomotor (III or VI nerve) neuropathy.

2566. Which is the most frequently involved cranial nerve in diabetes?

Harrison's 20th Ed. Chapter 438, Page 3212

A. III
B. IV
C. VI
D. VII

In regard to cranial mononeuropathies, a seventh nerve palsy is most common, followed by third nerve, sixth nerve, and, less frequently, fourth nerve palsies.

2567. Which of the following is not a feature of diabetic third nerve palsy?

Harrison's 20th Ed. Chapter 438, Page 3212

A. Abrupt in onset
B. Intense retro-orbital pain
C. Bilateral ptosis
D. Restriction of medial gaze & upgaze

Diabetic III nerve palsy is abrupt in onset, heralded by intense retro-orbital pain, double vision, unilateral ptosis & restriction of medial gaze & upgaze.

2568. Which of the following is not a feature of diabetic third nerve palsy?

Harrison's 20th Ed. Chapter 438, Page 3212

A. Abrupt in onset
B. Intense retro-orbital pain
C. Dilated pupil
D. Improve spontaneously in 3–6 months

Pupil is nearly always spared in diabetic III nerve palsy as pupillomotor fibers are present on the outer layers of III nerve fascicle, and an ischemic lesion tends to involve the center of the fascicle. Thus, diabetic third nerve palsies are characteristically pupil-sparing.

2569. Trigeminal neuropathy occurs in which of the following illnesses?

Harrison's 20th Ed. Chapter 433, Page 2556, 3168

A. Systemic sclerosis (Scleroderma)
B. Sjögren syndrome
C. Leprosy
D. All of the above

In Systemic sclerosis (SSc), the central nervous system is generally spared, sensory trigeminal neuropathy due to fibrosis or vasculopathy can occur. Other causes include Sjögren syndrome, systemic lupus erythematosus, mixed connective tissue disease, herpes zoster (acute or postherpetic) and leprosy.

2570. Which of the following is related to insulin treatment for diabetes?

Curr Diabetes Rev. 2013 9(3):267-74

A. Diabetic truncal radiculoneuropathy
B. Diabetic amyotrophy
C. Insulin neuritis
D. All of the above

Insulin neuritis or "treatment induced neuropathy" is a reversible painful neuropathy seen with initiation of insulin treatment for diabetes.

2571. Which of the following about diabetic neuropathic cachexia is false?

Curr Diabetes Rev. 2013 9(3):267-74

A. Unintentional weight loss
B. Acute symmetrical painful peripheral neuropathy, no weakness
C. Burning pain in lower limbs & allodynia
D. None of the above

"Diabetic neuropathic cachexia" is a rare disorder associated with poor diabetic control that presents with large amounts of unintentional weight loss associated with an acute symmetrical painful peripheral neuropathy without weakness. Pain is characteristically burning in nature with predominant lower limb involvement and allodynia.

2572. Which of the following is a finding in Sjögren's syndrome?

Harrison's 20th Ed. Chapter 438, Page 3213

A. Sicca complex of xerophthalmia & xerostomia
B. Length-dependent axonal sensorimotor neuropathy
C. Trigeminal neuropathy
D. All of the above

Sjögren's syndrome is characterized by sicca complex of xerophthalmia, xerostomia & dryness of other mucous membranes, length-dependent axonal sensorimotor neuropathy, small-fiber neuropathy, trigeminal neuropathy, or sensory neuronopathy/ganglionopathy.

2573. Which of the following causes vasculitic neuropathy?

Harrison's 20th Ed. Chapter 438, Page 3213

A. Polyarteritis nodosa (PAN)
B. Churg-Strauss syndrome (CSS)
C. Rheumatoid arthritis
D. All of the above

Diagnosis of suspected vasculitic neuropathy is made by a combined nerve & muscle biopsy, with serial section or skip-serial techniques.

2574. Which of the following causes necrotizing vasculitis?

Harrison's 20th Ed. Chapter 438, Page 3213

A. Extrapulmonary pneumocystosis
B. Eosinophilic granulomatosis with polyangiitis (EGPA)
C. Malignant hypertension
D. All of the above

2575. Which of the following causes small-vessel venulitis isolated to the skin?

Harrison's 20th Ed. Chapter 456, Page 2589

A. Systemic lupus erythematosus
B. Rheumatoid arthritis
C. Sjögren's syndrome
D. All of the above

Systemic lupus erythematosus, rheumatoid arthritis, inflammatory myositis, relapsing polychondritis, and Sjögren's syndrome cause small-vessel venulitis isolated to the skin.

2576. In sarcoidosis, most common cranial nerve involved is?

Harrison's 20th Ed. Chapter 438, Page 3214

A. Third nerve
B. Fifth nerve
C. Seventh nerve
D. Twelfth nerve

In sarcoidosis, most common cranial nerve involved is seventh nerve, which can be affected bilaterally.

2577. In celiac disease, which of the neurologic finding may be present?

Harrison's 20th Ed. Chapter 438, Page 3214

A. Ataxia
B. Peripheral neuropathy
C. Neuromyotonia
D. All of the above

In celiac disease, various neurologic complications including ataxia, generalized sensorimotor polyneuropathy, pure motor neuropathy, multiple mononeuropathies, autonomic neuropathy, small-fiber neuropathy, and neuromyotonia have been reported.

2578. Which of the following drugs can cause peripheral neuropathy?

Harrison's 20th Ed. Chapter 438, Page 3214

A. Tumor necrosis blockers
B. Leflunomide
C. Metronidazole
D. All of the above

2579. Which of the following can complicate arteriovenous shunts created in arm for dialysis?

Harrison's 20th Ed. Chapter 438, Page 3214

A. Lymphedema
B. Ischemic monomelic neuropathy
C. Steal syndrome
D. All of the above

The most important complications of fistulae for HD are lymphedema, infection, aneurysm, stenosis, congestive heart failure, steal syndrome, ischemic neuropathy and thrombosis.

2580. Weakness developing in critically ill patients while in ICU is caused by?

Harrison's 20th Ed. Chapter 438, Page 3214

A. Critical illness polyneuropathy (CIP)
B. Critical illness myopathy (CIM)
C. Prolonged neuromuscular blockade
D. Any of the above

Most common causes of acute generalized weakness leading to admission to medical ICU are GBS & myasthenia gravis. Weakness that develops in critically ill patients while in ICU is caused by critical illness polyneuropathy (CIP) or critical illness myopathy (CIM) or by prolonged neuromuscular blockade.

2581. Neurologic finding in a case of critical illness polyneuropathy (CIP) include?

Harrison's 20th Ed. Chapter 301, Page 2083

A. Diffuse weakness, decreased reflexes
B. Distal sensory loss
C. Electrophysiologic studies show axonal degeneration
D. All of the above

2582. Carpal tunnel syndrome can be a presentation of which of the following illnesses?

Harrison's 20th Ed. Chapter 438, Page 3214

A. Familial amyloid polyneuropathy (FAP)
B. Hypothyroidism
C. Uremic neuropathy
D. All of the above

2583. Clinical presentation can mimic Guillain-Barré syndrome in?
N Engl J Med. 2012;366:2294-304

A. Porphyria
B. Sarcoidosis
C. Arsenic neuropathy
D. All of the above

2584. Acute, severe sensorimotor polyneuropathy can resemble Guillain-Barré syndrome in?
N Engl J Med. 2012;366:2294-304

A. Nitrofurantoin
B. Inflammatory bowel disease
C. Uremic neuropathy
D. All of the above

2585. Mycobacterium leprae causes?
Harrison's 20th Ed. Chapter 438, Page 3214

A. Mononeuropathy
B. Mononeuropathy multiplex
C. Polyneuropathy
D. Plexopathy

M. leprae causes mononeuropathy multiplex affecting peripheral nerves in cooler regions of body.

2586. Peripheral nerves are affected in which type of leprosy?
Harrison's 20th Ed. Chapter 438, Page 3214

A. Tuberculoid
B. Lepromatous
C. Borderline
D. All of the above

Peripheral nerves may be affected in all three types of leprosy. Neuropathies are most common in patients with borderline leprosy.

2587. In leprosy, sensory loss does not occur in all except?
Harrison's 20th Ed. Chapter 116, Page 869

A. Groin
B. Axilla
C. Pinnae of ears
D. Scalp

In leprosy, sensory loss spares midline of trunk anteriorly, groin, axilla & scalp - the warmer regions of the body.

2588. Which of the following cranial nerves is involved in leprosy?
Harrison's 20th Ed. Chapter 438, Page 3214

A. III
B. V
C. VI
D. XI

V & VII cranial nerves, greater auricular nerve in neck, median & ulnar nerves, and peroneal nerves are involved in leprosy.

2589. Lyme disease is caused by?
Harrison's 20th Ed. Chapter 438, Page 3215

A. Borrelia recurrentis
B. Borrelia burgdorferi
C. Borrelia hermsii
D. Borrelia turicatae

Lyme disease is caused by infection with Borrelia burgdorferi, a spirochete usually transmitted by the deer tick Ixodes dammini.

2590. Which of the following about Lyme disease is false?
Harrison's 20th Ed. Chapter 438, Page 3215

A. Facial neuropathy is common
B. Asymmetric polyradiculoneuropathy or multiple mononeuropathies
C. EDx is suggestive of a primary axonopathy
D. None of the above

2591. Diphtheritic neuropathy develops how many months after the initial infection?
Harrison's 20th Ed. Chapter 438, Page 3215

A. 1 or 2 months
B. 2 or 3 months
C. 3 or 4 months
D. 4 or 5 months

A generalized polyneuropathy may manifest 2 or 3 months following the initial diphtheritic infection. Early treatment with antitoxin and antibiotics does not alter natural history of associated peripheral neuropathy which resolves after several months.

2592. HIV-infected individuals develop a neuropathy due to?
Harrison's 20th Ed. Chapter 438, Page 3215

A. Direct result of the virus itself
B. Other associated viral infections (CMV)
C. Neurotoxicity secondary to antiviral medications
D. All of the above

2593. Which of the following is the presentation of nerve involvement in HIV infection?
Harrison's 20th Ed. Chapter 438, Page 3215

A. Polyradiculopathy
B. Distal symmetric polyneuropathy (DSP)
C. Inflammatory demyelinating polyneuropathy
D. Any of the above

Major presentations of peripheral neuropathy associated with HIV infection include distal symmetric polyneuropathy (DSP), inflammatory demyelinating polyneuropathy (GBS & CIDP), multiple mononeuropathies (vasculitis, CMV-related), polyradiculopathy (CMV-related), autonomic neuropathy, and sensory ganglionitis.

2594. Most common form of peripheral neuropathy associated with HIV infection is?
Harrison's 20th Ed. Chapter 438, Page 3215

A. Distal symmetric polyneuropathy (DSP)
B. Inflammatory demyelinating polyneuropathy
C. Autonomic neuropathy
D. Sensory ganglionitis

DSP is the most common form of peripheral neuropathy associated with HIV infection and usually is seen in patients with AIDS.

2595. Which of the following Anti-HIV drug is neurotoxic & causes a painful sensory neuropathy?
Harrison's 20th Ed. Chapter 438, Page 3215

A. Dideoxycytidine
B. Dideoxyinosine
C. Stavudine
D. All of the above

2596. Anti-HIV drug not associated with neuropathy is?

Harrison's 20th Ed. Chapter 438, Page 3215

A. Zidovudine
B. Lamivudine
C. Abacavir
D. All of the above

Zidovudine, lamivudine and abacavir are not associated with neuropathy. Dideoxycytidine, dideoxyinosine & stavudine are neurotoxic and can cause a painful sensory neuropathy.

2597. Which of the following neuropathy usually develops at the time of seroconversion in HIV infection?

Harrison's 20th Ed. Chapter 438, Page 3215

A. HIV-associated polyradiculoneuropathy
B. Acute inflammatory demyelinating polyneuropathy (AIDP)
C. Chronic inflammatory demyelinating polyneuropathy (CIDP)
D. HIV-related multiple mononeuropathies

Acute inflammatory demyelinating polyneuropathy (AIDP) usually develops at the time of seroconversion, whereas CIDP can occur any time in the course of the HIV infection.

2598. Lumbosacral polyradiculopathy in patients with AIDS is due to?

Harrison's 20th Ed. Chapter 438, Page 3215

A. Herpes zoster
B. CMV infection
C. Tuberculosis
D. Lymphoma

Lumbosacral polyradiculopathies are usually due to CMV infection in patients with AIDS.

2599. Which of the following can be caused by HIV infection?

Harrison's 20th Ed. Chapter 438, Page 3215

A. Distal symmetric polyneuropathy (DSP)
B. Inflammatory demyelinating polyradiculoneuropathy
C. Progressive polyradiculopathy
D. All of the above

2600. Which of the following can be caused by HIV infection?

Harrison's 20th Ed. Chapter 438, Page 3215

A. Multiple mononeuropathies
B. Inflammatory demyelinating polyradiculoneuropathy
C. Sensory neuronopathy/ganglionopathy
D. All of the above

2601. Which of the following about peripheral neuropathy due to herpes varicella-zoster (HVZ) infection is false?

Harrison's 20th Ed. Chapter 438, Page 3215

A. Due to reactivation of latent virus
B. Due to a primary infection
C. 25% of affected patients have postherpetic neuralgia (PHN)
D. HVZ vaccine recipients has no effect on PHN

Postherpetic neuralgia (PHN) is reduced by 67% in those who have received HVZ vaccine.

2602. Most common malignancy causing neuropathies is?

Harrison's 20th Ed. Chapter 438, Page 3215

A. Lung cancer
B. Carcinoma breast
C. Carcinoma ovary
D. Carcinoma stomach

Most common malignancy causing neuropathy is lung cancer. Neuropathies also complicate carcinoma of breast, ovaries, stomach, colon, rectum.

2603. Paraneoplastic encephalomyelitis/sensory neuronopathy (PEM/SN) usually complicates which of the following malignancies?

Harrison's 20th Ed. Chapter 438, Page 3216

A. Small cell lung carcinoma
B. Carcinoma breast
C. Carcinoma ovary
D. Carcinoma stomach

Paraneoplastic encephalomyelitis/sensory neuronopathy (PEM/SN) usually complicates small cell lung carcinoma.

2604. Autoantigen found in sera / CSF of patients with paraneoplastic PEM/SN is?

Harrison's 20th Ed. Chapter 438, Page 3216

A. Amphiphysin
B. Hu protein
C. Gephyrin
D. Cyclin B1

Polyclonal antineuronal antibodies (IgG) directed against Hu antigen are found in sera or CSF in the majority of patients with paraneoplastic PEM/SN.

2605. Which of the following is beneficial in PEM/SN?

Harrison's 20th Ed. Chapter 438, Page 3216

A. Plasmapheresis
B. Intravenous immunoglobulin
C. Immunosuppressive agents
D. None of the above

Treatment of the underlying cancer generally does not affect the course of PEM/SN. However, occasional patients may improve following treatment of the tumor.

2606. Which of the following is a potentially neurotoxic drug?

Harrison's 20th Ed. Chapter 438, Page 3216

A. Isoniazid
B. Disulfiram
C. Pyridoxine
D. All of the above

Nitrofurantoin, isoniazid, disulfiram and pyridoxine are potentially neurotoxic drugs. They cause a sensory greater than motor length-dependent axonal neuropathy or neuronopathy/ganglionopathy.

2607. What dose of Chloroquine causes neuromyopathy?

Harrison's 20th Ed. Chapter 438, Page 3216

A. 500 mg/day for one year
B. 1000 mg/day for one year
C. 500 mg/day for two years
D. 1000 mg/day for two years

Signs & symptoms of chloroquine neuropathy & myopathy are reversible with its discontinuation.

2608. Which of the following can cause neuromyopathy similar to chloroquine & hydroxychloroquine?

Harrison's 20th Ed. Chapter 438, Page 3216

A. Amiodarone
B. Thalidomide
C. Colchicine
D. All of the above

Amiodarone neuromyopathy, similar to chloroquine & hydroxychloroquine neuromyopathy, typically appears after patients have taken Amiodarone for 2–3 years. Inclusions in muscle & nerve biopsies may persist for ~2 years following discontinuation of Amiodarone.

2609. Thalidomide is used to treat?

Harrison's 20th Ed. Chapter 438, Page 3217

A. Multiple myeloma (MM)
B. GVHD
C. Leprosy
D. All of the above

Thalidomide is an immunomodulating agent used to treat MM, GVHD & leprosy.

2610. What dose of Pyridoxine (Vitamin B6) can cause toxicity?

Harrison's 20th Ed. Chapter 438, Page 3217

A. 100 mg/day
B. 106 mg/day
C. 110 mg/day
D. 116 mg/day

At high doses of Pyridoxine (116 mg/day), patients can develop a severe sensory neuropathy with dysesthesias and sensory ataxia.

2611. Toxic effects of which of the following drugs continue even after stopping the drug?

Harrison's 20th Ed. Chapter 438, Page 3217

A. Chloroquine
B. Hydroxychloroquine
C. Thalidomide
D. All of the above

Even after stopping Thalidomide for 4–6 years, ~50% patients continue to have significant symptoms.

2612. Which of the following is inhibited by isoniazid (INH) resulting in pyridoxine deficiency and neuropathy?

Harrison's 20th Ed. Chapter 438, Page 3217

A. Pyridoxal phosphate
B. Pyridoxal 5'-phosphate
C. Pyridoxal kinase
D. Pyridoxal phosphokinase

INH inhibits pyridoxal phosphokinase, resulting in pyridoxine deficiency and consequent neuropathy. Prophylactic administration of pyridoxine 100 mg/day can prevent this neuropathy. Pyridoxine (Vitamin B6) refers to a family of compounds that include pyridoxine, pyridoxal, pyridoxamine, and their 5'-phosphate derivatives.

2613. Coasting effect refers to?

Harrison's 20th Ed. Chapter 438, Page 3219

A. Response to drug varies is same patient
B. Drug effect amplified by addition of another drug
C. Drug effect reduced by addition of another drug
D. Adverse effects of drug continue even after stopping medication

Severity of neuropathy increases with duration of treatment & progression stops once drug treatment is completed. Platinum compounds are an exception where sensory loss may progress for several months after cessation of treatment - The coasting effect.

2614. Which of the following about hexacarbons is false?

Harrison's 20th Ed. Chapter 438, Page 3219

A. n-Hexane and methyl n-butyl ketone
B. Water-insoluble industrial organic solvent
C. Leads to covalent cross-linking between axonal neurofilaments
D. None of the above

2615. Most common presentation of lead poisoning is?

Harrison's 20th Ed. Chapter 438, Page 3219

A. Sensory neuropathy
B. Motor neuropathy
C. Autonomic neuropathy
D. Encephalopathy

Most common presentation of lead poisoning is an encephalopathy. Motor neuropathy can also occur. Sensation is generally preserved. Autonomic nervous system can be affected.

2616. In lead poisoning, serum levels of which of the following is elevated?

Harrison's 20th Ed. Chapter 438, Page 3219

A. Alpha fetoprotein
B. Ceruloplasmin
C. Coproporphyrin
D. Prolactin

Serum coproporphyrin level is elevated in lead poisoning.

2617. In lead poisoning, chelation therapy with which of the following is beneficial?

Harrison's 20th Ed. Chapter 438, Page 3220

A. Calcium disodium ethylene-diaminetetraacetic acid (EDTA)
B. British anti-Lewisite (BAL)
C. Penicillamine
D. All of the above

2618. In mercury toxicity, the primary site of neuromuscular pathology is in?

Harrison's 20th Ed. Chapter 438, Page 3220

A. Motor neurons
B. Lateral spinothalamic tract
C. Medical longitudnal fasciculus
D. Dorsal root ganglia

In mercury toxicity, the primary site of neuromuscular pathology is in the dorsal root ganglia.

2619. Potassium ferric ferrocyanide II is useful in intoxication with which of the following?

Harrison's 20th Ed. Chapter 438, Page 3220

A. Mercury
B. Arsenic
C. Lead
D. Thallium

With acute intoxication, potassium ferric ferrocyanide II may be effective in preventing absorption of thallium from the gut.

2620. Which of the following is not helpful in Thallium toxicity?

Harrison's 20th Ed. Chapter 438, Page 3220

A. Potassium ferric ferrocyanide II
B. Adequate diuresis
C. Chelating agents
D. All of the above

2621. Mee's lines are related to which of the following?

Harrison's 20th Ed. Chapter 438, Page 3220

A. Organophosphates
B. Thallium
C. Hexacarbons
D. Lithium

2622. Mee's lines are related to which of the following?
Harrison's 20th Ed. Chapter 438, Page 3220

A. Mercury
B. Arsenic
C. Lead
D. Gold

Mee's lines are transverse lines at the base of fingernails & toenails. Mee's lines are seen in arsenic toxicity and also in thallium poisoning.

2623. Which of the following in arsenic toxicity is not diagnostically helpful?
Harrison's 20th Ed. Chapter 438, Page 3220

A. Arsenic levels in serum
B. Arsenic levels in urine
C. Arsenic levels in hair
D. Arsenic levels in fingernails

Because arsenic is cleared from blood rapidly, serum level of arsenic is not diagnostically helpful.

2624. Diagnosis of vitamin B12 deficiency is made by?
Harrison's 20th Ed. Chapter 438, Page 3220

A. Low serum cobalamin levels
B. Raised levels of methylmalonic acid
C. Raised levels of homocysteine
D. All of the above

Serum methylmalonic acid & homocysteine, the metabolites that accumulate when cobalamin-dependent reactions are blocked, are elevated.

2625. Which of the following anesthetic agent can produce acute cobalamin deficiency neuropathy?
Harrison's 20th Ed. Chapter 438, Page 3220

A. Halothane
B. Nitrous oxide
C. Isoflurane
D. Methoxyflurane

Use of nitrous oxide as an anesthetic agent can produce acute cobalamin deficiency neuropathy and subacute combined degeneration of cord.

2626. Beriberi in Singhalese language means?
Harrison's 20th Ed. Chapter 438, Page 3220

A. I'm sick, I'm sick
B. I can't, I can't
C. I'm tired, I'm tired
D. I want to be alone, I want to be alone

Beriberi means "I can't, I can't" in Singhalese, the language of natives of Sri Lanka. Dry beriberi refers to neuropathic symptoms. The term wet beriberi is used when cardiac manifestations predominate (in reference to edema).

2627. Erythrocyte transketolase activity is reduced in the blood of which nutritional neuropathy?
Harrison's 20th Ed. Chapter 438, Page 3220

A. Thiamine (Vitamin B1)
B. Pyridoxine (Vitamin B6)
C. Cobalamin (Vitamin B12)
D. Riboflavin

Blood & urine assays for thiamine are not reliable for diagnosis of deficiency. Erythrocyte transketolase activity and the percentage increase in activity (in vitro) following the addition of thiamine pyrophosphate (TPP) are more accurate & reliable.

2628. The term vitamin E is usually used for?
Harrison's 20th Ed. Chapter 438, Page 3221

A. α-tocopherol
B. β-tocopherol
C. γ-tocopherol
D. δ-tocopherol

Term vitamin E is usually used for α-tocopherol, most active of the four main types of vitamin E.

2629. Vitamin E deficiency usually occurs secondary to?
Harrison's 20th Ed. Chapter 438, Page 3221

A. Abetalipoproteinemia
B. Short-bowel syndromes
C. Cystic fibrosis
D. All of the above

Vitamin E deficiency usually occurs secondary to lipid malabsorption or in uncommon disorders of vitamin E transport like Abetalipoproteinemia, cystic fibrosis, as a consequence of various cholestatic and hepatobiliary disorders as well as short-bowel syndromes.

2630. Abetalipoproteinemia is characterized by?
Harrison's 20th Ed. Chapter 438, Page 3221

A. Pigmentary retinopathy
B. Acanthocytosis
C. Progressive ataxia
D. All of the above

Abetalipoproteinemia is a rare autosomal dominant disorder characterized by steatorrhea, pigmentary retinopathy, acanthocytosis and progressive ataxia.

2631. The main clinical feature of Vitamin E deficiency is?
Harrison's 20th Ed. Chapter 438, Page 3221

A. Pancytopenia and aplastic anemia
B. Subacute combined degeneration of cord
C. Spinocerebellar ataxia
D. Autonomic instability

2632. Clinical features of vitamin E deficiency resemble those of?
Harrison's 20th Ed. Chapter 438, Page 3221

A. Subacute combined degeneration of spinal cord
B. Friedreich's ataxia
C. Pellagra
D. Tabes dorsalis

The main clinical features of Vitamin E deficiency are spinocerebellar ataxia and polyneuropathy, resembling Friedreich's ataxia or other spinocerebellar ataxias. Patients manifest progressive ataxia & signs of posterior column dysfunction (impaired joint position & vibratory sensation). Because of the polyneuropathy, there is hyporeflexia, but plantar responses may be extensor as a result of the spinal cord involvement. Other neurologic manifestations may include ophthalmoplegia, pigmented retinopathy, night blindness, dysarthria, pseudoathetosis, dystonia and tremor.

2633. Drug that acts as pyridoxine (Vitamin B6) antagonist is?
Harrison's 20th Ed. Chapter 438, Page 3221

A. Isoniazid
B. Cycloserine
C. Penicillamine
D. All of the above

Isoniazid, cycloserine and penicillamine act as pyridoxine antagonists by combining to aldehyde moiety of vitamin B6. Vitamin B6 deficiency is most commonly seen in patients treated with isoniazid or hydralazine.

2634. Measurement of xanthurenic acid after tryptophan loading helps in the diagnosis of?

Molecular Aspects of Medicine (2016), doi: 10.1016/j.mam.2016.08.001

A. Thiamine (Vitamin B1) deficiency
B. Pyridoxine (Vitamin B6) deficiency
C. Cobalamin (Vitamin B12) deficiency
D. Riboflavin deficiency

Measurement of xanthurenic acid after tryptophan loading can help confirm the diagnosis of pyridoxine (Vitamin B6) deficiency.

2635. Strachan's syndrome is characterized by?

Rev Neurol. 1997;25:1950-1956

A. Painful sensory neuropathy
B. Orogenital dermatitis
C. Amblyopia and deafness
D. All of the above

Strachan's syndrome is characterized by a painful sensory neuropathy associated with orogenital dermatitis, amblyopia and deafness.

2636. Which of the following is a feature of copper deficiency?

Harrison's 20th Ed. Chapter 438, Page 3221

A. Lower limb paresthesias, spasticity and gait difficulties
B. Microcytic anemia
C. Neutropenia, pancytopenia
D. All of the above

2637. Excess of which of the following is an established cause of copper deficiency?

Harrison's 20th Ed. Chapter 438, Page 3221

A. Vitamin E excess
B. Vitamin B6 excess
C. Zinc excess
D. Iron excess

Excess zinc is an established cause of copper deficiency. Zinc upregulates enterocyte production of metallothionine, which results in decreased absorption of copper.

2638. Which of the following damage neurons in dorsal root ganglion?

Harrison's 20th Ed. Chapter 438, Page 3217 Table 438-7

A. Cisplatin
B. Varicella zoster virus (VZV)
C. Vitamin E deficiency
D. All of the above

Others that damage neurons in dorsal root ganglion include Mercury toxicity, Vitamin B6 deficiency, Nitrofurantoin, INH, Etoposide, Cisplatin, Ataxia Telangiectasia, Friedreich's Ataxia.

2639. Which of the following is toxic to dorsal root ganglia neurons?

Harrison's 20th Ed. Chapter 438, Page 3217 Table 438-7

A. Cisplatin
B. Paclitaxel
C. Vincristine
D. Thalidomide

Cisplatin is toxic to dorsal root ganglia neurons, producing a dose-related large-fiber sensory neuropathy (neuronopathy).

2640. Which of the following is not a feature of cisplatin toxicity?

Harrison's 20th Ed. Chapter 438, Page 3217

A. Hearing loss
B. Lhermitte's sign
C. Sensory ataxia
D. Decrease in motor strength

Small-fiber sensation (pain & temperature) and motor strength are spared in cisplatin toxicity (asymmetric proprioceptive sensory loss without weakness).

2641. Which of the following is a median neuropathy?

Harrison's 20th Ed. Chapter 438, Page 3222

A. Pronator teres syndrome
B. Anterior interosseous neuropathy
C. Carpal tunnel syndrome
D. All of the above

2642. The number of tendons in carpal tunnel is?

A. 7
B. 8
C. 9
D. 10

2643. In carpal tunnel syndrome (CTS), nocturnal paresthesia is common in?

Harrison's 19th Ed. 49

A. Thumb
B. Index finger
C. Middle finger
D. All of the above

2644. Systemic diseases associated with carpal tunnel syndrome include?

Harrison's 20th Ed. Chapter 438, Page 3222

A. Hypothyroidism
B. Rheumatoid arthritis
C. Diabetes mellitus
D. All of the above

Other diseases include Uremic neuropathy, AL primary amyloidosis, Familial amyloid polyneuropathy (FAP), Acromegaly, Systemic Sclerosis,

2645. Which of the following signs relate to diagnosis of mononeuropathy of upper limb?

Harrison's 20th Ed. Chapter 438, Page 3222

A. Tinel's sign
B. Phalen's sign
C. Froment sign
D. All of the above

In carpal tunnel syndrome (CTS), sensation of tingling can be reproduced when a percussion hammer is tapped over wrist (Tinel's sign) or wrist is flexed for 30–60 sec. (Phalen's sign). Froment sign indicates thumb adductor weakness and consists of flexion of thumb at the interphalangeal joint when attempting to oppose the thumb against lateral border of the second digit. This is seen in cubital tunnel syndrome.

2646. The root value of median nerve is?

Harrison's 20th Ed. Chapter 22, Page 141

A. C5 - T1
B. C6 - T1
C. C7 - T1
D. C8 - T1

2647. The root value of ulnar nerve is?
Harrison's 20th Ed. Chapter 22, Page 141

A. C5 - T1
B. C6 - T1
C. C7 - T1
D. C8 - T1

2648. The root value of radial nerve is?
Harrison's 20th Ed. Chapter 22, Page 141

A. C5 - T1
B. C6 - T1
C. C7 - T1
D. C8 - T1

2649. Which of the following nerve is involved if the site of lesion is 'Cubital tunnel'?
Harrison's 20th Ed. Chapter 438, Page 3222

A. Radial nerve
B. Ulnar nerve
C. Median nerve
D. All of the above

Ulnar nerve passes through the condylar groove between the medial epicondyle and the olecranon. Ulnar neuropathy at the elbow is called "Cubital Tunnel Syndrome" (tardy ulnar palsy).

2650. Which of the following nerve is involved in Saturday night palsy?
Harrison's 20th Ed. Chapter 438, Page 3222

A. Radial nerve
B. Ulnar nerve
C. Median nerve
D. All of the above

2651. Meralgia paresthetica relates best to?
Harrison's 20th Ed. Chapter 438, Page 3222

A. Radial neuropathy
B. Lateral femoral cutaneous neuropathy
C. Ulnar neuropathy at the elbow
D. Peroneal neuropathy

The neuropathy affecting lateral femoral cutaneous nerve is also known as meralgia paresthetica.

2652. Which of the following neuropathies occur during pregnancy?
Harrison's 20th Ed. Chapter 438, Page 3222

A. Peroneal neuropathy
B. Meralgia paresthetica
C. Carpal tunnel syndrome
D. All of the above

Compressive mononeuropathies during pregnancy and delivery are peroneal neuropathy, meralgia paresthetica, carpal tunnel syndrome, femoral neuropathy, isolated obturator neuropathy. There is a clear association between pregnancy and an increased frequency of idiopathic facial palsy (Bell's palsy). Restless leg syndrome is the most common peripheral nerve and movement disorder in pregnancy.

2653. Peroneal neuropathy needs to be distinguished from?
Harrison's 20th Ed. Chapter 438, Page 3222

A. L5 radiculopathy
B. Pott's disease
C. Diabetic radiculopathy
D. Sciatic neuropathy

Peroneal neuropathy needs to be distinguished from L5 radiculopathy. In L5 radiculopathy, ankle invertors and evertors are weak and needle EMG reveals denervation.

2654. Which of the following is false for Brachial Plexus?
Harrison's 20th Ed. Chapter 438, Page 3223

A. Four roots
B. Three trunks
C. Two divisions per trunk
D. Three cords

Brachial plexus is composed of five roots, three trunks (upper, middle, & lower), with two divisions (anterior & posterior) per trunk. Trunks divide into three cords (medial, lateral, & posterior).

2655. Parsonage-Turner syndrome relates best with?
Harrison's 20th Ed. Chapter 438, Page 3223

A. Brachial plexus
B. Lumbosacral plexus
C. Radiation-Induced plexopathy
D. Peroneal neuropathy

Immune-mediated brachial plexus neuropathy (IBPN) is also called acute brachial plexitis, neuralgic amyotrophy and Parsonage - Turner syndrome.

2656. Pain in immune-mediated brachial plexus neuropathy (IBPN) is at?
Harrison's 20th Ed. Chapter 438, Page 3223

A. Neck
B. Shoulder
C. Arm
D. Hand

IBPN usually presents with an acute onset of severe pain in the shoulder region.

2657. Out of the following, which is most commonly involved in IBPN?
Harrison's 20th Ed. Chapter 438, Page 3223

A. Root
B. Trunk
C. Division
D. Cord

Most common pattern of IBPN involves the upper trunk or a single or multiple mononeuropathies primarily involving the suprascapular, long thoracic, or axillary nerves.

2658. Which of the following surgical procedures is the most common cause of brachial plexopathy?
Harrison's 20th Ed. Chapter 438, Page 3223

A. Reduction of subluxated shoulder
B. Repair of fracture of neck of humerus
C. Median sternotomy
D. Repair of fracture of clavicle

Most common surgical procedures associated with brachial plexopathy as a complication are those that involve median sternotomies.

2659. Which of the following is false about electrodiagnostic features of demyelination?
Harrison's 20th Ed. Chapter 438, Page 3207

A. Slowing of nerve conduction velocity (NCV)
B. Dispersion of evoked compound action potentials
C. Conduction block & prolongation of distal latencies
D. None of the above

2660. Electrodiagnostic studies (EDx) help to diagnose which of the following neuropathies?

Harrison's 20th Ed. Chapter 438, Page 3207

A. Axonal
B. Demyelinating
C. Neuronal
D. All of the above

Electrodiagnostic studies help to classify neuropathy into either axonal, demyelinating or neuronal.

2661. Mononeuropathy multiplex syndrome may be a manifestation of all except?

Harrison's 20th Ed. Chapter 438, Page 3214

A. Leprosy
B. Sarcoidosis
C. Syphilis
D. NeuroAIDS

2662. Mononeuropathy multiplex syndrome may be a manifestation of?

Harrison's 20th Ed. Chapter 438, Page 3214

A. Eosinophilic granulomatosis with polyangiitis
B. Rheumatoid vasculitis
C. Tangier disease (ABCA I deficiency)
D. All of the above

2663. Sensory neuronopathy (or ganglionopathy) is best related to?

Harrison's 20th Ed. Chapter 22, Page 142

A. Amyloidosis
B. Sarcoidosis
C. Sjogren's syndrome
D. Gaucher disease Type 1

2664. Example of motor neuronopathies include?

Harrison's 20th Ed. Chapter 90, Page 673

A. Lower-motor form of amyotrophic lateral sclerosis
B. Poliomyelitis
C. Hereditary spinal muscular atrophies
D. All of the above

2665. Which of the following is a motor-predominant neuropathy?

Am Fam Physician. 2010;81(7):887-892

A. Acute intermittent porphyria
B. Diphtheritic neuropathy
C. Lead neuropathy
D. All of the above

2666. Which of the following is a neuronal neuropathy?

Am Fam Physician. 2010;81(7):887-892

A. Sjögren's syndrome
B. Cisplatin toxicity
C. Pyridoxine toxicity
D. All of the above

2667. Which of the following is not a demyelinating neuropathy?

Am Fam Physician. 2010;81(7):887-892

A. Guillain-Barré syndrome
B. Multifocal motor neuropathy (MMN)
C. HIV neuropathy
D. Diphtheria neuropathy

2668. Which of the following is not a axonal neuropathy?

Am Fam Physician. 2010;81(7):887-892

A. Toxic
B. HIV
C. Charcot-Marie-Tooth 2 (CMT2)
D. All of the above

Most toxic neuropathies are distal axonal degenerations. In HIV, length-dependent axonal degeneration of sensory fibers without nerve-fiber regeneration occurs.

2669. Which of the following is a acute onset neuropathy?

Am Fam Physician. 2010;81(7):887-892

A. Porphyria
B. Diphtheria
C. Guillain-Barré syndrome
D. All of the above

2670. Which of the following is a recurrent neuropathy?

Am Fam Physician. 2010;81(7):887-892

A. Porphyria
B. Refsum's disease
C. Hereditary neuropathy with pressure palsies (HNPP)
D. All of the above

2671. Example of motor neuronopathies include?

Harrison's 20th Ed. Chapter 90, Page 673

A. Lead intoxication
B. Dapsone intoxication
C. Porphyria
D. All of the above

2672. Peripheral neuropathy includes disorders of?

Am Fam Physician. 2010;81(7):887-892

A. Peripheral nerves
B. Dorsal or ventral nerve roots
C. Dorsal root ganglia
D. All of the above

Peripheral neuropathy includes disorders of peripheral nerves, dorsal or ventral nerve roots, dorsal root ganglia, brachial or lumbosacral plexus, cranial nerves (except I & II) & other sensory, motor, autonomic or mixed nerves.

2673. Which of the following is false about peripheral neuropathy?

Am Fam Physician. 2010;81(7):887-892

A. Sensory symptoms precede motor symptoms
B. Small-fiber neuropathies present with paresthesias
C. Large-fiber neuropathies present as gait disturbance
D. None of the above

2674. Term ataxic-neuropathy is used for?

Am Fam Physician. 2010;81(7):887-892

A. Small-fiber sensory neuropathies
B. Large-fiber sensory neuropathies
C. Motor-predominant neuropathies
D. Autonomic neuropathies

2675. Which of the following is not a small-fiber sensory neuropathy?

Ann Indian Acad Neurol. 2008;11(2):89–97

A. Amyloidosis
B. Sjogren's syndrome
C. Hereditary sensory and autonomic neuropathy
D. Friedreich's ataxia

Causes of small fiber neuropathy include Diabetes, Amyloidosis, Fabry's disease, Tangier's disease, Hereditary sensory and autonomic neuropathy, Sjogren's syndrome & Chronic idiopathic small fiber sensory neuropathy.

2676. Which of the following is not a large-fiber sensory neuropathy?

Ann Indian Acad Neurol. 2008;11(2):89–97

A. Sjögren's syndrome
B. Fabry's disease
C. Cisplatin neuropathy
D. Pyridoxine toxicity

Guillain-Barré Syndrome and Other Immune-Mediated Neuropathies

2677. Guillain-Barré syndrome was first described in which year?
N Engl J Med. 2012;366:2294-304

A. 1869
B. 1898
C. 1916
D. 1934

Guillain–Barré syndrome, characterized by acute areflexic paralysis with albuminocytologic dissociation (elevated protein in CSF and normal cell counts), was described in 1916.

2678. Miller Fisher syndrome was first reported in which year?
N Engl J Med. 2012;366:2294-304

A. 1923
B. 1943
C. 1956
D. 1966

Miller Fisher syndrome, characterized by ophthalmoplegia, ataxia & areflexia, was reported in 1956 as a likely variant of Guillain–Barré syndrome, because the CSF of affected patients showed albuminocytologic dissociation.

2679. Feature not typical of Guillain-Barre syndrome is?
Harrison's 20th Ed. Chapter 439, Page 3225

A. Acute onset
B. Males & females are at equal risk
C. Autoimmune
D. Polyradiculoneuropathy

Males are at 1.5-fold higher risk for GBS than females. Adults are more frequently affected than children.

2680. Facial diparesis is present in what proportion of GBS patients?
Harrison's 20th Ed. Chapter 439, Page 3225

A. 10%
B. 20%
C. 50%
D. 80%

Facial diparesis is present in 50% of GBS patients.

2681. Bilateral facial nerve palsy occurs in which of the following?
Harrison's 20th Ed. Chapter 439, Page 3214

A. Leprosy
B. Sarcoidosis
C. Sjogren's syndrome
D. All of the above

Facial palsy that is often bilateral occurs in sarcoidosis and in Guillain-Barre syndrome.

2682. GBS manifests as?
Harrison's 20th Ed. Chapter 439, Page 3225

A. Rapidly evolving areflexic ascending motor paralysis
B. With or without sensory disturbance
C. Autonomic involvement is common
D. All of the above

2683. Which of the following about GBS is false?
Lancet. 2016;388:717-27

A. Annual incidence rate of GBS increases with age
B. Estimated lifetime risk of developing GBS <1 in 1000
C. Post-infectious, rapidly progressive, monophasic disorder
D. None of the above

2684. Which of the following is not typical of Guillain-Barre syndrome?
Harrison's 20th Ed. Chapter 439, Page 3225

A. Fever & constitutional symptoms are absent at onset
B. Lower cranial nerves are frequently involved
C. DTRs disappear within first few days of onset
D. Bladder dysfunction is a prominent feature

Presence of fever & constitutional symptoms at onset cast doubt on the diagnosis of GBS. Transient bladder dysfunction may occur in severe GBS. If bladder dysfunction is a prominent & early in the course, GBS is unlikely.

2685. In GBS, clinical worsening reaches a plateau in how many weeks of onset?
Harrison's 20th Ed. Chapter 439, Page 3225

A. 1 week
B. 4 weeks
C. 8 weeks
D. 12 weeks

Clinical worsening stops and GBS patient reaches a plateau almost always within 4 weeks of onset.

2686. Limited or regional GBS syndromes include?
Harrison's 20th Ed. Chapter 439, Page 3225

A. Acute motor axonal neuropathy (AMAN)
B. Acute motor sensory axonal neuropathy (AMSAN)
C. Miller Fisher syndrome (MFS)
D. All of the above

Limited or regional GBS syndromes are Miller Fisher syndrome, pure sensory forms, ophthalmoplegia with anti-GQ1b antibodies (severe motor-sensory GBS), GBS with severe bulbar & facial paralysis associated with cytomegalovirus (CMV) infection & anti-GM2 antibodies & acute pandysautonomia.

2687. Which of the following is the most common form of GBS?
Harrison's 20th Ed. Chapter 439, Page 3225

A. Acute inflammatory demyelinating polyradiculoneuropathy
B. Acute axonal motor disorder
C. Acute sensory & motor axonal neuropathy
D. Miller Fisher syndrome (MFS)

In Europe & North America ~95% of GBS are acute inflammatory demyelinating polyradiculoneuropathy. ~5% are AMAN & AMSAN.

2688. Nationality of Charles Miller Fisher was?

A. Canadian
B. American
C. British
D. Brazilian

Charles Miller Fisher was a Canadian stroke specialist.

2689. Which of the following is a demyelinating disorder?
Harrison's 20th Ed. Chapter 439, Page 3226 Table 439-1

A. Acute motor axonal neuropathy (AMAN)
B. Acute motor sensory axonal neuropathy (AMSAN)
C. Miller Fisher syndrome (MFS)
D. All of the above

Acute motor axonal neuropathy (AMAN) and acute motor sensory axonal neuropathy (AMSAN) subtypes are axonal variants of Guillain-Barré syndrome (GBS).

2690. Which of the following is a regional variant of GBS?
Harrison's 20th Ed. Chapter 439, Page 3225

A. Pure sensory form
B. GBS with severe bulbar & facial paralysis
C. Acute pandysautonomia
D. All of the above

Regional variants of GBS include pure sensory forms, ophthalmoplegia with anti-GQ1b antibodies as part of severe motor-sensory GBS, GBS with severe bulbar & facial paralysis, sometimes associated with antecedent cytomegalovirus (CMV) infection and anti-GM2 antibodies and acute pandysautonomia.

2691. Organisms involved in antecedent infections in Guillain-Barre syndrome include?
Harrison's 20th Ed. Chapter 439, Page 3225, N Engl J Med. 2012;366:2294-304

A. Campylobacter jejuni
B. Human herpes virus
C. Cytomegalovirus
D. All of the above

~70% of GBS occur 1–3 weeks after an acute infectious process (respiratory or gastrointestinal). Antecedent infection or reinfection with Campylobacter jejuni, human herpes virus infection, CMV, Epstein-Barr virus, HIV, hepatitis E, Zika, chikungunya, Mycoplasma pneumoniae & swine influenza vaccine have been identified. Case clusters are rare. Presence of sialylated lipopolysaccharides on C. jejuni strains is a form of molecular mimicry that promotes autoimmune recognition of sialylated cell surface molecules on axons. Asymptomatic Campylobacter infection also may trigger Guillain-Barre syndrome.

2692. Which of the following is false if preceding infection in GBS case is C. jejuni?
Lancet. 2016;388:717–27

A. A pure motor axonal form of GBS occurs
B. Seropositivity against GM1 & GD1a gangliosides
C. Poorer outcome
D. None of the above

2693. Which of the following vaccinations could predispose to Guillain-Barre syndrome?
Harrison's 20th Ed. Chapter 439, Page 3225

A. Swine influenza vaccine
B. Influenza A vaccine
C. Older type rabies vaccine
D. All of the above

Immunizations with swine influenza vaccine, influenza A vaccines and older-type (Semple) rabies vaccine are implicated as a trigger of GBS. There is no increased risk of GBS with meningococcal vaccinations.

2694. Guillain-Barre syndrome occurs more frequently in patients with following diseases except?
Harrison's 20th Ed. Chapter 439, Page 3225

A. Hodgkin's disease
B. Chronic myeloid leukemia
C. HIV-seropositive individuals
D. Systemic lupus erythematosus

GBS also occurs more frequently in patients with lymphoma (Hodgkin's disease), HIV-seropositive individuals and in patients with SLE.

2695. Which of the following statements is false about GBS?
Harrison's 20th Ed. Chapter 439, Page 3226

A. Both cellular & humoral immune mechanisms involved
B. Analogous to experimental allergic neuritis (EAN)
C. Molecular mimicry mechanism
D. None of the above

2696. Which of the following is the critical event in the development of GBS?
N Engl J Med. 2012;366:2294-304

A. B cells recognize glycoconjugates on C. jejuni
B. Activation of B cells T cell
C. Escape of activated B cells from Peyer's patches into regional lymph nodes
D. All of the above

In the immunopathogenesis of GBS, a critical event in the development of GBS is the escape of activated B cells from Peyer's patches into regional lymph nodes.

2697. Which of the following is a functional region of myelinated axons?
Harrison's 20th Ed. Chapter 439, Page 3226 Figure 439-1

A. Internodes
B. Paranode
C. Juxtaparanodes
D. All of the above

Myelinated axons are divided into four functional regions. They are the nodes of Ranvier, paranodes, juxtaparanodes & internodes.

2698. Which of the following antiganglioside antibody is common in GBS?
Harrison's 20th Ed. Chapter 439, Page 3228 Table 439-2

A. Anti GM1
B. Anti GM2
C. Anti GM3
D. Anti GM4

Anti GM1, an antiganglioside antibody is common in GBS (20–50%), particularly in those preceded by C. jejuni infection.

2699. Which of the following is most relevant to Gangliosides?
N Engl J Med. 2012;366:2294-304

A. Lectin
B. Heparan
C. Ceramide
D. Mannose

Gangliosides are composed of a ceramide attached to one or more sugars (hexoses) and contain sialic acid (N-acetylneuraminic acid) linked to an oligosaccharide core. Gangliosides are important components of the peripheral nerves.

2700. Which of the following is a Ganglioside?
N Engl J Med. 2012;366:2294-304

A. GM1
B. GD1a
C. GT1a
D. All of the above

GM1, GD1a, GT1a, and GQ1b are gangliosides.

2701. Which of the following gangliosides is strongly expressed at the nodes of Ranvier?

Harrison's 20th Ed. Chapter 439, Page 3228 Table 439-2, N Engl J Med. 2012;366:2294-304

A. GM1
B. GT1a
C. GQ1b
D. All of the above

Gangliosides GM1 and GD1a are strongly expressed at the nodes of Ranvier, where voltage-gated sodium (Nav) channels are localized. Contactin associated protein (Caspr) & voltage-gated potassium (Kv) channels are present at paranodes and juxtaparanodes respectively. IgG anti-GM1 or anti-GD1a autoantibodies bind to the nodal axolemma, leading to membrane-attack complex (MAC) formation. This results in disappearance of Nav clusters and detachment of paranodal myelin, which can lead to nerve-conduction failure and muscle weakness.

2702. IgG autoantibodies to GQ1b cross-react with which of the following?

N Engl J Med. 2012;366:2294-304

A. GM1
B. GD1a
C. GT1a
D. All of the above

IgG autoantibodies to GQ1b, which cross-react with GT1a, are strongly associated with the Miller Fisher syndrome, its incomplete forms (acute ophthalmoparesis and acute ataxic neuropathy), and its CNS variant, Bickerstaff's brainstem encephalitis (acute ophthalmoplegia, ataxia, and impaired consciousness after an infectious episode).

2703. The anti-GQ1b antibody syndrome includes which of the following?

N Engl J Med. 2012;366:2294-304

A. Bickerstaff's brainstem encephalitis
B. Miller Fisher syndrome
C. Pharyngeal-cervical-brachial weakness
D. All of the above

The anti-GQ1b antibody syndrome includes the Miller Fisher syndrome, acute ophthalmoparesis, acute ataxic neuropathy, Bickerstaff's brainstem encephalitis, and pharyngeal–cervical–brachial weakness.

2704. GQ1b is strongly expressed in which of the following cranial nerves?

N Engl J Med. 2012;366:2294-304

A. Oculomotor nerve
B. Trochlear nerve
C. Abducens nerve
D. All of the above

GQ1b is strongly expressed in the oculomotor, trochlear, and abducens nerves, as well as muscle spindles in the limbs. Glossopharyngeal and vagus nerves strongly express GT1a and GQ1b, possibly accounting for dysphagia.

2705. Which of the following is false about Miller Fisher syndrome?

N Engl J Med. 2012;366:2294-304

A. Anti-GQ1b antibodies are found in > 90% patients
B. IgG titers are highest early in the course
C. Areflexia of limbs without weakness
D. None of the above

Anti-GQ1b IgG antibodies are found in >90% of patients with MFS, and titers of IgG are highest early in the course. Anti-GQ1b antibodies are not found in other forms of GBS unless there is extraocular motor nerve involvement.

2706. Which of the following is not found in Miller Fisher syndrome?

N Engl J Med. 2012;366:2294-304

A. Ataxia
B. Areflexia of limbs
C. Weakness of limbs
D. Ophthalmoplegia

Miller Fisher's syndrome is an ocular variant of Guillain-Barre syndrome. It produces ophthalmoplegia with areflexia and mild ataxia, reflexes are normal. Antiganglioside antibodies (GQlb) can be detected in about 50% of cases.

2707. Which of the following is false about Miller Fisher syndrome?

N Engl J Med. 2012;366:2294-304

A. Rapidly evolving ataxia
B. Areflexia of limbs without weakness
C. Ophthalmoplegia often with pupillary paralysis
D. None of the above

2708. MFS is strongly associated with which of the following antibodies?

N Engl J Med. 2012;366:2294-304

A. GQ1a
B. GQ1b
C. GQ1c
D. GQ1d

Miller Fisher syndrome (MFS) presents as rapidly evolving ataxia & areflexia of limbs without weakness, and ophthalmoplegia, often with pupillary paralysis. MFS is strongly associated with antibodies to ganglioside GQ1b.

2709. Which of the following is a central nervous system variant of Miller Fisher syndrome?

N Engl J Med. 2012;366:2294-304

A. Anti-Hu–associated paraneoplastic encephalitis (PEM)
B. Bickerstaff's brainstem encephalitis
C. Post–infectious brainstem encephalitis
D. All of the above

Antibodies against ganglioside GQ1b have also been detected in patients with Bickerstaff's brainstem encephalitis. Bickerstaff's encephalitis is characterized by ophthalmoplegia and ataxia but is also accompanied by pyramidal and sensory tract findings and cerebrospinal fluid pleocytosis.

2710. In demyelinating GBS, basis for flaccid paralysis & sensory disturbance is?

Harrison's 20th Ed. Chapter 439, Page 3227

A. Conduction block
B. Neurodegeneration
C. Apoptosis
D. All of the above

In demyelinating forms of GBS, basis for flaccid paralysis & sensory disturbance is conduction block. Secondary axonal degeneration usually occurs in severe cases.

2711. CSF findings in Guillain-Barre syndrome include all except?

Harrison's 20th Ed. Chapter 439, Page 3227

A. Elevated CSF proteins
B. CSF protein elevated by end of first week
C. No pleocytosis
D. CSF is normal when symptoms are present for < 6 hours

CSF is often normal when symptoms have been present for 48 hours. By the end of first week the level of protein is usually elevated without accompanying pleocytosis. Sustained CSF pleocytosis suggests an alternative diagnosis (viral myelitis, unrecognized HIV infection, leukemia or lymphoma with infiltration of nerves or neurosarcoidosis.

2712. Cytoalbuminologic dissociation best relates to?
Lancet. 2016;388:717–27

A. Normal CSF protein level & CSF TLC > 5 cells/μL
B. Raised CSF protein level & CSF TLC < 5 cells/μL
C. Normal CSF protein level & CSF TLC > 50 cells/μL
D. Raised CSF protein level & CSF TLC < 50 cells/μL

Cytoalbuminologic dissociation implies elevation of CSF protein level above laboratory normal value and CSF total white cell count <50 cells/μL).

2713. Electrodiagnostic feature of GBS is?
Harrison's 20th Ed. Chapter 439, Page 3227

A. Prolonged F-wave latencies
B. Prolonged distal latencies
C. Reduced amplitudes of compound muscle action potentials
D. All of the above

Edx features are mild or absent in the early stages of GBS and lag behind the clinical evolution. In AIDP, the earliest features are prolonged F-wave latencies, prolonged distal latencies and reduced amplitudes of compound muscle action potentials (CMAPs).

2714. Which of the following criteria is used for the diagnosis of Guillain-Barre syndrome?
Harrison's 20th Ed. Chapter 439, Page 3227

A. Amsel criteria
B. CASPAR criteria
C. Research Domain Criteria (RDoCs)
D. Brighton Criteria

Brighton criteria. Brain 137:33,2014.

2715. In CSF of GBS patient, increase in which of the following reflects axonal damage & predicts a residual deficit?
Harrison's 20th Ed. Chapter 439, Page 3227

A. Tau
B. Amyloid precursor protein (APP)
C. Chymotrypsin
D. Apolipoprotein E

Tau & 14-3-3 protein levels are elevated early in some cases of GBS. Tau increases in CSF may reflect axonal damage & predict a residual deficit.

2716. Which of the following can cause ptosis?
Harrison's 20th Ed. Chapter 28, Page 190

A. Guillain-Barre syndrome
B. Miller Fisher syndrome
C. Lambert-Eaton syndrome
D. All of the above

2717. Which of the following can cause ptosis without ophthalmoparesis?
Harrison's 20th Ed. Chapter 441, Page 3240 Table 441-1

A. Myotonic dystrophy
B. Congenital myopathies
C. Neuromuscular junction disorders
D. All of the above

2718. Differential diagnosis of Guillain-Barré syndrome includes?
Harrison's 20th Ed. Chapter 439, Page 3228

A. Hypokalemia
B. Polymyositis
C. Porphyria
D. All of the above

Differential diagnosis of Guillain-Barré syndrome include transverse myelitis & neuromyelitis optica, Lyme polyradiculitis, porphyria, vasculitic neuropathy, poliomyelitis, West Nile virus, CMV polyradiculitis, critical illness neuropathy or myopathy, myasthenia gravis, botulism, poisonings with organophosphates, thallium, or arsenic, paralytic shellfish poisoning, severe hypophosphatemia.

2719. Which of the following must be considered in the differential diagnosis of Guillain Barre syndrome?
Harrison's 20th Ed. Chapter 148, Page 1107

A. Adult botulism
B. Tick paralysis
C. Eaton Lambert syndrome
D. All of the above

Adult botulism, myasthenia gravis, stroke syndromes, Eaton Lambert syndrome and tick paralysis must be considered in the differential diagnosis of cases include Guillain Barre syndrome (GBS).

2720. Type of respiratory failure in GBS is?
Harrison's 20th Ed. Chapter 293, Page 2026

A. I
B. II
C. III
D. IV

Type II respiratory failure is a consequence of alveolar hypoventilation and results from the inability to eliminate carbon dioxide effectively due to impaired CNS drive to breathe, impaired strength with failure of neuromuscular function in the respiratory system and increased load(s) on the respiratory system. Reduced strength can be due to impaired neuromuscular transmission as in myasthenia gravis, Guillain-Barre syndrome, amyotrophic lateral sclerosis or respiratory muscle weakness (e.g. myopathy, electrolyte derangements, fatigue).

2721. What length of time after the first motor symptoms in GBS, immunotherapy is no longer effective?
Harrison's 20th Ed. Chapter 439, Page 3229

A. 3 days
B. 14 days
C. 30 days
D. 60 days

Each day counts in the treatment of GBS. ~2 weeks after first motor symptoms, immunotherapy is no longer effective.

2722. What percentage of patients with GBS require ventilatory assistance?
Harrison's 20th Ed. Chapter 439, Page 3229

A. ~ 10%
B. ~ 20%
C. ~ 30%
D. ~ 40%

~30% of patients with GBS require ventilatory assistance, sometimes for prolonged periods of time.

2723. Which of the following about treatment of GBS is false?
Harrison's 20th Ed. Chapter 439, Page 3229

A. High-dose IVIg & plasmapheresis are equally effective
B. Combination of IVIg & plasmapheresis offers no advantage
C. After successful treatment of GBS, relapse may occur in II or III week
D. None of the above

IVIg is administered as five daily infusions for a total dose of 2 g/kg body weight. A course of plasmapheresis usually consists of 40–50 mL/kg plasma exchange (PE) four to five times over a week. Glucocorticoids have not been found to be effective in GBS.

2724. Guillain-Barre syndrome best relates to which of the following?
Harrison's 20th Ed. Chapter 344, Page 2497

A. Autoimmune lymphoproliferative syndrome (ALPS)
B. Hemophagocytic lymphohistiocytosis (HLH)
C. Hyper-IgM (HIGM) Syndromes
D. Wiskott-Aldrich Syndrome

Autoimmune lymphoproliferative syndrome (ALPS) is characterized by nonmalignant T and B lymphoproliferation causing splenomegaly and enlarged lymph nodes. 70% of patients also display autoimmune manifestations like autoimmune cytopenias, Guillain-Barre syndrome, uveitis & hepatitis.

2725. Which of the following statements about Gullain-Barre syndrome (GBS) is false?
Harrison's 20th Ed. Chapter 439, Page 3229

A. Escape of activated B cells from Peyers patches into regional lymph nodes
B. Anti GQ1b IgG antibodies are found in >90% of patients with Miller Fisher subtype of GBS
C. Glucocorticoids are effective in GBS
D. Severe proximal motor & sensory axonal damage is a poor prognostic sign

Glucocorticoids have not been found to be effective in GBS. CIDP responds to glucocorticoids, whereas GBS does not.

2726. Factor that worsen the outlook for recovery in GBS is?
Harrison's 20th Ed. Chapter 439, Page 3230

A. Severe proximal motor & sensory axonal damage
B. Fulminant or severe attack
C. Delay in the onset of treatment
D. All of the above

2727. Patient characteristic consistently related to poor prognostic outcome in GBS is?
Harrison's 20th Ed. Chapter 439, Page 3230, Lancet. 2016;388:717–27

A. Age > 40 years
B. Preceding diarrhea (or C. jejuni infection in past 4 weeks)
C. High disability at nadir
D. All of the above

Factors that worsen the outlook for recovery in AIDP are patients with severe proximal motor and sensory axonal damage, advanced age, a fulminant or severe attack and a delay in the onset of treatment.

2728. What percentage of patients with GBS achieve a full functional recovery?
Harrison's 20th Ed. Chapter 439, Page 3230

A. ~ 65%
B. ~ 75%
C. ~ 85%
D. ~ 95%

~85% of patients with GBS achieve a full functional recovery within several months to a year.

2729. In optimal settings, mortality rate in patients with GBS is?
Harrison's 20th Ed. Chapter 439, Page 3230

A. <1%
B. <3%
C. <5%
D. <7%

In optimal settings, mortality rate in patients with GBS is <5%. Death usually results from secondary pulmonary complications.

Chronic Inflammatory Demyelinating Polyneuropathy

2730. Which of the following is false about chronic inflammatory demyelinating polyneuropathy (CIDP)?

Harrison's 20th Ed. Chapter 439, Page 3230

A. Initial attack is indistinguishable from that of GBS
B. Acute-onset form of CIDP may mimic GBS
C. CIDP should be considered if it deteriorates >9 weeks after onset or relapses at least three times
D. None of the above

2731. Which of the following is false about chronic inflammatory demyelinating polyneuropathy (CIDP)?

Harrison's 20th Ed. Chapter 439, Page 3230

A. Onset is usually gradual over a few months
B. Motor & sensory symptoms present
C. Death from CIDP is uncommon
D. None of the above

2732. Lewis-Sumner Syndrome is?

Harrison's 20th Ed. Chapter 439, Page 3230, N Engl J Med. 2005;352:1343-56

A. Multifocal acquired demyelinating sensory & motor neuropathy
B. Multifocal motor neuropathy
C. Distal acquired demyelinating symmetric neuropathy
D. Motor neuron disease

Lewis-Sumner syndrome is also called multifocal acquired demyelinating sensory and motor (MADSAM) neuropathy. It is a variant of CIDP in which discrete peripheral nerves are involved.

2733. Lewis-Sumner Syndrome is characterized by all except?

Harrison's 20th Ed. Chapter 439, Page 3230, N Engl J Med. 2005;352:1343-56

A. Motor and sensory deficits
B. Discrete peripheral nerves are involved
C. Asymmetrical presentation of symptoms
D. Poor response to intravenous immune globulin in presence of antibodies to gangliosides

Weakness of the limbs is usually symmetric in CIDP, but can be strikingly asymmetric in Lewis-Sumner syndrome.

2734. Classic chronic inflammatory demyelinating polyneuropathy is characterized by all except?

N Engl J Med. 2005;352:1343-56

A. Symmetrical weakness in proximal muscles
B. Symmetrical weakness in distal muscles
C. Weakness progressively increases for > 2 months
D. Not associated with impaired sensation

2735. Which of the following electrodiagnostic findings is not a feature of classic chronic inflammatory demyelinating polyneuropathy?

N Engl J Med. 2005;352:1343-56

A. Partial motor-nerve conduction block
B. Reduced motor-nerve conduction velocity
C. Prolonged distal motor latencies
D. Absent F-wave latencies

Edx findings in CIDP reveal variable degrees of conduction slowing, prolonged distal latencies, distal and temporal dispersion of CMAPs, and conduction block as the principal features. Presence of conduction block is a certain sign of an acquired demyelinating process. Evidence of axonal loss, presumably secondary to demyelination, is present in >50% of patients.

2736. Chronic inflammatory demyelinating polyneuropathy may be associated with all of the following except?

Harrison's 20th Ed. Chapter 439, Page 3230

A. HIV
B. SLE
C. Diabetes mellitus
D. Hypothyroidism

In all patients with presumptive CIDP, it is also reasonable to exclude vasculitis, collagen vascular disease (SLE), chronic hepatitis, HIV infection, amyloidosis, diabetes mellitus, inflammatory bowel disease and lymphoma.

2737. Which of the following is related to CIDP?

Harrison's 20th Ed. Chapter 439, Page 3230

A. Contactin-1 (CNTN1)
B. Contactin-associated protein-1 (CASPR1)
C. Neurofascin-155 (NF155)
D. All of the above

2738. Presence of IgG4 CNTN1 antibodies in CIDP patients leads to?

Harrison's 20th Ed. Chapter 439, Page 3230

A. Early axonal damage & severe distal motor involvement
B. Sensory ataxia with tremor
C. Poor response to IVIg
D. All of the above

Antibodies of IgG4 isotype directed against contactin-1 (CNTN1) or neurofascin-155 (NF155) are associated with early axonal damage, severe distal motor involvement or sensory ataxia with tremor, and a poor response to IVIg. CNTN1 and its partner contactin-associated protein-1 (CASPR1) interact with NF155 at paranodal axoglial junctions.

2739. Patients with clinical features of CIDP may also have?

Harrison's 20th Ed. Chapter 439, Page 3230

A. Monoclonal gammopathy of undetermined significance
B. POEMS syndrome
C. Churg-Strauss syndrome
D. Sjögren's syndrome

As many as 25% of patients with clinical features of CIDP also have a monoclonal gammopathy of undetermined significance (MGUS).

2740. Which of the following treatments is effective in CIDP?

Harrison's 20th Ed. Chapter 439, Page 3230

A. High-dose IVIg
B. Plasma exchange (PE)
C. Glucocorticoids
D. All of the above

High-dose IVIg, PE & glucocorticoids are all more effective than placebo in CIDP. Patients who fail therapy with IVIg, PE & glucocorticoids may benefit from treatment with azathioprine, methotrexate, cyclosporine, cyclophosphamide, and anti-CD20 (rituximab).

2741. Intravenous immune globulin has been established to be efficacious in?

N Engl J Med. 2001;345:747

A. Guillain-Barré syndrome
B. Chronic inflammatory demyelinating polyneuropathy
C. Myasthenia gravis
D. All of the above

2742. Intravenous Immunoglobulin (IVIg) has been used successfully in which of the following diseases?

N Engl J Med. 2001;345:747

A. Kawasaki disease
B. Graft-versus-host disease
C. Multiple sclerosis
D. All of the above

Intravenous Immunoglobulin (IVIg) has been used successfully to block reticuloendothelial cell function and immune complex clearance in various immune cytopenias such as immune thrombocytopenia. In addition, IVIg is useful for prevention of tissue damage in certain inflammatory syndromes such as Kawasaki disease and as Ig replacement therapy for certain types of immunoglobulin deficiencies. Use of IVIg in selected patients with graft-versus-host disease, multiple sclerosis, myasthenia gravis, Guillain-Barre syndrome and chronic demyelinating polyneuropathy is established.

2743. Intravenous immune globulin has been established to be efficacious in?

N Engl J Med. 2001;345:747

A. Corticosteroid-resistant dermatomyositis
B. Kawasaki's syndrome
C. GVHD prevention in allogeneic BM transplants
D. All of the above

IVIg blocks reticuloendothelial cell function and immune complex clearance in immune thrombocytopenia. In addition, IVIg is useful for prevention of tissue damage in certain inflammatory syndromes such as Kawasaki disease and as Ig replacement therapy for certain types of immunoglobulin deficiencies. IVIg is also useful in selected patients with graft-versus-host disease, multiple sclerosis, myasthenia gravis, Guillain-Barré syndrome, and chronic demyelinating polyneuropathy.

2744. The mode of action of immune globulin involves?

N Engl J Med. 2001;345:747

A. Modulation of expression & function of Fc receptors
B. Interference with activation of complement & cytokines
C. Provision of antiidiotypic antibodies
D. All of the above

2745. The half-life of infused immune globulin in immunocompetent persons is?

N Engl J Med. 2001;345:747

A. Two weeks
B. Three weeks
C. Four weeks
D. Five weeks

2746. Most natural autoantibodies in adult serum are of?

N Engl J Med. 2001;345:747

A. IgG class
B. IgM class
C. IgA class
D. All of the above

2747. Which of the following about total dose of Intravenous immune globulin is true?

N Engl J Med. 2012;366:2294-304

A. 1 grams per kilogram over 3 days
B. 1 grams per kilogram over 5 days
C. 2 grams per kilogram over 3 days
D. 2 grams per kilogram over 5 days

Intravenous immune globulin has replaced plasma exchange as the treatment of choice in GBS patients who are not able to walk unaided. Immune globulin is given at a total dose of 2 grams per kilogram of body weight over a period of 5 days.

2748. Which of the following is true regarding definition of partial nerve conduction block?

N Engl J Med. 2005;352:1343-56

A. Drop of 20% or more in negative peak area
B. Drop of 20% or more in peak-to-peak amplitude
C. Change of <15% in duration between proximal & distal site stimulation
D. All of the above

2749. Which of the following is false about Multifocal Motor Neuropathy?

N Engl J Med. 2005;352:1343-56

A. Symmetric weakness
B. Relative sparing of sensory fibres
C. Starts in distal arm muscles
D. A partial motor-conduction block at multiple sites

Multifocal motor neuropathy (MMN) presents as slowly progressive motor weakness & atrophy evolving over years in the distribution of selected nerve trunks, associated with sites of persistent focal motor conduction block in the same nerve trunks. Sensory fibers are relatively spared. The arms are affected more frequently than the legs, and >75% of all patients are male.

2750. Which of the following is effective in the treatment of Multifocal Motor Neuropathy?

N Engl J Med. 2005;352:1343-56

A. Corticosteroids
B. Plasma exchange (PE)
C. Immune globulin therapy
D. Methotrexate

2751. Which of the following is effective in the treatment of Multifocal Motor Neuropathy?

N Engl J Med. 2005;352:1343-56

A. Corticosteroids
B. Plasma exchange (PE)
C. Cyclophosphamide
D. Methotrexate

Most patients with Multifocal motor neuropathy (MMN) respond to high-dose IVIg. Refractory patients may respond to rituximab or cyclophosphamide. Glucocorticoids and PE are not effective.

Myasthenia Gravis and Other Diseases of the Neuromuscular Junction

2752. Who was the first person to describe clinical features of MG?

A. Howard Wolfe
B. Amato Beeson
C. Nicolle Gilhus
D. Thomas Willis

A physiologist by the name of Thomas Willis was the first to describe the clinical features of MG in 1672. He wrote of a woman who, when she tried to talk for a prolonged period, "temporarily lost her power of speech and became mute as a fish."

2753. Myasthenia gravis (MG) is a neuromuscular disorder involving?

Harrison's 20th Ed. Chapter 440, Page 3232

A. Skeletal muscle
B. Smooth muscle
C. Cardiac muscle
D. All of the above

MG is a neuromuscular disorder characterized by weakness & fatigability of skeletal muscles.

2754. At neuromuscular junctions in myasthenia gravis, the defect in acetylcholine receptors (AChRs) is?

Harrison's 20th Ed. Chapter 440, Page 3232

A. Decrease in their number
B. Decrease in their size
C. Alteration in their shape
D. All of the above

In MG, underlying pathogenetic defect is decrease in number of available AChRs at neuromuscular junctions due to antibody-mediated autoimmune attack. This was first demonstrated by the use of a radioactively labeled snake toxin, α-bungarotoxin, which binds specifically, quantitatively, and irreversibly to acetylcholine receptors of skeletal muscles.

2755. Which of the following is false about neuromuscular junction in MG?

Harrison's 20th Ed. Chapter 440, Page 3233 Figure 440-1

A. Normal nerve terminal
B. Flattened, simplified postsynaptic folds
C. Widened synaptic space
D. None of the above

In MG, NM junction has a normal nerve terminal, reduced number of AChRs (stippling), flattened, simplified postsynaptic folds, & widened synaptic space.

2756. ACh from how many vesicles is released when action potential reaches nerve terminal?

Harrison's 20th Ed. Chapter 440, Page 3232

A. 5 to 20
B. 50 to 100
C. 150 to 200
D. 500 to 800

When an action potential travels down a motor nerve & reaches nerve terminal, acetylcholine (Ach) from 150 to 200 vesicles is released and combines with AChRs that are densely packed at peaks of postsynaptic folds.

2757. Structure of AChR consists of?

Harrison's 20th Ed. Chapter 440, Page 3232

A. 1-alpha, 2-beta, 1-delta, and 1-gamma or epsilon
B. 1-alpha, 1-beta, 2-delta, and 1-gamma or epsilon
C. 1-alpha, 1-beta, 1-delta, and 2-gamma or epsilon
D. 2-alpha, 1-beta, 1-delta, and 1-gamma or epsilon

Structure of nicotinic AChR consists of five subunits - 2-alpha, 1-beta, 1-delta, and 1-gamma or epsilon arranged around a central pore. Each of the two α subunits has an acetylcholine-binding site that is located extracellularly & centered around amino acids 192 and 193.

2758. Which of the following about Myasthenia gravis is false?

Harrison's 20th Ed. Chapter 440, Page 3232

A. Acetylcholine receptor consists of five subunits - 1-alpha, 2-beta, 1-gamma, 1-delta or 1-epsilon
B. Pathologic antibodies are IgG & are T cell dependent
C. Absence of anti AChR antibodies does not exclude diagnosis
D. Mycophenolate mofetil is useful

2759. SNARE stands for?

Mol Cell Neurosci. 2012 ;50(1):58–69

A. Soluble N-ethylmaleimide-sensitive fusion protein attachment protein receptors
B. Soluble N-ethylmaleimide-sensitive fusion protein adherent protein receptors
C. Soluble N-ethylmaleimide-sensitive fusion protein assembly protein receptors
D. Soluble N-ethylmaleimide-sensitive fusion protein absorbing protein receptors

In exocytosis/neurosecretion, SNAREs (soluble N-ethylmaleimide-sensitive fusion protein attachment protein receptors) play a role in vesicle docking, priming, fusion & synchronization of neurotransmitter release. Neurotransmitter release at neuronal synapses is directed by action potentials, whereas in sensory synapses, release is driven by receptor potentials that direct graded exocytosis. SNARE proteins associated with the vesicles are termed vesicle-SNAREs (v-SNAREs) and those on the presynaptic plasma membrane are called target-SNAREs (t-SNAREs).

2760. Which of the following is the most abundant protein of neuronal synaptic vesicles?

Mol Cell Neurosci. 2012 ;50(1):58–69

A. Synapsin
B. Actin
C. Synaptotagmin 4
D. Synaptobrevin

Synaptobrevin is the most abundant protein of neuronal synaptic vesicles. Others include synapsin, actin, and synaptotagmin 4. Synaptotagmins are the vesicle-bound calcium sensors. Complexins act as calcium-dependent switches.

2761. Which of the following is a criteria that provides supporting evidence for an antibody-mediated process?

N Engl J Med. 1994; 330:1797-1810

A. Presence of antibody
B. Antibody interacts with target antigen

C. Passive transfer reproduces disease features

D. All of the above

Myasthenia gravis is a disease due to an antibody-mediated autoimmune attack directed against acetylcholine receptors at neuromuscular junctions. The supporting evidence satisfies a set of five criteria that define the pathogenesis of autoantibody-mediated disorders. First, antibody is present. Second, antibody interacts with target antigen, acetylcholine receptor. Third, passive transfer reproduces disease features. Fourth, immunization with antigen produces a model disease. Fifth, a reduction of antibody levels ameliorates disease.

2762. Number of available acetylcholine receptors in NMJ is reduced by antibodies through?

N Engl J Med. 1994; 330:1797-1810

A. Accelerated endocytosis & degradation of receptors

B. Functional blockade of acetylcholine-binding sites

C. Complement-mediated damage to acetylcholine receptors

D. All of the above

2763. The first step in vesicle fusion at NMJ is?

Mol Cell Neurosci. 2012 ;50(1):58–69

A. Docking

B. Tethering

C. Priming

D. Fusion

The first step in vesicle fusion is tethering followed by docking, priming and fusion.

2764. Which of the following is a protein in SNARE complex?

Mol Cell Neurosci. 2012 ;50(1):58–69

A. Synaptobrevin

B. Syntaxin

C. SNAP-25/23 (synaptosomal-associated proteins)

D. All of the above

2765. With the opening of the channel in AChR, which of the following cation gains rapid entry?

Harrison's 20th Ed. Chapter 440, Page 3232

A. Sodium

B. Potassium

C. Calcium

D. Magnesium

ACh combines with binding sites on alpha subunits of AChR to open the channel permitting rapid entry of cations, chiefly sodium.

2766. Acetylcholinesterase (AChE) rapidly terminates the action of ACh by?

Harrison's 20th Ed. Chapter 440, Page 3232

A. Oxidation

B. Reduction

C. Hydrolysis

D. Phosphorylation

Acetylcholinesterase (AChE) rapidly terminates the action of acetylcholine (ACh) by hydrolysis.

2767. Which of the following about myasthenia gravis is false?

Harrison's 20th Ed. Chapter 440, Page 3232

A. ACh is released normally

B. Decrease in number of available ACh receptors

C. Increased presynaptic rundown

D. Thymus abnormal in ~ 75% of patients

Amount of ACh released per impulse normally declines on repeated activity (presynaptic rundown). In MG, this "normal" rundown along with decreased efficiency of NM transmission results in weakness or myasthenic fatigue. Thymus is abnormal in ~75% of patients with MG.

2768. In MG, the autoimmune antibody is targeted against?

Harrison's 20th Ed. Chapter 440, Page 3232

A. Acetylcholine

B. Acetylcholine receptor (AChR)

C. Acetylcholinesterase (AChE)

D. All of the above

In MG, specific anti-AChR autoimmune antibody is targeted against Acetylcholine receptor (AChR).

2769. In MG, anti-AChR antibodies reduce the number of available AChRs at NM junctions by which mechanism?

Harrison's 20th Ed. Chapter 440, Page 3232

A. Cross-linking & rapid endocytosis of AChR receptors

B. Blockade of the active site of AChR

C. Damage to postsynaptic muscle membrane

D. All of the above

Anti-AChR antibodies reduce the number of available AChRs at NM junctions by accelerated turnover of AChRs by its rapid endocytosis, blockade of the active binding site of AChR, and damage to postsynaptic muscle membrane by the antibody + complement.

2770. What is the role of protein muscle-specific kinase (MuSK)?

Harrison's 20th Ed. Chapter 440, Page 3232

A. AChR activation at NMJ

B. AChR blocking at NMJ

C. AChR clustering at NMJ

D. All of the above

An immune response to muscle-specific kinase (MuSK), a protein involved in AChR clustering at neuromuscular junctions, can also result in MG, with reduction of AChRs.

2771. Which of the following is involved in the pathogenesis of MG?

Harrison's 20th Ed. Chapter 440, Page 3232, 3233

A. Antibodies against agrin

B. Muscle-specific kinase (MuSK)

C. Antibodies against low-density lipoprotein receptor related protein 4 (LRP4)

D. All of the above

2772. Pathogenic anti-AChR antibody in myasthenia gravis is which immunoglobulin type?

Harrison's 20th Ed. Chapter 440, Page 3232

A. IgA

B. IgG

C. IgM

D. IgE

Anti-MuSK antibody occurs in about 40% of patients without AChR antibody. A small proportion of patients whose sera are negative for both AChR and MuSK antibodies have antibodies to another protein at the neuromuscular junction-low-density lipoprotein receptor related protein 4 (LRP4) - that is important for clustering of AChRs. The pathogenic antibodies are IgG and are T cell dependent. Antibodies against agrin have recently been found in some patients with MG. Agrin is a protein derived from motor nerves that normally binds to LRP4 and thus may also interfere with clustering of AChRs at neuromuscular junctions.

2773. Thymus is abnormal in what proportion of patients with MG?

Harrison's 20th Ed. Chapter 440, Page 3232

A. 25%

B. 50%

C. 75%

D. 100%

Thymus is abnormal in 75% of patients with MG. In 65%, thymus is "hyperplastic" though not necessarily enlarged. 10% of patients have thymic tumors (thymomas). Muscle-like cells within the thymus (myoid cells), which bear AChRs on their surface, may serve as a source of autoantigen and trigger the autoimmune reaction within thymus gland.

2774. Thymoma along with which of the following is called Good's syndrome?

Arch Intern Med. 1985;145:1704–7

A. Pure red cell aplasia

B. Hypogammaglobulinemia

C. Systemic lupus erythematosus

D. Ulcerative colitis

Thymoma with hypogammaglobulinemia also is called Good's syndrome.

2775. Hypogammaglobulinemia is observed in association with?

Harrison's 20th Ed. Chapter 344, Page 2496, 502

A. Thymoma

B. Chronic lymphocytic leukemia (CLL)

C. Myeloma

D. All of the above

2776. Individuals with hypogammaglobulinemia are at particular risk of?

Harrison's 20th Ed. Chapter 117, Page 881

A. C. difficile colitis

B. Giardiasis

C. Septic shock caused by P. aeruginosa

D. All of the above

Individuals with hypogammaglobulinemia are at particular risk of C. difficile colitis and giardiasis.

2777. WHIM syndrome consists of all except?

Harrison's 20th Ed. Chapter 60, Page 398

A. Warts

B. Hypogammaglobulinemia

C. Infections

D. Myelofibrosis

WHIM syndrome consists of warts, hypogammaglobulinemia, infections & myelokathexis (retention of WBCs in marrow). WHIM syndrome is caused by dominant gain-of-function mutation of CXCR4, resulting in cell retention in bone marrow.

2778. Paraneoplastic syndrome associated with thymic tumors presents as?

Harrison's 20th Ed. Chapter 74, Page 553

A. Myasthenia gravis

B. Pure red cell aplasia

C. Hypogammaglobulinemia

D. Any of the above

2779. Staging system for thymomas is named after?

Harrison's 20th Ed. Chapter 74, Page 554 Table 74-14

A. Atkin

B. Falkson

C. Masaoka

D. Tomaszek

The staging system for thymoma was developed by Masaoka and colleagues.

2780. Thymoma and / or myasthenia gravis is associated with which of the following?

Harrison's 20th Ed. Chapter 55, Page 357

A. Pemphigus vulgaris

B. Pemphigus foliaceus

C. Paraneoplastic pemphigus

D. Bullous pemphigoid

2781. Which of the following muscles are typically involved early in the course of MG?

Harrison's 20th Ed. Chapter 440, Page 3233

A. Chewing muscles

B. Facial muscles

C. Lids & extraocular muscles

D. Palate, tongue & pharyngeal muscles

In MG, due to early involvement of lids & extraocular muscles (EOMs), diplopia & fluctuating fatigable ptosis are common initial complaints.

2782. Involvement of extraocular muscles leads to all except?

Harrison's 20th Ed. Chapter 440, Page 3233

A. Diplopia

B. Ophthalmoplegia

C. Ptosis

D. Nystagmus

Most frequently affected muscle in MG is levator palpebrae superioris. Its weakness leads to ptosis, with or without Cogan's lid twitch. Ptosis may first ocur one eye, it almost always becomes bilateral with time.

2783. Which of the following is best related to ptosis?

A. Inverse-care law

B. Hering's law of equal innervation

C. Sutton's law

D. Hy's law

Heing's law, or the law of equal innervation, states that the same amount of innervation goes to an extraocular muscle and to its yoked fellow. The amount of innervation to the yoked pair is always determined by the fixating eye. Hering's law is important in understanding the topic of primary and secondary deviations.

2784. Which of the following about myasthenia gravis is false?

Harrison's 20th Ed. Chapter 440, Page 3233

A. Women more affected than men

B. Lids & extraocular muscles involved early

C. Limb weakness is proximal and asymmetric

D. Deep tendon reflexes diminished

Women are affected more frequently than men, in a ratio of ~3:2. Cranial muscles, particularly lids & extraocular muscles are involved early in MG. Diplopia & ptosis are common initial complaints. Limb weakness is proximal & asymmetric. Deep tendon reflexes are preserved.

2785. Dysarthric "mushy" quality speech in MG is due to?

Harrison's 20th Ed. Chapter 440, Page 3233

A. Weakness of the palate
B. Weakness of the tongue
C. Weakness of the pharynx
D. All of the above

In MG, speech has a nasal timbre caused by weakness of the palate or dysarthric "mushy" quality due to tongue weakness.

2786. In MG, when patient attempts to smile, facial weakness manifests as?

Harrison's 20th Ed. Chapter 440, Page 3233

A. "Elfin" facies
B. "Snarling" expression
C. "Chipmunk" facies
D. Leonine facies

Facial weakness produces a vertical myasthenic "snarling" expression when patient attempts to smile.

2787. Which of the following is related to myasthenia gravis?

DeJong's The Neurologic Examination, 7th Ed. Page 323

A. Dropped Head Syndrome
B. Ectropion
C. Trident tongue
D. All of the above

Causes of dropped head syndrome (head ptosis, floppy head, camptocormia) are inflammatory myopathy, ALS, and myasthenia gravis.

2788. Weakness out of proportion to wasting occurs in?

DeJong's The Neurologic Examination, 7th Ed. Page 479

A. Inflammatory myopathy
B. Myasthenia gravis
C. Periodic paralysis
D. All of the above

Weakness out of proportion to wasting occurs in inflammatory myopathy, myasthenia gravis, and periodic paralysis.

2789. Oculomasticatory myorhythmia is characteristic of which of the following?

Harrison's 20th Ed. Chapter 171, Page 1225

A. Leigh's disease
B. Lambert-Eaton syndrome
C. CNS Whipple's disease
D. Guillain-Barré syndrome

Oculomasticatory myorhythmia refers to pendular vergence movements of eyes synchronous with contractions of masticatory muscles. It is characteristic for CNS Whipple's disease.

2790. Which of the following is not a feature of Rowland Payne syndrome?

DeJong's The Neurologic Examination, 7th Ed. Page 315

A. Unilateral Horner syndrome
B. Ipsilateral vocal cord paralysis
C. Ipsilateral paralysis of hemidiaphragm
D. Ipsilateral deviation of tongue

Rowland Payne syndrome is a triad of unilateral Horner syndrome, ipsilateral vocal cord paralysis, and ipsilateral paralysis of hemidiaphragm. It is due to disruption of the oculosympathetic nerve, vagus nerve, and phrenic nerve in anterior neck (tumour, trauma).

2791. To grade clinical severity of myasthenia gravis, which of the following scale is used?

N Engl J Med. 1994; 330:1797-1810

A. Nicole scale
B. Wolfe scale
C. Gilhus scale
D. Osserman scale

Osserman scale: grade I involves focal disease (restricted to ocular muscles); grade II, generalized disease that is either mild (IIa) or moderate (IIb); grade III, severe generalized disease; and grade IV, a crisis, with life-threatening impairment of respiration. MGFA (Myasthenia Gravis Foundation of America) is also used to classify MG.

2792. Which of the following weakness is prominent in MuSK antibody positive MG?

Harrison's 20th Ed. Chapter 440, Page 3233

A. Facial weakness
B. Bulbar weakness
C. Lids & extraocular muscle weakness
D. Tongue weakness

Bulbar weakness is prominent in MuSK antibody positive MG.

2793. In MG, weakness becomes generalized, affecting limb muscles in what proportion of cases?

Harrison's 20th Ed. Chapter 440, Page 3233

A. ~ 55%
B. ~ 65%
C. ~ 75%
D. ~ 85%

In ~85% of patients, the weakness becomes generalized, affecting the limb muscles as well.

2794. MG muscle weakness will not become generalized if it remains restricted to extraocular muscles for?

Harrison's 20th Ed. Chapter 440, Page 3233

A. 6 months
B. 1 year
C. 2 years
D. 3 years

In MG, if muscle weakness remains restricted to extraocular muscles for 3 years (ocular MG), it is unlikely to become generalized.

2795. Which of the following is false about MG?

Harrison's 20th Ed. Chapter 440, Page 3233

A. No loss of reflexes
B. No impairment of sensation
C. No HMF neurologic defect
D. None of the above

MG is characterized by typical distribution of skeletal muscle weakness & fatigability, without loss of reflexes or impairment of sensation or other neurologic function.

2796. At which place is an ice-pack applied in ice-pack test (IPT) for NMJ defect?

Harrison's 20th Ed. Chapter 440, Page 3233, N Engl J Med. 2016;375:e39

A. Ear
B. Tongue
C. Eye
D. Any of the above

If ptosis is due to an NMJ defect, application of a pack of ice over the ptotic eye often results in improvement due to less depletion of quanta of AChR in cold & reduced activity of AChE at NMJ. However, IPT is limited by the need for ptosis and is therefore not suitable for all cases of MG. It is useful in cardiac patients and the elderly, where use of anticholinestrase agents is contraindicated.

2797. Ice is applied over the eye for how many minutes in ice pack test?

Neurol India 2016;64:1173-4

A. 1 minute
B. 2 minutes
C. 3 minutes
D. 4 minutes

Ice pack test consists of application of ice to eyes for 2 minutes, ensuring that eyes are covered to prevent burns. Reduction in muscle fiber temperature <22°C reduces the contractile force of muscle leading to a false negative result.

2798. Ice pack test is considered positive when there is an increase in palpebral fissure of?

Neurol India 2016;64:1173-4

A. 1 mm
B. 2 mm
C. 3 mm
D. 4 mm

Ice pack test is considered positive when there is an increase in palpebral fissure of 2 mm or more of the palpebral fissure on removal of the ice pack.

2799. Which of the following is a nonpharmacological test for evaluation of MG?

Neurol India 2016;64:1173-4

A. Ice pack test
B. Rest test
C. Sleep test
D. All of the above

For the rest test, patient is asked to close eyes for 5 minutes, and then improvement in ptosis is measured. For sleep test, patient is asked to lie down with eyes closed for 30 minutes in a quiet, dark room. Improvement in ptosis & ophthalmoparesis is then assessed.

2800. Pain in the head or eye in association with diplopia occurs in?

DeJong's The Neurologic Examination, 7th Ed. Page 204

A. Posterior communicating aneurysm
B. Ophthalmoplegic migraine
C. Tolosa-Hunt syndrome
D. All of the above

Pain in head or eye in association with diplopia occurs in diabetic third nerve palsy, posterior communicating aneurysm, ophthalmoplegic migraine, Tolosa-Hunt syndrome (painful ophthalmoplegia) & giant cell arteritis.

2801. Simpson´s test refers to?

Neurol India 2016;64:1173-4

A. Increased ptosis on sustained down gaze
B. Increased ptosis on sustained up gaze
C. Increased ptosis on sustained lateral gaze
D. Any of the above

In Simpson test, the patient is asked to maintain upgaze for 2–3 minutes testing for fatigue induced ptosis.

2802. Which of the following test is used to diagnose MG?

Arch. Ophthalmol. 1979;97:678, Arch. Neurol. 1981;31:531

A. 'Peek' sign
B. Gorelick´s test
C. Cogan's lid twitch sign
D. All of the above

The earliest manifestation of ocular MG is slowing of saccadic movement on rapid refixation. The 'peek' sign occurs when palpebral fissure widens after a period of voluntary eyelid closure. Gorelick´s test is for bilateral asymmetrical ptosis. Finger elevation of opposite side eyelid while patient looks up, causes decreased ptosis on contralateral side. Cogan's lid twitch sign is characteristic of MG. It consists of a brief overshoot twitch of lid retraction following sudden return of eyes to primary position after a period of downgaze. Curtain sign or seesaw ptosis is elicited by manually raising the more ptotic lid. It causes the eye with less or no ptosis to suddenly crash.

2803. In myasthenia gravis (MG), which of the following about "trident tongue" is false?

DeJong's The Neurologic Examination, 7th Ed. Page 331

A. Occurs in long-standing disease
B. Tongue atrophy
C. Triple furrowed, grooves along median sulcus on each side
D. None of the above

Except for MG, neuromuscular junction disorders & myopathies rarely involve tongue to clinically significant degree. Tongue weakness & fatigability occurs in MG but generally only with severe involvement.

2804. Lingua plicata is characteristic of?

DeJong's The Neurologic Examination, 7th Ed. Page 38

A. Myasthenia gravis
B. Melkersson-Rosenthal syndrome
C. Myxedema
D. Down's syndrome

A triple furrowed tongue is seen in myasthenia gravis. Lingua plicata is seen in Melkersson-Rosenthal syndrome while macroglossia is typical of amyloid, myxedema & Down's syndrome.

2805. Which of the following is a cause of jaw drop?

DeJong's The Neurologic Examination, 7th Ed. Page 238

A. Myasthenia gravis (MG)
B. ALS
C. Kennedy's disease
D. All of the above

2806. Acquired autoimmune channelopathies include?

DeJong's The Neurologic Examination, 7th Ed. Page 791

A. Myasthenia gravis (MG)
B. Lambert-Eaton syndrome
C. Neuromyotonia & paraneoplastic cerebellar degeneration
D. All of the above

2807. Genetic channelopathies include?

DeJong's The Neurologic Examination, 7th Ed. Page 791

A. Periodic paralysis
B. Myotonia congenita, paramyotonia
C. Congenital myasthenia syndromes
D. All of the above

Genetic channelopathies include periodic paralysis, myotonia congenita, paramyotonia, the congenital myasthenia syndromes, malignant hyperthermia (MH), familial hemiplegic migraine, familial episodic ataxia, and the idiopathic generalized epilepsies.

2808. "Look of perpetual surprise" is a characteristic facial expression in?

DeJong's The Neurologic Examination, 7th Ed. Page 37

A. Progressive supranuclear palsy
B. Pseudobulbar palsy
C. Myasthenia gravis
D. Athetosis and dystonia

2809. "Immobile face with precipitate laughter & crying" is a characteristic facial expression in?

DeJong's The Neurologic Examination, 7th Ed. Page 37

A. Progressive supranuclear palsy
B. Pseudobulbar palsy
C. Myasthenia gravis
D. Athetosis and dystonia

Fixed ("masked") face is typical of parkinsonism. Look of perpetual surprise is seen in progressive supranuclear palsy, immobile face with precipitate laughter & crying is seen in pseudobulbar palsy, grimacing is typical of athetosis & dystonia. Ptosis & weakness of facial muscles is seen in some myopathies & myasthenia gravis.

2810. In seronegative MG, antibodies can be found against?

Harrison's 20th Ed. Chapter 440, Page 3233

A. Muscle-specific tyrosine kinase
B. Myasthenia-specific tyrosine kinase
C. Membrane-specific tyrosine kinase
D. None of the above

Presence of anti-AChR antibodies is diagnostic of MG, but a negative test does not exclude MG. Antibodies to muscle-specific tyrosine kinase (MuSK) are present in ~40% of AChR antibody-negative patients with generalized MG.

2811. Anti-AChR antibodies are detectable in what percentage of all myasthenic patients?

Harrison's 20th Ed. Chapter 440, Page 3233

A. ~ 45%
B. ~ 65%
C. ~ 85%
D. ~ 99%

2812. Anti-AChR antibodies are detectable in what percentage of ocular MG patients?

Harrison's 20th Ed. Chapter 440, Page 3233

A. ~ 25%
B. ~ 50%
C. ~ 75%
D. ~ 99%

Anti-AChR antibodies are detectable in ~85% of all MG patients & in only ~50% of ocular MG patients.

2813. Anti-MuSK antibodies are found in what percentage of AChR antibody-negative patients with generalized MG?

Harrison's 20th Ed. Chapter 440, Page 3233

A. ~ 10%
B. ~ 40%
C. ~ 80%
D. ~ 100%

~40% of AChR antibody-negative patients with generalized MG have anti-MuSK antibodies.

2814. Anti MuSK antibodies are present in what percentage of AChR antibody-positive MG patients?

Harrison's 20th Ed. Chapter 440, Page 3233

A. Rare
B. 25%
C. 50%
D. 80%

2815. Anti MuSK antibodies are present in what percentage of patients with MG limited to ocular muscles?

Harrison's 20th Ed. Chapter 440, Page 3233

A. Rare
B. 25%
C. 50%
D. 80%

MuSK antibodies are rarely present in AChR antibody-positive MG patients or in patients with MG limited to ocular muscles.

2816. Which of the following statements about antibodies to muscle-specific kinase (MuSK) is false?

Harrison's 20th Ed. Chapter 440, Page 3233

A. Found in ~40% of AChR antibody-negative generalized MG
B. Not present in AChR antibody-positive patients
C. Not present in MG limited to ocular muscles
D. None of the above

2817. It is best to test which of the following muscles in repetitive nerve stimulation for evidence of MG?

Harrison's 20th Ed. Chapter 440, Page 3234

A. Proximal muscle groups
B. Distal muscle groups
C. Interosseous muscles
D. Any of the above

It is best to test weak muscles or proximal muscle groups in repetitive nerve stimulation for evidence of MG. Anti-AChE medication must be stopped 6–24 hours before testing.

2818. In myasthenic patients, rapid reduction of what proportion in amplitude of evoked responses is noted?

Harrison's 20th Ed. Chapter 440, Page 3234

A. > 10%
B. > 20%
C. > 30%
D. > 50%

In repetitive nerve stimulation for evidence of MG, electric shocks are delivered at a rate of three per second (3 Hz) to the appropriate nerves, and action potentials are recorded from muscles. In myasthenic patients there is a rapid reduction of > 10% in the amplitude of the evoked responses. (Normal <10%).

2819. In myasthenia gravis, which of the following spirometric statement is false?

Harrison's 20th Ed. Chapter 279, Page 1950

A. Normal FRC
B. Low TLC
C. Elevated RV
D. Normal FVC

In MG, FRC remains normal, as both lung recoil & passive chest wall recoil are normal. TLC is low and RV is elevated, as respiratory muscle strength is insufficient. Caught between the low TLC and the elevated RV, FVC and FEV1 are reduced as "innocent bystanders." As airway size and the lung vasculature are unaffected, both airways resistance (R_{aw}) and DL_{CO} are normal.

2820. Type of respiratory failure in MG is usually?

Harrison's 20th Ed. Chapter 293, Page 2026

A. Type I
B. Type II
C. Type III
D. Type IV

In myasthenia gravis, reduced strength due to impaired neuromuscular transmission results in type II respiratory failure i.e. alveolar hypoventilation and inability to eliminate carbon dioxide effectively.

2821. Fluctuating ptosis that worsens late in the day is typical of?
Harrison's 20th Ed. Chapter 28, Page 190

A. Myasthenia gravis
B. Glaucoma
C. Optic nerve glioma
D. Orbital cellulitis

Fluctuating ptosis that worsens late in the day is typical of myasthenia gravis.

2822. Which of the following is a cause of myogenic ptosis?
Harrison's 20th Ed. Chapter 28, Page 190

A. Myasthenia gravis
B. Chronic progressive external ophthalmoplegia
C. Oculopharyngeal dystrophy
D. All of the above

2823. Which of the following muscles open the eyelid?
Harrison's 20th Ed. Chapter 28, Page 190

A. Tenon's muscle
B. Müller's muscle
C. Zinn muscle
D. All of the above

Two muscles that open the eyelid are Müller's muscle & levator palpebrae superioris.

2824. Which of the following is an eye-related finding in myasthenia gravis?
Harrison's 20th Ed. Chapter 28, Page 190

A. Pupils are always normal
B. Diplopia is intermittent & variable
C. Diplopia is not confined to any single ocular motor nerve
D. All of the above

MG is a major cause of painless diplopia which is intermittent, variable, and not confined to any single ocular motor nerve distribution. Pupils are always normal. Fluctuating ptosis may be present.

2825. Cause of episodic generalized weakness is?
Harrison's 20th Ed. Chapter 21, Page 138

A. Myasthenia gravis
B. Lambert-Eaton myasthenic syndrome
C. Multiple sclerosis
D. All of the above

Causes of episodic generalized weakness include electrolyte disturbances (hypokalemia, hyperkalemia, hypercalcemia, hypernatremia, hyponatremia, hypophosphatemia, hypermagnesemia), muscle disorders (periodic paralyses, metabolic defects of muscle), neuromuscular junction disorders (myasthenia gravis, Lambert-Eaton myasthenic syndrome), central nervous system disorders (transient ischemic attacks of brainstem, transient global cerebral ischemia, multiple sclerosis).

2826. The edrophonium test is now used in which of the following patients of suspected MG?
Harrison's 20th Ed. Chapter 440, Page 3235

A. Who have negative antibody
B. Who have negative electrodiagnostic testing
C. Who have negative ice-pack test
D. All of the above

2827. Which of the following drug must be kept at hand while conducting Edrophonium anticholinesterase test?
Harrison's 20th Ed. Chapter 440, Page 3235

A. Atropine
B. Neostigmine
C. Adrenaline
D. All of the above

Atropine (0.6 mg) should be drawn up in a syringe, ready for IV use if nausea, diarrhea, salivation, fasciculations, syncope or bradycardia develop following IV edrophonium.

2828. Apart from Edrophonium which drug can be used for Anticholinesterase Test?
Harrison's 20th Ed. Chapter 440, Page 3235

A. Atropine
B. Neostigmine
C. Adrenaline
D. All of the above

A longer acting drug like neostigmine (orally) may be used for anticholinesterase test, as it permits more time for detailed evaluation of strength.

2829. Which of the following diseases can cause false-positive Edrophonium anticholinesterase test?
Harrison's 20th Ed. Chapter 440, Page 3235

A. Amyotrophic lateral sclerosis
B. Hodgkin lymphoma
C. Charcot-Marie-Tooth disease
D. Creutzfeldt-Jakob disease (CJD)

False-positive Edrophonium anticholinesterase test occur in occasional patients with amyotrophic lateral sclerosis, and in placebo-reactors.

2830. Which of the following is a cause of autoimmune MG?
Harrison's 20th Ed. Chapter 440, Page 3235

A. Congenital myasthenic syndromes (CMS)
B. Treatment with penicillamine
C. Kearns-Sayre syndrome
D. Botulism

Treatment with penicillamine and check point inhibitors for cancer may result in autoimmune MG.

2831. Drugs that can exacerbate weakness in myasthenic patients are all except?
Harrison's 20th Ed. Chapter 440, Page 3235

A. Penicillamine
B. Aminoglycoside antibiotics
C. Procainamide
D. Diazepam

Drugs that may exacerbate MG include aminoglycosides (streptomycin, tobramycin, kanamycin), Quinolones (ciprofloxacin, levofloxacin, ofloxacin, gatifloxacin), macrolides (erythromycin, azithromycin), Nondepolarizing muscle relaxants (D-Tubocurarine, pancuronium, vecuronium, atracurium), Beta-blockers (Propranolol, atenolol, metoprolol), Local anesthetics (Procaine, Xylocaine), Procainamide, Botulinum toxin, Quinine derivatives (Quinine, quinidine, chloroquine, mefloquine), Magnesium, Penicillamine.

2832. Which of the following drugs contain a thiol group in their chemical structure?
Harrison's 20th Ed. Chapter 55, Page 357

A. Penicillamine
B. Captopril
C. Enalapril
D. All of the above

Drugs containing a thiol group in their chemical structure are penicillamine, captopril, enalapril. They are most commonly associated with drug-induced pemphigus.

2833. Which of the following component of the neuromuscular junction may be affected in congenital myasthenic syndromes (CMS)?

Harrison's 20th Ed. Chapter 440, Page 3235

A. Presynaptic nerve terminal
B. Various subunits of AChR
C. Various subunits of AChE
D. All of the above

Congenital myasthenic syndromes (CMS) are disorders of neuromuscular junction that are not autoimmune but are due to genetic mutations in which virtually any component of the neuromuscular junction may be affected. Alterations in function of presynaptic nerve terminal or in various subunits of the AChR or AChE have been identified in different forms of CMS.

2834. Which of the following statements about congenital myasthenic syndromes (CMS) is false?

Harrison's 20th Ed. Chapter 440, Page 3235

A. Due to genetic mutations, not autoimmune
B. Symptoms begin in infancy or childhood
C. AChR antibody tests are consistently negative
D. A subunit of AChR is affected in ~75% of cases

CMS should be suspected when symptoms of myasthenia begin in infancy or childhood & AChR antibody tests are consistently negative. CMS that involve AChR, ε subunit is affected in ~75%.

2835. Double seronegative MG i.e. absence of AChR & MuSK antibodies occurs in what percentage of generalized MG patients?

Harrison's 20th Ed. Chapter 440, Page 3235

A. ~ 2%
B. ~ 5%
C. ~ 8%
D. ~ 10%

Double seronegative MG i.e. absence of AChR & MuSK antibodies occurs in ~10% of generalized MG patients.

2836. Which of the following CMS patients worsen with AChE inhibitors?

Harrison's 20th Ed. Chapter 440, Page 3235

A. Slow channel syndrome
B. AChE deficiency
C. DOK-7 related CMS
D. All of the above

2837. Myasthenia gravis is related to which of the following?

Harrison's 20th Ed. Chapter 440, Page 3235

A. Neuromyelitis optica (NMO)
B. M component on electrophoretic analysis
C. Hyperthyroidism
D. All of the above

2838. Disorders associated with myasthenia gravis include?

Harrison's 20th Ed. Chapter 440, Page 3235

A. Hashimoto's thyroiditis
B. Graves' disease
C. Systemic lupus erythematosus
D. All of the above

Disorders associated with Myasthenia Gravis are thymoma, thymus hyperplasia, Hashimoto's thyroiditis, Graves' disease, rheumatoid arthritis, lupus erythematosus, skin disorders, family history of autoimmune disorder. Hyperthyroidism or hypothyroidism, occult infection, medical treatment for other conditions may exacerbate myasthenia gravis. Tuberculosis, diabetes, peptic ulcer, gastrointestinal bleeding, renal disease, hypertension, asthma, osteoporosis, obesity are disorders that may interfere with therapy.

2839. Which of the following is false about Lambert-Eaton myasthenic syndrome (LEMS)?

Harrison's 20th Ed. Chapter 440, Page 3235

A. Presynaptic disorder of neuromuscular junction
B. Proximal muscles of lower limbs most commonly affected
C. Normal deep tendon reflexes
D. Incremental responses on repetitive nerve stimulation

LEMS is a presynaptic disorder of NM junction. Proximal muscles of lower limbs are most commonly affected. Ptosis & diplopia occur in ~70% of patients. Patients with LEMS have depressed or absent reflexes, experience autonomic changes such as dry mouth and impotence, and have incremental responses on repetitive nerve stimulation.

2840. Which of the following is false about Lambert-Eaton myasthenic syndrome (LEMS)?

Harrison's 20th Ed. Chapter 440, Page 3235

A. Autoantibodies against P/Q type calcium channels
B. Associated small-cell carcinoma of lung
C. Plasmapheresis ineffective
D. 3,4 Diaminopyridine (3,4-DAP) helpful

LEMS is caused by autoantibodies directed against P/Q type calcium channels at the motor nerve terminals impairing release of ACh & are detected in ~85% of LEMS patients. Small cell lung carcinoma is common in LEMS. Treatment of LEMS involves plasmapheresis & immunosuppression, 3,4-Diaminopyridine (3,4-DAP) & pyridostigmine.

2841. Muscle testing reveals "jerky release" or "give-away weakness" in which of the following?

Harrison's 20th Ed. Chapter 440, Page 3235

A. Lambert-Eaton myasthenic syndrome (LEMS)
B. Botulism
C. Hyperthyroidism
D. Neurasthenia

Muscle testing reveals "jerky release" or "give-away weakness" characteristic of non-organic disorders like Neurasthenia - a myasthenia-like fatigue syndrome without an organic basis.

2842. Which of the following cause weakness of somatic musculature due to presynaptic neuromuscular junction abnormality?

Harrison's 20th Ed. Chapter 440, Page 3235

A. Lambert-Eaton myasthenic syndrome (LEMS)
B. Botulism
C. Congenital myasthenic syndromes (CMS)
D. All of the above

CMS are not due to autoimmune but due to genetic mutations presynaptic nerve terminal or in subunits of AChR or AChE. In Botulism, bacterial toxin interferes with release of acetylcholine from presynaptic nerve terminal.

2843. Morvan's syndrome consists of?

Harrison's 20th Ed. Chapter 440, Page 3236

A. Encephalitis
B. Autonomic dysfunction
C. Neuromyotonia
D. All of the above

Morvan's syndrome consists of encephalitis, insomnia, confusion, hallucinations, autonomic dysfunction and neuromyotonia.

2844. Myasthenic patients have an increased incidence of?

Harrison's 20th Ed. Chapter 440, Page 3236

A. Hyperthyroidism
B. Systemic lupus erythematosus
C. Rheumatoid arthritis
D. All of the above

2845. Myasthenic patients have an increased incidence of?

Harrison's 20th Ed. Chapter 440, Page 3236

A. Neuromyelitis optica
B. Rippling muscle disease
C. Chronic inflammatory demyelinating polyneuropathy
D. All of the above

Myasthenic patients have an increased incidence of neuromyelitis optica, neuromyotonia, Morvan's syndrome (encephalitis, insomnia, confusion, hallucinations, autonomic dysfunction, and neuromyotonia), rippling muscle disease, granulomatous myositis/myocarditis & CIDP.

2846. Rippling muscle disease is associated with?

Journal of Clinical Neuroscience 2006;13(5):576-578

A. Caveolin-3
B. Connexin 26
C. MYO7A
D. TMC1

Caveolin-3 protein is expressed exclusively in muscle cells and forms scaffolding on cytoplasmic surface of sarcolemmal membrane. Improper caveolin-3 oligomerization results in skeletal muscle T-tubule system derangement, sarcolemmal membrane alterations, and large subsarcolemmal vesicle formation. Caveolin-3 mutations can result in four muscle disease phenotypes: limb girdle muscular dystrophy, rippling muscle disease, distal myopathy, and hyperCKemia.

2847. Botulinum toxin is produced by?

Harrison's 20th Ed. Chapter 148, Page 1105

A. Clostridium botulinum
B. Clostridium argentinense
C. Clostridium butyricum
D. All of the above

Botulinum toxin is produced by four recognized species of clostridia namely Clostridium botulinum, Clostridium argentinense, Clostridium baratii, and Clostridium butyricum.

2848. Which serotype of botulinum toxin produces the most severe syndrome?

Harrison's 20th Ed. Chapter 148, Page 1106

A. Serotype A
B. Serotype B
C. Serotype E
D. Serotype F

2849. Clinical syndrome of botulism consists of?

Harrison's 20th Ed. Chapter 148, Page 1106

A. Bilateral cranial-nerve palsies
B. Respiratory compromise
C. Bilateral descending flaccid paralysis of voluntary muscles
D. All of the above

Clinical syndrome of botulism consists of bilateral cranial-nerve palsies, respiratory compromise, bilateral descending flaccid paralysis of voluntary muscles and even death.

2850. Which of the following illnesses is considered in the differential diagnosis of adult botulism?

Harrison's 20th Ed. Chapter 148, Page 1107

A. Miller Fisher syndrome
B. Myasthenia gravis
C. Eaton-Lambert syndrome
D. All of the above

2851. The universally accepted method for confirmation of botulism is?

Harrison's 20th Ed. Chapter 148, Page 1108

A. Muscle biopsy
B. Nerve stimulation studies
C. Mouse bioassay
D. HPLC

The universally accepted method for confirmation of botulism is the mouse bioassay.

2852. Muscarinic side effects of anticholinesterase medication include all except?

Harrison's 20th Ed. Chapter 440, Page 3237

A. Diarrhea
B. Abdominal cramps
C. Dry mouth
D. Nausea

Muscarinic side effects of anticholinesterase medication are diarrhea, abdominal cramps, salivation and nausea.

2853. Thymoma is suspected if thymus is enlarged after?

Harrison's 20th Ed. Chapter 440, Page 3237

A. > 10 years
B. > 20 years
C. > 30 years
D. > 40 years

Thymic shadow on CT is normal in young adulthood, but thymus enlargement in a patient >40 years is highly suspicious of thymoma.

2854. By consensus, thymectomy should be done in all patients with generalized MG between?

Harrison's 20th Ed. Chapter 440, Page 3237

A. Puberty and 55 years
B. 30 and 55 years
C. 40 and 65 years
D. 50 and 75 years

It is the consensus that thymectomy should be carried out in all patients with generalized MG who are between puberty and at least 55 years of age.

2855. Which of the following patients may not benefit from thymectomy?

Harrison's 20th Ed. Chapter 440, Page 3237

A. Ocular myasthenia
B. MuSK-positive MG
C. Seronegative MG
D. All of the above

2856. Which of the following statements about MG is false?

Harrison's 20th Ed. Chapter 440, Page 3237

A. Patients with anti-MuSK MG get less benefit from anticholinesterase agents
B. Patients with anti-MuSK - positive MG respond less well to thymectomy
C. Rituximab is effective in MG patients with MuSK antibody
D. None of the above

2857. If immediate improvement is essential, which of the following is used to manage MG?

Harrison's 20th Ed. Chapter 440, Page 3237

A. Thymectomy
B. High-dose cyclophosphamide
C. Glucocorticoids
D. Intravenous immunoglobulin (IVIg)

In MG, if immediate improvement is essential, IVIg is given or plasmapheresis instituted.

2858. Which of the following produce clinical improvement within a period of 1–3 months?

Harrison's 20th Ed. Chapter 440, Page 3237

A. Glucocorticoids
B. Cyclosporine
C. Tacrolimus
D. All of the above

For the intermediate term goal of improvement, glucocorticoids, cyclosporine or tacrolimus produce clinical improvement within a period of 1–3 months.

2859. Which of the following immunosuppressive agents is preferred (toxicity & cost) in treatment of MG?

Harrison's 20th Ed. Chapter 440, Page 3237

A. Azathioprine
B. Cyclosporine
C. Mycophenolate mofetil
D. Cyclophosphamide

2860. Beneficial effect of azathioprine takes how long to appear?

Harrison's 20th Ed. Chapter 440, Page 3237

A. 7 – 21 days
B. 1 – 3 months
C. 3 – 6 months
D. 18 months

Beneficial effects of azathioprine & mycophenolate mofetil begin after many months (up to a year) because mycophenolate mofetil does not kill or eliminate preexisting autoreactive lymphocytes.

2861. Which of the following is used in MG patients refractory to optimal treatment with immunosuppressive agents?

Harrison's 20th Ed. Chapter 440, Page 3237

A. Tacrolimus
B. High-dose cyclophosphamide
C. Mycophenolate mofetil
D. Intravenous immunoglobulin (IVIg)

Patient with MG refractory to optimal treatment with conventional immunosuppressive agents, high-dose cyclophosphamide may induce long-lasting benefit by "rebooting" the immune system.

2862. Drug of choice for long-term treatment of myasthenic patients is?

Harrison's 20th Ed. Chapter 440, Page 3238

A. Azathioprine
B. Mycophenolate mofetil
C. Cyclosporine
D. Tacrolimus

2863. In patients taking azathioprine, which out of the following drugs should not be used?

Harrison's 20th Ed. Chapter 440, Page 3238

A. Paracetamol
B. Allopurinol
C. Cephalosporins
D. Terfenadine

In patients taking azathioprine, allopurinol should never be used to treat hyperuricemia, because due to a common degradation pathway, severe bone marrow depression may occur.

2864. Which of the following may be used as indications of adequacy of azathioprine dosage?

Harrison's 20th Ed. Chapter 440, Page 3238

A. Increase in hemoglobin
B. Decrease in ESR
C. Increase in hematocrit
D. Increase of RBC mean corpuscular volume

Reduction of lymphocytes to <1000/μL and/or an increase of MCV may be used as indications of adequacy of azathioprine dosage.

2865. Which of the following drug is useful in the treatment of anti-MuSK antibody positive MG?

Harrison's 20th Ed. Chapter 440, Page 3238

A. Tacrolimus
B. Rituximab
C. Cyclophosphamide
D. Azathioprine

Rituximab, a monoclonal antibody that depletes CD20 B cells, is useful in the treatment of anti-MuSK antibody positive MG.

2866. Which of the following has been found beneficial in MG patients?

Harrison's 20th Ed. Chapter 440, Page 3238

A. Trastuzumab
B. Eculizumab
C. Tocilizumab
D. Bevacizumab

Eculizumab is an anti-C5 complement inhibitor.

2867. Eculizumab is used in the treatment of?

Harrison's 20th Ed. Chapter 440, Page 3238

A. Paroxysmal nocturnal hemoglobinuria
B. Familial (Atypical) Hemolytic-Uremic Syndrome (aHUS)
C. Acute cellular rejection (ACR)
D. All of the above

2868. Most common cause of myasthenic crisis is?

Harrison's 20th Ed. Chapter 440, Page 3238

A. Hyperthyroidism
B. Hypothyroidism
C. Intercurrent infection
D. Drug underdose

The most common cause of myasthenic crisis is intercurrent infection.

2869. Which of the following is useful to assess MG patient's clinical status?

Cleveland clinic J of Med. 2013;80(11):711-21

A. Forward arm abduction time (5 min)
B. Forced vital capacity
C. Time to development of ptosis on upward gaze
D. All of the above

Most useful clinical tests to assess MG patient's clinical status include forward arm abduction time (up to a full 5 min.), forced vital capacity, range of eye movements, and time to development of ptosis on upward gaze. Patient's AChR antibody level also provides clinically valuable confirmation of the effectiveness of treatment.

2870. Which of the following is false about Myasthenia gravis?

Cleveland clinic J of Med. 2013;80(11):711-21

A. Age of onset has a bimodal distribution
B. Fluctuating muscle weakness with fatigue
C. Generalized fatigue without objective weakness
D. Ptosis alternating from one eye to the other

In MG, age of onset has a bimodal distribution, with an early incidence peak in the second to third decade with a female predominance and a late peak in the 6th to the 8th decade with a male predominance. Generalized fatigue without objective weakness is inconsistent with myasthenia gravis. Ptosis alternating from one eye to the other is fairly characteristic of myasthenia gravis.

2871. Myasthenia gravis is commonly associated with?

Cleveland clinic J of Med. 2013;80(11):711-21

A. Hypothyroidism
B. Hyperthyroidism
C. Rheumatoid arthritis
D. All of the above

Myasthenia gravis is commonly associated with hypothyroidism, hyperthyroidism, systemic lupus erythematosus, rheumatoid arthritis, vitiligo, diabetes and neuromyelitis optica.

2872. Which of the following is an AChR antibody subtype?

Cleveland clinic J of Med. 2013;80(11):711-21

A. Binding
B. Blocking
C. Modulating
D. All of the above

There are three AChR antibody subtypes : binding, blocking, and modulating. Binding antibodies are present in 80% to 90% of patients with generalized myasthenia gravis and 50% of those with ocular myasthenia gravis. Testing for blocking and modulating AChR antibodies increases the sensitivity by less than 5% when added to testing for binding antibodies.

2873. MuSK stands for?

Cleveland clinic J of Med. 2013;80(11):711-21

A. Membrane-specific kinase (MuSK)
B. Muscle-specific kinase (MuSK)
C. Membrane-specific tyrosine kinase (MuSK)
D. Muscle-specific tyrosine kinase (MuSK)

In most cases of myasthenia gravis the patient has autoimmune antibodies against constituents of the neuromuscular junction, specifically acetylcholine receptor (AChR) and muscle-specific tyrosine kinase (MuSK).

2874. Which of the following about MuSK is false?

Cleveland clinic J of Med. 2013;80(11):711-21

A. Transmembrane component of postsynaptic neuromuscular junction
B. Activated through binding of agrin to lipoprotein-related protein 4
C. Antibodies against MuSK activate complement system
D. MG with MuSK antibodies is rarely associated with thymoma

Like AChR, MuSK is a transmembrane component of the postsynaptic neuromuscular junction. During formation of the neuromuscular junction, MuSK is activated through the binding of agrin (a nerve-derived proteoglycan) to lipoprotein-related protein 4 (LRP4, receptor for agrin), after which complicated intracellular signaling promotes the assembly and stabilization of AChR. Unlike AChR antibodies, antibodies against MuSK do not activate the complement system, and complement fixation is not essential for clinical myasthenic symptoms to appear. Also, myasthenia gravis with MuSK antibodies is rarely associated with thymoma. MuSK antibodies block the binding of MuSK to acetylcholinesterase. MuSK antibody-positive myasthenia gravis tend to respond poorly to acetylcholinesterase inhibitors. Most MuSK antibody-positive patients have a favorable response to immunosuppressive therapy.

2875. Decremental response on repetitive nerve stimulation studies can be seen in?

Cleveland clinic J of Med. 2013;80(11):711-21

A. Myasthenia gravis
B. Motor neuron disease
C. Lambert-Eaton myasthenic syndrome
D. All of the above

Repetitive nerve stimulation studies use a slow rate (2 - 5 Hz) of repetitive electrical stimulation. The study is positive if the motor response declines by >10%. Decremental response may be seen in myasthenia gravis, motor neuron disease or Lambert-Eaton myasthenic syndrome.

2876. Medication that can exacerbate weakness in myasthenia gravis is?

Cleveland clinic J of Med. 2013;80(11):711-21

A. Penicillamine
B. Procainamide
C. Aminoglycosides
D. All of the above

Medications that can exacerbate weakness in myasthenia gravis are penicillamine, interferons, procainamide, quinidine, and antibiotics, including quinolones and aminoglycosides.

Muscular Dystrophies and Other Muscle Diseases

2877. Clinical findings of a myopathy include all except?

Harrison's 20th Ed. Chapter 441, Page 3239

A. Proximal limb weakness
B. Symmetric limb weakness
C. Depressed reflexes
D. Preserved sensation

Clinical findings of a myopathy are proximal, symmetric limb weakness (arms or legs) with preserved reflexes and sensation.

2878. Muscular dystrophies are characterized by the progressive loss of muscle in accordance with?

Current Opinion in Genetics and Development. 2003;13(3):231-238

A. Age of onset
B. Severity
C. Group of muscles affected
D. All of the above

2879. Which of the following is not a childhood muscular dystrophy?

doi:10.1155/2012/485376

A. Limb-girdle muscular dystrophy
B. Duchenne muscular dystrophy (DMD)
C. Becker muscular dystrophy (BMD)
D. Emery-Dreifuss muscular dystrophy (EDMD)

Duchenne muscular dystrophy (DMD), Becker muscular dystrophy (BMD) and Emery-Dreifuss muscular dystrophy (EDMD) have their first clinical manifestations during childhood. Laminopathies such as myotonic dystrophy or limb-girdle muscular dystrophy appear during adulthood.

2880. Which of the following is not a cause of intermittent weakness of muscles?

Harrison's 20th Ed. Chapter 441, Page 3240

A. Myasthenia gravis
B. Polymyositis
C. Myophosphorylase deficiency
D. Carnitine palmitoyltransferase deficiency

Disorders causing intermittent muscle weakness include myasthenia gravis, periodic paralyses (hypokalemic, hyperkalemic), and metabolic energy deficiencies of glycolysis (myophosphorylase deficiency), fatty acid utilization (carnitine palmitoyltransferase deficiency), and some mitochondrial myopathies.

2881. Which of the following about limb-girdle weakness is false?

Harrison's 20th Ed. Chapter 441, Page 3240

A. Proximal muscles are weaker than the distal
B. Symmetrically affected
C. Facial muscles are spared
D. None of the above

2882. Which of the following is characteristic of facioscapulohumeral dystrophy (FSHD)?

Harrison's 20th Ed. Chapter 441, Page 3240

A. Difficulty with eye closure
B. Impaired smile
C. Scapular winging
D. All of the above

Facial weakness manifesting as difficulty with eye closure and impaired smile along with scapular winging are characteristic of facioscapulohumeral dystrophy (FSHD).

2883. Which of the following is virtually diagnostic of myotonic dystrophy type 1?

Harrison's 20th Ed. Chapter 441, Page 3240

A. Facial weakness
B. Distal limb weakness
C. Hand grip myotonia
D. All of the above

Facial & distal limb weakness associated with hand grip myotonia is virtually diagnostic of myotonic dystrophy type 1.

2884. Ptosis or extraocular muscle weakness is caused by?

Harrison's 20th Ed. Chapter 441, Page 3240

A. Neuromuscular junction disorders
B. Oculopharyngeal muscular dystrophy
C. Mitochondrial myopathies
D. All of the above

Ptosis or extraocular muscle weakness can be caused by neuromuscular junction disorders, oculopharyngeal muscular dystrophy, mitochondrial myopathies, and some congenital myopathies.

2885. Which of the following is characteristic of inclusion body myositis?

Harrison's 20th Ed. Chapter 441, Page 3240

A. Atrophy and weakness of wrist flexors
B. Atrophy and weakness of finger flexors
C. Atrophy and weakness of quadriceps muscles
D. All of the above

A pathognomonic pattern characteristic of inclusion body myositis (IBM) is atrophy & weakness of wrist flexors, finger flexors and quadriceps muscles, often asymmetric.

2886. Which of the following can have a presentation of "dropped head syndrome"?

Harrison's 20th Ed. Chapter 441, Page 3240

A. Myasthenia gravis
B. Amyotrophic lateral sclerosis
C. Hyperparathyroidism
D. All of the above

Dropped head syndrome indicates selective neck extensor muscle weakness. Neuromuscular diseases associated with this pattern of weakness include myasthenia gravis, amyotrophic lateral sclerosis, late-onset nemaline myopathy, hyperparathyroidism, focal myositis, and some forms of inclusion body myopathy.

2887. Pathologic fatigability occurs in which of the following?

Harrison's 20th Ed. Chapter 441, Page 3241

A. Disorders of neuromuscular transmission
B. Disorders of defects in glycolysis
C. Chronic myopathies
D. All of the above

Pathologic fatigability refers to inability to maintain or sustain a force. It occurs in disorders of neuromuscular transmission and in disorders altering energy production (glycolysis, lipid metabolism, or mitochondrial energy production), chronic myopathies.

2888. Muscle cramps often occur in which of the following neurogenic disorders?

Harrison's 20th Ed. Chapter 441, Page 3241

A. Motor neuron disease
B. Radiculopathies
C. Polyneuropathies
D. All of the above

Muscle cramps often occur in neurogenic disorders, especially motor neuron disease, radiculopathies, and polyneuropathies. They are not a feature of most primary muscle diseases. There are no pathologic reflexes in myopathies.

2889. Which of the following is false in myopathies?

Harrison's 20th Ed. Chapter 441, Page 3241

A. There are no pathologic reflexes
B. There is no sensory loss
C. There is no bowel & bladder dysfunction
D. None of the above

2890. Fixed contracture is a distinctive feature of?

Harrison's 20th Ed. Chapter 441, Page 3242

A. Motor neuron disease
B. Stiff-Person syndrome
C. Emery-Dreifuss muscular dystrophy
D. Paramyotonia congenita (PC)

In Emery-Dreifuss muscular dystrophy and Bethlem myopathy, fixed contractures are an early and distinctive feature.

2891. Which of the following is a chloride channel disorder?

Harrison's 20th Ed. Chapter 441, Page 3242

A. Paramyotonia congenita (PC)
B. Myotonic muscular dystrophy type 1 (DM1)
C. Myotonic muscular dystrophy type 2 (DM2)
D. Myotonia congenita

2892. In which of the following myotonia, muscle weakness is not prominent?

Harrison's 20th Ed. Chapter 441, Page 3242

A. Paramyotonia congenita (PC)
B. Myotonic muscular dystrophy type 1 (DM1)
C. Myotonic muscular dystrophy type 2 (DM2)
D. Myotonia congenita

2893. Which of the following is related to stiff-Person syndrome?

Harrison's 20th Ed. Chapter 441, Page 3242

A. Serum antibodies against PMP22
B. Serum antibodies against ornithine decarboxylase
C. Serum antibodies against dopa decarboxylase
D. Serum antibodies against glutamic acid decarboxylase

Serum antibodies against glutamic acid decarboxylase are present in approximately two-thirds of stiff-Person syndrome cases. This disorder is characterized by progressive muscle rigidity, stiffness & painful spasms mostly of lower extremity, triggered by auditory, sensory, or emotional stimuli. Sometimes, only one extremity is affected (stiff-limb syndrome).

2894. Which of the following antibodies are associated with Stiff-Person syndrome?

Harrison's 20th Ed. Chapter 441, Page 673

A. GAD
B. Amphiphysin
C. GlyR
D. All of the above

The three main targets of autoantibodies in patients with Stiff-Person spectrum disorders are presynaptic proteins GAD and amphiphysin, and postsynaptic glycine receptor (GlyR). Presence of amphiphysin antibodies indicates a paraneoplastic etiology related to SCLC and breast cancer. GAD antibodies are much more frequently present in nonparaneoplastic disorders. GlyR antibodies are also detectable in patients with PERM.

2895. Which of the following is false about Stiff-Person Syndrome?

Harrison's 20th Ed. Chapter 441, Page 673

A. Muscle stiffness & superimposed spasms
B. Involves jaw
C. Associated with cancers
D. Serum antibody against glutamic acid decarboxylase present

Rigidity mainly involves lower trunk & legs, but it can affect the upper extremities & neck. Sometimes, only one extremity is affected when it is called Stiff Limb syndrome.

2896. Acquired neuromyotonia is also called?

Harrison's 20th Ed. Chapter 441, Page 3242

A. Rett syndrome
B. Munchausen's syndrome
C. Isaacs syndrome
D. Andersen-Tawil syndrome

Peripheral nerve hyperexcitability (neuromyotonia, or Isaacs' syndrome) is characterized by spontaneous and continuous muscle fiber activity of peripheral nerve origin.

2897. Which of the following is false about 'Neuromyotonia'?

Harrison's 20th Ed. Chapter 441, Page 3242

A. Muscle stiffness at rest & during sleep
B. Distal limb muscles most severely affected
C. Myokymia
D. None of the above

2898. Which of the following is a feature of Isaacs syndrome?

Harrison's 20th Ed. Chapter 441, Page 674

A. Hypertrophic muscles
B. Paresthesias
C. Hyperhidrosis
D. All of the above

2899. Drugs that cause true myalgia include?

Harrison's 19th Ed. 462e-4 Table 462e-3

A. Cimetidine
B. Labetalol
C. Statins
D. All of the above

Drugs that cause true myalgia include Cimetidine, Cocaine, Cyclosporine, Danazol, Emetine, Gold, Heroin, Labetalol, Methadone, d-Penicillamine, Statins, L-Tryptophan, Zidovudine.

2900. Which of the following is a painful muscle condition?

Harrison's 20th Ed. Chapter 441, Page 3243

A. Paramyotonia congenita
B. Amyotrophic lateral sclerosis
C. Fibromyalgia
D. All of the above

Painful muscle conditions not associated with muscle weakness include fibromyalgia and polymyalgia rheumatica.

2901. Which of the following is associated with polymyalgia rheumatica?

Harrison's 20th Ed. Chapter 13, Page 86

A. Takayasu's arteritis
B. Henoch-Schönlein purpura
C. Temporal arteritis
D. Granulomatosis with polyangiitis (Wegener's)

Giant cell arteritis, also referred to as cranial arteritis or temporal arteritis, is an inflammatory disorder of medium- and large-sized arteries, may accompany polymyalgia rheumatica.

2902. Which of the following enzymes is not found in muscles?

Harrison's 20th Ed. Chapter 441, Page 3243

A. Creatine kinase (CK)
B. Aldolase
C. Lactic dehydrogenase (LDH)
D. Gamma-glutamyl transferase (GGT)

Creatine kinase (CK), aspartate aminotransferase (AST), alanine aminotransferase (ALT), aldolase, and lactic dehydrogenase (LDH) are enzymes sharing an origin in both muscle and liver. Gamma-glutamyl transferase (GGT) has a liver origin and is not found in muscle.

2903. Which of the following enzyme is not found in muscle?

Harrison's 20th Ed. Chapter 441, Page 3243

A. Aspartate aminotransferase (AST)
B. Alanine aminotransferase (ALT)
C. Lactic dehydrogenase (LDH)
D. g-glutamyl transferase (GGT)

Enzymes AST, ALT, aldolase and LDH originate in both muscle & liver. Origin of GGT is liver and is not found in muscle.

2904. Which of the following is helpful in differentiating myopathies from neuropathies & neuromuscular junction diseases?

Harrison's 20th Ed. Chapter 441, Page 3243

A. EMG
B. Repetitive nerve stimulation
C. Nerve conduction studies (NCS)
D. All of the above

2905. Which of the following is the gold standard for diagnosing patients with hereditary myopathies?

Harrison's 20th Ed. Chapter 441, Page 3243

A. Muscle biopsy
B. Genetic testing
C. Electrodiagnostic studies
D. All of the above

Genetic testing is the gold standard for diagnosing patients with hereditary myopathies. Muscle biopsy is extremely helpful in evaluation of acquired myopathies but is performed less frequently in suspected hereditary myopathies as genetic testing has become more widely available.

2906. Which of the following is accompanied by myoglobinuria?

Harrison's 20th Ed. Chapter 441, Page 3243

A. Myasthenia gravis
B. Polymyositis
C. Paramyotonia congenita
D. Myoadenylate deaminase deficiency

The states of metabolic energy deficiencies of glycolysis (myophosphorylase deficiency), fatty acid utilization (carnitine palmitoyltransferase deficiency), cause activity-related muscle breakdown accompanied by myoglobinuria, appearing as light-brown- to dark-brown-colored urine.

2907. Mutations affecting nuclear membrane proteins are responsible for?

Harrison's 20th Ed. Chapter 441, Page 3247 Figure 441-6

A. LGMD
B. Distal myopathies
C. EDMD
D. All of the above

2908. Mutations in genes that encode for sarcomeric and Z-disk proteins cause?

Harrison's 20th Ed. Chapter 441, Page 3247 Figure 441-6

A. Myofibrillar myopathy
B. Hereditary inclusion body myopathy
C. Nemaline rod myopathy
D. All of the above

Mutations in genes that encode for sarcomeric & Z-disk proteins cause forms of LGMD & distal myopathies like myofibrillar myopathy, forms of hereditary inclusion body myopathy, also, nemaline rod myopathy & other congenital myopathies. Mutations affecting nuclear membrane proteins cause most forms of EDMD.

2909. Nationality of Guillaume Benjamin Amand Duchenne de Boulogne was?

Journal of the History of Medicine and Allied Sciences. 2000;55(2):158-178

A. Polish
B. French
C. German
D. Danish

2910. Who discovered dystrophin gene?

Cell. 1987;51(6):919-28

A. Little
B. Gowers
C. Kunkel
D. Meryon

2911. The largest known human gene is?

Harrison's 20th Ed. Chapter 456, Page 3358

A. GNAS1
B. CFTR
C. Dystrophin
D. Emerin

2912. Which of the following is not a cytoskeletal protein?

Harrison's 20th Ed. Chapter 252, Page 1763

A. Desmin
B. Myosin
C. Laminin
D. Vinculin

Cytoskeletal proteins are desmin, cardiac myosin and vinculin while lamininis a nuclear membrane protein.

2913. Dilated cardiomyopathy is associated with?

Harrison's 20th Ed. Chapter 252, Page 1763

A. Duchenne's muscular dystrophy
B. Becker's muscular dystrophy
C. Limb-Girdle muscular dystrophies
D. All of the above

2914. Duchenne muscular dystrophy is present at?

Harrison's 20th Ed. Chapter 441, Page 3244

A. Birth
B. 1–2 years
C. 3–5 years
D. 5–7 years

Duchenne dystrophy is present at birth, but it usually becomes apparent between ages 3 & 5.

2915. Which of the following about Duchenne Muscular Dystrophy is false?

Harrison's 20th Ed. Chapter 441, Page 3244

A. X-linked recessive muscular dystrophy
B. Affects 1 in 3000 male births
C. Caused by mutations in dystrophin gene
D. None of the above

2916. Patients with Duchenne dystrophy are typically in a wheelchair by the age of?

Drug Des Devel Ther. 2017; 11: 533–545

A. 8
B. 10
C. 12
D. 14

Patients with Duchenne dystrophy are typically in wheelchair by age of 12.

2917. Which of the following virus can cleave dystrophin?

Harrison's 20th Ed. Chapter 254, Page 1780

A. Echovirus
B. Epstein-Barr virus
C. Coxsackie virus
D. West Nile virus

Abnormal dystrophin can be acquired when the coxsackie virus cleaves dystrophin during viral myocarditis.

2918. Clinical picture of which of the following resembles that of Duchenne muscular dystrophy?

Harrison's 20th Ed. Chapter 254, Page 1780

A. Tay-Sachs disease
B. Amyotrophic lateral sclerosis (ALS)
C. Pompe's disease
D. Gaucher disease

In the childhood form of α-glucosidase, or acid maltase, deficiency (type II glycogenosis) or Pompe's disease, clinical picture resembles Duchenne muscular dystrophy with delayed motor milestones resulting from proximal limb muscle weakness and involvement of respiratory muscles with calf muscle hypertrophy.

2919. The most important endocrine alteration in DMD/BMD patients is?

doi:10.1155/2012/485376

A. Hypothyroidism
B. Hypogonadism
C. Type II diabetes mellitus
D. Addison's syndrome

The most important endocrine alteration in DMD/BMD patients is hypogonadism. Consequences are delayed puberty, growth failure, osteoporosis, and metabolic abnormalities.

2920. Which of the following diseases can also cause Duchenne muscular dystrophy?

American Journal of Human Genetics. 1987;40(3):212-227

A. Pyruvate kinase deficiency
B. Glycerol kinase deficiency (GKD)
C. Adenosine kinase deficiency
D. Mevalonate kinase deficiency

Glycerol kinase deficiency (GKD) is an X-linked recessive enzyme defect. The responsible gene lies in a region containing genes in which deletions can cause Duchenne muscular dystrophy and adrenal hypoplasia congenita. Combinations of these three genetic defects are addressed as Complex GKD.

2921. 'Gowers' maneuver' is diagnostic of?

Harrison's 20th Ed. Chapter 441, Page 3242 Table 441-4

A. Duchenne muscular dystrophy (DMD)
B. Limb-Girdle muscular dystrophy
C. Emery-Dreifuss muscular dystrophy
D. Facioscapulohumeral muscular dystrophy

2922. Gowers' sign is due to weakness of which group of muscles?

Harrison's 20th Ed. Chapter 441, Page 3242 Table 441-2

A. Knee extensor muscles
B. Hip muscles
C. Anterior compartment of leg muscles
D. Posterior compartment of leg muscles

Gowers' sign refers to the inability to get up from the floor without climbing up the extremities. Weakness is in the hip, thigh, and trunk muscles.

2923. In DMD, which of the following muscle groups are preferentially involved?

DeJong's The Neurologic Examination, 7th Ed. Page 481

A. Distal limb muscles
B. Neck flexors
C. Neck extensors
D. Anterior abdominal muscles

Loss of muscle strength is progressive, with predilection for proximal limb muscles and neck flexors.

2924. Which of the following muscles undergo pseudohypertrophy in DMD?

DeJong's The Neurologic Examination, 7th Ed. Page 481

A. Supraspinatus
B. Infraspinatus
C. Latissimus dorsi
D. Serratus anterior

Pseudohypertrophy is common in Duchenne & Becker dystrophy. Calf muscles & infraspinatus are often strikingly enlarged due to pseudohypertrophy. Wasting of axillary folds is also seen.

2925. Kocher-Debré-Semelaigne (infant Hercules) syndrome is best related to?

DeJong's The Neurologic Examination, 7th Ed. Page 482

A. Hypothyroidism
B. Hyperthyroidism
C. Polymyositis
D. Central core disease

Kocher-Debré-Semelaigne (infant Hercules) syndrome is diffuse muscular hypertrophy due to hypothyroidism, early in life. Hoffman syndrome refers to hypertrophic myopathy due to hypothyroidism in adults.

2926. Muscle enlargement may occur in?

DeJong's The Neurologic Examination, 7th Ed. Page 482

A. Cysticercosis
B. Sarcoidosis
C. Amyloidosis
D. All of the above

Muscle enlargement may occur due to interstitial infiltrates, as in cysticercosis, trichinosis, sarcoidosis & amyloidosis.

2927. Which of the following about DMD is false?

doi:10.1155/2012/485376

A. Due to mutation in dystrophin gene
B. Dystrophin is the largest identified human gene
C. Dystrophin is on X chromosome
D. Mostly due to gene duplication

DMD is caused by a mutation of gene encoding 427-kDa dystrophin protein on the inner surface of sarcolemma. Dystrophin gene is one of the largest identified human genes (>2000 kb) on the short arm of X chromosome (Xp21). Most common gene mutation is a deletion. Less often, Duchenne's dystrophy is caused by a gene duplication or point mutation.

2928. Which of the following is an uncommon cause of death in Duchenne's muscular dystrophy?

doi:10.1155/2012/485376

A. Pulmonary infection
B. Aspiration of food
C. Acute gastric dilation
D. Cardiac cause (cardiomyopathy)

By age 16–18 years, patients of DMD are predisposed to serious, sometimes fatal pulmonary infections. Other causes of death include aspiration of food and acute gastric dilation. Cardiac cause of death is uncommon despite the presence of a cardiomyopathy in almost all patients.

2929. Which of the following statements about serum CK levels in DMD is false?

doi:10.1155/2012/485376

A. Invariably elevated
B. Serum CK levels are abnormal at birth
C. Decline late in the disease
D. None of the above

In DMD, serum CK levels are invariably elevated (20 to 100 times). Levels are abnormal at birth but decline late in the disease because of inactivity & loss of muscle mass.

2930. The most common gene mutation in DMD is?

Harrison's 20th Ed. Chapter 441, Page 3255

A. Deletion
B. Duplication
C. Point mutation
D. Any of the above

The most common gene mutation is a deletion. The size varies but does not correlate with disease severity. Deletions are not uniformly distributed over the gene but rather are most common near the beginning (5' end) and middle of the gene.

2931. Which of the following about dystrophin gene is false?

doi:10.1155/2012/485376

A. > 2000 kb in size
B. Localized to short arm of X chromosome at Xp21
C. Most common gene mutation is a deletion
D. None of the above

2932. Which of the following about dystrophin is false?

doi:10.1155/2012/485376

A. 427-kDa protein
B. Localized to inner surface of sarcolemma of muscle fiber
C. Western blot analysis of muscle biopsy helps in revealing abnormalities of dystrophin protein
D. None of the above

2933. Muscle biopsy of a patient of DMD shows which of the following?

doi:10.1155/2012/485376

A. Muscle fibers of varying size
B. Small groups of necrotic and regenerating fibers
C. Connective tissue & fat replace lost muscle fibers
D. None of the above

2934. Dystrophin binds to which of the following in sarcolemma?

Harrison's 20th Ed. Chapter 441, Page 3247 Figure 441-6

A. Laminin
B. Alpha-dystroglycan
C. F-actin
D. Caveolin-3

Dystrophin is part of a large complex of sarcolemmal proteins and glycoproteins. Dystrophin binds to F-actin at its amino terminus and to beta-dystroglycan at the carboxyl terminus.

2935. In essence, the key defect in DMD due to abnormal dystrophin protein is?

Harrison's 20th Ed. Chapter 441, Page 3247 Figure 441-6

A. Physical weakening of the sarcolemma
B. Disruption of Golgi apparatus
C. Abnormal mitochondria
D. Abnormal extracellular matrix (ECM)

Dystrophin-glycoprotein complex confer stability to the sarcolemma. Disruption of dystrophin-glycoprotein complexes weakens sarcolemma, causing membrane tears and a cascade of events leading to muscle fiber necrosis and eventually muscular dystrophy.

2936. Which of the following significantly slows progression of Duchenne's dystrophy?

Harrison's 20th Ed. Chapter 441, Page 3244

A. Azathioprine
B. Glucocorticoids
C. Cyclosporine
D. IVIg

Glucocorticoids (prednisone 0.75 mg/kg per day), significantly slows progression of Duchenne's dystrophy for up to 3 years.

2937. First and currently only FDA-approved drug for DMD is?

Drug Des Devel Ther. 2017; 11: 533–545

A. Apalutamide
B. Tecovirimat
C. Eteplirsen
D. Stiripentol

Eteplirsen is beneficial for DMD patients with deletions ending at exon 50 and starting at exon 52. It acts to promote dystrophin production by restoring the translational reading frame of DMD through specific skipping of exon 51 in defective gene variants.

2938. Becker's Muscular Dystrophy resembles which of the following muscular dystrophy?

Harrison's 20th Ed. Chapter 441, Page 3239

A. Duchenne's muscular dystrophy
B. Limb-Girdle muscular dystrophy
C. Emery-Dreifuss muscular dystrophy
D. Myotonic dystrophy

Becker's muscular dystrophy is a less severe and 10 times less frequent form of X-linked recessive Duchenne's muscular dystrophy.

2939. Most patients with Becker's muscular dystrophy first experience difficulties at what age?

Harrison's 20th Ed. Chapter 441, Page 3240

A. Birth
B. 1–2 years
C. 3–5 years
D. 5–15 years

Most patients with Becker's dystrophy first experience difficulties between ages 5 and 15 years.

2940. Calpains are Ca^{++} dependent?

N Engl J Med. 2005;352:2413-23

A. Cysteine proteases
B. Arginine proteases
C. Methionine proteases
D. Leucine proteases

2941. Tissue-specific calpains have been implicated in?

N Engl J Med. 2005;352:2413-23

A. Diabetes
B. Multiple sclerosis
C. Limb-girdle muscular dystrophy type 2A (LGMD2A)
D. All of the above

2942. Which of the following statements about Calpain is false?

N Engl J Med. 2005;352:2413-23

A. Calpain activity is regulated by calpastatin
B. Calpains are involved in apoptosis
C. Calpain is a cytoplasmic protease
D. None of the above

2943. Which of the following is a type of adult-onset LGMD?

Harrison's 20th Ed. Chapter 441, Page 3247

A. Calpainopathy
B. Fukutin-related protein (FKRP) deficiency
C. Anoctaminopathy
D. All of the above

The most common types of adult-onset LGMD are calpainopathy (LGMD2A), Fukutin-related protein (FKRP) deficiency (LGMD2I), and anoctaminopathy (LGMD2L).

2944. Which of the following statements is false?

Harrison's 20th Ed. Chapter 441, Page 3244 Table 441-3

A. Abnormal protein associated with LGMD1A is Myotilin
B. Abnormal protein associated with LGMD1B is Lamin A/C
C. Abnormal protein associated with LGMD1C is Caveolin-3
D. Abnormal protein associated with LGMD1D is Desmin

Abnormal protein associated with LGMD1D is DNAJB6 while abnormal protein associated with LGMD1E is Desmin.

2945. Abnormal protein Calpain-3 is associated with?

Harrison's 20th Ed. Chapter 441, Page 3244 Table 441-3

A. LGMD1F
B. LGMD1G
C. LGMD1H
D. LGMD1I

2946. Gower sign, calf hypertrophy & rippling muscles are clinical features of?

Harrison's 20th Ed. Chapter 441, Page 3244 Table 441-3

A. LGMD1A
B. LGMD1B
C. LGMD1C
D. LGMD1D

2947. Which of the following about LGMD2A is false?

Harrison's 20th Ed. Chapter 441, Page 3247

A. Marked scapular winging
B. Calf muscle hypertrophy
C. Lack of cardiac involvement
D. Lack of lung involvement

LGMD2A is associated with marked scapular winging, lack of calf muscle hypertrophy, and lack of cardiac and lung involvement.

2948. LGMD2A is caused by gene mutations in?

Harrison's 20th Ed. Chapter 441, Page 3245 Table 441-4

A. Calpain-1
B. Calpain-2
C. Calpain-3
D. Calpain-4

2949. LGMD2B is due to defect in?

Harrison's 20th Ed. Chapter 441, Page 3245 Table 441-4

A. Dysferlin
B. Emerin
C. Telethonin
D. Titin

2950. Which of the following is a variant of LGMD2B?

Harrison's 20th Ed. Chapter 441, Page 3245 Table 441-4

A. Welander distal myopathy
B. Tibial muscular dystrophy (Udd)
C. Laing distal myopathy
D. Miyoshi myopathy

Miyoshi's myopathy is variant of LGMD2B with calf muscles affected at onset.

2951. In which of the following gastrocnemius muscles are preferentially affected at onset?

Harrison's 20th Ed. Chapter 441, Page 3245, Table 441-4

A. Welander distal myopathy
B. Tibial muscular dystrophy (Udd's)
C. Laing distal myopathy
D. Miyoshi myopathy

In dysferlinopathies (LGMD2B) there is a predilection for early atrophy of gastrocnemius muscles. Miyoshi myopathy is unique in that gastrocnemius muscles are preferentially affected at onset.

2952. Which of the following muscular dystrophy has its onset in infancy?

Harrison's 20th Ed. Chapter 441, Page 3245 Table 441-4

A. Muscle-eye-brain disease
B. Walker-Warburg syndrome
C. Fukuyama congenital muscular dystrophy
D. All of the above

Merosin deficiency, Fukitin-related protein deficiency, Fukuyama congenital muscular dystrophy, Muscle-eye-brain disease, Walker-Warburg syndrome are congenital muscular dystrophies that have an onset at birth. Clinically, Walker-Warburg syndrome is more severe, with death by 1 year.

2953. Which of the following is a lipid myopathy?

DeJong's The Neurologic Examination, 7th Ed. Page 773

A. Carnitine deficiency
B. McArdle's disease
C. Phosphofructokinase deficiency
D. Kearnes-Sayre syndrome

2954. Which of the following statements is false?

Harrison's 20th Ed. Chapter 441, Page 3245 Table 441-4

A. Abnormal protein associated with LGMD2A is Calpain-3
B. Abnormal protein associated with LGMD2B is Dysferlin
C. Abnormal protein associated with LGMD2C is Telethonin
D. None of the above

Abnormal protein associated with LGMD2C is γ sarcoglycan.

2955. Which of the following is clinically similar to Duchenne or Becker dystrophies?

Harrison's 20th Ed. Chapter 441, Page 3245 Table 441-4

A. LGMD2G
B. LGMD2H
C. LGMD2I
D. LGMD2J

LGMD2C, D, E, F and I are clinically similar to Duchenne or Becker dystrophies.

2956. Udd type distal myopathy is due to deficiency of?

Harrison's 20th Ed. Chapter 441, Page 3245 Table 441-4

A. Desmin
B. Titin
C. Plectin 1
D. Fukutin

2957. Which of the following is best related to congenital myasthenic syndrome?

Harrison's 20th Ed. Chapter 441, Page 3245 Table 441-4

A. Dermatitis herpetiformis
B. Cicatricial pemphigoid
C. Epidermolysis bullosa
D. Pemphigus foliaceus

LGMD2Q has onset in infancy to fourth decade. Presentation may includes proximal weakness, ptosis & extraocular weakness with epidermolysis bullosa (a congenital myasthenic syndrome).

2958. Which of the following LGMD has Hutterite descent?

Harrison's 20th Ed. Chapter 441, Page 3245 Table 441-4

A. LGMD2P
B. LGMD2Q
C. LGMD2R
D. LGMD2S

Hutterites, Amish and Mennonites are ethno-religious, isolated groups that have their origins from early 16th century.

2959. Which of the following distal myopathy begins in hands?

Harrison's 20th Ed. Chapter 441, Page 3246 Table 441-5

A. Welander distal myopathy
B. Tibial muscular dystrophy
C. Nonanka distal myopathy
D. Miyoshi myopathy

In autosomal dominant Welander's distal myopathy, onset is in 5th decade, weakness begins in hands and slowly progresses to involve distal lower extremities. Lifespan is normal.

2960. Which of the following distal myopathies begin in lower limbs?

Harrison's 20th Ed. Chapter 441, Page 3246 Table 441-5

A. Tibial muscular dystrophy
B. Nonanka distal myopathy
C. Miyoshi myopathy
D. All of the above

2961. Serum CK is elevated most in which of the following distal myopathies?

Harrison's 20th Ed. Chapter 441, Page 3246 Table 441-5

A. Welander distal myopathy
B. Tibial muscular dystrophy
C. Nonanka distal myopathy
D. Miyoshi myopathy

Serum CK level is is very elevated in Miyoshi myopathy. In other distal myopathies, serum CK is only slightly increased.

2962. Which of the following gene mutation is the most common cause of X-linked EDMD?

Harrison's 20th Ed. Chapter 441, Page 3247

A. FHL1
B. Lamin A/C
C. Nesprin-1
D. Emerin

Emerin mutations are the most common cause of X-linked EDMD.

2963. Which of the following gene mutation is the most common cause of autosomal dominant EDMD?

Harrison's 20th Ed. Chapter 441, Page 3247

A. FHL1
B. Lamin A/C
C. Nesprin-1
D. Emerin

2964. Autosomal dominant EDMD is also known as?

Harrison's 20th Ed. Chapter 441, Page 3247

A. LGMD1A
B. LGMD1B
C. LGMD1C
D. LGMD1D

2965. Autosomal dominant EDMD can occur with mutations in?

Harrison's 20th Ed. Chapter 441, Page 3247

A. Nesprin-1 gene
B. Nesprin-2 gene
C. TMEM43 gene
D. All of the above

2966. In EDMD, which of the following precedes muscle weakness?

Harrison's 20th Ed. Chapter 441, Page 3247

A. Cardiomyopathy
B. Atrial fibrillation
C. Atrioventricular heart block
D. Contractures

2967. In EDMD, prominent contractures are present at?

Harrison's 20th Ed. Chapter 441, Page 3248

A. Elbows
B. Ankles
C. Neck
D. All of the above

2968. In which of the following myopathies, fixed contractures occur early & are a distinctive feature of the disease?

Harrison's 20th Ed. Chapter 441, Page 3242

A. Facioscapulohumeral (FSH) Muscular Dystrophy
B. Bethlem myopathy
C. Nemaline (rod) myopathy
D. Fukuyama congenital muscular dystrophy (FCMD)

in Emery-Dreifuss muscular dystrophy and Bethlem myopathy, fixed contractures occur early and represent distinctive features of the disease.

2969. Which of the following is caused by mutations in LMNA gene?

Harrison's 20th Ed. Chapter 441, Page 3357

A. Lipodystrophies
B. Emery-Dreifuss muscular dystrophy
C. Progeria syndromes
D. All of the above

LMNA gene encodes nuclear lamins A and C. Autosomal dominant and autosomal recessive disorders are caused by mutations in LMNA gene. They include several forms of lipodystrophies, Emery-Dreifuss muscular dystrophy, progeria syndromes, a form of neuronal Charcot-Marie-Tooth disease (type 2B1), and a group of overlapping syndromes.

2970. Proximal myotonic myopathy (PROMM) is best related to?

Harrison's 20th Ed. Chapter 441, Page 3248

A. Myotonic dystrophy type 1 (DM1)
B. Myotonic dystrophy type 2 (DM2)
C. Myotonic dystrophy type 3 (DM3)
D. Myotonic dystrophy type 4 (DM4)

Myotonic dystrophy type 2 (DM2) is also called proximal myotonic myopathy (PROMM).

2971. "Hatchet-faced" appearance is typical of which of the following conditions?

Harrison's 20th Ed. Chapter 441, Page 3248

A. Facioscapulohumeral (FSH) Muscular Dystrophy
B. Myotonic dystrophy
C. Emery-Dreifuss muscular dystrophy
D. Limb-Girdle muscular dystrophy

Patients with myotonic dystrophy have a typical "hatchet-faced" appearance due to temporalis, masseter and facial muscle atrophy and weakness. Frontal baldness is also a characteristic feature.

2972. Footdrop is a feature of?

Harrison's 20th Ed. Chapter 441, Page 3248

A. Facioscapulohumeral (FSH) muscular dystrophy
B. Myotonic dystrophy type 1 (DM1)
C. Type 1 lepra reactions
D. All of the above

Besides the above, also Welander, Udd, and Markesbery-Griggs type distal myopathies cause footdrop.

2973. Hypersomnia is a feature of?

Harrison's 20th Ed. Chapter 441, Page 3248

A. Myotonic dystrophy type 1 (DM1)
B. Paraneoplastic encephalomyelitis and focal encephalitis
C. Acute radiation central nervous system (CNS) toxicity
D. All of the above

2974. In Myotonic dystrophy, involvement of which of the following muscles leads to dysarthria and dysphagia?

Harrison's 20th Ed. Chapter 441, Page 3248

A. Palatal
B. Pharyngeal
C. Tongue
D. All of the above

2975. Trinucleotide expansion is best related to?

Harrison's 20th Ed. Chapter 441, Page 3356

A. Fragile X syndrome
B. Huntington's disease
C. X-linked spinobulbar muscular atrophy
D. All of the above

Trinucleotide expansion is a a cause of the fragile X syndrome, Huntington's disease, X-linked spinobulbar muscular atrophy, and myotonic dystrophy.

2976. Which of the following is due to a CTG repeat expansion?

Harrison's 20th Ed. Chapter 441, Page 3155

A. SCA6
B. SCA7
C. SCA8
D. SCA17

Spinocerebellar ataxia1, SCA2, SCA3 (Machado-Joseph disease), SCA6, SCA7, and SCA17 are caused by CAG triplet repeat expansions in different genes. SCA8 is due to an untranslated CTG repeat expansion, SCA12 is linked to an untranslated CAG repeat, and SCA10 is caused by an untranslated pentanucleotide repeat. Myotonic dystrophy type 1 (DM1) is transmitted by an intronic mutation consisting of an unstable expansion of a CTG trinucleotide repeat in a serine-threonine protein kinase gene - DMPK.

2977. Which of the following is an "antimyotonia drug"?

Harrison's 20th Ed. Chapter 441, Page 3248

A. Mexiletine
B. Amiodarone
C. Flecainide
D. Sotalol

Phenytoin & mexiletine are the preferred antimyotonia drugs.

2978. Which of the following is the initial manifestation of FSHD?

Harrison's 20th Ed. Chapter 441, Page 3248

A. Scapular winging
B. Footdrop
C. Facial weakness
D. Nerve deafness

Facial weakness is the initial manifestation in FSHD appearing as an inability to smile, whistle, or fully close eyes.

2979. Scapular winging becomes apparent with attempts at?

Harrison's 20th Ed. Chapter 441, Page 3248

A. Abduction and forward movement of arms
B. Adduction and forward movement of arms
C. Abduction and backward movement of arms
D. Adduction and backward movement of arms

Scapular winging becomes apparent with attempts at abduction & forward movement of arms.

2980. Which of the following muscles is relatively spared in Facioscapulohumeral (FSH) muscular dystrophy?

Harrison's 20th Ed. Chapter 441, Page 3248

A. Facial
B. Biceps
C. Triceps
D. Deltoid

Weakness of shoulder girdles brings patient to the doctor. Scapular winging is common. Biceps, triceps, wrist extensors & muscles weakness of anterior compartment muscles of legs are severely affected, with relative sparing of deltoid muscles.

2981. Coats' disease is a disorder consisting of?

Harrison's 20th Ed. Chapter 441, Page 3248, Indian J Ophthalmol. 2010;58(2):119-124.

A. Retinal telangiectasia
B. Intra- and/or subretinal exudation
C. Retinal detachment
D. All of the above

The hallmark lesion of Coats' disease is idiopathic retinal telangiectasia which appears as 'light bulb appearance' on fluorescein angiography. Other features include irregular retinal vessel dilatations, retinal vessel tortuosity, areas of capillary non-perfusion, intra- and/or subretinal exudation and retinal detachment.

2982. Which of the following gene is related to FSHD1?

Harrison's 20th Ed. Chapter 441, Page 3249

A. MYO7A
B. SIX1
C. GJB2
D. DUX4

FSHD1 is associated with deletions of tandem 3.3-kb repeats at 4q35. Within these repeats lies DUX4 gene, which usually is not expressed after early muscle development. In patients with FSHD1 these deletions lead to toxic expression of DUX4 gene. In FSHD2, there is no deletion, but a mutation in SMCHD1, leading to permissive expression of DUX4 gene.

2983. Which of the following is false about oculopharyngeal muscular dystrophy (OPMD)?

Harrison's 20th Ed. Chapter 441, Page 3249

A. Progressive external ophthalmoplegia
B. Normal pupillary reactions for light & accommodation
C. No diplopia
D. None of the above

2984. Muscle fibers with rimmed vacuoles is a feature of?

Harrison's 20th Ed. Chapter 441, Page 3249

A. Welander distal myopathy
B. Oculopharyngeal muscular dystrophy (OPMD)
C. Tibial muscular dystrophy (Udd)
D. All of the above

On electron microscopy, a distinctive feature of OPMD is the presence of 8.5 nm tubular filaments in muscle cell nuclei.

2985. Which of the following gene is related to OPMD?

Harrison's 20th Ed. Chapter 441, Page 3249

A. WFS1
B. TECTA
C. COCH
D. PABP2

The molecular defect in OPMD is an expansion of a polyalanine repeat tract in a poly-RNA-binding protein (PABP2) gene.

2986. Muscle fibers with rimmed vacuoles is a feature of all except?

Harrison's 20th Ed. Chapter 441, Page 3249

A. Miyoshi myopathy
B. Inclusion body myositis (IBM)
C. Markesbery-Griggs distal myopathy
D. GNE myopathy

2987. Large deposits of myosin heavy chain in muscle fibers is a feature of?

Harrison's 20th Ed. Chapter 441, Page 3249

A. Laing distal myopathy
B. Miyoshi myopathy
C. Williams myopathy
D. Tibial muscular dystrophy (Udd)

2988. Which of the following is not a late-onset distal myopathy?

Harrison's 20th Ed. Chapter 441, Page 3249

A. Welander distal myopathy
B. Tibial muscular dystrophy (Udd)
C. Markesbery-Griggs distal myopathy
D. Laing distal myopathy

Laing distal myopathy has its onset in childhood or early adult life while rest appear after 40 years of age.

2989. Which of the following has autosomal recessive inheritance?

Harrison's 20th Ed. Chapter 441, Page 3249

A. Welander distal myopathy
B. Miyoshi myopathy
C. Tibial muscular dystrophy (Udd)
D. Markesbery-Griggs distal myopathy

GNE myopathy (Nonaka distal myopathy) and Miyoshi myopathy have autosomal recessive inheritance.

2990. Which of the following produce prominent anterior tibial weakness?

Harrison's 20th Ed. Chapter 441, Page 3249

A. GNE myopathy
B. Williams myopathy
C. Laing distal myopathy
D. All of the above

2991. In which of the following gastrocnemius muscles are preferentially affected at onset?

Harrison's 20th Ed. Chapter 441, Page 3249

A. Welander distal myopathy
B. Tibial muscular dystrophy (Udd's)
C. Laing distal myopathy
D. Miyoshi myopathy

2992. Serum CK levels are markedly elevated in?

Harrison's 20th Ed. Chapter 441, Page 3249

A. Welander distal myopathy
B. Tibial muscular dystrophy (Udd's)
C. Laing distal myopathy
D. Miyoshi myopathy

2993. Which of the following is not a congenital myopathy?

Harrison's 20th Ed. Chapter 441, Page 3240 Table 441-1

A. Central core disease
B. Nemaline (rod) myopathy
C. Miyoshi myopathy
D. Centronuclear (myotubular) myopathy

Miyoshi myopathy is a type of distal myopathy. Minicore myopathy (multi-minicore disease), fingerprint body myopathy, and sarcotubular myopathy are also congenital myopathies.

2994. Patients with which of the following congenital myopathies are susceptibile to malignant hyperthermia?

Harrison's 20th Ed. Chapter 64, Page 433

A. Central core disease
B. Nemaline (rod) myopathy
C. Centronuclear (myotubular) myopathy
D. All of the above

Malignant hyperthermia during anesthesia may occur in central core disease. C-terminal mutations of the RYR1 gene (ryanodine receptor gene on chromosome 19q) predispose to this complication.

2995. Severe brain impairment is seen in which of the following congenital muscular dystrophies?

Harrison's 20th Ed. Chapter 441, Page 3249

A. Fukuyama congenital muscular dystrophy (FCMD)
B. Muscle-eye-brain (MEB) disease
C. Walker-Warburg syndrome (WWS)
D. All of the above

Congenital muscular dystrophy with severe brain impairment are FCMD, MEB disease & WWS. In MEB & WWS, but not in FCMD, vision is impaired. WWS is the most severe congenital muscular dystrophy.

2996. Which of the following is a principal source of energy for skeletal muscles?

Harrison's 20th Ed. Chapter 441, Page 3249

A. Amino acid
B. Fatty acid
C. Lactic acid
D. All of the above

Fatty acids and glucose are the two principal sources of energy for skeletal muscles.

2997. Alpha-glucosidase or acid maltase deficiency is also called?

Harrison's 20th Ed. Chapter 441, Page 3249

A. Leigh's syndrome
B. Kearns-Sayre syndrome (KSS)
C. Pompe's disease
D. McArdle's disease

Alpha-glucosidase or acid maltase deficiency is also called Pompe's Disease. It is caused by mutations of the α-glucosidase gene.

2998. Which out of the following is the most common alpha-glucosidase, or acid maltase deficiency?

Harrison's 20th Ed. Chapter 441, Page 3249

A. Infantile form
B. Childhood form
C. Adult form
D. None of the above

There are three clinical forms of alpha-glucosidase, or acid maltase deficiency (type II glycogenosis). The infantile form is the most common, with onset of symptoms in the first 3 months of life.

2999. Which of the following about Pompe's disease is false?

Harrison's 20th Ed. Chapter 441, Page 3249

A. Autosomal recessive disorder
B. Caused by mutations of the alpha-glucosidase gene
C. Enzyme replacement tt beneficial in infantile-onset type
D. None of the above

Enzyme replacement therapy (ERT) with IV recombinant human alpha-glucosidase is beneficial in infantile-onset type.

3000. De-branching enzyme deficiency is also called?

Harrison's 20th Ed. Chapter 441, Page 3249

A. Type I glycogenosis
B. Type II glycogenosis
C. Type III glycogenosis
D. Type IV glycogenosis

α-glucosidase, or acid maltase, deficiency is called type II glycogenosis. De-branching enzyme deficiency is called type III glycogenosis while branching enzyme deficiency is called type IV glycogenosis.

3001. von Gierke's disease is also called?

Ann Neurol. 2014;76(6):891-898

A. Type I glycogenosis
B. Type II glycogenosis
C. Type III glycogenosis
D. Type IV glycogenosis

Type 0 glycogen storage disease (GSD) is called Lewis' disease. The names of various other GSD's are Type I (von Gierke's disease), Type II (Pompe's disease), Type III (Forbes-Cori disease), Type IV (Andersen's disease), Type V (McArdle's disease), Type VI (Hers' disease), Type VII (Tarui's disease), Type XI (Fanconi-Bickel syndrome).

3002. Which of the following is a disorder of glycolysis causing exercise intolerance?

Harrison's 20th Ed. Chapter 441, Page 3250

A. Myophosphorylase deficiency
B. Phosphofructokinase deficiency
C. Lactate dehydrogenase deficiency
D. All of the above

Disorders of glycolysis causing exercise intolerance include myophosphorylase deficiency (type V glycogenosis), phosphofructokinase deficiency (type VII glycogenosis), phosphoglycerate kinase deficiency (type IX glycogenosis), phosphoglycerate mutase deficiency (type X glycogenosis), lactate dehydrogenase deficiency (glycogenosis type XI), and beta-enolase deficiency. These glycolytic defects are associated with recurrent myoglobinuria.

3003. Which of the following is called McArdle's disease?

Harrison's 20th Ed. Chapter 441, Page 3250

A. Myophosphorylase deficiency
B. Phosphofructokinase deficiency
C. Lactate dehydrogenase deficiency
D. Beta-enolase deficiency

Myophosphorylase deficiency is also called McArdle's disease and is the most common of the glycolytic defects associated with exercise intolerance.

3004. McArdle disease caused by mutations in?

Harrison's 20th Ed. Chapter 441, Page 3250

A. KCNQ4 gene
B. EYA4 gene
C. ACTG1 gene
D. PYGM gene

McArdle disease caused by mutations in the PYGM gene leading to myophosphorylase deficiency.

3005. Seizure disorder with mental retardation is a feature of which of the following?

Harrison's 20th Ed. Chapter 441, Page 3250

A. Myophosphorylase deficiency
B. Phosphofructokinase deficiency
C. Phosphoglycerate kinase deficiency
D. Beta-enolase deficiency

In McArdle's disease, exercise tolerance is enhanced by warm-up or brief periods of rest. Hemolytic anemia accompany deficiencies of phosphofructokinase & phosphoglycerate kinase. Seizure disorder with mental retardation is the usual clinical presentation in phosphoglycerate kinase deficiency.

3006. Which of the following is a X-linked recessive disorder?

Harrison's 20th Ed. Chapter 441, Page 3250

A. Myophosphorylase deficiency
B. Phosphofructokinase deficiency
C. Phosphoglycerate mutase deficiency
D. Phosphoglycerate kinase deficiency

Myophosphorylase deficiency, phosphofructokinase deficiency & phosphoglycerate mutase deficiency are inherited as autosomal recessive disorders. Phosphoglycerate kinase deficiency has X-linked recessive inheritance.

3007. Which of the following statements about lipid as energy source is false?

Harrison's 20th Ed. Chapter 441, Page 3250

A. Fatty acids are derived from circulating VLDL in blood
B. Fatty acids are derived from triglycerides in muscle fibers
C. Oxidation of fatty acids occurs in mitochondria
D. None of the above

3008. To enter mitochondria, a fatty acid must first be converted to?

Harrison's 20th Ed. Chapter 441, Page 3250

A. Enoyl–acyl carrier
B. Acyl-NADH
C. Acyl-CoA
D. Amino-acyl-tRNA

Oxidation of fatty acids occurs in mitochondria. To enter mitochondria, a fatty acid must first be converted to an "activated fatty acid," acyl-CoA.

3009. Acyl-CoA must be linked to which of the following for transport into mitochondria?

Harrison's 20th Ed. Chapter 441, Page 3250

A. Acyl-CoA dehydrogenase
B. Cystinosin
C. Carnitine
D. Carnitine palmitoyltransferase (CPT) I

Acyl-CoA must be linked with carnitine by enzyme carnitine palmitoyltransferase (CPT) I for transport into mitochondria.

3010. Enzyme carnitine palmitoyltransferase (CPT) I is present on?

Harrison's 20th Ed. Chapter 441, Page 3250

A. Outer side of outer mitochondrial membrane
B. Inner side of outer mitochondrial membrane
C. Outer side of inner mitochondrial membrane
D. Inner side of inner mitochondrial membrane

Carnitine palmitoyltransferase (CPT) I is present on inner side of outer mitochondrial membrane.

3011. Enzyme carnitine palmitoyltransferase (CPT) II is present on?

Harrison's 20th Ed. Chapter 441, Page 3250

A. Outer side of outer mitochondrial membrane
B. Inner side of outer mitochondrial membrane
C. Outer side of inner mitochondrial membrane
D. Inner side of inner mitochondrial membrane

Carnitine is removed by CPT II, an enzyme attached to the inside of inner mitochondrial membrane, allowing transport of acyl-CoA into the mitochondrial matrix for beta-oxidation.

3012. Myoglobinuria in CPT2 deficiency is precipitated by?

Harrison's 20th Ed. Chapter 441, Page 3250

A. Prolonged exercise
B. Fasting
C. Infections
D. All of the above

CPT2 deficiency is much more common in men than women (5:1) and is the most common recognizable cause of recurrent myoglobinuria. Muscle pain and myoglobinuria can be precipitated by prolonged exercise, fasting or infections.

3013. Which of the following is false about human mitochondrial DNA (mtDNA)?

Harrison's 20th Ed. Chapter 441, Page 3250

A. Double-stranded circular molecule
B. Codes for transfer & ribosomal RNAs & polypeptides
C. Directly inherited from cytoplasm of oocyte mainly
D. None of the above

Each mitochondrion possesses a DNA genome that is distinct from that of nuclear DNA. Human mitochondrial DNA (mtDNA) consists of a double-strand, circular molecule comprising 16,569 base pairs. It codes for 22 transfer RNAs, 2 ribosomal RNAs, and 13 polypeptides of the respiratory chain enzymes. Genetics of mitochondrial diseases differ from genetics of chromosomal disorders. DNA of mitochondria is directly inherited from the cytoplasm of gametes, mainly oocyte. Sperm contributes very little. Thus, mitochondrial genes are derived almost exclusively from mother.

3014. Which of the following is a mitochondrial myopathy?

Harrison's 20th Ed. Chapter 441, Page 3250

A. Chronic progressive external ophthalmoplegia (CPEO)
B. Skeletal muscle - CNS syndromes
C. Pure myopathy
D. All of the above

Mitochondrial myopathies include chronic progressive external ophthalmoplegia (CPEO), skeletal muscle - CNS syndromes & pure myopathy.

3015. Which of the following about Kearns-Sayre Syndrome (KSS) is false?

Harrison's 20th Ed. Chapter 441, Page 3250

A. Onset before 20 years of age
B. CPEO
C. Pigmentary retinopathy
D. Diplopia

In CPEO, varying degrees of ptosis & weakness of extraocular muscles are seen, usually in the absence of diplopia, a point of distinction from myasthenia gravis. Triad of clinical findings in KSS includes onset before age 20, CPEO, and pigmentary retinopathy, plus one or more of the following features: complete heart block, cerebrospinal fluid protein >100 mg/dL, or cerebellar ataxia.

3016. Which of the following is the most common endocrine abnormality in Kearns-Sayre Syndrome?

Harrison's 20th Ed. Chapter 441, Page 3250

A. Diabetes mellitus
B. Addison's disease
C. Hypoparathyroidism
D. Hyperaldosteronism

Diabetes mellitus occurs in 13% of KSS patients.

3017. Which of the following about KSS is false?

Harrison's 20th Ed. Chapter 441, Page 3250

A. Sporadic disorder
B. Caused by single mtDNA deletions
C. Spontaneous deletion occur in ovum or zygote
D. Spontaneous deletion occur in spermatozoa

KSS is a sporadic disorder. The disease is caused by single mtDNA deletions arising spontaneously in the ovum or zygote. The most common deletion removes 4,977 bp of contiguous mtDNA.

3018. Which of the following is false about progressive external ophthalmoplegia (PEO)?

Harrison's 20th Ed. Chapter 441, Page 3250

A. Due to mtDNA mutations
B. Inherited in a Mendelian fashion
C. Onset is usually after puberty
D. Ragged red fibers seen in muscle biopsy

PEO is caused by nuclear DNA mutations affecting mtDNA copy number & integrity. It is inherited in a Mendelian fashion. Onset is usually after puberty. CSF protein is normal. Ragged red fibers are prominently seen in muscle biopsy.

3019. Which of the following chromosome is affected in autosomal dominant form of CPEO?

Harrison's 20th Ed. Chapter 441, Page 3250

A. 4q35
B. 10q24
C. 15q22–26
D. All of the above

Autosomal dominant form of CPEO is linked to loci on 3 chromosomes - 4q35, 10q24 & 15q22–26.

3020. "Twinkle" is the gene product of?

Harrison's 19th Ed. 462e-16

A. 4q35
B. 10q24
C. 15q22–26
D. All of the above

In chromosome 10q–related CPEO, mutations occur in C10orf2 gene. Its gene product is twinkle, named for its punctate, starlike staining properties. It co-localizes with mtDNA and is critical for lifetime maintenance of mitochondrial integrity.

3021. Enzyme important in mtDNA replication is?

Harrison's 20th Ed. Chapter 441, Page 3251

A. Carnitine palmitoyltransferase (CPT) I
B. Acid maltase
C. Myoadenylate deaminase
D. POLG

In CPEO mapped to chromosome 15q, a mutation affects the gene encoding mtDNA polymerase (POLG), an enzyme important in mtDNA replication.

3022. Characteristic feature of myoclonic epilepsy with ragged red fibers (MERRF) is?

Harrison's 20th Ed. Chapter 441, Page 3251

A. Myoclonic epilepsy
B. Cerebellar ataxia
C. Progressive muscle weakness
D. All of the above

Characteristic features include myoclonic epilepsy, cerebellar ataxia, and progressive muscle weakness in a limb-girdle distribution. Other more variable features include dementia, peripheral neuropathy, optic atrophy, hearing loss, and diabetes mellitus.

3023. To be called ragged red fiber, which of the following is abnormal in a muscle cell?

Harrison's 20th Ed. Chapter 441, Page 3250

A. Golgi apparatus
B. Mitochondria
C. Cell membrane
D. Nucleus

Term ragged red fibers was coined by Olson (1972) to describe muscle fibers with significant numbers of abnormal mitochondria (enlarged, bizarrely shaped with crystalline inclusions) highlighted with modified trichrome stain.

3024. Which of the following is caused by maternally inherited point mutations of mitochondrial tRNA gene?

Harrison's 20th Ed. Chapter 441, Page 3251

A. Kearns-Sayre syndrome (KSS)
B. MERRF
C. Pompe's disease
D. All of the above

MERRF & MELAS are caused by maternally inherited point mutations of mitochondrial tRNA genes.

3025. Which of the following about Mitochondrial Myopathy, Encephalopathy, Lactic Acidosis, and Stroke like Episodes (MELAS) is false?

Harrison's 20th Ed. Chapter 441, Page 3251

A. Cerebral lesions conform to a vascular distribution
B. Partial motor or generalized seizures
C. Serum lactic acid is elevated
D. Muscle biopsies show ragged red fibers

In MELAS, the term stroke like is appropriate because cerebral lesions do not conform to a strictly vascular distribution. Like KSS, onset is before age 20. Seizures are partial motor or generalized. Cerebral insults cause hemiparesis, hemianopia, and cortical blindness. Serum lactic acid is typically elevated. CSF protein is increased. Muscle biopsies show ragged red fibers.

3026. Which of the following about Mitochondrial Myopathy, Encephalopathy, Lactic Acidosis, and Stroke like Episodes (MELAS) is false?

Harrison's 20th Ed. Chapter 441, Page 3251

A. Focal lesions in frontal lobes
B. Basal ganglia calcification
C. Vascular territories are not respected
D. Cerebral angiography essentially normal

IN MELAS, neuroimaging shows basal ganglia calcification. Focal lesions mimiking infarction are seen mainly in occipital & parietal lobes. Strict vascular territories are not respected, and cerebral angiography does not show lesions of the major cerebral blood vessels.

3027. Which of the following is caused by maternally inherited point mutations of mitochondrial tRNA gene?

Harrison's 20th Ed. Chapter 441, Page 3251

A. Kearns-Sayre syndrome (KSS)
B. MELAS
C. Pompe's disease
D. Mitochondrial DNA depletion syndrome (MDS)

MERRF & MELAS are caused by maternally inherited point mutations of mitochondrial tRNA genes.

3028. Which of the following point mutation is most common in MELAS?

Harrison's 20th Ed. Chapter 441, Page 3251

A. A3243G point mutation in tRNALeu(UUR)
B. 3252G point mutation in tRNALeu(UUR)
C. 3256T point mutation in tRNALeu(UUR)
D. 3271C point mutation in tRNALeu(UUR)

In MELAS, A3243G point mutation in tRNALeu(UUR) is the most common (80%).

3029. Which of the following is a calcium channelopathy?

Harrison's 20th Ed. Chapter 441, Page 3251

A. Hypokalemic periodic paralysis
B. Hyperkalemic periodic paralysis
C. Paramyotonia congenita
D. Andersen-Tawil syndrome

3030. Which of the following is a potassium channelopathy?

Harrison's 20th Ed. Chapter 441, Page 3251

A. Hypokalemic periodic paralysis
B. Hyperkalemic periodic paralysis
C. Paramyotonia congenita
D. Andersen-Tawil Syndrome

3031. Hypokalemic periodic paralysis type 1 is caused by mutation in which of the following gene?

Harrison's 20th Ed. Chapter 441, Page 3251

A. CALCL1A1
B. CALCL1A2
C. CALCL1A3
D. CALCL1A4

HypoKPP type 1 is inherited as an autosomal dominant disorder with incomplete penetrance. It is due to mutations in voltage-sensitive, skeletal muscle calcium channel gene, CALCL1A3. HypoKPP type 2 is due to mutations in voltage-sensitive sodium channel gene (SCN4A). The muscle cell depolarizes when potassium levels are low.

3032. Onset of hypokalemic periodic paralysis (HypoKPP) is at?

Harrison's 20th Ed. Chapter 441, Page 3251

A. Childhood
B. Adolescence
C. Adulthood
D. Middle age

Onset of hypokalemic periodic paralysis (Hypokpp) occurs at adolescence. Episodic weakness with onset after age 25 is almost never due to periodic paralyses.

3033. In hypokalemic periodic paralysis, preferred vehicle for administration of IV potassium is?

Harrison's 20th Ed. Chapter 441, Page 3251

A. Normal saline
B. GDW
C. Ringer lactate
D. Mannitol

Treatment of hypokalemic periodic paralysis is oral KCl (0.2–0.4 mmol/kg), every 30 minutes. Should IV therapy become necessary (swallowing problems or vomiting), Mannitol is the preferred vehicle for administration of IV potassium as glucose solution may further reduce serum potassium levels.

3034. Hyperkalemic periodic paralysis (HyperKPP) is caused by mutation in which of the following gene?

Harrison's 20th Ed. Chapter 441, Page 3252

A. SCN1A
B. SCN2A
C. SCN3A
D. SCN4A

HyperKPP is an autosomal dominant disorder due to mutations of voltage-gated sodium channel SCN4A gene.

3035. Attacks of muscle weakness are induced by cold in which of the following?

Harrison's 20th Ed. Chapter 441, Page 3252

A. Thomsen's disease
B. Becker's disease
C. Paramyotonia congenita
D. All of the above

In paramyotonia congenita (PC), the attacks of weakness are cold-induced or occur spontaneously. Myotonia in chloride channel disorders - Thomsen's disease and Becker's disease is worsened by cold and improved by activity.

3036. Long QT syndrome is a feature of which of the following?

Harrison's 20th Ed. Chapter 441, Page 3252

A. Thomsen's disease
B. Becker's disease
C. Paramyotonia congenita
D. Andersen-Tawil Syndrome

Autosomal dominant Andersen-Tawil Syndrome is a potassium channel disorder characterized by episodic weakness, cardiac arrhythmias (long QT, ventricular ectopy, bidirectional ventricular arrhythmias), and dysmorphic features (short stature, scoliosis, clinodactyly, hypertelorism, small or prominent low-set ears, micrognathia, and broad forehead). It is caused by mutations of the inwardly rectifying potassium channel (Kir 2.1) gene that heighten muscle cell excitability.

3037. Serum CK level is most conspicuously elevated in which of the following endocrine myopathies?

Harrison's 20th Ed. Chapter 441, Page 3252

A. Hyperthyroidism
B. Hypothyroidism
C. Hyperparathyroidism
D. Diabetes mellitus

In hypothyroidism, serum CK level is elevated (up to 10 times normal), even when there is minimal clinical evidence of muscle disease. EMG is typically normal.

3038. Characteristic prolongation of relaxation phase of muscle stretch reflexes in hypothyroidism is best observed in?

Harrison's 20th Ed. Chapter 441, Page 3252

A. Triceps reflex
B. Biceps reflex
C. Supinator reflex
D. Knee reflex

Relaxation phase of muscle stretch reflexes is characteristically prolonged in hypothyroidism and is best observed at the ankle or biceps brachii reflexes.

3039. Which class of the following lipid-lowering agents cause myopathy?

Harrison's 20th Ed. Chapter 441, Page 3253

A. Fibrates
B. HMG-CoA reductase inhibitors (statins)
C. Niacin (nicotinic acid)
D. All of the above

All classes of lipid-lowering agents have been implicated in muscle toxicity, including fibrates (clofibrate, gemfibrozil), HMG-CoA reductase inhibitors (statins), niacin (nicotinic acid) & ezetimibe.

3040. "Acute quadriplegic" myopathy best relates to?

Harrison's 20th Ed. Chapter 441, Page 3253

A. Glucocorticoid related myopathy
B. Lipid-lowering agent related myopathy
C. Vitamin D related myopathy
D. Vitamin E related myopathy

Glucocorticoid myopathy occurs with chronic treatment or as "acute quadriplegic" myopathy secondary to high-dose IV glucocorticoid use. Acute quadriplegic myopathy can also occur in sepsis.

3041. Which of the following glucocorticoid pose a high risk for myopathy?

Harrison's 20th Ed. Chapter 441, Page 3253

A. Triamcinolone
B. Betamethasone
C. Dexamethasone
D. All of the above

Fluorinated glucocorticoids like triamcinolone, betamethasone and dexamethasone pose a high risk for myopathy.

3042. Which of the following medication can cause mitochondrial myopathy with ragged red fibers?

Harrison's 20th Ed. Chapter 441, Page 3253 Table 441-6

A. Zidovudine
B. D-penicillamine
C. Glucocorticoids
D. Vitamin D

Zidovudine myopathy produces muscle atrophy affecting thigh & calf muscles. Muscle biopsy shows ragged red fibers with minimal inflammation.

3043. Drug-related inflammatory or antibody-mediated myopathy is caused by which of the following medications?

Harrison's 20th Ed. Chapter 441, Page 3253 Table 441-6

A. Zidovudine
B. D-penicillamine
C. Glucocorticoids
D. Vitamin D

Drug-related inflammatory or antibody-mediated myopathy is most consistently caused by D-penicillamine. Myasthenia gravis and polymyositis can also occur with D-penicillamine.

Chronic Fatigue Syndrome

3044. Which of the following is not a characteristic of Chronic fatigue syndrome (CFS)?
Harrison's 20th Ed. Chapter 442, Page 3254

A. Persistent fatigue
B. Unexplained fatigue
C. Fatigue alleviated by rest
D. Severe impairment in daily functioning

Chronic fatigue syndrome (CFS) is a disorder characterized by persistent & unexplained fatigue resulting in severe impairment in daily functioning. CFS is a constellation of symptoms with no pathognomonic features and remains a diagnosis of exclusion.

3045. Institute of Medicine has renamed CFS as?
Harrison's 20th Ed. Chapter 442, Page 3254

A. Fatigue syndrome
B. Exhaustion malady
C. Systemic weariness complex
D. Systemic exercise intolerance disease

The Institute of Medicine has changed the diagnostic criteria & proposed the name of CFS as systemic exercise intolerance disease (SEID).

3046. Which of the following is a characteristic of fatigue in CFS?
Harrison's 20th Ed. Chapter 442, Page 3254 Table 442-1

A. Lasts for at least 6 months
B. Not the result of organic disease or of continuing exertion
C. Not alleviated by rest
D. All of the above

3047. In CFS, which of the following symptoms is concurrently present for 6 months?
Harrison's 20th Ed. Chapter 442, Page 3254 Table 442-1

A. Tender cervical or axillary lymph nodes
B. Impaired memory or concentration
C. Sore throat
D. All of the above

In CFS, four or more of the following symptoms are concurrently present for 6 months: impaired memory or concentration, sore throat, tender cervical or axillary lymph nodes, muscle pain, pain in several joints, new headaches, unrefreshing sleep, or malaise after exertion.

3048. Which of the following is included in the exclusion criteria of CFS?
Harrison's 20th Ed. Chapter 442, Page 3254 Table 442-1

A. Alcohol or substance abuse
B. Severe obesity
C. Schizophrenia
D. All of the above

Exclusion Criteria for defining CFS include medical condition explaining fatigue, major depressive disorder (psychotic features) or bipolar disorder, schizophrenia, dementia, or delusional disorder, anorexia nervosa, bulimia nervosa, alcohol or substance abuse and severe obesity (body mass index >40).

3049. Which of the following about CFS is false?
Harrison's 20th Ed. Chapter 442, Page 3254

A. Prevalence is higher among women
B. Associated with an increase in mortality from suicide
C. Mean age of onset is between 29 & 35 years
D. None of the above

3050. Which of the following infection state acts as a precipitating factor for CFS?
Harrison's 20th Ed. Chapter 442, Page 3254

A. Lyme disease
B. Mononucleosis
C. Q fever
D. All of the above

Mononucleosis, Q fever, Lyme disease act as the trigger of fatigue in CFS.

3051. Excessive production of which of the following induces asthenia?
Harrison's 20th Ed. Chapter 442, Page 3255

A. Interleukin 1
B. Interleukin 4
C. Interleukin 8
D. Interleukin 17

Excessive production of interleukin 1 induces asthenia and other flulike symptoms.

3052. Which of the following is beneficial in CFS?
Harrison's 20th Ed. Chapter 442, Page 3256

A. Cognitive-behavioral therapy (CBT)
B. Community reinforcement approach (CRA)
C. Contingency management (CM)
D. Motivational enhancement therapy (MET)

Cognitive-behavioral therapy (CBT) and graded exercise therapy (GET) are the only beneficial interventions in CFS.

Biology of Psychiatric Disorders

3053. Psychiatric disorder is characterized by disturbance in?

Harrison's 20th Ed. Chapter 443, Page 3256

A. Emotion

B. Cognition

C. Socialization

D. All of the above

Psychiatric disorders are central nervous system diseases characterized by disturbances in emotion, cognition, motivation & socialization. They are highly heritable, with genetic risk comprising 20–90% of disease vulnerability.

3054. Which of the following is a diagnostic scheme for classification of psychiatric illnesses?

Harrison's 20th Ed. Chapter 443, Page 3256

A. Beers criteria

B. Research domain criteria (RDoC)

C. STOPP criteria

D. Wells' criteria

Research Domain Criteria (RDoC) is proposed by National Institute of Mental Health to provide a causal framework for classification of behavioral disturbance.

3055. Which of the following is an intellectual disability syndrome?

Harrison's 20th Ed. Chapter 443, Page 3257

A. Fragile X

B. Rett syndrome

C. Tuberous sclerosis

D. All of the above

Intellectual disability syndromes include fragile X, Rett syndrome and tuberous sclerosis.

3056. Which of the following genes is related to autism spectrum disorders (ASD)?

Harrison's 20th Ed. Chapter 443, Page 3257

A. PTEN

B. TSC1

C. TSC2

D. All of the above

Genes TSC1, TSC2, and PTEN are negative regulators of signaling through the target of rapamycin complex 1 (TORC1), which regulates protein synthesis. Rapamycin is a selective inhibitor of TORC1.

3057. Fragile X syndrome is related to which of the following?

Harrison's 20th Ed. Chapter 443, Page 3257

A. CACNA1C

B. CACNB2

C. FMR1

D. MECP2

Fragile X syndrome is a cause of inherited autism and mental disability. It is due to mutations in FMR1 that result in loss of encoded fragile X mental retardation protein (FMRP). FMRP is a polyribosome-associated mRNA binding protein that represses translation of a subset of all mRNAs, several of which encode proteins that comprise postsynaptic density, including metabotropic glutamate receptor 5 (mGluR5).

3058. Copy number variants (CNVs) best relate to?

Harrison's 20th Ed. Chapter 443, Page 3257

A. Deletions

B. Duplications

C. Deletions and duplications

D. All of the above

There is striking overlap among submicroscopic deletions and duplications, called copy number variants (CNVs). They carry large risks for ASD, schizophrenia, and bipolar disorders, as well as epilepsy and intellectual disability.

3059. CHRNA5-A3-B4 nicotinic acetylcholine receptor gene cluster on chromosome 15 is associated with?

Harrison's 20th Ed. Chapter 443, Page 3257

A. Alcohol addiction

B. Cocaine addiction

C. Marijuana addiction

D. Phencyclidine addiction

CHRNA5-A3-B4 nicotinic acetylcholine receptor gene cluster on chromosome 15 is associated with nicotine and alcohol addiction.

3060. Mutations in which of the following genes can cause obsessive-compulsive & attention-deficit hyperactivity disorders?

Harrison's 20th Ed. Chapter 443, Page 3257

A. MECP2

B. FMR1

C. TSC1

D. NRXN1

Mutations in MECP2 gene can cause obsessive-compulsive & attention-deficit hyperactivity disorders.

3061. Which of the following neurotransmitter is affected in nicotine abuse?

Harrison's 20th Ed. Chapter 443, Page 3259 Table 443-1

A. GABA

B. Glutamate

C. Acetylcholine

D. Serotonin

3062. Which of the following neurotransmitter is affected in ethanol abuse?

Harrison's 20th Ed. Chapter 443, Page 3259 Table 443-1

A. GABA

B. Glutamate

C. Acetylcholine

D. All of the above

3063. Which of the following neurotransmitter is affected in cocaine abuse?

Harrison's 20th Ed. Chapter 443, Page 3259 Table 443-1

A. Endorphin

B. Glutamate

C. Dopamine

D. Serotonin

3064. Which of the following is a noncompetitive antagonist of N-methyl-D-aspartate (NMDA) glutamate receptors?

Harrison's 20th Ed. Chapter 443, Page 3259

A. Imipramine
B. Lithium
C. Tranylcypromine
D. Ketamine

Ketamine is a noncompetitive antagonist of N-methyl-D-aspartate (NMDA) glutamate receptors.

3065. Which of the following is related to morphine use?

Harrison's 20th Ed. Chapter 443, Page 3260

A. Nociceptin/orphanin
B. μ-opioid receptors
C. δ-opioid receptors
D. κ-opioid receptors

Acute activation of μ-opioid receptors by morphine activates Gi/o proteins, leading to inhibition of adenylyl cyclase (AC), resulting in reduced cyclic AMP production, protein kinase A (PKA) activation, and activation of transcription factor CREB. Other known opioid receptors are kappa, delta, and nociceptin/orphanin.

3066. Which of the following is the rate-limiting enzyme in catecholamine biosynthesis?

Harrison's 20th Ed. Chapter 443, Page 3260 Figure 443-2

A. 11β-hydroxylase
B. Tyrosine hydroxylase
C. Lysyl hydroxylase
D. Tryptophan hydroxylase

3067. Which of the following provides dopaminergic input to the limbic structures?

Harrison's 20th Ed. Chapter 443, Page 3261 Figure 443-3

A. Nucleus accumbens (NAc)
B. Ventral tegmental area (VTA)
C. Locus coeruleus (LC)
D. All of the above

Ventral tegmental area (VTA) provides dopaminergic input to all of the limbic structures.

3068. Norepinephrine best relates to which of the following?

Harrison's 20th Ed. Chapter 443, Page 3261 Figure 443-3

A. Locus coeruleus (LC)
B. Dorsal raphe (DR)
C. Arcuate nucleus
D. All of the above

3069. Arcuate nucleus releases which of the following?

Harrison's 20th Ed. Chapter 443, Page 3261 Figure 443-3

A. Norepinephrine
B. β-endorphin
C. Serotonin
D. Orexin

Arcuate nucleus releases β-endorphin and melanocortin.

3070. In schizophrenia, there is reduction of cortical & subcortical gray matter in?

Harrison's 20th Ed. Chapter 443, Page 3260

A. Frontal lobes
B. Temporal lobes
C. Limbic system
D. All of the above

3071. Neuropil includes?

Harrison's 20th Ed. Chapter 443, Page 3260

A. Axons
B. Dendrites
C. Glial cell processes
D. All of the above

The reduction in cortical thickness in schizophrenia is associated with increased cell packing density & reduced neuropil (axons, dendrites & glial cell processes) without an apparent change in neuronal cell number.

3072. The principal inhibitory neurotransmitter in the brain is?

Harrison's 20th Ed. Chapter 443, Page 3260

A. Glutamate
B. γ-aminobutyric acid (GABA)
C. Acetylcholine
D. Dopamine

Enzyme glutamic acid decarboxylase 1 (GAD1) is involved in the synthesis of γ-aminobutyric acid (GABA), GABA is the principal inhibitory neurotransmitter in the brain.

3073. Which of the following is strongly associated with schizophrenia risk?

Harrison's 20th Ed. Chapter 443, Page 3261

A. Complement component 1
B. Complement component 2
C. Complement component 3
D. Complement component 4

3074. Drugs of abuse alter neurotransmission through initial actions at?

Harrison's 20th Ed. Chapter 443, Page 3261

A. Ion channels
B. Neurotransmitter receptors
C. Neurotransmitter transporters
D. All of the above

Psychiatric Disorders

3075. Which of the following provides framework for classification of behavioral disturbance?

Harrison's 20th Ed. Chapter 444, Page 3262

A. DSM-5
B. ICD-10
C. RDoC
D. All of the above

Diagnostic and Statistical Manual of Mental Disorders (DSM-5) of the American Psychiatric Association, tenth revision of the International Classification of Diseases (ICD-10) and Research Domain Criteria (RDOC) proposed by National Institute of Mental Health are used to classify behavioral disturbances.

3076. DSM-IVTR was released in which year?

Harrison's 20th Ed. Chapter 445, Page 3280

A. 2000
B. 2001
C. 2002
D. 2004

Diagnostic and Statistical Manual of Mental Disorders of the American Psychiatric Association, 4th edition, text revision (DSM-IVTR) was released in year 2000.

3077. DSM-V was released in which year?

Harrison's 20th Ed. Chapter 444, Page 3280

A. 2008
B. 2010
C. 2012
D. 2013

3078. General medical condition leading to mental disorders is denoted by which of the following in the multiaxial system of classification?

Harrison's 18th Ed. 3529

A. Axis I
B. Axis II
C. Axis III
D. Axis IV

3079. In DSM-IV-PC, axis III disorders refer to?

Harrison's 18th Ed. 3529

A. Presence or absence of a major mental disorder
B. Any underlying personality disorder
C. General medical condition
D. Psychosocial and environmental problems

The revised fourth edition for use by primary care physicians of the Diagnostic and Statistical Manual (DSM-IV-PC) provides the current multiaxial system of classification. Presence or absence of a major mental disorder (axis I), any underlying personality disorder (axis II), general medical condition (axis III), psychosocial and environmental problems (axis IV), and overall rating of general psychosocial functioning (axis V).

3080. The most prevalent psychiatric illnesses in the general community is?

Harrison's 20th Ed. Chapter 444, Page 3262

A. Anxiety disorders
B. Personality disorders
C. Feeding and eating disorders
D. Somatic symptom disorders

Anxiety disorders are the most prevalent psychiatric illnesses in the general community, present in 15-20% of medical clinic patients.

3081. Subjective sense of unease best relates to?

Harrison's 20th Ed. Chapter 444, Page 3262

A. Anxiety
B. Panic attack
C. Obsessive-compulsive disorder
D. All of the above

Anxiety is defined as a subjective sense of unease, dread, or foreboding.

3082. Which of the following is not an anxiety disorder?

Harrison's 20th Ed. Chapter 444, Page 3262

A. Obsessive-compulsive disorder
B. Phobic disorder
C. Bipolar disorder
D. Stress disorder

3083. Which of the following about panic disorder is false?

Harrison's 20th Ed. Chapter 444, Page 3262

A. Diagnostic criteria require at least 1 month history
B. Sudden onset, usually resolving in an hour
C. First attack is usually outside the home
D. None of the above

3084. Agoraphobia commonly accompanies?

Harrison's 20th Ed. Chapter 444, Page 3263

A. Bipolar disorder
B. Panic disorder
C. Obsessive-compulsive disorder
D. All of the above

Agoraphobia occurs commonly in patients with panic disorder. It is an acquired irrational fear of being in places where one might feel trapped or unable to escape.

3085. Which of the following medical disorders can present as an attack of panic disorder?

Harrison's 20th Ed. Chapter 444, Page 3263

A. Pheochromocytoma
B. Thyrotoxicosis
C. Hypoglycemia
D. All of the above

3086. Which of the following can evoke an attack of panic disorder?

Harrison's 20th Ed. Chapter 444, Page 3263

A. Intravenous infusion of sodium lactate
B. Carbon dioxide inhalation
C. Cholecystokinin tetrapeptide (CCK-4)
D. All of the above

IV sodium lactate, alpha2-adrenergic antagonist yohimbine, cholecystokinin tetrapeptide (CCK-4), and carbon dioxide inhalation evoke a panic attack in panic disorder patients by activating a pathway involving noradrenergic neurons in locus coeruleus and serotonergic neurons in dorsal raphe. Agents that block serotonin reuptake can prevent attacks.

3087. Which of the following SSRIs has very long half-life?

Harrison's 20th Ed. Chapter 444, Page 3264 Table 444-1

A. Fluoxetine
B. Citalopram
C. Paroxetine
D. Sertraline

3088. Which of the following is a serotonin-norepinephrine reuptake inhibitor (SNRI)?

Harrison's 20th Ed. Chapter 444, Page 3263

A. Fluoxetine
B. Venlafaxine
C. Paroxetine
D. Sertraline

Fluoxetine, paroxetine, sertraline are selective serotonin reuptake inhibitors (SSRIs), and venlafaxine is a serotonin-norepinephrine reuptake inhibitor (SNRI).

3089. Which of the following is the most noradrenergic of SNRIs?

Harrison's 20th Ed. Chapter 444, Page 3264 Table 444-1

A. Vortioxetine
B. Levomilnacipran
C. Mirtazapine
D. Duloxetine

3090. Which of the following tricyclic antidepressants (TCA) is best tolerated, especially by elderly?

Harrison's 20th Ed. Chapter 444, Page 3264 Table 444-1

A. Amitriptyline
B. Nortriptyline
C. Imipramine
D. Doxepin

3091. MAOIs should not be used concomitantly with?

Harrison's 20th Ed. Chapter 444, Page 3263

A. Selective serotonin reuptake inhibitors (SSRIs)
B. Serotonin-norepinephrine reuptake inhibitor (SNRI)
C. Tricyclic antidepressants (TCA)
D. All of the above

MAOIs should not be used concomitantly with SSRIs, because of the risk of serotonin syndrome, or with TCAs, because of possible hyperadrenergic effects.

3092. Antidepressants typically take how much time to become effective?

Harrison's 20th Ed. Chapter 444, Page 3263

A. 24–36 hours
B. 5–10 days
C. 1–3 weeks
D. 2–6 weeks

Antidepressants typically take 2–6 weeks to become effective.

3093. In treatment resistant panic disorder cases, which of the following is efficacious?

Harrison's 20th Ed. Chapter 444, Page 3263

A. Aripiprazole
B. Divalproex sodium
C. Pindolol
D. All of the above

In treatment resistant panic disorder cases, short-term augmentation with aripiprazole, divalproex sodium or pindolol is efficacious.

3094. In panic disorders, following recovery, drug treatment should be continued for what length of time?

Harrison's 20th Ed. Chapter 444, Page 3263

A. 3–6 months
B. 1–2 years
C. 2–5 years
D. Life long

In panic disorders, once patients have achieved a satisfactory response, drug treatment should be maintained for 1–2 years to prevent relapse.

3095. Which of the following is a mixed norepinephrine/serotonin reuptake inhibitors and receptor blocker?

Harrison's 20th Ed. Chapter 444, Page 3264 Table 444-1

A. Venlafaxine
B. Duloxetine
C. Mirtazapine
D. All of the above

Venlafaxine, Desvenlafaxine, Duloxetine, Mirtazapine, Vilazodone, Vortioxetine and Levomilnacipran are mixed norepinephrine/serotonin reuptake inhibitors (SNRI) and receptor blockers.

3096. Which of the following is a monoamine oxidase inhibitor (MAOI)?

Harrison's 20th Ed. Chapter 444, Page 3264 Table 444-1

A. Amoxapine
B. Bupropion
C. Phenelzine
D. Trazodone

Phenelzine, Tranylcypromine, Isocarboxazid, and selegiline are MAOIs.

3097. Extrapyramidal symptoms can appear with the use of?

Harrison's 20th Ed. Chapter 444, Page 3264 Table 444-1

A. Amoxapine
B. Bupropion
C. Phenelzine
D. Trazodone

3098. Which of the following is to be avoided when monoamine oxidase inhibitors (MAOIs) are used?

Harrison's 20th Ed. Chapter 444, Page 3263

A. Tobacco
B. Coffee
C. Wine
D. Whisky

Patients taking monoamine oxidase inhibitors (MAOIs) need to maintain a low-tyramine die, i.e. avoidance of cheese and wine.

3099. Which of the following is a weak, reversible monoamine oxidase inhibitor?

Harrison's 20th Ed. Chapter 139, Page 1055

A. Rifamycin
B. Colistin
C. Linezolid
D. Nitrofurantoin

Linezolid is a weak, reversible monoamine oxidase inhibitor and coadministration with sympathomimetics and foods rich in tyramine should be avoided. Linezolid has been associated with serotonin syndrome when coadministered with selective serotonin-reuptake inhibitors.

3100. Which of the following is contraindicated to use along with monoamine oxidase inhibitor?

Harrison's 20th Ed. Chapter 422, Page 3103

A. Tyramine containing foods
B. Decongestants
C. Meperidine
D. All of the above

3101. Which of the following is a monoamine oxidase inhibitor?

Harrison's 20th Ed. Chapter 217, Page 1563

A. Mebendazole
B. Halofantrine
C. Furazolidone
D. Ivermectin

Furazolidone is a monoamine oxidase (MAO) inhibitor. Furazolidone inhibits MAOs gradually over several days, so the risks are small if treatment is limited to a 5-day course.

3102. Anorgasmia/impotence occurring as side effect of antidepressant medication is managed with?

Harrison's 20th Ed. Chapter 444, Page 3265 Table 444-2

A. Cyproheptadine
B. Bupropion
C. Amantadine
D. Any of the above

3103. Diarrhea occurring as side effect of antidepressant medication is managed with?

Harrison's 20th Ed. Chapter 444, Page 3265 Table 444-2

A. Cyproheptadine
B. Bupropion
C. Fluoxetine
D. Famotidine

3104. Which of the following anxiolytic drugs has no active metabolite?

Harrison's 20th Ed. Chapter 444, Page 3266 Table 444-4

A. Oxazepam
B. Temazepam
C. Clonazepam
D. All of the above

Oxazepam, Temazepam, Clonazepam, Lorazepam, and Triazolam have no active metabolites. Diazepam, Alprazolam, Chlordiazepoxide, and Buspirone have active metabolites.

3105. Which of the following benzodiazepines is difficult to withdraw?

Harrison's 20th Ed. Chapter 444, Page 3266 Table 444-4

A. Alprazolam
B. Clonazepam
C. Chlordiazepoxide
D. Oxazepam

3106. Which of the following benzodiazepines is a prodrug?

Harrison's 20th Ed. Chapter 444, Page 3266 Table 444-4

A. Flurazepam
B. Triazolam
C. Lorazepam
D. Temazepam

3107. Many patients with generalized anxiety disorder (GAD) also suffer from?

Harrison's 20th Ed. Chapter 444, Page 3263

A. Major depression
B. Dysthymia
C. Social phobia
D. All of the above

3108. Which of the following complaints are relatively rare in generalized anxiety disorder (GAD)?

Harrison's 20th Ed. Chapter 444, Page 3263

A. Shortness of breath
B. Palpitations
C. Tachycardia
D. All of the above

Unlike panic disorders, complaints of shortness of breath, palpitations, and tachycardia are relatively rare in generalized anxiety disorder (GAD).

3109. Which of the following statements is false?

Harrison's 20th Ed. Chapter 444, Page 3263

A. All anxiogenic agents act on GABA-A receptor/chloride ion channel complex
B. Serotonin (5-HT) has a role in anxiety
C. 3α-reduced neuroactive steroids has a role in anxiety
D. None of the above

All anxiogenic agents act on the γ-aminobutyric acid (GABA)A receptor/chloride ion channel complex.

3110. Which of the following is a GABA-A type II receptor site?

Harrison's 20th Ed. Chapter 444, Page 3263

A. Hippocampus
B. Striatum
C. Neocortex
D. All of the above

Benzodiazepines bind two separate GABA-A receptor sites: type I, has wide neuroanatomic distribution, and type II, which is concentrated in hippocampus, striatum & neocortex.

3111. Sedation & memory impairment of benzodiazepines is related to?

Harrison's 20th Ed. Chapter 444, Page 3263

A. Alpha 1 subunit of GABA-A receptor
B. Alpha 2 subunit of GABA-A receptor
C. Alpha 3 subunit of GABA-A receptor
D. All of the above

Anti-anxiety effects of benzodiazepines are influenced by their relative binding to alpha 2 & 3 subunits of GABA-A receptor, and sedation and memory impairment to the alpha 1 subunit.

3112. Which of the following is a 5-HT1A agonist?

Harrison's 20th Ed. Chapter 444, Page 3263

A. Lorazepam
B. Buspirone
C. Oxazepam
D. Alprazolam

Buspirone and tandospirone are 5-HT1A agonists.

3113. Which of the following is a 5-HT2A & 5-HT2C receptor antagonist?

Harrison's 20th Ed. Chapter 444, Page 3263

A. Mirtazapine
B. Nefazodone
C. Lorcaserin
D. Pimavanserin

Mirtazapine is a 5-HT2A receptor antagonist. Lorcaserin is a selective 5-HT2C receptor agonist. Pimavanserin is an inverse agonist of serotonin 5-HT2A receptor.

3114. Benzodiazepines should not be prescribed for more than how many weeks to avoid risk of abuse and dependence?

Harrison's 20th Ed. Chapter 444, Page 3264

A. 1–2 weeks
B. 2–3 weeks
C. 3–4 weeks
D. 4–6 weeks

Benzodiazepines should not be prescribed for >4–6 weeks because of the development of tolerance and the risk of abuse & dependence.

3115. Which of the following is not a long-acting benzodiazepine?

Harrison's 20th Ed. Chapter 444, Page 3264

A. Diazepam
B. Alprazolam
C. Flurazepam
D. Clonazepam

Longer-acting benzodiazepines are diazepam, chlordiazepoxide, flurazepam, and clonazepam. Shorter-acting benzodiazepines are alprazolam, lorazepam and oxazepam. It is more difficult to taper patients off shorter-acting benzodiazepines.

3116. Which of the following is a non-benzodiazepine anxiolytic agent?

Harrison's 20th Ed. Chapter 444, Page 3265

A. Diazepam
B. Buspirone
C. Flurazepam
D. Clonazepam

Buspirone is a nonbenzodiazepine anxiolytic agent. It is nonsedating, does not produce tolerance or dependence, does not interact with benzodiazepine receptors or alcohol, and has no abuse or disinhibition potential. But, requires several weeks to take effect and thrice-daily dosing.

3117. Which of the following is contraindicated during pregnancy?

Harrison's 20th Ed. Chapter 118, Page 887

A. Live-virus vaccines
B. Clarithromycin
C. Primaquine
D. All of the above

Pregnancy is not a contraindication to administration of inactivated vaccines, but should be avoided.

3118. Which of the following is contraindicated during pregnancy?

Harrison's 20th Ed. Chapter 264, Page 1831

A. Angiotensin converting enzyme (ACE) inhibitors
B. Angiotensin receptor blockers
C. Endothelin-receptor blockers
D. All of the above

3119. Which of the following is contraindicated during pregnancy?

Harrison's 20th Ed. Chapter 264, Page 1831

A. Miltefosine
B. IFN-based therapy
C. Ribavirin
D. All of the above

3120. Which of the following is contraindicated during pregnancy?

Harrison's 20th Ed. Chapter 444, Page 3265

A. Methotrexate
B. Leflunomide
C. Benzodiazepines
D. All of the above

Benzodiazepines are contraindicated during pregnancy and breast-feeding.

3121. Which of the following is contraindicated during breast-feeding?

Harrison's 20th Ed. Chapter 444, Page 3265

A. Treatment for TB
B. Live-virus or other vaccines
C. Warfarin
D. None of the above

Treatment for TB, live-virus or other vaccines & warfarin are not contraindicated in breast-feeding women. Breast-feeding is not contraindicated in women with hepatitis B. Breast-feeding does not increase the risk of HCV infection between an infected mother and her infant.

3122. Which of the following is contraindication for breast-feeding?

Harrison's 20th Ed. Chapter 444, Page 3265

A. HIV
B. Diloxanide furoate
C. Furazolidone
D. All of the above

Pregnancy and breast-feeding are absolute contraindications to radioiodine treatment. Also, use of Atovaquone-proguanil & ivermectin should be avoided.

3123. Which of the following anticonvulsants with GABAergic properties is beneficial in anxiety-related syndromes?

Harrison's 20th Ed. Chapter 444, Page 3265

A. Gabapentin
B. Pregabalin
C. Divalproex
D. All of the above

Anticonvulsants with GABAergic properties like gabapentin, oxcarbazepine, tiagabine, pregabalin, and divalproex are beneficial in anxiety-related syndromes.

3124. Which of the following about phobic disorders is false?

Harrison's 20th Ed. Chapter 444, Page 3265

A. Marked & persistent fear of objects or situations
B. Usually experience anxiety only in specific situations
C. Processing of fear stimulus occurs in lateral nucleus of amygdala
D. None of the above

Processing of fear stimulus occurs through lateral nucleus of the amygdala, extending through central nucleus & projecting to periaqueductal gray region, lateral hypothalamus & paraventricular hypothalamus.

3125. Which of the following is useful in treatment of "performance anxiety"?

Harrison's 20th Ed. Chapter 444, Page 3265

A. Benzodiazepines
B. Propranolol
C. MAOIs
D. All of the above

Beta blockers like propranolol, 20–40 mg orally 2 hours before the event, are effective in the treatment of "performance anxiety".

3126. Which of the following is useful in treatment of social anxiety?

Harrison's 20th Ed. Chapter 444, Page 3265

A. Paroxetine
B. Sertraline
C. Venlafaxine
D. All of the above

3127. Risk factor for the development of Posttraumatic Stress Disorder (PTSD) is?

Harrison's 20th Ed. Chapter 444, Page 3266

A. Past psychiatric history
B. High neuroticism
C. Extroversion
D. All of the above

3128. Which of the following is related to PTSD?

Harrison's 20th Ed. Chapter 444, Page 3266

A. Central tegmental area (VTA)
B. Locus coeruleus
C. Nucleus accumbens (NAc)
D. All of the above

In PTSD, there is excessive release of norepinephrine from locus coeruleus in response to stress & increased noradrenergic activity at projection sites in hippocampus & amygdala.

3129. Which of the following may be beneficial in preventing development of PTSD?

Harrison's 20th Ed. Chapter 444, Page 3267

A. Hydrocortisone
B. Intranasal oxytocin
C. Morphine
D. All of the above

3130. Comorbid alcoholism in PTSD is best treated with?

Harrison's 20th Ed. Chapter 444, Page 3267

A. Nefazadone
B. Topiramate
C. Naltrexone
D. Mirtazepine

Comorbid alcoholism in PTSD is best treated with naltrexone.

3131. In obsessive-compulsive disorder (OCD), obsession pertains to?

Harrison's 20th Ed. Chapter 444, Page 3267

A. Thoughts
B. Actions
C. Behavior
D. All of the above

Obsessive-compulsive disorder (OCD) is characterized by obsessive thoughts and compulsive behaviors that impair everyday functioning.

3132. Which of the following is the most frequent comorbid condition in OCD?

Harrison's 20th Ed. Chapter 444, Page 3267

A. Depression
B. Eating disorders
C. Tics
D. All of the above

In OCD, comorbid conditions are common, the most frequent being depression, other anxiety disorders, eating disorders, and tics.

3133. Obsessive-compulsive disorder (OCD) is related to which of the following clinical conditions?

Harrison's 20th Ed. Chapter 444, Page 3268

A. Wilson's disease
B. Myoclonus
C. Tourette's syndrome
D. Parkinson's disease

Family studies show an aggregation of OCD with Tourette's disorder. Both are more common in males and in first-born children.

3134. Anatomy of obsessive-compulsive behavior includes?

Harrison's 20th Ed. Chapter 444, Page 3268

A. Orbital frontal cortex
B. Caudate nucleus
C. Globus pallidus
D. All of the above

3135. Which of the following part of the brain is responsible for acquisition and maintenance of habit and skill learning?

Harrison's 20th Ed. Chapter 444, Page 3268

A. Hippocampus
B. Amygdala
C. Caudate nucleus
D. Mammillary bodies

Anatomical localization of obsessive-compulsive behavior is to orbital frontal cortex, caudate nucleus, & globus pallidus. Caudate nucleus is involved in acquisition & maintenance of habit & skill learning.

3136. Which of the following is useful in the treatment of obsessive-compulsive disorder (OCD)?

Harrison's 20th Ed. Chapter 444, Page 3268

A. Clomipramine
B. Fluoxetine
C. Fluvoxamine
D. All of the above

3137. In treatment resistant cases of OCD, which of the following is added to treatment?

Harrison's 20th Ed. Chapter 444, Page 3268

A. Buspirone
B. Neuroleptic
C. Benzodiazepine
D. Any of the above

Clomipramine, fluoxetine, fluvoxamine, and sertraline are useful in the treatment of OCD. In treatment-resistant cases, augmentation with buspirone, neuroleptic or benzodiazepine is beneficial and in severe cases deep brain stimulation is effective.

3138. Which of the following about Obsessive-Compulsive Disorder is false?

N Engl J Med. 2014;371:646-53

A. Male:female sex ratio is approximately 1:1
B. Onset after 30 years of age is unusual
C. Hyperactivity in orbitofrontal cortex & caudate
D. None of the above

Studies have consistently shown hyperactivity in the orbitofrontal cortex and caudate in OCD. Other key implicated regions suggesting abnormalities in functional or structural connections include anterior cingulate cortex, thalamus, amygdala, and parietal cortex.

3139. Obsessions are?

N Engl J Med. 2014;371:646-53

A. Recurrent thoughts
B. Recurrent urges
C. Recurrent images
D. All of the above

Obsessions are recurrent thoughts, urges, or images that are experienced, at some time, as intrusive and unwanted. Compulsions are repetitive behaviors (hand washing, ordering, and checking) or mental acts (praying and counting) that the person feels driven to perform in response to an obsession. The diagnosis of OCD requires that a person have obsessions, compulsions, or both.

3140. Persons with OCD may have which of the following?

N Engl J Med. 2014;371:646-53

A. Hallucinations
B. Smell disorder
C. Color blindness
D. Tic disorder

Up to 30% of persons with OCD have a tic disorder. Its presence is associated with a poor response to pharmacotherapy for OCD in children & adolescents. An early age at OCD onset, more severe OCD, coexisting tics, and hoarding symptoms have all been associated with a poor response to clomipramine and SSRIs.

3141. Which of the following is not a selective serotonin-reuptake inhibitor (SSRI)?

N Engl J Med. 2014;371:646-53

A. Paroxetine
B. Fluvoxamine
C. Clomipramine
D. Sertraline

Clomipramine is a tricyclic antidepressant. Paroxetine, fluvoxamine, fluoxetine, citalopram, escitalopram, and sertralineor are selective serotonin-reuptake inhibitor (SSRI) and in OCD are the first-line pharmacologic treatment.

3142. Mood disorders are characterized by a disturbance in the regulation of?

Harrison's 20th Ed. Chapter 444, Page 3268

A. Mood
B. Behavior
C. Affect
D. All of the above

Mood disorders are characterized by a disturbance in the regulation of mood, behavior, and affect.

3143. Which of the following is a mood disorder?

Harrison's 20th Ed. Chapter 444, Page 3268

A. Depressive disorders
B. Bipolar disorders
C. Depression in association with medical illness or alcohol and substance abuse
D. All of the above

3144. Which of the following about major depressive disorder (MDD) is false?

Harrison's 20th Ed. Chapter 444, Page 3268

A. Absence of manic or hypomanic episode in MDD
B. MDD more frequent in families of bipolar individuals
C. Bipolar disorder more frequent in families of MDD individuals
D. None of the above

3145. Depressive symptoms can be triggered by which of the following group of drugs?

Harrison's 20th Ed. Chapter 444, Page 3268

A. Antihypertensive drugs
B. Anticholesterolemic drugs
C. Antiarrhythmic drugs
D. All of the above

3146. Iatrogenic depression can be caused by which of the following group of drugs?

Harrison's 20th Ed. Chapter 444, Page 3268

A. Glucocorticoids
B. Antimicrobials
C. Systemic analgesics
D. All of the above

Iatrogenic depression can be induced by antihypertensives, anticholesterolemics, antiarrhythmics, glucocorticoids, antimicrobials, systemic analgesics, antiparkinsonian medications, and anticonvulsants.

3147. Which of the following occurs in patients with depression?

Harrison's 20th Ed. Chapter 444, Page 3268

A. Reduced parasympathetic nervous system activity
B. Increased platelet aggregation
C. Increased risk of subsequent diagnosis of Alzheimer's disease
D. All of the above

3148. Which of the following can produce hyperglycemia and carbohydrate craving?

Harrison's 20th Ed. Chapter 444, Page 3268

A. MAOI
B. TCAs
C. SSRIs
D. All of the above

MAOIs can induce hypoglycemia and weight gain, while TCAs can produce hyperglycemia and carbohydrate craving. SSRIs, like MAOIs, may reduce fasting plasma glucose.

3149. Major depression is defined as depressed mood on a daily basis for?

Harrison's 20th Ed. Chapter 444, Page 3268

A. A minimum duration of 1 week
B. A minimum duration of 2 weeks
C. A minimum duration of 4 weeks
D. A minimum duration of 6 weeks

Major depression is defined as depressed mood on a daily basis for a minimum duration of 2 weeks.

3150. In patients with depression, mood is worse in?

Harrison's 20th Ed. Chapter 444, Page 3269

A. Morning
B. Afternoon
C. Evening
D. Night

Major depression is defined as depressed mood on a daily basis for a minimum duration of 2 weeks. Patients with depression often notice a diurnal variation in mood, worse in morning hours.

3151. Presence of which of the following significantly increases near-term suicidal risk in depressed patients?

Harrison's 20th Ed. Chapter 444, Page 3269

A. Anxiety
B. Agitation
C. Panic
D. All of the above

Presence of anxiety, panic, or agitation significantly increases near-term suicidal risk in depressed patients. ~4–5% of all depressed patients will commit suicide.

3152. Dysthymic disorder best relates to?

Harrison's 20th Ed. Chapter 444, Page 3269

A. Seasonal affective disorder
B. Persistent depressive disorder
C. Pseudodementia
D. Cyclothymic disorder

Dysthymic disorder refers to a persistent depressive disorder that consists of a pattern of chronic (at least 2 years), ongoing depressive symptoms that are usually less severe and/or less numerous than those found in major depression, but the functional consequences may be equivalent to or even greater. The two conditions can occur together and it is labeled as "double depression".

3153. Which of the following about depression is false?

Harrison's 20th Ed. Chapter 444, Page 3269

A. Men : women ration in depression is ~1 : 2
B. Incidence of depression increases with age in both sexes
C. Major depression of early onset is largely genetic in origin
D. None of the above

3154. Which of the following about unipolar depressive disorders is false?

Harrison's 20th Ed. Chapter 444, Page 3269

A. Usually begin in early adulthood
B. Recur episodically
C. Best predictor of future risk is the number of past episodes
D. None of the above

3155. Seasonal affective disorder best relates to?

Harrison's 20th Ed. Chapter 444, Page 3269

A. Seasonal pattern of depression
B. Depression in seasoned individuals
C. Depression in other members of family
D. Any of the above

A seasonal pattern of depression, which is more common in women, is called seasonal affective disorder. It manifests with onset & remission of episodes at predictable times of the year. The prevalence of depression increases with distance from equator, and improvement may occur by altering light exposure.

3156. Neuro-endocrine abnormality that reflect neuro-vegetative signs & symptoms of depression is?

Harrison's 20th Ed. Chapter 444, Page 3269

A. Increased cortisol & CRH secretion
B. Blunted response of TSH level to infusion of TRH
C. Decreased inhibitory response of glucocorticoids to dexamethasone
D. All of the above

Neuroendocrine abnormalities that reflect the neurovegetative signs & symptoms of depression include increased cortisol and corticotropin-releasing hormone (CRH) secretion, decreased inhibitory response of glucocorticoids to dexamethasone and blunted response of thyroid-stimulating hormone (TSH) level to infusion of thyroid-releasing hormone (TRH). Antidepressant treatment normalizes these abnormalities. Major depression is also associated with an upregulation of proinflammatory cytokines, and neurotrophins, an increase in measures of oxidative stress & cellular aging, telomere shortening & mitochondrial dysfunction.

3157. Sleep abnormality in patients with major depression is?

Harrison's 20th Ed. Chapter 444, Page 3269

A. Decrease in REM sleep
B. Increase in REM density
C. Decrease in stage IV delta slow-wave sleep
D. All of the above

Patients with major depression show a decrease in rapid eye movement (REM) sleep onset (REM latency), an increase in REM density, and, a decrease in stage IV delta slow-wave sleep.

3158. Which of the following is an ideal antidepressant?

Harrison's 20th Ed. Chapter 444, Page 3270

A. SSRI
B. TCA
C. MAOI
D. None of the above

There is no ideal antidepressant. No current compound combines rapid onset of action, moderate half-life, a meaningful relationship between dose & blood level, a low side effect profile, minimal interaction with other drugs, and safety in overdose.

3159. Which tricyclic antidepressant carries the greatest risk in overdose?

Harrison's 20th Ed. Chapter 444, Page 3270

A. Desipramine
B. Imipramine
C. Nortriptyline
D. Amitriptyline

Overdoses of tricyclic agents can be lethal, with desipramine carrying the greatest risk. TCAs are contraindicated in patients with serious cardiovascular risk factors.

3160. Which of the following is false about serotonin syndrome?

Harrison's 20th Ed. Chapter 444, Page 3270

A. Myoclonus
B. Abdominal cramping
C. Hyperpyrexia
D. Hypotension

MAOIs used concomitantly with SSRIs can lead to serotonin syndrome that results from hyperstimulation of brainstem 5HT1A receptors and is characterized by myoclonus, agitation, abdominal cramping, hyperpyrexia, hypertension, and potentially death.

3161. Akathisia refers to?

Harrison's 20th Ed. Chapter 444, Page 3270

A. Phobias for high pitched sounds
B. Inner sense of restlessness and anxiety
C. Obsession for cleanliness
D. Transient blindness

Akathisia refers to an inner sense of restlessness and anxiety.

3162. SSRI induced sexual dysfunction can be ameliorated by?

Harrison's 20th Ed. Chapter 444, Page 3270

A. Amantadine
B. Bethanechol
C. Buspirone
D. All of the above

All SSRIs impair sexual function. Sexual dysfunction can be ameliorated by lowering dose, weekend drug holidays, or by treatment with amantadine, bethanechol, buspirone, or bupropion.

3163. Principal active metabolite of Fluoxetine is?

Harrison's 20th Ed. Chapter 444, Page 3270

A. Isofluoxetine
B. Parfluoxetine
C. Norfluoxetine
D. Metafluoxetine

Principal active metabolite of Fluoxetine is Norfluoxetine.

3164. Which of the following is the most noradrenergic of the SNRI?

Harrison's 20th Ed. Chapter 444, Page 3271

A. Mirtazapine
B. Desvenlafaxine
C. Levomilnacipran
D. Vortioxetine

Levomilnacipran is the most noradrenergic of the SNRIs and theoretically may be appropriate for patients with more severe fatigue and anergia.

3165. Which of the following gene relates to serotonin transporter?

N Engl J Med. 2009;360:957

A. PCDH10
B. SHANK3
C. 5-HTT/SLC6A4
D. OXTR

In CNS, serotonin synthesis is catalyzed by Tph2. It is released at neural synapses, and its reuptake is controlled by 5-HTT. Circulating serotonin does not cross blood–brain barrier, so all its activity in brain is mediated by synthesis, reuptake, and binding to a 5-HT receptor (Htr). Pharmacologic inhibition of 5-HTT by SSRIs enhances serotonin activity.

3166. Which amino acid is the precursor of serotonin?

Harrison's 20th Ed. Chapter 80, Page 604

A. Tryptophan
B. Leucine
C. Isoleucine
D. Arginine

Serotonin (5-HT) is synthesized from tryptophan.

3167. Which of the following is a biologic effect of serotonin?

Harrison's 20th Ed. Chapter 80, Page 604

A. Stimulating intestinal secretion with inhibition of absorption
B. Stimulating increases in intestinal motility
C. Stimulating fibrogenesis
D. All of the above

3168. Which of the following about Mirtazapine is false?

Harrison's 20th Ed. Chapter 9, Page 56, 3271

A. Sedating, antiemetic and anxiolytic
B. Increases noradrenergic & serotonergic neurotransmission
C. Strongly antihistaminic
D. Weight loss

Mirtazapine is an antagonist at the postsynaptic serotonin receptors.

3169. Which of the following is a nonamphetamine psychostimulant with minimal abuse potential?

Harrison's 20th Ed. Chapter 9, Page 56

A. Dextroamphetamine
B. Methylphenidate
C. Modafinil
D. Pemoline

Pemoline is a nonamphetamine psychostimulant with minimal abuse potential.

3170. Which of the following SSRI is preferred in a patient in whom fatigue is a major symptom?

Harrison's 20th Ed. Chapter 9, Page 57

A. Paroxetine
B. Fluoxetine
C. Citalopram
D. Sertraline

For a patient in whom fatigue is a major symptom, a more activating SSRI (fluoxetine) is appropriate. For a patient in whom anxiety & sleeplessness are major symptoms, a sedating SSRI (paroxetine) is appropriate.

3171. Which of the following antidepressants can cause priapism?

Harrison's 20th Ed. Chapter 9, Page 57

A. Paroxetine
B. Trazodone
C. Bupropion
D. Sertraline

Antidepressant Trazodone is sedating, can cause orthostatic hypotension and priapism.

3172. Which of the following SSRI is associated with significant risk of sexual dysfunction?

Harrison's 20th Ed. Chapter 390, Page 2818

A. Escitalopram
B. Bupropion
C. Nefazodone
D. Mirtazapine

Among the SSRIs, paroxetine & escitalopram are associated with the highest risk of sexual dysfunction.

3173. Which of the following is a postsynaptic agonist of serotonin receptor 1A and antagonist of serotonin receptor 2A?

Harrison's 20th Ed. Chapter 390, Page 2818

A. Cyproterone acetate
B. Safinamide
C. Alprostadil
D. Flibanserin

Flibanserin, a postsynaptic agonist of serotonin receptor 1A and antagonist of serotonin receptor 2A, increases sexual desire and reduces resultant stress in women with HypoSexual Desire Disorder (HSDD)

3174. Which of the following SSRIs has no specific inhibitory effects on the P450 system?

Harrison's 20th Ed. Chapter 444, Page 3271

A. Sertraline
B. Escitalopram
C. Fluoxetine
D. Paroxetine

With the exception of citalopram & escitalopram, each of the SSRIs inhibits one or more cytochrome P450 enzymes.

3175. Which of the following is useful in managing treatment-resistant depression?

Harrison's 20th Ed. Chapter 444, Page 3271

A. Repetitive transcranial magnetic stimulation (rTMS)
B. Vagus nerve stimulation (VNS)
C. Deep brain stimulation (DBS)
D. All of the above

Electroconvulsive therapy, Transcranial magnetic stimulation (TMS), Vagus nerve stimulation (VNS) and Deep brain stimulation (DBS) are useful in managing treatment resistant depression.

3176. Response to treatment of depression should be evaluated after how many months?

Harrison's 20th Ed. Chapter 444, Page 3271

A. 1 month
B. 2 months
C. 3 months
D. 6 months

Regardless of the modality of treatment for depression, response should be evaluated after 2 months.

3177. Which of the following distinguish bipolar I mania from bipolar II hypomania?

N Engl J Med. 2011;364:51-9

A. Suicidal tendancy
B. Voluntarily produced physical symptoms of illness
C. Severity of elevated mood
D. Intentionally produced deficit symptoms

The greater severity of elevated mood and associated functional disability distinguish bipolar I mania (which is characterized by psychosis, the need for urgent care or hospitalization, or marked impairment) from bipolar II hypomania.

3178. Montgomery and Åsberg Depression Rating Scale (MADRS) ranges from?

N Engl J Med. 2011;364:51-9

A. 0 to 20
B. 0 to 40
C. 0 to 60
D. 0 to 80

Montgomery and Åsberg Depression Rating Scale [MADRS] ranges from 0 to 60.

3179. Which of the following is a feature of bipolar disorders?

Harrison's 20th Ed. Chapter 444, Page 3271

A. Mania
B. Hypomania
C. Depression
D. All of the above

Bipolar disorder is characterized by unpredictable swings in mood from mania (or hypomania) to depression.

3180. Which of the following is not a feature of mania?

Harrison's 20th Ed. Chapter 444, Page 3271

A. Increased psychomotor activity
B. Excessive social extroversion
C. Increased need for sleep
D. Impulsivity

3181. Mania in its pure form is associated with?

Harrison's 20th Ed. Chapter 444, Page 3271

A. Increased psychomotor activity
B. Impulsivity and impairment in judgment
C. Decreased need for sleep
D. All of the above

Mania in its pure form is associated with increased psychomotor activity, excessive social extroversion, decreased need for sleep, impulsivity and impaired judgment and expansive, grandiose mood.

3182. Which of the following is a feature of cyclothymic disorder?

Harrison's 20th Ed. Chapter 444, Page 3271

A. Many hypomanic periods usually of relatively short duration
B. Clusters of depressive symptoms
C. Manifestations present for at least 2 years
D. All of the above

In cyclothymic disorder, there are many hypomanic periods of short duration, alternating with clusters of depressive symptoms that do not meet the criteria of major depression. Mood fluctuations are chronic and should be present for at least 2 years before the diagnosis is made.

3183. Term rapid cycling is used for patients who have how many episodes of either depression or mania in a given year?

Harrison's 20th Ed. Chapter 444, Page 3271

A. One or more
B. Two or more
C. Three or more
D. Four or more

Term rapid cycling is used for patients, mostly women, who have four or more episodes of either depression or mania in a given year.

3184. Secondary mania may be induced by?

Harrison's 20th Ed. Chapter 444, Page 3272

A. Stimulant or sympathomimetic drugs
B. Hyperthyroidism
C. Huntington's or Wilson's disease
D. All of the above

Secondary mania may be induced by stimulant or sympathomimetic drugs, hyperthyroidism, AIDS, Huntington's or Wilson's disease and cerebrovascular accidents.

3185. Risk genes for bipolar disorder include?

Harrison's 20th Ed. Chapter 444, Page 3272

A. CACNA1C
B. Teneurin transmembrane protein 4 (ODZ4)
C. Neurocan (NCAN)
D. All of the above

Bipolar disorder concordance rate for monozygotic twins is ~80%. Risk genes identified include CACNA1C, teneurin transmembrane protein 4 (ODZ4), ankryn 3 (ANK3), neurocan (NCAN), and tetratricopeptide repeat and ankyrin repeat containing 1 (TRANK1).

3186. Drug for treatment of bipolar disorders include?

Harrison's 20th Ed. Chapter 444, Page 3272

A. Lithium carbonate
B. Sodium valproate
C. Olanzapine
D. All of the above

3187. Which of the following about lithium therapy is false?

Harrison's 20th Ed. Chapter 444, Page 3272

A. Side effects include polyuria & weight gain
B. Lithium exerts an antithyroid effect
C. No prophylactic effect in prevention of recurrent mania
D. Excreted mainly by kidneys

3188. Lithium carbonate is of use in which of the following?

Harrison's 20th Ed. Chapter 444, Page 3272

A. Acute mania
B. Prophylactically to prevent recurrent mania
C. Prevention of recurrent depression
D. All of the above

Lithium carbonate is the mainstay of treatment in bipolar disorder. Lithium also has a prophylactic effect in prevention of recurrent mania and, to a lesser extent, in prevention of recurrent depression.

3189. Which of the following about lithium therapy is false?

Harrison's 20th Ed. Chapter 310, Page 2525, 303, 2157 Table 310-1, 2162

A. Can induce lupus-like disease
B. Can cause chronic tubulointerstitial nephritis
C. Can cause nephrogenic diabetes insipidus
D. None of the above

3190. Which of the following about lithium therapy is false?

Harrison's 20th Ed. Chapter 56, Page 365

A. Can cause multifocal myoclonus
B. Can restore myelopoiesis in patients with neutropenia due to impaired production
C. Can induce onychomadesis
D. None of the above

3191. Which of the following about lithium therapy is false?

Harrison's 20th Ed. Chapter 54, Page 341, 342, 364

A. Can induce acne
B. Can exacerbate plaque psoriasis
C. Can cause alopecia
D. None of the above

3192. Which of the following about lithium therapy is false?

Harrison's 20th Ed. Chapter 240, Page 193, 1728 Table 240-1

A. Can decrease anionic gap (AG)
B. Can cause downbeat nystagmus
C. Can cause bradycardia & atrioventricular block
D. None of the above

3193. Concomitant administration of which of the following with lithium can result in increased serum levels of lithium?

Harrison's 20th Ed. Chapter 139, Page 1055

A. Benzodiazapine
B. Olanzapine
C. Metronidazole
D. Valproic acid

Concomitant administration of metronidazole with lithium can result in increased serum levels of lithium and associated toxicity.

3194. What proportion of a given dose of lithium carbonate is excreted unchanged through kidneys within 24 hours?

Harrison's 20th Ed. Chapter 444, Page 3272

A. 25%
B. 50%
C. 75%
D. 95%

~95% of a given dose of lithium carbonate is excreted unchanged through the kidneys within 24 hours.

3195. Which of the following is not a side effect of lithium therapy?

Harrison's 20th Ed. Chapter 444, Page 3272

A. Weight loss
B. Alopecia
C. Antithyroid effect
D. Polyuria

Side effects of lithium include gastrointestinal discomfort, nausea, diarrhea, polyuria, weight gain, skin eruptions, alopecia, edema, and antithyroid effect.

3196. In bipolar disorders, which of the following is effective in the depressed phase?

Harrison's 20th Ed. Chapter 444, Page 3272

A. Lithium carbonate
B. Sodium valproate
C. Olanzapine
D. Lamotrigine

Lithium carbonate is the mainstay of treatment in bipolar disorder. Sodium valproate & olanzapine are equally effective in acute mania, as is lamotrigine in the depressed phase.

3197. Therapeutic blood levels of lithium in the treatment of acute mania is?

Harrison's 20th Ed. Chapter 444, Page 3272

A. 0.4–0.8 mEq/L
B. 0.8–1.2 mEq/L
C. 1.4–2.2 mEq/L
D. 2.5–3.2 mEq/L

In the treatment of acute mania, lithium is initiated at 300 mg bid or tid. Dose is titrated every 2–3 days to achieve blood levels of 0.8–1.2 mEq/L.

3198. Therapeutic blood levels of valproic acid is?

Harrison's 20th Ed. Chapter 444, Page 3272 Table 444-9

A. 50–125 μg/mL
B. 100–225 μg/mL
C. 200–350 μg/mL
D. 380–525 μg/mL

3199. Therapeutic blood levels of carbamazepine is?

Harrison's 20th Ed. Chapter 444, Page 3272 Table 444-9

A. 1–4 μg/mL
B. 4–12 μg/mL
C. 12–22 μg/mL
D. 25–42 μg/mL

3200. Stevens-Johnson syndrome can occur with all except?

Harrison's 20th Ed. Chapter 444, Page 3272 Table 444-9

A. Lithium
B. Valproic acid
C. Carbamazepine
D. Lamotrigine

3201. Which of the following drugs is appropriate for patients who experience rapid cycling?

Harrison's 20th Ed. Chapter 444, Page 3272

A. Lithium carbonate
B. Sodium valproate
C. Olanzapine
D. Lamotrigine

Valproic acid is better for patients who experience rapid cycling (> 4 episodes a year) or who present with a mixed or dysphoric mania.

3202. Blood level of lithium is increased by all except?

Harrison's 20th Ed. Chapter 444, Page 3272 Table 444-9

A. Thiazides
B. Verapamil
C. Tetracyclines
D. NSAIDs

Blood level of lithium is increased by thiazides, tetracyclines, and NSAIDs, decreased by bronchodilators, verapamil, and carbonic anhydrase inhibitors.

3203. Which of the following is effective in bipolar disorder?

Harrison's 20th Ed. Chapter 444, Page 3272

A. Social rhythm therapy
B. ECT
C. Light therapy
D. All of the above

3204. In somatization disorder, which of the following is true to fulfill the diagnostic criteria?

Harrison's 20th Ed. Chapter 444, Page 3273

A. 2 pain, 2 GI, 2 sexual, & 2 pseudoneurologic symptom
B. 3 pain, 2 GI, 2 sexual, & 1 pseudoneurologic symptom
C. 3 pain, 2 GI, 1 sexual, & 2 pseudoneurologic symptom
D. 4 pain, 2 GI, 1 sexual, & 1 pseudoneurologic symptom

Formal diagnostic criteria for somatization disorder requires the recording of at least four pain, two gastrointestinal, one sexual, and one pseudoneurologic symptom.

3205. Munchausen's syndrome best relates to?

Harrison's 20th Ed. Chapter 444, Page 3273

A. Factitious disorder
B. Hypochondriasis
C. Conversion disorder
D. Feeding & eating disorder

Munchausen's syndrome is characterized by dramatic, chronic, or severe factitious illness.

3206. In conversion disorder, deficit symptoms involve?

Harrison's 20th Ed. Chapter 444, Page 3273

A. Motor
B. Sensory
C. Psychological
D. All of the above

In conversion disorder, deficit symptoms are not intentionally produced or simulated and involve motor or sensory function & psychological factors that initiate or exacerbate medical presentation.

3207. Which of the following best relates to hypochondriasis?

Harrison's 20th Ed. Chapter 444, Page 3273

A. Voluntarily produced physical symptoms of illness
B. Belief of serious medical illness
C. Intentionally produced deficit symptoms
D. Simulated deficit symptoms

In factitious disorder (malingering), patient consciously & voluntarily produces physical symptoms of illness. Essential feature in hypochondriasis is a belief of serious medical illness that persists despite reassurance & appropriate medical evaluation.

3208. Which of the following is required for the diagnosis of borderline personality disorder?

N Engl J Med. 2011;364:2037-42

A. Interpersonal hypersensitivity
B. Impulsivity
C. Affective dysregulation
D. All of the above

3209. Most distinctive characteristic of patients with BPD is?
N Engl J Med. 2011;364:2037-42

A. Excessive involvement in pleasurable activities
B. Decreased need for sleep
C. Hypersensitivity to rejection
D. Inflated self-esteem or grandiosity

Most distinctive characteristics of patients with BPD are their hypersensitivity to rejection and their fearful preoccupation with expected abandonment.

3210. Which of the following has the highest mortality among psychiatric conditions?
Harrison's 20th Ed. Chapter 444, Page 3274

A. Anorexia nervosa
B. Schizophrenia
C. Bipolar disorders
D. Posttraumatic stress disorder

Untreated anorexia nervosa has a mortality of 5.1/1000 which is highest among psychiatric conditions.

3211. Which of the following is false about anorexia nervosa?
Harrison's 20th Ed. Chapter 444, Page 3274

A. Extreme weight loss
B. Behavior of dieting/food restriction (self-starvation)
C. Excessive exercise (obsession with having a thin body)
D. None of the above

Anorexia nervosa (AN) is a highly distinctive disorder at the brain-body interface. A defining characteristic of anorexia nervosa is that the individual denial of the problem and ambivalence to take treatment.

3212. Which of the following is seen in blood picture of a patient of anorexia nervosa?
Harrison's 20th Ed. Chapter 444, Page 3274

A. Leukopenia with lymphocytosis
B. Elevated blood urea nitrogen
C. Metabolic alkalosis and hypokalemia
D. All of the above

3213. Endocrine disturbances seen in anorexia nervosa include?
Harrison's 20th Ed. Chapter 444, Page 3274

A. Hypogonadism
B. Growth hormone resistance
C. Hypercortisolemia
D. All of the above

3214. ARFID refers to?
N Engl J Med. 2017;376:2377-86

A. Appetite restrictive food intake disorder
B. Anxiety restrictive food intake disorder
C. Avoidant restrictive food intake disorder
D. Acute restrictive food intake disorder

ARFID is defined by the presence of avoidant or restrictive eating that results in persistent failure to meet nutritional needs.

3215. Purging in a patient of anorexia nervosa is suggested by?
N Engl J Med. 2005;353:1481-8

A. Enlargement of the salivary glands (chubby cheeks)
B. Eroded dental enamel
C. Scars on dorsum of hands from repeated, induced vomiting
D. All of the above

Anorexia nervosa occurs in two types: food restricting, and binge eating and purging.

3216. Which of the following treatment plan has proved to be effective in anorexia nervosa?
Harrison's 20th Ed. Chapter 444, Page 3274

A. CAT
B. CBT-E
C. MANTRA
D. SSCM

In 2017, the National Institute for Health and Care Excellence (NICE) has recommended Maudsley Anorexia Nervosa Treatment for Adults (MANTRA) as a first line treatment for adults with anorexia nervosa.

3217. Psychiatric conditions that coexist with anorexia nervosa include?
Harrison's 20th Ed. Chapter 444, Page 3274

A. Major depression or dysthymia
B. Anxiety disorders
C. Obsessive - compulsive disorder
D. All of the above

3218. Transition from bulimia nervosa to anorexia occurs in what percentage of cases?
Harrison's 20th Ed. Chapter 444, Page 3274

A. 2–5%
B. 10–15%
C. 20–30%
D. 30–50%

3219. Which of the following is not a feature of personality disorders?
Harrison's 20th Ed. Chapter 444, Page 3274

A. Characteristic patterns of thinking & feeling
B. Relative flexibility
C. Significant functional impairment
D. Subjective distress

Personality disorders are characteristic patterns of thinking, feeling & interpersonal behavior that are relatively inflexible & cause significant functional impairment or subjective distress.

3220. Obsessive-compulsive personality types is grouped in which personality cluster disorder?
Harrison's 20th Ed. Chapter 444, Page 3274

A. Cluster A
B. Cluster B
C. Cluster C
D. Any of the above

3221. Paranoid personality type is grouped in which personality cluster disorder?
Harrison's 20th Ed. Chapter 444, Page 3274

A. Cluster A
B. Cluster B
C. Cluster C
D. Any of the above

3222. Antisocial personality type is grouped in which personality cluster disorder?

Harrison's 20th Ed. Chapter 444, Page 3274

A. Cluster A
B. Cluster B
C. Cluster C
D. Any of the above

Personality disorders are grouped into 3 overlapping clusters. Cluster A includes paranoid (unjustified pervasive mistrust & suspiciousness), schizoid, and schizotypal personality disorders. Cluster B disorders include antisocial, borderline, histrionic & narcissistic types (impulsive behavior, excessively emotional, erratic). Cluster C includes avoidant, dependent & obsessive-compulsive personality types.

3223. In Mini Mental Status Examination, scoring is done out of?

Harrison's 20th Ed. Chapter 25, Page 155

A. 20
B. 30
C. 40
D. 50

3224. Depressive episodes that occur in conjunction with manic episodes are called?

N Engl J Med. 2005;353:1819-34

A. Anxiety disorders
B. Schizophrenic disorders
C. Bipolar disorders
D. Major depressive disorders

3225. "Dysthymia" is the term used for?

N Engl J Med. 2005;353:1819-34

A. Persistent, residual depressive symptoms
B. Generalized weakness
C. Absence of sweating
D. Difficulty in swallowing

3226. As regards risk of problems in depressed patients, which of the following statements is true?

N Engl J Med. 2005;353:1819-34

A. Suicide
B. Heart disease
C. Stroke
D. All of the above

3227. Which of the following about depression is false?

N Engl J Med. 2005;353:1819-34

A. Elevated cortisol levels
B. Higher levels of N-acetyl aspartate
C. Deficiencies of serotonin, norepinephrine, dopamine & GABA
D. Overactivity of acetylcholine, corticotropin-releasing factor, and substance P

3228. Disordered neurocircuitry in depression is observed in which of the following structures?

N Engl J Med. 2005;353:1819-34

A. Anterior and posterior cingulate cortex
B. Ventral, medial, and dorsolateral prefrontal cortex
C. Insula
D. All of the above

3229. Disordered neurocircuitry in depression is observed in which of the following structures?

N Engl J Med. 2005;353:1819-34

A. Ventral striatum
B. Hippocampus
C. Medial thalamus
D. All of the above

3230. Tricyclic antidepressants have greater efficacy than SSRIs in?

N Engl J Med. 2005;353:1819-34

A. Severe major depressive disorder
B. Depression with melancholic features
C. Depression in which physical symptoms or pain are prominent
D. All of the above

3231. Which of the following drugs has no direct action on the serotonin system?

N Engl J Med. 2005;353:1819-34

A. Bupropion
B. Venlafaxine
C. Duloxetine
D. Milnacipran

3232. Monoamine oxidase (MAO) is the enzyme involved in?

N Engl J Med. 2005;353:1819-34

A. Norepinephrine breakdown
B. Epinephrine breakdown
C. Dopamine breakdown
D. All of the above

3233. Mirtazapine blocks?

N Engl J Med. 2005;353:1819-34

A. Alpha2-adrenergic autoreceptors
B. Serotonin 5-HT2A and 5-HT3 receptors
C. Histamine H1 receptors
D. All of the above

Mirtazapine is a TCA. It increases noradrenergic & serotonergic neurotransmission through a blockade of central α2-adrenergic receptors and postsynaptic 5HT2 and 5HT3 receptors. It is also strongly antihistaminic and may produce sedation.

3234. Which of the following are classified as mood stabilizers?

N Engl J Med. 2005;353:1819-34

A, Lithium
B. Lamotrigine
C. Divalproex
D. All of the above

Mood Stabilizers include lithium, valproic acid, carbamazepine/oxcarbazepine & lamotrigine.

3235. ECT can be a first-line treatment for patients who have?

N Engl J Med. 2005;353:1819-34

A. Severe major depressive disorder with psychotic features
B. Psychomotor retardation
C. Medication resistance
D. All of the above

3236. Akinetic mutism can be caused by?

Harrison's 20th Ed. Chapter 300, Page 2069

A. Damage of the medial thalamic nuclei
B. Damage of the frontal lobes
C. Hydrocephalus
D. All of the above

3237. Milder form of akinetic mutism is called?

Harrison's 20th Ed. Chapter 300, Page 2069

A. Agnosia
B. Abulia
C. Akathesia
D. None of the above

Abulia describes a milder form of akinetic mutism characterized by mental & physical slowness & diminished ability to initiate activity, usually the result of damage to frontal lobes & its connections.

3238. Hypomobile and mute syndrome associated with a major psychosis is?

Harrison's 20th Ed. Chapter 300, Page 2069

A. Catatonia
B. Abulia
C. Agnosia
D. Akathesia

Catatonia is a hypomobile & mute syndrome that occurs as part of a major psychosis, usually schizophrenia or major depression.

3239. Beclouded dementia refers to?

Dement Geriatr Cogn Disord. 1999;10:310-314

A. Acute medical problem, or a poorly tolerated medication supervenes in a mildly demented patient
B. Transient confusion & drowsiness with febrile infection
C. Awake but unresponsive state
D. Awake but cannot produce speech

3240. MASA syndrome includes all except?

European Journal of Human Genetics. 1995;3(5):273-84

A. Mental retardation
B. Aphasia
C. Syncope
D. Adducted thumbs

MASA syndrome (Mental retardation, Aphasia, Spastic paraplegia, Adducted thumbs) is a historical term used to describe a phenotype now considered to be part of the X-linked L1 clinical spectrum (L1 syndrome), CRASH syndrome or Gareis-Mason syndrome.

3241. Asperger's syndrome best relates to?

Reviews in Neurological Diseases. 2006;3(1):1-7

A. Autism spectrum disorders (ASD)
B. Schizophrenia
C. Mood disorders
D. Substance use disorders

Individuals with autism-like symptoms (delays or abnormal functioning in social interactions, language as used in social communication, and symbolic or imaginative play, with onset prior to age 3) with relatively preserved cognitive functioning and language skills have Asperger's syndrome.

Schizophrenia

3242. Out of the following, who performed original research in schizophrenia?

A. Maurer D

B. Sachs GS

C. Kraepelin E

D. Kohn R

Dementia praecox, a term used by Emil Kraepelin, was replaced by Eugen Bleuler who called those closely related diseases characterized not by deterioration of intellect but by splitting of cognitive sides of personality from the affective or emotional sides by the name of schizophrenia. Kraepelin and Bleuler were the first to suggest that schizophrenia is an organic brain disease with significant cognitive deficits.

3243. Schizophrenia presents typically in?

Harrison's 20th Ed. Chapter 444, Page 3275

A. Early childhood

B. Late adolescence

C. Middle age

D. Old age

Schizophrenia presents typically in late adolescence and early adulthood as a lifelong phenomenon.

3244. Which of the following is a pathognomonic feature of schizophrenia?

Harrison's 20th Ed. Chapter 444, Page 3275

A. Perturbations of language

B. Perturbations of perception

C. Perturbations of thinking

D. None of the above

There are no pathognomonic features of schizophrenia.

3245. Major symptom cluster seen in schizophrenia is?

Harrison's 20th Ed. Chapter 444, Page 3275

A. Positive

B. Negative

C. Cognitive

D. All of the above

Three major symptom clusters seen in schizophrenia are positive (conceptual disorganization, hallucinations & delusions), negative (loss of function, anhedonia, decreased emotional expression, impaired concentration, and diminished social engagement), and cognitive symptoms (disabling deficits in working memory & cognitive control of behavior). Delusions & hallucinations of schizophrenia are more complex, bizarre, and threatening than those of dementia.

3246. Which of the following is false about the negative symptoms of schizophrenia?

Harrison's 20th Ed. Chapter 444, Page 3275

A. Carry a poor long-term outcome

B. Respond inadequately to drug treatment

C. Predominate in one-third of the schizophrenic population

D. None of the above

Negative symptoms carry a poor long-term outcome and a respond inadequately to drug treatment. Negative symptoms develop prior to positive symptoms.

3247. Patients with symptoms of schizophrenia and independent periods of mood disturbance are called?

Harrison's 20th Ed. Chapter 444, Page 3275

A. Schizoaffective disorder

B. Schizophreniform disorder

C. Schizocognitive disorder

D. Schizopolar disorder

Patients with symptoms of schizophrenia and independent periods of mood disturbance are termed to have schizoaffective disorder. Schizophreniform disorder describes patients who meet the symptom requirements but not the duration requirements for schizophrenia. Schizotypal and schizoid personality disorders refers to individuals who show a lifetime pattern of social & interpersonal deficits (inability to form close interpersonal relationships, eccentric behavior, and mild perceptual distortions).

3248. What percentage of schizophrenic patients commit suicide?

Harrison's 20th Ed. Chapter 444, Page 3275

A. 10%

B. 20%

C. 30%

D. 40%

About 10% of schizophrenic patients commit suicide.

3249. Worldwide lifetime prevalence of schizophrenia is?

Harrison's 20th Ed. Chapter 444, Page 3275

A. 1.5%

B. 3.8%

C. 5.2%

D. 7.6%

Schizophrenia is a sporadic or familial mental disorder of yet unknown etiology. It occurs in all ethnic populations with a worldwide lifetime prevalence of ~1–1.5%. Schizophrenia affects males & females roughly equally.

3250. Which of the following about schizophrenia is false?

Harrison's 20th Ed. Chapter 444, Page 3275, 3114

A. Equal prevalence rates in men & women

B. Peak age of onset is in III decade of life

C. Rate of completed suicide is about 10%

D. None of the above

Schizophrenia & bipolar disorders are equally frequent in both men and women. There may be sex differences in symptoms though. Schizophrenia has an earlier age of onset (II & III decades) and is associated with intact memory.

3251. Which of the following neurologic findings may be seen in untreated patients of schizophrenia?

Harrison's 20th Ed. Chapter 444, Page 3275

A. Motor rigidity

B. Tremor

C. Dyskinesias

D. All of the above

Neurologic examination in patients with schizophrenia is usually normal, but motor rigidity, tremor, and dyskinesias are noted in one-quarter of untreated patients of schizophrenia.

3252. Which out of the following prescription medications is frequently associated with symptoms of schizophrenia?

Harrison's 20th Ed. Chapter 444, Page 3275

A. Clonidine
B. Lorazepam
C. Tizanidine
D. Reserpine

Most common prescription medications associated with symptoms of schizophrenia are clonidine, quinacrine, and procaine derivatives.

3253. Risk factors for schizophrenia include all except?

Harrison's 20th Ed. Chapter 444, Page 3275

A. Summer birth
B. Increasing paternal age
C. Prenatal nutritional deficiency
D. Intrauterine exposure to viral infection.

Risk factors for schizophrenia include urban birth, winter birth, migration, increasing paternal age, fetal hypoxia, maternal-fetal Rhesus blood-group incompatibility, prenatal nutritional deficiency & intrauterine exposure to viral infection.

3254. Among monozygotic twins, the incidence of schizophrenia is?

Harrison's 20th Ed. Chapter 444, Page 3275

A. ~ 25%
B. ~ 50%
C. ~ 75%
D. ~ 100%

Among twins, the incidence of schizophrenia is ~10% in dizygotic twins of affected individuals, and ~50% in monozygotic twins.

3255. If both parents are affected with schizophrenia, the risk for offspring is?

Harrison's 20th Ed. Chapter 444, Page 3275

A. 20%
B. 40%
C. 60%
D. 80%

If both parents are affected with schizophrenia, the risk for offspring is 40%.

3256. Alleles of which of the following genes is associated with both ASDs and schizophrenia?

Harrison's 20th Ed. Chapter 443, Page 3257

A. MeCP2
B. NRXN1
C. TSC 1 & 2
D. FMR1

Mutations in MeCP2, FMR1 and TSC1&2 can cause mental retardation without autism spectrum disorders (ASDs), and alleles of NRXN1 is associated with both ASDs and schizophrenia. Polymorphisms in CACNA1C are strongly associated with both schizophrenia & bipolar disorder.

3257. Which of the following is with both schizophrenia?

Harrison's 20th Ed. Chapter 443, Page 3257

A. Alleles of NRXN1
B. Common polymorphisms in CACNA1C
C. Duplication of chromosome 16p
D. All of the above

3258. In schizophrenia, reduction of cortical & subcortical gray matter is seen in?

Harrison's 20th Ed. Chapter 443, Page 3260

A. Frontal lobe
B. Temporal lobe
C. Limbic system
D. All of the above

In schizophrenia, reduction of cortical & subcortical gray matter is seen in frontal and temporal lobes and in the limbic system.

3259. The best-established neuropathologic finding in schizophrenia is?

Harrison's 20th Ed. Chapter 443, Page 3260

A. Cerebral hemisphere asymmetry
B. Reduced number of gyri & sulci
C. Enlargement of lateral ventricles
D. Increase in cortical thickness

The best-established neuropathologic finding in schizophrenia is enlargement of the lateral ventricles of the cerebral hemispheres accompanied by a reduction in cortical thickness.

3260. Which of the following is a neuropathological finding in brain of schizophrenia patients?

Harrison's 20th Ed. Chapter 443, Page 3260

A. No change in neuronal cell number
B. Increased cell packing density & reduced neuropil
C. Reduction in cortical thickness
D. All of the above

In schizophrenia, reduction in cortical thickness is associated with increased cell packing density & reduced neuropil (axons, dendrites, and glial cell processes) with no reduction in neuronal cell number.

3261. Current antipsychotic drugs are efficacious for which symptom cluster seen in schizophrenia?

Harrison's 20th Ed. Chapter 444, Page 3275

A. Positive
B. Negative
C. Cognitive
D. All of the above

Positive symptoms cluster seen in schizophrenia responds to current antipsychotic drugs that generally lack efficacy for negative and cognitive symptoms.

3262. Which of the following is not a typical feature of schizophrenia?

Harrison's 20th Ed. Chapter 444, Page 3275

A. Bizzare psychosis
B. Frequent mood disturbances
C. Hypervigilance
D. Altered short term memory

Features that preclude the diagnosis of schizophrenia are significant mood symptoms, any relevant medical disease, temporal-lobe epilepsy, evidence of substance abuse and drug reaction. Delusions & hallucinations of schizophrenia are more complex & bizarre than those of dementia.

3263. Anhedonia refers to?

Harrison's 20th Ed. Chapter 65, Page 441

A. Depressed mood
B. Loss of reality
C. Loss of interest in pleasure
D. Loss of self-esteem

Anhedonia refers to loss of interest in pleasure or decreased ability to experience pleasure.

3264. Which of the following diseases can begin with schizophrenia-like features?

Harrison's 20th Ed. Chapter 423, Page 3114

A. Frontotemporal dementia
B. Huntington's disease
C. Alzheimer's disease
D. All of the above

FTD, HD, vascular dementia, Dementia with Lewy bodies (DLB), AD, or leukoencephalopathy can begin with schizophrenia-like features.

3265. Which of the following is not a schizophrenia subtype?

N Engl J Med. 2003;349:1738-49

A. Catatonic
B. Atonic
C. Paranoid
D. Residual

Four subtypes of schizophrenia are catatonic, paranoid, disorganized, and residual.

3266. In which of the following subtypes of schizophrenia, negative symptomatology exists in the absence of delusions, hallucinations, or motor disturbance?

N Engl J Med. 2003;349:1738-49

A. Catatonic
B. Disorganized
C. Paranoid
D. Residual

In residual-type subtype of schizophrenia, negative symptomatology exists in the absence of delusions, hallucinations, or motor disturbance.

3267. Echolalia or echopraxia is a feature of which of the following subtypes of schizophrenia?

N Engl J Med. 2003;349:1738-49

A. Catatonic
B. Disorganized
C. Paranoid
D. Residual

Catatonic subtype patients have profound changes in motor activity, negativism & echolalia or echopraxia.

3268. Which of the following is related to schizophrenia?

N Engl J Med. 2003;349:1738-49

A. Split personality
B. Multiple-personality
C. 'Functional' psychosis
D. None of the above

3269. Which of the following term was used to address schizophrenia in past?

N Engl J Med. 2003;349:1738-49

A. Frontotemporal dementia
B. Dementia with Lewy bodies
C. Dementia praecox
D. Conversion reaction

3270. Mostly, people do not get schizophrenia after the age of?

N Engl J Med. 2003;349:1738-49

A. 15 years
B. 25 years
C. 35 years
D. 45 years

Mostly, people do not get schizophrenia after the age of 45 years.

3271. Area of the brain that are predominantly and consistently affected in schizophrenia is?

N Engl J Med. 2003;349:1738-49

A. Amygdala
B. Anterior & medial nuclei of thalamus
C. Dorsolateral prefrontal cortex (DLPFC)
D. All of the above

3272. Which of the following cortical layers is thinner than normal in schizophrenia?

N Engl J Med. 2003;349:1738-49

A. I
B. II
C. IV
D. V

Cortical layers II and III are thinner than normal in schizophrenia.

3273. Which of the following is not a structural abnormality in brain of schizophrenia individuals?

N Engl J Med. 2003;349:1738-49

A. Ventricular enlargement
B. Absence of glial proliferation
C. Reduction in neuropil
D. Decreased volume of Nucleus accumbens

3274. Which of the following recreational drugs can mimic symptoms of schizophrenia in healthy individuals?

N Engl J Med. 2003;349:1738-49

A. Amphetamine
B. Phencyclidine (PCP)
C. Lysergic acid diethylamide (LSD)
D. All of the above

3275. Which of the following is related to the increased occurrence of schizophrenia?

N Engl J Med. 2003;349:1738-49

A. Tsunami
B. Plague epidemic
C. Nuclear holocaust in Japan
D. Dutch hunger winter

During severe famine, pregnant mothers tend to deliver children who have an increased incidence of schizophrenia later in their life. This observation stems from the experiences of the "Dutch hunger winter" during 1944 – 1945.

3276. The most prevalent excitatory transmitter in brain is?
N Engl J Med. 2003;349:1738-49

A. GABA
B. Glutamate
C. Serotonin
D. Dopamine

Most prevalent transmitter in the human brain is glutamate. It is mostly excitatory at synapses.

3277. Most prevalent inhibitory transmitter in brain is?
N Engl J Med. 2003;349:1738-49

A. GABA
B. Glutamate
C. Serotonin
D. Dopamine

Neurotransmitter is γ-amino-butyric acid (GABA) is mostly inhibitory at the synapses.

3278. Serotonergic neurons in the CNS are found primarily in?
N Engl J Med. 2003;349:1738-49

A. Midline raphe nuclei
B. Locus coeruleus
C. Striatum
D. Thalamus

Serotonergic neurons in the CNS are found primarily in the midline raphe nuclei, located in the brain stem from the midbrain to the medulla.

3279. Principal site for synthesis of norepinephrine in human brain is?
N Engl J Med. 2003;349:1738-49

A. Midline raphe nuclei
B. Locus coeruleus
C. Striatum
D. Thalamus

Locus coeruleus is the principal site for synthesis of norepinephrine (NE) that has an excitatory effect on most of the brain.

3280. Which of the following is a dopamine pathway in the brain?
N Engl J Med. 2003;349:1738-49

A. Mesolimbic
B. Mesocortical
C. Nigrostriatal
D. All of the above

Dopamine pathways in the brain are mesolimbic, mesocortical, nigrostriatal & tuberoinfundibular.

3281. Dopaminergic fibers in brain arise in which of the following?
N Engl J Med. 2003;349:1738-49

A. Amygdala
B. Hippocampus
C. Ventral tegmental area (VTA)
D. Nucleus accumbens

Dopaminergic fibers in brian arise in the ventral tegmental area (VTA).

3282. Which of the following dopamine receptor subtype is excitatory?
N Engl J Med. 2003;349:1738-49

A. D1
B. D2
C. D3
D. D4

Dopamine receptor subtypes D1 and D5 are excitatory while D2, D3 and D4 are inhibitory.

3283. Which of the following dopamine receptor subtype is most abundant in nucleus accumbens?
N Engl J Med. 2003;349:1738-49

A. D1
B. D2
C. D3
D. D4

D3 receptors are mainly present in nucleus accumbens while D4 receptors express themselves in frontal cortex. D1 receptors tend to be distributed in cortical regions, while D2 are subcortical.

3284. Schizophrenia is characterized by?
N Engl J Med. 2003;349:1738-49

A. Hypodopaminergia in mesocortical neurons
B. Hyperdopaminergia in mesocortical neurons
C. Hypodopaminergia in mesolimbic neurons
D. None of the above

Schizophrenia is characterized by hypodopaminergia in mesocortical neurons and hyperdopaminergia in mesolimbic neurons.

3285. Which of the following is an ionotropic glutamate receptor?
N Engl J Med. 2003;349:1738-49

A. AMPA
B. Kainate
C. NMDA
D. All of the above

Ionotropic glutamate receptors (iGluRs) are AMPA (a-amino-3-hydroxy-5-methyl-4-isoxazole propionic acid), kainate, and NMDA.

3286. AMPA-receptor subunits are derived from which of the following genes?
N Engl J Med. 2003;349:1738-49

A. GluR4
B. GluR5
C. GluR6
D. GluR7

AMPA-receptor subunits are derived from GluR1, GluR2, GluR3 and GluR4 genes. Kainate receptors are derived from GluR5, GluR6, GluR7 and KA1, KA2 genes. NMDA receptor subunits are encoded by NR1, NR2A, NR2B, NR2C, NR2D genes.

3287. Glycine co-agonist essential for glutamatergic transmission is?
N Engl J Med. 2003;349:1738-49

A. Tyrosine
B. Serenine
C. Melanin
D. D-serine

3288. Serotonin is produced from?
N Engl J Med. 2003;349:1738-49

A. Arginine
B. L-tryptophan
C. Histidine
D. Leucine

Serotonin is produced by decarboxylation & hydroxylation of L-tryptophan.

3289. Which of the following hallucinogen is a 5-HT agonist?

N Engl J Med. 2003;349:1738-49

A. Amphetamine
B. LSD (lysergic acid diethylamide)
C. Ketamine
D. All of the above

Hallucinogen LSD (lysergic acid diethylamide) is a 5-HT agonist.

3290. GABA is synthesized from?

N Engl J Med. 2003;349:1738-49

A. Glutamic acid
B. Butyric acid
C. Sialic acid
D. Glycine

GABA is synthesized from glutamic acid by removal of alpha-carboxl group from glutamate by the action of glutamic acid decarboxylase (GAD).

3291. Which of the following scales is used for severity of clinical symptoms of schizophrenia?

N Engl J Med. 2003;349:1738-49

A. ESRS
B. BAS
C. PANSS
D. LNS

Positive and Negative Syndrome Scale (PANSS) is used for severity of clinical symptoms of schizophrenia. Brown–Peterson procedure and the Letter-Number Sequencing (LNS) task are measures of verbal working memory. Extrapyramidal Symptom Rating Scale (ESRS) and the Barnes Akathisia Scale (BAS) are used to assess movement disorders that occur with antipsychotic medication of schizophrenia.

3292. Reduction in volume of which of the following correlate with positive symptoms of schizophrenia?

N Engl J Med. 2003;349:1738-49

A. Medial temporal lobes (MTL)
B. Superior temporal gyrus (STG)
C. Hippocampus
D. Amygdala

Reduction in volume of superior temporal gyrus correlate with positive symptoms of schizophrenia while MTL reductions correlate with memory impairment.

3293. Term neuroleptic in Greek means?

N Engl J Med. 2003;349:1738-49

A. To straighten the neuron
B. To clasp the neuron
C. To thin the neuron
D. To energise the neuron

Term neuroleptic in Greek means "to clasp the neuron".

3294. Which of the following is not a typical antipsychotic drug?

Harrison's 20th Ed. Chapter 444, Page 3276 Table 444-10

A. Haloperidol
B. Risperidone
C. Chlorpromazine
D. Thiothixene

3295. Which of the following is not an atypical antipsychotic drug?

Harrison's 20th Ed. Chapter 444, Page 3276 Table 444-10

A. Ziprasidone
B. Perphenazine
C. Asenapine
D. Aripiprazole

First-generation or "typical" antipsychotic agents include Chlorpromazine, Perphenazine, Trifluoperazine, Thiothixene and Haloperidol. Second-generation or "atypical" antipsychotic agents are Clozapine, Risperidone, Olanzapine, Quetiapine, Ziprasidone, Aripiprazole and Amisulpride. Intramuscular depot preparations available are Fluphenazine decanoate, Haloperidol decanoate, Flupentixol decanoate and Risperidone microspheres.

3296. Agranulocytosis is a side effect of which of the following antipsychotic drug?

Harrison's 20th Ed. Chapter 444, Page 3276 Table 444-10

A. Olanzapine
B. Clozapine
C. Quetiapine
D. Chlorpromazine

3297. In UK, Clozaril Patient Monitoring Services (CPMS) monitors patient's?

N Engl J Med. 2003;349:1738-49

A. Hematological profile
B. Weight gain
C. Lenticular opacities
D. Myocarditis

In UK, it is mandatory for all patients receiving Clozapine to register with Clozaril Patient Monitoring Services (CPMS) that monitors patient's hematological profile.

3298. Which of the following antipsychotic drug is unlikely to increase prolactin levels?

Harrison's 20th Ed. Chapter 444, Page 3276

A. Aripiprazole
B. Clozapine
C. Ziprasidone
D. None of the above

3299. In schizophrenia, if antipsychotic medications are completely discontinued, the relapse rate is?

Harrison's 20th Ed. Chapter 444, Page 3276

A. 1% per month
B. 5% per month
C. 10% per month
D. 20% per month

If antipsychotic medications are completely discontinued in schizophrenia, the relapse rate is 60% within 6 months or 10% per month, until eventually almost all patients undergo relapse.

3300. Use of which of the following is least likely to cause hyperglycemia, weight gain, and hypertriglyceridemia?

Harrison's 20th Ed. Chapter 444, Page 3276

A. Clozapine
B. Ziprasidone
C. Olanzapine
D. Quetiapine

Clozapine, olanzapine & quetiapine cause hyperglycemia, weight gain & hypertriglyceridemia more than Ziprasidone.

3301. Which of the following may reduce tardive dyskinesia with the use of antipsychotic agents if given early in the syndrome?

Harrison's 20th Ed. Chapter 444, Page 3276

A. Vitamin E
B. Vitamin B12
C. Zinc
D. Calcium

Vitamin E may reduce abnormal involuntary movements with the use of antipsychotic agents, if given early in the syndrome.

3302. Which of the following is most commonly involved in tardive dyskinesia (TD)?

Harrison's 20th Ed. Chapter 444, Page 3276

A. Tongue
B. Trunk
C. Limbs
D. Respiratory muscles

TD comprises of choreiform movements involving mouth, lips & tongue. In severe cases trunk, limbs & respiratory muscles may be affected.

3303. Sleep disturbance in chronic schizophrenia includes?

Harrison's 20th Ed. Chapter 444, Page 3276

A. Day-night reversal
B. Sleep fragmentation
C. Insomnia
D. All of the above

3304. Which of the following anti-malarials should not be prescribed to patients of schizophrenia?

Harrison's 20th Ed. Chapter 444, Page 3276

A. Quinine
B. Lumefantrine
C. Mefloquine
D. Primaquine

Mefloquine should not be prescribed to patients with depression, generalized anxiety disorder, psychosis, schizophrenia, and seizure disorder.

3305. Dysthymia best relates to?

Harrison's 20th Ed. Chapter 444, Page 3276

A. Depressive disorder
B. Bipolar disorder
C. Seizure disorder
D. Schizophrenia

Mood disorders can be either depressive or bipolar disorders. Depressive disorders include the major & minor depressive disorders and dysthymia

3306. Neurovegetative symptoms best relate to?

Harrison's 20th Ed. Chapter 444, Page 3260

A. Depressive disorder
B. Bipolar disorder
C. Posttraumatic stress disorder (PTSD)
D. Schizophrenia

Symptoms of depression are referred to as neurovegetative symptoms.

3307. Deep brain stimulation (DBS) of which of the following elevates mood in normal and depressed individuals?

Harrison's 20th Ed. Chapter 444, Page 3260

A. Subgenual area 23
B. Subgenual area 24
C. Subgenual area 25
D. Subgenual area 26

Deep brain stimulation (DBS) of either nucleus accumbens or subgenual area 25 elevates mood in normal and depressed individuals.

3308. Which of the following is a broad group of psychoses?

N Engl J Med. 2018;379:270-80

A. Idiopathic psychoses
B. Psychoses due to medical conditions
C. Toxic psychoses
D. All of the above

3309. Psychosis due to SLE begins at what age?

N Engl J Med. 2018;379:270-80

A. Late second or third decade
B. Middle age
C. Senescence
D. Any age

Schizophrenia, bipolar disorder & depression with psychotic symptoms, begin in late II or III decade of life. Delusional disorders more often develop in middle age. Psychoses due to neurodegenerative diseases begin during senescence. Psychotic symptoms caused by drug abuse or prescribed medications & symptoms caused by medical disorders like SLE, seizures, or fevers can occur at any age.

3310. Diagnosis of secondary psychosis is favoured by which of the following?

N Engl J Med. 2018;379:270-80

A. Absence of a family history of psychotic disorders
B. A history of headaches, seizures, or hallucinations
C. An abrupt onset of symptoms without clear precipitants
D. All of the above

Features that suggest a secondary psychosis (toxic psychosis or psychosis due to medical conditions) rather than idiopathic type include a rapid decline in functional capacity from premorbid levels, an abrupt onset of symptoms without clear precipitants, a history of headaches, seizures, or hallucinations (visual, olfactory, or tactile) and an absence of a family history of psychotic disorders. Idiopathic psychotic disorders (schizophrenia & schizoaffective disorder, usually evolve through premorbid, prodromal, syndromal, progressive, and chronic stages.

3311. Persons with psychotic disorders are at risk for?

N Engl J Med. 2018;379:270-80

A. Suicide
B. Substance abuse
C. Committing acts of violence
D. All of the above

Persons with psychotic disorders are at risk for complications & derivative effects of psychosis like suicide attempts (lifetime prevalence, 34.5%), substance abuse (lifetime prevalence, 74%), homelessness (annual prevalence, 5%), victimization by others (prevalence over a 3-year period, 38%), and committing acts of violence.

3312. The most common genetic abnormality associated with a psychotic disorder is?

N Engl J Med. 2018;379:270-80

A. Chromosome 19q11.2 microdeletion
B. Chromosome 20q11.2 microdeletion
C. Chromosome 21q11.2 microdeletion
D. Chromosome 22q11.2 microdeletion

Chromosome 22q11.2 deletion syndrome (velocardiofacial syndrome or the DiGeorge syndrome) occurs in ~1 in 4000 live births. It is associated with cardiac, facial & limb abnormalities, and ~25% of affected patients have symptoms of schizophrenia or schizophrenia-like features that are indistinguishable from idiopathic schizophrenia.

Primary and Metastatic Tumors of the Nervous System

3313. Which is the most common primary CNS tumor?

Harrison's 20th Ed. Chapter 86, Page 643

A. Glial tumors
B. Meningiomas
C. Schwannomas
D. Pituitary adenoma

Glial tumors account for 30% of all primary brain tumors, meningiomas for 35%, vestibular schwannomas for 10%, & central nervous system (CNS) lymphomas ~2%.

3314. Brain tumors usually present with?

Harrison's 20th Ed. Chapter 86, Page 643

A. Progressive focal neurologic deficits
B. Seizure
C. Non-focal neurologic disorder
D. Any of the above

Brain tumors may present with subacute progression of a focal neurologic deficit, seizure, or nonfocal neurologic disorder like headache, dementia, personality change or gait disorder. All seizures that arise from a brain tumor will have a focal onset.

3315. Features of headache due to increased ICP include all except?

Harrison's 20th Ed. Chapter 86, Page 643

A. Frontal
B. Episodic
C. Frequency more than once a day
D. Develop rapidly, subside quickly

Headaches due to increased ICP are usually holocephalic.

3316. Which of the following is a MRI feature of malignant brain tumors?

Harrison's 20th Ed. Chapter 86, Page 643

A. Enhance with gadolinium
B. May have central areas of necrosis
C. Surrounded by edema of neighboring white matter
D. All of the above

Malignant brain tumors (primary or metastatic) typically enhance with gadolinium and may have central areas of necrosis. They are characteristically surrounded by edema of the neighboring white matter.

3317. Fluid-attenuated inversion recovery (FLAIR) MRI best appreciates which of the following?

Harrison's 20th Ed. Chapter 86, Page 643

A. Low-grade gliomas
B. Meningiomas
C. Metastatic brain tumors
D. Dural lymphoma

Low-grade gliomas usually do not enhance with gadolinium and are best appreciated on fluid-attenuated inversion recovery (FLAIR) MRIs.

3318. Which of the following is useful to diagnose a brain tumor?

Harrison's 20th Ed. Chapter 86, Page 643

A. Cerebral angiogram
B. Electroencephalogram (EEG)
C. Lumbar puncture
D. None of the above

3319. Which of the following helps in distinguishing brain tumor progression from necrotic tissue?

Harrison's 20th Ed. Chapter 86, Page 643

A. Fluid-attenuated inversion recovery (FLAIR) MRI
B. Positron emission tomography (PET)
C. MR perfusion and spectroscopy
D. All of the above

MR perfusion & spectroscopy provides information on blood flow or tissue composition. It also helps in distinguishing tumor progression from necrotic tissue as a consequence of treatment with radiation & chemotherapy.

3320. Headache as a presenting symptom is least common in?

Harrison's 20th Ed. Chapter 86, Page 644 Table 86-1

A. High-grade glioma
B. Low-grade glioma
C. Meningioma
D. Metastases

3321. Hemiparesis as a presenting symptom is most common in?

Harrison's 20th Ed. Chapter 86, Page 644 Table 86-1

A. High-grade glioma
B. Low-grade glioma
C. Meningioma
D. Metastases

3322. Impaired cognitive function as a presenting symptom is most common in?

Harrison's 20th Ed. Chapter 86, Page 644 Table 86-1

A. High-grade glioma
B. Low-grade glioma
C. Meningioma
D. Metastases

3323. Seizures as a presenting symptom is most common in?

Harrison's 20th Ed. Chapter 86, Page 644 Table 86-1

A. High-grade glioma
B. Low-grade glioma
C. Meningioma
D. Metastases

3324. Antiepileptic drug that does not induce hepatic microsomal enzyme system is?

Harrison's 20th Ed. Chapter 86, Page 644

A. Levetiracetam
B. Topiramate
C. Lacosamide
D. All of the above

Antiepileptic drugs that do not induce hepatic microsomal enzyme system include levetiracetam, topiramate, lamotrigine, valproic acid and lacosamide.

3325. Exposure to ionizing radiation is a risk factor for?

Harrison's 20th Ed. Chapter 86, Page 644

A. Meningiomas
B. Gliomas
C. Schwannomas
D. All of the above

The only established risk factor for meningiomas, gliomas and schwannomas is exposure to ionizing radiation.

3326. The established risk factor for primary CNS lymphoma is?

Harrison's 20th Ed. Chapter 86, Page 644

A. Foods containing N-nitroso compounds
B. Immunosuppression
C. Exposure to electromagnetic fields (cellular telephones)
D. Positive family history

3327. Well-documented environmental risk factor for the development of gliomas is?

Harrison's 20th Ed. Chapter 86, Page 644

A. Benzene
B. Cadmium
C. Ionizing radiation
D. Ozone

For majority of primary brain tumors, the only established risk factors are exposure to ionizing radiation (meningiomas, gliomas, and schwannomas) and immunosuppression (primary CNS lymphoma).

3328. Which of the following is associated with increased risk for deep vein thrombosis & pulmonary embolism?

Harrison's 20th Ed. Chapter 86, Page 644

A. Leptomeningeal metastases
B. Brain metastases
C. Medulloblastoma
D. All of the above

High-grade gliomas & brain metastases are associated with increased risk for DVT & PE because these tumors secrete procoagulant factors.

3329. Hereditary syndromes associated with an increased risk of brain tumors includes all except?

Harrison's 20th Ed. Chapter 86, Page 645 Table 86-2

A. Li-Fraumeni syndrome
B. Turcot syndrome
C. Werner syndrome
D. Pearson syndrome

Pearson syndrome is a mitochondrial disease consisting of pancreatic insufficiency, pancytopenia and lactic acidosis.

3330. Pheochromocytoma is associated with which of the following hereditary syndrome?

Harrison's 20th Ed. Chapter 86, Page 645 Table 86-2

A. Li-Fraumeni syndrome
B. Turcot syndrome
C. Werner syndrome
D. von Hippel-Lindau syndrome

3331. Lhermitte-Duclos disease is best related to?

Harrison's 20th Ed. Chapter 86, Page 645 Table 86-2

A. Gardner's syndrome
B. Gorlin syndrome
C. Cowden's syndrome
D. Werner's syndrome

3332. Which of the following about Foster Kennedy syndrome is false?

DeJong's The Neurologic Examination, 7th Ed. Page 141

A. Anosmia
B. Unilateral ipsilateral optic atrophy
C. Contralateral papilledema
D. None of the above

Foster Kennedy syndrome consists of anosmia accompanied by unilateral ipsilateral optic atrophy & contralateral papilledema, classically due to a large tumor involving orbitofrontal region (olfactory groove meningioma). It was first described by Sir William Gowers, later and more thoroughly by R. Foster Kennedy.

3333. Which of the following is absent in pseudo - Foster Kennedy syndrome?

DeJong's The Neurologic Examination, 7th Ed. Page 141

A. Anosmia
B. Unilateral ipsilateral optic atrophy
C. Contralateral papilledema
D. Anterior ischemic optic neuropathy

Ophthalmologic picture similar to Foster Kennedy syndrome, without anosmia, is more often due to anterior ischemic optic neuropathy, involving first one eye, leading to atrophy, then the other, leading to disc edema is termed as the pseudo - Foster Kennedy syndrome.

3334. Which of the following is false about Cogan's rule?

DeJong's The Neurologic Examination, 7th Ed. Page 210

A. Asymmetric optokinetic nystagmus (OKN)
B. Etiology in parietal lobe
C. More likely to be a tumor
D. None of the above

With asymmetric optokinetic nystagmus (OKN), the lesion is more likely to reside in the parietal lobe, and more likely to be nonvascular, that is, a tumor (Cogan's rule).

3335. Which of the following is a tumor-suppressor gene?

Harrison's 20th Ed. Chapter 86, Page 644

A. Epidermal growth factor receptor (EGFR)
B. Platelet-derived growth factor receptors (PDGFR)
C. Phosphatase and tensin homolog (PTEN)
D. All of the above

Tumor-suppressor genes include p53, cyclin-dependent kinase inhibitor 2A and 2B (CDKN2A/B) and phosphatase and tensin homolog on chromosome 10 [PTEN]). Proto-oncogenes include epidermal growth factor receptor (EGFR) and platelet-derived growth factor receptors (PDGFR).

3336. Molecular alterations in gliomas include?

Harrison's 20th Ed. Chapter 86, Page 644

A. Isocitrate dehydrogenase (IDH) mutations & 1p/19q codeletion
B. ATRX
C. p53
D. All of the above

3337. Which of the following is not a low-grade astrocytoma?

Harrison's 20th Ed. Chapter 86, Page 644

A. Astrocytoma
B. Pilocytic astrocytoma
C. Subependymal giant cell astrocytoma
D. Anaplastic astrocytoma

3338. Anaplastic astrocytoma belongs to which WHO prognostic grade of astrocytomas?

Harrison's 20th Ed. Chapter 86, Page 644

A. Grade I
B. Grade II
C. Grade III
D. Grade IV

3339. Out of the following, most common childhood brain tumor is?

Harrison's 20th Ed. Chapter 86, Page 644

A. Pilocytic astrocytoma
B. Subependymal giant cell astrocytoma
C. Pleomorphic xanthoastrocytoma
D. Glioblastoma multiforme

Pilocytic astrocytoma (spindle-shaped cells) is the most common childhood brain tumor and is typically benign. They occur typically in the cerebellum.

3340. Nervous system neoplasm seen in tuberous sclerosis is?

Harrison's 20th Ed. Chapter 86, Page 644

A. Astrocytoma
B. Schwannoma
C. Medulloblastoma
D. Hemangioblastoma

Subependymal giant cell astrocytoma mostly occurs in tuberous sclerosis.

3341. Which of the following is the preferred drug for high-grade astrocytomas?

Harrison's 20th Ed. Chapter 86, Page 645

A. Temozolomide
B. Carmustine (BCNU)
C. Lomustine (CCNU)
D. Vincristine

3342. Resistance to temozolomide best relates to?

Harrison's 20th Ed. Chapter 86, Page 645

A. Histone deacetylases (HDAC)
B. Ataxia telangiectasia mutated (ATM) gene
C. O6-methylguanine-DNA methyltransferase (MGMT)
D. Cyclic AMP response element binding (CREB) protein

Patients whose tumor contains DNA repair enzyme O6-methylguanine-DNA methyltransferase (MGMT) are relatively resistant to temozolomide and have a worse prognosis compared to those whose tumors contain low levels of MGMT as a result of silencing of the MGMT gene by promoter hypermethylation.

3343. Most important adverse prognostic factor in patients with glioblastoma is?

Harrison's 20th Ed. Chapter 86, Page 646

A. Older age
B. Absence of IDH mutations
C. Unresectable tumor
D. All of the above

Most important adverse prognostic factors in patients with glioblastomas are older age, absence of IDH mutations, unmethylated MGMT promoter, poor Karnofsky performance status, and unresectable tumor.

3344. Fried-egg appearance best relates to?

Harrison's 20th Ed. Chapter 86, Page 646

A. Ependymoma
B. Glioblastoma
C. Oligodendroglioma
D. Gliomatosis cerebri

3345. Oligodendrogliomas with deletions of which chromosome always respond to chemotherapy?

Harrison's 20th Ed. Chapter 86, Page 646

A. 1 p
B. 2 p
C. 3 p
D. 4 p

Oligodendrogliomas with deletions of chromosome 1p always respond to chemotherapy.

3346. Systemic combination chemotherapy (PCV) for oligodendrogliomas includes all except?

Harrison's 20th Ed. Chapter 86, Page 646

A. Procarbazine
B. Lomustine
C. Temozolomide
D. Vincristine

Oligodendrogliomas respond well to systemic combination chemotherapy with procarbazine, lomustine, and vincristine (PCV), or to temozolomide.

3347. In adults, ependymomas of spinal canal are mostly located in?

Harrison's 20th Ed. Chapter 86, Page 646

A. Cervical region
B. Thoracic region
C. Lumbosacral region
D. All of the above

In adults, myxopapillary histologic type is the most frequent ependymoma, which typically arises from the filum terminale of the spinal cord and appears in the lumbosacral region.

3348. Which of the following is associated with medulloblastoma?

Harrison's 20th Ed. Chapter 86, Page 645 Table 86-2

A. Gorlin syndrome
B. Turcot syndrome
C. Li-Fraumeni syndrome
D. All of the above

3349. Homer-Wright rosettes are best related to?

Harrison's 20th Ed. Chapter 86, Page 647

A. Meningioma
B. Primary central nervous system lymphoma (PCNSL)
C. Acoustic neuroma
D. Medulloblastoma

Histologically, medulloblastomas are highly cellular tumors with abundant dark staining, round nuclei, and rosette formation called Homer-Wright rosettes.

3350. Which of the following molecular subgroup of medulloblastoma has the worst outcome?

Harrison's 20th Ed. Chapter 86, Page 647

A. WNT-activated
B. SHH-activated
C. Non-WNT/non-SHH, group 3
D. Non-WNT/non-SHH, group 4

3351. Patients of medulloblastoma present with?

Harrison's 20th Ed. Chapter 86, Page 647

A. Headache
B. Ataxia
C. Signs of brainstem involvement
D. All of the above

Regardless of subtype, patients of medulloblastoma present with headache, ataxia, and signs of brainstem involvement.

3352. Meningiomas are more common in?

Harrison's 20th Ed. Chapter 86, Page 648

A. Women
B. In patients with neurofibromatosis type 2 (NF2)
C. In patients with a past history of cranial irradiation
D. All of the above

Meningiomas are the most common primary brain tumor. They are more common in women, in patients with neurofibromatosis type 2 (NF2) and in patients with a past history of cranial irradiation.

3353. Which of the following is the main in differential diagnosis of meningioma?

Harrison's 20th Ed. Chapter 86, Page 648

A. Hemangiopericytoma
B. Solitary fibrous tumors
C. Dural metastasis
D. Schwannoma

The main differential diagnosis of meningioma is a dural metastasis. Hemangiopericytomas and solitary fibrous tumors resemble meningiomas.

3354. On MRI, dural tail is seen in?

Harrison's 20th Ed. Chapter 86, Page 648

A. Meningioma
B. Dural metastases
C. Dural lymphoma
D. All of the above

3355. Neurofibromatosis type 1 (NF1) is associated with an increased incidence of schwannomas of?

Harrison's 20th Ed. Chapter 86, Page 648

A. Trigeminal nerve
B. Facial nerve
C. Eighth cranial nerve
D. Spinal nerve roots

Neurofibromatosis type 1 is associated with an increased incidence of schwannomas of spinal nerve roots.

3356. Schwannoma most frequently involves which cranial nerve?

Harrison's 20th Ed. Chapter 86, Page 648

A. II
B. III
C. V
D. VIII

3357. Cranial nerve where Schwannoma never occur is?

Harrison's 20th Ed. Chapter 86, Page 648

A. II
B. III
C. VIII
D. XI

Schwannomas are most frequent in the vestibular division of VIII cranial nerve, fifth cranial nerve is the second most frequent site. Schwannomas are not found in optic & olfactory nerves as they are myelinated by oligodendroglia rather than by Schwann cells.

3358. Radiographically, which of the following resemble lipomas?

Harrison's 20th Ed. Chapter 86, Page 649

A. Dysembryoplastic neuroepithelial tumors (DNTs)
B. Colloid cyst
C. Dermoid cyst
D. Epidermoid cyst

3359. Which of the following occurs in cerebellopontine angle?

Harrison's 20th Ed. Chapter 86, Page 649

A. Dysembryoplastic neuroepithelial tumors (DNTs)
B. Colloid cyst
C. Dermoid cyst
D. Epidermoid cyst

3360. Bruns' nystagmus best relates to?

DeJong's The Neurologic Examination, 7th Ed. Page 622

A. Occipital lobe
B. Temporal lobe
C. Cerebellopontine angle
D. Medulla oblongata

When a tumor of the cerebellopontine angle is present, nystagmus is coarse on looking toward the side of lesion and fine & rapid on gaze to the opposite side (Bruns' nystagmus).

3361. High-dose methotrexate is used in the treatment of?

Harrison's 20th Ed. Chapter 86, Page 649

A. Craniopharyngioma
B. Schwannoma
C. Primary central nervous system lymphoma
D. Oligodendroglioma

3362. NF1 gene is on chromosome?

Harrison's 20th Ed. Chapter 86, Page 649

A. 1
B. 4
C. 9
D. 17

Tumor-suppressor NF1 gene on chromosome 17. Its mutation causes von Recklinghausen's disease. It encodes protein neurofibromin. NF2 gene is on chromosome 22q, & encodes neurofibromin 2, schwannomin, or merlin (moesin, ezrin, radixin-like protein).

3363. Mutations of NF1 result in?

Harrison's 20th Ed. Chapter 86, Page 649

A. Optic nerve gliomas
B. Astrocytomas
C. Meningiomas
D. All of the above

Mutations of NF1 result in neurofibromas, plexiform neurofibromas, optic nerve gliomas, astrocytomas and meningiomas.

3364. Manifestation of NF1 (von Recklinhausen's disease) is?

Harrison's 20th Ed. Chapter 86, Page 649

A. Cafe-au-lait spots
B. Axillary freckling
C. Lisch nodules
D. All of the above

In addition to neurofibromas, which appear as multiple, soft, rubbery cutaneous tumors, other cutaneous manifestations of NF1 include cafe-au-lait spots and axillary freckling. NF1 is also associated with hamartomas of the iris termed Lisch nodules, pheochromocytomas, pseudoarthrosis of the tibia, scoliosis, epilepsy and mental retardation.

3365. Lisch nodules relate best to?

Harrison's 20th Ed. Chapter 86, Page 649

A. Ocular lens
B. Iris
C. Retina
D. Conjunctiva

Hamartomas of the iris are called Lisch nodules.

3366. NF2 is characterized by all except?

Harrison's 20th Ed. Chapter 86, Page 649

A. Bilateral vestibular schwannomas
B. Multiple meningiomas
C. Periungual fibromas
D. Astrocytomas

NF2 is characterized by bilateral vestibular schwannomas in over 90% of patients, multiple meningiomas and spinal ependymomas and astrocytomas.

3367. Bourneville's disease is also called?

Harrison's 20th Ed. Chapter 86, Page 649

A. Meningioma
B. Tuberous sclerosis
C. Ependymoma
D. Primary CNS lymphoma

Tuberous sclerosis is also called Bourneville's disease.

3368. TSC stands for?

Harrison's 20th Ed. Chapter 86, Page 649

A. Tuberous sclerosis complex
B. Tuberous sclerosis candidate
C. Tuberous sclerosis compound
D. Tuberous sclerosis combination

Tuberous sclerosis is caused by mutations in either TSC1 gene (9q34) and encodes hamartin, or TSC2 gene (16p13.3) and encodes the protein tuberin.

3369. Shagreen patches are best related to?

Harrison's 20th Ed. Chapter 86, Page 649

A. Secondary syphilis
B. Neurofibromatosis Type 1
C. Tuberous sclerosis
D. Von Hippel–Lindau syndrome

Shagreen patches are yellowish thickenings of skin over lumbosacral region of the back, seen in tuberous sclerosis.

3370. Tuberous sclerosis is characterized by all except?

Harrison's 20th Ed. Chapter 86, Page 649

A. Cutaneous lesions
B. Seizures
C. Deafness
D. Mental retardation

Tuberous sclerosis is characterized by cutaneous lesions, seizures, and mental retardation.

3371. Cutaneous lesions in tuberous sclerosis include all except?

Harrison's 20th Ed. Chapter 86, Page 345

A. Adenoma sebaceum
B. Ash leaf - shaped hypopigmented macules
C. Lentigo
D. Shagreen patches

In tuberous sclerosis, earliest cutaneous sign is an ash leaf spot. Other manifestations include adenoma sebaceum (facial angiofibromas), shagreen patch, hypomelanotic macules, periungual fibromas, renal angiomyolipomas, and cardiac rhabdomyomas. These patients have an increased incidence of subependymal nodules, cortical tubers, and subependymal giant-cell astrocytomas (SEGAs).

3372. Most effective therapy for subependymal giant-cell astrocytomas (SEGAs) is?

Harrison's 20th Ed. Chapter 86, Page 649

A. Alemtuzumab
B. Antithymocyte globulin
C. Sirolimus
D. Mycophenolate mofetil

3373. Hemangioblastomas in Von Hippel-Lindau syndrome are seen in?

Harrison's 20th Ed. Chapter 86, Page 666

A. Retina
B. Cerebellum
C. Spinal cord
D. All of the above

VHL syndrome consists of retinal, cerebellar, and spinal hemangioblastomas, which are slowly growing cystic tumors.

3374. Hemangioblastomas in Von Hippel-Lindau syndrome produce which hormone?

Harrison's 20th Ed. Chapter 86, Page 666

A. Parathyroid hormone (PTH)
B. Calcitonin
C. Erythropoietin
D. Antidiuretic hormone

Erythropoietin produced by hemangioblastomas results in polycythemia.

3375. Which of the following is the most common origin of brain metastases?

Harrison's 20th Ed. Chapter 86, Page 649

A. Ca. lung
B. Ca. ovary
C. Ca. thyroid
D. Ca. prostate

Lung cancers (primary & metastatic) are the most common origin of brain metastases.

3376. Breast cancer has a propensity to metastasize to?

Harrison's 20th Ed. Chapter 86, Page 649

A. Leptomeninges
B. Dura
C. Spinal cord
D. All of the above

3377. Breast cancer has a propensity to metastasize to?

Harrison's 20th Ed. Chapter 86, Page 649

A. Anterior pituitary gland
B. Posterior pituitary gland
C. Hypothalamus
D. Hippocampus

Breast cancer (esp. ductal carcinoma) has a propensity to metastasize to the cerebellum and the posterior pituitary gland.

3378. Which of the following cancers rarely metastasize to brain?

Harrison's 20th Ed. Chapter 86, Page 649

A. Prostate cancer
B. Ovarian cancer
C. Hodgkin's disease
D. All of the above

Prostate & ovarian cancer & Hodgkin's disease rarely metastasize to brain.

3379. Breast cancer that metastasizes to which of the following tends not to metastasize to brain?

Harrison's 20th Ed. Chapter 86, Page 649

A. Pleura
B. Bone
C. Lung
D. Liver

3380. Which of the following cancer has the greatest propensity to intracranial metastases with hemorrhage?

Harrison's 20th Ed. Chapter 86, Page 649

A. Melanoma
B. Thyroid cancer
C. Kidney cancer
D. All of the above

Melanoma, thyroid and kidney cancer have the greatest propensity to intracranial metastases hemorrhage.

3381. Ommaya reservoir best relates to?

Harrison's 20th Ed. Chapter 86, Page 651

A. Bone marrow transplantation
B. Ventriculoperitoneal shunt
C. Intraventricular cannula
D. Spinal cord compression

Ommaya reservoir is an intraventricular cannula to deliver chemotherapy intrathecally.

3382. Brain tumor metastases that spread to spinal cord via CSF pathways are termed?

Surg Neurol 1991;35:377-80

A. Pin metastases
B. Hanging metastases
C. Drop metastases
D. Confluent metastases

Intradural extramedullary spinal metastases that arise from intracranial lesions are called drop metastases.

3383. Which of the following is a cellular marker for proliferation?

Harrison's 20th Ed. Chapter 75, Page 560

A. Ki-66
B. Ki-67
C. Ki-68
D. Ki-69

Ki-67 protein (also known as MKI67) is a cellular marker for proliferation. Proliferation index (mitotic activity) can be determined with monoclonal antibody Ki-67 which recognizes a histone protein expressed in proliferating but not quiescent cells.

3384. Which of the following is a germ cell tumor?

Harrison's 20th Ed. Chapter 86, Page 640

A. Teratoma
B. Yolk sac tumor
C. Choriocarcinoma
D. All of the above

Malignant germ cell tumors include dysgerminomas, yolk sac tumors, immature teratomas, embryonal & choriocarcinomas.

3385. What level of 'Karnofsky performance status' have a poor prognosis in patients with brain tumor?

Harrison's 20th Ed. Chapter 65, Page 438 Table 65-4

A. < 70
B. < 80
C. < 90
D. < 100

Karnofsky performance scale and Eastern Cooperative Oncology Group (ECOG) performance scale are meant to assess patients with brain tumors. A Karnofsky score ≥ 70 indicates that patient is ambulatory & independent in self-care activities.

3386. Differential diagnosis of ring-enhancement lesions include?

Harrison's 20th Ed. Chapter 135, Page 1014

A. Glioblastoma
B. Brain abscess stage 3
C. L. monocytogenes meningoencephalitis
D. All of the above

3387. Differential diagnosis of ring-enhancement lesions include?

Harrison's 20th Ed. Chapter 197, Page 1450, 1445

A. Actinomycosis
B. CNS lymphomas
C. Toxoplasmosis
D. All of the above

3388. In vegetative state which of the following persists?

Harrison's 20th Ed. Chapter 300, Page 2068

A. Yawning
B. Coughing
C. Swallowing
D. All of the above

Encephalitis

3389. Sporadic cases of encephalitis in immunocompetent adults are mostly caused by?

Harrison's 20th Ed. Chapter 132, Page 992

A. HSV
B. West Nile virus (WNV)
C. St. Louis encephalitis virus
D. La Crosse virus

Most important viruses causing sporadic cases of encephalitis in immunocompetent adults are HSV, VZV and EBV. Epidemics of encephalitis are caused by arboviruses.

3390. Which of the following is a member of Flaviviruses?

Harrison's 20th Ed. Chapter 132, Page 992

A. Eastern equine encephalitis virus
B. Western equine encephalitis virus
C. West Nile virus (WNV)
D. California encephalitis virus

Epidemics of encephalitis are caused by arboviruses of which there are several groups like Alphaviruses (Eastern equine encephalitis virus, Western equine encephalitis virus), Flaviviruses (WNV, St. Louis encephalitis virus, Powassan virus), and Bunyaviruses (California encephalitis virus serogroup, La Crosse virus).

3391. Which of the following is a togavirus?

Harrison's 20th Ed. Chapter 132, Page 992

A. Toscana
B. Nipah
C. Chikungunya
D. Human parechovirus 3 (HPeV3)

3392. Viral "hemorrhagic" encephalitis can be seen in?

Harrison's 20th Ed. Chapter 132, Page 992

A. HSV
B. Colorado tick fever virus
C. California encephalitis virus
D. All of the above

~20% of patients with encephalitis have RBC's (>500/µL) in CSF tap (hemorrhagic encephalitis) which is also seen with HSV, Colorado tick fever virus and California encephalitis virus.

3393. Which of the following seizure type occurs in a case of severe viral encephalitis?

Harrison's 20th Ed. Chapter 132, Page 992

A. Absence (petit mal)
B. Tonic-clonic (grand mal)
C. Myoclonic
D. Any of the above

Virtually every possible type of focal neurologic disturbance can occur in viral encephalitis.

3394. Which of the following focal neurological findings is commonly encountered in viral encephalitis?

Harrison's 20th Ed. Chapter 132, Page 992

A. Aphasia
B. Ataxia
C. Involuntary movements
D. All of the above

Most common focal findings in viral encephalitis are aphasia, ataxia, hemiparesis, involuntary movements & cranial nerve deficits.

3395. "Atypical lymphocytes" in CSF of viral encephalitis are commonly seen in?

Harrison's 20th Ed. Chapter 132, Page 992

A. EBV
B. CMV
C. HSV
D. Enteroviruses

Atypical lymphocytes in CSF may be seen in EBV infection and less commonly with other viruses like CMV, HSV and enteroviruses.

3396. CSF PCR is most sensitive for which of the following viruses causing viral encephalitis?

Harrison's 20th Ed. Chapter 132, Page 993

A. WNV
B. HSV
C. Enterovirus
D. VZV

Sensitivity is ~98% & specificity is ~94% of CSF HSV PCR.

3397. Presence in CSF of which class of antibody against WNV indicates WNV encephalitis?

Harrison's 20th Ed. Chapter 132, Page 993

A. IgA
B. IgG
C. IgM
D. IgE

Demonstration of WNV intrathecally synthesized IgM antibodies is diagnostic of WNV encephalitis. They do not cross blood-brain barrier.

3398. Which of the following about HSV-1 encephalitis is false?

Harrison's 20th Ed. Chapter 132, Page 993

A. Focal findings in MRI
B. Invariably negative CSF cultures
C. Most sensitive CSF HSV PCR
D. None of the above

Focal findings in encephalitis raises the possibility of HSV encephalitis. Cultures are invariably negative in cases of HSV-1 encephalitis. CSF HSV PCR has a sensitivity of ~98%.

3399. In MRI, which cortical lobe of brain is most affected in HSV encephalitis?

Harrison's 20th Ed. Chapter 132, Page 993

A. Frontal
B. Temporal
C. Parietal
D. Occipital

~10% of patients with PCR-documented HSV encephalitis have normal MRI, although ~90% will have abnormalities in the temporal lobe.

3400. In MRI of viral encephalitis, abnormalities involving deep brain structures like thalamus, basal ganglia, and brainstem rather than cortex indicate infection with which of the following viruses?

Harrison's 20th Ed. Chapter 132, Page 993

A. HSV
B. VZV
C. WNV
D. All of the above

MRI abnormalities of patients with WNV encephalitis involve deep brain structures like thalamus, basal ganglia & brainstem rather than cortex. Presentation is therefore with prominent movement disorders (tremor, myoclonus) or Parkinsonism. Patients with WNV infection can also present with acute poliomyelitis-like areflexic paralysis.

3401. In MRI of viral encephalitis, areas of hemorrhagic infarction reflect infection with which of the following viruses?

Harrison's 20th Ed. Chapter 132, Page 993

A. HSV
B. VZV
C. WNV
D. All of the above

Patients with VZV encephalitis show areas of hemorrhagic infarction pointing towards a CNS vasculopathy rather than a true encephalitis.

3402. Which of the following bacterial infection can mimic viral encephalitis?

Harrison's 20th Ed. Chapter 132, Page 993

A. Listeria
B. Bartonella
C. Mycoplasma
D. All of the above

Bartonella infection is the most common bacterial infection mimicking viral encephalitis.

3403. In viral encephalitis, infection with which of the following can present as acute ascending paralysis resembling Guillain-Barre' syndrome?

Harrison's 20th Ed. Chapter 132, Page 993

A. HIV infection
B. Rabies
C. WNV
D. All of the above

Acute ascending paralysis resembling Guillain-Barre' syndrome but associated with CSF pleocytosis can occur with HIV infection, rabies, and WNV infection.

3404. Abnormalities in MRI are found in which of the following regions of the brain in viral encephalitis caused by rabies?

Harrison's 20th Ed. Chapter 132, Page 993

A. Brainstem
B. Hippocampus
C. Hypothalamus
D. All of the above

In rabies, CSF lymphocytic pleocytosis with areas of increased T2 signal abnormality in brainstem, hippocampus & hypothalamus are seen.

3405. PCR amplification of viral nucleic acid for diagnosis of viral encephalitis caused by rabies can be done from?

Harrison's 20th Ed. Chapter 132, Page 994

A. CSF
B. Saliva
C. Tears
D. All of the above

PCR amplification of viral nucleic acid from CSF and saliva or tears may also enable diagnosis.

3406. Enzyme in HSV, VZV, and EBV that phosphorylates acyclovir to produce acyclovir-5` monophosphate is?

Harrison's 20th Ed. Chapter 132, Page 995

A. 2`deoxyguanosine
B. 3`deoxyguanosine
C. Deoxypyrimidine kinase
D. Pyrimidine kinase

HSV, VZV, & EBV encode enzyme, deoxypyrimidine (thymidine) kinase, that phosphorylates acyclovir to produce acyclovir-5`-monophosphate.

3407. Which of the following metabolite of acyclovir acts as an antiviral agent by inhibiting viral DNA polymerase?

Harrison's 20th Ed. Chapter 132, Page 995

A. Monophosphate
B. Biphosphate
C. Triphosphate
D. Any of the above

Infected host cell enzymes phosphorylate acyclovir-5`-monophosphate to form a triphosphate derivative which acts as an antiviral agent by inhibiting viral DNA polymerase & by causing premature termination of nascent viral DNA chains.

3408. In adults suffering from HSV encephalitis, duration of intravenous acyclovir therapy should be for a minimum period of?

Harrison's 20th Ed. Chapter 132, Page 995

A. 3 days
B. 7 days
C. 10 days
D. 14 days

3409. In neonates suffering from HSV encephalitis, duration of intravenous acyclovir therapy should be for a minimum period of?

Harrison's 20th Ed. Chapter 132, Page 995

A. 5 days
B. 10 days
C. 14 days
D. 21 days

Adults should receive a dose of 10 mg/kg of acyclovir IV 8 hourly (30 mg/kg/day) for at least 14 days. Neonates with HSV encephalitis receive 20 mg/kg of acyclovir 8 hourly (60 mg/kg/day) for at least 21 days.

3410. Which of the following is not a side effect of IV acyclovir?

Harrison's 20th Ed. Chapter 132, Page 995

A. Hemolysis
B. Elevations in BUN & creatinine
C. Thrombocytopenia
D. Neurotoxicity

Complications of acyclovir therapy are elevations in BUN & creatinine levels (5%), thrombocytopenia (6%), GI toxicity (7%) & neurotoxicity (lethargy, obtundation, disorientation, confusion, agitation, hallucinations, tremors, seizures) (1%). Hemolysis, with resulting anemia, is a major side effect of IV ribavarin therapy.

3411. Which of the following drug is effective in CMV-related CNS infections?

Harrison's 20th Ed. Chapter 132, Page 995

A. Ganciclovir
B. Foscarnet
C. Cidofovir
D. All of the above

Ganciclovir & foscarnet (often used in combination) are effective in CMV-related CNS infections. Cidofovir may provide an alternative in patients who fail to respond to ganciclovir and foscarnet.

3412. Which of the following drugs is useful for treatment of WNV encephalitis?

Harrison's 20th Ed. Chapter 132, Page 995

A. Ganciclovir
B. Foscarnet
C. Cidofovir
D. None of the above

3413. Incidence & severity of sequelae in patients surviving viral encephalitis is more in infections with?

Harrison's 20th Ed. Chapter 132, Page 995

A. Eastern equine encephalitis virus
B. EBV
C. California encephalitis virus
D. Venezuelan equine encephalitis virus

In Eastern equine encephalitis virus infection, ~80% of survivors have severe neurologic sequelae. Severe sequelae are unusual in EBV, California & Venezuelan equine encephalitis.

3414. Incidence & severity of sequelae of viral encephalitis depends on which of the following?

Harrison's 20th Ed. Chapter 132, Page 996

A. Age of patient
B. Level of consciousness at time of initiation of therapy
C. Amount of HSV DNA in CSF at time of presentation
D. All of the above

Incidence & severity of sequelae are directly related to age of patient & level of consciousness at initiation of therapy. Clinical outcome following treatment correlates with amount of HSV DNA in CSF at presentation.

3415. Most common pathogen causing fungal meningitis is?

Harrison's 20th Ed. Chapter 132, Page 995

A. Coccidioides immitis
B. Histoplasma capsulatum
C. Cryptococcus neoformans
D. Candida

The most common pathogen causing fungal meningitis is C. neoformans.

3416. Which of the following cranial nerve is most frequently involved in T. pallidum invasion of CNS?

Harrison's 20th Ed. Chapter 132, Page 996

A. II
B. III
C. VII
D. XII

Cranial nerves VII and VIII are most frequently involved in syphilis.

3417. Negative result of which of the following does not rule out neurosyphilis?

Harrison's 20th Ed. Chapter 132, Page 996

A. CSF VDRL
B. CSF FTA-ABS
C. MHA-TP
D. All of the above

A negative CSF VDRL does not rule out neurosyphilis. A negative CSF FTA-ABS or MHA-TP rules out neurosyphilis.

3418. In tuberculous meningitis, which sample of CSF is best for detecting acid-fast bacilli (AFB)?

Harrison's 20th Ed. Chapter 132, Page 996

A. First tube
B. Middle tube
C. Last tube
D. Any of the above

In TBM, last tube of CSF collected at LP is the best tube to send for a smear for AFB. If there is a pellicle in CSF or a cobweb-like clot on surface of fluid, AFB is demonstrated in smear of clot / pellicle.

3419. Eosinophils in the CSF are found in meningitis due to?

Harrison's 20th Ed. Chapter 132, Page 996

A. L. monocytogenes
B. T. pallidum
C. C. immitis
D. La Crosse virus

Eosinophils in the CSF are found in C. immitis meningitis.

3420. The most common complication of fungal meningitis is?

Harrison's 20th Ed. Chapter 132, Page 996

A. Seizure
B. Amnesia
C. Hydrocephalus
D. Hearing loss

The most common complication of fungal meningitis is hydrocephalus.

3421. In progressive multifocal leukoencephalopathy, which of the following is not involved?

Harrison's 20th Ed. Chapter 132, Page 997

A. Frontal cortex
B. Cerebellum
C. Midbrain
D. Spinal cord

In PML, multifocal areas of demyelination distributed throughout the brain but sparing spinal cord and optic nerves are seen.

3422. Which of the following is false about progressive multifocal leukoencephalopathy?

Harrison's 20th Ed. Chapter 132, Page 997

A. Occurs in immunosuppressed population
B. Only known manifestation of JC virus infection
C. Late manifestation of AIDS
D. None of the above

3423. Which of the following is useful for the diagnosis of progressive multifocal leukoencephalopathy?

Harrison's 20th Ed. Chapter 132, Page 997

A. EEG
B. CT scan of brain
C. Positive CSF PCR for JCV DNA
D. Serologic studies for JC virus

Positive CSF PCR for JCV DNA with typical MRI lesions in appropriate clinical setting is diagnostic of PML.

3424. Typical visual deficit seen in progressive multifocal leukoencephalopathy is?

Harrison's 20th Ed. Chapter 132, Page 997

A. Achromatopia
B. Homonymous hemianopia
C. Cortical blindness
D. Amaurosis fugax

Patients of progressive multifocal leukoencephalopathy present with visual deficits, typically homonymous hemianopia.

3425. Subacute sclerosing panencephalitis occurs after a latent interval of how many years after measles infection?

Harrison's 20th Ed. Chapter 132, Page 997

A. 1–2 years
B. 2–4 years
C. 4–6 years
D. 6–8 years

SSPE occurs after a latent interval of 6–8 years after measles infection.

3426. Which of the following is not a manifestation of subacute sclerosing panencephalitis?

Harrison's 20th Ed. Chapter 132, Page 997

A. Fever and headache
B. Progressive intellectual deterioration
C. Focal and/or generalized seizures
D. Ataxia

Signs of a CNS viral infection - fever & headache do not occur in SSPE.

3427. Which of the following diagnostic modalities are useful in SSPE?

Harrison's 20th Ed. Chapter 132, Page 997

A. EEG
B. CSF
C. MRI
D. All of the above

3428. CSF finding in SSPE is?

Harrison's 20th Ed. Chapter 132, Page 997

A. Acellular
B. Elevated gamma globulin level
C. Elevated CSF antimeasles antibody level
D. All of the above

In SSPE, CSF is acellular with markedly elevated gamma globulin level (>20% of total CSF protein). CSF antimeasles antibody levels are invariably elevated & oligoclonal antimeasles antibodies are present.

3429. Which of the following drugs is used in the treatment of SSPE?

Harrison's 20th Ed. Chapter 132, Page 997

A. Acyclovir
B. Isoprinosine
C. Cytarabine
D. Foscarnet

Isoprinosine (100 mg/kg/day), alone or in combination with intrathecal or intraventricular α-interferon prolongs survival with clinical improvement.

Acute Meningitis: Bacterial Meningitis

3430. In meningoencephalitis, which of the following is involved in the inflammatory reaction?

Harrison's 20th Ed. Chapter 133, Page 998

A. Meninges
B. Subarachnoid space (SAS)
C. Brain parenchyma
D. All of the above

3431. In adults, organism most commonly responsible for community-acquired bacterial meningitis is?

Harrison's 20th Ed. Chapter 133, Page 998

A. N. meningitidis
B. Streptococcus pneumoniae
C. Group B streptococci
D. H. influenzae

Organisms responsible for community-acquired bacterial meningitis are S. pneumoniae (~50%), N. meningitidis (~25%), group B streptococci (~15%), Listeria monocytogenes (~10%) & H. influenzae Type B (<10%).

3432. Most important predisposing condition that increase risk of pneumococcal meningitis is?

Harrison's 20th Ed. Chapter 133, Page 998

A. Acute or chronic pneumococcal sinusitis
B. Alcoholism
C. Pneumococcal pneumonia
D. Splenectomy

The most important predisposing condition that increase the risk of pneumococcal meningitis is pneumococcal pneumonia. Other risk factors include coexisting acute or chronic pneumococcal sinusitis or otitis media, alcoholism, diabetes, splenectomy, hypogammaglobulinemia, complement deficiency & head trauma with basilar skull fracture and CSF rhinorrhea.

3433. The mortality rate in pneumococcal meningitis is?

Harrison's 20th Ed. Chapter 133, Page 998

A. ~ 2%
B. ~ 5%
C. ~ 10%
D. ~ 20%

The mortality rate in pneumococcal meningitis remains -20% despite antibiotic therapy.

3434. Quadrivalent meningococcal glycoconjugate vaccine does not contain which serogroup?

Harrison's 20th Ed. Chapter 133, Page 998

A. Serogroup A
B. Serogroup B
C. Serogroup C
D. Serogroup Y

Quadrivalent (serogroups A, C, W-135 and Y) meningococcal glycoconjugate vaccine does not contain serogroup B which is responsible for one-third of cases of meningococcal disease.

3435. Individuals with deficiencies of which of the following are highly susceptible to meningococcal infections?

Harrison's 20th Ed. Chapter 133, Page 998

A. Galectin-1
B. Properdin
C. Pentraxin
D. Cathelin

Complement components are important for bactericidal activity of serum. Individuals with deficiencies of any of the complement components, chiefly of the terminal complement components (C5-9), properdin or factor D are highly susceptible to meningococcal infections. Such a deficiency increases the risk of disease by up to 600-fold and may result in recurrent attacks.

3436. Infection acquired by ingesting "ready-to-eat" foods is due to?

Harrison's 20th Ed. Chapter 133, Page 998

A. Actinobacillus actinomycetemcomitans
B. Kingella kingae
C. Listeria monocytogenes
D. Streptococcus bovis

3437. Which of the following is present in relatively small amounts in normal CSF?

Harrison's 20th Ed. Chapter 133, Page 999

A. White blood cells (WBCs)
B. Complement proteins
C. Immunoglobulins
D. All of the above

Normal CSF contains few WBCs, relatively small amounts of complement proteins & immunoglobulins.

3438. Which of the following is a bacterial cell-wall component?

Harrison's 20th Ed. Chapter 133, Page 999

A. Lipopolysaccharide (LPS)
B. Teichoic acid
C. Peptidoglycan
D. All of the above

3439. Following intracisternal inoculation of LPS, which of the following cytokine is first to appear?

Harrison's 20th Ed. Chapter 133, Page 999

A. Interleukin 1α
B. Interleukin 1β
C. Interleukin 1γ
D. Interleukin 1δ

In meningitis, cytokines like tumor necrosis factor alpha (TNFα) and interleukin 1b (IL-1β) are present in CSF within 1–2 hours of intracisternal inoculation of LPS.

3440. Raised intracranial pressure in bacterial meningitis is due to?

Harrison's 20th Ed. Chapter 133, Page 999

A. Interstitial edema
B. Vasogenic edema
C. Cytotoxic edema
D. All of the above

The combination of interstitial, vasogenic, and cytotoxic edema leads to raised ICP and coma.

3441. Which of the following is not a feature of classic clinical triad of meningitis?

Harrison's 20th Ed. Chapter 133, Page 999

A. Fever
B. Headache
C. Vomiting
D. Nuchal rigidity

The classic clinical triad of meningitis is fever, headache & nuchal rigidity. Decreased level of consciousness occurs in >75% of patients. Nausea, vomiting & photophobia are also common complaints.

3442. Which of the following is the pathognomonic sign of meningeal irritation?

Harrison's 20th Ed. Chapter 133, Page 999

A. Fever
B. Headache
C. Photophobia
D. Nuchal rigidity

Nuchal rigidity ("stiff neck") is the pathognomonic sign of meningeal irritation.

3443. While eliciting Brudzinski's sign, which part of body is moved passively?

Harrison's 20th Ed. Chapter 133, Page 1000

A. Hip joint
B. Knee joint
C. Neck
D. Ankle joint

Brudzinski's sign is positive when passive flexion of neck results in spontaneous flexion of hips & knees.

3444. Kernig and Brudzinski's signs may be absent or reduced in?

Harrison's 20th Ed. Chapter 133, Page 1000

A. Very young patients
B. Elderly patients
C. Immunocompromised individuals
D. All of the above

Kernig and Brudzinski's signs may be absent or reduced in very young or elderly patients, immunocompromised individuals or patients with a severely depressed mental status.

3445. Which of the following sign is positive in meningitis?

DeJong's The Neurologic Examination, 7th Ed. Page 764

A. Kernig sign
B. Brudzinski's neck sign
C. Lasègue's sign
D. All of the above

The Kernig sign, Brudzinski's neck sign and Lasègue's sign (straight leg raising) are positive in meningitis. To avoid spinal flexion, patient with meningitis may sit in bed with hands placed far behind, head thrown back, hips & knees flexed, and the back arched (Amoss's, Hoyne's, or tripod sign).

3446. Which of the following is a sign for meningeal inflammation?

DeJong's The Neurologic Examination, 7th Ed. Page 765

A. Brudzinski's contralateral leg sign
B. Brudzinski's cheek sign
C. Brudzinski's symphysis sign
D. All of the above

In Brudzinski's cheek sign, pressure is applied against the cheeks on or just below the zygoma, which results in flexion at elbows with an upward jerking of the arms. In Brudzinski's symphysis sign, pressure is applied on symphysis pubis that causes flexion of both lower extremities.

3447. Resistance to elbow extension due to meningeal inflammation is?

DeJong's The Neurologic Examination, 7th Ed. Page 765

A. Guilland's sign
B. Bikele sign
C. Lomadtse sign
D. Schrijver-Bernhard reflex

In Bikele sign, with elbow flexed, shoulder abducted, elevated, and externally rotated, examiner attempts to passively extend the elbow. If meningeal inflammation is present or there is brachial plexitis, resistance is observed to elbow extension.

3448. Generalized seizure and status epilepticus in bacterial meningitis may be due to?

Harrison's 20th Ed. Chapter 133, Page 1000

A. Hyponatremia
B. Cerebral anoxia
C. Toxic effects of antimicrobial agents
D. All of the above

Generalized seizure activity & status epilepticus in bacterial meningitis may be due to hyponatremia, cerebral anoxia or less commonly, toxic effects of antimicrobial agents (high-dose penicillin).

3449. Over 90% of patients of bacterial meningitis have a CSF opening pressure of?

Harrison's 20th Ed. Chapter 133, Page 1000

A. > 100 mm H_2O
B. > 120 mm H_2O
C. > 160 mm H_2O
D. > 180 mm H_2O

More than 90% of patients will have a CSF opening pressure >180 mm H_2O.

3450. Signs of increased intracranial pressure (ICP) include?

Harrison's 20th Ed. Chapter 133, Page 1000

A. Deteriorating or reduced level of consciousness
B. Dilated poorly reactive pupils
C. Cushing reflex
D. All of the above

Signs of increased ICP include a deteriorating or reduced level of consciousness, papilledema, dilated poorly reactive pupils, sixth nerve palsies, decerebrate posturing, and the Cushing reflex.

3451. Cushing reflex in raised ICP relates to?

Harrison's 20th Ed. Chapter 133, Page 1000

A. Bradycardia
B. Hypertension
C. Irregular respirations
D. All of the above

Cushing reflex includes bradycardia, hypertension & irregular respirations.

3452. Petechiae due to meningococcemia are found on?

Harrison's 20th Ed. Chapter 133, Page 1000

A. Trunk and lower extremities
B. Mucous membranes and conjunctiva
C. Palms and soles
D. All of the above

Petechiae due to meningococcemia are found on trunk & lower extremities, in mucous membranes & conjunctiva, and occasionally on palms & soles.

3453. In bacterial meningitis, CSF/serum glucose ratio is?

Harrison's 20th Ed. Chapter 133, Page 1000

A. < 0.4
B. < 0.5
C. < 0.6
D. < 0.8

CSF/serum glucose ratio in bacterial meningitis is <0.4 in ~60% of patients.

3454. CSF glucose concentration is low when CSF/serum glucose ratio is?

Harrison's 20th Ed. Chapter 133, Page 1000

A. < 0.4
B. < 0.5
C. < 0.6
D. < 0.8

CSF glucose concentration is low when CSF/serum glucose ratio is <0.6.

3455. CSF/serum glucose ratio of <0.4 is seen in?

Harrison's 20th Ed. Chapter 133, Page 1000

A. Fungal meningitis
B. Tuberculous meningitis
C. Carcinomatous meningitis
D. All of the above

Besides bacterial meningitis, CSF/serum glucose ratio <0.4 is also seen in fungal, tuberculous, and carcinomatous meningitis.

3456. Limulus amebocyte lysate assay in CSF is diagnostic of?

Harrison's 20th Ed. Chapter 133, Page 1001

A. Gram-negative bacterial meningitis
B. Fungal meningitis
C. Tuberculous meningitis
D. Carcinomatous meningitis

Limulus amebocyte lysate assay detects gram-negative endotoxin in CSF & is diagnostic of gram-negative bacterial meningitis. (Specificity 85–100%; sensitivity 100%).

3457. In Rocky Mountain spotted fever (RMSF), skin rash typically begins in?

Harrison's 20th Ed. Chapter 133, Page 1001

A. Face and scalp
B. Wrists and ankles
C. Chest and abdomen
D. Neck

Skin rash in RMSF typically begins in wrist & ankles. It spreads distally & proximally rapidly to involve palms & soles.

3458. Noninfectious CNS disorder that can mimic bacterial meningitis is?

Harrison's 20th Ed. Chapter 133, Page 1001

A. Subarachnoid hemorrhage
B. Behçet's syndrome
C. Pituitary apoplexy
D. All of the above

Noninfectious CNS disorders that can mimic bacterial meningitis are subarachnoid hemorrhage, medication-induced hypersensitivity meningitis, chemical meningitis due to rupture of tumor contents into the CSF, carcinomatous or lymphomatous meningitis, meningitis associated with inflammatory disorders like sarcoid, systemic lupus erythematosus (SLE), and Behçet's syndrome, pituitary apoplexy and Vogt-Koyanagi-Harada syndrome.

3459. Vogt-Koyanagi-Harada syndrome refers to?

Harrison's 20th Ed. Chapter 133, Page 1001

A. Drug-induced hypersensitivity meningitis
B. Carcinomatous meningitis
C. Meningitis associated with sarcoid
D. Uveomeningitic syndromes

Vogt-Koyanagi-Harada syndrome refers to uveomeningitic syndromes.

3460. Which of the following causes a subacutely evolving meningitis?

Harrison's 20th Ed. Chapter 133, Page 1001

A. Mycobacterium tuberculosis
B. Cryptococcus neoformans
C. Treponema pallidum
D. All of the above

Subacutely evolving meningitis is caused by Mycobacterium tuberculosis, Cryptococcus neoformans, Histoplasma capsulatum, Coccidioides immitis and Treponema pallidum.

3461. Which of the following viral infections can mimic the clinical presentation of bacterial meningitis?

Harrison's 20th Ed. Chapter 133, Page 1001

A. Varicella-zoster virus
B. Herpes simplex virus
C. Cytomegalovirus
D. Enterovirus

3462. In bacterial meningitis, the goal is to begin antibiotic therapy within what time of patient's arrival?

Harrison's 20th Ed. Chapter 133, Page 1001

A. 1 hour
B. 3 hours
C. 6 hours
D. 12 hours

In bacterial meningitis, the goal is to begin antibiotic therapy within 60 minutes of patient's arrival in the emergency room.

3463. Which of the following cephalosporin is preferred in CNS infection with P. aeruginosa?

Harrison's 20th Ed. Chapter 133, Page 1002 Table 133-3

A. Ceftriaxone
B. Cefotaxime
C. Ceftazidime
D. None of the above

Meningitis due to P. aeruginosa should be treated with ceftazidime, cefepime, or meropenem.

3464. Close contacts of a patient of meningococcal meningitis should receive chemoprophylaxis with?

Harrison's 20th Ed. Chapter 133, Page 1002

A. Rifampin
B. Ciprofloxacin
C. Azithromycin
D. Any of the above

Close contacts of meningococcal meningitis patient should receive chemoprophylaxis with rifampin, ciprofloxacin, azithromycin or ceftriaxone.

3465. In meningococcal meningitis chemoprophylaxis, adult dose of rifampin is?

Harrison's 20th Ed. Chapter 133, Page 1002

A. 450 mg once a day for 1 day
B. 450 mg twice a day for 2 days
C. 600 mg once a day for 1 day
D. 600 mg twice a day for 2 days

In meningococcal meningitis chemoprophylaxis, rifampin is given as a 2-day regimen of 600 mg every 12 hour for 2 days in adults.

3466. Which antibiotic should be added to the empirical regimen in acute meningitis for coverage of L. monocytogenes?

Harrison's 20th Ed. Chapter 133, Page 1002

A. Ampicillin
B. Nafcillin
C. Penicillin G
D. Metronidazole

Ampicillin should be added to the empirical regimen for coverage of L. monocytogenes.

3467. Which of the following is false about vancomycin therapy in S. pneumoniae meningitis?

Harrison's 20th Ed. Chapter 133, Page 1002

A. Antibiotic of choice if cephalosporin MIC is >1 μg/mL
B. Rifampin produces synergistic effect to vancomycin
C. Vancomycin can be given by intraventricular route
D. None of the above

3468. Which of the following statements about duration of antimicrobial therapy in meningitis is false?

Harrison's 20th Ed. Chapter 133, Page 1002

A. 1 week course of IV penicillin is recommended for meningococcal meningitis
B. 2 week course of IV antimicrobial therapy is recommended for pneumococcal meningitis
C. 3 week course of ampicillin is recommended for L. monocytogenes meningitis
D. 4 week course of IV antibiotic is recommended for gram-negative bacilli meningitis

A 3-week course of IV antibiotic therapy is recommended for meningitis due to gram-negative bacilli.

3469. Dexamethasone exerts its beneficial effect by?

Harrison's 20th Ed. Chapter 133, Page 1002

A. Inhibiting the synthesis of IL-1β & TNF-α at mRNA level
B. Decreasing CSF outflow resistance
C. Stabilizing the blood-brain barrier
D. All of the above

Dexamethasone exerts its beneficial effect by inhibiting the synthesis of IL-1β and TNF-α at the mRNA level, decreasing CSF outflow resistance and stabilizing the blood-brain barrier.

3470. When should dexamethasone be given in acute bacterial meningitis?

Harrison's 20th Ed. Chapter 133, Page 1002

A. Before antibiotic therapy
B. Along with antibiotic therapy
C. After antibiotic therapy
D. Any of the above

Rationale for giving dexamethasone 20 minutes before antibiotic therapy is that it inhibits production of TNF by macrophages & microglia only if it is administered before these cells are activated by endotoxin.

3471. Benefit of dexamethasone therapy is not significant if started how many hours after antimicrobial therapy?

Harrison's 20th Ed. Chapter 133, Page 1003

A. > 1 hour
B. > 3 hours
C. > 6 hours
D. > 12 hours

Dexamethasone therapy is unlikely to be of significant benefit if started > 6 hours after antimicrobial therapy has been initiated.

3472. Benefits of dexamethasone therapy are most striking in patients with?

Harrison's 20th Ed. Chapter 133, Page 1003

A. Gram-negative bacterial meningitis
B. Pneumococcal meningitis
C. Meningococcal meningitis
D. Staphylococcal meningitis

3473. Mortality is higher in meningitis due to?

Harrison's 20th Ed. Chapter 133, Page 1003

A. H. influenzae
B. N. meningitidis
C. L. monocytogenes
D. S. pneumoniae

Mortality is 3–7% for meningitis caused by H. influenzae, N. meningitidis or group B streptococci. 15% for that due to L. monocytogenes and 20% for S. pneumoniae.

3474. Predictors of increased mortality in bacterial meningitis include?

Harrison's 20th Ed. Chapter 133, Page 1003

A. Onset of seizures within 24 hours of admission
B. CSF glucose concentration of < 40 mg/dL
C. CSF protein concentration of > 300 mg/dL
D. All of the above

Risk of death from bacterial meningitis increases with decreased level of consciousness on admission, onset of seizures within 24 hours of admission, signs of increased ICP, young age (infancy) & age >50, presence of shock and/or need for mechanical ventilation, delay in initiation of treatment, CSF glucose concentration <40 mg/dL and CSF protein >300 mg/dL.

3475. Common sequelae of bacterial meningitis include all except?

Harrison's 20th Ed. Chapter 133, Page 1003

A. Decreased intellectual function
B. Seizures
C. Visual loss
D. Hearing loss

Common sequelae of bacterial meningitis include decreased intellectual function, memory impairment, seizures, hearing loss & dizziness & gait disturbances.

Viral Meningitis

3476. Which of the following viruses has a nonseasonal prevalence in causing viral meningitis?

Harrison's 20th Ed. Chapter 133, Page 1003

A. Arboviruses
B. LCMV
C. Mumps
D. HSV

HSV & HIV viral meningitis have no seasonal predominance. Arboviruses & enteroviruses are frequent during summer/early fall. LCMV & mumps viruses cause viral meningitis during winter months.

3477. Which of the following is uncommon in viral meningitis?

Harrison's 20th Ed. Chapter 133, Page 1003

A. Fever
B. Headache
C. Meningeal irritation
D. Marked confusion

Viral meningitis presents as fever, headache, meningeal irritation and an inflammatory CSF profile. Fever may be accompanied by malaise, myalgia, anorexia, nausea and vomiting, abdominal pain, and/or diarrhea. Mild degree of lethargy or drowsiness may occur but more profound alterations in consciousness like stupor, coma, or marked confusion, should prompt consideration of alternative diagnoses.

3478. Which of the following is common in viral meningitis?

Harrison's 20th Ed. Chapter 133, Page 1003

A. Kernig's and Brudzinski's signs
B. Headache - frontal or retroorbital
C. Focal neurological deficits
D. Seizures

Headache in viral meningitis is usually frontal or retro-orbital with photophobia, pain on moving eyes & mild teminal nuchal rigidity. Evidence of severe meningeal irritation, such as Kernig's and Brudzinski's signs, is generally absent. Seizures or other focal neurologic signs or symptoms suggest involvement of the brain parenchyma and do not occur in uncomplicated viral meningitis.

3479. Which of the following viruses is a less common cause of viral meningitis?

Harrison's 20th Ed. Chapter 133, Page 1003

A. Enteroviruses
B. Arboviruses
C. Adenoviruses
D. HSV-2

Enteroviruses account for > 85% of aseptic meningitis cases. Viruses belonging to the Enterovirus genus are members of the family Picornaviridae and include the coxsackieviruses, echoviruses, polioviruses, and human enteroviruses 68 to 71. Adenoviruses rarely cause viral meningitis.

3480. Typical CSF profile in viral meningitis includes all except?

Harrison's 20th Ed. Chapter 133, Page 1003

A. Lymphocytic pleocytosis - 25 to 500 cells/μL
B. Normal or slightly elevated protein - 20 to 80 mg/dL
C. Reduced glucose concentration
D. Normal or mildly elevated pressure (100–350 mm H_2O)

Examination of CSF is the most important laboratory test in the diagnosis of viral meningitis. The typical profile is a lymphocytic pleocytosis (25 to 500 cells/μL), a normal or slightly elevated protein concentration (20 to 80 mg/dL), a normal glucose concentration, and a normal or mildly elevated opening pressure (100 to 350 mm H_2O).

3481. PMNs may predominate in CSF of viral meningitis in the first 48 hours of illness in which of the following infections?

Harrison's 20th Ed. Chapter 133, Page 1003

A. Echovirus 9
B. West Nile virus
C. Mumps
D. All of the above

PMNs may predominate in the first 48 hours of illness, especially in patients with infections due to echovirus 9, West Nile virus or Eastern equine encephalitis (EEE) virus, or mumps.

3482. Cell counts of several thousand per microliter are seen in viral meningitis due to which of the following?

Harrison's 20th Ed. Chapter 133, Page 1003

A. Echovirus 9
B. West Nile virus
C. Mumps
D. Arboviruses

3483. Cell counts of several thousand per microliter are seen in viral meningitis due to which of the following?

Harrison's 20th Ed. Chapter 133, Page 1003

A. Echovirus 9
B. West Nile virus
C. Lymphocytic choriomeningitis virus (LCMV)
D. Arboviruses

Total CSF cell count in viral meningitis is typically 25 to 500/μL, although cell counts of several thousand per microliter are occasionally seen, especially with infections due to lymphocytic choriomeningitis virus (LCMV) and mumps virus.

3484. Low CSF glucose concentration is seen in viral meningitis due to which of the following?

Harrison's 20th Ed. Chapter 133, Page 1003

A. Echovirus 9
B. West Nile virus
C. Lymphocytic choriomeningitis virus (LCMV)
D. Arboviruses

3485. Low CSF glucose concentration is seen in viral meningitis due to which of the following?

Harrison's 20th Ed. Chapter 133, Page 1003

A. CMV
B. West Nile virus
C. Mumps
D. EBV

The CSF glucose concentration is typically normal in viral infections, although it may be decreased in 10 to 30% of cases due to mumps as well as in cases due to LCMV.

3486. In CSF, lymphocytic pleocytosis with low glucose concentration should suggest which of the following?

Harrison's 20th Ed. Chapter 133, Page 1003

A. Fungal meningitis
B. Listerial meningitis
C. Tuberculous meningitis
D. All of the above

3487. In CSF, lymphocytic pleocytosis with low glucose concentration should suggest which of the following?

Harrison's 20th Ed. Chapter 133, Page 1003

A. Sarcoid
B. Neoplastic meningitis
C. Tuberculous meningitis
D. All of the above

As a rule, a lymphocytic pleocytosis with a low glucose concentration should suggest fungal, listerial, or tuberculous meningitis or noninfectious disorders (e.g., sarcoid, neoplastic meningitis).

3488. Which of the following is the most important method for diagnosing CNS viral infections?

Harrison's 20th Ed. Chapter 133, Page 1003

A. Neopterin
B. β2-microglobulin
C. LDH
D. PCR amplification of viral nucleic acid

Amplification of viral-specific DNA or RNA from CSF using PCR amplification is the single most important method for diagnosing CNS viral infections.

3489. At what temperature should CSF be stored for culture for diagnosis of viral infection (> 24 hours)?

Harrison's 20th Ed. Chapter 133, Page 1004

A. – 20 °C
B. – 40 °C
C. – 50 °C
D. – 70 °C

Beyond 24 hours, CSF specimens for viral isolation are stored in a (–)70°C freezer.

3490. Enteroviruses may be found in all except?

Harrison's 20th Ed. Chapter 133, Page 1004

A. Feces
B. Blood
C. Urine
D. Throat washings

Enteroviruses & adenoviruses may be found in feces, arboviruses & LCMV in blood, mumps & CMV, in urine and enteroviruses, mumps, and adenoviruses in throat washings.

3491. Serologic studies are a crucial diagnostic tool for which of the following viruses?

Harrison's 20th Ed. Chapter 133, Page 1004

A. West Nile virus (WNV)
B. HSV
C. VZV
D. CMV

For West Nile virus (WNV), serologic studies are a crucial diagnostic tool.

3492. Oligoclonal bands in CSF is not found in which of the following conditions?

Harrison's 20th Ed. Chapter 133, Page 1004

A. HIV infection
B. HSV infections
C. Subacute sclerosing panencephalitis (SSPE)
D. Progressive rubella panencephalitis

Oligoclonal bands in CSF are not seen with arbovirus, enterovirus, or HSV infections. But, seen in infections with HIV, HTLV type I, VZV, mumps, SSPE & progressive rubella panencephalitis.

3493. Oligoclonal bands are found in which of the following?

Harrison's 20th Ed. Chapter 133, Page 1004

A. Multiple sclerosis
B. Neurosyphilis
C. Lyme neuroborreliosis
D. All of the above

Oligoclonal bands are encountered in multiple sclerosis, neurosyphilis & Lyme neuroborreliosis.

3494. Which of the following viruses is the most common cause of viral meningitis?

Harrison's 20th Ed. Chapter 133, Page 1004

A. Enteroviruses
B. Arboviruses
C. Adenoviruses
D. HSV-2

3495. A case of viral meningitis with exanthemata, hand-foot-mouth disease, herpangina, pleurodynia, myopericarditis, and hemorrhagic conjunctivitis suggest the diagnosis of which infection?

Harrison's 20th Ed. Chapter 133, Page 1004

A. HSV-2 infection
B. EBV infection
C. LCMV infection
D. Enterovirus infection

Enteroviruses are the most common cause of viral meningitis. Occur in summer months, especially in children. Physical findings may include exanthemata, hand-foot-mouth disease, herpangina, pleurodynia, myopericarditis, and hemorrhagic conjunctivitis.

3496. A case of viral meningitis occuring in clusters during summer should prompt for infection with?

Harrison's 20th Ed. Chapter 133, Page 1004

A. HSV-2 infection
B. Arbovirus infection
C. LCMV infection
D. Enterovirus infection

Arbovirus infections typically occur in summer months and early fall, in both endemic & epidemic form, reflecting transmission through infected insect vectors. Arboviral meningitis should be considered when clusters of meningitis cases occur in a restricted geographic region during the summer or early fall.

3497. Which of the following arboviruses can cause meningitis & encephalitis?

Harrison's 20th Ed. Chapter 133, Page 1004

A. WNV
B. St. Louis encephalitis virus
C. California encephalitis group of viruses
D. All of the above

Most important causes of arboviral meningitis and encephalitis are WNV, St. Louis encephalitis virus and California encephalitis group of viruses.

3498. In WNV epidemics, which of the following may serve as sentinel infections for subsequent human disease?

Harrison's 20th Ed. Chapter 133, Page 1004

A. Avian deaths
B. Cattle deaths
C. Rodent deaths
D. All of the above

In WNV epidemics, avian deaths may serve as sentinel infections for subsequent human disease.

3499. 'Mollaret's meningitis' is due to?

Harrison's 20th Ed. Chapter 133, Page 1005

A. HIV

B. HSV

C. EBV

D. CMV

'Mollaret's meningitis' appear to be due to HSV.

3500. Which of the following viral infections commonly produces cranial nerve palsies?

Harrison's 20th Ed. Chapter 133, Page 1005

A. HIV

B. HSV

C. EBV

D. CMV

Cranial nerve palsies, most commonly involving cranial nerves V, VII or VIII are more common in HIV meningitis than in other viral infections.

3501. A case of viral meningitis along with orchitis, oophoritis, parotitis, pancreatitis should prompt for infection with?

Harrison's 20th Ed. Chapter 133, Page 1005

A. HSV-2 infection

B. Arbovirus infection

C. LCMV infection

D. Mumps infection

Mumps meningitis occurs in late winter or early spring, especially in males. The presence of orchitis, oophoritis, parotitis, pancreatitis, or elevations in serum lipase and amylase are suggestive of the diagnosis. Clinical meningitis occurs in 5% of patients with parotitis, but only 50% of patients with meningitis have associated parotitis. Mumps infection confers lifelong immunity, so a documented history of previous infection excludes this diagnosis.

3502. Aseptic meningitis occurring in winter, with a history of exposure to house mice excreta, leukopenia, thrombocytopenia and CSF pleocytosis suggest the diagnosis of which infection?

Harrison's 20th Ed. Chapter 133, Page 1005

A. HSV-2 infection

B. EBV infection

C. LCMV infection

D. Mumps

LCMV infection should be considered when aseptic meningitis occurs in late fall or winter, and in individuals with a history of exposure to house mice (Mus musculus) excreta, rash, pulmonary infiltrates, alopecia, parotitis, orchitis, or myopericarditis. Laboratory clues to the diagnosis of LCMV include leukopenia, thrombocytopenia, abnormal LFT, marked CSF pleocytosis (>1000 cells/μL) and hypoglycorrachia (<30%).

3503. A case of viral meningitis complicated by acute cerebellar ataxia should prompt for infection with?

Harrison's 20th Ed. Chapter 133, Page 1005

A. HSV-2 infection

B. Arbovirus infection

C. LCMV infection

D. VZV CNS infection

VZV meningitis should be suspected in the presence of concurrent chickenpox or shingles though up to 40% of VZV meningitis occur in the absence of rash. VZV can produce acute cerebellar ataxia. The syndrome of acute cerebellar ataxia and meningeal inflammation generally appears ~21 days after onset of the rash and rarely develops in the pre-eruptive phase.

3504. Acyclovir therapy is of benefit in patients with meningitis caused by?

Harrison's 20th Ed. Chapter 133, Page 1005

A. HSV-1 or -2

B. Severe EBV infection

C. Severe VZV infection

D. All of the above

Oral or intravenous acyclovir may be of benefit in patients with meningitis caused by HSV-1 or -2 and in cases of severe EBV or VZV infection.

Chronic and Recurrent Meningitis

3505. Chronic meningitis is diagnosed when?

Harrison's 20th Ed. Chapter 134, Page 1007

A. > 4 weeks duration
B. Persistent CSF WBC count > 5/μL
C. Chronic & persistent or recurrent & discrete headache
D. All of the above

3506. Which of the following can cause chronic meningitis?

Harrison's 20th Ed. Chapter 134, Page 1007

A. Autoimmune inflammatory disorders
B. Chemical meningitis
C. Parameningeal infections
D. All of the above

Five categories of disease cause most cases of chronic meningitis: meningeal infections, malignancy, autoimmune inflammatory disorders, chemical meningitis, and parameningeal infections.

3507. Which of the following is not a cardinal feature of chronic meningitis?

Harrison's 20th Ed. Chapter 134, Page 1007

A. Hydrocephalus
B. Radiculopathies
C. Cognitive or personality changes
D. All of the above

Persistent headache, hydrocephalus, cranial neuropathies, radiculopathies, and cognitive or personality changes are the cardinal features of chronic meningitis.

3508. Which of the following is best related to resorbption of CSF?

Harrison's 20th Ed. Chapter 134, Page 1007

A. Choroid plexus
B. Arachnoid villi
C. Virchow-Robin spaces
D. All of the above

CSF is produced by choroid plexus of cerebral ventricles, exits through narrow foramina into subarachnoid space surrounding brain & spinal cord, circulates around the base of brain and over cerebral hemispheres, and is resorbed by arachnoid villi projecting into superior sagittal sinus. Spread of infectious and other infiltrative processes from subarachnoid space into brain parenchyma may occur via the arachnoid cuffs that surround blood vessels that penetrate brain tissue (Virchow-Robin spaces).

3509. Recurrent meningitis is a feature of all except?

Harrison's 20th Ed. Chapter 134, Page 1008

A. Vogt-Koyanagi-Harada syndrome
B. Behçet's syndrome
C. Wegener's granulomatosis
D. Mollaret's meningitis

3510. Recurrent meningitis is a feature of?

Harrison's 20th Ed. Chapter 134, Page 1008

A. Neurocysticercosis
B. Drug hypersensitivity
C. Syphilis
D. Mumps

Exposure to ibuprofen, sulfonamides, isoniazid, tolmetin, ciprofloxacin, phenazopyridine lead to recurrent episodes with recurrent exposure. Improvement occurs after discontinuation of drug.

3511. Uveitis is a feature of?

Harrison's 20th Ed. Chapter 134, Page 1008

A. Vogt-Koyanagi-Harada syndrome
B. Sarcoid
C. CNS lymphoma
D. All of the above

Uveitis is a feature of Vogt-Koyanagi-Harada syndrome, sarcoid or CNS lymphoma.

3512. Iridocyclitis is a feature of?

Harrison's 20th Ed. Chapter 134, Page 1008

A. Systemic lupus erythematosus
B. CNS sarcoidosis
C. Wegener's granulomatosis
D. Behçet's syndrome

Iridocyclitis is a feature of Behçet's syndrome.

3513. Which of the following is a feature of Behçet's syndrome?

Harrison's 20th Ed. Chapter 134, Page 1008

A. Aphthous oral lesions
B. Genital ulcers
C. Hypopyon
D. All of the above

Aphthous oral lesions, genital ulcers and hypopyon suggest Behçet's syndrome.

3514. Fatal levels of raised ICP can occur without enlarged ventricles in?

Harrison's 20th Ed. Chapter 134, Page 1011

A. Lyme disease
B. CNS sarcoidosis
C. Cryptococcal meningitis
D. Chronic benign lymphocytic meningitis

In cryptococcal meningitis, fatal levels of raised ICP can occur without enlarged ventricles.

3515. Anti-Ro/SSA positivity is associated with?

Harrison's 20th Ed. Chapter 348, Page 2514

A. Sensorineural hearing loss
B. Raynaud's phenomenon
C. Congenital heart block
D. All of the above

Congenital heart block in newborn due to damage to developing conducting system of heart results from transfer of anti-Ro antibody from mother to child.

3516. Most useful empirical therapy for chronic meningitis is?

Harrison's 20th Ed. Chapter 134, Page 1013

A. Antituberculous therapy
B. Antifungal medication
C. Glucocorticoids
D. Ventricular-peritoneal shunt

Most useful empirical therapy for chronic meningitis is administration of glucocorticoids rather than antituberculous therapy.

Brain Abscess and Empyema

3517. Cerebritis is best related to?
Harrison's 20th Ed. Chapter 135, Page 1013

A. Encephalitis
B. Meningitis
C. Abscess
D. Thrombophlebitis

Focal bacterial, fungal or parasitic infections involving brain tissue are classified as either cerebritis or abscess, depending on the presence or absence of a capsule. When brain tissue is directly injured by a viral infection the disease is referred to as encephalitis.

3518. Which of the following is true for the capsule of a brain abscess?
Harrison's 20th Ed. Chapter 135, Page 1013

A. Fibrous
B. Vascularized
C. No capsule
D. All of the above

Brain abscess is a focal, suppurative infection within brain parenchyma, typically surrounded by a vascularized capsule. Term cerebritis refers to describe a nonencapsulated brain abscess.

3519. Predisposing conditions for brain abscess include?
Harrison's 20th Ed. Chapter 135, Page 1013

A. Paranasal sinusitis
B. Otitis media/mastoiditis
C. Dental infections
D. All of the above

Predisposing conditions for brain abscess include otitis media/mastoiditis, paranasal sinusitis, dental infections (direct contiguous spread); pyogenic infections (hematogenous spread); penetrating head trauma or neurosurgical procedures.

3520. In immunocompetent individuals the most common pathogen that causes brain abscess is?
Harrison's 20th Ed. Chapter 135, Page 1013

A. Streptococcus
B. Klebsiella
C. Staphylococcus
D. E. coli

3521. In immunocompromised hosts the most common pathogen that causes brain abscess is?
Harrison's 20th Ed. Chapter 135, Page 1013

A. Taenia solium
B. Mycobacterium tuberculosis
C. Nocardia
D. E. coli

In immunocompetent individuals the most important pathogens are Streptococcus spp., Enterobacteriaceae (Proteus spp., E. coli sp., Klebsiella spp.), anaerobes (Bacteroides spp., Fusobacterium spp.) and staphylococci. In immunocompromised hosts most brain abscesses are caused by Nocardia spp., Toxoplasma gondii, Aspergillus spp., Candida spp. and C. neoformans. In Latin America & in immigrants from Latin America, the most common cause of brain abscess is Taenia solium (neurocysticercosis). In India & East Asia, mycobacterial infection (tuberculoma) remains a major cause of focal CNS mass lesions.

3522. Otogenic abscesses occur predominantly in?
Harrison's 20th Ed. Chapter 135, Page 1013

A. Frontal lobe
B. Occipital lobe
C. Cerebellum
D. Pons

Otogenic abscesses occur predominantly in the temporal lobe (55–75%) and cerebellum (20 - 30%).

3523. Abscesses that develop as a result of dental infections are usually located in?
Harrison's 20th Ed. Chapter 135, Page 1013

A. Frontal lobe
B. Occipital lobe
C. Cerebellum
D. Pons

Abscesses that develop as a result of direct spread of infection from frontal, ethmoidal, or sphenoidal sinuses and those that occur due to dental infections are usually located in the frontal lobes.

3524. Which of the following is false about hematogenous brain abscesses?
Harrison's 20th Ed. Chapter 135, Page 1013

A. At the junction of gray & white matter
B. Predilection for MCA territory
C. Multiple
D. Encapsulated

Hematogenous abscesses account for ~25% of brain abscesses. Hematogenous abscesses are multiple, and multiple abscesses (50%) have a hematogenous origin. Hematogenous abscesses are poorly encapsulated.

3525. Late cerebritis stage is seen during?
Harrison's 20th Ed. Chapter 135, Page 1014

A. Days 1–3
B. Days 4–9
C. Days 10–13
D. Day 14 and beyond

3526. Which of the following is not a part of the classic clinical triad of brain abscess?
Harrison's 20th Ed. Chapter 135, Page 1014

A. Headache
B. Fever
C. Nuchal rigidity
D. Focal neurologic deficit

The classic clinical triad of brain abscess consists of headache, fever, and a focal neurologic deficit. Others include new onset of focal or generalized seizure activity, and focal neurologic deficits (hemiparesis, aphasia, or visual field defects). Presence of nuchal rigidity is unusual with brain abscess.

3527. Most common symptom of brain abscess is?
Harrison's 20th Ed. Chapter 135, Page 1014

A. Headache
B. Fever
C. Seizure
D. Focal neurologic deficit

Most common symptom in patients with a brain abscess is headache, occurring in >75% of patients.

3528. The clinical presentation of a brain abscess depends on?
Harrison's 20th Ed. Chapter 135, Page 1014

A. Its location
B. Nature of the primary infection, if present
C. Level of intracranial pressure (ICP)
D. All of the above

Clinical presentation of a brain abscess depends on its location, nature of the primary infection, if present, and the level of ICP.

3529. A temporal lobe abscess may present with?
Harrison's 20th Ed. Chapter 135, Page 1014

A. Hemiparesis
B. Upper homonymous quadrantanopia
C. Nystagmus
D. Ataxia

Hemiparesis is the most common localizing sign of a frontal lobe abscess. A temporal lobe abscess may present with a disturbance of language (dysphasia) or an upper homonymous quadrantanopia. Nystagmus & ataxia are signs of a cerebellar abscess. Signs of raised ICP (papilledema, nausea & vomiting, drowsiness or confusion) can be the dominant presentation of abscesses in cerebellum. Meningismus is not present unless abscess has ruptured into ventricle or infection has spread to subarachnoid space.

3530. When should a lumbar puncture performed in patients suspected of brain abscess?
Harrison's 20th Ed. Chapter 135, Page 1014

A. As early as possible
B. On day 3
C. On day 10
D. Should not be performed

LP should not be performed in those with known or suspected focal intracranial infections (abscess / empyema) as CSF analysis contributes nothing to diagnosis or therapy, & LP increases the risk of herniation.

3531. Conditions that can cause headache, fever, focal neurologic signs, and seizure activity include?
Harrison's 20th Ed. Chapter 135, Page 1014

A. Bacterial meningitis
B. Superior sagittal sinus thrombosis
C. Acute disseminated encephalomyelitis
D. All of the above

Conditions that can cause headache, fever, focal neurologic signs & seizures are brain abscess, subdural empyema, bacterial meningitis, viral meningoencephalitis, superior sagittal sinus thrombosis & acute disseminated encephalomyelitis.

3532. Medical therapy for treatment of brain abscess is for which of the following patients?
Harrison's 20th Ed. Chapter 135, Page 1015

A. Whose abscesses are neurosurgically inaccessible
B. Patients with small (<2–3 cm) abscesses
C. Patients with nonencapsulated abscesses (cerebritis)
D. All of the above

3533. All patients of brain abscess should receive parenteral antibiotic therapy for?
Harrison's 20th Ed. Chapter 135, Page 1015

A. A minimum of 2–4 weeks
B. A minimum of 4–6 weeks
C. A minimum of 6–8 weeks
D. A minimum of 8–12 weeks

All patients of brain abscess should receive a minimum of 6 - 8 weeks of parenteral antibiotic therapy.

3534. Anticonvulsant therapy is continued for at least how many months after resolution of brain abscess?
Harrison's 20th Ed. Chapter 135, Page 1015

A. 3
B. 6
C. 9
D. 12

Anticonvulsant therapy is continued for at least 3 months after resolution of the brain abscess.

3535. The mortality rate in patients of brain abscess is?
Harrison's 20th Ed. Chapter 348, Page 2514

A. <5%
B. <10%
C. <15%
D. <20%

The mortality rate in patients of brain abscess is <15%. Significant sequelae, including seizures, persisting weakness, aphasia, or mental impairment, occur in ≥20% of survivors.

3536. Most common parasitic disease of the CNS worldwide is?
Harrison's 20th Ed. Chapter 135, Page 1015

A. Neurocysticercosis
B. Toxoplasmosis
C. Schistosomiasis
D. Amebiasis

Neurocysticercosis is the most common parasitic disease of the CNS worldwide.

3537. Most common manifestation of neurocysticercosis is?
Harrison's 20th Ed. Chapter 135, Page 1015

A. New-onset partial seizures
B. New-onset generalized seizures
C. Focal neurologic deficit
D. Headache

Most common manifestation of neurocysticercosis is new-onset partial seizures with or without secondary generalization.

3538. Spinal cysticerci can mimic the presentation of?
Harrison's 20th Ed. Chapter 135, Page 1015

A. Chronic arachnoiditis
B. Cauda equina syndrome
C. Conus medullaris syndrome
D. Intraspinal tumors

Spinal cysticerci can mimic the presentation of intraspinal tumors.

3539. In MRI, lesions of neurocysticercosis with viable parasites appear as?
Harrison's 20th Ed. Chapter 135, Page 1015

A. Multiple lesions in the deep white matter
B. Nodular lesion surrounded by edema
C. Cystic lesions
D. Parenchymal brain calcifications

The lesions of neurocysticercosis with viable parasites appear as cystic lesions.

3540. In neurocysticercosis, a very early sign of cyst death is?

Harrison's 20th Ed. Chapter 135, Page 1015

A. Multiple lesions in the deep white matter
B. Hypointensity of vesicular fluid (T2) as compared to CSF
C. Nodular lesion surrounded by edema
D. Parenchymal brain calcifications

In neurocysticercosis, a very early sign of cyst death is hypointensity of the vesicular fluid on T2-weighted images when compared with CSF. Parenchymal brain calcifications are the most common finding and evidence that the parasite is no longer viable.

3541. Which of the following findings on neuroimaging calls for treatment with anticysticidal drugs?

Harrison's 20th Ed. Chapter 135, Page 1015

A. Cysticerci appearing as cystic lesions in brain
B. Cysticerci appearing as enhancing lesions in brain
C. Cysticerci appearing as enhancing lesions in subarachnoid space
D. All of the above

Cysticerci appearing as cystic lesions or as enhancing lesions in the brain parenchyma or in the subarachnoid space at the convexity of the cerebral hemispheres should be treated with anticysticidal therapy.

3542. Which of the following drug is used in the treatment of neurocysticercosis?

Harrison's 20th Ed. Chapter 135, Page 1015

A. Pentamidine isethionate
B. Pyrantel pamoate
C. Suramin
D. Praziquantel

Albendazole and praziquantel are used in the treatment of neurocysticercosis.

3543. The superior sagittal sinus drains into?

Harrison's 20th Ed. Chapter 135, Page 1018

A. Transverse sinus
B. Sigmoid sinus
C. Internal jugular vein
D. Cavernous sinus

Superior sagittal sinus drains into the transverse sinuses which becomes sigmoid sinus before draining into internal jugular vein.

3544. Which of the following communicates with the meningeal veins?

Harrison's 20th Ed. Chapter 135, Page 1018

A. Frontal superior cerebral veins
B. Parietal superior cerebral veins
C. Occipital superior cerebral veins
D. Diploic veins

Diploic veins, which drain into superior sagittal sinus, provide a route for the spread of infection from the meninges as they communicate with the meningeal veins.

3545. Which of the following can spread infection to the superior sagittal sinus?

Harrison's 20th Ed. Chapter 135, Page 1018

A. Bacterial meningitis
B. Subdural empyema (SDE)
C. Epidural abscess
D. All of the above

3546. Which of the following receive venous drainage from the middle ear and mastoid cells?

Harrison's 20th Ed. Chapter 135, Page 1018

A. Transverse sinus
B. Sigmoid sinus
C. Internal jugular vein
D. Cavernous sinus

3547. Which of the following sinuses is the most common site of primary infection resulting in septic cavernous sinus thrombosis?

Harrison's 20th Ed. Chapter 135, Page 1018

A. Frontal sinus
B. Maxillary sinus
C. Sphenoid sinus
D. All of the above

Sphenoid & ethmoid sinuses are the most common sites of primary infection resulting in septic cavernous sinus thrombosis.

3548. Which of the following does not pass through the cavernous sinus?

Harrison's 20th Ed. Chapter 135, Page 1018

A. III, IV & VI cranial nerves
B. Ophthalmic & maxillary branches of trigeminal nerve
C. Middle cerebral artery
D. Internal carotid artery

III, IV & VI and ophthalmic & maxillary branches of V cranial nerve, along with internal carotid artery pass through the cavernous sinus.

3549. Headache & earache are the most frequent symptoms of?

Harrison's 20th Ed. Chapter 135, Page 1018

A. Transverse sinus thrombosis
B. Internal jugular vein thrombosis
C. Superior sagittal sinus thrombosis
D. Cavernous sinus thrombosis

Headache and earache are the most frequent symptoms of transverse sinus thrombosis.

3550. Gradinego's syndrome is due to thrombosis in which of the following intracranial sinuses?

Harrison's 20th Ed. Chapter 135, Page 1018

A. Transverse sinus
B. Sigmoid sinus
C. Internal jugular vein
D. Cavernous sinus

Transverse sinus thrombosis may present with otitis media, sixth nerve palsy & retro-orbital or facial pain (Gradinego's syndrome).

3551. Retro-orbital pain is a feature of?

Harrison's 20th Ed. Chapter 135, Page 1018

A. Viral meningitis
B. Transverse sinus thrombosis
C. Cavernous sinus thrombosis
D. All of the above

Headache of viral meningitis is usually frontal or retroorbital and is often associated with photophobia & pain on eye movement. Retroorbital pain is also a feature of cluster headache, paroxysmal hemicrania, dengue, leptospirosis.

3552. Pott's puffy tumor best relates to?

Harrison's 20th Ed. Chapter 31, Page 210

A. Frontal sinusitis
B. Maxillary sinusitis
C. Sphenoid sinusitis
D. Ethmoid sinusitis

Patients with advanced frontal sinusitis can present with Pott's puffy tumor, with soft-tissue swelling & pitting edema over frontal bone from a communicating subperiosteal abscess.

Alcohol and Alcohol Use Disorders

3553. One typical alcohol drink produces blood levels of?
Harrison's 20th Ed. Chapter 445, Page 3278

A. ~ 10 mg/dL
B. ~ 20 mg/dL
C. ~ 30 mg/dL
D. ~ 40 mg/dL

Blood values of ~20 mg/dL result from ingestion of one typical drink.

3554. Which of the following is a congener in beverages?
Harrison's 20th Ed. Chapter 445, Page 3278

A. Methanol
B. Butanol
C. Acetaldehyde
D. All of the above

3555. Which of the following is a congener in beverages?
Harrison's 20th Ed. Chapter 445, Page 3278

A. Histamine
B. Iron
C. Lead
D. All of the above

Beverages have additional components called congeners that affect the drink's taste and might contribute to adverse effects on the body. Congeners include methanol, butanol, acetaldehyde, histamine, tannins, iron and lead.

3556. The major site of absorption of alcohol is?
Harrison's 20th Ed. Chapter 445, Page 3278

A. Mouth and esophagus
B. Stomach
C. Proximal small intestine
D. Large bowel

Alcohol is absorbed from mucous membranes of mouth & esophagus in small amounts, from stomach & large bowel in modest amounts. The major site of absorption is the proximal portion of small intestine.

3557. Alcohol is excreted directly through which of the following?
Harrison's 20th Ed. Chapter 445, Page 3278

A. Lungs
B. Urine
C. Sweat
D. All of the above

Between 2% and 10% of ethanol is excreted directly through lungs, urine, or sweat. Greater part is metabolized to acetaldehyde in liver.

3558. In liver, which of the following is responsible for metabolism of alcohol?
Harrison's 20th Ed. Chapter 445, Page 3278 Figure 445-1

A. Alcohol dehydrogenase (ADH)
B. Aldehyde dehydrogenase (ALDH)
C. Microsomal ethanol-oxidizing system (MEOS)
D. All of the above

Two pathways operate to metabolise alcohol in body. First pathway (~80%) occurs in cell cytosol where alcohol dehydrogenase (ADH) produces acetaldehyde, which is then rapidly destroyed by aldehyde dehydrogenase (ALDH) in cytosol and mitochondria to either Acetyl CoA or Acetate. Second pathway (~20%) is microsomal ethanol-oxidizing system or MEOS in smooth endoplasmic reticulum.

3559. Alcohol is devoid of which of the following?
Harrison's 20th Ed. Chapter 445, Page 3278

A. Minerals
B. Proteins
C. Vitamins
D. All of the above

Alcohol is devoid of nutrients such as minerals, proteins and vitamins.

3560. Alcohol affects levels of which of the following vitamins?
Harrison's 20th Ed. Chapter 445, Page 3278

A. Folate (folacin or folic acid)
B. Pyridoxine (B6)
C. Nicotinic acid (niacin, B3)
D. All of the above

Alcohol produces modest effects on folate (folacin or folic acid), pyridoxine (B6), thiamine (B1), nicotinic acid (niacin, B3) and vitamin A levels.

3561. Which of the following is false about alcohol ketoacidosis?
Harrison's 20th Ed. Chapter 445, Page 3278

A. Large anion gap
B. Increase in serum lactate
C. Increase in β-hydroxybutyrate/lactate ratio
D. None of the above

Alcohol ketoacidosis patients show an increase in serum ketones with mild increase in glucose but a large anion gap, a mild - moderate increase in serum lactate & increased β-hydroxybutyrate/lactate ratio of between 2:1 and 9:1 (normal 1:1).

3562. Intoxicating effect of alcohol is due to its action on?
Harrison's 20th Ed. Chapter 445, Page 3278

A. Neurotransmitters
B. Receptors
C. Transporters
D. All of the above

Intoxicating effect of alcohol is due to its action on several neurotransmitters, receptors & transporters.

3563. Alcohol affects which of the following neurochemical systems in the brain?
N Engl J Med. 2008;359:715-21

A. γ-aminobutyric acid (GABA)
B. Glutamate
C. Dopamine
D. All of the above

Neurochemical systems in brain influenced by alcohol are γ-aminobutyric acid (GABA), glutamate, dopamine, and opiate systems. GABA and glutamate are involved with alcohol stimulation, sedation, intoxication & many symptoms of alcohol withdrawal. Dopamine & opiate systems are involved with reinforcement, reward, some aspects of craving, sustained use of alcohol and potential relapse after prolonged abstinence in dependent person.

3564. Mutations in which of the following predisposes to the development of alcoholic liver disease?

Harrison's 20th Ed. Chapter 445, Page Table 335-1, N Engl J Med. 2018;378:270-80

A. Chromatin modifying protein 2B
B. Receptor expression enhancing protein 2
C. Patatin-like phospholipase domain-containing 3 (PNLAP3)
D. Patatin-like phospholipase domain-containing protein 6

Genetic mutations in patatin-like phospholipase domain-containing 3 (PNLAP3) & transmembrane 6 superfamily, member 2 (TM6SF2) predispose to the development of alcoholic liver disease/alcoholic cirrhosis.

3565. Which of the following is related to alcohol-use disorders?

N Engl J Med. 2008;359:715-21

A. Nucleus basalis of Meynert
B. Nucleus accumbens
C. Caudate nucleus
D. All of the above

Ethanol inhibits inhibitory neurons in midbrain ventral tegmental area (VTA) leading to increased dopamine release in nucleus accumbens. Blockade of dopamine in nucleus accumbens can terminate rewarding effects of addictive drugs.

3566. Which of the following is false about actions of alcohol?

Harrison's 20th Ed. Chapter 445, Page 3278

A. Alcohol inhibits GABA-A receptors
B. Alcohol inhibits NMDA receptors
C. Inhibition of uptake of adenosine
D. Increases synaptic serotonin levels

Alcohol acutely enhances actions at γ-aminobutyric acid A (GABA-A) receptors and inhibits N-methyl-D-aspartate (NMDA) excitatory glutamate receptors.

3567. Which of the following is false about actions of alcohol?

Harrison's 20th Ed. Chapter 445, Page 3278

A. Increases dopamine levels in ventral tegmentum
B. Increase in cortisol & adrenocorticotropic hormone (ACTH)
C. Release of beta endorphins
D. None of the above

3568. Which of the following is false about actions of alcohol?

Harrison's 20th Ed. Chapter 445, Page 3278

A. Increase in nicotinic acetylcholine system
B. Release of dopamine, GABA and glutamate in brain
C. Upregulation of serotonin receptors
D. None of the above

3569. A standard drink contains how many grams of ethanol?

N Engl J Med. 2013;368:365-73

A. 10 grams
B. 12 grams
C. 14 grams
D. 16 grams

A standard drink (12 oz of beer, 5 oz of wine, or 1.5 oz of 80-proof liquor) contains 14 grams of ethanol.

3570. "Legal intoxication" in USA requires a blood alcohol concentration of at least?

Harrison's 20th Ed. Chapter 445, Page 3279

A. 40 mg/dL
B. 80 mg/dL
C. 120 mg/dL
D. 160 mg/dL

"Legal intoxication" in USA requires a blood alcohol concentration of at least 80–100 mg/dL.

3571. Compensatory mechanism in alcohol tolerance is?

Harrison's 20th Ed. Chapter 445, Page 3279

A. Metabolic or pharmacokinetic tolerance
B. Cellular or pharmacodynamic tolerance
C. Learned or behavioral tolerance
D. All of the above

Alcohol tolerance involves compensatory mechanisms like metabolic or pharmacokinetic tolerance, cellular or pharmacodynamic tolerance and learned or behavioral tolerance.

3572. At low doses, alcohol can have which of the following beneficial effects?

Harrison's 20th Ed. Chapter 445, Page 3279

A. Decreased rates of myocardial infarction
B. Decreased rates of stroke
C. Decreased rates of gallstones
D. All of the above

Beneficial effects of low doses of alcohol are decreased rates of myocardial infarction, stroke, gallstones and vascular & Alzheimer's dementias.

3573. Health-promoting quality at low doses of red wine is due to?

Harrison's 20th Ed. Chapter 445, Page 3279

A. Flavinols
B. Dronabinol
C. Flavonoids
D. Aescin

3574. Which of the following occurs in chronic alcoholism?

Harrison's 20th Ed. Chapter 445, Page 3279

A. Episode of temporary anterograde amnesia
B. Deficiency in REM sleep
C. Exacerbation of sleep apnea
D. All of the above

Alcoholics may experience episodes of temporary anterograde amnesia (blackout), reduced rapid eye movement (REM) and deep sleep, exacerbated sleep apnea & prominent and disturbing dreams.

3575. Hangover syndrome consists of all except?

Harrison's 20th Ed. Chapter 445, Page 3279

A. Abdominal pain
B. Headache
C. Thirst
D. Fatigue

After heavy drinking, on the following day, hangover syndrome consists of headache, thirst, nausea, vomiting, and fatigue.

3576. Which of the following is a feature of Wernicke's syndrome?
Harrison's 20th Ed. Chapter 445, Page 3279

A. Ophthalmoparesis
B. Ataxia
C. Encephalopathy
D. All of the above

3577. Korsakoff's syndrome in alcoholics is due to the deficiency of?
Harrison's 20th Ed. Chapter 445, Page 3279

A. Methionine
B. Thiamine
C. Tryptophan
D. All of the above

3578. Korsakoff's syndrome in alcoholics is predisposed by the deficiency of?
Harrison's 20th Ed. Chapter 445, Page 3279

A. Acetylketolase deficiency
B. Paraketolase deficiency
C. Transketolase deficiency
D. Semiketolase deficiency

Wernicke's syndrome refers to ophthalmoparesis, ataxia & encephalopathy. Korsakoff's syndrome includes retrograde & anterograde amnesia. Both are due to thiamine deficiency, especially in those with transketolase deficiency.

3579. Alcohol-induced intense sadness is a component of?
Harrison's 20th Ed. Chapter 445, Page 3279

A. Alcohol-induced mood disorder
B. Alcohol-induced anxiety disorder
C. Alcohol-induced psychotic disorder
D. All of the above

3580. Alcohol can cause all except which of the following?
Harrison's 20th Ed. Chapter 445, Page 3280

A. Impairs gluconeogenesis in liver
B. Increases lactate production
C. Increases oxidation of fatty acids
D. Increases fat accumulation in liver cells

Alcohol impairs gluconeogenesis in liver, increases lactate production and decreases oxidation of fatty acids leading to increased fat accumulation in liver cells. Repeated exposure to ethanol leads to alcohol-induced hepatitis, perivenular sclerosis and cirrhosis.

3581. Alcohol increases the risk of which of the following cancer?
Harrison's 20th Ed. Chapter 445, Page 3280

A. Breast cancer in women
B. Oral and esophageal cancer
C. Rectal cancer
D. All of the above

Alcohol consumption increases risk of breast cancer (in women), oral, esophageal and rectal cancers.

3582. Alcohol is associated with increased risks of?
N Engl J Med. 2013;368:365-73

A. Oropharyngeal carcinoma
B. Esophageal carcinoma
C. Breast carcinoma
D. All of the above

Beverage alcohol is a carcinogen, and even light drinking is associated with increased risks of oropharyngeal, esophageal, and breast carcinomas.

3583. "Holiday heart" refers to?
Harrison's 20th Ed. Chapter 445, Page 3280

A. Dilation of all heart chambers in chronic alcoholics
B. Paroxysmal tachycardia after a drinking binge in individuals without heart disease
C. Finding of >25% decrease in heart rarte at times of leisure
D. Finding of >10% decrease in SBP at times of leisure

Atrial or ventricular arrhythmias, especially paroxysmal tachycardia, can occur after a drinking binge in individuals with no other evidence of heart disease (holiday heart syndrome").

3584. Features of 'Fetal alcohol syndrome' include all except?
Harrison's 20th Ed. Chapter 445, Page 3280

A. Epicanthal eye folds
B. Poorly formed concha
C. Small teeth with faulty enamel
D. Microglossia

3585. Features of 'Fetal alcohol syndrome' include all except?
Harrison's 20th Ed. Chapter 445, Page 3280

A. Atrial or ventricular septal defect
B. Aberrant palmar crease
C. Polydactyly
D. Microcephaly with mental retardation

Fetal alcohol syndrome (FAS) can include facial changes with epicanthal eye folds, poorly formed ear concha, small teeth with faulty enamel, cardiac atrial or ventricular septal defects, aberrant palmar crease & limitation in joint movement, and microcephaly with mental retardation.

3586. Polydactyly is a feature of?
Harrison's 20th Ed. Chapter 309, Page 2151

A. Meckel-Gruber syndrome
B. Bardet Biedl syndrome (BBS)
C. Laurence-Moon syndrome
D. All of the above

Other syndromes with a feature of polydactyly are Meckel-Gruber syndrome, Sensenbrenner's syndrome, Carpenter's syndrome, Bardet-Biedl syndrome (BBS), Laurence-Moon syndrome.

3587. Which of the following is a feature of fetal alcohol spectrum disorder (FASD)?
Harrison's 20th Ed. Chapter 445, Page 3280

A. Low birth weight
B. Lower IQ
C. Hyperactive behavior
D. All of the above

Features of fetal alcohol spectrum disorder (FASD) include low birth weight, a lower IQ, hyperactive behavior, and some modest cognitive deficits.

3588. Hormonal changes during heavy drinking include?
Harrison's 20th Ed. Chapter 445, Page 3280

A. Increase in cortisol levels
B. Inhibition of vasopressin secretion
C. Decrease in serum triiodothyronine (T3)
D. All of the above

Hormonal changes during heavy drinking include an increase in cortisol levels, inhibition of vasopressin secretion at rising blood alcohol concentrations & enhanced secretion at falling blood alcohol concentrations, reversible decrease in serum T4 and T3.

3589. How many life areas are included in defining alcohol use disorder (AUD)?

Harrison's 20th Ed. Chapter 445, Page 3280

A. 8
B. 9
C. 10
D. 11

Alcohol use disorder (AUD) is defined as repeated alcohol-related dificulties in at least 2 of 11 life areas that cluster together in the same 12 month period.

3590. What percentage of patients have an alcohol use disorder?

Harrison's 20th Ed. Chapter 445, Page 3281

A. 5%
B. 10%
C. 15%
D. 20%

3591. Blood tests useful in identifying individuals consuming six or more standard drinks per day include?

Harrison's 20th Ed. Chapter 445, Page 3281

A. γ-glutamyl transferase (GGT)
B. Carbohydrate-deficient transferrin (CDT)
C. Serum uric acid (>7 mg/dL)
D. All of the above

Laboratory tests that are likely to be abnormal in persons with regular alcohol consumption of 6 to 8 or more drinks per day are γ-glutamyl transferase (GGT) (>35 U), carbohydrate-deficient transferrin (CDT) (>20 U/L), high-normal MCVs (≥91 μm^3) and serum uric acid (>7 mg/dL).

3592. Alcohol withdrawal symptoms peak in intensity on day?

Harrison's 20th Ed. Chapter 445, Page 3282

A. 1–2
B. 2–3
C. 3–4
D. 4–5

Alcohol withdrawal symptoms begin within 5–10 hours of decreasing ethanol intake, peak in intensity on day 2 or 3, and improve by day 4 or 5.

3593. Delirium in delirium tremens includes all except?

Harrison's 20th Ed. Chapter 445, Page 3282

A. Mental confusion
B. Agitation
C. Hallucinations
D. Fluctuating levels of consciousness

Delirium tremens (DTs) is a state of intense acute alcohol withdrawal. It includes delirium (mental confusion, agitation, and fluctuating levels of consciousness) associated with a tremor & autonomic overactivity (tachycardia, hypertension, and tachypnea).

3594. Medication helpful in alcoholic rehabilitation include?

Harrison's 20th Ed. Chapter 445, Page 3283

A. Naltrexone
B. Acamprosate
C. Disulfiram
D. All of the above

Naltrexone is a mu opioid receptor antagonist given in doses of 50–150 mg/day. It decreases activity in dopamine-rich ventral tegmental reward system. Acamprosate in doses of 2 gm/day inhibits the actions of NMDA receptors. Disulfiram (250 mg/day) is an ALDH inhibitor. It produces an unpleasant reaction in presence of alcohol due to rapidly rising blood levels of acetaldehyde. Other drugs under investigation are selective 5-HT3 receptor antagonist ondansetron, anticonvulsant topiramate, nalmafene (opioid receptor antagonist) and cannabinol receptor antagonist ramonibant.

3595. Which of the following drugs is an opioid antagonist?

Harrison's 20th Ed. Chapter 445, Page 3283

A. Varenicline
B. Baclofen
C. Nalmefene
D. Topiramate

Additional drugs under investigation for the alcohol rehabilitation treatment phase include opioid antagonist nalmefene, nicotinic receptor agonist varenicline, serotonin antagonist ondansetron, α-adrenergic agonist prazosin, GABA-B receptor agonist baclofen, anticonvulsant topiramate, and cannabinol receptor antagonists.

3596. Which of the following is a toxic alcohol?

N Engl J Med. 2018;378:270-80

A. Methanol
B. Isopropanol
C. Propylene glycol
D. All of the above

Toxic alcohols include methanol, ethylene glycol, isopropanol, diethylene glycol, and propylene glycol. Isopropanol is directly toxic while others exert toxic effects from their metabolites.

3597. Which of the following statements is false?

N Engl J Med. 2018;378:270-80

A. Methanol is metabolized to formic acid
B. Ethylene glycol is metabolized to oxalic and glycolic acid
C. Propylene glycol is metabolized to D-lactic and L-lactic acid
D. None of the above

Methanol is metabolized to formic acid,3 ethylene glycol to oxalic and glycolic acid,3 diethylene glycol to 2-hydroxyethoxyacetic acid and glycolic acid,4 and propylene glycol to D-lactic and L-lactic acid.

3598. Which of the following about alcohol dehydrogenase is false?

N Engl J Med. 2018;378:270-80

A. It catalyzes the first oxidation of toxic alcohols
B. Fomepizole is a strong inhibitor of alcohol dehydrogenase
C. Fomepizole has an affinity for alcohol dehydrogenase 8000 times that of ethanol
D. None of the above

3599. Poisoning with which of the following leads to formation of oxalate crystals?

N Engl J Med. 2018;378:270-80

A. Methanol
B. Isopropanol
C. Propylene glycol
D. Ethylene glycol

3600. Which of the following leads to elevation of osmolal or anion gap?

N Engl J Med. 2018;378:270-80

A. Ketoacidosis
B. Chronic kidney disease
C. Sick cell syndrome
D. All of the above

An elevated osmolal or anion gap does not always indicate toxic alcohol poisoning. Lactic acidosis, ketoacidosis, chronic kidney disease, and the sick cell syndrome all may increase both gaps.

ANSWERS

1. D
2. D
3. D
4. D
5. B
6. D
7. D
8. D
9. D
10. D
11. D
12. D
13. A
14. D
15. D
16. C
17. D
18. A
19. C
20. C
21. C
22. C
23. C
24. C
25. B
26. D
27. D
28. D
29. B
30. D
31. D
32. D
33. D
34. A
35. A
36. A
37. D
38. A
39. C
40. C
41. D
42. D
43. D
44. D
45. D
46. D
47. D
48. D
49. D
50. D
51. D
52. A
53. A
54. B
55. A
56. C
57. D
58. A
59. D
60. B
61. D
62. D
63. C
64. D
65. D
66. D
67. B
68. C
69. A
70. D
71. B
72. C
73. B
74. D
75. B
76. C
77. D
78. B
79. C
80. D
81. A
82. A
83. D
84. D
85. B
86. D
87. B
88. C
89. A
90. D
91. C
92. D
93. A
94. D
95. D
96. D
97. D
98. D
99. D
100. D
101. B
102. C
103. C
104. D
105. C
106. D
107. C
108. D
109. A
110. C
111. D
112. D
113. D
114. D
115. D
116. D
117. A
118. B
119. D
120. D
121. D
122. D
123. D
124. B
125. B
126. D
127. D
128. A
129. D
130. D
131. D
132. D
133. D
134. D
135. A
136. C
137. D
138. C
139. B
140. D
141. D
142. D
143. A
144. A
145. C
146. D
147. A
148. D
149. D
150. A
151. C
152. D
153. D
154. C
155. D
156. D
157. C
158. A
159. C
160. D
161. D
162. D
163. D
164. B
165. D
166. D
167. D
168. D
169. D
170. D
171. D
172. D
173. B
174. D
175. D
176. D
177. D
178. D
179. C
180. B
181. D
182. A
183. C
184. C
185. A
186. D
187. D
188. C
189. D
190. D
191. A
192. C
193. B
194. A
195. A
196. B
197. A
198. D
199. A
200. A
201. D
202. C
203. A
204. B
205. D
206. A
207. B
208. B
209. C
210. D
211. B
212. D
213. D
214. D
215. C
216. C
217. B
218. D
219. D
220. C
221. B
222. D
223. A
224. B
225. B
226. B
227. B
228. A
229. D
230. C
231. A
232. A
233. B
234. D
235. D
236. A
237. B
238. C
239. A
240. B
241. B
242. D
243. D
244. D
245. D
246. C
247. B
248. D
249. D
250. D
251. D
252. D
253. C
254. A
255. A
256. A
257. C
258. D
259. D
260. C
261. D
262. D
263. D
264. C

ANSWERS

265. C
266. A
267. A
268. A
269. C
270. A
271. C
272. A
273. D
274. D
275. D
276. C
277. C
278. D
279. D
280. A
281. D
282. D
283. D
284. C
285. C
286. D
287. A
288. A
289. A
290. D
291. B
292. A
293. B
294. C
295. A
296. D
297. C
298. C
299. A
300. B
301. A
302. C
303. D
304. B
305. C
306. D
307. D
308. D
309. A
310. C
311. C
312. A
313. D
314. B
315. B
316. C
317. C
318. C
319. D
320. D
321. D
322. A
323. C
324. D
325. D
326. D
327. B
328. C
329. B
330. C
331. B
332. D
333. D
334. D
335. D
336. C
337. C
338. C
339. D
340. D
341. C
342. D
343. C
344. D
345. D
346. A
347. B
348. C
349. D
350. B
351. C
352. D
353. D
354. A
355. D
356. B
357. D
358. D
359. D
360. B
361. C
362. A
363. D
364. D
365. D
366. D
367. D
368. D
369. D
370. D
371. D
372. A
373. D
374. D
375. D
376. A
377. D
378. D
379. D
380. B
381. C
382. A
383. D
384. A
385. A
386. C
387. D
388. B
389. D
390. A
391. D
392. A
393. B
394. A
395. C
396. D
397. B
398. B
399. A
400. D
401. C
402. D
403. B
404. D
405. D
406. A
407. D
408. B
409. A
410. B
411. C
412. D
413. D
414. C
415. D
416. D
417. D
418. C
419. A
420. D
421. A
422. D
423. B
424. D
425. B
426. D
427. D
428. D
429. D
430. C
431. B
432. D
433. D
434. D
435. D
436. D
437. D
438. B
439. C
440. D
441. D
442. A
443. B
444. D
445. D
446. C
447. B
448. A
449. D
450. D
451. D
452. D
453. C
454. C
455. D
456. D
457. C
458. D
459. D
460. D
461. D
462. C
463. A
464. D
465. C
466. D
467. D
468. C
469. A
470. D
471. A
472. D
473. D
474. A
475. D
476. B
477. D
478. A
479. C
480. D
481. D
482. D
483. C
484. A
485. A
486. D
487. D
488. D
489. D
490. C
491. C
492. D
493. D
494. A
495. A
496. C
497. D
498. D
499. C
500. B
501. A
502. D
503. B
504. C
505. D
506. A
507. B
508. D
509. D
510. D
511. B
512. C
513. C
514. D
515. D
516. C
517. D
518. D
519. B
520. B
521. C
522. D
523. D
524. B
525. B
526. A
527. B
528. D

ANSWERS

529. A
530. B
531. D
532. D
533. C
534. D
535. A
536. D
537. C
538. D
539. D
540. C
541. B
542. B
543. B
544. C
545. B
546. B
547. D
548. B
549. D
550. D
551. D
552. D
553. B
554. B
555. C
556. B
557. C
558. A
559. D
560. D
561. D
562. D
563. D
564. C
565. C
566. C
567. C
568. D
569. D
570. D
571. B
572. D
573. D
574. B
575. B
576. C
577. D
578. B
579. C
580. D
581. D
582. C
583. C
584. B
585. C
586. C
587. C
588. D
589. C
590. C
591. B
592. B
593. C
594. C
595. A
596. C
597. C
598. D
599. A
600. A
601. D
602. C
603. D
604. D
605. D
606. C
607. D
608. D
609. D
610. A
611. D
612. B
613. D
614. D
615. A
616. B
617. A
618. C
619. D
620. D
621. A
622. A
623. B
624. C
625. B
626. D
627. D
628. D
629. B
630. B
631. A
632. B
633. A
634. B
635. A
636. B
637. D
638. D
639. A
640. C
641. D
642. C
643. B
644. B
645. D
646. D
647. C
648. A
649. B
650. A
651. B
652. C
653. D
654. D
655. A
656. D
657. D
658. A
659. B
660. C
661. D
662. B
663. C
664. A
665. A
666. B
667. D
668. D
669. D
670. D
671. D
672. B
673. D
674. C
675. C
676. D
677. D
678. D
679. D
680. D
681. A
682. D
683. C
684. D
685. C
686. C
687. D
688. D
689. C
690. C
691. D
692. C
693. A
694. C
695. C
696. D
697. C
698. D
699. D
700. D
701. D
702. D
703. D
704. D
705. D
706. D
707. D
708. D
709. D
710. D
711. D
712. D
713. D
714. B
715. A
716. D
717. D
718. D
719. D
720. D
721. B
722. B
723. D
724. B
725. D
726. C
727. C
728. C
729. A
730. D
731. D
732. B
733. D
734. D
735. B
736. D
737. C
738. D
739. A
740. A
741. B
742. B
743. B
744. D
745. D
746. D
747. D
748. D
749. C
750. D
751. B
752. C
753. B
754. D
755. D
756. C
757. D
758. C
759. D
760. C
761. B
762. D
763. D
764. C
765. A
766. A
767. D
768. C
769. D
770. D
771. D
772. C
773. D
774. C
775. B
776. D
777. A
778. A
779. A
780. C
781. B
782. C
783. D
784. D
785. D
786. C
787. B
788. B
789. D
790. A
791. A
792. A

ANSWERS

793. C
794. B
795. D
796. A
797. D
798. D
799. D
800. B
801. C
802. C
803. C
804. D
805. D
806. A
807. D
808. B
809. B
810. B
811. A
812. A
813. D
814. C
815. D
816. D
817. D
818. A
819. B
820. C
821. D
822. B
823. D
824. D
825. C
826. D
827. D
828. B
829. B
830. D
831. C
832. D
833. D
834. A
835. D
836. A
837. D
838. D
839. D
840. A
841. C
842. B
843. B
844. D
845. A
846. D
847. A
848. D
849. C
850. A
851. B
852. D
853. A
854. A
855. C
856. D
857. A
858. A
859. D
860. A
861. C
862. B
863. D
864. D
865. D
866. B
867. C
868. D
869. D
870. B
871. A
872. D
873. D
874. A
875. C
876. C
877. D
878. D
879. D
880. C
881. C
882. D
883. B
884. A
885. D
886. A
887. D
888. C
889. C
890. D
891. D
892. C
893. D
894. B
895. D
896. D
897. D
898. A
899. A
900. D
901. D
902. B
903. A
904. A
905. B
906. A
907. A
908. A
909. D
910. D
911. C
912. D
913. D
914. D
915. A
916. D
917. D
918. B
919. A
920. A
921. A
922. D
923. A
924. D
925. D
926. A
927. B
928. B
929. D
930. C
931. B
932. D
933. A
934. A
935. D
936. B
937. D
938. D
939. D
940. B
941. C
942. D
943. A
944. D
945. D
946. D
947. C
948. C
949. D
950. D
951. D
952. A
953. C
954. D
955. C
956. A
957. A
958. D
959. D
960. D
961. B
962. C
963. A
964. A
965. B
966. C
967. B
968. C
969. D
970. A
971. D
972. B
973. C
974. B
975. C
976. D
977. D
978. B
979. D
980. D
981. D
982. C
983. C
984. C
985. C
986. B
987. D
988. B
989. A
990. B
991. B
992. D
993. D
994. D
995. C
996. C
997. A
998. D
999. D
1000. D
1001. B
1002. D
1003. C
1004. C
1005. D
1006. D
1007. B
1008. D
1009. D
1010. C
1011. C
1012. C
1013. C
1014. D
1015. D
1016. D
1017. D
1018. D
1019. C
1020. D
1021. B
1022. B
1023. D
1024. A
1025. D
1026. A
1027. C
1028. C
1029. D
1030. A
1031. D
1032. D
1033. C
1034. B
1035. D
1036. C
1037. A
1038. D
1039. C
1040. D
1041. B
1042. A
1043. D
1044. A
1045. D
1046. B
1047. D
1048. C
1049. D
1050. D
1051. D
1052. D
1053. B
1054. D
1055. D
1056. D

ANSWERS

1057. B
1058. C
1059. C
1060. A
1061. B
1062. B
1063. C
1064. A
1065. B
1066. A
1067. A
1068. D
1069. B
1070. B
1071. A
1072. D
1073. A
1074. B
1075. D
1076. B
1077. A
1078. D
1079. D
1080. B
1081. C
1082. C
1083. B
1084. D
1085. A
1086. D
1087. D
1088. C
1089. B
1090. C
1091. C
1092. D
1093. D
1094. D
1095. A
1096. A
1097. D
1098. A
1099. A
1100. C
1101. D
1102. B
1103. B
1104. A
1105. D
1106. D
1107. A
1108. A
1109. B
1110. B
1111. B
1112. D
1113. D
1114. B
1115. D
1116. B
1117. B
1118. C
1119. C
1120. A
1121. D
1122. C
1123. C
1124. D
1125. B
1126. C
1127. B
1128. C
1129. D
1130. B
1131. C
1132. B
1133. A
1134. A
1135. A
1136. A
1137. B
1138. B
1139. A
1140. B
1141. D
1142. B
1143. D
1144. B
1145. C
1146. D
1147. C
1148. D
1149. D
1150. D
1151. D
1152. D
1153. D
1154. D
1155. D
1156. C
1157. A
1158. B
1159. D
1160. B
1161. D
1162. B
1163. B
1164. D
1165. A
1166. A
1167. D
1168. C
1169. C
1170. A
1171. D
1172. C
1173. B
1174. D
1175. C
1176. B
1177. A
1178. D
1179. A
1180. A
1181. D
1182. D
1183. C
1184. D
1185. C
1186. A
1187. C
1188. D
1189. A
1190. D
1191. B
1192. B
1193. C
1194. C
1195. A
1196. B
1197. D
1198. D
1199. D
1200. C
1201. D
1202. C
1203. C
1204. D
1205. A
1206. D
1207. D
1208. D
1209. A
1210. C
1211. B
1212. D
1213. D
1214. D
1215. D
1216. D
1217. D
1218. A
1219. D
1220. D
1221. A
1222. D
1223. C
1224. A
1225. D
1226. B
1227. C
1228. A
1229. B
1230. B
1231. B
1232. D
1233. D
1234. A
1235. C
1236. D
1237. C
1238. D
1239. A
1240. D
1241. D
1242. D
1243. D
1244. D
1245. D
1246. A
1247. C
1248. D
1249. D
1250. A
1251. B
1252. D
1253. B
1254. B
1255. D
1256. C
1257. B
1258. C
1259. C
1260. A
1261. D
1262. C
1263. D
1264. C
1265. B
1266. D
1267. D
1268. D
1269. D
1270. A
1271. B
1272. D
1273. C
1274. D
1275. D
1276. A
1277. D
1278. B
1279. A
1280. D
1281. D
1282. C
1283. D
1284. A
1285. C
1286. D
1287. C
1288. C
1289. C
1290. D
1291. D
1292. D
1293. D
1294. D
1295. A
1296. A
1297. C
1298. D
1299. D
1300. D
1301. C
1302. D
1303. D
1304. B
1305. D
1306. C
1307. C
1308. B
1309. D
1310. B
1311. D
1312. A
1313. D
1314. D
1315. C
1316. D
1317. D
1318. D
1319. A
1320. A

ANSWERS

1321. D
1322. C
1323. D
1324. D
1325. D
1326. D
1327. A
1328. D
1329. A
1330. B
1331. D
1332. D
1333. D
1334. D
1335. D
1336. D
1337. D
1338. D
1339. D
1340. D
1341. D
1342. A
1343. A
1344. D
1345. D
1346. D
1347. D
1348. C
1349. D
1350. A
1351. D
1352. C
1353. C
1354. A
1355. D
1356. B
1357. C
1358. D
1359. D
1360. C
1361. A
1362. C
1363. A
1364. D
1365. A
1366. C
1367. D
1368. D
1369. C
1370. C
1371. D
1372. D
1373. C
1374. D
1375. C
1376. D
1377. A
1378. D
1379. A
1380. D
1381. D
1382. D
1383. D
1384. B
1385. A
1386. C
1387. B
1388. D
1389. D
1390. D
1391. C
1392. D
1393. B
1394. B
1395. C
1396. D
1397. C
1398. D
1399. A
1400. D
1401. D
1402. C
1403. D
1404. C
1405. B
1406. D
1407. D
1408. A
1409. C
1410. D
1411. C
1412. C
1413. D
1414. D
1415. D
1416. A
1417. D
1418. B
1419. A
1420. B
1421. B
1422. A
1423. C
1424. C
1425. B
1426. D
1427. D
1428. C
1429. B
1430. D
1431. A
1432. D
1433. D
1434. B
1435. C
1436. A
1437. C
1438. B
1439. D
1440. B
1441. D
1442. D
1443. C
1444. D
1445. A
1446. D
1447. D
1448. D
1449. B
1450. D
1451. D
1452. D
1453. D
1454. B
1455. A
1456. D
1457. D
1458. D
1459. C
1460. D
1461. D
1462. D
1463. C
1464. B
1465. B
1466. B
1467. A
1468. A
1469. B
1470. C
1471. C
1472. D
1473. B
1474. D
1475. D
1476. B
1477. A
1478. D
1479. C
1480. D
1481. A
1482. D
1483. B
1484. D
1485. D
1486. D
1487. C
1488. D
1489. B
1490. A
1491. D
1492. B
1493. D
1494. B
1495. D
1496. D
1497. C
1498. D
1499. D
1500. D
1501. A
1502. D
1503. D
1504. D
1505. B
1506. D
1507. D
1508. C
1509. D
1510. B
1511. D
1512. D
1513. C
1514. A
1515. D
1516. C
1517. C
1518. C
1519. D
1520. B
1521. D
1522. D
1523. D
1524. B
1525. D
1526. D
1527. D
1528. C
1529. D
1530. D
1531. D
1532. D
1533. A
1534. C
1535. B
1536. C
1537. D
1538. C
1539. D
1540. A
1541. B
1542. D
1543. D
1544. C
1545. B
1546. D
1547. C
1548. C
1549. A
1550. B
1551. D
1552. D
1553. C
1554. D
1555. D
1556. D
1557. B
1558. D
1559. D
1560. B
1561. A
1562. D
1563. D
1564. B
1565. C
1566. A
1567. D
1568. D
1569. D
1570. C
1571. C
1572. A
1573. A
1574. B
1575. C
1576. D
1577. C
1578. C
1579. B
1580. C
1581. B
1582. D
1583. D
1584. B

Neurology

ANSWERS

1585. B	1629. D	1673. C	1717. D	1761. D	1805. C
1586. D	1630. B	1674. D	1718. D	1762. D	1806. D
1587. D	1631. D	1675. D	1719. B	1763. D	1807. D
1588. B	1632. C	1676. D	1720. C	1764. C	1808. C
1589. C	1633. D	1677. D	1721. D	1765. D	1809. A
1590. D	1634. C	1678. D	1722. D	1766. D	1810. D
1591. B	1635. C	1679. D	1723. B	1767. B	1811. D
1592. C	1636. D	1680. B	1724. D	1768. A	1812. A
1593. B	1637. B	1681. D	1725. D	1769. B	1813. A
1594. C	1638. D	1682. D	1726. D	1770. D	1814. D
1595. A	1639. B	1683. D	1727. B	1771. D	1815. C
1596. D	1640. D	1684. C	1728. D	1772. C	1816. B
1597. A	1641. C	1685. D	1729. C	1773. D	1817. C
1598. D	1642. B	1686. D	1730. B	1774. A	1818. D
1599. D	1643. B	1687. A	1731. D	1775. D	1819. D
1600. A	1644. D	1688. D	1732. C	1776. D	1820. B
1601. D	1645. D	1689. D	1733. C	1777. A	1821. C
1602. A	1646. C	1690. D	1734. A	1778. C	1822. D
1603. B	1647. B	1691. D	1735. C	1779. A	1823. D
1604. C	1648. B	1692. D	1736. A	1780. A	1824. C
1605. A	1649. B	1693. A	1737. A	1781. D	1825. C
1606. C	1650. B	1694. D	1738. A	1782. B	1826. B
1607. B	1651. A	1695. D	1739. D	1783. D	1827. D
1608. D	1652. A	1696. A	1740. D	1784. D	1828. D
1609. D	1653. D	1697. C	1741. D	1785. D	1829. D
1610. C	1654. C	1698. D	1742. D	1786. A	1830. D
1611. D	1655. D	1699. D	1743. D	1787. D	1831. D
1612. A	1656. D	1700. D	1744. D	1788. B	1832. D
1613. D	1657. A	1701. D	1745. D	1789. B	1833. D
1614. C	1658. B	1702. C	1746. C	1790. D	1834. A
1615. C	1659. B	1703. D	1747. C	1791. D	1835. A
1616. B	1660. C	1704. D	1748. D	1792. D	1836. D
1617. D	1661. C	1705. D	1749. B	1793. C	1837. D
1618. B	1662. D	1706. D	1750. D	1794. A	1838. A
1619. D	1663. D	1707. D	1751. B	1795. D	1839. C
1620. D	1664. C	1708. D	1752. C	1796. C	1840. D
1621. D	1665. C	1709. D	1753. C	1797. D	1841. C
1622. C	1666. D	1710. A	1754. D	1798. B	1842. D
1623. D	1667. D	1711. B	1755. D	1799. A	1843. D
1624. B	1668. D	1712. C	1756. A	1800. D	1844. C
1625. B	1669. D	1713. A	1757. A	1801. D	1845. C
1626. D	1670. B	1714. D	1758. D	1802. A	1846. D
1627. D	1671. A	1715. C	1759. B	1803. D	1847. D
1628. D	1672. D	1716. C	1760. B	1804. D	1848. D

ANSWERS

1849. D
1850. A
1851. C
1852. D
1853. D
1854. C
1855. C
1856. B
1857. D
1858. D
1859. D
1860. B
1861. D
1862. A
1863. B
1864. C
1865. A
1866. B
1867. C
1868. B
1869. D
1870. D
1871. A
1872. D
1873. D
1874. C
1875. B
1876. D
1877. D
1878. B
1879. B
1880. C
1881. B
1882. C
1883. D
1884. D
1885. B
1886. C
1887. C
1888. D
1889. C
1890. B
1891. D
1892. C
1893. C
1894. D
1895. D
1896. D
1897. B
1898. D
1899. B
1900. A
1901. D
1902. D
1903. D
1904. A
1905. D
1906. C
1907. B
1908. C
1909. D
1910. A
1911. A
1912. A
1913. D
1914. B
1915. D
1916. B
1917. D
1918. D
1919. A
1920. A
1921. D
1922. D
1923. C
1924. D
1925. D
1926. D
1927. B
1928. B
1929. B
1930. B
1931. D
1932. D
1933. D
1934. A
1935. D
1936. D
1937. D
1938. D
1939. C
1940. B
1941. D
1942. A
1943. D
1944. D
1945. D
1946. D
1947. C
1948. B
1949. D
1950. B
1951. A
1952. A
1953. D
1954. B
1955. B
1956. D
1957. D
1958. B
1959. B
1960. A
1961. D
1962. D
1963. C
1964. D
1965. D
1966. B
1967. B
1968. C
1969. D
1970. A
1971. D
1972. B
1973. D
1974. D
1975. A
1976. D
1977. D
1978. C
1979. A
1980. A
1981. D
1982. A
1983. D
1984. D
1985. C
1986. D
1987. C
1988. A
1989. D
1990. A
1991. C
1992. B
1993. D
1994. D
1995. D
1996. D
1997. C
1998. D
1999. D
2000. D
2001. C
2002. D
2003. C
2004. B
2005. B
2006. D
2007. A
2008. B
2009. C
2010. C
2011. A
2012. D
2013. C
2014. B
2015. B
2016. D
2017. D
2018. D
2019. A
2020. D
2021. B
2022. D
2023. A
2024. D
2025. D
2026. D
2027. C
2028. D
2029. D
2030. B
2031. B
2032. D
2033. C
2034. C
2035. C
2036. D
2037. D
2038. D
2039. C
2040. A
2041. D
2042. C
2043. D
2044. D
2045. A
2046. A
2047. B
2048. D
2049. D
2050. B
2051. A
2052. D
2053. C
2054. D
2055. D
2056. C
2057. D
2058. B
2059. A
2060. D
2061. C
2062. B
2063. C
2064. D
2065. D
2066. C
2067. C
2068. C
2069. C
2070. D
2071. B
2072. D
2073. D
2074. D
2075. D
2076. D
2077. B
2078. D
2079. D
2080. C
2081. D
2082. D
2083. D
2084. D
2085. D
2086. D
2087. B
2088. D
2089. D
2090. D
2091. A
2092. B
2093. C
2094. D
2095. D
2096. D
2097. A
2098. A
2099. A
2100. B
2101. B
2102. D
2103. A
2104. D
2105. D
2106. D
2107. D
2108. D
2109. C
2110. C
2111. B
2112. B

ANSWERS

2113. C
2114. D
2115. D
2116. A
2117. C
2118. A
2119. B
2120. A
2121. B
2122. A
2123. D
2124. D
2125. D
2126. D
2127. D
2128. B
2129. D
2130. D
2131. B
2132. B
2133. A
2134. C
2135. D
2136. A
2137. C
2138. D
2139. D
2140. B
2141. A
2142. C
2143. D
2144. D
2145. B
2146. A
2147. B
2148. D
2149. C
2150. C
2151. C
2152. A
2153. C
2154. C
2155. B
2156. C
2157. C
2158. B
2159. C
2160. B
2161. D
2162. D
2163. D
2164. D
2165. D
2166. A
2167. A
2168. D
2169. D
2170. D
2171. B
2172. B
2173. D
2174. C
2175. C
2176. C
2177. D
2178. C
2179. C
2180. D
2181. B
2182. D
2183. B
2184. D
2185. D
2186. C
2187. C
2188. C
2189. C
2190. B
2191. B
2192. D
2193. D
2194. A
2195. D
2196. D
2197. B
2198. D
2199. D
2200. D
2201. D
2202. D
2203. D
2204. D
2205. D
2206. A
2207. B
2208. D
2209. A
2210. D
2211. D
2212. D
2213. D
2214. D
2215. D
2216. C
2217. D
2218. D
2219. D
2220. D
2221. A
2222. A
2223. D
2224. D
2225. C
2226. B
2227. D
2228. D
2229. D
2230. D
2231. D
2232. D
2233. C
2234. D
2235. D
2236. D
2237. D
2238. B
2239. D
2240. B
2241. C
2242. D
2243. B
2244. A
2245. B
2246. C
2247. D
2248. A
2249. B
2250. C
2251. D
2252. A
2253. B
2254. C
2255. A
2256. B
2257. C
2258. D
2259. A
2260. A
2261. D
2262. D
2263. C
2264. A
2265. A
2266. D
2267. C
2268. B
2269. D
2270. D
2271. D
2272. D
2273. D
2274. B
2275. D
2276. D
2277. B
2278. D
2279. D
2280. D
2281. C
2282. D
2283. D
2284. D
2285. A
2286. A
2287. B
2288. A
2289. B
2290. B
2291. A
2292. D
2293. D
2294. C
2295. D
2296. D
2297. D
2298. D
2299. C
2300. D
2301. C
2302. D
2303. D
2304. C
2305. A
2306. A
2307. D
2308. D
2309. A
2310. D
2311. B
2312. D
2313. B
2314. B
2315. A
2316. B
2317. D
2318. C
2319. D
2320. C
2321. D
2322. A
2323. D
2324. A
2325. A
2326. B
2327. A
2328. A
2329. C
2330. B
2331. B
2332. D
2333. A
2334. A
2335. A
2336. A
2337. D
2338. C
2339. C
2340. B
2341. B
2342. C
2343. B
2344. B
2345. B
2346. A
2347. D
2348. D
2349. D
2350. B
2351. D
2352. B
2353. A
2354. C
2355. D
2356. D
2357. B
2358. C
2359. C
2360. B
2361. A
2362. A
2363. D
2364. D
2365. D
2366. D
2367. D
2368. C
2369. D
2370. D
2371. D
2372. A
2373. A
2374. A
2375. B
2376. A

ANSWERS

2377. C
2378. D
2379. D
2380. A
2381. D
2382. D
2383. D
2384. D
2385. C
2386. D
2387. B
2388. A
2389. D
2390. B
2391. A
2392. D
2393. B
2394. B
2395. B
2396. D
2397. D
2398. C
2399. D
2400. D
2401. D
2402. D
2403. D
2404. B
2405. D
2406. D
2407. D
2408. D
2409. A
2410. B
2411. D
2412. D
2413. D
2414. B
2415. A
2416. B
2417. D
2418. B
2419. B
2420. D
2421. A
2422. A
2423. D
2424. A
2425. D
2426. A
2427. D
2428. D
2429. D
2430. C
2431. D
2432. B
2433. D
2434. C
2435. B
2436. B
2437. A
2438. D
2439. D
2440. D
2441. C
2442. B
2443. D
2444. D
2445. B
2446. A
2447. C
2448. D
2449. D
2450. D
2451. D
2452. C
2453. D
2454. C
2455. A
2456. D
2457. A
2458. D
2459. A
2460. D
2461. D
2462. D
2463. B
2464. A
2465. B
2466. D
2467. C
2468. D
2469. D
2470. A
2471. A
2472. B
2473. C
2474. D
2475. D
2476. D
2477. D
2478. C
2479. C
2480. B
2481. D
2482. A
2483. A
2484. B
2485. D
2486. C
2487. C
2488. D
2489. D
2490. C
2491. B
2492. D
2493. D
2494. D
2495. D
2496. D
2497. D
2498. B
2499. A
2500. D
2501. D
2502. D
2503. A
2504. D
2505. A
2506. B
2507. B
2508. A
2509. C
2510. C
2511. B
2512. B
2513. D
2514. C
2515. D
2516. D
2517. D
2518. D
2519. B
2520. A
2521. B
2522. C
2523. A
2524. D
2525. D
2526. A
2527. C
2528. D
2529. D
2530. D
2531. D
2532. D
2533. B
2534. C
2535. D
2536. B
2537. A
2538. D
2539. C
2540. D
2541. D
2542. D
2543. D
2544. A
2545. B
2546. A
2547. D
2548. D
2549. A
2550. D
2551. C
2552. D
2553. B
2554. D
2555. D
2556. D
2557. D
2558. D
2559. D
2560. C
2561. D
2562. A
2563. A
2564. A
2565. D
2566. D
2567. C
2568. C
2569. D
2570. C
2571. D
2572. D
2573. D
2574. D
2575. D
2576. C
2577. D
2578. D
2579. D
2580. D
2581. D
2582. D
2583. D
2584. D
2585. B
2586. D
2587. C
2588. B
2589. B
2590. D
2591. B
2592. D
2593. D
2594. A
2595. D
2596. D
2597. B
2598. B
2599. D
2600. D
2601. D
2602. A
2603. A
2604. B
2605. D
2606. D
2607. A
2608. A
2609. D
2610. D
2611. C
2612. D
2613. D
2614. D
2615. D
2616. C
2617. D
2618. D
2619. D
2620. C
2621. B
2622. B
2623. A
2624. D
2625. B
2626. B
2627. A
2628. A
2629. D
2630. D
2631. C
2632. B
2633. D
2634. B
2635. D
2636. D
2637. C
2638. D
2639. A
2640. D

ANSWERS

2641. D
2642. C
2643. D
2644. D
2645. D
2646. B
2647. D
2648. A
2649. B
2650. A
2651. B
2652. D
2653. A
2654. A
2655. A
2656. B
2657. B
2658. C
2659. D
2660. D
2661. C
2662. D
2663. C
2664. D
2665. D
2666. D
2667. C
2668. D
2669. D
2670. D
2671. D
2672. D
2673. D
2674. B
2675. D
2676. B
2677. C
2678. C
2679. B
2680. C
2681. B
2682. D
2683. D
2684. D
2685. B
2686. C
2687. A
2688. A
2689. C
2690. D
2691. D
2692. D
2693. D
2694. B
2695. D
2696. C
2697. D
2698. A
2699. C
2700. D
2701. A
2702. C
2703. D
2704. D
2705. D
2706. C
2707. D
2708. B
2709. B
2710. A
2711. D
2712. D
2713. D
2714. D
2715. A
2716. D
2717. D
2718. D
2719. D
2720. B
2721. B
2722. C
2723. D
2724. A
2725. C
2726. D
2727. D
2728. C
2729. C
2730. D
2731. D
2732. A
2733. D
2734. D
2735. D
2736. D
2737. D
2738. D
2739. A
2740. D
2741. D
2742. D
2743. D
2744. D
2745. B
2746. A
2747. D
2748. D
2749. A
2750. C
2751. C
2752. D
2753. A
2754. A
2755. D
2756. C
2757. D
2758. A
2759. A
2760. D
2761. D
2762. D
2763. B
2764. D
2765. A
2766. C
2767. C
2768. B
2769. D
2770. C
2771. D
2772. B
2773. C
2774. B
2775. D
2776. D
2777. D
2778. D
2779. C
2780. B
2781. C
2782. C
2783. B
2784. D
2785. B
2786. B
2787. D
2788. D
2789. C
2790. D
2791. D
2792. B
2793. D
2794. D
2795. D
2796. C
2797. B
2798. B
2799. D
2800. D
2801. B
2802. D
2803. D
2804. B
2805. D
2806. D
2807. D
2808. A
2809. B
2810. A
2811. C
2812. B
2813. B
2814. A
2815. A
2816. D
2817. A
2818. A
2819. D
2820. B
2821. A
2822. D
2823. B
2824. D
2825. D
2826. D
2827. A
2828. B
2829. A
2830. B
2831. D
2832. D
2833. D
2834. D
2835. D
2836. D
2837. D
2838. D
2839. C
2840. C
2841. D
2842. D
2843. D
2844. D
2845. D
2846. A
2847. D
2848. A
2849. D
2850. D
2851. C
2852. C
2853. D
2854. A
2855. D
2856. D
2857. D
2858. D
2859. A
2860. C
2861. B
2862. B
2863. B
2864. D
2865. B
2866. B
2867. D
2868. C
2869. D
2870. C
2871. D
2872. D
2873. D
2874. C
2875. D
2876. D
2877. C
2878. D
2879. A
2880. B
2881. D
2882. D
2883. D
2884. D
2885. D
2886. D
2887. D
2888. D
2889. D
2890. C
2891. D
2892. D
2893. D
2894. D
2895. B
2896. C
2897. D
2898. D
2899. D
2900. C
2901. C
2902. D
2903. D
2904. D

ANSWERS

2905. B
2906. D
2907. C
2908. D
2909. B
2910. C
2911. C
2912. C
2913. D
2914. A
2915. D
2916. C
2917. C
2918. C
2919. B
2920. B
2921. A
2922. B
2923. B
2924. B
2925. A
2926. D
2927. D
2928. D
2929. D
2930. A
2931. D
2932. D
2933. D
2934. C
2935. A
2936. B
2937. C
2938. A
2939. D
2940. A
2941. D
2942. D
2943. D
2944. D
2945. D
2946. C
2947. B
2948. C
2949. A
2950. D
2951. D
2952. D
2953. A
2954. C
2955. C
2956. B
2957. C
2958. D
2959. A
2960. D
2961. D
2962. D
2963. B
2964. B
2965. D
2966. D
2967. D
2968. B
2969. D
2970. B
2971. B
2972. D
2973. D
2974. D
2975. D
2976. C
2977. A
2978. C
2979. A
2980. D
2981. D
2982. D
2983. D
2984. D
2985. D
2986. A
2987. A
2988. D
2989. B
2990. D
2991. D
2992. D
2993. C
2994. A
2995. D
2996. B
2997. C
2998. A
2999. D
3000. C
3001. A
3002. D
3003. A
3004. D
3005. C
3006. D
3007. D
3008. C
3009. C
3010. B
3011. D
3012. D
3013. D
3014. D
3015. D
3016. A
3017. D
3018. A
3019. D
3020. B
3021. D
3022. D
3023. B
3024. B
3025. A
3026. A
3027. B
3028. A
3029. A
3030. D
3031. C
3032. B
3033. D
3034. D
3035. D
3036. D
3037. B
3038. B
3039. D
3040. A
3041. D
3042. A
3043. B
3044. C
3045. D
3046. D
3047. D
3048. D
3049. D
3050. D
3051. A
3052. A
3053. D
3054. B
3055. D
3056. D
3057. C
3058. C
3059. A
3060. A
3061. C
3062. D
3063. C
3064. D
3065. B
3066. B
3067. B
3068. A
3069. B
3070. D
3071. D
3072. B
3073. D
3074. D
3075. D
3076. A
3077. D
3078. C
3079. C
3080. A
3081. A
3082. C
3083. D
3084. B
3085. D
3086. D
3087. A
3088. B
3089. B
3090. B
3091. D
3092. D
3093. D
3094. B
3095. D
3096. C
3097. A
3098. C
3099. C
3100. D
3101. C
3102. D
3103. D
3104. D
3105. A
3106. A
3107. D
3108. D
3109. D
3110. D
3111. A
3112. B
3113. B
3114. D
3115. B
3116. B
3117. D
3118. D
3119. D
3120. D
3121. D
3122. D
3123. D
3124. D
3125. B
3126. D
3127. D
3128. B
3129. D
3130. C
3131. A
3132. A
3133. C
3134. D
3135. C
3136. D
3137. D
3138. D
3139. D
3140. D
3141. C
3142. D
3143. D
3144. C
3145. D
3146. D
3147. D
3148. B
3149. B
3150. A
3151. D
3152. B
3153. D
3154. D
3155. A
3156. D
3157. D
3158. D
3159. A
3160. D
3161. B
3162. D
3163. C
3164. C
3165. C
3166. A
3167. D
3168. D

ANSWERS

3169. D
3170. B
3171. B
3172. A
3173. D
3174. B
3175. D
3176. B
3177. C
3178. C
3179. D
3180. C
3181. D
3182. D
3183. D
3184. D
3185. D
3186. D
3187. C
3188. D
3189. D
3190. D
3191. D
3192. D
3193. C
3194. D
3195. A
3196. D
3197. B
3198. A
3199. B
3200. A
3201. B
3202. B
3203. D
3204. D
3205. A
3206. D
3207. B
3208. D
3209. C
3210. A
3211. D
3212. D
3213. D
3214. C
3215. D
3216. C
3217. D
3218. B
3219. B
3220. C
3221. A
3222. B
3223. B
3224. C
3225. A
3226. D
3227. B
3228. D
3229. D
3230. D
3231. A
3232. A
3233. D
3234. D
3235. D
3236. D
3237. B
3238. A
3239. A
3240. C
3241. A
3242. C
3243. B
3244. D
3245. D
3246. D
3247. A
3248. A
3249. A
3250. D
3251. D
3252. A
3253. A
3254. B
3255. B
3256. B
3257. D
3258. D
3259. C
3260. D
3261. A
3262. B
3263. C
3264. D
3265. B
3266. D
3267. A
3268. D
3269. C
3270. D
3271. D
3272. B
3273. D
3274. D
3275. D
3276. B
3277. A
3278. A
3279. B
3280. D
3281. C
3282. A
3283. C
3284. A
3285. D
3286. A
3287. D
3288. B
3289. B
3290. A
3291. C
3292. B
3293. B
3294. B
3295. B
3296. B
3297. A
3298. D
3299. C
3300. B
3301. A
3302. A
3303. D
3304. C
3305. A
3306. A
3307. C
3308. D
3309. D
3310. D
3311. D
3312. D
3313. B
3314. D
3315. A
3316. D
3317. A
3318. D
3319. C
3320. C
3321. D
3322. D
3323. B
3324. D
3325. D
3326. B
3327. C
3328. B
3329. D
3330. D
3331. C
3332. D
3333. A
3334. D
3335. C
3336. D
3337. D
3338. C
3339. A
3340. A
3341. A
3342. C
3343. D
3344. C
3345. A
3346. C
3347. C
3348. D
3349. D
3350. C
3351. D
3352. D
3353. C
3354. D
3355. D
3356. D
3357. A
3358. C
3359. D
3360. C
3361. C
3362. D
3363. D
3364. D
3365. B
3366. C
3367. B
3368. A
3369. C
3370. C
3371. C
3372. C
3373. D
3374. C
3375. A
3376. D
3377. B
3378. D
3379. B
3380. D
3381. C
3382. C
3383. B
3384. D
3385. A
3386. D
3387. D
3388. D
3389. A
3390. C
3391. C
3392. D
3393. D
3394. D
3395. A
3396. B
3397. C
3398. D
3399. B
3400. C
3401. B
3402. D
3403. D
3404. D
3405. D
3406. C
3407. C
3408. D
3409. D
3410. A
3411. D
3412. D
3413. A
3414. D
3415. C
3416. C
3417. A
3418. C
3419. C
3420. C
3421. D
3422. D
3423. C
3424. B
3425. D
3426. A
3427. D
3428. D
3429. B
3430. D
3431. B
3432. C

ANSWERS

3433. D
3434. B
3435. B
3436. C
3437. D
3438. D
3439. B
3440. D
3441. C
3442. D
3443. C
3444. D
3445. D
3446. D
3447. B
3448. D
3449. D
3450. D
3451. D
3452. D
3453. A
3454. C
3455. D
3456. A
3457. B
3458. D
3459. D
3460. D
3461. B
3462. A
3463. C
3464. D
3465. D
3466. A
3467. D
3468. D
3469. D
3470. A
3471. C
3472. B
3473. D
3474. D
3475. C
3476. D
3477. D
3478. B
3479. C
3480. C
3481. D
3482. C
3483. C
3484. C
3485. C
3486. D
3487. D
3488. D
3489. D
3490. C
3491. A
3492. B
3493. D
3494. A
3495. D
3496. B
3497. D
3498. A
3499. B
3500. A
3501. D
3502. C
3503. D
3504. D
3505. D
3506. D
3507. D
3508. B
3509. C
3510. B
3511. D
3512. D
3513. D
3514. C
3515. C
3516. C
3517. C
3518. B
3519. D
3520. A
3521. C
3522. C
3523. A
3524. D
3525. B
3526. C
3527. A
3528. D
3529. B
3530. D
3531. D
3532. D
3533. C
3534. A
3535. C
3536. A
3537. A
3538. D
3539. C
3540. B
3541. D
3542. D
3543. A
3544. D
3545. D
3546. A
3547. C
3548. C
3549. A
3550. A
3551. D
3552. A
3553. B
3554. D
3555. D
3556. C
3557. D
3558. D
3559. D
3560. D
3561. D
3562. D
3563. D
3564. C
3565. B
3566. A
3567. D
3568. D
3569. C
3570. B
3571. D
3572. D
3573. A
3574. D
3575. A
3576. D
3577. B
3578. C
3579. A
3580. C
3581. D
3582. D
3583. B
3584. D
3585. C
3586. D
3587. D
3588. D
3589. D
3590. D
3591. D
3592. B
3593. C
3594. D
3595. C
3596. D
3597. D
3598. D
3599. D
3600. D